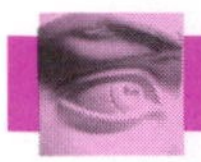

NURSING MANAGEMENT OF PULMONARY ALTERATIONS

Ineffective Airway Clearance Related to Excessive Secretions or Abnormal Viscosity of Mucus, p. 722

Ineffective Breathing Pattern Related to Decreased Lung Expansion, p. 723

Ineffective Breathing Pattern Related to Musculoskeletal Fatigue or Neuromuscular Impairment, p. 724

Inability to Sustain Spontaneous Ventilation Related to Respiratory Muscle Fatigue or Metabolic Factors, p. 724

Impaired Gas Exchange Related to Ventilation/Perfusion Mismatching or Intrapulmonary Shunting, p. 725

Impaired Gas Exchange Related to Alveolar Hypoventilation, p. 726

Risk for Aspiration, p. 727

Dysfunctional Ventilatory Weaning Response (DVWR) Related to Physical, Psychologic, or Situational Factors, p. 728

NURSING MANAGEMENT OF NEUROLOGIC ALTERATIONS

Altered Cerebral Tissue Perfusion Related to Vasospasm or Hemorrhage, p. 842

Decreased Adaptive Capacity: Intracranial Related to Failure of Normal Intracranial Compensatory Mechanisms, p. 843

Unilateral Neglect Related to Perceptual Disruption, p. 844

Impaired Verbal Communication: Aphasia Related to Cerebral Speech Center Injury, p. 845

NURSING MANAGEMENT OF RENAL ALTERATIONS

Fluid Volume Deficit Related to Absolute Blood Loss, p. 914

Fluid Volume Deficit Related to Relative Loss, p. 915

Fluid Volume Excess Related to Renal Dysfunction, p. 915

Altered Renal Tissue Perfusion Related to Decreased Renal Blood Flow, p. 916

NURSING MANAGEMENT OF GASTROINTESTINAL ALTERATIONS

Impaired Swallowing Related to Neuromuscular Impairment, Fatigue, and Limited Awareness, p. 976

NURSING MANAGEMENT OF ENDOCRINE ALTERATIONS

Fluid Volume Excess Related to Increased Secretion of ADH, p. 1048

Fluid Volume Deficit Related to Decreased Secretion of ADH, p. 1049

Hyperthermia Related to Increased Thyroid Hormone, p. 1049

Hypothermia Related to Decreased Thyroid Hormone, p. 1050

NURSING MANAGEMENT RELATED TO TRAUMA

Dysreflexia Related to Excessive Autonomic Response to Noxious Stimuli (e.g. Distended Bladder, Distended Bowel, Skin Irritation) Occurring in Patients with Cervical or High Thoracic (T7 or Above) Spinal Cord Injury, p. 1093

NURSING MANAGEMENT OF SHOCK

Decreased Cardiac Output Related to Sympathetic Blockade, p. 1118

Risk for Infection, p. 1119

NURSING MANAGEMENT OF TRANSPLANTATION

Risk for Infection Risk Factor: Immunosuppressive Drugs Required to Prevent Rejection of Transplanted Organ, p. 1216

CRITICAL CARE NURSING

DIAGNOSIS AND MANAGEMENT

THIRD EDITION

CRITICAL CARE NURSING

DIAGNOSIS AND MANAGEMENT

Lynne A. Thelan, RN, MN
Critical Care Consultant and Lecturer
Mercer Island, Washington

Linda D. Urden, RN, DNSc, CNA
Administrative Director
Patient Care Services
Butterworth Hospital
Grand Rapids, Michigan

Mary E. Lough, RN, MS, CCRN
Critical Care Cardiovascular Clinical Nurse Specialist
Sequoia Hospital
Redwood City, California
and
Associate Clinical Professor
University of California at San Francisco
San Francisco, California

Kathleen M. Stacy, RN, MS, CCRN
Critical Care Clinical Nurse Specialist
Cardiopulmonary Clinical Outcomes Manager
Tri-City Medical Center
Oceanside, California
and
Adjunct Faculty
San Diego State University School of Nursing
San Diego, California

With 516 illustrations

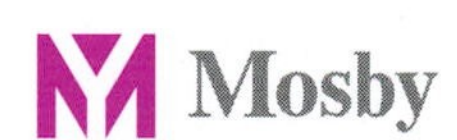

St. Louis Baltimore Boston Carlsbad Chicago Minneapolis New York Philadelphia Portland
London Milan Sydney Tokyo Toronto

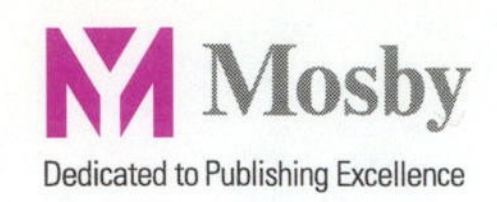

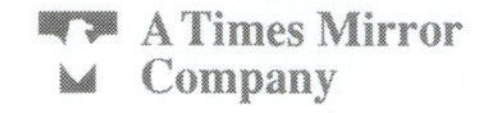

Publisher: Nancy L. Coon
Editor: Barry Bowlus
Senior Developmental Editor: Nancy C. Baker
Project Manager: Deborah L. Vogel
Production Editor: Sarah E. Fike
Designer: Pati Pye
Manufacturing Supervisor: Don Carlisle

A NOTE TO THE READER:
The author and publisher have made every attempt to check dosages and nursing content for accuracy. Because the science of pharmacology is continually advancing, our knowledge base continues to expand. Therefore we recommend that the reader always check product information for changes in dosage or administration before administering any medication. This is particularly important with new or rarely used drugs.

THIRD EDITION

Printed in the United States of America
Composition by Graphic World, Inc.
Lithography/color film by Graphic World, Inc.
Printing/binding by World Color Book Services

Mosby, Inc.
11830 Westline Industrial Drive
St. Louis, Missouri 63146

Library of Congress Cataloging-in-Publication Data

Critical care nursing : diagnosis and management / Linda D. Urden . . .
[et al.]—3rd ed.
p. cm.
Includes bibliographical references and index.
ISBN 0-8151-3692-7
1. Intensive care nursing. 2. Emergency nursing. I. Urden, Linda Diann.
[DNLM: 1. Critical Care—nurses' instruction. WY 154 C93296 1998]
RT120.I5C752 1998
610.73′61—dc21
DNLM/DLC
for Library of Congress 97-33345
CIP

97 98 99 00 01 / 9 8 7 6 5 4 3 2 1

Contributors

Carlotta A. Beebe, RN, MSW, MS
Lecturer
Pediatric Critical Care and Acute Care Pediatric Nurse Practitioners Programs
University of Michigan
and
Child Family Psychiatric Social Worker
Private Practice
Ann Arbor, Michigan

Jamie D. Blazek, RN, MPH, FNP
Senior Clinical Transplant Coordinator
Ochsner Transplant Center
Ochsner Clinic
New Orleans, Louisiana

Jennifer Bloomquist, RN, MN
Cardiac Rehabilitation Clinical Nurse Specialist
Naval Medical Center
San Diego, California

JoAnn M. Clark, RN, MSN, CFNP, CGNP
Assistant Clinical Professor
and
Coordinator, Gerontological Nurse Practitioner Program
School of Medicine, Division of Graduate Nursing Education
University of California, San Diego
LaJolla, California

Beverly Means Carlson, RN, MS, CCRN
Research Associate and Outcomes Management Consultant
Health Services Research and Development
Sharp Healthcare
San Diego, California

Beverly A. Deliyanides, RN, MSN, CPAN
Staff Educator
Post Anesthesia Care Unit
Butterworth Hospital
Grand Rapids, Michigan

Joni Dirks, RN, MS, CCRN
Clinical Nurse Specialist
Department of Veteran Affairs Medical Center
Palo Alto, California

Marilyn Kuhel Douglas, RN, DNSc, CCRN
Nurse Researcher/Clinical Nurse Specialist, MICU/CCU
Department of Nursing Service
Veterans Affairs Palo Alto Health Care System
Palo Alto, California

Lorraine Fitzsimmons, RN, DNSc, FNP, CS
Graduate Program Chair
Advanced Practice Nursing of Adults and the Elderly
San Diego State University School of Nursing
San Diego, California

Jeannine Forrest, RN, MS
Teaching Associate
Medical Surgical Nursing
University of Illinois at Chicago
Chicago, Illinois

Judith K. Glann, RN, MSN, CCRN
Critical Care/Cardiovascular Clinical Nurse Specialist
St. Vincent Hospital
Santa Fe, New Mexico

Ruth N. Grendell, RN, DNSc
Assistant Chair and Professor
Department of Nursing
Point Loma Nazarene College Department of Nursing
San Diego, California

Mary Gritzmaker Schira, RN, PhD
Faculty
School of Nursing
University of Texas at Arlington
Arlington, Texas

Lynne Jett, RN, MSN, C
Professional Development Specialist
Education Department
Tri-City Medical Center
Oceanside, California

Karen L. Johnson, RN, MSN, CCRN
Doctoral Student
College of Nursing
University of Kentucky
Lexington, Kentucky

Jacqueline L. Kartman, RN, MS, CS, CCRN, APNP
Advanced Practice Nurse
Cardiothoracic Surgery
Gunderson Lutheran Medical Center
La Crosse, Wisconsin

Julene B. Kruithof, RN, MSN, CCRN
Staff Educator
Adult Critical Care and Cardiothoracic Telemetry Unit
Butterworth Hospital
Grand Rapids, Michigan

Martha J. Love, RN, MN
Staff Nurse
MICU/CCU
Veterans Administration Medical Center
San Diego, California

Helen Luikart, RN, MS
Nurse Educator/Transplant Coordinator
Department of Cardiothoracic Surgery
Stanford University
Stanford, California

Jeanne M. Maiden, RN, MS, CCRN
Professional Development Specialist
Education Department
Tri-City Medical Center
Oceanside, California

Nancy McLaughlin, RN, MSN, CCRN
Clinical Nurse Specialist-SICU
Critical Care/Emergency Services/Burns and Trauma Nursing
University of Alabama University Hospital
Birmingham, Alabama

Kathleen A. Mendez, RN, MS, CCRN
Neuroscience Clinical Outcomes Manager
Tri-City Medical Center
Oceanside, California

Bobbie J. Monroe, RN, BSN, CCRN, CNRN, JD
Staff Nurse
Critical Care Nursing
St. Luke's Episcopal Hospital
Houston, Texas

Mary Courtney Moore, RN, RD, PhD
Research Assistant Professor
Department of Molecular Physiology and Biophysics
Vanderbilt University
Nashville, Tennesee

Mimi O'Donnell, RN, MS, CS
Cardiovascular Clinical Nurse Specialist
Massachusetts General Hospital
Boston, Massachusetts

Mariann R. Piano, RN, PhD
Assistant Professor
College of Nursing
University of Illinois at Chicago
Chicago, Illinois

Donna Prentice, RN, MSN(R), CS, CCRN
Critical Care Clinical Nurse Specialist
Barnes-Jewish Hospital at Washington University
St. Louis, Missouri

Elizabeth A. Remsburg-Bell, RN, MSN
Clinical Nurse Specialist
Department of Obstetrics
Butterworth Hospital
Grand Rapids, Michigan

Debra L. Ryan, RN, MN, CCRN
Clinical Nurse Specialist
Surgical Critical Care Services
Butterworth Hospital
Grand Rapids, Michigan

Julie A. Shinn, RN, MA, CCRN, FAAN
Cardiovascular Clinical Nurse Specialist
Department of Nursing
Stanford Health Services
Stanford, California

Susan Windham, RN, MN
Kidney Transplant Coordinator
California Pacific Medical Center
San Francisco, California

Sharon E. Witmer, RN, MSN, CCRN
Educational Nurse Specialist
Pediatric/Perinatal Nursing
University of Michigan Health System
Ann Arbor, Michigan

Acknowledgments for Previous Contributors

Wendy Bodwell, RN, MSN, CCRN

Karen Brasfield, RN, MSN

Dorothy Brundage, RN, PhD, FAAN

Rebecca Wills Butler, RN, MN

Katherine M. Fortinash, RNCS, MSN

Susan Frye, RN, MSN, JD

Sheana Whelan Funkhouser, RN, DNSc

Colleen O'Donnell, RN, MS, CCRN

Angela S. Paloma, RN, MN

Jeanne Raimond, RN, MSN, CCRN

Kate Relling-Garskof, RN, MSN, CS

Linda M. Valentino, RN, BSN

Helen Vos, RN, MS

Reviewers

Kathyrn S. Bizek, RN, MSN, CS, CCRN
Clinical Nurse Specialist, Critical Care
Detroit Receiving Hospital and University Health Center
Associate Graduate Faculty, College of Nursing
Wayne State University
Detroit, Michigan

Vicki Bungy, RN, MN, CNCC, (C)
Program Head, Critical Care Nursing Specialty
British Columbia Institute of Technology
Vancouver, British Columbia, Canada

Kay Knox Greenlee, RN, MSN, CCRN
Clinical Nurse Specialist—Surgical/Special Care
St. Cloud Hospital
St. Cloud, Minnesota

Cynthia Hermey, RN, MN, CCRN
Nurse Manager, Critical Care and Progressive Care
Oconee Memorial Hospital
Seneca, South Carolina

Ruth M. Kleinpell, RN, PhD, CCRN
Associate Professor
Rush University College of Nursing
Chicago, Illinois

Nora E. Ladewig, RN, MSN, CCRN
Clinical Practice Nurse V
St. Luke's Medical Center
Milwaukee, Wisconsin

Deborah S. Lammert, RN, C, MSN, CCRN-P
Clinical Nurse Specialist
The Children's Hospital at Saint Francis
Tulsa, Oklahoma

Marijo Letizia, RN, C, BSN, MS, PhD
Assistant Professor of Nursin
Loyola University
Chicago, Illinois

Margo McCaffery, RN, MS, FAAN
Consultant in the Nursing Care of Patients with Pain
Los Angeles, California

Joy W. Thompson, RN, MSN, CCRN
Staff Nurse
St. Louis University Hospital
St. Louis, Missouri

Linda Waite, RN, MN, CCRN
Nursing Administration
Fairview Southville Hospital
Edina, Minnesota

To

Mom

with love

L.D.U.

To

Jim Stevens

Husband Extraordinaire

M.E.L.

To James and Sherrie-Anne

for all their love

To Lorraine and Beverly

for all their encouragement

To Lynne, Kathy, Jeanne, and Sharon

for all their support

To Cindy

for her continuing friendship

K.M.S.

User's Preface

We are most grateful to the many students and nurses who made the previous editions of this book successful. The success has validated our commitment to proclaim the outstanding contributions of critical care nurses and to promote research-based nursing in the complex critical care environment. We actively solicited feedback from users of the previous editions and eagerly incorporated their comments and suggestions regarding format, content, and organization. And so, with this third edition, we again present to you a book that is thorough in all that is most pertinent to critical care nurses in a format that is organized for clarity and comprehension.

ORGANIZATION

The book's nine units are again organized around alterations in dimensions of human functioning that span biopsychosocial realms.

The content of Unit 1, ***Foundations of Critical Care Nursing,*** forms the basis of practice regardless of the physiologic alterations of the critically ill patient. Although chapters in the book may be studied in any sequence, we recommend that Chapter 1, ***Coordination of Care for the Critically Ill,*** be studied first because it clarifies the major assumptions on which the entirety of the book is based. Chapter 2, ***Ethical Issues,*** delineates ethical theories and strategies for dealing with the ethical dilemmas that arise on a daily basis in critical care. Chapter 3, ***Legal Issues,*** provides a basis of information to help the critical care nurse be cognizant of practice issues that may have legal implications. Teaching and learning theory, strategies to best meet the learning needs of critical care patients, and sample teaching plans are delineated in Chapter 4, ***Patient Education.*** Chapter 5, ***Psychosocial Alterations,*** examines the theoretic basis and nursing process for alterations in self-concept and coping. Chapter 6, ***Sleep Alterations,*** examines a perennial problem in critical care. Chapter 7, ***Nutritional Alterations and Management,*** examines the nutritional needs of the critically ill patient and provides specific recommendations for different disorders. The concepts of pain and sedation management in the critically ill are discussed in Chapter 8, ***Pain and Sedation.*** Unit II, ***Special Populations,*** addresses the needs of the critically ill pediatric, obstetric, and geriatric patient in the critical care unit as well as managing the recovery of the perianesthesia patient.

Unit III, ***Cardiovascular Alterations;*** Unit IV, ***Pulmonary Alterations;*** and Unit V, ***Neurologic Alterations;*** are each structured with the following chapters:

- Anatomy and Physiology
- Clinical Assessment
- Diagnostic Procedures
- Disorders
- Therapeutic Management
- Nursing Diagnosis and Management

This organization permits easy retrieval of information for students and clinicians and provides for flexibility for the instructor to individualize teaching methods by assigning chapters that best suit student needs. Unit VI, ***Renal Alterations;*** Unit VII, ***Gastrointestinal Alterations;*** and Unit VIII, ***Endocrine Alterations,*** are organized similarly. However, in these units the assessment parameters, such as clinical and diagnostic procedures, are discussed in one chapter. In addition, disorders and therapeutic management are combined into one chapter.

Unit IX, ***Multisystem Alterations,*** covers disorders that affect multiple body systems and necessitate discussion as a separate category. Unit IX consists of five chapters:

- **Trauma**
- **Shock**
- **Systemic Inflammatory Response Syndrome and Multiple Organ Dysfunction Syndrome**
- **Burns**
- **Transplantation**

Finally, five appendixes are included, which contain useful information for all students and practitioners of critical care. Appendix A, ***North American Nursing Diagnosis Association's (NANDA) Taxonomy I Revised,*** contains all diagnostic categories. Appendix B, ***Nursing Interventions Classification (NIC),*** contains the organizing framework of research-based nursing interventions formulated by nurse researchers at the University of Iowa. Appendix C, ***Advanced Cardiac Life Support (ACLS) Guidelines,*** presents the American Heart Association's decision trees for use in treating life-threatening dysrhythmias, administering emergency drugs, and defibrillation during cardiopulmonary resuscitation. Appendix D, ***Physiologic Formulas for Critical Care,*** features commonly encountered hemodynamic, oxygenation, and other calculations and is presented in easily understood formulas. Recommendations for nutritional supplement are also included. Examples of clinical pathways and algorithms are presented in Appendix E, ***Interdisciplinary Plans of Care.***

NURSING DIAGNOSIS AND MANAGEMENT

A dominant theme of the book continues to be nursing diagnosis and management, reflecting the strength of critical care nursing practice. The power of research-based critical care practice is incorporated into nursing interventions. To foster critical thinking and decision making, a boxed "menu" of nursing diagnoses complete with specific etiologic or related factors accompanies each medical disorder and major medical treatment discussions and directs the learner to the section in the book where appropriate nursing management is detailed. To facilitate student learning, the nursing management plans incorporate nursing diagnosis definition, etiologic or related factors, clinical manifestations, and intervention with rationale. The nursing management plans are liberally cross-referenced throughout the book for easy retrieval by the reader.

NURSING RESEARCH ABSTRACTS, LEGAL REVIEWS, AND CULTURAL INSIGHTS

Research Abstracts are integrated throughout the book to encourage incorporation of research findings into clinical practice. The abstracts are derived from published research in research, critical care, and specialty journals and are distinguished by having at least one nurse author.

Reviews of medical malpractice case law pertinent to critical care are highlighed throughout the book to focus on the importance of safe delivery of patient care and to illustrate actions for which the nurse may be liable.

The importance of recognizing cultural diversity and implications for practice are reflected in Cultural Insight boxes throughout the text. These boxes provide information and strategies to address various multicultural issues in critical care.

NEW TO EDITION

We have incorporated an illustration of an eye on the cover as well as throughout this entire text. This unique design element symbolizes the "vision" that critical care nurses embody every day in their profession. This vision includes utilizing a holistic approach, working with other health care professionals to offer the best care, being forever attentive to the needs of patients and their families, and keeping an eye on the future to ensure a continuum of top-notch, quality care.

New to this edition are the following chapters:

- **Coordination of Care for the Critically Ill**
- **Pain and Sedation**
- **The Pediatric Patient in the Adult Critical Care Unit**
- **High Risk and Critical Care Obstetric Issues**
- **Perianesthesia Management**

Also new to this edition is the inclusion of *NIC boxes* in the Therapeutic Management chapters. These boxes list the important nursing actions for a variety of nursing interventions that would be commonly incorporated in the management of a critically ill patient requiring a specific therapeutic treatment, such as mechanical ventilation. *Pharmacology boxes* have also been added to the Therapeutic Management chapters. These boxes outline the common medications, along with any special considerations, used in treatment of the different disorders presented in the text. *Patient Education boxes* have been added to the Disorders chapters. These boxes list the special topics that should be taught to the patient and family to prepare them for discharge. Information that should be included as part of the patient's history has been incorporated into *Data Collection boxes* located in the Clinical Assessment chapters. Through the *new links feature* (∞) the chapters are "linked" to assist the reader in pulling different concepts together to understand the total management of the critically ill patient. In addition, the links serve as a mechanism for cross-indexing complex concepts in more depth. They also help stimulate critical thinking and assist the learner to explore the material as a basis for deeper understanding.

LEARNER ENHANCEMENTS

In addition to the new links feature, learner enhancements from previous editions are continued in this text. The case studies enhance student learning and promote critical thinking by illustrating the clinical course of a patient experiencing the history, clinical manifestations, treatment, and outcomes discussed in the related unit or chapter. Case studies are organized in the following manner: clinical history, current problems, medical and nursing diagnoses, plan of care, medical and nursing management and patient outcome, and revised plan of care.

Finally, the teaching and learning package accompanying this book has been revised for this edition. The *Instructor's Resource Manual* provides a variety of aids to help enhance the course instruction. Provided for each chapter in the text is an overview, objectives, concepts, content outline, and detailed teaching strategies paralleling the chapter content. Student review sheets for each chapter focus on analysis and critical thinking. A separate section includes work sheets and exercises that enhance and complement the use of multimedia within the course. A comprehensive NCLEX coded test bank presenting approximately 650 multiple-choice questions is included. Guidelines for integrating multimedia components with text and classroom instruction help to enhance the content presentation. Adapted course outlines provide content recommendations for varying course lengths and settings. In addition to the *Manual,* an IBM *Computerized Testbank* is available for exam generation. A *Multimedia Learning Guide* includes the critical thinking activities relating to the text and multimedia components. Fifty two-color *Transparency Acetates* complete the comprehensive teaching and learning package.

MULTIMEDIA CURRICULUM

Content in this edition of *Critical Care Nursing* correlates with Mosby's Critical Care Nursing Teaching and Learning System. Instructors can augment with the text through the use of *Mosby's Critical Care Nursing Video Series and Critical Care Nursing—Critical Thinking: An Interactive Video Series.* The multimedia icon ( ) in this text guides readers to specific correlations between the text and the two video series.

The *Video Series* consists of eight tapes that are correlated in content in *Critical Care Nursing.* The tapes are as follows:

- Introduction to Critical Care Nursing
- Concepts of Mechanical Ventilation
- Nursing Management of the Patient on Mechanical Ventilation
- Clinical Assessment and Evaluation of Oxygenation Status
- Concepts of Hemodynamic Pressure Monitoring
- Nursing Management of the Patient Undergoing Hemodynamic Pressure Monitoring
- Intracranial Pressure Monitoring: Concepts and Nursing Management
- Ethical Issues in Critical Care Nursing

Critical Care Nursing—Critical Thinking: An Interactive Video Series, developed by Fuld Institute for Technology in Nursing Education (FITNE) in cooperation with Mosby, correlates to content in *Critical Care Nursing.* The program consists of four one-sided discs. Disc 1, "Orientation to Critical Care Nursing," contains an orientation to the program and a critical thinking segment that reviews use of the nursing process in critical care nursing. With the other three discs, "Cardiovascular Care," "Pulmonary Care" and "Neurologic Care," the student can study via a tutorial component that reviews and provides exercises on related critical care concepts, techniques, equipment, and nursing diagnoses. Students can also learn via a case study format that allows them to make a variety of critical thinking decisions about patients as they progress through their stay in the critical care unit.

Critical Care Nursing: Diagnosis and Management represents our continued commitment to bringing you the best in all things a textbook can offer: the best and brightest in contributing and consulting authors; the latest in scientific research befitting the current state of health care and nursing; an organizational format that exercises diagnostic reasoning skills and is logical and consistent; and outstanding artwork and illustrations that enhance student learning. We pledge our continued commitment to excellence in critical care education.

Linda D. Urden
Mary E. Lough
Kathleen M. Stacy

Acknowledgments

A project of this book's magnitude is never merely the work of its authors. The concerted talent, hard work, and inspiration of a multitude of people have produced *Critical Care Nursing: Diagnosis and Management,* third edition, and have helped to make it the state-of-the-science text we affirm it to be. A "tradition of publishing excellence" has been evident throughout our partnership with Mosby. We deeply appreciate the assistance of our acquisition editor, Barry Bowlus, and senior developmental editor, Nancy C. Baker, who have helped us document and refine our ideas and transform our book into a reality. Their creativity, expertise, availability, and generosity of time and resources have been invaluable to us throughout this endeavor. We are also grateful to Sarah Fike, production editor, for her scrupulous attention to detail. We remain indebted to artists George J. Wassilchenko and Donald O'Connor for their extraordinary talent. Their detailed work appears throughout the text, and its beauty is in itself an inspiration to learning. Finally we wish to thank those authors who contributed work to the first and second editions of this book. Without the foundation they provided, a third edition would not have been born.

A SPECIAL THANKS FROM LYNNE A. THELAN

Many years ago, when Joe Davie, Linda Urden, and I started the first edition of *Critical Care Nursing: Diagnosis and Management,* we knew we were providing a service to the critical care nursing profession. Little did we know that by this edition, our readers would have made this text No. 1 and the standard by which all other critical care books are measured.

I am grateful to the many readers who have made our title a success, and I am most pleased that this edition, under the editorship of Linda Urden, Kate Stacy, and Mary Lough builds on the strong foundation established in the two previous editions. Today, as I turn my focus toward raising my family, I know that this book's tradition of excellence is in good hands. Linda, Kate, and Mary have found new ways to present critical care nursing material while keeping with the quality of information for which we are known. Congratulations to all who have made this book the text of choice.

Contents

UNIT I
FOUNDATIONS OF CRITICAL CARE NURSING

1 Coordination of Care for the Critically Ill, 3
2 Ethical Issues, 19
3 Legal Issues, 35
4 Patient Education, 49
5 Psychosocial Alterations, 63
6 Sleep Alterations, 103
7 Nutritional Alterations and Management, 121
8 Pain and Sedation, 169

UNIT II
SPECIAL POPULATIONS

9 The Pediatric Patient in the Adult Critical Care Unit, 205
10 High Risk and Critical Care Obstetric Issues, 243
11 Gerontologic Alterations and Management, 271
12 Perianesthesia Management, 297

UNIT III
CARDIOVASCULAR ALTERATIONS

13 Cardiovascular Anatomy and Physiology, 331
14 Cardiovascular Clinical Assessment, 355
15 Cardiovascular Diagnostic Procedures, 377
16 Cardiovascular Disorders, 483
17 Cardiovascular Therapeutic Management, 529
18 Cardiovascular Nursing Diagnosis and Management, 585

UNIT IV
PULMONARY ALTERATIONS

19 Pulmonary Anatomy and Physiology, 601
20 Pulmonary Clinical Assessment, 625
21 Pulmonary Diagnostic Procedures, 641
22 Pulmonary Disorders, 655
23 Pulmonary Therapeutic Management, 689
24 Pulmonary Nursing Diagnosis and Management, 719

UNIT V
NEUROLOGIC ALTERATIONS

25 Neurologic Anatomy and Physiology, 733
26 Neurologic Clinical Assessment, 763
27 Neurologic Diagnostic Procedures, 779
28 Neurologic Disorders, 791
29 Neurologic Therapeutic Management, 821
30 Neurologic Nursing Diagnosis and Management, 839

UNIT VI
RENAL ALTERATIONS

31 Renal Anatomy and Physiology, 849
32 Renal Clinical Assessment and Diagnostic Procedures, 865
33 Renal Disorders and Therapeutic Management, 877
34 Renal Nursing Diagnosis and Management, 911

UNIT VII
GASTROINTESTINAL ALTERATIONS

35 Gastrointestinal Anatomy and Physiology, 919
36 Gastrointestinal Clinical Assessment and Diagnostic Procedures, 931
37 Gastrointestinal Disorders and Therapeutic Management, 945
38 Gastrointestinal Nursing Diagnosis and Management, 973

UNIT VIII
ENDOCRINE ALTERATIONS

39 Endocrine Anatomy and Physiology, 977
40 Endocrine Clinical Assessment and Diagnostic Procedures, 989
41 Endocrine Disorders and Therapeutic Management, 1001
42 Endocrine Nursing Diagnosis and Management, 1045

UNIT IX
MULTISYSTEM ALTERATIONS

43 Trauma, 1051
44 Shock, 1097
45 Systemic Inflammatory Response Syndrome and Multiple Organ Dysfunction Syndrome, 1121
46 Burns, 1141
47 Transplantation, 1171

APPENDIXES

A North American Nursing Diagnosis Association's (NANDA) Taxonomy, A-1
B Nursing Interventions Classification (NIC) Taxonomy, B-1
C Advanced Cardiac Life Support (ACLS) Guidelines, C-1
D Physiologic Formulas for Critical Care, D-1
E Interdisciplinary Plans of Care, E-1

INSIDE FRONT COVER

Quick reference guide for:

Nursing Management Plans

INSIDE BACK COVER

Quick reference guide for:

Data Collection Boxes
Pharmacology Tables
Case Study Boxes
Legal Reviews
Cultural Insights
Research Abstracts
Nursing Interventions Classification (NIC) Boxes

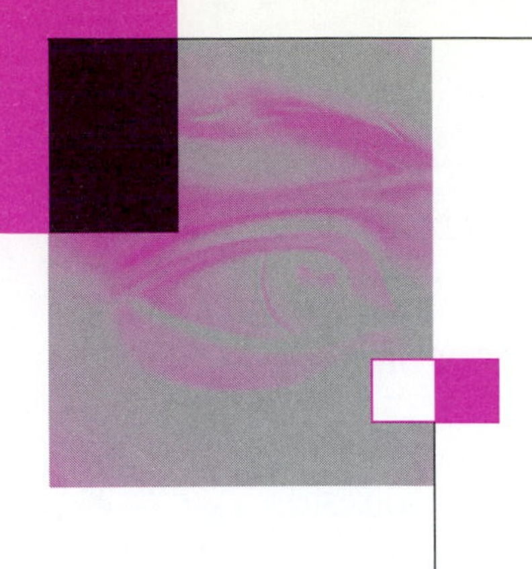

Detailed Contents

UNIT I
FOUNDATIONS OF CRITICAL CARE NURSING, 1

1 Coordination of Care of the Critically Ill, 3
Nursing's Unique Role in Health Care, 3
The Nursing Process, 4
Interdisciplinary Planning for Care, 10

2 Ethical Issues, 19
Morals and Ethics, 19
Ethical Theories, 19
Ethical Principles, 20
Withholding and Withdrawing Treatment, 24
Medical Futility, 25
Ethics as a Foundation for Nursing Practice, 26
Ethical Decision Making in Critical Care, 28
Strategies for Promotion of Ethical Decision Making, 31
Summary, 32

3 Legal Issues, 35
Critical Care Nursing Practice: Legal Obligations Overview, 35
Tort Liability, 36
Administrative Law and Licensing Statutes, 38
Negligence and Malpractice, 38
Nurse Practice Acts, 41
Specific Patient Patient Care Issues, 42

4 Patient and Family Education, 49
Challenges for Patient and Family Education in Critical Care, 49
Adult Learning Theory, 50
Teaching-Learning Process, 50
Teaching Toward Transfer From Critical Care, 57
Sample Written Teaching Tool, 58

5 Psychosocial Alterations, 63
Effects of Stress on Mind/Body Interactions, 64
Significance to Nursing, 65
Self-Concept, 67
Powerlessness, 71
Hopelessness, 72
Mental Status Changes Requiring Medical Evaluation, 74
Care of Specific Populations, 82
Summary, 84

6 Sleep Alterations, 103
Physiology of Sleep, 103
Sleep Changes with Age, 106
Sleep Changes with Chronic Illness, 107
Circadian Desynchronization, 107
Pharmacology and Sleep, 107
Sleep Deprivation, 109
Recovery Sleep, 110
Sleep Disorders, 110
Assessment of Sleep Pattern Disturbance, 114
Case Study, 114

7 Nutritional Alterations and Management, 121
Nutrient Metabolism, 121
Implications of Undernutrition for The Sick or Stressed Patient, 124
Assessing Nutritional Status, 124
Nutrition and Cardiovascular Alterations, 126
Nutrition and Pulmonary Alterations, 133
Nutrition and Neurologic Alterations, 135
Nutrition and Renal Alterations, 137
Nutrition and Gastrointestinal Alterations, 143

Nutrition and Endocrine Alterations, 149
Nutrition and Hematomimmune Alterations, 152
Administering Nutrition Support, 155
Evaluating Response to Nutrition Support, 162

8 Pain and Sedation, 169

Pain, 169
Physiology of Pain, 169
Types of Acute Pain, 176
Pain Assessment, 176
Pain Management, 180
Sedation, 188
Assessment, 190
Levels of Sedation, 190

UNIT II SPECIAL POPULATIONS, 203

9 The Pediatric Patient in the Adult Critical Care Unit, 205

Respiratory System, 205
Cardiovascular System, 216
Nervous System, 224
Gastrointestinal System/Fluids/Nutrition, 229
Pain Management, 230
Psychosocial Issues of the Child and Family, 232

10 High Risk and Critical Care Obstetric Issues, 243

Fetal Development, 243
Placental Development and Function, 244
Physiologic Alterations in Pregnancy, 246
Cardiac Disease, 251
Resuscitation, 254
Hypertensive Disease, 255
HELLP, 256
Disseminated Intravascular Coagulation, 258
Pulmonary Dysfunction, 259
Diabetic Ketoacidosis, 262
Trauma, 262
Neurologic Dysfunction, 266
Summary, 268

11 Gerontologic Alterations and Management, 271

Studies on Aging, 271
Cardiovascular System, 272
Respiratory System, 276
The Renal System, 279
The Gastrointestinal System, 280
The Liver, 280
The Central Nervous System, 282
Immune System, 286
Physical Examination and Diagnostic Procedures, 288
Summary, 291

12 Perianesthesia Management, 297

General Anesthesia, 297
The Perianesthesia Assessment, 304
Care of the Postanesthesia Patient, 309
Management of Postanesthesia Problems and/or Emergencies, 312

UNIT III CARDIOVASCULAR ALTERATIONS, 329

13 Cardiovascular Anatomy and Physiology, 331

Anatomy, 331
Physiology, 344

14 Cardiovascular Clinical Assessment, 355

History, 355
Physical Examination, 355

15 Cardiovascular Diagnostic Procedures, 377

Laboratory Assessment, 377
Diagnostic Procedures, 384

16 Cardiovascular Disorders, 483

Coronary Artery Disease, 483
Myocardial Infarction, 490
Sudden Cardiac Death, 501
Heart Failure, 502
Cardiomyopathy, 507
Endocarditis, 508
Valvular Heart Disease, 510
Atherosclerotic Diseases of the Aorta, 514
Peripheral Vascular Disease, 517
Carotid Artery Disease, 519
Deep Vein Thrombosis, 521
Hypertensive Crisis, 523

17 Cardiovascular Therapeutic Management, 529

Temporary Pacemakers, 529
Cardiac Surgery, 541
Implantable Cardioverter Defibrillator, 550
Catheter Interventions for Coronary Artery Disease, 552
Balloon Valvuloplasty, 561
Thrombolytic Therapy, 561
Mechanical Circulatory Assist Devices, 567
Effects of Cardiovascular Drugs, 574

18 Cardiovascular Nursing Diagnosis and Management, 585

UNIT IV
PULMONARY ALTERATIONS, 599

19 Pulmonary Anatomy and Physiology, 601
Thorax, 601
Conducting Airways, 604
Respiratory Airways, 607
Pulmonary Blood and Lymph Supply, 610
Ventilation, 613
Respiration, 618
Ventilation/Perfusion Relationships, 618
Gas Transport, 620

20 Pulmonary Clinical Assessment, 625
History, 625
Physical Examination, 627
Assessment Findings of Common Disorders, 633

21 Pulmonary Diagnostic Procedures, 641
Laboratory Studies, 641
Diagnostic Procedures 647
Bedside Monitoring, 653

22 Pulmonary Disorders, 655
Acute Respiratory Failure, 655
Acute Respiratory Distress Syndrome, 660
Pneumonia, 663
Pulmonary Embolus, 668
Status Asthmaticus, 671
Air Leak Disorders, 673
Thoracic Surgery, 677
Long-Term Mechanical Ventilation, 681

23 Pulmonary Therapeutic Management, 689
Oxygen Therapy, 689
Artificial Airways, 692
Invasive Mechanical Ventilation, 703
Noninvasive Mechanical Ventilation, 710
Pharmacology, 713
New Frontiers in Treatment, 715

24 Pulmonary Nursing Diagnosis and Management, 719

UNIT V
NEUROLOGIC ALTERATIONS, 731

25 Neurologic Anatomy and Physiology, 733
Divisions of the Nervous System, 733
Microstructure of the Nervous System, 733
Central Nervous System, 736

26 Neurologic Clinical Assessment, 763
History, 763
Physical Examination, 763
Rapid Neurologic Examination, 774

27 Neurologic Diagnostic Procedures, 779
Radiologic Procedures, 779
Cerebral Blood Flow Studies, 784
Electrophysiology Studies, 786
Lumbar Puncture, 787

28 Neurologic Disorders, 791
Coma, 791
Persistent Vegetative State, 795
Brain Death, 798
Cerebrovascular Accident, 798
Guillain-Barré Syndrome, 812
Craniotomy, 814

29 Neurologic Therapeutic Management, 821
Assessment of Intracranial Pressure, 821
Management of Intracranial Hypertension, 826
Herniation Syndromes, 832
Pharmacologic Agents, 834
New Frontiers in Treatment, 834

30 Neurologic Nursing Diagnosis and Management, 839

UNIT VI
RENAL ALTERATIONS, 847

31 Renal Anatomy and Physiology, 849
Macroscopic Anatomy, 849
Vascular Anatomy, 849
Microscopic Structure and Function, 850
Neural Innervation, 852
Processes of Urine Formation, 852
Functions of the Kidneys, 854
Fluid Balance, 856
Factors Controlling Fluid Balance, 859
Electrolyte Balance, 860

32 Renal Clinical Assessment and Diagnostic Procedures, 865
History, 865
Physical Examination, 865
Additional Assessment Parameters, 869
Laboratory Assessment, 872
Radiologic Assessment, 875

33 **Renal Disorders and Therapeutic Management, 877**

Acute Renal Failure, 877
Acute Tubular Necrosis, 878
Assessment and Diagnosis, 879
Dialysis, 886
Pharmacology, 903

34 **Renal Nursing Diagnosis and Management, 911**

UNIT VII
GASTROINTESTINAL ALTERATIONS, 917

35 **Gastrointestinal Anatomy and Physiology, 919**

Role of the Brain, 919
Gastrointestinal Tract, 919
Accessory Organs of Digestion, 926

36 **Gastrointestinal Clinical Assessment and Diagnostic Procedures, 931**

Clinical Assessment, 931
History, 931
Physical Examination, 931
Laboratory Studies, 935
Diagnostic Procedures, 936
Assessment Findings of Common Disorders, 940

37 **Gastrointestinal Disorders and Therapeutic Management, 945**

Acute Gastrointestinal Hemorrhage, 945
Acute Pancreatitis, 950
Acute Intestinal Obstruction, 958
Fulminant Hepatic Failure, 962
Therapeutic Management, 965

38 **Gastrointestinal Nursing Diagnosis and Management, 973**

UNIT VIII
ENDOCRINE ALTERATIONS

39 **Endocrine Anatomy and Physiology, 977**

The Pancreas, 979
Pituitary Gland and Hypothalamus, 982
The Thyroid Gland, 983

40 **Endocrine Clinical Assessment and Diagnostic Procedures, 989**

Clinical Assessment, 990
Pancreatic Laboratory Assessment, 990
Laboratory Assessment, 993
Diagnostic Procedures, 994

41 **Endocrine Disorders and Therapeutic Management, 1001**

Stress and Critical Illness, 1001
Diabetes Mellitus, 1001
Diabetic Ketoacidosis, 1003
Hyperglycemic Hyperosmolar Nonketotic Syndrome, 1015
Diabetes Insipidus/Hyposecretion of Antidiuretic Hormone, 1021
Syndrome of Inappropriate Antidiuretic Hormone/Hypersecretion of Antidiuretic Hormone, 1027
Thyrotoxic Crisis, 1031
Myxedema Coma, 1038

42 **Endocrine Nursing Diagnosis and Management, 1045**

UNIT IX
MULTISYSTEM ALTERATIONS

43 **Trauma, 1051**

Mechanisms of Injury, 1051
Phases of Trauma Care, 1052
Specific Trauma Injuries, 1057
Spinal Cord Injuries, 1064
Maxillofacial Injuries, 1071
Thoracic Injuries, 1073
Abdominal Injuries, 1079
Genitourinary Injuries, 1083
Pelvic Fractures, 1084
Lower Extremity Orthopedic Injuries, 1086
Complications of Trauma, 1087
Hypermetabolism, 1087
Infection, 1087
Sepsis, 1088
Pulmonary Complications, 1088
Pain, 1089
Gastrointestinal Complications, 1089
Renal Complications, 1089
Vascular Complications, 1090
Missed Injury, 1090
Multiple Organ Dysfunction Syndrome, 1091

44 **Shock, 1097**

Shock Syndrome, 1097
Hypovolemic Shock, 1100
Cardiogenic Shock, 1102
Anaphylactic Shock, 1105
Neurogenic Shock, 1109
Septic Shock, 1111

45 Systemic Inflammatory Response Syndrome and Multiple Organ Dysfunction Syndrome, 1121

The Inflammatory Response, 1121
Multiple Organ Dysfunction Syndrome, 1124
Experimental Pharmacologic Approaches in SIRS and MODS, 1135

46 Burns, 1141

Anatomy and Functions of the Skin, 1141
Pathophysiology and Etiology of Burn Injury, 1142
Classification of Burn Injuries, 1142
Initial Emergency Burn Management, 1146
Special Management Considerations, 1149
Burn Nursing Diagnosis and Management, 1151
Resuscitation Phase, 1152
Acute Care Phase, 1158
Rehabilitation Phase, 1168
Stressors of Burn Nursing, 1169

47 Transplantation, 1171

Immunology of Transplant Rejection, 1171
Heart Transplantation, 1179
Heart and Lung Transplantation, 1184
Single- and Double-Lung Transplantation, 1188
Liver Transplantation, 1191
Kidney Transplantation, 1199
Pancreas Transplantation, 1205

Appendix A *North American Nursing Diagnosis Association's (NANDA) Taxonomy, A-1*

Appendix B *Nursing Interventions Classification (NIC) Taxonomy, B-1*

Appendix C *Advanced Cardiac Life Support (ACLS) Guidelines, C-1*

Appendix D *Physiologic Formulas for Critical Care, D-1*

Appendix E *Interdisciplinary Plans of Care, E-1*

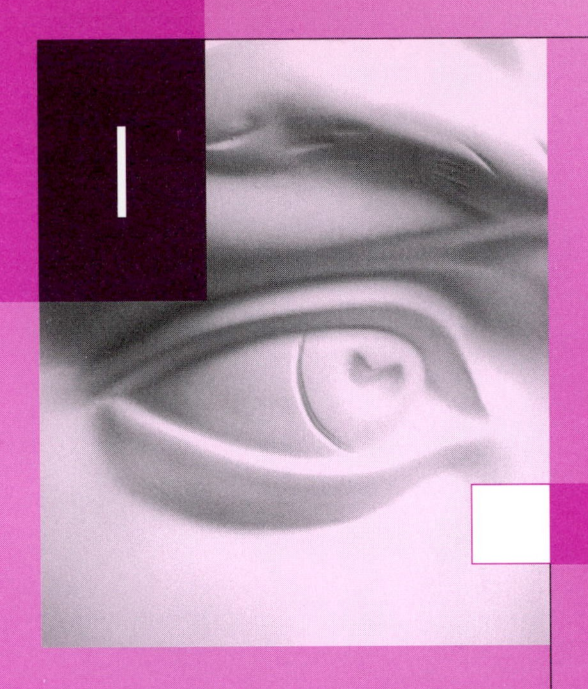

FOUNDATIONS OF CRITICAL CARE NURSING

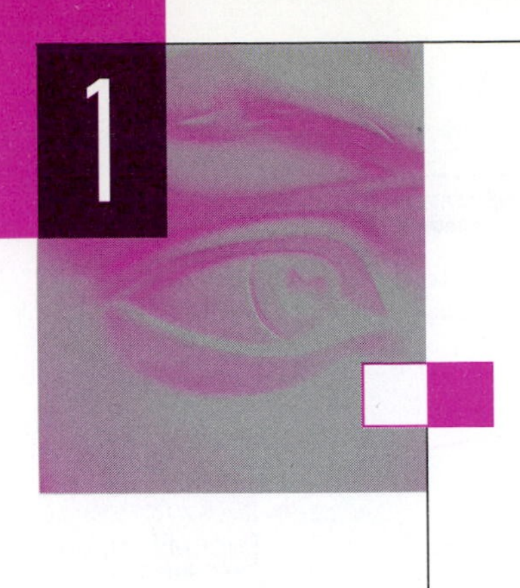

Coordination of Care for the Critically Ill

HEALTH CARE IS undergoing dramatic change at a speed that makes it almost impossible to remain current and be proactive. The chaos and multiple challenges facing health care providers and consumers are evident in critical care, where new treatment modalities and technology interface with a continued strive for quality and positive outcomes. Efficiency and cost-effectiveness in relation to health care services are now commonly discussed and emphasized to all health care practitioners. To some, it appears that quality patient care has taken the back seat to the new emphasis on cost containment and that quality and cost-effectiveness are not congruent. It is incumbent on all critical care health care providers to face these challenges both from their individual discipline scope of practice and collectively from collaborative and interdisciplinary approaches.

The purpose of this chapter is to provide an overview of planning of care and services for critically ill patients. Specifically, nursing's unique role in critical care is described, along with various nursing classifications that delineate nursing diagnoses, interventions, and outcomes. In addition, the importance of collaborative interdisciplinary planning for outcomes is discussed. Finally, the design and implementation of care management via case management and outcomes management are delineated with examples of tools, such as clinical pathways, algorithms, and protocols.

NURSING'S UNIQUE ROLE IN HEALTH CARE

Nursing is dynamic and responds to the changing nature of societal needs.[1] Four features of contemporary nursing practice have been described as:[1]

- *Attention to the full range of human experiences and responses to health and illness without restriction to a problem-focused orientation*
- *Integration of objective data with knowledge gained from an understanding of the patient's or group's subjective experience*
- *Application of scientific knowledge to the processes of diagnosis and treatment*
- *Provision of a caring relationship that facilitates health and healing*

The phenomena of concern to nurses are human experiences and responses to birth, illness, and death. Specifically, the following areas are those for which nursing care is focused:[1]

- *Physiologic and pathophysiologic processes*
- *Care and self-care processes*
- *Physical and emotional comfort, discomfort, and pain*
- *Emotions related to experiences of birth, health, illness, and death*
- *Meanings ascribed to health and illness*
- *Decision- and choice-making abilities*
- *Perceptual orientations*
- *Relationships, role performance, and change processes within relationships*

Today's health care environment necessitates a nursing framework that is flexible and responsive to the needs of the public who are served.[1] Although nursing has both independent and dependent nursing actions, it is essential that an interdependence with all health care professionals is actualized. It is through such collaborative efforts and exchange of knowledge and ideas about care delivery that quality patient outcomes are made evident.[1,2]

The American Association of Critical Care Nurses (AACN) has described a vision for the future health

BOX 1-1 Essential Attributes of the Critical Care Nurse

- Autonomous decision maker
- Research-based practitioner
- Expert in planning patient care
- Able to articulate the unique role of nursing
- Expert delegator
- Able to understand and integrate economic implications of care into goals and outcomes of practice
- Systems thinker with broad perspectives on care provision
- Focused on outcome-driven practice
- Manager, facilitator, and coordinator of patient experiences
- Possessor of excellent interpersonal skills
- Role model for caring practices

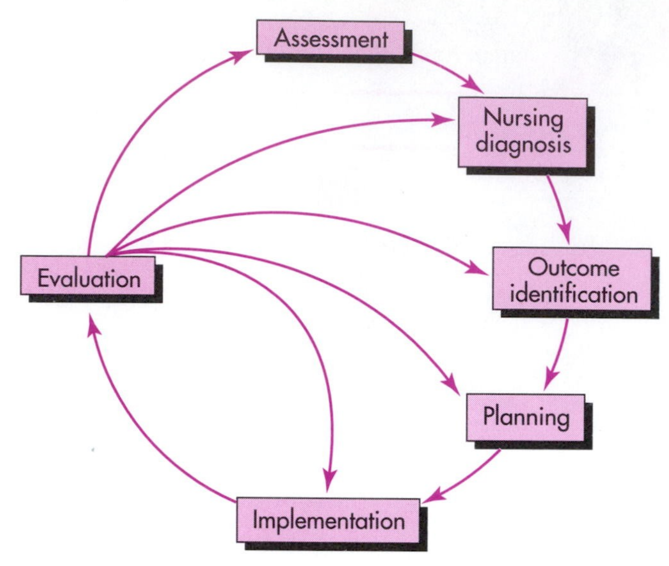

FIGURE 1-1. Cyclical nature of the nursing process. (Modified from Fortinash K, Holoday-Worret P: *Psychiatric nursing care plans,* ed 2, St Louis, 1995, Mosby.)

care system that is driven by the needs of patients and families.[3] The association identified characteristics for the nurse of the future that foster support of the patient-driven care system. These characteristics are summarized[3] in part in Box 1-1. Many of these attributes are important qualities that can be extended to all health care professionals.

THE NURSING PROCESS

The nursing process is a method for making clinical decisions. It is a way of thinking and acting in relation to the clinical phenomena of concern to nurses. Classically, the nursing process comprises five phases or dimensions: assessment, nursing diagnosis, planning, implementation, and evaluation. More recently, the nursing process has been revised to a six-step process.[4] *Outcome identification* was added as a separate step, which follows after nursing diagnosis but comes before the planning stage (see Figure 1-1).

The nursing process is a systematic decision making model that is cyclic, not linear. By virtue of its evaluation phase, the nursing process incorporates a feedback loop that maintains quality control of its decision-making outputs.

The nursing process is indeed a method for solving clinical problems, but it is not merely a problem-solving method. Similar to a problem-solving method, the nursing process offers an organized, systematic approach to clinical problems. Unlike a problem-solving method, the nursing process is continuous, not episodic. The six phases constitute a continuous cycle throughout the nurse's moment-to-moment data interpretation and management of patient care.

Assessment

By virtue of nursing's unique orientation and commitment to holism, nurses collect an enormous amount of data about a patient's biopsychosocial health status. And by virtue of an array of technophysiologic monitoring devices, critical care nurses process an additional layer of data in the form of physiologic parameter measurements. Consequently, in the process of assembling this data base, the critical care nurse needs some place to file the information as it is collected. Ideally, this storage system would contain compartments, which could keep the data separated and organized. Such a system is called an *assessment* or *organizational framework.* Organizational frameworks can also serve as guides for assessment, and their compartments consist of headings corresponding to the attributes the nurse accepts as constituting the nature of humans, health, illness, and nursing.

Assessment frameworks. Assessment frameworks are necessary to process the volume of information nurses accrue in the assessment of a patient. Frameworks facilitate diagnostic reasoning by guiding data collection and organizing it into manageable parts. Organizing incoming information in this way increases its availability for retrieval and facilitates subsequent identification of relationships among the

TABLE 1-1 Comparison of Selected Organizational Frameworks

Medicine	Nursing	
BODY SYSTEMS	**NANDA TAXONOMY I REVISED**	**FUNCTIONAL HEALTH PATTERNS**
Cardiovascular	Exchanging	Health perception-Health management
Respiratory	Communicating	Nutritional-Metabolic
Neurologic	Relating	Elimination
Endocrine	Valuing	Activity-Exercise
Metabolic	Choosing	Sleep-Rest
Hematopoietic	Moving	Cognitive-Perceptual
Integumentary	Perceiving	Self-perception-Self-concept
Gastrointestinal	Feeling	Role-Relationship
Genitourinary	Knowing	Sexuality-Reproductive
Reproductive		Coping-Stress tolerance
Psychiatric		Value-Belief

data. The selection of any one framework over another, as long as it is designed to organize nursing data, is an individual choice.

Body systems. Assessment frameworks are neither new nor unique to nursing. Traditionally, nursing used medicine's body system's assessment framework for the collection and organization of data, but as nursing's knowledge base and conceptual orientation became increasingly differentiated and complex, the biologic, mechanistic scheme of medicine was found to be insufficiently comprehensive for its use by nurses as a tool for holistic assessment. The assessment framework for generalist medical practice and two frameworks for nursing practice are shown in Table 1-1.

Functional health pattern typology. Developed by Marjory Gordon, functional health patterns are categories of human biologic, psychologic, developmental, cultural, social, and spiritual assessments. Health patterns, or sequences of health behavior across time, are identified and interpreted by the nurse and determined to be either functional or dysfunctional. Functional health patterns are the patient's strengths; dysfunctional health patterns form the basis for the patient's nursing diagnoses.[5]

NANDA Taxonomy. In 1986 at the Seventh Conference of the North American Nursing Diagnosis Association (NANDA), a classification system for nursing diagnoses was endorsed. Named Taxonomy I, now "Revised," this classification system is based on a unitary person framework (NANDA's conceptual framework) and replaces the alphabetized listing of diagnoses used previously.[6] See Appendix A for a complete list of NANDA nursing diagnoses.

Nursing Diagnosis

Historically, nursing interventions tended to be disjointed and episodic. The nurse often considered each piece of assessment data as a separate, discrete entity, neither seeking nor perceiving relationships between groups of symptoms. Intervention strategies were planned and carried out in relation to what were considered to be series of independent findings.

With nursing diagnosis as a component of our decision-making methods, we necessarily become more systematic in the collection and interpretation of data and accomplish a change in the substance of our clinical operations, from symptom management to problem solving.

At its Ninth Conference, the NANDA assembly endorsed the following working definition of nursing diagnosis[6]:

> A nursing diagnosis is a clinical judgment about individual, family or community responses to actual or potential health problems/life processes. Nursing diagnoses provide the basis for selection of nursing interventions to achieve outcomes for which the nurse is accountable.

The most essential and distinguishing feature of any nursing diagnosis is that it describes a health condition *primarily resolved by nursing interventions or therapies.*

Nursing diagnoses most commonly identified in critical care[7] are delineated in Table 1-2. All approved diagnoses have accompanying definitions to better explain the health state they represent. These definitions are important because they clarify more about the health state than is apparent from the label alone.

TABLE 1-2 Commonly Identified Nursing Diagnoses in Critical Care*

Nursing Diagnosis	Percent of Time Identified
Pain	93
Risk for Infection	92
Impaired Gas Exchange	92
Decreased Cardiac Output	91
Risk for Impaired Skin Integrity	90
Fluid Volume Excess	89
Altered Cardiopulmonary Perfusion	88
Ineffective Airway Clearance	87
Anxiety	84
Ineffective Breathing Pattern	81
Sleep-pattern Disturbance	81
Risk for Fluid Volume Deficit	81
Fluid Volume Deficit	78
Sensory Overload	75
Risk for Injury	74
Impaired Skin Integrity	73
Risk for Activity Intolerance	73
Activity Intolerance	73
Knowledge Deficit	70
Bathing/Hygiene Self-Care Deficit	70

*Top 20 diagnoses based on nurses' ratings of "nearly always" and "frequently present" in their critical care practice.

Some nursing diagnoses need accompanying qualifiers or specifiers based on the characteristics of the health problem as it manifests itself in a particular patient. For example, the diagnosis Fear needs specification as to the object of the patient's particular fear, such as death, pain, disfigurement, or malignancy. Examples of nursing diagnoses and qualifying statements are shown in Table 1-3.

Guidelines for ETIOLOGIC/RELATED FACTORS

In many instances, NANDA's etiologies are broad categories or examples needing to be made specific, based on characteristics of the health state and the patient being treated. For example, one of several possible etiologies for the diagnosis Fluid Volume Excess is *compromised regulatory mechanism.* Considering this the cause of the fluid excess in a particular patient, the nurse needs to specify the regulatory mechanism and in what way it is compromised (for example, inappropriate ADH secretion by the neurohypophysis) before the diagnosis can be formally stated.

TABLE 1-3 Examples of Nursing Diagnoses and Qualifying Statements

Nursing Diagnosis	Qualifying Statement
Altered Nutrition	Less Than Body Requirements
Knowledge Deficit	Disease Process/Symptom Management
Fear	Disfigurement/Change in Bodily Functions
Risk for Infection	Risk Factor: Immunosuppression
Fluid Volume Deficit	Blood Loss

Nursing diagnostic labels may rightfully serve as etiologies for other diagnoses. Examples are Anxiety R/T* knowledge deficit, and Activity Intolerance R/T decreased cardiac output.

The treatment plan formulated for a given diagnosis must include interventions aimed at resolution or management of the etiologic factors, as well as the health state. In fact, in some instances nursing treatment is directed exclusively at the etiology of a diagnosis, with the logical expectation that, if the causative factors are reduced in influence, the problem should begin to resolve. This is true especially in instances where a nursing diagnosis has as its etiology another nursing diagnosis. Consider treatment approaches to the diagnosis Ineffective Breathing Pattern R/T high abdominal incision pain. Predictably, little effectiveness is shown if the interventions are focused solely on reviewing the rationale for slow, deep, symmetrical breathing; demonstrating the technique; and encouraging the patient in its performance without some plan for manipulation of the pain variable.

Citing a medical condition or diagnosis as the etiology is conceptually inadvisable if the diagnostic statement is to retain its identity as a health problem primarily resolved by nursing therapies. See Table 1-4 for examples of nursing diagnoses and etiologies.

Guidelines for DEFINING CHARACTERISTICS

As with diagnostic labels and statements of etiology, defining characteristics cited for diagnoses are in nonspecific form and often need to be modified to reflect the particular situation presented by the patient being diagnosed. For example, the diagnosis Impaired Gas Exchange has as one of its possible defining char-

*Related to.

TABLE 1-4 Examples of Nursing Diagnoses and Etiologies

Nursing Diagnosis	Etiology (related to)
Ineffective Airway Clearance	Excessive secretions or abnormal viscosity of mucus
Altered Cerebral Tissue Perfusion	Vasospasm or hemorrhage
Decreased Cardiac Output	Sympathetic blockade
Anxiety	Treat to biologic, psychologic, or social integrity
Ineffective Family Coping	Critically ill family member

acteristics *abnormal blood gases.* In the nurse's formulation of this diagnostic statement for clinical use, the specific blood gas value used to diagnose the problem should be cited in the statement (e.g., Po_2: 54 mm Hg and/or Pco_2: 50 mm Hg) versus the nonspecific sign category, abnormal blood gases.

Guidelines for DIAGNOSING RISK STATES

Predicting a potential health problem in a given patient involves an estimation of probability. The potential for an event or pattern of response to occur can truly be said to exist in almost any situation. An appraisal of the patient's health status and the identification of risk factors that place him or her at higher risk for the health problem than the general population is completed. All nurses have a tacit understanding of this risk, and monitoring and intervention are carried out as part of routine nursing management to avert the problem; hence there is no need to state the problem. The diagnosis indicating this potential and its risk factors would be stated so that additional and/or more intensified interventions, over those that are routine, can be planned. Risk nursing diagnoses have only two parts to the statement: the *health problem at risk* and the *risk factors* (e.g., Risk for Ineffective Individual Coping; risk factors: malignant biopsy results, absence of interpersonal support system, and history of alcohol abuse). See Box 1-2 for examples of the format for nursing diagnoses.

Outcome Identification

The emphasis on patient outcomes has become increasingly important in the provision of quality care and services. It is important that nurse-sensitive outcomes are delineated so that nursing care and services can be described and understood by all health care professionals, consumers, and payors.[8,9] Outcome statements consist of highly specific indicators that will be used by the nurse in the evaluation phase as criteria that either (1) the actual diagnosis has been resolved or reduced or (2) the risk diagnosis has not occurred. An outcome statement is a projection of the expected influence that the nursing intervention will have on the patient in relation to the identified diagnosis.

As shown in Figure 1-2, outcome criteria for an *actual* diagnosis are developed from the signs and symptoms of the nursing diagnosis. In other words, the assessment findings that were used to certify the existence of a diagnosis should also be used to establish its resolution or improvement. Outcome criteria for a

BOX 1-2 Format for Nursing Diagnoses

ACTUAL PROBLEM (THREE-PART STATEMENT)

Part 1: Nursing diagnosis

Altered Tissue Perfusion: Myocardial

Part 2: Etiologic Factors (related to):

Acute myocardial ischemia secondary to coronary artery disease (CAD)

Part 3: Defining characteristics

Angina > 30 min but < 6 hr
ST-segment elevation on 12-lead ECG
Elevation of CK and CK-MB enzymes
Apprehension

RISK PROBLEM (TWO-PART STATEMENT)

Part 1: Nursing diagnosis

Risk for Aspiration

Part 2: Etiologic factors (related to):

Impaired laryngeal sensation or reflex
Impaired laryngeal peristalsis or tongue function
Impaired laryngeal closure or elevation
Increased gastric volume
Increased intragastric pressure
Decreased lower esophageal sphincter pressure
Decreased antegrade esophageal propulsion

CAD, Coronary artery disease; *CK,* creatine kinase; *CK-MB,* MB isoenzyme of creatine kinase.

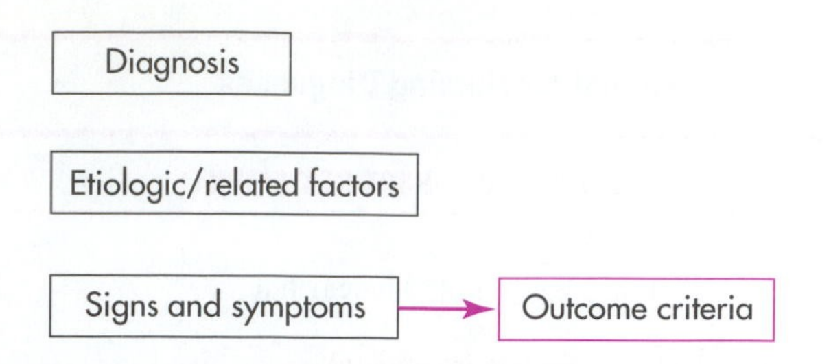

FIGURE 1-2. Developing outcome criteria for an actual diagnosis.

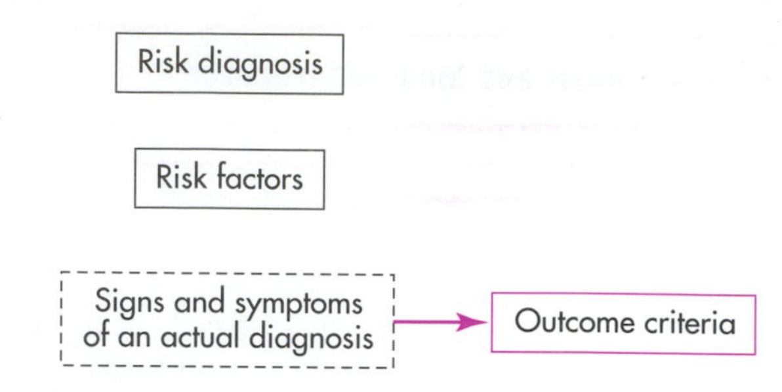

FIGURE 1-3. Developing outcome criteria for a risk diagnosis.

risk diagnosis differ only in that, being a two-part statement, clinical manifestations will be absent from the diagnostic statement. Figure 1-3 illustrates how the outcome criteria are developed from what would be the signs and symptoms of the risk problem *were it to become actual.*

Outcome criteria should be measurable, desirable, and, given full consideration to the resources of the patient and those of the nurse, attainable.

Measurable outcome criteria consist of patient behaviors, statements, and/or physiologic parameters that are recognizable on their occurrence. Many of the phenomena critical care nurses diagnose and treat are readily measurable, such as adequacy of spontaneous ventilation, cardiac output, and tissue perfusion. Many, however, are not readily measurable and thus present a challenging task to care planning in general and outcome criteria development specifically. Phenomena such as anxiety, powerlessness, disturbed body image, and ineffective coping involve the patient's subjective perception and, as such, resist the nurse's quantification.

Outcome statements are made further measurable by indicating the date and time of anticipated attainment. Projecting outcome attainment seems in some situations to be an arbitrary exercise, such as predicting the date or hour for the return of clear lung fields. However, the importance of this aspect of outcome criteria development lies in the fact that a specific deadline for evaluation of outcome attainment has been designated. Evaluating attainment of the outcome at designated intervals ensures that certain problems do not persist beyond acceptable time periods.

The desirability and attainability of patient outcome criteria are other important aspects of planning nursing management. Individual patient baseline and patterns and nurse and patient resources are the dominant considerations given to a projection of desired outcome, versus normative values. See Table 1-5 for examples of correct and incorrect outcome criteria statements for assorted nursing diagnoses.

Planning

During the planning phase, comprehensive planning of all care and services for the patient is done. The process consists of collaboration by the nurse with all appropriate health care providers, patients, and family members/significant others. Priorities for care are identified, with an emphasis on effective, timely interventions to positively influence patient outcomes. Coordination of some care activities and responsibilities may be delegated to others according to the care team member's expertise and specific scope of practice. It is during this stage that interdisciplinary planning of care is done so that a comprehensive plan of care is formulated (refer to the discussion on interdisciplinary planning later in this chapter).

Nursing interventions. Also known as *nursing orders* or *nursing prescriptions,* nursing interventions constitute the treatment approach to an identified health alteration. Interventions are selected to satisfy the outcome criteria and prevent or resolve the nursing diagnosis. It is important to link diagnostic labels with interventions and nurse-sensitive outcomes so that a consistent framework is available for evaluating nursing interventions and outcomes.[10,11]

Intervention strategies that consist solely of monitoring, measuring, checking, obtaining physician orders, documenting, reporting, and notifying do not fulfill criteria for the treatment of a problem. Nursing interventions for nursing diagnoses designate therapeutic activity that assists the patient in moving from one state of health to another. Exciting advances in nurse management of such phenomena as ventilation-perfusion inequalities, excessive preload and afterload, increased intracranial pressure, and sensory-perceptual alterations associated with critical illness

TABLE 1-5 Correct and Incorrect Outcome Criteria Statements

Nursing Diagnosis	Incorrect Outcome	Correct Outcome
Fluid Volume Deficit	Improved hydration Patient will be offered 100 ml fluid q 2 hr	Systolic blood pressure ≥100 mm Hg 24 hr fluid intake ≥body surface area fluid requirements Skin turgor ≤3 seconds
Decreased Cardiac Output	Hemodynamic stability	Cardiac index 2.5-4.0
Pain	Patient will have a reduction in pain	Pain ≤ "4/10" min after IV narcotic
Powerlessness	Patient will perceive greater control over situation	Patient will make five decisions regarding his or her care

afford the critical nurse the opportunity to incorporate potency into treatment plans.

Interventions have the greatest impact when they are directed at the etiologic/related factors of the diagnosis, or, in the case of a risk diagnosis, the risk factors. This stipulates that the etiologic factors of a problem be modifiable by nursing management. To achieve the most favorable patient outcome, the multiple etiologic factors of a problem must be studied carefully and interventions selected to modify each. Planned interventions must provide clarity, specificity, and direction to the spectrum of nurses implementing care for a patient.

Medically delegated actions, such as administering medications and initiating ventilator setting changes, are included in the interventions but with the emphasis placed squarely on the assessments and judgments the nurse makes in evaluating their effectiveness, patient tolerance, safety, dosage, titration, and discontinuance.

Nursing interventions classification. A research team at the University of Iowa has developed and refined a classification system of nursing interventions that is research-based and clinically driven. The Nursing Interventions Classification (NIC) framework contains 433 nursing interventions that are categorized into 27 classes and 6 domains.[11] See Appendix B for a listing of all of the NIC interventions. Interventions consist of both direct care and indirect care nursing interventions. Many nursing interventions are directly linked with NANDA nursing diagnoses. *Nurse-initiated treatments* are those interventions initiated by the nurse in response to a nursing diagnosis.[12] The use of the NIC framework facilitates clinical decision making and provides a standardized language that describes the core of essential nursing interventions. In addition, the research base provides a method to link diagnoses with outcomes in the evaluation of care and services.[11]

Frequently used nursing interventions in critical care[11] are delineated in Box 1-3. The interventions were identified from a sample of practicing critical care nurses. Of the possible nursing interventions (433), 226 interventions are used at least once monthly by 50% of the nurses surveyed. The interventions in Box 1-3 were reported as being used at least once every day by a majority of the respondents. An example of a NIC nursing intervention is presented in Box 1-4. NIC boxes are interspersed throughout this text, as appropriate. An example of how NANDA nursing diagnostic categories link with NIC interventions is presented in Box 1-5.

Implementation

Implementation is the action component of planning. It is the phase of the nursing process in which the nursing treatment plan is carried out. Assessment and evaluation are continuous throughout this phase.

Evaluation

Evaluation of attainment of the expected patient outcomes occurs formally at intervals designated in the outcome criteria. Informal evaluation occurs continuously. The evaluation phase and the activities that take place within it are perhaps the most important dimensions of the nursing process (see Figure 1-1). Evaluation of patient progress against a standard of nursing management incorporates accountability into the process—accountability to the standard of care. Lack of progress in outcome attainment or lack of

BOX 1-3 Frequently Used Nursing Interventions in Critical Care

MEDICATION MANAGEMENT
Medication Administration
Medication Administration: Parenteral
Analgesic Administration
Medication Administration: Oral

RESPIRATORY MANAGEMENT
Oxygen Therapy
Respiratory Monitoring
Airway Suctioning
Airway Management
Artificial Airway Management
Mechanical Ventilation
Ventilation Assistance
Aspiration Precautions

TISSUE PERFUSION MANAGEMENT
Intravenous Therapy
Fluid Monitoring
Fluid Management
Circulatory Care
Dysrhythmia Management
Hemodynamic Regulation
Invasive Hemodynamic Monitoring

SKIN/WOUND MANAGEMENT
Skin Surveillance
Pressure Management
Pressure Ulcer Prevention

ELECTROLYTE AND ACID-BASE MANAGEMENT
Fluid and Electrolyte Management
Acid-base Monitoring
Electrolyte Monitoring
Acid-Base Management
Electrolyte Management
Electrolyte Management: Hypokalemia

THERMOREGULATION
Temperature Regulation

IMMOBILITY MANAGEMENT
Positioning
Bed Rest Care

PHYSICAL COMFORT PROMOTION
Pain Management
Environmental Management: Comfort

SELF-CARE FACILITATION
Oral Health Maintenance
Bathing
Energy Management

RISK MANAGEMENT
Vital Signs Monitoring
Infection Control
Infection Protection
Environmental Management: Safety
Fall Prevention

COMMUNICATION
Active Listening
Communication Enhancement

COPING ASSISTANCE
Emotional Support
Presence
Touch

HEALTH SYSTEM MANAGEMENT
Technology Management
Specimen Management
Tube Care

progress in problem solving is readily identified and kept in check, and alternate solutions can then be proposed. The nursing process depicting an actual and a risk diagnosis format is illustrated in Figure 1-4.

INTERDISCIPLINARY PLANNING FOR CARE

The growing managed care environment has forced emphasis on examining methods of care delivery and processes of care by all health care professionals. Partnerships have been formed or strengthened, with a focus on increasing quality of care and services while containing or decreasing costs.[2,13-15] Coordination of care in critical care units has been demonstrated to significantly influence patient outcomes.[16] It is now more important than ever to create and enhance partnerships because the resulting interdependence and collaboration among disciplines is essential to achieve positive patient outcomes.

NURSING INTERVENTION CLASSIFICATIONS

BOX 1-4 Acid-Base Management

DEFINITION: Promotion of acid-base balance and prevention of complications resulting from acid-base imbalance

ACTIVITIES:

Maintain patent IV access
Maintain a patent airway
Monitor ABG and electrolyte levels, as available
Monitor hemodynamic status, including CVP, MAP, PAP, and PCWP levels if available
Monitor for loss of acid (e.g., vomiting, nasogastric output, diarrhea, and diuresis), as appropriate
Monitor for loss of bicarbonate (e.g., fistula drainage and diarrhea), as appropriate
Position to facilitate adequate ventilation (e.g., open airway and elevate head of bed)
Monitor for symptoms of respiratory failure (e.g., low Pao_2 and elevated $Paco_2$ levels and respiratory muscle fatigue)
Monitor respiratory pattern
Monitor determinants of tissue oxygen delivery (e.g., Pao_2, Sao_2, and hemoglobin levels and cardiac output), if available
Provide oxygen therapy, if necessary
Provide mechanical ventilatory support, if necessary
Monitor determination of oxygen consumption (e.g., Svo_2 and $avDo_2$ levels), if available
Obtain ordered specimen for laboratory analysis of acid-base balance (e.g., ABG, urine, and serum levels), as appropriate
Monitor for worsening electrolyte imbalance with correction of the acid-base imbalance
Reduce oxygen consumption (e.g., promote comfort, control fever, and reduce anxiety), as appropriate
Monitor neurological status (e.g., level of consciousness and confusion)
Administer prescribed alkaline medication (e.g., sodium bicarbonate) as appropriate, based on ABG results
Provide frequent oral hygiene
Instruct the patient and/or family on actions instituted to treat the acid-base imbalance
Promote orientation

From McCloskey JC, Bulechek GM: *Nursing interventions classification,* ed 2, St Louis, 1996, Mosby.
ABG, Arterial blood gas; *CVP,* central venous pressure; *MAP,* mean arterial pressure; *PAP,* pulmonary arterial pressure; *PCWP,* pulmonary capillary wedge pressure.

NURSING INTERVENTION CLASSIFICATIONS

BOX 1-5 Linking NANDA Diagnosis With NIC Interventions
Sleep Pattern Disturbance

DEFINITION: Disruption of sleep time causes discomfort or interferes with desired lifestyle

SUGGESTED NURSING INTERVENTIONS FOR PROBLEM RESOLUTION:

Dementia Management
Environmental Management
Environmental Management: Comfort
Medication Administration
Medication Management
Medication Prescribing
Security Enhancement
Simple Relaxation Therapy
Sleep Enhancement
Touch

ADDITIONAL OPTIONAL INTERVENTIONS:

Anxiety Reduction
Autogenic Training
Bathing
Calming Technique
Coping Enhancement
Energy Management
Energy Promotion
Exercise Therapy: Ambulation
Kangaroo Care
Meditation
Music Therapy
Nutrition Management
Pain Management
Positioning
Progressive Muscle Relaxation
Self-Care Assistance: Toileting
Simple Massage
Urinary Incontinence Care: Enuresis

From McCloskey JC, Bulechek GM: *Nursing interventions classification,* ed 2, St Louis, 1996, Mosby.

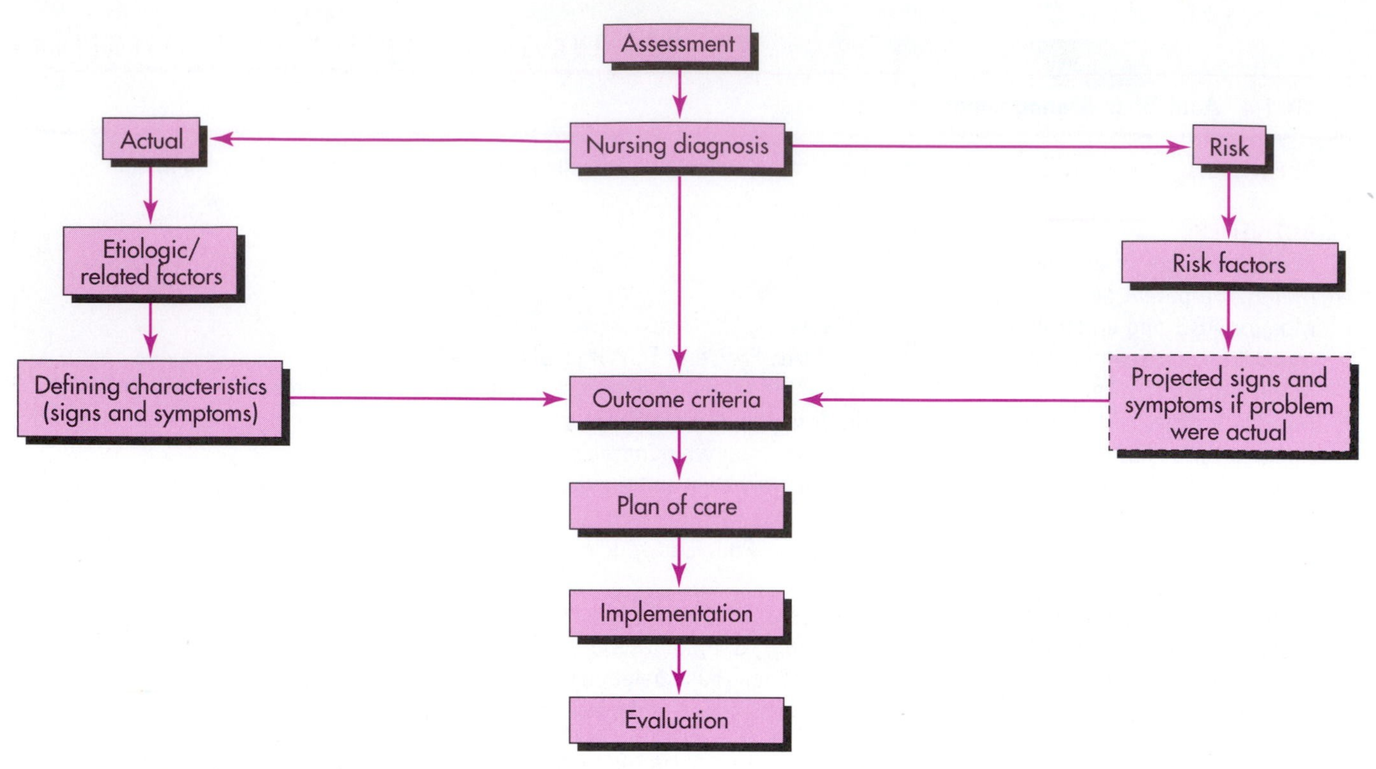

FIGURE 1-4. Nursing process depicting an actual and a risk diagnosis format of the six-step process. (Adapted from Fortinash K, Holoday-Worret P: *Psychiatric nursing care plans,* ed 2, St Louis, 1995, Mosby.)

Interdisciplinary Care Management Models

There are several different models of care delivery and care management used in health care. An overview of the various terms and models are presented in this chapter. The reader is encouraged to seek additional resources and consultation for a more in-depth explanation of the models.

Care management. *Care management* is a system of integrated processes designed to enable, support, and coordinate patient care throughout the continuum of health care services. Care management takes place in many different settings; care is delivered by various professional health care team members and nonlicensed providers, as appropriate. Actual coordination of care and services may be done by health care staff or insurance/payor staff. Care management must be patient-focused, continuum-driven, based on a team approach, and results-oriented. Another term associated with this model of care is *disease state management,* which connotes the process of managing a population's health over a lifetime. In disease state management, however, there is a focus on managing complex and chronic disease states, such as diabetes or congestive heart failure, over the entire continuum.

Case management. *Case management* is the process of overseeing the care of patients and organizing services in collaboration with the patient's physician or primary health care provider. The case manager may be a nurse, allied health care provider, or the patient's primary care provider. Case managers are usually assigned to a specific population group and facilitate effective coordination of care services as patients move in and out of different settings. Ideally, the case manager oversees the care of the patient across the continuum of care.

Outcomes management. *Outcomes management* refers to a model aimed at managing the outcomes of care by the use of various tools, quality improvement processes, and interdisciplinary team involvement and action. Specifically, there is an emphasis on consistent standards of care; measurement of disease-specific clinical outcomes, as well as patient functioning and well-being; and assessment of clinical and outcome data for the specific conditions.[17] Outcomes management also takes place in multiple settings across the continuum of care. Professional nurse outcomes managers ensure variances that form the plan of care are addressed in a timely manner, and they also examine aggregate information with the team for quality improvement in the interdisciplinary plan of care.

 **RESEARCH ABSTRACT** 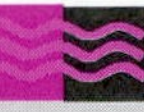

Facilitating the recovery of open heart surgery patients through quality improvement efforts and CareMAP implementation.

Griffith D and others: *Amer J Crit Care* 5(5):346, 1996.

PURPOSE

The purpose of this study was to illustrate how care coordination and implementation of standard protocols can affect outcomes for open heart surgery patients.

DESIGN

Descriptive, explorative.

SAMPLE

The pilot project examined activity and ventilator weaning of open heart surgery patients. The intervention study used 49 open heart surgery patients who were 70 years or younger, hemodynamically stable, had no prior use of pulmonary medicines, maintained ejection fractions of 30% or greater, and had creatinine levels of 2 mg/dL or less.

PROCEDURE

Variance analysis from an open heart surgery CareMAP revealed frequent respiratory alterations. These variations served as the basis for a pilot study to examine the variances with the implementation of a revised weaning protocol. Arterial blood gas (ABG) sampling decreased from an average of 5.8 per patient to 3.9; invasive lines and catheters were removed sooner; the level of patient activity increased; and length of stay (LOS) decreased for all open heart surgery patients. A rapid recovery–continuous quality improvement team was formed and focused on three areas: an aggressive activity regimen, quicker ventilator weaning, and quicker transfer to the step-down unit.

RESULTS

Ventilator time decreased by 4.4 hours to an average of 5.1 hours; overall LOS decreased for all patients; average postoperative hospital LOS decreased by 2.4 days to 4.7 days; no reintubations occurred.

DISCUSSION/IMPLICATIONS

The quality improvement process using the CareMAP pathway tool and weaning protocol positively affected the outcomes of open heart surgery patients in this study. The synergy of using the pathway with a protocol enhanced the ventilation weaning process and entire surgical hospital experience. Quality was maintained, and costs were lowered because of a decrease in hospital days. It is through collaborative team efforts such as this process and program that critical care quality can be enhanced in a cost-effective and efficient manner.

Care Management Tools

There are many quality improvement tools available to providers for care management. Four tools are addressed in this chapter: clinical pathways, algorithms, practice guidelines, and protocols.

Clinical pathway. The *clinical pathway* presents an overview of the entire multidisciplinary plan of care for routine patients. It focuses on the critical elements in the care of certain patient populations and may track variances from the pathway. Pathways are developed by a multidisciplinary team, based on a specific diagnosis or condition and integrated with latest research and best practices from the literature. Pathways are ideal for high-volume diagnosis groups that are amenable to standardization. Many pathways are incorporated into the medical record or are computerized, making them a permanent part of the clinical record.

Clinical pathways have been demonstrated to decrease patients' length of stay and overall costs, while maintaining or increasing quality of care.[18-22] Length of stay (LOS) is an outcome variable tracked by health care team members, as well as payors. The pathway target LOS for a particular condition or diagnosis-related group (DRG) may be determined by using external references or guidelines that are published by insurance companies. Milliman and Robertson has annual publications that recommend LOSs for inpatient and outpatient care. These references are used by many utilization management staff as the standard practice. Variances from the recommended days are discussed with physicians for rationales and action. LOS for disorders in this text are described, as appropriate, using the geometric mean length of stay (GMLOS). The GMLOS is calculated without the outliers that would greatly skew the data.[23]

See Figure 1-5 for an example of a congestive heart failure (CHF) pathway. The pathway delineates essential care/treatment categories in the first column, with specific functions listed on the appropriate day in the second through sixth columns. This pathway is initiated in the emergency department and is based on an expected

Butterworth
HEALTH SYSTEM
Grand Rapids, MI 49503

CONGESTIVE HEART FAILURE CLINICAL PATH (DRG 127)

This pathway is only a guideline. Patient care will vary on their individual needs. Please refer to CPM Guidelines of Care and Education Record for the Congestive Heart Failure Patient.

Ejection Fraction: ____
NYHA Functional Class:
Admit ______ Discharge ______
I-no limits II-Limit w/activity
III-SOB w/ADLs IV-symptoms@ rest

Please fill in dates and check all boxes that apply, write NA over boxes that do not apply.

Stamp with addressograph

Length of stay will vary for each patient. Pathway is based on average stay. Less complicated and younger patients may have shorter than average length of stays. Some patients may stay longer than the average if their condition is more severe.

Dates	ER	DAY 1	DAY 2	DAY 3	DAY 4	OUTCOMES
Consults (*see criteria on back)	☐Consider cardiology NP ☐Consider cardiology ☐ Consider MSW	☐Consider Cardiac Rehab ☐Consider cardiology NP ☐Consider cardiology ☐Consider Dietary ☐Consider Pharmacy				☐ Follow up established with PCP/ cardiology
Assessment & Interventions	☐VS/strict I & O ☐Consider BiPAP/CPAP ☐Assess oxygen/O2 protocol ☐Bronchodilator protocol ☐Old records/echos ☐Cardiac monitor ☐Foley/Inter. Infusion Device	**☐VS/strict I & O** **☐Daily weight** ☐ Continue O2 assessment	**☐VS/strict I & O** **☐ Patient weighs self and logs their weight** **☐Use same scale if possible** ☐Consider d/c monitor, foley	**☐VS/strict I & O** **☐Patient weighs self and logs their weight** **☐Use same scale if possible**	**☐VS/strict I & O** **☐Patient weighs self and logs their weight** **☐ Use same scale if possible**	☐ Patient keeps log of their weight daily and notifies MD/NP with weight gain as per education record teaching. ☐ F & E status WDL for this patient
Medications	☐Pre-admission meds ☐IV diuretics ☐Consider digoxin, ACE inhibitors, nitrates, inotropes	☐Adjusting of meds ☐ Consider ACE inhibitor ☐Sq heparin if not on coumadin	☐Change to po meds ☐Consider adjusting ACE inhibitor ☐D/C sq heparin if OOB	☐Stabilization of meds ☐Consider adjusting ACE inhibitor ☐D/C sq heparin if OOB		☐ Patient verbalizes purpose of medications, doses, side effects, etc., per ed record
Diet	**☐Fluid restriction** ☐NPO except ice chips	**☐Fluid restriction** ☐Sodium restriction	**☐Fluid restriction** ☐Sodium restriction	**☐Fluid restriction** ☐Sodium restriction	**☐Fluid restriction** ☐Sodium restriction	☐ Patient verbalizes understanding of cardiac diet and fluid restriction
Activity	☐Bedrest with BRP	☐Bedrest with BRP ☐Physical therapy prn	☐OOB	☐OOB		☐ Cardiac rehab or exercise program in place prn
Tests	☐CXR, EKG, U/A ☐CPK/MB, SMA + lytes, Mg++, plts, CBC, TSH - if a-fib/new onset CHF ☐PT/PTT if on coumadin/hep ☐Digoxin level if on digoxin	☐ Chem 7	☐Consider repeat CXR ☐Chem 7	☐Chem 7	☐Consider CXR prior to d/c ☐Chem 7	☐ Diagnostic studies WDL for pt
Education (see Ed Record)	☐See CHF Ed Record	☐Reinforce CHF Ed Record ☐Smoking counseling/**Smoking cessation program initiated prn** **☐Provide copy of CHF book/CHF kit - review w/pt**	☐See Ed Record ☐Smoking counseling **☐Review CHF book w/pt**	☐See Ed Record ☐Smoking counseling **☐Review CHF book w/pt**	☐See Ed Record ☐Smoking counseling **☐Review CHF book w/pt**	☐ Patient d/c with copy of the CHF book/kit and verbalizes understanding as per ed record ☐ **Smoking cessation program initiated prn**
Discharge Planning	☐Assess support systems/home environment ☐Identify pot. barriers to d/c	☐Assess support systems/home environment ☐Identify pot. barriers to d/c ☐Assess need for cardiac rehab after d/c	☐Assess need for home care ☐Assess need for assistive devices (i.e. 02)	☐RN review discharge plan. ☐Assess need for assistive devices (i.e. 02)	☐Discharge plans per preprinted d/c instruction sheet ☐Support services in place (i.e.: O2, rehab, home nursing)	☐ Patient has home care and assistive devices in place prn ☐ Able to verbalize d/c plan ☐ Document d/c NYHA Funcitonal class
Signatures (Name/Time)	________	________	________	________	________	________

This report is prepared pursuant to but not limited to (P.A.368 of 1978). This report is a review function and as such is confidential and shall be used only for the purpose provided by law and shall not be a public record and shall not be available for court subpoena.

R:\NURSING\PATHS\CHF.DOC 12/16/96 2:20 PM ©Butterworth Hospital (616-391-1276) XO2763 **Return to Mail Code 16 when completed**

FIGURE 1-5. CHF pathway. (Courtesy Butterworth Health Systems, Grand Rapids, MI.)

length of stay of 4 days. Expected outcomes are delineated in the last, or seventh, column. The second page of the pathway lists criteria for the various referrals described in the pathway. There is a coding system to track variances so that the pathway also serves as a quality improvement tool for the team to examine and make changes in practice, as appropriate. Other examples of clinical pathways are included in Appendix E.

Algorithm. An *algorithm* is a step-wise decision-making flowchart for specific care process(es). Algorithms are more focused than clinical pathways and guide the clinician through the "if, then" decision-making process, addressing patient responses to particular treatments.[22] Well-known examples of algorithms are the Advanced Cardiac Life Support (ACLS) algorithms published by the American Heart Association (see Appendix C).

Algorithms may be used with clinical pathways and are particularly helpful when patients develop variances from the pathway that are amenable to a concise decision-making guide.[24] Schriefer describes the synergy that develops when algorithms are combined with pathways.[22] Whenever "bottlenecks" to a pathway occur, algorithms are considered an enhancement (see Figure 1-6). Weaning, medication selection, medication titration, individual practitioner variance, and appropriate patient placement algorithms have been developed to give practitioners additional standardized decision-making abilities. See Figure 1-7 for an example of an algorithm that has been useful in the management of atrial fibrillation developing after a coronary artery bypass graft (CABG). Other examples of algorithms are found in Appendix E.

Criteria for Medical Social Work Referral	Criteria for Cardiology NP Consult	Criteria for Cardiac Rehab Referral/PT
Increased anxiety	New onset CHF	Decreased mobility/lack of ability to perform ADLs
Depressed Mood/Affect	Readmission within 30 days	Lack of knowledge of ways/activities to decrease tissue oxygen demands
Caregiver of a dependent spouse	NYHA function class III or IV	New diagnosis
Socially Isolated/limited support system	Needs CHF education	History of smoking/smoking cessation referrals
Inadequate financial resources to meet needs		Secondary diagnosis of Ischemic Heart Disease

Criteria for Dietary Consult	Criteria for Pharmacy Consult
Serum albumin <3.0	Patient on 7 or more medications
Diet for discharge is new to patient or different from diet prior to admission	Patient on two medications of same class
Admission weight gain of ten pounds or greater over last discharge weight	Serum Creatinine > 2.5 mg/dl excluding admission creatinine
	Serum potassium > 5.6 or < 3.0 mEq/liter
	Medication related admission (eg: Digoxin toxicity)

Instructions: Please indicate any significant variances that may prolong the stay in the boxes to the right. Write in the variance code, the date the variance occurred, comments and your initials. Your comments for improving the care for this population or the pathways format are appreciated.

CODES FOR COMMON VARIANCES:

Code	Issue	Code	Issue	Code	Issue
427.9	Arrhythmia	P1	Lives alone/lack of home support	S1	Pathway documentation incomplete
786.50	Chest pain	P2	Pt education not complete	S2	Imprinted Orders not used
787.02	Nausea	P4	Anxiety	S3	Discharge instructions not used
787.01	Vomiting	P6	Unexpected transfer to ICU	S6	Delay in PT consult
		P8	Abnormal lab values	S8	Delay in MSW consult
		P25	Activity intolerance	S9	Delay in dietitian consult

Pathway Variance/ Exception Code	Date	Comments	Initials

Ideas for improving care for this population:	Ideas for improving format of this pathway:

This report is prepared pursuant to but not limited to (P.A.368 of 1978). This report is a review function and as such is confidential and shall be used only for the purpose provided by law and shall not be a public record and shall not be available for court subpoena.

R:\NURSING\PATHS\CHF.DOC 12/16/96 2:20 PM ©Butterworth Hospital (616-391-1276) XO2763 Return to Mail Code 16 when completed

FIGURE 1-5 CONT'D. For legend see p. 14.

Practice guideline. *Practice guidelines* are usually developed by professional organizations (e.g., American Association of Critical Care Nurses, Society of Critical Care Medicine, American College of Cardiology or government agencies such as the Agency for Health Care Policy and Research [AHCPR]). Practice guidelines are generally written in text prose style rather than in the flowchart format of pathways and algorithms. Practice guidelines are used as resources in formulating the pathway or algorithm. Of particular interest to the critical care practitioner is the AHCPR clinical practice guideline *Heart Failure: Evaluation and Care of Patients with Left Ventricular Systolic Dysfunction.*[25,26] There are three components: the complete guideline, a quick reference guide for clinicians, and a patient and family guide. These publications have been used to develop pathways and teaching guides for patients with congestive heart failure and are excellent examples of nationally developed guidelines.

Protocol. A *protocol* is a very common tool in research studies. Protocols are more directive and rigid than pathways or guidelines, and providers are not supposed to vary from a protocol. Patients are screened carefully for specific entry criteria before being started on a protocol. There are many national research protocols, such as those for cancer and chemotherapy studies. Protocols are helpful when built-in "alerts" signal the provider to potentially serious problems. Computerization of protocols assists providers in being more proactive to dangerous drug interactions, abnormal laboratory values, and other untoward effects that are preprogrammed into the computer.

Managing and Tracking Variances

It is essential that all variances are addressed and managed in a timely manner by the health care team members.[27] All of the previously described care management tools provide methods to track variances.

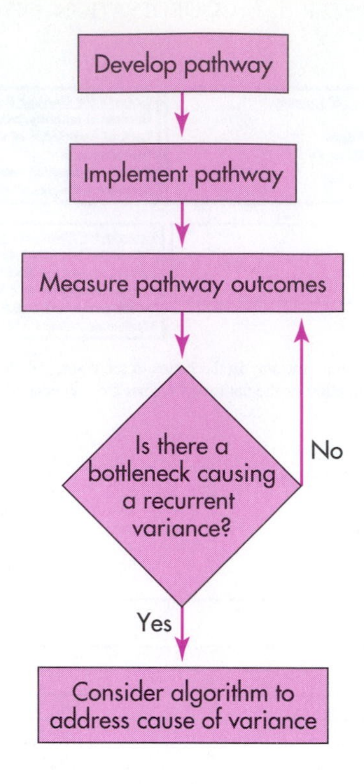

FIGURE 1-6. Combining an algorithm with a pathway. (From Schriefer J: The synergy pathways and algorithms: two tools work better than one, *Jt Comm J Qual Improv* 20(9):485-499, 1994.)

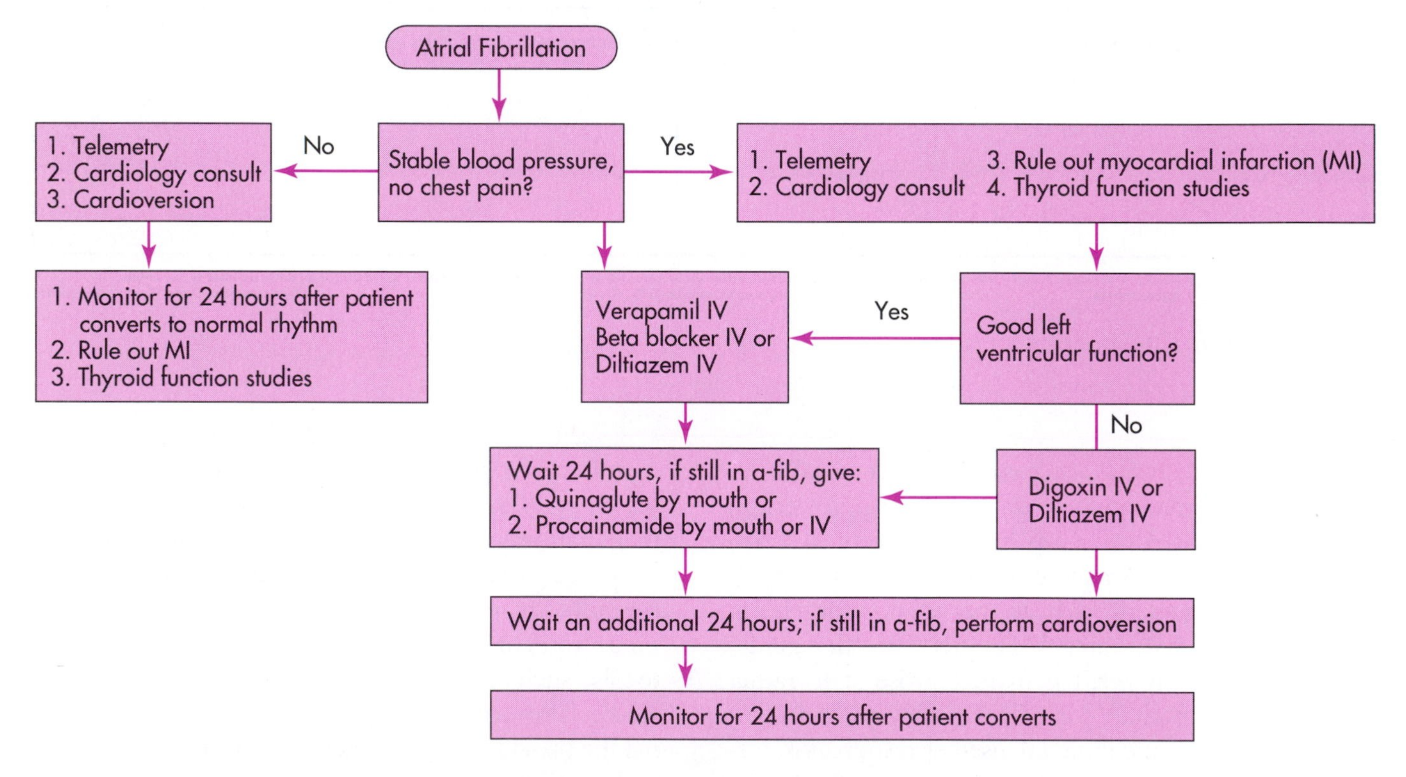

Doses*

Verapamil 6 mg IVP (over 2 min) q 5 min (max: 15 mg)
Metropolol 6 mg IVP q 5 min (max: 15 mg)
Diltiazem 20 mg IVP; mr 25 mg IVP x1; then, if necessary 10-15 mg/hr IV drip x 24h
Digoxin 0.5 mg IVP; then 0.25 mg IVP a 6h x 2 doses then qd
Quinidine gluconate 324 mg PO tid
Procainamide SR 750 mg PO q 6h or 10 mg/kg (</=1 gm) IV over 1h then 2 mg/min IV

*Doses are guidelines and may require adjustment based on specific patient parameters

FIGURE 1-7. Atrial fibrillation algorithm. (From Schriefer J: The synergy pathways and algorithms: two tools work better than one, *Jt Comm J Qual Improv* 20(9):485-499, 1994.)

Whether variance coding is included on a pathway (see Figure 1-5) or is tracked by another quality improvement method, both individual and aggregate data must be assessed and analyzed. Except for protocols, which are more rigid and research-based, algorithms, pathways, and guidelines can be used according to the practitioner's discretion. Tracking variances from the expected standard is one method to determine the utility of the tools in particular settings and patient populations. There needs to be a link between the care management system and the quality improvement program so that changes, as appropriate, can be made to positively affect the outcomes of care and services.

REFERENCES

1. American Nurses Association: *Nursing's social policy statement,* Washington DC, 1995, The Association.
2. White KR, Begun JW: Profession building in the new health care system, *Nurs Adm Q* 20(3):79-85, 1996.
3. American Association of Critical Care Nurses: *The nurse of the future position statement,* Aliso Viejo, Calif, 1993, The Association.
4. American Nurses Association: *American Nurses Association standard of practice,* Kansas City, Mo, 1991, The Association.
5. Gordon M: *Manual of nursing diagnosis 1997-1998,* St Louis, 1997, Mosby.
6. Kim MJ, McFarland GK, McLane AM: *Pocket guide to nursing diagnoses,* ed 7, St Louis, 1997, Mosby.
7. Gordon M, Hiltunen E: High frequency: treatment priority nursing diagnoses in critical care, *Nurs Diagn,* 6(4):143-154, 1995.
8. Brooten D, Naylor M: Nurses' effect on changing patient outcomes, *Image J Nurs Sch* 27(2):95-99, 1995.
9. Himali U: A unified nursing language: the missing link in establishing nursing-sensitive patient outcomes, *Am Nurse,* 27(2):23, 1995.
10. Chase S, Leuner J: Do clinicians use diagnostic labels to direct intervention selection? *Nurs Diagn,* 7(1):33-39, 1996.
11. Titler M, Bulechek GM, McCloskey JC: Use of nursing interventions classification by critical care nurses, *Crit Care Nurse,* 16(4):38-54, 1996.
12. McCloskey JC, Bulechek GM, editors: *Nursing interventions classification (NIC),* ed 2, St Louis, 1996, Mosby.
13. Society of Critical Care Medicine and American Association of Critical Care Nurses: *Essential provisions for critical care in health care system reform (joint position statement),* Anaheim, Calif, Aliso Viejo, Calif, 1994, The Associations.
14. Lumsdon K, Hagland M: Mapping care, *Hosp Health Netw,* 67(20):34-40, 1993.
15. Grady G, Wojner A: Collaborative practice teams: the infrastructure of outcomes management, *AACN Clin Issues Crit Care Nurs,* 7(1):153-158, 1996.
16. Knaus W and others: An evaluation of outcome from intensive care in major medical centers, *Ann Intern Med* 104:410-418, 1986.
17. Wojner A: Outcomes management: an interdisciplinary search for best practice, *AACN Clin Issues Crit Care Nurs* 7(1):133-145, 1996.
18. Redick E, Stroud A, Kurack T: Expanding the use of critical pathways in critical care, *DCCN,* 13(6):316-321, 1994.
19. Capuano T: Clinical pathways—practical approaches, positive outcomes, *Nurs Manage* 26(1):34-37, 1995.
20. Rudisill P, Phillips M, Payne C: Clinical paths for cardiac surgery patients: a multidisciplinary approach to quality improvement outcomes, *J Nurs Care Qual* 8(3):27-33, 1994.
21. Philibin and others: Does QI work? The management to improve survival in congestive heart failure (MISCHF) study, *Jt Comm J Qual Improv* 22(11):721-733, 1996.
22. Schriefer J: The synergy of pathways and algorithms: two tools work better than one, *Jt Comm J Qual Improv* 20(9):485-499, 1994.
23. Lorenz E, Jones M: *St. Anthony's DRG Guidebook,* Reston, Va, 1997, St. Anthony Publishing.
24. Maxam-Moore V, Goedecke R: The development of an early extubation algorithm for patients after cardiac surgery, *Heart Lung* 25(1):61-68, 1996.
25. Dunbar S, Dracup K: Agency for health care policy and research: clinical practice guidelines for heart failure, *J Cardiovasc Nurs* 10(2):85-88, 1996.
26. Agency for Health Care Policy and Research: *Heart failure: evaluation and care of patients with left-ventricular systolic dysfunction,* Rockville, Md, 1994, US Department of Health and Human Services.
27. Mateo M, Newton C: Managing variances in case management, *Nurs Case Manage* 1(1):45-51, 1996.

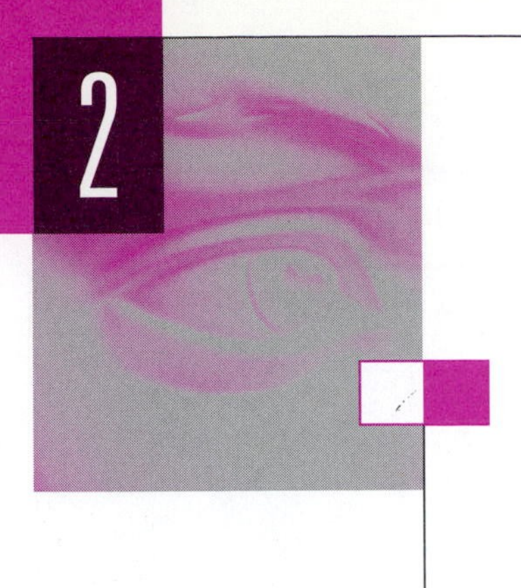

Ethical Issues

THE CONTEMPORARY CRITICAL care nurse is confronted with moral and ethical conflicts on a frequent, sometimes daily, basis and is the health care professional who is most involved with all persons affected by the ethical decisions made.[1] It is essential that the critical care nurse have an understanding of professional nursing ethics and ethical theories and principles and that he or she is able to use a decision-making model to guide nursing actions. The purpose of this chapter is to provide an overview of ethical theories and principles and professional nursing ethics. An ethical decision-making model is described and illustrated. In addition, recommendations are given about methods to discuss ethical issues in the critical care setting. (Ethical Issues in Critical Care)

MORALS AND ETHICS

Morals Defined

The word *moral* is derived from the Latin *moralis,* which is defined as "good or right in conduct or character . . . making the distinction between right and wrong . . . principles of right and wrong based on custom."[2] Morals are the "shoulds," "should nots," "oughts," and "ought nots" of actions and behaviors and have been related closely to sexual mores and behaviors in Western society. Religious and cultural values and beliefs largely mold one's moral thoughts and actions. Morals form the basis for action and provide a framework for evaluation of behavior.

Ethics Defined

The word *ethics* is derived from the Greek *ethos,* which is defined as "the system or code of morals of a particular person, religion, group, or profession . . . the study of standards of conduct and moral judgment."[2] The term *ethics* is sometimes used interchangeably with the word *morals.* However, ethics is more concerned with the "why" of the action rather than with whether the action is right or wrong, good or bad.[3] Ethics implies that an evaluation is being made that is theoretically based on or derived from a set of standards. *Normative ethics* is the division of ethics that focuses on "norms or standards of behavior and value and their ultimate application to daily life"[4] with an emphasis on evaluation for purposes of guiding moral action. *Bioethics* incorporates all aspects of life but most often refers to health care ethics and the application of ethical principles to individual cases.

ETHICAL THEORIES

Philosophers have described ethical theories to be the combination of thinking processes, related principles, and rationales. The approach is normative, because it attempts to provide a basis for action. There are two traditional ethical theories briefly discussed in this chapter: teleologic and deontologic.

Teleologic Theory (Consequentialism)

The focus of this theoretic approach is on the consequence of an action. Individuals are obligated to provide the greatest amount of happiness for the greatest number or the least amount of harm to the greatest number. According to Fowler, utilitarian ethics is the most important teleologic theory for use in health care today.[4] Two common aphorisms summarize the utilitarian approach: "the greatest good for the greatest number" and "the end justifies the means."[3]

Philosophers Jeremy Bentham and John Stuart Mill professed the utilitarian theory and presented arguments for the approach with what has been described as "calculus morality." The outcomes of all alternative actions on the welfare of present and future generations are calculated. Rather than determining utility of an action on a single situation or act (act utilitarianism), rule utilitarians judge actions on moral rules, which leads to the greatest good for the greatest number.[4]

The effect of consequences on present and future conditions of persons and groups takes precedence in utilitarianism.[5,6] Given the scarce resources of health care dollars, this approach for ethical decision making may be increasingly important. Future productivity of patients may serve to determine the types and amount of treatment or health care services that they receive.[5,6] Emergency situations may require a standard to be violated, such as omitting a sterile procedure to save a life or safely triage patients. According to utilitarian theory, truth-telling may not be upheld if it is determined not to be in the best interest of the patient.[5,7]

Deontologic Theory (Formalism)

The focus of the deontologic approach to ethical problems is on the rules that determine the rightness or wrongness of the action.[4,6] Immanuel Kant, a German philosopher, has been credited with the formulation of this approach. Democratic principles or laws are stressed, and universality is the basis for decisions.[6] Past moral or ethical judgments are considered, and value is assigned to significant relationships, commitments, and promises. Actions are independently assessed for their own value, and the consequences are not part of the decision.[5]

Kant espoused the belief that moral actions would supercede all other reasons for action and issued a "categorical imperative" that only actions that should become universal law be demonstrated.[7] Categorical imperatives are unconditional commands that are morally necessary and required under any circumstances. One has a duty to obey categorical imperatives with no exceptions and under all circumstances. The aphorism inherent in formalism is "the end does not justify the means." Decisions based on formalism are normally congruent with one's moral convictions and serve to validate one's strong sense of duty when acting out of principle regardless of consequences.[5,8] Strict adherence to rules, policies, and standards may stifle creativity and examination of alternatives in the fast-paced health care environment of today.

ETHICAL PRINCIPLES

There are certain ethical principles that were derived from classic ethical theories that are used in health care decision making.[5] Principles are general guidelines that govern conduct, provide a basis for reasoning, and direct actions. The six ethical principles that are discussed in this chapter are autonomy, beneficence, nonmaleficence, veracity, fidelity, and justice/allocation of resources (Box 2-1).

BOX 2-1 Ethical Principles in Critical Care

- Autonomy
- Beneficence
- Nonmaleficence
- Veracity
- Fidelity
  - Confidentiality
  - Privacy
- Justice/Allocation of Resources

Autonomy

The concept of autonomy appears in all ancient writings and early Greek philosophy. Immanuel Kant described an ethical person as one who is guided and motivated in response to one's own inward obedience, free from coercion, desire, or fear of future consequences.[7] Persons are not to be treated as a means to an end but rather as an end themselves.[9] In health care, autonomy can be viewed as the freedom to make decisions about one's own body without the coercion or interference of others. Autonomy is a freedom of choice or a self-determination that is a basic human right. It can be experienced in all human life events.

The obligation for health care professionals is to respect the values, thoughts, and actions of patients and not to let their own values or morals influence treatment decisions.[10] Fry described this as a respect for the "unconditional worth of the individual."[9] Often there is a conflict between the values of the patient and the health care professionals when dealing with life-sustaining matters in critical care. For patient autonomy to be maintained, patient decisions regarding treatments—such as resuscitation—must be supported.[11]

The critical care nurse is often "caught in the middle" in ethical situations, and promoting autonomous decision making is one of those situations. As the nurse works closely with patients and families to promote autonomous decision making, another crucial element becomes clear. Patients and families must have all of the information about a certain situation to make a

NURSING INTERVENTION CLASSIFICATIONS

BOX 2-2 Decision-Making Support

DEFINITION: Providing information and support for a patient who is making a decision regarding health care

ACTIVITIES:
Determine whether there are differences between the patient's view of own condition and the view of health care providers
Inform patient of alternative views or solutions
Help patient identify the advantages and disadvantages of each alternative
Establish communication with patient early in admission
Facilitate patient's articulation of goals for care
Obtain informed consent, when appropriate
Facilitate collaborative decision making
Be familiar with institution's policies and procedures
Respect patient's right to receive or not to receive information
Provide information requested by patient
Help patient explain decision to others, as needed
Serve as a liaison between patient and family
Serve as a liaison between patient and other health care providers
Refer to legal aid, as appropriate
Refer to support groups, as appropriate

From McCloskey JC, Bulechek GM: *Nursing interventions classification,* ed 2, St Louis, 1996, Mosby.

decision that is best for them. Not only should they be given all of the information and facts, but they must also have a clear understanding of what was presented. This is where the nurse is a most important member of the health care team—that is, as patient advocate, providing more information, clarifying points, reinforcing information, and providing support during the process.[10] See Box 2-2 for nursing intervention activities that facilitate decision making. The legal implications of informed consent are discussed in Chapter 3. The Patient Self-Determination Act (PSDA) legislates that patients are informed of their right to designate health care treatments (see Chapter 3).[12]

Beneficence

The concept of doing good and preventing harm to patients is a *sine qua non* for the nursing profession. However, the ethical principle of beneficence—which requires that one promote the well-being of patients—points to the importance of this duty for the health care professional. The principle of beneficence presupposes that harms and benefits are balanced, leading to positive or beneficial outcomes.

In approaching issues related to beneficence, there is commonly conflict with another principle, that of autonomy. *Paternalism* exists when the nurse or physician makes a decision for the patient without consulting or including the patient in the decision process. *Paternalism* is "making people do what is good for them" and "preventing people from doing what is bad for them."[7] Jameton[7] described two types of paternalists: strong paternalists who make decisions for obviously competent persons and weak paternalists who make decisions for persons who are mentally or physically unable to make their own decisions.

Traditional health care has been based on a paternalistic approach to patients. Many patients are still more comfortable in deferring all decisions about care and treatment to their health care provider. Active involvement by various organizations and agencies regarding health care has demonstrated a trend toward the public's need and desire for more information about health care and alternative treatments and providers. Paternalism, or maternalism in the case of female providers, may always be a possibility in the health care setting, but enlightened consumers are changing this practice of health care professionals.

In the critical care setting, there are many instances and possibilities for paternalistic actions by the nurse. Postoperative care, which is designed to assist the patient with a quick recovery, is a good example of paternalistic action by the nurse. Encouraging the patient to turn, cough, and deep breathe and increasing activity in the form of dangling, sitting in a chair, and ambulating are all paternalistic when the patient is in pain, sleep-deprived, and wanting to be left alone. However, there are times when the priorities of benefits and harms must be balanced. In this instance, the duty to do no harm—which is the next principle to be discussed—takes precedence over paternalistic actions. When there are conflicts in ethical principles, one must weigh all of the benefits and choose the best one.

Nonmaleficence

The ethical principle of nonmaleficence, which dictates that one prevent harm and remove harmful situations, is a *prima facie* duty for the nurse. Thoughtfulness and care are necessary, as is balancing risks and benefits, which was discussed earlier with beneficence. Beneficence and nonmaleficence are on two ends of a continuum and are often carried out differently, depending on the views of the practitioner. A practitioner using a utilitarian approach will consider long-term consequences and the good to society as a whole. The practitioner operating from a deontologic basis will consider the principle and its effect on the single individual in the situation.

Such complex situations as quality of life versus sanctity of life are always difficult to analyze in the critical care setting as well as in non–critical care settings. Flynn described decisions such as withholding and withdrawing treatments as being based on not one ethical principle alone, but rather on a balance of all ethical principles so that the most appropriate moral decision can be made.[13] Nonmaleficence must serve as the guide for practice of health care professionals.[5]

Veracity

Veracity, or truth-telling, is an important ethical principle that underlies the nurse-patient relationship. In 1860 Florence Nightingale described veracity with patients: "Far more now than formerly does the medical attendant tell the truth to the sick who are really desirous to hear it about their own state."[14] Nightingale's philosophy was not agreed on by other health care providers of the time (i.e., physicians), but she was sensitive to the needs of patients who sought information about their own conditions.

Veracity is important in soliciting informed consent, so that the patient is aware of all potential risks and benefits from specific treatments or their alternatives. Once again, the critical care nurse can be in the middle of a situation where all of the facts and information about a particular treatment option are not disclosed. Sometimes information has been given accurately but has been delivered with bias or in a way that is misleading. In this case and other instances with veracity, the ethical principle of autonomy has been violated.[15] Veracity must guide all areas of practice for the nurse, that is, colleague relationships and employee relationships, as well as the nurse-patient relationship.

Fidelity

Another ethical principle that is closely related to autonomy and veracity is fidelity. Fidelity, or faithfulness and promise-keeping to patients, is also a *sine qua non* for nursing. It forms a bond between individuals and is the basis of all relationships, both professional and personal. Regardless of the amount of autonomy that patients have in the critical care areas, they still depend on the nurse for a multitude of types of physical care and emotional support. A trusting relationship that establishes and maintains an open atmosphere is one that is positive for all involved.[16]

Aroskar[15] pointed out that making a promise to a patient is voluntary for the nurse, whereas respect for a patient's decision making is a moral obligation. She described the critical care nurse as experiencing a great deal of moral conflict. "Fidelity to patients in 'high-tech' care units may require that nurses question the use of specific technologies for a specific patient or even the admission of a hopelessly ill patient . . . to such a unit."[15]

As do all the other principles, fidelity extends to the family of the critical care patient. When a promise is made to the family that they will be called if an emergency arises or that they will be informed of other special events, the nurse must make every effort to follow through on the promise. Not only will fidelity be upheld for the nurse-family relationship, but there will also be a positive reflection on the nursing profession as a whole and on the institution in which the nurse is employed.

Confidentiality is one element of fidelity that is based on traditional health care professional ethics. According to Veatch and Fry,[17] the nursing and medical professions have established ethical codes that allow no patient-centered reasons for breaking the principle of confidentiality. Confidentiality is described as a right whereby patient information can only be shared with those involved in the care of the patient. An exception to this guideline might be when the welfare of others is at risk by keeping patient information confidential. Again in this situation, the nurse must balance ethical principles and weigh risks with benefits. Special circumstances, such as mandatory reporting laws, will guide the nurse in certain situations.

Privacy has also been described as inherent in the principle of fidelity. It may be closely aligned with confidentiality of patient information and a patient's right to privacy of his or her person, such as maintaining privacy for the patient by pulling the curtains around the bed or making sure that he or she is adequately covered.

Justice/Allocation of Resources

The principle of justice is often used synonymously with the concept of allocation of scarce resources. Contrary to the belief of many people, health care is not a right guaranteed by the Constitution of the United States. Rather, *access* to health care should be provided to all people. With escalating health care costs, expanded technologies, an aging population with its own special health care needs, and (in some instances) a scarcity of health care personnel, the question of health care allocation becomes even more complex.

The application of the justice principle in health care is concerned primarily with divided or portioned allocation of goods and services, which is termed *distributive justice.*[18] According to Jameton, distributive justice appears at three levels of health care: national policies and budget, state or local distribution of resources, and distribution in the individual health care settings.[7] Traditionally, six criteria for making decisions about allocation of resources have been used.[7,19] Distribution has been based on the following:

- Equality for all persons
- Individual merit
- Societal contribution
- Free market acquisition
- Individual need
- Similar treatment for similar cases

Equality for all persons. Equality for all persons has been a traditional stance of health care and has been evidenced in ethical codes and in the practices of professionals. With equality, all persons are given equal treatments and resources, such as access to health care, technologies, specialists, personnel to perform necessary care and treatment, and support for physical and emotional needs during the process.

Individual merit. Distribution of services based on individual merit has not been a traditional practice of health care professionals and is an area that may be subtle to observe. Individual merit might be based on that which has already been achieved or that which is expected to occur in the future, such as in the case of an infant or child or a person who may have potential for success in some endeavor. Basically, the issue at hand is whether this type of person deserves a particular treatment. The decision is based on values that are subjective and not driven by a set of rules or principles.

Societal contribution. Decisions based on the societal contribution of the individual examine the worth of that individual in society and are subjective and value-based. Using this as a framework for making decisions causes elderly persons,[20] young persons, those who have conditions that are socially undesirable such as alcoholism or mental diseases, and those who are handicapped to be considered as having no worth to society.

Free market acquisition. Justice determined by free market acquisition is guided by money and what individuals can acquire with their money. Persons both in the past and in the present who have unlimited money are able to receive the ultimate in services and are able to quickly search for and find services to meet their needs and desires. They are usually limited only by the technologies and services available. However, when time is not crucial, money will pay for technologies or services that can be developed if money is available to support such efforts.

Individual need. Jameton described individual need as most applicable to health care in deciding allocation of resources.[7] The dilemma arises when one considers one individual's need for heart transplantation or other technologies versus the possibility of using those resource dollars for early education on preventing heart disease for many people. In delineating problematic areas in the determination of individual needs, Levine-Ariff asserted that level and type of need should be identified.[19] If harm would come to the individual were the need not met, the need takes precedence and should be met.

Similar treatment for similar cases. The concept of similar treatment for similar cases expands on the concept of equality and applies the same basic principle at the societal level. However, consideration of contribution to society is also inherent in this method of decision. For instance, criteria may be established that designate that all who have a certain condition and who are under a certain age will be given the treatment, surgery, or service. This allows equal access of all who meet those criteria but disallows others who do not meet the criteria. Decisions based on this standard cover groups of people, whereas decisions based on individual need hold only for that one person.

Allocation of Scarce Resources in Critical Care

Major factors influencing health care ethics are rapid health care inflation and the shrinking allocation of public funds to both primary and secondary care. In addition, the number of uninsured persons is increasing, and there is a trend toward the distribution of health care resources to high cost–individual care. End-of-life spending continues to rise, with 28% of Medicare directed at 5% of persons in the last year of life and 40% to persons in the last month of life.[21] The era has changed to one that now does more with less. However, clinical judgment regarding whether specific interventions are beneficial to patient outcomes must still be important in treatment decisions.[22] As health care resources become increasingly more scarce, allocation of resources to certain programs and rationing of resources within certain programs will become more evident.[23] Allocation of resources brings ethical challenges to the daily clinical realities facing health care practitioners.[24]

Allocation of Technologies and Treatments

Limitations of resources force society and the critical care health professionals to reexamine the goals of critical care for patients. Once considered experimental, coronary artery bypass surgery, magnetic resonance imaging, kidney dialysis, and heart transplantation are now widely accepted and funded by payors.[23] Because the possibilities and number of organ transplants are increasing, there are not enough available organs. To increase the availability of donated organs, most states have enacted "required request" laws, which mandate that families must be approached about donation of organs on the death of their loved ones.[25-27] Procurement of organs has posed new ethical dilemmas for health care professionals, who must now act in accordance with state laws.

Other technologies found in critical care that were considered experimental only a few years ago are the intraaortic balloon pump (IABP)[28] and the left ventricular assist device (LVAD). Essential in the use of all technologies and critical care treatments are veracity, autonomy, and informed consent,[28] which have been discussed earlier in this chapter. Legal implications about informed consent are discussed in Chapter 3. In cases in which research protocols are used with patients in the critical care units, all ethical principles apply.[29]

Quality of life is an issue that should be considered when examining the use of technologies. It is an area that is personal and value-laden and one that will be different for all involved and dependent on the content.[30,31] Quality of life has dual dimensions of both objectivity and subjectivity. Objectivity examines the person's functionability, whereas subjectivity analyzes his or her psychosocial state. An evaluation of quality of life issues can take place only after one has received the technology and "lived" that "new" life.[32]

Allocation of Health Care Energy

Knaus stated that "access to an expensive and complex resource like intensive care can never be absolute."[33] Critical care nurses are faced with rationing of critical care beds and nursing staff on a daily basis. Strengths and weaknesses of the staff must be balanced with the needs of the patient. Orientation and other special circumstances—such as designation for charge nurse, trauma nurse, and code nurse—must be considered when scheduling staff and making assignments. Any inexperienced staff, float staff, or registry staff must be given appropriate orientation and backup during the shift.

There is commonly a triage system for critical care units that is called on when there are more admissions than available beds. The critical care nurse is instrumental in assisting the medical director to determine patient selection for transfer, if appropriate. Some hospitals use a set of standards, criteria, or guidelines for determining patient admission and transfer to and from critical care areas. The *Guidelines for Admission/Discharge Criteria in Critical Care* developed by the American Association of Critical Care Nurses[34] are provided in Box 2-3. These guidelines can serve as the basis for development of criteria specific to the critical care nurse's institution.

WITHHOLDING AND WITHDRAWING TREATMENT

The technologic support of life at all costs has recently come to be questioned by both health care professionals and health care consumers. Physicians and nurses who are closest to the issues have debated the moral and ethical implications and have looked to ethicists for guidance and legal opinion. Both medical and nursing associations have developed guidelines for their practitioners about withholding and withdrawing treatments. The American Association of Critical Care Nurses position statement *Withholding and/or Withdrawing Life-Sustaining Treatment*[35] is presented in Box 2-4.

The decision not to employ aggressive measures or to discontinue treatments that have been in place is always difficult and stressful for all involved in the decision, particularly those who continue to care for the patient on a daily basis.[36] Legal implications for withholding or withdrawing treatments and orders not to resuscitate the patient are delineated in Chapter 3.

LEGAL REVIEW 

Understaffing and Nursing Liability

Application of the professional malpractice standard to critical care nursing and increased recognition afforded to nurses by state and federal legislation and the judiciary have extended nursing liability into new areas. These include overwork, understaffing, and "floating" nurses into unfamiliar care settings, all of which potentially compromise patient care. The resulting legal dilemma is that, although hospitals and nurse supervisors can be derelict in their staffing decisions, it is the staff nurse who may be liable in tort or subject to sanctions by the state for the results of those decisions.

As a general rule, nurses do not have statutory protection against understaffing or excessive consecutive number of hours worked. However, many states have regulations that address the minimal competency and training requirements for nurses who "float" or are assigned to unfamiliar areas.

The ANA *Code for Nurses* addresses nursing accountability for individual judgment and actions and criteria for accepting responsibilities, delegating activities to others, and seeking consultation. Nurse supervisors have legal duties (1) to supervise, (2) to properly assign tasks, and (3) to allocate and assign sufficient numbers of trained staff.

In the case of *Leavitt v. St. Tammany Parish Hospital,* the plaintiff-patient fell after the staff failed to respond to her call for help. The defendant-hospital was found liable for failure to have on duty a sufficient number of staff members to respond to the patients' needs. In this particular case, nurses were not named as defendants. However, the court stated in its opinion that the nurses knew of the patient's debilitated condition, yet despite this knowledge failed to take measures to prevent a foreseeable injury. The court concluded that the nurses breached their duty of reasonable care owed to the plaintiff.

It is inadvisable to document inadequate staffing in the medical record. However, nurses subject to understaffing and assignments in unfamiliar units should be thoroughly familiar with their state board of nursing position statement on the issue and their hospital's policies and procedures. Nurses should also keep notes of all efforts taken to remedy the problem, consistently communicate the problem to their superiors, and refuse to acquiesce to a pattern of understaffing or assignments to patient care areas with which they are unfamiliar.

The 1974 amendments to the National Labor Relations Act (NLRA) extended the jurisdiction of the National Labor Relations Board (NLRB) to voluntary and nonprofit hospitals. In *Misericordia Hosp. Medical Center v. NLRB,* the NLRB ordered the reinstatement of a nurse terminated for submitting data that described nursing staff shortages in a Joint Commission on Accreditation of Health Care Organizations (JCAHO) report. The court upheld the jurisdiction extended to the NLRB and the protections the agency gave nurses from dismissal and termination as a result of efforts to improve their working conditions.

See Hoffman NA: Nursing and the future of health care: the independent practice imperative, *Specialty L Dig.: Health Care* 160:7, 1992; *Leavitt v. St. Tammany Parish Hosp.,* 396 So. 2d 406 (La App 1981); *Misericordia Hosp Medical Center v NLRB,* 623 F2d 808 (2d Cir 1980); and Politis EK: Nurses' legal dilemma: when hospital staffing compromises professional standards, *USFL Rev* 18(1):109, 1983.

There appears to be more reluctance to withdraw treatments, which is reflective of ethical and moral conflicts within each of the practitioners. Withholding usually means that there is no hope for success from the onset, whereas withdrawing means surrendering hope. Also, difficult discussions must take place between the health care professionals and the family. The nurse must be sure to examine the treatment with regard for the patient's best interests and wishes and to act accordingly.[36-38]

MEDICAL FUTILITY

The concept of medical futility has resulted in various discussions and proposed criteria or formulas to predict outcomes of care.[21, 39-41] Medical futility has both a qualitative and a quantitative basis and can be defined as "any effort to achieve a result that is possible but that reasoning or experience suggests is highly improbable and that cannot be systematically reproduced."[42]

Therapy or treatment that achieves its predictable outcome and desired effect is, by definition, effective. But effect must be distinguished from benefit. If that predictable and desired effect is of no benefit to the patient, it is nonetheless futile. It is suggested that when physicians conclude from either personal or colleague experiences or from empiric data that a particular treatment in the most recent 100 cases in which it has been used has been useless, the treatment should be

BOX 2-3 Admission/Discharge Guidelines in Critical Care

CRITERIA ARE BASED ON THE FOLLOWING DATA AND RESOURCES:

- Standards of nursing care for the critically ill
- Current unit admission and discharge patterns
- Available resources within the critical care unit: level and quantity of nursing care, expertise and qualifications of personnel, and equipment and technology
- Number and distribution of critical care beds within the institution
- Institutional occupancy trends
- Data provided by existing measurement tools in the institution (e.g., patient classification tools, severity of illness indexes)
- Alternative institutional and community resources available for discharged or triaged patients

CRITERIA ADDRESS THE FOLLOWING ELEMENTS:

- Physiologic parameters that define the need for critical care
- Physiologic parameters that define readiness for discharge
- Definition of unit-specific patient population
- Frequency and type of medical evaluation and/or treatment required by the patient's condition
- Frequency and type of critical care nursing assessments and interventions needed by the patient
- Technologic monitoring and intervention only available in the critical care setting
- Requirements by external regulatory bodies
- Institutional policies that mandate or preclude critical care for specific patient populations
- Designation of the health team member(s) accountable for admission/discharge decisions
- A plan for triage when the need exceeds available physical and human resources
- A plan for conflict resolution between health care team members using the admission/discharge criteria

considered futile.[42] It is incumbent on physicians to make optimal use of health-related resources in a technically appropriate and effective manner. Therefore in this era of escalating health care costs and limited resources, the physician has a particular responsibility to avoid futile treatment.[42]

ETHICS AS A FOUNDATION FOR NURSING PRACTICE

Traditional theories of professions include a code of ethics as the basis for the practice of professionals. The moral foundation of nursing is discussed in the literature by various authors who describe the unique relationship of the professional nurse with the patient, which establishes a caring, trusting approach.[43,44] It is by adherence to a code of ethics that the professional fulfills an obligation for quality practice to society.

A professional ethic is based on three elements: the professional code of ethics, the purpose of the profession, and the standards of practice of the profession. The need for the profession and its inherent promise to provide certain duties form a contract between nursing and society. The code of ethics developed by the professionals is the delineation of its values and relationships with and among members of the profession and society. The professional standards describe specifics of practice in a variety of settings and subspecialties. Each element is dynamic, and ongoing evaluations are necessary as societal expectations change, technologies increase, and the profession evolves.

Nursing Code of Ethics

The American Nurses Association (ANA) provides the major source of ethical guidance for the nursing profession.[43] According to the preamble of the *Code for Nurses,* "When individuals become nurses, they make a moral commitment to uphold the values and special moral obligations expressed in their code."[44] The 11 statements of the Code are found in Box 2-5. They are based on the underlying assumption that nursing is concerned with protection, promotion, and restoration of health; prevention of illness; and the alleviation of suffering of patients.[44]

The *Code for Nurses* was adopted by the ANA in 1950 and has undergone revisions over the years. It provides a framework for the nurse in ethical decision making and provides society with a set of expectations of the profession. The Code is "not open to negotiation in employment settings, nor is it permissible for individuals or groups of nurses to adapt or change the language of this code."[44] The ANA also suggests that the requirements of the Code may not be in concert with the law and that it is the nurse's obligation to uphold the Code, because of the societal commitment inherent in nursing.

BOX 2-4 AACN Position Statement: *Withholding and/or withdrawing life-sustaining treatment*

ADVANCES IN HEALTHCARE technology have dramatically increased the ability to prolong life. Because of these advances, ethical and legal dilemmas arise when complex therapy is instituted to sustain vital functions, even when there is no hope of reversing the disease processes.

The American Association of Critical Care Nurses recognizes that critical care nurses have a significant role in supporting a patient's preferences and beliefs about ending treatments of this type.

THEREFORE, AACN resolves that when choices about withholding and/or withdrawing life-sustaining treatments are being considered, critical care nurses should collaborate with individual patients or their surrogates, physicians and other healthcare providers. This should happen in an atmosphere that promotes reasoned deliberation and communication of a patient's preferences and best interests.

To support this resolution, AACN believes that the following elements are essential for nursing practice:

- Critical care nurses will participate in ongoing assessment of a patient's ability to make decisions about their own health care.
- Critical care nurses will participate in discussions exploring the patient's beliefs about end of life care at the earliest appropriate time. The best time for discussions and decision-making about withholding and/or withdrawal of life-sustaining treatment is before entry into the health care system.
- When patients cannot make decisions for themselves, their preferences may be determined from advanced directives (such as living wills or durable power of attorney for health care), previous spoken or written information, and personal lifestyle.
- Critical care nurses, as patient advocates, will initiate and promote the decision-making process and assure that nursing care goals are consistent with patient preferences or best interests.
- In the event that life-sustaining treatment is withheld or withdrawn, critical care nurses will participate in planning, implementing, and evaluating supportive care. Supportive care includes providing comfort, hygiene, safe surroundings and emotional support for patients and the family.

Thus AACN believes that health care institutions must have policies that direct a process to withhold and/or withdraw life-sustaining treatment. These policies should include:

- A process for ongoing review of treatment goals and interventions. The scope of the care the patient will receive should be specified in writing.
- A process for designating a surrogate when the patient does not have decision-making capacity.
- A process for dispute resolution among patients, surrogates, and health care team members when there is disagreement about the decision-making process.
- A process for transferring care of a patient to another qualified critical care nurse, when a decision to withhold and/or withdraw life-sustaining treatment conflicts with the nurse's personal beliefs and values.

This position on withholding and/or withdrawing life-sustaining treatment is based on these beliefs and ethical principles:

1. Individuals have a moral and legal right and responsibility to make decisions about their health care and the use of life-sustaining treatment.
2. There is no moral or legal difference between withholding and withdrawing treatment. Considerations that justify not initiating treatment also justify withdrawing treatment.
3. A person's capacity to make decisions is shown by their ability to understand relevant information, reason, and deliberate about choices, reflect on information according to their individual values and preferences, and communicate their decision to health care providers.
4. The process for decision-making on behalf of incapacitated patients should be directed by the established standards of substituted judgment or best interests.

DEFINITIONS

Advance directives

A document in which a person gives advance directions about medical care or designates who should make medical decisions on their behalf if they should lose decision-making capacity. There are two types of advance directives: treatment directives, such as living wills, and proxy directives, such as durable power of attorney for health care.

Best interest standard

This standard gives priority to the protection of the patient's welfare. In these cases the designated surrogate tries to make a choice on the patient's behalf that seeks to implement what is in the patient's best interests by reference to more objective, societally shared criteria.

Substituted judgment

The doctrine of substituted judgment requires that the surrogate attempt to reach the decision that the incapacitated person would make if he/she were able to choose. This standard preserves the patient's interest in self-determination.

BIBLIOGRAPHY

American Association of Critical Care Nurses (1989). *Role of the critical care nurse as a patient advocate.* Newport Beach, Ca: Author.

American Nurses' Association (1985). *Code for nurses with interpretive statements.* Washington, DC: Author.

President's Commission for the Study of Ethical Problems in Medicine and Biomedical and Behavioral Research (March 1983). Washington, DC: Government Printing Office.

The Hastings Center (1987). *Guidelines on the termination of life-sustaining treatment and the care of the dying.* Briarcliff Manor, NY: Author.

Adopted by AACN Board of Directors, February 1990.

From American Association of Critical Care Nurses.

BOX 2-5 Code of Ethics For Nurses

1. The nurse provides services with respect for human dignity and the uniqueness of the client, unrestricted by considerations of social or economic status, personal attributes, or the nature of health problems.
2. The nurse safeguards the client's right to privacy by judiciously protecting information of a confidential nature.
3. The nurse acts to safeguard the client and the public when health care and safety are affected by the incompetent, unethical, or illegal practice of any person.
4. The nurse assumes responsibility and accountability for individual nursing judgments and actions.
5. The nurse maintains competence in nursing.
6. The nurse exercises informed judgment and uses individual competence and qualifications as criteria in seeking consultation, accepting responsibilities, and delegating nursing activities to others.
7. The nurse participates in activities that contribute to the ongoing development of the profession's body of knowledge.
8. The nurse participates in the profession's efforts to implement and improve standards of nursing.
9. The nurse participates in the profession's efforts to establish and maintain conditions of employment conducive to high quality nursing care.
10. The nurse participates in the profession's effort to protect the public from misinformation and misrepresentation and to maintain the integrity of nursing.
11. The nurse collaborates with members of the health professions and other citizens in promoting community and national efforts to meet the health needs of the public.

From American Nurses Association: *Code for nurses with interpretive statements,* Washington, DC, 1985, The Association.

The Nurse as Patient Advocate

Winslow[45] described the evolution of nursing ethics from traditional loyalty to physicians to contemporary advocacy of patient rights. The loyalty ethic was based on a military model; advocacy is based on a legal model. He further discussed areas of concern for the nurse when serving in an advocacy role. Patients and their families are sometimes not ready or willing to accept the nurse as an advocate. Advocacy is commonly associated with controversy, and the nurse may experience conflict between interests and loyalties.[45,46] Advocacy "involves an act of free will and a studied choice to view ourselves in a particular way in our relationship to others."[46] Active advocacy reflects the nurse's responsibility and obligation to the patient and incorporates both personal and professional values and standards.[4,47,48] There are five important conditions for advocacy. First, the members of the profession must communicate to clarify obligations and responsibilities. Second, open lines of communication among professionals about patient rights must be maintained. Third, it is essential for trust to be established and maintained between the nurse and the patient. Fourth, the nurse must be aware of all conditions and situations related to the health care decision. The fifth condition is that the nurse must remain educated about current legal and ethical trends.

The American Association of Critical Care Nurses adopted a position statement regarding patient advocacy.[49] The position statement is found in Box 2-6 and can be used as a guideline for the critical care nurse in any setting.

The critical care nurse is in a key position to respond to the needs of patients and families and serve as advocate for them. Respect for individual values, expressed needs, quality-of-life concerns, privacy, inclusion in decision making, autonomy, and personal dignity contributes to patient- and family-centered care.[50,51] Marsden[52] describes family-centered care in critical care as an obligation, not an option. The nurse–patient–family relationship needs to be examined for uniqueness to critical care in which the nurse advocates for the patient and family. Humanizing care, particularly that in critical or terminal situations, is important in upholding these principles.[52,53]

ETHICAL DECISION MAKING IN CRITICAL CARE

The Nurse's Role

As discussed earlier in this chapter, the critical care nurse encounters ethical issues on a daily basis. Although the nurse may feel powerless regarding the ability to influence ethical decisions,[54] this need not be the case. Because the nurse is on the "front line" with such issues as do not resuscitate (DNR) orders, response to treatments, and application of new technologies and new protocols, he or she may be the one who best knows the patient's and/or family's wishes about treatment prolongation or cessation.

BOX 2-6 **AACN Position Statement**
Role of the critical care nurse as patient advocate

THE AMERICAN ASSOCIATION of Critical Care Nurses believes that patient advocacy is an integral component of critical care nursing practice. Therefore, definitions of advocacy and the behaviors that typify advocacy are essential.

WHEREAS, the *Code for Nurses* (American Nurses' Association, 1985) requires that nurses safeguard the patient and the public when health care and safety are affected by the incompetent, unethical, or illegal practice of any person, and

WHEREAS, many definitions of advocacy exist, and

WHEREAS, critical care nurses are confronted with situations that require them to act immediately on the patient's behalf, and

WHEREAS, personal and professional risks are associated with being a patient advocate, and

WHEREAS, state nurse practice acts may require the nurse to be a patient advocate, and

WHEREAS, the process of informed consent mandates that the patient or the patient's surrogate be informed fully and give consent freely, and

WHEREAS, the continuum of advocacy is not limited to the individual but may extend to societal concerns,

THEREFORE, BE IT RESOLVED THAT the American Association of Critical Care Nurses believes the critical care nurse is a patient advocate,

AND THAT the American Association of Critical Care Nurses defines advocacy as respecting and supporting the basic values, rights, and beliefs of the critically ill patient.

BE IT FURTHER RESOLVED THAT the American Association of Critical Care Nurses believes that as a patient advocate, the critical care nurse shall do the following:

1. Respect and support the right of the patient or the patient's designated surrogate to autonomous informed decision making.
2. Intervene when the best interest of the patient is in question.
3. Help the patient obtain necessary care.
4. Respect the values, beliefs, and rights of the patient.
5. Provide education and support to help the patient or the patient's designated surrogate make decisions.
6. Represent the patient in accordance with the patient's choices.
7. Support the decisions of the patient or the patient's designated surrogate or transfer care to an equally qualified critical care nurse.
8. Intercede for patients who cannot speak for themselves in situations that require immediate action.
9. Monitor and safeguard the quality of care the patient receives.
10. Act as liaison between the patient, the patient's family, and health care professionals.

BE IT RESOLVED THAT the American Association of Critical Care Nurses recognizes that health care institutions are instrumental in providing an environment in which patient advocacy is expected and supported.

ALSO, BE IT FURTHER RESOLVED THAT as patient advocate, critical care nurses initiate and promote actions to improve the health care of the critically ill through social change.

REFERENCE

American Nurses Association (1985). *Code for nurses with interpretive statements.* Washington, DC: Author.

Adopted by AACN Board of Directors, August 1989.

From American Association of Critical Care Nurses.

Therefore it is important that the nurse be included as part of the health care team that determines ethical dilemma resolution.[55,56]

What is an Ethical Dilemma?

In general, ethical cases are not always clear-cut or black and white, but rather arise in settings and circumstances that involve innumerable side issues and distractions.[57,58] The most common ethical dilemmas encountered in critical care are foregoing treatment and allocating the scarce resource of critical care. But how does one know that a true ethical dilemma exists?

Before the application of any decision model, a decision must be made about the existence of a true ethical dilemma. Thompson and Thompson[59] delineated the following criteria for defining moral and ethical dilemmas in clinical practice:

1. Awareness of different options
2. An issue with different options
3. Two or more options with true or "good" aspects and the choice of one over the other compromises the option not chosen

Krekeler asserted that ethical situations arise when "the moral decision of one person conflicts with the moral decision of another. Both decisions may be good for each individual in question and undoubtedly are made according to their traditional values."[5] What complicates this process is when there is a third person involved, as is the case in most treatment care decisions in the critical care areas.

Steps in Ethical Decision Making

To facilitate the ethical decision process, a model or framework must be used so that all involved will consistently and clearly examine the multiple ethical issues that arise in critical care. Steps in ethical decision making are listed in Box 2-7.

BOX 2-7 Steps in Ethical Decision Making

1. Identify the health problem.
2. Define the ethical issue.
3. Gather additional information.
4. Delineate the decision maker.
5. Examine ethical and moral principles.
6. Explore alternative options.
7. Implement decisions.
8. Evaluate and modify actions.

Step one. First, the major aspects of the medical and health problem must be identified. In other words, the scientific basis of the problem, potential sequelae, prognosis, and all data relevant to the health status must be examined.

Step two. The ethical problem must be clearly delineated from other types of problems. Systems problems—that is, those resulting from failures and inadequacies in the organization and operation of the health care facility and the health care system as a whole—are often misinterpreted as being ethical issues. Occasionally, a social problem that stems from conditions existing in the community, state, or country as a whole is also confused with ethical issues. Social problems can lead to a systemic problem, which can constrain responses to ethical problems.

Step three. Although categories of necessary additional information will vary, whatever is missing in the initial problem presentation should be obtained. If not already known, the health prognosis and potential sequelae should be clarified. Usual demographic data—such as age, ethnicity, religious preferences, and educational and economic status—may be considered in the decision process. The role of the family or extended family and other support systems needs to be examined. Any desires that the patient may have expressed either in writing or in conversation about treatment decisions are essential to obtain.

Step four. The patient is the primary decision maker and autonomously makes these decisions after receiving information about the alternatives and sequelae of treatments or lack of treatments. However, in many ethical dilemmas, the patient is not competent to make a decision, as occurs when he or she is comatose or otherwise physically or mentally unable to make a decision. It is in these situations that surrogates are designated or court appointed, because the urgency of the situation requires a quick decision. Although the decision process and ultimate decision are more important than who makes the decision, delineating the decision maker is an important step in the process.[59]

Others who are involved in the decision also need to be identified at this time, such as family, nurse, physician, social worker, clergy, and any other members of disciplines having close contact with the patient. The role of the nurse must be examined. There may not be a need for a nurse decision; rather the nurse may provide additional information and support to the decision maker.

Step five. Personal values, beliefs, and moral convictions of all involved in the decision process need to be known. Whether actually achieved through a group meeting or through personal introspection, values clarification facilitates the decision process. (See Box 2-8 for values clarification activities).

Professional ethical codes of the nurse and physician will serve as a foundation for future decisions. At this time, legal constraints or previous legal decisions for circumstances at hand will need to be assessed and acknowledged.

General ethical principles need to be examined in relation to the case at hand. For instance, are veracity, informed consent, and autonomy promoted? Beneficence and nonmaleficence will be analyzed as they relate to the patient's condition and desires. Close examination of these principles will reveal any compromise of ethical or moral principles for either the patient or the health care provider and assist in decision making.

Step six. After the identification of alternative options, the outcome of each action must be predicted. This analysis helps one to select the option with the best "fit" for the specific situation or problem. Both short-range and long-range consequences of each action must be examined, and new or creative actions must be encouraged. Consideration also must be given to the "no action" option, which is also a choice.[59]

Step seven. When a decision has been reached, it is usually after much thought and consideration, and rarely does complete agreement occur among all interested persons.[59] Krekeler recommended following the action until the actual results of the decision can

NURSING INTERVENTION CLASSIFICATIONS

BOX 2-8 Values Clarification

DEFINITION: Assisting another to clarify her/his own values in order to facilitate effective decision-making

ACTIVITIES: Think through the ethical and legal aspects of free choice, given the particular situation before beginning the intervention
Create an accepting, nonjudgmental atmosphere
Use appropriate questions to assist the patient in reflecting on the situation and what is important personally
Use a value sheet clarifying technique (written situation and questions), as appropriate
Pose reflective, clarifying questions that give the patient something to think about
Encourage patient to make a list of what is important and not important in life and the time spent on each
Encourage patient to list values that guide behavior in various settings and types of situations
Help patient define alternatives and their advantages and disadvantages
Encourage consideration of the issues and consequences of behavior
Help patient to evaluate how values are in agreement with or conflict with those of family members/significant others
Support patient's decision, as appropriate
Use multiple sessions, as directed by the specific situation
Avoid use of the intervention with persons with serious emotional problems
Avoid use of cross-examining questions

From McCloskey JC, Bulechek GM: *Nursing interventions classification,* ed 2, St Louis, 1996, Mosby.

be seen.[5] Fowler stated that the decision may need to be modified to meet legal or policy requirements.[60]

Step eight. Evaluation of an ethical decision serves to both assess the decision at hand and use it as a basis for future ethical decisions. If outcomes are not as predicted, it may be possible to modify the plan or to use an alternative that was not originally chosen.

STRATEGIES FOR PROMOTION OF ETHICAL DECISION MAKING

The complexity of health care and frequent ethical dilemmas encountered in clinical practice demand the establishment of mechanisms to address ethical issues found in hospitals and health care facilities. Four types of mechanisms are discussed briefly: institutional ethics committees, inservice and education, nursing ethics committees, and ethics rounds and conferences.

Institutional Ethics Committees (IECs)

Although not required by law, many health care facilities have developed IECs as a way to review ethical cases that are problematic for the practitioner.[61-64] The three major functions of IECs are education, consultation, and recommendation to policy-making bodies. Kemp[65] identified three models of IECs. In the *optional-optional model,* committees serve as consultants and make recommendations that are not binding. The *optional-mandatory model* requires that health care providers consult with the committees when there is an ethical problem, but recommendations are again not binding. The *mandatory-mandatory model* requires that ethical dilemmas be presented to the committees, and recommendations must be followed.

IECs very often comprise executive medical staff. Membership may include staff physicians, administrators, legal counsel, nurses, social workers, clergy, and community public volunteers. To fulfill its requirement for consultation, the committee must include members that not only have expertise, but also are representative of various groups. Regardless of the type of committee model, consultation and support become available to the practitioners.

Inservice and Education

Basic education about ethical principles and decision making is an important first step in facilitating ethical decision making among nursing staff in the critical care area.[66] It is important for nurses to examine their own values, beliefs, and moral convictions. Nurses need to know and use the ANA *Code for Nurses* in their daily clinical practice. Treatment choices for patients and ethical issues involving patients, nurses, and medical colleagues need to be explored and discussed in the classroom setting where no time constraints or extraneous distractions exist to interrupt the decision process.

Nursing Ethics Committees

Nursing ethics committees provide a forum in which nurses can discuss ethical issues that are pertinent to nurses at the individual, unit, or department level.[67] Unlike the IEC, which involves treatment choices of patients, the nursing committee may or may not involve a patient situation. Depending on the specific goals of the committee, it can also serve as a resource to nursing staff, make recommendations to a policy-making body about a variety of professional issues, or actually formulate policies. It may also serve to educate the department on ethical and professional issues. Membership usually comprises representatives from all major clinical areas or divisions, educators, clinical nurse specialists, administrators, and other specialty staff. Some departments such as critical care may have their own unit or division committee.

Ethics Rounds and Conferences

Ethics rounds at the unit level regarding patients in the unit can be done by nurses on a weekly or otherwise established basis. Rounds educate the staff to problems and serve to be "preventive" when facilitated appropriately.[59] During the discussions, potential problems may be identified early and actions taken to decrease or prevent a future problem. An individual patient ethics conference can be scheduled to include only the nursing staff or to include a multidisciplinary group to discuss unit issues. A patient ethics conference may function either as a liaison with the IEC or as an end in itself.

SUMMARY

The emergence of critical care as a specialty and the introduction of sophisticated technologic innovations into critical care units have had a great impact on health care professional practices. Ethical dilemmas are encountered daily in the practice of critical care. The criticality of the situation and speed that is required to make decisions often prevent practitioners from gaining insight into the desires, values, and feelings of patients. The practitioner is often left with no clear ethical or legal guidelines, particularly in the fast-paced modern critical care unit. By assuming a solely technologic approach, practitioners will violate the rights of patients and their professional codes of ethics.

By using an ethical decision-making process, the rights of the patient will be protected and logical analysis of the case will lead to a decision that is made in the best interests of the patient. It is through moral reasoning and examining, weighing, justifying, and choosing ethical principles that patient rights and individuality will be upheld. The practice of nursing is built on a foundation of moral and ethical caring, and the critical care nurse is pivotal in identifying ethical patient situations and can participate in the decision-making process.

REFERENCES

1. Aroskar MA: Ethical decision-making in patient care, *Am Nurse* 26(3):10, 1994.
2. Guralnik D, editor: *Webster's new world dictionary of the American language,* New York, 1981, Simon & Shuster.
3. Catalano JT: Systems of ethics: a perspective. *Crit Care Nurse* 14(6):91, 1992.
4. Fowler M: Introduction to ethics and ethical theory: a road map to the discipline. In Fowler M, Levine-Ariff J, editors: *Ethics at the bedside,* Philadelphia, 1987, JB Lippincott.
5. Krekeler K: Critical care nursing and moral development, *Crit Care Nurse* 10(2):1, 1987.
6. Young S: The nurse manager: clarifying issues in professional role responsibility, *Pediatr Nurs* 13(6):430, 1987.
7. Jameton A: Duties to self: professional nursing in the critical care unit. In Fowler M, Levine-Ariff J, editors: *Ethics at the bedside,* Philadelphia, 1987, JB Lippincott.
8. Luckenbill-Brett J, Stuhler-Schlag M: Mandatory reporting: legal and ethical issues, *J Nurs Adm* 17(12):32, 1987.
9. Fry S: Autonomy, advocacy, and accountability: ethics at the bedside. In Fowler M, Levine-Ariff J, editors: *Ethics at the bedside,* Philadelphia, 1987, JB Lippincott.
10. Singleton KA, Dever R: The challenge of autonomy: respecting the patient's wishes, *DCCN* 10(3):160, 1991.
11. Ott B, Nieswiadomy RM: Support of patient autonomy in the do not resusitate decision, *Heart Lung* 20(1):66, 1991.
12. Omery A: The new patient self-determination act: increasing emphasis on patient autonomy, *DCCN* 10(3):123, 1991.
13. Flynn P: Questions of risk, duty, and paternalism: problems in beneficence. In Fowler M, Levine-Ariff J, editors: *Ethics at the bedside,* Philadelphia, 1987, JB Lippincott.
14. Nightingale F: *Notes on nursing,* Toronto, 1969, Dover Publications.
15. Aroskar M: Fidelity and veracity: questions of promise keeping, truth telling and loyalty. In Fowler M, Levine-Ariff J, editors: *Ethics at the bedside,* Philadelphia, 1987, JB Lippincott.
16. Washington G: Trust: a critical element in critical care nursing, *Focus Crit Care* 17(5):418, 1990.
17. Veatch R, Fry S: *Case studies in nursing ethics,* Philadelphia, 1987, JB Lippincott.
18. Omery A: A healthy death, *Heart Lung* 20(3):310, 1991.
19. Levine-Ariff J: Justice and the allocation of scarce nursing resources in critical care nursing. In Fowler M, Levine-Ariff J, editors: *Ethics at the bedside,* Philadelphia, 1987, JB Lippincott.

20. Baltz J, Wilson JL: Age-based limitation for ICU care: is it ethical? *Crit Care Nurse* 15(6):65, 1995.
21. Miles S: Health-care reform and clinical ethics: old values for new times. *AACN Clin Issues Crit Care Nurs* 5(3):299, 1994.
22. Bryan-Brown CW, Dracup K: Doing more with less. *Am J Crit Care* 5(5):320, 1996.
23. White J: Rationing health care resources, *Nurs Connect* 4(1):22, 1991.
24. Terry P, Rushton CH: Allocation of scarce resources: ethical challenges, clinical realities. *Am J Crit Care* 5(5):326, 1996.
25. Norris MK: Required request: why it has not significantly improved the donor shortage, *Heart Lung* 19(6):685, 1990.
26. Vernale C, Packard S: Organ donation as gift exchange, *Image J Nurs Sch* 22(4):239, 1990.
27. Vernale C: Critical care nurses' interactions with families of potential organ donors, *Focus Crit Care* 18(4):335, 1991.
28. Birkholz G: IABP: legal and ethical issues, *DCCN* 4:285, 1985.
29. Davison R, Davison L: Medical experimentation: ethics in high technology, *Crit Care Nurse* 10:27, 1987.
30. Oleson M: Subjectively perceived quality of life, *Image J Nurs Sch* 22(3):187, 1990.
31. Kleinpell RM: Concept analysis of quality of life, *DCCN* 10(4):223, 1991.
32. O'Mara R: Dilemmas in cardiac surgery: artificial heart and left ventricular assist device, *Crit Care Nurse* 10:48, 1987.
33. Knaus W: Rationing, justice, and the American physician, *JAMA* 255:1176, 1986.
34. American Association of Critical Care Nurses: *Guidelines for admission/discharge criteria in critical care,* 1987, Aliso Viejo, Calif, The Association.
35. American Association of Critical Care Nurses: *Withholding and/or withdrawing life-sustaining treatment,* 1990, Aliso Viejo, Calif, The Association.
36. Dalinis P, Henkelman WJ: Withdrawal of treatment: ethical issues. *Nurs Manage (Critical Care Edition)* 27(9):32AA, 1996.
37. Gilligan T, Raffin TA: How to withdraw mechanical ventilation: more studies are needed, *Am J Crit Care* 5(5):323, 1996.
38. Baggs JG, Schmitt MH: Intensive care decisions about level of aggressiveness of care, *Res Nurs Health* 18:345, 1995.
39. Noland LR: Medical futility: a bedside perspective. *AACN Clin Issues Crit Care Nurs* 5(3):366, 1994.
40. Montague J.: A futile-care formula may ease end-of-life issues, *Hosp Health Netw* Aug 4:176, 1994.
41. Taylor C: Medical futility and nursing. *Image J Nurs Sch* 27(4):301, 1995.
42. Schneiderman LJ, Jecker NS, Jonsen AR: Medical futility: its meaning and ethical implications, *Ann Intern Med* 112(12):949, 1990.
43. Curtin L: Collegial ethics of a caring profession, *Nurs Manage* 25(8):28, 1994.
44. American Nurses Association: *Code for nurses with interpretive statements,* Kansas City, Mo, 1985, The Association.
45. Winslow G: From loyalty to advocacy: a new metaphor for nursing, *Hastings Cent Rep* 14:32, 1984.
46. Nelson M: Advocacy in nursing, *Nurs Outlook* 36:136, 1988.
47. Evans SA: Critical care nursing: the ordinary is extraordinary, *Heart Lung* 20(3):21A, 1991.
48. Johanson WL: A scarce and available resource, *Heart Lung* 20(5):19A, 1991.
49. American Association of Critical Care Nurses: *Role of the critical care nurse as patient advocate,* 1989, Aliso Viejo, Calif, The Association.
50. Gordon S: Inside the patient-driven system, *Crit Care Nurse Suppl* 14(3):3, 1994.
51. Rushton CR: The critical care nurse as patient advocate. *Crit Care Nurse* 14(3):102, 1994.
52. Marsden C: Family centered critical care: an option or obligation? *Am J Crit Care* 1(3):115, 1991.
53. Dracup K, Bryan-Brown CW: Humane care in inhumane places, *Am J Crit Care* 4(1):1, 1995.
54. Erlen JA, Frost B: Nurses' perceptions of powerlessness in influencing ethical decisions, *West J Nurs Res* 13(3):397, 1991.
55. (No author listed): Nurses bring holistic view to ethical decision making, *Medical Ethics Advisor* 9(5):49, 1993.
56. Holly C, Lyons M: Increasing your decision-making role in ethical situations, *DCCN* 12(5):264, 1993.
57. Broom C: Conflict resolution strategies: when ethical dilemmas evolve into conflict, *DCCN* 10(6):354, 1991.
58. Wicclair MR: Differentiating ethical decisions from clinical standards, *DCCN* 10(5):280, 1991.
59. Thompson J, Thompson H: *Bioethical decision-making for nurses,* Norwalk, Conn, 1985, Appleton-Century-Crofts.
60. Fowler M: Piecing together the ethical puzzle: operationalizing nursing's ethics in critical care. In Fowler M, Levine-Ariff J, editors: *Ethics at the bedside,* 1987, Philadelphia, JB Lippincott.
61. Bushy A, Raub JR: Implementing an ethics committee in rural institutions, *JONA* 21(12):18, 1991.
62. Bartels D, Youngner S, Levine J: Ethics committees: living up to your potential, *AACN Clin Issues Crit Care Nurs* 5(3):313, 1994.
63. Bosek MS: A comparison of ethical resources, *MEDSURG Nursing* 2(4):332, 1993.
64. Feutz-Harter SA: Ethics committees: a resource for patient care decision-making, *JONA* 21(4):11, 1991.
65. Kemp V: The role of critical care nurses in the ethical decision-making process, *DCCN* 4:354, 1985.
66. Corley MC, Selig P: Prevalence of principled thinking by critical care nurses, *DCCN* 13(2):96, 1994.
67. Buchanan S, Cook L: Nursing ethics committees: the time is now, *Nurs Manage* 23(8):40, 1992.

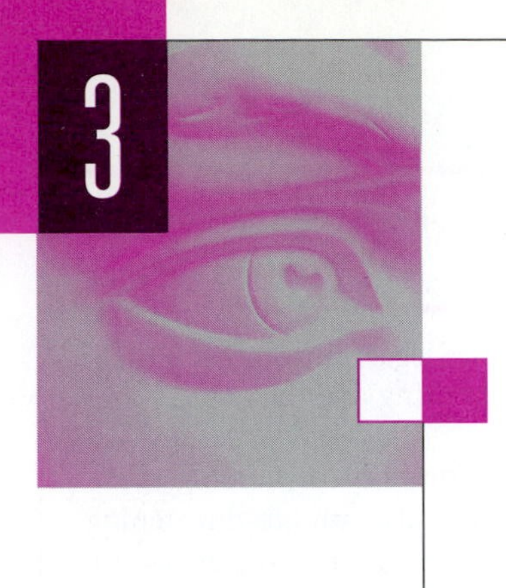

3 Legal Issues

CRITICAL CARE NURSING PRACTICE: LEGAL OBLIGATIONS OVERVIEW

Claims of negligence and malpractice against nurses are steadily increasing. Critical care nurses are confronted with a potential risk of liability for malpractice on a daily basis. The various tasks and procedures involved in the care of the critically ill can quite often be harmful if not performed with the utmost care. In addition, nurses must not lose sight of the fact that, more often than not, they are the overall protector and primary caregiver of the patients admitted to the critical care unit. Therefore nurses must take the reasonable steps necessary to minimize the chances of being named in a lawsuit.[1] The American Nurses Association (ANA) *Code for Nurses* offers guidelines[2] that relate to minimizing lawsuits (Box 3-1).

The American Association of Critical Care Nurses (AACN) has defined the scope of critical care nursing practice as follows[3]:

> Critical care nursing practice is a dynamic process, the scope of which is defined in terms of the critically ill patient, the critical care nurse and the environment in which critical care nursing is delivered; all three components are essential elements for the practice of critical care nursing. The critically ill patient is characterized by the presence of real or potential life-threatening health problems and by the requirement for continuous observation and intervention to prevent complications and restore health. The concept of the critically ill patient includes the patient's family and/or significant others. The critical care nurse is a registered professional nurse committed to ensuring that all critically ill patients receive optimal care.

In *Nursing: A Social Policy Statement,* the ANA defines nursing as the diagnosis and treatment of human problems.[4] Critical are nursing is that specialty within nursing that deals specifically with human responses to life-threatening problems.[5] The AACN has developed standards of practice specifically for the care of critically ill persons.[6] These standards and definitions raise important legal and professional issues[6] (Box 3-2).

Legal Relationships

When a nurse commences employment in a critical care facility and assumes the care of a patient, a relationship is created between patient and nurse and between employer and nurse. Every state has a law mandating entry-level educational requirements to become licensed to practice nursing. Thus the act of licensing creates a legal relationship between the nurse and the state.

These relationships impose legal obligations. For example, the nurse owes a patient the duty of reasonable and prudent care under the circumstances. The nurse owes the employer the duty of competency and the ability to follow policies and procedures; other contractual duties may exist as well. The nurse owes the state and public the duty of safe, competent practice as legally defined by practice standards.

The critical care nurse's legal duties are enforceable, and the nurse can be held legally accountable for breach or violation through a variety of laws and legal processes. Boxes 3-3 and 3-4 list sources of law and systems of enforcement. Nurses, hospitals, patients, and other health care providers are involved in a variety of legal disputes, including negligence and professional malpractice, incompetence, unauthorized practice, unprofessional or illegal conduct, workers' compensation, and contract and labor disputes.[7]

Membership in professional associations obliges the nurse to subscribe and adhere to standards defined by

BOX 3-1 Guidelines to Minimize Legal Risk

- Nurses assume accountability and responsibility for individual nursing judgments and actions.
- Nurses exercise informed judgments and use individual competence and qualifications as criteria for seeking consultation, accepting responsibility and delegating nursing activities to others.
- Nurses collaborate with others to meet the health needs of their patients.
- Nurses maintain the professional image and integrity of the nursing profession.
- Nurses maintain employment conditions conducive to high quality nursing care and strive to implement and improve nursing standards.
- Nurses engage in ongoing professional development.
- Nurses respect their patients' right to privacy and provide patients with protection and safeguards.

From American Nurses Association: *Code for nurses with interpretive statements,* Washington, DC, 1985, The Association.

BOX 3-2 Legal and Professional Issues for Critical Care Nurses

- The critical care nurse has legal obligations to the patient, the critical care setting and the environment.
- The ANA and AACN definitions of nursing speak to the fact that the nurse deals with life-threatening health problems. In this context, nursing errors are quite likely to cause substantial injuries, if not death, to a patient. Risk of liability is significant.
- The nurse has an obligation to provide continuous observation and intervention.
- The patient includes more than the individual for whom care is being provided; the family or significant other must also receive attention.
- The nurse is licensed by the state and has legal obligations to the public to perform her or his duties in a safe and competent manner.
- The critical care nurse's legal duties are those of a specialist, one with specialized knowledge and skill. These duties involve a higher standard of care, and the courts are applying with increasing frequency the professional malpractice standard in claims alleging nursing negligence.

the associations. For example, in addition to its own standards for nursing care, the AACN advises the critical care nurse to adhere to the *Code of Ethics* of the ANA.

Nurses' professional duties are further delineated and clarified by the practice standards of professional associations to which nurses belong and by the policies and procedures of the employing institution. For example, state nurses' associations are required to enforce the ANA *Code for Nurses* and have established standards of nursing practice. Likewise, the AACN, Association of Operating Room Nurses (AORN), Emergency Department Nurses Association (EDNA), American Association of Pediatric Nurse Practitioners (AAPNP), and myriad other professional organizations have identified standards of practice and guidelines in a variety of areas. Many of these organizations offer certification after completion of a specialized course of study and an examination. Certification is renewed periodically on satisfaction of academic and/or clinical practice requirements.

The scope of legal issues in nursing is broad. For example, in the past 2 decades health law as a specialty has evolved, embracing more than 60 subspecialty areas of practice.[8] Nurses need to seek their own legal advice and counsel for any questions and concerns and not rely on the overview of material provided in this chapter.

TORT LIABILITY

The area of civil law is divided into many categories, two of which are *contracts* and *torts.* The law of contracts contains a set of rules governing the creation and enforcement of an agreement between two or more parties (entities or individuals). A tort is a type of civil wrong, meaning that a dispute resulted from an occurrence between the parties. Tort law is generally divided into intentional and unintentional torts, strict liability, and specific torts. Box 3-5 classifies torts and lists examples within each category.

Intentional torts involve (1) intent and (2) an act. Intent exists when the actor intends to achieve a particular outcome and consequence. Assault, battery, false imprisonment, trespass, and infliction of emotional distress are all examples of intentional torts. In each of these torts, a specific act is required, and there is intentional interference with a person or property.

In *assault,* the act is behavior that places the plaintiff (the one being wronged who later sues) in fear or apprehension of offensive physical contact. In civil law the person being sued for wronging another is referred

BOX 3-3 Sources of Law

- Federal and state statutes/legislation (Statutory law)
- Federal and state rules and regulations (Administrative law)
- Federal and state constitutions (Constitutional law)
- Federal and state judicial opinions (Case law or Common law)

BOX 3-4 Law Enforcement Systems

- Civil
- Criminal
- Administrative (regulatory administration)

to as the *defendant. Battery* is the unlawful or offensive touching of or contact with the plaintiff or something attached to the plaintiff. *False imprisonment* is detaining, confining, or restraining another against his or her will. There are two types of *trespass:* one type involves a person's land, and the other involves his or her personal property. These acts are defined as unauthorized entry onto land of another or unauthorized handling of another's personal property. In addition, the law protects a person's interest in peace of mind through the tort claim of *infliction of mental or emotional distress.* The act here, however, must be one of extreme misconduct or outrageous behavior.

Nurses can avoid allegations of such torts by doing the following:

1. Reasonably assuring patients that the nursing care is part of an acceptable treatment plan.
2. Asking patients for their consent before giving care. (In addition, many hospital policies require that the nurse validate that the patient's physician has also obtained informed consent for medical treatment.)
3. Determining whether and when the patient needs self-protection or needs to be restrained to protect others from harm, and taking steps to protect the patient or others by following established protocols, hospital policies, and state regulations governing the use of restraints. (It is important to note that an erroneous decision regarding the use of physical restraints may lead to allegations of malpractice, failure to obtain informed consent, false imprisonment, or battery. It is the nurse's responsibility to exercise independent judgment in making a nursing diagnosis in which restraints may be clinically indicated. In some jurisdictions a physician's order may also be required. The nurse must also assess whether the patient has the capacity to give or withhold informed consent. One must determine whether the patient has been legally declared incompetent or whether the patient has a guardian or surrogate decision maker. Most jurisdictions apply the "least restrictive alternative" standard. The nurse needs to know the institutional policy and procedure for the use of restraints and request that the patient who refuses restraints sign a release of liability.[9])
4. Handling the patient's personal effects in a safe, secure manner and following hospital policies regarding patient valuables.
5. Avoiding extreme, outrageous behavior by delivering care according to generally accepted standards of care.

BOX 3-5 Classification of Torts

INTENTIONAL TORTS

Assault
Battery
False imprisonment
Trespass
Infliction of emotional distress

SPECIFIC TORTS

Defamation
  Slander
  Libel
Invasion of privacy

UNINTENTIONAL TORTS

Negligence
Medical/nursing treatment torts
  Professional malpractice
Abandonment

STRICT LIABILITY

Products liability

Unintentional torts involve failures or breach of nursing duties that lead to harm, including negligence, malpractice, and abandonment. *Negligence* is the failure to meet an ordinary standard of care, resulting in injury to the patient or plaintiff. *Malpractice* is a type of professional liability based on negligence and includes professional misconduct, breach of a duty or standard of care, illegal or immoral conduct, or failure to exercise reasonable skill, all of which lead to harm. A more complete discussion of the elements of these torts is found later in this chapter. *Abandonment* is a type of negligence in which a duty to give care exists, is ignored, and results in harm to a patient. It is the absence of care and the failure to respond to a patient that may give rise to an allegation of abandonment.

Nurses can avoid allegations of unintentional torts by doing the following:

1. Identifying the duty owed, knowing what the duty consists of, and providing nursing care that meets that duty or standard of care.
2. Applying the nursing process to patient care problems: consistent and timely assessment, diagnosis, plan and implementation, and evaluation.
3. Documenting the care that was delivered and participating in activities that minimize the opportunity for patient harm and exposure to liability. (These are commonly known as risk management strategies, several of which are discussed later in this chapter.)

Specific torts involve privacy interests and interests one has in his or her reputation. Invasion of privacy and defamation are both examples of such torts. *Defamation* is composed of two torts, *slander* (oral defamation) and *libel* (written defamation). Defamation is not the mere statement or writing of words that injures one's reputation or good name; the words must be communicated to another. If the words are true, this may provide a defense against a defamation claim. *Invasion of privacy* involves the violation of a person's right to privacy. Nurses can invade another's privacy by revealing confidential information without authorization or by failing to follow the patient's health care decisions.

Nurses can avoid allegations of these specific claims by (1) making statements about another's reputation only when necessary and substantiated by fact and (2) respecting another's privacy and autonomy and maintaining a confidential relationship with the patient.

ADMINISTRATIVE LAW AND LICENSING STATUTES

A second type of law and legal process in which nurses are involved is administrative law and the regulatory process. This area of law governs the nurse's relationship with the government, either state or federal. Administrative law involves the rules of the government's activities in regulating health care delivery and practice, and the rules of investigation, procedure, and evidence differ from the civil and criminal law. Several government health care agencies are involved in such regulation.

A state has the power to regulate nursing because the state is responsible for the health, safety, and welfare of its citizens. Therefore establishing minimal entry-level requirements, standards of nursing practice, and educational requirements are acceptable state actions. State legislatures create laws governing nursing practice (generally termed *nurse practice acts*), and a unit of the state government within the executive branch is responsible for the enforcement of nursing laws. This unit is often called the State Board of Nursing or Board of Nurse Examiners; however, names vary by states. Standards also vary by state, which is another important reason that nurses seek advice from counsel licensed to practice law in their own state.

NEGLIGENCE AND MALPRACTICE

As defined earlier, negligence is an unintentional tort involving a breach of duty or failure (through an act or an omission) to meet a standard of care, causing patient harm. Malpractice is a type of professional liability based on negligence in which the defendant is held accountable for breach of a duty of care involving special knowledge and skill. These torts have several elements, all of which the plaintiff has the burden of proving.

Definition of Elements

The law recognizes the following four elements of negligence and malpractice (Box 3-6). A *duty,* or legal obligation, requires the actor to conform to a certain standard of conduct for the protection of others against unreasonable risks.[10] The critical care nurse's legal duty is to act in a reasonable and prudent manner, as any other critical care nurse would act under similar circumstances. The standard is that of a critical care nurse—one with special knowledge and skill in critical care. The standard is one that is owed at the time the incident or injury occurred, not at the time of litigation. In most jurisdictions the standard of care is a national standard, as opposed to a local or community standard. Box 3-7 lists general critical care nursing duties as implied by statute and administrative rules and regulations, and as stated explicitly in judicial decisions.

Breach of duty involves a failure on the actor's part to conform to the standard required. *Causation,* the third element, involves proving that the actor's breach

BOX 3-6 Essential Elements of Negligence and Malpractice

- Duty and standard of care
- Breach of duty
- Causation
- Injury or damages

was reasonably close or causally connected to the resulting injury. This is also referred to as *proximate cause.* The fourth element, *injury or damages,* must involve an actual loss or damage to the plaintiff or his or her interest. A plaintiff may claim different types of damages, such as compensatory and/or punitive. Patient injury can range in value, depending on what happened to the patient. The plaintiff must produce evidence of the damages and their value. If the nurse breaches a standard of care that leads to injury, the plaintiff must show what amount of money will compensate for his or her injuries. The goal of the compensation is to provide the amount of money that will place the plaintiff back in the position he or she was in before the injury occurred.

Res ipsa loquitur is a rule of evidence used by plaintiffs in negligence or malpractice litigation. It literally means "the thing speaks for itself." It is a rebuttable presumption or inference of negligence by the defendant, which arises on plaintiff's proof that (1) the injury is one that ordinarily does not happen in the absence of negligence and (2) the instrumentality causing the injury was in the defendant's exclusive management and control. The burden then shifts to the defendant to prove absence of negligence. For example, negligence can be inferred when muscle ischemia and necrosis occur as a result of improper body positioning and the application of splints or restraints. Negligence can also be inferred from a foreign object left in a patient's body cavity after surgery.

Because critical care nurses deal with life-threatening situations, patient injury is potentially severe or may result in death. Should this occur as a result of negligence, the nurse may be held liable for the patient's death and also for the resulting loss to surviving family members. All states have wrongful death acts, and a number of states have both death acts and survival acts, which are prosecuted concurrently. With the two causes of action, the expenses, pain and suffering, and loss of earnings of the decedent up to the time of death are allocated to the survival action, and the loss of benefits to the survivors is allocated to the wrongful death action.

BOX 3-7 Legal Duties

Critical care nurses have a legal duty to do the following:

- Observe
- Assess
- Conduct ongoing observations and assessments
- Recognize significance of information
- Report
- Plan, implement, and evaluate care
- Respond to changes
- Interpret and carry out orders
- Take reasonable measures to ensure patient safety
- Exercise professional judgment
- Properly perform procedures
- Follow hospital policies and procedures
- Record and document

Box 3-8 illustrates specific examples of critical care nursing actions that have resulted in litigation. In cases such as these, the nurse's action is central to the lawsuit. However, nurses are named as sole or codefendants in a comparatively small percentage of cases. Although this pattern is changing, physicians and hospitals are generally named as defendants.

Typically, nursing negligence cases involve breach or failure in six general categories, which are listed in Box 3-9. The first category includes the use of defective equipment or the failure to perform safety and maintenance assessments. Nurses commonly make errors in drug identification, administration, and dosages. Nurses have failed to timely report to physicians changes in patient status and have also failed to communicate to supervisors a physician's failure to respond to the nurse's communication. Failure to supervise and assist patients who subsequently fall is also a source of nursing negligence. Improper wound care with resulting infection and incorrect instrument and sponge counts in the surgical setting are areas of practice that have also led to patient injury and lawsuits.

Legal Doctrines and Theories of Liability

In tort law there are several theories of liability under which the nurse's action may be examined and legal duties defined:

1. Personal
2. Vicarious: *respondeat superior*
3. Corporate

BOX 3-8 Examples of Critical Care Nursing Actions Involved in Negligence Lawsuits

GENERAL

- Failure to advise physician and/or supervisor of change in patient's health status
- Failure to monitor patients at requisite intervals
- Failure to adhere to established institutional protocols
- Failure to adequately assess clinical status
- Failure to respond to alarms
- Failure to maintain accurate, timely, and complete medical records
- Failure to properly carry out treatment and evaluate results of treatment
- Failure to use safe, functional equipment

SPECIFIC

- Failure to provide supplemental oxygen when the ventilator cannot be promptly reattached
- Failure to properly use intravenous infusion equipment, causing extensive extravasation of fluid
- Failure to monitor intravenous infusions, recognize infiltration, and discontinue intravenous therapy
- Failure to recognize signs of intracranial bleeding
- Failure to investigate patient's complaint of pain and discover hematoma under blood pressure cuff

BOX 3-9 Common Areas of Nursing Negligence

- Improper administration of treatments
- Improper administration of medications
- Inadequate or false written and verbal communication
- Insufficient supervision of patients
- Improper postoperative treatment and wound care
- Incorrect perioperative instrument and sponge counts

4. Other doctrines (e.g., temporary or borrowed servant; captain of the ship)

Under the theory of *personal liability,* each individual is responsible for his or her own actions. This includes the critical care nurse, the supervisor, the physician, the hospital, and the patient. Each has responsibilities that are uniquely his or her own. In contrast to personal liability, one may be afforded the protection of personal immunity.

In certain health care situations, Congress or state legislatures have determined that nurses do not have personal liability and are therefore immune from liability. Again, it is wise to seek advice to review what employment settings and laws apply to a particular situation.

As a general rule in most jurisdictions, mandatory reporting statutes include personal immunity provisions. For example, child abuse and dependent adult abuse statutes provide that a nurse who makes a good faith report will not be liable for making that report or the consequences of the report. Similarly, physicians, nurses, and hospitals mandated to report communicable and infectious diseases to state or federal authorities are immune from liability for good faith reporting in a confidential manner. Also, nurses who in good faith render voluntary emergency care in the field to a stranger are immune from liability for negligence under state Good Samaritan laws. Finally, federally employed nurses are protected by immunity provisions under the Federal Tort Claims Act.[11] However, many states have greatly restricted immunity at state and local levels. Certain personal immunities are not a guarantee against lawsuits; rather, they are potential defenses.

Vicarious liability is indirect responsibility—for example, the liability of an employer for the acts of the employee. Under the doctrine of *respondeat superior,* a master is liable for certain wrongful acts of a servant, as is a principal for those of an agent. An employer may be liable for an employee's acts that are performed within the legitimate scope of employment. In critical care, the nurse typically is an employee of a hospital. However, nurses may be independent contractors with the hospital through critical care nursing agencies or businesses. If the latter is the case, the nurse is not an employee of the hospital and the hospital is not vicariously liable for the nurse's action.

Critical care nurses who are hospital employees are given work assignments and provided equipment and supplies to perform those assignments by the employer's agent, a supervisor. As a general rule, the hospital is responsible for the patient census and staffing on the critical care unit as well as clinical orientation of the staff. Because of these responsibilities, the hospital-employer generally is responsible for the employee's performance within the parameters determined by the employer. Thus it would appear unjust to hold the individual nurse solely responsible for errors as a result of patient care assignments and staffing patterns controlled primarily by the hospital. However, sometimes that is the case.

Corporate liability is the liability attached to the corporate entity (e.g., the hospital) for its own corporate activities and decisions.

Other doctrines, such as *temporary or borrowed servant* and *captain of the ship,* may apply to the critical care nurse and the critical care unit. These doctrines are used when the plaintiff argues that the physician is responsible for the nurse's actions, even though the nurse is an employee of the hospital, not of the physician. If it can be shown that the nurse acted under the direction and control of the physician, it is possible that the physician may be accountable for the nurse's actions. However, these doctrines are becoming increasingly uncommon. What viability remains is typically found in cases involving nurse anesthetists and operating room nurses.

Risk Management and Reduction

Critical care nurses can minimize patient harm and subsequent claims of malpractice in a variety of ways. The hallmarks of risk reduction are knowledge of the professional standards of care, delivery and documentation of that care, and a consistent showing that the standards are met. Many of these sources are admissible as evidence in negligence and malpractice litigation. For these sources to serve as measuring sticks of nursing action or inaction, the question "Did the nurse breach the professional standard of care and the duty owed?" must be applied.

Another important component is the individual institution's risk management (RM) program. Nurses should be acutely aware of potential harms to patients and take affirmative steps to avoid and to correct deficiencies identified through the RM program. For example, many hospital RM programs require that reports or other documentation be completed for unusual incidents. Institutional policy defines which incidents are to be reported.

It behooves nurses to consider obtaining their own professional liability insurance as an RM strategy. Insurance is a mechanism whereby one can shift to another the potentially devastating economic burden of a lawsuit in which one is found to have been negligent or to have committed malpractice.

Insurance is a contract between the insured (the nurse) and the insurer (the insurance company). Therefore the written agreement between these parties must be examined carefully. It spells out the premium, the coverage, the terms, and the requirements the nurse must fulfill if he or she is sued. For example, most policies state that the insurance company will pay the nurse's legal fees, expenses related to litigation, and the final award. However, the nurse is obligated to notify the insurance company within a reasonable time of knowledge of a possible or pending lawsuit and to cooperate in the defense. The nurse also must know what type of policy he or she has: "occurrence" coverage or "claims made" coverage.

Self-insurance has serious drawbacks if it encourages plaintiffs to name nurses as defendants instead of or in addition to hospitals. Traditionally, nurses have not insured themselves, but instead have relied on their employers' (usually the hospitals') liability insurance. However, the judicial trend toward rendering a nurse's liability as nursing malpractice has made this reliance uncertain and hazardous. Today many hospital liability policies have exclusionary clauses by which the insurer disclaims liability for malpractice claims brought against the insured hospital. This means the insurer may have no contractual duty to defend nurse malpractice actions or pay awards for plaintiff verdicts.

Peer review and quality assurance programs are also important processes that can minimize patient harm and nursing liability. Peer review involves self-review, self-evaluation, and the audit of others' actions and records. Similarly, an accurate, timely, and complete medical record is imperative. Patient medical records are legal documents admissible in court as evidence of negligence or malpractice. As a general rule, peer review records and incident reports remain confidential and are inadmissible as evidence.

Other risk management techniques include strengthening communication skills and improving public relations. Risk management experts emphasize prompt reporting of an accident or injury and direct communication to the patient involved. The underlying rationale is that straightforward communication about the incident and what is being done to correct or alleviate the injury often decreases the patient's likelihood of suing. Maintaining the patient's trust is critical to reducing exposure to liability and to managing risk.

NURSE PRACTICE ACTS

The practice of nursing is regulated by the state. As a general rule, the state's police power to regulate prevails, as long as the state's actions are not arbitrary or capricious. All nurses must be licensed to practice under their individual state's licensure statutes. Licensure authorizes (1) the right to practice and (2) access to employment. Therefore licensure is a property right that is constitutionally protected.[12] Every state has legislation that defines the legal scope of nursing practice and defines unprofessional and illegal conduct that may lead to investigation and disciplinary action by the state and sanctions on the right to practice. The state nurse practice act establishes entry requirements, definitions of practice, and criteria for discipline. Although licensure is mandatory for registered nurses, statutory content varies among the states.

Generally, state law contains two definitions of nursing: one for the registered (or professional) nurse and one for the licensed practical (or vocational or technical) nurse. These definitions determine titles that may be used by nurses, the scope of nursing practice, and requirements for entering the nursing profession. In some states, advanced registered nursing practice, prescriptive authority for certain nurses, and third-party reimbursement are also defined by statute. Mandatory continuing education requirements are also defined by statute in most states. The state authorizes its board of nursing to monitor practice, implement standards of care, enforce rules and regulations, and issue sanctions. Sanctions include additional education, restricted practice, supervised practice, license suspension, and license revocation. Some form of disciplinary action generally occurs as a result of unauthorized practice, negligence or malpractice, incompetence, chemical or other impairment, criminal acts, or violations of specific nurse practice act provisions.

The scope of medical practice is also statutorily defined, and in most states a physician is given broad discretion to delegate tasks to others. Physicians may delegate to critical care nurses through written protocols or standing orders, which must be written, dated, and signed by the physician; standing orders and protocols must be updated regularly. The nurse must be adequately prepared to follow the protocol and perform with a reasonable degree of skill, care, and diligence as performed by similar nurses under similar circumstances. Protocol and standing orders need to identify unambiguously the corresponding roles of hospital administrators, nurses, and doctors. However, one must keep in mind that, within a state's jurisdiction, the scope of medical practice and the scope of nursing practice often overlap because each practice may authorize the same functions. Such overlapping creates problems at the regulatory level and will surely extend as the role of nursing continues to evolve.

Because it is afforded constitutional protection, the right to practice cannot be violated without due process of the law. The amount of due process in administrative law differs from other legal processes. Due process involves notice to the nurse that a complaint has been filed (voluntarily or by mandate); the notice is written and contains the charges against the nurse. Nurses in this situation should seek independent legal counsel immediately; the state will not provide it. The nurse must be given an opportunity to be heard, often in more than one forum, and be given the right to present his or her own evidence.

Chemical impairment is a common reason for disciplinary action. In some states, the impaired nurse may avoid serious sanctions by voluntarily suspending practice and entering a rehabilitation program. This must be done with the advice of counsel (the nurse's own lawyer). Generally, this option is available as long as no patient has been harmed because of the nurse's impairment.

SPECIFIC PATIENT CARE ISSUES

Myriad legal issues and controversies exist in the field of critical care. Concerns commonly arise in the areas of (1) informed consent and authorization for treatment and (2) the patient's right to accept or refuse medical treatment.

Informed Consent and Authorization for Treatment

The common law right not to be touched without giving consent has existed since the early eighteenth century. In the 1914 case of *Schloendorff v. Society of New York Hospital,* a court held that every adult of sound mind has a right to determine what shall be done with his or her own body, including the right to give consent and the right to refuse consent to treatment.[13] Most states now have informed consent statutes, and the body of case law on this subject has developed impressively since the early days of Schloendorff. Intrinsic to the doctrine of informed consent is the physician's legal duty to disclose certain information to the patient and the patient's legal right to *informed consent* and to subsequently refuse or accept medical treatment. Central to critical care nursing is the issue of the extent to which the nurse is involved in obtaining consent. As a general rule, the physician cannot delegate this function entirely to a registered nurse, and the nurse's exposure to liability increases if the nurse accepts full responsibility for obtaining the patient's consent. It is common nursing practice to witness and document the procedure and to obtain the patient's signature after the physician has disclosed the required information. However, the nurse should be thoroughly familiar with the state's informed consent statute and the individual institution's policy and procedure for obtaining informed consent. General exceptions to this common practice are the higher standards to which nurse anesthetists, nurse midwives, and nurse researchers are held.[14]

There are two types of consent: express and implied. *Express consent* may be written or verbal and is the consent given specifically for nonroutine procedures. *Implied consent* may be implied in fact, an assumption based on patient behavior (e.g., the patient extending an arm for venipuncture or nodding approval), or it may be implied in law (e.g., an unconscious, hemorrhaging patient in the emergency department). The following discussion summarizes the elements of valid informed consent, the adequacy of consent and negligent nondisclosure, and exceptions to consent requirements and the duty to disclose.

Valid consent must be (1) voluntary, (2) obtained, and (3) informed. Although consent can be either verbal or written, most hospital policies require that informed, voluntary consent to nonroutine procedures be obtained and confirmed in writing: signed and dated by the patient, physician, and witness (if required). Most informed consent statutes provide that a consent, in writing, to a medical or surgical procedure that meets the consent and disclosure requirements of the statute creates a legal presumption that informed consent was given.

In the vast majority of jurisdictions the decision maker (the one giving the consent) must be a legally competent adult (i.e., having reached majority or, in most states, the age of 18 years). Competence is a legal judgment, and as a general rule, there is a legal presumption of patient competence.[15] One is mentally incompetent (thereby rendering a consent invalid) if adjudicated incompetent. One must likewise have the capacity (a medical and nursing judgment) to give consent: the patient must be oriented and understand what he or she has been told; medications the patient is taking must be documented. In those adults legally adjudicated incompetent, the guardian may give consent if the guardian has been given this authority.

Minors are legally incompetent, and consent is obtained from the parent or guardian. However, in many jurisdictions there are two important exceptions to this rule: (1) mature minors may consent to treatment for substance abuse, sexually transmitted disease, and matters involving contraception and reproduction; and (2) emancipated minors may consent to treatment in general (minors are considered emancipated if married or divorced before the age of majority, if in the military service, or if living independently with parental consent).

Consent must also be informed and timely. The physician has a duty to disclose the following: diagnosis; condition; prognosis; material risks and benefits associated with the treatment or procedure; explanation of the treatment; providers of the treatment (who is performing, supervising, and/or assisting in the procedure); material risks and benefits of alternative therapy; and the probable outcome (including material risks and benefits) if the patient refuses the treatment or procedure. Failure to disclose such information or inadequate disclosure with resultant injury may constitute negligence and give rise to tort claims of malpractice, battery, negligent nondisclosure, and abandonment. Consent is generally valid for 7 to 30 days. However, the time at which consent expires must be explicitly stated in the institutional policy and procedure manual.

There are many exceptions to consent requirements and the duty to disclose, and clearly the exceptions vary according to jurisdiction. Emergencies constitute one exception, unless the patient refuses treatment or has previously made a competent and informed refusal. States vary significantly in the following treatment situations: endangered fetal viability, alcohol or other drug detoxification, emergency blood transfusions, caesarean sections, and substance abuse during pregnancy. Jurisdictions also vary on the issue of sources of consent (informal directives) for the incompetent patient or the patient in an emergency who has no legal guardian. Alternatives include consensus from as many next of kin as possible, with evidence that (1) the treatment is reasonable and necessary and (2) the family's decision would not be contrary to the patient's wishes (this is known as substituted judgment made by a surrogate decision maker). Another alternative is a court order for treatment. In the absence of substituted judgment, many courts use what is known as the *best interests standard.*

Lawsuits involving informed consent and the duty to disclose generally require three elements: (1) proof that the health care provider failed to disclose an existing material risk unknown to the patient or alternatives to the proposed treatment, (2) proof that the patient would not have consented if the risk had been disclosed (in other words, that disclosure of the risk would have led a reasonable patient in the plaintiff's position to refuse the procedure or choose a different course of treatment), and (3) proof of injury occurring as a result of the failure to disclose.[14,16]

The Right to Accept or Refuse Medical Treatment and the Law of Advance Directives

The right to consent and informed consent includes the right to refuse treatment. In most cases a competent adult's decision to refuse even life-sustaining treatment is honored.[17-21] The underlying rationale is that the patient's right to withdraw or withhold treatment is not outweighed by the state's interest in preserving life.

There are some situations in which the right to refuse treatment is not honored. These include, but are not limited to, the following situations:

1. The treatment relates to a contagious illness that threatens the health of the public (e.g., immunizations are required, even over religious objections, if there is substantial danger to the community).
2. Innocent third parties will suffer (e.g., a parent's wish to refuse a blood transfusion most likely would be overruled to save the life of a child; these cases are often decided on a case-by-case basis, and legal counsel must always be sought).
3. The refusal violates ethical standards (e.g., a Massachusetts court held that a hospital was not required to compromise its ethical principles by following a patient's decision, but must cooperate in the transfer of the patient to a hospital that is willing to cooperate.[22] However, a New Jersey court ruled to the contrary. A patient indicated that she did not want to be fed if she became incapacitated; the hospital opposed this. The court upheld the patient's right and refused to order her transfer.[23] Again, obtaining legal counsel in these instances is highly advisable).
4. Treatment must be instituted to prevent suicide and to preserve life. (Courts have clearly indicated, however, that terminally ill and/or comatose patients with no hope of recovery do not intend suicide when treatment has been refused.)

When patients refuse treatment, complex ethical, legal, and practical problems arise. Hospitals should have specific policies to guide nurses in these areas, and nurses' participation in hospital ethics committees or institutional ethics committees is strongly advisable.

Withholding and Withdrawing Treatment

As indicated earlier, an adult has the right to refuse treatment, even treatment that sustains life. This right means that the critical care nurse may participate in the withholding or withdrawing of treatment. Historically, the distinction between withholding and withdrawing treatments was considered the issue of importance, but that is no longer the case. Health care decisions become most complex when patients lose competency and capacity to personally make their own decisions.

Orders Not to Resuscitate and Other Orders

Hospital policies that address orders to withhold or withdraw treatment should exist in all critical care units. For example, orders not to resuscitate—commonly referred to as do-not-resuscitate (DNR) orders—should be governed by written policies, including, but not limited to, the following:

1. DNR orders should be entered in the patient's record with full documentation by the responsible physician about the patient's prognosis and the patient's agreement (if he or she is capable) or, alternatively, the family's consensus.
2. DNR orders should have the concurrence of another physician designated in the policy.
3. Policies should specify that orders are reviewed periodically (some policies require daily review).
4. Patients with capacity must give their informed consent.
5. For patients without capacity, that incapacity must be thoroughly documented, along with the diagnosis, prognosis, and family consensus.
6. Judicial intervention before writing a DNR order is usually indicated when the patient's family does not agree or there is uncertainty or disagreement about the patient's prognosis or mental status. As a general rule, however, in the absence of conflict or disagreement, DNR orders are legal in a majority of jurisdictions if executed clearly and properly.
7. Policies should specify who is to be contacted and notified within the hospital administration.

Other orders to withhold or withdraw treatment may involve mechanical ventilation, dialysis, nutritional support, hydration, and medications such as antibiotics. The legal and ethical implications of these orders for each patient must be carefully considered. Hospitals should have written policies on all orders to withhold and withdraw treatment. Policies must cover how decisions will be made: who will decide and what the roles of patient, family, health care providers, and the institution will be. Policies must be developed that consider state laws and judicial opinions.

Advance Directives and the Patient Self-Determination Act (OBRA 1990)

Rarely has a case so galvanized public opinion as the case of Nancy Cruzan.[24-31] The tragic experience

LEGAL REVIEW 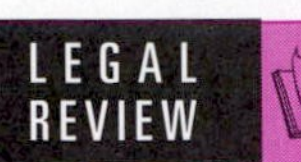 **The Durable Power of Attorney for Health Care**

The durable power of attorney for health care is the second and most recently developed advance directive. Approximately 30 states have statutes or pending legislation on this document.

As a general rule, the durable power of attorney for health care is more flexible than is the living will and has broader application: it is not restricted to traditional life-sustaining procedures, nor is it restricted to terminally ill patients.

The document authorizes the agent (attorney in fact) to make health care decisions for the principal when the principal is unable to make those decisions. The principal is the competent adult who executes the power of attorney document and designates the agent to make decisions on his or her behalf.

Similar to the living will, the durable power of attorney for health care is written, signed, dated, witnessed, and notarized. It is part of the medical record. As a general rule, it may be revoked at any time and in any manner. If the nurse's state has a statute governing this document, the nurse must also be familiar with (1) witness disqualifier provisions, (2) agent disqualifier provisions, (3) guardian preemption provisions, (4) revocation conditions, (5) effect on life insurance policies, if any, (6) the effect of out-of-state documents, and (7) immunity provisions.

See *In Re Estate of Greenspan,* 558 N.E.2d 1194 (Ill. 1990); *The durable power of attorney for health care law: a Catholic perspective,* Iowa Catholic Conference, 818 Insurance Exchange Building, Des Moines, Ia, 50309, 515-243-6256; Pozgar GD: *Legal aspects of health care administration,* ed 4, Rockville, Md, 1990, Aspen Systems.

and hardships of Nancy Cruzan and her family left an indelible mark in American jurisprudence, legislation, and health care.

In *Cruzan* the issue before the U.S. Supreme Court was to consider whether Cruzan had a federal constitutional right that would require the hospital to withdraw life-sustaining treatment from her under the circumstances. The court rejected the request for authority to withdraw artificial nutrition and hydration and held that the U.S. Constitution did not prohibit the state of Missouri from requiring clear and convincing evidence of Cruzan's wishes before treatment withdrawal.

The court stated that when a person is incompetent and unable to exercise the right to refuse treatment and a surrogate must act on his or her behalf, the state may institute procedural safeguards to ensure that the surrogate honors the wishes expressed by the person while competent. The court also held that the U.S. Constitution does not require a state to accept the substituted judgment of the family; the state may recognize only a personal right to make such health care decisions. A state may choose to defer only to the person's express wishes, rather than relying on the family's decision.

Perhaps more important, the court also held that a competent adult has a federal constitutional right to refuse medical treatment, including life-sustaining hydration and nutrition. This right falls under the Fourteenth Amendment due process clause and is not a fundamental privacy right under the First Amendment. The Cruzan decision quickly mobilized the U.S. Congress to pass landmark legislation known as the Patient Self-Determination Act/Omnibus Budget Reconciliation Act of 1990.[32-41] The statute requires that all adults must be provided written information on an individual's rights under state law to make medical decisions, including the right to refuse treatment and the right to formulate advance directives.

The 1990 law mandates that providers of health care services under Medicare and Medicaid must comply with requirements relating to patient advance directives, which are written instructions recognized under state law for provisions of care when persons are incapacitated. Providers may not be reimbursed for the care they provide unless the requirements of this provision are met.

Providers must have written policies and procedures to (1) inform all adult patients at the time treatment is initiated of their right to execute an advance directive and of the provider's policies on the implementation of that right, (2) document in medical records whether an individual has executed an advance directive, (3) not condition care and treatment or otherwise discriminate on the basis of whether a patient has executed an advance directive, (4) comply with state laws on advance directives, and (5) provide information and education to staff and the community on advance directives. The provisions became effective in December 1991.

Patients themselves can provide clear direction by preparing in advance written documents that specify their wishes. These documents are termed advance directives and include the living will and durable power of attorney for health care. To be effective in a jurisdiction, both of these directives must be statutorily or judicially recognized. The living will specifies that if certain circumstances occur, such as terminal illness, the patient will decline specific treatment, such as cardiopulmonary resuscitation and mechanical ventilation. The living will does not cover all treatment. For example, in some states nutritional support may not be declined through a living will. The durable power of attorney for health care is a directive through which a patient designates an agent—someone who will make decisions for the patient if the patient becomes unable to do so. Critical care nurses whose patients have executed advance directives must follow state law provisions and the hospital's policies.

Some states have also passed laws providing that a county, municipality, region, or medical center may establish a substitute medical decision-making board composed of health care professionals and lay persons. The board acts as a substitute decision maker if the patient does not have his or her own surrogate. It is of utmost importance that the critical care staff consult with hospital legal counsel in the event the patient has a designated surrogate or has executed one or more advance directives and also has had a court-appointed guardian in the past. Various statutory provisions in the context of guardianship are incongruous with many of the new laws relating to surrogate or substitute decision making and the laws of advance directives. The staff must know without question who has primary legal authority for the patient, and this information must be documented unambiguously.

REFERENCES

1. Hellinghausen MA: Providers face more liability as duties grow, *Nursing & Allied Health Week* 1(15):1, 1996.
2. American Nurses Association Committee on Ethics: *Code for nurses with interpretative statements,* Washington, DC, 1985, American Nurses Association.
3. American Association of Critical Care Nurses Board of Directors: *AACN position statement: scope of critical care nursing practice,* Newport Beach, Calif, 1986, American Association of Critical Care Nurses.
4. American Nurses Association: *Nursing: a social policy statement,* Washington, DC, 1980, The Association.
5. American Association of Critical Care Nurses: *Position statement: definition of critical care nursing,* Newport Beach, Calif, 1984, The Association.
6. American Association of Critical Care Nurses: *Standards for nursing care of the critically ill,* ed 2, Norwalk, Conn, 1989, Appleton & Lange.
7. Northrop CE, Kelly ME: *Legal issues in nursing,* St Louis, 1987, Mosby.
8. Christoffel T: *Health and the law: a handbook for health professionals,* 1982, New York, Macmillan.
9. Feutz-Harter SA: Legal implications of restraints, *J Nurs Adm* 20(10):8, 1990.
10. Prosser WL and others: *The law of torts,* ed 5, St Paul, Minn, 1988, West.
11. 28 U.S.C. Secs. 2671-80 (1986).
12. Walker DJ: Nursing 1980: new responsibility, new liability, *Trial* 16(12):43, 1980.
13. *Schloendorff v. Soc'y of N.Y. Hosp.,* 105 N.E. 92 (1914), *overruled on other grounds.*
14. Murphy EK: Informed consent doctrine: little danger of liability for nurses, *Nurs Outlook* 39(1):48, 1991.
15. Northrop CE: Nursing practice and the legal presumption of competency, *Nurs Outlook* 36(2):112, 1988.
16. *Pauscher v. Iowa Methodist Med. Center,* 408 N.W.2d 355 (Iowa 1987).
17. *Bouvia v. Superior Court,* 225 Cal. Rptr. 297; 179 C.A.3d 1127, *review denied* (Cal. App. 1986).
18. *In Re Farrell,* 529 A.2d 404 (N.J. 1987).
19. *McKay v. Bergstedt,* 801 P.2d 617 (Nev. 1990).
20. *State v. McAfee,* 385 S.E.2d 651 (Ga. 1989).
21. Wilson-Clayton ML, Clayton MA: Two steps forward, one step back: *McKay v. Bergstedt, Whittier L Rev* 12:439, 1991.
22. *Brophy v. New England Sinai Hosp.,* 497 N.E.2d 626 (Mass. 1986).
23. *In Re Requena,* 517 A.2d 869 (N.J. App. Div. 1986).
24. *Cruzan v. Director, Missouri Dept. of Health,* 110 S. Ct. 2841 (U.S. S. Ct. 1990).
25. *Cruzan v. Director, Missouri Dept. of Health* and the right to die: a symposium, *Ga L Rev* 25:1139, 1991.
26. *Cruzan v. Missouri,* USLW 58:4916, 1990.
27. Guarino KS, Antoine MP: The case of Nancy Cruzan: the Supreme Court's decision, *Crit Care Nurse* 11(1):32, 1991.
28. Kyba F: Decisions at the end of life: implications following Cruzan, *Tex Nurse* 65(2):13, 1991.
29. Morgan RC: How to decide: decisions on life-prolonging procedures, *Stetson L Rev* 20:77, 1990.
30. Quill T: Death and dignity, *N Engl J Med* 324(10):691, 1991.
31. Right to die symposium, *Issues Law Med* 7:169, 1991.
32. Iowa Hospital Association, Iowa Medical Society, Iowa State Bar Association: *Advance directives for health care: deciding today about your care in the future,* 1991, author.
33. American Hospital Association: *Put it in writing: a guide to promoting advance directives,* American Hospital Association, 840 North Lake Shore Drive, Chicago, Ill, 60611, 800-242-2626.
34. Cate FH, Gill BA: *The Patient Self-Determination Act: implementation issues and opportunities,* Washington, DC, 1991, The Annenberg Washington Program.

35. Choice in Dying: *Advance directive protocols and the Patient Self-Determination Act: a resource manual for the development of institutional protocols,* Choice in Dying, 200 Varick Street, New York, NY, 10014, 212-366-5540, 1991 (formerly Society for the Right to Die/Concern for Dying, 250 West 57th Street, New York, NY, 10107, 212-246-6962).
36. Emanuel L, Emanuel E: The medical directive: a new comprehensive advance care document, *JAMA* 261(22):3, 288, 1989.
37. Iowa Hospital Association: *The Patient Self-Determination Act of 1990: implementation in Iowa hospitals,* Iowa Hospital Association, 100 East Grand, Suite 100, Des Moines, Ia, 50309, 515-288-1955, 1991.
38. National Hospice Organization: *Advance medical directives,* National Hospice Organization, 1901 North Moore Street, Suite 901, Arlington, Va, 22209, 703-243-5900, 1991.
39. National Health Lawyers Association: *The patient self-determination directory and resources guide,* National Health Lawyers Association, 1620 Eye Street NW, Suite 900, Washington, DC, 20006, 202-833-1100, 1991.
40. Patient Self-Determination Act/Omnibus Budget Reconciliation Act of 1990, Pub L No 101-508, Sec. 4206; 42 U.S.C. Sec. 1395cc(a)(1) (1990).
41. Unisys Corp: *Advance directives,* informational release general no 122, Unisys Corp, PO Box 10394, Des Moines, Ia 50306, 800-776-6045, 1991.

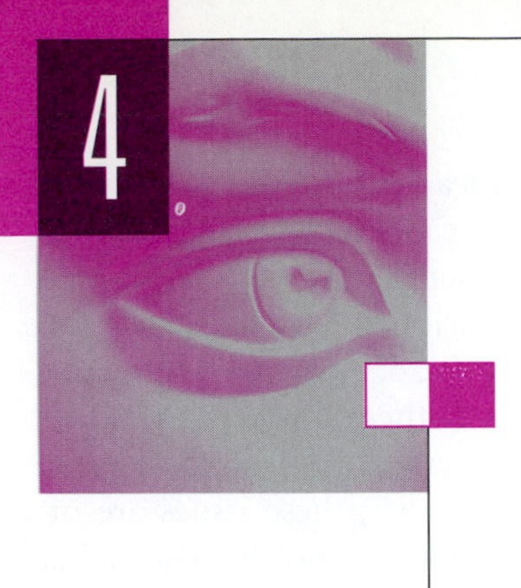

4

Patient and Family Education

CHALLENGES FOR PATIENT AND FAMILY EDUCATION IN CRITICAL CARE

PERSONS ENTERING THE health care system bring with them unique medical, social, and educational histories that affect their interactions with health care providers. Often, the illness or medical event creates new requirements in the area of life-style change or modification. Learning needs arise out of the new requirements. Therefore it is essential that nurses incorporate educational strategies into the plan of care for all patients. There have been tremendous changes in the delivery and complexity of health care: spiraling health care costs; increasing patient acuity resulting from advanced technology and new treatment regimens; decreasing lengths of hospital stay; and an increasing elderly population.[1,2] As the result of earlier hospital discharge, plans of care have more complicated treatment regimens and require new approaches to providing information for life-style changes.[3,4] Because of these changes, it is even more important that patients and families are provided with the information needed to make informed decisions and choices about health care alternatives.[1]

Priorities set by the critical care nurse must place maintenance of immediate physical and psychologic safety above the health promotion and educational needs. However, when the patient's clinical condition allows, the education plan can be initiated with continuation across the hospital stay into discharge. Box 4-1 delineates information that all patients and families must receive. Time constraints and the necessity to set priorities of care may limit the actual amount of time available for educating patients and families. The critical care unit offers unique challenges in that it is often a foreign and threatening environment to the patient and family. In addition, many patients and families may be experiencing denial and crisis related to the hospitalization and prognosis of the condition. Therefore assessment of readiness to learn must be an important consideration when planning educational sessions.

Along with a belief in the patient's right to know, the patient's right not to know must also be recognized in some cases. The patient's right not to know must be respected in those cases in which patients prefer not to learn about their illnesses. Simple basic

BOX 4-1 What Every Patient Should Know

- Orientation to room/environment: call light, bed controls, etc
- Orientation to unit routines: visiting hours, frequency of monitoring and nurse assessments, lab draws, daily weights, special shift routines, etc
- Explanations regarding reasons for equipment, monitors and associated alarms (e.g., cardiac monitor, ventilator, intravenous (IV) lines, IV pumps, pacemaker, pulse oximetry, etc)
- Orientation to the various care providers and services that they deliver
- Explanation of all procedures, both in the unit and off the unit
- Medications: names, and why the patient is receiving them
- Transition to next level of care: reason for transfer, environment, staffing, availability of care providers
- Discharge plan: medications, diet, activity, pathophysiology of disease, symptom management, special procedures and associated equipment, when to call health care provider, community resources

information about monitors and unit policy, for example, usually suffices in these cases. Indeed, more information than can be processed and integrated can greatly increase anxiety and may result in slower recovery. Individuals have the right to accept, adopt, or reject the information provided in educational encounters, however frustrating this may be to the nurse.

ADULT LEARNING THEORY

Central to successful implementation of an educational plan in the critical care and telemetry environment is the incorporation of the principles of adult learning theory. An educational plan that does consider the uniqueness of the adult population can potentially fail. It is beneficial for the nurse to have an understanding of this theory before planning or implementing the educational plan of care. Knowles described several assumptions on adult learning theory that differ from those of children.[5] Adults must be ready to learn, having moved from one developmental or educational task to the next. They need to know why it is important to learn something before they can actually learn it. Inherent in their attitudes is a responsibility for their own decisions. Consequently, they may resent when others try to force different beliefs on them. Adults bring a wealth of experience to the learning environment that must be recognized and promoted in educational techniques. Their orientation to learning is life-centered, so that tasks being taught should focus on current problem resolution. Finally, motivation for the adult learner arises out of internal pressures such as self-esteem and quality of life.

TEACHING-LEARNING PROCESS

The teaching-learning process used in the health care setting incorporates the dynamics of adult learning theory. The learner must be both physically and emotionally ready and able to learn.[5] The volume and complexity of information needed by persons facing new health challenges can be very confusing. In addition, there can be a significant loss of the capacity to focus and concentrate during periods after treatment and physiologic changes.[6] Patients and families may have different perceptions regarding the importance of information and whether that information was effectively communicated.[7,8] Box 4-2 describes steps of the teaching-learning process.

Assessment

The assessment step in patient teaching involves gathering a data base to assist the nurse in meeting the patient's and family's learning needs.[5] It is a vital part of any successful educational plan. Among the components of this assessment in the critical care unit are identification of the various physiologic, psychologic, environmental, and sociocultural stressors present; the patient's response to these stressors and adaptation to illness; and an examination of motivation and readiness to learn. In reality, these issues are often related to one another and cannot be assessed as separate entities. For ease of illustration, however, they are discussed separately.

Stressors

Physiologic stressors. One main physiologic stressor for the critically ill patient is the illness, often life-threatening, for which the patient was admitted. In addition, other physiologic changes in critically ill patients act as further stressors. These may include pain, hypoxia, cardiac dysrhythmias, hypotension, fluid and electrolyte imbalances, infection, fever, or neurologic deficits. The presence of the illness and other stressors may completely consume the patient's available energy and leave none for any type of orientation to stimuli or education.

A physical assessment will yield information about physiologic reactions to stress. The following factors should be considered:

- Is the patient in pain or some other type of distress?
- What is the patient's level of consciousness and orientation?
- Has the patient been sedated?
- Is the patient hypoxic or hypercapnic?
- Are the heart rate, blood pressure, cardiac output, and perfusion adequate?
- Can the patient see and hear?

These questions add to the data base for formulation of an effective educational plan.

Psychologic stressors. Serious illness affects a patient not only physically, but also psychologically. Intense emotions can alter a person's normal way of coping and ability to learn and retain information. Psychologic stressors often present in the critically ill person include helplessness, powerlessness, loneliness, changes in role in the family and at work, changes in body image, fear of future life-style changes, and fear of death. These and other psychologic stressors not only can result in physiologic changes, but also can trigger behavior consistent with anxiety, denial, and depression.

The psychologic assessment is also important in determining the patient's ability to respond to the teaching-learning experience. An important factor is the patient's stage in adaptation to illness during the time teaching is undertaken. The general characteris-

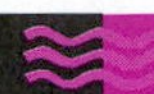 **RESEARCH ABSTRACT** 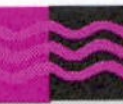

Coronary artery bypass graft (CABG) discharge information addressing women's recovery

Moore S: *Clinical Nursing Research* 5(1):97, 1996.

PURPOSE

Two research questions were asked: (1) What are the concerns, emotions, and physical sensations of women during the first month of recovery after CABG? (2) What actions are most helpful to female CABG patients in managing their concerns, emotions, and physical sensations during the first month of recovery?

DESIGN

Descriptive, survey.

SAMPLE

The convenience sample consisted of 20 women who had undergone their first CABG surgery with no major complications. The mean age was 66.9 years; 80% were Caucasian; 40% were married; 65% were retired; and they averaged 11.3 years of education. The average length of hospitalization after surgery was 9.5 days.

PROCEDURE

Subjects were interviewed 1 day before discharge, 48 hours after discharge, and 3 weeks after discharge. Face-to-face interviews were conducted for the first session; telephone interviews were conducted for the remaining two sessions. An investigator developed–structured interview guide, based on Johnson's recommendations for the design of cognitive information for patient coping with potentially stressful situations, directed the questions.

RESULTS

At discharge, the most commonly reported sensations were those associated with the chest incision; breathing; eating; energy level; sleep; breast, shoulder, and neck muscles; and the leg incision. The most commonly reported symptom was chest incision discomfort. Discomfort around the chest incision gradually decreased throughout the recovery period, but lasted as long as 3 weeks. About 20% of the women reported that they had a lump at the top of their chest incision that lasted 3 weeks after discharge. Housework was done during the recovery period, but not walking exercises. Many women reported extreme fatigue at all interview points. They also reported concerns regarding who would take care of them, since most of them lived alone.

DISCUSSION/IMPLICATIONS

This study is important since it described women's experiences; much research historically has not included women and therefore little information exists regarding women's unique needs. Although the sample size in this study was small, there were recovery experiences identified that are not routinely addressed in traditional CABG teaching and discharge information. Findings from this study provide a basis for further investigation that addresses all a patient's informational needs. In addition, there are clinical implications for the development of valid patient education and presurgery preparation teaching materials.

BOX 4-2 The Teaching-Learning Process

- Assess learning needs and readiness to learn
- Formulate teaching plan
- Implement teaching plan
- Evaluate attainment of learning objectives

tics of the *stages of adaptation to illness* are outlined in Table 4-1 with corresponding applications for the teaching-learning process. Salient points are reviewed here. It needs to be noted that each individual moves at his or her own pace through the stages, and it is not uncommon to skip or move back and forth through the stages. Because of individual variations, the stages can be encountered in both the critical care and telemetry units. The nurse must also consider that the family goes through stages of adaptation to their loved one's illness as well. Family members may or may not progress at the same rate as the patient, so teaching strategies may need modification to ensure meeting the individual needs of both the patient and the significant others.

The first response to acute illness is generally *disbelief and denial.* Although this response has some psychologic benefit for the patient, it acts as a barrier to learning. During this stage it is acceptable for the nurse to allow denial if it does not put the patient in danger. Teaching is focused on the present, and comments referring to the future must be avoided.

After a few days the denial mechanism usually breaks down and the patient moves into the stage of *developing awareness.* The patient must accept that he

TABLE 4-1 Teaching-Learning Process in Adaptation to Illness

Stage of Adaptation	Characteristic Patient Response	Implications for Teaching-Learning Process
Disbelief	Denial	Orient teaching to present. Teach during other nursing activities. Reassure patient about safety. Explain all procedures and activities clearly and concisely.
Developing awareness	Anger	Continue to orient teaching to present. Avoid long lists of facts. Continue to foster development of trust and rapport through good physical care.
Reorganization	Acceptance of sick role	Orient teaching to meet patient needs. Teach whatever patient wants to learn. Provide necessary self-care information; reinforce with written material.
Resolution	Identification with others with same problem; recognition of loss	Use group instruction. Use patient support groups and visits by recovered patients with same problem.
Identifying change	Definition of self as one who has undergone change and is now different	Answer patient's questions as they arise. Recognize that as basic needs are met more mature needs will arise.

or she is ill. This stage generally coincides with the assumption of the sick role. At this time a patient may respond with anger or guilt. If these emotions are turned inward, he or she may experience depression. If emotions are expressed outwardly, behavior may be hostile toward persons and things in the environment, including the nurse. It is important at this time to listen to the expressions of anger but not to argue with the patient. The nurse must remember that the patient is reacting to factors other than the nurse. Teaching during this time continues to be oriented to the present but may relate more to the disease process, which is now recognized by the patient. The patient is still too anxious to learn and assimilate lists of facts but may be interested in the meaning of symptoms and treatments as they relate to his or her experience at the moment.

The third stage of adaptation to illness is *reorganization.* At this time the patient has begun to work through the anger and guilt and to reorganize his or her self-concept and relationships with others consistent with the acceptance of the sick role. During this time the nurse teaches whatever the patient wants to learn, thus helping the patient to achieve the reorganization necessary to move on to adaptation.

The final stages of adaptation are *resolution* and *identity change.* They occur late in recovery. During these times the patient is more receptive to teaching based on objectives and to learning about long-term needs. Group instruction that includes the spouse and significant others can be an effective method at this time.

Also included in the psychologic assessment of the patient is an assessment of the patient's coping style. Coping can affect learning.[9] It is important for the nurse to recognize the patient's coping style and respect it during educational efforts.[10]

Environmental stressors. The physical surroundings in a critical care unit contribute to the stress of the experience for a patient. Factors such as sleep deprivation, observation of other patients, loss of privacy, bright lights, unfamiliar noises, unpleasant odors, and loss of contact with loved ones contribute to stress. Management and control of these factors have become important nursing functions, especially in the creation of a learning environment.

Sociocultural stressors. Variables such as age, gender, ethnic origin, economic status, religious beliefs, level of education, and occupation may add to the stress of illness and alter learning ability.[11-13] The nurse-patient interaction must be structured to recognize the effects of these variables on the process and outcome of the teaching-learning experience.

Assessment of Readiness to Learn

Assessment of motivation and readiness to learn is an important part of the teaching-learning process. This assessment incorporates an analysis of multiple factors that have previously been discussed. These include an appreciation of multiple stressors and their response and the patient's stage of adaptation to illness. In addition, an examination of motivation theory is helpful. One well-known and important theory describing human behavior motivation is Maslow's hierarchy of needs, which provides background for the discussion of motivation to learn.

Maslow described a number of needs that were postulated as motivating all behavior. According to this theory, human beings have a number of needs that are interrelated and hierarchic. In other words, the lower-level needs must be met before higher-level needs can emerge and be satisfied.

The need to know and understand are among the highest-level needs. During a time of critical illness, a patient's energy is often consumed by the lower-level physiologic and safety needs and it would be impossible for the patient to attend to learning interactions. Attempting to teach a patient who fears for his or her life and safety is of little use unless the patient is being taught that he or she is safe and in no immediate danger of dying. Once the lower-level needs are met and the patient feels out of danger, he or she will be more ready to learn and higher-level needs can be addressed. Therefore if the assessment discloses significant needs in lower areas, the nurse must address those needs before attempting any teaching. Once met, these needs cease to be the primary motivators of behavior and the patient can attend to his or her learning and other higher-level needs.

Formulate the Teaching Plan

The assessment of the multitude of factors that have been discussed assists the critical care nurse in the establishment of an adequate data base from which to formulate nursing diagnoses and devise an educational plan of care. In this plan of care, expected outcomes and behavioral objectives are identified. Nursing Management Plans for Knowledge Deficit are included at the end of this chapter. Also, various teaching content areas commonly identified in the critical care unit are presented here for review. Strategies for successful teaching described by Seley[3] are summarized in Box 4-3.

Determine teaching content. Determination of the content presented in the critical care unit depends on the patient's clinical and emotional status and varies with each patient. The nurse sets learning needs priorities based on the assessment as soon as possible. However, at times an acute event precludes full assessment at the time of admission. In this case, behavior crucial to the patient's treatment and his or her participation in care can be taught as soon as appropriate. The teaching must be guided by the patient and family—that is, teach what they want to know when they want to know it. If the patient's questions and concerns are left unanswered during this time of high anxiety, the unmet needs will serve as a block to further communication and prevent the patient from focusing his or her energy appropriately.

Although the specific content taught varies, depending on the condition for which the patient is admitted, certain areas need to be covered with any patient who is conscious. *Environmental factors* in a critical care unit can be frightening to patients and must be explained as soon as possible. Cardiac monitors, oxygen equipment, indwelling lines and catheters, frequent laboratory tests, and vital signs checks may cause the patient undue anxiety unless their purpose or function is understood. The reason for procedures, as well as their associated sensations or discomfort, need to be briefly explained. This information may not be retained and may require several repetitions, but it will assist in decreasing anxiety and providing a sense of control for the moment.

BOX 4-3 Teaching Tips

- Assess patient and family learning needs
- Assess patient and family readiness to learn
- Set realistic and measurable goals
- "Clump" information together in the most simple and understandable manner
- Provide opportunity for demonstration and practice of new skill(s)
- Provide written, simple, clear instructions; consider videotape or other alternative presentation format as appropriate to patient/family learning style and teaching material
- Provide feedback and opportunity for review of information
- Individualize regimen to patient life-style and preferences
- Reinforce new knowledge and behaviors
- Ensure appropriate followup (e.g., community resources, support groups, home health care, etc)

From Seeley JJ: *Am J Nurs* 10:63, 1994.

NURSING INTERVENTION CLASSIFICATIONS

BOX 4-4 Teaching: Disease Process

DEFINITION: Assisting the patient to understand information related to a specific disease process

ACTIVITIES:

Appraise the patient's current level of knowledge related to specific disease process
Explain the pathophysiology of the disease and how it relates to the anatomy and physiology, as appropriate
Describe common signs and symptoms of the disease, as appropriate
Describe the disease process, as appropriate
Identify possible etiologies, as appropriate
Provide information to the patient about condition, as appropriate
Avoid empty reassurances
Provide the family/significant other(s) with information about the patient's progress, as appropriate
Provide information about available diagnostic measures, as appropriate
Discuss life-style changes that may be required to prevent future complications and/or control the disease process
Discuss therapy/treatment options
Describe rationale behind management/therapy/treatment recommendations
Encourage the patient to explore options/get a second opinion, as appropriate or indicated
Describe possible chronic complications, as appropriate
Instruct the patient on measures to prevent/minimize side effects of the disease, as appropriate
Explore possible resources/support, as appropriate
Refer the patient to local community agencies/support groups, as appropriate
Instruct the patient on which signs and symptoms to report to health care provider, as appropriate
Provide the phone number(s) to call if complications occur
Reinforce information provided by other health care team members, as appropriate

From McCloskey JC, Bulechek GM: *Nursing intervention classifications*, ed 2, St Louis, 1996, Mosby.

Most of the time it is appropriate to give *information about the illness or diagnosis* in the critical phase of care. Nursing activities for teaching the disease process are found in Box 4-4. The nurse must often interpret and explain information provided by physicians. Despite the denial often present, some patients want to know about their illness, prognosis, complications, and reason for admission to the critical care unit. A patient may ask whether he or she is going to die. This is a traumatic question for both the patient and the nurse. Nurses may reluctantly talk about death with colleagues or a family but are often very uncomfortable in discussing it with patients. It is important for the nurse to remember that the entire experience of the critical care unit, although routine for the staff, is frightening for the patient who may be confronting mortality for the first time. Questions must be answered as honestly, compassionately, and sensitively as possible and be followed by supportive care as necessary.

Patients in critical care units experience many stressful *medical and nursing procedures* during the course of their care, including radiologic procedures, placement of vascular access or monitoring devices, intubation, suctioning, spinal taps, and many others. Educational and psychologic preparation for these procedures can decrease anxiety and increase patient cooperation with care. Two types of information can be offered to patients in preparation for these procedures. *Procedural information* refers to what will be done, when and where it will happen, and who will provide the service. *Sensory information* refers to what the patient can expect to feel during and after the procedure.[14] When time permits, allowing the patient to ask questions, see equipment that will be used, and practice movements or body positions that will be required can be very helpful in reducing anxiety. In addition, teaching the patient basic relaxation techniques, such as deep breathing or guided imagery, can be effective in helping patients relax during a stressful or uncomfortable procedure.[14,15] When these procedures must occur on an emergent basis without time for patient preparation, the nurse will explain what happened and why as soon as the patient stabilizes and is able to understand the information.

Another important educational consideration in the critical care environment is that the patient learns not only by what is said directly, but also by inadvertent comments or nonverbal cues. Nurses need to be especially attuned to staff or physician discussions at the patient's bedside, where information heard by the patient can be misinterpreted and possibly lead to increased anxiety and misinformation. In addition, if nonverbal cues from the nurse do not coincide with the reality of the situation or the severity of the patient condition, mistrust can ensue and alter the nurse-patient therapeutic relationship. These dynamics can also affect educational efforts with the family.

Formulate objectives. Inherent in any educational plan of care is careful consideration of desired objectives. Objectives state the desired behaviors expected from the implementation of the plan.[16] They are based on the patient's learning needs and serve as a guide for the teaching-learning process. Objectives are written in behavioral terms that are measurable and are stated in terms of what the patient is to learn, rather than what the nurse is to teach. Terms such as "to know," "understand," "be familiar with," "realize," and "appreciate" are open to many interpretations and are difficult to measure. Rather, active verbs such as *"identify," "state," "list," "describe,"* or *"demonstrate"* need to be used, because they are readily understood by all and easily lend themselves to evaluation.

Both long-term and short-term objectives are appropriate, although in many cases it takes days, weeks, or even months of repetition and practice for a new skill to be mastered. Indeed, time constraints in both the critical care and telemetry units may indicate considering only those needs identified as important and realistic to the patient with follow-up education after discharge.[17] However, a nurse in the critical care setting needs to identify goals that surpass the critical care phase, because the educational plan of care continues as the patient improves and is transferred to the telemetry unit. Generalized objectives have been developed for teaching programs used for large numbers of patients, such as cardiac teaching plans for patients recovering from myocardial infarctions. Standardized plans can be useful resource materials in developing a teaching plan but must not take the place of individualized, specific objectives designed for each patient.

Implement the Teaching Plan

Design the teaching-learning experience. Patients in the critical care environment are educated in many informal interactions with the nurse, and knowledge gained fosters patient understanding and well-being. Educational opportunities can be present during various nursing care activities, such as bathing and administration of medication. Each encounter with the patient and family must be viewed as a teaching opportunity. There are times, however, during the hospitalization when more formal or structured educational experiences are in order. Structured educational approaches have been found to be beneficial for immediate knowledge gain.[9] Included in this discussion are techniques in creating a learning environment and various teaching activities or methods that can be used to accomplish the desired outcomes based on the patient's individual learning objectives.

Create a learning environment. Patient barriers to learning related to physiologic, emotional, and motivational factors have been discussed. To structure a successful teaching-learning experience in a critical care area, the nurse must also carefully assess the environmental and iatrogenic barriers that affect the interaction. Bright lights, unpleasant odors, unfamiliar noises, and untidy surroundings can distract patients and add to cognitive impairment. Control of these factors can facilitate the learning process. Factors that cannot be controlled must be explained to the patient to alleviate anxiety and facilitate a trusting relationship between patient and nurse.

Teaching methods. There are three basic methods of teaching: lecture, discussion, and demonstration. The selection of the methods will be determined by various factors, including patient clinical status, readiness to learn, cognitive abilities, learning style, instructional time, and availability of teaching materials and resources. In addition, innovative methods of teaching and presentation of educational materials must be developed and used efficiently to maximize existing resources.[18]

Lecture. Lecture is the presentation of information in a highly structured format to a group. In this method the teacher provides a great deal of material but may not provide ample opportunities for teacher-learner interaction. This style of teaching is inappropriate for acutely ill individuals in the critical care unit. However, it may be useful in the telemetry unit. Optimally, the group size should be arranged to enable the learners to ask questions and get appropriate feedback on content presented.

Discussion. Discussion is less structured than is lecturing and allows an exchange and feedback between the teacher and learner. The teacher can adapt the material to meet the needs of the individual or group. Discussion groups can be effective with hospitalized

NURSING INTERVENTION CLASSIFICATIONS

BOX 4-5 Teaching: Psychomotor Skill

DEFINITION: Preparing a patient to perform a psychomotor skill

ACTIVITIES:

Demonstrate the skill for the patient
Give clear, step-by-step directions
Instruct the patient to perform the skill one step at a time
Inform the patient of the rationale for performing the skill in the specified manner
Guide patients' bodies so that they can experience the physical sensations that accompany the correct motions, as appropriate
Provide written information/diagrams, as appropriate
Provide practice sessions (spaced to avoid fatigue, but often enough to prevent excessive forgetting), as appropriate
Provide adequate time for task mastery
Observe patient return demonstrate the skill
Provide frequent feedback to patients on what they are doing correctly and incorrectly, so that bad habits are not formed
Provide information on available assistive devices that may be used to facilitate performance of the required skill, as appropriate
Instruct the patient on the assembly, use, and maintenance of assistive devices, as appropriate
Include the family/significant others, as appropriate

From McCloskey JC, Bulechek GM: *Nursing intervention classifications,* ed 2, St Louis, 1996, Mosby.

patients when a group with similar problems and at similar stages of adaptation can be gathered. Individual discussion with patients and families is appropriate and valuable during the acute phase of illness, because it allows them to express their feelings and interpretations.

Demonstration. Demonstration involves acting out a procedure while giving appropriate explanations to provide the learner with a clear idea of how to perform a task. The patient can then practice the skill and be given feedback about his or her performance. This method is often used in the acute care setting, such as when coughing and deep breathing or taking one's own pulse is taught. Nursing activities for teaching psychomotor skills are found in Box 4-5.

Other methods of instruction. In addition to the three basic methods just presented, several other approaches to delivering or augmenting information in a patient teaching program are available. They include commercially prepared or custom-designed printed materials, bedside videotape programs, and computer-assisted patient education programs. *Computer programs,* relatively new to health education, have been used in community-based education programs, hospital waiting rooms, designated teaching rooms, and, in some cases, at the bedside with microcomputers on transportable carts.[19] These programs allow the learner to set the program pace and are generally presented in an attractive, colorful format.[20]

Written materials can be very useful tools in patient and family education. They allow repetition and reinforcement of content and provide basic information in printed form for reference at a later time. To be useful, however, the content must be accurate and current and the patient and family must be able to read and understand it.[21]

It is estimated that the median literacy level of the U.S. population is at the tenth grade level, with about 20% of the population having reading skills at the fifth grade level or lower.[16] Other research indicates that approximately 50% of health care clients have serious difficulty reading instructional materials written at the fifth grade level.[22] The vast majority of patient education materials are written at or above the eighth grade level.[22] To ensure that the reading level of the educational material and the learner are well-matched, the patients need to be questioned about the last grade level completed in school. Because this level may not equal the grade level in reading ability, written material two to four grade levels below that must be selected.[22] Box 4-6 depicts examples of an instruction written at various reading levels.

BOX 4-6 Samples of Different Reading Levels

COLLEGE READING LEVEL

Consult your physician immediately with the onset of chest discomfort, shortness of breath, or increased perspiration.

TWELFTH GRADE READING LEVEL

Call your physician immediately if you experience chest discomfort, shortness of breath, or increased sweatiness.

EIGHTH GRADE READING LEVEL

Call your doctor immediately if you start having chest pain or shortness of breath or feel sweaty.

FOURTH GRADE READING LEVEL

Call your doctor right away if you start having chest pain, can't breathe, or feel sweaty.

In recent years the use of *educational videotapes* at the bedside or in group settings has gained increasing popularity. A review of the literature on the use of videotapes verifies that the medium can be used to address the basic and repetitive aspects of patient education and that it is effective for short-term knowledge gain.[23] The use of videotapes, however, is not a substitute for individualized patient teaching, and it is most effective when it is promoted by staff as reinforcing other educational activities.[23,24] It is essential that the nurse realize that audiovisual accessories are an adjunct to teaching but do not replace the central role of the nurse in objective accomplishment. Indeed, the credibility of the nurse or educational care plan can be seriously affected when discrepancy exists between the videotapes and information that is reinforced.

Closed-circuit television (CCTV) is becoming a common service in many health care settings. It also is best used as one component of a comprehensive educational program and is not intended to be used alone. CCTV allows for the viewing of the session to take place at the time that best suits the patient and family and can be stopped, restarted, or repeated as necessary. It ensures a consistent standard in presentation of routine educational topics.[25]

Evaluate Attainment of Learning Objectives

Evaluation of the educational plan of care focuses on the ability of the plan to attain the objectives and outcomes developed in the planning phase. This includes the documentation of the effectiveness of the teaching-learning process with measurement of the knowledge gain and behavior changes identified.[26]

In addition to the traditional evaluation of the educational plan based on objectives, other subtle effects of patient education can be identified. If the nurse in the critical care setting limits measurement of teaching effectiveness to long-term behavior changes, many critical educational activities necessary for the well-being of the patient will be judged failures. If the teaching meets a momentary need, the effect is no less valuable and successful. Less concrete but equally valuable outcomes, such as signs of relaxation when the information provided decreases anxiety or increases participation in self-care, also document beneficial effects of the educational plan. This does not negate the fact that in many situations written, measurable objectives are necessary and useful, but it does mean that they must not be the sole measures of educational success.[27] A good example of this is the interaction that occurs when a patient is taught about the cardiac monitor on admission to the critical care unit. In teaching the reason for and function of this equipment, the nurse not only increases the patient's knowledge about cardiac monitoring, but may also decrease the patient's anxiety about the critical care setting, thereby promoting rest and healing.

TEACHING TOWARD TRANSFER FROM CRITICAL CARE

Transfer from the critical care unit to a telemetry or another acute care area can be an anxiety-producing time for patients. During the stay in the critical care unit, constant interaction with the nurse, monitoring devices, and controlled environment has offered security to the patient. To avoid anxiety, nurses prepare patients for imminent or eventual transfer—that is, teach toward transfer. To do this, the nurse points out early in the stay that the patient will be there only temporarily until his or her condition improves and stabilizes, and these improvements will be made known to the patient on an ongoing basis. As the time for transfer approaches, careful explanations can reassure patients and families that close observation and monitoring are no longer necessary. When possible, tubes, machines, and equipment used in the critical care unit—which the patient may see as important to survival—need to be removed gradually rather than discontinued all at once. This will alleviate feelings of dependence on equipment.

BOX 4-7 Medication Card Format

GENERAL CONSIDERATIONS

1. Use simple, layman's language.
2. Keep information clear and concise.
3. Give medication information to patient in advance of discharge so that material can be absorbed and questions asked.

PERTINENT POINTS TO INCLUDE ON CARD

1. Basic physiology of how the medication works
2. Action of medication (i.e., why the patient is taking the medication)
3. Importance of taking medication exactly as described
   Include information on timing (i.e., before or after meals, before bedtime, before other medications taken)
4. Aids to medication administration
   Calendar
   Wallet ID
   Medic-alert band
   Small plastic boxes to organize the day's medications
5. Possible side effects
   Most common side effects
   Side effects or symptoms that require notification of physician
6. Prevention of complications
   Activities that should be avoided while on the medication
   Drug interactions
   Food interactions
   Special monitoring, such as blood work

At the time of transfer, patients can be told how care will change and what changes in activity, self-care, and visiting hours to expect. It is helpful to emphasize that the transfer represents an improvement in patient condition and, contrary to common references to a "step-down" unit, telemetry units are, in fact, a "step-up." The critical care unit nurse accompanies the patient to the new floor and introduces the new staff members to the patient. The patient can be told that a complete report on his or her condition will be given and that nursing management needs at this stage of recovery will be met in the new setting. Family members should be contacted and informed of the transfer. The management plan and educational plan developed in the critical care area must accompany the patient to the floor, and the new nurses are informed about current short-term and long-term goals and the patient's progress.

Although careful preparation and planning for transfer are always desirable, a patient may be transferred unexpectedly to make room for a more critically ill patient. When this situation occurs, the patient to be moved from the unit must be notified and prepared for the possibility of a quick transfer. Tangible evidence of improvement, such as more favorable vital signs or need for fewer medications or tubes, can be helpful in pointing out advances in condition before unplanned transfers.

SAMPLE WRITTEN TEACHING TOOL

Box 4-7 describes a format for the construction of a medication card, which is one method of illustrating key points for medications. Box 4-8 is a sample medication card, which can be useful in preparing a patient for discharge. There are many sources of "packaged" patient medication information materials that can be purchased for use in the health care settings.

BOX 4-8 Sample Medication Card

DIGOXIN

Digoxin is a medication ordered by your doctor to improve and strengthen the pumping action of your heart. It also is used to control heart rate and to promote regular heart rhythm. Overall, the effect is to help blood circulation.

Digoxin can be toxic if not taken properly and as prescribed by your doctor. Take it at the same time each day, even if you feel well. If a dose is forgotten and not remembered within 12 hours, do not double the dose the next time. However, if you remember within 12 hours, take the dose as soon as you remember.

Possible side effects

Because digoxin is a potent drug, it is important to recognize the possible signs of overdosage:

- Extreme fatigue
- Muscle weakness
- Loss of appetite
- Nausea or vomiting
- Lower stomach pain
- Diarrhea
- Slow or irregular heartbeat
- Blurred vision
- Seeing green, yellow, or white halos around objects
- Confusion

If you notice these side effects, call your doctor immediately.

Prevention of complications

Do not stop taking this medication without asking your doctor.

Do not take other medications (including nonprescription drugs) unless ordered by your doctor, because they can interfere with this medication.

If you are also taking a diuretic ("water pill"), ask your doctor about the need to eat foods high in the electrolyte potassium. Potassium is lost frequently when taking a water pill, and sometimes a low potassium level can cause digoxin overdosage.

Talk with your doctor about the need to weigh yourself daily. Also, ask whether you should check your pulse daily before taking digoxin, since this drug can affect your heart rate.

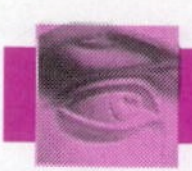

NURSING MANAGEMENT PLAN

KNOWLEDGE DEFICIT

DEFINITION:

Absence or deficiency of cognitive information related to specfic topic.

Knowledge Deficit_______________(Specify) Related to Cognitive/Perceptual Learning Limitations (e.g., sensory overload, sleep deprivation, medications, anxiety, sensory deficits, language barrier)

DEFINING CHARACTERISTICS

- Verbalized statement of inadequate knowledge of skills
- Verbalization of inadequate recall of information
- Verbalization of inadequate understanding of information
- Evidence of inaccurate follow-through of instructions
- Inadequate demonstration of a skill
- Lack of compliance with prescribed behavior

OUTCOME CRITERIA

- Patient participates actively in necessary and prescribed health behaviors.
- Patient verbalizes adequate knowledge or demonstrates adequate skills.

NURSING INTERVENTIONS AND *RATIONALE*

1. Continue to monitor the assessment parameters listed under "Defining Characteristics."
2. Determine specific cause of patient's cognitive or perceptual limitation. (See also table of contents for Impaired Verbal Communication, Anxiety, Sleep Pattern Disturbances, Sensory/Perceptual Alterations.)
3. Provide uninterrupted rest period before teaching session ***to decrease fatigue and encourage optimal state for learning and retention.***
4. Manipulate environment as much as possible ***to provide quiet and uninterrupted learning sessions:***
   Ensure lights are bright enough to see teaching aids but not too bright.
   Close door if necessary ***to provide quiet environment.***
   Schedule care and medications ***to allow uninterrupted teaching periods.***
   Move patient to quiet, private room for teaching *if possible.*
5. Adapt teaching sessions and materials to patient's and family's levels of education and ability to understand:
   Provide printed material appropriate to reading level.
   Use terminology understood by the patient.
   Provide printed materials in patient's primary language *if possible.*
   Use interpreters during teaching sessions *when necessary.*
6. Teach only present-tense focus during periods of sensory overload.
7. Determine potential effects of medications on ability to retain or recall information. Avoid teaching critical content while patient is taking sedatives, analgesics, or other medications affecting memory.
8. Reinforce new skills and information in several teaching sessions. Use several senses when possible in teaching session (e.g., see a film, hear a discussion, read printed information, and demonstrate skills related to self-injection of insulin).
9. Reduce patient's anxiety:
   Listen attentively and encourage verbalization of feelings.
   Answer questions as they arise in a clear and succinct manner.
   Elicit patient's concerns and address those issues first.
   Give only correct and relevant information.
   Continually assess response to teaching session and discontinue if anxiety increases or physical condition becomes unstable.
   Provide nonthreatening information before more anxiety-producing information is presented.
   Plan for several teaching sessions so information can be divided into small manageable packages.

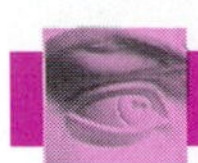

NURSING MANAGEMENT PLAN

Knowledge Deficit_____________(Specify) Related to Lack of Previous Exposure to Information

DEFINING CHARACTERISTICS

- Verbalized statement of inadequate knowledge or skills
- New diagnosis or health problem requiring self-management or care
- Lack of prior formal or informal education about the specific health problem
- Demonstration of inappropriate behaviors related to management of health problem

OUTCOME CRITERIA

- Patient verbalizes adequate knowledge about or performs skills related to disease process, its causes, factors related to onset of symptoms, and self-management of disease or health problem.
- Patient actively participates in health behaviors required for performance of a procedure or in those behaviors enhancing recovery from illness and preventing recurrence or complications.

NURSING INTERVENTIONS AND *RATIONALE*

1. Continue to monitor the assessment parameters listed under "Defining Characteristics."
2. Determine existing level of knowledge or skill.
3. Assess factors affecting the knowledge deficit:
   Learning needs, including patient's priorities and the necessary knowledge and skills for safety
   Learning ability of client, including language skills, level of education, ability to read, preferred learning style
   Physical ability to perform prescribed skills or procedures; consider effect of limitations imposed by treatment such as bedrest, restriction of movement by intravenous or other equipment, or effect of sedatives or analgesics
   Psychologic effect of stage of adaptation to disease
   Activity tolerance and ability to concentrate
   Motivation to learn new skills or gain new knowledge
4. Reduce or limit barriers to learning:
   Provide consistent nurse-patient contact ***to encourage development of trusting and therapeutic relationship.***
   Structure environment ***to enhance learning;*** control unnecessary noise, interruptions.
   Individualize teaching plan ***to fit patient's current physical and psychologic status.***
   Delay teaching until patient is ready to learn.
   Conduct teaching sessions during period of day when patient is most alert and receptive.
   Meet patient's immediate learning needs as they arise (e.g., give brief explanation of procedures when they are performed).
5. Promote active participation in the teaching plan by the patient and family:
   Solicit input during development of plan.
   Develop mutually acceptable goals and outcomes.
   Solicit expression of feelings and emotions related to new responsibilities.
   Encourage questions.
6. Conduct teaching sessions, using the most appropriate teaching methods:
   Discussion
   Lecture
   Demonstration/return demonstration
   Use of audiovisual or printed educational materials
7. Repeat key principles and provide them in printed form ***for reference at a later time.***
8. Give frequent feedback to patient when practicing new skills.
9. Use several teaching sessions when appropriate. ***New information and skills should be reinforced several times after initial learning.***
10. Initiate referrals for follow-up if necessary:
    Health educators
    Home health care
    Rehabilitation programs
    Social services
11. Evaluate effectiveness of teaching plan, based on patient's ability to meet preset goals and objectives, and determine need for further teaching.

REFERENCES

1. Aliberti LC: Managing patient education: a perspective for the 1990s, *Gastroenterology Nursing* 12:148, 1991.
2. Harvey CV, Hanchek K: Interdisciplinary patient teaching plans: design and implementation, *Orthop Nursing* 10(2):55, 1991.
3. Seley JJ: 10 strategies for successful patient teaching, *Am J Nurs* 10:63, 1994.
4. Barnason S, Zimmerman L: A comparison of patient teaching outcomes among postoperative coronary artery bypass graft (CABG) patients, *Prog Cardiovasc Nurs* 10(4):11, 1995.
5. Moss VA: Assessing learning abilities, readiness for education, *Seminars in Perioperative Nursing* 3(3):113, 1994.
6. Cimprich B: A theoretical perspective on attention and patient education, *ANS Adv Nurs Sci* 14(3):39, 1992.
7. Reiley P and others: Discharge planning: comparison of patients' and nurses' perceptions of patients following hospital discharge, *Image* 28(2):143, 1996.
8. Duryee R: The efficacy of inpatient education after myocardial infarction, *Heart Lung* 21(2):217, 1992.
9. Murphy MC and others: Education of patients undergoing coronary angioplasty: factors affecting learning during a structured educational program, *Heart Lung* 18(1):36, 1989.
10. Creamer-Bauer C, Webber M: Patient teaching strategies for peripheral laser procedures, *Health Educ Q* 12(3):135, 1985.
11. Barnes LP: The illiterate client: strategies in patient teaching, *MCN Am J Matern Child Nurs* 17(3):127, 1992.
12. Price JL, Cordell B: Cultural diversity and patient teaching, *Journal Contin Educ Nurs* 25(4):163, 1994.
13. Stewart B: Teaching culturally diverse populations, *Seminars in Perioperative Nursing* 3(3):160, 1994.
14. Williams CL, Kendall PC: Psychological aspects of education for stressful medical procedures, *Health Educ Q* 12(3):135, 1985.
15. Frenn M, Fehring R, Kartes S: Reducing the stress of cardiac catheterization by teaching relaxation, *DCCN* 5(2):108, 1986.
16. Redman BK: *The process of patient teaching in nursing,* ed 7, St Louis, 1993, Mosby.
17. Chan V: Content cardiac teaching: patient's perceptions of the importance of teaching content after myocardial infarction, *J Adv Nurs* 15(10):1139, 1990.
18. Barnes LP: Meeting goals with limited financial resources, *MCN Am J Matern Child Nurs* 17(3):267, 1992.
19. Bell JA: The role of microcomputers in patient education, *Comput Nurs* 4(6):255, 1987.
20. Dobberstein K: Computer-assisted patient education, *Am J Nurs* 87(5):697, 1987.
21. Bernier MJ: Developing and evaluating printed education materials: a prescriptive model for quality, *Orthop Nurs* 12(6):39, 1993.
22. Albright J and others: Readability of patient education materials: implications for clinical practice, *J Appl Nursing Research* 9(3):139, 1996.
23. Neilson E, Sheppard MA: Television as a patient education tool: a review of its effectiveness, *Patient Educ Couns* 11:3, 1988.
24. Durand RP, Counts CS: Developing audio-visual programs for patient education, *Am Neph Nurs Assoc* 13(3):158, 1986.
25. Chan V: Closed-circuit TV: an effective patient education tool, *Canadian Journal of Nursing Administration* Sept/Oct:20, 1992.
26. Weaver J: Patient education: an innovative computer approach, *Nurs Manage* 26(7):78, 1995.
27. Billie DA: Process oriented patient education, *DCCN* 2:2, 1983.

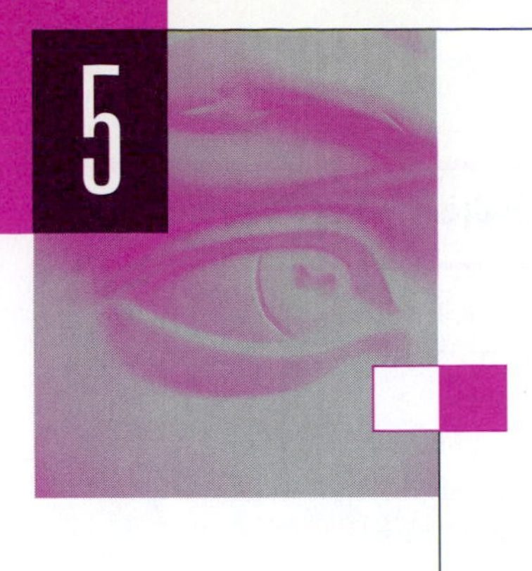

Psychosocial Alterations

Exemplar: Nancy Donovan, a 32-year-old single mother of two boys ages 5 and 8, was admitted to the Critical Care Burn Unit with second- and third-degree burns over 40% of her body—affecting portions of her face, anterior chest, arms, and legs. She had been using cleaning fluid near a gas water heater in the garage. She appears highly anxious and in intense pain, and she has symptoms of shock. Because of potential airway problems, she has been intubated and placed on a ventilator. Her prognosis is guarded. Her parents live in a small town 20 miles away. They have been notified and are on their way to the hospital. A neighbor activated the 911 emergency response system. The children, who were in school at the time of the accident, are staying with the neighbor until the grandparents arrive.

As initial treatment is directed toward physical stabilization, Nancy's psychologic responses to this crisis must also receive prompt attention. Recognizing that high anxiety levels begin a cyclic process of increased physical and psychologic pain and stress, it is essential to provide adequate pain and antianxiety relief and emotional support. Severe burn injuries pose a major coping challenge to any person, even if the individual is considered to be "psychologically healthy." Reactions to a burn injury are multiple and complex, and profound psychosocial issues are involved.[1] It is important for the nurse when preparing the plan of care to do an in-depth assessment of the patient's and family's coping skills. Another major task for the critical care nurse at this time is to help Nancy develop trust in her caregivers, because she is suddenly and totally dependent on others. Several potential alterations in self-concept and coping challenges can be suggested from this scenario. Take a moment to consider as many psychosocial issues that you can identify. This exemplar will be revisited periodically to relate additional information on self-concept and adaptation.

Patients requiring critical care must cope with a variety of stressors. A patient's response to these stressors depends on individual differences, such as age, gender, social supports, cultural background, medical diagnosis, current hospital course, and prognosis. The person's perception of self and relationships with others, spiritual values, and self-competency in social roles also play a major role in responses to stress and illness. The purpose of this chapter is to provide a theoretical basis for understanding these various issues and to provide the nurse with additional insight in implementing holistic nursing care.

The human self-concept is a major concern for nurses, because nursing interventions that do not consider the individual in his or her wholeness—including the self-concept—will probably not be effective. The self-concept comprises attitudes about oneself; perceptions of personal abilities, body image, and identity; and a general sense of worth. The stressors imposed by physical illness, trauma, and surgical procedures can cause disturbances in the self-concept. A person's response to these stressors depends upon a variety of individual differences, as previously mentioned.

Included in this chapter are discussions of the nursing diagnoses related to self-concept disturbances and alterations in coping patterns imposed by critical stages of illness—that is, Body Image Disturbance, Self-Esteem Disturbance, Altered Role Performance,

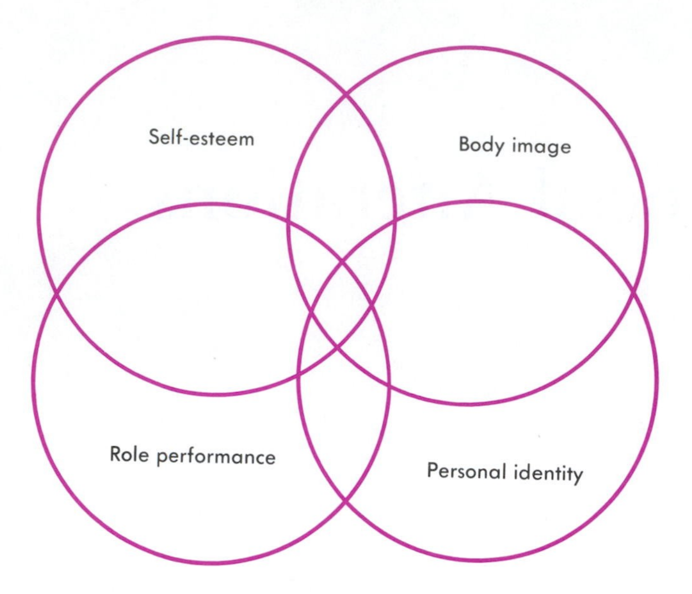

FIGURE 5-1. Four subcomponents of the human self-concept.

Powerlessness, Hopelessness, and Ineffective Coping (Individual and Family). The four subcomponents of the human self concept—Body Image, Self-Esteem, Role Performance, and Personal Identity are depicted in Figure 5-1. The nursing diagnosis, Personal Identity Disturbance, included as a subcomponent of the human self-concept by the North American Nursing Diagnosis Association (NANDA), is omitted because it is not yet sufficiently developed for useful application to clinical practice. Some of the various stressors experienced in the critical care setting are depicted in Box 5-1.

Each nursing diagnosis in this chapter is defined and then discussed in terms of specific characteristics, expected outcomes, and interventions. The problems common to critical care nursing are delineated in this chapter. Delirium, or acute confusion, which is frequently experienced by the critical care patient, is also discussed. Specific nursing roles as patient advocate, manager of care, and liaison with other health care providers are presented, as well as the mutual involvement with patient and family/support persons in the plan of care. The psychosocial needs of specific populations such as the elderly, chronically ill persons with acute exacerbations, and transplant recipients also are addressed. In addition, as previously mentioned, the exemplar of the young woman with severe burns is interspersed throughout the chapter to illustrate the potential psychosocial alterations and coping measures experienced by a patient in a critical care setting and to stimulate critical decision making.

BOX 5-1 Stressors in the Critical Care Setting

Patients' experience of critical illness and care varies. However, each patient must cope with at least some of the following stressors:

- Threat of death
- Threat of survival, with significant residual problems related to the illness/injury
- Pain or discomfort
- Lack of sleep
- Loss of autonomy over most aspects of life and daily functioning
- Loss of control over environment, including loss of privacy and exposure to light, noise, and general activity of the critical care unit, including the care of other patients
- Daily hassles or common frustrations
- Loss of usual role and with that, the arena in which usual coping mechanisms serve the patient
- Separation from family and friends
- Loss of dignity
- Boredom, broken only by brief visits, threatening stimuli, and frightening thoughts
- Loss of ability to express self verbally when intubated

Effects and response to the stressors are dependent on the individual's perception of the intensity of the stress and the following:

- Acute/chronic duration of stressors
- Cumulative effect of simultaneous stressors
- Sequence of stressors
- Individual's previous experience with stressors and coping effectiveness
- Amount of social support

EFFECTS OF STRESS ON MIND/BODY INTERACTIONS

Stress—whether biologic, psychologic, social, or positive or negative—elicits the same physical responses.[1] Extensive literature exists describing the relationship between the mind/body interactions and immune response to stress. All personal resources can be depleted by exposure to severe or prolonged stress. Several studies have shown the effects of different life events (e.g., bereavement, divorce, clinical depression, environmental disasters) as precursors or influencing factors in physical and mental illnesses.[2,3] Illness has been described as an unexpected stressful event that interrupts a person's usual pattern of living.[4,5] An illness that necessitates hospitalization can be a crisis event that can be further compounded when placement in a Critical Care Unit becomes necessary.

Three of the principal stress theories proposed by scientists describe stress as a stimulus, a response, and a transaction.[6-8] Hans Selye's[8] pioneer work portrayed the body responses to stress as the General Adaptation Syndrome (GAS). The three major phases are the alarm reaction, the stage of resistance, and stage of exhaustion. Stimulation of the sympathetic nervous branch of the autonomic nervous system and the release of endocrine hormones occur in the initial stage, which is commonly referred to as the "fight or flight" response. Elevations in blood pressure, tachycardia, increased muscle tone, increased alertness, and "free floating" anxiety are some of the responses. During the stage of resistance, energy resources continue to be used. The stage of exhaustion occurs when all strength reserves have been depleted; the person may become ill or die without replenishment of these resources. Reversal of these processes can be accomplished through use of medications, nutrition, stress reduction measures, and psychotherapy.

Neurnberger[7] proposed that a person can also respond to stress by "shutting down" via stimulation of the parasympathetic branch of the autonomic nervous system, the counterbalance to the sympathetic branch. He labeled this reaction as the General Inhibition Syndrome (GIS), or the "possum response." Both responses are designed as protective measures. Imbalances of either system can be detrimental. Overstimulation of the parasympathetic branch can lead to depression and is associated with diseases such as asthma; dominance of the sympathetic branch is associated with cardiovascular problems. Neurnberger also stated that the primary source of stress is the person's internal state of mind, or the emotional reaction to a perceived threat.

The work of Lazarus and Folkman[6] provides the foundation for transactional theories on stress. The person confronted by stress first makes a *cognitive appraisal* of its intensity. Response to the stressor is dependent on the perceived degree of threat imposed. A *secondary appraisal* determines what the response will be or the coping method to use to minimize the threat. The way that people cope with stress may be more important to overall morale, social function, and health/illness states than the frequency and severity of stress episodes.

Adaptation is an ongoing process involving both cognitive and physiologic neural-chemical and endocrine processes. The individual's sensitivity and vulnerability to the stressor are the determining factors of emotional and behavioral responses.[2] Therefore what may be an acutely stressful event to one person is not necessarily perceived as stressful by another. A person may employ different coping mechanisms to various stressors or to the same stressor at different times. A mechanism that is ineffective in one situation may be appropriate in another. Shedding tears may be a release of frustration; denial can, sometimes, help a person maintain morale.[4,9] Mental and physical health or disequilibrium—or homeostasis, and illness—are closely intertwined. Each person comes to an illness with a history and knowledge of the particular situation and its impact on life. Interpretation of the event and the responses are dependent on this history, which changes with each new encounter.

SIGNIFICANCE TO NURSING

Theoretical Basis

Four major concepts comprise the guidelines for nursing theories, research, education, and practice. These are (1) the *bio-psycho-social person;* (2) *health status;* (3) the *environment,* which includes significant others, culture, and economics; and (4) *nursing interventions* that assist individuals to promote, maintain, or restore an optimum level of health.[9] Holistic nursing care requires consideration of all factors, individual and environmental, that affect the patient's well-being and the ability to cope with crises such as illness. The nurse must have a sound knowledge base of anatomy and physiology, disease processes, remedial measures, and human responses to nursing interventions. The critical care nurse should be able to work with technology and to "know the patient" in order to humanize and individualize care. Decisions for interventions are based on an understanding of the patient's experiences, behavior patterns, feelings, and preferences[9-12] (Table 5-1). The critical care environment can be frightening. Technologic equipment can control one's breathing and prevent speaking. Invasive procedures, abrupt or continual noises, loss of privacy, sleep interruptions, pain, medications, and isolation or minimal contact with significant support persons create feelings of powerlessness and loss of control. Disorientation, which is common for patients in the critical care unit, is influenced by several factors that include the severity of the physical problem, chemical imbalances, overstimulation or deprivation, previous experiences with the health care system, and patient variables (e.g., age, gender, roles, fear, anxiety, confusion, and depression).[9,4] For others, the critical care unit is perceived as a safe environment where life-saving procedures are immediately at hand and administered by highly competent caregivers.

Nurse as Advocate

Patients and their families often rely on the nurse to intervene as an advocate on their behalf. The nurse

TABLE 5-1 Paradigm of Nursing in the Implementation of Holistic Patient-Centered Care

Assessment	Nursing Actions	Expected Outcomes
PERSON **Biologic Characteristics:** Age, gender, developmental phase Body functions (balance/imbalance) (includes internal environmental factors) **Psychologic Characteristics:** Self-concept components Spiritual beliefs/values Locus of control Coping mechanisms Role competency/role conflict Perception of current illness Intellect **Social Aspects:** Interrelationships Availability of support system	Focus all actions toward total strengths/needs of patient, including aspects related to environment and health status; use theoretical knowledge base for comparison purposes Identify person's perception of current illness, control of events, and availability of appropriate support system Identify coping mechanisms with previous stressors Assess and support ability to learn new self-care techniques Provide positive, honest feedback; establish trust	Continuity of care will be provided Patient will have realistic expectations of outcomes from current illness and its impact on physical and mental health Patient will use effective coping mechanisms in response to illness-related stressors Patient will participate in self-care, learn new psychomotor skills to achieve confidence in skill performance Patient will place trust in caregivers and verbalize satisfaction with care or express need for changes
ENVIRONMENT Cultural/ethnic/societal influences Area of residence, condition of living quarters/work place Access to available community resources—transportation, food, sanitation, support services, etc Access to recreation facilities Membership/attendance at religious/social functions Availability of significant others in social support system	Identify influencing factors in external environment that facilitate/inhibit patient's coping with current health problem Collaborate with health care team members in providing holistic care Provide safe, comfortable environment that is as stress-free as possible during hospitalization Encourage positive interactions with significant others	Inhibiting factors will be minimized; facilitative factors will be enhanced Collaborative team efforts will promote holistic approach to decision making; family will be included in decisions Hospital environment will be modified to provide safe, secure atmosphere Significant others will have central role in providing social support; patient will not be isolated
HEALTH Current and past mental/spiritual/physical health status Life-style practices Type of coping mechanisms Attitude toward life	Encourage positive interactions with significant others Instruct person and family on self-care activities Involve family in patient-centered activities as early as possible; support family members	Patient and family will have knowledge about illness and prognosis and can plan realistically for future Family caregivers will recognize own limits and seek help

may serve as interpreter when patients or families/significant others do not understand explanations because of the use of technical medical language. The advocate is needed to protect their rights; to inform them about their rights; and to help them make the correct decisions about treatment, set personal goals, and be involved in their own care. The advocate must also recognize that patients and families/significant others must agree to receive the information, and must face the fact that some families/significant others do not want a patient to receive the information.[13]

Individuals under stress may not verbally express their true needs, or needs may change under different circumstances. People in crisis may not recognize what their needs are and can misinterpret attitudes of caregivers as indifference. The role of advocate can be difficult when patient decisions seem inappropriate to the health professional. Underlying beliefs of patient advocacy include the following: the individual's right to select values that sustain life, to exercise personal judgment, and to make decisions without coercion.

The nurse advocate must, first, be able to advocate for himself or herself. The nurse needs self-knowledge about nursing and health care or needs to know what sources are available to assist patients in their decision making. Advocacy should be a process, not an event, and has been cited as a mark of nursing excellence.[14,15] According to Beyers,[16] research-based care is a form of advocacy that closes the gap between research, education, and practice. The nurse advocate champions for health, access to health care, and good use of resources.

Nurse as Manager of Care

The case management model of delivering patient care originated in response to the restrictions on the length of stay in hospitals and the amount of care during the stay allotted by the Diagnosis-Related Groups (DRG).[14,17] The model is outcome-based and is designed to maintain quality of care while streamlining costs. The nurse, as case manager, must be skilled in leadership and management and proficient in clinical skills. Beyers[16] states that effective nurses know how to design and manage services and are highly capable of forming and sustaining relationships. The nurse clinician who is the coordinator of the care provided by a multidisciplinary team is crucial to the outcome for the patient. Meeting a patient's emotional needs can also be cost-effective since failure to meet these needs may negatively affect the patient's adherence to the prescribed regimen and participation toward the desired outcome. Latini[18] describes in an article innovative critical pathways for trauma patients that have been designed by a transdisciplinary (multidisciplinary) team. Each pathway addresses the holistic patient care to be provided from prehospitalization to surgery and during critical care, rehabilitation, and home care. A 3-year evaluation has demonstrated the increased effectiveness in patient care, reduction of costs, patient satisfaction, and staff satisfaction. The vision of the American Association of Critical Care Nurses (AACN) is for nurses to work with other disciplines in a health care environment that is driven by the needs of patients and their families—an environment in which critical care nurses can make their optimal contribution in providing holistic care.[14]

SELF-CONCEPT

Some controversy exists among social scientists whether the construct of self-concept is unidimensional or multidimensional. Before 1980, much of the research was not theoretically based, and it was considered to be a global construct. The terms self-concept and self-esteem were often used synonymously. Since then, theoretical models have been used in the development of measurements, and the self-concept term is referred to as a broad definition that includes cognitive, affective, and behavioral aspects; whereas self-esteem is believed to be a narrower evaluative component of the broader term. Self-esteem is closely linked to one's sense of self-worth. Self-confidence; physical, intellectual, spiritual, and artistic selves; and self-roles in family and society are all considered as dimensions of the self-concept. However, many of the studies have relied on self-reports, and scientists have not been able to provide clear-cut definitions. Some scientists still prefer the global schema.[19]

The nursing discipline has chosen a multidimensional construct of self-concept that is useful for understanding individuals and their behavior (see Figure 5-1). Although self-concept is relatively stable, it can be modified. It influences how one reacts to and manages problems in daily life. A physical disfigurement may be more threatening to the adolescent who is seeking self-identity or be perceived as a greater detriment to a career or family role by a young adult than by a more mature individual.[4,9]

Three major subcomponents of the self-concept are discussed in this chapter: body image, self-esteem, and role performance. Alterations in self-concept may involve any or all of these interrelated components, and as previously mentioned, are dependent on multiple factors, including value of self-worth, interpersonal relationships, past experiences and achievements/failures, biochemical changes, and health status.

The self-concept is what one believes about oneself; the self-report is what one is willing to share about oneself. When assessing the self-concept of the critically ill patient, an understanding of the stages of illness and a person's behavioral responses is useful. The various stages of illness have been described by a number of scientists.[4,13,20,21] There is general agreement on three to four major stages. The initial, or impact stage, consists of the person experiencing symptoms; an interpretation of what they might mean; and an emotional response, such as fear or anxiety. The person may attempt some sort of self-care, consult family or another nonprofessional for advice, or contact a physician. The next stage consists of diagnosis and assumption of the dependent sick role that may be marked by denial, frustration, anger, increased anxiety, hostility, and passive behavior. On the other hand, the person may seek information and do everything possible to assist in recovery. Patients in critical care units usually do not have time to adjust to the illness and may exhibit signs of shock and numbness, avoid reality, and be unable to clearly understand the implications of the situation. The patient usually has been transferred to an intermediate unit before a true acknowledgment phase occurs. The final stage encompasses recovery or rehabilitation, transition to chronic illness, or death.

These stages are complex, highly individualized, and require adjustments in the self-concept, including changes in body image and interpersonal relationships and the limitations imposed by the person's condition. An individual with an acute problem, such as a heart attack, may panic if he or she believes that help will not arrive in time and may exhibit excessive demands or be suspicious of motives and methods of the caregivers. Depression and anxiety are common reactions as the person experiences a loss of control and worries over outcomes. During the illness acceptance stage, the individual may be preoccupied with symptoms and their treatment or be resistant to dependency on caregivers and express anger and resentment. In the convalescent stage, the person must relinquish the dependent role and, perhaps, make major changes in life-style and role performance. The disturbances of self-concept and their adaptations are examined individually in this chapter. It must be remembered, however, that although each subcomponent has unique characteristics, some characteristics are shared with several or all the other subcomponents.

Body Image Disturbance

Body image has received considerable attention in the nursing literature.[1,9,22-25] This body of knowledge forms the basis for interventions with patients experiencing the losses associated with altered body image. Body image is the mental picture an individual has of his or her body and its physical functioning at any given time. It is based on past and present perceptions and includes one's attitudes and feelings about one's body in appearance, build, health, performance ability, and gender-related concepts. The body image develops over time from internal sensation–postural changes, contact with persons and objects in the environment, emotional experiences, and fantasies.[4,5,19] Although the body image is a stable part of the self-concept, changes are influenced by cognitive growth and physical changes in the body.[26] Men and women may view body changes differently and may use differing coping mechanisms in adjusting to old age.[24] Stein,[27] Cross, and Markus[28] suggest that the ability to project possible images of self in the future that are highly desirable or feared can play a powerful role in motivating and regulating goal-directed behavior. A woman who has breast cancer may envision herself as a fortunate survivor after a mastectomy or may focus only on the disfigurement caused by the surgery and destruction of her feminine body image.

Changes to the body's appearance, structure, and/or function may be caused by disease, trauma, or surgery. Disturbances in body image arise when the person fails to perceive or adapt to the changes. A disturbance may have a biophysical, cognitive-perceptual, cultural, or spiritual basis. In some instances, the person may feel betrayed by the body, which no longer seems "normal." Such disturbances are manifested by verbal or nonverbal responses to the actual or perceived changes.[9] Some patients must extend their body image to incorporate environmental objects.[29] For example, the patient temporarily requiring assisted respirations must extend his or her body image to include the ventilator and its accessories. In this situation explanations to patient and family of the equipment being used and their purpose are helpful.

Exemplar: In addition to her burn pain, Nancy no longer has control of her breathing and cannot verbally communicate with her caregivers, thus increasing her anxiety. Explaining the purpose of the ventilator, continuing to monitor pain levels, and providing adequate analgesics and sedation are primary tasks at this time.

Another example is when a patient admitted to a surgical critical care unit after a traumatic amputation awakes to find his or her leg missing with no prior knowledge of the cause for the loss. Reliving the accident and receiving explanations about the need for the amputation are priorities for such a patient. Similar interventions are necessary after any disfiguring trauma or surgery, such as severe burns, a radical neck dissection, a mastectomy, or a colostomy. Body image may also be altered by the need to incorporate a prosthetic device or a donated body part.[1,30] The disease or problem may be corrected by surgery and treatments; however, whenever the result is visible to the patient and others, the change in body image can arouse intense feelings of anger, frustration, depression, and powerlessness.

The critical care nurse often begins the process of helping the patient live with this permanent alteration. Interventions by the nurse and others on the health team focus on helping the patient manage the physical changes and the psychosocial alterations. Helping the patient recognize, accept, and live with the resultant changes requires recognition that self-esteem and role performance may also be affected. The meaning of the alteration (appearance, structure, or function) varies with the individual. What is lost? What value is placed on it? What did the body part or function enable the person to enjoy or accomplish? What disability results? The values of the culture are important; wholeness, independence, and attractiveness are important in society today. The person's ability to cope, perception of the responses from others significant to him or her, and the help available to the individual and to the family are important factors in the outcome of body image disturbances.

Examplar: Nancy, the burn patient, faces several changes in body image. Scars, changes in skin texture, possible contractures, and altered function will all be sources for grieving the loss of physical beauty and will produce feelings of anger and depression. Fear of rejection by others may also occur if she perceives that others are appalled by her appearance.[1] When Nancy's parents, Mr. and Mrs. Morrison, arrive the nurse (or psychiatric nurse consultant) will help prepare them for the change in their daughter's appearance and condition before they come into the unit. (Family members may experience even more emotional strain than the patient and may not recognize that they, too, are in crisis.) The nurse will also gather more information on Nancy's personal history, coping abilities, and family interactions, when the time is appropriate. It is important for the parents, and for Nancy, that they be included as early as possible in planning her recovery.

Self-Esteem Disturbance

Self-esteem, or self-measurement of one's worth, develops as a part of self-concept through the reflected appraisals of significant others.[1,26] The way such information is interpreted is probably more important than is the content. Self-esteem is only partly related to material, economic, or social conditions. The need for self-esteem is a part of the hierarchy of human needs postulated by Maslow.[31] Having high self-esteem helps one deal with the environment and face more easily the maturational and situational crises of life. Overall, the goal is to maintain a high positive regard for oneself in the midst of everchanging views of oneself. This goal, when met, contributes to the quality of life of the individual. Persons with a well-developed self-esteem are at less risk for disturbances of self-esteem than those with poorly developed self-esteem.[32] Illness can rob a person of perspective and shrinks both the familiar world and the one of possibility, often leading to low self-esteem, powerlessness, helplessness, and depression.[9] A low self-regard impairs one's ability to adapt. The person may refuse to participate in self-care, exhibit self-destructive behavior, or be too compliant—asking no questions and permitting others to make all decisions.[1]

Self-esteem has been studied frequently in a variety of contexts and is an important concept for nurses who have a significant impact on ill patients.[1,14,26,29,31,33-36] When the illness is critical, a patient's self-esteem level may be imperiled. Perhaps the patient caused the accident that injured him or her and others, including family members; alcohol or drugs may have been a causal factor; or the person might be subject to arrest if he or she survives. Perhaps he or she will lose his or her job or be unable to return to his or her previous occupation.

Topics that make the nurse uncomfortable are frequently avoided. Patients and families can easily get the message not to discuss them. The nurse who expresses negative reactions to a patient, either openly or covertly, will reinforce a patient's low self-esteem. Attitudes of the caregiver can be misinterpreted as indifference. An aloof, insensitive, or superficial relationship with a patient who has acquired immunodeficiency syndrome

(AIDS), for example, can cause the patient to feel rejected, humiliated, and stigmatized.[37]

A person's self-image and self-esteem are strongly threatened when an ostomy is required for diversion of the intestinal or urinary tract. Many of the socially accepted values related to elimination needs have been instilled since childhood. The person fears the embarrassment of accidents, odors, and possible rejection by one's sexual partner. Resentment over the daily necessity to handle ostomy equipment and the change in life-style are constant reminders of the threat to self-image and self-esteem. An ostomy can also represent the loss of a body part and its prescribed function. The person may feel ashamed of his or her body.

The antecedents of self-esteem were the focus of Coopersmith's book.[38] He identified four major factors that contribute to the development of self-esteem: (1) the amount of acceptance and love from significant persons in one's life, (2) past successes and social position, (3) past reactions to devaluing situations, and (4) commitment to values and aspirations for oneself. Of special importance to the development of high self-esteem are three conditions: total or near-total acceptance of the child by the family; clearly defined limits that are reasonable, rational, and enforced; and respect and allowance for individual actions within the defined limits.

In old age a person faces loss of autonomy; losses related to changes in health status and sensory impairment (e.g., vision/hearing); loss of work role through retirement; and death of loved ones, all of which may lower self-esteem. Changes in the expectations of others for one's behavior and capacity may occur. If caregivers are impatient with performance deficits, the patient may feel inadequate and guilty. If patients are treated as children, they may believe themselves burdens and react with resentment. Failure to include them in decision making may cause them to feel useless and rejected. On the other hand, people with a strong sense of self-worth are likely to be adjusted, happy, and competent.[39,40] Defensive self-esteem is used to defend against the person's perception of a gap between his or her real self and ideal self. High self-esteem is associated with a low need for social approval, comfort with intimacy and self-disclosure, and the ability to acknowledge personal failures.

A person's level of self-esteem is an important factor in the response to a critical illness, and behavior during illness may be negatively affected by lowered self-esteem. Patients with severe burns may interpret the avoidance behavior of nurses and family who are appalled by their appearance and the odor in their room as a devaluation of themselves. They may refuse to cooperate with the treatment regimen and may judge themselves as failures and be unable to see a future that involves a return to a productive life. Anticipatory interventions that assist the staff and family members in their care of these patients would help to prevent such a situation. Nurses must communicate acceptance, genuine interest, and concern and avoid being judgmental.

Altered Role Performance

Interactions with others that create and modify roles are an important part of the self-concept. The roles one chooses reflect one's beliefs and feelings. Persons have primary, secondary, and tertiary roles. Primary roles are those associated with gender, age, and developmental stage. Secondary roles are those of daughter, sister, and so forth. Tertiary roles are those assumed by choice, such as scout leader or churchgoer. Illness, when it occurs, disrupts secondary and tertiary roles, and responses can be affected by primary role characteristics.

Role performance alterations are those problems that arise when a person experiences difficulties in making life transitions. Causative factors include lack of significant role models, inability to learn new roles because of life transitions, and cognitive-perceptual difficulties. See Box 5-2 for manifestations of altered role performance.[41]

Meleis[42,43] examined role theory from a nursing perspective and pointed out that nurses deal with persons who are experiencing transitions—that is, a change in role status. They may be completing a transition or about to begin one. Such transitions involve loss and addition to role relationships and may involve developmental, situational, or health-status–related events. Each of the types of transition can have implications for nursing practice. Examples include the teen-age girl who becomes pregnant (developmental), a young adult whose father dies (situational), and an older adult who experiences an acute onset of illness (health-illness event). All these transitions require changes in roles of the persons and families involved. The individuals concerned must incorporate new knowledge, alter behaviors, and change their self-concepts.

Nurses are often involved with situations that include alterations in role performance for individuals and families.[1,37,44] The rapid and potentially drastic changes that accompany critical illness may seriously

BOX 5-2 Manifestations of Altered Role Performance

- Change in self-perception of role
- Denial of role
- Change in other persons' perception of role
- Conflict in roles
- Change in physical capacity to resume role
- Lack of knowledge about role
- Change in usual patterns of responsibility

interfere with role relationships and expectations or abilities in role performance. The male patient after a myocardial infarction wonders about his roles as husband, breadwinner, and worker. If the patient is unable to resume previous roles, he may refuse to accept the new roles associated with the chronic cardiac condition. The psychosocial needs of the patient in such a situation depend on age, gender, occupation, family roles, previous experience with illness, suddenness of onset of illness, extent of illness, and prognosis.

For example, Mrs. B., age 23 years (para 1, gravida 1), is admitted to the medical critical care unit on her second postpartum day. She has pregnancy-induced hypertension complicated by the "HELLP syndrome," an acronym for *h*emolysis, *e*levated *l*iver enzymes, and a *l*ow *p*latelet count. Her baby boy, who was almost full-term, is doing well. The need for this admission means separation during the crucial first days of a new role. Her assumption of the mothering role is delayed. Photographs of the baby, brief visits so she can see him, and assurance that he is being well-cared for are important interventions to help her bridge this important transition. (For further discussion of critical care of high-risk pregnancy, see Chapter 10.)

The patient may be unable to meet the demands of the required role changes and thus experience role insufficiency.[42] The use of role supplementation is an approach nurses can use in such a situation. As described by Meleis,[42] this intervention involves both preventive and therapeutic efforts. By communicating and interacting with the patient and family, nurses may convey information or experiences that increase the awareness of the new roles and interrelationships necessary because of the role transition. In another example, role insufficiency may be displayed in behaviors that reflect fear of moving from the critical care unit to the intermediate care unit. A variety of nursing activities can anticipate and facilitate this transition.

Exemplar: Nancy faces many months of hospitalization and rehabilitation because of the severity of her burns. Her role as mother and wage-earner must be put aside, and other family members' roles will also be altered. Her mother has agreed to move into Nancy's home and care for the children so that they can remain in their familiar environment. Her father, who works in construction, will visit on weekends. Unfortunately, Nancy's job as a cashier in a grocery store may not remain open for an extended time period or she may not be physically capable of working. The children's roles will be affected as they adjust to the changes in their lives, as well. (Concerns about the role of the children's father are discussed in a later section.) Nancy and her family have many challenges before them.

POWERLESSNESS

Powerlessness as a nursing diagnosis is defined as the perception of the individual that one's own action will not significantly affect an outcome.[41] Unrelieved powerlessness may result in hopelessness, which is discussed in the next section.

The causes of powerlessness include factors in the health care environment, interpersonal interactions, one's cultural and religious beliefs, illness-related regimen, and a life-style of helplessness. A severe level of powerlessness may be manifested by a person's verbal expressions of having no control or influence over the situation, the eventual outcome, or over self-care. Powerlessness can also be manifested by depression over physical deterioration that occurs despite the patient's compliance with regimens, or by passivity and apathy. The range in levels of powerlessness varies and is dependent on the person's perceived control of situations, the amount of losses experienced, and the availability of social support. Powerlessness can be manifested by refusal to participate in self-care, delayed decision making or refusal to make decisions, and expressions of self-doubt in role performance. Frustration, anger, and resentment over the dependency on others often occurs with verbal expressions regarding dissatisfaction with care.

Most people expect to have the power to participate in making decisions that affect them. Both actual and perceived control over present or impending events are important.[45] When patients feel their choices are limited, they may act against their own best interests.[44,46-48] Given enough frustration, any exercise of control—even one with negative outcomes, such as signing out of the hospital against medical advice (AMA)—can become attractive.

Individuals vary in the amount of control they prefer. Important variables in this regard are the illness; values, traits, attitudes, and experiences; the hospital setting; and social displacement. Personality, age, religion, occupation, income, residence, and race may all be pertinent factors, also. Apparently there is an increase in variability in the amount of control preferred as people age.[24] The critical care unit routines may oppose or preclude any control by the patient. The person to whom control is important should be helped to continue to control as many areas of life as possible. On the other hand, a patient must be given the opportunity to choose not to control.[48]

Rotter's[47] research on human behavior and perception of control has been particularly helpful in explaining the variability of responses people have in similar situations. He proposed two major concepts—internal locus of control versus external locus of control. Individuals who have internal locus of control perceive themselves to be responsible for the outcome of events. Individuals with external locus of control believe their actions will have no effect on outcomes of a situation. The scale to measure internal/external locus of control developed by Rotter is useful in assessing this personality trait, which is a relatively stable tendency.

However, situations exist that can alter one's perception of control. A person with internal locus of control may experience a major illness such as a myocardial infarction or lung cancer even though major life-style changes had been made to avoid the illness. This experience forces that person to recognize that the illness could not be prevented simply by his or her own actions.

Another aspect of powerlessness is *learned helplessness*, or *excessive dependence*.[4,9] This occurs when a person who repeatedly experiences uncontrollable situations loses the motivation for making decisions about life events. Some people assume a martyr role and accept the illness state as their fate, thus doing nothing to improve their status. Others may find the sick role a gratifying means for gaining control over others by using their symptoms to receive attention.[13] Setting limits on these behaviors, encouraging independence and participation in self-care, counseling, and involving family members in establishing realistic goals are helpful strategies in assisting the person to abandon this manipulative behavior.

The patient's perception of control is affected by the interaction of the environment and limitations imposed by the disease process on the patient's physical and psychologic status. Critically ill patients generally experience a rapid onset of illness without time to acquire the illness role. A sense of powerlessness in such situations is not unexpected. If control is defined as the ability to determine the use of time, space, and resources, admission to a critical care unit strips away control of this power. Upon admission, persons lose their independent status; they become patients. Use of clothes and other personal belongings is usually restricted in a critical care unit. Patients cannot decide who enters the room, who provides personal care, or who intrudes with painful treatments. Hospital rules usually are not open to modification. Patients may feel anxious because they are separated from a familiar environment and have restrictions on visitors.

Poor interaction with the health care providers may make the situation worse. Patients may react aggressively, may try bargaining, or may refuse to comply with diagnostic and treatment regimens. They may resent the close scrutiny of the nurses and physicians and invasion of their privacy. They may fear death or permanent loss of function and may feel guilty if they have contributed to the cause of their illness or injury. By virtue of their experiences of critical illness and care, these patients may lose sight of areas of influence they do retain over themselves, because so much control is taken from them. Nursing emphasizes this intact influence on control and thus helps to preserve it.[45,49,50]

HOPELESSNESS

Hopelessness is a subjective state in which an individual sees limited or no alternatives or personal choices available and is unable to mobilize energy on his or her own behalf.[41] To help clarify this nursing diagnosis, a definition of hope is included—a feeling that provides comfort while enduring life threats and personal challenges and that what is wanted will happen; a desire that is accompanied by anticipation or expectation.[24,51,52] Most persons agree that an element of hope must be maintained no matter how hopeless things appear. Hope is a force that helps one survive. It is an attitude toward the future, and it occupies a key position between the present and future. The absence of hope is a serious situation.[24,52,53]

Causative factors related to hopelessness include (1) prolonged activity restriction, creating isolation; (2) a failing or deteriorating physiologic condition; (3) long-term stress; (4) abandonment; and (5) a lost belief in transcendent values or in God.[41]

Hopelessness is defined in terms of negative expectations concerning oneself and one's future life.[54] Motivation is lost; a decision is made not to want anything, to give up, and not to try to get something. The future seems dark, vague, and uncertain. Hope often arises in the presence of crisis, and instills vigorous resistance to giving up. The help of others in the situation supports the patient's belief. Caregivers who label hope-reflecting behavior in the critically or terminally ill patient as denial are less than helpful.[31,50] Hope wards off despair, mental anguish, disorganization, helplessness, and hopelessness.[55]

For example, a female patient with cancer who is receiving chemotherapy develops pneumonia and is placed on neutropenia precautions in the medical critical care unit. She may believe she has no chance of recovery, since she feels isolated from staff and family and believes that her body will not fight the infection successfully because the drugs for the cancer have lowered her ability to combat infection. She may despair and become desperate and despondent. What causes these feelings in critically ill patients? Why do they feel helpless? Their bodies have lost control or betrayed them. No longer do their physiologic mechanisms adapt to changes. They need external help.

Hopelessness can take control and immobilize the patient. The sense of impossibility can block attempts to change the situation. A system of negative expectancies about oneself and the future may result in a sense of overwhelming defeat. The hopeful person can imagine a future and that the storm will pass. The hopeless one gives up.

Exemplar: Feelings of powerlessness and hopelessness are inevitable throughout the long rehabilitation process for Nancy and her family. Being isolated from her usual surroundings and the need to relinquish her parenting role forces dependence on others. Her former husband, Bill, has shared custody of the children. He feels that he should take the children to his home, which is in another city; however, she does not believe his new wife will be good for the children, and she does not want their usual routine disrupted. She also fears that he will attempt to gain full custody of the children, claiming she is an "unsafe" mother. She feels helpless and powerless that her wishes may not be considered in the decision.

When individuals expect something to happen, they usually act in ways that increase the likelihood that the expectations will be met.[27] The expectation, whether positive or negative, becomes stronger the more times the "reinforcing circle" occurs.[56] This process is defined as a self-fulfilling prophecy. This idea is important in instances of hopelessness. Staff members may feel helpless when patients do not respond to their care; they may label patients as hopeless. Patients recognize this attitude and react to confirm this expectancy by giving up. Engel[57] identified the "giving up-given up" syndrome and included hopelessness as one component. Other components were a depreciated self-image; lack of gratification from roles and role relationships; interference with continuity of the past, present, and future; and reawakened painful memories.

Acutely ill persons are highly susceptible to such situations. Illness influences hopelessness by threatening internal resources (one's ability to cope) and external resources (one's perceptions of who can help). A patient's autonomy, self-esteem, independence, strength, and integrity may be at risk.

The critically ill patient is a multiproblem patient. Nurses and physicians are tempted to focus on the crisis and use of technical equipment and overlook the patient in his or her totality. The health care team may stereotype patients and underestimate their individual strengths.[9] The very nature of the critical care unit is frightening and increases the patient's sense of vulnerability and the fear of death.

The patient's degree of hopelessness is related to the perception and duration of his or her powerlessness. Thus feelings of hopelessness are not uncommon in critical care units. It is therefore important to foster a realistic sense of hope.[55,58] Science has progressed and can accomplish many things. Even if long-term survival is not likely, patients can be helped to plan to live the remaining life to the fullest. The critical care nurse can project an attitude of hope and identify some aspect of the situation in which hope is warranted, no matter how grave the situation, and attempt to channel feelings toward some positive outcome.

Families also need hope. To have hope has been identified in a number of studies as the most important need of families of critically ill patients.[12,59-61]

Miller[62] proposes a model of nursing strategies to inspire hope in families, believing that if family hope is developed and maintained, the patient's hope will be developed and maintained. See Box 5-3 for Miller's model of hope-inspiring strategies that can assist families in crisis situations.[63]

BOX 5-3 Strategies to Inspire Hope in Families of Critically Ill Patients

Hope-inspiring strategies include activities that assist families to accomplish the following:
- Maintain caring relationships
- Clarify distorted thinking
- Provide opportunities to be with the patient
- Decrease uncertainty
- Increase patient comfort and well-being
- Project feelings of hope
- Avoid unrealistic expectations
- Consider spiritual needs
- Decrease environmental hazards
- Explore the meaning of the crisis
- Use social support
- Consider the use of humor
- Support unique modes of personal comfort
- Expand the coping repertoire of the family

Adapted from Miller JF: *AACN Clin Issues in Crit Care Nurs* 2(2):307, 1991.

MENTAL STATUS CHANGES REQUIRING MEDICAL EVALUATION

Two medical diagnoses are associated with mental status changes that should be distinguished from ineffective coping. These clinical states, delirium and major depression, call for a medical and/or nurse specialist psychiatric evaluation and medical intervention.

Acute Confusion

Acute confusion, which encompasses global cognitive impairment, has not been clearly or consistently defined.[63] Synonyms include delirium (the medical term), critical care unit psychosis, postcardiotomy delirium, and acute brain failure.[40] Additional terms are acute mental status change, acute organic reaction, metabolic encephalopathy, and reversible cognitive dysfunction. There is loss of orientation to person, time, or place and the ability to reason, follow directions, process incoming stimuli, or maintain concentration.[64] Confused persons may be aware of these disturbances and fear that they are "losing their minds." The confused state is a secondary response to organic causes (e.g., hypoxia, drugs, or fluid and electrolyte imbalances) or to inorganic causes (e.g., stress or sleep deprivation). Onset is abrupt, and duration can be shortened if early diagnosis and treatment are initiated. It is estimated that confusion develops in 50% of hospitalized elderly patients; however, it is often misdiagnosed because of inaccurate assessment and assumptions that a mental deterioration is a result of the effects of aging.[40,61] More than 80% of confused statuses for the elderly are attributed to organic causes. Behavioral symptoms may be subtle and varied. Prodromal symptoms include insomnia, distractibility, drowsiness, anxiety, and nightmares. Symptoms of acute confusion resemble those of dementia, which makes differentiation between the two conditions more difficult. However, dementia, which cannot be reversed, has a gradual onset and is of long duration.

Approximately 10% to 15% of all hospitalized medical-surgical patients experience symptoms of acute confusion. This percentage is increased by 30% to 40% in the critical care setting. Hospital stays are prolonged for this population, with the average increase in stay 13 days.[63] An increased level of confusion may be the first indicator of a biologic problem or it may be a result of environmental stressors. The nurse must continually assess cognitive function. Several tools are available. The Mini-Mental State Examination (MMSE) developed by Folstein in 1988 is the most popular and easy to administer.[65] Items included on the examination relate to orientation, comprehension, recall, and following command.[65] (The full mental status examination is discussed in the assessment section later in this chapter.)

Etiology. There are many causes or contributors to acute confusion, which can occur for anyone at any given time. Three predisposing contributors to development of acute confusion are age 60 years or older; presence of brain damage; and presence of a chronic brain disorder, such as Alzheimer's.[63] Cognitive dysfunctions are believed to occur when "there is a widespread reduction of cerebral oxidative metabolism and an imbalance of neurotransmission."[63]

Drugs that are commonly used in the critical care unit are contributing factors to acute confusion. Some of these are digitalis, antibiotics, steroids, beta-blockers, and respiratory stimulants. Additional causes include sleep deprivation, sensory underload or overload, and immobilization, which are all common events encountered in the critical care unit.

The patient in the critical care unit is robbed of the restorative benefits of deep sleep and the rapid eye movement (REM) phase because of frequent interruptions by equipment noises, voices, and procedures. Constant bright overhead lights, the absence of day-night cycles, immobility, pain, and medications contribute to the patient's disorientation to time and place. Daytime napping, complaints of fatigue, slurred speech, depression, cognitive impairment, and hallucinations can result. Delayed recovery, increased length of stay, and the seriousness of sleep deprivation are closely related.[21] A number of hospitals across the nation have introduced physical changes in the environment of the critical care unit to reduce noise levels (e.g., installation of acoustic tiles, carpets, and private rooms). Team members have also suggested several corrective measures to keep noise levels to a minimum, such as scheduling procedures to avoid waking the patient as infrequently as possible, lowering lighting at intervals, and holding conversations/shift reports away from the patient's hearing distance.[12] The introduction of distraction measures such as soft music in the critical care unit has also served as a means for orienting individuals, as a stimulus, and as a calming effect.[66] (Refer to Chapter 6 for further discussion on sleep.)

The literature reports more than 30 separate terms for the confusion syndrome.[63] Many of the terms are misleading, are narrow in scope, and give cause for overlooking all possible reasons for the behaviors. "The classification of mental disorders of the *Diagnostic and Statistical Manual (DSM-IV)* utilizes the term *delirium* as the only official designation for this syndrome and has established specific criteria to be used for diagnosis."[65,67] (See the Nursing Management Plan for acute confusion at the end of the chapter.)

Assessment. Three forms of acute confusion have been identified: hyperactive, hypoactive, and a mixture of both forms.[40,63] The patient with the hyperactive form may remove intravenous lines, dressings, and catheters; be extremely restless and try to get out of bed; pick at things in the air; and call out to persons who are not there. Sympathetic nervous system responses of tachycardia, dilation of pupils, diaphoresis, and facial flushing are evident. In the hypoactive form, persons complain of extreme fatigue, are slow to respond, and have hypersomnolence that can progress to loss of consciousness. At times, these individuals are absorbed in a dreamlike state, mumble to themselves, experience vivid hallucinations, and make inappropriate gestures. The third form is a mixture of agitation and hypoactive behaviors that can vary throughout the day. Symptoms and hallucinations seem to worsen during nighttime hours, with more lucid intervals occurring during the day.

The mental status examination. The mental status examination is a full, criteria-based assessment of the patient's cognitive function and thought processes. Although the examination is rarely conducted in its entirety in the critical care setting, knowledge of its main components will enhance the nurse's effectiveness in collecting data to document findings using accepted terminology and to identify issues that need further assessment. The tool can be useful in evaluating the nursing diagnoses of "Knowledge Deficit," "Sensory-Perceptual Alterations," and "Altered Thought Processes."

Components of the mental status examination. The following discussion is organized around theoretical concepts presented by Barry.[1] Also, see Box 5-4 for categories of measurement.

Orientation and level of awareness. A common measurement for evidence of confusion is asking patients whether they know who they are and where they are, as well as having them state the day of the week, month, and year. Many times, mild to moderate confusion can actually be masked by patients who appear oriented.

Appearance and behavior. General observations include the patient's appearance and behaviors in terms of his or her consistency with a normal range in age and station in life, general health, and nutritional status. Recording this information supplies a basis for later comparison data should there be a change in the patient's condition.

Speech and communication. Speech may be garbled, slurred, distinct, rapid, or slow. Nonverbal communication such as eye contact, gestures, and posture are indicators of the patient's mood and thought formation, and the content of the intended message. It is important to evaluate the match between verbal and nonverbal communication patterns.

Mood/affect. The patient may seem normal in communication with caregivers and family, or there may be wide swings in emotions. Anxiety, fear, depression, or apathy may be apparent through verbal expressions or behaviors.

Thinking process. Disturbances in thought processes may be indicated by illogical statements, rapid speaking with quick shifts from one idea to another (flight of ideas), disconnected mixture of unrelated words (word salad), delusions, hallucinations, or obsessive behavior. Memory impairment may be masked by the patient unconsciously filling the gaps of memory with untrue statements, or "little white lies."

Memory. Recent memory is the first to be impaired and is most often seen in persons with a chronic

BOX 5-4 The Mental Status Examination

GENERAL OBSERVATIONS

- Appearance
- Reaction to interviewer
- Behavior and psychomotor activity

SENSORIUM AND INTELLIGENCE

- Level of consciousness
- Orientation
- Memory
- Intellectual function
- Judgment
- Comprehension

THOUGHT PROCESSES

- Form of thought
- Content of thought
- Mood
- Affect
- Insight

organic mental disorder (which is irreversible) in acute organic mental disorders, and in persons with depression when cognitive abilities are temporarily slowed. Recent memory refers to recall of events that have occurred during the immediate past and up to 1 or 2 previous weeks. Recent memory is assessed by asking the orientation questions related to person, time, and place. Long-term memory is assessed by asking individuals to describe events of their childhood. Long-term memory need not be affected by a deficit in recent memory. Questions can be asked conversationally without causing patients to feel they are being "cross-examined."

Perception. Perception of self, environment, and relationships with others is derived through the senses of vision, hearing, touch, and smell. Defense mechanisms during times of stress or illness can distort perceptions of a person's reality. The major type of perceptual distortion for hospitalized or critical care patients is hallucinations. These can be visual (picking at objects in the air, which may be perceived as insects); auditory (hearing voices, bells, or other sounds that are nonexistent); or tactile (feeling objects or sensations that are not evident). A hypnagogic hallucination is a type of false sensory perception that occurs during the twilight period between wake and sleep. This can be a common occurrence in well persons, especially during times of severe stress or fatigue.

An illusion is a distortion in perception of an actual stimulus. For example, a critical care patient may view the intravenous tubing as a snake crawling up his or her arm. Depersonalization and derealization are two perceptual dysfunctions in which the person feels a detachment from oneself and has a sense of unreality about the environment. Again, these are common manifestations in persons under extreme stress or fatigue.

Abstract thinking and judgment. A person with abstract thinking ability is able to reach a conclusion from a logical reasoning process. A person who thinks concretely interprets what is seen and heard exactly as they are sensed. A change to concrete thinking by a person who normally thinks in an abstract manner may be an indication of an organic mental dysfunction. Judgment has been defined as a "person's ability to behave in a socially appropriate manner." A person's judgment may be assessed by requesting that person to provide a solution to a hypothetical problem. For example, "What would you do if you found an expensive watch in a public restroom?" A hospitalized person's social judgment can be observed informally during interactions with staff, family, and other patients.

Assessment of suicide potential. Depression and hopelessness are common precursors to suicidal ideation. Caregivers are often reticent to question a person about suicide intent for fear of introducing the idea. However, *suicidal ideation stems from hopelessness and not from suggestion.* Most patients find the thoughts of wishing to die to be distressing and are ashamed to admit them. Questioning can relieve their concerns, because they can feel that staff are sensitive to their feelings.

Medical and nursing management of mental status changes. Sedation is prescribed for patients with hyperactive delirium. Neuroleptic drugs such as haloperidol, droperidol, and chlorpromazine commonly used for neurotic and personality disorders are also useful in the treatment of delirium. Currently, haloperidol is considered to be the drug of choice, and a regular dosing schedule is preferred rather than waiting until symptoms reoccur. A combination of haloperidol and lorazepam, a benzodiazepine drug, allows lower doses of each drug to be given, is very effective, and produces fewer side effects. When delirium is considered to be secondary to pain, narcotics can be administered. However, the paradoxic effects of depressed respirations and cardiac output can exacerbate the delirium. The use of barbiturates is no longer recommended as routine treatment, but they are used in the treatment of barbiturate withdrawal–induced delirium. Finally, neuromuscular blocking agents are sometimes used for severely agitated patients who are receiving mechanical ventilation; these agents decrease oxygen consumption, promote synchrony with the ventilator, and increase tissue oxygenation. These complex drugs can be dangerous and do not affect consciousness, cognition, or pain levels, thus necessitating the addition of sedatives or analgesics.[63]

Understanding the causes and symptoms of acute confusion, knowing the characteristics of persons at risk for developing acute confusion, and using appropriate measures to minimize causal factors are primary aspects of the critical care nurse role. Reducing noise levels and sensory overload, providing appropriate sensory stimulation (such as background music), promoting sleep and rest times, and permitting liberal visitation with family and significant others are appropriate interventions, especially in the critical care unit. Ongoing assessment of the patient's behavior and subtle biologic changes are of prime importance. A full bladder, pain, or medication side effects can cause agitation. Monitoring and correcting fluid and electrolyte levels, nutritional needs, oxygenation, and bowel and bladder function are all major tasks of the critical care nurse role. These factors can be potential causes of delirium, and delirium can contribute to deficiencies in these areas.

Providing safety measures is also of prime importance. The risk of falls and injuries can be minimized by using siderails, lowering the bed position, placing motion alarms on beds, observing the patient closely, and removing harmful objects. The use of restraints can add to the person's agitation and must be used only when necessary to protect the patient from harming self or others. A better solution is to have someone sit with the patient. Family members can be used for this purpose whenever possible, because their presence can have a calming effect. The family may be frightened as they observe their loved one's behavior. The nurse must assure them that the patient's condition is temporary. The use of touch; a calm, unhurried manner; and therapeutic communication are useful tools as the nurse interacts with delirious patients and their families. (Refer to the Nursing Management Plan on acute confusion at the end of this chapter.)

Major Depressive Episode

A major depressive episode is a mood disorder of at least 2 weeks' duration, characterized by depressed mood, diminished interest or pleasure in usual activities, insomnia, poor appetite, psychomotor retardation or agitation, and loss of energy. Patients will also report feelings of hopelessness, worthlessness, and guilt. Recurrent thoughts of death, loss of interest in life, and recurrent suicidal ideation may be present.[67]

A major depressive episode is not a natural consequence of a major medical illness. It is a psychiatric disorder that may complicate the patient's course. Apathy and hopelessness may lead the patient to refuse essential medical and nursing management.[68] Major depression may also complicate the underlying medical illness. Depressed patients have been shown to have a significantly higher mortality from cardiovascular disease than the nondepressed population.

The nurse who suspects that the patient is depressed can ask about the patient's thought content (see the section on assessment of mental status earlier in this chapter). If expressions of hopelessness, worthlessness, guilt, or suicidal ideation accompany a depressed mood, a psychiatric evaluation is indicated. Management generally consists of antidepressant medications. Unfortunately, a therapeutic effect is not seen until several weeks after therapeutic blood levels have been reached. Stimulants such as methylphenidate (Ritalin) may also be used for their antidepressant effect in the medically ill patient. Benzodiazepines are occasionally prescribed to treat the associated anxiety, if present. Antipsychotic medication is prescribed if the patient's depression has psychotic features.

The nurse can listen empathetically and convey that recovery from the depression is expected while realizing that the patient's depression cannot be overcome by cheerfulness or reassurance. If the patient is on suicide precautions, the nurse safeguards according to department policy and procedure, and alerts all on the health care team and the family. The nurse also informs the patient that precautions are being taken to safeguard the patient until his or her mood improves.

Exemplar: Depression is a common reaction to severe burns, because of the prolonged and painful rehabilitation period and possible disfiguring burns, especially of the face, neck, chest, arms, or hands.[5] Over the course of her hospitalization, Nancy has experienced severe depression and has expressed that she wished she had died in the fire. Because of the many psychosocial issues and their effects on Nancy, her family, and her caregivers, a psychiatric consultant is recommended to become an active participant on the health care team.

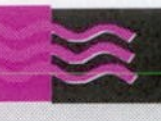

RESEARCH ABSTRACT

Definition and management of anxiety, agitation, and confusion.

Grossman S and others: *Nursing Connections* 9(2):49, 1996.

PURPOSE

Three research questions were the basis for this study: (1) What subjective and objective data do nurses collect to help them determine how to manage sedation needs? (2) What actions are most commonly used and in what order for managing sedation needs? (3) What outcomes of these actions are most often observed?

DESIGN

Prospective, descriptive.

SAMPLE

Twenty-seven medical intensive care unit (MICU) nurses volunteered to complete questionnaires about their process for assessing patients' sedation needs, formulating interventions, and evaluating patient outcomes. The average age of the nurses was 29 years, with 6 years of nursing experience; educational background varied. The surveys took into account 55 patients who had medical diagnoses typical of a MICU population. Patient age ranged from 22 to 84 years.

PROCEDURE

A Sedation Assessment Tool, consisting of open-ended questions, was developed by the investigators, pilot-tested, and refined before the data collection period. Data were collected during a 3-month period. Patients in the study were coded so that duplicate data collection would not take place; only one assessment per patient was included in the study. Investigators used content analysis to analyze data and determined their interrater reliability to be .89.

RESULTS

More objective data than subjective data were identified for each behavior category. The most commonly identified nursing actions were assessment to differentiate between pain, anxiety, agitation, and confusion; personal reassurances; relaxation and other comfort measures; administration of prescribed medications; collaboration with the physician to identify cause; and administration of additional medication. Outcome goals identified as effective were stable vital signs, normal oxygen saturation, progression with ventilator weaning, return to baseline level of orientation, and a quiet and arousable state.

DISCUSSION/IMPLICATIONS

Through this study, definitions of anxiety, agitation, and confusion were identified by the nursing staff of the MICU. By having a framework with commonly understood definitions, more consistent assessment and interventions can be done for this patient population. Since the majority of patients were intubated, objective data were used more often for assessing and planning interventions. Since this study used a small sample size and was specific to one patient population, findings cannot be generalized outside of this setting. Similar assessments could be done in other settings. In addition, further research could explore the relationship of the assessments, interventions, and outcomes.

Patients requiring critical care must cope with a variety of stressors (see Box 5-1). As mentioned earlier, each patient's response to these stressors is unique and depends on a variety of environmental factors and individual differences. The nurse's knowledge of assessment, diagnosis, and intervention in effective coping will also affect how well the patient copes.

Several theories of coping are presented here. According to White,[69] coping is an adaption strategy. People use coping when faced with serious problems that they cannot master with familiar behaviors. Uncomfortable affects such as anxiety or grief can accompany coping.

Lazarus and Folkman[6] define coping as a dynamic process involving cognitive and behavioral efforts to manage specific internal and/or external demands that are perceived to be exceeding the person's resources. Aguilera[70] states that coping activities encompass all the diverse behaviors that people use to meet actual or potential demands. The available coping mechanisms are those behaviors that a person draws upon that have been found to be effective in the past.

Weissman sees coping as a problem-solving process that draws on cognition, judgment, memory, and defense mechanisms.[71] He describes a variety of coping skills that people tend to use, including the steps for problem solving, the defense mechanisms, interpersonal strategies such as sharing concerns, and conscious coping mechanisms including distraction or laughing off a problem. Weissman emphasizes that no one strategy is superior. The key to effective coping is using the best strategy or mix of strategies in a given situation.[71]

NANDA[72] defines Ineffective Individual Coping as "the impairment of adaptive behaviors and problem-solving abilities of a person meeting life's demands and roles." The defining characteristics of Ineffective Individual Coping usually associated with critical illness include the following: the verbalization of inability to cope or to ask for help and being unable to meet personal basic needs. The person exhibits inappropriate use of defense mechanisms, is unable to problem solve, and may display destructive behavior to self and others.

Coping Mechanisms

When a patient copes effectively, what he or she is doing to cope often goes unnoticed. Emotionally the patient seems relatively comfortable, is a cooperative recipient of care, and exhibits nonproblematic behavior. The patient may be using multiple appropriate coping mechanisms that help manage a problem or stressful situation. The following discussion covers several coping mechanisms that may or may not be effective, depending on the degree that they are used. Some authors differentiate coping mechanisms that relate to adjusting, adapting, and successfully meeting a challenge from defense mechanisms that are automatic self-protective measures that develop in response to an internal or external stressor.[1] Examples of the latter include denial, acting-out behavior, avoidance, hypochondriasis, passive-aggressive behavior, and projection. The exemplar of Nancy Donovan, the burn patient, continues in the following comments.

Regression. *Regression* is an unconscious defense mechanism that involves a retreat, in the face of stress, to behavior characteristic of an earlier developmental level.[54] Regression allows the patient to give up his or her usual role, autonomy, and privacy to become the passive recipient of medical and nursing management. In fact, the patient who does not regress jeopardizes his or her own care. For example, John Bryan may insist on conducting business from the bedside or demand bathroom privileges when getting out of bed would be unsafe. Conversely, the patient who becomes too regressed presents another problem. Regression is a normal reaction to severe burns. Nancy Donovan may become childlike in interactions with staff, whine, cling to staff, and attempt to keep the nurse at the bedside constantly. In both cases, the patient requires the setting of limits on behavior to receive essential care. The patient is best served when limits are set in a supportive manner.

Although the behavior of these patients can provoke confrontations or reprimands, these responses must be avoided. Such responses from staff may only worsen a situation in which a patient is already struggling with issues of dependence and autonomy.

Suppression. *Suppression* is a conscious, intentional process in which patients push ideas, problems, or desires out of their conscious thoughts.[54] Patients often use suppression when their problems are overwhelming and they are in no position to resolve them. Weissman describes strategic suppression as a conscious attempt to focus only on the problems patients can solve in the present.[1] For example, before the accident, Nancy had been struggling to make her house payments on time, but now she uses suppression to postpone worry over losing the home until she is further along in recovery.

Denial. According to NANDA, *denial* includes both conscious and unconscious attempts to disavow knowledge or the meaning of an event.[72] In this text, the psychoanalytic definition of denial, "an unconscious defense mechanism that reduces anxiety by eliminating or reducing the seriousness of the perceived threat," is used to allow for the distinction between denial and suppression. When used by a critically ill patient, denial reduces the anxiety and the threat of the illness.[9] The degree to which denial is used varies among patients and may vary in the same patient at different times.

Patients may also deny different aspects of the illness. Some deny the probable medical significance of symptoms, as in the case of the 55-year-old cardiologist who interprets severe substernal chest pain as indigestion or the quadriplegic who cheerfully insists he will be back on his feet in no time. Other patients are unable to recognize signs of illness that are obvious to others, as in the case of the patient who cannot "see" the gangrenous foot requiring amputation.[4]

Other persons cannot readily influence the beliefs of a patient using denial. For example, the patient who is denying a myocardial infarction (MI) is not convinced of its occurrence by being shown the cardiogram interpretation or laboratory reports. The patient is best served by the nurse who recognizes the need for denial at the present time but who observes for cues that indicate readiness to accept the reality of the medical diagnosis. (Nancy may refuse to look at her body, avoid mirrors, and fear rejection by others because of her appearance. Forcing her to look at herself before she is ready can be extremely detrimental.)

Trust. *Trust* manifests itself in the critical care patient as the belief that the staff will get him or her through the illness, managing any untoward event that might occur. Trust is an unconscious process in which the patient transfers the trust learned in early significant relationships onto caregivers in the present.[13] For example, Nancy must learn to trust her caregivers. Her intense fear of pain or of falling when being moved from a stretcher to the Hubbard tank can affect other coping skills, as well.

Hope. Although hope has long been recognized as a significant factor in patient recovery and survival, the phenomenon receives little attention until the patient becomes hopeless. *Hope* is the expectation that a desire will be fulfilled. It can exist even in the face of a realistic appraisal of a grim situation.[58] Hope supports the patient and helps him or her endure the physical and psychologic insults that are a part of the daily experience.

Religious beliefs and practices. Religious beliefs and practices may provide the patient with some measure of acceptance of an illness, a sense of mastery and control, a source of hope and trust beyond the limits the staff can provide, and the strength to endure the current stress. A patient may discuss religious beliefs and concerns openly or view the subject as a private and personal matter. Patients who rely on religious beliefs benefit from the nurse who is accepting and respectful of those beliefs and who remains sensitive to the patient's willingness or reluctance to discuss those beliefs.[15,73,74]

Use of family support. The patient can use the presence of a supportive family to cope with critical illness. The patient with a supportive family knows that family members share a past and hope for a future with the patient. They love the patient as a person and member of the family. The patient also realizes that family members know him or her in ways the staff cannot. With them, the patient may know that his or her experience is truly understood, even when little is said. Family members can also be involved in the patient's personal care and attend to the practical problems the patient cannot, such as managing finances.[75]

Sharing concerns. Sharing concerns with a caring and understanding listener can relieve some of the patient's emotional distress. The patient is consoled knowing that he or she is not alone and that someone knows and cares about what is being experienced (as mentioned earlier with suicidal ideation).[1] The patient may share concerns with family members. On the other hand, the patient may be reluctant to upset loved ones further or may have a family in which such communication is not the norm. A patient who relies on this coping mechanism will benefit from a nurse who recognizes when a patient needs to talk and who knows how to listen.

Coping Assessment

Ineffective coping may be suggested in patient behaviors. Overt hostility, severe regression, or noncompliance with treatment may suggest ineffective coping. The patient may also report problems such as severe anxiety or despondence. The nurse who suspects that coping is ineffective needs to review the patient's medical history, mental status, and associated psychosocial factors.

It is not always clear whether coping is truly ineffective or whether intervention is indicated. Witnessing problematic behavior can be very uncomfortable, especially when that behavior is directed at the caregiver(s). Careful evaluation of one's reaction to the behavior is needed to discover whether patient care can continue to be provided objectively, or whether consultation with others on the team is needed to alleviate the problem.[1]

Coping Enhancement

Although the delivery of physical care is essential for patient survival and recovery, "caring for patients' psychological and social needs can be one of the most challenging aspects of nursing."[1] Several essential techniques for effective interventions include having an attitude of caring, openness and warmth and withholding judgment until you "know" the patient—have an understanding of the individual's perception about self—the current illness or problem, and the type of social support available. Assessment skills are essential, as well as a willingness to become involved when there is the potential or actual use of ineffective coping mechanisms.

Teaching the patient new coping skills may be an impossibility, since individuals have a repertoire of defense and coping mechanisms—conscious and unconscious—that are brought into play when facing stressful situations. A person who is experiencing extreme psychologic stress cannot learn new methods to manage these defense mechanisms. However, the nurse may help to reduce the level of anxiety by active listening, by encouraging support from family members and other caregivers, and by introducing changes in the environment, as appropriate. In doing so, the nurse can facilitate the changes the patient must make. It is extremely important that the patient recognize a personal need for help.[1]

A patient's trust in the nurse's competence in the physical and technical aspects of care aids in the patient's participation. Hope is instilled when the nurse and other caregivers display a sense of optimism regarding the patient's progress. It is essential that patients receive honest feedback, for patients are keen observers of their caregivers, and they read them well. Trust and hope are easily lessened when inappropriate information is given.

Supporting family members. Patient-centered care is also family-centered care. Consideration of nonbiologic or nonlegal partners of the patient as members of the patient's support system is also necessary in providing holistic care. The nurse's support of family members at the bedside can enhance the value of the visits for the patient. Patients often look to the family for love, understanding, support, and care of matters to which they cannot attend themselves. Although the nurse cannot perform full family assessment and give ongoing support to all family members, the critical care nurse can observe the quality of the patient-family interaction and formulate interventions that will aid the family in supporting the patient.[11,60,76-78]

As mentioned earlier, an illness of a family member can be a hardship on the total family. The illness (or death) of a patient can affect the health of other family members—particularly an elderly spouse.[79,80] Reactions to the stress are similar to the emotions experienced by the patient. The extended waiting time between visits with the patient; lack of information or misinterpretation of information; disruption in family roles and routines; being in an unfamiliar and challenging environment; and worry over outcomes, finances, and additional responsibilities can be overwhelming. Disorganization and emotional turmoil may result. Sleep deprivation is a common experience, leading to confusion and inability to make decisions.

Family members may also react to the crisis with expressions of anger and hostility toward the patient or staff, or be immobilized.[81] The family member may be at a loss for what to say or do during visits with the patient. The nurse might find some words to put the family member at ease and offer a suggestion for what to say to his or her loved one. For example, the nurse who observes a family member staring helplessly at an intubated, confused patient might say, "You can take his hand and tell him you are here."

If the family member is so upset that he or she completely loses composure, a brief attempt at supporting this family member away from the bedside may be adequate. In doing so, the nurse may determine that the family member needs the assistance of a consistent outside source of support and consult with other members of the health care team, such as a psychiatric nurse consultant, pastor/chaplain, or social worker.

Family members need understanding, respect, and emotional support. A recent study of patients' perspectives on health care revealed that their definition of patient-centered care included early involvement of their families in their care and decision making; support; accommodation/respect for their family and friends; and accurate, updated information.[11]

Families must frequently deal with the impending death of a loved one when there is deterioration in the patient's condition in spite of all efforts. Anticipatory grief is a process that is filled with emotional upheaval that can be as intense as when the loved one actually dies.[79,80] At this time, they are particularly sensitive to the nurse's words and actions, and may misinterpret them as signs of indifference. This may be particularly true for the nontraditional family members. It is essential that the health care team convey understanding and acceptance of the patient and his or her family. Some of the interventions that are meaningful to the family are reassuring them that the patient is receiving adequate pain medication, telling them what to expect as the dying process progresses, and helping them to comfort the patient with their presence. After the death, allow the family members to spend some time alone with the patient, be supportive of them as they work through their grief. Recognition of cultural and religious factors and incorporating them into the plan of care are also beneficial.

In Warren's[61] study of the perceptions of nurses' caring behaviors by families of critically ill patients, the following were identified: the nurse oriented them to the unit; informed the family about the patient's condition and what to expect; and encouraged them to ask questions. The nurse listened to their stories about the patient and enhanced the spirit of the family. They were treated as individuals, and a sense of bonding took place. The nurse used touch, comforted them, showed compassion, nurtured, and had an intuitive knowledge of subtle changes in the patient's condition.

Supporting spiritual care. Spiritual distress has been defined as the disruption in the life principle that pervades a person's entire being and that integrates and transcends one's biologic and psychosocial nature.[41] Separation from religious rituals and ties and intense suffering can induce spiritual distress for patients and their families. Probing questions such as, "How can a caring God let this happen?" or, "Why me?" or, "Am I being punished for some wrong that I have done?" are common indicators of spiritual distress. Some individuals may question their very existence and may even display anger toward religious representatives. Others may accept their illness as fate or just punishment, and resist help, give up, and wait to die.

Religious practices can directly affect caregiving practices such as diet; hygiene; and rituals surrounding birth, death, and medical interventions. The nurse needs to have a basic understanding of the various religious tenets of Eastern and Western philosophies and how they may affect a patient's plan of care.[82]

Patients easily succumb to feelings of helplessness and powerlessness in the technologic impersonalized environment of the critical care unit. Including a pastor or chaplain on the health care team is also an important aspect of holistic care. The chaplain may be the best person to assess spiritual needs and to assist patients and their families with coping with the crisis. Providing access to religious rituals, prayer, and scriptures are meaningful strategies in alleviating stress. The patient, with the help of the chaplain or pastor, can identify inner resources of strength, meaning, and purpose for the crisis event. The religious leader is also a valuable asset in ethical decisions such as termination of life support and can be of great assistance to health care team members as their personal resources are drained from the sustained or cumulative assistance of others in crisis.[83]

Spiritual health has been found to be associated with hardiness, a composite measure composed of commitment, challenge, a sense of control, and a mark of psychologic health.[83] Spiritual well-being can also refer to one's valuing of goodness, love and relatedness to others, or a general feeling of having a purposeful and fulfilled life. A study of 100 participants with diagnoses of human immunodeficiency virus (HIV), acquired immunodeficiency syndrome (AIDS), or AIDS-related complex (ARC) indicated that those who found meaning and purpose in life were hardier and survived longer. Coping techniques included prayer, visualization, meditation, attendance at church and spiritual retreats, and reading religious literature. Participants represented a variety of faiths including Catholic, Protestant, and Jewish denominations.[83]

A case study related to the several psychosocial alterations of the burn patient is included at the end of this chapter.

CARE OF SPECIFIC POPULATIONS

Chronically-Ill Persons in the Critical Care Unit

According to White and others[75] there are 110 million people in the United States who have one or more chronic diseases. These conditions have a direct effect on a successful outcome of a critical illness incident. The typical length of stay in the critical care unit is 2 or 3 to 4 days; however, this time may be extended for 1 or more weeks for a chronically ill patient who becomes acutely ill.[84] Usually, this type of patient is older and has multiple system problems such as cardiac, respiratory, and renal disturbances as well as nutritional deficits—diminished reserves resulting from the prolonged stress of coping with the primary problem. These individuals are at risk for developing episodes of mental confusion or delirium. They frequently have difficulty adjusting to the critical care environment, isolation from family, and reactions to medications. Sensory deficits in hearing and vision may also complicate their course of recovery. Whenever possible, these patients must be allowed to have their hearing aids and glasses.

Care of these patients can be very costly, and approximately fewer than 50% live to be discharged. Two recent and similar longitudinal studies[84,85] compared the effects of care provided for critically chronically ill patients in traditional critical care units and in low technology special care units (SCUs). Outcomes of complications, length of stay, costs, recovery and survival rates, and patient/family satisfaction were examined. Patients were carefully selected for placement in the two groups. The average age of the participants was 64 years, and respiratory and cardiac illness were the common chronic problems. The average hospital stay was 32.2 days.

The SCUs were designed with private rooms to ensure privacy and to promote sleep, and a nursing management model that included experienced staff was used. The family-oriented units allowed unlimited visiting hours and arrangements for overnight stays, if desired. Care in the critical care units followed the traditional protocols, limited visits with family, and used a primary care model under the supervision of physicians. Few significant differences in care were found in either study. However, costs were drastically lower in the SCUs, primarily because of the reduction in diagnostic costs and use of high technologic equipment other than mechanical ventilators.

According to Rudy and others[85] chronically ill patients survive one complication only to succumb to another. When complications do occur, the patient and family must make difficult decisions regarding extending aggressive treatment or restricting treatment, such as do not resuscitate orders. The frequent and close contact with the health care team and the friendlier environment of the SCU would facilitate in making those decisions.

Both studies demonstrated the efficacy of care in the SCU was equal to the care provided in the critical care unit. Satisfaction with care was implied. These studies contribute to the early body of knowledge that carefully selected, and highly vulnerable, patients can be appropriately cared for outside the critical care unit. These studies also back up social support theories to include patients and their families in making decisions regarding treatment choices.

Nurses caring for these patients have to be especially aware of their particular needs, observe for early signs of disorders, and act promptly to prevent major complications. Patience, excellent therapeutic communication skills, and a solid foundation in geriatric nursing are valuable attributes.

Care of Elderly Trauma Patients

By the year 2000, it is estimated there will be more than 35 million senior adults (older than 65 years) in the United States. As this population increases, the number of trauma injuries for this population will also increase. Trauma injuries resulting from falls, burns, and motor vehicle accidents are the fifth leading cause of traumas for elderly persons, and the mortality rate is significantly higher for this population than for younger persons.[86] Causative factors include polypharmacy, chronic illnesses, sensory deficits (e.g., diminished vision, hearing, sense of touch, and slowing of psychomotor and cognitive responses), and osteoporosis. Osteoporosis makes these individuals more susceptible to fractures of the extremeties (especially of the hip) and spinal cord injuries. (See Chapter 11.)

The critical care and perioperative nurses must carefully evaluate the geriatric trauma patient for fluid and electrolye imbalances; signs of impaired renal, respiratory, and circulatory function; and pain. All of these factors can contribute to psychosocial alterations. Because of the potential delay in elimination of medications, these patients may have mental status changes related to the many drug and narcotic side effects.[86,87]

Care of Patients Who Require Transplants

The advances in technology have contributed to the belief that any organ can be replaced. People often have unrealistic expectations about what can or cannot be done to help them.[9] Waiting for a donor to die can be like living with a time bomb. The potential recipient can experience guilt from waiting for someone to die, but at the same time realize that one's own death may come before an organ is available. These patients and their families experience a gamut of emotions. Concerns include worry over the financial burden, stress for the family, anxiety over the possible rejection of the organ, and the threat of taking immune-suppressant drugs for the remainder of their lives. The constant fear of infections is ever present, since an illness may delay or deny their suitability for the surgery.

Persons receiving bone marrow transplants experience a complex process involving repeated hospital stays of various lengths. Coping with prolonged isolation and side effects of immune-suppressant drugs and body radiation can be very taxing. The fear of rejection is a major concern. The donor, who is commonly a family member, may experience guilt feelings if the graft fails. The nurse's role is critical in maintaining hope during these periods. Demonstrating patience and empathy to the patient's and family's array of emotions is very important.[30,88]

The number of persons awaiting kidney transplants has increased during the last several years. Success rates of the surgery range between 91% and 97%, and costs have slowed to one third of the cost of dialysis. Most individuals awaiting kidney transplants must endure dialysis several times a week for many months or years, which is extremely costly, time-consuming, and stress-producing. Providing dialysis care for 90,000 patients in the United States in 1991 cost an estimated $4 billion.[30] The availability of donor organs is much less than the demand. Psychologic evaluation is an essential component of the preoperative work up to determine the patient's ability to cope with the lifelong medical regimen and to accept the donated organ as a part of the body. Living donors are also evaluated psychologically. The donor must offer the kidney freely, without coercion, and fully understand the risks and benefits of the procedure. Most kidney transplant patients will experience at least one episode of rejection. The threat of rejection can cause much anxiety. A second kidney transplant may be possible if a suitable organ can be found. However, progression of the disease process may preclude the patient's chances of survival during the waiting period.

Psychosocial nursing management for these patients is challenging, because they face the varied emotions of hope or hopelessness, anxiety and despair, grief, helplessness, and depression.[30,89]

DePalma and Townsend[90] report that approximately 39,000 people in the United States were waiting for organ transplants in 1995. More than 3000 died during the waiting period. During that time 5000 suitable organs were not donated. Criteria for a heart transplant candidate include an age limit of 20 to 50 years, a duration of illness of less than 5 years, no severe kidney or liver impairment, no diabetes, no infection, and adequate pulmonary function. Many heart transplant candidates lose their eligibility because of the long waiting period, or they die before a heart becomes available. Many ethical issues surround the persons involved in the process. A health care team consisting of the nurse, chaplain, psychiatric consult, and social services representative is extremely helpful in resolving these issues and in making decisions.

The study by Jalowiec and others[91] identified 39 preoperative stressors for patients awaiting a heart transplant. The 10 worst stressors were (1) the need for a transplant, (2) having end-stage heart disease, (3) experiencing the symptoms of the illness, (4) being a burden on the family, (5) waiting, (6) having an uncertain future, (7) fatigue, (8) having less control over life, (9) depending on others, and (10) financial concerns. Worry over increased cost of medical care as the physical condition deteriorated was a major concern. Other stressors during the waiting period included always "being on call" and wearing a pager so that the transplant candidate could be admitted within 2 hours of the page. Disruptions in work, family, and personal roles also affected one's self-concept and self-esteem.

Concerns during hospitalization after the surgery included the classic stressors experienced by patients in the critical care unit, as well as the threat of the body rejecting the donated organ and the patient being able to psychologically accept the new body part. The health care team caring for transplant patients work closely together to intervene in case of rejection, infection, and/or complications resulting from medications. Nurses are the primary teachers and prepare the patient and family for the long-term self-care needs.

SUMMARY

Several authors have emphasized the caring aspect of nursing. The critical care environment is not always conducive to more than the management of the physiologic needs of critically ill patients. However, as demonstrated by the discussion in this chapter, it is paramount that nurses consider the mind-body links in providing holistic nursing management and promoting recovery. One aspect of critical care nursing is knowing what emotional and behavioral responses are to be expected in a given patient care situation and recognizing atypical responses. The placement of these responses within a theoretical context has been presented as an important tool in assessment and for providing appropriate interventions. As health care teams have gained prominence during the last few years, some emphasis has been made on the need for group collaboration in providing quality care. Major psychosocial nursing diagnoses related to the self-concept, self-esteem, and self-image have been discussed as well as those of delirium (acute confusion), depression, spiritual distress, and ineffective individual and family coping. Nursing management for specific psychosocial alterations are included at the end of the chapter.

CASE STUDY

NURSING MANAGEMENT PLAN FOR BURN PATIENT NANCY DONOVAN

Psychosocial Alterations

DEFINING CHARACTERISTICS

Early Posttrauma Phase (First Several Weeks)

- Shock, terror, fear of dying. *Sample statements:* "What happened to me?" "How did it happen?" "How did I get here?" "Will I die?" "I'm so afraid!"
- Fear/anxiety related to endotracheal tube and inability to verbally communicate and breathe on her own. Examples: tries to move head, attempts to pull at tube, attempts to fight ventilator's pace, restless.
- Alterations in comfort resulting in pain. *Examples:* cries out when touched or moved, moans, displays nonverbal responses (tense, guarded posture, grimacing, restlessness, agitation.)
- Anticipatory pain between medications or before treatments/dressing changes. *Examples:* sleeplessness, restlessness; verbalizes fear—bargains for delay in treatments or continually asks for pain relief medications (when off ventilator).
- Spiritual distress. *Sample statements:* "Why did God let this happen?" "Why didn't I die and get it over with?" "What did I do wrong that I'm being punished like this?"
- Guilt (cause of accident because of own carelessness). *Sample statements:* "Why was I so stupid?" "I'll probably lose my job, my home, and my kids because I was so dumb." "I will be such a burden on my parents."
- Ineffective coping and depressed state. *Sample statements:* "I've never had anything like this happen before. What am I to do?" "I'm no good to anyone, even myself."
- Overdependence on caregivers because of prolonged hospitalization and inability to care for self because of severe burns on hands and arms, weakness, and repeated dressing changes. *Sample statements:* "I can't do anything for myself. You attend to my needs so well. Why should I learn how to change dressings? Besides, my fingers are so painful that I can't handle things well." "I'm too tired to do anything for myself."

Late Posttrauma Phase

- Loss of control. *Sample statements:* "I'm so tired of this routine. Can't I have any say in what's done for me?" Expressions of anger and frustration because visits with family/friends are so limited.
- Disturbance in body image. *Examples:* refusal to look at self in mirrors or to participate in self-care; frequent verbal and nonverbal expressions of disgust over appearance; not interested in improving appearance, "because nothing would do any good, anyhow."
- Use of defense mechanisms such as regression, denial, and withdrawal evidenced by immature behavior (e.g., crying, screaming, and swearing during treatments or when demands are not met as quickly as desired); sullen attitude; refusal to speak to caregivers, pretending to be asleep or sleeping for long periods during the day; refusing visitors, then complaining of being bored and feeling that no one cares.
- Fear over future surgeries and treatments. *Sample statements:* "I dread more surgery. It is always so painful." "Will I ever recover from this mess and be free of pain?"
- Anxiety about being discharged from unit. *Examples:* overdependence on specific caregivers and displaying manipulative behaviors; acting-out behavior that would delay transfer from acute care setting.

OUTCOME CRITERIA

- Patient begins to accept the situation.
- Patient agrees to be an active participant in care and cooperates with health care providers.
- Patient informs caregivers regarding needs.
- Patient accepts support from family.
- Patient uses appropriate problem-solving skills and coping mechanisms.
- Patient sets realistic goals for self and expresses feeling of hope for recovery/future.
- Patient gains sense of control; diminished feelings of hopelessness and helplessness are evident.

NURSING INTERVENTIONS AND *RATIONALE*

1. Continue to monitor the assessment parameters under "Defining Characteristics."
2. Use active listening and therapeutic communication techniques. ***These interventions aid in establishing trust and permit the patient to express concerns.***

Continued

CASE STUDY—CONT'D

NURSING MANAGEMENT PLAN FOR BURN PATIENT NANCY DONOVAN

NURSING INTERVENTIONS AND *RATIONALE*—cont'd

3. Use calming techniques. Instruct why the endotracheal tube must be inserted. Establish a method for her to express her needs. ***Loss of control over breathing and expression can be frightening. Fear and anxiety can contribute to pain.***
4. Perform ongoing assessment of pain intensity, frequency, and precipitating factors. Anticipate pain control needs. Give analgesic before painful procedures. Instruct in nondrug remedies (e.g., imaging, biofeedback, music therapy) ***Nondrug therapies aid patient to have some control over pain. (Patient-controlled anesthesia pumps are also useful.) Amount of sedation is decreased and risks for mental status changes are reduced.***
5. Explore cultural, religious beliefs/practices, perception of meaning of life, and interrelationships. Consult with family, psychiatric nurse, or chaplain on health care team. Nurse can also pray with patient, read scriptures, etc. ***Spiritual distress can lead to depression, guilt, low self-esteem. Spiritual well-being has been linked with psychologic health.***
6. Suggest effective coping strategies to help patient cope with emotional responses to stressors. ***Identification of appropriate responses to stress aids patient in decisions about what coping strategies to use.*** If depression includes suicidal ideation, question patient about plans. Seek consult if deemed appropriate. ***Patients often feel relieved that others have noticed how they feel. Guilt over such emotions is lessened. Help can become available.***
7. Set limits. Encourage patient to participate in self-care activities, even if in minimal ways. Instruct patient in ways that she can do things for herself. ***Persons commonly make excuses for not doing tasks because they feel embarrassed, or self-esteem is threatened if they cannot perform skills successfully.***
8. Allow patient to have some control over schedule of procedures. ***Feeling in control aids in lessening feelings of helplessness and hopelessness. Patient will be more willing to participate in care and will use more effective coping skills.***
9. Don't force patient to look into mirrors. Monitor readiness. Actively listen to concerns. Consult with social worker/psychiatric consultant. Provide honest positive feedback. Make contact with person who has survived a similar experience. ***There is a great threat to body image. Patients mourn the loss of attractiveness and may fear intimacy with significant other and contacts with others for fear of being rejected and ridiculed.***
10. Meet with health care team to plan outcomes. Include patient and family in decisions. ***Providing information about future therapies and realistic outcomes aids in setting appropriate goals, and including patient/family in decisions aids in compliance with plan of care.***

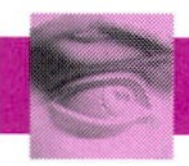

NURSING MANAGEMENT PLAN

BODY IMAGE DISTURBANCE

DEFINITION:

Disruption in the way subjects perceive their body image.

Body Image Disturbance Related to Functional Dependence on Life-Sustaining Technology (ventilator, dialysis, IABP, halo traction)

DEFINING CHARACTERISTICS

- Actual change in function requiring permanent or temporary replacement
- Refusal to verify actual loss
- Verbalization of the following: feelings of helplessness, hopelessness, powerlessness, fear of failure to wean from technology

OUTCOME CRITERIA

- Patient verifies actual change in function.
- Patient does not refuse or fight technologic intervention.
- Patient verbalizes acceptance of expected change in lifestyle.

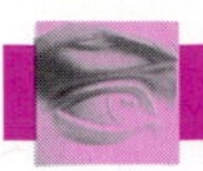
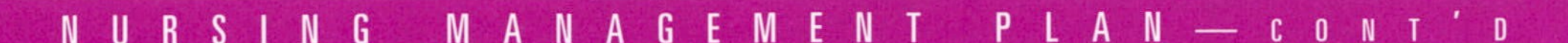

NURSING MANAGEMENT PLAN—CONT'D

BODY IMAGE DISTURBANCE

Body Image Disturbance Related to Functional Dependence on Life-Sustaining Technology (ventilator, dialysis, IABP, halo traction)

NURSING INTERVENTIONS AND *RATIONALE*

1. Continue to monitor the assessment parameters listed under "Defining Characteristics." In addition, assess patient's response to the technologic intervention.
2. Assess responses of family and significant others. ***Body image is derived from the "reflected appraisals" of family and significant others.***
3. Provide information needed by patient and family.
4. Promote trust, security, comfort, and privacy.
5. Recognize anxiety. Allow and encourage its expression. ***Anxiety is the most predominant emotion accompanying body image alterations.***
6. Assist patient to recognize his or her own functioning and performance in the face of technology. For example, assist the patient to distinguish spontaneous breaths from mechanically delivered breaths. ***This activity will assist in weaning the patient from the ventilator when feasible. To establish realistic, accurate body boundaries, a patient needs help to separate himself or herself from the technology that is supporting his or her functioning. Any participation or function on the part of the patient during periods of dependency is helpful in preventing and/or resolving an alteration in body image.***
7. Plan for discontinuation of the treatment (e.g., weaning from ventilator). Explain procedure that will be followed, and be present during its initiation.
8. Plan for transfer from the critical care environment.
9. Document care, ensuring an up-to-date management plan is available for all involved caregivers.

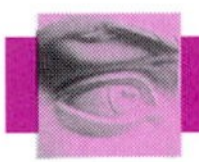

NURSING MANAGEMENT PLAN

Body Image Disturbance Related to Actual Change in Body Structure, Function, or Appearance

DEFINING CHARACTERISTICS

- Actual change in appearance, structure, or function
- Avoidance of looking at body part
- Avoidance of touching body part
- Hiding or overexposing body part (intentional or unintentional)
- Trauma to nonfunctioning part
- Change in ability to estimate spatial relationship of body to environment
- Verbalization of the following:
  - Fear of rejection or reaction by others
  - Negative feelings about body
  - Preoccupation with change or loss
  - Refusal to participate in or to accept responsibility for self-care of altered body part
- Personalization of part or loss with a name
- Depersonalization of part or loss by use of impersonal pronouns
- Refusal to verify actual change

OUTCOME CRITERIA

- Patient verbalizes the specific meaning of the change to him or her.
- Patient requests appropriate information about self-care.
- Patient completes personal hygiene and grooming daily with or without help.
- Patient interacts freely with family or other visitors.
- Patient participates in the discussions and conferences related to planning his or her medical and nursing management in the critical care unit and transfer from the unit.
- Patient talks with trained visitors (support group representatives) at least twice about his or her loss.

NURSING INTERVENTIONS AND *RATIONALE*

1. Continue to monitor the assessment parameters listed under "Defining Characteristics." In addition, assess patient's mental, physical, and emotional state; recognize assets, strengths, response to illness, position in Lee's phases, coping mechanisms, past experience with stress, and support systems.
2. Appraise the response of family and significant others. ***Body image is derived from the "reflected appraisals" of family and significant others.***
3. Determine the patient's goals and readiness for learning.
4. Provide the necessary information to help the patient and family adapt to the change. Clarify misconceptions about future limitations.
5. Permit and encourage the patient to express the significance of the loss or change; note nonverbal behavioral responses.
6. Allow and encourage the patient's expression of anxiety. ***Anxiety is the most predominant emotional response to a body image disturbance.***

Continued

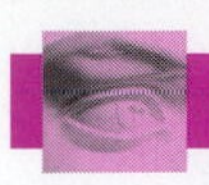

NURSING MANAGEMENT PLAN—CONT'D

Body Image Disturbance Related to Actual Change in Body Structure, Function, or Appearance

NURSING INTERVENTIONS AND *RATIONALE*—cont'd

7. Recognize and accept the use of denial as an adaptive defense mechanism when used early and temporarily.
8. Recognize maladaptive denial as that which interferes with the patient's progress and/or alienates support systems. Use confrontation.
9. Provide an opportunity for the patient to discuss sexual concerns.
10. Touch the affected body part ***to provide patient with sensory information about altered body structure and/or function.***
11. Encourage and provide movement of altered body part ***to establish kinesthetic feedback. This enables the person to know his or her body as it now exists.***
12. Prepare the patient to look at the body part. Call the body part by its anatomical name (e.g., stump, stoma, limb) as opposed to "it" or "she." ***The use of impersonal pronouns increases a sense of fantasy and depersonalization of the body part.***
13. Allow the patient to experience excellence in some aspect of physical functioning—walking, turning, deep breathing, healing, self-care—and point out progress and accomplishment. ***This helps to balance the patient's sense of dysfunction with function.***
14. Avoid false reassurance. Acknowledge the difficulty of incorporating the altered body part or function into one's body image. ***This evidences the nurse's sensitivity and promotes trust.***
15. Talk with the patient about his or her life, generativity, and accomplishments. ***Patients with disturbances in body image frequently see themselves in a distortedly "narrow" sense. Encouraging a wider focus of themselves and their life reduces this distortion.***
16. Help the patient explore realistic alternatives.
17. Recognize that incorporating a body change into one's body image takes time. Avoid setting unrealistic expectations and ***thereby inadvertently reinforcing a low self-esteem.***
18. Suggest the use of additional resources such as trained visitors who have mastered situations similar to those of the patient. Refer patient to a psychiatric liaison nurse or psychiatrist if needed.

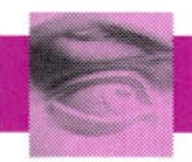

NURSING MANAGEMENT PLAN

SELF-ESTEEM DISTURBANCE

DEFINITION:

Negative self-evaluation/feelings about self or self-capabilities, which may be directly or indirectly expressed.

Self-Esteem Disturbance Related to Feelings of Guilt About Physical Deterioration

DEFINING CHARACTERISTICS

- Inability to accept positive reinforcement
- Lack of follow-through
- Nonparticipation in therapy
- Not taking responsibility for self-care (i.e., self-neglect)
- Self-destructive behavior
- Lack of eye contact

OUTCOME CRITERIA

- Patient verbalizes feelings of self-worth.
- Patient maintains positive relationships with significant others.
- Patient manifests active interest in appearance by completing personal grooming daily.

NURSING INTERVENTIONS AND *RATIONALE*

1. Continue to monitor the assessment parameters listed under "Defining Characteristics." In addition, assess the meaning of health-related situation. How does the patient feel about himself or herself, the diagnosis, and the treatment? How does the present fit into the larger context of his or her life?
2. Assess the patient's emotional level, interpersonal relationships, and feelings about himself or herself. Recognize the patient's uniqueness (how the hair is worn, preference for name used).
3. Help the patient discover and verbalize feelings and understand the crisis by listening and providing information.

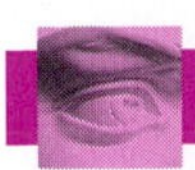

NURSING MANAGEMENT PLAN—CONT'D

SELF-ESTEEM DISTURBANCE

Self-Esteem Disturbance Related to Feelings of Guilt About Physical Deterioration

NURSING INTERVENTIONS AND *RATIONALE*—*cont'd*

4. Assist the patient to identify strengths and positive qualities that increase the sense of self-worth. Focus on past experiences of accomplishment and competency. Help the patient with positive self-reinforcement. Reinforce the obvious love and affection of family and significant others.
5. Assess coping techniques that have been helpful in the past. Help the patient decide how to handle negative or incongruent feedback about the situation.
6. Encourage visits from family and significant others. Facilitate interactions and ensure privacy. Help family members entering the critical care unit by explaining what they will see. Increase visitors' comfort with equipment; offer chairs and other courtesies.
7. Encourage the patient to pursue interest in individual or social activities, even though difficult in the critical care unit.
8. Reflect caring, concern, empathy, respect, and unconditional acceptance in nurse-patient relationships.
9. Remember that for the patient the nurse is a significant other who provides important appraisals of the patient and who can facilitate the change process.
10. Help the family support the patient's self-esteem.
11. Provide for continuity of nurse assignment to ensure consistent contacts that can ***facilitate support of the patient's self-esteem.***

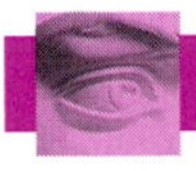

NURSING MANAGEMENT PLAN

POWERLESSNESS

DEFINITION:

Perception that one's own action will not significantly affect an outcome; a perceived lack of control over a current situation or immediate happening.

Powerlessness Related to Lack of Control Over Current Situation and/or Disease Progression

DEFINING CHARACTERISTICS

Severe

- Verbal expressions of having no control or influence over situation
- Verbal expressions of having no control or influence over outcome
- Verbal expressions of having no control over self-care
- Depression over physical deterioration that occurs despite patient's compliance with regimens
- Apathy

Moderate

- Nonparticipation in care or decision making when opportunities are provided
- Expressions of dissatisfaction and frustration about inability to perform previous tasks and/or activities
- Lack of progress monitoring
- Expressions of doubt about role performance
- Reluctance to express true feelings, fearing alienation from caregivers
- Passivity
- Inability to seek information about care
- Dependence on others that may result in irritability, resentment, anger, and guilt
- No defense of self-care practices when challenged

Low

- Passivity

OUTCOME CRITERIA

- Patient verbalizes increased control over situation by wanting to do things his or her way.
- Patient actively participates in planning care.
- Patient requests needed information.
- Patient chooses to participate in self-care activities.
- Patient monitors progress.

NURSING INTERVENTIONS AND *RATIONALE*

1. Continue to monitor the assessment parameters listed under "Defining Characteristics." In addition, assess the patient's feelings and perception of the reasons for lack of power and sense of helplessness.

Continued

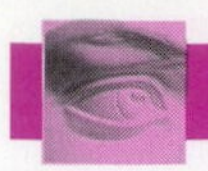
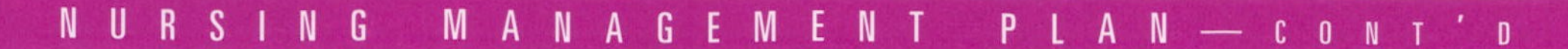

POWERLESSNESS

Powerlessness Related to Lack of Control over Current Situation and/or Disease Progression

NURSING INTERVENTIONS AND *RATIONALE*—*cont'd*

2. Determine as far as possible the patient's usual response to limited control situations. Determine through ongoing assessment the patient's usual locus of control (i.e., believes that influence over his or her life is exerted by luck, fate, powerful persons [external locus of control] or that influence is exerted through personal choices, self-effort, self-determination [internal locus of control]).
3. Support patient's physical control of the environment by involving him or her in care activities; knock before entering room if appropriate; ask permission before moving personal belongings. Inform the patient that, although an activity may not be to his or her liking, it is necessary. ***This gives the patient permission to express dissatisfaction with the environment and regimen.***
4. Personalize the patient's care using his or her preferred name. ***This supports the patient's psychologic control.***
5. Provide the therapeutic rationale for all the patient is asked to do for himself or herself and for all that is being done for and with him or her. Reinforce the physician's explanations; clarify misconceptions about the illness situation and treatment plans. ***This supports the patient's cognitive control.***
6. Include patient in care planning by encouraging participation and allowing choices wherever possible (e.g., timing of personal care activities and deciding when pain medicines are needed). Point out situations in which no choices exist.
7. Provide opportunities for the patient to exert influence over himself or herself and his or her body, thereby affecting an outcome. For example, share with the patient the nurse's assessment of his or her breath sounds and explain that they can be improved by self-initiated deep breathing exercises. ***Feedback that the patient has been successful in helping clear his or her lungs reinforces the influence he or she does retain.***
8. Encourage family to permit patient to do as much independently as possible ***to foster perceptions of personal power.***
9. Assist the patient to establish realistic short-term and long-term goals. ***Setting unrealistic or unattainable goals inadvertently reinforces the patient's perception of powerlessness.***
10. Document care to provide for continuity ***so that the patient can maintain appropriate control over the environment.***
11. Assist the patient to regain strength and activity tolerance as appropriate, ***thus increasing a sense of control and self-reliance.***
12. Increase the sensitivity of the health team members and significant others to the patient's sense of powerlessness. Use power over the patient carefully. Use the words "must," "should," and "have to" with caution, ***because they communicate coercive power and imply that the objects of "musts" and "shoulds" are of benefit to the nurse versus the patient.***
13. Plan with the patient for transfer from the critical care unit to the intermediate unit and eventually to home.

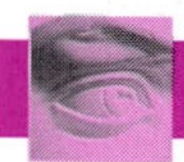

NURSING MANAGEMENT PLAN

ACUTE CONFUSION

DEFINITION:

The abrupt onset of a cluster of global, transient changes and disturbances in attention, cognition, psychomotor activity level of consciousness, and/or, sleep/wake cycle.

Acute Confusion Related to Sensory Overload, Sensory Deprivation, and Sleep Pattern Disturbance

DEFINING CHARACTERISTICS[61,65]

(At least two of the following)

Early symptoms

- Sudden onset of global cognitive function impairment (from hours to days)
- Restlessness, agitation, and combative behavior
- Drowsiness (can lead to loss of consciousness)
- Slurring of speech, inappropriate statements or "word salad," mumbling or inappropriate gestures
- Short attention span (needs questions repeated); inability to learn new material

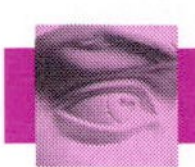

NURSING MANAGEMENT PLAN—CONT'D

ACUTE CONFUSION

Acute Confusion Related to Sensory Overload, Sensory Deprivation, and Sleep Pattern Disturbance

Early symptoms—cont'd

- Disordered awake-sleep cycle
- Disorientation to person, time, place, and situation
- Difficulty in separating dreams from reality (may experience bizarre dreams/nightmares)
- Anger at staff for continued questions about his or her orientation

Later symptoms

- Symptoms that tend to fluctuate throughout the day and night
- Early symptoms continue and may be more frequent and of longer duration
- Illusions
- Hallucinations
- Extreme agitation (e.g., attempts to climb out of bed, pull out catheters, rip off dressings)
- Calling out in loud voice, swearing, or attempting to bite or hit people who approach patient

CONTRIBUTING FACTORS[30,61]

- Fluid and electrolyte imbalances
- Potential for organ dysfunction (hepatic, renal, gastrointestinal, cardiac, respiratory) caused by inadequate oxygenation
- Delay in metabolism and excretion of drugs, thus prolonging half-life and increasing drugs' effect or interaction with other drugs
- Immune-suppressant drugs side effects
- Narcotic analgesics
- Hypersensitivity to drugs
- Surgical time (or time on bypass equipment) more than 4 hours of duration
- Stressors in critical care unit (see Box 5-1)
- Physical and mental status of patient before surgery (preexisting medical conditions such as diabetes, epilepsy, neoplasm)
- Withdrawal symptoms, such as those from alcohol, drugs, or amphetamines
- Availability of social/spiritual/family support

NURSING INTERVENTIONS AND *RATIONALE*

1. Continue to monitor the assessment parameters listed under "Defining Characteristics." In addition, determine and document the patient's dominant spoken language, his or her literacy, and the language(s) in which he or she is literate. Determine and document his or her premorbid degree of orientation, cognitive capabilities, and any sensory-perceptual deficits. ***It is sometimes the case that people are not literate in their spoken language or, less commonly, that they are literate only in their second language. These situations can result in unfortunate errors in the appraisal of patients' ability to communicate in writing and in estimating the extent of their orientation. Similarly, assuming that the patients were or were not fully oriented before critical care admission bases the nurse's assessment on possibly erroneous assumptions.***

For sensory overload

1. Initiate each nurse-patient encounter by calling the patient by name and identifying yourself by name. ***This fosters reality orientation and assists the patient in filtering irrelevant or impersonal conversation.***
2. Assess the patient's immediate physical environment from his or her viewpoint, and explain equipment, its sounds, and its therapeutic purpose. Demonstrate audible and visual alarms, and explain the possible alarm conditions. ***This decreases alienation of the patient from the technologic environment and reduces the inherent sense of fear and urgency accompanying alarm conditions.***
3. For each procedure performed, provide "preparatory sensory information" (i.e., explain procedures in relation to the sensations the patient will experience, including duration of sensations). ***Preparatory sensory information enhances learning and lessens anticipatory anxiety.***
4. Limit noise levels. Certainly, audible alarms cannot and must not be silenced, and many critical, albeit noisy, activities must take place in the critical care area. It has been shown, however, that noise levels produced by clinical personnel exceed those levels designated as "acceptable" and are often greater than those generated by technologic devices. Staff conversations must be kept soft enough that they are inaudible to the patient whenever possible. Critical care personnel are to assume that everything said at or around a patient's bedside is intended for that patient's awareness and that it will be interpreted as pertaining to him or her. ***As in the discussion that follows, conversations about the patient but not to him or her foster depersonalization and delusions of reference.***

Continued

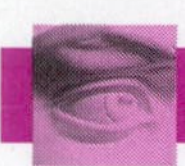

NURSING MANAGEMENT PLAN—CONT'D

ACUTE CONFUSION

Acute Confusion Related to Sensory Overload, Sensory Deprivation, and Sleep Pattern Disturbance

NURSING INTERVENTIONS AND *RATIONALE*—cont'd

For sensory overload—cont'd

5. Well-enforced noise limits need to exist for nighttime.
6. Readjust alarm limits on physiologic monitoring devices as the patient's condition changes (improves or deteriorates) ***to lessen unnecessary alarm states.***
7. Consider use of head phones and audio cassette or compact disk player with patient's favorite and/or subliminal or classical music. ***This can effectively filter out assaultive noise of the critical care environment and supplant it with familiar, soothing sounds and rhythms.***
8. Modify lighting. Day-night cycles need to be simulated with environmental lighting. At no time should overhead fluorescent lights be abruptly turned on without either warning the patient, assisting him or her out of the supine position, and/or shielding his or her eyes with gauze or a face cloth. ***Continuous bright lighting sustains anxiety and promotes circadian rhythm desynchronization.***
9. To the extent possible, shield patients from viewing urgent and emergent events in the critical care unit. ***Resuscitation efforts, albeit difficult to conceal, engender fear in the patient and a sense of instability and vulnerability (e.g., "I'm next").*** When such an event occurs, the nurse needs to elicit the patient's cognitive and emotional reaction; thoughts, impressions, and feelings need to be shared and misconceptions clarified. A useful approach for the nurse in this interchange is that of emphasizing the differences between the patient at hand and the one resuscitated (e.g., "He was considerably older," "more unstable," "had serious lung disease").
10. Ensure patients' privacy, their modesty, and, at the very least, their dignity. Physical exposure and nudity, although seeming to pale in importance alongside such priorities as physiologic assessment and stabilization, are primal indignities in all individuals. Patients must be kept minimally exposed. When, in the course of assessment and intervention, it becomes necessary to expose the patient, the nurse is to first verbally apologize for this necessity. ***To be naked is to feel vulnerable; to be vulnerable is to feel fearful. In this regard, fear is an emotion concomitant to critical care that is preventable through nursing intervention.***

For sensory deprivation

1. Provide reality orientation in four spheres (person, place, time, and situation) at more frequent intervals than when testing. Convey this information in the context of routine conversation. SAMPLE STATEMENTS: "Mr. Clark, this is Tuesday morning and you're in University Hospital. Your heart surgery was yesterday morning, and you're doing well. My name is Joe, and I'm your nurse today." ***The patient is made to feel patronized by repetitions such as, "Do you know where you are?"*** Given the effects of general anesthesia, narcotic analgesics, sedatives, and sleep, it is fully expected that some degree of disorientation will exist normally.
2. Ensure the patient's visual access to a calendar. (Of interest, the design of most state-of-the-art critical care units now reflects many of the principles of sensory stimulation. One such coronary care unit was designed with a large wall clock facing the patient. A patient who had spent more than 1 week in this unit later reflected that one of the most "distressing, frustrating" aspects of his stay in the coronary care unit was the monotonous, inescapable attention to the clock and its painfully slow documentation of the passing of time.)
3. Apprise the patient of daily news events and the weather.
4. Touch patients for the express purpose of communicating caring. Hold their hands, stroke their brows, rub the skin on an aspect of their arms. ***Touch is the universal language of caring. In the setting of critical care, in which there is considerable physical body manipulation, it is useful and important to contrast assaultive touch with comforting touch.*** Touch can be used as a technique for distraction from painful stimuli when used in conjunction with uncomfortable procedures. (IMPORTANT: See discussion of the use of touch in management of the patient experiencing hallucinations, p. 93.)
5. Foster liberal visitation by family and significant others. Encourage significant others to touch the patient as consistent with their individual comfort level and cultural norms.
6. Structure and identify opportunities for the patient to exercise decision-making skills, however small. ***Although not so designated, patients with sensory alterations experience a type of "cognitive deprivation" as well.***

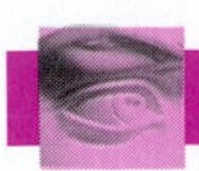

NURSING MANAGEMENT PLAN—CONT'D

ACUTE CONFUSION

Acute Confusion Related to Sensory Overload, Sensory Deprivation, and Sleep Pattern Disturbance

NURSING INTERVENTIONS AND *RATIONALE*—cont'd

For sensory deprivation—cont'd

7. Assist patients to find meaning in their experiences. Explain the therapeutic purpose of all that they are asked to do for themselves and all that is done with them and for them. Avoid statements such as, "Will you turn to that side for me?" or "I need you to swallow this medication." ***These statements implicitly convey that the maneuver has some value for the nurses versus the patients.*** Similarly, use "thank you" judiciously. ***This simple salutation, when used indiscriminately, suggests something was done to benefit the nurses and not the patients.*** Patients need to find meaning and to identify their roles in the experience of critical illness and critical care. The sensations that constitute this experience and those that do not are made bearable and intelligible when attached to the larger picture of their conditions, treatment, and progress.

For sleep pattern disturbances

For excellent management strategies of sleep pattern disturbance, see the sleep Nursing Management Plans in Chapter 6.

For management of the patient experiencing hallucinations

1. Approach the patient with a calm, matter-of-fact demeanor. ***The goal of this interaction is for the nurse to demonstrate external control. This helps decrease the anxiety and fear that generally accompany hallucinations and allows the patient to feel safe. Anxiety is transferrable.***
2. Address the patient by name. ***This is a useful presentation of reality because self-identity is the last sphere of orientation to vanish.***
3. In responding to the patient's description of the hallucination, DO NOT deny, argue, or attempt to disprove the existence of the perceived event. ***Statements such as, "There are no voices coming from that air vent" or, "Look, I'm brushing my hand across the wall, and there are no bugs" confuse the patient further, because the hallucination, although frightening, is his or her perceived reality.***
4. Express to the patient that your experiences are dissimilar, and acknowledge how frightening his or hers must be. SAMPLE STATEMENT: "I don't hear (see, etc.) what you do, but I know how frightening such an experience must be to you. I'm Joe, your nurse, and I'm going to stay with you until the voices (etc.) go away." Remain with any patient who is experiencing a hallucination. ***Feelings of fear and anxiety often accelerate when a patient is left alone. He or she needs someone to represent a nonthreatening reality. In addition, validating the patient's feelings demonstrates acceptance and sensitivity to the experience and promotes trust.***
5. DO NOT explore the content of the hallucination with the patient by asking about its nature or character. ***The nurse is the patient's link with reality. Pursuit of a detailed description of a hallucination may signify to the patient that the nurse accepts his or her sensory distortion as factual. This may further confuse the patient and distance him or her more from reality.**** The nurse can help bridge the gap between the patient's misperception and reality by addressing the feelings (e.g., fear, anxiety) and/or meanings (e.g., danger, death) engendered by the hallucination. Determination of how the misperception affects the patient emotionally; acknowledgment of those feelings, and a calm, controlled, matter-of-fact approach will provide the trust and comfort he or she needs to tolerate this frightening experience. In other words, deal with the intent more than the content of the hallucination. ***The resultant decrease in anxiety will enable the patient to focus more accurately on his or her immediate environment.***
6. Talk concretely with the patient about things that are really happening. SAMPLE STATEMENTS: "How does your chest incision feel this afternoon, Mr. Clark?" "Your sister Kate was here to see you, but you were sleeping. She went down to the cafeteria and will be back." "Your secretions are a little easier for you to cough up today." ***Interpretation of reality-based stimuli by the nurse encourages the patient to focus on actual circumstances and discourages a preoccupation with sensory misperceptions.***
7. There may be circumstances in which it is appropriate for the nurse simply to distract the patient by changing the topic. This tactic is useful in situations of escalating anxiety and confusion or when all else fails. Topics need to consist of basic themes that are universally understood and culturally congruent, such as music, food, or weather. They may also be topics of special interest to the patient, such as hobbies, crafts, or sports. Topics that evoke strong emotions, such as politics, religion, or sexuality, are to be avoided with most patients.

*An exception is the patient who the nurse suspects is experiencing auditory hallucinations (i.e., hearing "voice commands"). To ascertain that the voices are not telling the patient to harm himself or herself, it is appropriate for the nurse to ask simply and concretely, "What are the voices saying?"

Continued

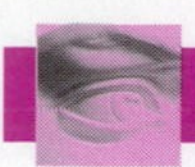

NURSING MANAGEMENT PLAN—CONT'D

ACUTE CONFUSION

Acute Confusion Related to Sensory Overload, Sensory Deprivation, and Sleep Pattern Disturbance

NURSING INTERVENTIONS AND *RATIONALE*—cont'd

For management of the patient experiencing hallucinations—cont'd

This is especially true of the patient with reality distortions; sometimes hallucinations and delusions are expressions of repressed conflicts associated with religious, sexual, or aggressive issues. Pursuit of such subjects could increase confusion and anxiety.

8. The use of touch: ***Touch presents a nonthreatening external reality and can therefore be useful in the management of patients with sensory alterations. However, in the patient experiencing hallucinations (as well as delusions and illusions), touch can be readily misinterpreted as, for instance, aggression or pain, or it can actually provide the basis for a tactile illusion.*** Therefore the use of touch as an intervention strategy is to be avoided in any patient who demonstrates escalating anxiety or paranoid, suspicious, or mistrustful thoughts.
9. Types of hallucinations include the following: auditory—voices or running commentaries, with self-destructive messages; visual—persons or images that appear threatening; olfactory—smells that may be interpreted as poisonous gases; gustatory—tastes that seem peculiar or harmful; and tactile—touch that feels unusual or unnatural.
10. Specific management strategies for patients experiencing hallucinations:
    - Auditory hallucinations
      a. Patient behaviors: Head cocked as if listening to an unseen presence; lips moving.
      b. Therapeutic nurse responses: "Mr. Clark, you appear to be listening to something." If patient acknowledges voices: "I don't hear any voices, but I know this is troubling you. The voices will go away. Nothing is going to harm you. I'm Joe, your nurse, and I'll be here with you."
      c. Nontherapeutic nurse responses: "Tell me about your conversations with these voices." "To whom do the voices belong—anyone you know?"
    - Visual hallucinations
      a. Patient behaviors: Staring into space as if focused on an unseen object; startled movements and anxious facial expression.
      b. Therapeutic nurse responses: "Mr. Clark, something seems to be troubling you. Tell me what it is." If patient states he visualizes people, images, or the devil in his environment and implies a sense of danger, respond, "There are only nurses and doctors here, Mr. Clark. I know this must be upsetting, but these images will go away. We're here with you in the hospital. Nothing will happen to you."
      c. Nontherapeutic nurse responses: "Describe the people you see. What are they wearing?" "What does the devil mean in your life? What about God?"

For management of the patient experiencing delusions

1. Explain all unseen noises, voices, and activity simply and clearly. ***They readily feed a delusional system.*** SAMPLE STATEMENTS: "That is Dr. Smith. He's come to see you and other patients here in the hospital." "The voices and activity you hear are from the bedside of the patient behind this curtain. He's being helped by one of the nurses."
2. Avoid the "negative challenge" (e.g., "Nobody here stole your belongings" or "Doctors and nurses do not harm people") of the patient's delusion. Similarly, avoid defending the referents of the patient's belief: "Nurses are good" and "Doctors mean well." ***Remember, a delusion is a belief, albeit false, that cannot be changed with logic. To attempt this change is to challenge the patient's belief system and thereby escalate his or her anxiety, further blurring the boundaries between reality and the patient's internally based "logic."***
3. For the patient with persecutory delusions who refuses food, fluids, or medications because of a belief they have been poisoned or tainted, permit the refusal unless it is a life-threatening event. Try again in 20 minutes; allow the patient to choose an alternative selection of food or to read the label on the unit's medication. Coercion, show of force, or engaging in complicated, logical justifications will only heighten the patient's suspiciousness and possibly reinforce the delusional belief. ***When the patient feels more in control, he or she need not rely on the "paradoxical" quality of the delusion to equip him or her with a false sense of power. His or her power instead is derived from making reality-based decisions.***
4. Staff members should be particularly careful not to engage in unnecessary laughter or whispering within view of the delusional patient. ***The delusional patient is hypervigilant, scanning the environment for evidence to corroborate or confirm his or her belief that staff members are colluding against him or her; clearly, laughter and whispers easily suggest this belief, this delusion of reference. This rationale pertains to the patient experiencing hallucinations and/or illusions as well.***

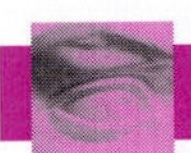

NURSING MANAGEMENT PLAN—CONT'D

ACUTE CONFUSION

Acute Confusion Related to Sensory Overload, Sensory Deprivation, and Sleep Pattern Disturbance

NURSING INTERVENTIONS AND *RATIONALE*—cont'd

For management of the patient experiencing delusions—cont'd

5. Observe the principles detailed in the third intervention under management of the patient experiencing hallucinations, p. 93.

For management of the patient experiencing illusions

1. As with the management of delusions, the nurse simply and briefly interprets reality-based stimuli for the patient in a calm, matter-of-fact manner. ***Seen and unseen noises, voices, activity, and people can provide the stimulus for a sensory misinterpretation, an illusion.***
2. The immediate environment of the patient must provide as low a level of stimulation as possible. Nursing interventions detailed previously under "Sensory Overload" are especially relevant here.
3. The theme of the nurse's verbal approach to the patient experiencing illusions is similar to that outlined for hallucinations and delusions: address the feelings and meanings associated with the experience, not the content of the sensory misinterpretation.
   - Patient behaviors: Eyes darting, startled movements; frightened facial expression. "I know who you are. You're the devil come to take me to hell."
   - Therapeutic nurse responses: "I'm Joe, your nurse. I know this experience is troubling for you. You're in the hospital, and no one here will harm you."
   - Nontherapeutic nurse responses: "There are no such things as devils or angels." "Do you think the devil would be dressed in white?" ***The first nontherapeutic nurse response carries a parental tone (i.e., "you know better than that"), thus infantilizing the patient and adding to his or her feelings of powerlessness over the environment. The second nontherapeutic response reflects obvious logic, which is not in the patient's sensory domain; therefore it cannot be processed and only adds to his or her confused state.***
4. Observe the principles detailed under the fifth item in management of the patient experiencing hallucinations, p. 93.

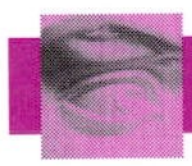

NURSING MANAGEMENT PLAN

INEFFECTIVE INDIVIDUAL COPING

DEFINITION:

Impairment of adaptive behaviors and problem-solving abilities of a person in meeting life's demands and roles.

Ineffective Individual Coping Related to Situational Crisis and Personal Vulnerability

DEFINING CHARACTERISTICS

- Verbalization of inability to cope. *Sample statements:* "I can't take this anymore." "I don't know how to deal with this."
- Ineffective problem solving (problem lumping). *Sample statements:* "I have to eliminate salt from my diet. They tell me I can no longer mow the lawn. This hospitalization is costing a mint. What about my kids' future? Who's going to change the oil in the car? This is an incredible amount of time away from work."
- Ineffective use of coping mechanisms.
  Projection: blames others for illness or pain.
  Displacement: directs anger and/or aggression toward family. Sample statement: "Get out of here. Leave me alone." Curses, shouts, or demands attention; strikes out or throws objects.
  Denial of severity of illness and need for treatment.
- Noncompliance. *Examples:* activity restriction; refusal to allow treatment or to take medications.
- Suicidal thoughts (verbalizes desire to end life).
- Self-directed aggression. *Examples:* disconnects or attempts to disconnect life-sustaining equipment; deliberately tries to harm self.
- Failure to progress from dependent to more independent state (refusal or resistance to care for self).

Continued

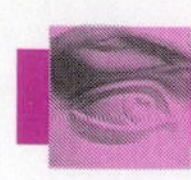

NURSING MANAGEMENT PLAN—CONT'D

INEFFECTIVE INDIVIDUAL COPING

Ineffective Individual Coping Related to Situational Crisis and Personal Vulnerability

OUTCOME CRITERIA

- Patient verbalizes beginning ability to cope with illness, pain, and hospitalization. *Sample statements:* "I'm trying to do the best I can." "I want to help myself get better."
- Patient demonstrates effective problem solving (lists and prioritizes problems from most to least urgent).
- Patient uses effective behavioral strategies to manage the stress of illness and care.
- Patient demonstrates interest or involvement in illness or environment. *Examples:* patient does the following:
  - Requests medications when anticipating pain.
  - Questions course of treatment, progress, and prognosis.
  - Asks for clarification of environmental stimuli and events.
  - Seeks out supportive individuals in his or her environment.
  - Uses coping mechanisms and strategies more effectively to manage situational crisis.
  - Demonstrates significant reduction in impulsive, angry, or aggressive outbursts (projection, shouting, cursing) directed toward family.
  - Verbalizes futuristic plans, with cessation of self-directed aggressive acts and suicidal thoughts.
  - Willingly complies with treatment regimen.
  - Begins to participate in self-care.

NURSING INTERVENTIONS AND *RATIONALE*

1. Continue to monitor the assessment parameters listed under "Defining Characteristics."
2. Actively listen and respond to patient's verbal and behavioral expressions. ***Active listening signifies unconditional respect and acceptance for the patient as a worthwhile individual. It builds trust and rapport, guides the nurse toward problem areas, encourages the patient to express concerns, and promotes compliance.***
3. Offer effective coping strategies to help the patient better tolerate the stressors related to his or her illness and care. Give permission to vent feelings in a safe setting. *Sample statements:* "I don't blame you for feeling angry or frustrated." "Others who are ill like you have expressed similar feelings." "I will listen to anything you want to share with me." "We don't have to talk; I'd like to sit here with you." "It's perfectly OK to cry." ***Individuals who are provided with opportunities to express their feelings will be better able to release pent-up emotions and derive a greater sense of relief and comfort. Thus they are less likely to resort to overly impulsive, aggressive acts, which may harm self or others.***
4. Inform the family of the patient's need to displace anger occasionally but that you will be working with the patient to help him or her release his or her feelings in a more constructive, effective way. ***Family members who are well-informed are better equipped to cope with their loved one's emotional anguish and outbursts. They are less likely to waste energy on feelings of guilt, fear, anger, or despair and can use their strength to help the patient in more constructive ways. The knowledge that their loved one is being cared for emotionally, as well as physically, will offer family members a greater sense of comfort and understanding. They will feel nurtured and respected by the nurse's attempt to include them in the process.***
5. With the patient, list and number problems from most to least urgent. Assist him or her in finding immediate solutions for most urgent problems; postpone those that can wait; delegate some to family members; and help him or her acknowledge problems that are beyond his or her control. ***Listing and numbering problems in an organized fashion help break them down into more manageable "pieces" so that the patient is better able to identify solutions for those that are solvable and to suppress those that are less relevant or not amenable to interventions.***
6. Identify individuals in the patient's environment who best help him or her to cope, as well as those who do not. Validate your observations with the patient. *Sample statements:* "I notice you seemed more relaxed during your daughter's visit." "After the clergy left, you were able to sleep a bit longer than usual; would you like to see him more often?" "Your grandson was a bit upset today; I'll be glad to talk to him if you like." ***Supportive persons can invoke a calming effect on the patient's physiologic and psychologic states. Conversely, well-meaning but nonsupportive individuals can have a deleterious effect on the patient's ability to cope and must be carefully screened and counseled by the nurse.***

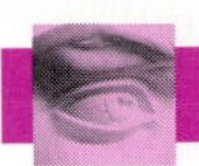
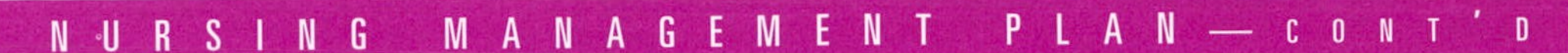

NURSING MANAGEMENT PLAN—CONT'D

INEFFECTIVE INDIVIDUAL COPING

Ineffective Individual Coping Related to Situational Crisis and Personal Vulnerability

NURSING INTERVENTIONS AND *RATIONALE*—cont'd

7. Teach the patient effective cognitive strategies to help him or her better manage the stress of critical illness and care. Help him or her construct pleasant thoughts, situations, or images that can simultaneously inhibit unpleasant realities. *Examples:* a day at the beach, a walk in the park, drinking a glass of wine, or being with a loved one. ***Pleasant thoughts or images constructed during critical illness and care tend to inhibit or reduce the intensity of the unpleasant, stressful effects of the experience.***
8. Assist the patient in using coping mechanisms more effectively so he or she can better manage his or her situational crisis:
   - Suppression of problems beyond his or her control.
   - Compensation for illness and its effects; focusing on his or her strengths, interests, family, and spiritual beliefs.
   - Adaptive displacement of anger, fear, or frustration through healthy, verbal expressions to staff.

   Effective use of coping mechanisms helps to assuage the patient's painful feelings in a safe setting. Thus the patient is strengthened and need not resort to the use of more ineffective defenses to eliminate anxiety.
9. Initiate a suicidal assessment if the patient verbalizes the desire to die, states that life is not worth living, or exhibits self-directed aggression. *Sample statement:* "We know this is a bad time for you. You're saying repeatedly that you want to die. Are you planning to harm yourself?" If the response is yes, remain with the patient, alert staff members, and provide for psychiatric consultation as soon as possible. Continue to express concern to the patient and protect him or her from harm. ***Suicidal thoughts as a result of ineffective coping or exhaustion of coping devices are not an uncommon occurrence in critically ill patients. If the mood state is distressing enough, a patient may seek relief by attempting a self-destructive act. Although the patient may not imminently have the energy to succeed in his or her attempt, voicing specific plans signifies a depressed mood state and a depletion of coping strategies. Thus immediate intervention is needed, since the attempt may be successful when the patient's energy is restored.***
10. Encourage the patient to participate in self-care activities and treatment regimen in accordance with his or her level of progress. Offer praise for his or her efforts toward self-care. ***Patients who take an active role in their own treatment and progress are less apt to feel like helpless or powerless victims. This greater sense of control over their illness and environment will guide them more swiftly toward becoming as independent as possible.***

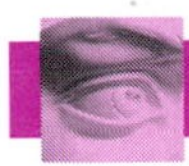

NURSING MANAGEMENT PLAN

INEFFECTIVE FAMILY COPING

DEFINITION:

Insufficient, ineffective, or compromised support, comfort, assistance, or encouragement—usually by a supportive primary person (family member or close friend); patient may need it to manage or master adaptive tasks related to his/her health challenge.

Ineffective Family Coping Related to Critically Ill Family Member

DEFINING CHARACTERISTICS

- Disruption of usual family functions and roles.
- Inability to accept or deal with crisis situation; use of defense mechanisms (e.g., denial, anger); unrealistic expectations of patient's outcome and care provided; judgmental toward health care providers.
- Nonrecognition that family is in state of crisis.
- Inappropriate emotional outbursts; arguments among family and with others; inability to respond to each other's feelings or support each other.
- Misinterpretation of information; short attention span with repeated questions about information already provided; members do not share information with each other.
- Inability to make decisions regarding changes in family structure or about course of care for ill member; noncooperation among family members.

Continued

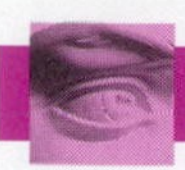

NURSING MANAGEMENT PLAN—CONT'D

INEFFECTIVE FAMILY COPING

Ineffective Family Coping Related to Critically Ill Family Member

DEFINING CHARACTERISTICS—cont'd

- Expressions of grief, hopelessness, powerlessness, and isolation; do not seek or respond to support services.
- Hesitancy to spend time with ill person in the critical care unit, or inappropriate behavior when visiting (may upset patient.)
- Neglect of own personal health; fatigue, apathy; refuse offers for respite time.

OUTCOME CRITERIA

- The family will express an understanding of course/prognosis of illness, therapies, and alternative measures.
- The family will diminish or resolve conflicts and cooperate in decision making.
- The family will develop trust and mutual support for each member and form a cohesive unit.
- The family will support ill person in making decisions (if capable) or respect prior wishes regarding provision of health care.
- Family efforts will be directed toward a purpose and readjust to changes in life patterns and role functions. Members will accept responsibility for changes.
- The family will identify and use effective coping strategies.
- The family will identify and use available resources as needed to facilitate resolution of the crisis.
- The family will have a sense of control and confidence in meeting personal and collective needs.

NURSING INTERVENTIONS AND *RATIONALE*

1. Identify family's perception of the crisis situation. Determine family structure; roles; developmental phase; and ethnic, cultural, and belief factors that may affect communication with family and the plan of care. Identify strengths of family. ***All initial nursing interventions should be directed toward resolving the crisis situation. Understanding and use of family theory principles will facilitate this process and individualize care.***
2. Provide honest and accurate information in language persons can understand. Give updated information as appropriate. Listen! ***This facilitates open communication between family and health care providers, projects a caring attitude and concern for them and patient, and assists family in making decision and being involved with the plan and goals of care.***
3. Encourage liberal visitation with patient. Prepare family for what they will observe in a technical environment before the visit. Inform them about patient's appearance, behaviors (etc.) that may be distressing to them. Explain the etiology of patient responses to stimuli, (e.g., pain, trauma, surgery, medication) and explain that these behaviors are being monitored and are usually temporary. Encourage them to touch patient and let patient know of their presence. ***This prevents a strong emotional reaction to an unfamiliar and frightening situation; involves family as support to each other and to patient; demonstrates the nurse's concern for them as persons; and facilitates satisfaction with care being provided for their loved one.***
4. Identify and support effective coping behaviors. ***This aids in family's sense of control and resolution of helplessness/powerlessness.***
5. Observe for signs of fatigue and the need for emotional/spiritual support and respite from hospital waiting routine. Encourage family to verbalize feelings. Provide information on available resources. Alert interdisciplinary team members (social, psychologic/spiritual) to family needs. Provide pager device (if available), or obtain phone numbers when family leaves hospital premises. ***This provides support, comfort; facilitates hope; resolves sense of isolation; gives sense of security; and diminishes guilt feelings for attending to personal needs.***
6. Instruct family in simple caregiving techniques and encourage participation in patient's care. ***This facilitates a sense of "normalcy" to experience, self-confidence, and assurance that good care is being provided.***
7. Serve as advocate for patient and family. Teach family how to negotiate with the health care delivery system and include them in health care team conferences when appropriate. ***This facilitates informed decision making; promotes control, satisfaction; and permits mutual goal setting.***
8. Consider nonbiologic or nonlegal family relationships. Encourage contact with patient and participation in care. ***This facilitates holistic care and support of emotional ties and demonstrates respect for the family unit and relationships.***
9. Provide emotional support, compassion when patient's condition worsens or deteriorates. ***The use of touch and expression of concern for the patient and family conveys comfort and trust in the health care provider and respect and assurance that the family's loved one will receive appropriate care and attention.***

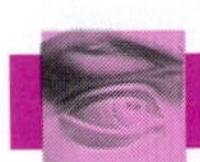

NURSING MANAGEMENT PLAN

ANXIETY

DEFINITION:

A vague, uneasy feeling, the source of which is often nonspecific or unknown by the individual.

Anxiety Related to Threat to Biologic, Psychologic, and/or Social Integrity

DEFINING CHARACTERISTICS

Subjective

- Verbalizes increased muscle tension
- Expresses frequent sensation of tingling in hands and feet
- Relates continuous feeling of apprehension
- Expresses preoccupation with a sense of impending doom
- States has difficulty falling asleep
- Repeatedly expresses concerns about changes in health status and outcome of illness

Objective

- Psychomotor agitation (fidgeting, jitteriness, restlessness)
- Tightened, wrinkled brow
- Strained (worried) facial expression
- Hypervigilance (scans environment)
- Startles easily
- Distractibility
- Sweaty palms
- Fragmented sleep patterns
- Tachycardia
- Tachypnea

OUTCOME CRITERIA

- Patient effectively uses learned relaxation strategies.
- Patient demonstrates significant decrease in psychomotor agitation.
- Patient verbalizes reduction in tingling sensations in hands and feet.
- Patient is able to focus on the tasks at hand.
- Patient expresses positive, futuristic plans to family and staff.
- Patient's heart rate and rhythm remain within limits commensurate with physiologic status.

NURSING INTERVENTIONS AND *RATIONALE*

1. Continue to monitor the assessment parameters listed under "Defining Characteristics."
2. Instruct the patient in the following simple, effective relaxation strategies:
   - If not contraindicated cardiovascularly, tense and relax all muscles progressively from toes to head.
   - Perform slow, deep-breathing exercises.
   - Focus on a single object or person in the environment.
   - Listen to soothing music or relaxation tapes with eyes closed.

   Progressive toe-to-head relaxation releases the muscular tension that may be a stress-related effect resulting from the threat or change in the patient's health status and outcome of illness. Deep-breathing exercises provide slow, rhythmic, controlled breathing patterns that relax the patient and distract him or her from the effects of his or her illness and hospitalization. Focusing on a single object or person helps the patient dismiss the myriad of disorienting stimuli from his or her visual-perceptual field, which can have a dizzying, distorted effect. A clear sensorium allows him or her to feel more in control of his or her environment. Music or words expressed in soft, low tones tend to produce soothing, relaxing effects that counteract or inhibit escalating anxiety and provide respites from the patient's situational crisis. Closed eyes eliminate distracting, visual stimuli and promote a more restful environment.
3. Actively listen to and accept the patient's concerns regarding the threats from his or her illness, outcome, and hospitalization. ***Active listening and unconditional acceptance validate the patient as a worthwhile individual and assure him or her that his or her concerns, no matter how great, will be addressed. Knowledge that he or she has an avenue for ventilation will assuage anxiety.***
4. Help the patient distinguish between realistic concerns and exaggerated fears through clear, simple explanations. *Sample statements:* "Your lab results show that you're doing OK right now." "The shortness of breath you're experiencing is not unusual." "The pain you described is expected, and this medication will relieve it." ***A patient who is informed about his or her progress and is reassured about expected symptoms and management of care will be better equipped to maintain a more realistic perspective of his or her illness and its outcome. Thus anxiety emanating from imagined or exaggerated fears will likely be assuaged or averted.***

Continued

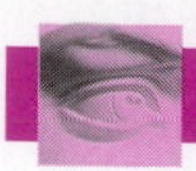

NURSING MANAGEMENT PLAN—CONT'D

ANXIETY

Anxiety Related to Threat to Biologic, Psychologic, and/or Social Integrity

NURSING INTERVENTIONS AND *RATIONALE*—cont'd

5. Provide simple clarification of environmental events and stimuli that are not related to the patient's illness and care. *Sample statements:* "That loud noise is coming from a machine that is helping another patient." "The visitor behind the curtain is crying because she's had an upsetting day." "That gurney is here to bring another patient to x-ray." ***Clarification of events and stimuli that are unrelated to the patient helps to disengage him or her from the extant anxiety-provoking situations surrounding him or her, thus avoiding further anxiety and apprehension.***
6. Assist the patient in focusing on building on prior coping strategies to deal with the effects of his or her illness and care. *Sample statements:* "What methods have helped you get through difficult times in the past?" "How can we help you use those methods now?" (See the Ineffective Individual Coping nursing management plan, pp. 95-97, for interventions that assist patients to use coping strategies effectively.) ***Use of previously successful coping strategies in conjunction with newly learned techniques arms the patient with an arsenal of weapons against anxiety, providing him or her with greater control over his or her situational crisis and decreased feelings of doom and despair.***
7. Give the patient permission to deny or suppress the effects of his or her illness and hospitalization with which he or she cannot cope or control. *Sample statements:* "It's perfectly OK to ignore things you can't handle right now." "How can we help ease your mind during this time?" "What are some things or tasks that may help distract you?" ***Adaptive denial can be helpful in reducing feelings of anxiety in patients with life-threatening illness.*** Bigus* reports that in studies of two groups of patients with myocardial infarction, the group that used adaptive denial demonstrated significantly fewer symptoms of state anxiety than those patients who failed to use it.

*From Bigus KM: *West J Nurs Res* 3:150, 1981.

REFERENCES

1. Barry P: *Psychosocial nursing: assessment and intervention in care of the physically ill,* ed 2, Philadelphia, 1989, JB Lippincott.
2. Glaser J, Glaser R: Perspective on psycho-immune response. In Adler R and others, editors: *Psychoneuroimmunology,* San Diego, 1991, Academic Press.
3. Grendell R: Psychologic aspects of physiologic illness. In Fortinash K, Holloday-Worrett P, editors: *Psychiatric-mental health nursing,* St. Louis, 1996, Mosby.
4. Benner P, Wrubel J: *The primacy of caring: stress and coping in health and illness,* Menlo Park, Calif, 1989, Addison-Wesley.
5. Weissman AD: Coping with illness. In Hackett TP, Cassem NH, editors: *Massachusetts General Hospital Psychiatry,* ed 2, Littleton, Mass, 1987, PSG Publishing.
6. Lazarus R, Folkman S: *Stress, appraisal, and coping,* New York, 1984, Springer.
7. Neurnberger P: *Freedom from stress: a holistic approach,* Honesdale, Penn, 1981, The Himalayan International Institute of Yoga Science and Philosophy.
8. Selye H: *Stress in health and disease,* Boston, 1976, Butterworth.
9. Benner P, Tanner C, Chesla C: *Expertise in nursing practice,* New York, 1996, Springer.
10. Geary P, Formella L, Tringali R: Significance of the insignificant, *Crit Care Nurs Q* 17(3):51-59, 1994.
11. Gerteis M and others, editors: *Through the patient's eyes: understanding and promoting patient-centered care,* San Francisco, 1993, Jossey-Bass.
12. Horrigan B: Critical care nurses make sure ICU experience for patients and their families is as positive as it can be, *Crit Care Nurs Q* Feb Suppl:11-13, 1994.
13. Kozier B, Erb G, Blais K: *Professional nursing practice: concepts and perspectives,* ed 3, Menlo Park, Calif, 1997, Addison-Wesley.
14. Gordon S: The patient driven system, *Crit Care Nurs Q* 14(3)(June suppl):3-28, 1994.
15. Millette B: Client advocacy and the moral orientation of nurses, *West J Nurs Res* 15(5):607-618, 1993.
16. Beyers M: The new reality, *JONA* 26(6):5-6, 1996.
17. Yoder Wise P: *Leading and managing in nursing,* St Louis, 1995, Mosby.
18. Latini E: Trauma critical pathways: a care delivery system that works, *Crit Care Nurs Q* 19(1):83-87, 1996.
19. Byrne B: *Measuring self-concept across the life span,* Washington DC, 1996, American Psychiatric Association.
20. Lee J: Emotional reactions to trauma, *Nurs Clin North Am* 5(4):577, 1970.

21. Smeltzer S, Bare B, editors: *Brunner and Suddarth's textbook of medical-surgical nursing,* ed 8, Philadelphia, 1996, JB Lippincott.
22. Baxley KO and others: Alopecia: effect on cancer patient's body image, *Cancer Nurs* 7(6):499, 1984.
23. Brundage D, Broadwell D: Altered body image. In Phipps W, Long B, Woods N, editors: *Medical-surgical nursing: concepts and clinical practice,* ed 5, St Louis, 1995, Mosby.
24. Janelli, L: Are there body image differences between older men and women? *West J Nurs Res* 15(3):327-329, 1993.
25. Murray, RLE: Symposium on the concept of body image, *Nurs Clin North Am,* 7(4):593, 1972.
26. Norris J, Kunes-Connell M: Self esteem disturbance, *Nurs Clin North Am,* 20(4):745, 1985.
27. Stein K: Schema model of the self-concept, *Image J Nurs Sch,* 27(3):187-192, 1995.
28. Cross S, Markus H: Self-schemas, possible selves and competent performance, *J of Ed Psychol* 86(3):423-438, 1994.
29. Smith S: Extended body image in the ventilated patient, *Intensive Care Nurs,* 5(1):31, 1989.
30. Wright J, Skelton B: *Desk reference for critical care nursing,* Boston, 1993, Jones & Bartlett.
31. Maslow H: *Motivation and personality,* New York, 1954, Harper & Row.
32. Hirst SP, Metcalf BJ: Promoting self-esteem, *J Gerontol Nurs* 10(2):72, 1984.
33. Coward, D: Self-transcendence and correlates in a healthy population, *Nurs Res* 45(2):116-121, 1996.
34. McFarland G, McCann J: Self-perception—self-concept. In Thompson JM and others, editors: *Mosby's clinical nursing,* ed 4, St Louis, 1997, Mosby.
35. Meisenhelder JB: Self-esteem: a closer look at clinical interventions, *Int J Nurs Stud* 22(2):127, 1985.
36. Meisenhelder JB: Self-esteem in women: the influence of employment and perception of husband's appraisals, *Image J Nurs Sch* 18(1):8, 1986.
37. Bennett MJ: Stigmatization: experiences of persons with acquired immunodeficiency syndrome, *Issues Ment Health Nurs* 11:141, 1990.
38. Coopersmith S: *The antecedents of self-esteem,* San Francisco, 1967, WH Freeman.
39. Herr K, Mobily P: Geriatric mental health, chronic pain and depression, *J of Psychosoc Nurs* 30(9):7-12, 1992.
40. Stanley M, Gauntlett-Beare P: *Gerontological nursing,* Philadelphia, 1995, FA Davis.
41. Kim M, McFarland GK, McLane AM: *Pocket guide to nursing diagnoses,* ed 7, St Louis, 1997, Mosby.
42. Meleis AI: Role insufficiency and role supplementation: a conceptual framework, *Nurs Res,* 24(4):264, 1975.
43. Meleis AI: The evolving nursing scholarliness. In Chinn PL, editor: *Advances in nursing theory development,* Rockville, Md, 1983, Aspen Systems.
44. Roberts SL, White BS: Powerlessness and personal control model applied to the myocardial infarction patient, *Progress Cardiovasc Nurs* 5(3):84, 1990.
45. Canaille L and others: A place to be yourself: empowerment from the client's perspective, *Image J Nurs Sch* 25(4):297-303, 1993.
46. Janis IL, Rodin J: Attribution, control, and decision-making: social psychology and health care. In Stone GC, Adler NC, editors: *Health psychology—a handbook,* San Francisco, 1979, Jossey-Bass.
47. Rotter JB: Generalized expectancies for internal versus external control of reinforcement, *Psych Monogr* 80(609):1, 1966.
48. Seligman ME: *Helplessness: on depression, development and death,* San Francisco, 1975, WH Freeman.
49. Radwin L: Knowing the patient: a process model for individualized interventions, *Nurs Res* 44(6):364-370, 1995.
50. Reiley P and others: Discharge planning: comparison of patients' and nurses' perceptions of patients following hospital discharge, *Image J Nurs Sch* (2):143-147, 1996.
51. Farran C, Salloway J, Clark D: Measurement of hope in a community-based older population, *West J Nurs Res* 12(1):42-59, 1990.
52. Herth K: Fostering hope in terminally ill people, *J of Adv Nurs Res* 15:1250-1259, 1990.
53. Herth K: Abbreviated instrument to measure hope: development and psychometric evaluation, *J of Adv Nurs Res* 17:1251-1259, 1992.
54. Beck AT and others: The measurement of pessimism: the hopelessness scale, *J Couns Clin Psych* 42(6):861, 1974.
55. Fryback J: Health for people with terminal diagnoses, *Nurse Sci Q* 6(3):147-159, 1993.
56. Simonton O, Simonton S, Creighton J: *Getting well again,* Los Angeles, 1978, Jeremy P Tarcher.
57. Engel GL: A life setting conducive to illness: the giving up-given up syndrome, *Ann Intern Med* 69:293, 1968.
58. Morse J, Doberneck B: Delineating the concept of hope, *Image J Nurs Sch* 27(4):277-278, 1995.
59. Czerwiec M: When a loved one is dying: families talk about nursing care, *AJN* 96(5):32-36, 1996.
60. Villaire M: Interview with Margaret Campbell: making an end-of-life difference, *Crit Care Nurs Q* 14(1):110-117, 1994.
61. Warren N: The phenomena of nurses' caring behaviors as perceived by the critical care family, *Crit Care Nurs Q* 17(3):67-72, 1994.
62. Miller JF: Developing and maintaining hope in families of the critically ill, *AACN Clin Issues in Crit Care Nurs* 2(2):307, 1991.
63. Geary S: Intensive care unit psychosis revisited: understanding and managing delirium in the critical care setting, *Crit Care Nurs Q* 17(1):51-63, 1994.
64. Strachan G, Glenner G: Delirium, dementia, amnestic and other cognitive disorders. In Fortinash K, Holloday-Worrett P, editors: *Psychiatric-mental health nursing,* St Louis, 1996, Mosby.
65. Fortinash K, Holloday-Worrett P, editors: *Psychiatric-mental health nursing,* St Louis, 1996, Mosby.
66. Johnston K, Rohaly-Davis J: An introduction to music therapy: helping oncology patients in the ICU, *Crit Care Nurs Q* 18(4):54-60, 1996.

67. American Psychiatric Association: *Diagnostic and statistical manual of mental disorders,* ed 4 (revised), Washington, DC, 1994, The Association.
68. Roose SP: Diagnosis and treatment of depression in the medical setting, *J Clin Psychiatry,* 51(suppl):3, 1990.
69. White RW: Strategies of adaption: an attempt at systematic description. In Monat A, Lazarus RS, editors: *Stress and coping: an anthology,* ed 2, New York, 1985, Columbia University Press.
70. Aguilera DC: *Crisis intervention: theory and methodology,* ed 7, St Louis, 1994, Mosby.
71. Weissman AD: *The coping capacity,* New York, 1984, Human Sciences Press.
72. North American Nursing Diagnosis Association: *Nursing Diagnosis: Definitions & Classifications,* St Louis, 1995-1996, The Association.
73. Armentrout D: Heart cry: a biblical model of depression, *J of Psychol and Christianity* 14(2):101-111, 1995.
74. Gillman J and others: Pastoral care in a critical care setting, *Crit Care Nurs Q* 19(1):10-20, 1996.
75. White N, Richter J, Fry C: Coping, social support and adaptation to chronic illness, *West J Nurs Res,* 14(2):211-224, 1992.
76. Astrom G, Norberg A, Hallberg I: Skilled nurses' experiences of caring, *J Prof Nurs* 11(2):110-118, 1995.
77. Villaire M: A day in the life of an ICU nurse, *Crit Care Nurs Q,* Feb suppl:14-15, 1994.
78. Villaire M: Interview with Toni Tripp-Reimer: crossing over the boundaries, *Crit Care Nurs Q* 14(3):134-141, 1994.
79. Buchanan H, Geubtner M, Snyder C: Trauma bereavement program: review of development and implementation, *Crit Care Nurs Q* 19(1):35-44, 1996.
80. Wheeler S: Helping families cope with death and dying, *Nursing* 26:25-30, July 1996.
81. Bomar P, editor, *Nurses and family health promotion: concepts, assessment and interventions,* Philadelphia, 1996, WB Saunders.
82. Specter R: *Cultural diversity in health and illness,* ed 4, Stamford, Conn, 1996, Appleton & Lange.
83. Carson V, Green, H: Spiritual well-being: a predictor of hardiness in patients with Acquired Immunodeficiency Syndrome, *J Prof Nurs* 8(4):209-220, 1992.
84. Douglas S and others: Survival experience of chronically critically ill patients, *Nurs Res* 45(2):73-77, 1996.
85. Rudy E and others: Patient outcomes for the chronically critically ill: special care unit versus intensive care unit, *Nurs Res,* 44(6):324-331, 1996.
86. Keough V, Letizia M: Perioperative care of elderly trauma patients, *AORNJ* 63(5):932-937, 1996.
87. Lazear S: Trauma across the lifespan, 1996, Sacramento, Calif, CME (Continuing Medical Education) Resource
88. Decker W: Psychosocial considerations for bone marrow transplant recipients, *Crit Care Nurs Q* 18(4):67-73, 1995.
89. Juneau B: Psychologic and psychosocial aspects of renal transplantation, *Crit Care Nurs Q* 7(4):62-66, 1995.
90. DePalma J, Townsend R: Ethical issues in organ donation and transplantation: are we helping a few at the expense of many? *Crit Care Nurs Q* 19(1):1-9, 1996.
91. Jalowiec A, Grady K, White-Williams C: Stressors in patients awaiting heart transplant, *Behav Med* 19(4):145-154, 1994.

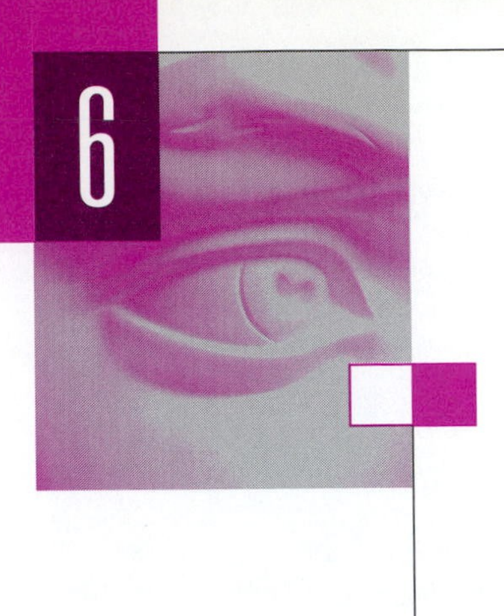

Sleep Alterations

William Shakespeare recognized early the therapeutic value of sleep: "O sleep, o gentle sleep, nature's soft nurse!" Because critical illness requires frequent treatments and 24-hour intensive monitoring, patients admitted to critical care units often suffer an altered sleep pattern. The inability to rest and sleep is one of the causes, as well as one of the outcomes, accompanying illness. Bahr[1] stated, "The phenomenon of sleep has the potential for relieving an individual of stress and responsibility when a break is needed to recharge the person's spirit, mind and body; or, it can remain maddeningly aloof when it is needed most." A lack of sleep can have disastrous results for the critically ill patient. The critical care nurse can promote recovery and healing through facilitating sleep for patients. To do this, the nurse must understand the physiology of normal sleep and recognize events that can potentially disrupt sleep in the critical care environment. The purpose of this chapter is to familiarize the reader with the phenomenon of sleep and the types of sleep pattern disturbances that may occur in critical care and to describe the assessment of sleep pattern disturbances and sleep disorders in critically ill patients.

PHYSIOLOGY OF SLEEP

Sleep has been defined as "a state of unconsciousness from which a person can be aroused by appropriate sensory or other stimuli."[2] Adults normally spend approximately one third of their lives asleep. Research involving simultaneous monitoring using the electroencephalogram (EEG), electrooculogram (EOG), and electromyogram (EMG) has shown that there are two distinct stages of sleep: *rapid eye movement (REM)* and *non-rapid eye movement (NREM)*.

NREM Sleep

NREM sleep is divided into four stages (NREM 1 through 4), which are associated with progressive relaxation. NREM stage 1 is a transitional state, with the EEG pattern being similar to that seen in the awake stage. Figure 6-1 shows EEG patterns of subjects who were awake. Stage 1 is the lightest level of sleep, lasting only 1 to 2 minutes (Figure 6-2). This stage is characterized by aimless thoughts; a feeling of drifting; and frequent myoclonic jerks of the face, hands, and feet. The individual is easily awakened during this stage.

NREM stage 2 differs from stage 1 in that the background wave frequency on the EEG is slower, with *sleep spindles* (characteristic waveforms) superimposed and high voltage spikes known as K-complexes (Figure 6-3).[3] This stage lasts from 5 to 15 minutes, during which the individual becomes more relaxed but is still easily awakened. Stages 1 and 2 in the average young adult constitute 50% to 60% of the total sleep time.

Stages 3 and 4 are characterized by large, slow-frequency delta waves on the EEG and are primarily differentiated by the relative percentage of these waves (Figures 6-4 and 6-5). Random stimuli do not arouse the individual from these deepest levels of sleep. The time spent in stages 3 and 4 varies from 15 to 30 minutes and constitutes approximately 20% of the total sleep time. During NREM sleep, the EOG gradually slows and eye movements cease. EMG patterns also decline, indicating profound muscle relaxation; however, they do not reach the low levels that they do in REM sleep. The parasympathetic nervous system predominates during NREM sleep. The cardiac and respiratory rates, the metabolic rate, and the blood pressure decrease to basal levels. Thus the supply/demand ratio of coronary blood flow is likely to improve.[4] NREM sleep may in fact have antidysrhythmic properties.

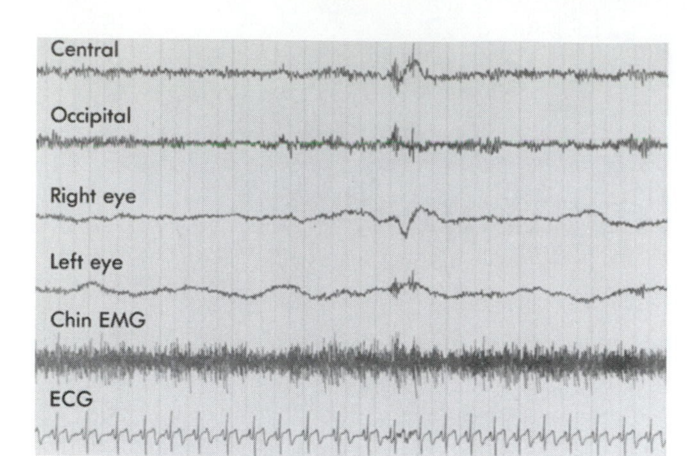

FIGURE 6-1. Awake.

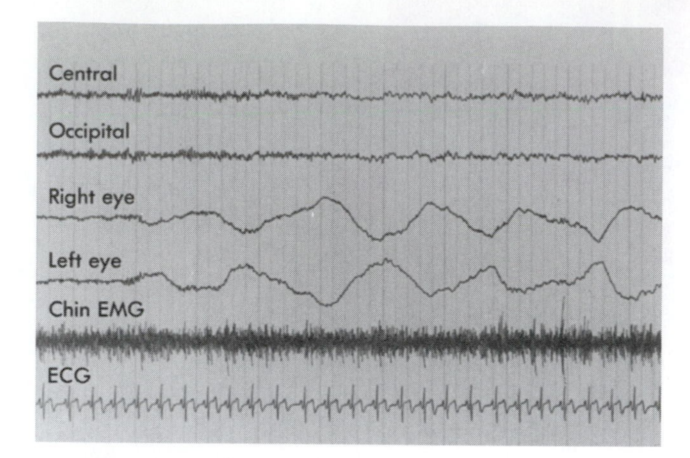

FIGURE 6-2. NREM stage 1 sleep.

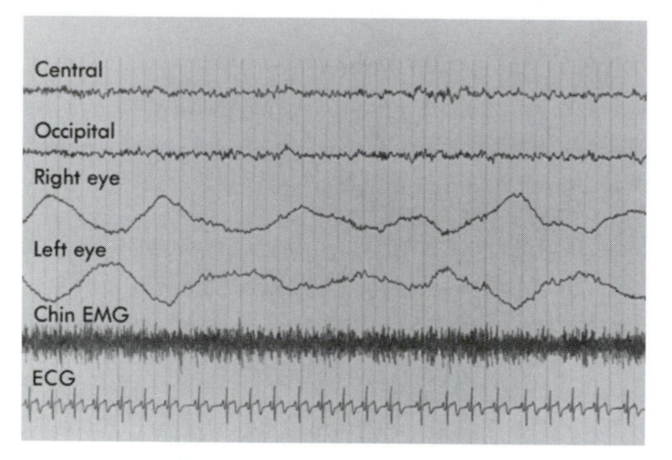

FIGURE 6-3. NREM stage 2 sleep.

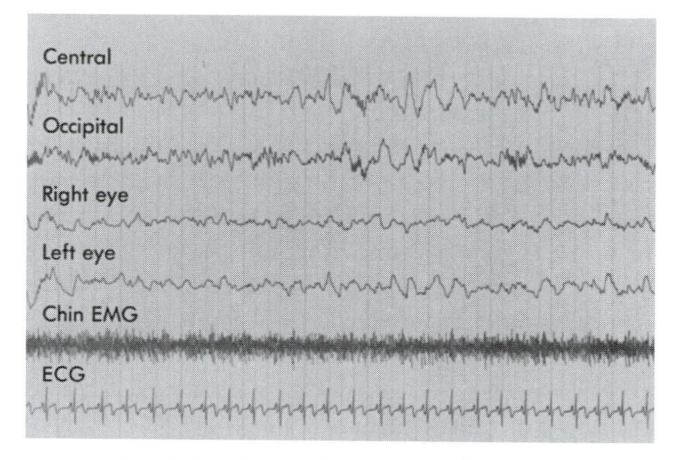

FIGURE 6-4. Delta sleep NREM stage 3.

In addition, during slow wave sleep, growth hormone (GH) is secreted by the anterior pituitary gland and functions to promote protein synthesis while sparing catabolic breakdown. Elevated GH and other anabolic hormones, such as prolactin and testosterone, imply that anabolism is taking place during NREM stage 4, particularly in tissues with a high protein content. Thus activities associated with NREM stage 4 include protein synthesis and tissue repair, such as the repair of epithelial and specialized cells of the brain, skin, bone marrow, and gastric mucosa.[5] NREM dreams are often realistic and thoughtlike, rarely in color, and often similar to a recent activity. These dreams are generally more difficult to remember than are REM dreams. NREM sleep, then, is a time of energy conservation and renewal.

REM Sleep

REM, or *paradoxical,* sleep constitutes 20% to 25% of the total sleep time in the young adult. This type of sleep is paradoxical in that some areas of the brain are quite active during REM sleep, while other areas are suppressed. During REM sleep, bursts of eye movements are seen on the EOG that are often associated with periods of dreaming. EMG patterns become essentially flat, indicating immobility and functional paralysis of the skeletal muscles. The cerebral cortical activity increases during REM so that the EEG patterns resemble those recorded during the waking state (Figure 6-6). During REM sleep, the individual is more difficult to awaken than in any other stage of sleep.[3] In this regard, REM sleep can be thought of as a "dissociative state."

The sympathetic nervous system predominates during REM sleep. Oxygen consumption increases, and cardiac output, blood pressure, heart rate, and respiratory rate may become erratic. An increase in premature ventricular contractions (PVCs) and tachydysrhythmias associated with respiratory pauses may occur during REM sleep.[4] Evidence suggests that the

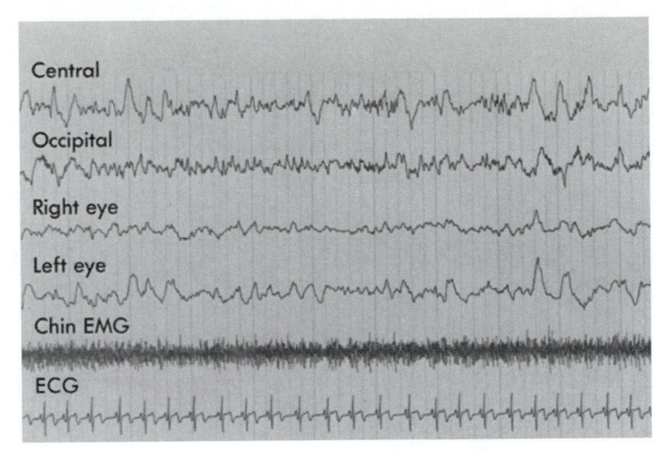

FIGURE 6-5. Delta sleep NREM stage 4.

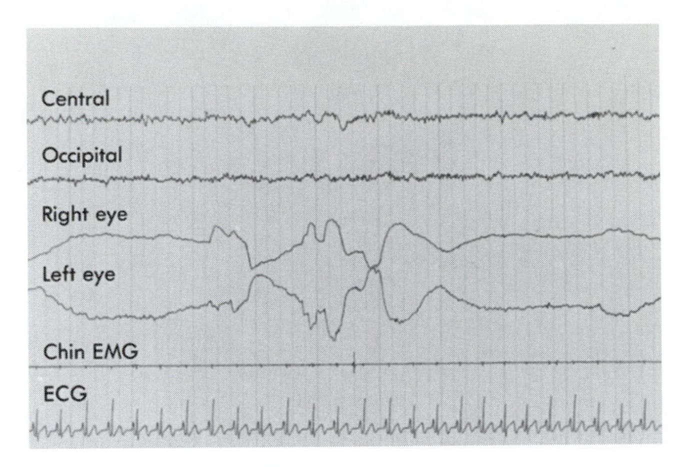

FIGURE 6-6. REM sleep.

adrenalin surge that more than doubles during REM sleep may be responsible for episodes of ischemia, sudden cardiac death, and strokes in the early morning hours.[5,6] Arterial pressure surge and increases in heart rate, coronary arterial tone, and blood viscosity could cause the combination of plaque rupture and hypercoagulability.[7] Serum cholesterol and antidiuretic hormone levels increase, and perfusion to the gray matter in the brain doubles. The dreams of REM sleep tend to be colorful, vivid, and implausible, often containing an element of paralysis. REM sleep filters information stored from the day's activities, sifting the important from the trivial, helping to psychologically integrate activities such as problem solving. REM sleep seems to facilitate emotional adaptation to the physical and psychologic environment and is needed in large quantities after periods of stress or learning. The adequacy of sleep is judged by the relative periods spent in each of the stages of sleep.[8]

REM sleep, like the other stages of sleep, is essential to physiologic and psychologic well-being. REM sleep is of great importance to nurses because as the patient is entering this stage of sleep, the nurse may notice a change in vital signs and become concerned that the patient's condition is worsening. If the nurse increases the monitoring of the patient, adjusts drips, and measures vital signs in response to this perceived change in condition, he or she may awaken the patient. Thus the patient may not get the sleep he or she needs. Further research must address the ways in which the nurse can assess sleep and all of its stages without unnecessarily disrupting the patient from the much-needed sleep. An accurate knowledge of sleep will assist nurses in monitoring patients safely while ensuring that they achieve optimal quality of sleep.

Cyclic Aspects

At the onset of sleep, the individual normally progresses through repetitive cycles beginning with NREM stages 1 through 4 and then backward again to stage 2. From stage 2, the individual enters REM. Stage 2 is then reentered, and the cycle repeats (Figure 6-7). These cycles occur at approximately 90-minute intervals, so that four or five cycles are normally completed in the sleep period. Early in the sleep period, NREM predominates. During the end of the sleep period, NREM periods tend to be longer than those of NREM sleep.

The rhythmic nature of sleep is not unique. The body experiences rhythms in temperature, blood pressure, heart rate, respiratory rate, and hormone secretion. This cyclic 24-hour rhythm has been termed the circadian rhythm. Within the central nervous system, the bilaterally paired suprachiasmatic nuclei are the major endogenous pacemaker for the circadian rhythms. Sleep normally occupies the low phase of the circadian rhythm, whereas wakefulness and activity normally occupy the higher phase. Although regular nighttime sleep is synchronized with other circadian rhythms such as hormone levels, temperature, and metabolic rate, the major determinants of human sleeping are external time cues, light/dark changes, and particular social events such as meal times.[9]

The cyclic nature of sleep and wakefulness is thought to be regulated by complex neurochemical reactions arising in the tissues of the brainstem that are known as the *reticular formation.* The sleep-wakefulness cycles, as well as the REM/non-REM cycle, are thought to be mediated by the neurotransmitters *serotonin, dopamine, norepinephrine,* and *epinephrine.* According to Fordham, "simple explanations or single controls of sleep do not fit with the

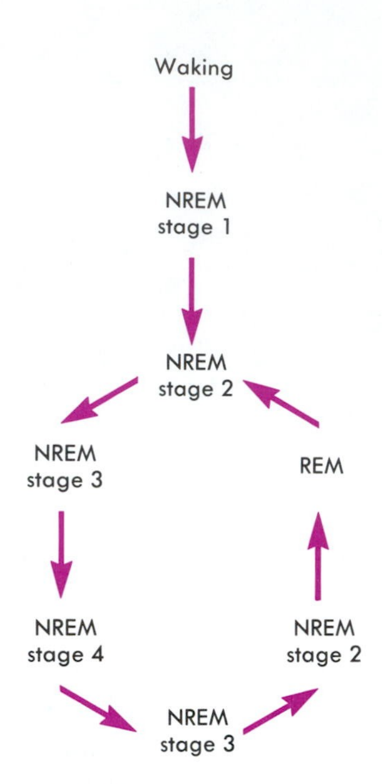

FIGURE 6-7. The cyclic nature of sleep.

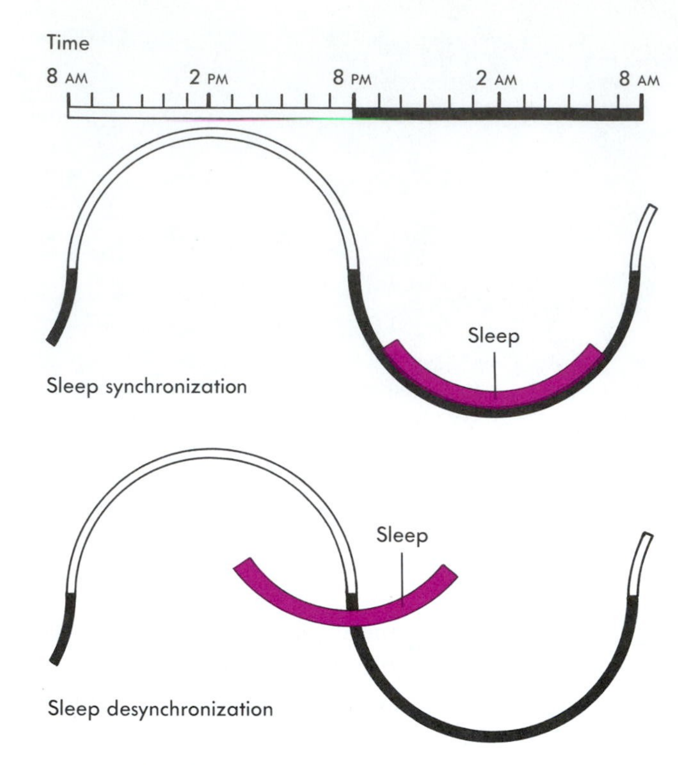

FIGURE 6-8. Sleep synchronization and desynchronization with circadian rhythm.

evidence." Current research suggests that the control of sleep is a very complex process not confined to one localized part of the brain.[10]

It is interesting to note that the neurotransmitters dopamine and serotonin are major determinants of mood and affect. The changes in mood and affect in persons with sleep deprivation and desynchronization may partially be explained by the functioning of these transmitters. It is also interesting to note in light of the major role of neurotransmitters in sleep, that sleep disorders are commonly seen in psychiatric illness; that is, early morning awakenings are classically found with major depressive disorders that are thought to be biochemically induced.

The sleep-wake cycle follows the circadian rhythm in a 24-hour cycle synchronized with other biologic rhythms. Nighttime sleep is the normal pattern for most adults. Serotonin, for example, is usually released around 8 PM to prepare the body for sleep. Conversely, adrenocorticotropic hormone (ACTH), corticotropin-releasing hormone (CRH), and cortisol all normally peak in the early morning hours to prepare the individual for the day's stresses. If a person is deprived of sleep, especially the deeper stages, these hormones will still be released, but at times that may or may not coordinate appropriately with the stresses he or she is about to face. Thus an abnormal sleep pattern will compromise the patient's ability to cope with the stress of critical illness, thereby complicating his or her recovery. When sleep occurs during the low phase of the circadian rhythm, circadian synchronization is present. Sleep that occurs during normal waking hours is out of phase or desynchronized (Figure 6-8). Desynchronized sleep is rated as poor-quality sleep and causes a decreased arousal threshold; therefore frequent awakenings are more likely. Irritability, restlessness, depression, anxiety, and decreased accuracy in task performance are characteristic effects of desynchronized sleep. Resynchronization with the circadian rhythm must occur whenever sleep has become desynchronized for the individual to establish a normal sleep-activity pattern. Although variable among individuals, the resynchronization process is thought to require a minimum of 3 days with a consistent sleep-wake schedule. During resynchronization, the individual often feels fatigued and unable to perform all of his or her activities of daily living.

SLEEP CHANGES WITH AGE

Of the factors that influence the quality of sleep, age is one of the most prominent. The sleep of a normal infant is divided into two types. The first is characterized by no eye or body movements and regular respirations. The second type is associated with eye and body movements and a predominant suck reflex. The first type of sleep develops into NREM sleep and the latter into REM sleep. The infant, unlike the adult, goes from wakefulness directly into REM sleep. By approximately 3 months of age, the full-term infant develops the normal adult pattern of falling from wakefulness into NREM sleep. Infants spend a relatively large proportion of their sleep time in REM sleep. For the full-term newborn this percentage is approximately 40% to 50% of total sleep time. By the age of 3 years, REM sleep is approximately one third of the total sleep time, and by late childhood, REM is one fourth of total sleep time.[11]

As the biologic systems change during the aging process, stress is placed on the human system, and the delicate mechanism of sleep is altered.[12] Hayter,[8] in a study of 212 healthy, noninstitutionalized older adults ages 65 to 93, found extreme variability in the sleep behaviors of different subjects within age-groups. Sleep behaviors between men and women had few differences, although women did report more difficulty getting to sleep and more frequent use of sleep aids than did men. The number of daytime naps and nighttime awakenings and variability in sleep behaviors increased with age. By age 75, the number of naps and length of naptime increased, resulting in a gradual increase in the total sleep time. Therefore both the time needed to fall asleep and the amount of time spent in bed increased with age. These changes—along with more fragmentation, increased sleep-onset problems, and frequent long periods of wakefulness at night—cause elderly persons to perceive an impairment in their quality of sleep. In caring for older persons, it is important to remember that individuals differ widely in terms of both the age of onset of these changes and individual adaptations.

Advanced age involves losses of functional capabilities, health, friends, spouse, and material belongings. Because these losses can lead to depression—a state that is relatively common in the older population—the relationship between depression and sleep disturbance is important for the nurse to consider when working with elderly persons. By disrupting the psychologic state of the elderly patient, these losses may compound existing sleep difficulties.

SLEEP CHANGES WITH CHRONIC ILLNESS

Chronic illnesses tend to increase the frequency and severity of sleep problems. The amount, quality, and consistency of sleep may all decrease as sleep becomes dysfunctional. Although total sleep deprivation rarely occurs outside of the experimental setting, in the critical care unit, sleep is often interrupted and fragmented. When sleep is fragmented, patients spend a greater proportion of their sleep time in the transitional stages (i.e., NREM stages 1 and 2) and less time in the deeper stages of sleep. Illnesses that commonly affect sleep are arthritis, angina pectoris, chronic obstructive pulmonary disease (COPD), congestive heart failure, diabetes mellitus, peptic ulcers, alcoholism, parkinsonism, thyroid disorders, chronic pain, and depression. Both situational stress and long-term anxiety are causes of disrupted and restless sleep. As anxiety and depression increase, so does lack of sleep, and as sleep decreases, anxiety and depression increase—a vicious cycle resulting in disrupted sleep and not feeling rested on awakening.[9]

CIRCADIAN DESYNCHRONIZATION

Circadian disruption, or desynchronization, is a type of sleep-pattern disturbance that may affect critically ill patients. The loss of rhythmicity may result from external stressors, which then alters the timing relationships of neural, hormonal, and cellular systems. Animals and humans respond to stressors, such as surgery, immobilization, and pain, with increased levels and altered timing of adrenal and other hormones. Farr and others[13] reported that circadian levels; the timing of temperature, blood pressure, and heart rate; and urinary excretion of catecholamines, sodium, and potassium were altered after surgery in hospitalized patients. Nurses must closely observe patients for clinical manifestations of such alterations and anticipate problems such as poor responses to physiologic challenges, disruption of sleep, gastrointestinal disturbances, decreased vigilance and attention span, and malaise. Nursing interventions that maintain normal rhythmicity of the day-night cycle—such as opening window blinds, placing clocks and calendars within the patient's view, allowing the patient to retire and rise at familiar times, and following individual sleep-related rituals—should be encouraged. Attention must be given to minimizing disruption during rest periods.[13]

PHARMACOLOGY AND SLEEP

Patients hospitalized in critical care units often receive pharmacologic therapy, which may affect their quality of sleep and compound sleep disturbances. The critical care nurse must be aware of the effects that commonly used drugs have on sleep. In fact, hypnotic

TABLE 6-1 **Common Drugs That Affect Sleep**

Drug	Effect on Sleep	Comments
BARBITURATES		
Amobarbital	Increases NREM 2	Not considered drugs of choice because of toxicity and long-lasting effects
Pentobarbital Secobarbital	Suppresses REM	Often patients experience rebound insomnia, restless sleep, and frequent dreaming and nightmares when drugs are discontinued
Phenobarbital	Decreases REM in doses greater than 200 mg	REM rebound (increased REM in subsequent sleep) after withdrawal of phenobarbital
BENZODIAZEPINES		
Diazepam	Increases NREM 1 Decreases NREM 3 and 4 Decreases REM	NREM suppression is not dose related REM suppression is dose related May increase sleep apneic episodes
Flurazepam	Increases total sleep time Decreases NREM 2, 3, and 4 Decreases REM	Conflicting reports about effects on sleep Long half-life may produce daytime drowsiness
Midazolam	No reports available as of yet	
Triazolam	Decreases sleep latency (time it takes to get to sleep) Decreases awakenings Increases total sleep time	Drug has a short half-life; should not be used for a prolonged time because of decreased effectiveness; use decreased doses with elderly patients
MISCELLANEOUS		
Chloral hydrate	Thought to be an effective sedative that does not disrupt sleep	Drug has a short half-life and some reports of nightmares; increased daytime drowsiness
Chlordiazepoxide Methaqualone	Minimally disrupts sleep	
Morphine	Decreases NREM 3 and 4 Decreases REM	Results in increased spontaneous arousals and overall lighter sleep

drugs have been found to promote the lighter stages of sleep (i.e., NREM stage 2) and may, paradoxically, be the cause of night terrors, hallucinations, and agitation in the elderly.[8] This area has great potential for nursing research. Common drugs that affect sleep are described in Table 6-1.

Barbiturates, sedative-hypnotic, and analgesic medications may compound sleep disorders by further decreasing NREM stages 3 and 4 and REM sleep. Amobarbital, secobarbital, and pentobarbital reduce REM and increase NREM stage 2 sleep.

Diazepam increases NREM stage 1 and reduces NREM stages 3 and 4 and REM. REM suppression depends on the dose, with the larger doses leading to greater suppression. Flurazepam may be an effective hypnotic if administered in dosages equaling less than 60 mg/day. However, the long half-life of flurazepam may lead to morning drowsiness and may increase sleep apneic episodes in susceptible persons.[14] Chloral hydrate has been shown to be an effective sedative that does not simultaneously disrupt sleep. Chlordiazepoxide and methaqualone also minimally disrupt sleep. Triazolam is effective for short-term use in increasing the total sleep time and decreasing the number of nocturnal awakenings, although it decreases REM sleep during the first 6 hours of sleep. These REM changes have been predominantly noted in young adults. An early morning "hangover" may occur with triazolam, and rebound insomnia and retrograde amnesia may occur.[15] Morphine increases spontaneous arousals during sleep and shortens the sleep time by reducing REM and NREM stages 3 and 4, resulting in overall lighter sleep.[13]

The prolonged half-life of medications, coupled with altered metabolism or decreased excretion of the drug resulting from renal or liver disease that may occur in elderly persons, can cause the effects of sedatives to continue into the daytime, leading to confusion and sluggishness. Sedative and analgesic medications must not be withheld, but rather, decreased dosages of drugs that minimally disrupt sleep are to be used to complement comfort measures, with dosages reduced gradually as the medication is no longer necessary. It is the responsibility of the critical care nurse to assess the need for sedative and analgesic medications, to administer them in the most effective manner to promote sleep, and to monitor their effectiveness.

BOX 6-1 Effects of Selective Sleep Deprivation

SYMPTOMS OF NREM SLEEP DEPRIVATION

Fatigue
Anxiety
Increased illness

SYMPTOMS OF REM SLEEP DEPRIVATION

Restlessness
Disorientation
Combativeness
Delusions
Hallucinations

SLEEP DEPRIVATION

Much of what is known about the function of sleep has been learned from observations made when persons are deprived of sleep in the laboratory setting. Both physiologic and psychologic symptoms of sleep deprivation have been reported[15] (Box 6-1). These symptoms may be, but are not always, associated with the length of sleep deprivation. The symptoms vary among individuals with such factors as age, premorbid personality, motivation, and the environment.[10]

Selective *REM deprivation* leads to irritability, apathy, decreased alertness, and increased sensitivity to pain. Continued loss of REM sleep may lead to perceptual distortion and significant disturbance in mental-emotional function, often within 72 hours of REM deprivation. Manifestations of sleep deprivation range from disorientation and restlessness to frank auditory and visual hallucinations, with personality changes, including withdrawal and paranoia.[10]

Selective *NREM deprivation* is less well-studied, but it appears that fatigue is the primary result of NREM deprivation.[16] Because of the renewal, repair, and conservation functions of NREM sleep, deprivation may impair the immune system and depress the body's defenses, rendering the individual more vulnerable to disease and complications.

The critical care environment affects both the quantity and quality of sleep the critically ill patient receives. The patient admitted to the critical care unit is bombarded with combined sensory overload and deprivation. There are unfamiliar sights, sounds, people, and perceptions. Little time for sleep is available in the critical care unit; noise, lights, and patient care activities interfere with sleep patterns.[17,18] Such environmental conditions have been shown to be of primary importance in sleep deprivation in the critical care unit. Dlin and others[18] showed that the chief deterrents to sleep in the critical care unit in order of importance were (1) activity and noise, (2) pain and physical condition, (3) nursing procedures, (4) lights, (5) vapor tents, and (6) hypothermia. Woods and Falk[19] found that 10% to 17% of noises in the critical care unit were of a level capable of arousing patients from sleep (greater than 70 decibels).

Using EEGs, Hilton[20] documented quantity and quality of sleep of nine patients in a respiratory critical care unit. Total sleep time ranged from 6 minutes to 13.3 hours. Only 50% to 60% of the sleep occurred at night, and no patients had complete sleep cycles. NREM stage 1 sleep predominated, to the deprivation of all other stages. Significant deprivation of restorative sleep (NREM stages 3 and 4) was demonstrated, with only 4.7% to 10.5% of sleep time being spent in those stages (normally 30% to 35% of sleep time). Sleep-disturbing events validated by EEG were mainly staff and environmental noise, which occurred on the average of every 20 minutes. Quality and quantity of sleep were reported as poor in all subjects. Nightmares, hallucinations, restlessness, or other behavioral changes were observed in 60% of the patients in the sample. Simpson and others[21] in a study of 102 patients who underwent cardiac surgery showed that nurses can modify many of the factors that disturb sleep by promoting an environment that facilitates improved sleep.

Psychologic stresses and fear associated with the critical care environment and the critical illness make it difficult for patients to relax and fall asleep. Fear and stress precipitate sympathetic nervous system stimulation, which decreases the arousal threshold and results in frequent awakenings and sleep stage transitions.[14]

The relationship between sleep deprivation and delirium in the critical care unit has been shown to be significant. In a study of 62 patients in critical care units and surgical critical care units who ranged in age from 16 to 70 years, Helton and others[22] correlated mental status alterations (disorientation, combativeness, hallucinations, paranoia, and delusions) and sleep deprivation. A 33% increase in mental status alterations was found in severely sleep-deprived patients, defined as those who received less than 50% of their normal sleep time. Shaver, in a review of sleep research, noted that sleep deprivation is considered to be a contributing factor in postoperative psychosis.[23]

Mortality is higher in critical care patients who exhibit symptoms of delirium.[24] Perhaps persons experiencing hallucinations and paranoia (the most severe consequences of sleep deprivation) are in fact dreaming in the awake state. This hypothesis remains to be verified by research; however, caution needs to be taken in diagnosing a previously non–confused elderly patient as having organic mental disorder (OMD) until the possibility of sleep deprivation has been ruled out.

"There is substantial evidence to support the fact that 4 days of sleep deprivation results in a decreased production of adenosine triphosphate (ATP), the critical energy substance. Sleep returns this balance to normal."[25] An understanding of the stages of sleep and the effects of sleep deprivation assists the nurse in evaluating the quantity and quality of sleep that patients receive.

RECOVERY SLEEP

When an individual has been sleep deprived, the changes in physiologic and psychologic performance can be reversed through recovery sleep. Rosa and others[26] found that recall returned to baseline with 4 to 8 hours of recovery sleep after 40 to 64 hours of total sleep deprivation (Figure 6-9).

Deprivation of REM and NREM stage 4 results in rebounds in an attempt to compensate for "debts." The phenomenon of *REM rebound* occurs after selective REM deprivation. In an attempt to make up for lost REM and NREM stage 4 sleep, REM and NREM stage 4 periods quantitatively increase in the sleep periods after the deprivation. NREM stage 4 sleep is preferentially restored first, presumably because of its anabolic function. Because REM sleep is replenished last, it is more likely that REM debts will occur. REM rebound can exacerbate angina, dysrhythmias, duodenal ulcer pain, or sleep apneic episodes.[14] When a patient is exhibiting any of these symptoms and has had a period of sleep deprivation, REM rebound should be considered when determining the cause. Although the symptoms of angina, dysrhythmias, duodenal ulcer pain, and sleep apnea are treated as usual, further REM deprivation should be avoided.

SLEEP DISORDERS

Sleep Apnea Syndrome

Sleep apnea syndromes (SAS), or sometimes called sleep disordered breathing, can be further differentiated as periodic cessation of breathing that results from upper airway obstruction (*obstructive sleep apnea*), a lack of respiratory muscle activity (*central sleep apnea*), or a combination of both (*mixed apnea*).[27] Guilleminault and others[28] have suggested that in all populations except the elderly, more than 30 episodes of apnea per 7 hours of sleep or an *apnea index* (the number of apneas per hour) of five or greater is diagnostic of SAS. Because a relationship exists between advanced age and sleep apnea episodes, further research must be done to determine diagnostic criteria for every age-group. It has been shown that an apnea index exceeding 20 results in greater mortality. Treatment is recommended for patients with an apnea index of 5 to 20 if additional risk factors, such as smoking, hypercholesterolemia, or high blood pressure, are present. An apnea index less than 20 complicated by daytime sleepiness also requires treatment. SAS results in daytime somnolence, systemic or pulmonary hypertension, arterial blood gas abnormalities, life-threatening dysrhythmias, chronic respiratory failure, sexual dysfunction, and mental insufficiency. Hence it is clearly a life-threatening disorder that requires proper diagnosis and treatment.[29]

Obstructive sleep apnea

Definition. Obstructive sleep apnea (OSA) is the most common form of sleep apnea. OSA is characterized by cessation of air flow resulting from upper airway obstruction, although respiratory effort is exerted. Manifestations can range from a few mild symptoms to very severe symptoms that often constitute pickwickian syndrome. The syndrome most commonly affects men older than 50 years and postmenopausal women, with predominant symptoms being snoring and excessive daytime sleepiness. Patients often have associated obesity, large jowls, and thick necks.[30] Other symptoms include systemic and pulmonary hypertension, arterial blood gas abnormalities, life-threatening cardiac dysrhythmias, chronic respiratory failure, sexual dysfunction, and mental insufficiency. An understanding of OSA is helpful to the critical care nurse, because the physiologic effects of the syndrome can be life threatening.

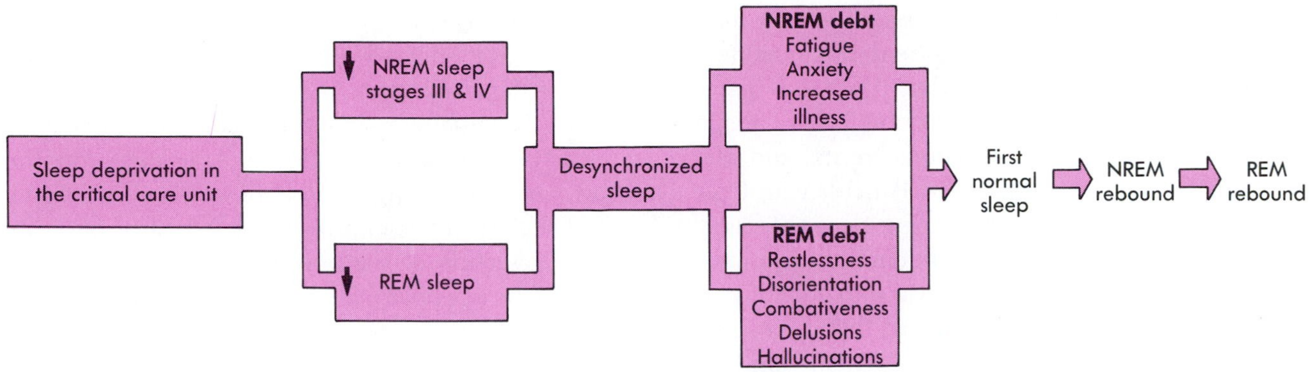

FIGURE 6-9. The effects of sleep deprivation on sleep cycling, debt, and rebound. (Modified from Slota M: *Focus Crit Care* 15(3):41, 1988.)

Etiologic factors. The cause of obstructive sleep apnea is not entirely understood; however, upper airway structure, hormonal balance, and neural control are implicated. Factors that contribute to OSA are (1) anatomic narrowing of the upper airway, (2) increased compliance of the upper airway tissue, (3) reflexes affecting upper airway caliber, and (4) pharyngeal inspiratory muscle function.[31] Computerized tomographies of awake subjects have shown that patients with SAS have narrower airways than do normal subjects. The narrower the airway, the more easily it becomes obstructed.

Upper airway patency is also affected by upper airway function, which is under the control of the respiratory motor neurons. During sleep, this control varies and causes decreased neural activity, thereby narrowing the airway. This effect is especially prevalent during REM sleep when the motor neurons are hypotonic. Unstable control of the respiratory nerves of the diaphragmatic, intercostal, and upper airway muscles can cause sleep apneas.[31] Hypothyroidism can alter respiratory controls and therefore contribute to obstructive sleep apnea. Other contributing disorders are exogenous obesity, kyphoscoliosis, and autonomic dysfunction.

Pathophysiology. Although the pathophysiology of OSA is unclear, hypotheses suggest that the various types of sleep apnea are all actually part of a disease continuum. Failure of the central respiratory rhythm control center to generate a stable rhythm is thought to be the basic defect responsible for sleep apnea syndrome. Cyclic oscillations occur with greater frequency at night and are further exacerbated by mouth breathing.[32]

The patient with obstructive sleep apnea develops cycles of hypoxemia, hypercapnia, and acidosis with each episode of apnea until he or she is aroused and air flow resumes. Alveolar hypoventilation accompanies each episode of apnea and results in hypercapnia. Between episodes, alveolar ventilation improves so that overall there is not retention of CO_2. Morning headaches may result from lingering hypercapnia.

All types of sleep apnea are accompanied by arterial desaturation and potentially by hypoxemia, which may cause pulmonary vasoconstriction and an increased systemic vascular resistance. However, desaturation and hypoxemia are most severe in the obstructive type. With obstruction, inspiratory subatmospheric intrathoracic pressures are abnormally elevated. This leads to a tendency for airways to collapse, resulting in both hemodynamic and electrocardiographic changes.

The extremely elevated pressures that occur in individuals with obstructive sleep apnea who have apneic spells in both REM and NREM stages cause systemic and pulmonary hypertension. Systemic pressures of 200/120 mm Hg (awake control: 130/80 mm Hg) and pulmonary artery pressures of 80/54 mm Hg (awake control: 30/20 mm Hg) have been reported.[32] Cardiac dysrhythmias associated with obstructive apnea include bradycardias, sinus arrest, and occasionally, second-degree heart blocks. After resumption of air flow, tachycardias commonly occur. Thus bradycardia-tachycardia syndrome is associated with obstructive sleep apnea. Careful monitoring can help the nurse identify this syndrome and assist in its diagnosis and treatment.

Assessment and diagnosis. The classic features of obstructive sleep apnea syndrome are daytime sleepiness and nocturnal snoring. Often the patient's sleep partner originally reports the disrupted sleep, because of episodes of apnea and loud, abrupt sounds as breathing resumes. Patients become excessively sleepy during the day because of sleep fragmentation. Daytime napping and dozing at inappropriate times may be reported. Morning headaches are a complaint of many patients with OSA. The headache is frontal and diffuse, disappearing in several hours. Patients with OSA have increased motor activity during sleep. Memory loss, poor judgment, decreased attention span, irritability, personality changes, exercise intolerance, and impotence often lead to employment difficulties and marital problems for sleep apnea patients. Examination of the throat typically reveals enlarged tonsils, uvula, or tongue or excessive pharyngeal tissue.

Diagnosis of obstructive sleep apnea syndrome is made by polysomnogram (PSG), a sleep study. The polysomnogram is used to determine the number and length of apnea episodes and sleep stages, number of arousals, air flow, respiratory effort, oxygen desaturation, and vital signs. This monitoring is done using the electroencephalogram, electrooculogram, electromyogram, and electrocardiogram. Respiratory air flow and effort are measured with nasal and oral thermistors and thoracic and abdominal strain gauges, respectively. Gas exchange is monitored with an ear oximeter or a transcutaneous SaO_2 (oxygen saturation) electrode.

After OSA is diagnosed, the patient's hematocrit (Hct) levels are checked for signs of hypoxia-induced polycythemia. Arterial blood gases are checked to assess for daytime hypoxia or hypercapnia. Thyroid function and the pharynx are evaluated for causes of sleep apnea that can possibly be medically or surgically corrected.

Medical management. Medical management includes mechanical and surgical approaches, as well as the use of medication. Treatment varies depending on the type and extent of the patient's illness. Weight loss for those who are overweight is extremely important in the treatment of obstructive sleep apnea. Alcohol should be avoided, particularly before bedtime.

Nasal continuous positive airway pressure (CPAP) has been the most exciting development in recent years in the treatment of obstructive sleep apnea and is currently the treatment of choice.[29] Positive pressure is delivered via a mask placed over the nose, splinting the airway open. This improves oxygenation and stimulates afferent impulses from the upper airways, resulting in reflex dilation of the upper airways and stimulation of ventilation. Obstructive sleep apnea is improved by nasal CPAP, which in turn improves the sleep pattern and decreases daytime hypersomnolence.

Uvulopalatopharyngoplasty (UPPP) is a surgical approach to the treatment of obstructive sleep apnea. This procedure is used when anatomic abnormalities are the cause of the obstruction and a surgical approach is indicated. Essentially, a large tonsillectomy is performed and redundant tissue is removed. After this procedure most patients no longer snore; however, only 50% experience sleep apnea improvement.[33] Because of the extensive resection of the posterior pharynx, regurgitation may be a problem for as many as 33% of patients. Patient selection by means of cephalometry of pharyngoscopy to identify the specific site of airway obstruction is important to the success of UPPP and other pharyngeal reconstructive surgeries.

Tracheostomy is rarely used in the treatment of obstructive sleep apnea since the development of nasal CPAP. Fewer than 5% of patients currently require tracheostomy.[29] It is indicated for severe apnea with life-threatening dysrhythmias, cor pulmonale, hypersomnolence, and failure of conservative treatment. The complications of tracheostomy are significant, including infection, bleeding, bronchitis, and granulation tissue, as well as the psychosocial complications of an altered body image.

Because obstructive sleep apnea is so well-treated by nasal CPAP, drug therapy is used only if CPAP is ineffective or unavailable. Protriptyline (Vivactil), a nonsedating tricyclic antidepressant, has been shown to decrease the number of apnea episodes and reduce daytime hypersomnolence by suppressing REM sleep when apneic episodes occur. Oxygen may be used to relieve hypoxemia and nocturnal desaturations. In general, drug therapy has been disappointing in the treatment of obstructive sleep apnea.

Nursing management. Nursing management for patients diagnosed with OSA includes educating the patient, monitoring the effects of drug therapy, providing preoperative teaching, and monitoring for and preventing postoperative complications of UPPP or tracheostomy (Box 6-2). Medroxyprogesterone stimulates alveolar hypoventilation but in the dosages required for sleep apnea may be too expensive for some patients, and it may have feminizing effects in men. For these reasons, patient compliance with therapy may be jeopardized. Protriptyline reduces daytime hypersomnolence and nocturnal apneas. In addition to these effects, however, it has the anticholinergic effects of urinary retention and tolerance with prolonged use. Oxygen, as with other drugs, needs careful monitoring to verify its effectiveness and proper dosage.

Nasal CPAP is most effective when patients are properly fitted with the nasal mask and have adequate

BOX 6-2 NURSING DIAGNOSIS AND MANAGEMENT

STATUS POST-UVULOPALATOPHARYNGOPLASTY (UPPP)

- Risk for Aspiration risk factors: impaired laryngeal sensation or reflex; impaired laryngeal closure or elevation; decreased lower esophageal sphincter pressure, p. 727
- Acute Pain related to transmission and perception of cutaneous, visceral, muscular, or ischemic impulses, p. 197
- Sleep Pattern Disturbance related to fragmented sleep, p. 118
- Anxiety related to threat to biologic, psychologic, and/or social integrity, p. 99
- Knowledge Deficit: Reportable Symptoms related to lack of previous exposure to information, p. 61

instruction in the application of the mask and blower. Allowing patients to develop comfort with the equipment facilitates the success of the therapy. If patients are admitted to the critical care unit with a history of obstructive sleep apnea, they need to use their home CPAP equipment as part of their regular sleep routine.

UPPP reduces the number of apneas. Complications of UPPP include hemorrhage, infection, swallowing difficulty, impaired speech, nasal reflux, dry mouth, increased gag reflex, and recurrence of snoring.[33] Patients need close postoperative observation of their airways because of airway edema (see Ineffective Airway Clearance in Chapter 24). Postoperative pain is common but manageable with analgesics. Precautions to prevent respiratory depression in this group of patients are imperative. Patients are to be observed for regurgitation phenomena and signs of infection.

In the event that a tracheostomy is indicated, patients need to be evaluated for their ability to care for the tracheostomy at home. Careful preoperative instruction includes airway management techniques, such as suctioning and routine tracheostomy changes; information about communication techniques with the tracheostomy; explanation of comfort measures, such as pain relief; and close nursing observation. Emphasis is placed on the relief of the apnea symptoms accomplished by the tracheostomy. Patients with UPPP may temporarily require a tracheostomy for airway management after the UPPP procedure. The critical care nurse must support the patient and family during the critical phase after the operation and be especially sensitive to long-term adjustments to changes in body image. In this case, the nurse can assist the patient to deal with possible disenchantment during convalescence.

Central sleep apnea

Definition, etiology, and pathophysiology. Central sleep apnea (CSA) is not a single disease, but rather a heterogenous group of disorders in which breathing ceases momentarily during sleep because of transient withdrawal of central nervous system (CNS) drive to the muscles of respiration.[34] Central sleep apnea is characterized by decreased respiratory output along with the absence of thoracic and abdominal muscle movements. Patients complain of disrupted sleep and of waking with a choking feeling. Snoring may be present. Central sleep apnea is a relatively rare disorder, occurring at perhaps 10% the rate of OSA. Patients tend to be older and have less pronounced oxygen desaturation and hemodynamic effects. The mechanisms involved in central sleep apnea include defects in the respiratory control mechanism or muscles, transient instabilities in respiratory drive, and reflex inhibition of central respiratory drive. Central sleep apnea can be viewed clinically by hypercapnic and nonhypercapnic responses. Hypercapnic CSA arises in the situation of central alveolar hypoventilation or respiratory neuromuscular disease. This type of CSA is associated with encephalitis, brainstem neoplasm or infarction, spinal cord injury, muscular dystrophy, myasthenia gravis, bulbar poliomyelitis, and postpolio syndrome. Nonhypercapnic CSA occurs most often in patients with Cheyne-Stokes respiration secondary to other medical disorders or as an idiopathic disorder.[34]

Assessment and diagnosis. Because the underlying mechanisms are heterogenous, the presenting symptoms are variable as well. Patients with hypercapnic CSA characteristically have symptoms of chronic respiratory failure. Patients with nonhypercapnic CSA demonstrate a pattern of breathing characterized by a waxing and waning of tidal volume. This type of CSA can occur in patients with congestive heart failure and in patients with renal/metabolic disturbances.

Medical management. Central sleep apnea associated with central alveolar hypoventilation is managed generally by noninvasive measures—such as advice not to use sedative medications—and supplemental O_2 at nighttime after an assessment has been made of gas exchange during both sleep and wakefulness. Respiratory stimulants such as medroxyprogesterone can improve ventilation during sleep in selected patients. If noninvasive and pharmacologic measures fail, consideration is given to a phrenic nerve pacemaker for nocturnal diaphragmatic stimulation or some form of assisted ventilation. Assisted ventilation may be intermittent positive pressure ventilation via a snug-fitting nasal mask or may require a tracheostomy. When there is associated neuromuscular weakness, supplemental O_2 and assisted ventilation with a nasal mask are generally very effective.[34]

Nursing management. The nursing management of the patient with central sleep apnea involves careful nighttime observation and assessment of breathing pattern. Anxiety about or fear of sleep because of apneic episodes is common and needs to be confronted. Patient reassurance of continuous nursing observation and monitoring is helpful.

For the patient with a chest cuirass, observation for upper airway collapse as a result of this treatment is essential. Supplemental oxygen may help some patients.[29]

ASSESSMENT OF SLEEP PATTERN DISTURBANCE

Assessment of the patient on admission to the critical care unit includes a description of the normal sleep pattern, including awakenings, naps, normal bedtime and waking time; customary habits that enhance sleep (e.g., number of pillows, extra blankets, nighttime clothing, bedtime rituals, and medications); any recent changes in the patient's normal pattern resulting from the acute illness; recent and more distant history of sleep disturbances; the severity, duration, and frequency of sleep disturbances; and history of chronic illnesses and physical conditions that may disturb sleep, such as COPD, bronchial asthma, bronchitis, arthritis, nocturnal angina, hyperthyroidism, hypertension, duodenal ulcer, or reflux esophagitis and nocturia.

The patient's response to the critical care environment should be assessed, along with the noise level in the patient's immediate environment. The critical care nurse needs to elicit any history of snoring because of its relationship to sleep apnea and sleep disturbances. One effective way to assess the quality of the patient's sleep is for the nurse to ask the patient how his or her sleep in the hospital compares with sleep at home. Because of the extreme variations in sleep behaviors, individual differences must be recognized and a flexible, individualized plan of care formulated to promote rest and sleep. Sleep, like pain, is a multidimensional process with considerable individual variations making the assessment of sleep a difficult process. For this reason, both qualitative and physiologic indices are needed to measure sleep.[35] The scientific standard for the measurement of sleep is the polysomnogram. While the PSG is generally considered a medical diagnostic tool, researchers have employed it to validate the results of observational and perceptual tools used to measure sleep. In normal, healthy individuals a high correlation exists between the person's subjective assessment of sleep recorded on a sleep log or questionnaire and PSG data. However, in hospitalized persons this correlation does not always exist.[6,36]

Another problem in the measurement of sleep is that nurses' observations of patients' sleep have demonstrated both overestimation and underestimation of sleep when compared with PSG recordings. When a tool with specific sleep criteria was used, however, the amount of time a patient actually spent awake during the night (a measure of sleep efficiency) was valid when compared with PSG data.[35]

Sleep efficiency is an important sleep variable—it is defined as the proportion of actual sleep time in the total sleep period. Usual adult sleep efficiency is 95% of actual sleep time, whereas in multisystem trauma patients in the critical care area, it may be as low as 65%.[26] Many patients are at risk for sleep pattern disturbance, including patients with invasive monitoring, those requiring hourly or more frequent assessments and interventions, patients whose illness will require an extended stay in critical care, patients in pain, patients requiring restraint, or patients exhibiting initial signs of sensory overload and sleep deprivation.[37] A nursing sleep record of a patient's sleep for 48 to 72 hours may assist in assessing actual quantity of sleep in addition to assessing necessary and unnecessary wakenings. The sleep record includes the date and time, whether the patient was awake or asleep, and any procedures that necessitated waking the patient. A 24-hour flow sheet such as is common in critical care units could include an area for documentation of sleep. Just as nurses document other data relevant to the patient's recovery, sleep periods of more than 90 minutes in duration, number and length of awakenings, and total possible sleep time need to be recorded and evaluated.

CASE STUDY

The case study is designed to illustrate clinical problem solving and patient care management occurring in actual patients. The case, reviewed retrospectively, demonstrates how medical and nursing diagnoses may be effectively used in critical care. The case study also

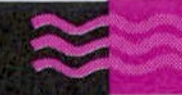

RESEARCH ABSTRACT

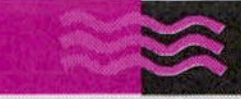

Effects of critical care unit noise on the subjective quality of sleep.

Topf M, Bookman M, Arand D: *Journal Advanced Nursing* 24:545, 1996

PURPOSE

The purpose of this study was to compare the subjective quality of sleep among subjects in two groups: a group that heard an audiotape recording of critical care unit (CCU) sounds and a group that did not hear the audiotape.

DESIGN

Post-test only control group experimental design.

SAMPLE

The sample consisted of 60 females with no hearing loss or sleep problems; the average age was 36 years; and the average education level was 18 years. There were no differences in sample characteristics between the two groups.

PROCEDURE

Subjects were randomly assigned to one of two groups. The experimental group heard an audiotape recording of CCU noises throughout the night; the audiotape was withheld from the control group (quiet group). Both groups were assigned to a sleep laboratory for the study. Subjects participated 1 night per week over 9 months. CCU noises were audiotaped in an eight-bed cardiothoracic CCU during a weekday night. This audiotape was played during the sleep hours for the experimental group. Subjects were given a self-rating questionnaire that assessed subjective sleep in the areas of how long it took to fall asleep, number of awakenings, number of minutes of sleep, and number of positive and negative adjectives regarding their sleep. They were also asked to describe dreams in detail.

RESULTS

There were significant differences between the groups for time to fall asleep ($p < .001$); time spent sleeping ($p < .01$); number of times awakened ($p < .01$); number of positive adjectives descriptive of sleep ($p < .001$); number of negative adjectives descriptive of sleep ($p < .01$); and quality of sleep compared with sleep at home ($p < .05$). There were no significant differences in the quality of dreams between the two groups.

DISCUSSION/IMPLICATIONS

Findings from this study indicate that persons exposed to CCU noises demonstrate poorer subjective sleep compared with those not exposed to CCU noises. Time to fall asleep for the experimental group was much greater than that of the quiet group (60 minutes vs 40 minutes), and number of times awakened was more than double that of the quiet group (7.75 times vs 3.2 times). Although the study consisted of a small sample size and was conducted in a controlled laboratory setting, it has implications for clinical practice. An environmental assessment of all of the sounds, as well as their loudness, can be conducted as quality improvement in sleep for patients. Research can be further developed for implementation in the clinical setting so that other variables affecting sleep in the clinical setting can be assessed.

demonstrates revisions to the plan of care and the nursing and medical management outcomes that are apt to occur during the course of a complicated hospitalization as the patient responds physiologically to treatment. Often, in a short case anecdote, such as presented in this chapter, the clinical answer may appear to be obvious from the day of admission. In practice, however, critical care patient management is sometimes investigative, and the "correct" diagnosis for an individual patient may not become apparent until midway in the hospitalization. Additionally, a patient with an apparently straightforward diagnosis may develop an unexpected complication, and the plan of care and potential outcomes will then require revision. Many of the case studies in this text demonstrate this principle.

The nursing management plans, which—unlike the case study—are not patient-specific, provide a basis nurses can use to individualize care for their patients. Use of the case study and management plans in this chapter can enhance the understanding and application of the *Sleep* content in clinical practice. See the nursing management plans at the end of this chapter.

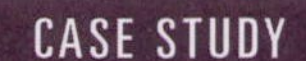

CASE STUDY

SLEEP

CLINICAL HISTORY

Mr. T is a 73-year-old, muscular, well-nourished, retired construction worker. He has a history of moderate restrictive lung disease. Also, he has had several cerebral vascular accidents, which affected Broca's speech area, but he is now without residual effects. He has a permanent VVI pacemaker for sick sinus syndrome.

CURRENT PROBLEMS

Mr. T arrived at the clinic with chest discomfort that did not radiate and shortness of breath with exertion. Echocardiogram evaluation showed a large aneurysm of the ascending aorta and aortic dilation, stenosis, and insufficiency.

EMERGENCY MEDICAL MANAGEMENT

Surgical intervention was recommended. Mr. T had an unstable intraoperative course that involved a 4-hour run on heart-lung bypass, including circulatory arrest with profound hypothermia (to 16° C) and retrograde cerebral perfusion for 63 minutes. He was admitted to the surgical intensive care unit. His postoperative course was complicated by excessive bleeding secondary to coagulopathy; this required massive blood product replacement. He also experienced pulmonary shunting, which required an FIO_2 of .80 with positive end-expiratory pressure (PEEP) of 15 cm H_2O to maintain adequate oxygenation. Three days postoperatively Mr. T was responsive to commands, although he required Versed at 1 mg/hr. Mr. T received Lasix per IV drip and as a result diuresed some of the 25-pound weight gain. He made slow but definite progress, with decreasing oxygen needs.

MEDICAL DIAGNOSIS

Elective resection and grafting of ascending aortic aneurysm complicated by coagulopathy and acute respiratory distress syndrome (ARDS)

NURSING DIAGNOSES

- Impaired Gas Exchange related to ventilation/perfusion mismatch
- Altered Nutrition: Less than Body Requirements related to lack of exogenous nutrients
- Sleep Pattern Disturbance risk factors: fragmented sleep and/or circadian desynchronization

PLAN OF CARE

1. Continue to monitor for impaired gas exchange.
2. Monitor for altered tissue perfusion.
3. Monitor for altered nutrition, including effects on healing, infection, and skin integrity.
4. Monitor for sleep pattern disturbance by initiating a sleep record to document actual sleep cycles.

MEDICAL AND NURSING MANAGEMENT AND PATIENT OUTCOME

Mr. T's cardiopulmonary status stabilized such that he could be weaned successfully from epinephrine, Levophed, and amrinone drips, requiring only a dobutamine drip. He started total parenteral nutrition on the fifth postoperative day. Mr. T continued to require mechanical ventilation; however, the FIO_2 he required could be decreased to .40 with PEEP of 5 cm H_2O. Mr. T continued to require sedation; every time it was decreased, he became so restless that there was danger of dislodging the endotracheal tube. A neurologist was consulted, and a CT scan documented a recent cerebral infarct. Mr. T was following commands with both sides of his body although the left side was weaker than the right. The sleep record indicated that for the past week Mr. T had potentially accomplished only two sleep cycles in any 24-hour period. Eleven days postoperatively, Mr. T began to show signs of extreme agitation. Haldol was ordered and scheduled to be administered q 4 hours.

MEDICAL DIAGNOSIS

Resolving ARDS and inability to wean from mechanical ventilation

NURSING DIAGNOSES

- Sleep Pattern Disturbance related to circadian desynchronization and fragmented sleep
- Activity Intolerance related to prolonged immobility

CASE STUDY—CONT'D

SLEEP

REVISED PLAN OF CARE

1. Modify environmental factors to promote sleep.
2. Assess patient's sleep history as reported by spouse. Assess bedtime rituals, daily routines, factors that contribute to comfort and relaxation.
3. Balance patient's activity with rest periods. Schedule activity to decrease 2 hours before bedtime.
4. Help patient maintain a consistent sleep/wake cycle.
5. Continue to document sleep pattern with periods of time awake.
6. Encourage patient to assist in his personal care. Begin with low energy ADLs, such as face washing and oral care.

MEDICAL AND NURSING MANAGEMENT AND PATIENT OUTCOME

Mr. T was moved to a private room. Designated times for rest were initiated, with one rest period in the morning and one in the afternoon. At home, Mr. T customarily had fallen asleep watching TV at 10:30 PM. His family brought in pictures of family members for his room and an afghan Mr. T used when he slept on the couch at home. Mr. T's agitation decreased. His sleep pattern was now four or five sleep cycles at night, with one consistent nap per day. He was gaining energy and was able to sit in a chair for 2 hours without tiring. He was able to wash his face and perform oral care with assistance. A tracheostomy was performed on the fourteenth postoperative day.

MEDICAL DIAGNOSIS

Same

NURSING DIAGNOSIS

Sleep Pattern Disturbance related to fragmented sleep and circadian desynchronization

REVISED PLAN OF CARE

1. Continue with measures to promote sleep.
2. Continue to encourage small increments of self-care. Teach strengthening exercises that patient can perform in bed.
3. Encourage participation in decision making related to care through use of a communication board.
4. Begin oral feedings with patient assisting as tolerated.

MEDICAL AND NURSING MANAGEMENT AND PATIENT OUTCOME

Mr. T continued to gain strength and maintained four or five sleep cycles per night. He was able to be weaned from the ventilator to a tracheostomy cradle at 40% oxygen. Tube feedings were continued at night to supplement a full liquid diet. Mr. T was transferred to the intermediate care area in good spirits and was able to communicate his wishes. He was making steady progress in his ability to ambulate to and from the chair in his room.

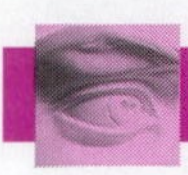

NURSING MANAGEMENT PLAN

SLEEP PATTERN DISTURBANCE

DEFINITION:

Disruption of sleep time causes discomfort or interferes with desired life-style.

Sleep Pattern Disturbance Related to Fragmented Sleep

DEFINING CHARACTERISTICS

- Decreased sleep during one block of sleep time
- Daytime sleepiness
- Sleep deprivation
  - Less than one half of normal total sleep time
  - Decreased slow-wave, or REM sleep
- Anxiety
- Fatigue
- Restlessness
- Disorientation and hallucinations
- Combativeness
- Frequent wakenings
- Decreased arousal threshold

OUTCOME CRITERIA

- Patient's total sleep time approximates patient's normal.
- Patient can complete sleep cycles of 90 minutes without interruption.
- Patient has no delusions, hallucinations, illusions.
- Patient has reality-based thought content.
- Patient is oriented to four spheres.

NURSING INTERVENTIONS AND *RATIONALE*

1. Continue to monitor the assessment parameters listed under "Defining Characteristics."
2. Assess normal sleep pattern on admission and any history of sleep disturbance or chronic illness that may affect sleep or sedative/hypnotic use. Promote normal sleep activity while patient is in critical care unit. Assess sleep effectiveness by asking patient how his or her sleep in the hospital compares with sleep at home. (See Chapter 5, Psychosocial Alterations, for management of acute confusion.)
3. Minimize awakenings ***to allow for at least 90-minute sleep cycles.*** Continually assess the need to awaken the patient, particularly at night. Distinguish between essential and nonessential nursing tasks. Organize nursing management to allow for maximum amount of uninterrupted sleep while ensuring close monitoring of the patient's condition. Whenever possible, monitor physiologic parameters without waking the patient. Coordinate awakenings with other departments, such as respiratory therapy, laboratory, and x-ray, ***to minimize sleep interruptions.***
4. Minimize noise, particularly that of the staff and noisy equipment. Reduce the level of environmental stimuli.
5. Plan nap times to assist in equilibrating the normal total sleep time. Discourage or prevent catnaps (sleep lasting longer than 90 minutes at a time) ***because these physically refresh the individual and thereby decrease the stimulus for longer sleep cycles in which REM sleep is obtained.*** Early morning naps, however, may be beneficial in promoting REM sleep ***because a greater proportion of early morning sleep is allocated to REM activity.***
6. Promote comfort, relaxation, and a sense of well-being. Treat pain. Eliminate stressful situations before bedtime. Use of relaxation techniques, imagery, backrubs, or warm blankets may be helpful. Other interventions may include increased privacy or a private room and providing the patient with his or her own garments or coverings. Individual patients may prefer quiet or may prefer the background noise of the television ***to best promote sleep.***
7. Be aware of the effects of commonly used medications on sleep. ***Many sedative and hypnotic medications decrease REM sleep.*** Sedative and analgesic medications should not be withheld, but rather, drugs that minimally disrupt sleep are to be used to complement comfort measures, with dosages reduced gradually as the medication is no longer necessary. Do not abruptly withdraw REM suppressing medications, ***because this can result in "REM rebound."***
8. Foods containing tryptophan (e.g., milk or turkey) may be appropriate ***because these promote sleep.***
9. Be aware that the best treatment for sleep deprivation is prevention.
10. Facilitate staff awareness that sleep is essential and health promoting. Assess the critical care unit for sleep-reducing stimuli and work to minimize them.
11. Document amount of uninterrupted sleep per shift, especially sleep episodes lasting longer than 2 hours. This can be effectively documented as part of the 24-hour flow sheet and reported routinely, shift to shift. ***Sleep pattern disturbance is diagnosed, treated, and resolved more efficiently when formally documented in this manner.***

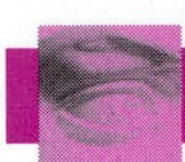

NURSING MANAGEMENT PLAN

Sleep Pattern Disturbance Related to Circadian Desynchronization

DEFINING CHARACTERISTICS

- Sleep is out of synchronization with biologic rhythms, resulting in sleeping during the day and awakening at night
- Anxiety and restlessness
- Decreased arousal threshold

OUTCOME CRITERIA

- Majority of patient's sleep time will fall during low cycle of the circadian rhythm (normally at night).

NURSING INTERVENTIONS AND *RATIONALE*

1. Continue to monitor the assessment parameters listed under "Defining Characteristics."
2. Assist patient to maintain normal day-night cycles by decreasing lighting, noise, and sensory stimulation at night and critically evaluating the need to awaken the patient at night. Maintain a regular schedule for external time cues, such as mealtimes and favorite television shows.
3. Increase activity during the daytime to stimulate wakefulness. Increased physical activity until 2 hours before bedtime is useful in ***promoting naturally induced sleep.*** Limiting caffeine intake after early afternoon will promote sleep in the evening.
4. Do not schedule routine procedures at night.
5. Be aware that cardiac dysrhythmias can be precipitated by the decreased arousal threshold secondary to desynchronization.
6. If desynchronization occurs, plan for resynchronization by maintaining constancy in day-night pattern for at least 3 days (may require 5 to 12 days to reacclimatize). Plan for activities during the day ***to stimulate wakefulness*** and use comfort measures (comfortable body position, warm blankets, backrub, etc.) ***to promote sleep*** at night. Resynchronization is characteristically associated with chronic fatigue, malaise, and a decreased ability to perform life tasks.

REFERENCES

1. Bahr R: Sleep-wake patterns in the aged, *J Gerontol Nurs* 9(10):534, 1983.
2. Guyton AC: *Medical physiology,* ed 8, Philadelphia, 1991, WB Saunders.
3. Rechtschaffen A, Kales A: *A manual of standardized terminology, techniques and scoring systems for sleep stages of human subjects,* Washington DC, 1968, US Department of Health, Education and Welfare.
4. Verrier RL, Kirby DA: Sleep and cardiac arrhythmias, *Ann N Y Acad Sci* 533:238, 1988.
5. Somers VL and others: Sympathetic/nerve activity during sleep in normal subjects, *N Engl J Med* 328(5):303, 1993.
6. Closs SJ: Assessment of sleep in hospitalized patients: a review of methods, *J Adv Nurs* 13:501, 1988.
7. Muller JE, Tofler MB, Stone PH: Circadian variation and triggers of onset of acute cardiovascular disease, *Circulation* 79(4):733, 1989.
8. Hayter J: Sleep behaviors of older persons, *Nurs Res* 32(4):242, 1983.
9. Hodgson L: Why do we need sleep: relating theory to nursing practice, *J Adv Nurs* 16:1503, 1991.
10. Fordham M: In Wilson Bennett J, Butemp L, editors: *Patient problems: a research base for nursing care,* London, 1988, Scutain Press.
11. Slota MC: Implications of sleep deprivation in the pediatric critical care unit, *Focus Crit Care* 15(3):35, 1988.
12. Wilse WB: Age related changes in sleep, *Clin Geriatr Med* 5(2):275, 1989.
13. Farr LA, Campbell-Grossman C, Mack JM: Circadian disruption and surgical recovery, *Nurs Res* 37(3):170, 1988.
14. Sanford S: Sleep and the cardiac patient, *Cardiovasc Nurs* 19(5):19, 1983.
15. Brewer MJ: To sleep or not to sleep: the consequences of sleep deprivation, *Crit Care Nurse* 5(6):35, 1985.
16. Wotring K: Using research in practice, *Focus Crit Care* 9(5):34, 1982.
17. Kido L: Sleep deprivation and intensive care unit psychosis, *Emphasis: Nurs* 4(1):23, 1991.
18. Dlin B, Rosen H, Dickstein K: The problems of sleep and rest in the intensive care unit, *Psychosomatics* 12:155, 1971.
19. Woods N, Falk S: Noise stimuli in the acute care area, *Nurs Res* 23:144, 1974.
20. Hilton B: Quantity and quality of patient's sleep and sleep disturbing factors in a respiratory intensive care unit, *J Adv Nurs* 1:453, 1976.
21. Simpson T, Rayshan LE, Cameron C: Patient's perceptions of environmental factors that disturb sleep after cardiac surgery, *Am J Crit Care* 5(3):173, 1996.

22. Helton M, Gordon S, Nunnery S: The correlation between sleep deprivation and ICU syndrome, *Heart Lung* 9(3):464, 1980.
23. Shaver JL, Giblin EC: Sleep, *Annu Rev Nurs Res* 4:71-93, 1989.
24. Noble M: Communication in the ICU: therapeutic or disturbing, *Nurs Outlook* 27:195, 1979.
25. Fabijan M, Gosselin M: How to recognize sleep deprivation in your ICU patient and what to do about it, *Can Nurse* 4:20, 1982.
26. Rosa R, Bonnet M, Warm J: Recovery of performance during sleep following sleep deprivation, *Psychophysiology* 20:152, 1983.
27. Noureddine S: Sleep apnea: a challenge in critical care, *Heart Lung* 25(1):37, 1996.
28. Guilleminault C, van den Hoed J, Milter M: Clinical overview of sleep apnea syndrome. In Guilleminault C, Dement WC, editors: *Sleep apnea syndromes,* New York, 1978, Alan R Liss.
29. Kryger MH, Roth T, Dement W: *Principles and practice of sleep medicine,* Philadelphia, 1994, WB Saunders.
30. Katz I and others: Do patients with obstructive sleep apnea have thick necks? *Am Rev Resp Disorders* 141:1228, 1990.
31. Hudgel DW: Mechanisms of obstructive sleep apnea, *Chest* 101:541, 1992.
32. Bjurstrom R, Schoene R, Pierson D: The control of ventilatory drives: physiology and clinical applications, *Respir Care* 31(11):1128, 1986.
33. Sanders M and others: The acute effects of uvulopalatopharyngoplasty on breathing during sleep in sleep apnea patients, *Sleep* 11(1):75, 1988.
34. Bradley TD, Phillipson EA: Central sleep apnea, *Clin Chest Med* 13(3):493, 1992.
35. Fontaine DK: Measurement of nocturnal sleep patterns in trauma patients, *Heart Lung* 18(4):402, 1989.
36. Richards KC, Bairnsfather L: A description of night sleep patterns in the critical care unit, *Heart Lung* 17(1):35, 1988.
37. Spenceley S: Sleep inquiry: a look with fresh eyes, *Image J Nurs Sch* 25(3):249, 1993.

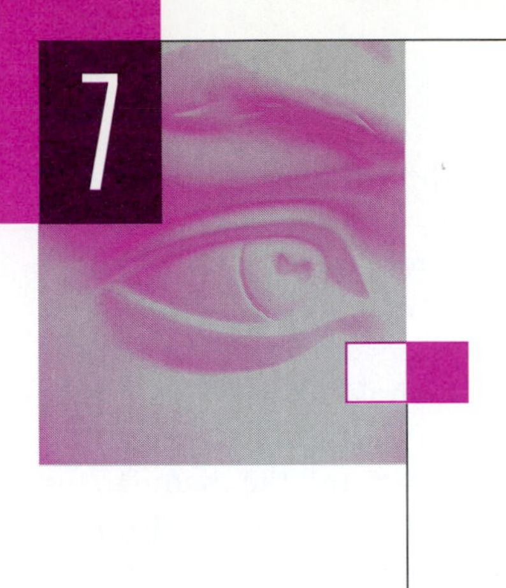

Nutritional Alterations and Management

NUTRIENT METABOLISM

Energy-yielding Nutrients

THE ENERGY-YIELDING nutrients are carbohydrates, proteins, and fats. They are composed mostly of carbon, hydrogen, and oxygen. For proper metabolic functioning, adequate amounts of vitamins, electrolytes, minerals, and trace elements also must be supplied. The process by which these nutrients are used at the cellular level is known as *metabolism.* The major purpose of nutrient metabolism is the production of energy and the preservation of lean body mass.

Carbohydrates. Through the process of digestion, carbohydrates are broken down into glucose, fructose, and galactose. After absorption from the intestinal tract, fructose and galactose are converted to glucose, the primary form of carbohydrate used at the cellular level. Glucose provides the energy needed to maintain cellular functions, including transport of substrates across cellular membranes, secretion of specific hormones, muscular contraction, and the synthesis of new substances. Most of the energy produced from carbohydrate metabolism is used to form adenosine triphosphate (ATP), the principal form of immediately available energy within the cytoplasm and nucleoplasm of all body cells. One gram of carbohydrate provides approximately 4 kcal of energy.

One form of carbohydrate that is poorly digested by the majority of the world's adults is lactose, or milk sugar. In *lactose intolerance,* the individual lacks lactase, the intestinal enzyme required for digestion of lactose. Consumption of lactose often causes abdominal cramping, bloating, and diarrhea. The individual with lactose intolerance may tolerate cheeses, yogurt, acidophilus milk, and buttermilk, since these products contain less lactose than unmodified milk. In addition, lactase enzyme supplements are available to be taken orally, and some markets now sell milk that has been treated with lactase.

Inside the cell, glucose is either stored as glycogen or lipid, or it is metabolized for the release of energy. Liver and muscle cells have the largest glycogen reserves. In addition to glucose obtained from glycogen, glucose can be formed from lactate, amino acids, and glycerol. This process of manufacturing glucose from nonglucose precursors is called *gluconeogenesis.* Gluconeogenesis is carried out at all times, but it becomes especially important in maintaining a source of glucose in times of increased physiologic need and limited exogenous supply. Only the liver and, to a lesser extent, the kidney are capable of producing significant amounts of glucose for release into the blood for use by other tissues; other tissues that store glycogen or perform gluconeogenesis use the carbohydrate to meet their own energy needs.

Proteins. Proteins are made up of chains of amino acids. Each amino acid consists of carbon, hydrogen, and oxygen, as well as nitrogen in the form of the amine group NH_2. Amino acids are the protein components that can be used at the cellular level.

Proteins have important structural and functional duties within the body. Proteins provide the structural basis of all lean body mass, such as the vital organs and skeletal muscle. Proteins are important for visceral (cellular) functions such as initiation of chemical reactions (hormones and enzymes), transportation of other substances (apoproteins and albumin), preservation of immune function (antibodies), and maintenance of osmotic pressure (albumin) and blood neutrality (buffers). Some amino acids are used for energy, providing approximately 4 kcal per gram.

Proteins constantly are synthesized, broken down into amino acids, and then resynthesized into new protein. This three-step process is called *protein turnover.* In very active tissues—such as those of the gut, liver, and kidney—protein turnover occurs every few days. The average turnover time of all body protein has been estimated at 80 days; the rate of turnover is fastest in enzymes and hormones involved in metabolic activities. If necessary, 90% of endogenous protein can be reused, with the diet providing the remaining 10% for protein synthesis. To preserve lean body mass, a constant supply of protein must be ensured.

Through digestion, complex proteins, which are too large to be absorbed intact, are broken down into amino acids and dipeptides or tripeptides (composed of two or three amino acids, respectively) that can be absorbed across the intestinal wall. Certain amino acids are *essential;* that is, they cannot be produced by the body and must be supplied through the diet. Essential amino acids include valine, leucine, isoleucine, lysine, phenylalanine, tryptophan, threonine, and methionine, as well as histidine and arginine in infants. Other amino acids are *nonessential;* they can be manufactured by the body under normal circumstances if the essential amino acids are in adequate supply.

The amine group is essential for protein synthesis, but it is the nonamine portion of the molecule (the "keto-acid") that is used in gluconeogenesis. If a keto-acid is used for gluconeogenesis, the amine group can be excreted in the urine as ammonia or urea. Therefore if the rate of gluconeogenesis rises, urinary nitrogen excretion also rises. In assessing protein nutrition, it is common to measure *nitrogen balance,* or the amount of nitrogen excreted compared with that consumed. The urinary route is ordinarily the major route of nitrogen excretion, so in determining nitrogen balance, urinary nitrogen excretion is measured (preferably over a 24-hour period). Nitrogen intake is recorded over the same time period, and losses of nitrogen from feces and other routes is usually estimated. Most healthy adults are in nitrogen equilibrium, excreting an amount equivalent to the amount they consume. Individuals who excrete less nitrogen than they consume are in *positive nitrogen balance;* this occurs during growth, pregnancy, and healing. Individuals who excrete more nitrogen than they consume are in *negative nitrogen balance;* this state is common in the early posttrauma or postoperative period. When the rate of gluconeogenesis is excessive, extensive loss of structural and visceral (cellular) proteins can occur. Visceral proteins, including immunoglobulins, albumin, and complement, are critical for survival. Preservation of body protein is therefore a key goal of nutritional support of critically ill patients.

Fat (lipids). Lipids include fatty acids, triglycerides (three fatty acids bound to a glycerol backbone), phospholipids (lipids containing phosphate groups), cholesterol, and cholesterol esters. Aside from their involvement in such functions as the maintenance of cell membranes and the manufacture of prostaglandins, lipids—primarily in the form of triglycerides—provide a stored source of energy. They are calorically dense molecules, providing more than twice the amount of energy per gram (9 kcal) as protein and carbohydrates.

Most dietary lipids—consisting primarily of triglycerides—are too large to be absorbed intact and are hydrolyzed in the intestine to form monoglycerides and diglycerides, which contain one or two fatty acids, respectively, bound to glycerol. Bile salts produced in the liver are detergents, and they promote the formation of micelles (emulsions of fatty acids, monoglycerides, and bile salts). Long-chain fatty acids, which contain more than 12 carbon atoms, are very insoluble in water; they are found mainly in the interior of the micelle. The external portion of the micelle is more water soluble than the interior portion. This allows the micelle to cross the unstirred water layer that coats the intestinal absorptive surface. Once inside the intestinal cells, monoglycerides and long-chain fatty acids rejoin to form triglycerides, and they are surrounded by specific proteins to form chylomicrons. These chylomicrons are transported out of the intestine through the lymphatic system, finally entering blood circulation through the thoracic duct. Some of the chylomicrons are taken up by the liver, but the majority are directly transported to other tissues. Short-chain fatty acids (less than 8 carbon atoms long) and medium-chain fatty acids (8 to 12 carbon atoms long) are more water soluble than longer fatty acids; triglycerides containing these fatty acids can be absorbed without hydrolysis and are soluble enough to be transported to the liver via the portal vein, without chylomicron formation (Figure 7-1). Short- and medium-chain fatty acids have advantages in nutritional care of patients who have insufficient bile salt formation or inadequate intestinal surface area for absorption of long-chain fatty acids.

With the aid of the enzyme *lipoprotein lipase,* triglyceride-containing chylomicrons are broken down outside the cell and enter the cell as fatty acids and glycerol. (Heparin stimulates lipoprotein lipase, and low doses of heparin are sometimes given to patients receiving intravenous lipid emulsions to improve lipid

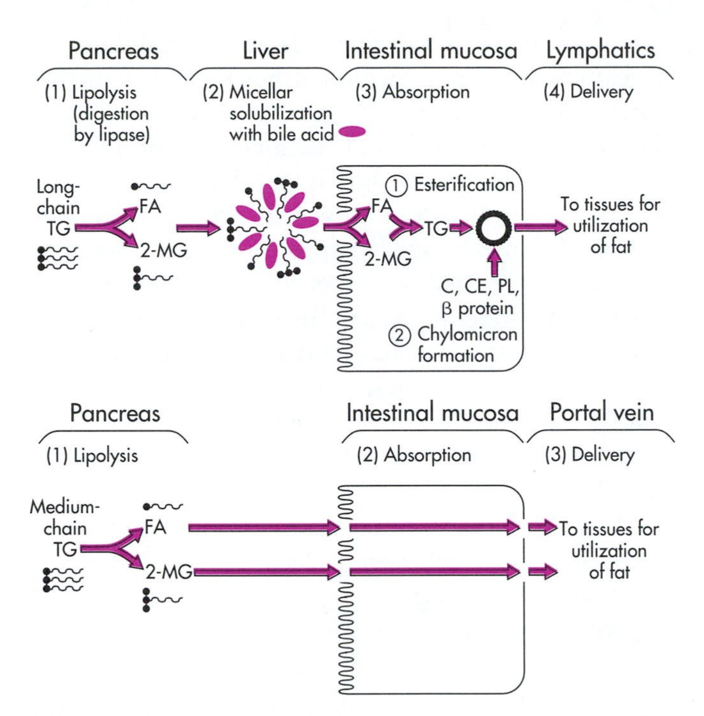

FIGURE 7-1. Digestion and absorption of fats. Long-chain fats must undergo micelle formation for absorption and must rejoin with monoglycerides (esterification) and be packaged with other lipids into chylomicrons to be soluble enough for transport through the body. Medium-chain fats can be absorbed without micelle formation. They are small enough to enter the blood stream without esterification or chylomicron formation. *TG,* Triglyceride; *FA,* fatty acid; *2-MG,* 2-monoglyceride; *C,* cholesterol; *CE,* cholesterol ester; *PL,* phospholipid; *β protein;* β-lipoprotein. (From Moore MC: *Pocket guide to nutritional care,* 1996, St Louis, Mosby; modified from Wilson FA, Dietschy JM: *Gastroenterology* 6:912, 1971).

use.) Insulin also stimulates the cellular uptake of triglycerides. Once inside the cell, the fatty acids are oxidized or reformed into triglycerides for storage. During an overnight fast, prolonged starvation, or metabolic stress when the carbohydrate supply is limited, the blood glucose level declines, and consequently, insulin levels decrease. In response, a process called *lipolysis* causes the breakdown of intracellular triglycerides, which provides fatty acids for energy production and glycerol for gluconeogenesis.

The fatty acids released from adipose tissue are used by either the liver or peripheral tissue. In the liver, fatty acids are degraded to ketones (betahydroxybutyrate, acetoacetate, and acetone). In the absence of glucose, fatty acid breakdown and ketone production are increased. Ketones can be directly oxidized by skeletal muscle and used for energy. During prolonged starvation, the brain—which normally uses glucose—converts to ketones as its primary energy source. This is a body defense mechanism to ensure a supply of energy when carbohydrate intake is low.

Protein-Calorie Malnutrition

Malnutrition results from the lack of necessary nutrients in the body or improper absorption and distribution of them. Although an inadequate supply of both macronutrients and micronutrients can lead to deficiencies and decreased functioning, the lack of protein and calories exacerbates the debilitation that may occur in response to critical illness—thus the use of the term *protein-calorie malnutrition.* To put it simply, an inadequate exogenous supply of calories for energy results in the breakdown of endogenous protein for gluconeogenesis, severely restricting the availability of protein and amino acids for maintenance of body proteins and healing. Malnutrition can be caused by simple starvation—the inadequate intake of nutrients (e.g., in the patient with anorexia related to cancer). It also can be the result of an injury that increases the metabolic rate beyond the supply of nutrients (hypermetabolism). In the seriously ill patient, if malnutrition occurs, usually it is the result of the combined effects of starvation and hypermetabolism.

Metabolic Response to Starvation and Stress

To understand the development of malnutrition in the hospitalized patient, the nurse must understand the metabolic response to starvation and physiologic stress. Changes in endocrine status and metabolism work together to determine the onset and extent of malnutrition. Nutritional imbalance occurs when the demand for nutrients is greater than the exogenous nutrient supply. The major difference between one who is starved and one who is starved and injured is that the latter experiences an increased reliance on endogenous protein breakdown to provide precursors for glucose production to meet increased energy demands.[1] Therefore although carbohydrate and fat metabolism are also affected, the main concern is with protein metabolism and homeostasis.

During an acute, nonstressed fast, blood levels of glucose and insulin fall, and glucagon levels rise. Glucagon promotes the use of glycogen reserves, which become quickly exhausted. Glucagon also stimulates gluconeogenesis, and skeletal muscle provides a large amount of the substrates required for gluconeogenesis. As fasting progresses, triglycerides are mobilized as the primary source of fuel, and consequently the blood ketone levels begin to increase. Once the circulating ketone level rises, the brain is able to use ketones for 70% of its energy, thereby decreasing the total body's reliance on glucose as a major energy source. As gluconeogenesis from protein precursors decreases, protein breakdown and nitrogen excretion also slow. Obligatory glucose users—such as blood cells, the renal medulla, and 30% of brain cells—still require a small amount of amino acids, because they continue to rely on glucose as their preferred source of fuel. However, endogenous protein stores are "spared" from use for gluconeogenesis to a major extent, and protein homeostasis is partially restored.

Of concern to those caring for critically ill patients is the combination of starvation and the physiologic stress resulting from injury, trauma, major surgery, and/or sepsis. This physiologic stress results in profound metabolic alterations that persist from the time of the stressful event until the completion of wound healing and recovery. Stress normally causes an increased metabolic rate (hypermetabolism) that necessitates a rise in oxygen consumption and energy expenditure.

Hormonal changes that occur at the initiation of the stressful event begin the hypermetabolic process. With stimulation of the sympathetic nervous system, the adrenal medulla releases catecholamines (epinephrine and norepinephrine). These in turn stimulate the body's metabolic response to stress. Also released in response to stress are adrenocorticotropic hormone (ACTH) and antidiuretic hormone (ADH), as well as glucocorticoids and mineralocorticoids. These hormonal changes tend to stimulate nutrient substrates, primarily amino acids, to move from peripheral tissues (e.g., skeletal muscle) to the liver for gluconeogenesis. Unfortunately, this mobilization of substrates occurs at the expense of body tissue and function at a time when the needs for protein synthesis (e.g., for wound healing and acute phase proteins) also are high. Hyperglycemia results from the effects of increased catecholamines, glucocorticoids, and glucagon. Again the body relies on its protein stores to provide substrates for gluconeogenesis, because glucose now becomes the major fuel source. Loss of protein results in a negative nitrogen balance and weight loss. The classic response to metabolic stress is the use of protein for fuel.[1]

IMPLICATIONS OF UNDERNUTRITION FOR THE SICK OR STRESSED PATIENT

Malnutrition is widespread among hospitalized patients. For example, recent reports indicate that as many as one third of patients hospitalized for major abdominal surgery and one half of general medical patients show evidence of malnutrition.[2-5] Although illness or injury is the major factor contributing to development of malnutrition, other possible contributing factors include lack of communication among the nurses, physicians, and dietitians responsible for the care of these patients; frequent diagnostic testing, which causes patients to miss meals or to be too exhausted for meals; medications and other therapies that cause anorexia, nausea, or vomiting and thus interfere with food intake; or inadequate use of tube feedings or total parenteral nutrition to maintain the nutritional status of these patients. Nutritional status tends to deteriorate during hospitalization unless appropriate nutrition support is started early and continually reassessed.[4]

Malnutrition is an ominous finding among very ill patients. Wound dehiscence, decubitus ulcers, sepsis, and pulmonary infections are more common among undernourished patients. Medical patients with evidence of undernutrition at hospital admission have longer hospital stays, as well as a trend toward greater mortality.[5]

ASSESSING NUTRITIONAL STATUS

A nutrition screening should be conducted on every patient admitted to a hospital or skilled nursing facility. A brief questionnaire to be completed by the patient or significant other, the nursing admission form, or the physician's admission note usually provides enough information to determine whether the patient is nutritionally at risk (Box 7-1). Any patient judged to be nutritionally at risk needs a more thorough nutrition assessment.

Nutrition assessment involves collection of four types of information—*A,* anthropometric measurements, *B,* biochemical (laboratory) data, *C,* clinical signs (physical examination), and *D,* diet and pertinent medical history. It provides a basis for identifying patients who are malnourished or at risk of malnutrition, determining the nutritional needs of individual patients, and selecting the most appropriate methods of nutritional support for patients with or at risk of developing nutritional deficits. Nutrition support (the provision of specially formulated or delivered enteral or intravenous nutrients to prevent or treat malnutrition)[6] provides a method of coping with the nutritional problems of very ill patients both in the hospital and at home. The assessment can be performed by or under the supervision of a registered dietitian or by a nutrition care specialist (e.g., a nurse with specialized expertise in nutrition).[7]

BOX 7-1 Patients Who Are at Risk of Malnutrition

Adults who exhibit any of the following:

- Involuntary loss or gain of a significant amount of weight (>10% of usual body weight in 6 months, >5% in 1 month), even if the weight achieved by loss or gain is appropriate for height
- Weight 20% more or less than ideal body weight, or body mass index <19 or >27
- Chronic disease
- Chronic use of a modified diet
- Increased metabolic requirements
- Illness or surgery that may interfere with nutritional intake
- Need for enteral tube feeding or parenteral nutrition
- Inadequate nutrition intake for > 7 days
- Regular use of three or more medications
- Poverty

Infants and children who exhibit any of the following:

- Low birth weight
- Small-for-gestational age
- Weight loss of 10% or more
- Weight-for-length or weight-for-height <10th percentile or >90th percentile
- Increased metabolic requirements
- Impaired ability to ingest or tolerate oral feedings
- Inadequate weight gain or a significant decrease in an individual's usual growth percentile
- Poverty

Anthropometric Measurements

Height and current weight are essential anthropometric measurements, and they are measured, rather than obtained through patient or family report. The most important reason for obtaining anthropometric measurements is to be able to detect changes in the measurements over time (e.g., response to nutritional therapy). They are also used as an indicator of underweight or overweight. The patient's measurements may be compared with standard tables of weight-for-height or standard growth charts for infants and children. Another simple and reliable tool for interpreting appropriateness of weight for height for adults and older adolescents is the body mass index (BMI).

$$\text{BMI} = \text{weight} \div \text{height}^2$$

Weight is measured in kilograms and height in meters. A BMI less than 19 is usually considered underweight, and a BMI greater than 27 is considered overweight. A nomogram is available for determination of BMI without performing any calculations (Figure 7-2).

It may be impossible to measure the height of some patients accurately. Total height can be estimated from knee height.[8] To measure knee height, bend the knee 90 degrees and measure from the base of the heel to the anterior surface of the thigh.

For men, height (cm) = 6419.0 − (0.04 × age) + (2.02 × knee height [cm])

For women, height (cm) = 84.88 − (0.24 × age) + (1.83 × knee height [cm])

Good judgment must be used in interpreting anthropometric data. As an example, edema may mask significant weight loss or underweight. Moreover, any history of recent weight change must be kept in mind. A woman who was obese 4 months ago and has lost 15 kg (33 lb) since then may be at nutritional risk, even if her current weight is appropriate for her height.

In addition to height and weight data, other measurements such as arm muscle circumference, skinfold thickness, and body composition (proportion of fat and lean tissue, determined by bioelectric impedance or other methods) are sometimes performed, but these measurements are not routine in all institutions. Also, edema can make these measurements inaccurate, and thus they have little value in many acutely ill patients.[9]

Biochemical Data

A wide range of laboratory tests can provide information about nutritional status. Those most often used in the clinical setting are described in Table 7-1. As the table emphasizes, there are no perfect diagnostic tests for evaluation of nutrition, and care must be taken in interpreting the results of the tests.

Clinical or Physical Manifestations

A thorough physical examination is an essential part of nutrition assessment. Box 7-2 lists some of the more common findings that may indicate an altered nutritional state. It is especially important for the nurse to check for manifestations of muscle wasting, loss of subcutaneous fat, skin or hair changes, and impairment of wound healing.

Diet and Relevant Health History

Information about dietary intake and significant variations in weight is a vital part of the history. Dietary intake can be evaluated in several ways, including a diet record, a 24-hour recall, and a diet history. The

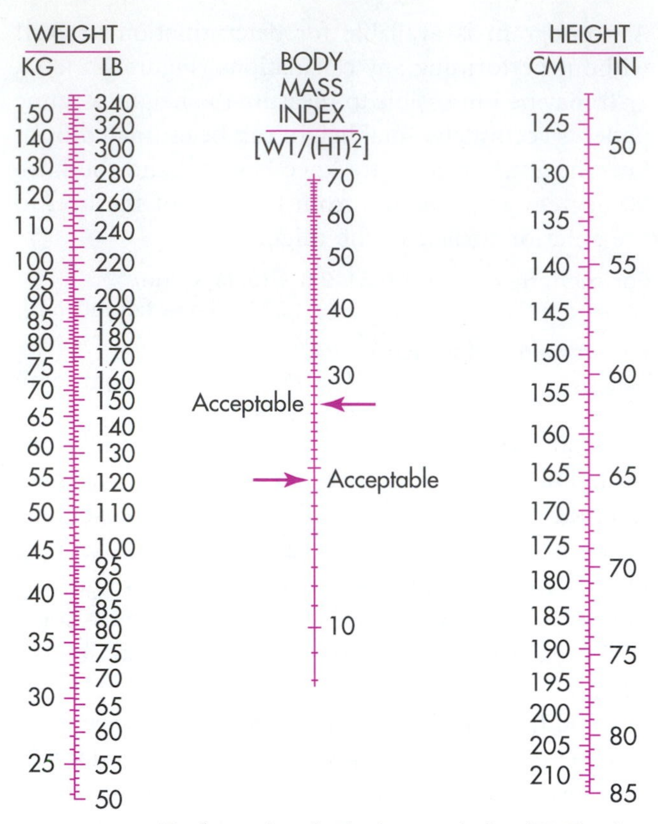

FIGURE 7-2. To determine the body mass index (BMI), place a straightedge across the figure, and connect the weight and height values. The BMI is at the point where the straightedge crosses the BMI line. (Modified from Wardlaw GM, Insel PM: *Perspectives in nutrition,* ed 2, New York, 1993, McGraw-Hill.)

diet record, a listing of the type and amount of all foods and beverages consumed for some period (usually 3 days), is useful for evaluating the patient's intake in the critical care setting if there is a question about the adequacy of intake. However, such a record reveals little about the patient's habitual intake before the illness or injury. The 24-hour recall of all food and beverage intake is easily and quickly performed, but it, too, may not reflect the patient's usual intake and thus has limited usefulness. The diet history consists of a detailed interview about the patient's usual intake, along with social, familial, cultural, economic, educational, and health-related factors that may affect intake. Although the diet history is time-consuming to perform and may be too stressful for the acutely ill patient, it provides a wealth of information about food habits over a prolonged period and provides a basis for planning specific patient teaching, if changes in eating habits are desirable. Other information to include in a nutrition history is listed in Table 7-2.

Evaluating Nutritional Assessment Findings

It is rare for a patient to exhibit a lack of only one nutrient. Usually nutritional deficiencies are combined, with the patient lacking adequate amounts of protein, calories, and possibly vitamins and minerals. A common form of combined nutritional deficit among hospitalized patients is protein-calorie malnutrition (PCM). Two types of PCM are *kwashiorkor* and *marasmus.*

Kwashiorkor is evidenced by low levels of the serum proteins albumin, transferrin, and prealbumin; low total lymphocyte count; impaired immunity; loss of hair or hair pigment; edema resulting from low plasma oncotic pressure caused by a loss of plasma proteins; and an enlarged, fatty liver. Marasmus is recognizable by weight loss, a decrease in skinfold measurements, loss of subcutaneous fat, muscle wasting, and low levels of creatinine excretion (an indicator of loss of muscle mass). Because PCM weakens musculature, increases vulnerability to infection, and can prolong hospital stays, the health care team should diagnose this serious disorder as quickly as possible so that appropriate nutritional intervention can be implemented.

Determining Nutritional Needs

Indirect calorimetry, a method by which energy expenditure is calculated from oxygen consumption and carbon dioxide production, is the most accurate method for determining caloric needs. Some ventilators are constructed so that they can perform indirect calorimetry. However, for most patients indirect calorimetry requires the use of a metabolic cart, which is not available in all institutions. In addition, information received from the metabolic cart is limited—measurements are conducted over a relatively brief period (often only 20 to 30 minutes) and may not be representative of energy expenditure over the whole day.

Calorie and protein needs of patients are often estimated by using formulas that provide allowances for increased nutrient usage associated with injury and healing. Commonly used formulas can be found in Appendix D.

NUTRITION AND CARDIOVASCULAR ALTERATIONS

Diet and cardiovascular disease may interact in a variety of ways. In one situation, excessive nutrient intake—manifested by overweight or obesity and a

TABLE 7-1 Diagnostic Tests Used in Nutrition Assessment

Area of Concern	Possible Deficiency	Comments
SERUM PROTEINS		
Decrease of serum albumin, transferrin (iron transport protein), or thyroxine-binding prealbumin*	Protein	These proteins are produced in the liver, are depressed in hepatic failure, and are falsely low in fluid volume excess and elevated in volume deficit. Albumin has a long half-life (14-20 days) and is slow to change in malnutrition and repletion; transferrin has a half-life of 7-8 days, but levels increase in iron deficiency, and prevalence of iron deficiency limits usefulness in diagnosing protein deficits; prealbumin half-life is 2-3 days, and levels fall in trauma and infection.
HEMATOLOGIC VALUES		
Anemia (decreased Hct, Hgb)		Hct and Hgb are falsely low in fluid volume excess and falsely high in fluid volume deficit.
Normocytic (normal MCV, MCHC)	Protein	
Microcytic (decreased MCV, MCH, MCHC)	Iron, copper	
Macrocytic (increased MCV)	Folate, vitamin B_{12}	
Total lymphocyte count (TLC = WBC × % lymphocytes) < 1200/mm³	Protein	TLC is decreased in severe debilitating disease.
URINARY CREATININE		
Creatinine excretion of < 17 mg/kg/day (women), < 23 mg/kg/day (men)	Protein (reflects lean body mass)	It is difficult to collect accurate 24-hr urine; creatinine excretion varies widely from day to day; levels decline with age as percentage of lean body mass declines.
NITROGEN BALANCE†		
Negative values	Protein, calories (during calorie deficit, protein is metabolized to provide calories)	Negative values occur when more nitrogen is excreted than is consumed (reflects inadequate intake or increased needs); positive values occur when more is consumed than lost (e.g., during nutrition repletion, growth, or pregnancy); normal healthy adults excrete exactly what they consume. Limitations: it is difficult to collect accurate 24-hr urine; retention of nitrogen does not necessarily mean that it is being used for tissue synthesis.

*Evaluation of at least one of these is a part of almost every nutritional assessment.

†Protein is 16% nitrogen. Thus nitrogen balance = [24-hr protein intake (g) × 0.16] − [24-hr urine urea nitrogen (g) + 4 g]. The 4 g is an estimate of fecal, skin, and other minor losses.

Hct, Hematocrit; *Hgb,* hemoglobin; *MCV,* Mean corpuscular volume; *MCHC,* mean corpuscular hemoglobin concentration; *MCH,* mean corpuscular hemoglobin.

BOX 7-2 Clinical Manifestations of Nutritional Alterations

Manifestations that may indicate protein-calorie malnutrition:
- Hair loss; dull, dry, brittle hair; loss of hair pigment
- Loss of subcutaneous tissue; muscle wasting
- Poor wound healing
- Hepatomegaly
- Edema

Manifestations often present in vitamin deficiencies:
- Conjunctival and corneal dryness (vitamin A)
- Dry scaly skin; follicular hyperkeratosis, in which the skin appears to have gooseflesh continually (vitamin A)
- Gingivitis; poor wound healing (vitamin C)
- Petechiae; ecchymoses (vitamins C or K)
- Inflamed tongue; cracking at the corners of the mouth (riboflavin [vitamin B_2], niacin, folic acid, vitamin B_{12}, or other B vitamins)
- Edema; congestive heart failure (thiamin [vitamin B_1])
- Confusion; confabulation (thiamin [vitamin B_1])

Manifestations often present in mineral deficiencies:
- Blue sclerae; pale mucous membranes; spoon-shaped nails (iron)
- Hypogeusia, or poor sense of taste; dysgeusia, or bad taste; eczema; poor wound healing (zinc)

Manifestations often observed with excessive vitamin intake:
- Hair loss; dry skin; hepatomegaly (vitamin A)

diet rich in cholesterol and saturated fat—is a risk factor for development of arteriosclerotic heart disease. Conversely, the consequences of chronic myocardial insufficiency can include malnutrition.[10]

Nutrition Assessment in Cardiovascular Alterations

A nutrition assessment provides the nurse and other members of the health care team the information necessary to plan the patient's nutrition care and teaching. Key points of the nutrition assessment of the cardiovascular patient are summarized in Table 7-3. The major nutritional concerns relate to appropriateness of body weight and the levels of serum lipids and blood pressure.

Nutrition Intervention in Cardiovascular Alterations

Myocardial infarction. The following guidelines will assist the nurse in providing appropriate nutritional care for the patient in the immediate postmyocardial infarction (MI) period:

1. Limit meal size for the patient with severe myocardial compromise or postprandial angina. Although a meal of typical size is less stressful than is a bed bath or shower for the patient with an uncomplicated condition, these meals increase cardiac index, stroke volume, heart rate, myocardial oxygen consumption, and whole-body oxygen consumption; thus they increase cardiac work. Five to six small meals daily are less likely than are three larger meals to increase myocardial work, promote ischemia, and cause angina.[11]
2. Monitor the effect of caffeine on the patient, if caffeine is included in the diet. Because caffeine is a stimulant, it might be expected to increase heart rate and myocardial oxygen demand. In the United States and in most industrial nations, coffee is the richest source of caffeine in the diet, with about 150 mg of caffeine per 180 ml (6 fluid oz) of coffee. In comparison, the caffeine content of the same volume of tea or cola is approximately 50 mg or 20 mg, respectively.
3. Use caution in serving foods at temperature extremes. Although most patients appear to tolerate cold fluids (ice water) well, a subset of patients manifest electrocardiographic changes after drinking ice water.[12] Very hot or very cold foods could potentially trigger vagal or other neural input and cause cardiac dysrhythmias. Monitor patients carefully if such foods are consumed.

Hypertension. A substantial number of individuals with hypertension are "salt sensitive," with their disorder improving when sodium intake is limited. Consequently restriction of sodium intake, usually to 2.5 g or less/day, is often advised to help control hypertension.[13] The primary sodium source in the American diet is salt (sodium chloride) added during food processing and preparation or at the table. One teaspoon of salt provides about 2.3 g of sodium. Most salt substitutes contain potassium chloride and may be used with the physician's approval by the patient who has no renal impairment. "Lite salt" is about half sodium chloride and half potassium chloride. If used, it must be used very sparingly to maintain an adequate restriction of sodium intake.

TABLE 7-2 Nutrition History Information

Area of Concern	Significant Findings	Nutrients of Special Concern
Inadequate intake of nutrients	Avoidance of specific food groups because of poverty or poor dentition	Protein, iron
	Alcohol abuse	Protein, vitamin B_1, niacin, folate
	Anorexia, nausea, vomiting	Most nutrients, particularly protein, electrolytes
	Confusion, coma	All nutrients
Inadequate absorption of nutrients	Previous GI surgeries:	
	Gastrectomy	Vitamin B_{12}, minerals, calories (if the patient experiences dumping syndrome)
	Ileal resection	Vitamins B_{12}, A, E; minerals; calories (in extensive small bowel resection)
	Certain medications:	
	Antacids, cimetidine (reduce upper duodenal acidity)	Minerals
	Cholestyramine (binds fat-soluble nutrients)	Vitamins A, D, E, K
	Corticosteroids	Protein
	Anticonvulsants	Calcium
Increased nutrient losses	Chronic or acute blood loss	Iron
	Severe diarrhea	Fluid, electrolytes
	Fistulas, draining abscesses, wounds	Protein, zinc
	Nephrotic syndrome	Protein, zinc
	Peritoneal dialysis or hemodialysis	Protein, zinc, water-soluble vitamins
Increased nutrient requirements	Fever*	Calories
	Surgery, trauma, burns, infection	Calories, protein, zinc, vitamin C
	Neoplasms (some types)	Calories, protein
	Physiologic demands (pregnancy, lactation, growth)	Calories, protein, iron

*Each 1° C (1.8° F) elevation in temperature increases caloric needs by approximately 13%.

Heart failure. Nutrition intervention in heart failure (HF) is designed to reduce fluid retained within the body and thus reduce the preload. Because fluid accompanies sodium, limitation of sodium is necessary to reduce fluid retention. Specific interventions include (1) limiting sodium intake, usually to 2 g/day or less and (2) limiting fluid intake as appropriate. If fluid is restricted, the daily fluid allowance is usually 1.5 to 2 L/day, to include both fluids in the diet and those given with medications and for other purposes. Some foods that are normally served as solids are actually liquids at body temperature. These include gelatins (100% water), custard (75% water), sherbet and fruit ices (50% water), and ice cream (33% water). (∞Heart Failure, p. 502.)

Cardiac cachexia. The severely malnourished cardiac patient often suffers from congestive heart failure (CHF).[10] Therefore sodium and fluid restriction, as previously described, are appropriate. It is important to concentrate nutrients into as small a volume as possible and to serve small amounts frequently, rather than three large meals daily, which may overwhelm the patient. The patient also can be given calorie-dense foods and supplements.

Because the patient is likely to tire quickly and to suffer from anorexia, enteral tube feeding or total parenteral nutrition (TPN) may be necessary. Most commonly used tube feeding formulas provide 1 calorie/ml, but more concentrated products are available to provide adequate nutrients in a smaller volume. Some

TABLE 7-3 Nutrition Assessment of the Cardiovascular Patient

Area of Concern	Significant Findings: History	Physical Assessment	Laboratory Data
Overweight/obesity	Excessive kcal intake Sedentary life-style	Weight >120% of desirable, or BMI >27	
Protein-calorie malnutrition (cardiac cachexia)	Chronic cardiopulmonary disease, causing: Decreased food intake related to angina, respiratory embarrassment, or fatigue during eating Malabsorption of nutrients caused by hypoxia of the gut Medications that impair appetite (e.g., digitalis, quinidine)	Weight <85% of desirable, or BMI <19 Muscle wasting Loss of subcutaneous fat	Serum albumin < 3.5 g/dL (or low transferrin or prealbumin level) Negative nitrogen balance Creatinine excretion of <17 mg/kg/day (women), <23 mg/kg/day (men)
Elevated serum lipid levels	Frequent or daily use of foods high in cholesterol and saturated fat Sedentary life-style Family history of hyperlipidemia Overweight or obesity	Xanthomas, or yellowish plaques, deposited in the skin (uncommon)	Serum cholesterol >200 mg/dL Low-density lipoprotein cholesterol >130 mg/dL
Elevated blood pressure	Daily use of high-sodium foods and salt at the table Consumption of >2 alcoholic drinks/day		

Modified from Moore MC: *Pocket guide to nutritional care,* ed 3, St Louis, 1996, Mosby.

examples of formulas for fluid-restricted patients are Magnacal (Sherwood Medical), Deliver 2.0 (Mead Johnson), TwoCal HN (Ross), and Resource Plus (Sandoz), which provide 1.5 to 2 calories/ml. During TPN, 20% lipid emulsions with 2 calories/ml provide a concentrated energy source. (The 10% emulsions, in contrast, contain only 1.1 calorie/ml.)

The nurse must monitor the fluid status of these patients carefully when they are receiving nutrition support. Assessment of breath sounds, presence and severity of peripheral edema, and changes in body weight are performed daily or more frequently. A consistent weight gain of more than 0.11 to 0.22 kg (0.25 to 0.5 lb) a day usually indicates fluid retention, rather than gain of fat and muscle mass.

Nutrition Teaching in Cardiovascular Alterations

Myocardial infarction. The patient recovering from MI must recognize the need for permanent changes in diet and life-style to reduce the risk of additional MIs. These changes include weight reduction, if the person is overweight, and control of cholesterol, fat, and saturated fat intake.

Weight reduction. Gradual loss of weight (no more than 0.45 to 0.9 kg [1 to 2 lb] per week) is the goal. This can be achieved through moderate exercise and reduction of dietary intake.

Control of cholesterol, fat, and saturated fat intake. The National Cholesterol Education Program has recommended intensive dietary therapy for individuals with LDL*-cholesterol levels of 160 mg/dL and higher and those with levels of 130 to 159 mg/dL who have definite coronary heart disease or two other risk factors (e.g., male gender, coronary heart disease before age 55 in a parent or sibling, diabetes mellitus, history of cerebrovascular or peripheral vas-

*LDL, Low-density lipoprotein.

TABLE 7-4 Dietary Therapy of High Blood Cholesterol

Nutrient	Recommended Intake: Step-One Diet	Recommended Intake: Step-Two Diet
Total fat	<30% of total calories	
Saturated fatty acids	<10% of total calories	<7% of total calories
Polyunsaturated fatty acids	Up to 10% of total calories	
Monounsaturated fatty acids	10% to 15% of total calories	
Carbohydrates	50% to 60% of total calories	
Protein	10% to 20% of total calories	
Cholesterol	<300 mg/day	<200 mg/day
Total calories	To achieve and maintain desirable weight	

From National Cholesterol Education Program: *Report of the Expert Panel on Detection, Evaluation, and Treatment of High Blood Cholesterol in Adults,* NIH Publ No 89-2925, Washington DC, 1989, US Department of Health and Human Services.

cular disease, and more than 30% overweight).[14] Individuals older than 70 years may not benefit from a cholesterol-lowering diet.[15]

A two-step program (Table 7-4) has been established to reduce saturated fat and cholesterol intake, and total fat intake is limited as well, to aid in weight reduction. Initially, the patient receives counseling about the Step-One Diet (Table 7-5), which reduces the most common and obvious sources of saturated fatty acids and cholesterol in the diet and can be implemented without drastic diet or life-style changes for most patients. If, after adhering to the diet for 3 months, the patient does not succeed in lowering LDL cholesterol to the desirable level, he or she may progress to the Step-Two Diet. Although the physician or nurse often can provide education about the Step-One Diet, referral to a dietitian is valuable for patients who have difficulty in adhering to the diet or who have a disappointing response to the diet. The dietitian's help is particularly needed by patients who progress to the Step-Two Diet.

Diet teaching should emphasize that changes do not have to result in a restrictive or unpalatable diet. Patients need to be encouraged to consume a diet rich in complex carbohydrates (starches and fibers), which are found primarily in breads, cereals, and fresh vegetables and fruits. Not only do carbohydrates help to replace fats in the diet, but also the "soluble fibers"—such as those in oat products, legumes, apples, and citrus fruits (but not the cellulose found in wheat bran)—are hypocholesterolemic. Animal protein intake needs to be limited to no more than approximately 6 oz/day; dried beans and peas are good meat substitutes for individuals seeking to lower their fat intake. Regular consumption of fish (at least one to two meals/week) helps to lower the risk of coronary heart disease; therefore fish intake needs to be encouraged. Use of fish oil supplements, however, has not been shown to lower LDL-cholesterol levels or the risk of MI and are not recommended. Because egg yolks are rich in both cholesterol and saturated fat, the person following the Step-One Diet must eat no more than three egg yolks/week, and the person following the Step-Two Diet must eat no more than one yolk/week. Egg whites, which are free of fat and cholesterol, can be used liberally. Fat intake must be limited to approximately 6 to 8 tsp/day, with the unsaturated vegetable oils being the most desirable dietary fats (see Table 7-5). Moderate alcohol intake usually is allowed, but excessive intake is to be discouraged—especially for obese or overweight individuals—because it is relatively high in calories.

Hypertension. The patient must understand the rationale for the necessary dietary changes, as well as the risks associated with noncompliance. Recommended dietary changes include the following:

1. Reduce weight, if overweight or obese. Even if the patient does not achieve the ideal weight, weight loss helps to control hypertension.
2. Restrict sodium intake. Although the patient with no renal impairment may use a salt substitute with the physician's approval, many patients do not care for the taste of the substitutes. The patient and/or the person normally responsible for the patient's food preparation can be encouraged to experiment with the use of low-sodium herbs and seasonings to replace salt. The patient may be encouraged to know that the taste for sodium declines after approximately 3 months if the low-sodium regimen is followed conscientiously.

   Almost all fresh fruits and vegetables are low in sodium and can be used to provide interest in the diet. These foods are also a good source of potassium, and evidence suggests that a high-potassium intake helps to prevent hypertension.[13]
3. Consume no more than 2 oz of alcohol daily. The equivalent of 1 oz of alcohol is 2 oz of

TABLE 7-5 Recommended Diet Modifications to Lower Blood Cholesterol: the Step-One Diet

Food Source	Choose	Decrease
Fish, chicken, turkey, and lean meats	Fish; poultry without skin; lean cuts of beef, lamb, pork or veal; shellfish	Fatty cuts of beef, lamb, pork; spare ribs, organ meats, regular cold cuts, sausage, hot dogs, bacon, sardines, roe
Skim and low-fat milk, cheese, yogurt, and dairy substitutes	Skim or 1% fat milk (liquid, powdered, evaporated)	Whole milk (4% fat); regular, evaporated, condensed; cream, half and half, 2% milk, imitation milk products, most nondairy creamers, whipped toppings
	Buttermilk	
	Nonfat (0% fat) or low-fat yogurt	Whole-milk yogurt
	Low-fat cottage cheese (1% or 2% fat)	Whole-milk cottage cheese (4% fat)
	Low-fat cheeses, farmer or pot cheeses (all of these should be labeled no more than 2-6 g fat/oz)	All natural cheeses (e.g., blue, Roquefort, Camembert, cheddar, swiss)
		Low-fat or "light" cream cheese, low-fat or "light" sour cream
		Cream cheeses, sour cream
	Sherbet	Ice cream
	Sorbet	
Eggs	Egg whites (2 whites = 1 whole egg in recipes), cholesterol-free egg substitutes	Egg yolks
Fruits and vegetables	Fresh, frozen, canned, or dried fruits and vegetables	Vegetables prepared in butter, cream, or other sauces
Breads and cereals	Homemade baked goods using unsaturated oils sparingly, angel food cake, low-fat crackers, low-fat cookies	Commercially baked goods: pies, cakes, doughnuts, croissants, pastries, muffins, biscuits, high-fat crackers, high-fat cookies
	Rice, pasta	Egg noodles
	Whole-grain breads and cereals (oatmeal, whole wheat, rye, bran, multigrain, and so on)	Breads in which eggs are major ingredient
Fats and oils	Baking cocoa	Chocolate
	Unsaturated vegetable oils: corn, olive, rapeseed (canola oil), safflower, sesame, soybean, sunflower	Butter, coconut oil, palm oil, palm kernel oil, lard, bacon fat
	Margarine or shortening made from one of the unsaturated oils listed above	
	Diet margarine	
	Mayonnaise and salad dressings made with unsaturated oils listed above	Dressings made with egg yolk
	Low-fat dressings	
	Seeds and nuts	Coconut

From National Cholesterol Education Program: *Report of the Expert Panel on Detection, Evaluation, and Treatment of High Blood Cholesterol in Adults,* NIH Publ No 89-2925, Washington, DC, 1989, US Department of Health and Human Services.

100-proof whiskey, 8 oz of wine, or 24 oz of beer. Alcohol has a direct pressor effect.[13]
4. Obtain regular, moderate exercise.[16]

Heart failure. Recommended dietary changes include the following:

1. Restrict sodium intake. This teaching is the same as that for the hypertensive patient.
2. Restrict fluid intake, if appropriate. The patient and family need help in learning to measure and record fluid intake, including those foods that are consumed as solids, such as ice cream, custard, and sherbet.
3. Consume a balanced, nutritious diet if cachectic or undernourished. Patients should be encouraged to avoid low-calorie foods and choose instead those with high-caloric density. Good choices include meats and poultry, cheeses, yogurt, frozen yogurt, and ice cream.

NUTRITION AND PULMONARY ALTERATIONS

Malnutrition has extremely adverse effects on respiratory function, decreasing both surfactant production, diaphragmatic mass, and vital capacity.[17] Patients with acute respiratory disorders find it difficult to consume adequate oral nutrients and can rapidly become malnourished. Ventilator dependency not only interferes with nutrient intake, but also energy expenditure, which was found to be greater in ventilator-dependent patients than in spontaneously breathing patients.[18] Patients with chronic disorders and long-term weight loss have proved challenging to rehabilitate nutritionally. Patients who do tolerate nutritional repletion demonstrate significant improvements in pulmonary function.[17,19] Patients with undernutrition and end-stage chronic obstructive pulmonary disease (COPD), however, are often unable to tolerate the increase in metabolic demand that occurs during refeeding. In addition, they are at significant risk for development of cor pulmonale and may fail to tolerate the fluid required for delivery of enteral or parenteral nutrition support.[20] Prevention of severe nutritional deficits, rather than correction of deficits once they have occurred, is the key to nutritional management of these patients. (∞Acute Respiratory Failure, p. 655; Prolonged Mechanical Ventilation, p. 681.)

Nutrition Assessment in Pulmonary Alterations

Nutrition assessment is summarized in Table 7-6. The patient with respiratory compromise is especially vulnerable to the effects of fluid volume and carbohydrate excess and must be assessed continually for these complications.

Nutrition Intervention in Pulmonary Alterations

Prevent or correct undernutrition and underweight. The nurse and dietitian work together to encourage oral intake in the undernourished or potentially undernourished patient who is capable of eating. Small frequent feedings are especially important, because a very full stomach can interfere with diaphragmatic movement. Mouth care needs to be provided before meals and snacks to clear the palate of the flavors of sputum and medications. Administering bronchodilators with food can help to reduce the gastric irritation caused by these medications.

Because of anorexia, dyspnea, debilitation, or need for ventilatory support, however, many patients will require tube feeding or TPN. It is especially important for the nurse to be alert to the risk of pulmonary aspiration in the patient with an artificial airway. To reduce the risk of pulmonary aspiration during tube feeding, the nurse must (1) keep the patient's head elevated at least 45 degrees during feedings, unless contraindicated; (2) discontinue feedings 30 to 60 minutes before any procedures that require lowering the head; (3) keep the cuff of the artificial airway inflated during feeding, if possible; (4) monitor the patient for increasing abdominal distention; and (5) check tube placement before each feeding (if intermittent) or at least every 4 to 8 hours if feedings are continuous.

Avoid overfeeding. Overfeeding of total calories or of carbohydrate or lipid alone can impair pulmonary function. The production of carbon dioxide (V_{CO_2}) increases when carbohydrate is relied on as the primary energy source.[19] This is unlikely to be significant in the patient who is eating foods. Instead, it is an iatrogenic complication of TPN, in which glucose is often the predominant calorie source, or occasionally of tube feeding in a patient with a very high carbohydrate formula. Excessive carbohydrate intake can raise Pa_{CO_2} sufficiently to make it difficult to wean a patient from the ventilator. There is some evidence that overfeeding of calories, regardless of the amount of carbohydrate in the feedings, produces excessive V_{CO_2}.[21] A balanced regimen with both lipids and carbohydrates providing the nonprotein calories is optimal for the patient with respiratory compromise, and the patient needs to be reassessed continually to ensure that caloric intake is not excessive.

Excessive lipid intake can impair capillary gas exchange in the lungs, although this is not usually sufficient to produce an increase in Pa_{CO_2} or decrease in

TABLE 7-6 **Nutrition Assessment of the Pulmonary Patient**

Area of Concern	Significant Findings: History	Physical Assessment	Laboratory Data
Protein-calorie malnutrition	Chronic lung disease: poor intake of protein and calories because of the following: Breathing difficulty from pressure of a full stomach on the diaphragm Unpleasant taste in the mouth from chronic sputum production Gastric irritation from bronchodilator therapy Increased energy expenditure from increased work of breathing	Muscle wasting Loss of subcutaneous fat Recent weight loss, weight measurement of <90% of desirable, or BMI <19	Serum albumin <3.5 g/dL, or low transferrin or prealbumin level Total lymphocyte count <1200/mm³ Creatinine excretion <17 mg/kg (women) or <23 mg/kg (men)
	Acute respiratory alterations: inadequate intake of protein and calories because of the following: Upper airway intubation Altered state of consciousness Dyspnea Increased protein and calorie requirements caused by increased work of breathing or acute pulmonary infections Catabolism resulting from corticosteroid use	Same as for chronic disease	Same as for chronic disease
Overweight/obesity (in patients with chronic lung disease)	Decreased caloric needs resulting from decreasing metabolic rate with aging (metabolic rate declines by 2%/decade after age 30) or decreased activity to compensate for impaired respiratory function	Weight >120% of desirable or BMI >27	
Elevated respiratory quotient (RQ)*	Use of glucose or other carbohydrate to provide 70% or more of nonprotein calories Consumption of excess calories	Tachypnea, shortness of breath	RQ ≥1 Elevated $\dot{V}O_2$ and $\dot{V}CO_2$ Elevated $PaCO_2$ (not always present)
Fluid volume excess	Administration of more than 35-50 ml fluid/kg/day Increased antidiuretic hormone (ADH) release resulting from stress and ventilator dependency	Dependent edema Pulmonary rales Bounding pulse Shortness of breath	Serum sodium <135 mEq/L BUN, hematocrit, and serum albumin decreased from previous values
Excess lipid intake	Administration of intravenous (IV) lipids		Serum triglyceride >150 mg/dL Low $\dot{V}A\dot{Q}$†

Modified from Moore MC: *Pocket guide to nutritional care,* ed 3, St Louis, 1996, Mosby.
BUN, blood urea nitrogen.
*RQ, or CO_2 produced ÷ O_2 consumed, is measured by indirect calorimetry, which is not available in all institutions.
†The defect is not usually sufficient to alter PaO_2 or $PaCO_2$, except in patients with the most severe lung disease.

PaO_2.[17,19] However, the patient with severe respiratory alteration may be further compromised by lipid overdose. If lipid intake is maintained at no more than 2 g/kg/day, lipid excess is rarely a problem. Lipids are available as 20 g/100 ml (20% lipid emulsion) and 10 g/100 ml (10% emulsion). Serum triglyceride levels greater than 150 mg/dL may indicate inadequate lipid clearance and a need to decrease the lipid dosage.

Prevent fluid volume excess. Pulmonary edema and failure of the right side of the heart, which may be precipitated by fluid volume excess, further worsen the status of the patient with respiratory compromise. Strict intake records must be maintained to allow for accurate totals of fluid intake. Usually the patient requires no more than 35 to 40 ml/kg/day of fluid. For the patient receiving nutrition support, fluid intake can be reduced by using 20% lipid emulsions as a source of calories, by using tube feeding formulas providing at least 2 calories/ml (the dietitian can recommend appropriate formulas), and by choosing oral supplements that are low in fluid. Some examples are cottonseed oil (Lipomul [Upjohn]), an oral lipid supplement providing 6 calories/ml, and powdered glucose polymers, which increase caloric intake without increasing volume. The nurse plays a valuable role in continually reassessing the patient's state of hydration and alerting other team members to changes that may dictate an increase or decrease in fluid intake.

Nutrition Teaching in Pulmonary Alterations

Teaching focuses on achieving or maintaining the desirable body weight and preventing nutritional deficits.

Undernourished patients and patients at risk of undernutrition. Undernourished patients are encouraged to follow the previously outlined suggestions concerning nutrition intervention. Specifically, they are to continue to eat frequent small meals and choose calorie-dense foods. They may need help in determining which foods are good calorie sources and in learning to increase calories by adding fat or by using nutritional supplements.

Overweight or obese patients. Some patients with chronic lung disease become overweight or obese, rather than underweight, primarily because they restrict their activity because of their disease. The nurse can help them learn how to make dietary changes that promote weight loss, which often improves their activity tolerance. In addition, with the physician's agreement, the nurse may recommend a graduated exercise program designed to assist the patient in increasing the metabolic rate and the number of calories used.

NUTRITION AND NEUROLOGIC ALTERATIONS

Because neurologic disorders tend to be long-term problems, they necessitate good nutritional care to prevent nutritional deficits and promote well-being.

Nutrition Assessment in Neurologic Alterations

Nutrition-related assessment findings vary widely in the patient with neurologic alterations, depending on the type of disorder present. Some common findings are shown in Table 7-7.

Nutrition Intervention in Neurologic Alterations

Prevention or correction of nutritional deficits

Oral feedings. Patients with dysphagia or weakness of the swallowing musculature often experience the greatest difficulty in swallowing foods that are dry or thin liquids, such as water, that are difficult to control. For these patients, the nurse and dietitian can work together to plan suitable meals and evaluate patient acceptance and tolerance. Some suggestions that may help the patient with dysphagia or weakness of the swallowing musculature include the following: (∞Cerebrovascular Accident, p. 798.)

1. Serve soft, moist foods.
2. Thicken beverages with infant cereal, yogurt, or ice cream if the patient has difficulty swallowing fluids or chokes on water and other thin liquids. Alternatively, fluid can be provided by gelatin, sherbet, sorbet, fruit ices, popsicles, and ice cream. Fruit nectars may be better tolerated than thinner juices.
3. Do not rush the patient who is eating, because this may increase the risk of pulmonary aspiration. Providing small amounts of food at frequent intervals, rather than larger amounts only at mealtimes, may help the patient feel less need to hurry. Keep suction equipment available in case aspiration does occur.
4. Place the patient in the Fowler position before feedings, if possible, to allow gravity to facilitate effective swallowing.

Tube feedings or TPN. Patients who are unconscious or unable to eat because of severe dysphagia, weakness, ileus, or other reasons will need tube feedings or TPN. Prompt initiation of nutrition support must be a priority in the patient with neurologic impairments. Needs for protein and calories are increased

TABLE 7-7 Nutrition Assessment of the Patient With Neurologic Alterations

Area of Concern	Significant Findings: History	Significant Findings: Physical Assessment	Significant Findings: Laboratory Data
DISORDERS OF PROTEIN AND CALORIE NUTRITURE			
Protein-calorie malnutrition	Decreased intake because of the following: Coma or confusion Feeding/swallowing difficulties such as dribbling of food and beverages from mouth, dysphagia, weakness of muscles involved in chewing and swallowing Ileus resulting from spinal cord injury or use of pentobarbital Anorexia resulting from depression Increased needs because of the following: Hypermetabolism and catabolism after head injury Catabolism resulting from corticosteroid use Trauma and surgical wounds Loss of protein from decubitus ulcers	Muscle wasting Loss of subcutaneous fat Weight <90% of desirable or BMI <19 Change in hair texture, loss of hair	Serum albumin <3.5 g/dL (or low transferrin or prealbumin value) Negative nitrogen balance Total lymphocyte count $<1200/mm^3$ Creatinine excretion <17 mg/kg/day (women) or <23 mg/kg/day (men)
Overweight/obesity	Decreased caloric needs resulting from inactivity Reliance on soft or pureed foods, which are often more dense in calories than higher fiber foods Increased food intake resulting from depression/boredom	Weight >120% of desirable or BMI >27	
VITAMIN AND MINERAL DEFICIENCIES			
Iron (Fe)	Poor intake of meats resulting from chewing difficulties (e.g., as occurs with myasthenia gravis) Loss of blood in trauma	Pallor, blue sclerae	Microcytic anemia (low Hct, Hgb, MCV, MCH, MCHC) Serum Fe <50 μg/ml
Zinc (Zn)	Poor intake of meat resulting from chewing problems Increased needs for healing decubitus ulcers, trauma, or surgical wounds	Hypogeusia, dysgeusia Diarrhea Seborrheic dermatitis Alopecia	Serum Zn <60 μg/ml
FLUID ALTERATIONS			
Fluid volume deficit	Poor intake resulting from difficulty in swallowing (e.g., as occurs with cerebrovascular accident) Inability to express thirst Fluid restriction in an effort to reduce intracranial edema	Poor skin turgor Decreased urinary output Dry, sticky mucous membranes	Serum sodium >145 mEq/L Serum osmolality >300 mOsm/kg Increased BUN and Hct levels Urine specific gravity >1.030

Modified from Moore MC: *Pocket guide to nutritional care,* ed 3, St Louis, 1996, Mosby.

by infection and fever, as may occur in the patient with encephalitis or meningitis. Needs for protein, calories, zinc, and vitamin C are increased during wound healing, as occurs in the trauma patient and the patient with decubitus ulcers.

Patients with neurologic deficits have an increased risk of certain complications, particularly pulmonary aspiration, during tube feeding and thus they require especially careful nursing management. Patients of most concern are (1) those with an impaired gag reflex, such as some patients with cerebral vascular accident; (2) those with delayed gastric emptying, such as patients in the early period after spinal cord injury and patients with head injury treated with barbiturate coma; and (3) patients likely to experience seizures. To help prevent pulmonary aspiration, the patient's head is kept elevated, if not contraindicated; when elevation of the head is not possible, administering feedings with the patient in the prone or lateral positions will allow free drainage of emesis from the mouth and decrease the risk of aspiration. (∞Aspiration Lung Disorder, p. 667.)

Although case reports in the literature suggest that formulas for enteral feeding can interfere with phenytoin absorption, one controlled investigation failed to find any effect on overall absorption of phenytoin.[22] Until this issue has been resolved, phenytoin levels should be monitored carefully in patients receiving enteral feedings.

Hyperglycemia is a common complication in patients receiving corticosteroids. Patients treated with these drugs are to have blood glucose levels monitored regularly and may require insulin to prevent substantial loss of glucose in the urine, as well as osmotic diuresis, loss of excessive amounts of potassium, and other fluid and electrolyte disturbances.

Prompt use of nutrition support is especially important for patients with head injuries, because head injury causes marked catabolism, even in patients who receive barbiturates, which should decrease metabolic demands.[23] Head-injured patients rapidly exhaust glycogen stores and begin to use body proteins to meet energy needs, a process that can quickly cause PCM. The catabolic response to head injury is partly a result of the corticosteroids often used in treatment. However, the hypermetabolism and hypercatabolism are also caused by dramatic hormonal responses to this type of injury.[23] Levels of cortisol, epinephrine, and norepinephrine increase, with levels of norepinephrine elevating as much as 7 times normal. These hormones increase the metabolic rate and caloric demands, causing mobilization of body fat and proteins to meet the increased energy needs. Furthermore, head-injured patients undergo an inflammatory response and may be febrile, creating increased needs for protein and calories. Improved survival has been observed in head-injured patients who receive adequate nutrition support early in the hospital course.[23] (∞Head Injuries, p. 1057.)

Prevention of overweight and obesity. Many stable patients with neurologic disorders are less active than their healthy counterparts and require fewer calories. Thus they may become overweight or obese if given normal amounts of calories for their age and gender. Within 1 or 2 months after spinal cord injury, substantial amounts of muscle atrophy and loss of body mass begin to occur as a result of denervation and disuse.[24] Consequently, body weight and caloric needs decline. Ideal body weights for paraplegics and quadriplegics are 4.5 kg and 9 kg, respectively, less than those for healthy adults of the same height.[25] Stable, rehabilitating paraplegics need approximately 27.9 calories/kg/day, and quadriplegics need approximately 22.7 calories/kg/day.[25] Patients with dysphagia or extreme swallowing musculature weakness may rely on very soft, easy-to-chew foods that are usually more dense in calories than are bulky, high-fiber foods. Thus they also may gain unneeded weight that will hamper their care and impede mobility. Decreased use of high-fat foods—such as shakes, ice cream, butter, margarine, and pastries—will help to reduce calorie intake.

Nutrition Teaching in Neurologic Alterations

The primary nutrition teaching needs of the patient and family are coping with dysphagia and preventing unwanted weight gain. The nurse can share with them the suggestions for dealing with dysphagia that are described in the section concerning nutrition interventions in neurologic alterations (p. 135). Dysphagia is frustrating and frightening for the patient and requires much understanding and patience by the family. Support and empathy on the part of the nurse can make their coping process easier. For the patient who is at risk of becoming overweight or obese, suggestions for reducing caloric intake are appropriate.

NUTRITION AND RENAL ALTERATIONS

Providing adequate nutritional care for the patient with renal disease can be extremely challenging. Although renal disturbances and their treatments can markedly increase needs for nutrients, necessary restrictions in intake of fluid, protein, phosphorus, and potassium make delivery of adequate calories, vitamins, and minerals difficult. Thorough nutrition

TABLE 7-8 Nutrition Assessment of the Renal Patient

Area of Concern	History	Physical Assessment	Laboratory Data
Protein-calorie malnutrition	Poor dietary intake because of the following: Dietary restrictions on protein-containing foods Anorexia caused by zinc deficiency (lost in dialysis or decreased in diet because of restrictions on meats, whole grains, legumes) Increased protein and amino acid losses from the following: Dialysis (hemodialysis losses ≈ 10-13 g/session; CAPD losses ≈ 5-15 g/day)* Tissue catabolism resulting from corticosteroid use Proteinuria (e.g., as occurs with nephrotic syndrome) Increased needs for protein and calories during peritonitis and other infections	Muscle wasting Loss of subcutaneous tissue Weight <90% of desirable or BMI <19 (Loss of weight and subcutaneous fat may be masked by edema) Loss of hair, change of hair texture	Serum albumin <3.5 g/dL or low transferrin or prealbumin level Total lymphocyte count <1200/mm^3 Negative nitrogen balance
Altered lipid metabolism	Nephrotic syndrome, with elevated cholesterol levels Excess carbohydrate (CHO) consumption from the following: Emphasis on CHO in the diet to replace some of the calories normally provided by protein Use of glucose as an osmotic agent in dialysis Oliguria or anuria		Serum cholesterol >250 mg/dL Serum triglyceride >180 mg/dL
Potential fluid volume excess	Patient knowledge deficit about or noncompliance with fluid restriction	Edema Hypertension Acute weight gain (≥1%-2% of body weight)	Hematocrit decreased from previous levels
DISORDERS OF MINERALS/ELECTROLYTES			
Phosphorus (P) excess	Oliguria or anuria	Tetany	Serum P >4.5 mg/dL Calcium × P product (Ca in mg/dL × P in mg/dL) >70
Zinc (Zn) deficit	Poor intake because of restriction of protein-containing foods Loss in dialysis	Hypogeusia, dysgeusia Alopecia Seborrheic dermatitis Diarrhea	Serum Zn <60 μg/ml
Iron (Fe) deficit	Decreased intake because of restriction of protein-containing foods Loss of blood in dialysis tubing	Fatigue Pallor, blue sclerae	Hematocrit <37% (women) or <42% (men); hemoglobin <12 g/dL (women) or <14 g/dL (men); low MCV, MCH, MCHC levels
Sodium excess	Oliguria or anuria	Edema Hypertension	

Modified from Moore, MC: *Pocket guide to nutritional care,* ed 3, St Louis, 1996, Mosby.
CAPD, continuous ambulatory peritoneal dialysis.
*Increased by 50%-100% in peritonitis.

TABLE 7-8 Nutrition Assessment of the Renal Patient—cont'd

Area of Concern	History	Physical Assessment	Laboratory Data
DISORDERS OF MINERALS/ELECTROLYTES—cont'd			
Potassium (K^+) excess	Oliguria or anuria	Weakness, flaccid muscles	Serum K^+ >5 mEq/L Elevated T wave and depressed ST segment on ECG
Aluminum (Al) excess	Use of aluminum-containing phosphate binders Al contamination of TPN constituents	Ataxia, seizures Dementia Renal osteodystrophy with bone pain and deformities	Plasma Al >100 μg/L
DISORDERS OF VITAMIN NUTRITURE			
A excess	Oliguria or anuria Daily administration of tube feedings, TPN, or oral supplement with vitamin A	Anorexia Alopecia, dry skin Hepatomegaly Fatigue, irritability	Serum retinol level of >80 μg/dL
C deficit	Loss in dialysis Decreased intake resulting from restriction of K^+-containing fruits and vegetables	Gingivitis Petechiae, ecchymoses	Serum ascorbate <0.4 mg/dL
B_6	Failure of the diseased kidney to activate vitamin B_6 Loss in dialysis	Dermatitis Ataxia Irritability, seizures	Plasma pyridoxal phosphate <34 nmol (normal levels not well-established)
Folic acid	Loss in dialysis Decreased intake resulting from restriction of meats, fruits, and vegetables	Glossitis (inflamed tongue) Pallor	Hematocrit <37% (women) or <42% (men), elevated MCV level Serum folate <6 ng/ml

assessment provides the basis for successful nutritional management in patients with renal disease.

Nutrition Assessment in Renal Alterations

Assessment is summarized in Table 7-8.

Nutrition Intervention in Renal Alterations

The goal of nutritional interventions is to administer adequate nutrients, including calories, protein, vitamins, and minerals, while avoiding excesses of protein, fluid, electrolytes, and other nutrients with potential toxicity.

Protein. Evidence suggests that a low-protein diet retards the progression of renal damage in selected patients. It is postulated that a high-protein intake increases glomerular flow and pressures, as the kidney attempts to excrete the urea and other nitrogenous products derived from the protein. The increase in glomerular pressures may hasten the death of the glomeruli.[26] Consequently, decreased protein intake (0.6 to 0.8 g/kg/day compared with the 0.8 g/kg/day recommended for the healthy person and the 1.7 g/kg/day actually consumed by the average American) is recommended for some patients with renal insufficiency who do not yet need dialysis. Women and patients with renal failure from diabetes or hypertension appear to benefit less from protein restriction than do men and patients with glomerulonephritis and interstitial nephritis.[26] Nutritional status of patients on a low-protein diet must be carefully monitored, because protein undernutrition is apt to occur.[27]

Although uremia necessitates control of protein intake, the patient with renal failure often has other physiologic stresses that actually increase protein/ amino acid needs: losses because of dialysis, wounds, and fistulae; use of corticosteroid drugs that exert a catabolic effect; increased endogenous secretion of catecholamines, corticosteroids, glucagon, and parathyroid hormone, all of which can cause or aggravate catabolism; and catabolic conditions, such as trauma, surgery, and sepsis associated or coincident with the renal disturbances. During hemodialysis and arteriovenous (A-V) hemofiltration, amino acids are freely filtered and lost, but proteins such as albumin and immunoglobulin are not. Both proteins and amino acids are removed during peritoneal dialysis, creating a greater nutritional requirement for protein.[28] Protein needs are estimated at approximately 1.2 g/kg/day for patients receiving hemodialysis or hemofiltration,[29] and 1.2 to 1.5 g/kg/day for those receiving peritoneal dialysis.[28,30] Although these amounts are greater than the recommended daily level for healthy adults, they are lower than the amount found in the diet of most adults, and thus many patients will perceive them as restrictions.

It is commonly recommended that at least 50% of protein be in the form of "high biologic value" protein. Foods containing protein of high biologic value—such as eggs, milk, beef, poultry, and fish—are richer in essential amino acids than are foods with lower biologic value protein—such as grains, legumes, and vegetables. The philosophy is to reduce urea formation by providing a diet in which the protein consists primarily of essential amino acids, those which the body cannot make, with the idea that the patient will form adequate amounts of nonessential amino acids via the process of transamination (transfer of amine groups from one carbon backbone, or keto acid, to another). Specialized products, in which almost all of the amino acids are essential, have been developed for enteral tube feeding and TPN. However, use of these products has not been found to improve patient outcome or nutritional status, in comparison with products with balanced amino acid mixtures.[31] During growth and severe stress or critical illness, a number of "nonessential" amino acids are needed in greater amounts than usual, and the need for these amino acids exceeds the body's ability to synthesize them. These amino acids are referred to as "conditionally essential," and they include arginine, glutamine, histidine, serine, taurine, cysteine, and tyrosine. Standard amino acid solutions, containing both essential and nonessential amino acids, are more effective at promoting healing, immune function, and optimal organ function than solutions of essential amino acids alone.[31] (∞Acute Renal Failure, p. 877.)

Fluid. The patient with renal insufficiency usually does not require a fluid restriction until urine output begins to diminish. Patients receiving hemodialysis are usually limited to a fluid intake resulting in a gain of no more than 0.45 kg (1 lb) per day on the days between dialysis. This generally means a daily intake of 500 to 750 ml plus the volume lost in urine.[28,30] With the use of continuous peritoneal dialysis, hemofiltration, or arteriovenous hemodialysis, the fluid intake can be liberalized. Most patients receiving peritoneal dialysis can tolerate 2000 ml per day.[28] This more liberal fluid allowance permits more adequate nutrient delivery, whether by oral, tube, or parenteral feedings. Enteral formulas containing 1.5 to 2 calories/ml or more provide a concentrated source of calories for tube-fed patients who require fluid restriction. Intravenous lipids, particularly 20% emulsions, can be used to supply concentrated calories for the TPN patient.

Calories. It is essential that the renal patient receive an adequate number of calories to prevent catabolism of body tissues to meet energy needs. Catabolism not only reduces the mass of muscle and other functional body tissues, but also releases nitrogen that must be excreted by the kidney. Adults with renal insufficiency need about 35 to 40 calories/kg/day, compared with the 25 to 30 calories/kg/day needed by healthy adults, to prevent catabolism and ensure that all protein consumed is used for anabolism rather than to meet energy needs. After renal transplantation, when the patient usually receives large doses of corticosteroids, it is especially important to ensure that caloric intake is adequate (usually 25 to 35 calories/kg/day) to prevent undue catabolism.

High-carbohydrate foods such as hard candies, sugar, honey, jelly, jellybeans, and gumdrops are often used as a means of supplying calories to the patient with renal failure, because these foods are low in sodium and potassium, which are retained in renal failure. However, hypertriglyceridemia is found in a substantial number of patients with renal disorders. This condition is worsened by excessive intake of simple refined sugars, such as sucrose (table sugar) or glucose. Glucose in the peritoneal dialysate may be a significant calorie source[32] and a contributing factor in hypertriglyceridemia. Approximately 70% of the glucose instilled during peritoneal dialysis to serve as an osmotic agent may be absorbed, and this must be considered part of the patient's carbohydrate intake.[33] The glucose monohydrate used in intravenous and dialysate solutions supplies 3.4 calories/g. Thus if the patient receives 4.25% glucose (4.25 g glucose/100 ml solution) in the dialysate, he or she receives the following:

$$42.5 \text{ g/L} \times 70\% \times 3.4 \text{ calories/g} = 101 \text{ calories/L of dialysate}$$

RESEARCH ABSTRACT

Nursing management of enteral tube feedings.

Mateo M: *Heart Lung* 25(4):318, 1996.

PURPOSE

The purpose of this study was to describe management practices of nurses who give care to patients receiving enteral tube feedings.

DESIGN

Descriptive survey

SAMPLE

The convenience sample consisted of 235 registered nurses who worked in critical care and medical-surgical units at a midwestern university medical center. There were 180 usable questionnaires for data entry.

PROCEDURE

The investigator-developed, 43-item questionnaire was based on a literature review and had questions regarding tube feeding flow rate checks, flushing the tubes, method of unclogging tubes, checking for residuals and administering medications. Questionnaires were distributed via nurses' mailboxes, with reminder letters sent one month later, and issuing a certificate of participation in a research study. Subjects were asked to answer the questions based on their practice for the previous 2 months.

RESULTS

Flow rates were checked between 1 and 4 hours by 70% of the nurses; 16% checked every 8 hours, and 14% checked every 12 hours or longer. Ninety-four percent indicated that they regularly flushed the enteral feeding tube: 29% before the feeding; 43% after each feeding; and 59% flushed the tube every 4 hours. Tap water, sterile water, and sterile normal saline solution were used as irrigants. The primary intervention used by most of the nurses (94%) to unclog tubes was an irrigant solution. The most frequently used solutions used were carbonated beverage (81%), sterile water (49%), dissolved papain (46%), and tap water (42%). Most RNs (95%) reported checking residuals every 4 hours; of these, 50% discarded the residual, whereas 49% readministered it. An amount equal to or greater than 100 ml was considered to be excessive by 50% of the nurses. Flushing the enteral tube with water was done before (47% of the time) and after (95%) giving medications. When multiple medications were given, 38% of the nurses reported flushing the tube between each medication.

DISCUSSION/IMPLICATIONS

Practices regarding management of enteral feedings vary widely among nurses in this sample and setting. Nurses' rationale for the difference in practice was not assessed, which may have revealed additional variables for analysis. Without consistency in enteral tube-feeding procedures, it is difficult to illustrate the impact of any practice on patient outcome. Procedures that are research-based and consistently used by all practitioners need to be formulated and placed into practice. Additional research is needed to demonstrate the impact of protocols and practice on the efficacy of patient care and outcomes.

To help control hypertriglyceridemia, only about 30% to 35% of the patient's calories should come from carbohydrates, including glucose from the dialysate, with the major portion of dietary carbohydrate coming from complex carbohydrates (starches and fibers).[28,30] Consuming at least 20 to 25 g of fiber daily helps to control triglyceride levels.[30] Sources of dietary fiber include 100% bran and raisin bran cereals (5 to 10 g/oz); cooked dried beans and peas (5 to 7 g fiber/0.5 cup); cereals containing whole grains (not 100% bran), berries, apples, oranges, pears, corn, and peas (3 to 5 g/serving); whole grain breads and most fruits and vegetables (1 to 2 g/serving). For the tube-fed patient, a formula containing dietary fiber can be chosen.

To help control hypertriglyceridemia, and to provide concentrated calories in minimal fluid, fat may need to supply as much as 40% of the patient's calories.[30] Hypercholesterolemia is commonly found in patients with renal failure, so unsaturated fats and oils (corn, soybean, sunflower, safflower, cottonseed, canola, and olive) are preferred over saturated fats (primarily from meats and dairy products), which tend to raise cholesterol levels. The necessary restriction of meat, milk, and other protein foods in the diet will help lower cholesterol and saturated fat intake. For patients who need a caloric supplement, Lipomul (Upjohn) is a palatable oral lipid supplement providing 6 calories/ml with minimal sodium and potassium. Intravenous lipids and the

TABLE 7-9 Daily Nutritional Recommendations for Adults With Renal Failure

Nutrient	Recommended Daily Nutrient Intakes	
	Healthy Adults	Adults in Renal Failure
Protein or amino acids (g/kg)	0.8	0.6-0.8 (renal insufficiency)* 1.2-1.4 (hemodialysis)* 1.2-1.5 (peritoneal dialysis)* 1.3-1.5 (immediately after transplant) 1.0 (stable after transplant)
Energy (calories/kg)	25-30	30-35 (renal insufficiency, dialysis—include calories from peritoneal dialysate)* 25-35 (after transplant; fat no more than 30% of calories)
Electrolytes and minerals†		
Sodium (mg; 1 mEq = 23 mg)	<2400 mg desirable	1000-3000 mg (renal insufficiency) 2000-3000 mg (hemodialysis) 2000-4000 mg (peritoneal dialysis, after transplant)
Potassium (mg/kg)	Not specified	Not restricted (renal insufficiency—unless glomerular filtration rate [GFR] <10 ml/min—peritoneal dialysis, after transplant) 40 (hemodialysis)*
Phosphorus (mg)	800-1200	8-12/kg (renal insufficiency)* <17/kg (dialysis)* Unrestricted, monitor (after transplant)
Calcium (mg)	800-1200	1200-1600 (renal insufficiency) Usually > 1000, depends on serum level (dialysis)
Iron (mg)	10-15	15+, as needed to prevent anemia (all groups)
Zinc (mg)	12-15	15+, as needed to prevent deficiency (all groups)
Vitamins‡		
C (mg)	60	60-100
B_6 (mg)	1.6-2.0	5.0-10
Folic acid (mg)	0.18-0.2	0.8-1.0

Data modified from Beto JA: *J Am Dietet Assoc* 95:898, 1995; Kopple JD: *Am J Kidney Dis* 24:1002, 1994; Coats KG and others: *J Am Dietet Assoc* 93:637, 1993; National Research Council: *Recommended dietary allowances,* ed 10, Washington, DC, 1989, National Academy of Sciences—National Research Council; and National Research Council: *Nutrition and your health: dietary guidelines for Americans,* ed 4, Washington, DC, 1995, USDA and USDHHS.
*Based on estimated dry weight or ideal body weight.
†Do not supplement with magnesium; monitor magnesium levels.
‡Daily supplement providing recommended daily allowance of B complex vitamins and vitamin C is appropriate, but do not supplement vitamin A.

long-chain fats found in most enteral formulas, except those prepared from blended foods, are primarily polyunsaturated.

Other nutrients. Table 7-9 summarizes the recommended nutrient intake for patients with renal disorders. The recommendations for healthy adults are included to provide a basis for comparison. Certain nutrients are restricted because they are excreted by the kidney. Phosphorus is one example: its restriction appears to delay progression of renal damage.[26] Phosphorus is found primarily in meat, milk, nuts, and whole grains, so that limitation of protein intake will also help lower phosphorus levels. (See Chapter 32, Renal Clinical Assessment and Diagnostic Procedures, and Chapter 33, Renal Disorders and Therapeutic Management.)

The patient has no specific requirement for the fat-soluble vitamins A, E, and K, because they are not removed in appreciable amounts by dialysis and restriction prevents development of toxicity. Elevated levels of vitamin A are a common finding in dialyzed patients. On the other hand, needs for several water-soluble vitamins and trace minerals are increased in the dialysis patient because they are small enough to pass freely through the dialysis filter. If the patient is not receiving supplements of the water-soluble vitamins listed in Table 7-9, or levels of trace elements are not being monitored, the nurse can consult with the physician about the need for such measures. Similarly, if the patient is receiving vitamin A-containing TPN or tube feeding daily, the nurse can discuss with the physician, pharmacist, and dietitian the desirability of devising nutrient solutions providing only the water-soluble vitamins.

Nutrition Teaching in Renal Alterations

The primary nutrition teaching for such a complex dietary regimen will normally be performed by the dietitian, but the nurse can reinforce and supplement the dietary instruction. In particular, an understanding of the need for a generous caloric intake may make the patient more cooperative in consuming meals and supplements or agreeing to more aggressive nutrition support when it is apparent that tube feeding or TPN is necessary. The nurse can help the patient and family learn to recognize sources of high and low biologic value protein and to select moderate amounts of the high biologic value protein, to measure all fluid intake and maintain daily records of all fluid intake, and to control sodium and potassium intake as necessary.

NUTRITION AND GASTROINTESTINAL ALTERATIONS

Because the gastrointestinal (GI) tract is so inherently related to nutrition, it is not surprising that catastrophic occurrences in the GI tract—hemorrhage, perforation, infarct, or related organ failure—have acute and severe adverse effects on nutritional status.

Nutrition Assessment in Gastrointestinal Alterations

Assessment is summarized in Table 7-10. The area and amount of the GI tract affected determine, to a large extent, the likelihood and degree of nutritional deficits, because each portion of the bowel has a role to play in absorption (Figure 7-3). The ileum is among the most nutritionally important areas. Bile salt absorption, which is necessary for optimal fat digestion and absorption, occurs in this area, as does absorption of vitamin B_{12}. Patients with ileal disease or resection are likely to become malnourished as a result of significant loss of calories (fat) in the feces, as well as loss of minerals and fat-soluble vitamins trapped in the fat. The ileocecal valve is especially critical in maintaining adequate nutrition. Not only does it slow entry of GI contents into the large bowel, allowing more time for absorption to take place in the small bowel, but it also helps prevent migration of the microorganisms from the large bowel into the small bowel. Proliferating microorganisms in the small bowel deconjugate the bile salts, further impairing fat absorption. Deconjugated bile salts also irritate the intestinal mucosa and raise the osmolality level within the bowel, promoting diarrhea.[34] The ileum can absorb most of the nutrients normally absorbed in the upper half of the small bowel, but it is impossible for the duodenum and jejunum to compensate for the loss of the ileum function.

Nutrition Intervention in Gastrointestinal Alterations

The GI tract is the preferred route for delivery of nutrients in GI disease, as it is in all other disease states. However, after damage or resection, enteral nutrition support may be inadequate or impossible, at least temporarily. Because hepatic failure and bowel dysfunction, including failure resulting from inflammatory bowel disease or bowel resection, are two of the most nutritionally challenging GI alterations, most of this discussion is devoted to them.

Hepatic failure. Hepatic failure is associated with a wide spectrum of metabolic alterations. Because the diseased liver has impaired ability to deactivate hormones, levels of circulating glucagon, epinephrine, and cortisol are elevated. These hormones promote catabolism of body tissues and cause glycogen stores to be exhausted. Release of lipids from their storage depots is accelerated, but the liver has decreased ability to metabolize them for energy. Furthermore, as many as half of the patients with hepatic failure may have malabsorption of fat because of inadequate production of bile salts by the liver.[35] Therefore body proteins are increasingly used for energy sources, producing tissue wasting. The branched-chain amino acids (BCAAs)—leucine, isoleucine, and valine—are especially well-used for energy, and their levels in the blood decline. Conversely, levels of the aromatic amino acids (AAAs)—phenylalanine, tyrosine, and tryptophan—rise as a result of tissue catabolism and impaired ability of the liver to clear them from the blood. Hyperammonemia is a feature of hepatic failure, but it may not be the causative agent in encephalopathy. The "false neurotransmitter" hypothesis suggests that AAAs cause encephalopathy. According

TABLE 7-10 Nutrition Assessment of the Patient With a Gastrointestinal Disorder

Area of Concern	History	Physical Assessment	Laboratory Data
Protein-calorie malnutrition	Decreased oral intake caused by the following: Fear of symptoms—pain, cramping, diarrhea—associated with eating (e.g., as occurs with peptic ulcer, dumping syndrome) Alcohol abuse Nausea, vomiting, anorexia Increased losses because of the following: Maldigestion or malabsorption (e.g., as occurs with inadequate bile salt production, increased loss of bile salts in short bowel syndrome, diarrhea, inadequate absorptive area in short bowel syndrome) GI bleeding Fistula drainage Increased requirements caused by the following: Needs for healing (e.g., surgical wounds, fistulae)	Muscle wasting Loss of subcutaneous fat Weight <90% of desirable, recent weight loss or BMI <19 Hair loss or change in hair texture	Serum albumin <3.5 g/dL or low transferrin level Total lymphocyte count < $1200/mm^3$ Creatinine excretion <17 mg/kg/day (women) or <23 mg/kg/day (men) Negative nitrogen balance Fecal fat >5 g/day or >5% of intake
Potential fluid volume deficit	Losses caused by severe vomiting or diarrhea (e.g., as occurs with GI obstruction, short bowel syndrome)	Poor skin turgor Dry, sticky mucous membranes Complaint of thirst Loss of ≥ 0.23 kg (0.5 pounds) in 24 hr	Hct >52% (men) or >47% (women) BUN >20 mg/dL Serum sodium >145 mEq/L Serum osmolality >300 mOsm/kg Urine specific gravity >1.030
DISORDERS OF MINERAL/ELECTROLYTE NUTRITURE			
Calcium (Ca)	Increased loss because of steatorrhea (Ca forms soaps with fat in the stool and thus becomes unabsorbable)	Tingling of fingers Muscular tetany and cramps Carpopedal spasm Convulsions	Serum Ca level of <8.5 mg/dL (severe deficits only)
Magnesium (Mg)	Inadequate intake because of poor diet in alcoholism Increased losses because of the following: Diarrhea or steatorrhea Loss of small bowel fluid (e.g., as occurs with short bowel syndrome, fistulae)	Tremor Hyperactive deep reflexes Convulsions	Serum Mg <1.5 mEq/L
Iron (Fe)	Blood loss Impaired absorption because of decreased upper GI acidity with gastrectomy or use of antacids and cimetidine Inadequate intake (e.g., restriction of protein foods in hepatic failure)	Pallor, blue sclerae Fatigue	Hct <42% (men) or <37% (women); Hgb <14 g/dL (men) or <12 g/dL (women); low MCV, MCH, MCHC Serum Fe <60 μg/dL

Modified from Moore MC: *Pocket guide to nutritional care*, ed 3, St Louis, 1996, Mosby.

TABLE 7-10 Nutrition Assessment of the Patient With a Gastrointestinal Disorder—cont'd

Area of Concern	History	Physical Assessment	Laboratory Data
Zinc (Zn)	Increased losses caused by the following: Diarrhea, steatorrhea Loss of small bowel fluid Diuretic use (in hepatic failure) Increased urinary losses (in alcoholism) Inadequate intake caused by the following: Protein restriction (in hepatic failure) Poor diet (in alcoholism)	Anorexia Hypogeusia, dysgeusia Seborrheic dermatitis	Serum Zn <60 μg/dL
Potassium (K^+)	Increased loss caused by the following: Diarrhea Diuretic use Hyperaldosteronism (in hepatic failure) GI suction	Muscle weakness, ileus Diminished reflexes	Serum K^+ <3.5 mEq/L
DISORDERS OF VITAMIN NUTRITURE			
A	Increased loss in steatorrhea (vitamin A dissolves in fatty stools) Impaired release of vitamin A from storage in the liver because of inadequate production of retinol-binding protein, the transport protein, in malnutrition or liver failure	Drying of skin and cornea Poor wound healing Follicular hyperkeratosis (resembles gooseflesh)	Serum retinol <20 μg/dL
K	Impaired absorption in steatorrhea Decreased production because of destruction of intestinal bacteria by antibiotic usage	Petechiae, ecchymoses Prolonged bleeding	Prothrombin time >12.5 sec (not always accurate in liver failure)

to this hypothesis, AAAs are transported across the blood-brain barrier where they are converted to false neurotransmitters, which compete with the normal neurotransmitters for binding sites. The net result is to impede normal neurotransmission and produce hepatic encephalopathy.[26] (∞Fulminant Hepatic Failure, p. 962.)

Monitoring of fluid and electrolyte status. Ascites and edema result from decreased colloid osmotic pressure in the plasma, because the diseased liver produces less albumin and other plasma proteins, increased portal pressure caused by obstruction, and renal sodium retention from secondary hyperaldosteronism. To control the fluid retention, restriction of sodium (usually 500 to 1500 mg, or 20 to 65 mEq, daily) and fluid (1500 ml or less daily) is generally necessary, in conjunction with administration of diuretics.[35] Patients must be weighed daily to evaluate the success of treatment. In addition, laboratory data and physical status must be closely observed for potassium deficits caused by diuretic therapy and hyperaldosteronism.

Provision of a nutritious diet and evaluation of response to dietary protein. Nutrition intervention in hepatic failure is based on the metabolic alterations. A diet with adequate protein helps to suppress catabolism and promote liver regeneration. Stable patients with cirrhosis usually tolerate 0.8 to 1 g protein/kg/day. Patients with severe stress or nutritional deficits have increased

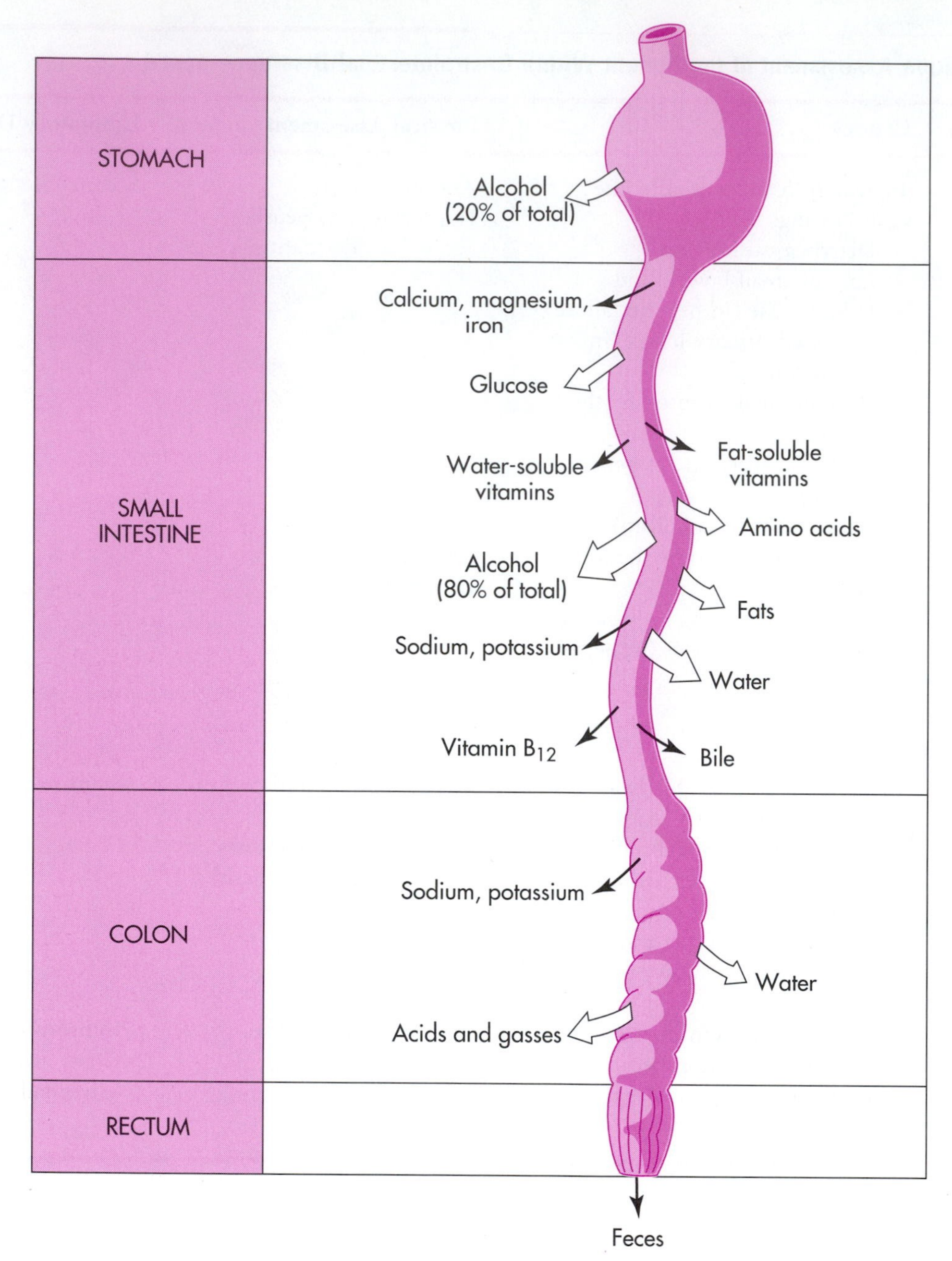

FIGURE 7-3. The GI tract's major absorption sites and their relative amount of absorption, indicated by the size of the arrow. (Modified from Wardlaw GM, Insel PM: *Perspectives in nutrition,* ed 2, New York, 1993, McGraw-Hill.)

needs—as much as 1 to 1.5 g/kg/day.[35] However, if encephalopathy occurs or appears to be impending, tolerance of protein is impaired and protein intake is reduced to 0.5 g/kg/day or less.[31] A diet adequate in calories (at least 30 calories/kg daily) is provided to help prevent catabolism and to prevent the use of dietary protein for energy needs.[35] Moderate amounts of fat are given, unless the patient has steatorrhea, in which case it is necessary to rely heavily on carbohydrates and medium-chain triglycerides (MCTs) to meet caloric needs. Soft foods are preferred, because the patient may have esophageal varices that might be irritated by high-fiber foods. Because alcoholism is often the cause of hepatic failure and the diets of alcoholics have been shown to be low in zinc, vitamin B complex, folate, and magnesium, supplements of these nutrients are usually provided daily.[36] Anorexia, malaise, and confusion may interfere with oral intake, and the nurse may need to provide much encouragement to the patient to ensure intake of an adequate diet. Small frequent feedings are usually better accepted by the anorexic patient than are three large meals daily. The nurse must assess the patient's neurologic status daily to evaluate tolerance of dietary protein. Increasing lethargy, confusion, or asterixis may signal a need for decreased protein intake. Anorexia—coupled with the unpalatable nature of the very low-sodium, low-protein diet required in impending coma—may result in a need for tube feedings.

BCAA-enriched products have been developed for enteral and parenteral nutrition of patients with hepatic disease. Theoretically, these products should benefit patients with severe hepatic disease by providing energy, decreasing muscle protein breakdown, increasing body protein synthesis, normalizing circulating amino acid levels, and decreasing the formation of false neurotransmitters. However, several clinical trials have failed to show clear-cut evidence that BCAA-enriched products improve cirrhosis or encephalopathy more than standard products with balanced amino acid composition. BCAA-enriched products are significantly more expensive than standard products, so their use does not seem justified in all patients with liver disease. In a subset of patients with encephalopathy who do not tolerate standard diets or nutrition support products, BCAA-enriched products may improve electroencephalogram results, arousal, and survival, as well as nutritional status.[31,35,36] Patients with liver failure often receive lactulose, which causes diarrhea. If oral or tube feedings are also administered, diarrhea from concurrent administration of lactulose is not to be confused with intolerance of the feedings.

The patient who undergoes successful liver transplantation is usually able to tolerate a regular diet with few restrictions. Intake during the postoperative period must be adequate to support nutritional repletion and healing; 1 to 1.2 g protein/kg/day and approximately 30 calories/kg/day are often sufficient. Immunosuppressant therapy (corticosteroids and/or cyclosporine) frequently contributes to glucose intolerance.[37] Dietary measures to control glucose intolerance include: (1) obtaining approximately 30% of dietary calories from fat; (2) emphasizing complex sources of carbohydrates; and (3) eating several small meals daily, with some of the day's carbohydrates in each meal. Moderate exercise often helps to improve glucose tolerance. (∞Liver Transplantation, p. 1191.)

Short bowel syndrome. The normal, healthy small bowel is estimated to be approximately 350 to 600 cm in length, depending on whether measurements are made during surgery, when the GI tract retains much of the muscle tonus, or on postmortem examination, when minimal tone is present.[38] It is difficult to estimate the amount remaining at the time of intestinal resection, and thus many patients undergo contrast radiographs when stable to determine the length of the remaining bowel. The major nutritional problems associated with bowel resection are loss of absorptive area, with increased fecal losses of fluids, electrolytes, fat, protein, and other nutrients; increased loss of bile salts, especially if the terminal ileum was resected, with further malabsorption of fat; and micronutrient deficiencies resulting from trapping of minerals and fat-soluble vitamins within the excreted fat.[34,38] After bowel resection, the remaining intestine undergoes marked hyperplasia, with increasing length of the remaining villi, which increases the available absorptive area. The result is improved absorption of water, electrolytes, and glucose.[38] The adaptive response may take up to 1 year to become complete, and it does not occur without the stimulus of nutrients within the gut.[38,39]

Administration of fluids and electrolytes. Extensive bowel resection is associated with marked gastric hypersecretion. The increase in gastric juices, coupled with the sudden loss of absorptive area, results in the loss of several liters of fluid daily, along with potassium, magnesium, and zinc. The nurse's role in management of these patients during the period immediately after extensive bowel resection includes (1) keeping strict intake and output records, including volume or weight of stools if they are frequent or loose; (2) continually assessing the patient's state of hydration; and (3) administering fluids and electrolytes and evaluating the patient's response—including daily weight measurements—to evaluate the adequacy of fluid replacement.

Administration of nutrition support. The extent of the resection is a determinant of the amount and type of nutrition support required. If more than 50% of the small bowel remains, few dietary changes may be needed.[34] With more extensive resection, leaving only 120 to 150 cm (4 to 5 feet) of small bowel, TPN is usually initiated during the early postoperative period. Small amounts of enteral feedings are begun as soon as possible to stimulate intestinal adaptation. Enteral feedings may consist of an elemental, or predigested, diet given by tube. Fat is the most difficult nutrient to absorb, and the formula will ordinarily be very low in fat or will be high in MCTs, which are more readily absorbed than are the long-chain triglycerides predominating in most foods (see Figure 7-1). Alternatively, a low-fat, high-starch diet may be given by mouth.[34] Lactose, or milk sugar, is often tolerated poorly by patients with bowel resection, but low-fat cheese and yogurt, which are relatively low in lactose, may be tolerated.[38] MCTs can be served in juice or used in food preparation to increase caloric intake. Alcohol and caffeine stimulate intestinal motility and may have to be avoided for at least 1 year after surgery. Patients receiving oral feedings often require much encouragement to eat, because they may associate eating with worsening of diarrhea. As more and more enteral intake is tolerated, TPN is gradually tapered. Some patients with 70% to 80% resection of the small bowel can eventually be maintained on enteral feedings only, especially if the terminal ileum and ileocecal valve are retained, but patients with less than 60 cm of small bowel or only the duodenum remaining usually require TPN indefinitely.[39] Many patients show an extraordinary degree of adaptation, even with very extensive resection, and thus gastrointestinal tolerance of enteral feedings is continually assessed. Careful records must be kept of all enteral and parenteral intake to determine when TPN can be decreased or discontinued.

Administration of medications. In some patients with short bowel syndrome, in whom diarrhea is prolonged or especially severe and causes anal excoriation or copious ostomy output, antidiarrheal agents, such as diphenoxylate with atropine or codeine, may be beneficial. Anticholinergic drugs, such as glycopyrrolate, can also be used to counteract the gastric hypersecretion.

Inflammatory bowel disease. Both Crohn's disease (regional ileitis) and ulcerative colitis can result in severe undernutrition. In Crohn's disease, inflammation extends through all layers of the bowel wall. It can affect any part of the GI tract but most often affects the terminal ileum. In acute exacerbations, abdominal pain, fever, nausea, and diarrhea occur. With chronic disease, weight loss, anorexia, anemia, and steatorrhea (recognized by stools that are difficult to flush away and that leave an oily layer on the water in the toilet) are common. In ulcerative colitis, congestion, edema, and ulcerations affect the mucosal and submucosal layers of the bowel. It usually involves the rectum and colon, and sometimes extends to the ileum. Bloody diarrhea, abdominal pain, weight loss, anorexia, and rectal pain are common.

Acute exacerbations of the disease. In addition to maintaining or improving nutritional status, enteral tube feedings or TPN induce remission of symptoms in 60% to 80% of patients with acute episodes of Crohn's disease. Enteral feeding is preferred, except where there is a high-output fistula or an intestinal obstruction in the upper small bowel.[39] Although nutrition support appears to be effective in acute exacerbations of Crohn's disease, there is no evidence that dietary manipulation alone will maintain remission of the disease over the long term.[39] Nutrition support does not cause remission of ulcerative colitis, but it may benefit patients by helping to maintain lean body mass and functional capability.[39]

Chronic disease. A low-fat diet often decreases steatorrhea, which is common with ileal involvement. A high-protein diet (1.5 to 2 g/kg/day) helps promote bowel regeneration and replace losses.[40] If areas of intestinal stenosis are present, a restricted fiber diet that eliminates berries, raw fruits except banana or avocado, raw vegetables, whole grains, and dried beans or peas is commonly recommended to reduce the potential for bowel obstruction.[40] Lactose intolerance is common in Crohn's disease, but some individuals may tolerate yogurt, buttermilk, and cheese. Lactase enzyme can be added to milk to hydrolyze the lactose.

Nutrition Teaching in Gastrointestinal Alterations

Teaching usually focuses on three areas: the rationale for dietary modifications and nutrition support, components of a nutritious and balanced diet, and the need to take vitamin/mineral supplements as ordered. Both the patient with hepatic failure and the one with bowel failure require high-calorie, high-protein diets during convalescence. In addition, the patient with short bowel syndrome must adhere to a low-fiber diet with generous amounts of fluids. Although fat is an excellent source of calories, fat malabsorption is a problem for patients with GI alterations. Even with intestinal adaptation and hyperplasia, fat absorption may never normalize in the patient with short bowel syndrome, and the patient may experience less diarrhea and discomfort if a low-fat diet is followed permanently. Fat restriction appears to be most beneficial for patients who still have a colon.[41] Hyperoxaluria (excessive oxalate secretion in the urine), which contributes to development of oxalate-containing renal stones, is common in short bowel syndrome because of excessive oxalate absorption.[34] In the normal individual, much of the dietary oxalate becomes complexed with calcium in the intestinal tract, and is unabsorbable. In the person with short bowel syndrome, calcium forms soaps with the unabsorbed fat and is unavailable to bind oxalate. Limiting dietary oxalate and taking a calcium supplement reduce the risk of renal stones.[34] Oxalate is found in beets, carrots, celery, eggplant, green beans, deep green leafy vegetables, chocolate, coffee, nuts, blackberries, plums, nuts, and whole wheat.

Glucose oligosaccharides (e.g., Polycose [Ross] and Moducal [Mead Johnson])—which can be added to beverages, cereals, or soups without increasing the sweetness—and MCT oil are two caloric supplements that also can be used. Patients with steatorrhea usually need daily oral water-miscible supplements of the fat-soluble vitamins A and E to prevent deficiencies. Supplements of calcium, zinc, and magnesium may also be needed, since these minerals are often trapped in the fat in the stool. If the terminal ileum was resected or is significantly affected by inflammatory bowel disease, vitamin B_{12} absorption is likely to be impaired, and supplementation is usually needed. In cases in which blood loss has been sufficient to cause anemia, iron supplementation is often provided. The nurse needs to ensure that the patient understands the dosage and is capable of administering these supplements.

In addition, patients who will be discharged while still receiving tube feedings or TPN (usually those with bowel dysfunction) must be taught the mechanics of administering their feedings and maintaining their feeding tube or catheter, as well as methods of preventing and coping with problems and complications. The need for long-term nutrition support may have severe emotional and financial effects. Providing emotional support and counseling are among the nurse's most important roles in assisting these patients. In an effort to encourage resumption of normal activity patterns, many patients are begun on cyclic feedings—usually administered nocturnally—as discharge is anticipated. The costs of long-term home nutrition support are high, although not nearly as high as continued hospitalization, and the social worker or financial counselor must be involved early in the patient's hospitalization in exploring routes of payment, as plans are made for discharge.

NUTRITION AND ENDOCRINE ALTERATIONS

Endocrine alterations have far-reaching effects on all body systems, and thus they affect nutritional status in a variety of ways.

Nutrition Assessment in Endocrine Alterations

The nutrition assessment process is summarized in Table 7-11. Because of the prevalence of non–insulin-dependent diabetes mellitus (NIDDM) patients among the hospitalized population, the nutritional problems most commonly noted in patients with endocrine alterations are overweight and obesity.

Nutrition Intervention in Endocrine Alterations

Underweight and malnourished patients. The most severely undernourished patients are usually those with pancreatitis, because of loss of pancreatic exocrine function. Pancreatic insufficiency—with inadequate release of trypsin, chymotrypsin, and pancreatic lipase and amylase—results in impaired digestion and subsequent loss of nutrients in the stool. Fat malabsorption is the most marked effect of pancreatic insufficiency. Fat lost in the stools is accompanied by calcium, zinc, and other minerals, along with the fat-soluble vitamins. Nutritional care in malabsorptive disorders is discussed more thoroughly in the section concerning nutrition in GI alterations. (∞Acute Pancreatitis, p. 950.)

Patients with insulin-dependent diabetes mellitus (IDDM) or endocrine dysfunction caused by pancreatitis often have weight loss and malnutrition as a result of tissue catabolism, because they cannot use dietary carbohydrates to meet energy needs. Although patients with NIDDM are more likely to be overweight than underweight, they too may become malnourished as a result of chronic or acute infections, trauma, major surgery, or other illnesses. Delivery of nutrition support in these patients, especially control of blood glucose, can be challenging. Blood glucose is monitored regularly, usually several times a day until the patient is stable. Regular insulin added to the solution is the most common method of managing hyperglycemia in the patient receiving TPN. The dosage required may be larger than the patient's usual subcutaneous dose, because some of the insulin adheres to glass bottles and plastic bags or administration sets.

In patients receiving enteral tube feedings, the transpyloric route (via nasoduodenal, nasojejunal, or jejunostomy tube) may be the most effective, since gastroparesis may make intragastric tube feedings impossible or inadequate. Transpyloric feedings are given continuously or by slow intermittent infusion, because dumping syndrome and poor absorption often occur if feedings are given rapidly into the small bowel. For the continuously tube-fed diabetic patient, control of blood glucose may be improved either with continuous insulin infusion or by use of a formula containing fiber, if such a formula is not contraindicated. Fiber may slow the absorption of the carbohydrate in the formula, producing a more delayed and sustained glycemic response.

TABLE 7-11 Nutrition Assessment of the Patient With an Endocrine Disorder

Area of Concern	History	Physical Findings	Laboratory Data
Underweight or protein-calorie malnutrition	Increased losses of calories in urine or feces caused by the following: Impaired glucose metabolism and glucosuria in type I diabetes mellitus Steatorrhea (in pancreatitis) Decreased intake because of the following: Discomfort with eating (in pancreatitis) Alcoholism (often a cause of pancreatitis)	Weight <90% of desirable or BMI <19 Recent weight loss Wasting of muscle and subcutaneous tissue	Urine glucose >0.5% Fecal fat >5 g/24 hr or <95% of intake Serum albumin <3.5 g/dL, or low transferrin or prealbumin level Total lymphocyte count <1200/mm^3 Creatinine excretion <17 mg/kg/day (women) or <23 mg/kg/day (men)
Overweight	NIDDM Sedentary life-style	Weight >120% of desirable or BMI >27	
Risk for fluid volume deficit	Diuresis (from diabetes insipidus or osmotic diuresis of HHNK or ketoacidosis)	Poor skin turgor Dry, sticky mucous membranes Thirst Loss of >0.23 kg (0.5 pound) in 24 hr Increased urine output	Serum glucose >250 mg/dL Urine glucose >0.5% Serum sodium >145 mEq/L Increasing Hct BUN >20 mg/dL
Risk for fluid volume excess	Fluid retention caused by SIADH	Edema (peripheral and/or pulmonary) Gain of >0.23 kg (0.5 pound) in 24 hr	Serum sodium <135 mEq/L Decreasing Hct
Potential zinc deficiency	Impaired absorption (in steatorrhea associated with pancreatitis) Increased urinary losses (in diuresis, diabetes mellitus, and alcoholism) Poor intake (in alcoholism)	Hypogeusia, dysgeusia Alopecia Seborrheic dermatitis Impaired wound healing	Serum zinc <60 μg/ml

Modified from Moore MC: *Pocket guide to nutritional care,* ed 3, St Louis, 1996, Mosby.
NIDDM, Non–insulin-dependent diabetes mellitus; *HHNK,* hyperglycemic hyperosmolar nonketotic (coma); *SIADH,* syndrome of inappropriate secretion of antidiuretic hormone.

Overweight patients. Aggressive attempts at weight loss are rarely warranted among very ill patients, although weight loss in overweight patients with NIDDM improves glucose tolerance. Instead of suggesting a low-calorie diet, nurses must encourage patients to select foods providing fiber and starches. Diets rich in complex carbohydrates have been reported to lower insulin requirements, increase the sensitivity of the peripheral tissues to insulin, and decrease serum cholesterol levels.[42]

Nutrition support should not be neglected simply because a patient is obese, because PCM develops even among such patients. When a patient is not expected to be able to eat for at least 5 to 7 days or inadequate intake persists for that period, the nurse needs to consult with the physician regarding initiation of tube feedings or TPN, if no steps have been taken to do so. No disease process benefits from starvation, and development or progression of nutritional deficits may contribute to complications (e.g., decubitus ulcers;

pulmonary or urinary tract infections; and sepsis, which prolong hospitalization, increase the costs of care, and may even result in death).

Severe vomiting or diarrhea in the insulin-dependent diabetic patient. When insulin-dependent patients experience vomiting and diarrhea severe enough to interfere significantly with oral intake or result in excessive fluid and electrolyte losses, adequate carbohydrates and fluids must be supplied. If patients are receiving oral feedings, they may not be able to adhere to their usual diet, but they generally are to consume 10 to 20 g of carbohydrates every 1 to 2 hours[43]; the physician usually provides guidelines as to the amount. Small amounts of liquids taken every 15 to 20 minutes are generally tolerated best by the patient with nausea and vomiting. Blood glucose and urine ketone levels are monitored frequently and the physician is notified of increasing hyperglycemia, ketonuria, difficulty retaining fluids, or signs of dehydration.

Nutrition Teaching in Endocrine Alterations

Most nutrition teaching in the patient with endocrine alterations focuses on understanding of the diet of the diabetic patient and on achieving the desirable body weight. The underweight or overweight patient must be helped to understand the need for weight changes. For example, weight loss in the obese diabetic individual improves glucose tolerance and may reduce or eliminate the need for insulin. In addition, it usually has beneficial effects on blood pressure and serum cholesterol levels.

Diet instruction for the diabetic patient is usually carried out by the dietitian, but the nurse needs to reinforce the information given. In addition to the importance of achieving and/or maintaining the desirable body weight, individuals with diabetes must understand the following key concepts:

1. Both hypoglycemia and hyperglycemia can have serious consequences. The patient needs to be aware of the precipitating factors and symptoms associated with each condition. Precipitating factors for hypoglycemia include failing to eat scheduled meals or snacks, eating meals or snacks late, vomiting or poor food intake during acute illness, prolonged or intense physical activity without a compensatory increase in carbohydrate intake or decrease in insulin dosage, impaired gluconeogenesis with alcohol intake, and impaired mentation and self-care skills resulting from alcohol intoxication or use of controlled drugs. Clinical manifestations include hunger; irritability; headache; shakiness; sweating; and altered neurologic status, ranging from drowsiness to unconsciousness and convulsions.
2. Diabetic ketoacidosis or hyperglycemic hyperosmolar nonketotic coma may result from uncontrolled hyperglycemia. Acute infectious illnesses or failure to take the prescribed dosage of insulin or oral hyperglycemia agents are common causes of severe hyperglycemia. Clinical manifestations of diabetic ketoacidosis include thirst; warm, dry skin; nausea and vomiting; "fruity"-smelling breath; pain in the abdomen; drowsiness; and polyuria. Excessive thirst, polyuria, dehydration, shallow respirations, and an altered sensorium often accompany hyperglycemic hyperosmolar nonketotic coma.
3. Hypoglycemia and excessive hyperglycemia can cause serious complications. Self-monitoring of the blood glucose level is a vital part of diabetic control. No planned meal or snack should ever be omitted, particularly if the patient is using insulin or an oral hypoglycemic agent. Meals and snacks must be eaten at regular times each day to avoid undue fluctuations in blood glucose. No foods can be added to the diet, unless hypoglycemia occurs or unless the patient is engaging in vigorous physical exertion. The best way to know whether increased food is needed during exercise is to monitor the blood glucose level. Alcohol inhibits gluconeogenesis and thus can contribute to hypoglycemia; it is best if consumption is limited to no more than 2 oz once or twice a week.[43]

   Good diabetic control (avoidance of hyperglycemia) is associated with a decreased risk of development of retinopathy, neuropathy, and other long-term sequelae of diabetes.[44]
4. Arteriosclerosis and hypertension are more common in individuals with diabetes than in the general population. Therefore control of cholesterol and saturated fat intake (see Table 7-5) and limitation of sodium intake to no more than 3 g/day are recommended.[42,43]
5. Dietary control is part of the management of every person with diabetes. Using the exchange lists for meal planning developed by the American Diabetes Association and American Dietetic Association is one way of managing the diet. Some individuals adhere more closely to their diets if taught the "carbohydrate counting"

method instead.[45] Carbohydrate is the main source of glucose in the diet, and counting the grams of carbohydrate in foods consumed, rather than considering carbohydrate, protein, and fat, provides a simplified way of regulating dietary intake. With carbohydrate counting, insulin-dependent individuals usually administer an amount of insulin determined by the carbohydrate content of their intake (e.g., 1 unit of insulin per 10 g carbohydrate).

6. "Dietetic" and "diabetic" foods are unnecessary. Labels containing these words do not always mean that foods are unsweetened. They may be sweetened with fructose, sorbitol, or other absorbable sweeteners. The patient who wishes to use these products must read the label carefully to determine exactly what dietetic or diabetic means in this context. Some "dietetic" cookies contain more calories than does the standard version of the product. Fruits canned in water or juice (with the juice drained before serving) are available in all supermarkets and are suitable for the diabetic patient. Also, fat-free or very low-fat products may have more carbohydrate than the regular, fat-containing versions of those products. The patient must take this extra carbohydrate into account.
7. Moderate exercise has many benefits for patients with NIDDM, including increased sensitivity of the tissues to the effects of insulin and improved glucose tolerance, weight control, reduced blood cholesterol levels, and lowered blood pressure.[45] If the physician approves, the patient can be encouraged to begin an exercise program, gradually increasing the length and intensity of the exercise sessions.

NUTRITION AND HEMATOIMMUNE ALTERATIONS

Malnutrition has well-known adverse effects on hematoimmune function. Generalized PCM, for example, depresses cell-mediated immunity, secretory immunity, complement levels, and phagocyte activity. Deficiencies of single nutrients—especially iron; zinc; selenium; folic acid; and vitamins B_{12}, B_6, C, and A—also impair immunologic function.[46,47] Therefore in the patient with an existing hematoimmune disorder, maintenance of adequate nutrition is essential to prevent additional immunologic deficits.

Nutrition Assessment in Hematoimmune Alterations

Assessment of the patient with a hematoimmune disorder is summarized in Table 7-12. Acquired immunodeficiency syndrome (AIDS) is the hematoimmune disorder most likely to have profound nutritional consequences. Unfortunately, generalized PCM is a common sequela of AIDS. There are multiple etiologic factors for the malnutrition. AIDS itself may be associated with a poorly understood enteropathy that causes diarrhea and malabsorption. Furthermore, opportunistic GI infections caused by various fungi, viruses, bacteria, and protozoas may cause diarrhea.[48] *Cryptosporidium,* a particularly resistant protozoa, can cause intractable, profuse, watery diarrhea lasting for months. Calorie and protein needs are elevated in persons with AIDS, because metabolic rate and catabolism increase as a result of infection, fever, and malignancies such as lymphoma and Kaposi's sarcoma. At the same time, oral intake is frequently suppressed by emotional reactions to the personal, family, and financial stresses imposed by AIDS; oral and esophageal pain from lesions of Kaposi's sarcoma, herpes, candidiasis, and/or chemotherapy; nausea, vomiting, and anorexia associated with antibiotic therapy, chemotherapy for malignancies, or antiviral agents used in the treatment of AIDS (Table 7-13); and impaired motor ability, confusion, and dementia caused by AIDS encephalitis or opportunistic central nervous system infections. AIDS patients often have marked weight loss; hypoalbuminemia; and low levels of zinc, selenium, and other minerals.[46,47]

Nutrition Intervention in Hematoimmune Alterations

Nutritional needs may be quite high in some patients with AIDS, particularly those with sepsis. It is estimated that AIDS increases calorie needs 20% to 60%,[5] and patients may require 1.2 to 1.8 g amino acids/kg/day to maintain a zero or positive nitrogen balance.[49] Ideally, nutrition intervention in patients with AIDS can be achieved via the GI tract. Enteral feedings (oral or tube) maintain the integrity of the gut mucosa, are relatively inexpensive, and are the most physiologic acceptable means of nutritional support.

Promotion of adequate oral intake. As mentioned, a host of factors may interfere with adequate oral intake in the individual with AIDS. With thorough assessment and careful planning to meet the needs of the individual, however, it is often possible to increase oral intake significantly. If nutritional supple-

TABLE 7-12 Nutrition Assessment of the Patient With a Hematoimmune Disorder

Area of Concern	History	Physical Findings	Laboratory Data
Protein-calorie malnutrition	Nutrient losses caused by malabsorption and diarrhea Increased needs caused by infection and fever Poor intake caused by the following: Anorexia (related to respiratory or other infections, emotional stress, medication side effects) Pain associated with eating (e.g., *Candida,* esophagitis, and endotracheal Kaposi's sarcoma) Dementia or CNS infections Dysphagia	Weight <90% of desirable or BMI <19 Recent weight loss Wasting of muscle and subcutaneous tissue	Serum albumin <3.5 g/dL, or low transferrin or prealbumin level Negative nitrogen balance Creatinine excretion <17 mg/kg/day (women) or <23 mg/kg/day (men)
DISORDERS OF MINERAL AND VITAMIN NUTRITURE			
Iron (Fe)	Poor intake of meats, whole-grain or enriched breads and cereals, and legumes because of the following: Anorexia Pain associated with eating	Pallor, blue sclerae Fatigue Tachycardia	Hct <37% (women) or <42% (men); Hgb <12 g/dL (women) or <14 g/dL (men); Low MCV, MCH, MCHC
Zinc (Zn)	Poor intake of meats, whole-grain or enriched breads and cereals, and legumes because of the following: Anorexia Pain associated with eating	Hypogeusia, dysgeusia Alopecia Dermatitis Impaired wound healing Diarrhea	Serum Zn <60 μg/dL
Vitamin B_{12}	Small intestinal disease with malabsorption Macrobiotic or other vegetarian diet that does not include vitamin B_{12} sources	Pallor Glossitis Neuropathy Psychiatric symptoms	Hct <37% (women) or < 42% (men); Hgb <12 g/dL (women) or <14 g/dL (men); increased MCV

Modified from Moore MC: *Pocket guide to nutritional care,* ed 3, St Louis, 1996, Mosby.

ments must be given to improve intake, it is usually best to choose those that are lactose-free. Patients with disease of the small bowel often have lactose intolerance, which causes diarrhea when lactose is ingested. Awareness of the effects of drugs on nutrient intake (see Table 7-13) helps the nurse to plan appropriate interventions and patient teaching to maximize oral intake.

Administration of nutrition support. Despite dietary modifications and encouragement, some patients may find consuming an adequate diet impossible. Temporary oral or esophageal disorders—such as candidiasis, which produces painful lesions—may temporarily impair oral intake. Other individuals may have such severe diarrhea and malabsorption that they are unable to maintain their nutritional state with oral feedings alone. Nasogastric, nasoduodenal, or nasojejunal feeding tubes can be used to administer tube feedings if the patient does not have severe oral or esophageal disease. Gastrostomy or jejunostomy tubes are used when long-term feedings are needed or when oral and/or esophageal complications prevent nasal intubation. Continuous feedings (given either 24 hours a day or only nocturnally) may improve absorption in

TABLE 7-13 Nutrition-Related Side Effects of Some Medications Used in Treatment of Patients with AIDS

Medication	Side Effect				
	Nausea/ Vomiting	Diarrhea	Sore Mouth/ Throat	Dry Mouth/ Unpleasant Taste	Anorexia
AIDS CHEMOTHERAPEUTIC AGENTS					
Acyclovir	x	x	x	x	
Didanosine	x	x	x		
Zalcitabine	x		x	x	x
Zidovudine (AZT)	x	x		x	x
ANTIFUNGAL, ANTIBACTERIAL, AND ANTIPROTOZOAL AGENTS					
Amphotericin B	x	x			x
Atovaquoné	x	x			
Fluconazole	x	x			
Ketoconazole	x				x
Nystatin	x	x			
Pentamidine					
IV or IM	x			x	x
Inhalable	x		x	x	x
Rifabutin	x			x	
Trimethoprim-sulfamethoxazole	x	x	x		x
ANTIVIRAL AND ANTITUMOR AGENTS					
Foscarnet	x	x			
Interferon alfa	x	x	x	x	x

Modified from Moore MC: *Pocket guide to nutritional care,* ed 3, St Louis, 1996, Mosby.

individuals with small bowel disease. For patients with malabsorption, elemental formulas often are used. These contain predigested nutrients, no lactose, and little fat, thereby maximizing absorption in the patient with impaired absorptive ability.

Parenteral nutrition is reserved for patients for whom enteral feeding is not feasible or beneficial. Strict asepsis is maintained to reduce the risk of catheter-related infection. Patients with sepsis often are glucose-intolerant, and therefore it is especially important to monitor their blood glucose levels frequently.

Nutrition Teaching in Hematoimmune Alterations

Nutrition teaching for the patient with AIDS should include the importance of good nutrition in maintaining strength and optimal functioning and in preventing additional deficits in immune function and wound healing. The patient must be discouraged from viewing nutrition itself as a panacea; its major role is in supportive care.

Consumption of an adequate diet. The AIDS patient must be encouraged to consume an adequate diet of regular foods, if at all possible. High-fat foods are a good source of calories. However, their intake may need to be limited or avoided if the patient has diarrhea and malabsorption, because they tend to exacerbate the problem. Frequent small feedings are often better tolerated than are a few larger daily meals. Many individuals with disease of the small bowel exhibit lactose intolerance. Patients with lactose intolerance may be able to tolerate yogurt, chocolate milk, and aged cheeses even if they experience symptoms (bloating, abdominal cramping, and diarrhea) when they consume liquid milk. Lactase enzyme, available at many pharmacies and supermarkets, can be added to liquid milk to allow such patients to digest the lactose, and lactase-treated milk is available in many markets. Lactose-free commercial supplements also can be used to promote calorie and protein intake in patients with lactose intolerance.

A multivitamin/mineral supplement providing 100% of the recommended dietary allowances (RDAs) is suggested for patients with inadequate diets, but there is no evidence that any particular vitamin or mineral has a beneficial effect in treating AIDS or its associated complications.[46,47]

Food safety. Individuals with AIDS are especially susceptible to infections caused by food-borne organisms. To prevent such infections, food must be stored, prepared, and served with scrupulous cleanliness. All individuals preparing food for the patient must be taught to avoid cross contaminating food (e.g., using a cutting board to slice meat when it has just been used to prepare raw vegetables). All raw fruits and vegetables must be washed well, and meat must be thoroughly cooked. Consumption of raw eggs, fish or shellfish (e.g., sushi or raw oysters), and meat must be avoided, as must unpasteurized milk. Leftover food must be promptly refrigerated and then discarded if not consumed within 3 days.

Food fads and medicinal uses of foods. As with patients suffering from other chronic and serious diseases, individuals with AIDS often adhere to alternative or "complementary" treatments. A variety of diets, special foods, and supplements are used by individuals with AIDS.[50] Some of the practices, such as use of megadoses of fat-soluble vitamins and minerals or use of a macrobiotic diet, can be harmful. There is no empiric evidence to show that any are helpful. While maintaining a nonjudgmental and accepting attitude, the nurse needs to encourage the patient to follow a balanced diet. Sometimes it is possible to help the patient devise ways to make the alternative diet practice more helpful (e.g., encouraging the addition of seafood to the macrobiotic diet).

Nutrition support modalities. Patients with AIDS need to be made aware of the nutrition support options available to them. With this information, the patient will have a basis for making an informed decision about initiating or continuing nutrition support. The patient's family or friends also may need this information to assist the health care team in making decisions about providing nonvolitional nutrition support in a patient with severe dementia.

ADMINISTERING NUTRITION SUPPORT

Enteral Nutrition Support

The enteral route is the preferred method of feeding whenever possible, because this route is generally safer, more physiologically acceptable, and much less expensive than is parenteral feeding. The GI tract plays an important role in maintaining the body's immunologic defenses. Some of the barriers to infection in the GI tract include the normal acidic gastric pH; peristalsis, which limits GI tract colonization by pathogenic bacteria; the normal gut microflora, which inhibit growth of or destroy some pathogenic organisms; rapid desquamation and regeneration of intestinal epithelial cells (with pathogenic organisms being excreted with the desquamated cells); the layer of mucus secreted by GI tract cells; bile, which detoxifies endotoxin in the intestine and also delivers immunoglobulin A to the intestine; and gut-associated lymphoid tissue.[51] All of these immune defenses are stimulated by the presence of food within the GI tract. Resting the GI tract by providing only parenteral nutrients has been demonstrated in animal models to contribute to "bacterial translocation" whereby bacteria normally found in the GI tract cross the intestinal barrier, are found in the regional mesenteric lymph nodes, and give rise to generalized sepsis. In humans the importance of bacterial translocation has not been fully defined, but it is noteworthy that in a group of 98 trauma patients randomized to receive enteral feedings or TPN, major infectious complications were significantly lower in those receiving enteral nutrition.[52] A meta-analysis confirmed that early enteral feedings, compared with TPN, reduced sepsis rates in postoperative patients.[53]

Some of the enterally delivered nutrients that may benefit critically ill patients include fiber and the amino acids glutamine and arginine. Fiber is not digested by the human but can be metabolized by gut bacteria to yield short-chain fatty acids, the primary fuel of the colon cells. Glutamine is the major fuel of the small intestinal cells; because of poor solubility, TPN solutions provide little glutamine, whereas the proteins contained in enteral feedings do provide glutamine. Arginine is involved in protein synthesis and also is a precursor of nitric oxide, a molecule that stimulates vasodilation in the gut and heart and mediates hepatic protein synthesis during sepsis.[54,55]

There are a variety of commercial enteral feeding products, some of which are designed to meet the specialized needs of very sick patients. Products designed for the stressed patient with trauma or sepsis are usually rich in glutamine; arginine; branched amino acids (a major fuel source, especially for muscle); and antioxidant nutrients, such as vitamins C, E, and A, and selenium. The antioxidants help to reduce oxidative injury to the tissues (e.g., from reperfusion injury).

Some products can be consumed orally, but it is difficult for the critically ill patient to consume enough orally to meet the increased needs associated with stress. Table 7-14 provides more information about the major categories of products.

Oral supplementation. For patients who can eat and have normal digestion and absorption but simply cannot consume enough regular foods to meet caloric and protein needs, oral supplementation may be necessary. Patients with mild to moderate anorexia, burns, or trauma sometimes fall into this category. To improve intake and tolerance of supplements, the critical care nurse needs to do the following:

1. Collaborate with the dietitian to choose appropriate products and allow the patient to participate in the selection process, if possible. Milk shakes made with ice cream and half-and-half; powdered milk added to cereal and fluid milk; and instant breakfast are often more palatable and economical than are commercial supplements. However, intolerance of lactose is common among adults, especially Blacks, Asians, Native Americans, and Inuits. Furthermore, many disease processes (e.g., Crohn's disease, radiation enteritis, AIDS, and severe gastroenteritis) can cause lactose intolerance. Individuals with this problem often require commercial lactose-free supplements.
2. Serve commercial supplements well-chilled or on ice, because this improves flavor.
3. Advise patients to sip formulas slowly, consuming no more than 240 ml over 30 to 45 minutes. These products contain easily digestable carbohydrates. If formulas are consumed too quickly, rapid hydrolysis of the carbohydrate in the duodenum can contribute to dumping syndrome, characterized by abdominal cramping, weakness, tachycardia, and diarrhea.
4. Record all supplement intake separately on the intake and output sheet so that it can be differentiated from intake of water and other liquids.

Enteral tube feedings. Tube feedings are used for patients who have at least some digestive and absorptive capability but are unwilling or unable to consume enough by mouth. Patients with profound anorexia and those experiencing severe stress that greatly increases their nutritional needs (e.g., those with major burns or trauma) often benefit from tube feedings.[39] Individuals who require elemental formulas because of impaired digestion or absorption or the specialized formulas for altered metabolic conditions (see Table 7-14) usually require tube feeding, because the unpleasant flavors of the free amino acids, peptides, or protein hydrolysates used in these formulas are very difficult to mask.

Location and type of feeding tube. Nasal intubation is the simplest and most commonly used route for gaining access to the GI tract; this method allows access to the stomach, duodenum, or jejunum. Using a small-bore, soft (e.g., polyurethane or silicone rubber) feeding tube promotes comfort. Tube enterostomy—a gastrostomy or jejunostomy—is used primarily for long-term feedings (6 to 12 weeks or more) and when obstruction makes the nasoenteral route inaccessible. Tube enterostomies may also be used for the patient who is at risk for tube dislodgement because of severe agitation or confusion. A conventional gastrostomy or jejunostomy is often performed at the time of other abdominal surgery. The percutaneous endoscopic gastrostomy (PEG) tube has become extremely popular because it can be inserted without the use of general anesthetics. Percutaneous endoscopic jejunostomy (PEJ) tubes are also used, but reported complication rates have been several times greater than those with PEGs.[56]

Transpyloric feedings via nasoduodenal, nasojejunal, or jejunostomy tubes are commonly used when there is a risk of pulmonary aspiration, because theoretically the pyloric sphincter provides a barrier that lessens the risk of regurgitation and aspiration. In one series of 100 patients (including 13 who had previously aspirated during oral or nasoenteral feeding), none of the patients aspirated the tube feeding formula when it was delivered via surgical jejunostomy.[26] On the other hand, other investigators reported the frequency of aspiration to be the same with nasoduodenal and nasogastric tubes.[57] In one series of 36 patients with PEJ tubes, pulmonary aspiration occurred in four patients; however, in all four cases the tube tips were found to have migrated into the stomach or the feeding ports on the tube were found to be in the duodenum at the time of aspiration.[56] Thus the data regarding aspiration and jejunal feedings remain inconclusive, but at the present it seems that having the feeding ports positioned distal to the ligament of Treitz may result in the least risk of pulmonary aspiration.[56]

Since transpyloric feedings can be given without regard to the rate of gastric emptying, they often have an advantage over intragastric feedings for patients with gastric atony, such as those with head injury, gastroparesis associated with uremia or diabetes, or postoperative ileus. Small bowel motility returns more quickly than gastric motility after surgery, and thus it

TABLE 7-14 Enteral Formulas

Formula Type	Nutritional Uses	Clinical Examples	Examples of Commercial Products (Manufacturer)
FORMULAS USED WHEN GI TRACT IS FULLY FUNCTIONAL			
Polymeric (standard): Contains whole proteins (10%-15% of calories), long-chain triglycerides (25%-40% of calories), and glucose polymers or oligosaccharides (50%-60% of calories); most provide 1 calorie/ml	Inability to ingest food Inability to consume enough to meet needs	Oral or esophageal cancer Coma, stroke Anorexia resulting from chronic illness Burns or trauma	Ensure (Ross) Nutren (Clintec) Isosource (Sandoz) Pediasure (Ross), for children ages 1-10 Attain (Sherwood) Isocal (Mead Johnson)
High-nitrogen: Same as polymeric except protein provides >15% of calories	Same as polymeric, plus mild catabolism and protein deficits	Trauma or burns Sepsis	Isotein HN (Sandoz) Osmolite HN (Ross) Ultracal (Mead Johnson)
Concentrated: Same as polymeric except concentrated to 2 calorie/ml	Same as polymeric, but fluid restriction needed	Congestive heart failure Neurosurgery COPD Liver disease	Deliver 2.0 (Mead Johnson) TwoCal HN (Ross) Magnacal (Sherwood) Nutren 2.0 (Clintec)
FORMULAS USED WHEN GI FUNCTION IS IMPAIRED			
Elemental or predigested: Contains hydrolyzed (partially digested) protein, peptides (short chains of amino acids), and/or amino acids, little fat (<10% of calories) or high MCT, and glucose polymers or oligosaccharides; most provide 1 calorie/ml	Impaired digestion and/or absorption	Short bowel syndrome Radiation enteritis Inflammatory bowel disease	Criticare HN (Mead Johnson) Vital High Nitrogen (Ross) Reabilan HN (Elan) Vivonex Pediatric (Sandoz), for children ages 1-10 yr Accupep HPF (Sherwood)
DIETS FOR SPECIFIC DISEASE STATES*			
Renal failure: Concentrated in calories; low sodium, potassium, magnesium, phosphorus, and vitamins A and D; low protein for renal insufficiency; higher protein formulas for dialyzed patients	Renal insufficiency	Predialysis	Suplena (Ross) Travasorb Renal (Clintec) Amin-Aid (Kendall McGaw), contains only essential amino acids and histidine
	Dialysis	Hemodialysis or peritoneal dialysis	Nepro (Ross)
Hepatic failure: Enriched in BCAA; low sodium	Protein intolerance	Hepatic encephalopathy	Travasorb Hepatic (Clintec) Hepatic-Aid II (Kendall McGaw)
Pulmonary dysfunction: Low carbohydrate, high fat	Respiratory insufficiency	Ventilator dependence	NutriVent (Clintec) Pulmocare (Ross)
Glucose intolerance: High fat, low carbohydrate (contains starch and fructose)	Glucose intolerance	Individuals with diabetes mellitus whose blood sugar is poorly controlled with standard formulas	Glucerna (Ross)
Critical care: High protein; most contain MCT to improve fat absorption; some have increased zinc and vitamin C for wound healing; some are high in antioxidants (vitamin E, β-carotene); some are enriched with arginine, glutamine, and/or omega-3 fatty acids	Critical illness	Severe trauma or burns Sepsis	Immun-Aid (Kendall McGaw) Protain XL (Sherwood) Impact (Sandoz) Perative (Ross) Replete (Clintec)

*These diets may be beneficial for selected patients, but there is no evidence that they are needed by all patients with these disease states.

is often possible to deliver transpyloric feedings within 1 to 2 days of trauma or surgery.[52,53]

Nursing management. The nurse's role in delivery of tube feedings usually includes insertion of the tube, if a temporary tube is used; maintenance of the tube; administration of the feedings; prevention and detection of complications associated with this form of therapy; and participation in assessment of the patient's response to tube feedings. Assessment of response is discussed later in this chapter.

Tube placement. Critical care nurses are usually familiar with tube insertion, and therefore this topic is not discussed in depth here. However, transpyloric passage of tubes deserves special mention. Tubes with mercury, stainless steel, or tungsten weights on the proximal end are often used when transpyloric tube placement is desired, in the belief that the weight will encourage transpyloric passage of the tube or that the weight will help the tube maintain its position once it passes into the bowel. However, unweighted tubes are either just as likely or more likely to migrate through the pylorus than weighted tubes.[38,58] Because the weights sometimes cause discomfort while being inserted through the nares, unweighted tubes may be preferable. Administration of metoclopramide or erythromycin before tube insertion increases the likelihood of tube passage through the pylorus.[58,59]

Correct tube placement must be confirmed before initiation of feedings and regularly throughout the course of enteral feedings. Radiographs are the most accurate way of assessing tube placement, but repeated radiographs are costly and can expose the patient to excessive radiation. The pH of fluid removed from the feeding tube can be used to confirm tube placement; some tubes are equipped with pH monitoring systems. If the pH is less than 4 in patients not receiving gastric acid inhibitors, or less than 5.5 in patients who are receiving acid inhibitors, the tube tip is likely to be in the stomach.[60] Intestinal secretions usually have a pH greater than 6, and respiratory tract fluids usually have a pH greater than 5.5. The esophagus may have an acid pH, which may cause confusion between esophageal and gastric placement. However, other clues can help in identifying a tube with its distal tip in the esophagus; it may be especially difficult to aspirate fluid out of the tube, a large portion of the tube may extend out of the body (but a tube inserted to the proper length could be coiled in the esophagus), and belching often occurs immediately after air is injected into the tube.[60] Food coloring (usually blue, which is unlikely to be confused with any body secretion) can be added to the formula as an aid to detection of formula in the respiratory system.

Tube maintenance and oral care. Maintenance of the tube includes regular irrigation of the tube to maintain patency, skin care around the insertion site, and mouth care. Small-bore (usually 8 or 10 French) "nonreactive" tubes made of polyurethane, silicone rubber, and similar materials are much more comfortable for the patient than are the older polyethylene or polyvinylchloride tubes (usually 12 to 16 French), which stiffen with age. Patient complaints of discomfort and nasal and skin erosion have decreased with the use of the "nonreactive" tubes. Unfortunately, these small tubes tend to clog readily. Regular irrigation helps to prevent tube occlusion. Generally, 30 to 60 ml of irrigant every 3 to 4 hours or after each feeding is appropriate. The volume of irrigant may have to be reduced during fluid restriction. The irrigant is usually water, but other fluids, such as cranberry juice or cola beverages, are sometimes used in an effort to reduce the incidence of tube occlusion. However, cranberry juice is inferior to, and cola beverages appear no better than, water for irrigating tubes.[61] Furthermore, once a tube has occluded, cranberry juice and cola are of little use in clearing the occlusion, but a solution of pancreatic enzymes may be effective.[59]

The skin around the tube should be cleaned at least daily, and the tape around the tube replaced whenever loosened or soiled. Secure taping helps to prevent movement of the tube, which may irritate the nares or skin or result in accidental dislodgement of the tube. Dressings are used initially around gastrostomy insertion sites. The dressing is changed daily and the skin cleansed with half-strength hydrogen peroxide. If leakage of gastric fluid occurs around a gastrostomy tube, the skin can be protected with karaya powder.

To prevent dryness of the mouth (a common complaint during tube feeding), the patient is encouraged to breathe through the nose as much as possible, drink and eat as much as desired (if compatible with the patient's nutrition orders), and suck sugar-free candies or chew sugar-free gum (if allowed); regular mouth care is also of benefit. Patients often report that they can "taste" the tube feedings, and frequent mouth care will clear the palate of unpleasant flavors from the formula, as well as clean the teeth, tongue, and oral mucous membranes.

Formula delivery. Careful attention to administration of tube feedings can prevent many complications. Very clean or aseptic technique in the handling and administration of the formula can help prevent bacterial contamination and a resultant infection.[52] The optimal schedule for delivery of feedings also is important. Tube feedings may be administered intermittently or continuously. Bolus feedings, which are intermittent feedings delivered rapidly into the stomach or small bowel, are likely to cause distention, vomiting, and dumping syndrome with diarrhea. Instead of using bolus feedings, nurses can gradually drip intermittent feedings, with each feeding lasting 20 to 30 minutes or longer, to promote optimal assimilation. The question of which feeding schedule—continuous or intermittent—is superior in critically ill patients remains unanswered. However, in one group of 24 mechanically ventilated intensive care patients receiving continuous nasogastric feedings but no routine antacids or H_2-receptor antagonists, 13 patients were observed to have a gastric pH that was always greater than 3.5; in the other 11 patients, pH was intermittently less than 3.5.[62] The patients with a pH greater than 3.5 were significantly more likely to develop pneumonia, and the mortality rate was high among patients developing pneumonia.[62] It appeared that patients with the high gastric pH had lost their natural defense against microorganisms in the stomach, and bacteria proceeded to colonize the trachea and subsequently cause pneumonia. Where continuous enteral feedings are desirable in very sick patients, it may be that transpyloric, rather than intragastric, feedings are preferable. (∞Pneumonia, p. 663.)

Prevention and correction of complications. Some of the more common complications of tube feeding are pulmonary aspiration, diarrhea, constipation, tube occlusion, and delayed gastric emptying. Nursing management of these problems is detailed in Table 7-15.

Total Parenteral Nutrition

Total parenteral nutrition (TPN) refers to the delivery of all nutrients by the intravenous route. It is used when the GI tract is not functional or when nutritional needs cannot be met solely via the GI tract. Likely candidates for TPN include patients who have a severely impaired absorption (as in short bowel syndrome, collagen-vascular diseases, or radiation enteritis); intestinal obstruction; peritonitis; or prolonged ileus. It may also be useful in selected patients who can benefit from a period of bowel rest, including those with moderate to severe pancreatitis or with enterocutaneous fistulae.[39] In both cases, enteral intake (which stimulates secretion of digestive enzymes) is likely to exacerbate the condition, whereas bowel rest may promote healing. In addition, some postoperative, trauma, or burn patients may need temporary TPN.

Routes for TPN. TPN may be delivered through either central or peripheral veins. Because it requires an indwelling catheter, central vein TPN carries an increased risk of sepsis, as well as potential insertion-related complications, such as pneumothorax and hemothorax.[39] Air embolism is also more likely with central vein TPN. However, central venous catheters provide very secure IV access and allow delivery of more hyperosmolar solutions than does peripheral TPN. TPN solutions containing 25% to 35% dextrose are commonly used via central veins, and this provides an inexpensive source of calories. Patients requiring multiple IV therapies and frequent blood sampling usually have multilumen central venous catheters, and TPN is often infused via these catheters. Some clinical studies have reported that catheter-related sepsis is higher with multilumen catheters; others have found no difference in comparison to single lumen catheters.[63] Clearly, patients requiring multilumen catheters are likely to be very ill and immunocompromised, and scrupulous aseptic technique is essential in maintaining multilumen catheters. The manipulation involved in frequent changes of IV fluid and obtaining blood specimens through these catheters increases the risk of catheter contamination. Peripherally inserted catheters (PICs) allow central venous access through long catheters inserted in peripheral sites. This reduces the risk of complications associated with percutaneous cannulation of the subclavian vein (e.g., subclavian vein laceration, pneumothorax, and chylothorax).

Peripheral TPN rarely is associated with serious infectious or mechanical complications, but it does require good peripheral venous access. Therefore it may not be appropriate for long-term nutrition support or for patients receiving multiple IV therapies.

Nursing management. Nursing management of the patient receiving TPN includes catheter care, administration of solutions, prevention or correction of complications, and evaluation of patient responses to IV feedings. Evaluation of patient response is discussed later in this chapter.

The indwelling central venous catheter provides an excellent nidus for infection.[63] The nurse has a major role in preventing this complication of TPN therapy. Catheter care includes maintaining an intact dressing at the catheter insertion site and manipulating the catheter and administration tubing with aseptic technique. Dressings for TPN catheters may consist of

TABLE 7-15 Nursing Management of Enteral Tube Feeding Complications

Complication	Contributing Factor(s)	Prevention/Correction
Pulmonary aspiration	Feeding tube positioned in esophagus or respiratory tract	Check tube placement before intermittent feeding and every 4-6 hr during continuous feedings by checking the pH of fluid aspirated from the tube (usually gastric juice pH is <3.5); be aware that an in-rush of air can sometimes be auscultated over the right upper quadrant even when the distal tip of the tube is in the esophagus or respiratory tract
	Regurgitation of formula	Elevate head to 45° during feedings unless contraindicated; if head cannot be raised, position patient in lateral (especially right lateral, which facilitates gastric emptying) or prone position to improve drainage of vomitus from the mouth; if head must be in a dependent position, discontinue feedings 30-60 min earlier and restart them only when the head can be raised
		Keep cuff of endotracheal or tracheostomy tube inflated during feedings, if possible
		Cisapride or metoclopramide may improve gastric emptying and decrease the risk of regurgitation
		Add food coloring to formula to facilitate diagnosis of aspiration
		Evaluate feeding tolerance every 2 hr initially, then less frequently as condition becomes stable; intolerance may be manifested by bloating, abdominal distention and pain, lack of stool and flatus, diminished or absent bowel sounds, tense abdomen, increased tympany, nausea and vomiting, residual volume >200 ml aspirated from an NG tube or >100 ml aspirated from a gastrostomy tube (but a high residual volume in the absence of other abnormal findings does not appear to be grounds for stopping feedings); use a 60 ml syringe to aspirate residual volumes to prevent collapse of the tube, which prevents full emptying of the stomach; (measuring residual volumes is a controversial practice; see the section on tube occlusion that follows); if intolerance is suspected, abdominal radiographs may be done to check for distended gastric bubble, distended loops of bowel, or air/fluid levels.
Diarrhea	Medications with GI side effects (antibiotics, digitalis, laxatives, magnesium-containing antacids, quinidine, caffeine, and many others)	Evaluate the patient's medications to determine their potential for causing diarrhea, consulting the pharmacist if necessary
	Hypertonic formula or medications (e.g., oral suspensions of antibiotics, potassium, or other electrolytes), which cause dumping syndrome	Evaluate formula administration procedures to be sure that feedings are not being given by bolus infusion; administer the formula continuously or by slow intermittent infusion
		Dilute enteral medications well

Data adapted from McClave SA and others: *JPEN J Parenter Enteral Nutr* 16:99, 1992; Powell KS and others: *JPEN J Parenter Enteral Nutr* 17:243, 1993; and Spapen HD and others: *Crit Care Med* 23:481, 1995.
NG, Nasogastric.

TABLE 7-15 Nursing Management of Enteral Tube Feeding Complications—cont'd

Complication	Contributing Factor(s)	Prevention/Correction
Diarrhea—cont'd	Bacterial contamination of the formula	Use scrupulously clean technique in administering tube feedings; prepare formula with sterile water if there are any concerns about the safety of the water supply or if the patient is seriously immunocompromised; keep opened containers of formula refrigerated and discard them within 24 hr; discard enteral feeding containers and administration sets every 24 hr; hang formula no more than 4-8 hr unless it comes prepackaged in sterile administration sets; be especially careful with feedings given to patients being fed transpylorically or those receiving cimetidine or antacids, because these patients lack the normal antibacterial barrier of the stomach's acid
	Fecal impaction with seepage of liquid stool around the impaction	Perform a digital rectal examination to rule out impaction; see guidelines for prevention of constipation that follow
Constipation	Low-residue formula, creating little fecal bulk	Consult with the physician regarding the possibility of using a fiber-containing formula
Tube occlusion	Medications administered via tube (which either physically plug the tube or coagulate the formula, causing it to clog the tube)	If medications must be given by tube, avoid use of crushed tablets; consult with the pharmacist to determine whether medications can be dispensed as elixirs or suspensions; irrigate tube with water before and after administering any medication; never add any medication to the formula unless the two are known to be compatible
	Sedimentation of formula	Irrigate tube every 4-8 hr during continuous feedings and after every intermittent feeding
	Aspirating gastric contents to measure residual volumes (acidified protein from the formula clots in the tube)	It has been suggested that aspiration of gastric residuals be avoided with small-bore feeding tubes (8 French) and that patient tolerance be assessed by physical examination; if residuals are measured, flush the tube thoroughly after returning the formula to the stomach and use a tube as large as is compatible with patient comfort (usually 10 French)
Gastric retention	Delayed gastric emptying related to head trauma, sepsis, diabetic or uremic gastroparesis, electrolyte balance, or other illness	The cause must be corrected if possible; consult with the physician about use of transpyloric feedings or metoclopramide or cisapride to stimulate gastric emptying; encourage patient to lie in right lateral position frequently, unless contraindicated

transparent film, gauze and tape, or hydrocolloid. A meta-analysis of seven prospective studies comparing transparent film and gauze/tape dressings revealed that catheter tip infections were more prevalent with the use of transparent dressings.[64] There are few studies available that examine skin cleansing agents for catheter insertion sites. In one randomized trial of povidone-iodine, alcohol, and chlorhexidine hydrochloride, the investigators determined that chlorhexidine was more effective than the other agents in reducing catheter-related infections.[65]

TPN solutions usually consist of amino acids, dextrose, electrolytes, vitamins, minerals, and trace elements. Although dextrose-amino acid solutions are commonly thought of as good growth media for microorganisms, they actually suppress the growth of most organisms usually associated with catheter-related sepsis, except yeasts. However, because the many manipulations required to prepare solutions increase the possibility of contamination, TPN solutions are best used with caution. They need to be prepared under laminar flow conditions in the pharmacy, with avoidance of additions on the nursing unit. Solution containers need to be inspected for cracks or leaks before hanging, and solutions must be discarded within 24 hours of hanging. An in-line 0.22 μm filter, which eliminates all microorganisms but not endotoxins, may be used in administration of solutions. Use of the filter, however, cannot be substituted for scrupulous aseptic technique, because there is no conclusive evidence that filters decrease sepsis rates.

In contrast to dextrose-amino acid solutions, IV lipid emulsions support the proliferation of many microorganisms. Furthermore, lipid emulsions cannot be filtered through an in-line 0.22 μm filter, because some particles in the emulsions have larger diameters than this. Lipid emulsions are handled with strict asepsis, and they must be discarded within 12 to 24 hours of hanging. There is a trend toward mixing lipid emulsions with dextrose-amino acid TPN solutions. Although this saves nursing time, the nurse must be extremely careful in administering these solutions. TPN solutions containing lipids cannot be filtered through an in-line 0.22 μm filter, and they support the growth of most bacteria and *Candida albicans* better than do dextrose-amino acid TPN solutions.

Prevention or correction of complications. Some of the more common and serious complications of TPN include catheter-related sepsis, air embolism, pneumothorax, central venous thrombosis, catheter occlusion, and metabolic imbalances such as hypoglycemia and hyperglycemia. These complications, along with nursing approaches to their management, are described in Table 7-16.

Nutrition Pharmacology

A variety of nutrients, hormones, and growth factors have potential for improving the outcome of critically ill patients. In addition to arginine, glutamine, and fiber or short-chain fatty acids, which have already been discussed, growth hormone has been observed to improve healing of donor sites in burn patients and to reduce the risk of sepsis in critically ill patients.[66] Insulin-like growth factor-1 (IGF-1) appears to have promise in preserving lean body mass of injured patients.[66] The effects of the "omega-3" or "n-3" fatty acids are also under investigation. These long-chain fatty acids derived primarily from fish oil are involved in synthesis of eicosanoids (molecules with hormone–like activity)—prostaglandins, prostacyclin, and leukotrienes—and thus may modulate the inflammatory response.[54] Improvement of cell-mediated immunity and T-lymphocyte function have been reported in patients receiving formulas supplemented with nucleotides (particularly ribonucleic acid [RNA]).[54-55]

EVALUATING RESPONSE TO NUTRITION SUPPORT

Assessment of response to nutrition support is an ongoing process that involves anthropometric measurements, physical examination, and biochemical evaluation. Table 7-17 summarizes some of the parameters that are used most frequently. Daily weighings and the maintenance of accurate intake and output records are especially crucial for evaluating nutritional progress and state of hydration in the patient receiving nutrition support. In addition, the nurse is the health care team member who has the most constant contact with the patient; therefore he or she is uniquely qualified to evaluate bowel function and feeding tolerance, for example, in determining whether the patient has enough diarrhea to preclude advancement of enteral feedings or whether the patient is at risk of pulmonary aspiration because of slow gastric emptying.

TABLE 7-16 **Nursing Management of TPN Complications**

Complication	Clinical Manifestations	Prevention/Correction
Catheter-related sepsis	Fever, chills, glucose intolerance, positive blood culture	Maintain an intact dressing, change if contaminated by vomitus, sputum, and so on; use aseptic technique when handling catheter, IV tubing, and TPN solutions; hang a bottle of TPN no longer than 24 hr, lipid emulsion no longer than 12-24 hr; use an in-line 0.22 μm filter with TPN to remove microorganisms; avoid drawing blood, infusing blood or blood products, piggybacking other IV solutions into TPN IV tubing, or attaching manometers or transducers via the TPN infusion line, if at all possible If catheter-related sepsis is suspected, remove catheter or assist in changing the catheter over a guidewire and administer antibiotics as ordered
Air embolism	Dyspnea, cyanosis, apnea, tachycardia, hypotension, "millwheel" heart murmur; mortality estimated at 50% (depends on quantity of air entering)	Use Luer-Lok syringe or secure all connections well; use an in-line 0.22 μm air-eliminating filter; have patient perform Valsalva maneuver during tubing changes; if the patient is on a ventilator, change tubing quickly at end expiration; maintain occlusive dressing over catheter site for at least 24 hr after removing catheter to prevent air entry through catheter tract If air embolism is suspected, place patient in left lateral decubitus and Trendelenburg's positions (to trap air in the apex of the right ventricle, away from the outflow tract) and administer oxygen and CPR as needed; immediately notify physician, who may attempt to aspirate air from the heart
Pneumothorax	Chest pain, dyspnea, hypoxemia, hypotension, radiographic evidence, needle aspiration of air from pleural space	Thoroughly explain catheter insertion procedure to patient, because when a patient moves or breathes erratically he or she is more likely to sustain pleural damage; perform x-ray examination after insertion or insertion attempt If pneumothorax is suspected, assist with needle aspiration or chest tube insertion, if necessary; chest tubes are usually used for pneumothorax of > 25%
Central venous thrombosis	Edema of neck, shoulder, and arm on same side as catheter; development of collateral circulation on chest; pain in insertion site; drainage of TPN from the insertion site; positive findings on venogram	Follow measures to prevent sepsis; repeated or traumatic catheterizations are most likely to result in thrombosis. If thrombosis is suspected, remove catheter and administer anticoagulants and antibiotics as ordered
Catheter occlusion or semiocclusion	No flow or a sluggish flow through the catheter	If infusion is stopped temporarily, flush catheter with saline or heparinized saline If catheter appears to be occluded, attempt to aspirate the clot; if this is ineffective, physician may order thrombolytic agent such as streptokinase or urokinase instilled in the catheter
Hypoglycemia	Diaphoresis, shakiness, confusion, loss of consciousness	Infuse TPN within 10% of ordered rate; observe patient carefully for signs of hypoglycemia after discontinuance of TPN If hypoglycemia is suspected, administer oral carbohydrate; if the patient is unconscious or oral intake is contraindicated, the physician may order a bolus of IV dextrose
Hyperglycemia	Thirst, headache, lethargy, increased urinary output	Administer TPN within 10% of ordered rate; monitor blood glucose level at least daily until stable; the patient may require insulin added to the TPN if hyperglycemia is persistent; sudden appearance of hyperglycemia in a patient who was previously tolerating the same glucose load may indicate onset of sepsis.

TABLE 7-17 Evaluating Response to Nutrition Support

Parameter	Frequency of Measurement*	Purpose/Comments
ANTHROPOMETRIC MEASUREMENTS		
Weight	Daily	Indicator of efficacy or of overfeeding; underweight patient should have steady gain, and normal weight or overweight patient should maintain current weight Detection of overhydration: a consistent gain of > 0.11-0.22 kg (0.25-0.5 lb)/day usually indicates fluid retention
PHYSICAL EXAMINATION		
State of hydration	Daily	Detection of overhydration: check for edema of dependent body parts, shortness of breath, rales in lungs, fluid intake consistently > output Detection of dehydration: look for poor skin turgor, dry mucous membranes, complaints of thirst, output > intake (measure stool volumes if liquid), > 10% difference between blood pressure when lying and standing
Bowel motility	Daily	Detect hypermotility or hypomotility; auscultate bowel sounds to be sure that peristalsis is present in patients receiving enteral feedings and to help determine when feedings can start in those not being enterally fed; evaluate stool consistency: hard, dry stools, decreased stool frequency, or < 3 stools/wk may indicate constipation in the tube-fed patient, although infrequent stools are expected in the patient who is receiving nothing by mouth; loose or liquid stools, increased frequency, or > 3 stools/day may indicate diarrhea
Gastric emptying (tube-fed patients)	Every 4-6 hr or as indicated	Detect gastric retention: measure gastric residual as described in the discussion of tube feeding complications
HEMATOLOGIC AND BIOCHEMICAL MEASUREMENT		
Serum albumin, transferrin, or prealbumin level	Weekly	Indicator of efficacy: levels should be maintained or improved if nutrition support is adequate
Serum glucose and electrolyte levels	Daily until stable, then 2-3/wk	Indicate whether intake is adequate or excessive
Blood urea nitrogen (BUN) level	1-2/wk	Increased level indicates inadequate fluid intake, renal impairment, or excessive protein intake
Serum calcium, phosphorous, and magnesium levels	1-2/wk	Measure of adequacy of intake
Serum triglyceride levels (patients receiving IV lipid emulsions)	After each increase in lipid dosage; then 2-3/wk when stable	Elevated levels indicate lipid clearance and possibly a need for reduction in lipid dosage
REE (resting energy expenditure)—measured by indirect calorimetry, not available in all institutions)	At beginning of nutrition support and as indicated	Permits accurate determination of energy expenditures, allowing the nutrition support regimen to be planned to avoid overfeeding or underfeeding

Modified from Moore MC: *Pocket guide to nutritional care,* ed 3, St Louis, 1996, Mosby.
*These are suggested frequencies only; individual patients may need more or less frequent assessment.

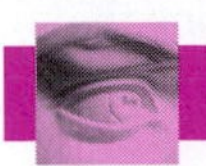

NURSING MANAGEMENT PLAN

ALTERED NUTRITION: LESS THAN BODY REQUIREMENTS

DEFINITION:

The state in which an individual experiences an intake of nutrients insufficient to meet metabolic needs.

Altered Nutrition: Less than Body Requirements Related to Lack of Exogenous Nutrients and Increased Metabolic Demand

DEFINING CHARACTERISTICS

- Unplanned weight loss of 20% of body weight within the past 6 months
- Serum albumin <3.5 g/dL
- Total lymphocytes <1500 mm^3
- Anergy
- Negative nitrogen balance
- Fatigue; lack of energy and endurance
- Nonhealing wounds
- Daily caloric intake less than estimated nutritional requirements
- Presence of factors known to increase nutritional requirements (e.g., sepsis, trauma, multiple organ dysfunction syndrome [MODS])
- Maintenance of NPO status for >7-10 days
- Long-term use of 5% dextrose intravenously
- Documentation of suboptimal calorie counts
- Drug or nutrient interaction that might decrease oral intake (e.g., chronic use of bronchodilators, laxatives, anticonvulsives, diuretics, antacids, narcotics)
- Physical problems with chewing, swallowing, choking, and salivation and presence of altered taste, anorexia, nausea, vomiting, diarrhea, or constipation

OUTCOME CRITERIA

- Patient exhibits stabilization of weight loss or weight gain of $^1/_2$ pound daily.
- Serum albumin is >3.5 g/dL.
- Total lymphocytes are <1500 mm^3.
- Patient has positive response to cutaneous skin antigen testing.
- Patient is in positive nitrogen balance.
- Wound healing is evident.
- Daily caloric intake equals estimated nutritional requirements.
- Increased ambulation and endurance are evident.

NURSING INTERVENTIONS AND *RATIONALE*

1. Monitor patient during physical care for signs of nutritional deficiencies.
2. Measure admission height and weight.
3. Weigh patient daily.
4. Ensure that specimens for biochemical tests of nutritional status are collected properly and on time.
5. Administer parenteral and enteral solutions as prescribed.
6. Control infusion rate of parenteral and enteral solutions through infusion control devices and check rate every hour.
7. Flush enteral feeding tubes every 4 hours ***to maintain patency.***
8. Document oral intake through calorie counts.
9. Perform serial assessments of patient's strength, endurance, conditions of wounds.

REFERENCES

1. Buckley S, Kudsk KA: Metabolic response to critical illness and injury, *AACN Clin Issues Crit Care Nurs* 5:443, 1994.
2. Coats KG and others: Hospital-associated malnutrition: a reevaluation 12 years later, *J Am Dietet Assoc* 93:27, 1993.
3. Detsky AS and others: Is this patient malnourished? *JAMA* 271:54, 1994.
4. McWhirter JP, Pennington CR: Incidence and recognition of malnutrition in hospital, *BMJ* 308:945, 1994.
5. Messner RL and others: Effect of admission nutritional status on length of hospital stay, *Gastroenterol Nurs* 13:202, 1991.
6. A.S.P.E.N. Board of Directors: Standards for nutrition support: hospitalized patients, *Nutr Clin Prac* 10:208, 1995.
7. JCAHO Board of Directors: *1995 comprehensive accreditation manual for hospitals,* Oakbrook, Ill, 1994, JCAHO.
8. Gianino S, St John RE: Nutritional assessment of the patient in the intensive care unit, *Crit Care Nurs Clin N Am* 5:1, 1993.
9. Manning EM, Shenkin A: Nutritional assessment in the critically ill, *Crit Care Clin* 11:603, 1995.
10. Freeman LM, Roubenoff R: The nutritional implications of cardiac cachexia, *Nutr Rev* 52:340, 1994.

11. Sidery MB: Meals lie heavy on the heart, *J R Coll Physicians Lond* 28:19, 1994.
12. Kirchoff KT and others: Electrocardiographic response to ice water, *Heart Lung* 19:41, 1990.
13. National Education Programs Working Group: Report on the management of patients with hypertension and high blood cholesterol, *Ann Intern Med* 114:224, 1991.
14. Summary of the second report of the National Cholesterol Education Program (NCEP) Expert Panel on Detection, Evaluation, and Treatment of High Blood Cholesterol in Adults (Adult Treatment Panel II), *JAMA* 269:3015, 1993.
15. Krumholz HM and others: Lack of association between cholesterol and coronary heart disease mortality and morbidity and all-cause mortality in persons older than 70 years, *JAMA* 272:1335, 1994.
16. Dwyer J: Overview: dietary approaches for reducing cardiovascular disease risks, *J Nutr* 125(3 suppl):656S, 1995.
17. Pezza M and others: Nutritional support for the patient with chronic obstructive pulmonary disease, *Monaldi Arch Chest Dis* 49(3 suppl 1):33, 1994.
18. Ireton-Jones CS, Borman KR, Turner WW Jr: Nutrition considerations in the management of ventilator-dependent patients, *Nutr Clin Prac* 8:60, 1993.
19. Pinard B, Geller E: Nutritional support during pulmonary failure, *Crit Care Clin* 11:705, 1995.
20. Schols AM and others: Energy balance in chronic obstructive pulmonary disease, *Am Rev Resp Dis* 143:1248, 1991.
21. Talpers SS and others: Nutritionally associated increased carbon dioxide production, *Chest* 102:551, 1992.
22. Marvel ME, Bertino JS Jr: Comparative effects of an elemental and a complex enteral feeding formulation on the absorption of phenytoin suspension, *JPEN J Parenter Enteral Nutr* 15:316, 1991.
23. Ott L, Young B: Nutrition in the neurologically injured patient, *Nutr Clin Prac* 6:223, 1991.
24. Shizgal HM and others: Body composition in quadriplegic patients, *JPEN J Parenter Enteral Nutr* 10:364, 1986.
25. Cox SAR and others: Energy expenditure after spinal cord injury: an evaluation of stable rehabilitating patients, *J Trauma* 25:419, 1985.
26. Weltz CR, Morris JB, Mullen JL: Surgical jejunostomy in aspiration risk patients, *Ann Surg* 215:140, 1992.
27. Brodsky IG and others: Effects of low protein diets on protein metabolism in insulin-dependent diabetes mellitus patients with early nephropathy, *J Clin Endocrinol Metab* 75:351, 1992.
28. Kopple JD: Effect of nutrition on morbidity and mortality in maintenance dialysis patients, *Am J Kidney Dis* 24:1002, 1994.
29. Hakim RM, Levin N: Malnutrition in hemodialysis patients, *Am J Kidney Dis* 21:125, 1993.
30. Beto JA: Which diet for renal failure: making sense of the options, *J Am Diet Assoc* 95:898, 1995.
31. Zaloga G, Ackerman MH: A review of disease-specific formulas, *AACN Clin Issues Crit Care Nurs* 5:421, 1994.
32. Kaiser BA and others: Growth of children following the initiation of dialysis: a comparison of three dialysis modalities, *Pediatr Nephrol* 8:733, 1994.
33. Grodstein GP and others: Glucose absorption during continuous ambulatory peritoneal dialysis, *Kidney Int* 19:564, 1981.
34. Grant JP and others: Malabsorption associated with surgical procedures and its treatment, *Nutr Clin Prac* 11:43, 1996.
35. Nompleggi DJ, Bonkovsky HL: Nutritional supplementation in chronic liver disease: an analytical review, *Hepatology* 19:518, 1994.
36. Gecelter GR, Comer GM: Nutritional support during liver failure, *Crit Care Clin* 11:675, 1995.
37. Plevak DJ and others: Nutritional support for liver transplantation: identifying calorie and protein requirements, *Mayo Clin Proc* 69:225, 1994.
38. Purdum PP III, Kirby DF: Short-bowel syndrome: a review of the role of nutrition support, *JPEN J Parenter Enteral Nutr* 14:93, 1991.
39. A.S.P.E.N. Board of Directors: Guidelines for the use of parenteral and enteral nutrition in adult and pediatric patients, *JPEN J Parenter Enteral Nutr* 17(suppl):5SA, 1993.
40. Lewis JD, Fisher RL: Nutrition support in inflammatory bowel disease, *Med Clin N Am* 78:1443, 1994.
41. Mobarhan S: Carbohydrate versus fat in the dietary treatment of short-bowel syndrome, *Nutr Rev* 52:354, 1994.
42. American Diabetes Association *Medical management of non-insulin-dependent (type II) diabetes,* ed 3, Alexandria, Va, 1994, The Association.
43. American Diabetes Association *Medical management of insulin-dependent (type I) diabetes,* ed 2, Alexandria, Va, 1994, The Association.
44. Strowig SM, Raskin P: Glycemic control and the complications of diabetes: after the Diabetes Control and Complications Trial, *Diabetes Res* 3:237, 1995.
45. American Diabetes Association: Position statement: nutrition recommendations and principles for people with diabetes mellitus, *Diabetes Care* 19(suppl 1):S16, 1996.
46. Beal JA, Martin BM: The clinical management of wasting and malnutrition in HIV/AIDS, *AIDS Patient Care and STDs* 9:66, 1995.
47. Berger DS: Combating malnutrition in HIV infection, *AIDS Patient Care and STDs* 10:94, 1996.
48. Bowers JM and others: Diarrhea in HIV-infected individuals: a review, *AIDS Patient Care and STDs* 10:25, 1996.
49. Suttmann U and others: Nitrogen balance in HIV-infected patients during total parenteral nutrition, *Int Conf on AIDS* 9:77, 1993, (abstract WSB344).
50. Bates BR, Kissinger P, Bessinger RE: Complementary therapy use among HIV-infected patients, *AIDS Patient Care and STDs* 10:32, 1996.
51. Lord LM, Sax HC: The role of the gut in critical illness, *AACN Clin Issues Crit Care Nurs* 5:450, 1994.

52. Heyland DK, Cook DJ, Guyatt GH: Enteral nutrition in the critically ill patient: a critical review of the evidence, *Intensive Care Med* 19:435, 1993.
53. Moore FA and others: Early enteral feeding, compared with parenteral, reduces postoperative septic complications: the results of a meta-analysis, *Ann Surg* 216:172, 1992.
54. Grant JP: Nutritional support in critically ill patients, *Ann Surg* 220:610, 1994.
55. Heyland DK, Cook DJ, Guyatt GH: Does the formulation of enteral feeding products influence infectious morbidity and mortality rates in the critically ill patients? *Crit Care Med* 22:1192, 1994.
56. Henderson JM, Strodel WE, Gilinsky NH: Limitations of percutaneous endoscopic jejunostomy, *JPEN J Parenter Enteral Nutr* 17:546, 1993.
57. Strong RM and others: Equal aspiration rates from postpylorus and intragastric-placed small-bore nasoenteric feeding tubes: a randomized, prospective study, *JPEN J Parenter Enteral Nutr* 16:59, 1992.
58. Lord LM and others: Comparison of weighted vs unweighted enteral feeding tubes for efficacy of transpyloric intubation, *JPEN J Parenter Enteral Nutr* 17:271, 1993.
59. Clevenger F, Rodriguez DJ: Decision-making for enteral feeding administration: the why behind where and how, *Nutr Clin Prac* 10:104, 1995.
60. Metheny N and others: pH testing of feeding-tube aspirates to determine placement, *Nutr Clin Prac* 9:185, 1994.
61. Metheny N, Eisenberg P, McSweeney M: Effect of feeding tube properties and three irrigants on clogging rates, *Nurs Res* 37:165, 1988.
62. Jacobs S and others: Continuous enteral feeding: a major cause of pneumonia among ventilated intensive care unit patients, *JPEN J Parenter Enteral Nutr* 14:353, 1990.
63. Collins E and others: Care of central venous catheters for total parenteral nutrition, *Nutr Clin Prac* 11:109, 1996.
64. Hoffmann KK and others: Transparent polyurethane film as an intravenous catheter dressing: a meta-analysis of the infection risks, *JAMA* 267:2072, 1992.
65. Maki DG, Ringer M, Alvarado CJ: Prospective randomized trial of povidone-iodine, alcohol, and chlorhexidine for prevention of infection associated with central venous and arterial catheters, *Lancet* 338:339, 1991.
66. Zeigler TR, Gatzen C, Wilmore DW: Strategies for attenuating protein-catabolic responses in the critically ill, *Annu Rev Med* 45:459, 1994.

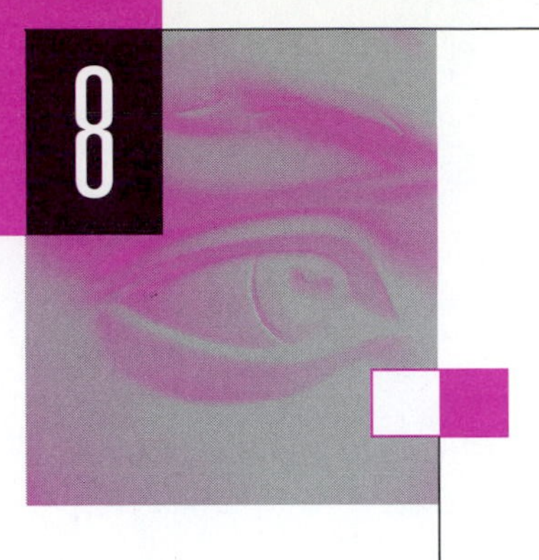

Pain and Sedation

PAIN

PAIN IS DEFINED in a number of ways. Pain is a warning signal from the body that an injury has occurred. Unlike other sensations, pain is the protective signal for a threat to survival.[1] Pain is an unpleasant sensory experience that is associated with actual and potential tissue damage. Pain is not simply a pure physiologic response to an injury but is associated with an emotional response to the sensation.[2] Pain is an extremely complex set of responses to a physical stimulus. The definition with the most clinical significance is that pain is whatever the person experiencing it says it is, and it occurs when that person says it does.[3] Pain is a common thread that binds critical care patients together. Whether the pain is from an elective procedure or trauma, its presence is ubiquitous.[4] Studies examining the ability of the critically ill surgical patient to sleep identified pain and the inability to get comfortable as the most commonly cited barriers to sleep.[5] Because of the significance of pain in the critically ill patient and the associated morbidity, pain was the first clinical problem chosen by the Agency for Health Care Policy and Research (AHCPR) for guideline development.[6] In addition, the American Association of Critical Care Nurses (AACN) identified pain as a priority area for nursing research, and many nursing professional organizations have developed pain management position statements.[7,8]

With the frequency of the diagnosis of pain and the professional responsibility to manage pain, the critical care nurse must understand the mechanisms, the assessment technique, and the appropriate therapeutic measures to manage the pain state. Unfortunately, studies of pain management reflect that the critical care patient is commonly undermedicated. On average the nurse administered only 30% to 36% of the maximum opioid dose ordered.[9] One study of critically ill patients revealed that the second most commonly recalled memory of their illness was that of a painful, uncomfortable experience.[10,11]

PHYSIOLOGY OF PAIN

The need to have a basic understanding of the pathophysiology of pain is necessary to understand the consequences of assessment and intervention. The pathophysiology of pain involves both the peripheral and central nervous systems.

Peripheral Nervous System

The peripheral nervous system contains a multitude of free nerve endings. The sensation of pain requires the activation of some of these free nerve endings. Other similar nerve endings are responsible for the transmission of sensations of touch, pressure, and warmth. The nerve endings responsible for pain, the nociceptors, are specialized. Because the role of pain in the body is protective, the nerve endings do not adapt to repeated painful stimuli. On the contrary, repeated stimulation heightens their sensitivity. The supersensitive state lowers the threshold for stimulation and increases the response to stimulation.[2] This phenomenon is responsible for the hypersensitive state of many critically ill patients. In this hypersensitive state, known as hyperalgesia, the slightest painful stimulus is interpreted as very painful.[12] Nociceptors are present in numerous organs in the body. They are primarily located in skin, joints, muscle, fascia, viscera, and the smooth muscle of the arterial walls. They are activated by thermal, mechanical,

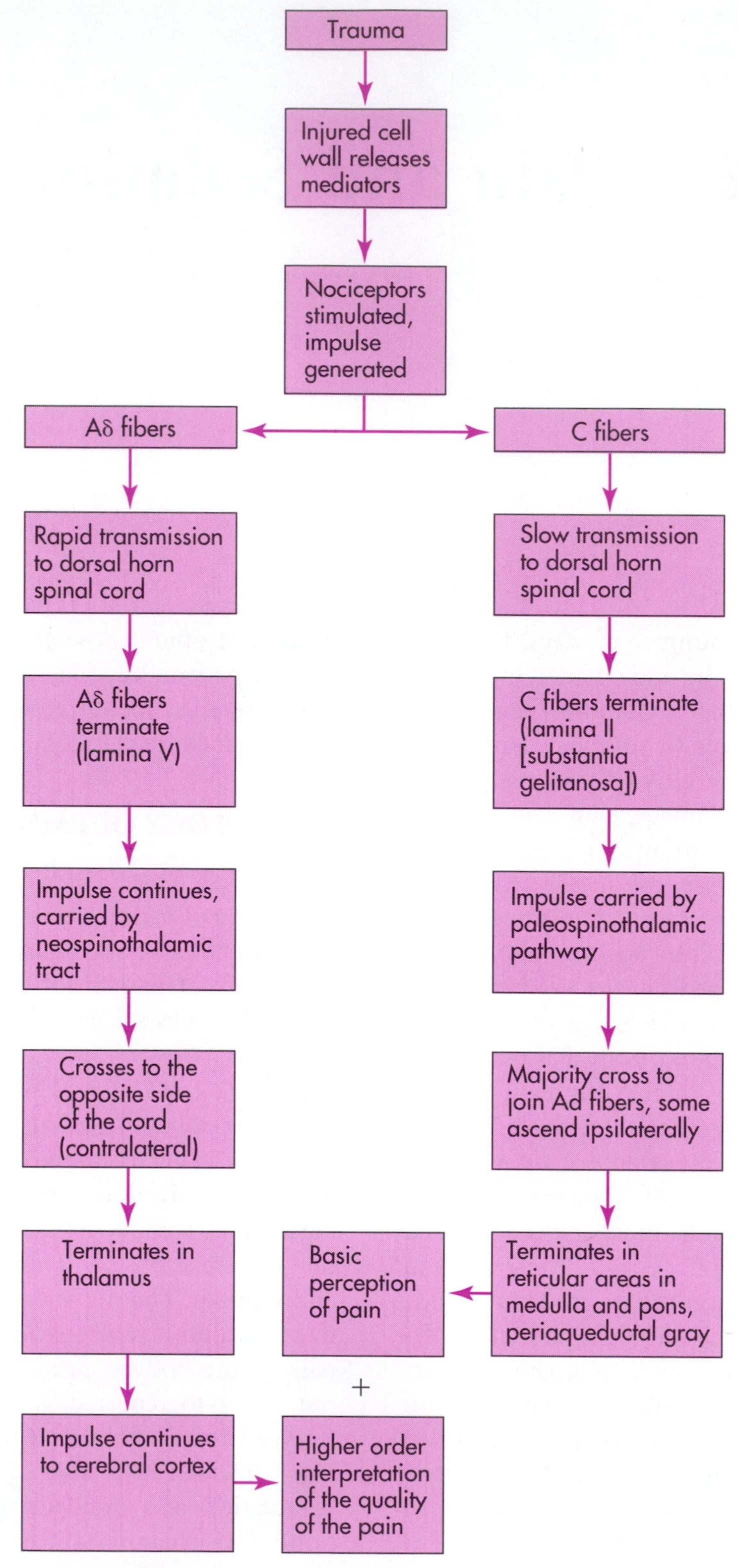

FIGURE 8-1. Dual pathways of pain transmission using the Aδ and C fibers for nociception.

and chemical stimuli. There are two types of afferent nerve fibers that transmit painful stimuli from the site of injury through distinct neural pathways. Figure 8-1 illustrates the dual pathways for pain transmission.

One type of fiber, Aδ, conducts the rapid acute pain sensation described as prickling, sharp, and fast. This type of fiber is activated by mechanical and thermal stimuli. The second type of nociceptor is the polymodal C fiber. C fibers are implicated in the trans-

TABLE 8-1 Selected Neurotransmitters

Neurotransmitter	General Locations	Effect on Pain Transmission
β-Endorphins	Hypothalamus/pituitary	Inhibits
Acetylcholine	CNS, PNS	Excites
Bradykinins	Plasma cells	Excites
Dynorphins	CNS	Inhibits
Enkephalins	Spinal cord	Inhibits
Gamma-aminobutyric (GABA)	Dorsal horn	Inhibits
Histamines	Plasma cells	Excites
Potassium	Plasma cells	Excites
Prostaglandins	Plasma cells	Enhances excitement
Serotonin	Platelets, brainstem, dorsal horn	Enhances inhibition
Substance P	Nerve terminals, spinal cord	Excites

TABLE 8-2 Nerve Fibers for Pain Transmission

Nerve Fiber (Description)	General Location	Type of Pain Transmitted	Patient Descriptors	Rate of Transmission
Aδ fibers (thinly myelinated)	Skin, cutaneous tissue	Mechanical, thermal stimulus; easily localized	Sharp, pricking, electric, acute	Rapid, within 0.1 sec; velocity 6-30 m/sec
C fibers (primitive, unmyelinated)	Subcutaneous tissue, fascia, tendons, joints, ligaments, muscles	Mechanical, chemical, or thermal stimulus; difficult to localize	Throbbing, aching, burning, gnawing, chronic	Slow, 1+ sec, increases slowly; velocity 0.5-2 m/sec

mission of pain described as dull, diffuse, prolonged, and delayed. These fibers are activated by chemicals released when cell damage occurs. Some of these chemicals, or neurotransmitters, are potassium, histamine, bradykinin, serotonin, and acetylcholine.[1,2] These chemical transmitters are responsible for irritating the nerve endings and for activating the peripheral nerve system for transmission of other neurotransmitters that are active in the inhibition of the transmission of pain. Table 8-1 lists some of the mediators and their role in pain. These mediators are released when there is tissue damage of any type. Depending on which of the mediators is active, there are other associated reactions at the site of injury, including vasoconstriction, vasodilatation, or altered capillary permeability.

Both the Aδ fibers and the C fibers have roots in the dorsal horn of the spinal column. They are the afferent arm of the ascending spinal pathways of pain. In the dorsal horn at the laminae, the nociceptor neurons release Substance P; Substance P has as excitatory effect on the spinal cord and enhances the transmission of pain.[13] This is the point of integration of the peripheral and central nervous systems for the transmission of the pain impulse (Table 8-2).

Central Nervous System

The central nervous system has two components used in the pain response, the ascending, or conducting, pathways and the descending, or modulating, pathways.

Ascending pain pathways. The ascending tracts synapse with primary Aδ and C afferent nerve fibers that terminate in laminae I through V of the spinal cord. Aδ terminal fibers have been found in laminae I and V. Type C fibers are predominantly found in the laminae II, which is also known as the substantia gelatinosa. Most C fiber transmission immediately synapses

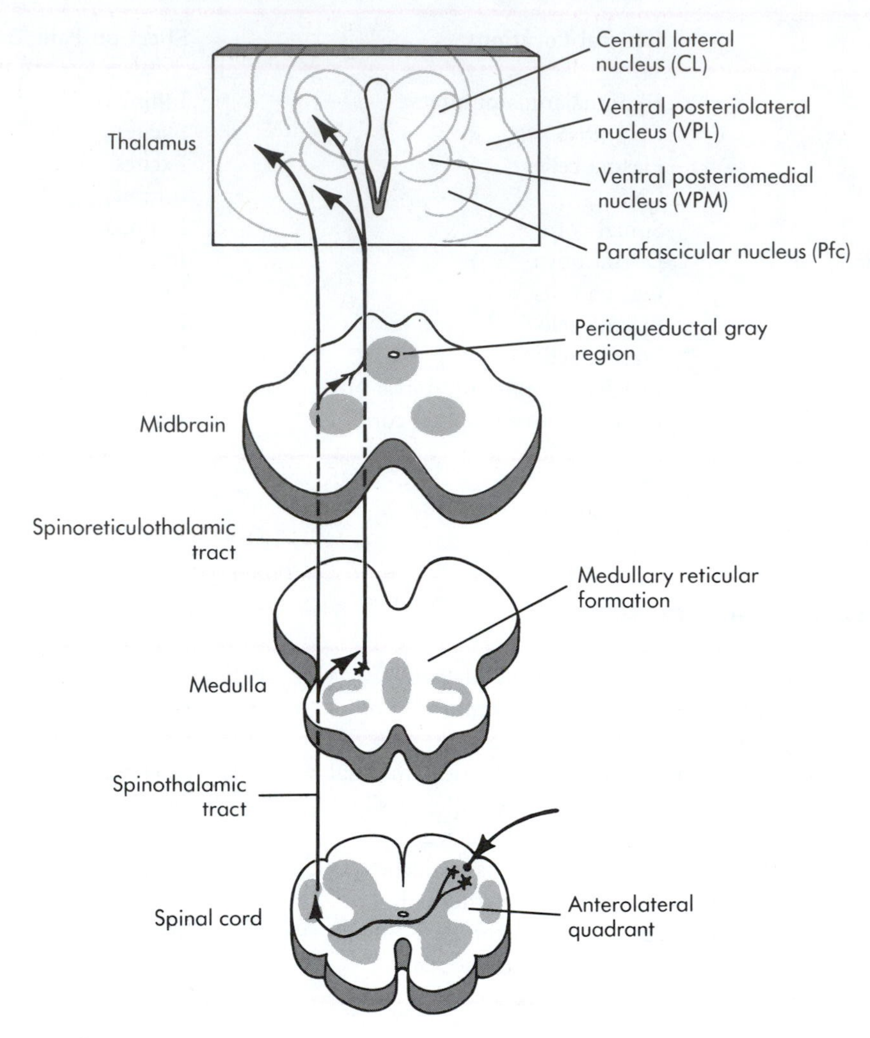

FIGURE 8-2. Ascending somatosensory system. (From Barker E: *Neuroscience nursing,* St Louis, 1994, Mosby.)

with neurons to ascend to the thalamus. The sensations are transmitted via the spinothalamic tract (Figure 8-2). Two other tracts are responsible for the transmission of nociceptor messages. The spinoreticular tract transmits to the brainstem reticular formation and terminates in the thalamus. The third nociceptor tract is the spinomesencephalic tract. This tract terminates in the midbrain reticular formation and the midbrain periaqueductal gray. This area of the brain is also responsible for strong inhibitory responses to the pain transmission. Nociception continues to the somatosensory cortex of the brain. Cortical interpretation of the stimulus is necessary to finalize the perception of the pain; to discretely locate the pain, identify its intensity, and interpret its meaning; and to add the emotional component. This cortical process underlies the patient's individual, unique perception of the pain.

Descending pain pathways. The other central nervous system component of pain is the descending analgesia system. This system is the endogenous pain modulation system, which is responsible for the body's attempt to intrinsically manage the pain.[14] The system consists of a series of neurons in the brain and spinal cord that synapse with the ascending neurons. Figure 8-3 illustrates the endogenous pain modification system. In the brain, the cortex and the hypothalamus activate the periaqueductal gray that influences fibers in the dorsal horns to release neurotransmitters that inhibit the action of the neurons that transmit pain impulses. These neurotransmitters that inhibit or modulate the transmission of pain are produced in the body at sites along the neural synapses. The sites are located in both the brain and the descending pathways. These neurotransmitters are the endogenous

CULTURAL INSIGHTS 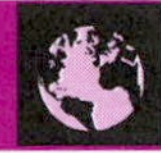 **Cultural Variations in Pain Behaviors**

Two female patients are admitted to the CCU (coronary care unit) within 30 minutes of each other with the diagnosis of rule out acute anterior myocardial infarction. The first patient is Mrs. Giovanni, a 71-year-old who has lived in "little Italy" since arriving in the United States many years ago. The second patient is Mrs. Yamaguchi, a 74-year-old who moved from Japan 5 years ago to live with her son and daughter-in-law in California. Both patients are limited in their ability to communicate in English.

Electrocardiograms show ST-segment elevation and T wave inversion in Leads V_2 through V_4 in both patients. Morphine 4 mg had been administered intravenously to both patients just before their transfer from the emergency department. Upon admission to the CCU, Mrs. Giovanni is crying, moaning, very restless, and clutching her chest. Her vital signs show an elevated systolic blood pressure, heart rate, and respiratory rate. The laboratory report indicates that her initial serum creatine phosphokinase (CPK) level is 927 mU/ml.

On the other hand, in the next bed, Mrs. Yamaguchi is lying very still, with her eyes closed and arms held rigidly at her side. The admitting nurse observes that her vital signs are also elevated. The laboratory reports that Mrs. Yamaguchi's CPK is 879 mU/ml, and her ECG is showing an increasing number of extra systoles. Further questioning by the nurse reveals that both patients are still experiencing chest pain and require further medication.

Physiologically, these cases are very similar. In the early stages of acute myocardial infarction, both patients are showing the classic physiologic signs of pain, yet their behaviors in the presence of this pain are vastly different. Several reasons are possible for this variation in response to pain, such as individual personality or psychologic status. But another possible explanation for this difference is the cultural background of each patient.

The pain response reflects the patient's attitude toward the pain and a learned behavior in response to the pain. The pain response is a behavior that reflects the values and priorities of the culture in which the patient was reared. The response is learned both through observation of how parents and other members of the immediate society responded to pain and through the experience of how parents reacted to children in pain.

Responses to pain have been described as either expressive or stoic. But this simple dichotomy is too restrictive to encompass the wide range of responses seen. It may be more helpful to imagine a continuum, with emotive (expressive) behaviors at one end and stoic behaviors at the other. As a working generality, pain responses of immigrants from Latin American countries, southern Europe, and the Middle East tend to lie closer to the emotive end of the scale. American Indians and those persons from cultures from northern Europe and Asia tend to be more stoic in responding to discomfort. There are, of course, numerous exceptions to these guidelines. Factors such as gender, degree of assimilation into mainstream American culture, socioeconomic status, age, and individual personality create considerable diversity within any one cultural group. Nevertheless, these guidelines can be a good starting point in evaluating the behavior of a given patient.

Before examining some of the reasons for an emotive or stoic response to pain and some possible interventions, it must be noted that there is no intrinsic right or wrong in either of these responses—the patient is behaving in a fashion that, because of cultural background, works under the given circumstances. There exists the danger that the nurse will project his or her own personal cultural beliefs onto the patient. It is not uncommon for the Anglo-American nurse, who has been taught to restrain the expression of pain and "act like a big boy or girl," to assume that those who express pain are being childlike or self-indulgent. This conclusion merely reflects the nurse's culture and has little to do with the motivation or motives of the patient. The behavior must be evaluated within the context of the patient's culture—not by comparison to American values and norms.

The stoic patient may seem ideal because of the congruence with the values of the dominant culture, but in reality, the concealment of pain can be detrimental to the patient. For one thing, pain inhibits healing. If the nurse does not know that the patient is in pain, the proper medications will not be administered and, in turn, the patient will not experience proper rest and its healing effects. In the case of acute myocardial infarction (AMI), pain can have more serious effects. The sympathetic response to pain, such as increased heart rate and systolic pressure; increased afterload, as reflected in higher peripheral vascular resistance; and increased tendency to ventricular ectopy places the patient at greater risk of lethal dysrhythmias, as well as increasing the myocardial oxygen demand. Effective pain management aimed at decreasing the sympathetic input on the cardiovascular system results in a decrease in myocardial oxygen demand and restores a more optimal supply/demand ratio.

Providing explanations to the patient who is afraid to take pain medications can be helpful in improving communication. Many immigrant patients are fearful that medications will become addictive and that too much will be given. Particularly, a person of Asian descent who has a small body stature may fear that the effects of the drug will put him or her out of control, or he or she may believe that pain is an essential part of the healing process.

Intervention in these cases obviously involves providing correct information about these concerns. It is particularly helpful for nurses to ask the patient to help them do their job by revealing the amount of pain, explaining that only in this way can the nurse, as the person responsible for the patient's well-being, do a good job. This approach, particularly in view of the Asian culture's emphasis on avoiding failure or embarrassment for all concerned, can have remarkable results.

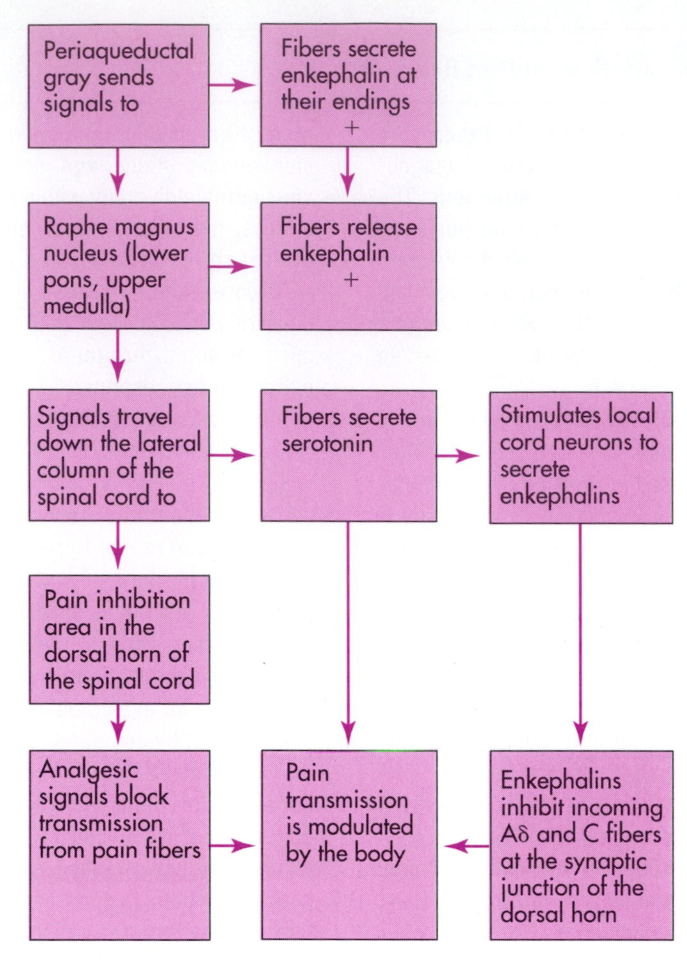

FIGURE 8-3. The body's endogenous pain modification, or analgesia, system.

opioid peptides known as the endogenous opioids and are considered morphine-like. There are primarily three types of endogenous opioids: dynorphins, β-endorphins, and enkephalins; all three are from different chemical families.[12] Upon release the endogenous opioids, or endorphins, bind to the nerve receptor sites located throughout the ascending pain transmission system and significantly modify the transmission of pain (Figure 8-4). The binding sites, or receptors, are generally classified as the mu (μ) effect, kappa (κ) effect, and delta (δ) effect. Each receptor type acts differently when stimulated. A knowledge of the individual responses contributes to the interpretation of physiologic findings in the assessment of pain and pain management responses. Some of the effects that are quantifiable are summarized in Table 8-3. Different levels of these pain-modifying endorphins in individuals are responsible for the difference in response to the same painful stimulus among individuals.

β-Endorphins are located primarily in the hypothalamus and the midbrain. They are the most morphine-like. Research indicates that the β-endorphins are released during accupuncture and transcutaneous stimulation.[2] They are also released in response to stress, fear, restraint, hypertension, and hypoglycemia. Endorphin release is well-documented during labor and delivery and exercise.[13] Endorphin release during stress accounts for a person's ability to perform normally or supranormally with an apparent unawareness of pain after an injury. This response is referred to as *stress analgesia.*

The enkephalins are located primarily in the limbic system and the hypothalamus, as well as periaqueductal gray. The endings of many of the nerves in these areas secrete enkephalins. In an associated response, fibers originating in the same area but with their endings in the dorsal horn secrete serotonin. The serotonin in turn acts on yet another set of neurons to incite the release of additional enkephalins.[13] The enkephalins block the presynaptic transmission of both Aδ and C fibers.[13] This inhibition can last from minutes to hours, providing analgesia for that period.

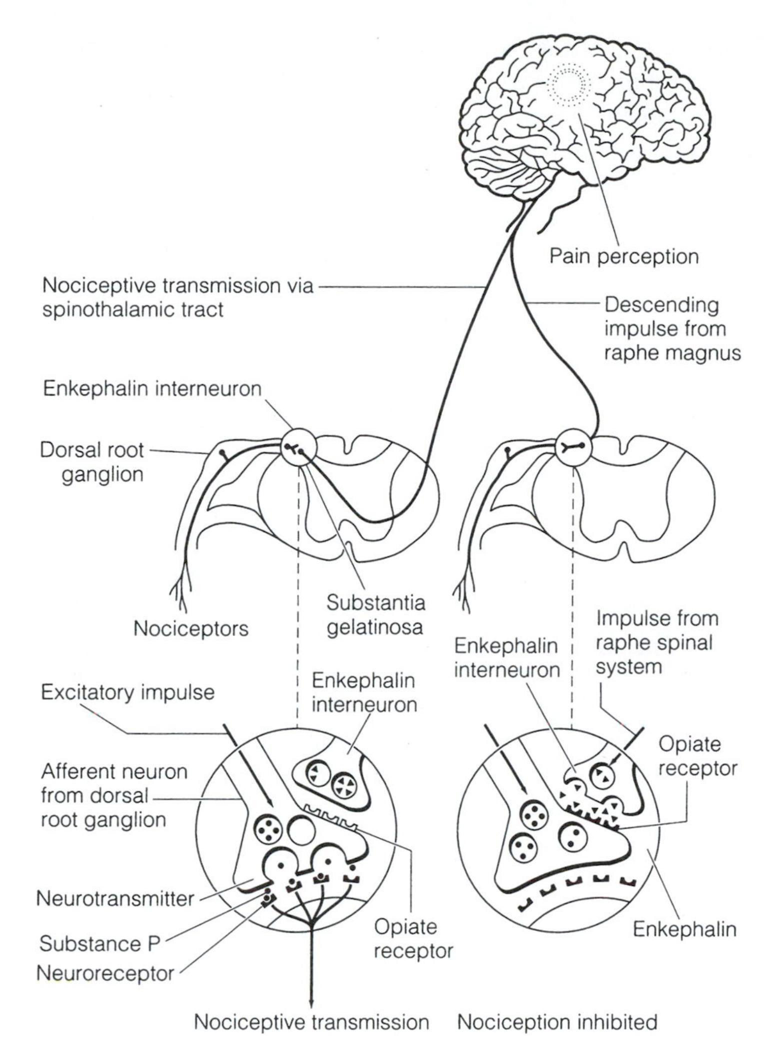

FIGURE 8-4. The role of enkephalin in pain management. (From Salerno E, Willens, J: *Pain management handbook: an interdisciplinary approach,* St Louis, 1996, Mosby.)

TABLE 8-3 Opiate Receptor Classification and Actions

Affected Area	μ Effect	δ Effect
Pupils	Miosis	Mydriasis
Respiratory system	Stimulates, then depresses	Stimulates
Heart	Bradycardia	Tachycardia
Temperature	Hypothermia	
Gastrointestinal (GI)	Constipation	Nausea

Adapted from: Willens J: Pain management in the trauma patient. In Cardona D, and others, editors: *Trauma nursing: from resuscitation through rehabilitation,* ed 2, Philadelphia, 1994, WB Saunders.

The dynorphins are found in minute quantities in the nervous system, primarily in the periaqueductal gray and the spinal cord. They are extremely powerful opiates; they appear to have as much as 200 times the pain-killing effect of morphine.

A second, less-discussed inhibitory pathway contributes to pain modification. This pathway is a nonopioid form of endogenous analgesia. It is the monoamine system. The primary neurotransmitters involved in this system are serotonin and norepinephrine.

Serotonin is a major pain-inhibiting factor from the medulla to the spinal cord descending pathway.[2,13,14] At the dorsal horn, serotonin is responsible for the release of enkephalins.[13] Norepinephrine's role in pain modulation is in its attachment to α_2-adrenergic receptors and the resulting inhibition of nociception.[2]

TYPES OF ACUTE PAIN

Although all pain uses primarily the same nociception, pain experts describe the type of pain by differentiating the location of the fibers that are sensitized. The fibers are most commonly grouped as cutaneous, somatic, visceral, and deafferentation.

Cutaneous Pain

Cutaneous, or superficial pain, begins with injury at the skin, such as an incision or insertion of a needle. This trauma to the tissue activates the nociceptors on the skin. The mediators histamine, bradykinin, potassium, or hydrogen ions are released into the extracellular fluid around the wound. The cell wall injury causes the release of serotonin from platelets, prostaglandins, and substance P. All of the active mediators will sensitize and activate the cutaneous fibers to transmit the noxious stimuli to the central nervous system.[1,2] The cutaneous Aδ fibers are now sensitive to noxious stimuli that would not ordinarily be interpreted as painful, such as touch, pressure, or stretch. Normally, the patient is able to discretely locate this type of pain.

Somatic Pain

Somatic pain originates in the subcutaneous tissue, the joints, tendons, muscles, and fascia. It is also associated with muscle ischemia and spasm.[2] Bradykinin and histamine release are associated with somatic pain. C fibers are responsible for the transmission of this type of pain. Somatic pain is difficult for the patient to locate. It can be either dull, aching, or diffuse.[1,2,11] In addition, deep somatic pain is associated with an autonomic nervous system response that may cause nausea; vomiting; and cold, clammy skin.

Visceral Pain

In general, the viscera has only sensory receptors for pain. The unique characteristic of visceral pain is that highly localized stimulation of pain receptors in the viscera can cause minimal discomfort. However, diffuse stimulation of multiple receptors can cause extreme pain.[13] Visceral pain results from compression, distention, or stretching of the viscera in the thoracic or abdominal cavity. The pain of myocardial ischemia or infarction is considered visceral. Visceral pain is described as pressure, deep, and squeezing. It is sometimes difficult to localize and is associated with referred pain. The visceral pain fibers are unique in that they travel to the spinal cord with the fibers of the sympathetic nervous system. This may account for the intense sympathetic nervous system response often seen with this type of pain.[2]

Deafferentation Pain

Deafferentation pain is seen most commonly in the cancer patient. The mechanism of this pain is an injury to either a central or peripheral nerve component from either the disease or its treatment. The injury is normally a consequence of tumor invasion, thermal damage from radiation, or chemical injuries from radiation.[1] This is also considered to be the type of pain stemming from a number of chronic pain syndromes. In this regard the origin of the pain may be peripheral or central. Neuralgia and phantom pain are peripheral deafferentation pains, in which thalamic lesions related to cerebrovascular accidents (CVAs) cause central deafferentation pain.[14]

PAIN ASSESSMENT

Adequate assessment of pain in the critically ill patient is made more difficult by the complexity of the critical care experience. For instance, there may be the complicating factor of altered communication, or the patient may be unconscious and unable to communicate pain. Pain assessment in the critically ill population has three major components: assessment technique, patient barriers to assessment, and nurse and/or physician barriers to complete or accurate assessment. The complexity of assessment requires the use of multiple strategies by critical care practitioners.

Multidimensional Assessment

Because pain is a multidimensional phenomenon, it requires a multidimensional assessment. Complete assessment involves the collection of subjective and objective data about the patient's physiologic, cognitive, and emotional response to the pain.[15] Because of the life/death immediacy of most actions in the critical care environment, assessment is normally one-dimensional.[16] The evaluation of pain includes type, location, intensity, aggravating factors, and alleviating factors. The most important consideration in assessment is that pain is an entirely subjective experience. Pain is whatever the patient says it is and however the patient describes it.[3,6] In the assessment of pain type, the verbal patient can give descriptive terms. The patient may describe the pain as dull, aching, or sharp and stabbing. This provides the nurse with data regarding the type of pain the patient is experiencing (i.e., visceral or cutaneous). The differentiation between types of pain may contribute to the determination of cause and management. A patient who has had defibrillation and cardiopulmonary resuscitation (CPR) after a heart attack may complain of chest pain that is prickling or stinging. This information would lead the nurse to investigate for cutaneous injuries, such as defibrillation burns. The same patient may describe a dull, aching pain with radiation that might lead the nurse to consider a visceral anginal pain from myocardial ischemia. A verbal description of pain is furthermore important because it provides a baseline description, allowing the critical care nurse to monitor changes in the type of pain, which could indicate a change in the underlying pathology.

Pain Assessment Tools

Intensity or severity of pain is a measurement that has undergone a great deal of recent investigation. Studies have shown that the consistent use of a visual tool aids both the patient and the practitioner in correctly identifying the intensity of the patient's pain.[3,6,10,17] Multiple visual analog scales are available (Figure 8-5). Many critical care units have identified a specific tool to be used. The use of a single tool provides consistency of assessment and documentation. The employment of a pain grading scale is also useful in the critical care environment.[16] Asking the patient to grade his or her pain on a scale of 1 to 10 is a consistent method and aids the nurse in objectifying the subjective nature of the patient's pain. The pain grading scale is also useful in establishing a baseline for comparison of future episodes of pain. A unique part of the assessment of pain is the need to have the patient identify exactly what amount or level of pain allows functionality and is acceptable to the patient. This level of acceptable pain is the target for subsequent pain management techniques.[3,6]

Pain Location

The next area of evaluation is the location of the patient's pain. Location is normally easy for the patient to identify, although visceral pain is more difficult for the patient to localize.[1,2] If the patient has difficulty naming the location, ask that he or she point to the location on himself or herself or on a simple anatomic drawing. This technique is also helpful in identifying multisites of pain.[18]

Asking the patient to identify factors that moderate pain is an important evaluation component for the critical care nurse. Position or movement as a component of pain may contribute significantly to the final evaluation of the pain occurrence; the example of deep breathing intensifying the chest pain because of pericarditis is an illustration of this. Moderating factors that reduce the pain or discomfort are also important findings. The moderation of pain continues after the patient leaves the critical care environment. A knowledge of any alleviation activities contributes to the patient's plan of care throughout the continuum of care.

The subjective data of intensity, type, location, and moderating factors form a single component of pain assessment. The critical care nurse also completes a physiologic assessment on any patient who reports pain. It is important to note that lack of a physiologic response to pain does not mean that the patient is reporting pain that does not exist.[3,10,12,18] A number of things may explain the lack of a physiologic response. Many of the therapies employed in the critical care area are designed to block the sympathetic nervous system response to stress, successfully blocking the same response to pain. If there is a response to pain, the nurse assesses for the following findings: tachycardia, hypertension, tachypnea, increased muscle tone in the area of pain, sweating, pallor, and hypervigilence. Any of the body's responses to sympathetic nervous system stimulation might be expected. Complicating this finding in the critical care patient is the possibility of the original illness or injury as the cause of the sympathetic response.[2,10]

Some critical care patients respond to pain or painful stimuli by simply withdrawing from the painful stimuli. This patient is able to perceive the pain, but the higher somatosensory cortical contribution of interpretation of the pain is absent. There are also patients who do not respond at all to painful stimuli. These patients lack integrity in the nociceptive system and are unable to perceive the pain. These phenomena are usually associated with pathologies in the brain or spinal cord that interrupt the system.

Behavioral Assessment

Certain behaviors may be manifested in the patient with pain. It is important to remember that not all patients have an observable behavioral response. Diligent observation of the patient experiencing pain may uncover behavioral cues. Table 8-4 lists behaviors associated with pain. These behaviors may indicate pain, or they may indicate an attempt to control pain with types of distraction.[12,16,18]

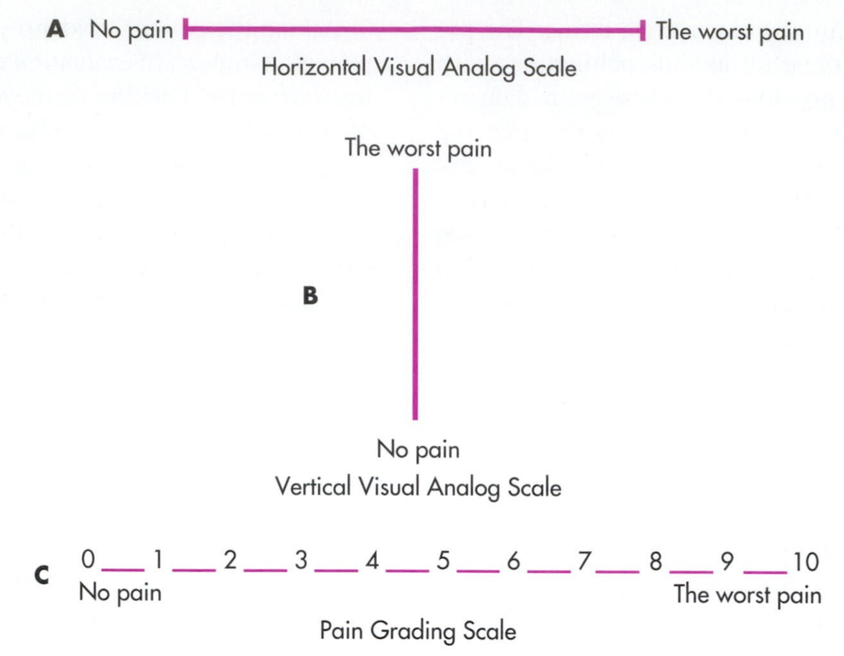

FIGURE 8-5. Visual analog scales. **A,** Horizontal Visual Analog Scale; **B,** Vertical Visual Analog Scale; **C,** Pain Grading Scale.

TABLE 8-4 Behaviors Associated With Pain

Type	Examples
Expression	Grimacing, frowning, eyes squeezed close, withdrawn expression, staring, crying, teeth clenched, wrinkled brow
Noises	Groaning, moaning, sighing, sobbing, grunting
Speech	Cussing, shouting, praying, calling for help, chanting
Body movements	Rocking, thrashing, tossing/turning
Behaviors	Guarding, protective posturing, massaging or applying pressure, reading, watching TV, wandering

Adapted from Salerno E, Willens J: *Pain management handbook,* St Louis, 1996, Mosby.

Patient Barriers to Pain Assessment

Communication. The most obvious patient barrier to the assessment of pain in the critical care population is an alteration in the ability to communicate. The patient who is intubated is unable to verbalize a description of the pain. If the patient is able to communicate in any way, then he or she may report the pain in that manner. If the patient is able to write a description, he or she may be able to thoroughly describe the pain in writing. It is the nonverbal patients whom the nurse relies on most intensely for nonverbal clues or behaviors to assess the presence and intensity of pain. Because the nurse cannot be assured of predictable pain behaviors, other sources of assessment need to be addressed. The patient's family can contribute significantly in the assessment of behavioral clues to pain. The family is intimately familiar with the patient's normal responses to pain and can assist the nurse in identifying such clues. If there is absolutely no observable evidence to support a diagnosis of pain, the practitioner needs to use the concept that if the trauma, disease, injury, or procedure is a painful one for most patients, it is painful for this patient.[3]

Altered level of consciousness. The presence of delirium, dementia, or altered mentation related to psychoactive therapies or disease states presents a unique pain assessment barrier. It has been erroneously thought that the confused patient would be unable to perceive pain. Research now supports that the patient with altered cognitive abilities is able to accurately report pain when questioned or upon the actual painful event. The limitation for this population is in pain recall and the ability to integrate the pain experience over time.[6] The critical care nurse needs to assess for pain frequently in cognitively impaired patients and not anticipate that these patients will initiate a pain discussion.

The patient in a coma presents a dilemma for the critical care nurse. Because pain relies on cortical response to provide recognition, there is the belief that the patient without higher cortical functioning has no perception of pain.[1,19] Conversely, the inability to interpret the nociceptive transmission does not negate the transmission. The critical care nurse can initiate a discussion with the other members of the health care team to formulate a plan of care for the coma patient's comfort.

Cultural influences. Another barrier to accurate pain assessment is the cultural influences on pain and pain reporting.[15,17,19,20] The cultural influences may be compounded by the patient who speaks another language than that of health team members. Although this chapter does not address specific cultural groups and their typical responses to pain, a few generalizations are made. The first consideration in assessing a patient from a different cultural group is to avoid the assumption that the patient will have a specific response to pain or exhibit a particular behavior because of culture. Patients are uniquely individual in their response to pain, and the health care practitioner might unjustly assign or expect behaviors that a patient will not exhibit. A second consideration that is commonly overlooked is the role of pain in the life of the patient. The nurse must communicate with the patient or the family to ascertain this role. Some cultures believe that God's test or punishment takes the form of pain. Persons of such cultures would not necessarily believe that the pain should be relieved. Other cultures perceive pain as being associated with an imbalance in life, hot and cold for instance. Persons of these cultures believe they need to manipulate the environment to restore balance to accomplish pain control.[20] The complexities and intricacies of cultural beliefs require much greater discussion. Many critical care units have established references or resources for dealing with cultural diversity in the critically ill patient. It is important for the nurse to support, whenever possible, the special beliefs and needs of the patient and his or her family to provide the most therapeutic environment for healing to occur. (∞Cultural Pain Responses, p 799.)

Knowledge deficit. A relatively overlooked patient barrier to accurate pain assessment is the public knowledge deficit regarding pain and pain management. Many patients and their families are scared by the risk of addiction to pain medication. They fear that addiction will occur if the patient is medicated frequently or with sufficient amounts of opiates necessary to relieve the pain. This belief is compounded by programs such as the "Just Say No to Drugs" campaign that increase the public's concern regarding drugs.[21] The concern is powerful enough for some that they will deny or deliberately underreport the frequency or intensity of pain. Another inaccurate belief on the part of some patients is the expectation that unrelieved pain is part of a critical illness or procedure.[22] As part of the patient plan for pain management the critical care nurse must teach both the family and patient the importance of pain control and the use of opioids in treating the critically ill patient.

Health Professional Barriers to Pain Assessment and Management

The health professional's beliefs and attitudes about pain and pain management are commonly a barrier to accurate and adequate assessment of pain that can lead to poor management practices.[3,6,9,10,12] It is well-documented that the study of pain assessment and management is lacking in most schools of nursing.[10,22] Multiple studies conducted by pain experts McCaffery and Ferrell (1989, 1991, 1992) have documented nurses' misconceptions or lack of knowledge regarding addiction, physiologic dependence, drug tolerance, and respiratory depression. The most problematic misconception on the part of nurses is the belief that the patient must have a physiologic and behavioral response to pain that matches the nurses' picture of what a patient in pain looks like (i.e., the patient must have a marked change in vital signs and be moaning, writhing, and crying to truly be in pain). This misbelief hampers appropriate management of the patient's pain. The critical care nurse must remember that pain is what the patient states it is and that no additional finding is necessary to treat the patient's pain.[3] When a patient is denied pain management based on the misconception that there is a certain behavior that always accompanies pain, an ethical conflict arises.[22,23]

Nursing concerns with addiction can contribute to misinterpretation of signs during the pain assessment process. Addiction rates for patients in acute pain who receive opioid analgesics are less than 1%.[3,24] Some of the misbeliefs that surround addiction result from lack of knowledge about the terms addiction and tolerance. *Addiction* is defined by Jacox and others "as a pattern of compulsive drug use that is characterized by an incessant longing for a drug and the need to use the drug for effects other than pain control." *Tolerance* is defined as a decreasing duration of opioid action.[3,25-27] Physical dependence and tolerance to opioids may develop if the drugs are given over a long period. If this is an anticipated problem, withdrawal may be avoided by simply weaning the patient from the opioid slowly to allow the brain to reestablish neurochemical balance in the absence of the opioid.[2] Tolerance to an opioid is a rare phenomenon in the critical care patient.

Another concern on the behalf of the health care professional is the fear that aggressive management of pain with opiates will cause critical respiratory depression.[6,13,28,29] Opioids can cause respiratory depression, but in the critically ill this is a rare phenomenon. Like addiction, the incidence is less than 1%.[24] Respiratory depression from the administration of opioids, though a concern, can be managed with diligent assessment practices.

PAIN MANAGEMENT

The management of pain in the critically ill patient is as multidimensional as the assessment and is a multidisciplinary task. The control of pain can be pharmacologic, nonpharmacologic, or a combination of the two therapies. The most commonly used course for pain control in critical care is in the pharmacologic domain.

Pharmacologic Control of Pain

The pharmacologic management of pain has infinite variety in the critical care unit. Although this is not an in-depth discussion of pharmacology, some commonly administered agents are discussed. Pain pharmacology is divided into four categories of action: opioid agonists (morphine, hydromorphone, fentanyl, and meperidine); partial agonists and agonist antagonists (buprenorphine, pentazocine); nonopioids (acetaminophen, nonsteroidal antiinflammatory drugs [NSAIDs]); and adjuvants (anticonvulsants, antidepressants). How the pain is approached and managed is a progression or combination of the available agents, the type of pain, and the patient response to the therapy.

Opioid analgesics. An agonist binds to an opiate receptor to fully activate the receptor response. A partial agonist initiates a partial response, an antagonist blocks the response, and an agonist antagonist enhances the response of one type of receptor while blocking the response of another.[26] The clinical response varies, based on the receptor involved and the mechanism of the drug.

Morphine. Morphine, an mu (μ) agonist, is the opioid most commonly prescribed in the critical care unit.[26,29] Morphine is a very effective opioid analgesic with manageable side effects, rapid onset, and a variety of delivery methods. It is the standard by which all other opioids are measured. It is also the agent that most closely mimics the endogenous opioids in the pain modification system. Morphine is indicated for severe pain. Morphine has the additional benefit of actions that are helpful for managing other symptoms. Morphine dilates peripherally, both veins and arteries, making it useful in reducing myocardial workload. Morphine is also viewed as an antianxiety agent, because of the calming effect it produces.[9,17,30] The most commonly reported side effects of morphine are fatigue, constipation, nausea, vomiting, and hypotension. A serious side effect requiring diligent monitoring is the respiratory depressant effect. Although an infrequent occurrence, the effect can have significant sequelae for the critically ill patient. There is a subset of patients at greater risk for this effect after the administration of morphine: the very old, those with a neuromuscular disorder, patients with chronic obstructive pulmonary disease, and patients who are opiate-naïve or receiving the first dose of the opiate.[12] The critical care nurse must monitor the patient intensively with the first dose. Normal tolerance to the respiratory effect of the drug develops over time.[31] If the patient exhibits sign of respiratory depression, it can be readily reversed with the administration of the opioid antagonist naloxone. The initial assessment finding of respiratory depression may be a drop in arterial oxygen saturation. There may be a change in mentation or level of consciousness that indicates an increase in sedation, which normally precedes the critical respiratory effect. There will be a decrease in the rate and depth of respirations. Most critical care units have a protocol that clearly defines respiratory depression (normally six to eight respirations/minute) and the treatment required. Critical respiratory depression is readily reversed with the administration of the opiate antagonist naloxone. The usual dose is 0.4 mg. This is considered full dosing. Naloxone is normally given in 0.1 mg increments while the patient is carefully monitored for reversal of the respiratory symptoms. It is important that the patient be given only enough naloxone to reverse the respiratory depression. If the patient is given a full dose, there can be an abrupt return of the pain, accompanied by nausea, vomiting, severe agitation, and anxiety.[30] It is important to know and carefully follow the unit protocol for respiratory depression secondary to the administration of opiates. (∞Pulse Oximetry, p. 653.)

Another caution in the use of morphine in the critically ill is the hypotensive effect. This can be particularly problematic in the hypovolemic patient. The vasodilatory effect of morphine is potentiated in the volume-depleted patient. Hemodynamic status must be carefully monitored.[31] In the event of a hypotensive response, volume resuscitation effectively restores blood pressure.

Fentanyl. Fentanyl is an opioid analgesic. It is also an mu (μ) agonist, and consequently the effects are similar to those of morphine. It is available in a variety of forms: intravenous, intraspinal, and transdermal. The transdermal form is commonly referred to as the Duragesic patch or the 72-hour patch. Fentanyl and the derivative sufentanil have historically been used as adjuncts to the induction and maintenance of anesthesia.[19] The use of fentanyl in the critical care unit is growing in popularity. Since the side effects of fentanyl are similar to those of morphine, the nurse must monitor carefully for respiratory effects. Fentanyl in higher doses has the additional hazard of creating muscle rigidity in the chest wall muscles. Patients receiving fentanyl analgesia require careful attention to the hemodynamic profile. There are occasional indications for the use of transdermal fentanyl in the critically ill patient. The customary use is for the chronic pain state or for the pain from cancer, and in critical care for the patient who requires extended pain control. Transdermal delivery requires 17 hours for onset of action and has a duration of 72 hours. If this delivery method is used, the patient will require other opioid management until the fentanyl takes effect.[19]

Meperidine. Meperidine (Demerol) is an effective opioid for short-term use. Its profile is similar to that of morphine. It is considered the weakest of the opioids and needs to be administered in large doses to be equivalent in action to morphine.[32] The duration of action is short, so dosing will be frequent. A major concern with the drug is the metabolite normeperidine. Normeperidine is a CNS neurotoxic agent. At high doses in the renal- or hepatic-compromised patient or in the elderly patient, it may induce a CNS toxicity. At the mildest, it will produce mood alterations including apprehension, anxiety, restlessness, sadness, and anger. In severe toxicity it can produce convulsions and myoclonus.[33] Meperidine is also implicated in significant tachycardias. Although meperidine is useful for short-term use in selected patients, it must be avoided in patients who require longer periods of analgesia.[26] Any patient receiving meperidine for pain control must be carefully monitored for the previously mentioned signs of toxicity. The AHCPR guidelines suggest its use be limited to those patients with a documented sensitivity or allergic response to other mu agonists.[6]

Hydromorphone. Hydromorphone is a semisynthetic mu (μ) opioid agonist that has a more rapid onset of action and a shorter duration than morphine. It is an effective opioid with multiple routes of delivery. Milligram-for-milligram it is more potent than morphine. Consequently, it is commonly the opioid of choice when the route is subcutaneous.

Codeine and hydrocodone are effective opioids that are well-absorbed after oral administration. Constipation is a significant effect of both drugs. Oxycodone, another oral agent, is considered a moderately strong opioid. All three of these agents are indicated for moderate pain states. They are normally combined with aspirin or acetaminophen. Patients must be cautioned to monitor any additional aspirin or acetaminophen intake.

Nonopioid analgesics. There is limited reference in the literature as to the role of nonopioid analgesics in the critical care unit.[16] Whether this is because of a lack of physician orders for the drugs or the perception that opioids are of more value in the critically ill patient is unclear. The nonopioids may indeed have more of a role in the management of pain in the critically ill.

Nonsteroidal antiinflammatory drugs. The use of nonsteroidal antiinflammatory drugs (NSAIDs) in combination with opioids is indicated in the patient with acute musculoskeletal and soft tissue inflammation.[25] The mechanism of action in the NSAIDs is the inhibition of the synthesis and release of the neurotransmitter prostaglandin. This action occurs in the peripheral nervous system component of pain, unlike the opioids, which act in the central nervous system. Although prostaglandins are implicated in pain and inflammation, they are also responsible for maintaining the integrity of the mucous lining of the gastric mucosa. An additional role of the prostaglandins in the body is the production of thromboxane. Thromboxane causes the aggregation and clumping of platelets, two side effects associated with the use of NSAIDs. There are two NSAIDs commonly used in the critical care unit: acetaminophen and ketorolac. Acetaminophen is commonly ordered for the relief of minor pain; ketorolac is used parenterally for short-term pain management and is particularly useful as a co-analgesic with an opioid. Since ketorolac is an NSAID, monitoring for clumping of platelets is of primary importance. Evaluate laboratory work for evidence of an increase in bleeding time, and assess the patient for any signs of abnormal bleeding. Of particular concern is any evidence of gastrointestinal (GI) bleeding.[34] It is important to consider the concurrent use of opioids and NSAIDs to affect pain modification at both areas of transmission. This combination of agents often significantly reduces the amount of opioids required for effective pain management. See Table 8-5 for more information on pharmacologic management of pain.

There are other pharmacologic agents used in the critical care unit. The most important factor in the management of pain with any pharmacologic agent is the careful assessment and reassessment of the patient's pain status during the administration of the drug. The need to adjust the dosage, increase the frequency, or change the agent will be based on assessment findings.

Delivery Methods

The most common route for drug administration is the intravenous route, via continuous infusion, bolus administration, or patient-controlled analgesia (PCA). Traditionally, the choice has been IV bolus administration. The benefits of this method are the rapid onset of action and the ease of titration. The major disadvantage is the rise and fall of the serum level of the opioid, leading to periods of pain control with periods of breakthrough pain.[35]

Continuous infusion of the opioids via an infusion pump provides constant blood levels of the ordered opioid; this promotes a consistent level of comfort. It is a particularly helpful method of administration during sleep because the patient awakens with an adequate level of pain relief.[36] It is important that the patient be given the loading dose that relieves the pain and raises the circulating dose of the drug. After the basal rate is established the patient maintains a steady state of pain control, unless there is additional pain from a procedure, an activity, or a change in the patient's condition. Orders for additional boluses of opioid need to be available.

Patient controlled analgesia. Patient controlled analgesia is a method of delivery, via an infusion pump, that allows the patient to self-administer small doses of analgesics. This method of medication delivery allows the patient to control the level of pain and sedation and to avoid the peaks and valleys of intermittent dosing by the health care professional. The patient can self-administer a bolus of medication the moment the pain begins, thus acting preemptively. See Box 8-1 for further information on patient controlled analgesia assistance.

Although a variety of routes can be used with PCA, it is traditionally administered via an IV route.[30] Certain patients are not candidates for PCA. Alterations in the level of consciousness or mentation preclude understanding the use of the equipment. The very elderly or patients with renal or hepatic insufficiency may require careful screening for PCA.

Allowing the patient to self-administer opioid doses does not diminish the role of the critical care nurse in pain management. The nurse advises for necessary changes to the prescription and continues to monitor the effects of the medication and doses. The patient is closely monitored during the first 2 hours of therapy and after every change in the prescription. If the patient's pain does not respond within the first 2 hours of therapy, a total reassessment of the pain state is essential. The nurse monitors the number of boluses the patient delivers. If he or she is bolusing more often than the prescription, the dose may be insufficient to maintain pain control. Naloxone must be readily available to reverse adverse opiate respiratory effects. Ideally, the patient undergoing an elective procedure requiring opioid analgesia postoperatively is instructed in the use of PCA during preoperative teaching. This allows the patient to become comfortable with the concept of self-medication before use.

Intraspinal pain control. Intraspinal anesthesia uses the concept that the spinal cord is the primary link in nociceptive transmission. The goal is to mimic the body's endogenous opioid pain modification system by interfering with the transmission of pain by providing an opiate receptor binding agent directly into the spinal cord. The benefits of the intraspinal route include good-to-excellent pain control with typically lower doses of opioids, increased patient mobility, minimal sedation, and typically, increased patient satisfaction.[30] There is also very little change in the hemodynamic status of the patient. Intraspinal anesthesia is particularly appropriate for pain in the thorax, the upper abdomen, and the lower extremities. There are two intraspinal routes: intrathecal and epidural (see Figure 8-6). Regardless of the route, the effects of the opioid agonist used will be the same so assessment parameters will mimic those used for other routes. See Box 8-2 for more information on intraspinal analgesia administration.

Intrathecal analgesia. Intrathecal (subarachnoid) opioids are placed directly into the cerebral spinal fluid and attach to spinal cord receptor sites. Opioids introduced at this site act quickly at the dorsal horn. The dural sheath is punctured, eliminating any barrier for pathogens between the environment and the cerebral spinal fluid. This creates the risk for serious infections. The intrathecal route is usually reserved for

TABLE 8-5 Selected Pharmacologic Agents Used for Pain Management

Drug	Dosage	Action	Special Considerations
Amitriptyline (Elavil)	PO 10 mg/day	Blocks reuptake of serotonins	Can be sedating
Bupivacaine (Marcaine)	Epidural 1-5 mg/hr	Local hydrophilic anesthetic; blocks C and Aδ fiber transmission	May be given alone or in combination with an opioid; monitor carefully for hypotension, respiratory depression
Butorphanol (Stadol)	1-2 mg q 3-4 hr IM or slow IV	Agonist-antagonist	Psychometric effects, anxiety, hallucinations, nightmares
Capsaicin	Topical 3-4 times/day	Causes release and depletion of Substance P	Effective for peripheral neuropathies, neuralgias
Codeine	15-30 mg q 4 hr	Weak μ agonist	Effective for minor pain; constipating
Diazepam (Valium)	IV 2-5 mg PO 2.5-10 mg	Adjuvant agent for pain; antilytic	Must not be given directly with an opioid, which can increase side effects, sedation
Fentanyl	IV 0.1 mg Epidural 25-250 μg or 10-25 μg/hr	Moderate-dose analgesia High-dose anesthesia opioid agonist	80 times as potent as morphine Transdermal onset 72 hours
Hydromorphone (Dilaudid)	PO 2 mg q 4 hr IM 1.5 mg	μ Agonist	Shorter duration of action than morphine
Ibuprofen (Advil, Motrin)	200-600 mg q 6 hr	NSAID	GI upsets, prolonged bleeding time
Ketorolac (Toradol)	15-30 mg IM qid	Parenteral NSAID; prevents production of prostaglandins	Platelet aggregation interrupted; inhibits maintenance of gastric mucosa
Meperidine (Demerol)	IM 75-150 mg q 4 hr	μ Agonist	Short half-life, very neurotoxic, limited use advised
Methadone (Dolophine)	PO 20 mg q 4 hr IV 5-10 mg	μ Agonist	Very efficient orally; accumulates with multiple dosing, causing serious sedation (2-5 days)
Oxycodone (Percocet, with Tylenol; Percodan, with aspirin)	PO 2 tabs (10 mg total) q 4 hr	Moderately strong μ agonist	Combination with aspirin, Tylenol blocks both peripheral and central pathways
Pentazocine (Talwin)	PO 50-100 mg q 3-4 hr SQ/IM 30-60 mg q 3-4 hr IV 30 mg	Mixed agonist-antagonist, blocks μ and activates κ receptors, considered a weak agent	Has ceiling effect, increases cardiac workload
Propoxyphene (Davrocet-N)	PO 1-2 tabs q 4 hr	Weak μ agonist	CNS toxic metabolite, not for long-term use, for minor pain
Morphine	IV 2-15 mg/hr bolus IV 1-10 mg/hr continuous infusion IM 5-15 mg q 3-4 hr SQ 5-15 mg q 3-4 hr Epidural 1-5 mg/hr bolus Epidural 0.5-2.0 mg/hr continuous infusion PO 8-20 mg q 4 hr	Analgesia, antianxiety, opioid agonist	Respiratory depression, hypotension, nausea, vomiting, sedation, pruritus; titrate to effect

NURSING INTERVENTION CLASSIFICATIONS

BOX 8-1 Patient-Controlled Analgesia (PCA) Assistance

DEFINITION: Facilitating patient control of analgesic administration and regulation

ACTIVITIES:
Collaborate with physicians, patient, and family members in selecting the type of narcotic to be used
Recommend administration of aspirin and nonsteroidal antiinflammatory drugs in conjunction with narcotics, as appropriate
Avoid use of Demerol
Ensure that patient is not allergic to analgesic to be administered
Teach patient and family to monitor pain intensity, quality, and duration
Teach patient and family to monitor respiratory rate and blood pressure
Establish nasogastric, venous, subcutaneous, or spinal access, as appropriate
Validate that the patient can use a PCA device: is able to communicate, comprehend explanations, and follow directions
Collaborate with patient and family to select appropriate type of patient-controlled infusion device
Teach patient and family members how to use the PCA device
Assist patient and family to calculate appropriate concentration of drug to fluid, considering the amount of fluid delivered per hour via the PCA device
Assist patient or family member to administer an appropriate bolus loading dose of analgesic
Teach the patient and family to set an appropriate basal infusion rate on the PCA device
Assist the patient and family to set the appropriate lockout interval on the PCA device
Assist the patient and family in setting appropriate demand doses on the PCA device
Consult with patient, family members, and physician to adjust lockout interval, basal rate, and demand dosage, according to patient responsiveness
Teach patient how to titrate doses up or down, depending on respiratory rate, pain intensity, and pain quality
Teach patient and family members the action and side effects of pain-relieving agents
Document patient's pain, amount and frequency of drug dosing, and response to pain treatment in a pain flow sheet
Recommend a bowel regimen to avoid constipation
Consult with clinical pain experts for a patient who is having difficulty achieving pain control

From McCloskey JC, Bulechek GM: *Nursing intervention classifications,* ed 2, St Louis, 1996, Mosby.

intraoperative use. Single bolus dosing provides short-term relief for pain that is short lived (e.g., the pain of labor and delivery is well-managed using this regimen).[36] Side effects of intrathecal pain control include postdural puncture headache and infection.

Epidural analgesia. Epidural analgesia is commonly used in the critical care unit after major abdominal surgery, nephrectomy, thoracotomy, and major orthopedic procedures.[24] Certain conditions preclude the use of this pain control method: systemic infection, anticoagulation, and increased intracranial pressure. Epidural delivery of opiates provides longer-lasting pain relief with less dosing of opiates. When delivered into the epidural space, 5 mg of morphine may be effective for 6 to 24 hours, compared with 3 to 4 hours when delivered intravenously. Opioids infused in the epidural space are more unpredictable than those administered intrathecally. The epidural space is filled with fatty tissue and is external to the dura mater. The fatty tissue interferes with uptake and the dura acts as a barrier to diffusion, making diffusion rate difficult to predict. The rapidity of the diffusion of the drug is determined by the type of drug used. The drugs are either hydrophilic or lipophilic. Hydrophilic drugs are water-soluble and penetrate the dura slowly, giving them a longer onset and duration of action. Morphine is hydrophilic. Lipophilic drugs are lipid-soluble; they penetrate the dura rapidly and therefore have a rapid onset of action and a shorter duration of action.[24] Fentanyl is lipophilic. The dura itself acts as a physical barrier and causes delay in diffusion, which in comparison to the intrathecal route allows more drug to be absorbed in the systemic circulation, requiring greater doses for pain relief.[30] Drugs delivered epidurally may be bolused or continuously infused. Epidural analgesia is experiencing increased usage in the critical care environment and requires careful monitoring. The nurse must assess the patient for respiratory

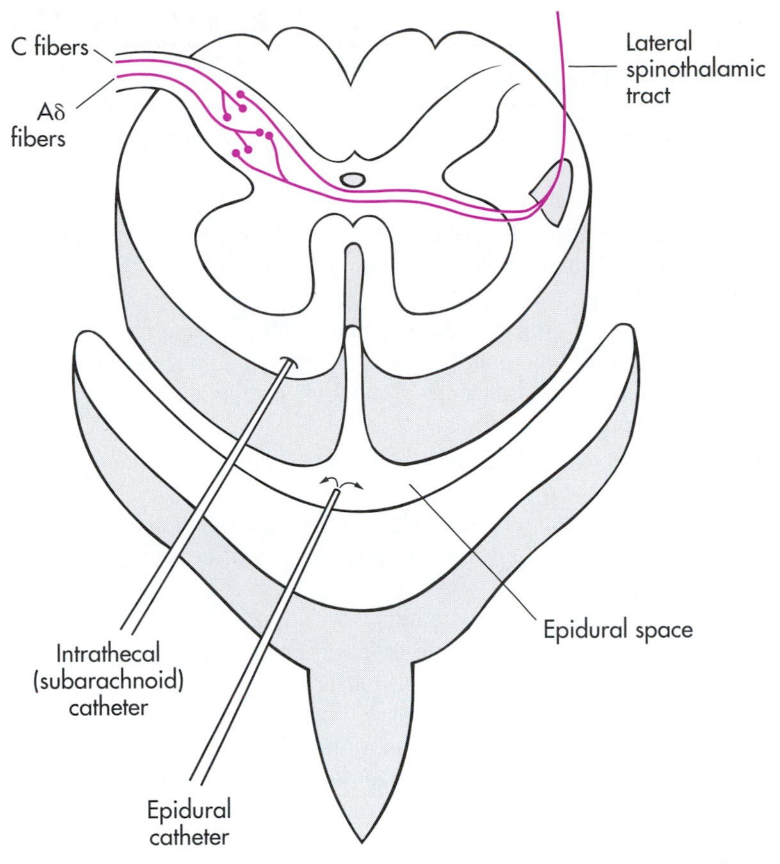

FIGURE 8-6. Intraspinal catheter placement in spinal cord cross section.

depression using the unit protocol. This phenomenon may occur early in the therapy or as late as 24 hours after initiation. The epidural catheter also puts the patient at risk for infection. The efficiency of this pain control method and the increased mobility of the patient does not diminish the nurse's responsibility to monitor and evaluate the outcomes of the pain management protocol in use.

Equianalgesia

At some point in the patient's recovery strong opioids are replaced by more moderate agents. In doing any conversion the goal is to provide equal analgesic effects with the new agents. This concept is referred to *as equianalgesia.* The critical care nurse is the practitioner most likely to convert the patient from parenteral medication to oral medication in preparation for a change in the level of care or in preparation for discharge. Studies have identified that nurses lack knowledge regarding equal doses between IV and oral administration. There is the misconception that when a patient is able to take oral medication the pain is less severe. The change to oral medications does not indicate a need for less medication. The nurse needs to practice equianalgesia when converting the patient. Because of the variety of agents and routes, the professional pain organizations have developed equianalgesia charts for use by the health care professional. All critical care units need to have a chart posted for easy referral. Table 8-6 is an equianalgesia chart used in clinical practice.[37]

Non-Pharmacologic Methods

There are numerous methods of pain management other than drugs that appear in the critical care literature.[25] In most instances these therapies augment and enhance the pharmacologic management of the patient's pain. Stimulating other non–pain sensory fibers present in the periphery modifies pain transmission. These fibers are stimulated by thermal changes, as in the application of heat or cold, by simple massage, or by the action of the transcutaneous electrical nerve stimulator (TENS). The use of massage has been a mainstay in the nursing management of the patient in pain. It is an appropriate pain management technique for most critically ill patients.

The use of TENS has contraindications in the critical care unit. Because the device is controlled by the

NURSING INTERVENTION CLASSIFICATIONS

BOX 8-2 Analgesic Administration: Intraspinal

DEFINITION: Administration of pharmacologic agents into the epidural or intrathecal space to reduce or eliminate pain

ACTIVITIES:

Check patency and function of catheter, port, and/or pump
Ensure that IV access is in place at all times during therapy
Label the catheter and secure it appropriately
Ensure that the proper formulation of the drug is used (e.g., high concentrating and preservation free)
Ensure narcotic antagonist availability for emergency administration and administer per physician order, as necessary
Start continuous infusion of analgesic agent after correct catheter placement has been verified, and monitor rate to ensure delivery of prescribed dosage of medication
Monitor temperature, blood pressure, respirations, pulse, and level of consciousness at appropriate intervals and record on flow sheet
Monitor level of sensory blockade at appropriate intervals and record on flow sheet
Monitor catheter site and dressings to check for a loose catheter or wet dressing, and notify appropriate personnel per agency protocol
Administer catheter site care according to agency protocol
Secure needle in place with tape and apply appropriate dressing according to agency protocol
Monitor for adverse reactions, including respiratory depression, urinary retention, undue somnolence, itching, seizures, nausea, and vomiting
Monitor orthostatic blood pressure and pulse before the first attempt at ambulation
Instruct patient to report side effects, alterations in pain relief, numbness of extremities, and need for assistance with ambulation if weak
Follow institutional policies for injection of intermittent analgesic agents into the injection port
Provide adjunct medications as appropriate (e.g., antidepressants, anticonvulsants, and nonsteroidal antiinflammatory agents)
Increase intraspinal dose, based on pain intensity score
Instruct and guide patient through nonpharmacologic measures (e.g., simple relaxation therapy, simple guided imagery, and biofeedback) to enhance pharmacologic effectiveness
Instruct patient about proper home care for external or implanted delivery systems, as appropriate
Remove or assist with removal of catheter according to agency protocol

From McCloskey JC, Bulechek GM: *Nursing intervention classifications,* ed 2, St Louis, 1996, Mosby.

patient, mentation must be intact. TENS is also contraindicated in patients with pacemakers or automatic implantable defibrillators because these devices may recognize and erroneously interpret the TENS electrical signal. TENS therapy is efficient, patient-controlled pain management for orthopedic, obstetric, and some postoperative pain states.

Using the cortical interpretation of pain as the foundation, there are a number of interventions known to reduce the patient's pain report. These modalities include cognitive techniques: patient teaching, relaxation, distraction, guided imagery, music therapy, and hypnosis.[25,38] (See Box 8-3 for patient education for pain management.)

Relaxation is a well-documented method for reducing the distress associated with pain.[39] While not a substitute for pharmacology, relaxation is an excellent adjunct to control pain. Relaxation decreases oxygen consumption and muscle tone and can decrease heart rate and blood pressure. Relaxation gives the patient a sense of control over the pain and reduces muscle tension and anxiety. Not all patients are interested in relaxation therapy. For those patients, deep-breathing exercises may be helpful and frequently lead to relaxation. Excellent references for thorough techniques in relaxation therapy are available.[3]

Guided imagery is a technique that uses the imagination to provide control over pain. It can be used to distract or relax. Guiding a patient to a place that is pain-free and relaxing takes a considerable time commitment on the part of the nurse. Although this may be difficult in the critical care environment, guiding a patient to a place in his or her imagination that is free from pain can be done rapidly and may be very beneficial.[25]

TABLE 8-6 Equianalgesia Chart

This chart is designed to assist the practitioner in identifying approximate doses of medication that will provide similar pain relief. All dosing of all drugs should be based on the patient's response to the medication. This chart is based on the recommendations of the American Pain Society. *Single IV doses are equivalent to 1/2 the IM dose.* All IM and PO doses in this chart are considered equivalent to 10 mg of morphine in clinical effect

Analgesic	IM Route (mg)	PO Route (mg)	Comments
Morphine	10	30-60	PO 3-6x IM dose Morphine is the gold standard to which the effect of other opiates is compared
Fentanyl	1		
Meperidine (Demerol)	75	300	PO 4x IM dose; neurotoxic metabolite; use with extreme caution
Hydromorphone (Dilaudid)	1.5	7.5	PO 5x IM dose; shorter duration than MS
Oxycodone		15-30	Effect may last up to 6 hr
Codeine	130	200	PO 1.3-1.5x IM dose; very constipating; high doses may cause nausea and vomiting
Nalbuphine (Nubain)	10		May precipitate withdrawal in opiate-dependent patients
Butorphanol (Stadol)	2		Same as above

Jacox and others: *Acute pain management: operative or medical procedures and trauma. Clinical practice guidelines, Publication 92-0032,* Rockville, Md, 1992, Agency for Health Care Policy and Research, US Department of Health and Human Services.
x, Times.

Music therapy is a commonly used intervention for relaxation. Music that is pleasing to the patient may have very soothing effects.[40] Ideally, the music should be supplied by a small set of very light headphones. This method also serves to minimize the distracting and anxiety-producing noises of a critical care unit.[41] It is important to educate the patient and family regarding the role of music in relaxation and pain control and also to provide music of the patient's choice.

The patient and family may provide information about other sources of distraction for the patient. Determining what distraction therapies the patient normally uses may provide a clue to which might work during the illness. Some persons are distracted by television; however, for others, television is a source of increased anxiety. Do not assume that the patient does or does not want to watch television until you determine whether it will be beneficial or harmful to the patient.

The key to success with any of these therapies is to understand their mechanism of action so that the therapy matches the needs of the patient. All of the previously mentioned interventions require the patient's cooperation. There must be some commitment on the part of the patient to the treatment. When handled efficiently non-pharmacologic tools can assist in pain management.

BOX 8-3 PATIENT EDUCATION

PAIN MANAGEMENT

- Role of pain in illness or injury
- Pain as a barrier to healing
- Responsibility for communicating pain experienced
- Role of positioning in pain management
- Pharmacologic agents being used
- Delivery method and implications of pharmacologic agents
- Facts regarding addiction of pharmacologic agents
- Role of relaxation and guided imagery in pain management

There are an increasing number of therapies appearing in the critical care research. It is important for the practitioner to be aware of the current literature to provide the most effective and current interventions to manage the patient's pain.

Today's health care environment mandates that patients experience positive outcomes as rapidly as possible. Since pain is a major barrier to early mobility and rapid return to a preillness state, pain management is of paramount importance to the critical care nurse. Since the critically ill patient is the most difficult to assess and manage, it is imperative that the critical care nurse develop the skill and intervention techniques necessary to manage the most difficult of the pain states. As patient advocate, the nurse assumes the responsibility for establishing pain control as a priority for the health care team.[42]

SEDATION

Sedation in the Critically Ill

One area of challenge for the critical care nurse is the management of patients who are agitated or anxious. Although much anxiety and agitation can be minimized by ongoing reassurance and orientation of the patient, pharmacologic sedation is also used to abate patient anxiety, decrease agitation, promote comfort, and facilitate diagnostic tests or procedures.[43] The critical care nurse is often the one who selects the most appropriate sedative from several alternatives prescribed by the physician. Consequently, the nurse needs to understand how to administer, monitor, and assess for sedative effects, taking into account patient factors, cost, and pharmacokinetics.[43]

Definitions. To understand concepts related to sedation, it is helpful to define some key terms. The terms *anxiety* and *agitation* describe clinical symptoms that are indicators of the need for sedation. Other descriptors are restlessness, delirium, fear, tension, and psychosis.

Sedation: Sedation is a nonspecific term used to describe the induction of a state in which the patient is calm, relaxed, and relatively pain-free. Sedation may be with or without a corresponding decrease in level of consciousness. Sedative agents commonly used in the critical care unit have no analgesic activity.[43,44]

Agitation: Agitation describes the process in which cognitive processes are impaired—manifested by disorientation, impaired short-term memory, altered perceptions, abnormal thought processes, and inappropriate behavior.[44]

Anxiety: Anxiety is a syndrome of altered cognitive function and confusion that is demonstrated by restless behavior.[45] Anxiety includes the emotions of fear, trepidation, helplessness, restlessness, and loss of control. It is associated with physiologic changes such as tachycardia and diaphoresis.[45,46]

Anxiolysis: Anxiolysis means to relieve anxiety.[45,46]

Delirium: Delirium is clinically defined as agitation characterized by global disorders of cognition and wakefulness and by impairment of psychomotor behavior. Because of cerebral insufficiency, cognitive dysfunction occurs. This dysfunction includes disordered perception and decreases in deductive reasoning, memory, attention, and orientation.[47] Delirium management is discussed in Box 8-4.

Causes of Anxiety

Critical care patients today tend to be older and more severely ill than those from previous decades because of advances in pharmacology, clinical interventions, and technology.[43,44,47] The critical care environment is stressful because of incessant noise, lights, and activity. Also, the patient is subjected to physiologic and psychologic stress, which may exacerbate an existing illness.[43,44] For example, insertion of an endotracheal tube decreases the ability to communicate or obtain normal sleep intervals and predisposes the patient to stress, anxiety, and agitation. The presence of the unfamiliar faces of health care professionals as well as the patient's dependence on others may increase feelings of apprehension and helplessness. Moreover, the same stress response can exacerbate an underlying disease process and create symptoms that mimic anxiety. Thus it is crucial to identify the cause of the patient's agitation to guide appropriate treatment.

Pathophysiology of Anxiety

It is important to understand the pathophysiology of anxiety and the clinical implications of neurohumoral reactions to stress. These factors will affect the clinician's choice of sedation.

Pathways

The neurohumoral response to stress involves neurotransmission by at least four kinds of chemical transmitters and their corresponding receptors. Acetylcholine, norepinephrine, dopamine, and serotonin are neurotransmitters involved in the anxiety response.[46] The effects of anxiety on the noradrenergic and dopaminergic neurotransmitters are briefly discussed.

NURSING INTERVENTION CLASSIFICATIONS

BOX 8-4 Delirium Management

DEFINITION: Provision of a safe and therapeutic environment for the patient who is experiencing an acute confusional state

ACTIVITIES:

Identify etiological factors causing delirium
Initiate therapies to reduce or eliminate factors causing the delirium
Monitor neurological status on an ongoing basis
Provide unconditional positive regard
Verbally acknowledge the patient's fears and feelings
Provide optimistic but realistic reassurance
Allow the patient to maintain rituals that limit anxiety
Provide patient with information about what is happening and what can be expected to occur in the future
Avoid demands for abstract thinking, if patient can think only in concrete terms
Limit need for decision making, if frustrating/confusing to patient
Administer PRN medications for anxiety or agitation
Encourage visitation by significant others, as appropriate
Recognize and accept the patient's perceptions or interpretation of reality (hallucinations or delusions)
State your perception in a calm, reassuring, and nonargumentative manner
Respond to the theme/feeling tone, rather than the content, of the hallucination or delusion
Remove stimuli, when possible, that create misperception in a particular patient (e.g., pictures on the wall or television)
Maintain a well-lit environment that reduces sharp contrasts and shadows
Assist with needs related to nutrition, elimination, hydration, and personal hygiene
Maintain a hazard-free environment
Place identification bracelet on patient
Provide appropriate level of supervision/surveillance to monitor patient and to allow for therapeutic actions, as needed
Use physical restraints, as needed
Avoid frustrating patient by quizzing with orientation questions that cannot be answered
Inform patient of person, place, and time, as needed
Provide a consistent physical environment and daily routine
Provide caregivers who are familiar to the patient
Use environmental cues (e.g., signs, pictures, clocks, calendars, and color coding of environment) to stimulate memory, reorient, and promote appropriate behavior
Provide a low-stimulation environment for patient in whom disorientation is increased by overstimulation
Encourage use of aids that increase sensory input (e.g., eyeglasses, hearing aids, and dentures)
Approach patient slowly and from the front
Address the patient by name when initiating interaction
Reorient the patient to the health care provider with each contact
Communicate with simple, direct, descriptive statements
Prepare patient for upcoming changes in usual routine and environment before their occurrence
Provide new information slowly and in small doses, with frequent rest periods
Focus interpersonal interactions on what is familiar and meaningful to the patient

From McCloskey JC, Bulechek GM: *Nursing intervention classifications,* ed 2, St Louis, 1996, Mosby.

Stress and noradrenergics. Stress produces an elevated sense of fear and anxiety. As a result, the release of norepinephrine increases in the limbic systems (hippocampus, amygdala, locus caeruleus) and in the cerebral cortex.[46,48] Because of the elevated levels of norepinephrine, the α-adrenergic receptors, which normally bind with norepinephrine, down-regulate. This means receptor sensitivity, or norepinephrine production, is reduced. In turn, there is an increased responsiveness of locus caeruleus neurons to excitatory stimulation, producing manifestations of anxiety and agitation.[47,48]

Stress and dopaminergics. Acute stress increases dopamine release and metabolism in several areas of the brain, particularly in the medial and dorsolateral prefrontal cortex. The dopaminergic neurons in the prefrontal cortex control attention and working memory of coping patterns for the stress response. Dopaminergic receptors become hypersensitized with single or repeated exposures to stress.[46] This increases the brain's ability to respond to stressful events but also heightens fear and anxiety.

ASSESSMENT

Differential Diagnosis of Agitation

The critical care nurse must be as knowledgeable in diagnosing agitation and anxiety as in diagnosing other system problems. For example, if a patient experiences pain, medication is administered. However, if the patient continues to be anxious or agitated, the nurse must reassess the source of the problem. A sedative is only administered after ruling out or treating acute physiologic disturbances such as hypotension, hypoglycemia, hypoxemia, sepsis, or pharmacologic drug interactions.[43]

Panic Attacks

Panic attacks—which include symptoms of diaphoresis, tachycardia, dyspnea, hyperventilation, acute $Paco_2$ increase, insomnia, accentuated startle response, autonomic hyperarousal, and hypervigilance—are common in the critical care unit.[43] Conditioned fear and panic attacks are experienced by many patients, especially those who have experienced emergency procedures. The symptoms of panic attacks, such as dyspnea, hyperventilation, and tachycardia, can also mimic acute heart failure, although the treatment regimen is radically different.

Dopaminergic hyperfunction impulses are transmitted via the meso limbic pathways from the cortical brain to the limbic system. This causes bizarre behavioral and cognitive symptoms that are often referred to as "sundown syndrome." This psychomotor agitation usually occurs at night and is diagnostic of agitated delirium induced by stress.[46,48,49]

Algorithm

An algorithm or other protocols can help to differentiate the need for sedative, anxiolytic, or analgesic therapy for the critically ill patient. Figure 8-7 demonstrates a systematic approach for diagnosis and treatment of anxiety and agitation.[50]

Measurement Tools

The Ramsey and Olsson scales are tools to assess a patient's need for sedation therapy (Box 8-5).[49] These scales are also useful for evaluating the side effects of sedative or analgesic medications. They can provide a standardized baseline for determining when to repeat sedation administration.

LEVELS OF SEDATION

There are several levels of sedation available, depending on the therapeutic goal of the health care provider.

Preemptive Analgesia and Sedation

Preemptive analgesia and sedation is the treatment of pain and anxiety before application of a stimulus to decrease the physiologic and pharmacologic changes that occur during invasive procedures. The presence of anxiety exacerbates pain. Thus sedation and analgesia working in concert can minimize the effects of painful stimuli. This type of treatment can also establish a baseline of pharmacologic management to prevent breakthrough pain from occurring.[51]

Light Sedation

Purpose. Light sedation is typically achieved by administering a single, nonintravenous dose of a long-acting agent.[44,51]

Administration. Licensed health care professionals are permitted to administer sedatives.

Risks. Light sedation is a medically controlled state of analgesia or anxiolysis (antianxiety) that has a minimal risk (less than 1%) for respiratory depression, airway obstruction, cardiovascular depression, or a markedly depressed level of consciousness.

Types. Midazolam (Versed) 2 to 5 mg IV is an example of a medication that can be used for light sedation (see Table 8-7 for other examples).

Deep Sedation

Purpose. Deep sedation is a medically controlled state of depressed consciousness, also known as unconsciousness, from which the patient is not easily aroused.[44,48,51]

Administration. Deep sedation may only be administered by anesthesiologists, nurse anesthetists, or nurses trained in the administration of such sedatives, since the state and risks of deep sedation are indistinguishable from those of general anesthesia.[44,51] An electroencephalogram (EEG) can be used to monitor patients receiving therapeutic paralysis or deep

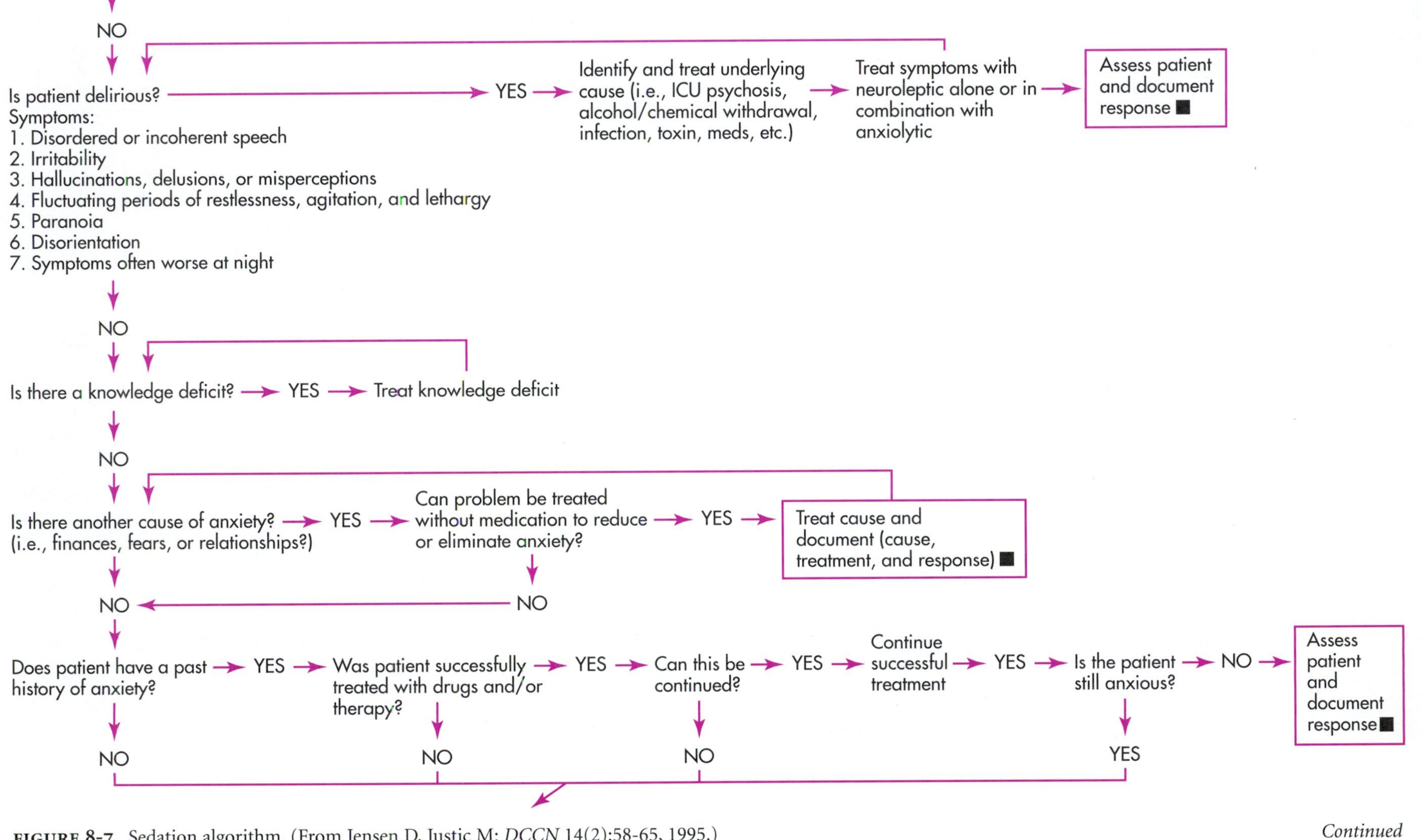

FIGURE 8-7. Sedation algorithm. (From Jensen D, Justic M: *DCCN* 14(2):58-65, 1995.)

Continued

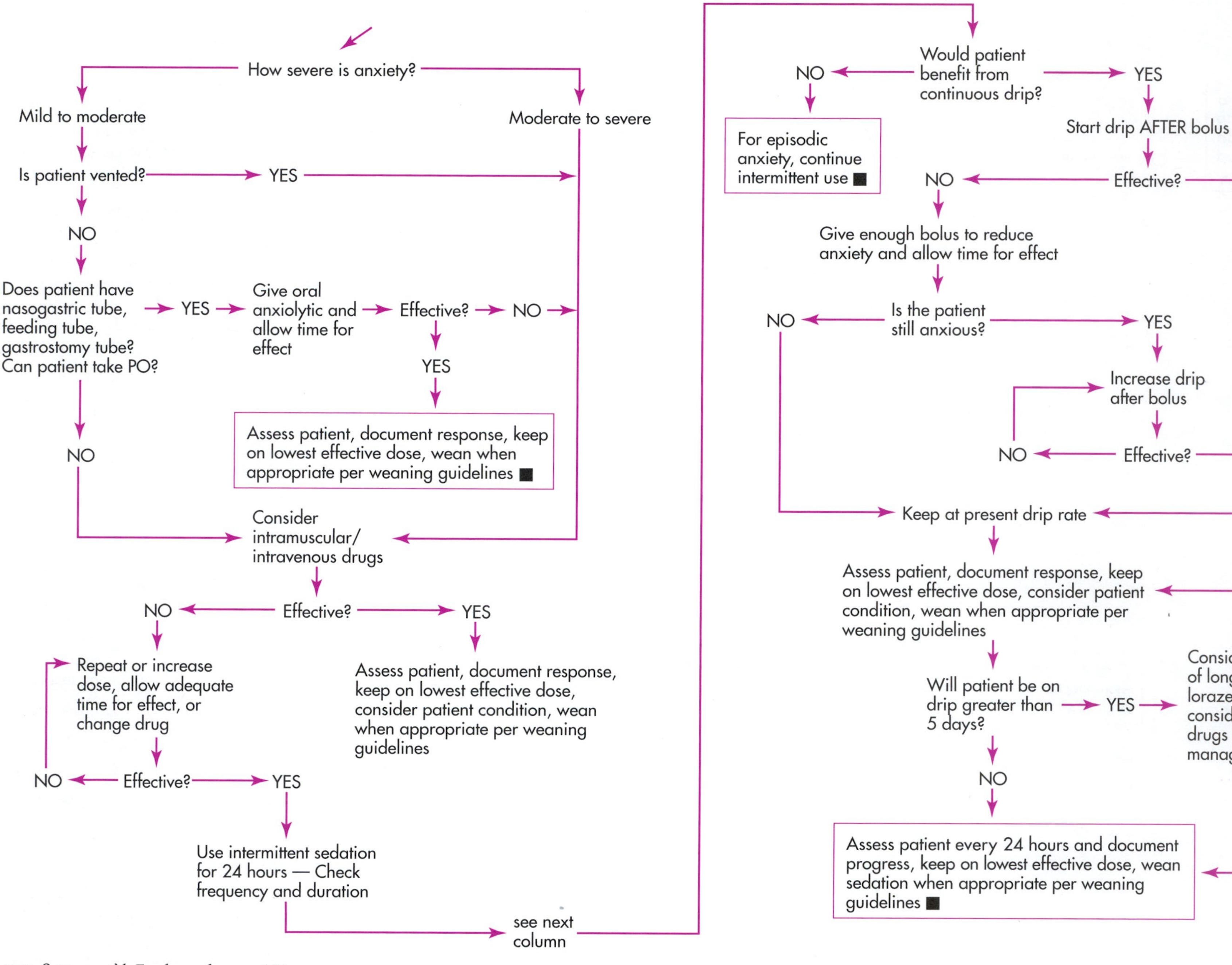

FIG. 8-7, cont'd. For legend see p. 191.

BOX 8-5 Modified Ramsey and Olsson Scales

MODIFIED RAMSEY SCALE

1. Anxious and agitated or restless
2. Cooperative, oriented, tranquil
3. Responds to commands only
4. Asleep but brisk response to glabellar tap or loud auditory stimulus
5. Asleep, sluggish response to glabellar tap or loud auditory stimulus
6. No response

MODIFIED OLSSON SCALE

1. Wide awake
2. Drowsy
3. Dozing intermittently, arouses easily
4. Mostly sleeping
5. Difficult to arouse

N/A Unable to assess

sedation. This monitor displays real-time recordings of neuronal activity and can be used to evaluate the effectiveness of sedation, as visualized by brain wave activity.

Risks. The patient undergoing deep sedation is at risk for the partial or complete loss of protective reflexes, the inability to maintain a patent airway, and the inability to respond purposefully to physical stimulation or verbal commands.

Types. Propofol is one example of a sedative used for deep sedation. Once reserved exclusively for the operating room, today this medication is commonly used in critical care units. It is administered as a continuous infusion, titrated to keep the patient unconscious (see Table 8-7). Propofol has a very short half-life, which is useful for patients who require deep sedation for a short period (e.g., after open heart surgery).

Conscious Sedation

Purpose. Conscious sedation is the condition produced by the administration of a drug or combination of drugs to relieve anxiety or pain during diagnostic or therapeutic procedures[48,51] (Box 8-6).

Administration. Conscious sedation is typically induced by repeatedly administering intravenous medications and titrating to the desired effect. The patient receiving conscious sedation has an altered level of consciousness, but retains the ability to maintain and protect a patent airway as well as respond purposefully to verbal commands and physical stimuli. It requires two health care providers: one to perform the procedure that requires sedation and a second to monitor the patient. Equipment that must be close at hand includes oxygen, bag-valve-mask resuscitator, suction equipment, cardiac monitor, pulse oximeter, blood pressure sphygmomanometer or arterial line, defibrillator, emergency drugs, and reversal agents. Table 8-8 lists the pharmacologic reversal agents for both opiates and benzodiazepines.

Risks. The administration of drugs for conscious sedation may have the unintended effect of compromising a patient's protective reflexes.[48,51]

Types. Benzodiazepines, such as diazepam (Valium) and midazolam (Versed), are among the most widely used agents employed for conscious sedation. Diazepam and midazolam provide a rapid onset of sedation when used intravenously and has a 1 to 2 hour period of recovery. Opiates, such as fentanyl or morphine, can also be used in conscious sedation (see Table 8-5).

Objectives. The goals and effects of conscious sedation include the following:

- *Alteration of mood:* A primary objective is to suppress patients' fear and anxiety. Verbal reassurance allows for a decrease in the use of opiates and sedatives.
- *Maintenance of consciousness:* The patient needs to be able to respond to commands and have all protective reflexes.
- *Cooperation:* The patient is awake enough to cooperate throughout the procedure.
- *Elevation of pain threshold:* Even with the use of local anesthetics for pain control at the operative site, sedatives are used to elevate the pain threshold.
- *Minor variation of vital signs:* Although protective reflexes are unaffected, the physiologic response must not be altered. With therapeutic conscious sedation there must be only slight changes in the blood pressure, heart rate, respiratory rate, and pulse oximetry readings.
- *Some degree of amnesia:* Some conscious sedation medications provide amnesic effects, based on the dose administered. The patient must never be rendered unconscious.

Associated effects. Conscious sedation can produce a range of desirable and undesirable effects in individual patients. Desirable effects include diminished verbal communication, cooperation, slightly slurred speech, and easy arousal from sleep. Undesirable effects include agitation, combativeness, severely slurred speech, respiratory depression, and unarousable sleep. If a deterioration in the patient's clinical condition

TABLE 8-7 Pharmacologic Agents Used for Sedation

Drug	Dosage	Action	Special Considerations
BENZODIAZEPINES			
(Anxiolytic)			
Diazepam (Valium)	Intermittent bolus 2-5 mg q 3-4 hrs; long duration	Depresses CNS at limbic subcortical levels of brain; suppresses seizure activity in the cortex, thalamus, limbic system	Adults 5-20 mg slow IV push 2-5 mg/min; may repeat q 5-10 min, up to max total dose of 20 mg Use 2-5 mg in elderly or debilitated patients
Lorazepam (Ativan)	Intermittent bolus 1-2 mg q 3-4 hr; continuous infusion 1-5 mg/hr	Depresses CNS at limbic subcortical levels of brain	Exerts less effect on respiratory and cardiovascular functions Liver disease causes variable effects
Midazolam (Versed)	.07-.08 mg/kg IM or .035 mg/kg IV (not >2.5 mg); short acting, rapid onset	Depresses CNS at limbic subcortical levels of brain	Use cautiously in patients with COPD, heart failure, renal disease Monitor BP, HR, RR, airway Amnesic effect
(Antipsychotic)			
Haldoperidol (Haldol)	Intermittent bolus 1-5 mg q 20 min; continuous infusion 0.5-20.0 mg/hr; onset 5-30 min	Depresses CNS at limbic subcortical levels of brain, midbrain, brainstem; inhibits catecholamine receptors; inhibits reuptake of neurotransmitters in brain	Adverse effects involve CNS Cardiovascular problems: tachycardia hypotension, dysrhythmias
Propofol (Diprivan)	Initial rate: 0.3 mg/kg/hr; continuous infusion: 0.3-3 mg/kg/hr; rapid acting, short half-life	Metabolized by hepatic conjugation to inactive metabolites by renal excretion; highly soluble lipid solution	Stopping infusion daily for neurologic assessment is important Decreased vascular tone, myocardial contractility, dysrhythmias, respiratory depression, anaphylactic reactions Not an analgesic; still need to give analgesia with it Use sterile technique when handling medication

COPD, Chronic obstructive pulmonary disease.

occurs, a patent airway must be maintained, ventilation supported, and cardiopulmonary resuscitation begun, if required.

Medical Management

The Society of Critical Care Medicine (SCCM) and the American College of Critical Care Medicine have recently developed clinical practice guidelines on pain and sedation.[47] These guidelines are helpful because they list the opiates and sedatives most commonly used in the critical care setting. For example, midazolam (Versed) or propofol (Diprivan) are the recommended agents if short-term sedation—lasting less than 24 hours,—is required. However, lorazepam (Ativan) is the drug of choice if long-term sedation is required. Haldoperidol (Haldol) is the preferred agent for the treatment of delirium in the critically ill adult.[49] Many drugs used for the treatment of anxiety and agitation are unpredictable in the critically ill patient. Patients with hepatic or renal insufficiency may require smaller doses because of heightened receptor sensitivity or reduced clearance of sedative agents.

NURSING INTERVENTION CLASSIFICATIONS

BOX 8-6 Conscious Sedation

DEFINITION: Administration of sedatives, monitoring of the patient's response, and provision of necessary physiological support during a diagnostic or therapeutic procedure

ACTIVITIES:

Review patient's health history and results of diagnostic tests to determine whether patient meets agency criteria for conscious sedation by a registered nurse
Ask patient or family about any previous experiences with conscious sedation
Check for drug allergies
Verify that patient has complied with dietary restrictions, as determined by agency criteria
Review other medications patient is taking and verify absence of contraindications for conscious sedation
Instruct the patient and/or family about effects of sedation
Evaluate the patient's level of consciousness and protective reflexes before conscious sedation
Obtain baseline vital signs
Obtain baseline oxygen saturation and EKG rhythm, as appropriate
Initiate an IV line, as appropriate
Administer medication as per physician's order or protocol, titrating carefully according to patient's response
Monitor the patient's level of consciousness and vital signs, as per agency protocol
Monitor oxygen saturation, as appropriate
Monitor the patient's EKG, as appropriate
Monitor the patient for adverse effects of medication, including agitation, respiratory depression, undue somnolence, hypoxemia, arrhythmias, apnea, or exacerbation of a preexisting condition
Restrain the patient, as appropriate
Ensure availability of and administer benzodiazepine receptor antagonist (flumazenil), as appropriate per physician's order or protocol
Ensure availability of and administer narcotic antagonists, as appropriate per physician's order or protocol
Determine whether the patient meets discharge or unit transfer criteria
Discharge or transfer patient, as per agency protocol
Document actions and patient response, as per agency policy

From McCloskey JC, Bulechek GM: *Nursing intervention classifications*, ed 2, St Louis, 1996, Mosby.

TABLE 8-8 Pharmacologic Reversal Agents for Drugs Used in Sedation

Drug	Dosage	Action	Special Considerations
OPIOID ANTAGONIST			
Naloxone (Narcan)	0.4-2 mg IV, IM, or SQ q 2-3 min	Displaces previously administered analgesics from receptors	Only effective in reversing respiratory depression caused by opiates Patient may relapse into respiratory depression May be administered continuous IV
BENZODIAZEPINE ANTAGONIST			
Flumazenil (Romazicon or Mazicon)	0.2 mg IV over 15 sec; if patient does not reach LOC after 45 sec repeat at 1-min intervals until 1 mg given	Inhibits benzodiazepine on the γ-aminobutyric acid–benzodiazepine receptor complex	Use cautiously in patient at risk for seizures Used to treat respiratory depression caused by diazepam and benzodiazepines Monitor patient for resedation after reversal of benzodiazepine effect

LOC, Loss of consciousness.

BOX 8-7 PATIENT EDUCATION

SEDATION

- Discuss the patient's pathophysiology, including the etiology of stress, anxiety, or agitation, as it applies
- Explain types of sedation and which kind that patient will receive
- Discuss the type of sedative that the patient is taking and its review mechanism of action, side effects, dosage, frequency, and duration
- Discuss non-pharmacologic ways to reduce anxiety and stress

Nursing Management

An understanding of the pathophysiology of anxiety, stress, and agitation helps the critical care nurse to effectively care for the anxious or agitated patient. Sedation tools can help provide a baseline for the effectiveness of pharmacologic and non-pharmacologic agents. Nurses focus on achieving an outcome that is comfortable for the patient, safe, and also cost-effective (Box 8-7).

Nurses can initiate or assist with many non-pharmacologic interventions. Biofeedback, relaxation, hypnosis, and music therapy are examples of activities that can increase serotonin production naturally within the body. This helps to naturally lower pain and anxiety. Music through a pair of light headphones can decrease pain and anxiety in critical care patients. Music can also enhance induction of the relaxation response because it provides a distraction from stress-producing stimuli, which directly affects the limbic system and may stimulate endorphin release.

Relaxation and uninterrupted sleep intervals also decrease the incidence of stress and produce a sedative effect. Deprivation of REM sleep for more than 24 hours is associated with psychologic disturbances, such as depression, illogical thinking, delusions, anxiety, confusion, and decreased pain tolerance. (∞REM Sleep, p. 104)

Even with excellent technique, emergencies arise with the administration of IV sedation. Nurses administering IV sedation medications must be familiar with institutional policies and procedures and the expected standard of care. Expertise in advanced cardiac life support (ACLS) is crucial for caring for the patient who receives IV conscious sedation. The skills acquired from ACLS—which address airway, breathing, and circulation—plus adjunctive therapies—such as intubation and interpretation of dysrhythmias—enable the critical care nurse to anticipate emergency situations, assist in stabilizing patients, and respond quickly when an emergency occurs. (See ACLS Algorithms, Appendix C.)

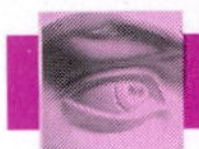

NURSING MANAGEMENT PLAN

ACUTE PAIN

DEFINITION:

The state in which an individual experiences and reports the presence of severe discomfort or an uncomfortable sensation.

Acute Pain Related to Transmission and Perception of Cutaneous, Visceral, Muscular, or Ischemic Impulses

DEFINING CHARACTERISTICS

Subjective

- Patient verbalizes presence of pain
- Patient rates pain on scale of 1 to 10 using a visual analog scale

Objective

- Increase in BP, pulse, and respirations
- Pupillary dilation
- Diaphoresis, pallor
- Skeletal muscle reactions (grimacing, clenching fists, writhing, pacing, guarding or splinting affected part)
- Apprehensive, fearful appearance
- May not exhibit any physiologic change

OUTCOME CRITERIA

NOTE: Outcome is highly variable, depending on individual patient and pain circumstance factors.

- Patient verbalizes that pain is reduced to a tolerable level or is removed.
- Patient's pain rating on scale of 1 to 10 is lower.
- BP, heart rate, and respiratory rate return to baseline 5 minutes after administration of IV narcotic or 20 minutes after administration of intramuscular (IM) narcotic.

NURSING INTERVENTIONS AND *RATIONALE*

1. Continue to monitor the assessment parameters listed under "Defining Characteristics." In addition, monitor postural vital sign changes; determine hydration status and manage fluid volume deficit, if indicated, before administering narcotic analgesic.
2. Modify variables that heighten the patient's experience of pain.
   - Explain to the patient that frequent, detailed, and seemingly repetitive assessments will be conducted ***to allow the nurse to better understand the patient's pain experience, not because the existence of pain is in question.***
   - Explain the factors responsible for pain production in the individual. Estimate the expected duration of the pain if possible.
   - Explain diagnostic and therapeutic procedures to the patient in relation to sensations the patient should expect to feel.
   - Reduce the patient's fear of addiction by explaining the difference between drug tolerance and drug addiction. Drug tolerance is a physiologic phenomenon in which a drug dose begins to lose effectiveness after repeated doses; drug dependence is a psychologic phenomenon in which narcotics are used regularly for emotional, not medical, reasons.
   - Instruct patient to ask for pain medication when pain is beginning and not to wait until it is intolerable.
   - Explain that the physician will be consulted if pain relief is inadequate with the present medication.
   - Instruct patient in the importance of adequate rest, especially when it reduces pain ***to maintain strength and coping abilities and to reduce stress.***
3. Pharmacologic interventions.
   - For postsurgical or posttraumatic cutaneous, muscular, or visceral pain, perform the following:
     a. Medicate with narcotic maximally to break the pain cycles as long as level of consciousness and vital signs are stable: check patient's previous response to similar dosage and narcotic.

     NOTE: First dose received postoperatively is usually reduced by one half ***to evaluate patient's individual response to medication.***

     b. Continuous pain requires continuous analgesia.
        (1) Establish optimal analgesic dose that brings optimal pain relief.
        (2) Offer pain medication at prescribed regular intervals rather than making patient ask for it ***to maintain more steady blood levels.***
        (3) Consider waking patient to avoid loss of opiate blood levels during sleep.

     c. If administering medication on prn basis, give it when patient's pain is just beginning, rather than at its peak. Advise patient to intercept pain, not endure it, or it may take several hours and higher doses of narcotics to relieve pain, leading

Continued

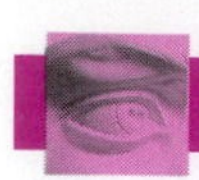

NURSING MANAGEMENT PLAN—CONT'D

ACUTE PAIN

Acute Pain Related to Transmission and Perception of Cutaneous, Visceral, Muscular, or Ischemic Impulses

to a cycle of undermedication and pain alternating with overmedication and drug toxicity.

d. Perform rehabilitation exercises (turn, deep breathe, leg exercises, ambulate) shortly before peak of drug effect ***because this will be the optimal time for the patient to increase activity with the least risk of increasing pain.***

e. When making the transition from one drug to another or from IM or IV to PO medications, the use of an equianalgesic chart is helpful. Equianalgesic means *approximately* the same pain relief. Many consider the IM and IV dose of medications equianalgesic; however, others recommend using one half the IM dose for the IV dose. To effectively use analgesics, each patient requires an individualized choice of drug, dose, time interval, and route. Close monitoring of the patient's response is needed to determine if the right analgesic choice was made.

f. To assess effectiveness of pain medication, do the following:
   (1) Reevaluate pain 5 minutes after IV and 20 minutes after IM medication administration, observe patient's behavior, and ask patient to rate pain on scale of 1 to 10.
   (2) Collaborate with physician to add or delete other medications that potentiate the action of analgesics, such as antiemetics, hypnotics, sedatives, or muscles relaxants.
   (3) Observe for indicators of undertreatment: report of pain not relieved; observed restlessness, sleeplessness, irritability, and anorexia; decreased activity level.
   (4) Observe for indicators of overtreatment: hypotension or bradycardia; respiratory rate <10/min; excessive sedation.

g. If IV patient-controlled analgesia (PCA) is used, perform the following:

(NOTE: Patient-controlled analgesia allows patients to administer small doses of their prescribed medication when they feel the need. Constant levels of the drug in the bloodstream mean lower doses can be used to obtain analgesia. Pain control is improved because the patient is in control and experiences less fear of unrelieved pain. Reduced net narcotic use is noted, as is less sedation. Critical care patients appropriate for patient-controlled analgesia are those who are alert, such as burn patients, trauma patients without head injury, and some postoperative patients.)
   (1) Instruct the patient on what the drug is, the dose, and how often it can be self-administered by pushing the button to activate the PCA machine. For example, "When you have pain, instead of asking the nurse to bring medication, push the button that activates the machine and a small dose of the pain medicine will be injected into your IV line. You can keep your pain under control by administering additional medicine as soon as your pain begins to return or increases. Also, push the button before undertaking a painful activity, such as ambulation. Try to balance your pain relief against sleepiness, and don't activate the machine if you start to feel sleepy. If your pain medicine seems to stop working despite pushing the button several times, call the nurse to check your IV. If you are not receiving adequate pain relief, the nurse will call your doctor."
   (2) Monitor vital signs, especially BP and respiratory rate, every hour for the first 4 hours, and assess postural heart rate and BP before initial ambulation.
   (3) Monitor respirations every 2 hours while patient is on patient-controlled analgesia.
   (4) If patient's respirations decrease to >10/min or if patient is overly sedated, anticipate IV administration to naloxone.

h. If epidural narcotic analgesia is used, do the following:

(NOTE: The delivery of narcotics, such as morphine or fentanyl, by epidural route to specific receptors in the spinal cord selectively blocks pain impulses to the brain for up to 24 hours. Effective analgesia can be obtained without many of the negative side effects or serum narcotic concentrations. Critical care patients appropriate for epidural analgesia include postsurgical and trauma patients.)
   (1) Keep patient's head elevated 30 to 45 degrees after injection ***to prevent respiratory depressant effects.***
   (2) Observe closely for respiratory depression up to 24 hours after injection. Monitor res-

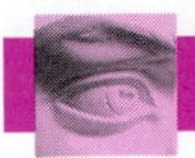

NURSING MANAGEMENT PLAN—CONT'D

ACUTE PAIN

Acute Pain Related to Transmission and Perception of Cutaneous, Visceral, Muscular, or Ischemic Impulses

piratory rate every 15 minutes for 1 hour; every 30 minutes for 7 hours; and every 1 hour for the remaining 16 hours.

(3) Assess for adequate cough reflex.

(4) Avoid use of other CNS depressants, such as sedatives.

(5) Observe for reports of pruritus, nausea, or vomiting.

(6) Anticipate administration of naloxone for respiratory depression (and smaller doses of naloxone for pruritus).

(7) Assess for and treat urinary retention.

(8) Assess epidural catheter site for local infection. Keep catheter taped securely ***to prevent catheter migration.***

- For peripheral vascular ischemic pain (hypothetical vascular occlusion of leg), do the following:
  a. Correctly identify and differentiate ischemic pain from other types of pain.

  NOTE: Ischemic pain is usually a burning, aching pain made worse by exercise and lessened or relieved by rest. Eventually the pain occurs at rest. Coldness and pallor of extremity may be noted, especially if the limb is elevated above the heart level. Rubor and mottling of the skin may be evident from prolonged tissue anoxia and inability of damaged vessels to constrict. Eventually cyanosis and gangrenous tissue will be evident. Chronic ischemia leads to trophic changes in the limb, such as flaking skin, brittle nails, hair, leg ulcers, and collulitis.

  b. Administer pain medications and evaluate their effectiveness as previously described. Remember that the pain of ischemia is chronic and continuous and can make the patient irritable and depressed.

  c. Treat the cause of the ischemic pain, and institute measures to increase circulation to the affected part.

4. Nonpharmacologic interventions.
   - Treat contributing factors; provide explanations (see intervention number 2 at beginning of this care plan).
   - Apply comfort measures.
     a. Use relaxation techniques, such as back rubs, massage, warm baths, music and aroma-therapy. Use blankets and pillows ***to support the painful part and reduce muscle tension.*** Encourage slow, rhythmic breathing.

     b. Encourage progressive muscle relaxation techniques.

     (1) Instruct patient to inhale and tense (tighten) specific muscle groups, then relax the muscles as exhalation occurs.

     (2) Suggest an order for performing the tension-relaxation cycle (e.g., start with facial muscles and move down body, ending with toes).

     c. Encourage guided imagery.

     (1) Ask patient to recall an experienced image that is very pleasurable and relaxing and involves at least two senses.

     (2) Have patient begin with rhythmic breathing and progressive relaxation, then travel mentally to the scene.

     (3) Have the patient slowly experience the scene —how it looks, sounds, smells, feels.

     (4) Ask patient to practice this imagery in private.

     (5) Instruct the patient to end the imagery by counting to three and saying, "Now I'm relaxed." If person does not end the imagery and falls asleep, the purpose of the technique is defeated.

     d. If TENS unit is prescribed by physician, do the following:

     (NOTE: TENS is a battery-operated unit that serves as a nerve stimulator. It produces mild, tingling sensations as it blocks incisional pain messages to the brain. It is sometimes used as part of the pain relief program for the postsurgical patient.)

     (1) Take the TENS unit, patient pamphlet, and teaching electrodes to the patient before surgery to explain the process.

     (2) Apply electrodes to skin, and instruct patient in proper use of unit. Let patient experience how the TENS unit should feel when activated. Refer to manufacturer's directions for proper application and operation of TENS unit.

     (3) Electrodes are usually placed by the physician on the skin alongside the operative incision at the close of the surgical procedure in the operating room. The unit is usually used for 3 to 5 days as an adjunct to medications.

Continued

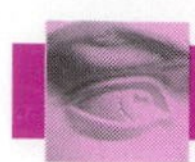

NURSING MANAGEMENT PLAN—CONT'D

ACUTE PAIN

Acute Pain Related to Transmission and Perception of Cutaneous, Visceral, Muscular, or Ischemic Impulses

(4) When the patient is awake and alert, readjust the amplitude or output of the TENS unit to the patient's comfort as necessary. Keep the TENS unit on continuously unless ordered otherwise. Occasionally, percutaneous epidural nerve stimulation is used when more than one nerve root is involved in producing pain. Again, patients are able to control their pain by adjusting the rate and frequency of a millivoltage electrical current stimulator affixed externally.

e. Assist with biofeedback, which represents a wide range of behavioral techniques that provide the patient with information about changes in body functions of which the person is usually unaware. For example, information used to reduce muscle contraction is obtained by an electromyogram recorded from body surface electrodes. Changes in blood flow are produced by monitoring skin temperature changes. The person using biofeedback tries to change the display of information in the desired direction by actions such as reducing muscle tension, by reducing or altering blood flow to a particular area. The critical care nurse should be familiar with the theoretic concepts of biofeedback and should support the patient in maximizing pain control through whatever techniques are successful for that patient.

REFERENCES

1. Caillet R: *Pain: mechanisms and management,* Philadelphia, 1993, FA Davis.
2. Puntillo K: Physiology of pain and its consequences in critically ill patients. In Puntillo K, editor: *Pain in the critically ill: assessment and management,* Gaithersburg, Md, 1991, Aspen.
3. McCaffery M, Beebe A: *Pain: clinical manual for nursing practice,* St Louis, 1989, Mosby.
4. Carson M, Barton D, Morrison C: Managing pain during mediastinal chest tube removal, *Heart Lung* 23(6):500-505, 1994.
5. Simpson T, Lee E, Cameron C: Patients' perceptions of environmental factors that disturb sleep after cardiac surgery, *Am J Crit Care* 5(2):173-181, 1996.
6. Jacox A and others: *Acute pain management: operative or medical procedures and trauma. Clinical practice guidelines, Publication 92-0032,* Rockville, Md, 1992, Agency for Health Care Policy and Research, US Department of Health and Human Services.
7. Lindquist R, Banasik J, Barnsteiner J: Determining AACN's research priorities for the 90s, *Am J Crit Care* 2:110-117, 1993.
8. American Nurses Association: Position statement: promotion of comfort and relief in the dying patient, 1992, Washington, DC, The Association.
9. Sun X, Weissman C: The use of analgesics and sedatives in the critically ill patient: physicians order versus medication administered, *Heart Lung* 23(2):169-176, 1994.
10. Alpen M, Titler M: Pain management in the critically ill: what do we know and how can we improve? *AACN Clin Issues Crit Care Nurs,* 5(2):159-168, 1994.
11. Maxam-Moore V, Wilkie D, Woods S: Analgesics for cardiac surgery patients in critical care: describing current practice, *Am J Crit Care* 3(1):31-39, 1994.
12. Willens J: Introduction to pain management. In Salerno E, Willens J, editors: *Pain management handbook: an interdisciplinary approach,* St Louis, 1996, Mosby.
13. Guyton A: *Textbook of medical physiology,* ed 8, Philadelphia, 1991, WB Saunders.
14. Barker E: *Neuroscience nursing,* St Louis, 1994, Mosby.
15. Jurf J, Nirschl A: Acute postoperative pain review and update, *Crit Care Nurs Q* 16(1):8-25, 1993.
16. McGuire D: Comprehensive and multidimensional assessment and measurement of pain, *J Pain Symptom Manage* 7(5):312-317, 1992.
17. Villaire M: An interview with Kathleen Puntillo. Pain: assessment, treatment and the coming thunder, *Crit Care Nurs* 12:159-168, 1995.
18. Voight L, Paice J, Pouilot J: Standardized pain flowsheet: impact on patient reported experiences after cardiovascular surgery, *Am J Crit Care* 4(4):308-312, 1995.
19. Halloran T, Pohlman A: Managing sedation in the critically ill patient, *Crit Care Nurs* suppl 1-16, 1995.
20. Bozeman M: Cultural aspects of pain management. In Salerno E, Willens J, editors: *Pain management handbook: an interdisciplinary approach,* St Louis, 1996, Mosby.
21. Douglas M: Cultural diversity in response to pain. In Puntillo K, editor: *Pain in the critically ill: assessment and management,* Gaithersburg, Md, 1991, Aspen.
22. Ulmer J: Identifying and preventing pain mismanagement. In Salerno E, Willens J, editors: *Pain management handbook: An interdisciplinary approach,* St Louis, 1996, Mosby.

23. Faucett J: Care of the critically ill patient. In Puntillo K, editor: *Pain in the critically ill: assessment and management,* Gaithersburg, Md, 1991, Aspen.
24. Puntillo K: Dimensions of procedural pain and its analgesic management in critically ill surgical patients, *Am J Crit Care* 3(2):116-122, 1994.
25. Gujol M: A survey of pain assessment and management practices among critical care nurses, *Am J Crit Care* 3(2):123-128, 1994.
26. Henknleman W: Inadequate pain management: ethical considerations, *Nurs Managem* 25(1):48a-48d, 1994.
27. Salerno E: Pharmacologic approaches to pain. In Salerno E, Willens J, editors: *Pain management handbook: An interdisciplinary approach,* St Louis, 1996, Mosby.
28. Watt-Watson J: Misbeliefs about pain. In Watt-Watson J, Donovan M, editors: *Pain management: nursing perspective,* St Louis, 1992, Mosby.
29. Spross J, Singer M: Patients with cancer. In Watt-Watson J, Donovan M, editors: *Pain management: nursing perspective,* St Louis, 1992, Mosby.
30. Dyble K: Epidural and intrathecal methods of analgesia in the critically ill. In Puntillo K, editor: *Pain in the critically ill: assessment and management,* Gaithersburg, Md, 1991, Aspen.
31. Paice J: Pharmacologic management. In Watt-Watson J, Donovan M, editors: *Pain management: nursing perspective,* St Louis, 1992, Mosby.
32. Wild L: Intravenous methods of analgesia for pain in the critically ill. In Puntillo K, editor: *Pain in the critically ill: assessment and management,* Gaithersburg, Md, 1991, Aspen.
33. Mather I, Denson D: Pharmacokinetics of systemic opioids for the management of pain. In Sinatra R and others, editors: *Acute pain:* mechanisms and management, St Louis, 1992, Mosby.
34. American Society of Hospital Pharmacists: *American hospital formulary service drug information '95,* Bethesda, Md, 1995, The Association.
35. McKenry L, Salerno E, editors: *Mosby's pharmacology in nursing,* ed 19, St Louis, 1995, Mosby.
36. Collins P, Spunt A, Huml M: Symptom management. In Salerno E, Willens J, editors: *Pain management handbook: an interdisciplinary approach,* St Louis, 1996, Mosby.
37. Kaiser K: Assessment and management of pain in the critically ill trauma patient, *Crit Care Nurs Q* 15(2):14-34, 1992.
38. McCaffery M, Ferrell B: Opioid analgesics: nurses' knowledge of doses and psychological dependence, *J Nurs Staff Dev* 8:72-84, 1994.
39. Herr K, Mobily P: Interventions related to pain, *Nurs Clinics North Am* 27(2):347-369, 1992.
40. Courts N: Non-pharmacologic approaches to pain. In Salerno E, Willens J, editors: *Pain management handbook: an interdisciplinary approach,* St Louis, 1996, Mosby.
41. Edgar L, Smith-Hanrahan C: Non-pharmacologic pain management. In Watt-Watson J, Donovan M, editors: *Pain management: nursing perspective,* St Louis, 1992, Mosby.
42. Meehan D and others: Analgesic administration, pain intensity, and patient satisfaction in cardiac surgical patients, *Am J Crit Care* 4(6):435-442, 1995.
43. Vitello J: Management of sedation: the nursing perspective, *Crit Care Nurse,* supplement 1-6, August 1996.
44. Carroll K, Magruder CC: The role of analgesics and sedatives in the management of pain and agitation during weaning from mechanical ventilation, *Crit Care Nurs Q* 15(4):68-77, 1993.
45. Miller B, Keane C: Encyclopedia and dictionary of medicine, nursing and allied health, ed 3, Philadelphia, 1983, WB Saunders.
46. Crippen D: Understanding the neurohumoral causes of anxiety in the ICU, *J Crit Illness* 10(8):550-560, 1995.
47. Shapiro B and others: Practice parameters for intravenous analgesia and sedation for adult patients in the intensive care unit: an executive summary, *Society of Critical Care Medicine* 23(9):1596-1600, 1995.
48. Crippen D: The role of sedation in the ICU patient with pain and agitation: pain management in the ICU, *Crit Care Clin* 5(2):369-390, 1990.
49. Bizek K: Optimizing sedation in critically ill mechanically ventilated patients, *Crit Care Nurs Clin North Am* 7(2):315-349, 1995.
50. Jensen D, Justic M: An algorithm to distinguish the need for sedative, anxiolytic, and analgesic agents, *DCCN,* 14(2):58-65, 1995.
51. Berger I, Waldhorn R: Analgesia, sedation and paralysis in the intensive care unit, *Am Fam Physician* 51(1):166-172, 1995.

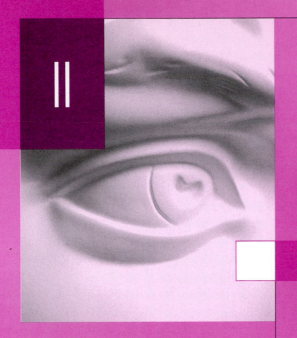

SPECIAL POPULATIONS

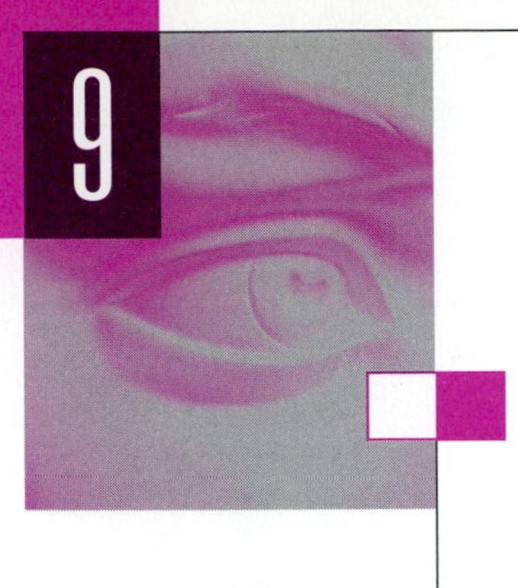

The Pediatric Patient in the Adult Critical Care Unit

As THE NUMBER of patients in managed care programs increases and the number of general hospital admissions decreases, more hospitals are admitting critically ill children to their adult critical care units. This chapter covers some of the developmental and physiologic differences between adults and children older than 1 month, along with some of the medical conditions that may result in an admission to an adult critical care unit and are assessed or treated differently from those experienced by adults. It must be emphasized that critically ill children must always be observed closely. During periods of stress, children are able to maintain physiologic stability for a period, but then they can decompensate quickly. Children are not "small adults." Many of the laboratory values, medications, blood product dosages and methods of administration, and other therapeutic modalities differ from those used with adults.[1-3]

Most children admitted to critical care units are younger than 5 years and therefore are less able to understand their circumstances and less able to verbalize their needs. Parents are the major sources of comfort for their children. They may also recognize subtle changes in their child's condition because they know their child better than anyone. Because of this, parental concerns must be addressed, and parents need to be present at the bedside as much as possible.

Even though some critically ill children can be managed in adult critical care units, there are certain situations in which children need the services of various pediatric subspecialties and/or pediatric intensivists and must be transferred to tertiary care pediatric critical care units. Some examples are children requiring high frequency ventilation, extracorporeal membrane oxygenation (ECMO), cardiac surgery, and treatment for some neurologic conditions requiring intracranial pressure (ICP) monitoring. In addition, transfer is considered for children who do not respond to treatment.

RESPIRATORY SYSTEM

Anatomy and Physiology

Upper airway. The upper airway of the infant and child is different from that of the adult. The epiglottis of the newborn is located at the level of cervical spine 1 and the older infant's is located at C3, as opposed to an adult's, which is located at C4 to C5. The infant's epiglottis is large and floppy, and because of its high placement, it can press against the pharyngeal soft palate on inspiration. The infant's tongue is also large, relative to head size, and fills the oral cavity. Because of this anatomy, the infant is generally an obligate nose breather until between 4 to 6 months of age, after which the larynx descends with growth.[4] Oral breathing is a very complex process for an infant, and it never occurs alone. Oronasal breathing is possible, but only up to 30% to 40% of ventilation can be provided orally. During sleep oranasal breathing can occur spontaneously and last for about 20 seconds. It can also occur when there is nasal obstruction, increased work of breathing, airway resistance, or crying.[5]

The larynx of the infant and young child, unlike that of the adult, is funnel-shaped, with the narrowest portion at the cricoid ring.[4] It also is pliable because of less developed cartilage, making it easier to collapse on inspiration or expiration. With changes in intrathoracic pressure, collapse can occur even with crying.[6] By 8 to 10 years of age the larynx has grown cylindrical; has assumed the narrowest portion at the glottic opening; and has increased in length, width, and internal diameter. By 12 years of age the diameter has grown to 1.8 cm.[3]

The submucosal layer of the larynx is also more loose in the infant and young child so that fluid can more easily accumulate in that space.[7] With the airway's "relatively" rigid confines, any accumulation of fluid encroaches into the airway space. Along with a shorter and narrower airway, any decrease in airway radius leads to a greater exponential increase in air-flow resistance, which increases the work of breathing.[8] Turbulent air flow, such as occurs with crying, doubles the already increased air-flow resistance.[8] Figure 9-1 illustrates the changes in airway diameter and air-flow resistance with obstruction from edema in an adult and in an infant. The soft palate and hypopharynx of the infant can narrow on inspiration during sleep, causing drops in oxygen saturation into the 80% or greater range.[9]

The infant or child with an abnormally small jaw and low-set ears must be considered as having a potentially difficult airway to manage and must have a consult with anesthesiology if airway management is required. Congenital malformations of the airway occur in utero at the same time these types of facial malformations occur.[4]

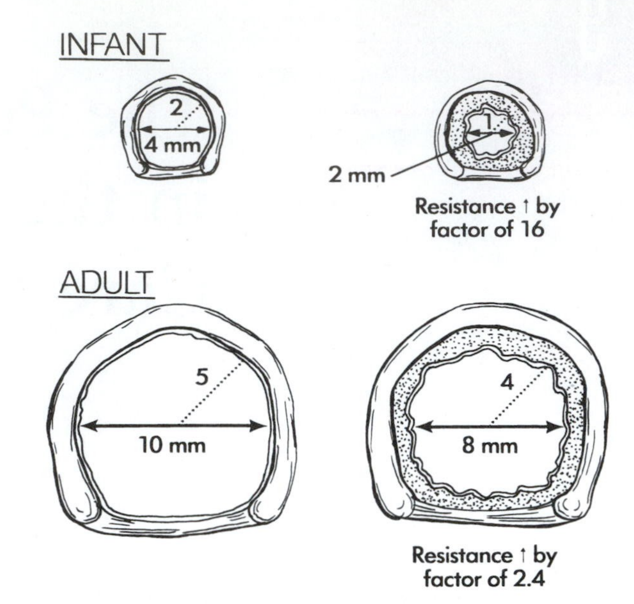

FIGURE 9-1 Effects of edema on airway resistance. Proportional increases in air-flow resistance with 1 mm of circumferential edema in the infant versus the adult. (From Zander J, Hazinski MF: Pulmonary disorders. In Hazinski MF, editor: *Nursing care of the critically ill child,* ed 2, St Louis, 1992, Mosby.)

Lower airway. Growth of distal airways lags behind growth of the proximal airways in the first 5 years of life.[10] The number and size of alveoli grow from 20 million alveolar sacs with a 2.8 m^2 surface area at birth to 300 million sacs with a 32 m^2 surface area by 8 years of age, compared with an adult's surface area of 75 m^2.[11] Alveolar collapse is more likely in the infant and young child because of the smaller alveolar size. Interalveolar pores appear between birth and 2 years,[12] and alveolar-bronchiole pores appear by 6 years.[13] The infant and young child are at greater risk for ventilation-perfusion mismatch and atelectasis without this collateral ventilation.

The infant's oxygen diffusing capacity across the alveolar-capillary membrane is only one third to one half the capacity of an adult's, even when controlling for surface area.[14] The infant and child have a higher metabolic rate than the adult; therefore oxygen consumption/kg is higher—6-8 ml/kg/minute versus the adult's 3-4 ml/kg/minute.[15] Hypoxemia, therefore, develops more rapidly in the context of respiratory compromise for the child than for the adult.[3]

Chest mechanics. The infant and young child's respiratory mechanics are very different from the older child's or adult's.[3,16] In the infant and young child the chest wall is more compliant because the bones are smaller and more cartilaginous. The ribs are more horizontally placed, providing less of a bellowing action on inspiration. Accessory muscles are less developed, so the external intercostals do not contribute to pulling the ribs up on inspiration. The diaphragm is more horizontal in the chest and tends to pull the lower ribs inward on inspiration. Because of these mechanics, the infant and toddler are almost totally dependent on diaphragm contraction for lung expansion. Anything that impedes diaphragmatic contractions can result in respiratory compromise. With any decrease in lung compliance, as with lung disease, diaphragmatic contractions, which cause decreased intrathoracic pressure, will produce intercostal and substernal retractions.[17,18] The greater the chest wall retractions, the more the diaphragm has to contract to offset the changes in intrathoracic pressure and be able to generate an adequate tidal volume.

The intercostal muscle tone in the infant is decreased during active rapid eye movement (REM) and quiet sleep. In the normal infant, apnea can occur as an indirect result of paradoxic chest movement (diaphragm contractions pushing the abdomen out with the chest wall sinking in). This produces decreased lung volumes, leading to hypoxemia. Increased diaphragmatic activity compensates for this paradoxic action but eventually fatigues, resulting in periods of apnea.[19] As with upper airway narrowing, oxygen saturation can periodically drop into the 80% or greater range during sleep. (∞Apnea, p. 214.)

Assessment and Oxygen Devices

The infant or child usually experiences respiratory failure more often than primary cardiac failure. Un-

TABLE 9-1 Significant Findings in the Infant or Child at Risk for Respiratory Failure

Assessment Area	Physical Findings	Discussion Points
Respiratory rate	• Infant: >60/min • Child: >40/min • Slow or irregular	Tachypnea usually first sign of distress in an infant; fatigue is a common contributing factor in respiratory failure
Mechanics	• Retractions (intercostal, supraclavicular, substernal) • Paradoxical movements (chest in and abdomen out)	
	• Grunting	Closing of the glottis to create "auto-PEEP" to keep alveoli open at end-expiration
	• Stridor	Sign of upper airway obstruction
	• Wheezing	Sign of lower airway obstruction
Air entry	• Changes in pitch, rather than volume of breath sounds	Chest expansion can sometimes be barely perceptible in a normal spontaneously breathing infant; the small, thin chest wall causes breath sounds from any area of the lungs to be easily referred throughout the chest, even over fluid or atelectasis; listen for bilateral breath sounds high in the axillae, because these are the two most separated points
Color/temperature	• Central coolness, pallor, or cyanosis	Peripheral changes may be normal in the infant or child
Heart rate	• <5 years: <60 or >180 bpm • 5-10 years: <60 or >160 bpm • >10 years: <50 or >140 bpm	The infant and child have limited ability to increase stroke volume, therefore with hypoxemia the heart rate increases to improve cardiac output; if bradycardia occurs with cardiorespiratory distress, arrest may be imminent
Neurologic	• Infant: hypotonia	Sign of hypoxia for infants
	• Child: irritability • Decreased level of consciousness	An early sign of hypoxia, often manifested as a decreased responsiveness to parents or to pain

PEEP, Positive end-expiratory pressure.

like the older adult who may have underlying cardiovascular disease, the infant and child tend to demonstrate bradycardia and apnea in cardiopulmonary failure and not ventricular dysrythmias.[3,20] For the infant or child who is conscious and needs supplemental oxygen, the device of comfort must be selected.[3] Minimizing anxiety and fear in the child is paramount to decrease the work of breathing. Table 9-1 outlines the assessment areas for the infant or child at risk for respiratory failure.[3]

Airway positioning. Knowledge of childhood anatomy is necessary in establishing a patent airway. The infant or toddler younger than 2 years, because of the large occiput, needs to have a small roll or towel placed under the upper shoulders with the jaw slightly extended into a "sniffing" position.[3] This displaces the tongue and lines up the posterior pharynx and tracheal opening for a clear airway. For the infant younger than 6 months, correct head positioning still may not prevent the large tongue from falling back into the posterior phaynx.[21] Oral airways must not be used unless the infant is unconscious, because the airway tip can stimulate laryngospasm as a result of the higher placement of the larynx.[22] Try side-lying placement, with the neck in a neutral position.[3] The older child needs to have a folded towel placed under the head, with the neck in an extended position to maintain a patent airway.[8] Figure 9-2 illustrates proper head positioning in the infant and child. The conscious child must be allowed to assume a position of choice for airway maintenance.

Supplemental oxygen devices. Many of the oxygen devices used with adults are also used with children. Some additions include oxygen hoods, for infants up to 1 year of age, which are clear plastic boxes that envelop the head and allow full vision of the head and access to the body; oxygen tents, which are used less often; and oxygen "blow-by," which uses oxygen tubing or a

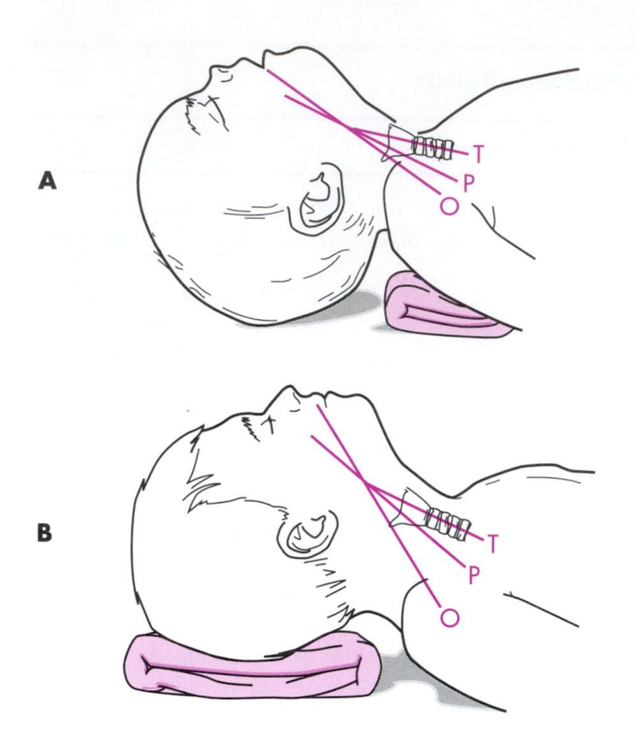

FIGURE 9-2 Correct airway positioning for ventilation of **A,** an infant and **B,** a child. Better air flow is provided with a straight alignment of the oropharynx *(O)*, pharynx *(P)*, and trachea *(T)*.

hose to blow oxygen toward the child's face without touching him or her. Oxygen masks can aggravate and upset the child and often are repeatedly pushed off.[23] In contrast, the child or parent can hold the blow-by tubing him or herself, ensuring greater compliance and resulting in oxygen saturations higher than those from oxygen masks.

An adult sized–self inflating resuscitation bag can be carefully used on an infant, providing only the force needed to cause appropriate chest expansion.[3] An appropriately sized bag minimizes the potential for overinflating the lungs. Bag sizes, along with other supplemental oxygen devices and oxygen administration, are outlined in Table 9-2. There must be no leaf-flap outlet valves when a self-inflating bag is used to assist spontaneous ventilation in an infant, because the infant is unable to generate enough negative inspiratory pressure to open the valve.[3] Bags equipped with spring-loaded positive end-expiratory pressure (PEEP) valves to provide constant positive airway pressure (CPAP) must not be used with the spontaneously breathing child for the same reason previously discussed.[3] Anesthesia ventilation bags have no flow valves that require opening on inspiration and therefore can be used to provide supplemental oxygen, PEEP, or CPAP to the spontaneously breathing infant or child.[3] Pressure manometers can be attached to the ventilation bags to measure peak inspiratory pressure. Ventilatory masks are measured in the child as in the adult—from the bridge of the nose to before the end of the chin.

Endotracheal Intubation

Procedure. Endotracheal tube (ETT) placement and management differs in the infant and young child than in the adult. Preoxygenation is especially important for the infant, who has higher resting oxygen demands.[29] The infant also has a smaller lung volume, allowing for smaller oxygen reserves. Intubation attempts, therefore, need to be shorter in duration (less than 30 seconds) with the infant than with the older child or adult.[3] Box 9-1 provides formulas for ETT measurements in the child. For the child younger than 2 years, there is no formula. Endotracheal tube size is matched to the infant's age (Table 9-3).[1-4,33]

When placed, the tip of the ETT should be 1 to 2 cm above the carina, about level with T2.[29] This level, confirmed on a chest radiograph, is just below where the clavicles connect to the spine, or at the third rib. Table 9-3 outlines approximate sizes for various intubation equipment for infants and children. After placement, bilateral breath sounds need to be assessed high in the axillae and over the abdomen in the infant.[3,4] The easy transmission of sounds in the chest of the child can be mistaken for breath sounds if there is accidental esophageal intubation.

ETT dislodgement can occur very easily in the infant or young child. The tip of the ETT is pulled upward with neck extension or when the head is turned completely to the side. Conversely, the ETT moves downward with neck flexion.[34] With the already shortened trachea of the young child, a more highly or lowly placed ETT can become dislodged or intubate the bronchus.

ETT obstruction can also occur with high placement, neck flexion, or head rotation, which can cause the bevel of the ETT to become pressed against the tracheal wall, occluding the lumen.[35] Secretions and mucous plugs may more easily occlude the lumen of a small diameter ETT.

Securing endotracheal/nasotracheal tubes. With the small infant or child there is less facial area for tape adherence for securing the tubes. A method with a low incidence of accidental extubation[36] uses two pieces of cloth tape, split halfway down the middle, creating a the shape of a *Y.* Figure 9-3 illustrates this technique.

TABLE 9-2 Supplemental Oxygen Devices and Oxygen Administration in Infants and Children

Device	Administration	Discussion Points
Nasal cannula	• Young infant[24,25] 0.5 L/min = 28% O_2 1.0 L/min = 32% O_2 2.0 L/min = 35% O_2 • Child Same as adult settings*	Minute volume, inspiratory/expiratory times, and amount of mouth breathing affects infant FiO_2 via a nasal cannula differently than for an adult given the same gas flow and O_2 percent.[24,26,27] Titrating O_2 can occur with as low as 0.125-0.25 L/min.
Oxygen hood[3]	• 10-15 L/min = nearly 100% O_2	Use with infants <1 year old
Oxygen blow-by	• 10-15 L/min = nearly 100% O_2	Better tolerated than oxygen masks Allow child or parent to hold tubing
Self-inflating resuscitation bag[28]	• Infant <3 months old: 1/4 L bag 3 months-4 years old: 1/2 L bag • Child 5-10 years old: 1 L bag >10 years old: 1.5 L bag	Do not use bags with leaf-flap outlet valves or with spring-loaded PEEP valves[3]
Anesthesia bag[29,3]	• Spontaneously breathing Flow rate 3 times minute ventilation • Nonspontaneously breathing <10 kg: 2 L/min flow rate 10-15 kg: 3.5-4 L/min flow rate >50 kg: 6 L/min flow rate	
PIP[30]	• ≤20-30 cm H_2O	
Ventilatory mask size[2]	• <6 months old: 0 • 6 months-3 years old: 1 • 3-6 years old: 2 • >6 years old: 3	Fit and placement on face same as for adult

*See Table 23-1, p. 690, for adult settings.
PIP, Peak inspiratory pressure.

BOX 9-1 Endotracheal Tube Measurements

ETT SIZE

- Formula >2 years old: **(age in years + 16) ÷ 4**
- Infant/toddler sizes based on age
- For any age: can compare circumference of child's little finger with external diameter size of ETT
- Cuffed tube: external diameter one half size smaller than appropriately sized uncuffed tube

ETT DEPTH OF INSERTION

- Formula (from teeth to midtrachea): **internal diameter ETT × 3**

ETT CUFF PRESSURE

- Allow for a barely sealed air leak

The skin of the child is more fragile than that of an adult's. Cloth tape can be irritating. Duoderm can be applied to the cheeks, with the securing tape attached on top of the Duoderm, or a zinc-oxide based "pink tape" can be used.

Mechanical ventilation. There are numerous types of unconventional mechanical ventilation used in the infant or child, such as inverse I:E ratio, high-frequency flow interruption, high-frequency positive pressure, high-frequency jet, high-frequency oscillation, and airway pressure release.[37] For most infants and children, standard means of positive pressure ventilatory support, using volume- or pressure-controlled ventilators, are used.[30,37]

The type of ventilation chosen depends on the child's size, minute ventilation requirements, and lung

TABLE 9-3 Approximate Sizes of Intubation Equipment and Tracheotomy Tubes for Infants and Children

Age Weight	3 mo 6 kg	6 mo 8 kg	1 yr 10 kg	3 yr 15 kg	6 yr 20 kg	8 yr 25 kg	12 yr 40 kg	16 yr 60 kg
ETT size (mm)*	3.0-3.5	3.5-4.0	4.0-4.5	4.5-5.0	5.0-5.5	6.0 c/u	7.0 c	7.0-8.0 c
Blade‡	0-1 s	0-1 s	1 s	2 s	2 s	2 s/c	3 s/c	3 s/c
Stylet F	6	6	6	6	14	14	14	14
Suction catheter F (fr)‡‡	6-8	8	8	8-10	10	10-12	12-14	12-14
Shiley Tracheotomy								
Shiley size (mm)	0	1	1-2	4	4	4	6	6
Internal diameter (mm ID)	3.4	3.7	3.7-4.1	5	5	5	7	7
Length (cm)	4	4.1	4.1-4.2	4.6	4.6	4.6	6.7	6.7

*Cuffed/uncuffed (c/u)
‡Straight or curved (s/c)
‡‡Catheter size twice the internal diameter size of any tracheal tube

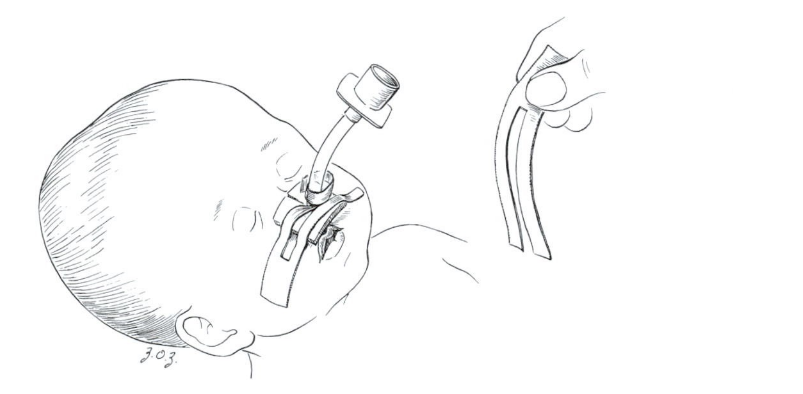
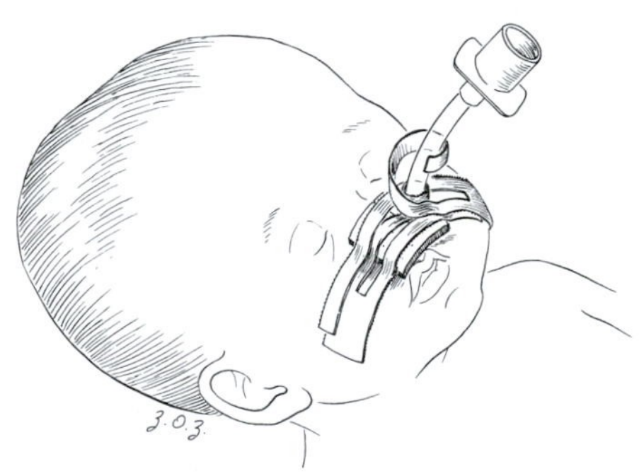

FIGURE 9-3. Securing of endotracheal tube with split taping. (Modified with permission from Zander J and Hazinski MF: Pulmonary disorders. In Hazinski MF, editor: *Nursing care of the critically ill child,* ed 2, St Louis, 1992, Mosby.)

compliance. There are several positive pressure ventilators available for the infant or small child, and adult ventilators can be made functional for the older child.[37,38] A continuous flow–time limited ventilator, in intermittent mandatory ventilation (IMV) mode, is commonly used with an infant or toddler. Continuous flow offsets the infant's inability to generate enough negative pressure to open an inspiratory demand valve.[37] The maximal size limit for using this ventilator is 15 kg because of the small flow limits that the machine provides.[37]

For the older child, noncontinuous flow–volume limited ventilation, in synchronized intermittent mandatory ventilation (SIMV) mode, is most often used.[30,37] Pressure support ventilation is also used in the child as the sole ventilatory mode if respiratory mechanics and work of breathing are stable[30] or to assist with spontaneous breathing, especially during the weaning process.[30,37] Table 9-4 outlines ventilator settings for initiating positive pressure ventilation for the infant and child.[37]

Ventilator-patient asynchrony can arise from several causes.[37,39] The Hering-Breuer reflex is a vagal reflex in which the child's sensing of positive lung inflation sets off immediate expiration, and lung deflation stimulates inspiration. Apnea, or active expiration during the ventilator's inspiratory cycle, also can cause asynchrony. The use of adult ventilators not appropriately adapted for the infant or child can cause asynchrony.[40] Since the small child decreases tidal volume and increases respiratory rate to deal with compromise, adult ventilators may not sense rapidly enough,

TABLE 9-4 Initiating Positive Pressure Ventilation in the Infant or Child

Parameter	Setting	Discussion Points
Rate of FiO_2	Age based to maintain PaO_2 >70 mm Hg	
Tidal volume	10-15 ml/kg	Includes compressibility of ventilator circuit tubing and dead space
I:E	Age specific, usually 1:2	Increase expiratory time with obstructive disease
Inspiratory time	0.4-0.5 seconds	
PEEP or CPAP	Starts at 3 cm H_2O and increases by 2-3 cm increments	Maintain PaO_2 >70 mm Hg with nontoxic O_2 levels (.40-.50) without causing circulatory depression; PEEP >15 cm warrants a pulmonary artery catheter to measure circulatory status; volutrauma must be addressed with pneumothorax suspicions

if at all, these spontaneous respiratory efforts, which then lead to increased work of breathing.[41,42] Asynchrony can lead to poor oxygenation or volutrauma.[39] Significant asynchrony may require sedation or sedation with neuromuscular blockade.

Criteria for weaning and extubation are much more extensive for the adult than for the child, but there are some guidelines. IMV or pressure support ventilation (PSV) is used to wean from positive pressure ventilation. PSV allows the child to have greater control over breathing, and asynchrony is not a problem.[37] It also decreases work of breathing[43,44] and diaphragmatic muscle fatigue,[45] both of which are a particular concern in the infant. Table 9-5 outlines guidelines for weaning and extubation.[37,46] Supplemental oxygen must be supplied after extubation via nasal cannula, ventilation mask, or oxygen hood at 5% to 10% more than what the child was receiving endotracheally.[46] Nasal or facial CPAP can also be given, but if the child fights this, it is best to remove it to minimize oxygen demands and prevent post-extubation complications.

Extubation complications. A post-extubation croup can occur in the small child, usually from 1 to 4 years of age.[47] The etiology is possibly from mechanical trauma[48] and from the absence of an air leak at 30 cm H_2O pressure from around the ETT.[49] Manifestations arising from airway edema include hoarseness, stridor, or a crowing cough that begins immediately or up to 3 hours post-extubation, peaking at 8 hours and resolving by 24 hours. Hoarseness can last for 72 hours.[47] Initial treatment consists of keeping the child calm. Procedures must be withheld if possible and crying averted to avoid increasing airway resistance. Hold supplemental humidified oxygen at the child's mouth immediately after extubation, and continue to provide cool mist.[47] More severe symptoms can be treated with racemic epinephrine and/or intravenous or inhaled steroid therapy.[47] Intubation equipment and intubation-qualified personnel need to be available for 4 hours after extubation.

Tracheotomies

Several types of tracheotomy tubes are available for the child, with the plastic, single cannula type the most popular for in-hospital care because of few complications.[33,53] Silastic tubes have been recommended for the infant and child because they are pliable and bend with tracheal movement. Uncuffed tubes are generally used for the infant and small child, allowing for a larger airway lumen.[29,33] A snug fit is necessary with a tube size of 0.5 mm larger than an appropriately sized ETT, because placement is below the cricoid ring.[29] Cuffed tubes can be used with the older child.[29] See Table 9-3 for tracheotomy tube sizes for the infant and child.

If accidental decannulation occurs in a new tracheotomy, pulling on the stay sutures in most instances allows for tube replacement. In the child who has had a long-term tracheostomy, usually for tracheal stenosis, reinserting a tracheal tube after accidental decannulation can be very difficult. Tracheomalacia with cricoid cartilage collapse can develop, resulting in upper airway obstruction once the tube is no longer in place.[54,55] In some cases, an airway can only be reestablished surgically. In others, a size-smaller ETT can be inserted into the stoma, or the child may have to be orally/nasally intubated.

TABLE 9-5 Guidelines for Discontinuing Positive Pressure Ventilation in the Infant or Child

Ventilatory Mode	Ventilatory Parameter	Discussion Points
Weaning		
Non-PSV	• Rate: decrease by 2-5 breaths/min (may be 1 breath/min in chronic conditions) Infant: down to minimum of 4 breaths/min Child: possibly down to spontaneous breathing with CPAP trials • PEEP/CPAP: decrease by 2-3 cm H_2O infant: down to 2-3 cm H_2O child: down to <5 cm H_2O • FiO_2: decrease by 5%-10%, to <.40-.50	Rapidity of each change can be variable, from hourly to every couple of weeks; for infants, rates must not go less than 4 breaths/min just before extubation, since ETT creates airway resistance, and the work of breathing may be increased too much with total spontaneous breathing[50,51] To maintain PaO_2 >70 mm Hg or SaO_2 >93%
PSV	• With SIMV: decrease rate first, down to CPAP • Pressure: to achieve tidal volume of 10-15 ml/kg, then decrease to 5 cm H_2O	See previous guidelines for rate and pressure changes
Extubation		
	• Vital capacity: Infant/toddler: >15 ml/kg when crying[52] Older child: >10-15 ml/kg • Negative inspiratory pressure: Infant/toddler: >45 cm H_2O when crying[52] Older child: >20-30 cm H_2O • Minute ventilation doubled • PaO_2 >60-70 mm Hg at an FiO_2 >0.4 • $PaCO_2$ 35-45 mm Hg	Positive gag/cough reflex Can tolerate own secretions

Bronchiolitis and Respiratory Syncytial Virus

Pathophysiology. Bronchiolitis is an acute inflammatory disease of the lower small airways, leading to obstruction.[56] It occurs in children younger than 2 years, most often in infants younger than 1 year, and is most severe in infants younger than 6 months.[56] Many different viruses can cause bronchiolitis, but *respiratory syncytial virus (RSV)* is the major cause.[56]

RSV occurs primarily from late fall to early spring.[57] It is highly contagious and spread by direct close contact through droplets.[57] The virus is shed for 3 to 8 days, but in young infants can occur for up to 4 weeks.[57] The virus can exist on environmental surfaces for many hours and on the hands for at least 1 half hour, resulting in high nosocomial spread by hospital staff.[57] Passive smoking has also been connected with RSV onset.[58] Reinfections occur frequently but are generally milder after infancy. Adults can also be infected, but they experience mild upper respiratory symptoms.[59]

RSV has an overall low mortality rate, but infants with congenital heart disease have a mortality rate of 37%.[60] Those with cystic fibrosis, bronchopulmonary dysplasia, or who are immunocompromised are also at greater risk for more serious disease and for occurrence beyond 1 year of age.[60] The chance of recovery from RSV can be excellent, but reactive airway disease is common for several years after infection. Up to 50% of infants who are infected with RSV develop asthma later in life.[61,62]

RSV typically involves inflammation of respiratory epithelium, leading to necrosis. The epithelium is replaced with nonciliated tissue. Submucosal edema forms with lymphocytic infiltrates and other alveolar debris. Obstruction occurs from mucous secretions and debris not being cleared because of the lack of ciliated epithelium. Epithelial basal layers regenerate after 3 to 4 days, and cilia regenerate after 15 days.[63]

Pathological pulmonary dynamics[63,64] usually involve lung hyperinflation almost two times normal. Obstruction occurs in a patchy distribution with complete obstruction, leading to atelectasis and partial obstruction, which results in hyperinflation. There are inspiratory and expiratory resistance, along with ventilation/perfusion mismatch, which lead to hypoxemia. Minute ventilation is usually increased significantly so that a normal $PaCO_2$ can be maintained. Respiratory failure ensues with a rising $PaCO_2$ (greater than 65 mm Hg), not because of obstruction, but because of fatigue.[65] Work of breathing can increase up to sixfold.[66] Apnea can develop, and this also results from a lack of respiratory effort.[67] The infant with RSV is usually hypervolemic because of increased antidiuretic hormone (ADH) and increased renin levels, causing hyperaldosteronism.[68]

Clinical assessment. The first symptoms to appear are those of an upper respiratory tract infection—sneezing and rhinorrhea. In many cases a family member has had a respiratory illness. After 2 to 3 days respiratory distress ensues, with increased respirations, coughing, nasal flaring, chest retractions, wheezing, irritability, and possible feeding difficulties.[63,64] Fever and lung rhonchi may or may not occur.[64] There is a linear relationship between increasing respirations and decreasing PaO_2,[69] and the infant usually is hypoxemic. The $PaCO_2$ remains normal until respirations reach 50-60/minute, and then it rapidly increases with tachypnea.[69] Oxygen saturation levels are the best predictor of severity of illness.[65,70] If respiratory failure ensues, it usually lasts 48-72 hours,[65] but impaired oxygenation can last several weeks, despite the apparent clinical recovery of the infant.[70] Once bronchiolar obstruction is evident, the illness is at its peak.[64] Improvement is gradual, and by 2 weeks the infant usually has recovered.[64]

Treatment. The overall treatment goal in RSV is supportive. Because of the highly contagious nature of RSV, place the infant in contact isolation, and other infants with RSV, as well as staff caring for them, must be cohorted together to prevent nosocomial spread of the infection.[57]

Oxygen continues to be the primary therapy[63,71] to decrease work of breathing and oxygen demands. Depending on the severity of illness, the infant can receive supplemental humidified oxygen via mask, tent, nasal CPAP (despite lung hyperinflation), or mechanical ventilation.[63,72] Inhaled $beta_2$ agonists may be tried because of the expiratory resistance, but the beneficial effects can be variable.[73,74] Unlike with asthma, corticosteroids show no improvement in lung function, acutely or later in the disease.[74,75]

Euvolemia must be maintained through careful use of diuretics and fluid restriction,[63] because pulmonary edema can occur from greater negative intrapulmonary pressures[76] or from fluid leaks with epithelial necrosis.[77]

Administration of an antiviral agent, ribavirin, is controversial.[60,78] It possibly has greater effect in the mechanically ventilated infant.[79] It is a broad-spectrum, aerosolized agent that traditionally has been administered for 12 to 20 hours/day for several days.[60] Newer protocols call for the administration of ribavirin over a 6-hour period.[80] When given to the mechanically ventilated infant, ribavirin crystallizes in ventilator and endotracheal tubes, necessitating meticulous attention to frequent ventilator tubing changes and ETT assessments for obstruction.[81,82]

In addition, the teratogenicity of ribavirin in humans has been questioned, although no effects have been reported in humans after 7 years of usage.[60] The drug can be absorbed through the respiratory tract from the environment, as it is released from respirator equipment, or from the infant's secretions.[60] The infant needs to be in contact isolation only because of the RSV, not because of the exposure to ribavirin. Standard surgical masks, gloves, or gowns provide no protection from the ribavirin. Caution must still be exercised, and pregnant staff must not provide care. Since ribavirin causes crystallization of particles, contact lenses can be damaged; however, close-fitting goggles can be worn. All staff and visitors need to be warned of the possible hazards of ribavirin.[60] The infant can be placed with other infants receiving ribavirin, and placement must be in a well-ventilated room with at least six air changes/hour.[60]

Status Asthmaticus

Pathophysiology. Asthma is a state of diffuse reversible air-flow obstruction that results from inflammation and edema, bronchoconstriction, and increased mucus secretion.[83] Status asthmaticus is moderate to severe air-flow obstruction that is refractory to intensive treatment with bronchodilators.[83] The majority of children with asthma experience its onset within the first 2 years of life; it can occur as young as a few weeks old.[83] Various nonspecific stimuli, such as allergens, pollutants, exercise, emotions, or infections, can set off a complex cascade of hyperreactivity in the airways.[63,83] In infants younger than 6 months, viral infections are the primary etiology.[83]

Clinical findings in status asthmaticus demonstrate[63,83,84] lung hyperinflation and air trapping, increased minute ventilation and ventilation/perfusion mismatch with hypoxemia and hypercapnia, metabolic and respiratory acidosis, right and left ventricular strain from increased pulmonary vasular resistance, and increased cardiac workload to maintain an elevated cardiac output in the face of increased afterload.

Sudden death can occur with status asthmaticus, resulting mostly from severe asphyxia and undertreatment.[85] A previous episode of respiratory failure in the child with asthma puts him or her at higher risk than other children with asthma for another life-threatening event.[83] Other risk factors for a life-threatening event include wide fluctuations in peak expiratory flow rate (PEFR), an increase less than or equal to 10% in PEFR or forced expiratory volume over 1 second (FEV_1) over emergency room measurement, a PEFR or FEV_1 of less than or equal to 25% of predicted value for age, a $Paco_2$ greater than or equal to 40 mm Hg, and an age of 1 year or younger.[83]

Clinical assessment. Assessing severe asthma in the infant versus the older child is different because of the anatomical and physiologic differences between them.[83] Physiologic changes can progress rapidly to respiratory failure in the infant. A peak flow meter used to measure PEFR or a spirometer for FEV_1 are the most objective measures of the degree of air-flow obstruction.[83] The methods require a child's full cooperation and generally are only used after 5 years of age.[83] Table 9-6 outlines guidelines for assessing severe asthma in infants and children.[83,84]

Treatment. Intensive care management of the child with status asthmaticus involves humidified oxygen to maintain an oxygen saturation of more than 95%, continuously nebulized selective $beta_2$ agonists, intravenous (IV) methylprednisolone, IV aminophylline, and possibly IV terbutaline.[83] If $Paco_2$ is more than 55 mm Hg or increasing greater than 5 to 10 mm Hg/hour, if pulsus paradoxus is greater than 30 mm Hg, or if acidosis or continual hypoxemia occurs, mechanical ventilation must be considered.[83] Chest percussion and vibration are contraindicated in status asthmaticus,[86] and are not useful for the patient recovering from severe asthma.[83,87,88]

Euvolemia is the goal,[83] since excessive hydration can cause fluid accumulation in bronchio-interstitial spaces secondary to the increased negative intrathoracic pressures.[76] Elevated ADH levels can also occur in status asthmaticus.[89]

Minimizing the child's anxiety is crucial. Sedating medications must be used very cautiously in the nonintubated child.[83] Environmental measures to promote comfort, decrease noxious stimuli, and enhance personal security (e.g., presence of parents) need to be used. (See the discussion of the child's experience of critical illness section on psychosocial issues of the child and family later in this chapter.

Apnea

Pathophysiology. Apnea most often occurs in the preterm infant and is a function of immaturity,[92] but it can occur in older infants as well. *Pathological apnea* in the full-term infant is defined as ineffective or absent respirations for more than 16 seconds, with or without hypotonia, cyanosis, or bradycardia.[93] This is to be differentiated from periodic or disorganized breathing. These conditions have shorter periods of apnea, interspersed with rapid or irregular breathing.[93] Some periodic breathing can be normal at any age.[94] Three types of apnea exist—central, obstructive, and mixed.[95] Central apnea involves failure of the respiratory centers in the brain to stimulate ventilation. Obstructive apnea involves a blocked airway; however, respiratory efforts can still be made, but they do not generate adequate gas exchange. Mixed apnea has both central and obstructive components and accounts for about 50% of cases.[96]

Aside from congenital etiologies, apnea may be a symptom of many reversible disorders.[97] Central apnea can occur with sepsis, electrolyte disorders, hypoglycemia, and hypothermia; cardiorespiratory disease involving hypoxemia or respiratory muscle fatigue; or CNS infections, seizures, hydrocephalus, or conditions related to increased intracranial pressure. Gastroesophageal reflux can also be a cause.[98]

Obstructive apnea can occur with tonsil and adenoid hypertrophy, abnormally large tongues, abnormally small mandibles, and vascular rings; after surgical correction for cleft palate; and with other forms of airway obstruction.[99]

Apnea may appear as an apparent life-threatening event (ALTE), which used to be referred to as near-miss SIDS. ALTE is defined as an event, that to the observer, was frightening coupled with an assumption that death would have occurred without intensive intervention. For instance, the child displayed some combination of apnea, color change,

TABLE 9-6 Guidelines for Assessing Severe Asthma in Infants and Children

Assessment Area	Physical Findings: Infant	Physical Findings: Child	Discussion Points
Respiratory rate	• Increase of >50% above normal	• Can range from normal to >95 percentile for age	Sleeping rates in infants and resting rates in children are good measures of obstruction; there is too much variability in awake or activity rates
Level of consciousness	• Decreased	• May be decreased	Assess response to parents and pain
Accessory muscle use	• Retractions in less-than-severe states	• Severe intercostal, tracheosternal, and sternocleidomastoid retractions and nasal flaring	In infants, compliant chest wall produces retractions earlier in course In children, retractions and flaring correlate well with degree of obstruction and with PEFR of <50% of predicted for age
Color	• Pallor, grayness, or cyanosis	• Possible cyanosis	
Dyspnea		• Can only speak single words or short phrases; cannot count to 10 in one breath	
Quality of cry	• Softer and shorter as FEV_1 decreases		
O_2 saturation	• <90% in less-than-severe states	• <90% on room air	Infants have greater ventilation/perfusion mismatch. In children, hypoxemia correlates well with degree of obstruction[90,91]
Breath sounds	• Wheezing, then becoming inaudible because of decreased air movement	• Same as in infant	Presence and volume of wheezing is the least-sensitive predictor of obstruction
$Paco_2$	• If >50 mm Hg or if rising 5-10 mm Hg/hr, consider mechanical ventilation	• Can range from <40 mm Hg with respiratory distress to >40 mm Hg as air movement significantly decreases	$Paco_2$ is best measure of ventilation in infants. A continually rising $Paco_2$ of >40 mm Hg in a child occurs when PEFR is <20% of predicted for age[91]
PEFR		• <50% of predicted for age or personal best	Best objective measure of obstruction; used in children >5 years of age; requires cooperation
Feeding/sucking ability	• Decreased or absent		

marked change in muscle tone, and/or choking or gagging.[100]

Monitoring. An episode of secondary central apnea can result from hospital procedures such as on suctioning or stimulating the larynx, passage of an NG tube, after lung hyperinflation, or with feedings.[93,96] Obstructive apnea can be brought on with neck flexion, pressure beneath the chin or on the lower rim of an applied face mask, or with supine positioning.[93,96]

Appropriate monitoring of the child experiencing apnea includes placement of an apnea monitor and alarms set at 16 to 20 seconds. Chest leads for separate apnea monitors are placed two fingerbreadths below the nipples at the midaxillary line.[101] A ventilation bag and a mask need to be at the bedside. Because ineffective respiratory efforts may be sensed as normal respirations, cardiac and/or pulse oximetry monitoring needs to be in place.

Treatment. Episodes of apnea must first be treated with gentle shaking of the infant or tapping the bottoms of the infant's feet while observing for return of effective respirations.[93,96] Slight extension of the neck to reopen the airway can be attempted. If recovery does not occur, manual ventilation with bag and mask at the infant's normal respiratory rate for age needs to be performed at the FiO_2 level the infant was previously receiving until normal respiratory pattern and heart rate return.[93,96] For frequent episodes (more than 2 to 3/hr) or for those that require prolonged manual ventilation, other treatments include[93,96] prone positioning, rocker beds, recurrent cutaneous stimulation, nasal CPAP (for mixed or obstructive apneas only), or a switch to continuous gavage feedings. Surgery may be necessary for obstructive apnea,[99] or CNS respiratory stimulants may be used when no other correctable cause of apnea exists.[96] Ultimately, mechanical ventilation may be needed.[93,96]

If there is no correctable cause, home monitoring may be necessary until the infant matures. This usually lasts until the infant has gone 2 to 3 months without apneic episodes requiring intervention.[100]

CARDIOVASCULAR SYSTEM

Anatomy and Physiology

The differences in cardiovascular function between children and adults are related to early physical development and the presence or absence of congenital cardiac disease. Congenital heart defects (CHDs) occur during the embryologic development of the heart, whereas acquired defects occur after birth. Some cases of CHDs are caused by single gene or chromosomal abnormalities and others are the result of exposure to teratogens such as the rubella virus, but in most cases the cause is unknown.[102] The heart develops from the third to eighth week of gestation, so development is complete before the woman may definitely know that she is pregnant.

Fetal circulation is designed to meet prenatal needs yet permit the modifications at birth that support the postnatal circulation.[102] Before the child is born, the lungs are essentially nonfunctional, the liver is partially functional, and the brain requires the highest oxygen concentration.[103] The structures that support fetal circulation and bypass the lungs and liver are the foramen ovale, ductus arteriosus, ductus venosus, the umbilical arteries, and the umbilical vein (Figure 9-4). After the child is born the lungs and liver begin normal function, so the structures of fetal circulation are no longer needed. The foramen ovale closes and the ductus arteriosus, ductus venosus, and the umbilical vessels become ligaments (Figure 9-5).

During fetal life, the patency of the ductus arteriosus is controlled by the low oxygen content and exogenous prostaglandins.[102] Thus postnatally, hypoxia maintains patency of the ductus arteriosus. Before repair of some congenital defects, it is essential that the ductus arteriosus remain open, so that the newborn receives a pulmonary vasculature vasodilator, such as prostaglandin E_1 (PGE_1) continuous IV drip. At birth, pulmonary resistance is high, but quickly falls to adult levels in the first few weeks of life. In newborns hypoxia, acidosis, and hypothermia may result in pulmonary vasoconstriction. This can lead to right-to-left (pulmonary-to-systemic) shunting of blood through the ductus arteriosus and foramen ovale. Treatment includes oxygenation, mechanical ventilation with hyperventilation to produce alkalosis, sedation, and keeping the newborn warm.

Assessment

Assessment of the cardiovascular (CV) system in the child includes the health history and physical assessment. As the pediatric data base is completed for the child with cardiac disease, the parents may report any of the following: poor feeding with fatigue noted during feeding, weight loss or inability to gain weight, respiratory problems such as dyspnea or tachypnea, frequent respiratory infections, cyanosis, and fatigue during play. Heart rate and blood pressure (BP) should be within normal range for age (Tables 9-7 and 9-8). Ascultate the heart for extra heart sounds and murmurs. (∞Cardiac Auscultation, p 365.)

Physiologic splitting of the second heart sound (S_2) is usually more pronounced in the pediatric patient. Sinus dysrhythmia is normal in the child, particularly during rest or sleep. To monitor perfusion, pedal pulses and capillary refill are evaluated hourly. Urine output must be at least 1 ml/kg/hr.

Hemodynamic Monitoring

Hemodynamic monitoring may be indicated in the critically ill pediatric patient. Issues in monitoring are related to the smaller size of the pediatric patient; fluid overload and blood loss are concerns. To accurately monitor intake, all fluid used for intravascular hemodynamic monitoring lines must be given by volume infusion pumps. Heparinized fluid is given in each line at 1 ml/hour in infants and 1 to 2 ml/hr in children.[1] A heparin concentration of 1 U/ml is sufficient to maintain catheter patency.[1] A two-syringe setup is used for drawing blood from arterial and central venous

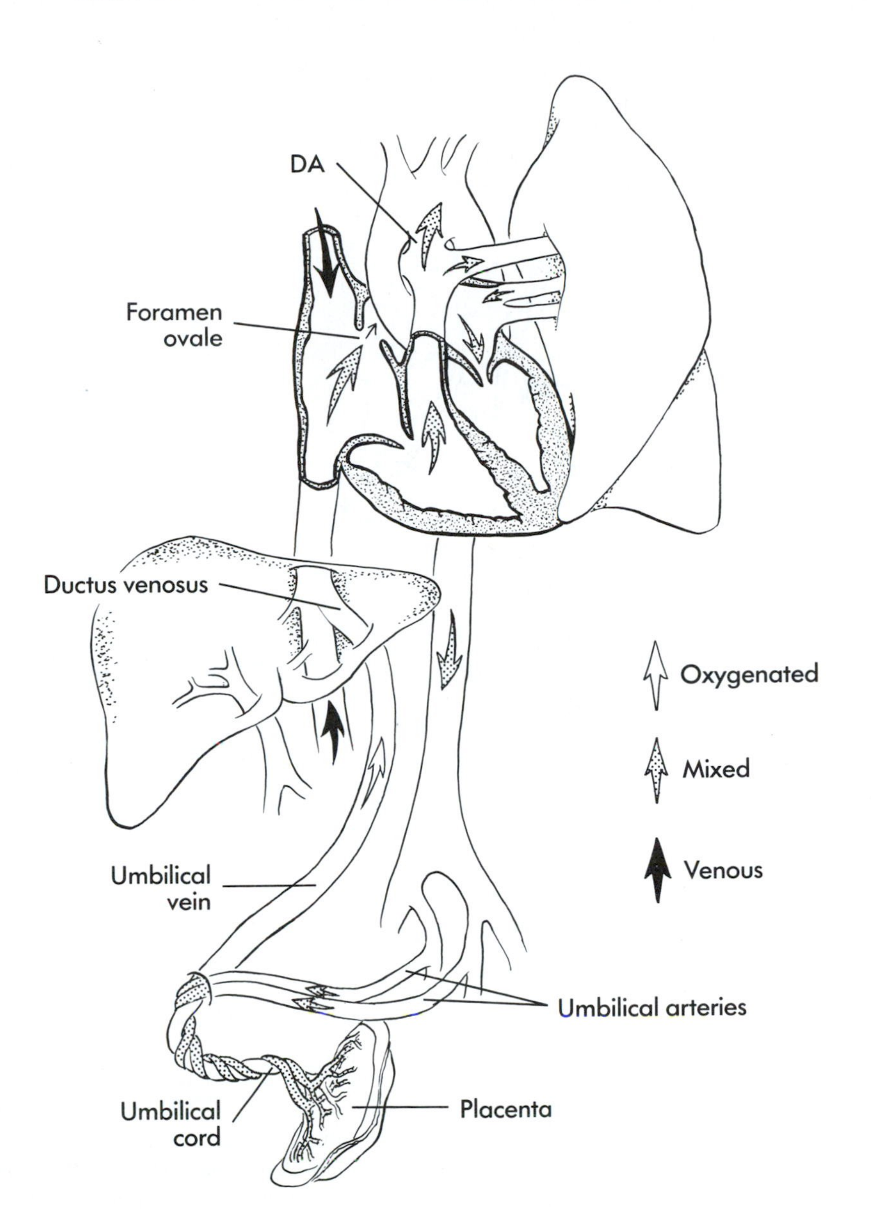

FIGURE 9-4. Fetal circulation. Fetal blood is oxygenated in the placenta (which is a less efficient oxygenator than the lungs). The oxygenated blood enters the fetus through the *umbilical vein* and enters the *ductus venosus,* bypassing the hepatic circulation and flowing into the inferior vena cava. When this blood reaches the right atrium, it is diverted by the *crista dividens* toward the atrial septum, and flows through the *foramen ovale* into the left atrium. The blood then passes through the left ventricle and ascending aorta to perfuse the head and upper extremities. This pathway allows the best-oxygenated blood from the placenta to perfuse the fetal brain. Venous blood from the head and upper extremities returns to the fetal heart through the superior vena cava, enters the right atrium and ventricle, and flows into the pulmonary artery. Since pulmonary vascular resistance is high, this blood is diverted through the *ductus arteriosus* (DA) into the descending aorta. Ultimately, much of this blood will return to the placenta through the *umbilical arteries.* (From Hazinski MF: *Nursing care of the critically ill child,* ed 2, St Louis, 1992, Mosby.)

pressure (CVP) lines (Figure 9-6). Before blood is drawn, the second syringe is filled with 2 ml of flush solution and blood is aspirated from the patient past the first syringe. The blood specimen is obtained from the first syringe and the line gently flushed with the second syringe (this process returns the aspirated blood to the patient). The port of the first syringe is flushed and recapped. Only small volumes of blood are drawn for laboratory tests. Each medical facility that cares for pediatric patients has policies for how much blood to draw for each test. All flush volumes are recorded as intake and an accurate record is kept

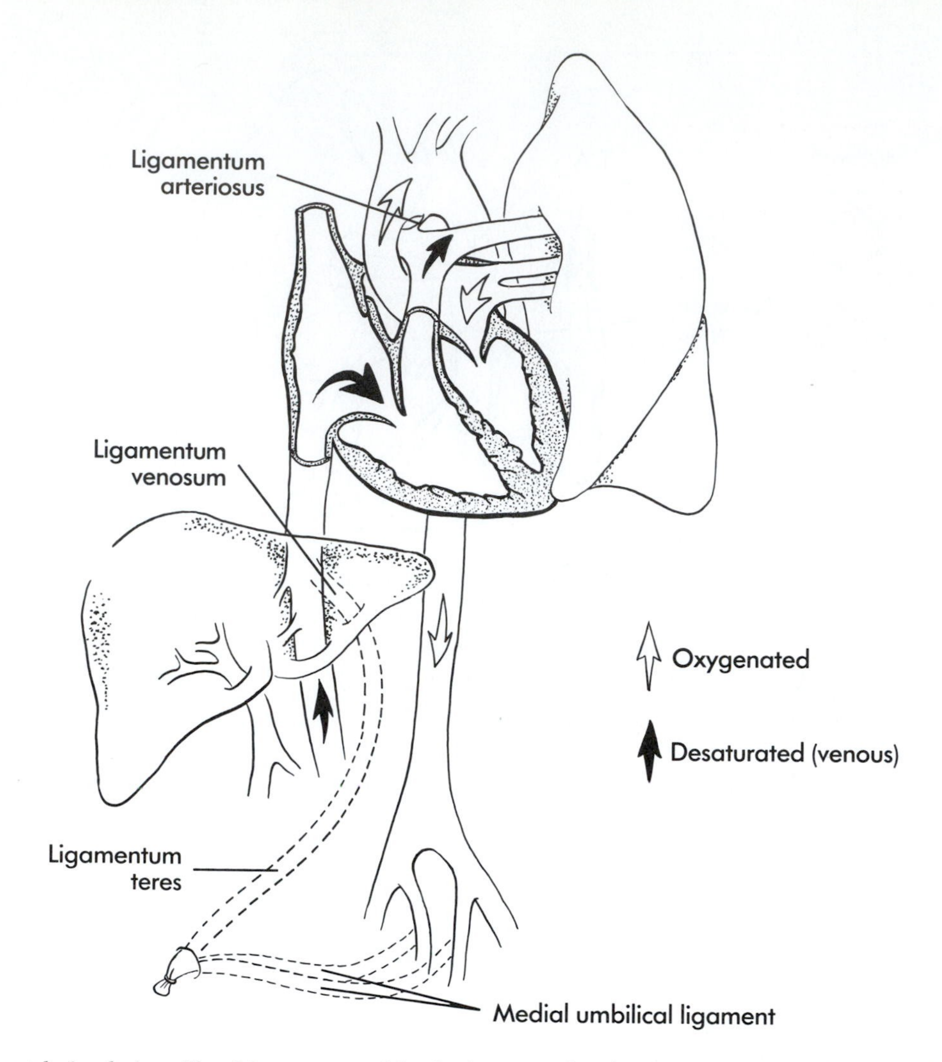

FIGURE 9-5. Postnatal circulation. Blood is oxygenated in the lungs, and pulmonary vascular resistance is low. Systemic venous (desaturated) blood returns to the heart through the superior and inferior vena cavae. This blood then flows through the right atrium and right ventricle, into the pulmonary artery, and ultimately into the pulmonary circulation. Oxygenated blood from the lungs returns to the left atrium through the pulmonary veins. This blood passes into the left ventricle and flows into the aorta and systemic arteries to perfuse the body. (From Hazinski MF: *Nursing care of the critically ill child,* ed 2, St Louis, 1992, Mosby.)

TABLE 9-7 Normal Heart Rates in Children

Age	Awake Heart Rate (Per Min)	Sleeping Heart Rate (Per Min)
Neonate	100-180	80-160
Infant (6 mo)	100-160	75-160
Toddler	80-110	60-90
Preschooler	70-110	60-90
School-age child	65-110	60-90
Adolescent	60-90	50-90

From Hazinski MF: *Nursing care of the critically ill child,* ed 2, St Louis, 1992, Mosby.

of the amount of blood lost, and periodically the child receives replacement. See Table 9-9 for pediatric blood volumes.

When continuously monitoring the blood pressure in the child, the arterial reading is considered more accurate than the cuff pressure.[1] Korotkoff's sounds are more difficult to hear when the BP is low. A size 4 or 5 French pulmonary artery catheter is used for the child. The child's vessel must be large enough to accept the 4 French catheter to initiate pulmonary artery monitoring. Since the smaller catheters have smaller balloons, refer to the catheter for balloon volume. To limit fluid intake, smaller volumes (usually 3

TABLE 9-8 Normal Blood Pressures in Children*

Age	Systolic Pressure (mm Hg)	Diastolic Pressure (mm Hg)
Birth (12 hr, <1000 g)	39-59	16-36
Birth (12 hours, 3 kg weight)	50-70	25-45
Neonate (96 hr)	60-90	20-60
Infant (6 mo)	87-105	53-66
Toddler (2 yr)	95-105	53-66
School age (7 yr)	97-112	57-71
Adolescent (15 yr)	112-128	66-80

*Blood pressure ranges taken from the following sources: **Neonate:** Versmold H and others: Aortic blood pressure during the first 12 hours of life in infants with birth weight 610-4220 gms, *Pediatrics* 67:107, 1981. 10th-90th percentile ranges used. **Others:** Horan MJ, chairman: Task Force on Blood Pressure Control in Children, report of the Second Task Force on Blood Pressure in Children, *Pediatrics* 79:1, 1987. 50th-90th percentile ranges indicated.
From Hazinski MF: *Nursing care of the critically ill child,* ed 2, St Louis, 1992, Mosby.

or 5 ml) of injectant are used for cardiac output studies. See Table 9-10 for cardiac output and stroke volume values. Left atrial, CVP, and pulmonary artery pressures in the child are comparable with adult values. (∞Hemodynamic Pressures, Table 15-14, p 447.)

Hemodynamic parameters are related to the body surface area of the child. The normal cardiac index for children is 3.5 to 5.5 $l/min/m^2$,[1] which is higher than that of adults. The right ventricular stroke work index of 5 to 7 g/m^2 is slightly less than the adult value.[1] When evaluating hemodynamic parameters, always relate the numbers to the clinical condition of the child. If the numbers do not correlate, revaluate calibration and zeroing of the monitoring equipment.

Congenital Heart Defects

Each year 0.8% of infants born are diagnosed with congenital heart defects.[104] Some CHDs can be diagnosed by ultrasound before birth, and some parents decide to deliver these babies at a tertiary center affiliated with a pediatric cardiac surgery program. Other newborns with cardiac anomalies are diagnosed after birth and transferred to tertiary care centers for further evaluation and often immediate surgery. Certain defects are totally repaired in the first few days of life, whereas other defects are repaired in stages. Infants with CHD may develop complications after discharge after a surgical procedure or while waiting for surgery and may be admitted to an adult critical care unit.

In the past, congenital heart defects were classified as cyanotic or acyanotic defects. In reality, though, children with acyanotic defects may develop cyanosis. Distinguishing the anomalies by hemodynamic pathophysiology is a more accurate method of classification. There are four defining pathophysiologic characteristics: (1) increased pulmonary blood flow, (2) decreased pulmonary blood flow, (3) mixed blood flow, and (4) obstruction of flow of blood out of the heart.[103,105] (Figure 9-7). At birth, pulmonary vascular resistance is high but decreases after the first few weeks of life. If a left-to-right (systemic-to-pulmonary) shunt is present, pulmonary blood flow increases and the child may develop congestive heart failure (CHF). Decreased pulmonary flow occurs when there is obstruction of blood flow from the right side of the heart to the pulmonary circulation or in the presence of a right-to-left (pulmonary-to-systemic) shunt. Children with CHDs are cyanotic. Mixed blood flow results from the mixing of oxygenated and deoxygenated blood. Obstruction of blood flow to the ventricles occurs with stenotic semilunar valves or a narrowed aorta. When caring for a child with surgical repair of cardiac defects, the nurse must know the actual circulation of blood, (e.g., has a palliative procedure been done, has total correction been done, or will this patient require additional stages of repair in the future). Complications of CHD include CHF, hypoxemia, dysrhythmias, endocarditis, shock, and cardiac arrest. Any of these complications may result in the admission of the child to the critical care unit.

Heart Failure

Heart failure (HF) may occur in children with CHD, after surgical repair of congenital defects, and in severe anemia.[106,107] Classifications and pathophysiology of HF are similar to that of the adult patient. Symptoms of HF are related to the pathophysiologic processes of left and right ventricular failure and high and low output failure (Chapter 16). (∞HF Description, p 502.)

Children usually exhibit manifestations of both right- and left-sided failure, rather than one or the other.[1] When infants exhibit HF, manifestations are specific to this age group.[103] The infant exhibits a change in responsiveness and may be lethargic or irritable. Respiratory distress is present with dyspnea; tachypnea; intercostal, substernal, sternal, supraclavicular, or substernal retractions; nasal flaring; or grunting.[103] Grunting occurs during expiration when the

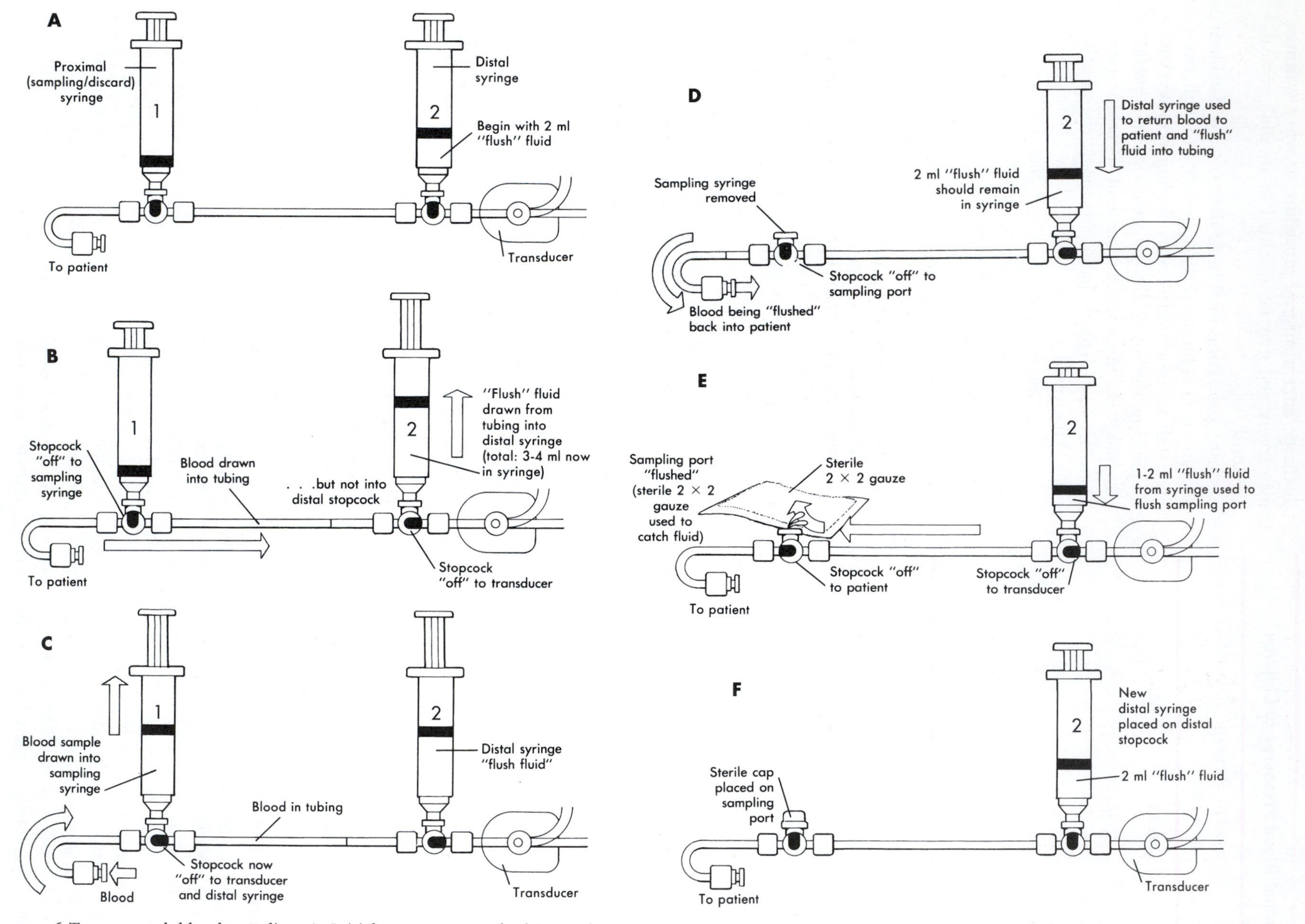

FIGURE 9-6 Two-stopcock blood sampling. **A,** Initial arrangement of tubing and syringes. Begin with exactly 2 ml of irrigation fluid in syringe 2 (near transducer). **B,** Turn syringe 2 stopcock "off" to the transducer and "open" to the catheter, and aspirate until patient blood is drawn into the tubing but *not* into syringe 2 or the stopcock. **C,** Turn stopcock 1 "off" to the transducer and syringe 2, and draw blood sample into syringe 1 (after discarding initial 0.1 ml). **D,** Turn stopcock 1 "off" to the sampling port and "open" between syringe 2 and the patient. Flush irrigation fluid from syringe 2 into tubing and patient, until blood is cleared from the tubing. Exactly 2 ml of irrigation fluid should remain in syringe 2. **E,** Turn stopcock 1 "off" to the catheter and "open" between the sampling port and transducer, and use the remaining fluid from syringe 2 to clear blood from the sampling port. **F,** Turn stopcock 1 "off" to the sampling port and cap it. Turn stopcock 2 "off" to the syringe port and refill irrigation syringe (with 2 ml fluid). Waveform should be visible on monitor. (From Hazinski MF: *Nursing care of the critically ill child,* ed 2, St Louis, 1992, Mosby.)

TABLE 9-9 Calculation of Circulating Blood Volume in Children

Age of the Child	Blood Volume (ml/kg)
Neonates	85-90
Infants	75-80
Children	70-75
Adults	65-70

From Hazinski, MF: *Nursing care of the critically ill child,* ed 2, St Louis, 1992, Mosby.

TABLE 9-10 Normal Pediatric Cardiac Output and Stroke Volume

Age	Cardiac Output (L/min)	Heart Rate	Normal Stroke Volume
Newborn	0.8-1.0	145	5 ml
6 mo	1.0-1.3	120	10 ml
1 yr	1.3-1.5	115	13 ml
2 yr	1.5-2.0	115	18 ml
4 yr	2.3-2.75	105	27 ml
5 yr	2.5-3.0	95	31 ml
8 yr	3.4-3.6	83	42 ml
10 yr	3.8-4.0	75	50 ml
15 yr	6.0	70	85 ml

From Hazinski MF: *Nursing care of the critically ill child,* ed 2, St Louis, 1992, Mosby.

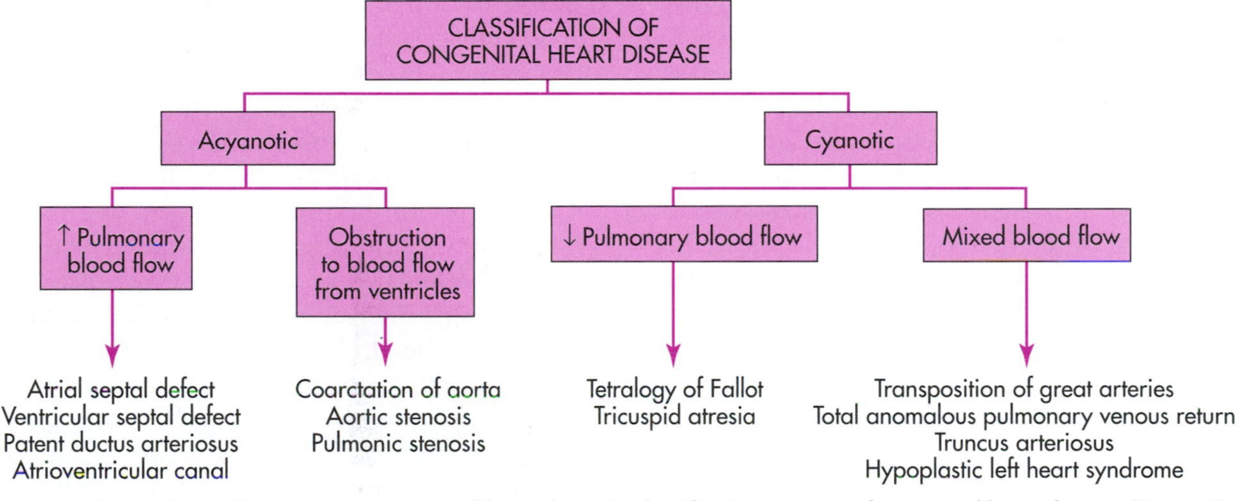

FIGURE 9-7 Comparison of acyanotic-cyanotic and hemodynamic classification systems of congenital heart disease. (From Wong D: *Whaley and Wong's nursing care of infants and children,* ed 5, St Louis, 1995, Mosby.)

infant breathes against a closed glottis to maintain positive end-expiratory pressure. Crackles usually are not ascultated in the infant.[1] During abdominal assessment, the liver may be palpated and is usually full and low in the infant with HF. With decreased cardiac output and perfusion, the infant's extremities are cool, pedal pulses are weak, capillary refill is slow, skin is mottled, and blood pressure is decreased. The infant is easily fatigued, feeds poorly, and may become dehydrated. Infants usually do not have fluid or sodium restrictions.

Digoxin is the inotropic drug of choice for HF.[106] The dosage is ordered in micrograms and is double-checked for accuracy. When the child is receiving digoxin, observe for signs of digitalis toxicity, and periodically monitor the child's digoxin level. Cardiac dysrhythmias may indicate toxicity. Bradycardia is most common, but any dysrhythmia may be noted.[1,106] Inotropic agents, vasodilators, and/or diuretics may be ordered. Serum potassium levels are closely monitored with diuretic therapy.

Hypoxemia

Cyanosis is present in children with certain congenital heart defects. Cyanosis is visible when there are 5 g of reduced hemoglobin per 100 ml of blood[1,108] and the arterial oxygen saturation is at or less than 75% to 85%.[1] Hypoxemia may be caused by respiratory or cardiac disease. Cyanosis that decreases with crying is thought to be respiratory in origin, whereas cyanosis that increases with crying is usually cardiac in origin.[1] Some children with CHD manifest hypercyanotic spells. This is most common in children with tetralogy of Fallot, and these episodes are often called "Tet spells." During these episodes, the child becomes very cyanotic, hypoxic, and tachypneic and may lose consciousness or develop seizures.[108] These spells are dangerous because the child may develop severe hypoxemia and possible cerebral hypoxia; cerebral vascular accidents or death may occur during these episodes.[108] Treatment of hypercyanotic spells includes soothing the child while placing the child in a knee-chest position and administering oxygen and physician-ordered morphine and fluid boluses. This child may need intubation, mechanical ventilation, and treatment of metabolic acidosis.

Dysrhythmias

Electrophysiology and electrocardiography principles are similar in the adult and pediatric patient. See Chapters 13 and 15. Differences include a faster heart rate in children and the variances in the PR and QT intervals related to the rapid heart rate. See Table 9-7 for normal pediatric heart rates. At birth the right ventricle is thicker than the left ventricle. Right ventricular dominance of the newborn period is replaced by left ventricular dominance in childhood and adulthood. Anatomical changes are most rapid in the first month, and by 6 months of age the left ventricle is dominant. With increasing age the heart rate decreases and the PR interval, QRS duration, and QT interval increase.[109]

In the pediatric patient, monitoring of respiratory rate and oxygen saturation is done concurrently with cardiac monitoring. It is important to recognize the manifestations of impending respiratory failure in the pediatric patient since respiratory failure precedes cardiac failure and potential cardiac arrest. Electrocardiogram (ECG) monitoring electrodes are placed along the nipple line on the chest to facilitate monitoring the cardiac rate and rhythm and the respiratory rate. Refer to the instructions for pediatric monitoring provided with the monitoring equipment.

Dysrhythmias are common in the child with underlying rhythm abnormalities and CHD and may occur in children with metabolic disorders. Other conditions that may cause dysrhythmias are abnormal potassium or calcium levels, hypoxia, acidosis, and hypothermia. A decrease in heart rate is an ominous sign in the pediatric patient. Asystole is the most common cardiac arrest rhythm, and bradycardia is the second-most common cardiac arrest–associated rhythm.[3] Ventricular fibrillation and pulseless ventricular tachycardia are uncommon pediatric rhythms.[3,104]

Supraventricular tachycardia. Supraventricular tachycardia (SVT) is the most common symptomatic tachydysrhythmia in children. P waves may or may not be seen, and the rate often exceeds 220 beats per minute (bpm). Wide QRS supraventricular tachycardia is relatively rare in children, so any wide QRS tachycardia must be treated as ventricular in origin until proved otherwise.[3] If the child in SVT is unstable and shows signs of decreased cardiac output, direct current (DC) cardioversion is indicated.[104,110] (The initial energy dose is 0.5 joules/kg, and if the tachydysrhythmia persists, the dose is doubled.[3]) In the stable child, procedures may include eliciting the diving reflex and other vagal maneuvers, pharmacologic therapy, and overdrive pacing. The drug of choice is adenosine.[2,104] The dose is 0.1 mg/kg rapid IV push and may be increased by 0.05 mg/kg increments every 2 minutes to a maximum of 0.25 mg/kg up to 12 mg or until termination of SVT.[2] IV verapamil is not recommended for young children because it has been associated with severe hypotension and cardiac arrest in infants younger than 1 year.[1,2]

Bradycardias. Bradycardias are the most common dysrhythmias in the pediatric patient and can result from hypoxia, acidosis, and/or hypothermia.[3] *Bradycardia* is defined as a cardiac rate less than the low limit for age. Bradydysrhythmias include sinus node dysfunction, heart block, and effects from pharmacologic therapy.[3] Treatment includes adequate oxygenation, epinephrine, atropine, transthoracic pacing, and chest compressions.[3] To initiate transthoracic pacing, adult electrodes are used if the child weighs more than 15 kg; if the child weighs less than 15 kg, use the small or medium pediatric electrodes.[111] The child may require sedation, intubation, and mechanical ventilation for successful transcutaneous pacing. The procedure results in mild to moderate discomfort, and it is seldom possible in the unsedated child.[111] The pacing pads cover a large area of the child's chest as compared with the adult. Pad placement is the same as with the adult, unless the child has dextrocardia. The condition of the skin is closely monitored.

Bacterial Endocarditis

Bacterial endocarditis may occur in children with CHD, but as in adults, may also occur in children with no history of cardiac disease. The most common causative organisms are *Streptococcus* and *Staphylococcus,* and rarely is the organism fungal. Manifestations in children are myalgias, arthralgias, headache, general malaise, fever, or the occurrence of an embolic event.[106] Most patients have a positive blood culture. Bacterial endocarditis must be recognized in children since the risk of death is great if antibiotics are not started early in the infective process. Antibiotic treatment usually lasts at least 6 weeks, and children usually stay in the hospital for treatment. The American Heart Association has published recommendations for bacterial endocarditis prophylaxis.[112]

Shock in Infants and Children

Shock is defined as decreased tissue perfusion resulting in cellular dysfunction.[113] Shock is classified as hypovolemic, cardiogenic, or distributive. Septic shock is the classification of distributive shock most common in children.

Hypovolemic shock. Hypovolemic shock may occur from severe vomiting or diarrhea and the resultant fluid loss or from blood loss caused by trauma or other bleeding problems. Treatment of hypovolemic shock is volume replacement. Albumin or other colloids may be given at 10 to 20 ml/kg.[106] Packed red cells are given for blood loss, starting with 10 ml/kg. Isotonic crystalloids (normal saline/Ringer's lactate) may be given initially in doses of 20 ml/kg rapidly IV. Crystalloids rapidly diffuse into the interstitial space, so only minimal volume is available in the intravascular space to increase circulating volume. The child must be closely monitored for tissue perfusion. (∞Hypovolemic Shock, p. 1100.)

Cardiogenic shock. Cardiogenic shock results from pump failure in congenital cardiac disease. The child develops tachycardia as a mechanism to increase cardiac output. Children have small stroke volumes, so increasing the heart rate increases cardiac output. The child will have decreased urine output (less than 0.5 to 1 ml/kg/hr), gain weight, and retain fluid. Crackles may be heard on lung ascultation, and frothy sputum may be present. Intubation and mechnical ventilation may be required. IV fluids may be given to optimize left ventricular end diastolic pressure, unless CVP or pulmonary artery wedge pressure (PAWP) is elevated. If fluid overload is present, inotropic support is provided. Vasodilators may also be required. These vasoactive medications are usually prepared using the rule of sixes (Box 9-2) and are infused in μg/kg/min in the pediatric patient. It is recommended that these drugs be infused through a central line.[3] A multilumen CVP catheter is often inserted to administer vasopressors, fluids, and other medications. (∞Cardiogenic Shock, p. 1102.)

BOX 9-2 Rule of Sixes for Preparing Variable Concentrations of Vasoactive Drugs

I. For drugs infused in doses of μg/kg/min (or multiples):
   A. Multiply weight (in kg) by 6; place this number of milligrams of drug in solution *totalling* 100 ml
   B. Then 1 ml/hr delivers 1 μg/kg/min
II. For drugs infused in doses of 0.1 μg/kg/min (or multiples):
   A. Multiply weight (in kg) by 0.6; place this number of milligrams of drug in solution *totalling* 100 ml
   B. Then 1 ml/hr delivers 0.1 μg/kg/min
III. For any concentration of a drug:

$$\text{Rate (ml/hr)} = \frac{\text{weight (kg)} \times \text{dose } (\mu\text{g/kg/min}) \times 60 \text{ min/hr}}{\text{concentration } (\mu\text{g/ml})}$$

From Hazinski, MF: (1992) *Nursing care of the critically ill child,* ed 2, St Louis, 1992, Mosby.

Sepsis/septic shock. Rule out sepsis may be an admitting diagnosis for the pediatric patient. Infants and very young children are at particular risk for developing sepsis or septic shock. This risk is increased when the patient has invasive monitoring lines, undergoes diagnostic testing, or has surgery. The child exhibits manifestations of the systemic inflammatory response syndrome (SIRS) or severe sepsis or septic shock. Instead of temperature elevation, the infant or child may have a low temperature or temperature instability. There is a change in level of consciousness, and the child may be irritable, restless, or lethargic. Urine output is decreased, the skin may be warm or mottled, and peripheral pulses may be strong and bounding. The child does not feed well, and decreased fluid intake may precipitate dehydration. Blood pressure is maintained within normal limits from activation of the body's compensatory mechanisms. Parents may remark that the child "does not seem right" or "something is different" with the child. Always listen to the parents' assessment of the child's status. (∞Septic Shock, Pathophysiology, p. 1111; Septic Shock Assessment and Diagnosis, p. 1113.)

Treatment of SIRS includes oxygen, fluids, and antibiotics, but the most effective treatment of SIRS is prevention. Handwashing before and after patient contact is essential. Sterile technique is maintained during suctioning, while managing invasive lines, and during dressing changes and wound care. (∞Systemic Inflammatory Response, p 1121.)

Severe sepsis or septic shock is diagnosed when perfusion decreases and the child becomes hypotensive. If the child is receiving inotropics, the BP may be normal, but there is a change in perfusion. The patient exhibits metabolic acidosis and hypoxemia, requiring intubation, mechanical ventilation, sedation, fluids, and vasopressor medications. Fluid replacement at 40 ml/kg has improved survival in septic shock.[114] Complications of septic shock include acute respiratory distress syndrome, acute renal failure, disseminated intravascular coagulation, and multiple organ dysfunction syndrome (MODS).

Cardiopulmonary Arrest

The pediatric patient must be assessed for manifestations of respiratory failure and sepsis, because failure to recognize these problems may result in the development of cardiopulmonary failure and respiratory or cardiac arrest. In the pediatric patient, respiratory arrest usually precedes cardiac arrest. In an arrest situation, oxygen is administered, and an airway established and maintained; see the section on airway management earlier in this chapter. For a cardiac arrest, compressions are started and an IV or intraosseous (IO) line established. Other interventions are based on the cardiac rhythm and cause of the arrest.

Pulseless arrest includes asystole, ventricular fibrillation, pulseless ventricular tachycardia, and electricomechanical dissociation (EMD).[3] Treatment of asystole includes cardiopulmonary resuscitation (CPR), airway maintenance with oxygenation and an IV or IO access. Epinephrine is the drug of choice. The first dose of epinephrine is 0.01 mg/kg (1:10,000, 0.1 ml/kg) given IV or IO, or if given endotracheally (ET), the dose is 0.1 mg/kg (1:1,000, 0.1 ml/kg). The second dose given IV, IO, or ET is 0.1 mg/kg (1:1,000, 0.1 ml/kg). Subsequent doses may be given IV or IO in a dose up to 0.2 mg/kg. It is important to note that the *volume* of epinephrine administered is 0.1 ml/kg whether conventional or high dose epinephrine is given. The dose of epinephrine is determined by the *concentration* of the drug (1:10,000 versus 1:1,000).[3]

Acidosis during resuscitation is corrected by effective ventilation and systemic perfusion. Sodium bicarbonate is considered only for documented severe acidosis associated with prolonged cardiac arrest, unstable hemodynamic state, hyperkalemia, or tricyclic antidepressant overdose.[3] It is uncertain as to whether atropine is useful in the treatment of asystole; clinical studies have failed to document its efficacy.[3] A vagolytic dose (0.2 mg/kg and a minimum dose of 0.1 mg/kg) may be given.[3] A dose smaller than the minimum dose may produce paradoxical bradycardia.[3] Defibrillation is not indicated for the treatment of asystole in the child. If EMD results in pulseless electrical activity, the cause should be determined and the treatment is the same as asystole.

For ventricular fibrillation or pulseless ventricular tachycardia, electrical defibrillation (2 joules/kg) is the treatment of choice. Defibrillate up to three times if needed (2 J/kg, 4 J/kg, 4 J/kg). If defibrillation is unsuccessful, epinephrine is given and lidocaine (1 mg/ kg) is helpful in preventing the recurrence of ventricular fibrillation[3]. Bretylium may also be used.

Bradydysrhythmias including sinus bradycardia, sinus node arrest with a slow junctional or ventricular escape rhythm, and various degrees of AV blocks are the most common terminal rhythms in children.[3] Hypoxemia, hypotension, and acidosis interfere with sinus node function and conduction of the cardiac impulse. CPR is required in the child if the heart rate is less than 60 and is associated with poor systemic perfusion. Vascular access is started, IV or IO. Epinephrine is given, as it is for pulseless arrest. Atropine may be given, and cardiac pacing may be indicated.

After arrest, the goals are to restore adequate blood pressure and effective perfusion and to correct hypoxia and acidosis. The inotropic agents dopamine, dobutamine, and epinephrine are used, but in the pediatric patient, epinephrine is the drug of choice.[3]

One other product that may be useful in pediatric arrest is the Broselow Pediatric Resuscitation Tape. This tape is color coded for each pediatric age group and provides resuscitation information based on the length and estimated weight of the child.[115,116]

NERVOUS SYSTEM

Anatomy

The nervous system grows rapidly before birth, and growth continues during infancy and childhood. One half of total brain growth occurs by 1 year, 75% by age 3, and 90% by age 6 or 7.[1,103] In comparison to the adult, the infant/toddler's head size is proportionally larger than the rest of the body. The skull is more flexible because the skull bones are not fused and are separated by spaces called the fontanelles. The anterior fontanelle is the junction of the coronal, sagittal, and frontal sutures, whereas the posterior fontanelle is the junction of the parietal and occipital bones.[103] By 3 months of age, the posterior fontanelle is usually closed, and the anterior fontanelle is closed by 20 months of age.[117]

Physiology

Both cerebral blood flow and oxygen consumption are increased in childhood in relation to increased metabolic needs. Hyperemia, tissue hypoxia, and acidosis result in cerebral arterial dilation and increased cerebral blood flow. Hyperventilation decreases cerebral blood flow, but severe hypercarbia may result in decreased oxygen consumption and use. The normal cerebral perfusion pressure (CPP) values are unknown in children. It is thought that CPP should be in the range of 40-60 mm Hg, but this figure may vary since perfusion is determined by blood flow and not blood pressure.[1] CPP must be maintained at a level to maintain blood flow.

Thermoregulation

Monitoring and maintaining the infant's temperature is a priority of pediatric nursing care. With a proportionally larger body surface and an increased metabolic rate, infants are predisposed to heat loss. The presence of minimal subcutaneous fat in the newborn results in increased heat loss in cold environments. Older children shiver to increase temperature, but the infant is unable to shiver effectively. In the newborn, heat is produced by a process called chemical (nonshivering) thermogenesis. Norepinephrine secreted in response to chilling stimulates fat metabolism in the vascular brown fat adipose tissue.[118] The internal heat produced is conducted through the blood to surface tissue.[118] Cold stress must be avoided because hypoxia, metabolic acidosis, or hypoglycemia may occur. Sudden infant temperature changes may also lead to apneic spells, especially during rapid rewarming. Nursing interventions to decrease heat loss include maintaining the infant in flexed position and avoiding heat transfer by radiation, convection, conduction, or evaporation. Infants may be placed in incubators or under radiant warmers.

Assessment

Cognitive function cannot be evaluated until the preschool and early childhood years, but level of consciousness (LOC), movement, and pupils can be evaluated in the pediatric patient. The Glasgow Coma Scale (GCS) is used for older children and has been modified for use in infants and younger children (Table 9-11). Evaluation of reflexes in children is comparable to adults, with a couple of exceptions. Although a positive Babinski reflex is an abnormal response in an adult, this response is normal in the child until age $1^1/_2$ to $2^1/_2$ years.[113,117] In the first few months of life, grasp is reflexive in the infant. With severe neurologic disease or injury, grasp may revert back to a reflex versus a purposeful response, so the grasp response may not indicate improvement of the child's neurologic status.

A situation referred to as the "talk and die phenomenon" may occur in both adults and children.[1] In this situation, the child with a closed head injury is awake and alert on admission to the hospital, but suddenly the child's condition deteriorates, and brainstem herniation and death result. Several hours after admission to the hospital, there is a change in LOC and the pupils dilate. The severity of the head injury is not initially recognized, but severe brain damage has occured and the child does not respond to treatment. The causes of death are cerebral herniation and ischemia. The pediatric patient with head injury requires careful assessment and ongoing frequent monitoring. (∞Trauma, Epidural Hematoma, p. 1060.)

Seizures

Seizures are brief manifestations of the brain's electrical system that result from cortical neuronal discharge. Seizures are the most commonly observed neurologic deficit in children and can occur with a variety of central nervous system (CNS) conditions (Box 9-3). Seizures are more common during the first 2 years of life. Brain injuries are the most common cause in the first few months of life, whereas infections are a common cause in older infants and toddlers. In preschoolers and older children, epilepsy is the most common cause. As children enter adolescence, hormonal and metabolic changes may alter the seizure threshold. The child who is in an unconscious state must be evaluated for a history of seizures since unconsciousness may be the result of a postictal state.

Clinical manifestations of seizures may be more subtle in the infant because of immaturity of the CNS. Some common behaviors seen with subtle seizures include (1) tonic horizontal deviations of the eyes with or without nystagmoid jerking; (2) repetitive blinking or fluttering of the eyelashes; (3) drooling, sucking, and/or tongue thrusting; and (4) swimming or rowing movements of the arms with occasional bicycling movements of the legs.[118] Apnea may also occur, so respiratory status must be closely monitored. Seizures

TABLE 9-11 Modified Glasgow Coma Scale for Infants and Children

	Child	Infant	Score
Eye opening	Spontaneous	Spontaneous	4
	To verbal stimuli	To verbal stimuli	3
	To pain only	To pain only	2
	No response	No response	1
Verbal response	Oriented, appropriate	Coos and babbles	5
	Confused	Irritable cries	4
	Inappropriate words	Cries to pain	3
	Incomprehensible words or nonspecific sounds	Moans to pain	2
	No response	No response	1
Motor response	Obeys commands	Moves spontaneously and purposefully	6
	Localizes painful stimulus	Withdraws to touch	5
	Withdraws in response to pain	Withdraws in response to pain	4
	Flexion in response to pain	Decorticate posturing (abnormal flexion) in response to pain	3
	Extension in response to pain	Decerebrate posturing (abnormal extension) in response to pain	2
	No response	No response	1

From Hazinski, MF: *Nursing care of the critically ill child,* ed 2, St Louis, 1992, Mosby.

must be differentiated from jitteriness in infants. With jitteriness, the predominant type of movements are tremors characterized by alternating rhythmic movements of equal rate and magnitude.[118] Both jitteriness and seizures may be observed in the infant with asphyxia, hypoglycemia, or hypocalcemia. Laboratory studies help determine the metabolic status of the infant.

Nursing management of seizures includes monitoring of respiratory status and perfusion, assessing for the cause of the seizure, determining methods to prevent additional seizures, providing a safe environment for the child, and documenting the seizure activity. Children admitted to the critical care unit may require intubation for respiratory complications of seizures, the sedative effects of anticonvulsants, or for status epilepticus.

Anticonvulsant therapy may be indicated for prolonged or recurrent seizures. Phenobarbital, phenytoin (Dilantin), and benzodiazepines (lorazepam, diazepam) may be ordered for the child.

Status Epilepticus

Status epilepticus is a medical emergency and is characterized by prolonged or repeated seizure activity.[119] Causes are high fever, meningitis, encephalitis, metabolic disorders, and abrupt stoppage of anticonvulsant drugs. There is an increase in cerebral blood flow, metabolic requirements, and oxygen needs. Cerebral edema may occur. An EEG may be required to confirm status epilepticus in patients in deep coma or with pharmacologic paralysis. Treatment includes short-term anticonvulsants, such as diazepam, lorazepam,[119] and midazolam[120]; airway maintenance, including intubation and oxygenation; barbiturate coma; or general anesthesia.[113] Nursing management includes monitoring the airway, perfusion, BP, heart rate, and neurologic status.

Bacterial Meningitis

Meningitis, an inflammation of the meninges and cerebral spinal fluid (CSF), is more common in children than in adults. Children younger than 5 years are more often affected, but school-age children and adolescents are also at risk. The causes of meningitis are septic (bacterial or fungal) or aseptic (viral),[117] but the information in this section pertains to bacterial meningitis. Common causative organisms are *Haemophilus influenzae* type B, *Streptococcus pneumoniae,* and *Neisseria meningitidis;* other causative organisms are Beta-hemolytic streptococcus, *Staphylococcus aureus, Escherichia coli, Pseudomonas,* and *Listeria monocytogenes.* Invasion of microorganisms triggers the inflammatory response, and a purulent exudate is

BOX 9-3 Etiology of Seizures in Children

NONRECURRENT (ACUTE)	RECURRENT (CHRONIC)
Febrile episodes	Idiopathic epilepsy
Intracranial infection	Epilepsy secondary to:
Intracranial hemorrhage	Trauma
Space-occupying lesions (cyst, tumor)	Hemorrhage
Acute cerebral edema	Anoxia
Anoxia	Infections
Toxins	Toxins
Drugs	Degenerative phenomena
Tetanus	Congenital defects
Lead encephalopathy	Parasitic brain disease
Shigella, Salmonella	Hypoglycemia injury
Metabolic alterations	Epilepsy—sensory stimulus
Hypocalcemia	Epilepsy-stimulating states
Hypoglycemia	Narcolepsy and catalepsy
Hyponatremia or hypernatremia	Psychogenic
Hypomagnesemia	Tetany from hypocalcemia, alkalosis
Alkalosis	Hypoglycemic states
Disorders of amino acid metabolism	Hyperinsulinism
Deficiency states	Hypopituitarism
Hyperbilirubinemia	Adrenocortical insufficiency
	Hepatic disorders
	Uremia
	Allergy
	Cardiovascular dysfunction or syncopal episodes
	Migraine

From Wong, D: Whaley & Wong's *Nursing care of infants and children*, ed 5, St. Louis, 1995, Mosby.

produced. There is decreased cerebral blood flow in meningitis, and aggressive hyperventilation may reduce cerebral blood flow below ischemic levels in children.[117]

Clinical manifestations include fever, chills, headache, vomiting, irritability or lethargy, photophobia, nuchal rigidity, and positive Kernig and/or Brudzinski signs. In meningococcemia, petechiae and purpura may be observed.[121] A sudden onset of meningococcemia is known as the Waterhouse-Friderichsen syndrome.[117] In this syndrome, the child develops severe septic shock, disseminated intravascular coagulation, and bilateral adrenal hemorrhage.[103] Lumbar puncture is the diagnostic test for meningitis. CSF studies show elevated white blood count, increased protein, and decreased glucose. The CSF/blood glucose ratio is usually less than 0.40.[117]

The child with meningitis is isolated during initial antibiotic treatment and for 24 hours after appropriate antibacterial therapy is started. Health care providers must use appropriate precautions because they are also at risk. Broad-spectrum antibiotics may be administered until the specific organism is identified, and then the appropriate drug is given. Antibiotics for meningitis are given in high doses and must be given at the scheduled times to maintain adequate blood levels. Acetaminophen may be given for elevated temperature; aspirin must not be used. Adequate hydration is maintained. Complications of bacterial meningitis include seizures; increased intracranial pressure (ICP); septic shock; cerebral ischemia, causing neurologic compromise; and possible loss of digits or distal parts of extremities in the case of meningococcemia.

Nursing management includes maintaining universal and isolation precautions; providing a quiet environment; monitoring neurologic, respiratory, and cardiovascular status; measuring and documenting head circumference in the child younger than 2 years; administering antibiotics and pain medications; and providing family education and support. The child may develop sequelae of meningitis, which include hearing loss, mental retardation, hydrocephalus, and death. There is now a vaccine for *Haemophilus influenzae* type B (HIB), and the first dose is given when an infant is 2 months of age.

Head Trauma

Trauma is the leading cause of death in the child older than 1 year, with head trauma a major determinant of pediatric mortality.[113,122,123] Head trauma is more common in males—results of motor vehicle accidents, falls, violence, or abuse.[12,103,124] The child in a motor vehicle accident may be an occupant of a vehicle or be a bicyclist or pedestrian. Falls are a common cause of head injuries in children younger than 2 years[122] because the child's head size is proportionally larger in relationship to total body size. Child abuse is the most common cause of head injury in the first year of life.[123]

Definitions and descriptions of the various types of head injuries are similiar to those for the adult. (∞Trauma, Head Injuries, p 1057.)

Though the pathophysiology of head injury is similar in adults and children, there are variations in the nursing assessment and management for the pediatric patient. During infancy, the most common causes of head injury are child abuse and falls.[122] The abused infant may be admitted to the critical care unit in serious condition with a severe head injury. One form of abuse in which there are no external signs of head injury is shaken baby syndrome. The patient exhibits changes in neurologic status that result from violent shaking. Diagnostic evaluations reveal subdural hematoma and retinal hemorrhage.[103] When completing the admission assessment, the nurse may find inconsistency in information provided about the injury or a history of injury that does not fit the described circumstances. There may be a history of emergency department visits and may be previous hospital admissions for evaluation of neurologic deficits. If child abuse is suspected, health care personnel have a legal obligation to report concerns to the appropriate child protection agency.

Falls occur in infants and children as they become more mobile. Infants can roll off beds, sofas, and changing tables. As the toddler begins to walk and climb, falls can result from an unsteady gait or a normal curiosity. Since the child's head is larger in proportion to the rest of the body, the child often lands head first in a fall. Motor vehicle accidents (MVAs) are the leading cause of death in the child older than 1 year.[103] Prevention is the best treatment for MVAs. Correct use of infant seats, seat belts, and helmets and caution when walking, playing near the street, or driving will decrease the incidence of head injury. The nurse is an advocate for child safety, providing information to parents on maintaining a safe environment to prevent injuries.

Firearms are the lethal weapons used in most homicides in older children and in most completed teenage suicides.[124] The child with a gunshot wound to the head is stabilized, a CT scan may be obtained, and the child is taken to surgery for debridement of the wound. Children who are victims of gunshot wounds to the head usually do not survive.

Complications of head injuries include hemorrhage, infections, cerebral bleeding, cerebral edema, seizures, and brain herniation. Treatment is based on the complication manifested by the patient. Both epidural and subdural hematoma occur in children, but epidural hematoma occurs less frequently in the infant or toddler.[103,113] This may be related to the fact that the middle meningeal artery is not embedded in the bony surface of the scalp until approximately 2 years of age.[103] Treatment for epidural hematoma is surgical intervention. Subdural hematoma is more common in children and may result from falls and abuse, including violent shaking.[103] Treatment of subdural hematoma may be frequent subdural taps or surgical intervention.

Children, especially infants, are at risk for infection after head injury. The child admitted to the critical care unit with a head injury must be constantly monitored for cerebral edema and signs of increased ICP. Continuous ICP monitoring may be initiated. (∞Assessment of ICP, p. 821; Management of Intracranial Hypertension, p. 826; Herniation Syndromes, p. 832; Diabetes Insipidus, p. 1021; SIADH, p. 1027.)

Two other potential complications of head injury—diabetes insipidus and syndrome of inappropriate antidiuretic hormone—are discussed in Chapter 41.

Nursing interventions include precise neurologic assessment, including using the GCS and monitoring for signs of increased ICP. The frequency of assessment is related to the severity of the injury. Observe behaviors in relationship to the developmental level and usual behavior of the child. Maintain IV fluid restriction (may be one half to two thirds of maintenance requirements)[117] and monitor respiratory status, ventilation parameters, and arterial blood gases. Provide pharmacologic paralysis or barbiturate coma if needed per the medical management plan. Administer diuretics, osmotic agents, antibiotics, pain medications, sedatives, and antipyretics. Children who survive severe head injury often require extended rehabilitation services. Involve the pediatric rehabilitation team in the care of the child while the child is in the critical care unit.

Working with the family of the child with a head injury is challenging. Information given to the parents must be accurate and consistent. The parents may be guilt-ridden, especially if they feel they might have been able to prevent the injury. Parents are encouraged to interact with the child soothingly and gently, even if the child cannot respond. Reading books, making a tape of home activities, and bringing in familiar toys or stuffed animals are ways to involve the family in the care of the child.

If the child is not expected to survive, the parents are informed. The child may be evaluated for brain death. Before the tests begin, the parents are offered the opportunity to spend time with the child. If brain death has occurred, the parents are told the test results. Parents may be asked to participate in the decision of when, but not if, to discontinue support. Special circumstances such as the impending arrival of a grandparent may influence the timing of the decision. Parents must be allowed to spend as much time as they desire with the child. (∞Brain Death, p. 798.)

GASTROINTESTINAL SYSTEM/FLUIDS/NUTRITION

Anatomy and Physiology

Coordination of sucking, swallowing, esophageal peristalsis, and breathing is established just after birth.[125] For the first 3 months of life, swallowing is a reflex activity that gradually becomes voluntary by 6 months of age.[126] Infant sucking, which is also a reflex, can be nutritive or nonnutritive.[127] Nonnutritive sucking involves no swallowing; occurs at a rapid rate; has self-soothing capacities,[128-130] which can also be used with the intubated infant; and affects the postprandial process.[131,132]

Nutritive sucking involves moving food from the mouth through the small intestines.[127] It involves bursts of about 10 to 30 sucks, interspersed with one to four swallows.[133] By 4 to 6 months of age this ability becomes stronger.[126]

Respirations are inhibited during swallowing.[126] The quality of nutritive sucking is one of several indicators of illness in the infant. The sucking involves a lot of motor activity and when changes in oxygen demand and consumption occur during illness, the infant will fatigue more readily and sucking will be weaker or even abate.[134]

Gastric volume for a term newborn is about 30 ml. By 3 months it increases to 150 to 180 ml, and by 12 months it is 240 ml,[135] compared with an adult's volume of 1500 ml.[136] The gastric emptying time in the infant or child can be variable, but generally occurs in about 2 hours.[137]

After birth, growth and maintenance of the small intestine require not only nutritional components, but the stimulation that comes from having food present in the gut lumen.[138,139] Even with good nutritional status, after 3 days of no gut stimulation,[138] decreased intestinal growth, mucosal atrophy, decreased cell turnover, poor brush-border activity, and blunted villi occur.[140,141]

The intestinal tract in the infant and young child is larger per body weight than the adult's.[142] Sodium and water conservation in the large intestine is immature in the infant, which accounts for the increased number of stools produced each day.[143] For the first 2 years of life, gut immunity is lower[144] and there is greater mucosal binding for bacterial toxins.[145] With these differences of immunity, sensitivity, and greater potential for fluid loss, the infant and toddler have a greater morbidity and mortality with enteric infections than does the adult.[146,147]

Total body water per weight is greater in the infant and child than in the adult because of differences in proportional organ sizes that have a high water content and greater proportion of interstitial lymph fluid.[148] Total body water ranges from 75% at birth to about 60% at 1 year of age, which is an adult level—with approximately 20% extracellular fluid (ECF) and 40% intracellular fluid (ICF).[148] Plasma volume is about 4% to 5% of body weight, making total blood volume about 85 ml/kg in the newborn, 75 ml/kg in the infant younger than 1 year, and 67 to 75 ml/kg in the child.[149]

Assessment and Treatment

The child's fluid requirements involve not only replacing output and insensible losses, but extra fluid for the production of new ICF and ECF during growth.[150] Fluid maintenance for the child with normal renal and cardiac status can be calculated using several formulas but these account only for basal metabolic needs and growth.[2,150] Table 9-12 provides formulas for normal fluid and electrolyte maintenance for the infant and child.[41,151,152] Box 9-4 provides adjustments to fluid maintenance based on level of activity or increased metabolic rate from disease.[151,153,154] Increased fluids for stress states related to critical care conditions (e.g., sepsis) is still controversial as to what those increases are and how to determine them.[155,156]

The infant and child also need more calories per body weight than the adult for energy expenditure, because of growth.[157] The Food and Nutrition Board's high-end ranges for recommended daily allowances for the normal, active child may be too generous for the critically ill child, because overfeeding can cause various pulmonary and metabolic complications in the already compromised child.[158] The first fluid formula listed in Table 9-12 can also be used for determining calories in the infant and child (substituting kcal for ml).[152] This formula already provides for a 30% increase in calories exceeding the basal metabolic rate needed for average hospital activity. Approximate daily weight gain in the growing child or adolescent is: 0 to 3 months of age—30 g/day; 3 to 12 months—15 g/day; 1 to 10 years—7 g/day; young adolescent—225 g/day; and older adolescent—300 g/day.[159,150] This needs to be taken into account when evaluating for fluid overload in the child.

Total parenteral nutrition. Providing needed calories in the face of fluid restrictions is a significant problem with the critically ill infant and child. Overfeeding with TPN can lead to deleterious effects[158,159] involving pulmonary gas exchange, pulmonary hypertension, and metabolic acidosis. Table 9-13 outlines daily dextrose, lipid, and amino acid amounts;

TABLE 9-12 Normal Fluid and Electrolyte Maintenance for Infants and Children

	Infant/Child Weight	Total Amount
Fluids	1-10 kg	(100 ml/kg/day)
	11-20 kg	(1000 ml + 50 ml/each kg over 10 days)
	>20 kg	(1500 ml + 20 ml/each kg over 20 days) or 100 ml/100 kcal/day can be used for children of any weight or 1500 ml/m^2/day can be used for children >10 g
Sodium		2-4 mEq/kg/day
Potassium		2-3 mEq/kg/day

BOX 9-4 Adjustments to Fluid Maintenance

Fever/hypothermia:	Increases/decreases 12% for each degree greater/less than 37.8° C rectal
Tachypnea:	Increases 25%-30%
Humidified mechanical ventilation:	Decreases 12%
Activity:	Noncritically ill resting child: increases 10% Restless/active child: increases 30%
Diaphoresis:	Increases 10%-25%
High humidity environment:	Decreases 25%-40%

administration rates; and intravenous line concentration limits for the infant and child on TPN.[159]

Dextrose solutions initially are titrated up over several days in reaching desired caloric levels to prevent hyperglycemia and to allow endogenous insulin secretions to adjust.[159,160] The seriously ill infant or child does better with lipids administered concomitantly with dextrose/amino acids over 24 hours, not only to decrease the solution's osmolarity[159] and increase longevity of cannulated vessels, but also to minimize fat intolerance.[159,161]

If TPN is to be cycled, the titration for a child less than 30 kg occurs over 2 hours, with the rate increased or decreased by half each hour.[159,162] If TPN is to be discontinued, the rate can be tapered over 24 hours without hypoglycemia occurring, as long as enteral nutrition is tolerated.[159] Enteral caloric intake generally increases ml for ml with TPN decreases. When the child can tolerate 75% of desired caloric hourly volume, TPN can be discontinued.[159]

Gavage feeding. There are many different formulas available for the infant and child, based on age, host factors, and nutritional requirements. Amounts for formula feeds are based on needed kcal/kg/day and tolerance.[159] For the full-term infant younger than 1 year, cow's milk (Enfami, Similac) or soy-based formulas (Isomil, ProSobee) are most commonly given. Human breast milk is highly recommended.[163,163a] For the child 1 to 6 years of age, Pediasure is designed specifically for this age group. Adult formulas can be given to the child older than 6 years. Osmolite and Isocal are preferred for their isotonicity and caloric and protein content.[164] It is not necessary to routinely dilute feedings. Full strength formulas can be given safely to the ill child.[159,165]

Continuous gavage feedings have advantages over bolus feedings. The risk for aspiration is less, particularly for the infant with reflux.[166] Increased gastrointestinal (GI) absorption[167] and increased growth can occur.[168] Diarrhea can also be managed with continuous feedings.[159,167]

Feeding tubes can be placed orally or nasally in the infant, but indwelling tubes are usually placed nasally. Determining the insertion length of a nasogastric tube in the child has traditionally been the same as that in the adult—nares to ear to xyphoid process.[169] It is possible that this measurement does not always allow for all the side holes of a feeding tube to be in the stomach.[170] Measuring to a point between the xyphoid and the umbilicus is a safer method. Table 9-14 provides guidelines for gavage feeding tube sizes and feeding rates in infants and children.[159]

Gavage feeding in the infant occurs with nonnutritive sucking during some portion of the feeding time, if possible.[159] The emotional and GI benefits of nonnutritive sucking have been discussed earlier in this chapter. In addition, the head of the bed or crib needs to be elevated for all infants receiving enteral formulas to minimize aspiration.

PAIN MANAGEMENT

It has been reported that many professionals believe that infants and children experience pain differently than adults.[171,172] Physicians have prescribed inade-

TABLE 9-13 **TPN Administration for Term Infants and Children***

	10-30 kg Child	<10 kg Child
DEXTROSE (need to calculate dextrose from all IV lines)		
Amount/rate	Initiate at 4-8 mg/kg/min	Same
	Maximum 10-17 mg/kg/min	Same
	Increase rate by 1.5-4 mg/kg/min or 2.5%-5% dextrose/day	0.3-0.8 mg/kg/min or 0.5%-1% dextrose/day
IV limits		
Peripheral	12.5% maximum	Same
Central	35% maximum	Same
LIPIDS		
Amount	1-4 g/kg/day	1-3 g/kg/day
(Minimum of 2%-4% of kcal/day of fat to prevent essential fatty acid deficiency)		
Rate	<0.25 g/kg/hour	Same
(Administer concomitantly with PN solution over 24 hours)		
AMINO ACIDS		
Amount/rate	Initiate at 1 g/kg/day	Same
	Maximum 1-2.5 g/kg/day	Same
	Increase rate by 0.5-1 g/kg/day	Same
MAXIMUM FLUID VOLUMES[160]	$4000\ ml/m^2/day$	200 ml/kg/day

*> 30 kg, use adult recommendations.
PN, Parenteral nutrition.

TABLE 9-14 **Guidelines for Gavage Feeding in Infants and Children**

Age	3 mo	6 mo	2 yr	5 yr	10 yr
Tube size	6 F	8 F	10 F	12 F	14 F

Method	Initial Volume/Rate	Advancement Volume/Rate
Bolus	2-5 ml/kg every 3-4 hr over 20 min	2-5 ml/kg every other feeding
Continuous	1-2 ml/kg/hr; initial volume not to exceed 55 ml/hr regardless of child's weight	1-2 ml/kg every 8-12 hr

quate dosages of analgesics,[173,174] and nurses have been unable to identify or have been reluctant to treat pain in children.[175,176] Even parents have been reluctant to treat their children's pain adequately and have held erroneous beliefs concerning potential drug addiction or future illicit drug usage.[177]

Physiology and Pharmacokinetics

Neurotransmitters and peripheral and central neural pathways for pain transmission are developed and are functional before birth.[178] The cardiorespiratory, hormonal, and metabolic responses to pain are the same in the child as in the adult.[178] The infant younger than 1 to 2 months may have a more immature blood-brain barrier, allowing greater permeability of water-soluble opioids, such as morphine.[179] The infant also has less protein binding with morphine,[180,181] allowing for greater free drug. In addition, the infant's liver cytochrome P_{450} system is immature, which is needed to biotransform the major opioids before excretion.[182] By 2 months of age, the elimination half-life and plasma drug clearance for morphine and its derivatives is equal to that of an adult.[183,184]

With fentanyl, plasma drug clearance is greater for the infant between 3 to 12 months of age than for the older child or adult, but the elimination half-life is longer.[185,186] The infant younger than 1 year has less available plasma protein binding for the fentanyl drug group than does the adult.[184]

The physiologic effects of untreated pain in the child can result in[187] (a) hyperglycemia from decreased insulin secretion with breakdown of carbohydrate and fat stores; (b) metabolic acidosis from increased use of fat; (c) increased corticosteroids, growth hormone, and catecholamines; (d) increased pulmonary vascular resistance; and (e) hypoxemia.

Assessment

Many of the factors that influence an adult's pain influence a child's. One of the differences, though, is the influence of parental anxiety and behavior regarding their child's overall experience of pain.[188] While most of the pain research has involved procedural pain, it is important to be cognizant of the acute and chronic pain and distress associated with the critical care unit and its repetitive procedures.

The child may not spontaneously express his or her need for pain treatment.[189] Staff need to be vigilant and actively explore a child's level of pain whenever there is the potential for pain to exist.[190] Self-report scales have been found to be the most accurate measurement of pain,[190] but these cannot be used with the preverbal child, the child who cannot comprehend the request to symbolically identify pain, or with the child who has a significantly altered level of consciousness. For the child up to 3 years old, behavioral scales are used as the primary source for pain assessment, with physiologic parameters secondary.[191] Crying, motor activity, and facial expression are the components that generally comprise behavioral scales.[192-194]

For the child at least 6 years old, self-reports are the primary assessment tool, with behavioral scales secondary.[191] For the child 3 to 6 years old, self-reports can be used but with a caveat. Many self-report scales have been tested as effective with this age-group[195-197] but the young child 3 to 4 years old may have difficulty using them.[198] Cognitive ability may not be advanced enough yet, or the child may have regressed in cognitive ability because of the illness. The child's rating may indicate a mood state and not pain. The child may refuse to comply with pain ratings out of fear of getting hurt even more,[199] to make the "scary" staff person go away, as the only means of control over the situation,[198] or because no relevance is seen between the rating request and what he or she is experiencing.[190] With this age-group, self-reports and behavioral scales may need to be used in tandem.

If obtaining a self-report of pain is not possible, numerical rating scales or behavioral assessments can be done by parents or staff.[190,200] Parental ratings of their child's pain are dependent on the parent-child relationship, the parents' beliefs about pain, and their own emotional state.[177,201] For parents who are in tune with their child, their ratings are used primarily. Their ratings often are consistent with how the child's rating would be,[200,202] but parents can overrate or underrate their child's pain.[203] Using behavioral scales to measure pain intensity may not always give a true reflection of a child's pain. Severe pain can be felt without any manifestation of expectable behaviors.[189,204] Figure 9-8 provides some pain scales for use with the infant and child.

Opioid Analgesics

The most commonly used narcotics in the child are morphine and fentanyl.[184] Methadone is used for weaning from iatrogenic narcotic dependency.[205] Meperidine is not a drug of choice because it causes depressed cardiac output and tachycardia, and its metabolite lowers seizure threshold and causes hyperexcitability with multiple dosing.[184] Opioids are given IVP, continuous infusion, or in epidurals and caudals. Because of the belief held by some that the older infant continues to be overly sensitive to the respiratory depressant effects of opioids beyond the neonatal period, some health care providers are hesitant to administer these drugs.[184] Respiratory depression is not a common side effect, and hesitancy in administering these drugs to an infant 2 months or older is unwarranted.[184] When given in age-appropriate dosages, no differences in incidence of respiratory depression have been reported.[179,185,206-208] The standard child dose of morphine is 0.1 mg/kg. The Acute Pain Management Guideline Panel[190] still suggests caution when administering morphine to a nonintubated infant younger than 6 months old and recommends one third of the regular child's dose (0.03 mg/kg). Table 9-15 outlines dosages of morphine and fentanyl for the infant and child.[184]

PSYCHOSOCIAL ISSUES OF THE CHILD AND FAMILY

Admissions to a critical care unit include children with illnesses, injuries, and imminent deaths that are

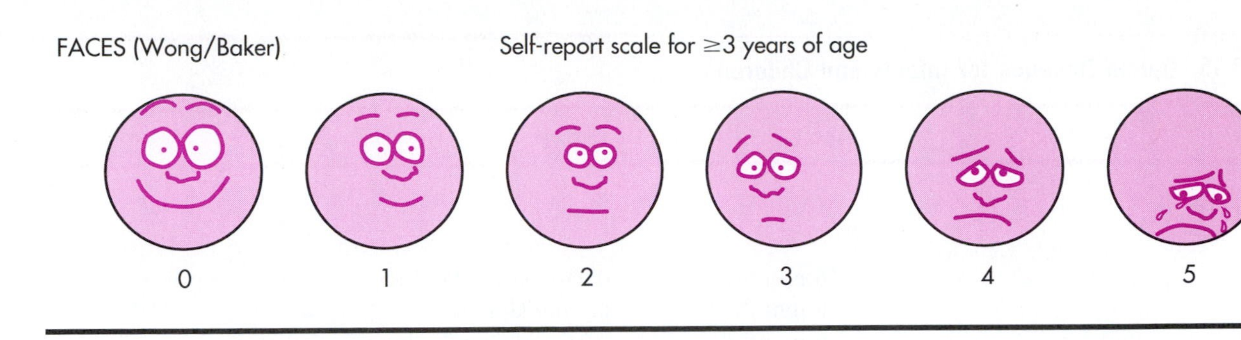

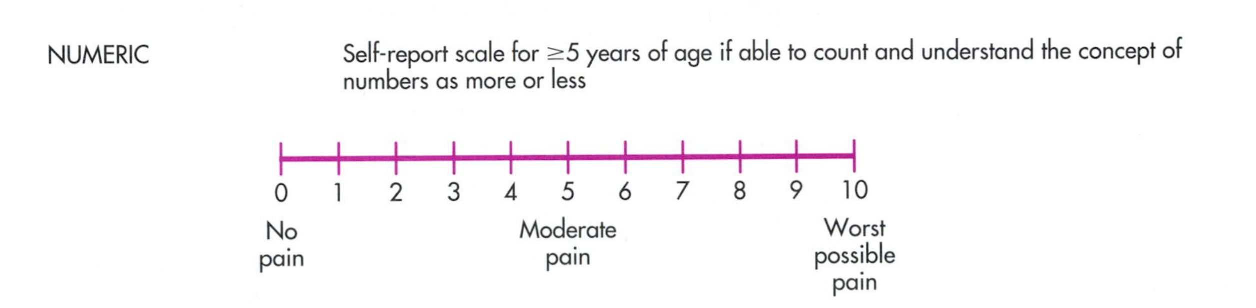

FLACC — Behavioral scale for infants or children

	0	1	2
Face	No particular expression or smile	Occasional grimace or frown, withdrawn, disinterested	Frequent to constant frown, clenched jaw, quivering chin
Legs	Normal position or relaxed	Uneasy, restless, tense	Kicking, or legs drawn up
Activity	Lying quietly, normal position, moves easily	Squirming, shifting back and forth, tense	Arched, rigid, or jerking
Cry	No cry (awake or asleep)	Moans or whimpers, occasional complaint	Crying steadily, screams or sobs, frequent complaints
Consolability	Content, relaxed	Reassured by occasional touching, hugging, or "talking to," distractable	Difficult to console or comfort

FIGURE 9-8 Pain rating scales for infants and children.
(FLACC courtesy Sandra I. Merkel and Terri Voepel-Lewis, University of Michigan Health Care Systems.)

often unanticipated by the family. With chronic illnesses, emotional reactions to stages of illness or death often occur in a stepwise fashion.[209,210] In a crisis situation, the parents can be very overwhelmed and be solely focused on the physiologic well-being of their child. If the child is conscious, he or she desperately needs the continual physical presence and emotional support from the parents; yet, this is a time when it can be very difficult for the parents to help their child emotionally.[211] Critical care staff need to be knowledgeable about childhood cognitive and emotional development and family dynamics to assist the family through this kind of crisis. This section can only introduce common issues.

TABLE 9-15 Opioid Dosages for Infants and Children

Agent	Age	Dosage
MORPHINE		
Route		
IVP	<6 months	0.03-0.05 mg/kg/dose
	>6 months	0.1 mg/kg/dose
Continuous infusion	<6 months	0.01-0.015 mg/kg/hour + IVP loading dose
	>6 months	0.02-0.03 mg/kg/hour + IVP loading dose
PCA		20 μg/kg/bolus; 6 boluses/hour; 8-10 min lockout or
		0.02-0.03 mg/kg/hr continuous + boluses
Epidural		0.03-0.1 mg/kg bolus q 6-12 hr
FENTANYL		
Route		
IV (short procedure)		2-3 μg/kg/dose (if sedation used: 1-2 μg/kg/dose)
Continuous infusion (intubated)		10 μg/kg loading dose + 2-5 μg/kg/hr
Epidural		0.2-2 μg/kg/hr, possibly with bupivacaine

IVP, Intravenous pyelography; *PCA,* patient controlled analgesia.

The Ill Child's Experience of Critical Illness

The emotional reactions of the child to hospitalization depend on the type and quantity of stress produced by the illness itself, the hospitalization experience, and the notions that the child has about the situation.[211-213] The final outcome is influenced, in part, by the child's age, level of development, adaptive capacity to control (within reason) the fears and anxieties that are provoked, the kinds of hospital procedures done, the attitude and reactions of parents and staff, and the environmental conditions of the hospital. A child in the critical care unit experiences significant stress,[214] and the important question is whether the child's capacity to cope, either physically or emotionally, in an age-appropriate fashion is exceeded.

The critically ill child needs, foremost, the physical presence of the parents (or primary caretaker) at the bedside. Twenty-four hours a day visitation for parents is imperative. They are the most reassuring persons in the child's eyes, and are needed psychologically by the child to believe that he or she will not be abandoned, left to be unsafe or left in pain and distress. The child, even more so than the adult patient, also needs to be protected from staff who would discuss the child's case at the bedside. Anxiety and fear are easily heightened when the child recognizes scary words or fills in ambiguities heard with his or her own distorted interpretations. For the child who is very ill and prostrate, anxieties may fester within the child, unknown to staff.

In the critically ill child it may be difficult to differentiate withdrawal from fatigue. Parental touch and verbalizations are extremely important to provide reassurance that the child is not alone. These are also needed for the child who is heavily sedated or unconscious, since some level of awareness may still exist. Other age-appropriate sensory stimuli such as soft objects for rubbing on the face, favorite snuggle toys from home, special objects that may have a feel or smell that the child can identify, audio cassettes of the mother's and/or family members' voices speaking to the child or reading a book, or a cassette with favorite music can be used as soothing measures for a child of any age. For the school-age child, repeated orientation to time, day, and place also can be reassuring, whereas, the younger child's primary concern is whether the parents are present.

Noxious procedures must be preceded by gently bringing the infant or child to a state of arousal. Even in depressed states of consciousness, gently speaking or stroking the child is done first. For the infant and toddler, someone (ideally the parent) needs to provide comfort and distraction during and after the procedure. A child of this age does not understand procedural explanations and apologies for performing them. An overall emotional tone of calmness and quiet soothing in body language and voice volume is most helpful in minimizing anxiety.[215,216]

The child 3 to 7 years old also needs this same emotional tone from staff and parents to assist him or her in tempering anxiety. A child this age also needs a brief explanation of what will be done. The purpose of the explanation is not to impart educational information, but rather to mute the sense of bodily assault by removing some of the surprise and by providing a working language for the child. The form of the explanation should be brief, only one or two sentences. Also, because of the underdeveloped sense of time, procedures are only spoken about just before they are to be done. By the same token, the child must not overhear from staff about procedures to be done in the future.

For the child 8 to 10 years old, the process is much the same, except that the older child can usually understand a fuller explanation of the procedure. Depending on how ill the child is, he or she may desire more rationale as a way of coping by using intellectual means. The child of this age feels he or she has more self-control over some aspects of illness or injury.[217] Understanding more about the relationship between symptoms, illness, and recovery is now possible intellectually, but is still relatively simplistic.[218,219] Acknowledgments of possible feelings after the procedure must also occur. Because of the child's greater ability of memory and in comprehending time, statements can now include reference to feelings about the repetition of procedures, the dread of future ones, the lack of control over them, or the child's wish to be able to make someone else the recipient of the procedures.

The older school-age child, while having a better understanding of his or her body and illness, still does not fully grasp what role the health care professional plays in recovery, since they are often seen as the purveyors of discomfort.[218] Despite this difficulty in fully understanding how treatment goals get accomplished because of the limits in logical reasoning of the child younger than 11 years, the bond between the health care professional and the child-patient can occur by helping to verbalize the child's feelings, without belittling or condemning him or her.

In the adolescent, any type of behavioral regression can occur that is seen in the younger child, but there is a different emphasis on the issues of privacy; boundaries; abandonment from family, peers, and pets; immobility; and body image. The young adolescent has a greater concern about separation from mother. Despite the ability for abstract reasoning, anxiety can bring on a cause-and-effect type of thinking. The adolescent, as does the younger child, fears pain and is very much threatened by invasive procedures.[220] With the adolescent's cognitive grasp of the finality of death, being surrounded by others who might or actually do die, the adolescent can worry deeply about his or her own mortality, even if it is not realistically at stake.[221] An adolescent may also fear recovery if hospitalization is felt to be a respite from intense family conflicts.

The Parents' Experience of a Child's Critical Illness

Parents of the critically ill child experience a great deal of stress and anxiety, regardless of the severity of the child's illness or length of stay in the critical care unit.

There are common issues that parents experience when their child is admitted to the critical care unit. With a sudden illness or injury, there often is denial. Parents may question the diagnosis or want to prove the physician wrong. The situation can feel very unreal, as if it were not happening to them. It may be difficult to grasp the totality of what has happened to their child. They can feel immobile and not know what they should do next. The parents may find it difficult to remember and process explanations given to them about what is happening with their child. This is usually a defense against pain. This forgetting can result in some parents feeling that staff do not explain very much to them. Other parents may feel that this is a sign of inadequacy on their own part. They may be reluctant to ask for repetitions out of embarrassment, especially after the first time. They may then ask their questions to others who may not be qualified to answer to their specific situation. Some parents may appear externally as very competent and composed during the height of the crisis. This must not be interpreted that they have less stress or anxiety.

Parents need to be reunited with their child, if this is their wish, as soon as they have been prepared about what to expect. Having them wait until all assessments are done and the room is cleaned up is unnecessary. But parents may be afraid to see their child. Changes in the child's appearance and in the child's emotional reactions can be very upsetting to parents.[222,223] If the child is conscious and relatively alert, the parents need to be informed that their child may show some form of regressive behavior, such as withdrawal or anger, which is expectable given the stress of the situation and the degree of illness or injury. Parents also can feel frightened about touching or talking to their child, believing this may harm the child. They must be told

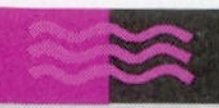

RESEARCH ABSTRACT

Reconciling technologic and family care in critical-care nursing.

Chelsa C: *Image* 28(3):199, 1996.

PURPOSE

The purpose of this naturalistic, interpretive study of general critical care nurses was to describe nursing practice with families.

DESIGN

Interpretive phenomenologic.

SAMPLE

The sample consisted of 130 nurses from neonatal, pediatric, and adult critical care units from seven tertiary and community hospitals; 98% of the subjects held a baccalaureate degree. The subjects' experience in nursing ranged from less than 1 year (novice practice, n = 25) to 5 or more years of experience (expert practice, n = 44), with 26 subjects who had practiced more than 5 years and were considered to be experienced, but not expert.

PROCEDURE

All nurses were interviewed three times in small groups. They were asked to describe recent clinical practice experiences in which they felt that they had made a difference or in which there was difficulty in the care. Clinical practice observations of 48 nurses at all levels of skill were conducted for at least 2 hours on three different episodes. All interviews and observations were tape recorded for subsequent transcription. Interpretation from 100 patient-care narratives was conducted for this portion of the study.

RESULTS

A range of practice with families was observed and categorized into four major themes. Organizational impediments to family involvement in care consisted of issues related to visiting and the families' access to their loved ones or the unit. In the second category, nursing practice with families, inconsistent practices were reported that differed according to the age and stage of illness of the patient. Taking up the technologic imperative was the third category, in which nurses dealt with the challenges of balancing technology with human needs. Nurses described the patients' families as meddlesome, an encumbrance in the unit; the ideal family was one that followed the rules and was cooperative. The last major category was that of balancing family concerns with the efforts to cure. Families were supported to participate in the care of their loved ones and were assisted to cope with the crisis of dealing with a critical situation.

DISCUSSION/IMPLICATIONS

Findings from this study demonstrated a wide range of skills and expertise nurses possess in working with families of the critically ill. Some nurses did not value including families in care and used multiple strategies to exclude them. Other nurses provided expert care using creative and innovative measures for family involvement in the highly technologic critical care environment. Although rationale and other possible reasons for nursing actions were not assessed in this study, there are implications for practice. Emphasis on patient-centered care is necessary in all health care delivery environments, and perhaps so that knowledge transfer can take place with all practicing nurses. Bedside nurses need to be supported in this area by education, consultation, and continuing acknowledgment and support for their efforts and outcomes of holistic care.

that it is OK to do this and if there are any concerns, staff will be right there in the room with them.

Intense anxiety is another emotion that can make parents question whether their reactions are normal. They wonder how other parents feel or behave. They can be extremely frightened by the intensity of their feelings and may wonder whether they will have a breakdown, or they may ward off crying because they fear they will never be able to stop.[210,224] These feelings are common in a crisis, and parents need to hear that their feelings are very understandable. And while they may feel like they will never stop crying or will go crazy, feeling it and having it happen are not the same thing. Some parents may behave with a lot of hostility toward staff or family members.[210] On the other hand, some may behave quite rigidly—visiting only briefly or not asking questions in an attempt to keep themselves intact.[210]

Guilt is another emotion that can torment parents greatly. They may feel responsible for their child's condition. Alternatively, now that the child is ill or injured, parents may feel troubled by previously held negative feelings toward the child. These may revolve around the normal exasperations of rearing a child, or the parents may have had ambivalence about having the child at all.

Anger is an emotion that usually takes its toll after the crisis period, usually with longer critical care unit stays. Destructive anger occurs when parents seek justification for their anger by blaming others for their child's condition. They are unreasonably critical of staff and feel belittled by them. An all too common occurrence is alienation between spouses. Either different coping styles or the blaming of one by the other prevents them from supporting each other.

Another situation that can occur with prolonged hospitalization of a child is the mother becoming totally devoted to the ill child. She will live at the hospital and be very involved in her child's care, but has abandoned interest in any other children at home or other family members. This is often a consequence of, and begets further, blame, anger, and alienation between the spouses. This situation requires intensive social work intervention and can result in a breakdown of the marriage.

REFERENCES

1. Hazinski MF: *Nursing care of the critically ill child,* ed 2, St Louis, 1992, Mosby.
2. The John Hopkins Hospital Department of Pediatrics, Barone M, editor: *The Harriet Lane handbook,* ed 143, St Louis, 1996, Mosby.
3. Chameides L, Hazinski MF: *Textbook of pediatric advanced life support,* Dallas, 1994, American Heart Association.
4. Backofen JE, Rogers MC: Emergency management of the airway. In Rogers MC, editor: *Textbook of pediatric intensive care,* ed 2, vol 1, Baltimore, 1992, Williams & Wilkins.
5. Miller MJ and others: Oral breathing in newborn infants, *J Pediatr* 107:465, 1985.
6. Wittenborg MH, Gyepes M, Crocker D: Tracheal dynamics in infants with respiratory distress, stridor, and collapsing trachea, *Radiology* 88:653, 1967.
7. Roberts KB: Upper airway obstruction. In Roberts KB, editor: *Manual of clinical problems in pediatrics,* ed 4, Boston, 1995, Little, Brown.
8. Cote CJ, Todres ID: The pediatric airway. In Cote CJ and others, editors: *A practice of anesthesia for infants and children,* ed 2, Philadelphia, 1993, WB Saunders.
9. Hudgel DW, Hendricks C: Palate and hypopharynx: sites of inspiratory narrowing of the upper airway during sleep, *Am Rev Resp Dis* 138:1542, 1988.
10. Hogg JC and others: Age as a factor in the distribution of lower airway conductance and in the pathologic anatomy of obstructive lung disease, *N Engl J Med* 282:1283, 1970.
11. Dunill MS: Postnatal growth of the lung, *Thorax* 17:329, 1962.
12. Macklem PT: Airway obstruction and collateral ventilation, *Physiol Rev* 51:368, 1971.
13. Boyden EA: Development and growth of the airways. In Hodson WA, editor: *Development of the lung,* New York, 1977, Marcel Dekker.
14. Nelson NM: Respiration and circulation after birth. In Smith CA, Nelson NM, editors: *The physiology of the newborn infant,* Springfield, Ill, 1976, Charles C Thomas.
15. Cross KW, Tizard JP, Trythall DA: The gaseous metabolism of the newborn infant, *Acta Paediatr* 46:265, 1957.
16. Papastamelos C and others: Developmental changes in chest wall compliance in infancy and early childhood, *J Appl Physiol* 78:179, 1995.
17. Muller NL, Bryan AC: Chest wall mechanics and respiratory muscles in infants, *Pediatr Clin North Am* 26:503, 1979.
18. Manno M: Cardiopulmonary arrest and resuscitation. In Roberts KB, editor: *Manual of clinical problems in pediatrics,* ed 4, Boston, 1995, Little, Brown.
19. Walsh-Sukys M: Apnea. In Blumer JL, editor: *A practical guide to pediatric intensive care,* ed 3, St Louis, 1991, Mosby.
20. Cummins RO: *Textbook of advanced cardiac life support,* Dallas, 1994, The American Heart Association.
21. Abernathy LJ, Allan PL, Drummond GB: Ultrasound assessment of the position of the tongue during induction of anesthesia, *Br J Anaesth* 65:744, 1990.
22. Schleien CL and others: Cardiopulmonary resuscitation. In Rogers MC, editor: *Textbook of pediatric intensive care,* ed 2, vol 1, Baltimore, 1992, Williams & Wilkins.
23. Amar D and others: An alternative oxygen delivery system for infants and children: the post-anesthesia care unit, *Can J Anaesth* 38:49, 1991.
24. Benaron DA, Benitz WE: Maximizing the stability of oxygen delivered via nasal cannula, *Arch Pediatr Adolesc Med* 148:294, 1994.
25. Fan LL, Voyles JB: Determinations of inspiratory oxygen delivered by nasal cannula in infants with chronic lung disease, *J Pediatr* 103:923, 1983.
26. Vain NE and others: Regulation of oxygen concentration delivered to infants via nasal cannulas, *Am J Dis Child* 143:1458, 1989.
27. Salyer JW, Brzoska MR: Oxygen administration. In Blumer JR, editor: *A practical guide to pediatric intensive care,* ed 3, St Louis, 1990, Mosby.
28. Lough MD, Doershuk CF, Stern PC: *Pediatric respiratory therapy,* Chicago, 1985, Year Book Medical.
29. Backofen JE, Rogers MC: Upper airway disease. In Rogers MC, editor: *Textbook of pediatric intensive care,* ed 2, vol 1, Baltimore, 1992, Williams & Wilkins.
30. Chatburn RL: Assisted ventilation. In Blumer JL, editor: *A practical guide to pediatric intensive care,* ed 3, St Louis, 1991, Mosby.
31. Blumer JL, editor: *A practical guide to pediatric intensive care,* ed 3, St Louis, 1991, Mosby.
32. Stenquist O, Bagge U: Cuff pressure and microvascular occlusion in the tracheal mucosa, *Acta Otolaryngol* 88:451, 1979.
33. Arnold J: Tracheotomy. In Blumer JL, editor: *A practical guide to pediatric intensive care,* ed 3, St Louis, 1991, Mosby.

34. Donn SM, Kuhns LR: Mechanisms of endotracheal tube movement with change of head position in the neonate, *Pediatr Radiol* 9:39, 1980.
35. Brasch RC, Heldt GP, Hecht ST: Endotracheal tube orifice abutting the tracheal wall: a case of infant airway obstruction, *Pediatr Radiol* 141:387, 1981.
36. Benjamin PK, Thompson JE, O'Rourke PP: Complications of mechanical ventilation in a children's hospital multidisciplinary care unit, *Respir Care* 35:873, 1990.
37. Martin LD and others: Principles of respiratory support and mechanical ventilation. In Rogers MC, editor: *Textbook of pediatric intensive care,* ed 2, vol 1, Baltimore, 1992, Williams & Wilkins.
38. Mushin WW and others: Bird ventilators; Bourns "adult volume" ventilator "Bear 1"; Bourns "infant pressure" ventilator BP 200; Bourns "infant volume" ventilator LS 104-150; Siemens-Elema "Servo" ventilator 900. In Mushin WW, editor: *Automatic ventilation of the lungs,* ed 3, St Louis, 1980, Blackwell Scientific.
39. Greenough A, Morley C, Davis J: Interaction of spontaneous respiration with artificial ventilation in preterm babies, *J Pediatr* 103:769, 1983.
40. Mushin WW and others: Clinical aspects of controlled respiration. In Mushin WW, editor: *Automatic ventilation of the lungs,* ed 3, Oxford, 1980, Blackwell Scientific.
41. Binda RE Jr, Cook DR, Fischer CG: Advantages of infant ventilators over adapted adult ventilators in pediatrics, *Anesth Analg* 55:769, 1976.
42. Martin LD and others: Inspiratory work and response times of a modified pediatric volume ventilator during synchronized intermittent mandatory ventilation and pressure support ventilation, *Anesthesiology* 71:977, 1989.
43. Fiastro JF, Habib MP, Quan SF: Pressure support compensation for inspiratory work due to endotracheal tubes and demand CPAP, *Chest* 93:499, 1988.
44. Kacmarek RM: The role of pressure support ventilation in reducing work of breathing, *Respir Care,* 33:99, 1988.
45. Brochard L and others: Inspiratory pressure support prevents diaphragmatic fatigue during weaning from mechanical ventilation, *Am Rev Resp Dis* 139:513, 1989.
46. Arnold J: Extubation. In Blumer JL, editor: *A practical guide to pediatric intensive care,* ed 3, St Louis, 1990, Mosby.
47. Koka BV and others: Postintubation croup in children, *Anesth Analg* 556:501, 1977.
48. Jordan WS, Graves CL, Elwyn RA: New therapy for post-intubation laryngeal edema and tracheitis in children, *JAMA* 212:585, 1970.
49. Kemper KJ, Benson, MS, Bishop MJ: Predictors of postextubation stridor in pediatric trauma patients, *Crit Care Med* 19:352, 1991.
50. LeSouef PN, England SJ, Bryan AC: Total resistance of the respiratory system in preterm infants with and without an endotracheal tube, *J Pediatr* 104:108, 1984.
51. Wall MA: Infant endotracheal tube resistance: effects of changing length, diameter, and gas density, *Crit Care Med* 8:38, 1980.
52. Shimada Y and others: Crying vital capacity and maximal inspiratory pressure as clinical indicators of readiness for weaning of infants less than a year of age, *Anesthesiology* 51:456, 1979.
53. Tepas JJ IV and others: Tracheostomy in neonates and small infants: problems and pitfalls, *Surgery* 89:635, 1981.
54. Azizkhan RG, Lacey SR, Wood RE: Anterior cricoid suspension and tracheal stomal closure for children with cricoid collapse and peristomal tracheomalacia following tracheostomy, *J Pediatr Surg* 28:169, 1993.
55. Ochi JW, Bailey CM, Evans JN: Pediatric airway reconstruction at Great Ormond Street: a ten year review. III. Decannulation and suprastomal collapse, *Ann Otol Rhinol Laryngol* 101:656, 1992.
56. Welliver J, Welliver R: Bronchiolitis, *Pediatr Rev* 14:134, 1993.
57. American Academy of Pediatrics: Summary of infectious diseases. In Peter G, editor: *Red book: report of the committee on infectious diseases,* ed 23, Elk Grove, Ill, 1994, American Academy of Pediatrics.
58. Reese AC and others: Relationship between urinary creatinine level and diagnosis in children admitted to hospital, *Am Rev Resp Dis* 146:66, 1992.
59. Hall CB and others: Respiratory syncytial virus infection within families, *N Engl J Med* 294:414, 1976.
60. American Academy of Pediatrics Committee of Infectious Disease: Use of ribavirin in the treatment of respiratory syncytial virus infection, *Pediatrics* 92:501, 1993.
61. McConnochie K, Roghmann K: Wheezing at 8 and 13 years: changing importance of bronchiolitis and passive smoking, *Pediatr Pulmonol* 6:138, 1989.
62. Weiss ST and others: The relationship of respiratory infections in early childhood to the occurrence of increased levels of bronchial responsiveness and atopy, *Am Rev Resp Dis* 131:573, 1985.
63. Helfaer MA and others: Lower airway disease: bronchiolitis and asthma. In Rogers MC, editor: *Textbook of pediatric intensive care,* ed 2, vol 1, Baltimore, 1992, Williams & Wilkins.
64. Roberts KB: Bronchiolitis. In Roberts KB, editor: *Manual of clinical problems in pediatrics,* ed 4, Boston, 1995, Little, Brown.
65. Downes JJ and others: Acute respiratory failure in infants with bronchiolitis, *Anesthesiology* 29:426, 1968.
66. Muller N and others: Diaphragmatic muscle fatigue in the newborn, *J Appl Physiol* 46:688, 1979.
67. Anas N and others: The association of apnea and respiratory syncytial virus infection in infants, *J Pediatr* 101:65, 1982.
68. Gozal D and others: Water, electrolyte, and endocrine homeostasis in infants with bronchiolitis, *Pediatr Res* 27:204, 1990.
69. Reynolds EOR: Arterial blood gas tensions in acute disease of the lower respiratory tract in infancy, *Br Med Bull* 1:1192, 1963.
70. Hall CB, Hall J, Speers DM: Clinical and physiological manifestations of bronchiolitis and pneumonia, *Am J Dis Child* 133:798, 1979.

71. Reynolds EOR: The affect of breathing 40 percent oxygen on the arterial gas tensions of babies with bronchiolitis, *J Pediatr* 63:1135, 1963.
72. Outwater KM, Crone RK: Management of respiratory failure in infants with acute viral bronchiolitis, *Am J Dis Child* 138:1071, 1984.
73. Alario A and others: The efficacy of nebulized metaproterenol in wheezing infants and young children, *Am J Dis Child* 146:412, 1992.
74. Wang EE and others: Bronchodilators for treatment of mild bronchiolitis: a factorial randomized trial, *Arch Dis Child* 67:289, 1992.
75. Leer JA and others: Corticosteroid treatment in bronchiolitis: a controlled collaborative study in 297 infants and children, *Am J Dis Child* 117:495, 1969.
76. Stalcup SA, Mellins RB: Mechanical forces producing pulmonary edema and acute asthma, *N Engl J Med* 197:592, 1977.
77. Becroft DMO: Bronchiolitis obliterans, bronchiectasis, and other sequelae of adenovirus type 21 infection in young children, *J Clin Pathol* 24:72, 1971.
78. Groothius JR and others: Early ribavirin treatment of respiratory syncytial viral infection in high-risk children, *J Pediatr* 117:792, 1990.
79. Smith DW and others: A controlled trial of aerosolized ribavirin in infants receiving mechanical ventilation for severe respiratory syncytial virus infection, *N Engl J Med* 325:24, 1991.
80. Englund JA and others: High-dose, short-duration ribavirin aerosol therapy compared with standard ribavirin therapy in children with suspected respiratory syncytial virus infection, *J Pediatr* 125:635, 1994.
81. Frankel LR and others: A technique for the administration of ribavirin to mechanically ventilated infants with severe respiratory syncytial virus infection, *Crit Care Med* 15:1051, 1987.
82. Wald ER: Respiratory syncytial virus and viral pneumonia. In Blumer JL, editor: *A practical guide to pediatric intensive care,* ed 3, St Louis, 1991, Mosby.
83. National Heart Lung & Blood Institute National Asthma Educational Program Expert Panel: Guidelines for the diagnosis and management of asthma, *J Allergy Clin Immunol* 88:425, 1991.
84. Stokes DC: Respiratory failure and status asthmaticus. In Roberts KB, editor: *Manual of clinical problems in pediatrics,* Boston, 1995, Little, Brown.
85. Malfino N and others: Respiratory arrest in near-fatal asthma, *N Engl J Med* 324:285, 1991.
86. Zander J, Hazinski MF: Pulmonary disorders. In Hazinski MF, editor: *Nursing care of the critically ill child,* ed 2, St Louis, 1992, Mosby.
87. Asher M and others: Effects of chest physical therapy on lung function in children recovering from acute severe asthma, *Pediatr Pulmonol* 9:146, 1990.
88. Sutton PP: Chest physiotherapy: time for reappraisal, *Br J Dis Chest* 82:127, 1988.
89. Baker JW, Yerger S, Segar WE: Elevated plasma antidiuretic hormone levels in status asthmaticus, *Mayo Clin Proc* 51:31, 1976.
90. Connett G, Lenney W: Use of pulse oximetry in the hospital management of acute asthma in children, *Pediatr Pulmonol* 15:345, 1993.
91. McFadden ER Jr, Lyons HA: Arterial blood gas tension in asthma, *N Engl J Med* 278:1029, 1968.
92. Ruggins N: Pathophysiology of apnea in preterm infants, *Arch Dis Child* 66:70, 1991.
93. Richardson DK, Alleyne CM: Management of the sick newborn. In Graef JW, editor: *Manual of pediatric therapeutics,* ed 4, Boston, 1988, Little, Brown.
94. American Academy of Pediatrics: Task force on prolonged infantile apnea, *Pediatrics* 76:129, 1985.
95. Finer N and others: Obstructive, mixed, and central apnea in the neonate: physiological correlates, *J Pediatr* 121:943, 1992.
96. Walsh-Sukys M: Apnea. In Blummer JL, editor: *A practical guide to pediatric intensive care,* ed 3, St Louis, 1990, Mosby.
97. Camfield P and others: Infant apnea syndrome: a prospective evaluation of etiologies, *Clin Pediatr* 21:604, 1982.
98. Plaxico DT, Loughlin GM: Nasopharyngeal reflux and neonatal apnea, *Am J Dis Child* 135:793, 1981.
99. Shaffner DH, Gioia FR: Neuromuscular disease and respiratory failure. In Rogers MC, editor: *Textbook of pediatric intensive care,* ed 2, vol 1, Baltimore, 1992, Williams & Wilkins.
100. National Institutes of Health Consensus Panel: Development conference of infantile apnea and home monitoring, Sept. 29 to Oct. 1, 1986, *Pediatrics* 79:292, 1987.
101. Wong DL, editor: Health problems during infancy. In *Whaley and Wong's Nursing care of infants & children,* ed 5, St Louis, 1995, Mosby.
102. Moore KL, Persaud TVN: *The developing human, clinically oriented embryology,* ed 5, Philadelphia, 1993, WB Saunders.
103. Wong DL, editor: *Whaley and Wong's Nursing care of infants and children,* ed 5, St Louis, 1995, Mosby.
104. Burton DA, Cabalka AK: Cardiac evaluation of infants, *Pediatr Clin North Am* 41:991, 1994.
105. Gaedke-Norris MK, Roland JA: Perioperative management of pulmonary circulation in children with congenital cardiac defects, *AACN Clin Issues Crit Care Nurs* 5:255, 1994.
106. Emmanouilides GC and others, editors: *Moss and Adams heart disease in infants, children and adolescents including the fetus and young adults,* ed 5, Baltimore, 1995, Williams & Wilkins.
107. Jensen C, Hill CS: Mechanical support for congestive heart failure in infants and children, *Crit Care Nurs Clin North Am* 6:165, 1994.
108. O'Brien P, Smith PA: Chronic hypoxia in children with cyanotic heart disease, *Crit Care Nurs Clin North Am* 6:215, 1994.
109. Park MK, Guntheroth WG: *How to read pediatric ECGs,* ed 3, St Louis, 1992, Mosby.

110. Hanisch DG, Perron L: Complex dysrhythmias in infants and children, *AACN Clin Issues Crit Care Nurs* 3:255, 1992.
111. Beland MJ: Noninvasive transcutaneous cardiac pacing in children. In Birkui MD, Trigano J, Zool P, editors: *Noninvasive transcutaneous cardiac pacing,* Mount Kisco, NY, 1993, Futura Publishing.
112. Committee on Rheumatic Fever, Endocarditis, and Kawasaki Disease of the Council of Cardiovascular Disease of the Young recommended by the AHA: Prevention of bacterial endocarditis, *JAMA* 264:2919, 1990.
113. Curley MAQ, Smith JB, Moloney-Harmon PA, editors: *Critical care nursing of infants and children,* Philadelphia, 1996, WB Saunders.
114. Carcillo JA and others: Role of early fluid resuscitation in pediatric septic shock, *JAMA,* 266:1242, 1991.
115. Hughes G and others: Tape measure to aid prescription in pediatric resuscitation, *Arch Emerg Med,* 7:21, 1990.
116. Luden RC and others: Length based endotracheal tube and emergency equipment in pediatrics, *Ann Emerg Med,* 8:900, 1992.
117. Menkes JH: *Textbook of child neurology,* ed 5, Baltimore, 1995, Williams & Wilkins.
118. Kenner C, Brueggemeyer A, Gunderson LP, editors: *Comprehensive neonatal nursing: a physiological perspective,* Philadelphia, 1993, WB Saunders.
119. Lacroix J and others: Admissions to a pediatric intensive care unit for status epilepticus: a ten year experience, *Crit Care Med* 22:827, 1994.
120. Rivera R and others: Midazolam in the treatment of status epilepticus in children, *Crit Care Med* 21:991, 1993.
121. Carno M: Meningococcemia: recognizing and reducing complications in pediatric patients, *AACN Clin Issues Crit Care Nurs* 5:278, 1994.
122. Altimier LB: Pediatric central neurological trauma: issues for special patients, *AACN Clin Issues Crit Care Nurs* 3:31, 1992.
123. Dandrinos-Smith S: The epidemiology of pediatric trauma, *Crit Care Nurs Clin North Am* 3:387, 1991.
124. Moloney-Harmon PA, Czerwinski SJ: Caught in the crossfire: children, guns, and trauma, *Crit Care Nurs Clin North Am* 6:525, 1994.
125. Weaver LT: Anatomy and embryology. In Walker WA and others, editors: *Pediatric gastrointestinal disease: pathophysiology, diagnosis, management,* ed 2, vol 1, St Louis, 1996, Mosby.
126. Milla PJ: Feeding, tasting, sucking. In Walker WA and others, editors: *Pediatric gastrointestinal disease,* vol 1, Philadelphia, 1991, BC Decker.
127. Herbst JJ: Development of suck and swallow, *J Pediatr Gastroenterol Nutr* 2:S131, 1983.
128. Miller H, Anderson G: Non-nutritive sucking: effects on crying and heart rate in intubated infants requiring assisted mechanical ventilation, *Nurs Res* 42:305, 1993.
129. Schwartz R and others: A meta-analysis of critical outcome variables in non-nutritive sucking in preterm infants, *Nurs Res* 36:292, 1987.
130. Woodson R, Drinkwin J, Hamilton C: Effects of non-nutritive sucking on state and activity: term-preterm comparisons, *Infant Behav Dev* 8:435, 1985.
131. Bernbaum JC and others: Non-nutritive sucking during gavage feeding enhances growth and maturation in preterm infants, *Pediatrics* 71:41, 1983.
132. Szabo JS, Hillemeier C, Oh W: Effect of non-nutritive and nutritive suck on gastric emptying in premature infants, *J Pediatr Gastroenterol Nutr* 4:348, 1985.
133. Gryboski JD: Suck and swallow in the premature infant, *Pediatrics* 43:96, 1969.
134. Wong DL, editor: The high risk newborn and family. In *Whaley and Wong's nursing care of infants and children,* ed 5, St Louis, 1995, Mosby.
135. Barness LA, Curran JS: Nutritional requirements. In Behrman R, Kliegman RM, Arvin AM, editors: *Nelson textbook of pediatrics,* ed 15, Philadelphia, 1996, WB Saunders.
136. Williams PL, editor: *Gray's anatomy: the anatomical basis of medicine and surgery,* ed 38, New York, 1995, Churchill Livingstone.
137. Seibert JJ, Byrne WJ, Euler AR: Gastric emptying in children: unusual patterns detected by scintography, *Am J Radiol* 141:49, 1983.
138. Hughes CA, Dowling RH: Speed of onset of adaptive mucosal hypoplasia and hypofunction in the intestines of parentally fed rats, *Clin Sci* 59:317, 1980.
139. Lucas A, Bloom SR, Aynsley-Green A: Metabolic and endocrine consequences of depriving preterm infants of enteral nutrition, *Acta Paediatr Scand* 72:245, 1983.
140. Lebenthal E, Young CM: Effects of intrauterine and postnatal malnutrition on the ontogeny of gut function, *Prog Food Nutr Sci* 10:315, 1986.
141. Levine GM and others: Role of oral intake in maintenance of gut mass and disaccharidase activity, *Gastroenterol* 67:975, 1974.
142. Motil K: Development of the gastrointestinal tract. In Wyllie R, Hyams J, editors: *Pediatric gastrointestinal disease,* Philadelphia, 1993, WB Saunders.
143. Weaver LT: Anatomy and embryology. In Walker WA and others, editors: *Pediatric gastrointestinal disease,* vol 1, Philadelphia, 1991, BC Decker.
144. Udall JN, Watson RR: Development of immune function. In Walker WA and others, editors: *Pediatric gastrointestinal disease,* vol 1, Philadelphia, 1991, BC Decker.
145. Chu SH, Walker WA: Bacterial toxin interaction with the developing intestine, *Gastroenterol* 104:916, 1993.
146. Ho MS, Glass RI, Pinsky PF: Diarrheal deaths in American children: are they preventable? *JAMA* 260:3281, 1988.
147. Laney DW, Cohen MB: Approach to the pediatric patient with diarrhea, *Gastroenterol Clin North Am* 22:499, 1993.
148. Friis-Hansen B: Body composition during growth. In vivo measurements and biochemical data correlation to differential anatomical growth, *Pediatrics* 47(suppl 2):264, 1971.

149. Luban NLC: Blood groups and blood component transfusion. In Miller DR, editor: *Blood diseases of infancy and childhood,* ed 7, St Louis, 1995, Mosby.
150. Simmons CF Jr, Ichikawa I: External balance of water and electrolytes. In Ichikawa I, editor: *Pediatric textbook of fluids and electrolytes,* Baltimore, 1990, Williams & Wilkins.
151. Besunder JB: Abnormalities in fluids, minerals, and glucose. In Blumer JL, editor: *A practical guide to pediatric intensive care,* ed 3, St Louis, 1991, Mosby.
152. Holliday MA, Segar WE: The maintenance need for water in parenteral fluid therapy, *Pediatrics* 19:823, 1957.
153. Adelman RD, Solhung MJ: Fluid therapy. In Behrman RE, Kliegman RM, Arvin AM, editors: *Nelson textbook of pediatrics,* ed 15, Philadelphia, 1996, WB Saunders.
154. Harmon WE: Fluid and electrolytes. In Graef JW, editor: *Manual of pediatric therapeutics,* ed 4, Boston, 1988, Little, Brown.
155. Chwals WJ and others: Measured energy expenditure in critically ill infants and young children, *J Surg Res* 44:467, 1988.
156. Pollack MM: Nutritional support of children in the intensive care unit. In Suskind RM, Lewinter-Suskind L, editors: *Textbook of pediatric nutrition,* ed 2, New York, 1993, Raven Press.
157. Deutschman CS: Nutrition and metabolism in the critically ill child. In Rogers MC, editor: *Textbook of pediatric intensive care,* ed 2, vol 2, Baltimore, 1992, Williams & Wilkins.
158. Chwals W: Overfeeding the critically ill child: fact or fiction, *New Horiz* 2:147, 1994.
159. Kovacevich DS, editor: *Parenteral and enteral nutrition manual,* ed 7, Ann Arbor, Mich, 1994, University of Michigan Medical Center.
160. Kerner JA: Parenteral nutrition. In Walker WA and others, editors: *Pediatric gastrointestinal disease: pathophysiology, diagnosis, management,* ed 2, vol 2, St Louis, 1996, Mosby.
161. American Academy of Pediatrics Committee on Nutrition: Use of intravenous fat emulsions in pediatric patients, *Pediatrics* 68:738, 1981.
162. Reed MD: Principles of total parenteral nutrition. In Blumer JL, editor: *Practical guide to pediatric intensive care,* ed 3, St Louis, 1991, Mosby.
163. Hamill PVV: *National Center for Health Statistics: growth charts for children birth-18 years, United States, vital & health statistics series 11,* No 165, DHEW Pub No 78-1650, Washington DC, 1977, DHEW.
163a. American Academy of Pediatrics Committee on Nutrition: *Pediatric nutrition handbook,* ed 3, Chicago, 1993, American Academy of Pediatrics.
164. Sinden AA, Dillard VL, Sutphen JL: Enteral nutrition. In Walker WA and others, editors: *Pediatric gastrointestinal disease: pathophysiology, diagnosis, management,* ed 2, vol 2, St Louis, 1996, Mosby.
165. Gottschlick M and others: Diarrhea in tube-fed burn patients: incidence, etiology, nutritional impact, and prevention, *JPEN J Parent Ent Nutr* 12:338, 1988.
166. Berger R, Adams L: Nutritional supplement in the critical care setting (Part II), *Chest* 96:372, 1989.
167. Orenstein SR: Enteral versus parenteral therapy for intractable diarrhea of infancy: a prospective, randomized trial, *J Pediatr* 109:277, 1986.
168. Yahov J and others: Assessment of intestinal and cardiorespiratory function in children with congenital heart disease on high-calorie formulas, *J Pediatr Gastroenterol Nutr* 4:778, 1985.
169. Wong DL, editor: Pediatric variations of nursing interventions. In *Whaley and Wong's nursing care of infants and children,* ed 5, St Louis, 1995, Mosby.
170. Welch JA and others: Staff nurses' experience as co-investigators in a clinical research project, *Pediatr Nurs* 16:364, 1990.
171. Anand KJ: Neonatal stress responses to anesthesia and surgery, *Clin Perinatol* 17:201, 1990.
172. McGrath PJ, Craig KD: Developmental and psychological factors in children's pain, *Pediatr Clin North Am* 36:823, 1989.
173. Altimier L and others: Post-operative pain management in preverbal children: the prescription and administration of analgesics with and without caudal analgesia, *J Pediatr Nurs* 9:226, 1994.
174. Schecter NL, Allen D: Physicians' attitudes toward pain in children, *J Dev Behav Pediatr* 7:350, 1986.
175. Hall SJ: Pediatric pain assessment in intensive care units, *Crit Care Nurs* 11:20, 1995.
176. Romsing J and others: Post-operative pain in children: comparison between ratings of children and nurses, *J Pain Symptom Manage* 11:42, 1996.
177. Finley GA and others: Parents' management of childrens' pain following "minor" surgery, *Pain* 64:83, 1996.
178. Anand KJS, Hickey PR: Pain and its effects in the human neonate and fetus, *N Engl J Med* 317:1321, 1987.
179. Way WL, Costley EC, Way EL: Respiratory sensitivity of the newborn infant to meperidine and morphine, *Clin Pharmacol Ther* 6:454, 1965.
180. Bhat R and others: Pharmacokinetics of a single dose of morphine in preterm infants during the first week of life, *J Pediatr* 117:477, 1990.
181. Kupferberg HJ, Way EL: Pharmacologic basis for the increased sensitivity of the newborn rat to morphine, *J Pharmacol Exp Ther* 141:105, 1963.
182. Wood M: Opioid agonists and antagonists. In Wood M, Wood AJJ, editors: *Drugs and anesthesia: pharmacology for anesthesiologists,* Baltimore, 1990, Williams & Wilkins.
183. Pokela ML and others: Age related morphine kinetics in infants, *Dev Pharmacol Ther* 20:26, 1993.
184. Yaster M and others: Pain, sedation, and post-operative anesthetic management in the pediatric intensive care unit. In Rogers MC, editor: *Textbook of pediatric intensive care,* ed 2, vol 2, Baltimore, 1992, Williams & Wilkins.
185. Hertzka RE and others: Fentanyl induced ventilatory depression: effects of age, *Anesthesiology* 70:213, 1989.
186. Singleton MA, Rosen JI, Fisher DM: Plasma concentrations of fentanyl in infants, children, and adults, *Can J Anesth* 34:152, 1987.

187. Anand KJS, Carr DB: The neuroanatomy, neurophysiology, and neurochemistry of pain, stress and analgesia in newborns and children, *Pediatr Clin North Am* 36:795, 1989.
188. Schechter NL and others: Individual differences in children's response to pain: role of temperament and parental characteristics, *Pediatrics* 82:171, 1991.
189. Hamers JPH and others: The influence of children's vocal expression, age, medical diagnosis, and information obtained from parents on nurses' pain assessment and decisions regarding intervention, *Pain* 65:53, 1996.
190. Acute Pain Management Guideline Panel: *Acute pain management: operative or medical procedures and trauma. Clinical practice guideline,* AHCPR Pub No 92-0032, Rockville, Md, 1992, Agency for Health Care Policy and Research, Public Health Service, US Department of Health and Human Services.
191. McGrath PJ and others: Report of the subcommittee on assessment and methodological issues in the management of pain in childhood cancer, *Pediatrics* 86:816, 1990.
192. Attia I and others: Measurement of post-operative pain and narcotic administration in infants using a new clinical scoring system, *Anesthesiology* 67:a532, 1987.
193. McGrath PA and others: CHEOPS: a behavioral scale for rating post-operative pain in children. In Felds HL and others, editors: *Advances in pain research and therapy,* New York, 1985, Raven Press.
194. Taddio A and others: A revised measure of acute pain in infants, *J Pain Symptom Manage* 10:456, 1995.
195. Beyer JE: *The Oucher: a user's manual and technical report,* Denver, 1984, University of Colorado.
195a. Eland JM: The child who is hurting, *Semin Oncol Nurs* 1:116, 1985.
195b. Hester NO: The pre-operational child's reaction to immunization, *Nurs Res* 29:250, 1979.
196. Van Cleve LJ, Savedra MC: Pain location: validity and reliability of body outline markings by 4 to 7 year old children who are hospitalized, *Pediatr Nurs* 19:217, 1993.
197. Wong DL, Baker C: Pain in children: comparison of assessment scales, *Pediatr Nurs* 14:9, 1988.
198. Hester NO: Personal correspondance, October 20, 1994.
199. McGrath PJ, Unruh A: Pain in children and adolescents, Amsterdam, *Elsevier* 1:351, 1987.
200. McGrath PA: Pain in the pediatric patient: practical aspects of assessment, *Pediatr Ann* 24:126, 1995.
201. Manne SL and others: Adult-child interaction during invasive medical procedures, *Health Psychol* 11:241, 1992.
202. Stein PR: Indices of pain intensity: construct validity among preschoolers, *Pediatr Nurs* 21:119, 1995.
203. Hester NO and others: *Measurement of children's pain by children, parents, and nurses: psychometric and clinical issues related to the poker chip tool and the pain ladder. Generalizability of procedures assessing pain in children: final report,* Grant No NR01382, Washington DC, 1989, National Center for Nursing Research.
204. Beyer JE, McGrath PJ, Berde CB: Discordance between self-report and behavioral pain measures in children aged 3-7 years after surgery, *J Pain Symptom Manage* 5:350, 1990.
205. Anand KJS, Arnold JA: Opioid tolerance and dependence in infants and children, *Crit Care Med* 22:334, 1994.
206. Farrington EA and others: Continuous intravenous morphine infusion in postoperative newborn infants, *Am J Perinatol* 10:84, 1993.
207. Lynn AM and others: Respiratory effects of intravenus morphine infusions in neonates, infants, and children after cardiac surgery, *Anesth Analg* 77:695, 1993.
208. Nichols DG and others: Disposition and respiratory effects of intrathecal morphine in children, *Anesthesiology* 79:733, 1993.
209. Friedman SB and others: Behavioral observation on parents anticipating the death of a child, *Pediatrics* 32:610, 1963.
210. Lindemann E: Symptomatology and management of acute grief, *Am J Psychiatry* 101:141, 1944.
211. Freud A: The role of bodily illness in the mental life of children, *Psychoanal Study Child* 7:69, 1952.
212. Caty S, Ellerton ML, Ritchie JA: Coping in hospitalized children: analysis of published case studies, *Nurs Res* 33:277, 1984.
213. Vernon DTA: *The psychological responses of children to hospitalization and illness,* Springfield, Ill, 1965, Charles C Thomas.
214. Rothstein P: Psychological stress in families of children in a pediatric intensive care unit, *Pediatr Clin North Am* 27:613, 1980.
215. Wolfer JA, Visintainer MA: Pediatric surgical patients' and parents' stress responses and adjustment, *Nurs Res* 24:244, 1975.
216. Mahaffy PR: The effects of hospitalization on children admitted for tonsillectomy and adenoidectomy, *Nurs Res* 14:12, 1965.
217. Neuhauser C and others: Children's concepts of healing: cognitive development and locus of control factors, *Am J Orthopsychiatry* 48:325, 1978.
218. Brewster AB: Chronically ill hospitalized children's concepts of their illness, *Pediatrics* 69:355, 1982.
219. Steward M, Regalbuto G: Do doctors know what children know? *Am J Orthopsychiatry* 45:146, 1975.
220. Stevens M: Adolescents' perception of stressful events during hospitalization, *J Pediatr Nurs* 1:303, 1986.
221. Schowalter J: Psychological reactions to physical illness and hospitalization in adolescents, *Child Psychiatry Hum Dev* 16:500, 1977.
222. Carter MC and others: Parental environmental stress in pediatric intensive care units, *DCCN* 4:180, 1985.
223. Curley MA: Effects of the nursing mutual participation model of care on parental stress in the pediatric intensive care unit, *Heart Lung* 17:682, 1988.
224. Affonso DD and others: Stressors reported by mothers of hospitalized premature infants, *Neonatal Network* 11:63, 1992.

High Risk and Critical Care Obstetric Issues

During the past 10 years, the worlds of critical care and obstetrics have seen a new emphasis on collaboration and integration. Traditionally, the two specialties have been separated, in part because of the typical normalcy and health-oriented approach of obstetrics and the crisis and illness orientation of critical care. During the past decade many factors have influenced the current integration we now see. Societal trends have had a significant impact. Many women are planning childbirth experiences at a later age, in part because of careers, educational plans, or second marriages. Technologic advances have had an impact in several ways. Advances have allowed women with congenital diseases to survive to childbearing age. Technology has also made it possible for more women to survive the antepartal experience. Advances in infertility have also played a role in the advent of critical care obstetrics.

It is important to recognize that critical care obstetrics encompasses two distinct populations: women with preexisting disease who become pregnant and women with normal pregnancies that become compromised by critical illness or injury. There are management considerations that are unique to pregnant critically ill women, some of which have been recently recognized (Box 10-1).

It would be impossible to discuss every aspect of management of the critically ill obstetric patient in one chapter. Instead, the focus and goal of this chapter is twofold: first, to provide a synopsis of the more commonly seen conditions or concerns in the realm of critical care obstetrics, and second, to emphasize the collaborative nature of this emerging field, recognizing that the manifestations and management are typically identical in pregnant and nonpregnant patients, although there must be consideration of the data value changes associated with pregnancy. Nursing management, unless unique to the critically ill obstetric patient, is not detailed.

FETAL DEVELOPMENT

Key to understanding the fetus is an appreciation for the timing of morphologic and functional development.[1] There are three defined stages in fetal development:[2]

Preembryonic stage: first 14 days of human development.

Embryonic stage: day 15 through 8 weeks. It is a period of tissue differentiation and essential organ development. Key developments in this period are at 4 weeks, as the fetal heart begins beating, and at 6 weeks, as the fetal circulation is established.

Fetal stage: 8 weeks through 40 weeks/delivery. It is a period in which structures are refined and function is perfected. Between 8 and 12 weeks, all organs are formed.

Factors that influence embryonic and fetal development include exposure to teratogens, maternal nutrition, and adequate maternal circulation. Developmental defects may be genetic or environmental in cause. Drug exposure accounts for 2% to 3% of all birth defects, genetic causes account for 25%, and the remaining causes may be multifactorial and are classified as "unknown."[2] The embryo is especially vulnerable to teratogens during organ system development. Figure 10-1 shows sensitive or critical periods in human development. The major risks of radiation exposure are fetal demise, growth retardation, congenital malformations, mental retardation, and sterility. Exposure to ionizing radiation is usually not of

BOX 10-1 Primary Goals in Managing a Critically Ill Obstetric Patient

- Optimizing maternal physiologic functioning
- Recognizing and treating potential or actual complications early
- Supporting fetal growth and development
- Supporting the maternal and family experience

concern until more than 50 to 100 (1×10^{-5} Gy [5 to 10 rads]) have been exceeded.[3,4] Use of proper shielding techniques and selective ordering of studies assists in decreasing risks to the mother and fetus. Static images generally create less radiation exposure than dynamic images such as computed tomography (CT) and angiography. Table 10-1 lists radiation exposure of common radiologic studies.[3,4]

Medication use in critically ill obstetric patients requires analysis of the risk-benefit ratio. Often the benefit may outweigh the potential fetal risk when all factors are considered. It is important to remember the influence that drug exposure can have on the developing fetus. See Box 10-2 for FDA labels regarding a drug's risk to a fetus.

Technologic advances, improvements in maternal-fetal diagnostics, and aggressive neonatal interventions have improved the survival of preterm infants. The minimum age for fetal survival is not clearly defined and at times controversial. *Viability* is defined as the ability of the fetus to survive in a defined environment, with fetal development being the ultimate determinate. Current research places minimum viability parameters between 23 to 26 weeks gestation and fetal weight between 500 to 1000 g (0.5 to 1.0 kg). Clinical outcomes improve dramatically when the fetus is 25 weeks or older and more than 1000 g, because of the advancing development of fetal organ systems.[1] Critical care clinicians may encounter situations when extrauterine viability, fetal outcomes, and maternal stability are uncertain. Clinical decisions must be made in light of the maternal fetal–risk benefit ratio. Personal, cultural, spiritual, and social beliefs regarding viability may affect the clinical decision-making process. Parental and family beliefs and desires may conflict with those of the health care team. When confronting the dilemma of viability, the parameters of gestational age, fetal weight, parental desires, and maternal-fetal mortality must be considered.

PLACENTAL DEVELOPMENT AND FUNCTION

Pregnancy is a time of major maternal physiologic and metabolic adaptations. These adaptations are necessary for the optimal growth and survival of the fetus. There are three mechanisms by which the fetoplacental unit influences maternal physiology and metabolism (Box 10-3).

Knowledge of the function and anatomy of the placenta provides insight into the pathology of pregnancy.[5] The placenta is generally regarded as an organ with the primary functions of oxygen transport, nutrition, and waste removal between the fetal and maternal circulation. There is a fetal side, where the chorionic villus circulation occurs, and a maternal side, where the placental bed forms and the uretoplacental vessels are found. Placental development begins at approximately 3 weeks gestation and develops at the site of embryo implantation. Growth continues to 20 weeks when it covers about one half of the inside of the uterus. After 20 weeks, the placenta only becomes thicker versus enlarging to cover more uterine surface.

The placenta also has endocrine functions and immunologic properties. Placental function depends on adequate maternal circulation. Blood flow to the uterus is dependent on systemic blood pressure, condition of blood vessels, maternal position, and uterine contractions. Contractions cause a decrease in uterine blood flow that is proportional to intensity and duration.

When the placenta is fully developed, fetal blood in the villi and maternal blood in the intervillous spaces are separated by a thin layer of tissue. Fetal blood flows through two umbilical arteries to the villi, and oxygenated blood flows through the umbilical vein to the fetus. Maternal blood, rich with oxygen and nutrients, enters the intervillous spaces where maternal-fetal exchange occurs. Figure 10-2 shows the vascular arrangement of the placenta.

The placental membranes manage transfer activity of substances via five major mechanisms.[6] Simple diffusion moves substances such as water, oxygen, carbon dioxide, and electrolytes from an area of high to low concentration. Facilitated diffusion moves substances requiring a carrier system, such as glucose and some oxygen, from an area of higher concentration to an area of lower concentration. Active transport moves substances such as amino acids, calcium, iron, iodine, and water-soluble vitamins from an area of low concentration to high concentration. Pinocytosis is necessary for transport of large molecules such as albumin and immune gamma globulin. Hydrostatic and

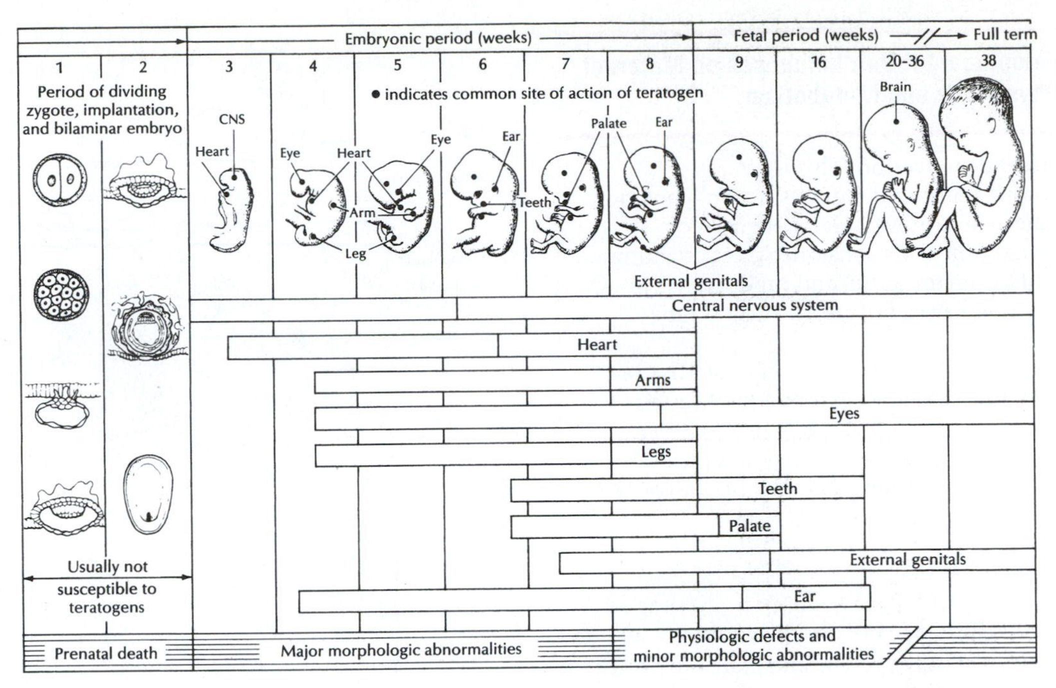

FIGURE 10-1 Sensitive, or critical, periods in human development. (From Lowdermilk D, Perry S, Bobak I: *Maternity & Women's Health Care,* ed 6, St Louis, 1996, Mosby.)

TABLE 10-1 Radiation Dose from Radiologic Studies

Radiologic Study Exposure	Estimated Fetal Radiation (1×10^{-5} Gy)
Chest x-ray	8
Skull x-ray	4
Cervical spine x-ray	2
Thoracic spine x-ray	402
Lumbar spine x-ray	275
Abdominal x-ray	185
IV/retrograde pyelography	585
Upper GI x-ray	330
Lower GI x-ray	465
Pelvimetry	750
Hip x-ray	100
Lower extremity x-ray	1

BOX 10-2 The FDA Categories of Labeling for Drug Use in Pregnancy

- Category A-Controlled studies in women fail to demonstrate risk to the fetus in the first 12 weeks. Possibility of fetal harm is remote.
- Category B-Animal studies do not indicate a risk to the fetus. Well-controlled studies with pregnant mothers fail to demonstrate a risk to the fetus.
- Category C-Studies have shown teratogenic effects in animal studies. There are no controlled studies in women.
- Category D-Evidence of fetal risk exists, but benefits in life-threatening or serious disease may make use acceptable despite risks.
- Category X-Studies demonstrate fetal abnormalities, or there is evidence of risk from human experience. The risk clearly outweighs the benefit.

Modified from G Briggs, R Freeman, S Yaffe: *Drugs in pregnancy and lactation,* ed 4, Baltimore, 1995, Williams & Wilkins.

osmotic pressure allow the majority of water flow. Factors that affect transport rate include size of the molecule, maternal-fetal-placental blood flow, placental area, blood saturation with oxygen and nutrients, and diffusion distance.

The fetus has inherent mechanisms to maintain adequate oxygenation in the presence of maternal hypoxia. The maternal PaO_2 needs to be greater than 60 mm Hg to promote release of oxygen from the red blood cells. Placental blood flow and the fetal hemoglobin level must also be adequate. The fetus is initially able to adapt to hypoxia because of its high hematocrit level and the hemoglobins' increased affinity for oxygen. The fetus can also shunt blood flow to the brain and heart to protect vital functions. Figure 10-3 shows alterations of fetal heart rate patterns by favorable and unfavorable physiologic responses to hypoxia.

BOX 10-3 Fetoplacental Unit Influences on Maternal Physiology and Metabolism

- Uteroplacental circulation: This is a massive arteriovenous shunt that requires major adaptation of the maternal cardiovascular system.
- Fetoplacental unit: This consumes great quantities of nutrients, excretes waste, and produces substances that have a hormonal effect on the mother.
- Developing fetus: Fetus and enlarging uterus exert pressure on the surrounding organs and vessels.

Adapted from DiSaia PJ: Radiation in gynecology. In Scott J and others, editors: *Danforth's obstetrics and gynecology,* ed 7, Philadelphia, 1994, JB Lippincott.

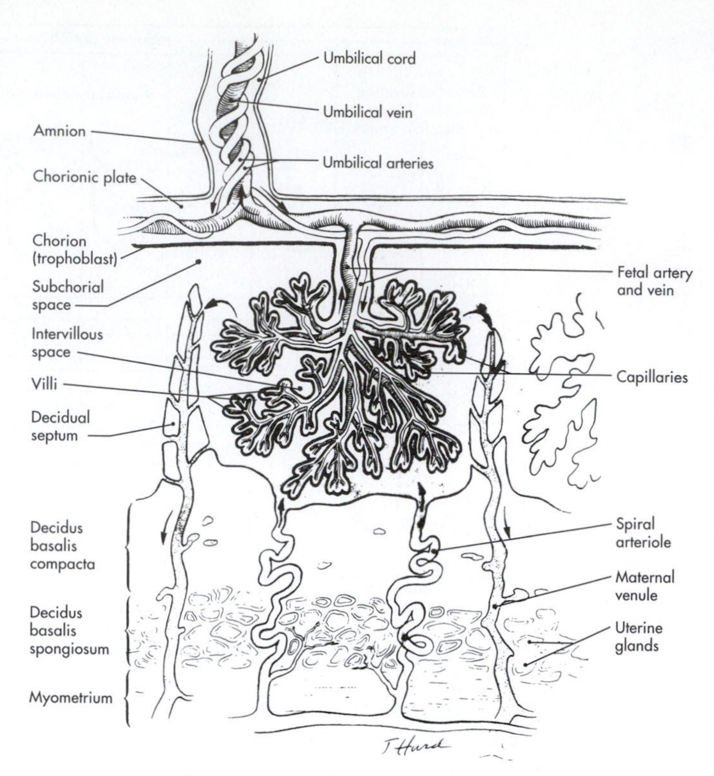

FIGURE 10-2 Cross section through placenta. *Arrows* indicate direction of blood flow. (From Bobak I, Jensen M: *Maternity and gynecologic care,* ed 5, St Louis, 1993, Mosby.)

The endocrine functions of the placenta are also essential to the survival of the fetus. The placenta produces several key hormones. Human chorionic gonadotropin (HCG) feeds the corpus luteum until the placenta fully develops and causes secretion of small amounts of testosterone. Human placental lactogen (HPL) stimulates changes in maternal metabolic processes and assists with protein and glucose uptake to the fetus. Progesterone allows for implantation to occur and decreases contractility of the uterus. Estrogen, secreted by the placenta as estriol, increases vascularity and promotes vasodilation in the villous capillaries.

Critically ill obstetric patients must be considered as part of a maternal-fetal-placental unit. Disease states or conditions that impair the transport of oxygen and nutrients or have the potential for fetal morbidity require corrective efforts. Pregnancies considered at risk for uteroplacental insufficiency carry a serious threat for intrauterine growth retardation (IUGR), intrauterine fetal death (IUFD), or fetal distress.[7] Corrective efforts to improve uterine blood flow include maternal positioning, oxygen therapy, hydration therapy, blood replacement products, and delivery of the fetus from an unfavorable environment.

PHYSIOLOGIC ALTERATIONS IN PREGNANCY

During pregnancy, the woman's body undergoes profound physiologic changes. These changes are necessary to maintain the pregnancy and to allow for fetal growth and development. So dramatic are the changes that they would probably be considered pathologic in the nonpregnant woman. Adaptations occur in nearly every organ system, beginning during the first week of gestation and continuing until up to 6 weeks after delivery. The only system where there are no documented characteristic changes is the nervous system. Understanding the physiologic adaptations is important to the management of the critically ill pregnant woman. In the limited space of this text there is not room for an exhaustive description of each adaptation. Physiologic changes are summarized, with special attention given to those areas that affect or are affected by critical illness or injury. The authors refer the reader to a comprehensive obstetric text for expanded detail.

Endocrine System

Hormonal changes are critically important to the initiation and maintenance of pregnancy. Maintenance of adequate estrogen and progesterone levels is essential (Box 10-4). During pregnancy, estrogen production increases approximately one thousandfold.[8] Progesterone is essential for maintenance of pregnancy and is first produced by the corpus luteum, then by the placental unit. HPL promotes maternal breakdown of lipids, causing increased levels and use of free fatty acids, and has an anti-insulin effect, contributing to hyperglycemia. HPL also contributes to breast growth and development, preparing the breasts for lactation.

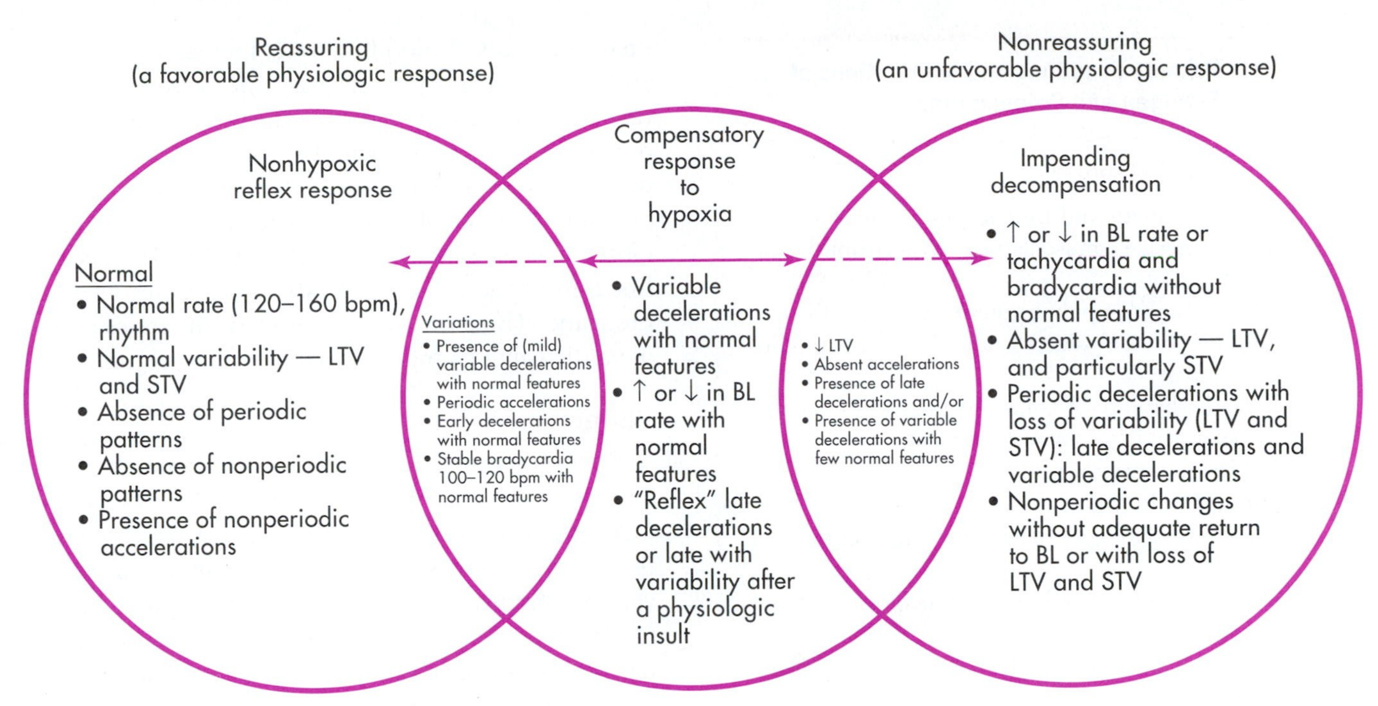

FIGURE 10-3 Alterations of fetal heart rate patterns by dynamic physiologic response. *LTV,* Long-term variability; *STV,* short-term variability; *BL,* baseline. (Modified from Adelsperger D: *Fetal heart monitoring: principles and practice,* Washington DC, 1993, AWHONN)

Thyroid enlargement and stimulation occur during pregnancy, causing an increase of approximately 25% in the maternal basal metabolic rate.

Reproductive System

Reproductive organs undergo remarkable changes during pregnancy. The uterus increases in weight 20 times and alters its capacity from 10 ml to 4.5 to 5 liters. The uterus grows out of the pelvic cavity, displacing intestines laterally and superiorly. When the pregnant woman assumes a supine position, the gravid uterus may compress the inferior vena cava and aorta, decreasing venous return to the heart.

Uterine blood flow increases dramatically as pregnancy progresses, from 50 ml/minute at 10 weeks to 500 ml/minute at 40 weeks.[9,10] Major expansion of the uterine vascular bed contributes to the development of decreased systemic vascular resistance.

Cardiovascular System

Pregnancy is characterized as a hyperdynamic (high flow), low-resistance state. This is facilitated through adaptations in blood volume, cardiac structure, cardiac output, vascular resistance, and heart rate.

Blood volume changes

- Total blood volume increases approximately 30% to 40%, or 1 to 1.5 L
- Blood volume maximizes between the 26th and 34th weeks
- Red blood cell volume increases approximately 20%
- Plasma volume increases 45% to 50%
- Total body water increases by approximately 6 to 8 L
- Colloid oncotic pressure (COP) decreases

Cardiac structural changes

- Heart is displaced to the left and upward and rotates slightly anteriorly
- No characteristic electrocardiographic changes
- Left axis deviation may occur because of mechanical displacement
- Cardiac volume increases slightly because of increased volume and hypertrophy

Cardiac ausculatory changes

- Physiologic S_1 (first heart sound) split
- S_3 (third heart sound) development is considered normal
- Systolic murmurs develop in 90% of all pregnant women
- Diastolic murmurs develop in 20% of all pregnant women
- Murmurs are physiologic in nature and disappear after delivery

Blood pressure variations may occur during pregnancy. Blood pressure may decrease slightly during the first trimester, reach a low point in the second trimester, and then return to normal for the duration of the pregnancy. Postural hypotension may occur with sudden position changes or supine positioning.

BOX 10-4 Primary Functions and Implications of Estrogen and Progesterone

FUNCTIONS OF ESTROGEN:

- Promotes growth and function of the uterus
- Causes uterine musculature hypertrophy and hyperplasia
- Increases blood supply to uteroplacental unit
- Promotes breast (ductal, alveolar, and nipple) development
- Increases pliability of connective tissue
  - Relaxes pelvic joints and ligaments
  - Allows for cervical softening
- Promotes sodium and water retention
- Produces psychologic changes, leading to emotional lability
- Decreases gastric secretion of hydrochloric acid and pepsin
- Increases sensitivity to carbon dioxide levels in the blood
- Produces integumentary changes
  - Hyperpigmentation
  - Stria gravidarum
- Affects blood component concentrations
  - Increases fibrinogen (factor I) concentration
  - Decreases plasma protein concentration
  - Causes leukocytosis

FUNCTIONS OF PROGESTERONE:

- Decreases maternal smooth muscle contractility
  - Uterus: prevents contractility
  - GI tract: contributes to nausea, heartburn, and constipation
  - Renal: contributes to urinary dilation, leading to urinary stasis
  - Vascular: dilates vessels and contributes to peripheral edema
- Produces metabolic effects
  - Resets hypothalamus up approximately 0.2° C (0.5° F)
  - Promotes fat storage
- Stimulates respiratory center to decrease CO_2 retention
- Stimulates secretion of sodium in the urine, thereby stimulating aldosterone production
- Promotes breast development and inhibits the action of prolactin

Cardiac output (CO) changes begin early in the first trimester, peak at the end of the second trimester, and remain elevated until term. Cardiac output increases 30% to 50% during pregnancy, with normal levels usually 6 to 7 L/minute.[11] Changes are attributed to increased blood volume, increased heart rate, and decreases in systemic vascular resistance. Heart rate increases 10 to 15 beats/minute during the second trimester and returns to normal 6 weeks postpartum. CO varies markedly depending on maternal position[12] (Table 10-2). The American College of Obstetricians and Gynecologists (ACOG) have defined indications for hemodynamic monitoring in pregnancy (Box 10-5). Table 10-3 summarizes hemodynamic value changes associated with pregnancy.[11,13]

Pulmonary System

Pulmonary physiologic changes are essential to provide adequate oxygenation for the mother's increased metabolic demands, as well as for the dependent fetus. As the uterus grows, it causes diaphragmatic elevation of approximately 4 cm, decreasing lung length. Compensatory and hormonal changes cause lower rib flaring and thoracic cage enlargement of 5 to 7 cm.[10,13]

Oxygen consumption increases approximately 15% to 25% throughout pregnancy. To meet these needs for additional oxygen, ventilatory changes (Figure 10-4) must occur. Vital capacity remains unchanged during pregnancy; however, there is an increase in tidal volume and slight increase in respiratory rate. Together, these account for an increase in minute ventilation by approximately 50% at term. Hyperventilation is normal and is primarily mediated by the effects of progesterone on the respiratory center. Hyperventilation causes a normal decrease in Pa_{CO_2} levels to approximately 28 to 32 mm Hg.[10,13] The resulting alkalosis is compensated by increased renal excretion of bicarbonate. Normal maternal Pa_{O_2} is 101 to 108 mm Hg.[10,13] The maternal oxyhemoglobin dissociation curve shifts to the right, facilitating the exchange of carbon dioxide from the fetus to the mother and the exchange of oxygen from the mother to the fetus.

Gastrointestinal System/Genitourinary System

There are both functional and structural gastrointestinal/genitourinary (GI/GU) system changes in pregnancy. Physiologic adaptations of the GI system are summarized in Table 10-4. Genitourinary structural changes include slight enlargement of the kidneys; dilation of pelvic, caliceal, and ureteral structures; bladder displacement forward and upward, and impaired blood and lymph drainage after the second trimester. Increases in blood volume and cardiac output, lowered systemic vascular resistance, and hormonal effects contribute to the primary physiologic functional changes summarized in Table 10-5. The greater increase in glomerular filtration rate over renal plasma flow increases the proportion of filtered

TABLE 10-2 Positional Cardiac Output Changes in Pregnancy

Maternal Position	Cardiac Output Range (L/min)
Knee-chest	6.9 (+/−2.1)
Right lateral	6.8 (+/−1.3)
Left lateral	6.6 (+/−1.4)
Sitting	6.2 (+/−2.0)
Supine	6.0 (+/−1.4)
Standing	5.4 (+/−2.0)

Clark S and others: *Am J Obstet Gynecol* 164(3):883, 1991.

BOX 10-5 ACOG Indications for Hemodynamic Monitoring in Pregnancy

- Severe pregnancy induced hypertension with persistent oliguria or pulmonary edema
- Massive hemorrhage or volume replacement needs
- Acute respiratory distress syndrome
- Shock of unknown etiology
- Sepsis with oliguria or refractory hypotension
- Cardiovascular decompensation during intrapartum or intraoperative periods
- Chronic disease during labor or intraoperatively (NYHA* Class III or IV cardiac disease)
- Pulmonary edema, oliguria, or heart failure refractory to treatment or of unknown etiology

**NYHA*, New York Heart Association.
Modified from American College of Obstetricians and Gynecologists: *Technical Bulletin Number* 121, 1988.

TABLE 10-3 Summary of Hemodynamic Value Changes Associated with Term Pregnancy

Parameter	Pregnancy (Normal Value)	Change
Mean arterial pressure (mm Hg)	90 (+/−6)	No significant change
Central venous pressure (mm Hg)	8 (+/−2)	No significant change
Pulmonary artery wedge pressure (mm Hg)	4 (+/−3)	No significant change
Heart rate (beats/min)	83 (+/−10)	17% increase
Cardiac output (L/min)	6.2 (+/−1.0)	43% increase
Systemic vascular resistance (dynes/sec/cm^5)	1210 (+/−266)	21% decrease
Pulmonary vascular resistance (dynes/sec/cm^5)	78 (+/−22)	34% decrease
Serum colloid oncotic pressure (mm Hg)	18 (+/−1.5)	14% decrease
Left ventricular stroke work index (g/m/m^2)	48 (+/−6)	No significant change

Modified from Clark S and others: *Am J Obstet Gynecol* 161:1439-1442, 1989; and Lee W, Cotton D: Cardiorespiratory changes during pregnancy. In Clark S and others: *Critical care obstetrics,* ed 2, Boston, 1991, Blackwell Scientific Publications.

plasma. This lowers serum plasma protein concentration and colloid oncotic pressure. The increase in filtration also enhances the renal clearance of many substances, causing decreased plasma levels. Urea and creatinine are excreted more efficiently, and therefore normal adult values signify decreased renal function in the pregnant patient. Normal pregnant serum creatinine levels are 0.46 mg/dL and blood urea nitrogen (BUN) levels are 8.2 mg/dL.[9,14]

Glycosuria and mild proteinuria are common in pregnancy but may be indicative of underlying pathology. While glomerular filtration is increased, tubular reabsorption of glucose and protein are unable to increase proportionately, resulting in glycosuria and proteinuria. Both occurrences warrant further investigation in pregnancy.

Changes During Labor and Delivery

Labor and delivery bring additional stresses to the maternal system, most notably in the cardiopulmonary systems. During labor, uterine contractions produce cyclical autotransfusions of approximately 300 to 500 ml. Delivery of the fetus produces a final autotransfusion of approximately 1000 ml into the maternal vascular system.[10] This occurs because of the contracted uterus shunting its blood, sudden removal

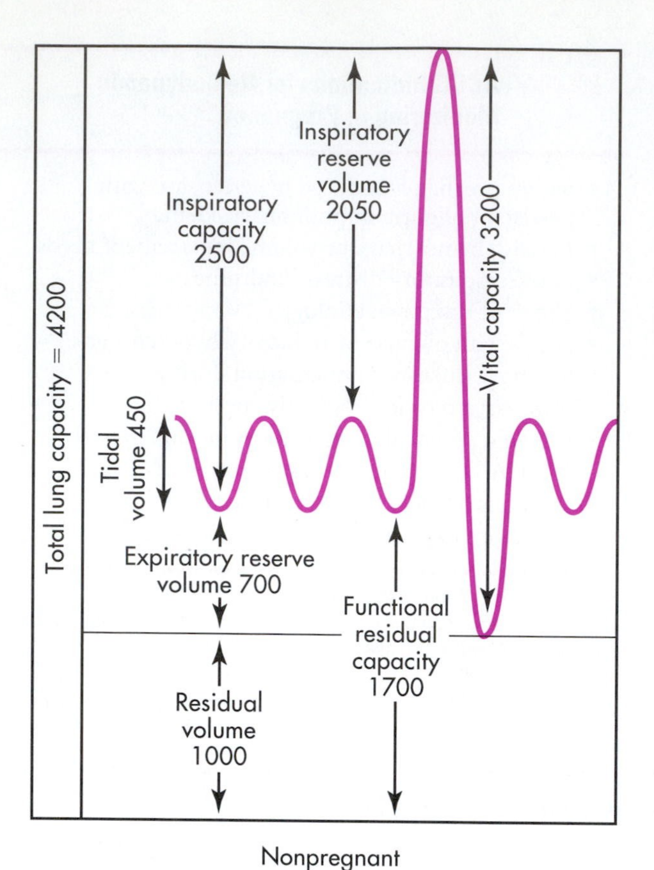

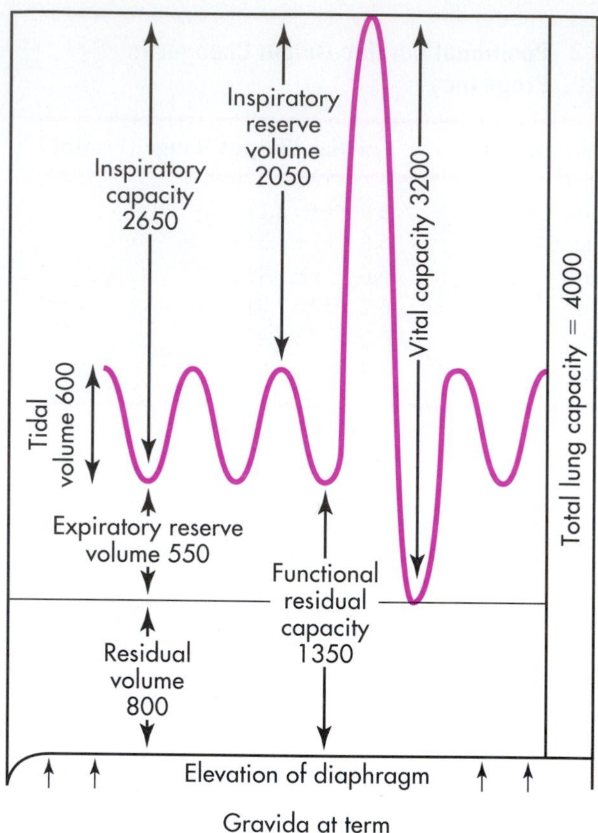

FIGURE 10-4 Pulmonary volumes and capacities during pregnancy, labor, and the postpartum period. (From Bonica JJ: *Principles and practice of obstetric analgesia and anesthesia,* 1967, Philadelphia, FA Davis.)

TABLE 10-4 Physiologic Adaptations of the GI System During Pregnancy

GI Function Change	Presumed Cause
Heartburn	Progesterone and estrogen; size of gravid uterus impeding gastroesophageal junction
Bleeding gums	Hyperemia
Constipation	Progesterone, causing decreased motility and intestinal secretion; enhanced water absorption
Hemorrhoids	Hyperemia; pelvic congestion; obstruction of venous return
"Morning sickness" or nausea	Increased levels of estrogen and HCG
Risk for aspiration	Displacement of lower esophageal sphincter; reduced gastric motility
Gallstones	Decreased gallbladder activity; impaired emptying

HCG, Human chorionic gonadotropin.

TABLE 10-5 Renal Physiologic Changes in Pregnancy

Parameter	Percent Change	Normal in Pregnancy
Renal blood flow	25%-50% increase	1250-1500 ml/min
Glomerular filtration rate	50% increase	140-170 ml/min
Renal plasma flow	35% increase	700-900 ml/min

of fetal supply demands, and resolution of vena caval compression. Table 10-6 summarizes the cardiac output changes in labor and delivery.

Normal blood loss from a vaginal birth is 300 to 500 ml[14,15]; blood loss from cesarean births usually is 1000 ml. Oxygen consumption increases approximately 200% to 300% during the labor and delivery process.[10] The cardiopulmonary changes occurring

TABLE 10-6 Cardiac Output Changes in Labor and Delivery

Stage of Labor/Delivery	Change in Cardiac Output
Early first stage of labor	15% increase, plus additional 15% with each contraction
Late first stage of labor	30% increase, plus additional 15% with each contraction
Second stage of labor	45% increase, plus additional 15% with each contraction
First 5 min postpartum	65% increase, secondary to autotransfusion
First hour postpartum	40% increase

Modified from: Lee W, Cotton D: Cardiorespiratory changes during pregnancy. In Clark S and others: *Critical care obstetrics*, ed 2, Boston, 1991, Blackwell Scientific Publications; and Troiano NH: Cardiac diseases in pregnancy. In Mandeville LK, Troiano NH, editors: *High-risk intrapartum nursing*, Philadelphia, 1992, JB Lippincott.

during labor and delivery are of significant concern since they occur over a short time, and maternal decompensation may occur.

In summary, maternal physiology is profoundly and rapidly affected by pregnancy. Adaptations begin early in the pregnancy and continue through the postpartum period, gradually returning to prepregnant states over 6 weeks. Understanding the physiologic stresses uniquely presented during pregnancy allows the clinician to provide comprehensive care to the pregnant woman experiencing critical illness or injury.

CARDIAC DISEASE

There are several general considerations in the care of the pregnant woman with cardiac disease. Cardiac disease during pregnancy may be a result of preexisting conditions, such as congenital diseases, or may be a result of primary cardiac disease arising during pregnancy. Prepregnancy counseling is highly recommended for women with known cardiac disease. Counseling includes determining the New York Heart Association[16] (NYHA) functional class (see Chapter 16) of the woman, as well as determining the maternal and fetal risks associated with the pregnancy (Table 10-7). Major fetal risks include fetal development of congenital heart disease, prematurity, IUGR, and IUFD. During the prenatal period, anticoagulant therapy is frequently recommended secondary to the already hypercoagulable state of pregnancy or preexisting conditions. Anticoagulant therapy using heparin is

TABLE 10-7 Maternal Mortality Associated with Pregnancy

Mortality Group	Condition
Group 1: Mortality <1%	• Atrial septal defect • Ventricular septal defect • Patent ductus arteriosus • Pulmonic tricuspid disease • Tetralogy of Fallot, corrected • Bioprosthetic valve • Mitral stenosis, NYHA Classes I and II
Group 2: Mortality 5%-15%	2A • Mitral stenosis, NYHA Classes III and IV • Aortic stenosis • Coarctation of aorta, without valvular involvement • Uncorrected tetralogy of Fallot • Previous myocardial infarction • Marfan's syndrome with normal aorta 2B • Mitral stenosis with atrial fibrillation • Artificial valve
Group 3: Mortality 25%-50%	• Pulmonary hypertension • Coarctation of aorta, with valvular involvement • Marfan's syndrome with aortic involvement

Modified from American College of Obstetricians and Gynecologists: *Technical Bulletin Number* 168, 1992.

recommended because of the teratogenic effects of oral agents.[12] Method and timing of delivery are primarily decided by obstetric considerations, taking into account the woman's ability to tolerate the labor process and associated physiologic changes. Selection of anesthesia techniques involves weighing risks and benefits of the procedures. As a general rule, most patients tolerate epidural anesthesia more favorably than general anesthesia. (∞Cardiovascular Disorder, p. 483.)

Pregnancy with Preexisting Heart Disease

Much progress has been made during the past 2 decades in managing pre-existing cardiac disease in the pregnant woman. Women in NYHA Class I or II generally have a favorable prognosis in pregnancy;

however, the dramatic physiologic changes present a significant confounding variable.

Atrial septal defect. Atrial septal defect (ASD) is the most common congenital anomaly seen during pregnancy, and the majority of women with ASD tolerate pregnancy, labor, and delivery without complications. The decrease in SVR lessens the degree of left-to-right shunt, whereas the hypervolemic state may slightly worsen the shunt and increase right ventricular workload. The most common complications seen with ASD are dysrhythmias, congestive heart failure, and thromboembolism.

Ventricular septal defect. The outcome of the pregnant woman with ventricular septal defect (VSD) and resultant left-to-right shunt is dependent on the size of the defect, with larger defects producing a less favorable prognosis. In the absence of significant symptoms and pulmonary hypertension, pregnancy is typically well-tolerated. Therapy is aimed at early recognition and treatment of signs of cardiac failure. Common complications include tachycardias, congestive heart failure, and development of pulmonary hypertension. (∞Cardiovascular Disorders, pp. 502, 510.)

Patent ductus arteriosus. Generally, patent ductus arteriosus (PDA) is well-tolerated during pregnancy, labor, and delivery. Precautions against the risks of infective endocarditis and thromboembolism may be taken. Severe PDA can produce large left-to-right shunts, producing pulmonary hypertension that is associated with significant maternal mortality.

Pulmonic/tricuspid disease. Isolated pulmonic or tricuspid valvular disease is uncommon but may be seen during the peripartum period. Because of the right-sided nature of the lesions, pregnancy, labor, and delivery are generally well-tolerated in spite of the hypervolemic state. The mainstay of treatment focuses on cautious fluid administration and balance.

Valve prosthesis. Management of the pregnant woman with a prosthetic valve focuses on maintenance of adequate anticoagulation to prevent thromboembolism and on infective endocarditis prophylaxis. Pregnant women with biologic valves usually do not require anticoagulation during pregnancy, unless evidence of thromboembolic disease or atrial fibrillation is present. Biologic valves are associated with slightly lowered mortality risks since anticoagulation is normally not required with their use.

Mitral stenosis. The presence of a stenotic mitral valve is the most common rheumatic valve disease. The primary concern with mitral stenosis during pregnancy is the impedance to ventricular filling, which produces a relatively fixed cardiac output. Additional risks include thromboembolism and dysrhythmias, especially atrial fibrillation. Cardiac output in the face of mitral stenosis is determined by two primary factors: length of diastolic filling and left ventricular preload. The length of diastolic filling may be negatively affected because of the normal hypervolemic state of pregnancy. In addition, discomfort or anxiety associated with labor may produce tachycardia, which can drastically impede ventricular filling, producing an even lower cardiac output with resultant cardiac failure and pulmonary edema. Tachycardia is commonly managed with beta-blockade therapy.

Maintenance and management of left ventricular preload is the second important consideration in mitral stenosis. Patients may require high normal or slightly elevated left ventricular filling pressures to maintain adequate flow across the stenotic mitral valve. Caution must be used when employing therapies that decrease preload, such as diuresis or epidural anesthesia. Invasive hemodynamic monitoring may be indicated to carefully tailor therapy. (∞Hemodynamic Monitoring, p. 442.)

In the immediate postpartum period, careful monitoring is essential because of the massive fluid shifts and large increases in cardiac output. Authorities recommend that optimal predelivery pulmonary artery wedge pressures be maintained at 14 mm Hg or less to accommodate the increase in wedge pressure of up to 16 mm Hg that can be associated in the immediate postpartum period.[17]

Aortic stenosis. Aortic stenosis (AS) is often accompanied by other valvular disease, especially disease affecting the mitral valve. The hallmark of AS is decreased left ventricular ejection. Mild AS is usually well-tolerated during pregnancy because of the natural hypervolemic state. Significant AS can produce left ventricular hypertrophy and dilation. Thromboembolic prophylaxis is advised. Critical to successful management is maintenance of cardiac output through prevention of hypovolemia, especially at the time of delivery. Any factor that diminishes venous return or produces hypotension worsens the effects of AS and significantly reduces cardiac output. The overall reported range for mortality is 17%.[17]

Tetralogy of Fallot. The four primary lesions associated with tetralogy of Fallot include VSD, overriding aorta, right ventricular hypertrophy, and pulmonary stenosis. Women with corrected tetralogy of Fallot are generally able to tolerate pregnancy well. While rare, if the congenital anomalies are not corrected, maternal mortality and fetal complications increase significantly. Cardiopulmonary function must be maximized by measures including the treatment of dysrhythmias and the use of prophylaxis for endocarditis. Considerations during labor and delivery include maintenance of adequate preload and blood pressure.

Previous myocardial infarction. The outcome of the pregnant woman with previous myocardial damage is dependent on many factors. The length of time between the myocardial event and delivery is especially important. Consideration must be given to the increased myocardial oxygen demands during pregnancy, and therapy is usually supportive in nature. Careful attention to preload is essential to prevent burdening the heart and producing congestive failure. (∞Congestive Heart Failure, p. 502.)

Marfan's syndrome. Marfan's syndrome is characterized by connective tissue weakness that can lead to aortic root and wall weakness. Mitral valve prolapse is commonly seen. Prognosis is based on aortic root diameter, with most authorities citing 4.0 cm as maximum, after which significant increases in mortality occur.[18,19] Prevention of tachydysrhythmias and hypertension is recommended, along with endocarditis prophylaxis. Beta-blockade therapy may be initiated for cardiac rate control and to decrease pressure on the weakened aortic wall. Goals of management include maintenance of cardiac output to meet physiologic needs without producing undo stress on the aortic wall. Careful blood pressure maintenance is essential. Differential diagnosis of chest and back pain is essential, along with recognition of other signs of aortic dissection. (∞Aortic Dissection, p. 515.)

Pulmonary hypertension and Eisenmenger's syndrome. Pulmonary hypertension during pregnancy may be primary or idiopathic. Eisenmenger's syndrome develops when, in the presence of a congenital left-to-right shunt (a result of ASD, VSD, or PDA), progressive pulmonary hypertension leads to shunt reversal or bidirectional shunting.[17] Regardless of the cause, the risk of sudden death because of pulmonary hypertension in pregnancy is 50%, and deaths have been reported up to 4 to 6 weeks postpartum.[18,20] Avoidance or termination of pregnancy is commonly recommended. If pregnancy is continued, therapeutic management is directed at avoidance of pulmonary vasoconstrictors, thromboembolism, and hypotension; maintenance of adequate preload and oxygenation; fetal surveillance; and reduction of stress at the time of delivery.

Coarctation of the aorta. Coarctation of the aorta may occur in isolation, or most often, in combination with valvular or septal anomalies. Patients with uncomplicated coarctation of the aorta who are relatively asymptomatic (NYHA Class I or II) have demonstrated good prognosis and minimal risk of complications or death.[17] Intrapartal management focuses on the prevention of hypertension to avoid aortic wall stress. Careful management of fluid balance and left ventricular function must occur to prevent congestive heart failure and to promote adequate perfusion.

Cardiac Disease Arising During Pregnancy

Peripartum cardiomyopathy. Women who have no evidence of previous cardiac disease but have cardiac failure during the last month of pregnancy or within the first 6 months postpartum are considered to have peripartum cardiomyopathy. To confirm the diagnosis, other causes of cardiac failure must be ruled out. Peripartum cardiomyopathy accounts for less than 1% of all cardiac problems associated with pregnancy[21] and carries mortality ranging from 25% to 50%.[17] Controversy continues regarding exact etiologies of peripartum cardiomyopathy, with viral and immune etiologies the leading suspected causes.

Symptomatology is identical to classic cardiac failure, as is the treatment of rest, sodium and fluid restriction, inotropes, diuretics, and afterload reduction. Anticoagulation is commonly employed to prevent thromboembolism. Treatments specific to the suspected cause, such as immunosuppressive therapy, may be employed as well.

Acute myocardial infarction. While acute myocardial infarction (AMI) is rare during pregnancy, mortality ranges from 35% to 45%, depending on the timing of the myocardial event, with increased mortality if delivery occurs within 2 weeks of infarction.[22] The dramatic physiologic demands throughout pregnancy challenge the woman's cardiovascular system and can cause ischemia, leading to infarction. Clinical diagnostics are similar to standard AMI detection, although diagnosis must be made with consideration of the normal physiologic cardiovascular changes. Treatment of AMI during pregnancy is focused on balancing myocardial oxygen supply and demand. Management may include nitrate and/or beta-blockade therapy, cardiac monitoring, oxygen therapy, management of pain and anxiety, and afterload reduction. Special consideration is given to the maternal physiologic demands required during the labor and delivery processes. Operative delivery interventions, such as forceps or cesarean section, may be necessary. (∞Myocardial Infarction, p. 490.)

Shock. *Shock* is best defined as tissue hypoxia that is a result of decreased perfusion. Because pregnancy is a hyperdynamic, low-resistance state with increased oxygen delivery and consumption requirements, the management of shock in the pregnant patient necessitates a different approach than with the nonpregnant patient. Normal physiologic adaptations that occur during pregnancy alter ranges in vital signs and laboratory values. Frequently the clinician may be obtaining data from and managing two patients, both mother and fetus. Finally, there are causes for shock in pregnancy and immediately postpartum that must be considered in addition to routine causes. (∞Shock, p. 1097.)

Hemorrhagic, septic, and cardiogenic shock are most commonly seen in pregnancy; neurogenic shock is an infrequent occurrence. Causes of hemorrhagic shock unique to pregnancy include abruptio placentae, ectopic pregnancy, placenta previa, and postpartum hemorrhage.[23] Postpartum hemorrhage can be attributed to uterine atony, genital tract lacerations, hematoma formation, retained placenta, and uterine prolapse.[24] Unique causes of septic shock in the pregnant patient include chorioamnionitis, septic abortion, and postpartum pyelonephritis.[23] Cardiogenic shock is most frequently a result of the presence of severe valve disease. Regardless of the cause, whether specific to pregnancy or not, the occurrence of shock requires aggressive intervention with treatment of the underlying cause.

Management of shock in pregnancy focuses on optimizing maternal stability in an effort to provide the most stable in-utero environment. Clinical judgments include assessment of the risks and benefits of therapeutic interventions and fetal viability. Consideration must be given to the potential vasoconstrictive nature of some pharmacotherapeutics and the potential for uteroplacental insufficiency.

RESUSCITATION

The occurrence of cardiopulmonary arrest during pregnancy is relatively rare. Successful management of the pregnant patient requires integration of physiologic changes present during pregnancy and adaptations for those from standard resuscitative guidelines. Fetal outcomes are directly related to the mother's condition and well-being. The interrelationship between fetal and maternal well-being may present unique ethical dilemmas for health care providers and family members. Etiologies, predisposing factors, and accompanying rationale for cardiopulmonary arrest during pregnancy are summarized in Table 10-8.

Basic Cardiac Life Support

American Heart Association recommendations[25] include only minor deviations from usual procedure. Critically important is the facilitation of venous return. This is accomplished through lateral displacement of the uterus, either through manual manipulation or through use of a wedge under the woman's hip. Airway management includes early intubation if possible because of the increased physiologic demands for oxygen delivery and the increased risk of aspiration. Because of the hyperemic nature of pregnancy and the risk for bleeding, nasal intubation must be avoided. No differences are required in compression ratio or depth. Physiologic adaptations in pregnancy place the woman at greater risk for complications from cardiopulmonary resuscitation, such as fractured ribs and sternum, hemothorax, hemopericardium, and internal organ damage. Specific organs of concern include the uterus, spleen, and liver.

Evaluation of fetal tolerance of the mother's condition is essential during cardiopulmonary arrest. Fetal hypoxia may develop because of decreased uteroplacental perfusion. Fetal gestational age is a prime consideration when determining course of action. Before the 24th week of gestation, resuscitative efforts are primarily focused on maternal outcome. After the 24th week of gestation, evaluation includes both maternal and fetal response to resuscitative efforts. Emergent cesarean section may be undertaken for fetal distress or to improve maternal status, although consideration also must be given to the stress that cesarean section produces. In late pregnancy, maternal and fetal outcomes are enhanced if delivery is accomplished within 15 minutes of cardiac arrest.[26]

Advanced Cardiac Life Support

There are no specific alterations of advanced life support guidelines for resuscitation during pregnancy. Pharmacologic and electrical therapeutic interventions are carried out as usual, although there are minor considerations in the case of pregnancy. Epinephrine may decrease uteroplacental perfusion because of its vasoconstrictive nature; however, the benefits outweigh the risks of administration. Lidocaine crosses the placenta but in therapeutic levels does not have adverse fetal or uteroplacental effects. If maternal toxicity occurs, fetal cardiac and central nervous system depression may occur. Fetal bradycardia is associated with bretylium administration; therefore careful fetal monitoring is recommended. There are no contraindications for use of atropine in pregnancy. Administration of sodium bicarbonate is to be undertaken cautiously. Maternal

TABLE 10-8 Etiologies of Cardiopulmonary Arrest in Pregnancy

Cause	Discussion
Preexisting cardiac disease	Dramatic volume changes and cardiac output requirements may be greater than diseased heart's ability to tolerate
Acute cardiac disease	May occur during pregnancy related to increased myocardial demands
Pregnancy induced hypertension	May induce multisystem dysfunction
Anaphylaxis/laryngeal edema	May occur as reaction to medications used to treat urinary infections
Preexisting asthma	Stress induced by pregnancy may compromise maternal ability to maintain adequate oxygenation
Aspiration pneumonia	May occur because of gastrointestinal sphincter incompetence
Pulmonary embolism	Hypercoagulable nature of pregnancy; venous stasis
Hypermagnesemia	Therapeutically used for seizure prevention; increased levels depress reflexes and may cause respiratory depression and subsequent arrest
Anesthesia	Complications from local, spinal, epidural, or general anesthesia used to facilitate delivery
Assorted other causes	Sepsis; trauma; amniotic fluid embolism; drug overdose

acidosis increases uteroplacental adrenergic reactivity and must be avoided, although maternal alkalosis may impair oxygen exchange to the fetus. Electrical therapies such as defibrillation, cardioversion, and pacing are not contraindicated in pregnancy. (See Appendix C, ACLS Algorithms.)

HYPERTENSIVE DISEASE

Hypertensive disease is a potentially life-threatening complication of pregnancy affecting 5% to 10% of all pregnancies and is the second leading cause of death in childbearing women.[27,28] Maternal complications include pathologic compromise of the cardiovascular, pulmonary, renal, neurologic, and hepatic systems (Table 10-9). Fetal complications result from decreased uteroplacental perfusion and include IUGR, prematurity, abruptio placentae, placental infarctions, hypoxia, and IUFD.

Hypertensive disease in pregnancy is most commonly seen in the younger or older patient. There is an increased incidence in primigravidas, as well as in mothers from low socioeconomic groups.[29] There appears to be a genetic predisposition. Current understanding of hypertensive disease in pregnancy is based on (1) a classification according to manifestations and time of onset in relation to gestation; (2) the fact that pregnancy can induce hypertension in women without a history of high blood pressure; and (3) the fact that elevated blood pressure in pregnancy can occur without the presence of generalized edema or proteinuria (transient hypertension). Proper diagnosis of hypertensive complications is critical and requires in-depth knowledge of disease pathophysiology to prevent or decrease the risk of maternal/fetal compromise.

ACOG Classification of Hypertension

The ACOG committee on terminology has established definitions for hypertension in pregnancy. This definition was reaffirmed by the National High Blood Pressure Education Working Group in 1990. According to ACOG, *hypertensive disease in pregnancy* is defined as a blood pressure (BP) greater than 140/90 mm Hg observed on at least two different occasions at least 6 hours apart after the 20th week of pregnancy. Box 10-6 shows the classification system for hypertensive disease during pregnancy.[30] *Preeclampsia* is the presence of hypertension with proteinuria, defined as 2+ on a dipstick from two samples, and/or edema, defined as a weight gain of greater than 5 pounds in 1 week. *Severe preeclampsia* is defined as a BP greater than 160/100 mm Hg, 3+ to 4+ proteinuria, and edema. Manifestations of severe preeclampsia include visual disturbances; right upper quadrant (RUQ) pain; epigastric pain; headache; pulmonary edema; impaired renal and/or liver function; and the *h*emolysis, *e*levated *l*iver enzymes, and *l*ow *p*latelet count (HELLP) syndrome. *Eclampsia* is the occurrence of maternal seizures or coma with absence of underlying neurologic condition and the presence of hypertension, proteinuria, and/or

TABLE 10-9 Complications of Hypertensive Disease in Pregnancy

Body System	Complications
Cardiovascular	Dysrhythmias; congestive heart failure; severe hypertension
Pulmonary	Pulmonary edema; acute airway obstruction
Renal	Oliguria; renal failure; ATN
Neurologic	Cerebral edema; eclampsia; cerebral hemorrhage; coma
Hepatic	Necrosis; rupture; periportal and subcapsular hemorrhage
Hematologic	DIC; hemolysis; thrombocytopenia

ATN, Acute tubular necrosis; *DIC,* disseminated intravascular coagulation.
Modified from Clark S and others: *Handbook of critical care obstetrics,* Boston, 1994, Blackwell Scientific Publications.

BOX 10-6 ACOG Classification System for Hypertensive Disease During Pregnancy

- Pregnancy Induced Hypertension (PIH)
- Transient (Gestational) Hypertension
  - Preeclampsia
    - Mild
    - Severe
  - Eclampsia
- Chronic Hypertension Preceding Pregnancy
- Chronic Hypertension with Superimposed:
  - PIH
  - Preeclampsia
  - Eclampsia

From American College of Obstetricians and Gynecologists: *Technical Bulletin Number* 219, 1996.

edema. These definitions have proven useful in establishing consistent guidelines for patient management.

Pregnancy Induced Hypertension

Pregnancy induced hypertension (PIH) is characterized by vasospasms in the venous and arterial systems that result in endothelial damage, platelet aggregation, and decreased vascular volume. The widespread arteriolar vasospasms result from abnormal sensitivity to vasoconstrictor substances of vascular smooth muscle, leading to injury of the endothelial lining. These generalized cyclic vasospasms lead to tissue ischemia and eventually end organ dysfunction (Figure 10-5). PIH can involve one or more organ systems and is thought to begin as early as implantation, but it is not expressed as a disease until late in gestation. Many theories to define the cause of hypertensive disease in pregnancy have been proposed. Despite years of research, the pathogenesis of PIH remains a debated topic. Current research focuses on four etiologic mechanisms: a placentation disorder, vasospasm, vessel spasm, and genetic predisposition.

Patients with PIH or chronic hypertension may have a significant decrease in circulating plasma volume as a result of damage done by vasospasms.[15] These vasospasms are the result of an imbalance of sensitivity to vasoconstrictive substances such as angiotensin II, prostacyclin, and thromboxane.[31] It is theorized that patients with hypertensive disease have a higher cardiac output and lower systemic vascular resistance in early pregnancy, which precedes an elevation in blood pressure and the classic manifestations of PIH.[32,33] This theory suggests that patients with PIH progress from a high cardiac output–low resistance state to a low cardiac output–high resistance state, leading to multisystem organ dysfunction. Approximately 50% of all PIH patients are intravascularly volume depleted, 30% demonstrate normal hemodynamic functioning, and the remaining 20% have intravascular volume overload.

Patients with PIH demonstrate a decrease in circulating plasma volume, renal perfusion, and glomerular filtration rate.[15,34] Proteinuria develops as a result of damage to the glomerulus. Laboratory analysis reveals an elevation in uric acid, creatinine, and BUN. Creatinine clearance may decrease, and oliguria develops as the disease progresses. Total urine protein of more than 5 g in a 24-hour period is associated with increased fetal mortality. Acute tubular necrosis (ATN) is rare, but may be seen in cases of severe PIH.

HELLP

HELLP is an associated syndrome of severe PIH and affects 4% to 12% of patients with preeclampsia-eclampsia.[15,34] Patients are critically ill and may require invasive hemodynamic monitoring. Maternal mortality ranges from 3.5% to 24.2%, whereas perinatal mortality ranges from 7.7% to 60%.[33,35] Clinical manifestations are related to damage done by cyclic arterial vasospasms and include RUQ pain, nausea with or without vomiting, epigastric pain, and general malaise. Hemolysis of red blood cells occurs as the cells are lysed, resulting in microangiopathic hemolytic anemia. Microemboli find their way to the hepatic vascular bed, causing ischemia and tissue damage. Platelets are

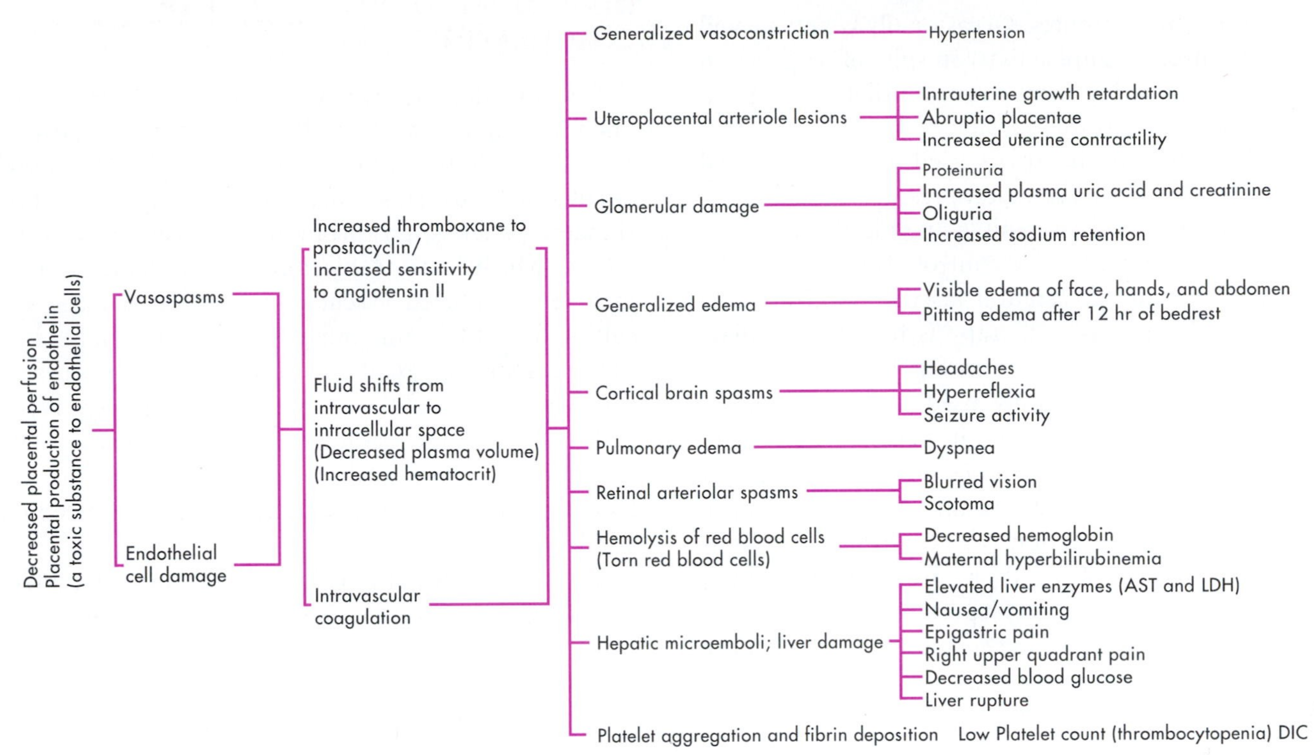

FIGURE 10-5 Pathophysiologic changes of preeclampsia. (From Gilbert E, Harmon J: *Manual of high risk pregnancy and delivery,* St Louis, 1993, Mosby.)

then consumed with resulting thrombocytopenia. Approximately 10% to 20% of pregnant patients with HELLP **will not** have elevated blood pressure diagnostic of hypertensive disease.[15]

The clinical manifestations of HELLP syndrome may suggest a multitude of other clinical diagnoses. Misdiagnosis is common and may result in a delay of correct treatment. Therefore any pregnant woman demonstrating clinical manifestations must be diagnosed with HELLP syndrome. Complications of HELLP include abruptio placentae, liver hematoma, disseminated intravascular coagulation (DIC), pulmonary edema, liver rupture, and acute renal failure.[36]

The treatment goals of severe preeclampsia are to prevent seizures, decrease arterial spasms, and effect prompt delivery of the fetus. Magnesium sulfate ($MgSO_4$) is the standard treatment for prevention and control of seizure activity in preeclampsia-eclampsia. Typical anticonvulsant therapies such as phenytoin, phenobarbital, or diazepam are not used because they primarily address neurologic dysfunction rather than vasospastic disease. $MgSO_4$ is used to decrease the excitability of smooth muscle fibers and amount of acetylcholine release in the central nervous system (CNS). A transient decrease in blood pressure may be seen, but it is of short duration. Serum magnesium levels of 4 to 7 mEq/L are felt to be therapeutic for prevention of seizure activity. A loading dose of 4 to 6 g is given via infusion pump over 15 to 20 minutes, followed by a maintenance infusion of 2 to 3 g/hour. Effects of magnesium toxicity are listed in Table 10-10.[15]

TABLE 10-10 Effects of Magnesium Toxicity

Blood Level	Effect
4-7 mEq/L	Therapeutic
10-12 mEq/L	Loss of DTR
15 mEq/L	Respiratory paralysis
25 mEq/L	Cardiac arrest

DTR, Deep tendon reflex.

Patients who are oliguric are at increased risk for magnesium toxicity and must be monitored closely for decreasing reflexes and respiratory drive. Serum magnesium levels are monitored every 6 to 8 hours. Calcium gluconate is used to reverse magnesium toxicity.

Control of eclamptic seizures is accomplished through administration of 4 to 6 g of intravenous $MgSO_4$ over 5 to 10 minutes. This bolus is followed by a continuous infusion of 2 to 3 g/hour. If a patient has a recurrent seizure, another 2 to 4 g bolus can be given over 3 to 5 minutes. Occasionally, a patient will have continuing seizure activity in spite of magnesium therapy, necessitating intubation, ventilatory support, and consideration of delivery.[33,37]

Antihypertensive therapy is used to reduce arterial vasospasms and decrease blood pressure, reducing left ventricular workload and enhancing placental and renal perfusion. Hypertensive control also decreases the potential for maternal cerebral vascular accidents. The goal of antihypertensive therapy is to maintain diastolic pressures less than 90 mm Hg.[15]

Hydralazine is commonly used as first-line management of hypertensive crisis in patients with severe preeclampsia-eclampsia. Hydralazine causes relaxation of arterial smooth muscle, resulting in vasodilation. Intravenous onset of action is 15 to 20 minutes. Typical dosing is 5 to 10 mg IV push every 20 minutes, to a total dose of 40 mg.[15,38] Hypertension that remains refractory to hydralazine necessitates the use of more potent antihypertensive agents.

Labetalol is a beta-blocker that causes a decrease in SVR and therefore blood pressure. Intravenous labetalol has an onset of action of 10 minutes. The initial dose is 10 mg, followed by an increase in dose every 10 minutes to a maximum of 300 mg.[15,38] Sodium nitroprusside is rarely used antepartally or intrapartally, but it may be administered to the severe preeclamptic-eclamptic patient when first-line drugs have failed. It is only considered when delivery is imminent or during the postpartum period since thiocyanide is the metabolite. Nifedipine is a calcium channel blocker that must be used cautiously when given concurrently with $MgSO_4$, because exaggerated hypotension may occur.

Collaborative management for patients with severe preeclampsia-eclampsia or HELLP syndrome is key to the stabilization of mother and fetus. Accurate initial assessment of the mother and documentation of baseline blood pressure are critical. Ongoing maternal assessment for manifestations of HELLP syndrome is crucial. Continuous assessment of the cardiovascular, renal, central nervous, and pulmonary systems provides early indications of worsening maternal condition. Fetal surveillance may include continuous fetal monitoring, biophysical profile, and fetal lung maturity testing. Delivery of the fetus may be indicated because of maternal condition or presence of fetal compromise. The goal of the health care team is to accurately monitor ongoing organ system dysfunction and prevent further damage leading to end organ failure and maternal-fetal mortality.

DISSEMINATED INTRAVASCULAR COAGULATION

Disseminated intravascular coagulation is a secondary complication of another disease process, which results in widespread formation of clots in the microcirculation. This causes massive consumption of fibrinogen, platelets, prothrombin, and Factors V, VIII, and X, which leads to bleeding. Precipitating factors include generalized vascular endothelial damage resulting from toxic, inflammatory, hypoxic, and/or immune responses; vascular disorders; and hemorrhage. Clotting abnormalities associated with pregnancy and/or DIC are the leading cause of maternal mortality.[6] DIC can cause fetal hypoxia and death, and potential neonatal sequelae include intracranial bleeding and brain death.[39]

Obstetric causes of DIC include abruptio placentae, preeclampsia-eclampsia, dead fetus syndrome, septic abortion, and amniotic fluid embolus. Pathophysiologic mechanisms are summarized in Figure 10-6. Primary treatment goals include identification of the underlying disorder; removal of the triggering event; and volume replacement, including blood component therapy. Secondary treatment may include anticoagulation therapy. (See Chapter 45).

Abruptio Placentae

Abruptio placentae is the most common obstetric cause of DIC. Twenty percent of mothers experiencing abruption have a significant clotting defect, with one fourth of this group experiencing postpartum hemorrhage.[4,15] The basic elements of treatment include the removal of blood clots from the uterus, blood component therapy, and fluid volume resuscitation.

Preeclampsia

DIC is occasionally seen in women with severe preeclampsia. Thrombocytopenia develops in 10% of women with severe preeclampsia-eclampsia,[4,15] placing them at risk for thromboembolic disease. Clinical evidence supports the concept that a majority of women with severe preeclampsia have a subclinical consumptive coagulopathy. Current research is evaluating the use of low dose heparin prophylaxis after surgical delivery of the fetus in the severe preeclamptic woman.

Dead Fetus Syndrome

Dead fetus syndrome is consistent with a true chronic DIC condition. The onset is gradual over 2 to 4 weeks. Eighty percent of women have spontaneous onset of labor after fetal demise. Treatment of the sta-

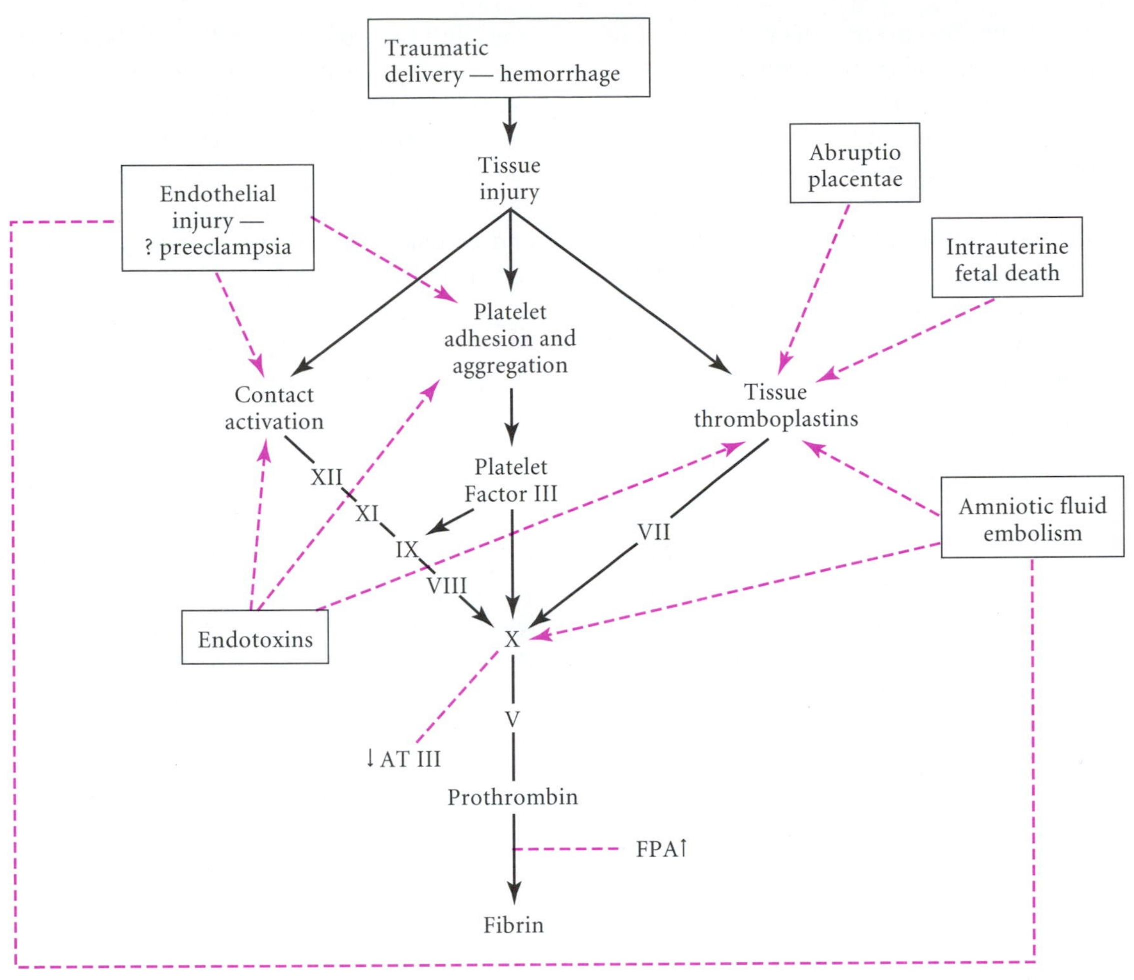

FIGURE 10-6 Pathophysiologic mechanisms in obstetric disseminated intravascular coagulation (DIC). (From Clark S and others: *Handbook of critical care obstetrics,* Boston, 1994, Blackwell Scientific Publications.)

ble patient is delivery of the fetus. Heparin may be used for women with associated coagulopathy.

Septic Abortion

Septic abortion is another well-documented cause of obstetric DIC. Bacterial endotoxins are the most likely initiating mechanism. The clinical findings of gram-negative septic shock are applicable to this condition. There appears to be a high correlation between the severity of the disease and the degree of coagulopathy. Aggressive antibiotic therapy and evacuation of the uterus are the front-line therapies for patients who are hemodynamically stable. Heparin therapy remains controversial.

PULMONARY DYSFUNCTION

Pulmonary dysfunction carries clinical significance because of the normally slightly hyperoxygenated condition associated with the physiologic changes in pregnancy. Compromise of respiratory function places both the mother and fetus at risk for harm. Maternal hypoxia can be the end result of several conditions, including pneumonia, asthma, trauma, acute respiratory distress syndrome (ARDS), and pulmonary embolism. Contributing factors (e.g., smoking, drug use, preexisting disease states), manifestations, and management differ very little from that which is seen in the nonpregnant individual (see Chapter 22). Common to these respiratory disorders is the issue of maternal-fetal hypoxia. *Maternal hypoxia* is defined by a PaO_2 less than 100 mm Hg, an SpO_2 less than 95%, a $PaCO_2$ greater than 35 mm Hg, a pH less than 7.40, and an SvO_2 less than 60%. Hyperventilation, shortness of breath, and dyspnea are commonly seen in pregnancy and must be differentiated from the usual maternal complaints.

Asthma

Although asthma often can be easily managed, it is associated with an increased incidence of hyperemesis gravidum, preeclampsia, chronic hypertension, preterm labor, perinatal mortality, spontaneous abortion, complicated labor, and low birthweight.[15,40] Some symptoms of asthma may actually lessen during pregnancy because of smooth muscle relaxation. Decreased cell mediated immunity and an increased level of corticosteroids may assist in diminishing the inflammatory response. Increased cyclic adenosine monophosphate (AMP) levels are also present and aid in maintaining an ongoing energy supply to cells. At the same time, other factors may contribute to worsening of symptoms. Nasal congestion, decreased functional residual volume, anxiety, failure to take medications, stress, and smoking can contribute to exacerbation of asthma symptoms. The decrease in cell-mediated immunity may predispose the mother to viral infections. Current practice recommendations include use of a peak flow meter twice a day to assist in objectively measuring maternal pulmonary function. If peak flow rates fall to 50% to 80% of the patient's norm, a review of symptoms and reevaluation of the management plan is performed. Flow rates less than 50% of the patient's norm signal the need for rapid assessment and intervention.[40]

Pneumonia

Pneumonia can result from a variety of factors and is often associated with asthma. Prior respiratory disease, concurrent illness, tobacco use, and anemia have all been linked with an increased maternal risk of pneumonia. Physiologic changes of pregnancy decrease the mother's ability to clear secretions and place her at increased risk for gastric aspiration. The severity of aspiration correlates directly to aspirate amount, particulate content, and pH. A variety of organisms can be seen in pneumonia, with some of the most common pathogens identified being *Streptococcus pneumoniae, Haemophilus influenzae, Mycoplasma,* and influenza viruses.[41]

Acute Respiratory Distress Syndrome

ARDS in pregnancy is often the result of a variety of conditions, including tocolytic administration leading to pulmonary edema, preeclampsia-eclampsia, abruptio placentae, postpartum hemorrhage, and amniotic fluid embolism (AFE). Some of the most common causes of ARDS in the perinatal patient are sepsis resulting from pyelonephritis, chorioamnionitis, IUFD, septic abortion, and postpartum endometritis. Women at risk for development of ARDS need to be assessed for early signs of worsening or changing dyspnea and tachypnea. As ARDS evolves there is a rapid deterioration in pulmonary function over a 24-hour period. Symptoms, including diffuse or basilar rales, bilateral opacities on the chest x-ray, and a deteriorating PaO_2 with increasing FiO_2 demands, need to be excluded from other etiologies, such as fluid overload and cardiac failure that can sometimes be seen in the last trimester. (∞ARDS, p. 660.)

Management of Respiratory Failure

Management of maternal hypoxia includes restoration and maintenance of the hypervolemic state without inducing fluid overload and further compromising cardiopulmonary function. Since colloidal osmotic pressure is decreased, great care must be taken to prevent the development of pulmonary edema when providing fluid replacement therapy. Oxygen is administered at a high flow rate via mask to achieve an optimal PaO_2 greater than 100 mm Hg and an SpO_2 greater than 95%. If intubation is required, placement of an orotracheal tube is more desirable than a nasotracheal tube because of hyperemic nasal passageways. If nasotracheal intubation is required, the smallest tube possible that will still allow adequate ventilation is used. Gastric decompression is instituted with a small-bore nasal or orogastric tube. When initiating mechanical ventilation the settings selected need to take into consideration the normal tachypnea, increased tidal volume (6 to 8 ml/kg lean body weight[42]) and decreased functional residual volume occurring in pregnancy. Caution must be taken to maintain the maternal $PaCO_2$ of 30 to 32 mm Hg, since respiratory alkalosis can lead to decreased uterine blood flow. Pharmacologic therapies must take into consideration maternal-fetal risk and benefits. Table 10-11 summarizes obstetric concerns of common drugs used in pulmonary dysfunction.[40,43]

Pulmonary Embolism

Thromboembolic disorders, including pulmonary embolism (PE), occur secondary to a variety of reasons, many of which are related to the physiologic changes in pregnancy. The greatest risk for developing PE is in the immediate postpartum period, especially after a cesarean section.[44] Two thirds of the patients who die from PE expire within 30 minutes of the initial event.[45] Assessment, management, and complications associated with PE are essentially no different than in the nonpregnant women; however, differential diagnosis of amniotic fluid embolism must be considered. Implantation of a venal caval filter may be

TABLE 10-11 Common Drugs Used for Pulmonary Dysfunction During Pregnancy

Drug	Considerations
Antibiotics	• Cephalosporins and erythromycin are generally well-tolerated
Inhaled corticosteroids	• Beclomethasone is generally considered safe
Systemic corticosteroids	• Documentation of decreased birthweights and increase in small-for-date babies • Majority of drug is metabolized by placental enzymes before entering fetal circulation • Small amount of steroid may cross into breast milk, yet it is still considered safe to breastfeed
Non-steroidal antiinflammatory agents	• Cromolyn and nedocromil are generally considered safe • Not associated with increased risks to fetus
Adrenergic agonists	• Epinephrine and isoproterenol may contribute to maternal-fetal tachycardia • Albuterol and terbutaline have fewer side effects and may have the additional benefit of tocolytic actions
Theophylline	• Not commonly used because of maternal side effects • Recommended that serum levels be maintained between 5-12 mg/ml to prevent complications of toxicity
Analgesics	• Morphine and meperidine must be avoided in active labor, since they can worsen bronchospasm • Will cross the placenta; this must be considered when completing a fetal assessment • Fentanyl may be a better agent to use • Epidural analgesia is considered safe
Beta mimetic tocolytics	• Contraindicated since can worsen maternal lung damage
Labor induction agents	• Oxytocin is the drug of choice • Prostaglandin F_{2a} must be avoided since it is a bronchoconstrictor
Neuromuscular blockade	• Can be administered safely as long as peripheral nerve testing is conducted to monitor drug dosages • Will cross the placenta, and this must be considered when assessing fetal activity

performed, but a suprarenal position is selected to prevent restriction of venous blood coming from the left ovary and draining into the left renal vein. (∞Pulmonary Embolism, p. 668.)

Amniotic Fluid Embolism

Amniotic fluid embolism is rare, yet it is associated with mortality rates of 80% to 90%, with the majority of deaths occurring in the first 2 hours after the event.[15,46,47] The most common precipitating factors associated with AFE are a large fetus, maternal age greater than 32 years, multiparity, premature separation of the placenta, IUFD, tumultuous labor, and small tears in the endocervical veins that may occur during normal labor. Placental abruption is seen in almost half the cases, with fetal death having occurred before the AFE.

There are many similarities between AFE, anaphylactic shock, and septic shock. Cellular mediators such as prostaglandins, histamines, and leukotrienes are associated with many of the manifestations of AFE. It is theorized that the amniotic membranes tear, releasing fluid into the maternal venous circulation, which then travels to the lungs. Transient pulmonary hypertension resulting from vasospasm occurs, which leads to right ventricular failure, pulmonary edema, and severe hypoxia. Left ventricular failure may also occur and further contributes to pulmonary failure. DIC is common and is thought to be a result of the activation of the fibrinolytic system by the amniotic fluid.

Sudden onset of symptoms during or immediately after delivery can lead to the suspicion of an AFE. Acute respiratory distress, shock out of proportion to blood loss, chills, fever, shivering, sweating, and cardiovascular collapse are seen. In a small percentage of patients a grand mal seizure may be the initial symptom. Pulmonary edema is present and is followed by acute cardiovascular collapse. Chest pain and bronchospasm are uncommon. More then 50% of patients die within the first hour, while 40% of survivors develop DIC.[15,46]

Diagnosis is confirmed by the presence of fetal squamous cells, lanugo, vernix caseosa, meconium, and mucin from blood aspirated from the pulmonary artery. Chest x-rays may show pulmonary edema, effusions, and cardiac enlargement. Management consists of maintaining oxygenation and supporting cardiac function. Inotropic support, fluid replacement, and administration of blood components are performed. Other therapies such as low dose heparin, bronchodilators, and steroids may also be used.

DIABETIC KETOACIDOSIS

Diabetic ketoacidosis (DKA) associated with pregnancy carries significant risk for maternal and fetal mortality. Fetal loss rates are reported from 50% to 90%.[15] Ten percent of pregnant diabetic patients experience DKA, with maternal mortality rates reported between 1% to 15%.[15,48] DKA may be precipitated by stress, improper insulin intake, infection, and beta-sympathomimetic agents.

Ketoacidosis occurs in pregnant diabetic patients more rapidly and at lower blood glucose levels than in nonpregnant persons with diabetes.[4] The insulin antagonistic properties of certain pregnancy hormones result in higher circulating blood glucose levels. The kidneys compensate by excreting additional bicarbonate to control maternal pH. This response results in the pregnant diabetic patient having diminished pH buffering capabilities. The diagnosis of DKA is made by monitoring manifestations of the pregnant diabetic patient and through laboratory analysis. Usual patient complaints include general malaise, thirst, polyuria, headache, disorientation, nausea, and weight loss. Diagnostic laboratory values include a serum blood glucose level greater than 300 mg/dL, a pH less than 7.25 to 7.30, and a bicarbonate level less than 10 mEq/L. Early manifestations of DKA may be subtle in the pregnant diabetic patient, and ketoacidosis may begin with blood glucose levels of 150 to 300 mg/dL.[15,48,49]

Successful management of DKA in pregnancy is dependent on identification of the underlying cause and the return of maternal baseline homeostasis. Goals of treatment include correction of fluid deficit, electrolyte imbalance, acidemia, and glucose imbalance and maternal-fetal stability. Careful attention must be given to the potential of maternal infection as the underlying cause. Fetal assessment includes careful monitoring during treatment if the fetus has reached a potentially viable gestational age. Delivery is delayed until the mother is stable and acidosis corrected. This may create a situation in which maternal stability takes precedence over fetal viability and requires continuous consideration of risks and benefits. Signs of fetal compromise may disappear once maternal stability has been achieved. Beta-mimetic therapy, such as terbutaline or ritodrine, for tocolysis is contraindicated for pregnant diabetic patients because it can induce DKA. Provision of maternal and family emotional support for the potential loss of a previable fetus or for fetal compromise is essential. (∞DKA, p. 1003.)

TRAUMA

The incidence of trauma in the pregnant person has been estimated to be around 6% to 7%, although a precise number is difficult to obtain since injuries can range from minor to life threatening.[50] The risk of injury increases with each trimester. Approximately 10% of injuries occur in the first trimester, 40% occur in the second trimester, and 50% occur in the third trimester.[15,39] As women continue to work late into their pregnancies and become involved in higher risk activities, the type and severity of injuries may begin to increase. The potential for domestic violence as the cause for injuries must also be considered. There are no different mechanisms that produce injuries in pregnant patients as compared with nonpregnant women.

Management of trauma during pregnancy and in the first 6 weeks postpartum is essentially, with a few exceptions, no different than the management of any other trauma patient (see Chapter 43). Normal physiologic changes associated with pregnancy may mask assessment findings and therefore affect decisions about interventions that are provided (Table 10-12). A critical point to remember is that the first priority is to provide whatever interventions would normally be provided to the nonpregnant individual, with the goal being to keep the mother alive. Keeping the mother alive is the best thing that can be done for the fetus, even though some of the interventions may produce transient alterations in fetal blood flow. Hesitation in providing necessary interventions increases the risk of harming both the mother and fetus. An exception to this situation may occur after the fetus has reached the state of viability and the mother is at risk for immediate demise. In this situation the decision may be made to perform an emergent cesarean section to save the infant.

TABLE 10-12 Initial Assessment and Management of Obstetric Trauma

PRIMARY SURVEY	
Assessment	**Management/Rationale**
AIRWAY	
Signs of Obstruction	
• Same as for nonpregnant patient	• Remove visible debris with caution because of increased hyperemia of nasal/oral area • Decrease risk of aspiration (resulting from enlarged uterus and effects of progesterone) by lateral tilt or by inserting NG/OG tube • Emergency cricoid thyrotomy/tracheotomy, if performed, is done above usual site because of upward displacement of thoracic structures
BREATHING	
Signs of Ineffective Respiration	

• Same as for nonpregnant patient with exception of the following:
  • ABGs
    • $SpO_2 < 95\%$
    • $PaO_2 < 100$ mm Hg
    • $PaCO_2 > 30$ mm Hg
    • pH < 7.40
  • Tidal volume < 800 ml
  • Labored respirations
  • RR < 20 bpm or > 24 bpm
	• 100% oxygen by mask since nasal passages tend to be hyperemic and there is a tendency for breathing through the mouth
	• Elevate HOB, if possible, to decrease pressure on thoracic structures resulting from elevated diaphragm
	• Oral intubation using smaller size (5.5-7.0) endotracheal tubes to decrease risk of bleeding because of increased vascularity of nasal area
	• Gastric decompression with OG tube or small NG tube (if patient does not tolerate OG tube placement) since prone to ileus and gastric reflux
	• Physiologic monitoring (RR, SpO_2, $EtCO_2$)
	• Obtain ABG, CXR
	• Emergent needle decompression/chest tube insertion for hemopneumothorax; may need to reassess entry point, because of upward/outward displacement of thorax

SIGNS OF INEFFECTIVE CIRCULATION	

• Same as for nonpregnant patient with exception of the following:
  • SBP < 100 mm Hg
  • MAP < 60 mm Hg
  • CVP < 4 mm Hg
  • Pale, moist, cool skin
	• DPL can be performed; open technique is usually preferred
	• Assess for possible placental abruption
	• Normally hypervolemic; skin is warm and slightly moist because of progesterone; may mask signs of hypoperfusion
	• Place CVC or large-bore IV in upper extremity sites since there is a potential for impeded venous return from lower extremities
	• Fluid resuscitation
	  • LR solution recommended since it has the potential to metabolize into bicarbonate via intrinsic body pathways; cannot administer blood products through same IV line
	  • 0.9 NS may decrease risk of developing maternal alkalosis (as compared with LR); can administer blood products through same IV line
	  • O negative blood can be given until type/cross done
	  • Replace 3 ml/1 ml of blood lost to compensate for hypervolemia associated with pregnancy
	  • Use caution because of increased risk for pulmonary edema resulting from decreased colloidal osmotic pressure
	• May apply MAST, but DO NOT inflate abdominal compartment
	• Tilt patient to side, even if on back board, to maximize venous return

NG/OG, Nasogastric/orogastric; *HOB,* head of bed; *CXR,* chest x-ray film; *DPL,* diagnostic peritoneal lavage; *SBP,* systolic blood pressure; *MAP,* mean arterial pressure; *CVC,* central venous catheter; *CVP,* central venous pressure; *LR,* lactated Ringer's; *NS,* normal saline; *MAST,* military antishock trousers.

Continued

TABLE 10-12 Initial Assessment and Management of Obstetric Trauma—cont'd

SECONDARY SURVEY	
Assessment	**Management/Rationale**
FOCUSED OBSTETRIC HISTORY	
• Gestational age • Single versus multiple pregnancy • Number of pregnancies, live births, abortions • Name of obstetrician • Rh factor • Prenatal complications • Past vaginal drainage, bleeding, clots • Past abdominal pain/uterine contractions	• Keep mother alive • Keep baby where it is • Vaginal examination to determine fetal presentation, status of amniotic membrane, presence of fetal parts or umbilical cord in vagina • Avoid manipulating cord—may lead to spasms • Emergent delivery—vaginal versus cesarean section, live versus postmortem
MATERNAL STUDIES	
Unexpected Diagnostic Study Results	

• Same as for nonpregnant patient with exception of the following:
  • CBC:
    • WBC count >18,000/mm³
    • RBC count <6,500,000/mm³
    • Hg <12g/100 ml
    • Hct <32%
    • Platelets <200,000
  • Fibrinogen >400
  • Chemistries:
    • BUN > or <9 mg/dL
    • Creatinine >0.5 mg/dL
    • Na slightly increased
    • Glucose slightly decreased
	• Insert urinary foley catheter with caution; rule out bleeding that may result from increased pelvic vascularity; consider using a smaller size catheter
	• Consider significance of positive toxicology results—is the fetus at risk for issues such as drug withdrawal or fetal alcohol syndrome
	• Hct/Hg results that are less than those identified may put both the mother and fetus at risk for hypoxia
	• Use caution when performing rectal examination to assist in determining fetal position/traumatic damage—pelvic vascular congestion contributes to development of hemorrhoids and predisposes mother to bleeding from this site
	• Obtain radiologic studies as needed; however, implement measures to decrease risk to fetus
	• May see left axis deviation on 12-lead ECG as a normal variant

FETAL STUDIES	
Signs of Fetal Distress	

• FHR <100-110
• Nonreassuring patterns on fetal monitoring
• Fundal height not appropriate for gestational age
• Vaginal drainage, bleeding, clots present
• Abdominal pain, uterine firmness, contractions present
• Amniocentesis
  • Presence of RBCs
  • L/S ratio and presence of phosphatidylgycerol
  • Kleihauer-Betke test to detect presence of fetal blood in maternal blood stream
	• Ultrasound to evaluate fetus
	• Assess fundal height, firmness, contractions q 30 min
	• Fetal monitoring (with pocket Doppler, ultrasound, or fetal monitor) as allowed based on interventions provided to mother
	• Differentiate uterine pain/contractions from other sources of abdominal pain
	• Administer tocolytics as needed
	• L/S ratio and presence of PG to determine fetal lung maturity
	• Kleihauer-Betke—indicates a break in the integrity of placental circulation if fetal cells are present

FHR, Fetal heart rate; *L/S,* lecithin/sphingomelin; *Pg,* phosphatidylglycerol.

TABLE 10-12 Initial Assessment and Management of Obstetric Trauma—cont'd

TERTIARY SURVEY	
Aspect of Care	**Purpose**

• Administer "follow-up medications"	Prophylactic measures
	• Antibiotics—choose broad-spectrum, nonteratogenic agents
	• Tetanus—does not cross placenta
	• Rh negative mothers:
	  • Can become Rh immunized within 72 hr
	  • Administer Rh_o(D) immune globulin (RhoGAM) (300 μg/15 ml fetal blood) if:
	    • Possibility of mother having received Rh positive blood
	    • Breach in integrity of the placenta of an Rh positive fetus as evidenced by positive Kleihauer-Betke test

Types of Injuries

Types of injuries can vary with the stage of pregnancy. In the first trimester, common injuries are associated with falls resulting from fainting from fatigue, hypoglycemia, and normal physiologic changes. The fetus is usually well-protected from external trauma since the uterus is located within the pelvis and is protected by bony structures. In the second trimester, as the enlarging uterus expands up out of the pelvis, maternal abdominal organs are displaced upward and laterally. Some protection is provided to the maternal abdominal organs since the uterus/fetus now occupies much of the abdominal cavity; however, the growing fetus becomes more vulnerable to injury. By the third trimester the fetus has begun to settle into the pelvis in preparation for birth. Hyperventilation and fainting are common as the fetus grows and demands greater metabolic needs from the mother. As relaxin secretion increases, the end effect of relaxed pelvis ligaments can lead to lordosis and pelvic tilt. This produces a change in gait and in the center of gravity/balance, which can increase the risk of falls.

Specific Body System Injuries

Cardiovascular. Manifestations related to cardiovascular injury may be masked because of normal physiologic changes in pregnancy. The hypervolemic, low systemic–resistance state that occurs during pregnancy can mask shock since up to 30% of blood volume can be lost before the classical manifestations are seen.[51] Lower extremity wounds may bleed more vigorously than might be expected because of venous congestion of the lower extremities.

Pulmonary. The most common ribs fractured are the middle ribs (5 to 9). The upper ribs (1 to 4) are associated with potential damage to the great vessels and the spine. The lower ribs (10 to 12) are associated with diaphragmatic, liver, and spleen damages. Consideration needs to be given to the fact that as the pregnancy progresses that chest anteroposterior diameter increases and the length decreases and that abdominal organs shift.

Neurologic injuries. New spinal cord injuries (SCIs) may contribute to spontaneous abortion or stillbirth. If the area of the SCI is above the 10th thoracic vertebra, the uterus is able to contract normally, although the mother will not experience labor pain. Complete SCI lesions above the fifth or sixth thoracic vertebra may lead to the development of hyperreflexia with the onset of labor. If severe irreversible brain damage or maternal brain death occurs, it is possible that the fetus may remain viable and continue to develop in utero. The issue of pregnancy maintenance in an irreversibly brain damaged or brain dead mother remains a controversial ethical issue.

Abdomen/pelvis. Failure to wear or improper use of seat belts can lead to blunt abdominal injury. Penetrating abdominal injuries also are seen, with gunshot wounds being the most common cause of abdominal injury. Since the uterus displaces maternal abdominal structures, the traditional assessment findings and sites of referred pain may be altered. Diagnostic peritoneal lavage (DPL) may be performed; however, the open technique using direct visualization is preferred. Peritoneal signs such as tenderness, rigidity, and rebound tenderness are unreliable indicators because of stretching of the abdominal wall. Bowel sounds may be absent since pregnant women are prone to ileus. All of these factors can contribute to delayed detection of abdominal injuries. Pelvic fractures can potentially injure the reproductive and urinary structures, although pelvic injury is not an absolute contraindication to vaginal delivery. Additional studies must be obtained before a final decision is made.

Reproductive system. Until 12 weeks of gestation the uterus is a pelvic organ. As the uterus enlarges it can assist in protecting other organs, but it becomes more vulnerable to injury. Direct trauma to the uterus/placenta reverses protective hemostasis by releasing an increased concentration of placental thromboplastin, a plasminogen activator, from the myometrium. The uteroplacental bed functions as a dilated passive, low-resistance system that lacks autoregulation and therefore has few if any compensatory mechanisms. The body perceives the uterus as a peripheral or nonvital organ. Since the uteroplacental system receives 20% to 30% of maternal cardiac output, maintenance of adequate circulating blood volume is essential to ensure adequate blood flow. The abdomen must be palpated to assess uterine position, size, and firmness; the presence of contractions; and the fetal position. Abruptio placentae, commonly seen with pelvic fractures, may occur immediately, within 48 hours, or up to 5 days after injury. Uterine damage/rupture is rare, but if it occurs, it is commonly at the site of a previous cesarean section. Even if there were no identifiable damage to the reproductive system, there may be an increased risk for premature rupture of membranes (PROM), premature labor, fetal/maternal hemorrhage, or fetal damage or demise. It is generally recommended that pregnant patients with trauma be admitted to the hospital for 24 to 48 hours of fetal monitoring since there may be latent injuries or the need for tocolytics.

Fetal injuries. The fetus is usually well-cushioned by amniotic fluid, the gravid uterus, and the abdominal wall, which all serve to distribute the force of injury. The most common cause of fetal death is maternal death. The second most common cause is skull fracture and intracranial hemorrhage secondary to engagement of the fetal head into the pelvis. Predictors of fetal demise include increased injury severity score (ISS), decreased maternal bicarbonate level on admission to the hospital, maternal acidosis, low Glascow Coma score, increasing fluid requirements, maternal abdominal injuries, and maternal hypoxia.[52]

NEUROLOGIC DYSFUNCTION

There are no known neurologic changes that are associated with pregnancy, yet women may have preexisting neurologic conditions. There are a large variety of neurologic conditions, (see Chapter 28) but only those conditions associated with the potential to place the mother and fetus at risk are discussed in this chapter.

Epilepsy

Some of the most common maternal neurologic disorders are seizures, although seizures do not appear to increase risk of PIH, premature delivery, or other common complications. The frequency of seizures during pregnancy, with preexisting epilepsy, has been known to increase as much as 45%.[53] This is thought to be a result of reduced plasma concentrations and altered pharmacokinetics secondary to impaired absorption, fluid retention, electrolyte changes, increased renal clearance, respiratory alkalosis, and hormonal changes that alter hepatic enzyme systems responsible for drug metabolism.[53] Efforts must be made to differentiate neurologic etiologies (i.e., epileptic) from nonneurologic etiologies (i.e., PIH), since management is significantly different. The major goals in managing the epileptic patient are to keep the mother seizure-free and to minimize the risk of fetal teratogenic effects from anticonvulsant medications. Consideration may be given to stop anticonvulsant drugs if the electroencephalogram (EEG) shows lack of ectopic activity and if the patient has been seizure-free on long term—low dose drugs. The discontinuance of medications must be carefully balanced against the potential development of seizures, since fetal damage resulting from hypoxia during seizures can occur.

Management focuses on identifying the minimal drug dose required to prevent seizures and drugs that pose the least risk for fetal harm. Although most anticonvulsant drugs have been associated with fetal abnormalities, studies have shown that 95% of fetuses are unaffected.[53] Polypharmacotherapy with multiple anticonvulsant agents must be avoided since this practice is associated with an increased risk of fetal damage. During the last month of pregnancy supplemental vitamin K may be administered to protect the newborn against bleeding caused by vitamin K depletion.[53] As maternal physiology gradually returns to the nonpregnant state, drug doses may need to be reduced in the first 2 to 3 weeks postpartum.[53]

LEGAL REVIEW 

Nursing Diagnosis and Advanced Nursing Practice Legislation

It is well-accepted that application of the nursing process to patient problems, with associated statements of nursing diagnosis, is a standard of professional nursing practice for all patients regardless of medical diagnosis.

The nursing diagnosis is now part of the definition of nursing in a typical state nurse practice act and is integral to the nursing regulatory framework as well. The nursing diagnosis has also been the subject of judicial commentary and analysis, as the following case illustrates.

In the case of *Sermchief v. Gonzales,* two nurse practitioners were sued by the Missouri State Board of Registration For the Healing Arts for the unauthorized practice of medicine. Both nurses had postgraduate training in obstetrics and gynecology. Their functions, among others, under standing orders and protocols included performing breast and pelvic examinations, obtaining Papanicolaou smears, dispensing certain medications and contraceptive devices, treating vaginitis and other conditions, inserting intrauterine devices, and providing counseling and education to patients.

The court held in favor of the nurses, stating their conduct constituted professional nursing as defined by the state's nurse practice act and did not constitute the unauthorized practice of medicine. The court noted that the language of the statute reflected legislative intent to expand the scope of authorized nursing practices and avoid statutory constraints on the evolution of new nursing functions. The court further concluded that the nurses' functions were the types of acts the legislature contemplated when it gave nurses the legal right to make assessments and nursing diagnoses. Of particular interest was the court's statement that the nurse undertakes only a nursing diagnosis, as opposed to a medical diagnosis, when he or she finds or fails to find clinical manifestations described by physicians in protocols and standing orders for the purpose of administering care and treatment prescribed by physicians in such protocols and orders.

Kim MF, McFarland GK, McFarlane AM: *Pocket guide to nursing diagnosis,* ed 7, St Louis, 1997, Mosby; Lounsbury P, Frye SJ: *Cardiac rhythm disorders: an introduction using the nursing process approach,* ed 2 St. Louis, 1992, Mosby; North American Nursing Diagnosis Association: *Classification of nursing diagnoses: proceedings of the eighth conference, North American Nursing Diagnosis Association,* Philadelphia, 1989, JB Lippincott; North American Nursing Diagnosis Association: *Taxonomy I Revised 1990 with official nursing diagnoses,* St Louis, 1990, The Association; *Sermchief v Gonzales,* 660 S.W.2d 683 (Mo. 1983); Tucker SM and others: *Patient care standards: collaborative practice planning,* ed 6, St Louis, 1996, Mosby.

Intracranial Hemorrhage

The most common cause of intracranial hemorrhage (ICH) in pregnancy is subarachnoid hemorrhage secondary to a ruptured cerebral aneurysm or arteriovenous malformation.[54] Mortality rates for pregnant patients with ICH are estimated to be 43%.[15] Patients with PIH and associated ICH may account for up to 60% of deaths associated with eclampsia.[15] Although it has been theorized that physiologic changes of pregnancy place increased strain on previously weakened cerebral vessels, clinical data has not supported this. Management of ICH is only slightly different in the pregnant patient. Hypotensive agents such as sodium nitroprusside are commonly used to maintain the blood pressure within a desired range but must be used with great caution if the patient has not yet delivered. Hypotension and toxic effects of nitroprusside can pose significant risk to the fetus.

Myasthenia Gravis

One third of patients with myasthenia gravis (MG) experience a deterioration in their condition during pregnancy, whereas the condition in the remaining two thirds remains unchanged or improves.[55] Management includes the recognition that interventions may be required in the second stage of labor when the abdominal muscles are required for pushing. There is increased maternal sensitivity to medications such as narcotics, CNS depressants, neuromuscular blockers, some anesthetics, and tocolytic agents. A myasthenic crisis may occur if magnesium sulfate is administered. Epidural medications may be safely used to decrease pain and fatigue during labor. It may be necessary to use forceps or vacuum-assisted delivery if the mother is unable to effectively push with contractions.[56] Maternal antibodies to neurotransmitters may cross the placenta and cause the fetus to have transient symptoms of

MG, manifested by respiratory depression, poor tone, weak cry, and poor sucking.

SUMMARY

Caring for the critically ill obstetric patient presents multiple challenges. Obstetric patients may be critically ill secondary to preexisting disease or the advent of critical illness or injury during pregnancy. Central to optimal care is the persistent application of physiologic changes of pregnancy to normal adult values. It is essential to remember that symptomatology may be altered because of the pregnant state. Understanding the intricate maternal-fetal relationship provides practitioners with a focus of maintaining maternal stability to enhance uteroplacental perfusion and an optimal in utero environment. All potential therapeutic interventions must be weighed in light of the risk/benefit ratio to maternal-fetal status. Critical situations may bring personal, cultural, social, spiritual, and/or ethical values into conflict. Decision making must be done in collaboration with family and health care team members and take into account all options. Finally, determining an appropriate environment for care can be a challenge. Some institutions have created dedicated obstetric intensive care units, whereas others provide care in either the obstetric care unit or critical care unit. Regardless of the location, the key factor is collaboration between specialties to optimize maternal-fetal outcomes and facilitate the family experience.

REFERENCES

1. Little GA: Fetal growth and development. In Eden RD, Boehm FH, editors: *Assessment and care of the fetus,* Norwalk, Conn, 1990, Appleton & Lange.
2. Niebyl J: Teratology and drug use during pregnancy and lactation. In Scott J and others, editors: *Danforth's obstetrics and gynecology,* ed 7, Philadelphia, 1994, JB Lippincott.
3. DiSaia PJ: Radiation in gynecology. In Scott J and others, editors: *Danforth's obstetrics and gynecology,* ed 7, Philadelphia, 1994, JB Lippincott.
4. Reece EA and others: *Handbook of medicine of the fetus and mother,* Philadelphia, 1995, JB Lippincott.
5. DeLia J, Bendon R: Normal and abnormal placental development. In Scott J and others, editors: *Danforth's obstetrics and gynecology,* ed 7, Philadelphia, 1994, JB Lippincott.
6. Olds SB and others: *Maternal-newborn nursing,* ed 4, Redwood City, Calif, 1992, Addison Wesley.
7. Huddleston JF and others: Antepartum assessment of the fetus. In Knupple R, Drukker J, editors: *High risk pregnancy,* Philadelphia, 1993, WB Saunders.
8. May K, Mahlmeister L: *Maternal and neonatal nursing: family-centered care,* ed 3, Philadelphia, 1994, JB Lippincott.
9. Cunningham FG and others: *Williams obstetrics,* ed 19, Norwalk, Conn, 1993, Appleton & Lange.
10. Harvey MG: Physiologic changes of pregnancy. In Harvey CJ: *Critical care obstetrical nursing,* Gaithersburg, Md, 1991, Aspen.
11. Clark S and others: Central hemodynamic observations in normal third trimester pregnancy, *Am J Obstet Gynecol* 161:1439-1442, 1989.
12. Briggs G, Freeman R, Yaffe S: *Drugs in pregnancy and lactation,* ed 4, Baltimore, 1995, Williams & Wilkins.
13. Lee W, Cotton D: Cardiorespiratory changes during pregnancy. In Clark S and others, editors: *Critical care obstetrics,* ed 2, Boston, 1991, Blackwell Scientific Publications.
14. Monga M, Creasy R: Cardiovascular and renal adaptation to pregnancy. In Creasy R, Resnik R, editors: *Maternal-fetal medicine: principles and practice,* ed 3, Philadelphia, 1994, WB Saunders.
15. Clark S and others: *Handbook of critical care obstetrics,* Boston, 1994, Blackwell Scientific Publications.
16. Criteria Committee of the New York Heart Association: *Nomenclature and criteria for diagnosis of disease of the heart and great vessels,* ed 6, Boston, 1964, Little, Brown.
17. Clark SL: Structural cardiac disease in pregnancy. In Clark S and others, editors: *Critical care obstetrics* ed 2, Boston, 1991, Blackwell Scientific Publications.
18. Jelsema R, Cotton D: Cardiac disease. In James DK and others, editors: *High risk pregnancy: management options,* London, 1994, WB Saunders.
19. Rutherford JD, Hands M: Pregnancy with preexisting heart disease. In Douglas PS, editor: *Cardiovascular health and disease in women,* Philadelphia, 1993, WB Saunders.
20. Shabetai R: Cardiac disease. In Creasy R, Resnik R, editors: *Maternal-fetal medicine: principles and practice,* ed 3, Philadelphia, 1994, WB Saunders.
21. James KB: Heart disease arising during pregnancy. In Douglas PS, editor: *Cardiovascular health and disease in women,* Philadelphia, 1993, WB Saunders.
22. Clark SL: Cardiac disease in pregnancy, *Am J Obstet Gynecol* 19:237-253, 1987.
23. Cashion K: Shock in the pregnant patient. In Harvey C, editor: *Critical care obstetrical nursing,* Gaithersburg, Md, 1991, Aspen.
24. Pozaic S: Hemorrhagic complications in pregnancy. In Harvey CJ, editor: *Critical care obstetrical nursing,* Gaithersburg, Md, 1991, Aspen.
25. American Heart Association: *Textbook of advanced cardiac life support,* Dallas, 1994, The Association.
26. Baird SM, McCoy G: Cardiopulmonary resuscitation during pregnancy, *NAACOG's Clinical Issues in Perinatal Women's Health Nurs* 3(3):548-549, 1992.
27. Atrash H and others: Maternal mortality in the United States, 1979-1986, *Am J Obstet Gynecol* 76:1055-1060, 1990.

28. Saftlas A and others: Epidemiology of preeclampsia and eclampsia in the United States, 1979-1986, *Am J Obstet Gynecol* 163:460-465, 1990.
29. Roberts J: Current perspectives on preeclampsia, *J Nurse Midwifery* 39(2):70-90, 1994.
30. American College of Obstetricians and Gynecologists: Hypertension in pregnancy, *ACOG Technical Bulletin* 219, 1996.
31. Walsh S: Preeclampsia: an imbalance in placental prostacyclin and tromboxane production, *Am J Obstet Gynecol* 152:335-340, 1985.
32. Easterling T, Benedetti J: Principles of invasive hemodynamic monitoring in pregnancy. In Clark S and others, editors: *Critical care obstetrics,* ed 2, Cambridge, Mass, 1991, Blackwell Scientific Publications.
33. Sibai B, Mabie C: Hemodynamics of preeclampsia, *Clin Perinatol* 18(4):727-747, 1991.
34. Martin J and others: The natural history of HELLP syndrome: patterns of disease progression and regression, *Am J Obstet Gynecol* 164:1500-1513, 1991.
35. Barton J, Sibai B: Care of the pregnancy complicated by HELLP syndrome, *Obstet Gynecol Clin North Am* 18(2):165-179, 1991.
36. Dildy G and others: Complications of pregnancy-induced hypertension. In Clark S and others, editors: *Critical care obstetrics,* ed 2, Boston, 1991, Blackwell Scientific Publications.
37. Villar M, Sibai B: Eclampsia, *Obstet Gynecol Clin North Am* 15(2):355-377, 1988.
38. Walker J: Hypertensive drugs in pregnancy: antihypertensive therapy in pregnancy, preeclampsia, and eclampsia, *Clin Perinatol* 18(4):845-873, 1991.
39. Gilbert E, Harmon J: Manual of high risk pregnancy and delivery, ed 2, St Louis, 1997, Mosby.
40. Mabie WC: Asthma in pregnancy, *Clin Obstet Gynecol* (39)1:56-69, 1996.
41. Rigby FB, Pastorek II JG: Pneumonia during pregnancy, *Clin Obstet Gynecol* (39)1:107-119, 1996.
42. Deblieux PM, Summer WR: Acute respiratory failure in pregnancy, *Clin Obstet Gynecol* (39)1:143-152, 1996.
43. Hornby PJ, Abrahams TP: Pulmonary pharmacology, *Clin Obstet Gynecol* (39)1:17-35, 1996.
44. Poole J: Pulmonary embolism, *NAACOG's Clinical Issues in Perinatal and Women's Health Nurs* (3)3:461-468, 1992.
45. Brown HL, Hiett AK: Deep vein thrombosis and pulmonary embolism, *Clin Obstet Gynecol* (39)1:87-100, 1996.
46. Martin RW: Amniotic fluid embolism, *Clinical Obstet and Gynecol* (39)1:101-106, 1996.
47. Sisson MC: Amniotic fluid embolism, *NAACOG's Clincal Issues in Perinatal and Women's Health Nurs* (3)3:469-474, 1992.
48. Miller E: Metabolic management of diabetes in pregnancy, *Semin Perinatol* 18(5):414-431, 1994.
49. Mandeville L: Diabetic ketoacidosis, *NAACOG's Clinical Issues in Perinatal and Women's Health Nurs* 3(3):514-520, 1992.
50. Maull KI, Pedigo RE: Injury to the female reproductive system. In Moore EE and others, editors: *Trauma,* ed 2, Norwalk, Conn, 1991, Appleton & Lange.
51. Harvey MG, Troiano NH: Trauma during pregnancy, *NAACOG's Clinical Issues in Perinatal and Women's Health Nurs* (3)3:521-529, 1992.
52. Hoft WS and others: Maternal predictors of fetal demise in trauma in pregnancy, *Surg Gynecol Obstet* 172:175, 1991.
53. Kochenour NK: Epilepsy. In Queenan JT, Hobbins JC, editors: *Protocols for high risk pregnancies,* ed 3, Cambridge, Mass, 1996, Blackwell Science Publications.
54. Gonik B, Allan SJ: Intracranial hemorrhage in pregnancy. In Clark S and others, editors: *Critical care obstetrics,* ed 2, Boston, 1991, Blackwell Scientific Publications.
55. Plauche WC: Myasthenia gravis in mothers and their newborns, *Clin Obstet Gynecol* (34)1:82-99, 1991.
56. Burke ME: Myasthenia gravis and pregnancy, *J Perinatal Neonatal Nurs* (7)1:1-21, 1993.

Gerontologic Alterations and Management

MORE THAN 50% OF critical care patients are older than 65 years.[1] Patients older than 65 years are also hospitalized for longer periods in the critical care unit.[1,2] Henning and others[2] found the average length of stay in the critical care unit (CCU) for an elderly person (i.e., older than 59.5 years) was 3.7 days, compared with 2.1 days for younger adults (i.e., 56.5 years of age). The survival rate for the former group was 81%, compared with 98% for the latter group.[1]

It was once thought that age was a predictor of clinical outcomes after CCU stay. Recent reports indicate severity of CCU illness, length of stay, prior CCU admission, and functional status are better predictors of CCU outcome, rather than age.[3,4] In addition, quality of life assessed at 1, 6, and 12 months after hospital discharge was not significantly different between young and old patients.[4] These data suggest that old age is not linked to functional recovery after CCU stay.

In the United States, individuals who are older than 65 years account for 12% of the total population. It is expected that in the next decade, such individuals will account for at least 20% of the general population.[5] Individuals older than 85 years are the fastest growing cohort of the elderly population. The overall life expectancy for a person born in 1913 is 74.9 years of age.[6] Currently the terms *senescent* and *elderly* apply to individuals 65 years and older. The term *young-old* is used to describe individuals 65 to 75 years old, *old-old* refers to persons 75 to 84 years old, and *oldest-old* describes those who are 85 or older.[5]

Advancing age is accompanied by physiologic changes in the cardiovascular, respiratory, renal, gastrointestinal, hepatic, integumentary, immune, and central nervous systems. With advancing age the incidence of disease increases, with cardiovascular and neoplastic diseases being the most common causes of death.[7] However, although physiologic decline and disease processes influence each other, physiologic decline occurs independently of disease. Therefore changes in physiologic function are important to consider when caring for the elderly patient.[7] The purpose of this chapter is to acquaint the critical care nurse with literature and research on the age-associated changes in physiologic function in healthy older adults and to describe implications for this population in critical care.

STUDIES ON AGING

Most of our information on aging is derived from studies on animals and prospective longitudinal studies in healthy elderly persons. Interestingly, many studies were conducted between 1974 and 1985, which corresponds to the establishment of the National Institute on Aging (NIA), which is part of the National Institutes of Health.[8] Most of our knowledge of age-related cellular and subcellular changes in various organ systems has come from animal models of aging. Ethical constraints and considerations have prevented the rigorous investigation of cellular and subcellular changes in the organ systems of aging humans. In addition, because of the increased incidence of disease with aging, it becomes difficult to recruit healthy elderly subjects. Some current areas of research supported by the NIA include clinical problems of the geriatric population that are associated with increased morbidity and mortality, clinical problems of nursing home patients, control of gene expression in aging, and genetic theories of aging.[8]

CARDIOVASCULAR SYSTEM

Advancing age has many effects on the cardiovascular system. With advancing age both the myocardium and the vascular system undergo a multitude of anatomic, cellular, and genetic changes that alter the function of both the myocardium and peripheral vascular system.[9]

Age-Related Morphologic Changes in the Myocardium

Myocardial collagen content increases with age.[10,11] Collagen is the principal noncontractile protein occupying the cardiac interstitium.[12] There are two types of collagen, Type I and Type III. The increase in myocardial stiffness in the aging heart probably results from an increase in Type I collagen, which is associated with scar-tissue formation and has a higher tensile strength.[12] Type III collagen is different from Type I in that it is a "softer" type and is associated with the reparative process of wound healing. Increased myocardial collagen content renders the myocardium less compliant. The decrease in myocardial compliance can adversely affect diastolic filling (through decreased distensibility and dilation) and myocardial relaxation. Consequently, the left ventricle must develop a higher filling pressure for a given increase in ventricular volume. The functional consequence could be an increase in myocardial oxygen consumption. Under normal physiologic conditions, an increase in myocardial oxygen demand is met with a corresponding increase in coronary artery blood flow. However, in the presence of coronary artery disease, coronary artery blood flow can be limited because of atherosclerotic-mediated narrowing of the coronary arteries. Hence the patient is at risk for developing myocardial ischemia and/or infarction. Clinical manifestations of myocardial ischemia include electrocardiographic (ECG) changes and chest pain. However, the sensation of chest pain is altered in the elderly person. Muller and others[13] found that complaints of chest pain were absent in 75% of elderly patients (older than 85 years) who sustained a myocardial infarction. Others[14] have also reported that chest pain in the elderly is less intense and of shorter duration and originates in other areas of the chest besides the substernal region.

The aging heart undergoes a modest degree of hypertrophy that is similar to pressure-overload–induced hypertrophy. Such hypertrophy entails a thickening of the left ventricular wall without appreciable changes in left ventricular cavity size.[15] The increase in left ventricular wall thickness is primarily a result of myocyte hypertrophy (increase in cell size). In elderly individuals, the myocardial hypertrophy may be caused by corresponding increases in aortic impedance and systemic vascular resistance.[16]

Functional Changes: Myocardial Contraction and Relaxation

When measured under similar experimental conditions, the developed contractile tension of isolated papillary muscle strips removed from aged and young adult animals is the same.[17] However the duration of contraction is prolonged in the aged animal. For example, twitch contractile recordings from adult (7-month) and aged (24-month) rats show that the duration of the contraction in the adult muscle strip is 350 msec, as compared with 500 msec in the aged muscle strip. Peak contractile force is 7.5 (g/mm^2) in each preparation.[18]

Myocardial contractility depends on numerous factors. However, the most important determinants of myocardial contraction are the intracellular level of free calcium and the sensitivity of the contractile proteins for calcium.[19] Since peak contractile force in the senescent myocardium is unaltered, this suggests that neither the amount of intracellular free calcium during systole nor the sensitivity of the contractile proteins for calcium is altered.

The prolonged duration of contraction (systole) is caused in part by a slowed or delayed rate of myocardial relaxation.[9,20] Myocardial relaxation depends on removal of calcium from the cell by uptake into the sarcoplasmic reticulum (SR) and extrusion of calcium across the plasma membrane (sarcolemma) by the action of the sarcolemmal sodium-calcium exchanger and sarcolemmal Ca^{2+}-ATPase pump.[19] In heart cells the decrease in intracellular calcium ion concentration at the start of diastole results primarily from uptake into the SR and, to a lesser extent, from efflux out of the cell via the sarcolemmal sodium-calcium exchanger and Ca^{2+}-ATPase pump. The age-associated decrease in the rate of relaxation may be partly the result of a reduced rate of calcium uptake (sequestration) by the SR.[21,22] Calcium uptake by the SR occurs via a Ca^{2+}-ATPase pump, which is embedded in the membrane of the SR. Investigators have found a decrease in the amount of messenger ribonucleic acid (mRNA) coding for the SR Ca^{2+}-ATPase pump in the aging myocardium.[23] Messenger RNA is the complementary nucleotide sequence transcribed from a gene sequence located along a deoxyribonucleotide (DNA) strand.[24] A decrease in mRNA or message for the synthesis of SR Ca^{2+}-ATPase pumps

TABLE 11-1 **Age-Related Changes in the Senescent Myocardium**

Change and Underlying Mechanism	Clinical Consequence
Increase in the duration of myocardial contraction and decrease in the rate of relaxation (diastole is shorter) A decrease in the rate of SR Ca^{2+} uptake	Diastole is shorter and therefore the time for coronary artery perfusion is shorter
Myosin isoform switching A different myosin heavy chain isoform is expressed, which is associated with reduced myosin ATPase activity and reduced velocity of shortening.	This isoform switching has been primarily found in animal models of aging; the increased expression of the β-myosin heavy chain isoform could represent an adaptational change that is associated with a decrease in the speed and extent of muscle shortening and therefore myocardial oxygen consumption
Decrease in β-adrenergic inotropic and chronotropic effects No change in b-adrenoreceptor density or affinity The attenuated b-adrenergic effect may be related to changes in postreceptor events, such as adenylyl cyclase activity and cyclic adenosine monophosphate production Decrease in catecholamine content of the heart, as well as a decrease in adrenergic nerve density	Decreased heart rate response to exercise and stress Decreased chronotropic and inotropic response to exogenously administered catecholamines
Decreased inotropic response to ouabain Decrease in the activity of the sarcolemmal Na-Ca exchanger Decrease in number of sarcolemmal Na^+-K^+-ATPase pumps	To date there are no reports on the inotropic effects of the cardiac glycoside digoxin in the aged human heart; however, based on data from animal studies there may be a similar attenuated inotropic effect

Data modified from Gerstenblith G and others: *Circ Res* 44:517, 1979; Guarnieri T and others: *Am J Physiol* 239:H501, 1980; Lakatta EG and others: *J Clin Invest* 55:61, 1975; Maciel LM and others: *Circ Res* 67(1):230, 1990; Scarpace PJ: *Fed Proc* 45:51, 1986; and Spurgeon HA, Steinbach MF, Lakatta EG: *Am J Physiol* 244:H513, 1983.
SR, Sarcoplasmic reticulum. *Ca^{2+}*, calcium; *ATP,* adenosine triphosphate.

may result in a decreased number of SR Ca^{2+}-ATPase pumps or decreased amount of Ca^{2+}-ATPase enzyme protein. These findings may in part explain the reduced uptake of calcium by the SR during relaxation and delayed rate of relaxation. Table 11-1 summarizes the age-associated changes in contraction and relaxation, as well as the effects of inotropic agents in the myocardium.[21,23,25-30] (∞Cardiac Physiology: Electrical Activity, p. 344.)

Changes in Myocardial Gene Expression

Some of the age-related changes in myocardial function are possibly the result of altered gene expression. Genes are a specific sequence of nucleotides located along the DNA strand that specify the amino acid sequence of a protein molecule. Gene expression refers to the transcription of a gene sequence along the DNA strand into a complementary mRNA strand.[31] Messenger RNA contains the genetic message for protein translation (protein synthesis), which occurs in the cytosol in association with free ribosomes or ribosomes attached to the endoplasmic reticulum. As previously noted, some of the changes in the older myocardium may be related to altered expression of proteins such the SR Ca^{2+}-ATPase.[23] In the hearts of senescent animals there are reports of the change in the contractile protein myosin.[31,32] Myosin contains the actin-binding site and myosin ATPase.[19] In the adult animal myocardium and in the human myocardium, two forms of the myosin are expressed: α-myosin heavy chain (α-MHC) and the β-myosin heavy chain (β-MHC). In animal models of aging, investigators have found an increase in the expression of the β-MHC isoform, which is associated with low myosin ATPase activity and reduced shortening velocity.[31,32] The significance of this isoform switch is not completely understood. Changes in gene expression and subsequent protein expression may represent an adaptive or protective response. On the other hand, some alterations in gene expression that occur in other tissue types are associated with abnormal tissue growth or carcinogenesis.[24]

Age-Associated Changes in Hemodynamics and the Electrocardiogram

Resting (supine) heart rate decreases with age.[33,34] Cinelli and others[33] reported a decrease in the resting heart rate from 78.8 beats/minute in young adults to 62.3 beats/minute in elderly adults. Heart rate is an important determinant of cardiac output (CO), and the normal resting heart beats approximately 70 times a minute. At rest or with minimal activity, the elderly person probably will not experience any untoward cardiovascular effect (i.e., a decrease in CO) with a heart rate of 62 beats/ minute. However, if the heart rate response is attenuated during exercise, the elderly person's capacity for exercise may be limited.

Intrinsic heart rate decreases with aging.[35] The *intrinsic heart rate* is the heart rate in the absence of parasympathetic and sympathetic influences. In healthy resting individuals, parasympathetic (cholinergic) influences predominate, which cause a heart rate of approximately 70 beats/minute.[19] In the absence of both parasympathetic and sympathetic influences, the heart rate of young adults averages about 100 beats/ minute (intrinsic heart rate). Jose[35] found that the intrinsic heart rate (in the presence of both sympathetic and parasympathetic blockers) in a 20-year-old person was 100 beats/minute, as compared with a heart rate of 74 beats/minute in an 80-year-old man. This decrease in intrinsic heart rate may in part explain the decrease in the resting (supine) heart rate that occurs with aging.

Resting CO and stroke volume are not changed with advancing age. Rodeheffer and others[36] studied subjects without coronary artery disease or other types of illnesses over a 30- to 80-year period (Baltimore Longitudinal Study of Aging) and found no changes in the resting CO or the cardiac index in participants.[36] At rest, left ventricular end-diastolic volume (preload), end-systolic volume (the volume of blood remaining in the ventricle after systole), and the ejection fraction are not affected by age.[37] In the elderly human myocardium, the early diastolic filling period and isovolumic phase of myocardial relaxation are prolonged.[38,39] However, these changes, although suggestive of diastolic dysfunction, do not translate into decreases in end-diastolic volume or stroke volume.[38,39] Finally, aging is associated with a moderate increase in pulmonary artery pressure.[40]

Advancing age produces changes in the ECG. R-wave and S-wave amplitude significantly decrease in persons older than 49 years, whereas Q-T duration increases (Table 11-2).[41] The increase in the duration of the Q-T interval is reflective of the prolonged rate of relaxation.[41] There is also a downward shift in the frontal plane axis from 48.93 to 38.83 degrees between the ages of 30 and 49 years, which is suggestive of a modest degree of cardiac enlargement or hypertrophy.[41]

The incidence of asymptomatic cardiac dysrhythmias increases in elderly patients.[42] The most common dysrhythmia occurring in elderly individuals is the premature ventricular contraction (PVC). Camm and others[43] and Fleg and Kennedy[44] report that 70% to 80% of all patients older than 60 years experience PVCs. In a healthy geriatric population (60 to 85 years old), 24-hour ambulatory electrocardiographic recordings revealed that 80% of the 98 subjects studied experienced asymptomatic ventricular ectopic beats. The findings of this study suggest that aging per se is associated with an increase in the occurrence of PVCs. Other common types of dysrhythmias are sinus node dysfunction (atrial fibrillation, atrial flutter, or paroxysmal supraventricular tachycardia) and atrioventricular conduction disturbances.[41,42] Because the majority of patients are asymptomatic, the use of antidysrhythmics is generally not recommended. The side effects and toxic effects of antidysrhythmics impose more of a risk, as compared with the risk of mortality or morbidity related to the dysrhythmia.[42] In contrast, in patients who are symptomatic and have malignant ventricular dysrhythmias (sustained ventricular tachycardia and/or fibrillation), pharmacologic therapy is warranted.[42] (∞Ventricular Dysrythmias, p 415.)

Age-Related Changes in Baroreceptor Function

Baroreceptor-reflex function is altered with aging.[45] Baroreceptors are mechanoreceptors that respond to stretch and other changes in the blood vessel wall and are located at the bifurcation of the common carotid artery and aortic arch.[19] Impulses arising in the baroreceptor region project to the vasomotor center (nucleus of tractus solitarius) in the medulla. Abrupt changes in blood pressure caused by increases in peripheral resistance, CO, or blood volume are sensed by the baroreceptors, resulting in an increase in the impulse frequency to the vasomotor center within the medulla. This increase inhibits vasoconstrictor impulses arising from the vasoconstrictor region within the medulla.[19] The result is a decrease in heart rate and peripheral vasodilation; both of these effects return the blood pressure to within normal limits. The baroreflex can be tested by measuring the heart rate

TABLE 11-2 **Age-Related Changes in Electrocardiographic Variables**

ECG Variable	<30 Years	30-39 Years	40-49 Years	>49 years
R-wave amplitude (mm)	10.43	10.53	9.01	9.25
S-wave amplitude (mm)	15.21	14.21	12.22	12.42
Frontal plane axis (degrees)	48.93	48.13	36.50	38.83
P-R duration (ms)	15.89	16.23	16.04	16.25
QRS duration (ms)	7.64	7.51	7.36	8.00
Q-T duration (ms)	37.83	37.50	37.99	39.58
T-wave amplitude (ms)	5.21	4.57	4.31	4.42

Data from Bachman S, Sparrow D, Smith LK: *Am J Cardiol* 48:513, 1981.

response (i.e., increase or decrease in heart rate) after the administration of either a pressor or depressor agent and by changing a person's position from lying to standing. Yin and others[46] and Elliott and others[47] found an attenuated increase in heart rate response in elderly subjects after the infusion of phenylephrine, an α_1-adrenoreceptor agonist that produces vasoconstriction and increases the blood pressure. Likewise, the baroreflex-mediated tachycardia response to depressor agents is also attenuated in elderly subjects.[46] There are several reports of an attenuation in the heart rate response of elderly subjects after changes in position (supine to standing).[48,49]

When an individual changes his or her position from supine to standing, the distribution of blood volume changes. This can result in a reduction in CO and hence blood pressure.[19] However, when a person changes position, there are simultaneous baroreceptor-mediated increases in the heart rate that maintain blood pressure by increasing CO. The baroreceptor-reflex response also mediates changes in the peripheral resistance and force of myocardial contraction, which likewise serve to offset the drop in blood pressure. It was once thought that postural hypotension occurred more frequently in elderly subjects and was an age-related phenolase. However, recent studies have shown that the prevalence of postural hypotension is quite low in elderly persons.[50,51] The prevalence of orthostatic hypotension is greater in institutionalized elderly patients who are receiving antihypertensive medications.[49]

Left Ventricular Function in Elderly Persons During Exercise

In most individuals, aging is associated with a decline in exercise performance. Exercise performance depends on a multitude of physiologic variables. Cardiac performance and the ability of the heart to increase and maintain CO is critical for increasing oxygen delivery to the peripheral tissues. During exercise, CO is increased by several mechanisms; however, the most important mechanisms include an increased heart rate, an increased inotropic state of the myocardium, and a decreased aortic impedance.[36] Some reports suggest that changes in exercise performance are related to a decrease in the maximal cardiac output achieved with exercise. However, Rodeheffer and others[36] reported that the elderly person's diminished ability to exercise is not because of the maximal CO that can be achieved during exercise. These investigators found no difference in CO response to different levels of exercise in subjects from the Baltimore Longitudinal Study on Aging.[36] With advancing age, the maximal heart rate achieved during exercise is attenuated; however, the decreased heart rate response is accompanied by an increase in left ventricular end diastolic volume (LVEDV) and stroke volume (SV). This augmentation in LVEDV and SV offsets the attenuated heart rate response and maintains CO in exercise. Changes in aortic impedance have not been studied in elderly individuals; however, in animal models, blood pressure and systemic vascular resistance are increased during exercise in senescent, but not young adult, animals.[52] In summary, in healthy older individuals there is no age-associated decline in cardiac output during exercise; however, other factors such as neural functioning, skeletal and joint functioning, as well as pulmonary function, may limit an older individual's ability to exercise.

The Peripheral Vascular System

The effects of aging on the peripheral vascular system are reflected in the gradual, but linear, rise in systolic blood pressure.[53,54] Diastolic blood pressure is less affected by age and generally remains the same or decreases.[54] Important determinants of systolic blood pressure include the compliance of the vasculature and the blood volume within the vascular system. Similar to the heart, the compliance of the vasculature is determined by its cell-type and tissue composition. With advancing age, the intimal layer thickens, principally because of an increase in smooth muscle cells (which have migrated from the medial layer), and the amount of connective tissue (collagen and elastic tissue) increases.[53] These changes occur in the intima of the large and distal arteries. This gradual decrease in arterial compliance or "stiffening of the arteries" is sometimes referred to as *arteriosclerosis.* Arteriosclerotic changes are also accompanied by changes caused by atherosclerosis, which is the accumulation of lipoproteins and fibrinous products—such as platelets, macrophages, and leukocytes—within a vessel.[55] The consequences of arteriosclerotic and atherosclerotic processes are that the arteries become progressively less distensible and the vascular pressure-volume relationship is altered. These changes are clinically significant, because small changes in intravascular volume are accompanied by disproportionate increases in systolic blood pressure.[56] The decrease in arterial compliance and disproportionate increase in systolic blood pressure may lead to an increase in afterload and the development of concentric (pressure-induced) ventricular hypertrophy in the elderly patient.[56]

It is well-recognized that increased serum lipoprotein levels are risk factors in the development and progression of atherosclerosis.[55] Lipoprotein levels increase with advancing age. However, innumerable factors can influence serum lipoprotein levels, making it very difficult to determine whether such changes contribute to the aging of the peripheral vascular system.[57,58] Serum lipoproteins are particles that contain varying amounts of cholesterol, triglycerides, phospholipids, and apoproteins.[55] There are five principal serum lipoproteins: chylomicrons, low-density lipoproteins (LDLs), very low-density lipoproteins (VLDLs), intermediate-density lipoproteins (IDLs), and high-density lipoproteins (HDLs). The lipoprotein classification is based on the lipoprotein's size and relative concentration of cholesterol, triglycerides, and apoproteins.[55] In men, the serum total cholesterol level (all of the lipoproteins combined) increases progressively from 150 to 200 mg/dL between the ages of 20 and 50 years and remains relatively unchanged until the age of 70 years.[58] As would be predicted, the age-related changes in serum LDL levels parallel the changes in the total serum cholesterol level. All lipoprotein fractions transport cholesterol; however, in healthy people, three fourths of the total cholesterol is transported within the LDL.[55] There are relatively few age-related changes in VLDL and HDL levels in men. In men, serum triglyceride levels peak at approximately age 40 and then decrease.[57,58]

In women, serum total cholesterol levels are low between the ages of 20 and 50 years.[57,58] However, between the ages 55 to 60 years, serum total cholesterol levels progressively increase, usually simultaneously with changes in the hormonal production of estrogen.[58] The increase in total serum cholesterol levels is primarily the result of an increase in the LDL fraction and, to a lesser extent, the VLDL and HDL fractions, which do not change appreciably with age in women. In women, serum triglyceride levels progressively increase with age.[58] (∞Laboratory Assessment: Serum Lipid Studies, p. 383.)

Arterial pressure is also governed by the amount of blood volume, which in turn is regulated by plasma levels of sodium and water and the activity of the renin-angiotensin system (RAS).[59] Plasma renin activity declines with age, and aging per se has no appreciable effect on sodium and water homeostasis.[60,61] However, as noted earlier, there are age-related changes in tubular function, as well as a decrease in the glomerular filtration rate (GFR), both of which can affect overall sodium and water homeostasis. Circulating levels of sodium-regulating hormones—such as natriuretic hormone, aldosterone, and antidiuretic hormone (ADH)—are not appreciably altered by advancing age.[61,62] However, a delayed natriuretic response after sodium loading and plasma volume expansion and diminished renal response to ADH secretion have been reported in elderly persons.[62]

RESPIRATORY SYSTEM

Many of the changes in the pulmonary system that occur with aging are reflected in tests of pulmonary function and include changes in thoracic wall expansion and respiratory muscle strength, morphology of alveolar parenchyma, and decreases in arterial oxygen tension (Pa_{O_2}) (Tables 11-3 and 11-4).[63] These changes occur progressively as age advances and should not alter the elderly person's ability to breathe effortlessly. However, factors such as repeated exposure to environmental pollutants, cigarette smoking, and frequent pulmonary infections can accelerate age-related changes, thereby making it difficult to identify the age-associated changes in pulmonary function. Interestingly, Thurlbeck[64] did not find age-related morpho-

TABLE 11-3 Age-Related Changes in Commonly Performed Pulmonary Function Tests

Pulmonary Function Test	Description	Standard Lung Volume and Capacity (ml)	Age-Related Change (ml)
Total lung capacity	Vital capacity plus residual volume	6000	No change
Vital capacity	Amount of air exhaled after a maximal inspiration	5000	↓ 3750
Tidal volume (VT)	Amount of air inhaled or exhaled with each breath	500	No change
Residual volume (RV)	Amount of air left in lungs after forced exhalation	1200	↑ 1800
Inspiratory reserve volume (IRV)	Amount of air that can be forcefully inhaled after inspiring a normal VT	3100	↓ 2800
Expiratory reserve volume (ERV)	Amount of air that can be forcefully exhaled after expiring a normal VT	1200	↓ 1000
Forced expiratory volume in 1 sec (FEV_1)	Volume exhaled in the first second of a single forced expiratory volume; expressed as a percent of the forced vital capacity	80%	↓ 75%

TABLE 11-4 Progressive Changes in Arterial Oxygen Tension (Pao_2) and Carbon Dioxide Tension ($Paco_2$)

Age-Group	Pao_2 (mm Hg)	$Paco_2$ (mm Hg)
<30 years	94	39
31-40	87	38
41-50	84	40
51-60	81	39
>60	74	40

Adapted from Sorbini CA and others: *Respiration* 25:3, 1968.

logic changes in the lung tissue of aging mice raised in a pollution-free and infection-free environment, suggesting the immense effect of environmental variables on pulmonary function.

Thoracic Wall and Respiratory Muscles

With advancing age, the chest wall (thoracic skeleton) and vertebrae undergo a small degree of osteoporosis, and at the same time the costal cartilages that connect the rib cage together become calcified and stiff. These changes may produce kyphosis and reduce chest wall compliance, respectively (Figure 11-1).[63,65,66] The functional effect is a decrease in thoracic wall excursion. Other factors, such as an increase in abdominal girth and change in posture, also decrease thoracic excursion. These anatomic structural changes are reflected by an increase in residual volume and decrease in vital capacity (see Table 11-3).

There is a gradual decrease in the strength of the respiratory muscles: the diaphragm and both the external and internal intercostal muscles. The diaphragm is the most important inspiratory muscle, because its movement accounts for 75% of the change in intrathoracic volume during quiet respiration.[67] The respiratory muscles are composed of skeletal muscle fibers.[67] During aging, skeletal muscle progressively atrophies and its energy metabolism decreases, which may partially explain the declining strength of the respiratory muscles.[68,69] In addition, there is an age-associated decrease in the effectiveness of the cough reflex, which is possibly caused by a decrease in ciliary responsiveness and motion.[70] These changes underscore the importance of deep breathing and coughing for the bedridden elderly patient in the critical care unit. (∞Muscles of Ventilation, p. 603.)

As noted previously, the age-associated changes in pulmonary function do not alter the elderly person's ability to breathe effortlessly. However, the decrease in respiratory muscle strength may be a limiting factor during exercise, because the respiratory muscles—specifically the accessory inspiratory muscles (sternocleidomastoid, scalene, and trapezius)—facilitate

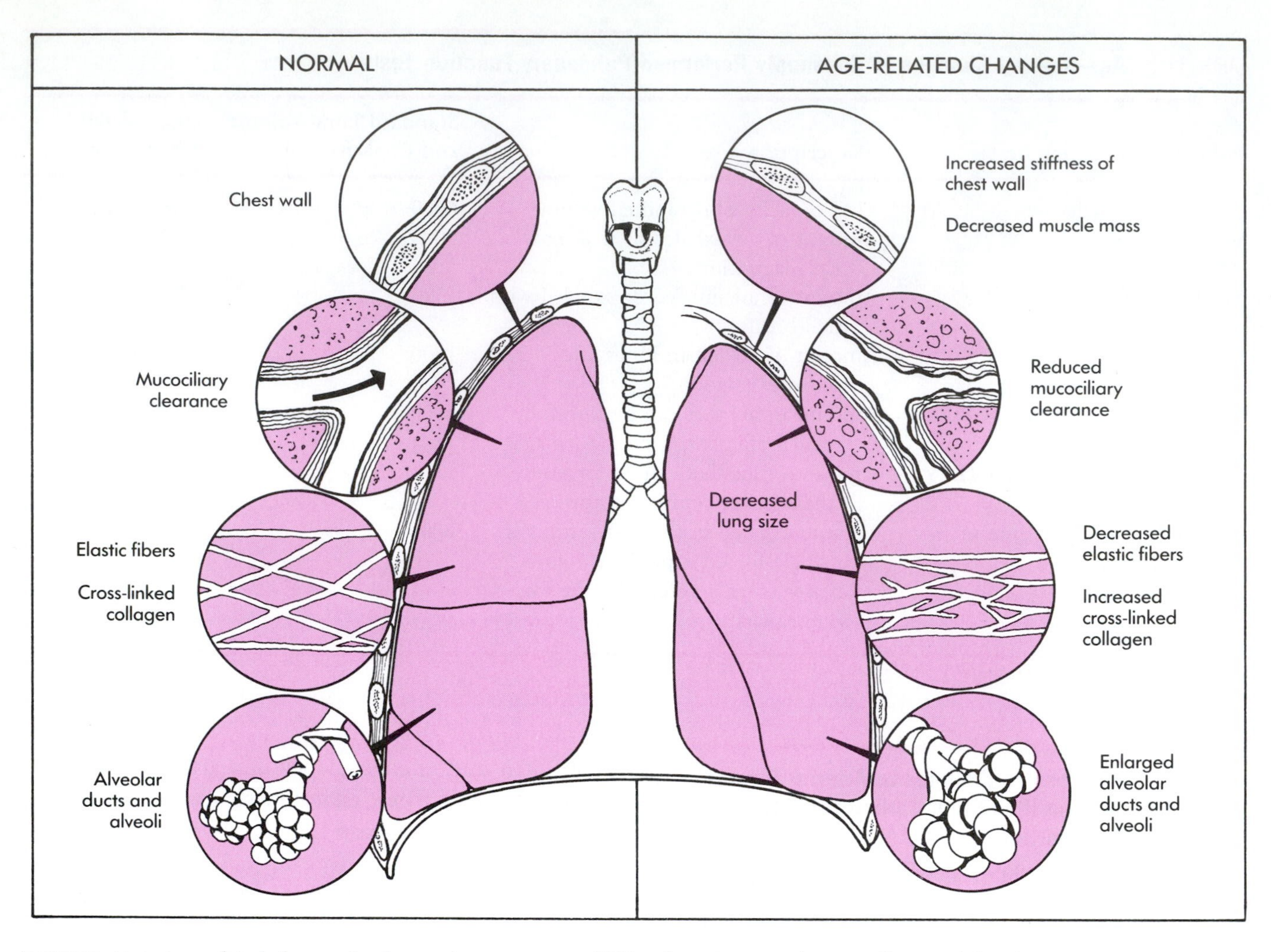

FIGURE 11-1 Age-related changes in the respiratory system. With advancing age, the compliance of the chest wall and lung tissue changes. There is also a reduced clearance of mucus by the cilia that line the pulmonary tree and an enlargement of the alveolar ducts and alveoli. More age-related changes in respiratory function are described in the text.

inspiration during exercise. However, this theory is not supported by the findings of Belman and Gaesser,[71] who reported that although ventilatory muscle strength improved after elderly men and women received ventilatory muscle training, neither submaximal or maximal exercise tolerance improved.

Alveolar Parenchyma

With advancing age a diminished recoil (or increased compliance) of the lung occurs.[72] The reduced recoil results from the increase in the ratio of elastin to collagen content that occurs with advancing age.[73] Collagen, elastin, and reticulin are the primary connective tissue proteins of the lung tissue.[74,75] They are responsible for the elasticity and performance of the airways of the lung. Whereas total lung collagen remains unaltered, the amount of elastin increases with age in the interlobular septa and pleura and possibly within the bronchi and their vessels.[74,75] These anatomic structural changes are reflected by an increase in residual volume and a decrease in forced expiratory volume. An additional anatomic structural change is the increase in the size of the alveolar ducts, which occurs after 40 years of age.[63] The bronchial enlargement displaces inhaled air volume away from the alveoli that line the alveolar ducts (see Figure 11-1).[63] Ventilation and the process of oxygen and carbon dioxide exchange (diffusion) depend on numerous factors, one of which is the surface area available for diffusion. A displacement of inhaled air volume away from the alveoli limits the surface area available for gas exchange. This may in part explain the progressive and linear decrease in the pulmonary diffusion capacity, which depends on both the surface area and capillary blood volume. There are reports that capillary blood volume and surface area decrease with advancing age.[76] (∞Respiration, p. 618.)

Pulmonary Gas Exchange

The arterial oxygen tension (Pa_{O_2}) decreases with age, such that the median Pa_{O_2} for healthy persons older than 60 years is 74.3 mm Hg, as compared with 94 mm Hg for younger adults.[77] In contrast, arterial carbon dioxide (Pa_{CO_2}) does not change with advancing age (see Table 11-4).[77] The decrease in Pa_{O_2} may be the result of an increase in the closing volume in the dependent lung zones during resting tidal breathing in older subjects.[78,79] Consequently, dependent lung zones may be ventilated intermittently, leading to regional differences in ventilation. It is possible that alterations in blood volume and vascular resistance within the pulmonary circulation may also contribute to ventilation/perfusion (V/Q) mismatching. Other factors, such as smoking and pulmonary disease, also have an impact on the level of arterial oxygenation. (∞Ventilation/Perfusion Relationships, p. 618.)

Lung Volumes and Capacities

With advancing age, total lung capacity and tidal volume do not change[65] (see Table 11-3). Residual volume (RV) increases with age, paralleling the decrease in chest wall compliance and reduced strength of the respiratory muscles (see Table 11-3).[63] The increase in RV may also add to the diminished strength of the inspiratory muscles by stretching the diaphragm and altering the tension-length relationship. Results from studies are conflicting with regard to age-related changes in functional residual capacity (FRC), which is the volume of air in the lungs at the normal resting end-expiratory position. There are reports of no change[80] and decreases[65] in FRC in elderly persons. The balance of two opposing forces, the elastic recoil of the lung and the outward recoil of the chest wall, determine the FRC.[67] These factors change in opposite directions with age: the elastic recoil of the lung decreases, thereby increasing compliance, and the outward recoil of the chest wall decreases, thus decreasing the compliance of the chest wall. One would predict that because these factors change in opposite directions, FRC would remain unaltered. In fact, Knudson and others[80] found no change in FRC in elderly persons supporting this prediction.

Other lung volumes that decrease with age include the inspiratory reserve volume (IRV) and the expiratory reserve volume (ERV).[65] The decrease in the ERV is the result of an increase in the RV. The decrease in IRV, however, has been found only in studies reporting a corresponding increase in FRC. See Table 11-3 and Figure 11-1 for a summary of age-related changes in pulmonary function.

The following dynamic measurements of lung volume are decreased in aging: maximal expiratory flow rate, maximal midexpiratory flow rate, forced expiratory volume in 1 second (FEV_1), and the ratio of FEV_1 to forced vital capacity.[81] Dynamic measurements of lung volume reflect changes in air flow rate; air flow rate depends on the resistance of airways and chest wall compliance. Hence the age-related decrease in the dynamic lung volume is probably caused by decreased chest wall compliance, increased likelihood of small airways closing during forced expiratory efforts (increasing airway resistance), and decreased strength of expiratory muscles.[82] (∞Bedside Pulmonary Function Tests, p. 648.)

THE RENAL SYSTEM

Aging produces changes in renal structure and function, many of which begin at approximately 30 to 40 years of age.[83] One of the prominent changes is a decrease in the number and size of the nephrons, which begins in the cortical regions and progresses toward the medullary portions of the kidney.[84] The decrease in the number of nephrons corresponds to a 20% decrease in the weight of the kidney between 40 and 80 years of age.[84] Initially, this loss of nephrons does not appreciably alter renal function because of the large renal reserve: the kidney contains approximately 2 million to 3 million nephrons, all of which are not needed to maintain adequate fluid and acid-base homeostasis. However, with time the geriatric patient also loses this "renal reserve."[84] Nephron loss is caused by a gradual reduction in blood flow to the glomerular capillary tuft.[85] Total renal blood flow declines after the fourth decade of life[83] because of hyaline arteriolosclerosis.[85,86] The etiology of this vascular lesion within the glomerular tuft is unknown. By the eighth decade of life, 50% of the glomeruli are lost as a result of this arteriolar hyalinization.[84] (∞Kidneys and Urinary Tract: Anatomy, p. 849.)

The GFR decreases with advancing age.[83,84] The GFR is the volume of fluid traversing the glomerular membrane in a given period and is an important regulator of water and solute excretion. GFR depends on the permeability of the glomerular capillary and the surface area available for filtration, as well as the balance of pressure gradients between the glomerular capillary and Bowman's space.[59] In elderly persons, the decrease in GFR is most likely caused by the decrease in nephron number, as well as the decrease in renal blood flow.[83] (∞Kidneys and Urinary Tract: Functions of the Kidneys/Excretion of Nitrogen Wastes, p. 855.)

Even though the remaining nephrons adapt to the loss of nephrons by glomerular hyperfiltration and increased solute load per nephron, the reduced GFR predisposes the elderly patient to adverse drug reactions and drug-induced renal failure. Some drugs are excreted unchanged in the urine, whereas other drugs have active or nephrotoxic metabolites that are excreted in the urine. In addition, the senescent kidney is more susceptible to injury by hypotensive episodes, because of the age-related decrease in renal blood flow and reduced pressure gradient across the afferent arteriole.[87]

There are also age-related changes in tubular function. The functions that are primarily carried out in the renal tubules are sodium and water concentration and conservation and acidification of the urine.[59] These functions are governed by the amount of sodium and water delivered to the tubules and overall acid-base balance. The age-related changes in tubular function become apparent when there are extreme changes in the body fluid composition or acid-base balance. For example, with systemic acidosis the rate and amount of total acid excretion (bicarbonate, titratable acid, and ammonium) are reduced.[83,87] This predisposes the elderly patient to metabolic acidosis, volume depletion, and hyperchloremia. However, at a normal pH level, the kidney of an elderly person is able to maintain acid-base homeostasis.

There is a diminished ability of the senescent kidney to excrete a free water load, conserve water during periods of dehydration, and conserve sodium during periods of low salt intake.[83] There are also age-related changes in extrarenal mechanisms, such as the decreased activity and responsiveness of the senescent kidney to the sympathetic nervous system and renin-angiotensin-aldosterone system, which are important in integrating overall fluid homeostasis and maintaining blood pressure in response to changes in body position.[60]

THE GASTROINTESTINAL SYSTEM

Age-related gastrointestinal changes occur in the processes of swallowing, motility, and absorption.[88,89] Swallowing may be difficult for the elderly person because of incomplete mastication of food.[89] Deteriorating dentition, diminished lubrication (secondary to salivary dysfunction), and ill-fitting dentures result in insufficient mastication of food within the oral cavity, thereby predisposing the elderly patient to aspiration.[88] In addition, the number and velocity of the peristaltic contractions of the elderly person's esophagus decrease and the number of nonperistaltic contractions increases.[89] (∞Mouth, p. 919.)

These changes in esophageal motility are referred to as presbyesophagus. These changes may predispose the patient to erosion of the esophageal wall (recurrent esophagitis), because food remains in the esophagus longer. In addition, bedrest and reclining in a supine position for a prolonged period can cause esophageal reflux, which also can lead to esophagitis. (∞Esophagus, p. 920.)

The aging process produces thinning of the smooth muscle within the gastric mucosa.[90] The epithelial layer of the gastric mucosa, which contains the chief and parietal cells, undergoes a modest degree of atrophy, resulting in the hyposecretion of pepsin and acid, respectively.[91] However, with aging there is a prevalence of gastritis-induced achlorhydria (decreased acid secretion). Therefore it remains unknown whether the changes in gastric acid secretion are a result of age-related changes or a disease process such as gastritis. (∞Stomach, p. 920.)

Mucin secretion from the mucus cells decreases, thereby altering the protective function of the gastric mucosal (bicarbonate) barrier. Because of this, the stomach wall is more susceptible to acid injury, thus increasing the incidence of gastric ulcerations.[92] Aging does not appreciably alter gastric emptying of solid foods. However, Moore and others[93] found a delay in the emptying of liquids from the stomach in elderly persons.

To our knowledge, there are no reported changes in small intestinal peristalsis or segmental movements with aging.[94] Alterations within the small intestine include a decrease in intestinal weight after the age of 50 and a flattening and shortening of jejunal villi.[94] Age produces no change in the small intestine's absorption of fats and proteins; however, decreased carbohydrate absorption has been reported.[95,96] There is essentially no change in vitamin or mineral absorption, except for a decrease in calcium absorption from the aged duodenum.[89] In summary, there are age-associated changes in gastrointestinal function; however, these changes are not of sufficient magnitude to produce malnutrition in healthy elderly humans.

THE LIVER

With advancing age, both hepatocyte number and liver weight decrease.[97] There is also a significant decrease in total liver blood flow, such that between 25 and 65 years of age there is a 50% decrease in total liver blood flow.[97-99] The liver has many complex functions, including carbohydrate storage, ketone body formation, reduction and conjugation of adrenal and gonadal steroid hormones, synthesis of plasma proteins, deamination of amino acids, storage of cholesterol, urea formation, and detoxification of toxins and drugs. However, despite changes in hepatocyte number and blood flow, liver function is not appreciably altered.[99] Several tests of liver function—such as serum bilirubin, alkaline phosphatase, and glutamic oxaloacetic transaminase levels—are not altered with advancing age. However, because of the decrease in total liver blood flow, there is some reduction in first-pass clearance of drugs. (∞Liver, p. 926.)

The most important age-related change in liver function is the decrease in the liver's capacity to metabolize drugs.[100,101] Although clinical tests of liver function do not reflect this change in metabolism, it is well-recognized that drug side effects and toxic effects occur more frequently in older adults than in young adults.[101] This reduced drug-metabolizing capacity is caused by a reduction in the activity of the drug-metabolizing enzyme system (MEOS) and decrease in total liver blood flow.[98,102]

Changes in Pharmacokinetics and Pharmacodynamics

There are many age-related changes in drug *pharmacokinetics,* which is the manner in which the body absorbs, distributes, metabolizes, and excretes a drug.[102,103] The aging process is associated with changes in gastric acid secretion, which can alter the ionization or solubility of a drug and hence its absorption (Table 11-5).[101,102]

Drug distribution depends on body composition, as well as the physiochemical properties of the drug. With advancing age, fat content increases, lean body mass decreases, and total body water decreases, which can alter the drug disposition.[102] For example, because of the increase in the ratio of body fat content to body weight, lipophilic drugs have a greater volume of distribution per body weight in elderly persons, as compared with younger adults. Other age-related factors[104] affecting drug disposition are listed in Table 11-5.

As noted previously, the senescent liver has a decreased ability to metabolize drugs, which also affects the clearance of some drugs. For example, there is a reduced clearance of loop diuretics in elderly patients, which reduces the peak plasma concentration of the diuretic, as well as decreases the magnitude of the diuretic response.[105] Other drugs—such as angiotensin II-converting enzyme (ACE) inhibitors—have delayed

TABLE 11-5 Age-Related Changes in Pharmacokinetics

Pharmacokinetic Parameter	Definition	Age-Related Changes
Absorption	Receptor-coupled or diffusional uptake of drug into tissue	Decreased absorptive surface area of small intestine Decrease in splanchnic blood flow Increase in gastric acid pH Decrease in gastrointestinal motility
Distribution	Theoretic space (tissue) or body compartment into which free form of drug distributes	Decreased lean body mass and total body water Increased total body fat Decreased serum albumin level Increased alpha$_1$-acid glycoprotein
Metabolism	Chemical change in drug that renders it active or inactive	Decreased liver mass Decrease in activity of microsomal drug-metabolizing enzyme system Decrease in total liver blood flow
Excretion	Removal of drug through an eliminating organ, which is often the kidney; some drugs are excreted in the bile or feces, in the saliva, or via the lungs	Decreased renal blood flow and GFR Decrease in distal renal tubular secretory function

Data from Gilman and others, editors: *Goodman and Gilman's the pharmacological basis of therapeutics,* London, 1990, Pergamon Press; and Vestal RE, Cusack BJ: Pharmacology and aging. In Schneider EL, Rowe JW, editors: *Handbook of the biology of aging,* San Diego, 1990, Academic Press.

excretion, increased serum concentration, and more prolonged duration of action because their excretion parallels GFR (which decreases with age).[106] See Table 11-5 for age-related changes in drug pharmacokinetics and Table 11-6[87,104,106-111] for the potential side effects, nursing interventions, and/or special considerations for frequently used pharmacologic agents in the elderly patient in the critical care unit.

There are reports of age-related changes in pharmacodynamics. *Pharmacodynamics* refers to the pharmacologic or physiologic response to a drug that occurs after the drug interacts with its receptor on the plasma membrane. The chronotropic and inotropic effects of beta-adrenergic agonists reportedly decrease in elderly patients.[112,113] There also are reports that age produces no change in heparin-stimulated increases in partial thromboplastin time, whereas there is a diminished effect of warfarin (Coumadin) (less of an increase in the prothrombin time). See Schwertz and Bushmann[103] for an extensive review of the pharmacologic considerations for the elderly patient in the critical care unit.

THE CENTRAL NERVOUS SYSTEM

Cognitive Functioning and Aging

Cognitive functioning involves the process of transforming, synthesizing, storing, and retrieving sensory input. Additional components include perception, attention, thinking, memory, and problem solving. For the aging individual, cognition is altered by the speed in which information is processed and retrieved.[114] Performance on timed tests declines slowly past the age of 20 years. Intelligence remains fairly stable past the age of 30 years until one reaches the mid-80s. Although the rate in which complex tasks are completed may be diminished, these age-related changes are not, however, synonymous with cognitive impairment. See Box 11-1 for additional information.

Marked deterioration of any component of cognitive functioning is not a normal expectation of the aging process.[115] Cognitive impairment in older adults more commonly results from acute and chronic etiologies. Acute problems such as infection, electrolyte imbalances, or pharmacologic toxicity are generally reversible once identified. Long-term chronic impairment develops from more organic causations such as multinfarct dementia or dementia of the Alzheimer's type.

Although dementia is pathology based and not to be an expected outcome of aging, there is a very high prevalance of chronic illness for individuals 85 years and older. It has been estimated that one fourth of individuals who are 85 or older are demented in the United States, and Alzheimer's disease accounts for two thirds of the etiology.[116] Alzheimer's disease is identified by amyloid-containing neuritic plaques in various areas of the cortex.[117] Alzheimer's disease is characterized by progressive short- and long-term memory loss. Marked decline in memory ultimately leaves the individual functionally impaired and physically dependent.

Changes in Structure and Morphology

The brain decreases approximately 20% in size between 25 and 95 years of age (Figure 11-2).[118] The reduced brain weight may be related in part to the overall decrease in the number of neurons that occurs with advancing age. Neurons are lost from the hippocampus, amygdala, and cerebellum, and from areas of the brainstem such as the locus ceruleus, the dorsal motor nucleus of the vagus, and the substantia nigra.[114,116] This is in contrast to areas such as the hypothalamus, where very few neurons disappear with advancing age.[118] In addition, portions of the cerebral cortex atrophy, principally the frontal and temporal cortical association areas (the superior frontal gyrus and superior temporal gyrus, respectively).[119]

The cerebral ventricles enlarge and develop an asymmetric appearance.[120] Cerebrospinal fluid (CSF) also accumulates in the ventricles; however, total brain CSF is not increased.[120] Accompanying the loss of neurons are changes in the ultrastructure and intracellular structures of the neuron.[121] The neuron is composed of a cell body, dendrite, and axon. Dendrites are long, spiny processes extending out from the cell body. One of the most ubiquitous changes in the aging brain is a decrease in the number of dendrite spines. Interestingly, between middle and late old age the length of the dendritic spines increases, but then decreases after late old age (older than 90 years).[118] There are also reports of large neuron shrinking and degenerative changes occurring in the cell bodies and axons of certain acetylcholine-secreting neurons. These changes may explain alterations in processing and receiving information.[118] (∞Microstructure of the Nervous System, p. 733.)

With advancing age, lipofuscins, neuritic plaques, and neurofibrillary bodies appear within the cytoplasm of the neuron.[118] Lipofuscins, or age pigment, are granules containing a dark fluorescent pigment. They are derived from lipid-rich membranes that have been partially disintegrated and oxidized. It is still not clear whether lipofuscin accumulation is harmful to

TABLE 11-6 Pharmacologic Agents Used in the Critical Care Unit and Frequent Side Effects Experienced by the Gerontologic Patient

Pharmacologic Agent	Drug Actions	Adverse Drug Effects*	Nursing Interventions and/or Special Considerations
ACE INHIBITORS			
Enalapril	Inhibits the conversion of angiotensin I to angiotensin II	Hypotension, especially in patients taking diuretics Hypokalemia	Monitor HR and BP Monitor serum creatinine level Monitor serum K^+ level Excreted by the kidney so the dosage is reduced if the GFR is reduced
DIURETICS			
Lasix	Inhibits Na^+ and Cl^- absorption from the proximal tubule and loop of Henle	Hypokalemia Volume depletion	Reduced rate of clearance and magnitude of the diuretic response
CARDIAC GLYCOSIDES			
Digoxin	Inhibits the sarcolemmal Na^+-K^+-ATPase	Digitalis toxicity	Monitor HR and serum K^+ and serum digoxin levels Verapamil, quinidine, and amiodarone increase serum digoxin levels
ANTIDYSRHYTHMICS			
Procainamide	Decreases myocardial conduction velocity and excitability and prolongs myocardial refractoriness	Procainamide toxicity	Procainamide is converted to its active metabolite, N-acetyl-procainamide (NAPA), in the liver; NAPA may accumulate and cause side effects, even though the procainamide plasma level is within therapeutic range
Lidocaine	Decreases automaticity (especially in Purkinje fibers) and prolongs conduction and refractoriness	Dizziness, paresthesia, and drowsiness at lower plasma concentrations	Can be administered only parenterally
CALCIUM CHANNEL BLOCKERS			
Verapamil	Blocks the entry of Ca^{2+} through voltage-dependent Ca^{2+} channels and decreases SA automaticity and AV conduction	Constipation May alter liver function	Monitor liver function tests Contraindicated in heart failure, sick sinus syndrome, or first-degree AV block
Nifedipine	Same as verapamil	Headaches, tachycardia, palpitations, flushing, and ankle edema	Calcium channel blockers have a negative inotropic effect, but nifedipine produces less of a negative inotropic effect as compared with verapamil
Diltiazem	Same as verapamil	Constipation	Monitor liver function tests Contraindicated in heart failure, sick sinus syndrome, or first-degree AV block

Continued

Data modified from Creasy WA and others: *J Clin pharmacol* 26:264, 1986; Gilman AG and others, editors: *Goodman and Gilman's the pharmacological basis of therapeutics,* London, 1990, Pergamon Press; Hockings N, Ajayi AA, Reid JL: *Br J Pharmacol* 21:341, 1986; Lynch RA, Horowitz LN: *Geriatrics* 46:41, 1991; Pederson KE: *Acta Med Scand* 697(suppl 1):1, 1985; Vidt GD, Borazanian RA: *Geriatrics* 46:28, 1991; Wall RT: *Clin Geriatr Med* 6:345, 1990; and Watters JM, McClaran JC: The elderly surgical patient. In Wilmore DW and others, editors: *In care of the surgical patient,* vol III, Special problems, New York, 1990, Scientific American.

*Not all side effects are listed for each drug.

AV, Atrioventricular node; *SA,* sinus node.

TABLE 11-6 Pharmacologic Agents Used in the Critical Care Unit and Frequent Side Effects Experienced by the Gerontologic Patient—cont'd

Pharmacologic Agent	Drug Actions	Adverse Drug Effects*	Nursing Interventions and/or Special Considerations
NARCOTIC ANALGESICS			
Meperidine	Blocks the transmission of pain and inhibits the release of substance P; site of action is within the CNS	Respiratory depression and oversedation Tremors and muscle twitches related to effects of the metabolite normeperidine	Accumulation of normeperidine can produce CNS hyperexcitability The volume of distribution for morphine is small; hence plasma and tissue levels are greater at a specific plasma concentration
Morphine	Synthetic analgesic; mechanism similar to meperidine	Respiratory depression and oversedation	

BOX 11-1 The Use of Physical Restraints on Elderly Patients in the Critical Care Unit

Physical restraints are commonly used in the critical care unit to reduce the risk of injury to the sick elderly patient or to prevent the patient from prematurely removing pacemakers, Swan-Ganz catheters, and so on. Physical restraints may be used in young, as well as elderly, patients. However, Catchen[122] found that physical restraints were more frequently used with elderly patients.

Previously, the most common rationale for the use of physical restraints was the prevention of injury to self or others.[123] More recently, Kapp[124] reported that nurses most often decide to restrain patients because of potential litigation resulting from injuries associated with falls or the premature removal of facilitative treatments. Among elderly people, falls represent a primary cause of injury, disability, and death.[125] Elderly patients experience the largest percentage of these falls in institutions, and the most frequent site is at the bedside.[125]

Nurses can use restraints intermittently, depending on the patient's level of alertness, or nurses can continuously restrain the patient. Interestingly, patients who were continually restrained fell more frequently than did those who were not, because the restraints produced more agitation and combative behavior.[123] In addition, several investigators have reported that patients lose their balance and steadiness and develop elimination problems when restraints are used.[122, 126] Of particular interest to critical care nurses is that elderly restrained patients are predisposed to aspiration pneumonia,[127] circulatory obstruction,[128] circulatory stress,[129] dehydration,[130] and orthostatic hypotension.[131] Other potential problems include discomfort, weakening and contracture of the affected limb, pressure sores, diminished respiratory excursion, and possible death from strangulation.[122]

Interestingly, once the medical order to use physical restraints is obtained, it is seldom discontinued. Restraints may magnify the patient's fear of losing control, diminish his or her sense of dignity, and distort others' future perceptions of the patient's mental competence.

Considering these deleterious effects of physical restraints, critical care nurses must carefully consider the risks and benefits of restraints. For example, it is well-recognized that premature removal of an arterial balloon pump catheter may produce excessive bleeding and cardiogenic shock. The best alternative to the use of physical restraints is continuous surveillance. However, this is not always feasible in a critical care unit, because of sudden emergencies or staffing conditions.

Protecting the patient from falls or inappropriate removal of treatments, such as catheters and intravenous tubing, can be achieved by limiting the movement of the patient's limbs or torso with the use of soft wrist/ankle restraints and a posey jacket, respectively. The nurse must observe the patient frequently and listen to his or her concerns. The call light should be within the patient's reach, and the nurse needs to encourage family and friends to visit frequently. In the event that physical restraints are deemed necessary, it is important to follow the institution's policy regarding the use of physical restraints. In addition, the nurse must release the restraints every hour to check color, motor skills, and sensation of torso and extremities and make an ongoing assessment about the necessity of using the restraints.

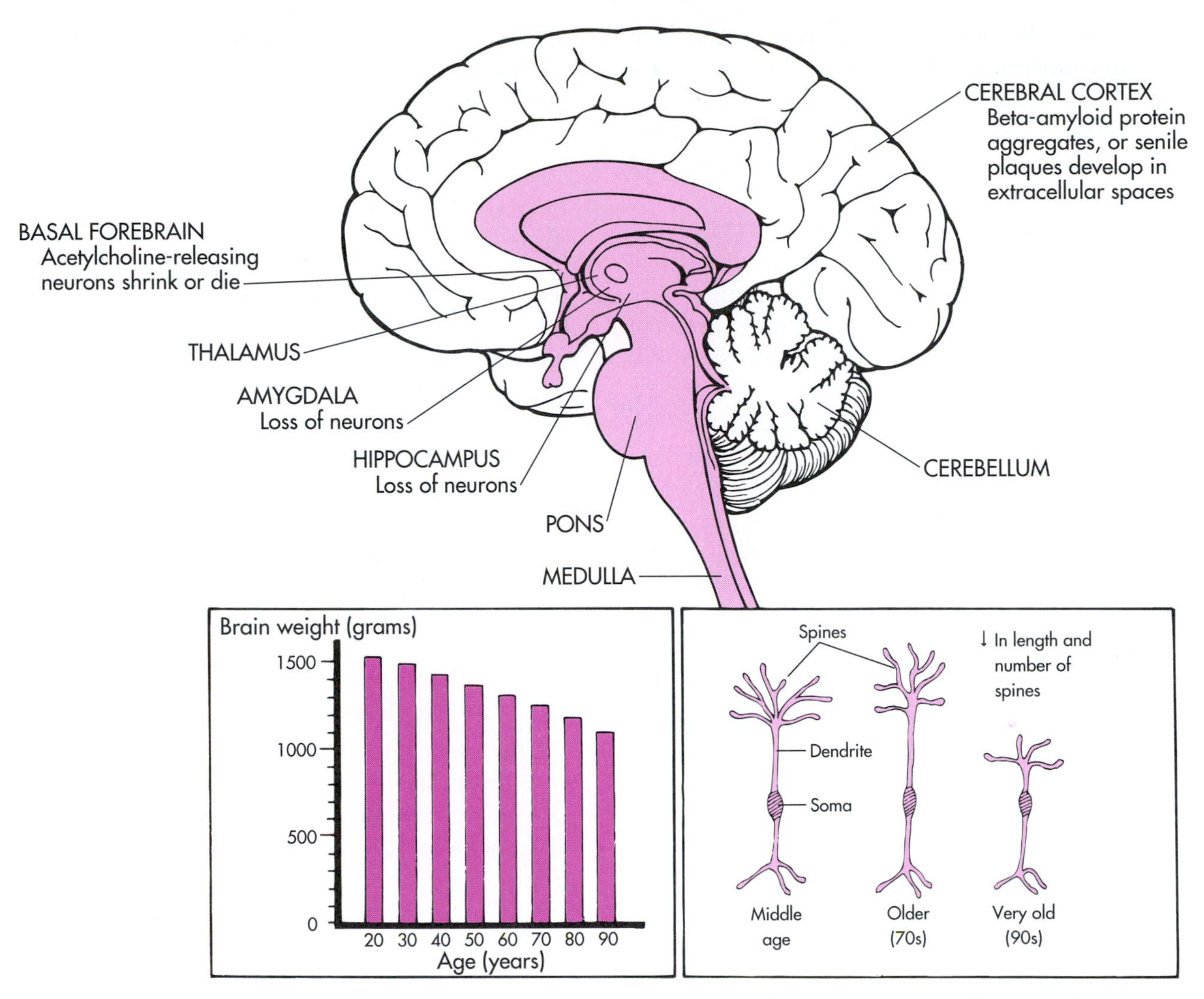

FIGURE 11-2 Summary of age-related changes in the brain. (From Soelkoe DJ: *Sci Am* 267:135, 1992.)

the brain.[118] Neuritic, or senile, plaques are aggregates of the beta-amyloid protein, and they also accumulate in the brain of normal senescent persons. Neuritic plaques are found in the hippocampus, cerebral cortex, and other brain regions.[118] Neurofibrillary tangles, which are bundles of helically wound protein filaments, occur in the hippocampus with advancing age in healthy persons.[119] However, they are present in larger numbers in persons with neuropathologic disorders such as Alzheimer's disease. It has been suggested that neurofibrillary tangles could interfere with neuronal signaling.[118]

In the senescent brain, synaptogenesis (synaptic regeneration) still occurs after partial nerve degeneration.[121] After a nerve fiber is damaged, neighboring undamaged neurons often sprout new fibers and form new connections. However, synaptogenesis occurs at a slower rate in the older brain.[121]

Neurotransmitter Synthesis

Advancing age is associated with changes in neurotransmitter function. Altered neurotransmitter function can result from changes in the available precursors for neurotransmitter synthesis, changes in the neurotransmitter receptor, and changes in the activity of the enzymes that synthesize and degrade the neurotransmitter. Different methods are used to examine changes in neurotransmitter function, and these methods include measuring neurotransmitter levels, neurotransmitter turnover, and receptor number and binding. Changes in neurotransmitter systems in the aging brain are equivocal, more than likely a result of the different methods employed to study neurotransmitter systems.[132] For example, in some studies, neurotransmitters have been quantified by measuring (1) the concentration of the neurotransmitters, (2) the breakdown or activation products, and (3) the activity of the enzyme responsible for the synthesis or breakdown of the neurotransmitters. To follow is a brief summary of age-related changes in the following neurotransmitters: acetylcholine (ACh), dopamine (DA), norepinephrine (NE), serotonin (5-HT), glutamate, and γ-aminobutyric acid (GABA).

With advancing age, the effect of ACh in the central nervous system (CNS) and the number of muscarinic receptors are both reduced.[133] DA levels in both the human and rat brains diminish with aging.[133] DA is the precursor for NE, and because of this, synthesis of NE may be affected by aging. However, there are reports of no change, and specifically no decrease, in NE. DA and ACh are also altered in two major age-related neurodegenerative disorders: Alzheimer's disease and Parkinson's disease. There are also reports of no change and no decreases in 5-HT levels.[133] These neurotransmitters have many functions within the CNS and are localized in different areas of the brain. Gottstein and Held[134] suggested that age-related changes in neurotransmitter levels may cause a "desynchronization" in neurotransmission, thereby affecting many neurologic functions.

Reports indicate that there are changes in the function of the neurotransmitters glutamate and GABA. In the central nervous system, glutamate is the major excitatory neurotransmitter, whereas GABA is the major inhibitory neurotransmitter.[135] There appears to be a decrease in the activity of the glutamate and GABA systems, possibly a result of decreases in the levels of both neurotransmitters and their receptor-binding properties. How these changes in glutamate and GABA systems affect elderly brain function is not well-understood.

Cerebral Metabolism and Blood Flow

Cerebral blood flow (CBF) decreases with advancing age. This decrease parallels the decrease in brain weight and is most likely caused by the reduction in neuron number and metabolic needs of the cerebral tissue.[134]

Pain and Aging

Although animal studies indicate decreases in neurotransmitter function and diminished concentrations of opioid receptors in various regions of the cortex (Hiller and others), there is little evidence to suggest that pain or its perception is altered in elderly people.[136,137] For the individual who is 60 years or older, pain often results from various chronic disease entities such as arthritis, osteoarthritis, cancer, and peripheral vascular disease.[138] In aging, pain is associated with a disease process, rather than being a phenomenon with senescence.[139,140] Unfortunately, myths and expectations still persist regarding aging and pain.

IMMUNE SYSTEM

There are several changes in immune function that render the elderly person more susceptible to infections.[139-144] Infections in the elderly population are associated with higher rates of mortality.[144] Common infections in the elderly include bacterial pneumonia, urinary tract infection, intraabdominal infections, gram-negative bacteremia, and decubitus ulcers (Box 11-2).[144] The reasons for the increased susceptibility are multifactorial and include changes in cell-mediated and humoral-mediated immunity; breakdown in physical barriers, such as the skin and oral mucosa; and changes in nutrition.

Cell-Mediated and Humoral-Mediated Immunity

Immune system function is dependent on many cell types with distinct functions. T cells are the primary effector of cell-mediated immunity, whereas bone marrow-derived B cells produce antibodies that are the effector cells of humoral-mediated immunity.[141,143] With aging there is a decline in cell-mediated immunity. Even though the total number of T cells remains unchanged with advancing age, there is a decrease in T cell function.[141,143] For example there is a decrease in T cell production of interleukin-2 (IL-2) and in differentiation of T cells into effector cells. IL-2 is essential for activating B cells, which eventually differentiate into antibody-secreting cells. Subsets of T cells mature into cytotoxic cells, while other T cells activate B cells and stimulate B cell proliferation. Changes in B lymphocytes function are less well-understood, even though with age there is a decline in the ability of B cells to produce antibodies into new antigens.[141] Changes in other cell types such as natural killer cells remains a controversial issue. Using animal models, there are reports that aging is associated with a decrease in NK cell function, whereas data regarding human NK cell function is less conclusive.[141] There are no reports of age-associated changes in the chemotaxis, phagocytic, or bactericidal action of neutrophils.[141]

Additional Risk Factors

Multiple concurrent chronic illnesses produce systemic stressors that ultimately diminish immune func-

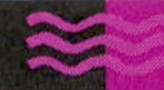 **RESEARCH ABSTRACT** 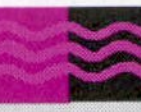

The assessment of discomfort in elderly confused patients: a preliminary study.

Miller J and others: *J Neurosci Nurs* 28(3):175, 1996.

PURPOSE

The purpose of this study was to explore the clinical utility, validity, and reliability of four different approaches to assessment of discomfort in the elderly: a question of discomfort; a discomfort thermometer; a discomfort screen; and the Discomfort Screen-Dementia Alzheimer Type (DS-DAT).

DESIGN

Descriptive

SAMPLE

The sample consisted of 46 patients with an average age of 83 years who had been admitted to a medical unit of a large southeast tertiary hospital. Patients were heavily dependent on staff members for assistance with the activities of daily living. They experienced severe confusion; 54% also had underlying chronic cognitive impairment. Most patients had more than one discomfort condition; 30% had arthritis, wounds, or decubitus ulcers.

PROCEDURE

Research assistants (RAs) assessed subjects daily for confusion and administered the discomfort instruments. Data collection took place between 8:30 AM and 1 PM. The discomfort question "Are you comfortable now?" was scored based on the patient's ability to respond. Patients were asked to evaluate their level of discomfort on the discomfort thermometer, a vertical analog scale. The RAs completed the discomfort screen, which consisted of medical record abstraction and patient observations. RAs also completed the DS-DAT, which consisted of patient observations.

RESULTS

Patients with less confusion were better able to answer the question regarding their *level of discomfort* ($p < .05$); 13% of patients were unable to respond to the question. Only 27% of the patients could respond to the scale; those having greater confusion were less able to respond. The discomfort screen demonstrated a low mean score (3.29, from a range of 0-9). The DS-DAT was a complex scale; three items were problematic to assess: relaxed body language, sad facial expression, and frown. The mean discomfort score was higher in the situations of likely discomfort (8.53) compared with situations of unlikely discomfort (4.64).

DISCUSSION/IMPLICATIONS

Current standards of practice for assessment of discomfort cannot be uniformly applied to all confused elderly patients. Findings from this study reveal that confused elderly patients have difficulty using the discomfort thermometer. The use of the word "pain" rather than "discomfort" might be easier for patients to understand. Because of a lack of interrater reliability and congruence with measurement of three items on the DS-DAT (relaxed body language, sad facial expression, and frown), the questions were eliminated from the assessment and the tool was modified. This tool has potential for use with acutely ill elderly patients as an observational measure of discomfort. However, it does not appear to be feasible for use in daily clinical practice because of its complexity and the amount of training needed for interrater reliability. The findings from this study suggest that a standard of practice in which patients self-report level of discomfort is not an adequate method of assessment with this population. It is important for nurses to anticipate the likelihood of discomfort as they assess and plan interventions for their elderly patients.

tioning. The critical care nurse must be aware that an exacerbation of preexisting illness such as diabetes or emphysema may present itself before infection is suspected. Introducing bacteria through invasive devices such as central lines or chest tubes may threaten an already suppressed immune system.

One must also consider how nutritional deficiencies, particularly protein malnutrition, are a common problem among the elderly. Inadequate protein intake can develop from prolonged anorexia and cognitive impairment. Protein malnutrition is associated with a shrinkage of lymphoid tissue, which then diminishes T cell functioning and cell-mediated immunity.[142] (∞Nutrition and Hematoimmune Alterations, p. 152.)

Furthermore, inadequate emptying of urine secondary to bedrest, obstruction, or side effects from anticholinergic medications can result in stagnation of urine and recurrent urinary tract infections. Long-term placement of urinary catheters are a significant source of bacteriuria. However, treatment with antibiotic therapy is not indicated unless the patient becomes symptomatic with anorexia, cognitive impairment, or has a history of diabetes.[144,145]

BOX 11-2 When to Say No to Life-Sustaining Antibiotic Treatment

In the case of a functionally and cognitively impaired elderly individual with repeated bouts of sepsis, the patient (when possible) along with family and primary health care providers needs to consider ethical issues and alternative options. One must understand that antibiotic treatment is optional. There comes a point when treatment is beyond routine and necessary, and health care providers must question whether management is pointed toward improving quality of life or prolonging an inevitable death. In 1983, the President's commission for the study of Ethical Problems in Medicine and Biomedical Research presented a statement that no particular treatment, including antibiotics, is universally warranted.[134a] Patients, family members, and caregivers should be informed of the option not to treat the source of infection. For many, pneumonia initiates the end of a longstanding, debilitating end-stage disease process. Therefore treating the pneumonia under this circumstance may prolong the dying process. Although difficult, there comes a time when antibiotics are no longer the appropriate choice, and we allow the continuum of life to run its course.

PHYSICAL EXAMINATION AND DIAGNOSTIC PROCEDURES

The various physiologic changes that occur with aging warrant special physical examination techniques.[146] The clinician must distinguish between changes in health caused by physiologic processes versus pathologic processes; therefore the nurse must ensure that the physical examination is conducted under optimal conditions. When beginning a physical examination, the clinician needs to consider the ability of the gerontologic patient to cooperate and hear, as well as his or her activity level. In addition, the patient's comfort and energy levels must be considered. Before beginning an examination, the nurse must ensure that the room's noise level and temperature and the patient's position in the bed are optimal and comfortable.[147]

Head and Neck

Normal funduscopic findings include a diminished pupillary response to penlight, a decrease in near and peripheral vision, and a loss of visual acuity to dim light. These changes result from an increase in opacity of the lens and a decrease in ciliary movement.[148] It is not uncommon to find irises that are pale blue or light gray, which stems from a decrease in melanocyte production.[148] Around the periphery of the iris, fat deposits may also be found, which are referred to as *arcus senilis.* The eyes also may appear sunken or recessed, because of a loss of subcutaneous tissue. These clinical manifestations may also be signs of dehydration; however, in elderly persons, these are normal findings. The pupils may appear small, which can be unrelated to changes in neurologic status or medication administration. The pupil at age 60 is one third the size of a pupil at age 20.[148] Patients may complain of dry, itching eyes, which result from a decrease in lacrimal activity.[148] Less remarkable deficits are noted in gerontologic patients' olfactory and gustatory senses.[149]

Loss of dentition is not a normal process of aging. It indicates poor nutrition and/or poor oral hygiene. Elderly patients commonly experience gradual hearing loss.[150] On physical examination, the elderly person may have a reduced ability to distinguish low and high sounds and may have difficulty in understanding high-pitched and rushed speech. The hearing loss is related to atrophy of the auditory nerve and the organ of Corti.[150]

Integumentary and Musculoskeletal Systems

As noted previously, the loss of elastic and connective tissue causes the skin to wrinkle; both skin wrinkles and sagging may be found over many areas of the body. The appearance and number of skin wrinkles also depends greatly on environmental agents and exposure to ultraviolet rays.[151] The nurse will also find that underlying structures, such as the veins and muscles, are more visible because of the transparency of the skin. Because of the loss of skin turgor, especially in the hands, the nurse assesses for dehydration by pinching the skin tissue over the sternum or forehead. (See Table 11-7 for age-related changes in the skin and their related nursing interventions.)

The nurse may also find multiple ecchymotic areas, because of decreased protective subcutaneous tissue layers, increased capillary fragility, and flattening of the capillary bed, which predispose elderly persons to developing ecchymosis.[152-154] In conjunction with frequent aspirin use, these physiologic factors result in increased bleeding tendencies and the appearance of ecchymotic areas. However, areas of ecchymosis may also indicate elder abuse. The nurse must assess for discrepancies between the patient's history and physical findings. Patients at high risk for abuse are those who require maximal physical assistance in the home

TABLE 11-7 Age-Related Changes in the Integumentary System

Skin Problem	Underlying Mechanisms	Nursing Interventions
Delayed wound healing	↓ Vascular supply to dermis ↓ Connective tissue layer ↓ SQ tissue layer Impaired inflammatory response ↓ New connective tissue proliferation	Use nonrestrictive dressings Weigh patient daily Support nutritional needs
Thermoregulation	↓ SQ tissue layer ↓ Number of capillary arterioles supplying skin ↓ Number of eccrine (sweat) glands	Monitor room temperature
Pressure ulcers	↓ Flattening of capillary bed ↓ Thinning of epidermis	Reposition patient every 2 hours Use pressure-relieving devices
IV infiltrations	↓ Connective tissue layer Vascular fragility	Monitor peripheral IV site hourly Discontinue IV at first sign of infiltration
Diminished skin turgor	↓ Connective tissue layer ↓ Eccrine and sebaceous gland activity	Bathe with tepid water Avoid use of deodorant soap

↓, Decreased.

setting.[155] Caregiver frustration may be expressed by physical assault.

Changes that occur in the musculoskeletal system are a decrease in lean body mass; a compression of the spinal column, which results from the thinning of cartilage between vertebra; and a decrease in the mobility of skeletal joints.[156, 157] Despite the ubiquitous finding of reduced joint mobility, no exact physiologic process gives rise to the altered mobility. It is possible that the reduced synovial fluid production that occurs with aging causes changes in function. There is also an increase in muscle rigidity, especially in the neck, shoulders, hips, and knees.[155] This may produce some changes in range of motion.

Bone demineralization afflicts both men and women as they age; however, it occurs 4 times more often in women than in men. *Bone demineralization* refers to an increase in osteoplast and osteoclast activity, which decreases calcium absorption into the bone.[157] Mineral loss (calcium and phosphorous), along with a decrease in bone mass, is referred to as *osteoporosis*.[157] Osteoporosis produces bones that are more "porous" or fragile. With extensive bone demineralization, an elderly patient may sustain multiple fractures. There is an accelerated incidence of osteoporosis in women, which occurs after the onset of menopause. A decrease in estrogen is implicated in this process, because estrogen replacement may arrest the osteoporosis process (although it will not reverse the process). The exact mechanism whereby estrogen affects bone mass is unknown. Recent evidence indicates estrogen stimulates intestinal absorption of calcium, and the loss of estrogen action after menopause may in part be related to postmenopausal osteoporosis.[157] Decreased intake of dietary calcium, immobility, excess glucocorticoid secretion, and smoking all contribute to the development of osteoporosis.

Respiratory and Cardiovascular Systems

Many of the physiologic changes that occur with aging and the mechanisms underlying them have been addressed previously. The physical correlates to these changes are only noted in this section. On inspection of the aging thorax, the nurse will find a greater anterior-posterior diameter and some degree of kyphosis. On initial auscultation, bibasilar crackles may be heard; however, with several deep breaths and coughing, they should be cleared. Bibasilar crackles that do not clear with deep inspirations are suggestive of pathology. There is also a diminished cough reflex, which predisposes the elderly patient to aspiration. No changes are noted with palpation, but the nurse needs to assess for areas of tenderness, which could be the result of old fractures. With percussion there is increased resonance. Changes in tests of pulmonary function are noted in Tables 11-3 and 11-4. (∞Pulmonary Physical Examination p. 627.)

There are relatively few modifications in the assessment of cardiovascular function and age-related physical findings in the elderly patient. As noted earlier, resting heart rate decreases and systolic blood pressure increases with age. Manifestations of left ventricular hypertrophy and aortic sclerosis may include a prominent cardiac apex impulse, a prominent S_4 (fourth heart sound) at the cardiac apex, a single S_2 (second heart sound) (with expiration), and a short early peaking systolic murmur.[156] (∞Cardiac Auscultation p. 365.)

Gastrointestinal and Renal Systems

On physical examination of the nonobese elderly patient, the abdominal organs are more easily palpated because of a decrease in subcutaneous tissue. Despite a change in gastrointestinal (GI) motility, bowel sounds are normoactive. There are no remarkable physical assessment considerations with the hepatic-biliary and renal systems and no age-related change in liver function tests. Blood urea nitrogen (BUN) and serum creatinine levels can be normal or decreased in elderly patients (Box 11-3). As noted earlier, the GFR decreases with age. In the hospital the GFR is estimated by the creatinine clearance. Endogenous creatinine is a metabolic by-product of muscle metabolism that is excreted by the kidney and is not reabsorbed. Usually the creatinine clearance is estimated by collecting a 24-hour urine sample to measure creatinine excretion. With advancing age, muscle mass decreases, thereby reducing the renal load of serum concentration of creatinine. Therefore, in the geriatric patient, neither the creatinine excreted nor the plasma creatinine level may reflect the change in GFR. In elderly patients, the Cockroft-Gault equation often is used to assess creatinine clearance (CrCl) and GFR (ml/min) because it incorporates serum creatinine levels, body weight, age, and gender as variables.[84] The Cockroft-Gault equation is as follows:

$$\text{CrCl (ml/min)} = (140 - \text{age}) \times \text{weight (kg)}$$

Box 11-3 lists the effects of aging on other laboratory tests that may or may not have clinical significance.[158]

BOX 11-3 Effects of Aging on Various Laboratory Values

VALUES THAT DO NOT CHANGE WITH AGE

Hemoglobin/hematocrit
Platelet count
White blood cell count with differential
Serum electrolytes
Coagulation profile
Liver function tests
Thyroid function tests
↔ or ↓ Blood urea nitrogen
↔ or ↓ Creatinine

VALUES THAT CHANGE WITH AGE BUT HAVE LITTLE CLINICAL SIGNIFICANCE

↓ Calcium
↑ Uric acid

VALUES THAT CHANGE WITH AGE AND HAVE CLINICAL SIGNIFICANCE

↓ Erythrocyte sedimentation rate
↓ Arterial oxygen pressure
↑ Blood glucose
↓ or ↑ Serum lipid profile
↓ Albumin

From Duthie EH, Abbasi AA: *Geriatrics* 46:41, 1991.
↔, No change; ↓, decreased; ↑, increased.

Neurologic System

Physical examination of the neurologic system begins with a review of the elderly patient's mental status. The nurse assesses the patient's level of consciousness, ability to communicate and follow commands, and short-term and long-term memory. In the critical care unit, parameters may be altered by hypoxia, electrolyte imbalances, or various medications. The practitioner may observe that the patient occasionally forgets minor details. Forgetfulness of important information—such as name, address, and marital status—is *not* part of the normal aging process. Although some elderly patients may have problems with short-term memory, long-term memory is intact. Elderly persons are commonly labeled "demented" or "confused." These cognitive syndromes have different etiologies and are not a normal part of aging. See Foreman, Gillies, and Wagner[159] for further review of impaired cognition in the elderly patient.

The neurologic examination for the geriatric patient always includes an assessment of muscle strength, reflexes, sensation, and cranial nerves.[160] There may be some changes in fine and gross motor skills. Handgrip strength declines with age and may correlate with a decreased ability to perform fine motor activity (e.g., tying a shoelace). Age diminishes the elderly patient's vibratory sense, primarily in the lower extremities. Reflexes are slowed, which is caused by neuronal loss.[160] Neurologic deficits may ultimately alter the patient's ability to perform self-care. In addition, changes in elderly patients' cognitive function may alter their ability to follow instructions and interpret patient-teaching instructions regarding their care in the critical care unit. Also, the critical care nurse evaluates the

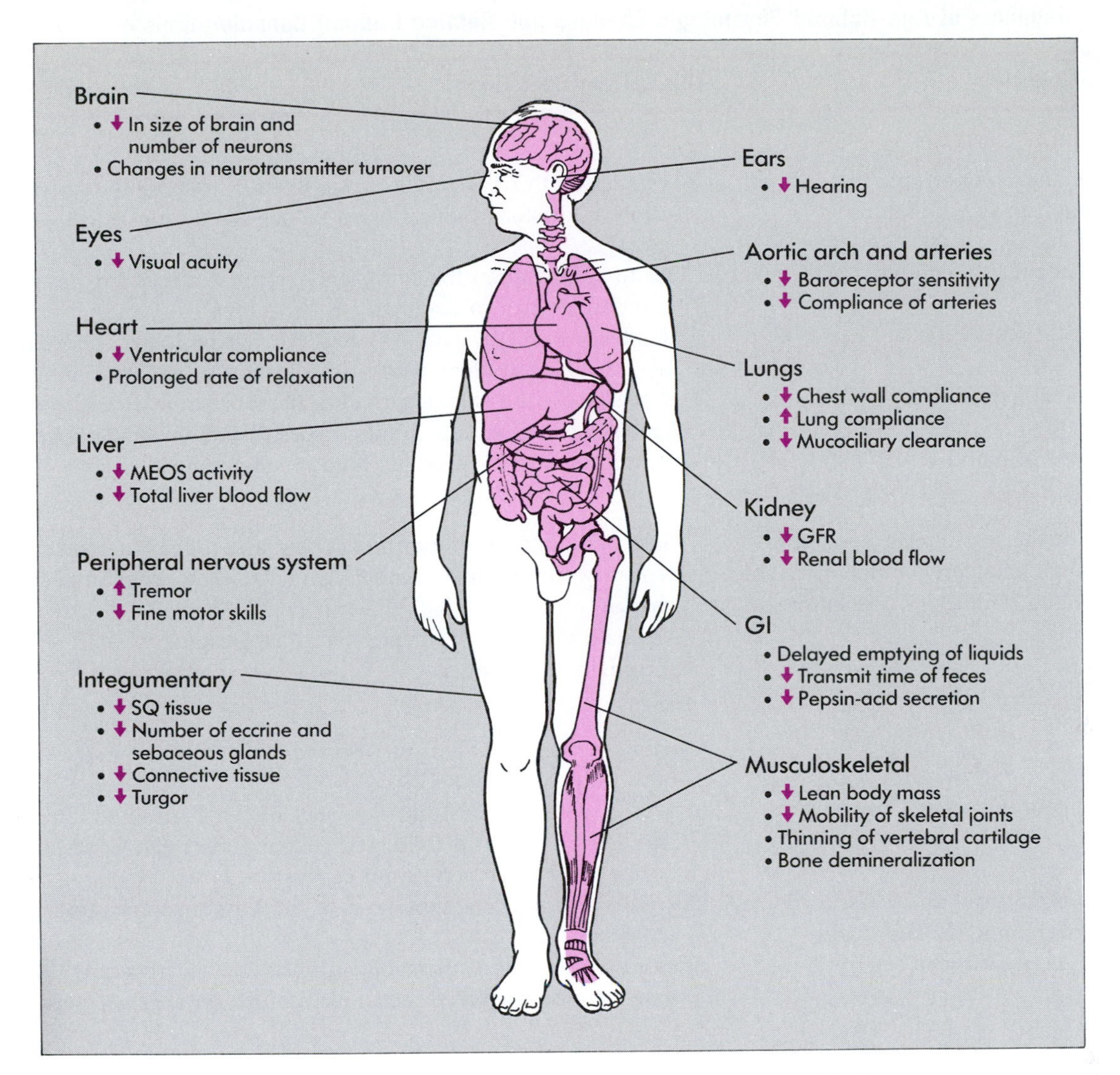

FIGURE 11-3 Summary of the physiologic changes that occur in all systems and that the critical care nurse must consider in caring for the elderly patient in the critical care unit. NOTE: *MEOS,* microsomal enzyme oxidative system; *GFR,* glomerular filtration rate; *GI,* gastrointestinal; *SQ,* subcutaneous.

patient's gait if the patient is ambulatory. (∞Neurologic Physical Examination, p. 763.)

Immune System

Infections in the older adult initially appear as an acute onset of mental status changes, anorexia, urinary incontinence, falls, or generalized weakness.[144,161] However, these may be signs of an urinary tract infection or pneumonia, two common infections in elderly persons. As noted earlier, the response of the immune system is attenuated, therefore signs such as fever and chills may initially be absent.

SUMMARY

The elderly patient requires more intense observation and consideration in the critical care unit, because his or her system has become less adaptable to stress and illness. Table 11-8 summarizes the major changes in the various systems, along with clinical considerations.[162] As shown in Figure 11-3, many physiologic changes occur with advancing age, and each change may render a particular system less adaptable to stress. In addition, the change in one system may affect another system in the presence of disease.

The critical care nurse must also be aware of socioeconomic factors that confront elderly patients, as well as life-style adjustments, such as the death of a spouse or friend. Changes in Medicare payment for hospitalization and medication have also placed a financial burden on such patients. To provide the best care and prevent iatrogenic complications, the critical care nurse must consider all physiologic and psychologic factors that affect the elderly patient.

TABLE 11-8 Summary of Age-Related Physiologic Changes and Related Clinical Considerations

Age-Related Effect	Clinical Considerations
CARDIOVASCULAR SYSTEM	
↓ Inotropic and chronotropic response of myocardium to catecholamine stimulation	The increase in CO achieved during stress or exercise is achieved by an increase in diastolic filling (increased dependence on Starling's law of the heart)
↑ Myocardial collagen content	Leads to a decrease in the compliance of the ventricle (higher filling pressures are needed to maintain stroke volume)
↓ Baroreceptor sensitivity	↑ Tendency for orthostatic hypotension after prolonged bedrest, or if patient is taking antihypertensive medication or has systolic hypertension
Prolonged rate of relaxation	May predispose the elderly patient to hemodynamic derangements in the presence of tachydysrhythmias, hypertension, or ischemic heart disease
↓ Compliance of blood vessels	↑ Peripheral vascular resistance and blood pressure
RESPIRATORY SYSTEM	
↓ Strength of the respiratory muscles, recoil of lungs, chest wall compliance, and efficiency and number of cilia in airways	↑ Susceptibility to aspiration, atelectasis, and pulmonary infection Patient may require more frequent deep breathing, coughing, and position change
↓ Pa_{O_2} level	↓ Ventilatory response to hypoxia and hypercapnia ↑ Sensitivity to narcotics
RENAL SYSTEM	
↓ GFR	Careful observation of patient when administering aminoglycosides, antibiotics, and contrast dyes
↓ Ability to concentrate and conserve water	May predispose patient to development of dehydration and hypernatremia, especially if patient is fluid restricted and insensible losses are high (e.g., during mechanical ventilation or fever)
↓ Ability to excrete salt and water loads, as well as urea, ammonia, and drugs	Observe for clinical manifestations of fluid overload and drug reactions
↓ Response to an acid load	After an acid load (i.e., metabolic acidosis) the elderly patient may be in a state of uncompensated metabolic acidosis for a longer period
LIVER	
↓ Total liver blood flow	Adverse drug reactions, especially with polypharmacy
GASTROINTESTINAL SYSTEM	
Diminished ability to swallow	May predispose elderly patient to aspiration pneumonia Assess for proper fit of dentures and ability to chew Flex head forward 45 degrees
Impaired esophageal motility	Develop awareness for complaints of food or medications "sticking in throat" Assess for complaints of heartburn or epigastric discomfort Avoid prolonged supine position
Delayed emptying of liquids	Examine abdomen for distention Investigate complaints of anorexia
↓ Stool weight and transit time	Obtain thorough bowel history, and note routine use of laxatives Increase intake of dietary fiber, and assess for fecal incontinence and impaction
NEUROLOGIC SYSTEM	
↑ Cranial dead space	Elderly persons may sustain a significant amount of hemorrhage before symptoms are apparent
↓ Number of neurons and dendrites and length of dendrite spines	Delayed or impaired processing of sensory and motor information
Delay in the rate of synaptogenesis	
Changes in neurotransmitter turnover	May cause desynchronization of neurotransmission

Modified from Rebenson-Piano M: *Crit Care Q* 12:1, 1989.

REFERENCES

1. Munoz E and others: Diagnosis-related groups, costs, and outcomes for patients in the intensive care unit, *Heart Lung* 18(6):627, 1989.
2. Henning RJ and others: Clinical characteristics and resource utilization of ICU patients: implications for organization of intensive care, *Crit Care Med* 15(3):264, 1987.
3. Rockwood K and others: One-year outcome of elderly and young patients admitted to intensive care units, *Crit Care Med* 21(5):687, 1993.
4. Chelluri L and others: Long-term outcome of critically ill elderly patients requiring intensive care, *JAMA* 269:3119, 1993.
5. Brock DB, Guralnik JM, Brody JA: Demography and epidemiology of aging in the United States. In Schneider EL, Rowe JW, editors: *Handbook of the biology of aging,* New York, 1990, Academic Press.
6. National Center for Health Statistics Health, United States, Bethesda, Md, 1991, Public Health Service.
7. Abrass IB: Biology of aging. In Wilson JD and others, editors: *Harrison's principles of internal medicine,* ed 12, New York, 1991, McGraw-Hill.
8. NIH Extramural Programs, US Department of Health and Human Services, 1988, Public Health Service.
9. Weisfeldt ML, Lakatta EG, Gerstenblith G: Aging and the heart. In Braunwald E, editor: *Heart disease,* Philadelphia, 1992, WB Saunders.
10. Eghbali M and others: Collagen accumulation in heart ventricles as a function of growth and aging, *Cardiovasc Res* 23:723, 1989.
11. Wegelius O, von Knorring J: The hydroxyproline and hexosamine content in human myocardium at different ages, *Acta Med Scand Suppl* 412:233, 1964.
12. Katz AM: Heart failure. In Fozzard HA and others, editors: *The heart and cardiovascular system,* New York, 1991, Raven Press.
13. Muller RT and others: Painless myocardial infarction in the elderly, *Am Heart J* 119:202, 1990.
14. Mukerji V, Holman AJ, Alpert MA: The clinical description of angina pectoris in the elderly, *Am Heart J* 117:705, 1989.
15. Gerstenblith G and others: Echocardiographic assessment of normal adult aging population, *Circulation* 56:273, 1977.
16. Walsh RA: Cardiovascular effects of the aging process, *Am J Med* 82:34, 1987.
17. Capasso JM and others: Effects of age on mechanical and electrical performance of rat myocardium, *Am J Physiol* 245:H72, 1983.
18. Wei JY, Spurgeon HA, Lakatta EG: Excitation-contraction in rat myocardium: alterations with adult aging, *Am J Physiol* 246H:784, 1984.
19. Opie LH: *The physiology of the heart and metabolism,* New York, 1991, Raven Press.
20. Lakatta, EG and others: Prolonged contraction duration in the aged myocardium, *J Clin Invest* 55:61, 1975.
21. Spurgeon HA, Steinbach MF, Lakatta EG: Prolonged contraction duration in senescent myocardium is prevented by exercise, *Am J Physiol* 244:H513, 1983.
22. Froehlich JP and others: Studies of sarcoplasmic reticulum function and contraction in young and aged rat myocardium, *J Mol Cell Cardiol* 10:427, 1978.
23. Maciel LM and others: Age-induced decreases in the messenger RNA coding for the sarcoplasmic reticulum Ca^{2+}-ATPase of the rat heart, *Circ Res* 67:230, 1990.
24. Moran LA and others: Biochemistry, Englewood Cliffs, NJ, 1994, Neil Patterson Publishers.
25. Lakatta EG and others: Diminished inotropic response of aged myocardium to catecholamines, *Circ Res* 36:262, 1975.
26. Guarnieri T and others: Contractile and biochemical correlates of beta-adrenergic stimulation of the aged heart, *Am J Physiol* 239:H501, 1980.
27. Scarpace PJ: Decreased beta-adrenergic responsiveness during senescence, *Fed Proc* 45:51, 1986.
28. Martinez JL and others: Age-related changes in the catecholamine content of peripheral organs in male and female FJ44 rats, *J Gerontol* 36:280, 1981.
29. Daly RN, Goldberg PB, Roberts J: Effects of age on neurotransmission at the cardiac sympathetic neuroeffector junction, *J Pharmacol Exp Ther* 245:798, 1988.
30. Gerstenblith G and others: Diminished inotropic responsiveness to ouabain in aged rat myocardium, *Circ Res* 44:517, 1979.
31. Capasso JM and others: Myocardial biochemical, contractile and electrical performance following imposition of hypertension in young and old rats, *Circ Res* 58:445, 1986.
32. Effron MB and others: Changes in myosin isoenzymes, ATPase activity, and contraction duration in rat cardiac muscle with aging can be modulated by thyroxine, *Circ Res* 60:238, 1987.
33. Cinelli P and others: Effects of age on mean heart rate variability, *Ageing* 10:146, 1987.
34. Ribera JM and others: Cardiac rate and hyperkinetic rhythm disorders in healthy elderly subjects: evaluation by ambulatory electrocardiographic monitoring, *Gerontology* 35:158, 1989.
35. Jose AD: Effect of combined sympathetic and parasympathetic blockage on heart rate and cardiac function in man, *Am J Cardiol* 18:476, 1966.
36. Rodeheffer RJ and others: Exercise cardiac output is maintained with advancing age in human subjects: cardiac dilation and increased stroke volume compensate for a diminished heart rate, *Circulation* 69:203, 1984.
37. Lakatta EG: Heart and circulation. In Schneider EL, Rowe JW, editors: *Handbook of the biology of aging,* San Diego, 1990, Academic Press.
38. Bonow RO and others: Effects of aging on asynchronous left ventricular regional function and global ventricular filling in normal human subjects, *JACC* 11:50, 1988.
39. Miller TR and others: Left ventricular diastolic filling and its association with age, *Am J Cardiol* 58:531, 1986.

40. Davidson WR, Fee WC: Influence of aging on pulmonary hemodynamics in a population free of coronary artery disease, *Am J Cardiol* 65:1454-1458, 1990.
41. Bachman S, Sparrow D, Smith LK: Effect of aging on the electrocardiogram, *Am J Cardiol* 48:513, 1981.
42. Horwitz LN, Lynch RA: Managing geriatric arrhythmias I. General considerations. *Geriatrics* 46:31, 1991.
43. Camm AJ and others: The rhythm of the heart in active elderly subjects, *Am Heart J* 99:598, 1980.
44. Fleg JL, Kennedy HL: Cardiac arrhythmias in 9 healthy elderly population: detection by a 24-hour ambulatory electrocardiography, *Chest* 81:638, 1982.
45. Docherty JR: Cardiovascular responses in ageing: a review, *Pharmacol Rev* 42:103, 1990.
46. Yin FCP and others: Age-associated decrease in ventricular response to haemodynamic stress during beta-adrenergic blockade, *Br Heart J* 40:1349, 1978.
47. Elliott HL and others: Effects of age in the responsiveness of vascular alpha-adrenoreceptors in man, *J Cardiovasc Pharmacol* 4:388, 1982.
48. Strogatz DS and others: Correlates of postural hypotension in a community sample of elderly blacks and whites, *JAGS* 39:562, 1991.
49. Applegate WB and others: Prevalence of postural hypotension at baseline in the systolic hypertension in the elderly program (SHEP) cohort, *JAGS* 39:1057, 1991.
50. Smith JJ and others: The effect of age on hemodynamic response to graded postural stress in normal men, *J Gerontol* 42:406, 1987.
51. Dambrink JHA, Wieling W: Circulatory response to postural change in healthy male subjects in relation to age, *Clin Sci* 72:335, 1987.
52. Yin FCP, Weisfeldt ML, Milnor WR: Role of aortic input impedance in the decreased cardiovascular response to exercise in aging dogs, *J Clin Invest* 68:28, 1981.
53. Bierman EL: Arteriosclerosis and aging. In Finch CE, Schneider EL, editors: *Handbook of the biology of aging,* New York, 1985, Van Nostrand Reinhold.
54. Schoenberger JA: Epidemiology of systolic and diastolic systemic blood pressure elevation in the elderly, *Am J Cardiol* 57:45c, 1986.
55. Lawn RM: Lipoprotein(a) in heart disease, *Sci Am* 266:54, 1992.
56. Rowe JW: Clinical consequences of age-related impairments in vascular compliance, *Am J Cardiol* 60:68G, 1987.
57. Kreisberg RA, Kasim S: Cholesterol metabolism and aging, *Am J Med* 82:54, 1987.
58. Davis CE and others: Lipoprotein-cholesterol distributions in selected North American populations: The Lipid Research Clinics Program Prevalence Study, *Circulation* 2:302, 1980.
59. Rose BD: *Clinical physiology of acid-base and electrolyte disorders,* New York, 1989, McGraw-Hill.
60. Hall JE, Coleman TG, Guyton AC: The renin-angiotensin system: normal physiology and changes in older hypertensives, *JAGS* 37:801, 1989.
61. Crane MG, Harris JJ: Effect of aging on renin activity and aldosterone excretion, *J Lab Clin Med* 87:947, 1976.
62. Sica DA, Harford, A: Sodium and water disorders in the elderly. In Zawada ET, Sica DA, editors: *Geriatric nephrology and urology,* Littleton, Mass, 1985, PSG Publishing.
63. Webster JR, Kadah H: Unique aspects of respiratory disease in the aged, *Geriatrics* 46:31, 1991.
64. Thurlbeck WM: Growth, ageing and adaptation. In Murray JF, Nadel JA, editors: *Textbook of respiratory medicine,* Philadelphia, 1988, WB Saunders.
65. Levitzky MG: Effects of aging on the respiratory system, *Physiologist* 27:102, 1984.
66. Mittman C and others: Relationship between chest wall and pulmonary compliance and age, *J Appl Physiol* 20:1211, 1965.
67. West JB: *Respiratory physiology, ed 5,* Baltimore, 1995, Williams & Wilkins.
68. Rizzato G, Marazzine L: Thoracoabdominal mechanisms in elderly men, *J Appl Physiol* 28:457, 1970.
69. Gutmann E, Hanzlikova V: Fast and slow motor units in ageing, *Gerontology* 22:280, 1976.
70. Pontoppidan HH, Beecher HK: Progressive loss of protective reflexes in the airway with advance of age, *JAMA* 1974:2209, 1960.
71. Belman MJ, Gaesser GA: Ventilatory muscle training in the elderly, *J Appl Physiol* 64:899, 1988.
72. Knudson RJ and others: Changes in the normal maximal expiratory flow-volume curve with growth and aging, *Am Rev Respir Dis* 127:725, 1983.
73. Turner JM, Mead J, Wohl ME: Elasticity of human lungs in relation to age, *J Appl Physiol* 25:664, 1968.
74. Pierce JA, Hocott JB: Studies on the collagen and elastin content of the human lung, *J Clin Invest* 39:8, 1960.
75. Pierce JA, Ebert RV: Fibrous network of the lung and its change with age, *Thorax* 20:469, 1965.
76. Semmens M: The pulmonary artery in the normal aged lung, *Br J Dis Chest* 64:65, 1970.
77. Sorbini CA and others: Arterial oxygen tension in relation to age in healthy subjects, *Respiration* 25:3, 1968.
78. LeBlanc P, Ruff F, Milic-Emili J: Effects of age and body position on "airway closure" in man, *J Appl Physiol* 28:448, 1970.
79. Holland J and others: Regional distribution of pulmonary ventilation and perfusion in elderly subjects, *J Clin Invest* 47:81, 1968.
80. Knudson RJ and others: Effect of aging alone on mechanical properties of the normal adult human lung, *J Appl Physiol* 43:1054, 1977.
81. Knudson RJ and others: The maximal expiratory flow-volume curve: normal standards, variability, and effects of age, *Am Rev Respir Dis* 113:587, 1976.
82. Wahba WH: Influence of aging on lung function: clinical significance of changes from age twenty *Anesth Analg* 62:764, 1983.
83. Weder AB: The renally compromised older hypertensive: therapeutic considerations, *Geriatrics* 46:36, 1991.

84. Gilbert BR, Vaughan ED: Pathophysiology of the aging kidney, *Clin Geriatr Med* 6(1):12, 1990.
85. Kasiske BL: Relationship between vascular disease and age-associated changes in the human kidney, *Kidney Int* 31:1153, 1987.
86. Anderson S, Brenner BM: Effects of aging on the renal glomerulus, *Am J Med* 80:435, 1986.
87. Watters JM, McClaran JC: The elderly surgical patient. In Wilmore DW and others, editors: *In care of the surgical patient,* (vol VII, Special Problems), New York, 1990, Scientific American.
88. Brandt LJ: Gastrointestinal disorders in the elderly. In Rossman I, editor: *Clinical geriatrics,* ed 3, Philadelphia, 1986, JB Lippincott.
89. Williams SA, Fogel RP: Common gastrointestinal problems in the elderly, *JAMA* 87:29, 1989.
90. Altman DF: Changes in gastrointestinal, pancreatic, biliary and hepatic function in aging, *Gastroenterol Clin North Am* 19:227, 1990.
91. Thomson AB, Keelan M: The aging gut, *Can J Physiol Pharmacol* 64:30, 1986.
92. Bansal SK and others: Upper gastrointestinal hemorrhage in the elderly: a record of 92 patients in a joint geriatric/surgical unit, *Age Ageing* 16:279, 1987.
93. Moore JG and others: Effect of age on gastric emptying of liquid-solid meals in man, *Dig Dis Sci* 28(4):340, 1983.
94. Schuster MM: Disorders of the aging GI system, *Hosp Prac* 11:95, 1976.
95. Curran J: Overview of geriatric nutrition, *Dysphagia* 5:72, 1990.
96. Ausman LM, Russel RM: Nutrition and aging. In Schneider EL, Rowe JW, editor: *Handbook of the biology of aging,* San Diego, 1990, Academic Press.
97. Sato TG, Miwa T, Tauchi H: Age changes in the human liver of the different races, *Gerontology* 16:368, 1970.
98. Bach B and others: Disposition of antipyrine and phenytoin correlated with age and liver volume in man, *Clin Pharmacokinet* 6:389, 1981.
99. Kampmann JP, Sinding J, Moller-Jorgensen I: Effect of age on liver function, *Geriatrics* 30:91, 1975.
100. Schmucker DL, Wang RK: Age-related changes in liver drug metabolism: structure versus function, *Proc Soc Exp Biol Med* 165:178, 1980.
101. Vestal RE, Cusack BJ: Pharmacology and aging. In Schneider EL, Rowe JW, editors: *Handbook of the biology of aging,* San Diego, 1990, Academic Press.
102. Yuen GJ: Altered pharmacokinetics in the elderly, *Clin Geriatric Med* 6:257, 1990.
103. Schwertz DW, Bushmann MT: Pharmacogeriatics, *Crit Care Q* 12:26, 1989.
104. Gilman AG and others, editors: *Goodman and Gilman's the pharmacological basis of therapeutics,* ed 8, London, 1990, Pergamon Press.
105. Mooradian AD: An update of the clinical pharmacokinetics, therapeutic monitoring techniques and treatment recommendations, *Clin Pharmacokinet* 18:165, 1988.
106. Creasy WA and others: Pharmacokinetics of captopril in elderly healthy male volunteers, *J Clin Pharmacol* 26:264, 1986.
107. Hockings N, Ajayi AA, Reid JL: Age and the pharmacodynamics of angiotension converting enzyme inhibitors, enalapril and enalaprilat, *Br J Pharmacol* 21:341, 1986.
108. Pederson KE: Digoxin interactions: the influence of quinidine and verapamil on the pharmacokinetics and receptor binding of digitalis glycosides, *Acta Med Scand* 697 (suppl 1):1, 1985.
109. Lynch RA, Horowitz LN: Managing geriatric arrhythmias, II. Drug selection and use, *Geriatrics* 46:41, 1991.
110. Vidt GD, Borazanian RA: Calcium channel blockers in geriatric hypertension, *Geriatrics* 46:28, 1991.
111. Wall RT: Use of analgesics in the elderly, *Clin Ger Med* 6:345, 1990.
112. Bertel O and others: Decreased beta-adrenoreceptor responsiveness as related to age, blood pressure and plasma catecholamines in patients with essential hypertension, *Hypertension* 2:130, 1980.
113. Kendall MJ and others: Responsiveness to beta-adrenergic receptor stimulation: the effects of age are cardioselective, *Br J Clin Pharmacol* 14:821, 1982.
114. Katzman R: Human nervous system. In Masoro EJ, editor: *Handbook of physiology: aging,* New York, 1995, Oxford University Press.
115. Foreman MD, Grabowski R: diagnostic dilemma: cognitive impairment in the elderly, *J Gerontologic Nurs* 18:5, 1992.
116. Evans DA and others: Prevalence of Alzheimer's disease in a community population of older persons, *JAMA* 162:2551, 1989.
117. Arriagada P and others: Neurofibrillary tangles but not senile plaques parallel duration and severity of Alzheimer's disease, *Neurology* 42:631, 1992.
118. Selkoe DJ: Aging brain, aging mind, *Sci Amer* 267:134, 1992.
119. Morris JC, McManus DQ: The neurology of aging: normal versus pathologic change, *Geriatrics* 46:47, 1991.
120. Lytle LD, Altar A: Diet, central nervous system, and aging, *Fed Proc* 38:2017, 1979.
121. Cotman CW: Synaptic plasticity, neurotropic factors and transplantation in the aged brain. In Schneider EL, Rowe JW, editors: *Handbook of the biology of aging,* San Diego, 1990, Academic Press.
122. Catchen H: Repeaters: inpatient accidents among the hospitalized elderly, *Nurs Res* 37:273, 1983.
123. Evans LK, Strumpf NE: Tying down the elderly. A review of the literature on physical restraint, *J Am Geriatr Soc* 1:65, 1989.
124. Kapp MB: Nursing home restraints and legal liability, *J Leg Med* 13:1, 1992.
125. Redford JB: Preventing falls in the elderly, *Hosp Med* 35:57, 1991.
126. Warshaw GA and other: Functional disability in the hospitalized elderly, *JAMA* 248:847, 1982.

127. Patrick ML: Care of the confused elderly, *Am J Nurs* 67:2536, 1967.
128. Gutheil T, Tardiff K: Indication and contraindication for seclusion and restraint. In Tardiff K, editor: *The psychiatric uses of seclusion and restraint,* Washington, DC, 1984. APA Press.
129. Robbins LJ and others: Binding the elderly: a prospective study of the use of mechanical restraint in an acute care setting, *J Am Geriatr Soc* 35:290, 1987.
130. Gerdes L: The confused or delirious patient, *Am J Nurs* 68:1228, 1968.
131. Miller M: Iatrogenic and nursigenic effect of prolonged immobilization of the ill aged, *J Am Geriatr Soc* 23:360, 1975.
132. Cooper JR, Bloom FE, Roth RH: *The biochemical basis of neuropharmacology,* ed 6, New York, 1991, Oxford University Press.
133. Morgan DG, May PC: Age-related changes in synaptic neurochemistry. In Schneider EL, Rowe JW, editors: *Handbook of the biology of aging,* San Diego, 1990, Academic Press.
134. Gottstein U, Held K: Effects of aging on cerebral circulation and metabolism in man, *Acta Neurol Scand Suppl* 72:54-55, 1979.
135. Cotman CW, Kahle JS, Korotzer AR: Maintenance and regulation in brain of neurotransmission, trophic factors and immune responses. In Masoro EJ, editor: *Handbook of physiology: aging,* New York, 1995, Oxford University Press.
136. Hiller JM, Fan L-Q, Simon EJ: Alterations in opioid receptor levels in discrete areas of the neocortex and in the globus pallidus of the aging guinea pig: a quantitative autoradiographic study, *Brain Res* 614:86, 1993.
137. Bonica JJ: *The management of pain,* Philadelphia, 1990, Lea & Febiger.
138. Egbert DA and others: Help for the hurting elderly: pain relief, *Postgraduate Medicine* 19:291, 1991.
139. Ferrell BR, Ferrell BA: Easing pain, *Geriatric Nurs* July/Aug:175, 1990.
140. Harkins SW, Kwentus J, Price DD: Pain and suffering in the elderly. In Bonica JJ, editor: *The management of pain,* Philadelphia, 1990, Lea & Febiger.
141. Miller RA: Immune system. In Masoro EJ, editor: *Handbook of physiology: aging,* New York, 1995, Oxford University Press.
142. Terpenning MS, Bradley SF: Why aging leads to increased susceptibility to infection, *Geriatrics* 46:77, 1991.
143. Miller RA: The aging immune system: primer and prospectus, *Science* 273:70, 1996.
144. McClure CL: Common infections in the elderly, *American Family Physician* 45:2691, 1992.

144a. President's Commission for the Study of Ethical Problems in Medicine and Biomedical and Behavioral Research: *Deciding to forgo life-sustaining treatment: a report on the ethical, medical and legal issues on treatment decisions,* 1993, Washington, DC, US Government County Office.

145. Jones SR: Infections in frail and vulnerable elderly patients, *Am J Med* 88:3C, 1990.
146. Fields SD: History-taking in the elderly: obtaining useful information, *Geriatrics* 46(8):26-35, 1991.
147. Geokas MC: The aging process, *Ann Int Med* 113:455, 1990.
148. Marmour MF: Management of elderly patients with impaired vision. In Ebaugh FG, editor: *Management of common problems in geriatric medicine,* Menlo Park, Calif, 1981, Addison-Wesley.
149. Bartoshuk LM: Taste: robust across the age span? *Ann NY Acad Sci* 561:65-75, 1989.
150. Goode RL: The effect of aging on the ear. In Ebaugh FG, editor: *Management of common problems in geriatric medicine,* Menlo Park, Calif, 1981, Addison-Wesley.
151. Lapiere CM: The ageing dermis: the main cause for the appearance of "old skin," *Brit J Dermatol* 122(Suppl 35):5, 1990.
152. Jones PL, Millman A: Wound healing and the aged patient, *Nurs Clin North Am* 25(1):263, 1990.
153. Kelly L, Mobily PR: Iatrogenesis in the elderly, *J Geron Nurs* 17(9):24, 1991.
154. Shenefelt PD, Fenske NA: Aging and the skin: recognizing and managing common orders, *Geriatrics* 45(10):57, 1990.
155. Exton-Smith AN: Mineral metabolism. In Finch CE, Schneider EL, editors: *Handbook of the biology of aging,* New York, 1985, Van Nostrand Reinhold.
156. Wenger NK: Cardiovascular disease in the elderly, *Curr Probl Cardiol* October:611, 1992.
157. Kalu DN: Bone. In Masoro EJ, editor: *Handbook of physiology: aging,* New York, 1995, Oxford University Press.
158. Duthie EH, Abbasi AA: Laboratory testing: current recommendations for older adults, *Geriatrics* 46:10, 1991.
159. Foreman MD, Gillies DA, Wagner D: Impaired cognition in the critically ill elderly patient: clinical implications, *Crit Care Q* 12:61, 1989.
160. Boss BJ: Normal aging in the nervous system: implications for SCI nurses, *SCI* 8(2):42, 1991.
161. Henshke PJ: Infections in the elderly, *Med J Aust* 158:830, 1993.
162. Piano MR: The physiologic changes that occur with aging, *Crit Care Q* 12:1, 1989.

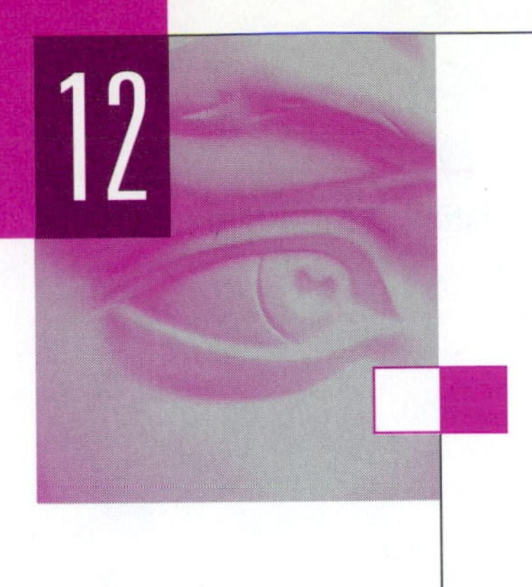

12

Perianesthesia Management

Caring for the critically ill patient who is emerging from anesthesia involves the assessment, diagnosis, treatment, and evaluation of perceived, actual, or potential physical or psychosocial problems that may result from the intrusion of anesthetic agents and techniques. The critical care nurse's unique knowledge base regarding anesthetic agents and techniques, physiologic and psychologic bodily responses to these intrusions, vulnerability of patients subjected to anesthesia, and medical interventions requiring anesthesia is coupled with all the principles of critical care nursing. Life-sustaining needs are of the highest priority, and constant vigilance is required because the postanesthesia needs of the patient are neither minimal nor episodic.[1]

GENERAL ANESTHESIA

The components of anesthesia are hypnosis, analgesia, muscle relaxation, sympatholysis, and amnesia. To anticipate how a patient will react when emerging from anesthesia, the nurse must have a thorough understanding of the pharmacologic concepts of anesthetic agents and adjuncts. Although the complexity of these agents, coupled with drug interactions and various levels of physical health, makes it difficult to predict the exact nature of each patient's emergence from anesthesia, an understanding of some general principles will prepare the nurse for the most commonly expected outcomes.

Factors in Selecting Type of Anesthetic Agent

Before administration of an anesthetic agent, and whether the anesthesia to be induced is general, regional, or local with level of sedation being conscious, deeply sedated, or unconscious, a number of factors have to be considered. These factors include the age and physical status of the patient, the type of surgery, the skills of the anesthesiologist and surgeon, and the patient's wishes. During the conscious state, the patient remains awake, protective reflexes remain intact, and the alteration in mood is minimal. During deep sedation, the patient is asleep but arousable, and there is minimal depression of protective reflexes. During the unconscious state, the patient is incapable of response to command, respirations are automatic, and there is minimal muscle tone lost. During general anesthesia, there is a controlled state of unconsciousness, the patient is not arousable, and there is partial or complete loss of protective reflexes.[2]

ASA Guidelines for Anesthesia

The American Society of Anesthesiologists (ASA) has formulated health categories as guidelines for anesthesia administration (Box 12-1).[3]

Ideal Anesthetic Characteristics

The ideal characteristics of anesthetic agents and adjuncts are listed in Box 12-2.[2]

Objectives and Stages of General Anesthesia

The objectives of general anesthesia are analgesia, unconsciousness, blocked reflexes, and skeletal muscle relaxation.

Stage I begins with the initiation of an anesthetic agent and ends with the loss of consciousness. It is commonly called the stage of analgesia. This stage has been described as the lightest level of anesthesia and represents sensory and mental depression. Stage I is the level of anesthesia used when nitrous oxide is employed. Patients are able to open their eyes on

BOX 12-1 ASA Categories

Category 1 - Normal, healthy patient
Category 2 - Patient with mild systemic disease
Category 3 - Patient with severe systemic disease (hypertension, dialectics)
Category 4 - Patient with severe systemic disease that is a threat to life
Category 5 - Patient with high morbidity
Category 6 - Brain death

BOX 12-2 Ideal Characteristics of Anesthetic Agents/Adjuncts

Rapid onset of action
Controllable duration of action
Identifiable levels of depths
Technically easy to administer
No untoward effects on vital signs
No toxic metabolites
Predictable elimination
High specificity of action
High margin of safety
Useful with all ages
Cost-effective
Rapid emergence

command, breathe normally, maintain protective reflexes, and tolerate mild painful stimuli.

Stage II starts with the loss of consciousness and ends with the onset of a regular pattern of breathing and the disappearance of the eyelid reflex. This is also called the stage of delirium. It is characterized by excitement, and because of this, many untoward responses such as vomiting, laryngospasm, and even cardiac arrest may take place during this stage. With the use of anesthetic agents that act much more rapidly than ether, this stage is passed rather quickly. In addition, the induction of anesthesia is usually facilitated by short acting barbiturates, which expedite a short duration of Stage II.

Stage III is the stage of surgical anesthesia. At this stage there is an absence of response to surgical incision. Patients experience a depression in all elements of nervous system function (i.e., sensory depression, loss of recall, reflex depression, and some skeletal muscle relaxation). Each anesthetic agent and adjunct affects the patient's clinical signs, such as blood pressure, differently. Consequently, monitoring levels of anesthesia depends on the particular properties of each agent.[4]

Inhalation Agents

The pharmacokinetics of inhalation anesthetics involve uptake, distribution, metabolism, and elimination. Basically this involves a series of partial pressure gradients starting in the anesthesia machine that travel to the patient's brain for induction and vice versa for emergence. The object of anesthesia is to achieve a constant and optimal partial pressure in the brain. The key to attaining anesthesia is having the alveolar partial pressure (PA) in equilibrium with the arterial partial pressure (Pa) and brain partial pressure (Pbr) of the inhaled anesthetic. The partial pressure of an inhalation anesthetic in the brain determines the depth of anesthesia. The more potent the anesthetic, the lower the partial pressure of the agent required to produce a certain depth of anesthesia.[5] The determination of the PA are the inspired partial pressure of the inhalation anesthetic, the characteristic of the anesthesia machine's delivery system, and the patient's alveolar ventilation.

The movement of the inhalation agent from the alveoli to the arterial blood depends on the blood gas partial coefficient and the cardiac output. The blood conveys the anesthetic agent to the tissues. Consequently, a normal cardiac output is needed to facilitate the movement of the inhalation anesthetic through the tissues to the brain. The partial pressure increases most rapidly in the tissues with the highest rates of blood flow. Of interest is the great variation in blood perfusion of certain tissues in the body. The body tissue compartments can be divided into four groups: (1) the vessel-rich group, which consists of the heart, brain, hepatoportal system, and endocrine glands; (2) the intermediate group of perfused tissues, which consists of muscle and skin; (3) the fat group, which includes marrow and adipose tissue; and (4) the vessel-poor group, which has the poorest circulation per unit volume and is composed of tendons, ligaments, connective tissue, teeth, bone, and other avascular tissue. The vessel-rich group of tissues receives 75% of the cardiac output; thus the brain becomes saturated rapidly with an anesthetic agent administered by inhalation. On termination of the anesthetic agent, the reverse takes place, and there is rapid removal of the agent from the brain.

The transfer of the inhalation anesthetic from the arterial blood to the brain is dependent on the blood-brain barrier coefficient of the agent and cere-

LEGAL REVIEW 

New or Investigational Drugs, Devices, Procedures, and Treatments

The federal Food and Drug Administration (FDA) regulates through licensing the prescription, administration, and use of investigational or experimental drugs and devices. This regulation is governed primarily by the 1938 Federal Food, Drug, and Cosmetic Act and the Medical Device Amendments of 1976. The Food, Drug, and Cosmetic Act is a valid exercise of Congressional power to control interstate commerce. The broad purpose of the statute and its amendments is to protect public health and safety by prohibiting in interstate commerce the sale or transport of misbranded, adulterated, defective, or unsafe products intended for human use or consumption.

The Medical Device Amendments of 1976 preempt state law regarding certain standards for warning of risks or labeling of a product. The amendments also govern certain areas of product design and design defect. In the case of *Slater v. Optical Radiation Corporation,* the plaintiff filed a products liability action alleging injury from a product rendered unsafe as a result of a design defect. The plaintiff had undergone cataract removal with subsequent implantation of an intraocular lens. The lens had not been approved by the FDA as safe and effective, but it had received an exemption under the experimental device exception of the Amendments to permit clinical trials of the lens. The plaintiff signed a consent form stating he had been advised that the lens was an experimental device. After pain and diminished vision in the affected eye resulted, the lens was removed but the plaintiff suffered permanent damage that had not been caused by the cataract.

The U.S. Court of Appeals, Seventh Circuit, ruled that the plaintiff's claim was preempted by the investigational device exemption, and the lawsuit was dismissed. The court reasoned that the investigational device exception is intended to encourage the study and development of medical devices by permitting controlled clinical trials of a product for which effectiveness and safety have not yet been established. The court stated that the Medical Device Amendments prohibit states from imposing by regulation, statute, or judicial ruling requirements for the safety and effectiveness of medical devices that differ from those established by the FDA. The court further noted that imposing liability for defective design on the manufacturer of a device (which had received investigational status by the FDA) would undermine the purpose and intent of the investigational device exception.

However, the Court stated that preemption by the Medical Device Amendments is limited to the issue of safety and effectiveness and does not preclude lawsuits alleging negligent implantation, removal, or contamination of a device, or failure to obtain informed consent to the use of an investigational device.

If the institution is funded in whole or in part by the federal government, human research involving investigational procedures, tests, or treatments is regulated generally under the authority of the Department of Health and Human Services (DHHS). Federal regulations were first established in 1975 and revised in 1981. Institutions sponsoring the research are required by regulation to establish institutional review boards (IRBs). The purpose of the IRB is to evaluate research proposals before implementation to determine whether human research subjects may be at risk, assess the risks involved, identify ways to protect human subjects, and approve or disapprove the proposal. Because IRBs' structure and role are defined by federal regulation, they operate similarly throughout the country.

The DHHS policy for protection of human research subjects contains the following salient provisions: (1) a description of the types of research governed by the regulations; (2) pertinent definitions, including definitions of research, human subject, and risk; (3) requirements for IRB membership; (4) duties and functions of the IRB; (5) review procedures for minimal risk research; (6) criteria for IRB approval of research proposals; (7) requirements for informed consent; and (8) procedures for documentation of informed consent.

It behooves the critical care nurse who participates in any form of clinical research, including the administration of FDA-unapproved or investigational drugs, to be familiar with these regulations and the sponsoring institution's IRB findings and recommendations on the research proposal.

See Federal Food, Drug, and Cosmetic Act, 21 U.S.C.A. Section 301 *et seq.* and Medical Device Amendments of 1976; Lynn JSR: Implantable medical devices: a survey of products liability case law, *Med Trial Tech Q* 38:44, 1991; Protection of Human Research Subjects, 45 C.F.R. Section 46.101 *et seq.* (1985); Shimm DS, Spece RG: Conflict of interest and informed consent in industry-sponsored clinical trials, *J Legal Med* 12:477, 1991; *Slater v. Optical Radiation Corp.,* No. 91-1544 (7th Cir. Apr. 22, 1992).

bral blood flow. The concentration gradient during induction of anesthesia is $P_A > Pa > Pbr$. During maintenance of surgical anesthesia, the brain tissue becomes saturated with the anesthetic agent, and the brain tissue is in equilibrium with the alveolar and arterial concentration. Consequently, $P_A = Pa = Pbr$. When the administration of the anesthetic agent is terminated, a reversal gradient takes place. In this instance, the P_A is almost zero, because only oxygen is administered during the emergence phase. The gradient that develops is PA < Pa < Pbr. The gradient favors the removal of the anesthetic agent from the brain tissue. Then the partial pressure in the tissues declines first, followed by that in the arterial blood. The agent returns to the lungs and is then eliminated into the atmosphere. The factors that affect the rate of elimination are the same ones that determine how rapidly an anesthetic agent takes a patient to surgical anesthesia. If a short procedure is performed (less than 1 hour), complete equilibrium among PA, Pa, and Pbr might not have occurred and the recovery from anesthesia will be more rapid. The reverse is true during long procedures in which equilibrium has occurred, and a prolonged emergence may be anticipated.

Table 12-1 lists the inhalation anesthetics presently used and their chief characteristics, effects, and nursing implications.[2]

Intravenous Anesthetics

The time-tested use of inhalation agents has proved that they possess some definite disadvantages. Because of the biotransformation hazards that have been reported with the halogenated inhalation anesthetics, other techniques have been sought to provide general anesthesia. Intravenous anesthetics are now providing a wide range of use in the perioperative period. Intravenous anesthetics are grouped by primary pharmacologic action into nonopioid and opioid intravenous agents. The nonopioid agents are further grouped into the barbiturates, nonbarbiturates, and tranquilizers. These drugs can be administered via intermittent intravenous bolus to induce anesthesia and/or be administered via continuous intravenous drip to maintain anesthesia.[6]

Nonopioid Intravenous Anesthetics

The nonopioid drugs appear to interact with gamma-aminobutyric acid (GABA) in the brain. GABA is an inhibitory neurotransmitter, and activation of the GABA receptors causes inhibition of the postsynaptic neuron and loss of consciousness. Barbiturates bind to GABA postsynaptic receptors, inhibiting neuronal activity and resulting in loss of consciousness. Tranquilizers, such as benzodiazepines, potentiate the action of GABA, leading to inhibition of neuronal activity. Conversely, etomidate (Amidate), a nonbarbiturate induction agent, antagonizes the muscarinic receptors in the central nervous system (CNS), resulting in loss of wakefulness.[7]

Table 12-2 presents the nonopioid intravenous anesthetics and their effects and nursing considerations.

Benzodiazepine antagonists. Physostigmine (Antilirium) is an anticholinesterase drug that inhibits the enzyme acetylcholinesterase. It results in an increase in the availability of acetylcholine at the receptor sites, which counteracts the negative effects of GABA thus reversing the CNS side effects of benzodiazepines, scopolamine and ketamine. Since this drug is a nonspecific agent, a number of vagally mediated cholinergic side effects can occur after its administration, including nausea, vomiting, salivation, bradycardia, bronchospasm, and seizures. Hence, because of its nonspecific properties, physostigmine is rarely used for the reversal of benzodiazepines.[2]

Flumazenil (Romazicon) antagonizes or reverses the effects of benzodiazepines, such as sedation, amnesia, anxiolysis, and muscle relaxation. However, flumazenil is not effective in the treatment of benzodiazepine-induced hypoventilation or respiratory failure. Flumazenil is specific for the benzodiazepine receptors and does not reverse the effects of barbiturates or opiates. Flumazenil must be used with great caution in patients who have a history of seizures or chronic benzodiazepine usage, because it can precipitate seizures. The incidence of postoperative nausea and vomiting is also increased.

Since flumazenil has a shorter duration of action than most of the benzodiazepines, the risk of sedation can occur after the initial dose is administered, especially when high doses of benzodiazepines are administered. Therefore the patient must be monitored for resedation and other residual effects. If the patient develops signs of resedation, flumazenil is repeated at 20 minute intervals. Flumazenil has proven to be a valuable asset in the care of the patient who has received an excessive dose of a benzodiazepine, such as midazolam or diazepam. Consequently, flumazenil is very useful intraoperatively, postoperatively, and in the intensive care unit.[7]

Opioid Intravenous Anesthetics

Anesthesia care now uses many new drugs and techniques to optimize patient outcomes. Opioid intravenous anesthetics constitute a major portion of the clinical anesthesia process, since these drugs enhance the effectiveness of inhalation agents by providing the analgesic portion of the anesthetic process. In addition, the use of opioids allows for a reduction in the concentration of the inhalation agent to be administered, resulting in a safer anesthetic process.

When opioids are administered into the body and bind to specific receptors, they produce a morphine-

TABLE 12-1 Inhalation Anesthetics

Drug	Characteristics	Effects	Nursing Considerations
Nitrous oxide	Light anesthetic; carrier for other inhalation agents; always given with oxygen	Anesthetic and analgesic; little pulmonary, cardiac, or CNS effects; increases intracranial pressure; amnesia	Eliminated via ventilation; nausea and vomiting; diffusion hypoxia; mild myocardial depression
Halothane (Fluothane)	Nonpungent, nonirritating odor; less likely to cause laryngospasms; pediatric agent	Bronchodilator; decreases mucociliary function and pharyngeal reflex	Myocardial depression; decreases SVR, contractility, and cardiac output; hepatotoxicity; "halothane shakes;" may trigger malignant hypothermia
Enflurane (Ethrane)	Used for deliberate hypotension cases	Vasodilator; marked cardiovascular stability; good operative analgesic; pleasant induction and emergence	Decreases SVR and seizure threshold; less nausea and vomiting
Isoflurane (Forane)	Pungent ether-like odor; low potential for toxicity; successful ambulatory agent	Higher cardiovascular stability; potentiates muscle relaxants	Mild depression of spontaneous ventilation; postoperative shivering; fewer dysrhythmias noted
Desflurane (Suprane)	Strong pungent odor; rapid onset; requires warmed vaporizer for administration	Minimal metabolism; respiratory depression; cardiovascular depression; no lingering analgesia	Observe for breath holding; coughing and laryngospasm; needs immediate analgesia
Sevoflurane (Ultane)	Little pungency; pediatric anesthetic	Minimal airway irritation; rapid elimination; great precision and control over anesthetic depth	May trigger malignant hypothermia; observe for breath holding

SVR, Systemic vascular resistance.

like or opioid agonist effect. The term *opioid* was derived because of the multitude of synthetic drugs with morphine-like actions, and with the advent of receptor physiology, it has replaced the term narcotic. *Narcotic* is derived from the Greek word for stupor and usually refers to both the production of the morphine-like effects and the physical dependence.

Because opioids are used to manage acute and chronic pain and are administered for general anesthesia, sedation, and pain relief during regional anesthesia, their implications are profound. It is imperative that the nurse be well-informed in all aspects of the pharmacology of the intravenous opioid agents.

Table 12-3 presents a summary of clinical uses and nursing implications for the most frequently used adjunctive opioids.

Opioid antagonists. Opioid antagonists are used to reverse the effects of opioids, particularly respiratory depression. The drug of choice in perianesthesia care is naloxone (Narcan). Naloxone reverses both the respiratory depressant effects and analgesics effects of opioids. Naloxone is titrated to the patient's response. The onset of action is 1 to 2 minutes, and if after 3 to 5 minutes inadequate reversal has been achieved, naxolone is repeated until reversal is complete. If the patient shows no sign of reversal, assessment of other pharmacologic agents administered is indicated. Drugs such as halothane, barbiturates, and muscle relaxants are not reversed by naloxone.

Naloxone's duration of action is 1 to 4 hours. If long-acting opioids are used, the patient must be monitored for respiratory insufficiency, because the

TABLE 12-2 **Nonopioid Intravenous Anesthetics**

Category	Drug	Characteristics	Effects	Nursing Considerations
Barbiturates	Thiopental (Pentothal)	Good patient acceptance; quick onset; very brief duration; no analgesia	CNS depression; spontaneous ventilation arrested; loss of laryngeal reflexes; causes histamine release (vasodilation, hypotension, and flushing)	IV administration painful; may cause myoclonus and hiccoughs; increased risk of aspiration
	Methohexital (Brevital)	Similar to thiopental but twice as potent; used in pediatric patients; no analgesia; hepatic metabolism	Similar to thiopental; lowers seizure threshold (epileptiform)	Similar to thiopental; burns when given intravenously
Nonbarbiturates	Etomidate (Amidate)	Agent of choice in patient with cardiovascular disease	Heart rate and cardiac output remain constant; minimal negative inotropic effects; suppression of adrenal function	May cause nausea and vomiting; burns when given intravenously; may cause myoclonus and hiccoughs
	Propofol (Diprivan)	No analgesic effect; avoid in patients with coronary stenosis, ischemia, and hypovolemia; antiemetic properties; hepatic metabolism	Patient wakes up clearly and quickly; myocardial depressant; may decrease blood pressure 20% to 25%	Rapid emergence may hasten pain awareness; low incidence of postoperative side effects; burns when given in small veins
Dissociative Anesthetic	Ketamine (Ketalar)	Profound analgesia and anesthesia; provides amnesia; may be used alone; may be given intravenously or intramuscularly	Produces cardiovascular and respiratory stimulation; may increase blood pressure and heart rate 10% to 50%; increases intracranial pressure	Monitor for and prevent emergent reactions; titrate pain medications
Butyrophenones	Haloperidol (Haldol)	Limited use in anesthesia because of long duration; antipsychotic; antiemetic		High incidence of extrapyramidal reactions

COPD, Chronic obstructive pulmonary disease.

depressant effects of the opioid may return. Often a low-dose continuous intravenous naloxone drip proves effective. One adverse effect to watch for when excessive doses of naloxone are given is an increase in blood pressure, which may be a response to pain. Too rapid reversal may induce nausea, vomiting, diaphoresis, or tachycardia. During the reversal procedure, vital signs are monitored closely. Naloxone must be used with caution in patients with cardiac irritability.

TABLE 12-2 Nonopioid Intravenous Anesthetics—cont'd

Category	Drug	Characteristics	Effects	Nursing Considerations
Butyrophenones —*cont'd*	Droperidol (Inapsine)	Major tranquilizer; works with CNS as dopamine antagonist; hepatic metabolism	Prevents and treats nausea and vomiting; neuroleptic, causing amnesia or indifference to surroundings; adrenergic blocker, causing extrapyramidal muscle movements, hypotension, and peripheral vasodilation	Postanesthetic dysphoria (internalized overwhelming fear); effects last longer than narcotics
Benzodiazepines	Diazepam (Valium)	Rapid onset; long half-life; potent amnesic; effective anxiolysis; renal excretion		Titrate pain medications; monitor vital signs for respiratory depression
	Midazolam (Versed)	Rapid onset; short duration; potent amnesic; effective anxiolysis; hepatic metabolism		Lower dose in elderly, debilitated, COPD, and liver disease patients; titrate pain medications; monitor vital signs
	Lorazepam (Ativan)	Slow onset of action; long duration; anticonvulsant action; renal excretion	Pronounced sedation; minimal cardiovascular effects	Poor IV compatibility; titrate pain medications; monitor vital signs and for respiratory depression; watch for orthostatic hypotension

Naloxone does not produce respiratory depression as does other narcotic antagonists, nor does it produce any significant side effects or pupillary constriction. Naloxone reverses natural or synthetic opioids, propoxyphene (Darvon), and the opioid-antagonist analgesic pentazocine. It must be administered with great caution in patients who are physically dependent on opioids, because reversal may precipitate acute withdrawal syndrome.[8]

Neuromuscular Blocking Agents

Neuromuscular blocking agents (NMBAs), or muscle relaxants, have contributed greatly to clinical anesthesia. Muscle relaxants are used to facilitate endotracheal intubation; procedures requiring skeletal muscle relaxation, such as intraperitoneal and thoracic surgery; and ophthalmic surgery to relax the extraocular muscles, and to terminate laryngospasm. They are also used to eliminate chest wall rigidity that may occur after the rapid injection of a potent opioid and to facilitate mechanical ventilation by producing total paralysis of the respiratory muscles.[9]

Skeletal muscle contraction occurs when acetylcholine is released from the motor neuron and binds to receptor sites on the muscle fiber (neuromuscular junction), resulting in repolarization. Skeletal muscle

TABLE 12-3 Opioid Adjunctive Agents

AGENTS		
Meperidine (Demerol) Morphine Fentanyl (Sublimaze) Sufentanil (Sufenta) Alfentanil (Alfenta) Pentazocine (Talwin)	Butoorphanol (Stadol) Nalbuphine (Nubain) Dezocine (Dalgan) Buprenorphine (Buprenex) Ketorolac (Toradol)	
Clinical Uses	**Nursing Implications**	**Nursing Considerations**
Preoperative sedation Induction of anesthesia Maintenance of anesthesia Postoperative pain management	Monitor for hypotension Monitor for bradycardia Monitor for respiratory depression May cause nausea and vomiting	Keep Narcan available Keep resuscitation equipment available Respiratory depressant effect may outlast analgesia

relaxation occurs when the release of acetylcholine ceases and any residual acetylcholine is destroyed by the enzyme acetylcholinesterase, resulting in depolarization. Neuromuscular blocking agents interfere with the relationship between acetylcholine and the nicotinic receptors. There are two general categories of skeletal muscle relaxants: nondepolarizing and depolarizing.[9,10]

Nondepolarizing NMBAs facilitate skeletal muscle relaxation by preventing repolarization from occurring. They bind to the receptor sites, thus blocking the binding of acetylcholine with them. Sustained muscle relaxation occurs, and voluntary control of skeletal muscle contraction is weakened or lost.[10]

The principal depolarizing skeletal muscle relaxant is succinylcholine (Anectine). Succinylcholine has the same effects as acetylcholine on the receptor sites. Once the succinylcholine attaches to the receptor, a brief period of depolarization occurs, which is manifested by transient muscular fasciculations. After depolarization takes place, succinylcholine promotes and maintains the receptor sites in a depolarized state and prevents repolarization. Succinylcholine has a brief duration of action because of the rapid hydrolysis by the enzyme pseudocholinesterase. The actions of succinylcholine cannot be pharmacologically reversed.[11]

Table 12-4 presents a pharmacologic overview of the commonly used skeletal muscle relaxants. There are a number of factors that can potentiate the effects of nondepolarizing NMBAs, as well as antagonize them; these factors are listed in Box 12-3.[9,10]

Neuromuscular blocking agent antagonists. The pharmacologic actions of nondepolarizing NMBAs can be reversed by anticholinesterase drugs, such as neostigmine. These drugs increase the amount of acetylcholine available at the receptor sites by preventing its destruction by acetylcholinesterase. This promotes more effective competition of acetylcholine with the nondepolarizing skeletal muscle relaxant that is occupying the receptor sites. Because of the increased availability and mobilization of the acetylcholine, the concentration gradient favors acetylcholine and the removal of the nondepolarizing agent from the receptors, resulting in the return of normal skeletal muscle repolarization and contraction.[9] These drugs also stimulate the muscarinic receptors, producing undesired side effects, such as miosis, bradycardia, bronchospasm, and enhanced peristalsis and secretions. To prevent or minimize these effects, antimuscarinic agents must be given with these reversal agents.[2,3]

Table 12-5 outlines the common NMBA reversal agents used in anesthesia and their nursing implications.

THE PERIANESTHESIA ASSESSMENT

Admission Observations

Physical assessment of the postanesthesia patient must begin immediately on admission to the unit. The anesthesiologist reports to the receiving nurse the patient's general condition, operation performed, type of

TABLE 12-4 Neuromuscular Blocking Agents

Long Acting	Intermediate Acting	Short Acting
Pancuronium (Pavulon) Gallamine (Flaxedil) Metocurine (Metubine) Doxacurium (Nuromax) Pipecuronium (Arduran)	Atracurium (Tracrium) Vecuronium (Norcuron)	Mivacurium (Mivacron) Alcuronium (Alloferin) Rocuronium (Zemuron) Succinylcholine (Anectine)—depolarizing agent
Characteristics	**Nursing Implications**	
	Depolarizing	**Nondepolarizing**
Compete with acetylcholine at the myoneural junction Shorter acting; most appropriate for anesthesia Provide surgical relaxation Facilitate intubation Assist in ventilatory support	Reversible only with time Use cautiously in patients with neuromuscular disease, such as myasthenia gravis or muscular dystrophy Adverse effects include bradycardia, tachycardia, ventricular dysrhythmias, asystole, hypertension, hyperkalemia Increases intraocular, intracranial, and intragastric pressure Precipitates muscle fasciculations and pain Prolongs respiratory depression Histamine release causes hypotension Use cautiously in patients with head injury, cerebral edema, trauma, burns, electrolyte imbalances, and renal or hepatic disease Be alert for manifestations of malignant hyperthermia	Reversible with time and anticholinesterase Use cautiously in patients with hepatic or renal disease, obesity, asthma, or COPD Adverse effects include tachycardia, hypertension, hypotension, bronchospasms, and flushing Rocuronium, vecuronium, and doxacurium cause minimal adverse effects and do not cause histamine release Atracurium's adverse effects include urticaria, pruritus, and rash When using atracurium monitor for hypothermia and acidosis Pancuronium is better suited for long-term indications Although more potent than pancuronium, pipecuronium's cardiovascular and histamine-induced adverse effects are less severe

anesthesia administered, estimated blood loss, and total intake and output during surgery. In addition, the nurse must be informed of any problems or complications encountered during the intraoperative period.[12]

Rapid assessment of the cardiorespiratory system is of initial concern. The patient's airway is assessed to ensure it is patent, and the patient's respirations are evaluated to ensure they are unlabored. The patient's blood pressure, pulse, rate of respiration, and oxygen saturation level are checked and recorded. All dressings and drains are quickly inspected for gross bleeding.[5] Once these initial observations are made, it is essential to systematically assess the patient's total condition.

Respiratory Function

Because postanesthesia patients have experienced some interference with their respiratory system, maintenance of adequate gas exchange is a crucial aspect of care in the immediate postoperative period. Any change in respiratory function must be detected early so that appropriate measures can be taken to ensure adequate oxygenation and ventilation.[13]

Respiratory function is evaluated by clinical assessment. Additionally, pulse oximetry is used to assess the adequacy of oxygenation, and capnography is used to assess the adequacy of ventilation. Arterial blood gas measurements may also be a part of the respiratory

BOX 12-3 Factors Influencing Neuromuscular Blockade

POTENTIATE

Hypocalcemia
Hypokalemia
Hyponatremia
Hypermagnesemia
Acidosis
Hypothermia
Antibiotics (gentamicin; tobramycin; amikacin; kanamycin; neomycin; polymyxin A, B, and E; clindamycin; tetracyclines; piperacillin; streptomycin)
Antidysrhythmics (procainamide, lidocaine, quinidine)
Beta-adrenergic blockers
Calcium-channel blockers
Diuretics (furosemide, thiazides)
Droperidol
Inhalation agents
Cyclosporine
Lithium
Dantrolene
Etomidate
Hepatic failure
Renal failure
Neuromuscular diseases

ANTAGONIZE

Phenytoin
Carbamazepine
Aminophylline
Theophylline
Sympathomimetic agents
Corticosteroids
Azathioprine

assessment. (∞Pulmonary Clinical Assessment, p. 625; Arterial Blood Gases, p. 641.)

Cardiovascular Function

The three basic components of the circulatory system that must be evaluated are the heart as a pump, the blood, and the arteriovenous system. Maintenance of good tissue perfusion depends on a satisfactory cardiac output; therefore most of the assessment is aimed at evaluating cardiac output.[14]

Cardiovascular function and perfusion are evaluated by clinical assessment. The patient's overall condition is observed, especially skin color and turgor. Peripheral cyanosis, edema, jugular venous distention, shortness of breath, and many other findings may be indicative of cardiovascular problems. In addition to checking all operative sites for blood loss, the amount of blood lost during surgery and the patient's most recent hemoglobin level are noted.

The patient's blood pressure (BP) must be assessed and correlated to the preoperative assessment, intraoperative course, and anesthetic course. BP can be measured noninvasively or invasively. Noninvasive methods include manual cuff measurements with a sphygmomanometer or automatically with an electronic blood pressure cuff. Invasively, the BP is measured via a catheter inserted into an artery, most commonly the radial artery.

Pulse pressure monitoring is an important determinant in the evaluation of perfusion. Rate and character of pulses are assessed bilaterally. Irregularities in pulses must be thoroughly investigated before therapy is initiated. Electrocardiographic (ECG) monitoring is also essential in the immediate postoperative recovery period. Dysrhythmias of any type may occur at any time and in any patient during the postoperative period.

Hemodynamic monitoring is commonly used with higher acuity patients in the postanesthesia recovery period. Hemodynamic monitoring is usually accomplished via a pulmonary artery catheter. (∞Bedside Hemodynamic Monitoring, p. 440.)

Central Nervous System Function

Assessment of the CNS in the immediate postanesthesia period generally involves only gross evaluation of behavior, level of consciousness, intellectual performance, and emotional status. A more detailed assessment of the CNS is necessary for patients who have undergone CNS surgery. (∞Neurologic Clinical Assessment, p. 773.)

Occasionally a patient becomes agitated and thrashes about; this behavior is referred to as *emergence delirium.* It seems to occur more often in adolescents and young adults than in patients of other age groups. Emergence delirium also tends to occur more commonly in patients who have undergone intraabdominal and intrathoracic procedures.[15]

Thermal Balance

The measurement of the patient's body temperature in the immediate postanesthesia recovery period is particularly important. Factors influencing the body temperature include type of anesthesia, preoperative medications, age of patient, site and temperature of intravenous fluids, body surface exposure, temperature of irrigations, temperature of the ambient air, and

TABLE 12-5 NMBA Reversal Agents

Drug	Characteristics	Effects	Nursing Considerations
Neostigmine (Prostigmin)	Binds with cholinesterase and inactivates it Preserves endogenous anticholinesterase	Antidote for nondepolarizing neuromuscular blockers Prevents postoperative distention and urinary retention Muscarinic effects cause bradycardia, bronchoconstriction, peripheral vasodilation, and coronary vasoconstriction	Does not cross blood-brain barrier Lasts 30-90 min May be given with atropine and glycopyrrolate to decrease muscarinic effects Use cautiously in patients with asthma or coronary disease
Pyridostigmine (Regonol)	Analog of neostigmine, with fewer adverse effects Only 20% as potent as neostigmine Increased onset of action (5-15 min)	Antidote for nondepolarizing neuromuscular blocking agents Muscarinic effects less severe than those of neostigmine	Longer half-life Lasts 120 min May be given with atropine and glycopyrrolate Use cautiously in patients with asthma, peptic ulcer, epilepsy, or pregnancy
Edrophonium (Tensilon)	Cholinergic Short-acting anticholinesterase	Parasympathetic effects: GI: salivation, dysphasia, nausea, vomiting, increased peristalsis CV: bradycardia, cardiac dysrhythmias, hypotension Respiratory: increased pharyngeal and tracheobronchial secretions EENT: Lacrimation, miosis, diplopia Skin: diaphoresis, flushing	Must be given with atropine Very rapid onset, but brief duration of action Use cautiously in presence of asthma, peptic ulcer, or bradycardia
Atropine	Anticholinergic Antimuscarinic Chronotropic stimulator in event of bradycardia	Preanesthetic medication to prevent or reduce respiratory tract secretions Restoration of cardiac rate during anesthesia Antidote for cholinesterase inhibitors Causes decreased sweating and predisposition to heat prostration	Crosses blood-brain barrier Ensures adequate hydration Provides temperature control to prevent hyperpyrexia
Glycopyrrolate (Robinul)	Similar to atropine Longer duration	Less incidence of dysrhythmias Slow increase in heart rate Protection against peripheral muscarinic effects of neostigmine and pyridostigmine	Does not cross blood-brain barrier Contraindicated in presence of glaucoma, peptic ulcer, or COPD

EENT, Eye(s), ear(s), nose, throat.

vasoconstriction (secondary to blood loss or anesthetic agents). Both hypothermia (temperature below 36° C) and hyperthermia (temperature above 38° C) are associated with physiologic alterations that may interfere with recovery.

The body maintains its temperature between a narrow range of 36° and 38° C. This is accomplished by a balance of heat production and heat loss that is controlled by the thermoregulation mechanisms in the CNS. These mechanisms receive input from various thermoreceptors located in the skin, nose, oral cavity, thoracic viscera, and spinal cord. These thermoreceptors then send sensory information in hierarchical order to the spinal cord, reticular formation, and the primary control center in the hypothalamic region of the brain.

The central temperature controls maintain body temperature via physiologic and behavioral responses. The physiologic thermoregulatory responses consist of sweating, shivering, and alterations in peripheral vasomotor tone. These responses fine-control the regulatory process of body temperature; consequently, heat is conserved via vasoconstriction and lost via vasodilation and sweating. The physiologic responses also can lower the metabolic rate to decrease heat production and increase muscle tone and shivering to increase heat production. Behavioral thermoregulation is accomplished by subjective feelings of discomfort or comfort. For example, in a hot environment a person seeks air conditioning, and in a cold environment a person seeks heat. It is a stronger response mechanism, but it can not fine-tune body temperature as the physiologic responses can.[5,16]

The accuracy of axillary, rectal, or oral measurements are frequently debated. Shell (skin) temperatures may be measured at the axilla or forehead with temperature strips. Invasive techniques that use the thermistor on a pulmonary artery catheter, the tympanic membrane or the bladder as a site for monitoring temperature are more accurate. The infrared tympanic thermometer has been found to accurately track core temperature. It is noninvasive, nontraumatic, and may be used with patients of all sizes. Whatever method, trending is essential in the immediate postanesthesia recovery period.[16]

Fluid and Electrolyte Balance

Evaluation of a patient's fluid and electrolyte status involves total body assessment. Imbalances readily occur in the postoperative patient, because of a number of factors, including the restriction of food and fluids preoperatively, fluid loss during surgery, and stress. The normal body response to stress is renal retention of water and sodium. In addition, postanesthesia patients often have abnormal avenues of fluid loss postoperatively.

Each patient must be evaluated to determine his or her baseline requirements and the fluid needed to replace abnormal loss. Most patients in the immediate postanesthesia recovery period receive intravenous fluids. It is important to know what fluids, if any, are to follow or whether the infusion is to be discontinued. All intravenous sites are checked regularly for signs of extravasation, phlebitis, and infection.

Oral intake must be prohibited after anesthesia until the laryngeal and pharyngeal reflexes are fully regained, as evidenced by the patient's ability to gag and swallow effectively. In addition, the management of postoperative nausea and vomiting remains critical.

Normal output in the average adult results from obligatory urinary output and insensible avenues of loss, including evaporation of water from the skin and exhalation during respiration. A lower-than-normal urinary output can be expected in the immediate postanesthesia recovery period as a result of the body's normal reaction to stress. Specific gravity determines whether to suspect dehydration, versus renal insufficiency. External losses from vomiting, nasogastric tubes, T-tubes, and wound drainage need to be assessed and monitored, also. Accurate measurement and recording of all intake and output is vital in the assessment of the patient's fluid and electrolyte status.[17]

Psychosocial Assessment

Assessment of the patient's psychosocial and emotional well-being is an important component of perianesthesia care. As with any other assessment, this must be made in the context of the whole patient. Almost all patients experience a degree of anxiety about anesthesia and the surgical procedure and a fear of postoperative pain. The physical manifestations include tachycardia; increased blood pressure; pale, cool skin; increased respiratory rate; hyperventilation; increased muscle tone; restlessness; agitation; and dilated pupils.[18]

The postanesthesia assessment must be comprehensive. Differentiation between normal physiologic function and the variety of pathologic symptoms in the immediate postanesthesia recovery period needs to be astute. Knowledgeable assessment of the postanesthesia patient is essential for the provision of safe and effective medical and nursing management.

CARE OF THE POSTANESTHESIA PATIENT

Stir-Up Regimen

The stir-up regimen is probably the most important aspect of perianesthesia nursing management. The basics of the regimen are aimed at the prevention of complications, primarily atelectasis and venous stasis. Five major activities—deep breathing exercises, coughing, positioning, mobilization, and pain management—constitute the stir-up regimen.[19]

Deep breathing exercises. The major factor contributing to postoperative pulmonary complications is low lung volumes resulting from a shallow, monotonous, sighless breathing pattern caused by general anesthesia, pain, and opioids. Therefore the patient must be stimulated to take three or four deep breaths every 5 to 10 minutes. Full lung expansion is important, and every effort must be made to enhance the patient's ability to do so.

The sustained maximal inspiration (SMI) maneuver is a method to enhance the lung volumes of postoperative patients. The SMI maneuver consists of having the patient inhale as close to lung capacity as possible and, at the peak of inspiration, having the patient hold that volume for 3 to 5 seconds before exhaling it. This maneuver has been more effective than simple deep breathing in preventing reduced lung volumes in the immediate postanesthesia period.[20] If the patient's vital capacity is inadequate or respiratory depression resulting from anesthesia is prolonged, deep breathing and the SMI maneuver may be augmented with a manual resuscitation bag connected to an oxygen source or with an intermittent positive-pressure breathing apparatus.

Incentive spirometry (IS) has become increasingly popular and is used to assist with preventing and treating atelectasis, promoting normal lung expansion, and improving oxygenation. IS devices allow patients visual feedback and observation of inspiratory volume. Instruction and practice before surgery provide patients with the opportunity to master the device and establish a baseline for themselves before anesthetic and surgical interventions.[19]

Coughing. The patient must be instructed to cough along with performing SMIs. The best way to clear the air passages of obstructive secretions is a purposeful cough. For the patient recovering from anesthesia, the cascade cough is the most effective cough maneuver. The patient is instructed to take a rapid, deep inhalation to increase the volume of air in the lungs, which will dilate the airways and allow air to pass beyond the retained secretions. On exhalation, the patient performs multiple coughs at succeedingly lower lung volumes. With each cough the length of airways undergoing dynamic compression increases, enhancing cough effectiveness.

Coughing is most effective with the patient sitting upright. Splinting of incisions and adequate analgesia facilitate coughing. If the patient is unable to sit upright, positioning the patient in a side-lying position with hips and knees flexed or in a semi-Fowler's position with the head and arms supported with pillows and knees flexed decreases abdominal tension and allows maximal movement of the diaphragm, thereby improving the effectiveness of the cough.

Between cascade cough maneuvers, the patient is encouraged to inhale and close the glottis. This dilates the airways, increases intrathoracic pressure, and compresses the smaller airways, as to "milk" the secretions toward the larger airways, where they can be expectorated in succeeding cough maneuvers.[21]

Positioning. When possible, patients recovering from anesthesia are maintained in a semiprone, side-lying position. The semiprone position promotes maintenance of a patent airway, prevents aspiration of emesis into the trachea, and permits optimal ventilation of the lower lung lobes. Frequent repositioning of patients (at least every hour) side to side is essential for the prevention of atelectasis and venous stasis. As soon as they are able, patients are encouraged to turn and change positions alone.

Mobilization. To prevent venous stasis, patients must be encouraged to move their legs and arms rhythmically, flexing and extending their extremities. Mobilization and flexion of the muscles aide venous return and improve cardiac output.[20]

Pain management. Achievement of the stir-up regimen's first four activities is difficult if adequate pain relief is not provided. Opioids depress the cough reflex and ciliary activity and may lower alveolar ventilation by direct depression of the respiratory center in the brain. They must not be used indiscriminately. If breathing is painful and splinting occurs, however, or if the patient refuses to cough or move because of pain, nothing is gained. (∞Pain Management, p. 180.)

Respiratory Function Management

The goal of oxygen is the optimal use of the oxygen-carrying capacity of arterial blood. All anesthetized patients experience some interference with their respiratory processes, and it is for this reason that most experts suggest routine oxygen administration. Pulse oximetry, a noninvasive technique, measures oxygen saturation of functional hemoglobin. Normal pulse oximetry values are 97% to 99%; however, preanesthetic baseline values must be noted. Some patients may normally have lower saturation values on room air, for a variety of reasons, and attempting to maintain higher oxygen saturation levels may result in prolonged oxygen therapy. (∞Oxygen Therapy, p. 689.)

Routine oxygen administration in the postanesthesia recovery period can be accomplished with nasal cannula (prongs) or face mask. Surgery and anesthesia often interrupt the normal functioning of the nose, so consideration of humidification and/or nebulization with oxygen delivery may be needed. Humidifiers convert water from the liquid to the gaseous state, whereas nebulizers produce tiny water particles. This is especially helpful at higher flow rates.[22]

Some patients recovering from anesthesia may require mechanical ventilation. Various modes, such as positive end-expiratory pressure (PEEP), continuous positive airway pressure (CPAP), and synchronized intermittent mandatory ventilation (SIMV), are used to improve the respiratory status of the patient. (∞Invasive Mechanical Ventilation, p. 703.)

When large amounts of secretions accumulate in the patient's lungs and they cannot be handled effectively by coughing, suctioning must be instituted. Suctioning must only be done when necessary and not routinely, because it is not without complications. (∞Suctioning, p. 701.)

Fluid and Electrolyte Balance Management

Postoperative parenteral fluid requirements vary with the patient's preoperative status and with the surgical procedure. Most disease processes, tissue injuries, and operative procedures greatly influence the physiology of fluids and electrolytes in the body. In the surgical patient, intravenous access to the circulatory system is necessary for the administration of anesthesia, resuscitation drugs, blood and blood products, and fluid and electrolyte solutions.

In deciding the type of fluid to use in the postanesthesia recovery period, one can differentiate between crystalloids and colloids, maintenance and replacement fluids, or fluids of differing tonicity. Because of the large variety of fluid solutions, some general guidelines are recommended in clinical practice. Crystalloids are generally used as maintenance fluids to compensate for insensible fluid losses and as replacement fluids to correct body fluid deficits (e.g., treatment of specific fluid and electrolyte disturbances). Colloids are generally used for fluid replacement, shock resuscitation, and fluid challenges. Maintenance fluid requirements are calculated according to body weight and are used to replace insensible losses from the lungs, skin, urine, and feces. Adults typically require 1.5 to 2 ml/kg/hr.[17]

One of the cardinal responsibilities during the immediate postanesthesia recovery period is the ability to evaluate in an orderly, logical, and expedient manner the fluid status of the patient. Choose an intravenous fluid solution appropriate to the patient's problem. When unsure, infuse a balanced salt solution. As with any therapeutic intervention, there can also be complications with fluid administration, such as fluid overload, acute heart failure, and edema formation. Box 12-4 outlines an example of one approach to fluid status assessment in the postanesthesia patient.[23]

The goal of fluid therapy in the immediate postanesthesia recovery period is the restoration of blood volume and tissue perfusion. Recovery after surgery is a dynamic process, and fluid reassessment is conducted periodically. Fluid challenges may be necessary in the hypovolemic patient or in the patient with clinical manifestations of hypoperfusion. The decision of whether to use crystalloids or colloids for fluid resuscitation is complex, controversial, often determined by personal preference and concern over expense, and may be inconsequential as long as fluids are infused appropriate to the needs of the patient.

Blood and blood components are reserved for specific patient situations. Red blood cells are indicated to increase oxygen-carrying capacity in patients with anemia. Platelets are used to treat bleeding associated with deficiencies in platelet number or function. Fresh frozen plasma is transfused to increase clotting factor levels in patients with demonstrated deficiencies. A good understanding of fluid types available, of a systematic approach to evaluating fluid depletion, and of the indications for blood component therapy allows one to make appropriate decisions when implementing fluid therapy in the immediate postanesthesia period.[23]

Pain Management

Adequate pain control is a major consideration in the recovering patient. Poorly controlled pain may have serious consequences in terms of hemodynamic responses to catecholamines and physical limitations on respiratory function. On the other hand, the medications used to control pain may in themselves have deleterious effects on hemodynamics and respiratory function.

BOX 12-4 Fluid Balance Evaluation

Volume status evaluation - assess heart rate, pulse quality, blood pressure, sitting and supine positions, skin color and turgor, mucous membrane moisture, and urine output
Concentration status - assess serum sodium concentration, serum osmolality
Composition status - assess arterial blood gas, serum electrolytes, blood urea nitrogen (BUN), and serum glucose level

Acute pain is an unpleasant sensation and emotional experience usually caused by damage to tissue or by noxious stimuli. Pain receptors, called nociceptors, are located mainly in the skin, blood vessels, subcutaneous tissue, foci, periosteum, and viscera, and are stimulated by noxious stimuli. Nociceptors act as transducers and convert the painful stimulus into impulses that are transmitted along peripheral fibers to the central nervous system. The degree of nociceptor input from the periphery to the central nervous system is influenced by temperature, sympathetic function, vasculature, and the chemical environment.[24] (∞Pain Management, p. 180.)

By activating the sympathoadrenal system, pain accelerates the cardiovascular system, as observed by the parameters of pulse and blood pressure. It has been suggested that pain, especially at upper abdominal and thoracic sites, decreases or, in fact, eliminates the normal sighing (yawn) mechanism. The absence of an appropriate sigh leads to reduced lung volumes and, ultimately, to the atelectasis/pneumonia sequelae. Again, appropriate pain relief in these patients may reduce the incidence of atelectasis and pneumonia postoperatively.[25]

Assessment of postoperative pain includes both behavioral and physiologic clues. Pain usually elicits an increased response by the sympathetic nervous system, which in turn produces a large amount of catecholamines, causing tachycardia, increased cardiac output, increased systemic vascular resistance, and ultimately an increase in blood pressure. Other assessment parameters of excessive sympathoadrenal activity resulting from acute pain include respiratory changes, excessive perspiration, changes in skin color, nausea, and vomiting. Other objective findings include generalized or local muscle tension or rigidity, unusual postures, knees drawn up to abdomen, restlessness, rubbing, and scratching. Finally, pain may affect the behavioral affect of the patient, so that the patient in acute pain may be irritable; depressed; withdrawn; or have behavioral reverses, such as hostility in an ordinarily quiet person.

Once the assessment has been made and it has been determined that the patient is indeed experiencing acute postoperative pain, certain interventions are suggested. If the patient has received an inhalation anesthetic, such as isoflurane, enflurane, or halothane, and demonstrates manifestations of acute pain, relief is instituted early in the postanesthetic period. Similarly, patients receiving a nitrous oxide–opioid technique are medicated early in the immediate postoperative period, particularly if the intraoperative opioids were of short duration. If medications such as sufentanil, meperidine, and morphine were used intraoperatively, opioids must be administered with caution to avoid respiratory depression as a result of the synergistic actions of the intraoperative and postoperative opioid agonists. Finally, if the patient was administered droperidol intraoperatively or preoperatively, great caution must be used because opioid agonists as well as barbiturates are significantly potentiated by this butyrophenone tranquilizer. Therefore the usual dosage of opioid agonists must be reduced by one third to one half during the first 8 to 10 hours postoperatively.[2]

General Comfort Management

General comfort and safety measures are important parts of postanesthesia care. For safety, there must always be at least two nurses (one of whom is a registered nurse) present whenever patients are recovering. An unconscious patient must never be left alone, and side rails must be raised on the bed whenever direct care is not being provided. The wheels of the bed must be locked to prevent sliding when care is being rendered.

General physical measures such as cleanliness must not be overlooked in the postanesthesia recovery period. Comfort measures, important to the total well-being of the patient, are often forgotten in the hustle of caring for postanesthesia patients. As soon as the patient is settled into the unit and assessment has been accomplished, all excess skin preparations and electrodes are removed; in addition to providing comfort, washing off excess skin preparations gives the nurse an excellent opportunity to further assess the patient's general condition. A back rub at this time may prevent later complaints of discomfort from positioning for long periods in the operating room. This is also a good time to change the patient's position, assist with range of motion exercises, and encourage deep breathing. Frequent position changes help prevent atelectasis, promote circulation, and prevent pressure sores from developing on the skin surfaces.

Mouth care is comforting to the patient who has not only had nothing by mouth but who has been medicated with an anticholinergic or glycopyrrolate to reduce secretions. When patients are fully conscious and their laryngeal reflexes have returned, they can rinse their mouths with mouthwash and water. Ice chips and small sips of water or juice may be offered to patients who can tolerate fluids. A petroleum-based ointment is applied to the lips after mouth care to prevent drying and consequent cracking.

Patients often complain of being cold when returning from the operating suite. This is a result in part of the effects of anesthesia and premedications and in part of the cool atmosphere of the operating suite. The normothermic patient may shiver or complain of feeling cold, so warm blankets may provide psychologic comfort. Blankets of any type must not, however, obscure the intravenous lines, arterial lines, or other monitoring apparatuses from the direct view of the attending nurse. The patient's temperature must be monitored closely to avoid overheating.

In addition to the physical comfort measures, remember to provide psychologic comfort. Reorientation, especially to time and place, is important to the postanesthesia patient, as is constant reassurance that the surgery is completed and that all went well. The nurse's presence at the bedside or gentle touch may also be comforting to the patient.[1]

MANAGEMENT OF POSTANESTHESIA PROBLEMS AND/OR EMERGENCIES

In the immediate postoperative period significant physiologic changes occur as the patient emerges from the effects of anesthesia. Factors that influence the development of problems are listed in Box 12-5.[26]

BOX 12-5 Factors Influencing the Development of Postoperative Problems

Intraoperative complications
Type of anesthetic technique
Preoperative condition of patient
Length and type of surgery
Urgency of surgery
Poorly controlled pain
Other drugs administered intraoperatively
Changes in fluid status and electrolyte balance
Alterations in body temperature

Respiratory Problems and/or Emergencies

Respiratory problems occur with some regularity in the postanesthesia period. Keep in mind that all general anesthetic agents and opioid analgesic drugs have respiratory depressant effects. Acute pain also impairs the ability to breathe deeply. Most respiratory problems are related to upper airway obstruction, though other problems can occur, including acute respiratory failure, aspiration, pulmonary edema, and respiratory arrest.[27]

Airway obstruction. Soft tissue obstruction occurs when the pharynx is blocked and air cannot flow in and out. The most common cause of soft tissue obstruction is the tongue. Clinical manifestations of an airway obstruction include snoring, stridor, flaring of the nostrils, retractions at the intercostal spaces and suprasternal notch, abnormal use of accessory muscles, asynchronous movements of the chest and abdomen, increased pulse rate, decreased oxygen saturation level, and decreased breath sounds.

Management of an airway obstruction begins with immediate recognition. Stimulation may be all that is necessary to relieve the obstruction and obtain a patent airway. With the nonreactive patient, the head tilt–chin lift maneuver or elevation of the mandible at its angles (jaw thrust) will displace the tongue and open the airway. If patency of the airway cannot be obtained by either of these methods, an oropharyngeal or nasopharyngeal airway is inserted. A nasopharyngeal airway is usually better tolerated, although it can occasionally cause nasal bleeding. Oropharyngeal airways must only be used in an unconscious patient because they can cause gagging, vomiting, and laryngospasm in the awake patient. The patient can also be turned on his or her side to a lateral position, which will facilitate the displacement of the tongue and drainage of secretions. If the obstruction is still unrelieved, positive pressure mask ventilation, intubation, tracheotomy, or cricothyrotomy is in order.[28]

Laryngeal edema. *Laryngeal edema* is defined as swelling of laryngeal tissue. This edema can cause varying degrees of airway obstruction. Manifestations include stridor, retractions, hoarseness, and a crouplike cough. Apprehension and restlessness can be present in the awake patient.

Management consists of placing the patient in the upright position; using cool, humidified oxygen; and administering nebulized racemic epinephrine. If the laryngeal edema is a result of an allergic reaction, the reaction must be managed with epinephrine, bronchodilators, and antihistamines. Reintubation is only performed if the patient's symptoms cannot be controlled with an inhalation treatment within 30 minutes, hypercarbia persists, or the patient appears to be in respiratory distress. If reintubation takes place, the endotracheal tube must be at least one size smaller than the previous tube used, and an air leak must be present around the cuff.[29]

Laryngospasm. Laryngospasm is caused by reflex contractions of the pharyngeal muscles, resulting in spasms of the vocal cords and the inability of the patient to take a breath. The spasms may result in either a partial or complete airway obstruction. Involvement of the intrinsic laryngeal muscles causes a reflex closure of the glottis, which results in an incomplete obstruction. Involvement of the extrinsic muscles causes a reflex closure of the larynx, which results in a complete airway obstruction. Manifestations include dyspnea, hypoxia, hypoventilation, absence of breath sounds, and hypercarbia. Crowing sounds may be heard if the spasm is incomplete. The chest does not expand normally and a rocking motion of the chest wall that stimulates abdominal breathing may be present. The patient panics if awake.

There are several factors that can help identify the patient at risk for a laryngospasm. Preoperatively, risks include a history of asthma, chronic obstructive pulmonary disease (COPD), or smoking. Intraoperatively, risks include the use of endotracheal tube (ETT), anesthetic agents, "light" anesthesia, multiple attempts at intubation, or surgical airway manipulation. Postoperatively, risks include coughing, "bucking" on the ETT, repeated suctioning, or excessive secretions in the nasopharyngeal area. Laryngospasm may also be precipitated by irritants and foreign bodies.

Laryngospasm is an emergency that requires an immediate response or the patient may rapidly deteriorate. Management is initiated by removing the stimulus, along with any irritants such as secretions, blood, or an airway that is too long. The patient's head must be hyperextended and positive pressure mask ventilation instituted on 100% oxygen. The anesthesiologist is notified immediately. If complete obstruction is unrelieved by positive pressure ventilations, a small dose of succinylcholine (10 to 20 mg) may be needed to relax the vocal cords to allow for ventilation. Positive pressure mask ventilation is continued until full muscle function has resumed. Endotracheal intubation is required if the laryngospasm persists or if refractory hypoxemia develops, though it may cause further irritation of the airway. Medications that may be used in the treatment of laryngospasm include lidocaine, steroids, and atropine.

After the spasm, the patient continues to receive supplemented oxygen until stable. It is also important at that time for the nurse to reassure the patient that the spasm has resolved. The patient's feelings of being unable to breathe during laryngospasm are intense, and emotional support from the nurse is imperative.[28,29]

Bronchospasm. Bronchospasm is a lower airway obstruction that is characterized by spasmodic contractions of the bronchial tubes. Bronchial airway constriction is a result of an increase in smooth muscle tone in the airways, and bronchospasms develop when the smooth muscles constrict and obstruct the airway. Inflammation has also been recognized as a fundamental component of bronchospasms.

Bronchiolar constriction may be centrally generated, as in asthma, or it may be a local response to airway irritation. Manifestations include wheezing, noisy shallow respirations, chest retractions, and use of accessory muscles. The patient can exhibit shortness of breath, coughing, and a prolonged expiratory phase of respiration. In addition, hypertension and tachycardia may be present. The patient's level of consciousness may range from lethargy to extreme anxiety.

Patients who smoke and those with chronic bronchitis have essentially irritable airways that react to stimulation. A preoperative history of asthma, a recent upper respiratory infection, severe emphysema, pulmonary fibrosis, or radiation pneumonitis are indicators of a greater risk of bronchospasm. Stimuli that produce a bronchospasm postoperatively include secretions, vomitus, and blood. Patients who have had laryngoscopies, bronchoscopies, or other surgical stimulation are also at increased risk of bronchospasm. There are also drugs that are believed to predispose the patient to developing bronchoconstriction resulting from cholinomimetic stimulation; these drugs include physostigmine, neostigmine, edrophonium, and barbiturates. Other histamine-releasing drugs such as tubocurarine, morphine, metocurine, and atracurium may potentially foster bronchospasm.

Bronchospasm is treated initially by removing any possible irritants or drugs. The first line of therapy consists of inhaled bronchodilators. These inhalants cause fewer cardiovascular side effects than systemically administered drugs. Common inhalant medications used are isoetharine, metaproterenol, albuterol, and beclomethasone. Systemic bronchodilators and antiinflammatory agents may also be required at times. Epinephrine or isoproterenol is occasionally needed as a continuous infusion. Methylprednisolone given intravenously manages the inflammatory aspect of bronchospasm. Cholinergics have been given by nebulizer to decrease secretions.[28,29] (∞Pulmonary Pharmacology, p. 713.)

Noncardiogenic pulmonary edema. *Pulmonary edema* may be defined simply as increased total lung water. Fluid can be accumulated in the interstitial spaces or in the alveoli, owing to cardiogenic or pulmonary capillary etiology. Noncardiogenic pulmonary edema in the postanesthesia recovery period can result from pulmonary aspiration, blood transfusion reaction, allergic drug reaction, upper airway obstruction, or sepsis. The causative factor seems to be most often an upper airway obstruction, usually laryngospasm. Often there had been a short episode of airway obstruction in the operating room. Noncardiogenic pulmonary edema has also occurred after the administration of naloxone to patients who have received general anesthesia. The reversal of the analgesics causes a rise in the level of adrenal catecholamines, which can lead to pulmonary hypertension and probably increased pulmonary vascular permeability.

During laryngospasm, the patient is inhaling against a closed glottis. This generates an increase in negative intrathoracic pressure. A tremendous subatmospheric transpulmonary pressure gradient is created that causes transudation, or leaking of fluid, from the pulmonary capillaries into the interstitium.

Pulmonary edema interferes with gas exchange by disrupting the diffusion pathway between the alveolus and the capillary. The partial pressure of oxygen in the alveolar gas is normally greater than the partial pressure of oxygen in the capillary blood. This difference promotes the oxygen diffusion. When fluid is present in the interstitial space, the distance the oxygen must be diffused is increased. This lack of diffusion of oxygen leads to hypoxemia. Carbon dioxide diffuses about 20 times more rapidly than oxygen and therefore can pass across a fluid-filled interstitial space much more easily. The patient with pulmonary edema may demonstrate hypoxemia without hypercarbia.

Manifestations of pulmonary edema include respiratory distress with tachycardia; shortness of breath; and the production of pink, frothy sputum. When auscultated, bilateral lung sounds demonstrate crackles and rhonchi. Oxygen saturation levels drop and arterial blood gases show hypoxia and hypercarbia. There is a decrease in lung compliance and the presence of pulmonary infiltrates via chest x-ray.

Management of the patient consists of maintenance of an unobstructed airway and supplemented oxygen to correct hypoxemia. Those patients who cannot maintain adequate oxygenation with a mask may require the use of CPAP or even mechanical ventilation with PEEP. The use of PEEP or CPAP improves hypoxemia by restoring the functional residual capacity. Vigorous pulmonary toilet may be required, as well as the use of hemodynamic monitoring, if the patient's blood pressure is labile and fluid balance is difficult to maintain.

Diuretics and fluid restriction are usually a part of the treatment regimen. Morphine can be titrated to relieve anxiety. Corticosteroid therapy can be used to decrease laryngeal edema and stabilize the pulmonary membrane. Noncardiogenic pulmonary edema occurs rapidly and requires early assessment and immediate intervention.[30]

Aspiration. *Aspiration* can be defined as the passage of regurgitate gastric contents or other foreign material into the trachea and down to the smaller air units. It can occur during the period of reduced protective airway reflexes. The most common and severest form of aspiration is the aspiration of gastric contents. The gastric acid in gastric contents damages the alveolar and capillary endothelial cells. Fluid rich with protein leaks into the interstitium and alveoli. This results in atelectasis and consolidation. Pulmonary compliance and functional residual capacity are decreased, and airway resistance and intrapulmonary shunting are increased, with hypoxemia resulting.

If aspiration is suspected, management begins with lowering the patient's head, if possible. The patient is positioned to the side or the head is turned to the side to permit gravity to pull secretions from the trachea. Management centers on promoting tissue oxygenation by maintaining arterial oxygenation via CPAP and supplemental oxygen. Positive pressure ventilation via mask can be applied if the patient is awake and able to protect his or her airway or via an ETT if the patient is unable to tolerate the mask or requires higher levels of airway pressure.[28,29] (∞Aspiration Lung Disorder, p. 667.)

Hypoxemia. Administration of oxygen by face mask to recovering patients is routine because of the many factors that can lead to hypoxemia in the postoperative patient. Respiratory depressant effects of residual agents may result in a shallow breathing pattern with increased dead space-to-tidal volume ratio. This is even more evident in patients after upper abdominal surgery, and the reduction in effective ventilation can have serious effects on oxygenation.[26]

The most common cause of hypoxemia is ventilation/perfusion mismatching. Atelectasis often occurs as a result of bronchial obstruction by secretions or blood. Reduction in functional residual capacity (FRC) is caused by the effects of anesthesia and, in the case of upper abdominal surgery, by the surgical procedure. When FRC falls below closing capacity, dependent alveoli occlude, leading to increased mismatching. Impairment of hypoxic pulmonary vasoconstriction by inhalation agents and some vasoactive drugs helps potentiate this effect.[29] (∞Acute Respiratory Failure, p. 655.)

Hypoventilation. Central respiratory depression is caused by all anesthetic agents. This may lead to significant hypoventilation and hypercarbia. Impaired respiratory muscle function, particularly after upper abdominal surgery, may contribute to the problem of carbon dioxide elimination. Incomplete reversal of neuromuscular blockade must also be considered. Other contributory factors may include tight dressings and body casts, obesity, and gastric dilation. In addition, increased carbon dioxide production may occur as a result of shivering or sepsis. This leads to hypercarbia in patients unable to increase ventilation enough to compensate.

Hypercarbia resulting from postoperative hypoventilation may cause hypertension and tachycardia, increasing the risk of myocardial ischemia in susceptible individuals. Hypoventilation, by itself or in combination with the other factors previously discussed, can cause hypoxemia. Very high levels of carbon dioxide may have sedative effects. Evaluation of suspected hypoventilation requires measurement of arterial blood gases.

Careful titration of opioid antagonists, such as naloxone, may be effective in improving ventilation without compromising pain relief. Planning ahead to provide adequate postoperative pain relief is essential for maintaining adequate postoperative ventilation, particularly in patients undergoing abdominal or thoracic procedures. Placing obese patients in a head-up position and relieving the effects of tight dressings and casts can also be important. Hypoventilation that cannot be improved sufficiently by noninvasive means requires intubation and mechanical ventilation until the patient is able to maintain adequate ventilation.[26,28]

Cardiovascular Problems and/or Emergencies

In the immediate postoperative period, cardiovascular complications causing an alteration in cardiac output can occur. These include anesthetic effects on cardiac function, myocardial dysfunction, dysrhythmias, hypertension, and hypotension. These conditions may occur individually or in combination.[31]

Anesthetic effects on cardiac function. In the immediate postoperative period the residual effects of anesthetic agents and their adjuncts must be considered in the evaluation of a patient who has cardiac dysfunction. Volatile anesthetic agents, such as halothane, enflurane, and isoflurane, can cause a dose-related reduction in myocardial function. Halothane causes a drop in blood pressure primarily because of a reduction in heart rate and myocardial contractility. It produces only a slight reduction in systemic vascular resistance (SVR). Enflurane not only decreases contractility but also reduces SVR. Isoflurane has the most significant hypotension action and the least negative inotropic effects of the three agents. The actions of these agents may be noted for several hours after the conclusion of surgery.[3,5] Nitrous oxide is an inhalation agent that demonstrates insignificant cardiac depression. The combined action of opioids given during emergence from nitrous oxide can result in marked cardiovascular depression, however.[5]

Therapy directed toward mitigating the myocardial depressant effects of inhalation anesthetic agents is primarily that of increasing preload. Elevation of the legs and a crystalloid fluid bolus are commonly sufficient treatment, but ephedrine or other positive inotropic agents may be needed.[2]

Individually, most opioids and benzodiazepines produce only moderate depression in cardiac function. Opioids reduce the sympathetic response and enhance vagal and parasympathetic tone. Benzodiazepines reduce SVR, as do most opioids because of histamine release. The combination of these medications may cause significant myocardial depression because of their sympathetic actions. Specifically, the overall reaction may include a lowered SVR, heart rate, ventricular contractility, catecholamine level, baroreceptor reflex, cardiac output, and blood pressure. Aggressive administration of crystalloid solutions may be required to counteract these effects. High-dose opioids combined with vecuronium produce a negative inotropic and chronotropic effect. Patients may require short-term vascular support until these medications dissipate.[8]

In contrast to most opioids, meperidine has a greater effect in diminishing myocardial contractility. Meperidine can cause histamine release, which can lower SVR and blood pressure. Sufentanil also has myocardial depressant effects, but with less hemodynamic instability than meperidine. Barbiturates depress the activity of the vasomotor center, causing peripheral vasodilation and hypotension. These actions are dose related and more marked in the presence of underlying cardiovascular disease. Ketamine has a direct myocardial depressant effect that is usually counterbalanced by its indirect effect on the autonomic nervous system to increase heart rate and blood pressure. In patients who are unable to mount a sympathetic response to stress, ketamine causes a net decrease in cardiac output. Propofol causes a dose-dependent decrease in blood pressure primarily because of a decrease in SVR. This must be considered when caring for patients who are hypovolemic or have minimal cardiac reserves.[28,32]

Local anesthetic agents may cause cardiovascular toxicity if inadvertently injected into the systemic circulation or if excessive dosage of the agent is used. A decrease in myocardial contractility, reduction in SVR, and diminished cardiac output have been observed secondary to these agents. The extent of cardiovascular compromise appears to occur in a dose-related fashion. Management of the cardiovascular complications associated with local anesthetic agents include measures to increase preload, namely elevation of legs and fluid administration. In refractory cases, ephedrine may also be needed.[3,5]

Myocardial dysfunction. During the immediate postoperative period, the causes of myocardial depression include pathologic processes and aberrant physiologic states, in addition to anesthetic side effects. These processes may occur alone or in combination and may be particularly hazardous in the presence of underlying cardiac disease.

Myocardial ischemia results from an imbalance of oxygen supply and demand. Commonly, ischemia is a result of a decrease in myocardial blood flow that is usually secondary to atherosclerosis, vasospasm, or hypotension. In the postoperative period, the stress of surgery and the action of certain anesthetic agents can increase myocardial ischemia.[31]

Dysrhythmias. In the immediate postanesthetic period, patients are predisposed to a variety of cardiac dysrhythmias. The most common dysrhythmias are sinus tachycardia, sinus bradycardia, premature ventricular contractions, supraventricular tachydysrhythmias, and ventricular tachycardia. If present, a thorough investigation, not just a reflex treatment, of the disturbance must be undertaken.

Accurate interpretation and identification of the dysrhythmia are essential because therapeutic intervention is based on diagnosis. Appropriate skin preparation and lead placement are extremely important to ensure clear, readable tracings, free from artifact. Additional 12-lead electrocardiographic capabilities need to be used if an interpretation cannot be made from bedside monitoring tracings.

The hemodynamic effects of the dysrhythmia also need to be thoroughly assessed. The clinical presentation of the dysrhythmia determines the severity of underlying cardiac disease and the type of treatment. Tachydysrhythmias shorten diastolic filling time and interfere with coronary artery perfusion. These two effects, coupled with an increase in myocardial oxygen consumption, may produce cardiac decompensation. Bradycardia can produce a clinically significant decrease in cardiac output if stroke volume is limited by underlying cardiac disease or if the venous return is reduced. Finally, the cause of the rhythm disturbance needs to be considered.[32]

The causes of postoperative dysrhythmias are variable. Circulatory instability; preexisting heart disease; an increase in vagal tone; drugs; pain; electrolytic disturbances; and alterations in acid-base balance, oxygenation, and ventilation are most common.

General anesthesia lowers the dysrhythmia threshold of the myocardium. Inhalation agents such as halothane, enflurane, and isoflurane sensitize the myocardium to catecholamines and depress sinoatrial (SA) and atrioventricular (AV) nodal function. Junctional rhythms and premature ventricular contractions are the most commonly seen dysrhythmias. Ketamine produces sympathetic stimulation, resulting in tachycardia and hypertension. Succinylcholine stimulates the cholinergic receptors, enhancing vagal tone, and it can produce sinus bradycardia or junctional escape rhythms. Opioids may cause bradycardia because of direct stimulation of the vagus nerve.

In addition, endogenous catecholamine levels in postoperative patients are elevated because of the pain and stress of surgery. Increased catecholamine levels increase sinus and AV node rates, as well as atrial and ventricular irritability. The direct result is tachydysrhythmias and atrial or ventricular premature contractions.[31,32]

Postoperative hypertension. Hypertension is not an unusual occurrence in the immediate postoperative period. The diagnosis of hypertension must be considered in the context of an elevated blood pressure in relation to the patient's preoperative and intraoperative blood pressure range. Most commonly, postoperative hypertension is related to fluid overload, heightened sympathetic nervous system activity, or preexisting hypertension. Postoperative hypertension, even as a transient episode, may have significant cardiovascular and intracranial consequences, and therefore aggressive diagnosis and treatment are indicated.

Increased sympathetic tone in the immediate postoperative period may be secondary to the stress of surgery; postoperative pain; anxiety or restlessness during emergence from anesthesia; bladder or bowel distention; or hypothermia. Stimulation of the autonomic nervous system can occur because of hypoxia or hypercarbia. These factors can occur alone or in combination.

Pain is one of the most common sources of increased sympathetic tone. Administering adequate amounts of analgesics, repositioning the patient for comfort, providing reassurance, and limiting environmental stimuli can contribute to alleviating postoperative pain and to lowering blood pressure. Hypothermia and shivering also contribute to postoperative hypertension and are easily treated with warm blankets, warming devices, warm intravenous fluids, and heated humidified oxygen. Bladder distention contributes to postoperative hypertension and must be alleviated. Placement of a urinary catheter may be needed. Hypoxia and hypercarbia must also be treated.

Pharmacologic treatment of postoperative hypertension includes the use of vasodilators, adrenergic inhibitors, and calcium channel blockers. The use of these agents is necessary when hypertension persists despite conservative measures previously mentioned.[27,31]

Postoperative hypotension. Maintenance of blood pressure depends on adequate preload, myocardial contractility, and afterload. Intravascular volume depletion because of inadequate replacement of blood loss, third space fluid loss, insensible loss, and urinary output is most often the cause of hypotension. Pulmonary embolism may also reduce preload by blocking flow of blood to the left side of the heart. Reduced myocardial contractility may be a result of the effects of anesthetic drugs, myocardial ischemia, or dysrhythmias. Reduced afterload in the form of low SVR may occur as a result of sepsis, hyperthermia, sympathectomy, or large arteriovenous shunts, as seen in chronic liver failure.

Prolonged hypotension can lead to serious ischemic organ damage. Prompt treatment is essential. If the underlying cause is not immediately apparent, the first treatment is an attempt to increase preload by placing the patient in the Trendelenburg position and infusing fluids. Examination of the ECG monitor for dysrhythmias or evidence of ischemia may help guide therapy. Examination of the lungs for evidence of pulmonary edema or tension pneumothorax must also be performed. Administration of vasopressors may be given to maintain perfusion while evaluation and establishment of additional monitoring modalities are undertaken. Insertion of a central venous catheter allows measurement of right ventricular filling pressure and may be used to guide fluid administration in patients with normal myocardial function. In the presence of left ventricular dysfunction or when the etiology remains unclear, a pulmonary artery catheter may be inserted to guide therapy through evaluation of left-sided filling pressure, cardiac output, and SVR. The use of additional fluids, inotropic agents, or vasoconstrictor or vasodilator drugs is determined by these measurements.[27,31] (∞Cardiac Pharmacology, p. 574.)

Thermoregulatory Problems and/or Emergencies

Patients recovering from anesthesia usually experience some form of thermoregulatory imbalance (i.e., a core body temperature that is outside the normothermic range of 36° to 38° C). Both hypothermia and hyperthermia can occur in the postoperative patient. Management of these alterations is important because they are associated with other physiologic alterations that may interfere with recovery.

Hypothermia. Hypothermia is a common occurrence both intraoperatively and postoperatively because the conditions associated with surgery and anesthesia typically inhibit the body's heat-generating mechanisms and favor its heat-loss mechanisms.[34] It occurs when systemic heat loss lowers core body temperature below 36° C. Causes of hypothermia include wound and skin exposure, respiratory gas exchange, fluid and blood administration, mechanical warming/cooling devices, chemical reactions, alterations in body temperature regulation, and disease states.[27] Clinical manifestations of hypothermia include bluish tint to skin (peripheral cyanosis); shivering and an increase in metabolic rate (early sign); dysrhythmias; and a decrease in metabolic rate (late sign), oxygen consumption, muscle tone, heart rate, and level of consciousness.

Hypothermia has several adverse effects, including discomfort, vasoconstriction, and shivering (Box 12-6). It depresses the myocardium and increases susceptibility to ventricular dysrhythmias. Significant hypothermia slows metabolic processes, leading to reduced drug biotransformation and impaired renal transport. This may prolong drug effects and delay emergence.[13]

Shivering. Shivering may be a result of either the compensatory response to hypothermia or the effects of anesthetic agents, and it can produce a 500% increase in the metabolic rate. Under these conditions, increased oxygen consumption and greater carbon

BOX 12-6 Physiologic Consequences of Hypothermia

Cardiovascular consequences
- Myocardial depression
- Ventricular dysrhythmias
- Increased blood viscosity
- Decreased effective blood volume
- Increased pulmonary and systemic vascular resistance

Neurologic consequences
- Decreased cerebral blood flow
- Impaired mentation
- Hypothalamic dysfunction

Renal consequences
- Decreased renal perfusion
- Increased renin secretion
- Decreased tubular reabsorption, producing "cold diuresis"
- Acute tubular necrosis

Gastrointestinal consequences
- Decreased intestinal motility/ileus
- Susceptibility to ulcerative changes

Metabolic consequences
- Decreased oxygen consumption
- Metabolic acidosis
- Decreased insulin production: hyperglycemia
- Electrolyte imbalances
- Altered hepatic clearing of substrates and drugs

Pulmonary consequences
- Depressed alveolar ventilation
- Alveolar edema
- Increased dead space ventilation

Modified from Vender JS, Speiss BD: *Post anesthesia care,* Philadelphia, 1992, WB Saunders.

dioxide production can increase the ventilatory requirements. If these requirements are not met, the $PaCO_2$ increases and the PaO_2 can decrease, especially if any significant intrapulmonary shunting co-exists. The demand for blood flow by the diaphragm can increase sharply, requiring cardiac output and myocardial workload to increase, resulting in an increase in myocardial oxygen consumption. This can result in myocardial ischemia, particularly in elderly patients or in patients with coronary artery disease.[34]

Peripheral vasoconstriction. Vasoconstriction, a particularly deleterious consequence of postoperative hypothermia, may be responsible for unexplained hypertension in the recovery room. Because vasoconstriction can increase systemic vascular resistance and myocardial workload, the potential for myocardial ischemia exists. In addition, vasoconstriction can mask hypovolemia, and sudden reductions in blood pressure can occur as the patient warms and vasodilates.[35]

Delayed drug clearance. Delayed drug clearance as a consequence of hypothermia is particularly significant in elderly patients who may already have impaired drug clearing mechanisms and a decreased metabolic rate. For example, the maximum rate of renal excretion of a drug can decline by 10% for every 0.6° C drop in body temperature.[33] In addition, elderly hypothermic patients are more likely to have residual paralysis because of muscle relaxants that are difficult to reverse pharmacologically.

Treatment. Management of the hypothermic patient is directed toward the restoration of normothermia. Rewarming prevents the thermoregulatory responses to cold, such as shivering. Management depends on the degree of temperature loss. If the patient's body temperature is between 36° and 37° C, the patient can simply be covered with warmed blankets, and heat lamps can be used to keep the patient adequately warm. If the patient's body temperature is less than 36° C, rapid rewarming is required to decrease the possible complications of hypothermia and the postanesthesia recovery time. Convective warming devices provide a safe and effective means of rewarming the patient. In patients with a normal metabolic rate, a setting of "low" or "medium" increases the mean body temperature at about 1° C per hour. A "high" setting increases the mean body temperature about 1.5° C per hour.[2,3] Other methods of rewarming are thermal mattresses, fluid and blood warming, and environmental warming.[34] Supplemental oxygen must be administered to meet the increased metabolic demand in shivering patients. Patients who are shivering may respond to a small dose of meperidine (Demerol).

Hyperthermia. By definition, hyperthermia occurs at any core body temperature above normal. Severe, clinically significant hyperthermia results when core temperature exceeds 40° C. Though not as common perioperatively as hypothermia, hyperthermia is nevertheless a serious complication of surgery. Postoperative temperature elevations may be caused by accidental overwarming of the patient during surgery, infection, sepsis, and transfusion reactions. As an elevated temperature increases oxygen demand and subsequently ventilatory and cardiac workload, a hyperthermia patient with poor cardiac reserve suffers serious consequences.

Postoperative fever must be distinguished from other hyperthermic syndromes. There is a fundamental difference between fever and specific hyperthermic states. In nonfever hyperthermic states, body temperature rises above normal despite the body's heat-dissipating mechanisms (e.g., vasodilation and sweating). Therefore excessive heat gain, secondary to either internal or external factors, exceeds the body's cooling capabilities with consequent rise in body temperature.[4,5]

In contrast, fever results from a resetting to a higher temperature from the normal set point. Until the body reaches its new set point temperature, heat-generating mechanisms (i.e., vasoconstriction and shivering) are activated. Once the new set point temperature is reached, there is an equilibrium between heat generation and heat loss. Unlike hyperthermia, with fever there is no physiologic activity to bring body temperature back to normal.

Factors that can contribute to raising core body temperature and fever during the perioperative period are listed in Box 12-7.[4,5,34]

Treatment. Primary therapy for hyperthermia includes cooling and decreasing thermogenesis. Cooling by either evaporative or direct external methods have proved effective. This includes ice packs, a cool environment, and cooling blankets. Gastric and bladder lavage have also proven effective.

Although physical cooling is an appropriate therapy for other hyperthermias, attempts to cool a febrile patient may be resisted by the thermoregulatory system. Consequently, the first cause of action is to restore normothermia with the use of antipyretic drugs. Antipyretics are useful because they have the ability to prevent prostaglandin synthesis in the hypothalamus. Measures to manage the febrile patient include using antipyretics (as indicated), providing a sponge bath with tepid water, keeping the environment cool, using a cooling blanket for sustained fever, and monitoring fluid and electrolyte balance as fluid needs increase during fever.[36] The possibility of malignant hyperthermia (MH) must always be considered.[17]

Malignant hyperthermia. Malignant hyperthermia is a genetically determined condition. MH is precipitated by certain general inhalation anesthetics, depolarizing skeletal muscle relaxants, local anesthetics, and stress. The incidence of MH ranges from 1 in 15,000 in children to 1 in 50,000 in adults. The onset of MH usually occurs during induction of anesthesia. However, there have been reports of it occurring up to 72 hours after the triggering agent is introduced. Because successful management of MH depends on early assessment and prompt intervention, the nurse must be knowledgeable in the pathophysiology and treatment of this syndrome.[33]

BOX 12-7 Factors Influencing Temperature and Fever

CAUSES OF ELEVATED CORE TEMPERATURE

Blood transfusion
Drug-induced fever
Overuse of techniques to prevent hypothermia
Hypothalamic injury
Malignant hyperthermia
Warm environment
Use of anticholinergics
Endocrine disorders
Neurogenic hyperthermia

CAUSES OF POSTOPERATIVE FEVER

Atelectasis
Wound infection
Abscess formation
Fat emboli after bone trauma
Drug reactions
Malignancy
Silent aspiration
Dehydration
Blood transfusion reaction
CNS damage
Urinary tract infections
Phlebitis/deep vein thrombosis
Pulmonary emboli

Identification of patients, before anesthesia, who may be susceptible to MH is of major therapeutic importance. On history and physical examination, MH-susceptible patients usually demonstrate some subclinical weakness or abnormality, such as deficient fine motor control. Many complain of muscle cramps that occur spontaneously, during an infectious illness, or during or after exercise. There may be a positive patient history or a positive genealogy going back two generations. Physical examination may reveal myopathies such as cryptorchidism, pectus carinatum, kyphosis, lordosis, ptosis, or hypoplastic mandible. Electromyographic changes are seen in fewer than half of MH-susceptible patients. Measurement of blood creatine phosphokinase (CPK) is usually about 70% reliable in determining susceptibility to MH.[3,4]

The most definitive test for detecting MH susceptibility is a biopsy of skeletal muscle. Samples are obtained from the quadriceps muscle and are subjected to isometric contracture testing. The skeletal muscle of the MH-susceptible patient has an increased isometric tension when exposed to caffeine or halothane.[37]

Pathophysiology. When a susceptible patient is exposed to a triggering agent, such as halothane, that causes MH to occur, the clinical features are produced by an excess of calcium ions in the myoplasm. With an elevated calcium ion concentration in the myoplasm, skeletal muscle contraction is intense and prolonged, leading to a hypermetabolic state of acid and heat production. More specifically, heat is produced by the accelerated and continued synthesis and use of adenosine triphosphate (ATP) during glycolysis. The metabolic by-product of glycolysis, lactic acid, is transported to the liver, where part of it is oxidized to provide the ATP necessary to help make glucose. This glucose, along with the glycogen, is released from the liver and transported back to the metabolically active muscle, where the cycle repeats. Respiratory and metabolic acidosis develop because of this hypermetabolic state, and symptoms such as tachycardia, tachypnea, ventricular dysrhythmias, and unstable blood pressure appear. Because of intense vasoconstriction, the skin is mottled and cyanotic. Box 12-8 lists the clinical manifestations of MH.

Elevated body temperature can actually be a late sign of MH. For this reason, the nurse must not prolong the assessment of the patient on the assumption that the patient's temperature must be significantly elevated before intervention is attempted. Once the patient's temperature begins to rise, it may increase at a rate of 0.5° C every 15 minutes and may approach levels as high as 46° C.[4]

Muscle rigidity occurs in about 75% of the patients who experience MH. This is especially true in MH-susceptible patients after the administration of succinylcholine. In fact, muscle rigidity may be so severe that the nurse cannot open the patient's mouth to insert an airway. The onset of skeletal muscle rigidity after the administration of succinylcholine could be a sign of impending development of MH.[4,36]

Triggers. Various environmental stimuli and pharmacologic agents can stimulate an acute episode of MH (Box 12-9). Fatigue, emotional upset, or very hot and humid weather can trigger a waking febrile episode. The anesthetic agents that may trigger MH seem to affect the sarcoplasmic reticulum. Because of their widespread use, halothane and succinylcholine are the most common triggering agents. Local anesthetics, such as lidocaine, are also triggering agents. It has been demonstrated that lidocaine causes the release of calcium ions into the mycoplasma in vitro. In MH-susceptible patients or in patients who have had an episode of MH in the operating room, all possible triggering agents must be stringently avoided. As another precaution, because emotional upsets trigger MH, nurses must provide a stress-free environment for their MH-susceptible patient.[33,36]

BOX 12-8 Signs and Symptoms of Malignant Hyperthermia

Hypoxemia
Metabolic acidosis
Respiratory acidosis
Hyperkalemia
Myoglobinuria
Elevated creatine phosphokinase
Tachycardia
Tachypnea
Ventricular dysrhythmias
Cyanosis
Skin mottling
Fever—hot, flushed skin
Rigidity
Profuse sweating
Unstable blood pressure

Modified from Drain CB, editor: *The post anesthesia care unit: a critical care approach to post anesthesia nursing,* ed 3, Philadelphia, 1994, WB Saunders.

BOX 12-9 Environmental and Pharmacologic Triggers of Malignant Hyperthermia

Environmental Stimuli
- Extensive skeletal muscle injury
- Emotional crisis
- Very hot and humid weather
- Strenuous and prolonged exercise

Pharmacologic Agents
- Halothane
- Enflurane
- Isoflurane (?)
- Succinylcholine
- *d*-Tubocurarine
- Gallamine (?)
- Amide local anesthetics—lidocaine, mepivacaine, bupivacaine, etidocaine
- Caffeine

From Drain CB, editor: *The post anesthesia care unit: a critical care approach to post anesthesia nursing,* ed 3, Philadelphia, 1994, WB Saunders.

Treatment. The cornerstone of the successful management of MH is early detection. If the patient develops acute MH, all inhalation anesthetics are stopped, the patient is hyperventilated with 100% oxygen, sodium bicarbonate (1 to 2 mg/kg) is administered, and dantrolene is given. It is important to know how to administer dantrolene. It must be diluted with sterile water, the starting dose is 2 mg/kg (there is only 20 mg per vial, so the average adult would need at least 7 to 10 vials to start), and repeat doses are likely, up to a dose of 10 mg/kg. Cooling measures, such as administering cold IV fluids, packing the patient in ice, and irrigating body cavities (e.g., stomach and bladder) with cold fluids, are initiated. Accurate intake and output records are essential because large amounts of fluids and diuretics are given. Laboratory tests, such as a complete blood count (CBC) and coagulation studies, are closely scrutinized for signs of bleeding or the onset of disseminated intravascular coagulation. Ongoing ECG and temperature monitoring are also essential. It is recommended that all emergency drugs be available on a special cart, either in the operating room or in the postanesthesia care unit.

Neurologic Problems and/or Emergencies

Almost all patients exhibit some level of arousal within 90 minutes of completion of the anesthetic. Although many factors are known to prolong anesthetic effects, most reports of delayed arousal and emergence delirium are anecdotal.

Delayed arousal. Delayed awakening after general anesthesia is a common and often easily explained problem. The etiology can usually be attributed to prolonged action of anesthetic drugs, metabolic causes, or neurologic injury. In most cases the prolonged sedation is the result of residual general anesthetic. Hypoventilation resulting from high concentrations of inhaled anesthetic limits the exhalation of the agent and prolongs its elimination. Opioids used as adjuncts may contribute to hypercarbia and sedation as well. Hypothermia, advanced age, hepatic dysfunction, and renal disease may contribute to prolonged recovery from anesthetics by heightening sensitivity, delaying elimination, or both. The use of premedication may also prolong recovery, especially if narcotics or benzodiazepines, particularly diazepam, are used.[38]

In addition to experiencing a slowing elimination of potent inhalation anesthetics, the hypoventilating patient may develop hypoxia and hypercapnia. The ensuing hypercapnia may cause significant narcosis, as well as potentiate the depressive effects of the anesthetics. In the diabetic patient, the administration of chlorpropamide or excessive insulin preoperatively may cause postoperative hypoglycemia, unconsciousness, or even coma.[39]

Severe electrolyte disturbances are most commonly seen after excessive water absorption during transurethral prostate surgery. The subsequent dilutional hyponatremia may manifest as sedation, coma, or hemiparesis. Dilutional hyponatremia may also be seen after the inappropriate release of antidiuretic hormone. Hypocalcemia after parathyroid surgery may result in delayed awakening. High magnesium levels after the prolonged administration of magnesium sulfate to the eclamptic or preeclamptic patient may also result in prolonged postoperative sedation, as well as muscle weakness after general anesthetic cesarean section.[17]

Neurologic injury and subsequent unconsciousness may be the result of an unsuspected cerebral vascular accident. Intracranial hemorrhage may result from hypertensive responses to anesthetic or surgical manipulations, especially in the patient receiving anticoagulant therapy. Paradoxical air emboli may cross a patent foramen ovale in the presence of a right-to-left shunt. Direct emboli from cardiac valves, intracardiac thrombi, and atherosclerotic vessels may also be a threat. Fat emboli may occur after massive long-bone or tissue damage and may not appear until during or after surgical manipulation or reduction of the fractures. Deliberate, induced hypotension in normal patients is not usually associated with neurologic damage. However, uncontrolled intraoperative hypotension may result in ischemia, especially in the patient with hypertension or carotid occlusive disease.[38] (∞Cerebrovascular Accident, p. 798.)

Treatment. The successful management of delayed arousal depends on careful consideration of the differential diagnosis. A thorough review of the patient's preoperative medical condition and the intraoperative course, both surgical and anesthetic, usually points to an etiology. If the cause of the sedation is not immediately obvious, the first consideration must be assessing the patient's oxygenation and ensuring adequate gas exchange. Pulse oximetry, end-tidal carbon dioxide measurement, and arterial blood gases can give an estimate of any ventilatory depression and rule out ongoing hypoxia and hypercarbia factors.[38,40]

If the cause is thought to be residual inhalation anesthetics, maintaining adequate ventilation should be sufficient treatment. If available, mass spectrophotometry can provide an estimate of exhaled anesthetic concentrations and confirm the diagnosis. Residual opioids can be reversed by naloxone, and anticholinergic CNS depression can be reversed by physostigmine. Physostigmine has been reported to reverse sedation from other hypnotics and general anesthetics as well. The benzodiazepine antagonist flumazenil has been shown to directly antagonize the CNS sedative and amnesic effects of the benzodiazepines.[4]

Body temperature is determined and warming instituted if hypothermia exists. Serum electrolytes and magnesium and calcium levels are checked if ion disturbance is suspected. Blood for a serum glucose assay may also be drawn, but the simple finger stick glucose determination is faster and accurate enough to exclude hypoglycemia from consideration if normal. Other laboratory tests may be useful as well if hepatic or renal disease is under consideration. Unless perioperative events point specifically to it, neurologic injury is usually a diagnosis of exclusion. If other causes of prolonged arousal have been excluded, a thorough neurologic consultation is obtained.[38]

Emergence delirium. Most patients emerge from general anesthesia in a calm, tranquil manner. Some patients, however, emerge in a state of "excitement," a condition characterized by restlessness, disorientation, crying, moaning, or irrational talking. In the extreme form of excitement, which is referred to as emergence delirium, the patient screams, shouts, and thrashes about wildly. It seems to be seen most frequently after tonsillectomy, thyroid surgery, circumcision, hysterectomy, and perineal and abdominal wall procedures.[40]

Hypoxia and resulting air hunger, as well as hypercarbia, may appear as restlessness, disorientation, slurred speech, and agitation. Hyponatremia, hypochloremia, and acid-base changes could all be seen during the immediate postoperative period and can be the cause of mental confusion. Pain is a common cause of restlessness and is commonly seen postoperatively.

Urinary bladder and gastric distention, which may cause considerable discomfort, are easily overlooked.[39,40]

Drug reactions are commonly implicated as the cause of postoperative agitation. Such reactions are less common than they once were, because the use of offending drugs is less prevalent. The most frequently implicated drugs are the anticholinergics, most notably scopolamine and atropine. They have been shown to have CNS toxic effects that can include psychotic behavior, delirium, and motor disturbances. Ketamine is also associated with a high incidence of unpleasant agitation. Neuroleptic drugs such as droperidol, especially in high doses, may be associated with the development of dyskinesia and involuntary muscle activity as well as postoperative confusion.[38]

The patient's state of apprehension or anxiety can have a marked effect on the appearance of emergence agitation, especially apprehensive patients and, conversely, those seemingly unconcerned about forthcoming major surgery. Factors such as fear of disfigurement or cancer and feelings of suffocation also increase the likelihood of emergence excitement. Young patients tend to have an increased incidence of postoperative excitation as do patients undergoing emergency procedures. Several psychiatric factors have been shown to increase the incidence of postoperative delirium, including a history of alcoholism, insomnia, depression, or debility.[40]

Treatment. If emergence delirium occurs, the patient's status is thoroughly evaluated. Management includes determining an etiology, initiating specific therapy, and protecting the patients from injuring themselves. When encountering a restless, confused postoperative patient, the first measure is to ensure that the agitation is not the result of hypoxia. Presuming pain to be the cause of agitation in a hypoxic patient and treating the excitement with opioids or sedatives may have disastrous consequences. Hypoxia must be quickly excluded from the differential diagnosis by pulse oximetry, arterial blood gas determination, or both.[2-4,39]

Hyponatremia may be suspected in the confused postprostate surgery patient, especially if the surgery was prolonged. A serum electrolyte determination can confirm the diagnosis. The treatment usually consists of fluid restriction, and rarely, hypertonic saline administration. Severe acid-base disturbances can be diagnosed and therapy directed by arterial blood gas determination. If pain appears to be the diagnosis after exclusion of hypoxia, intravenous opioids may be administered in small increments.

The CNS effects of the anticholinergics are usually dramatically reversed by the administration of physostigmine. The incidence of hallucinations with ketamine may be decreased by benzodiazepine or droperidol administration.[12] Gastric distention may be relieved by nasogastric aspiration, and urinary bladder distention is easily treated with catheterization.[2,3]

When dealing with perioperative anxiety, the best treatment is prevention. Some patients need reassurance that they will not experience intraoperative awareness and will receive pain medications, if needed, upon awakening.[41]

Occasionally, one is faced with a restless postoperative patient who does not seem to be getting relief from opioid administration. Small intravenous doses of a short-acting benzodiazepine such as midazolam may be warranted. The anxiolytics are administered in reduced doses, because their respiratory depressant effects may be cumulative with existing opioids, sedatives, and residual general anesthetics. If overt psychotic behavior is apparent, despite adequate treatment, psychiatric consultation needs to be obtained.[40]

The patient's respiratory function and airway patency is checked first, because restlessness is a well-known manifestation of hypoxia. Other causes of emergence delirium include a full bladder, cramped or sore muscles and joints from prolonged abnormal positioning on the operating table, pain, incomplete reversal of neuromuscular blocking agents, withdrawal from alcohol and other drugs, acid-base disturbances, and electrolyte abnormalities. The restless patient requires constant, careful observation. Gentle physical restraint may be required to prevent injury. Several nurses or other personnel may be needed. If hypoxia, pain, or a full bladder are ruled out, a change in positioning may have a quieting effect.[2,5]

Nausea and vomiting. Nausea and vomiting, though usually not life-threatening, are probably the most unpleasant and lasting memories many patients have of their anesthetic. Although the incidence has decreased in recent years, nausea and vomiting still result in significant postoperative morbidity and patient discomfort. *Nausea* is described as a subjective, unpleasant mental experience, usually leading to vomiting. Retching is the rhythmic muscular activity that usually precedes vomiting. *Vomiting* is defined as the forceful expulsion of gastrointestinal contents through the mouth.[42]

Decidedly unpleasant, vomiting can also be dangerous. The physical exertion may increase postoperative bleeding and disrupt delicate suture lines. Tearing or rupture of the esophagus is probably rare but must be a concern in patients with a history of esophageal pathology. Aspiration of emesis is a life-threatening complication in the patient whose airway protective reflexes are blunted by residual anesthetic or sedative drugs or damaged by surgical activity. If the vomiting is protracted, dangerous hypokalemia, hypochloremia, hyponatremia, and dehydration may develop. Nausea and vomiting are also the leading causes of unexpected hospitalization after surgery.[42,43]

The use of nitrous oxide is said to cause nausea and vomiting by gastric distention, sympathetic stimulation, and changes in middle ear pressure. Adjunct drugs given preoperatively or in conjunction with the inhalation anesthetics may themselves be suspected of contributing to the high rate of emetic sequelae. The opioids, when given as premedications, may contribute to nausea and vomiting. Meperidine has also been known to cause nausea and vomiting. Some of the newer general anesthetics have resulted in less nausea and vomiting than their predecessors. Halothane, in subanesthetic doses, may even be antiemetic. When administered alone or in conjunction with the opioids, the anticholinergics can act as potent antiemetics.[44]

Muscle relaxants are thought not to influence postoperative vomiting. The reversal of the muscle relaxants may contribute to postoperative vomiting, however. Neostigmine has potent muscarinic effects and may increase intestinal peristalsis and may even trigger spasm.[45]

Spinal anesthesia has long been known to trigger a significant incidence of nausea and vomiting. During spinal anesthesia, a systolic blood pressure less than 80 mm Hg results in significant incidence in emesis. The administration of 100% oxygen to these patients has significantly decreased the development of emesis.

Gastric distention and irritation causes nausea and vomiting by direct stimulation of the vomiting center. The stomach may become distended during anesthesia by manual insufflation via mask induction. The swallowing of air or blood may also result in significant stomach irritation. Acute appendicitis or bowel obstruction is notoriously associated with preoperative and postoperative emesis.

The site of the surgery may also influence the development of postoperative nausea and vomiting. Gastrointestinal procedures have a high frequency of postoperative emesis. Laproscopic, ophthalmic, and otologic procedures also have a high incidence. The duration of the procedure may also affect the frequency. Finally, pain triggers nausea and vomiting in many patients.[44]

Patients with a history of motion sickness are most likely to experience postoperative emetic sequelae with each subsequent anesthetic. A certain number of patients experience nausea after fasting, even before the administration of any drugs. Many patients develop nausea upon their first movement and thus may have emesis during transport.[5,43] The female gender is also said to be associated with high incidence of postoperative emesis. The incidence of nausea and vomiting tends to decrease with advancing age.[44]

Other circumstances may act to increase the likelihood of postoperative emesis in any given patient. Patients with a full stomach from either a recent meal or swallowed blood are more likely to vomit on induction of or on emergence from anesthesia. Alcohol intoxication or illicit drug use may also increase the frequency of emesis. Vigorous nasal or oropharyngeal suctioning can also elicit a strong gag reflex and trigger vomiting. In neurosurgical patients, especially those with closed head injury, increased intracranial pressure may trigger nausea and vomiting.[46]

Treatment. The most effective treatment of postoperative nausea and vomiting is prevention. Several maneuvers merit mention as being fairly simple to perform and effective in their usefulness. Avoidance of gastric insufflation is paramount. In addition, prevent the swallowing of blood during oral, pharyngeal, or nasal surgery. If distention is suspected, it is decompressed intraoperatively.[2,3,33] A nasogastric tube is placed to empty fluid and gases from the stomach. Unfortunately, its presence may trigger gagging and subsequent vomiting. An oral airway may elicit the same response in a partially conscious patient and is removed at the first signs of gagging to prevent vomiting and subsequent aspiration.[46]

Many drugs have been shown to possess antiemetic qualities. Some are most effective when given prophylactically. Many of the drugs, though, are associated with negative or undesirable side effects, and as a result prophylactic administration may be considered unjustified except under specific circumstances. Available antiemetics include anticholinergics, phenothiazines, antihistamines, butyrophenones, and antidopaminergics.[47]

It is important to remember the supportive care of the nauseated and vomiting patient. If vomiting is severe, electrolyte replacement must be considered. Prolonged vomiting may result in hypovolemia. Intravenous fluids may need to be increased to compensate for fluid losses. Opioids must never be withheld from the nauseated patient complaining of pain because pain itself may be the cause of the vomiting.[24,46]

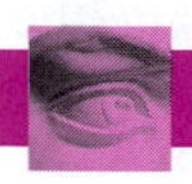

NURSING MANAGEMENT PLAN

HYPOTHERMIA

DEFINITION:

The state in which an individual's body temperature is reduced below normal range.

Hypothermia Related to Exposure to Cold Environment, Trauma, or Damage to the Hypothalamus

DEFINING CHARACTERISTICS

- Core body temperature below 35° C (95° F)
- Skin cold to touch
- Slurred speech, incoordination
- At temperature below 33° C (91.4° F):
  - Cardiac dysrhythmias (atrial fibrillation, bradycardia)
  - Cyanosis
  - Respiratory alkalosis
- At temperatures below 32° C (89.5° F):
  - Shivering replaced by muscle rigidity
  - Hypotension
  - Dilated pupils
- At temperatures below 28°-29° C (82.4-84.2° F):
  - Absent deep tendon reflexes
  - Hypoventilation (3 to 4 breaths/min to apnea)
  - Ventricular fibrillation possible
- At temperatures below 26°-27° C (78.8-80.6° F):
  - Coma
  - Flaccid muscles
  - Fixed, dilated pupils
  - Ventricular fibrillation to cardiac standstill
  - Apnea

OUTCOME CRITERIA

- Core body temperature is greater than 35° C (95° F).
- Patients are alert and oriented.
- Cardiac dysrhythmias are absent.
- Acid-base balance is normal.
- Pupils are normoreactive.

NURSING INTERVENTIONS AND *RATIONALE*

1. Continuously monitor core body temperature with a low-reading thermometer.
2. Intubation and mechanical ventilation may be needed. Heated air or oxygen can be added ***to help rewarm the body core.*** Because carbon dioxide production is low, do not hyperventilate the hypothermic patient because ***this action may induce severe alkalosis and precipitate ventricular fibrillation.***
3. Apply cardiopulmonary resuscitation (CPR) and advanced cardiac life support until core body temperature is up to at least 29.5° C before determining that patients cannot be resuscitated.
   a. Electrical defibrillation is usually successful in terminating ventricular fibrillation if the temperature is greater than 28° C.
   b. Administer cardiac resuscitation drugs sparingly ***because as the body warms, peripheral vasodilation occurs. Drugs that remain in the periphery are suddenly released, leading to a "bolus effect" that may cause fatal dysrhythmias.***

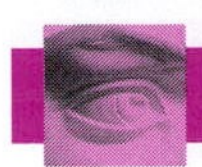

NURSING MANAGEMENT PLAN—CONT'D

HYPOTHERMIA

Hypothermia Related to Exposure to Cold Environment, Trauma, or Damage to the Hypothalamus

4. Monitor arterial blood gas (ABG) values to direct further therapy, and be sure that the pH, PaO_2, and $PaCO_2$ are corrected for temperature.
5. For abrupt-onset hypothermia (e.g., immersion in cold water; exposure to cold, wet climate; collapse in snow) rewarming can take place rapidly ***because the pathophysiologic changes associated with chronic hypothermia have not had time to evolve.***
   - Institute rapid, active rewarming by immersion in warm water (38°-43° C).
   - Apply thermal blanket at 36.6°-37.7° C. Some researchers suggest rewarming only the torso or trunk first, leaving the extremities exposed to room temperature. ***This is to prevent early peripheral vasodilation with abrupt redistribution of intravascular volume. This also prevents colder blood trapped in the extremities from returning to the body core before the heart is rewarmed.***
   - Perform rapid core rewarming with heated (37°-43° C) intravenous (IV) infusion, hemodialysis, peritoneal dialysis, and colonic or gastric irrigation fluids.
6. Monitor peripheral circulation because ***gangrene of the fingers and toes is a common complication of accidental hypothermia.***
7. For chronic hypothermia, the aggressiveness of treatment depends on the setting, underlying disease, and body temperature. Concurrent treatment of the underlying disease processes is indicated.
   - Core temperatures greater than 33° C may be rewarmed either slowly or rapidly.
   - Coma in patients with a temperature greater than 28° C is probably not caused by hypothermia. Look for other causes such as hypoglycemia, alcohol, narcotics, and head trauma, and treat accordingly.
   - If patients are hyperglycemic, remember that insulin is ineffective at body temperatures below 30° C.
   - Restore intravascular volume cautiously ***to avoid circulatory overloading of the hypothermic heart and to avoid precipitating pulmonary edema.*** As circulation and a more normal temperature are restored, patients may require large volumes of crystalloid and colloid fluids ***to refill the dilated vascular bed.***

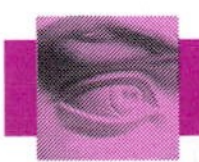

NURSING MANAGEMENT PLAN

HYPERTHERMIA

DEFINITION:

A state in which an individual's body temperature is elevated above his or her normal range.

Hyperthermia Related to Pharmacogenic Hypermetabolism (Malignant Hyperthermia)

DEFINING CHARACTERISTICS

Early signs

- BP >140/90 mm Hg
- Profuse diaphoresis
- Pulse rate >100 beats/min
- Masseter and general skeletal muscle rigidity and fasciculations
- Tachypnea
- Decreased level of consciousness

Late signs

- Increasing core body temperature up to 42°-43° C (107.6-109.4° F)
- Hot skin
- High-output left ventricular failure
  - Systemic BP <90 mm Hg
  - Pulse rate >100 beats/min and ventricular dysrhythmias
  - Cardiac index >4.0 L/min/m^2
  - Pulmonary artery wedge pressure (PAWP) and pulmonary artery diastolic (PAD) pressure >15 mm Hg; possible pulmonary edema
- Continued skeletal muscle rigidity and fasciculations
- PaO_2 <80 mm Hg
- Respiratory and metabolic acidosis

Continued

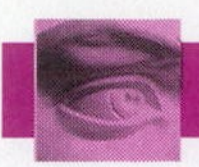

NURSING MANAGEMENT PLAN—CONT'D

Hyperthermia Related to Pharmacogenic Hypermetabolism (Malignant Hyperthermia)

Late signs—cont'd
- Fixed, dilated pupils
- Seizures/coma/decerebrate posturing
- Urinary output <30 ml/hr; reddish-brown (myoglobinuria)
- Prolonged bleeding (disseminated introvascular coagulation [DIC])

OUTCOME CRITERIA

- Core body temperature is below 38.3° C (101° F).
- Muscle rigidity and fasciculations are absent.
- Patient is alert and oriented.
- Pupils are normoreactive.

NURSING INTERVENTIONS AND *RATIONALE*

1. Continue to monitor assessment parameters listed under "Defining Characteristics."
2. Rapidly decrease metabolism.
   - It is recommended that health care institutions have an emergency malignant hyperthermia kit available that contains the items indicated in this box.
   - Administer dantrolene (Dantrium), ***which relaxes skeletal muscles by reducing the release of calcium from the sarcoplasmic reticulum.***
   - Observe for infiltration into surrounding tissues. ***Dantrolene is very alkaline and irritating to tissues.***
3. Initiate cooling measures.
   - Administer cold IV solutions (IV bag has been soaked in ice bath before administration).
   - Provide cool water sponge bath.
   - Apply cooling blanket until temperature within 1° to 3° F of desired level ***to avoid "overshoot" in which excessive cooling lowers the body temperature below the desired range.***
   - Institute iced saline solution lavages of stomach, rectum, and bladder.
   - Monitor core temperature continuously ***to avoid overcooling.***
4. Reverse metabolic and respiratory acidosis.
   - With physician's collaboration, administer sodium bicarbonate as necessary ***to treat metabolic acidosis.***
   - Initially hyperventilate patient with 100% oxygen; then ventilate with 15-20 ml/kg tidal volume at 15-20 breaths/min.
   - Assess arterial blood gas (ABG) values frequently, and make ventilatory adjustments as necessary ***to remedy hypoxemia and hypercarbia.***
5. Provide adequate nutrients to the tissues, and correct electrolyte imbalances.
   - With physician's collaboration, administer 50% dextrose and regular insulin ***to increase glucose uptake into liver to meet hypermetabolic needs of body and enhance the movement of potassium from extracellular fluid back into the cells.***
   - Monitor serum electrolytes ***to assess efficacy of previously mentioned action.***
   - Monitor blood urea nitrogen (BUN) and creatinine levels ***to evaluate for renal failure.***
   - Monitor serum enzyme levels, particularly creatine phosphokinase (CPK) elevations, ***for indication of degree of muscle hyperactivity.***
6. Correct cardiovascular instability and dysrhythmias.
   - Titrate vasoactive and inotropic drips per protocol to desired systemic BP, PAWP, and/or PAD.
   - Follow critical care emergency standing orders about the administration of antidysrhythmic agents.
7. Maintain a high urinary output (≥ 50 ml/hr). With physician's collaboration, perform the following:
   - Administer osmotic agents (mannitol) ***for excretion of excess fluid load and to increase urinary output to prevent renal failure.***
   - Administer diuretics (furosemide) ***to enhance secretion of myoglobin, potassium, sodium, and magnesium.***
   - Administer supplemental potassium chloride as indicated by serum potassium levels.
   - Possibly administer steroid (e.g., Solu-Cortef) ***for its mineralocorticoid effect of potassium excretion, to increase glomerular filtration rate, and to reduce cerebral edema.***
8. Correct hematologic abnormalities.
   - With physician's collaboration, administer heparin if DIC suspected.
   - Monitor coagulation studies ***for indications of DIC and for efficacy of heparin therapy.***
   - Assess stool/urinary/nasogastric (NG) drainage for occult blood.
9. Weigh patient daily ***to assist in assessment of hydration status.***

REFERENCES

1. DeFazia-Quinn D: *Post anesthesia nursing as a specialty.* In Drain CB, editor: *The post anesthesia care unit: a critical care approach to post anesthesia nursing,* ed 3, Philadelphia, 1994, WB Saunders.
2. Barash PG, Cullen BF, Stoetling RK, editors: *Clinical anesthesia,* ed 3, Philadelphia, 1996, JB Lippincott.
3. Miller R, editor: *Anesthesia,* ed 4, New York, 1995, Churchill Livingstone.
4. Drain CB, editor: *The post anesthesia care unit: a critical care approach to post anesthesia nursing,* ed 3, Philadelphia, 1994, WB Saunders.
5. Stoelting RK, Miller RD: *Basics of anesthesia,* ed 3, New York, 1994, Churchill Livingstone.
6. Longnecker D, Murphy F: *Dripps/Eckenhoff/Vandam introduction to anesthesia,* ed 8, Philadelphia, 1992, WB Saunders.
7. American Nurses Association: *Nurses drug facts: facts and comparisons,* St Louis, 1996, The Association.
8. Hodgson BB, Kizior RJ, Kingdon RT: *Nurse's drug handbook 1997,* ed 4, Philadelphia, 1997, WB Saunders.
9. Katz RL: Muscle relaxants: clinical considerations, *Semin Anesth* 14(1):1-70, 1995.
10. Katz RL: Muscle relaxants: new drugs and special situations, *Semin Anesth* 14(4):245, 1995.
11. Bevan DR, Donati F: Muscle relaxants. In Barash PG, Cullen BF, Stoetling RK, editors: *Clinical anesthesia,* ed 3, Philadelphia, 1996, JB Lippincott.
12. McGaffigan PA, Christoph SB: Assessment and monitoring of the post anesthesia patient. In Drain CB, editor: *The post anesthesia care unit: a critical care approach to post anesthesia nursing,* ed 3, Philadelphia, 1994, WB Saunders.
13. Stock CM: Respiratory function in anesthesia. In Barash PG, Cullen BF, Stoetling RK, editors: *Clinical anesthesia,* ed 3, Philadelphia, 1996, JB Lippincott.
14. Blank T, Lee DL: Cardiac physiology. In Miller R, editor: *Anesthesia,* ed 4, New York, 1995, Churchill Livingstone.
15. Drummond JC, Shapiro HM: Cerebral physiology. In Miller R, editor: *Anesthesia,* ed 4, New York, 1995, Churchill Livingstone.
16. Ferae D, Augustine SD: Hypothermia in PACU, *Crit Care Nurs Clin North Am* 3:135, 1991.
17. Tonnesen AS: Crystalloids and colloids. In Miller R, editor: *Anesthesia,* ed 4, New York, 1995, Churchill Livingstone.
18. Cook KG: Assessment and management of anxiety in recovery room patients, *Curr Rev Recov Room Nurses* 7(5):51-55, 1993.
19. O'Brien D: Care of the post anesthesia patient. In Drain CB, editor: *The post anesthesia care unit: a critical care approach to post anesthesia nursing,* ed 3, Philadelphia, 1994, WB Saunders.
20. Luce JM, Pierson DJ, Tyler ML: *Intensive respiratory care,* ed 2, Philadelphia, 1993, WB Saunders.
21. Thompson JM and others: *Mosby's clinical nursing,* ed 4, St Louis, 1997, Mosby.
22. Nortar ML: Difficult airway. In Healy T, Cohen P, editors: *A practice of anesthesia,* ed 6, New York, 1995, Edward Arnold.
23. Wansbrough SR, White PF: Sedation scales: measures of calmness or somnalence? *Anesth Analg,* 76:219, 1993.
24. Grove TM: Management of problems in the post anesthesia care unit. I. General considerations, pain, neurological problems, nausea and vomiting, *Curr Rev Post Anesth Care Nurses* 18:1, 1996.
25. Faut-Callahan M, Slach JF: Pain management. In Waugaman WR and others, editors: *Principles and practice of nurse anesthesia,* ed 2, Norwalk, Conn, 1992, Appleton & Lange.
26. Litwack K: *Post anesthesia care nursing,* ed 2, St Louis, 1995, Mosby.
27. Grove TM: Management of problems in the post anesthesia care unit. II. Respiratory, cardiovascular and thermal regulation problems, *Curr Rev Post Anesth Care Nurses* 18:9, 1996.
28. Odom JL: Airway emergencies in the post anesthesia care unit, *Nurs Clin North Am* 28:483, 1993.
29. Litwack K: *Post operative pulmonary complications,* Sacramento, 1995, CME Resource.
30. Ward D: Avoiding ventilatory emergencies, *Semin Anesth,* 15(2):183, 1996.
31. Bines AS, Landron SL: Cardiovascular emergencies in the post anesthesia care unit, *Nurs Clin North Am* 28:493, 1993.
32. Bratanow N, Atlee JL: Perioperative arrhythmias, *Semin Anesth,* 15(2):122, 1996.
33. Gravenstein N, Kirby R, editors: *Complications in anesthesiology,* Philadelphia, 1996, Lippincott-Raven.
34. Flacke WE, Flacke JW: Temperature: homeostasis and unintentional hypothermia. In Gravenstein N, Kirby R, editors: *Complications in anesthesiology,* Philadelphia, 1996, Lippincott-Raven.
35. Davies JM: Critical incidents during anesthesia. In Healy T, Cohen P, editors: *A practice of anesthesia,* ed 6, New York, 1995, Edward Arnold.
36. Gordon JJ, Westenfelder GD: Infectious diseases. In Vender JS, Speiss BD, editors: *Post anesthesia care,* Philadelphia, 1992, WB Saunders.
37. Black JW, Muldaon SM: Clinical perspectives on malignant hyperthermia, *Probl Anesth* 8:137, 1994.
38. Denlinger K: Prolonged emergence and failure to regain consciousness. In Gravenstein N, Kirby R, editors: *Complications in anesthesiology,* Philadelphia, 1996, Lippincott-Raven.
39. Benumof JL: *Airway management: principles & practice,* St Louis, 1996, Mosby.
40. Rosenberg H, Gildberg M: Postoperative emotional response. In Gravenstein N, Kirby R, editors: *Complications in anesthesiology,* Philadelphia, 1996, Lippincott-Raven.
41. Klock A, Roxzen MF: Anesthesiologist's role as perioperative physician, *Anesth Analg,* 83(4):67, 1996.

42. Mazze R, Wharton RS: Fluid and electrolyte problems. In Gravenstein N, Kirby R, editors: *Complications in anesthesiology,* Philadelphia, 1996, Lippincott-Raven.
43. Belatte RG: Common post anesthetic problems. In Vender JS, Speiss BD, editors: *Post anesthesia care,* Philadelphia, 1992, WB Saunders.
44. Watcha MF, White PF: Postoperative nausea and vomiting: its etiology, treatment, and prevention, *Anesthesiology* 77:162, 1992.
45. Kroft T, Upton P, Martz D: *Key topics in anesthesia,* St Louis, 1995, Mosby.
46. Orkin FK: Postoperative nausea and vomiting. In Gravenstein N, Kirby R, editors: *Complications in anesthesiology,* Philadelphia, 1996, Lippincott-Raven.
47. Feeley TW: The post anesthesia care unit. In Miller R, editor: *Anesthesia,* ed 4, New York, 1995, Churchill Livingstone.

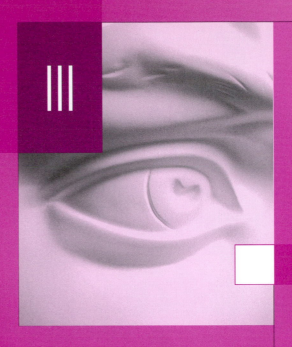

CARDIOVASCULAR ALTERATIONS

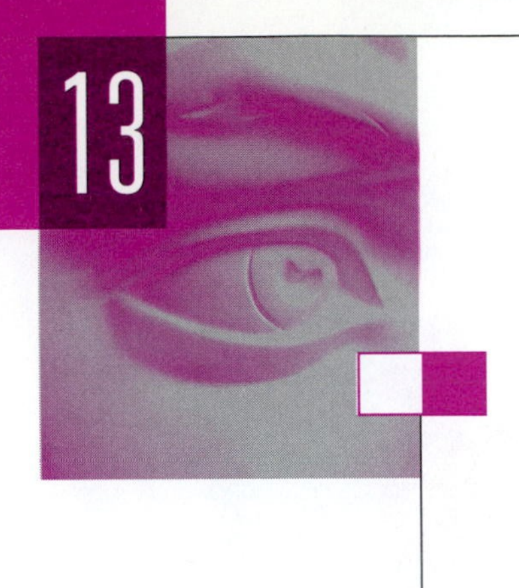

Cardiovascular Anatomy and Physiology

ANATOMY

DISCUSSION OF THE structure of the heart and blood vessels in this text begins on a macroscopic level and progresses to the cellular and molecular level.

Macroscopic Structure

Structures of the heart. The heart is situated in the anterior thoracic cavity, just behind the sternum (Figure 13-1). Posterior to the heart are several structures, including the esophagus, aorta, vena cava, and vertebral column. The position of the heart is such that the right ventricle constitutes the majority of the inferior (or diaphragmatic) and anterior surfaces, and the left ventricle makes up the anterolateral and posterior surfaces. The broader side (base) of the heart is superior, and the tip (apex) is inferior. The base of the heart includes not only the superior portion of the heart itself, but also the roots of the aorta, vena cava, and pulmonary vessels.

Size and weight of the heart. The average human heart is about the size of the clenched fist of that individual. In the adult, this averages 12 cm in length and 8 to 9 cm in breadth at the broadest part. In adult men, the weight of the heart averages 310 g, and that of women averages 255 g. Although there are no significant differences in ventricular wall thickness between men and women, mean values of heart weights increase in women between the third and tenth decades of life. In general, body weight appears to be a better predictor of normal heart weight than is body surface area or height.

Layers of the heart. There are four distinct layers of the heart.

Pericardium. The heart and roots of the great vessels are surrounded by a fibrous sac called the *pericardium,* also known as the *parietal pericardium.* The pericardium functions to hold the heart in a fixed position as well as to provide a physical barrier to infection.

Epicardium. The *epicardium* is tightly adhered to the heart and base of the great vessels and is sometimes referred to as the *visceral pericardium.* Together, the pericardium and epicardium form a sac around the heart. This sac normally contains a very small amount of pericardial fluid (approximately 10 ml) that serves as a lubricant between the pericardium and the epicardium. The pericardium is noncompliant to rapid increases in cardiac size or amount of fluid in the sac. For example, blood or serum can abnormally collect in this sac, as occurs in cardiac tamponade or pericardial effusion. If the fluid collection in the sac impinges on ventricular filling, ventricular ejection, or coronary artery perfusion, a clinical emergency may exist that would necessitate removal of the excess pericardial fluid to restore cardiac function.[1]

Myocardium. Next is the thick muscular layer—the *myocardium,* or mid-wall. This layer includes all of the atrial and ventricular muscle fibers necessary for contraction. The fibers of the myocardium are not organized along a single plane throughout the thickness of the ventricular wall, but they have a distinct arrangement such that the force of contraction is most efficient in ejecting blood toward the outflow tracts in a wringing motion (Figure 13-2). The myocardium is the muscle that is damaged by a "heart attack" or transmural myocardial infarction.[2]

The innermost layer is the *endocardium,* which is a thin layer of endothelium and connective tissue lining the heart. The endothelial lining is continuous with the blood vessels and includes intracardiac structures such as the papillary muscles and valves. Disruption

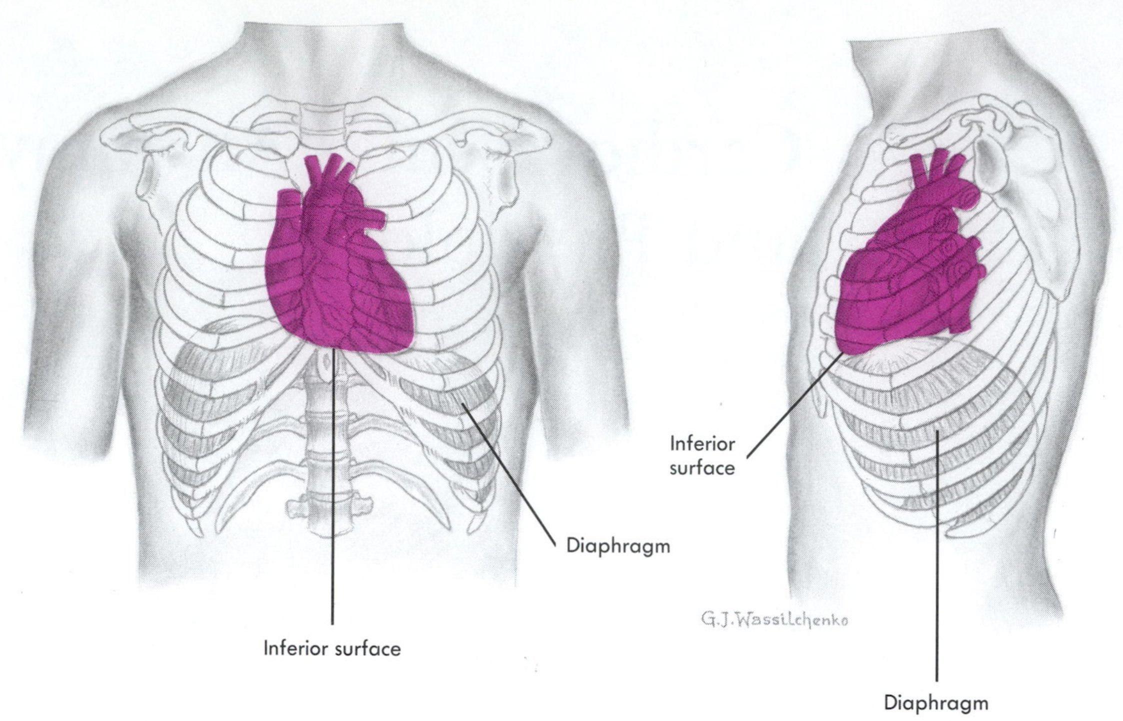

FIGURE 13-1. Anatomic location of the heart within the thoracic cavity.

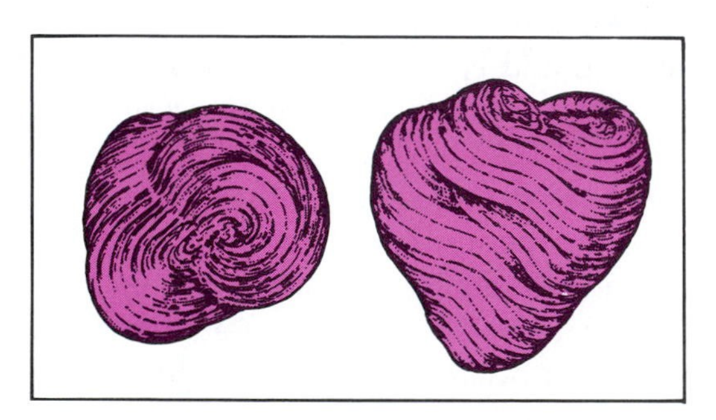

FIGURE 13-2. Macroscopic structure of the spiral musculature of the ventricular walls.

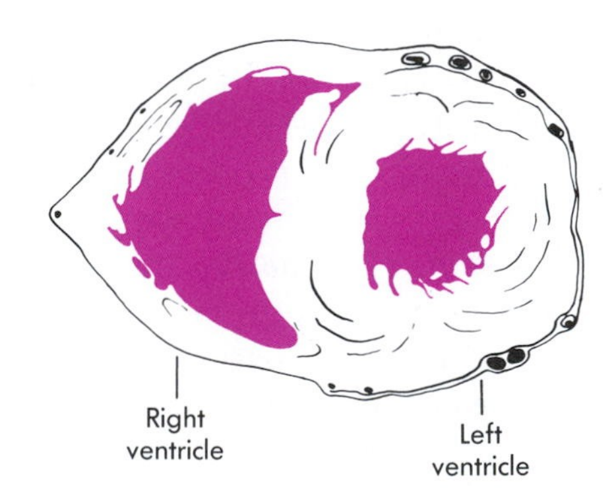

FIGURE 13-3. A transverse section of the ventricles of the adult heart. The right ventricle forms the greater part of the anterior surface of the heart, and the wall of the left ventricle is 3 times as thick as the wall of the right ventricle. (From Quaal S: *Comprehensive intraaortic balloon pumping,* St Louis, 1984, Mosby.)

in the endothelium as a result of surgery, trauma, or congenital abnormality can predispose the area to infection. This infective endocarditis is a devastating disease that, if left untreated, can lead to massive valve damage or sepsis and death.[3]

Cardiac chambers. The human heart has four chambers—the left and right atria and the left and right ventricles. The atria, or auricles, are thin-walled and normally low-pressure chambers. They function to receive blood from the vena cava and pulmonary arteries and to pump blood into their respective ventricles. Atrial contraction (also called *atrial kick*) contributes approximately 30% to ventricular filling, whereas the other 70% occurs passively during diastole. The ventricles are the main pumping forces of the heart. The right ventricle is approximately 3 mm thick, whereas the left ventricle is 10 to 13 mm thick (Figure 13-3). The right ventricle pumps blood into the low-pressured pulmonary circulation, which has a normal mean pressure of approximately 15 mm Hg. The left ventricle must generate tremendous force to eject blood into the aorta (normal mean pressure of approximately 100 mm Hg). Because of left ventricular thickness and the great force it must generate, the left ventricle is considered the major pump of the heart. When the left ventricular muscle thins out as the result of dilation or disease, the effective pumping pressure is diminished, leading to increased left atrial pressure,

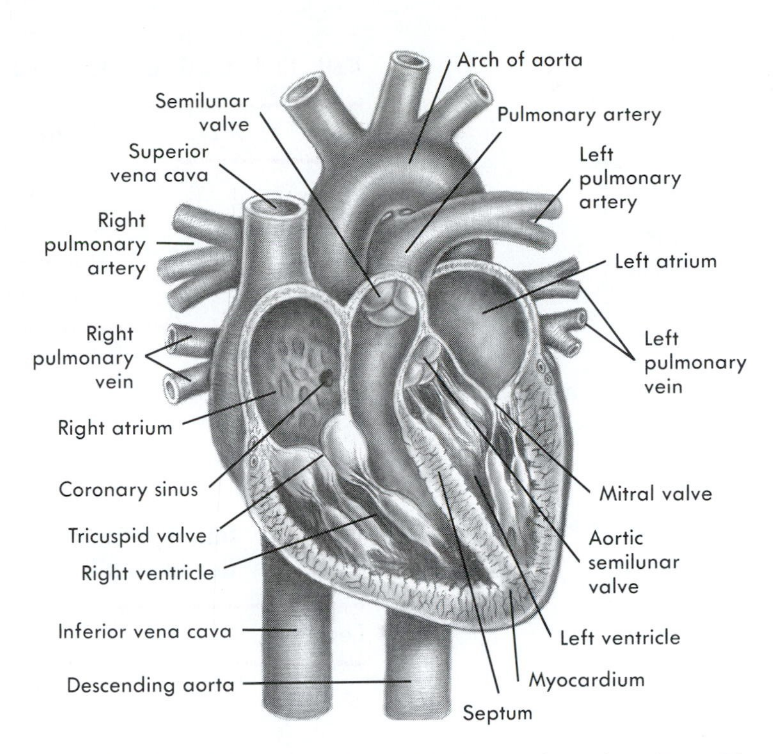

FIGURE 13-4. Cross-sectional view of the heart. Note the position of the four cardiac valves. (From Thompson JM and others: *Mosby's clinical nursing,* ed 3, St Louis, 1993, Mosby.)

pulmonary vasculature congestion, and ultimately systemic venous congestion.[4,5]

Cardiac valves. Cardiac valves are composed of flexible, fibrous tissue that is thinly covered by endocardium. The structure of the valves allows blood to flow in only one direction. The opening and closing of the valves is essentially passive and depends on pressure gradients on both sides of the valve. There are four cardiac valves, all of which are essential to proper cardiovascular function (Figure 13-4).

Atrioventricular valves. The two atrioventricular (AV) valves, so named for their location, are the *tricuspid* (three cusps) valve and the *mitral* (two cusps) valve. The AV valves prevent backflow of blood into the atria during ventricular contraction. The *chordae tendineae* and *papillary muscles,* which attach to the tricuspid and mitral valves, give the valves stability and prevent valve leaflet eversion during systole (Figure 13-5). Papillary muscles, located in the apical area of the endocardium, derive their blood supply from the coronary arteries. Each papillary muscle gives rise to approximately four to ten main chordae that divide into finer and finer cords as they approach the valve leaflets. The chordae tendineae are avascular structures covered by a thin layer of endocardium. A dysfunction of the chordae tendineae or of a papillary muscle can cause incomplete closure of an AV valve, which can result in a murmur. For example, after an acute myocardial infarction (AMI), the papillary muscles may be at risk for rupture as a result of inadequate blood supply from the coronary circulation. When a papillary muscle in the left ventricle ruptures, the mitral valve leaflets do not close completely. Clinically, this situation can cause a mitral regurgitation murmur that can potentially

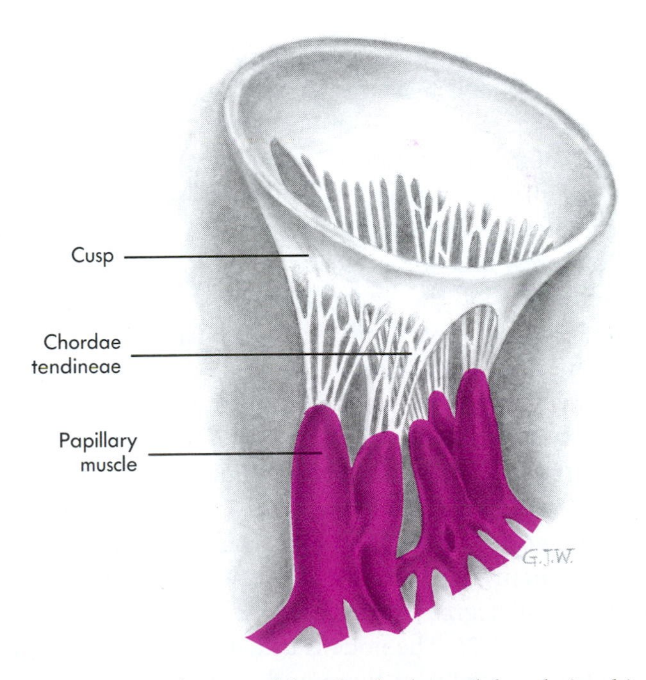

FIGURE 13-5. Diagram of the mitral valve and the relationships of the cusps, chordae tendineae, and the papillary muscles.

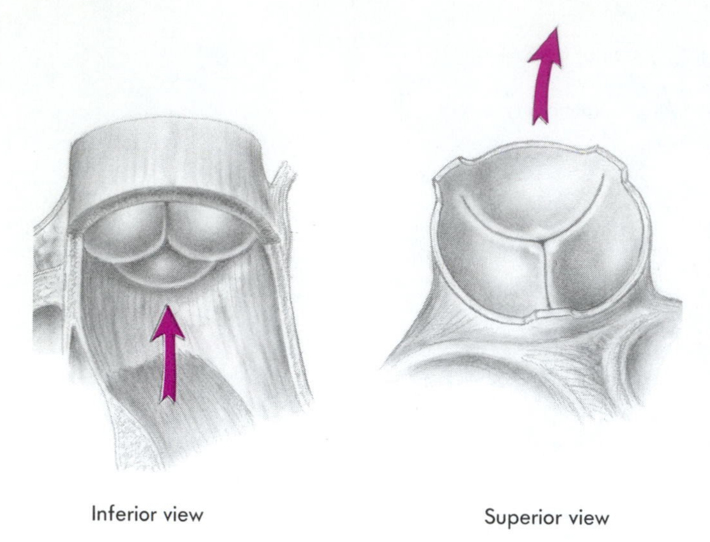

FIGURE 13-6. Diagram of the aortic valve and the cuplike leaflets.

TABLE 13-1 Cardiac Valves and Their Locations

Valve	Type	Situated Between
Tricuspid	AV	Right atrium, right ventricle
Pulmonic	SL	Right ventricle, pulmonary artery
Mitral	AV	Left atrium, left ventricle
Aortic	SL	Left ventricle, aorta

AV, Atrioventricular; *SL,* semilunar.

TABLE 13-2 Intrinsic Pacemaker Rates of Cardiac Conduction Tissue

Location	Rate (Beats/Min)
SA node	60-100
AV node	40-60
Purkinje's fibers	15-40

worsen the pulmonary congestion and lower cardiac output.[6]

Semilunar valves. The semilunar valves, the *pulmonic* and *aortic* valves, each has three cuplike leaflets (Figure 13-6). These valves separate the ventricles from their respective outflow arteries (Table 13-1). During ventricular systole, the semilunar valves open, allowing blood to flow out of the ventricles. As systole ends and the pressure in the outflow arteries exceeds that of the ventricles, the semilunar valves close, thus preventing blood regurgitation back into the ventricles.

The conduction system. Three main areas of impulse propagation and conduction—the sinoatrial (SA) node, the AV node, and the His/Purkinje fibers—are important in cardiac conduction.

The sinoatrial node. The sinoatrial node is considered the natural pacemaker of the heart, because it has the highest degree of automaticity or intrinsic heart rate (Table 13-2). The node is usually a spindle-shaped structure located near the mouth of the superior vena cava, on the posterior aspect of the right atrium. There is some normal variability in the position and shape of the node. The SA node contains two types of cells, the specialized pacemaker cells found in the node center and the border zone cells. Both the pacemaker cells and the border zone cells have inherent depolarization capabilities (they automatically depolarize 60 to 100 times/min). The cells in the nodal center are responsible for the actual pacemaking of the heart. The fibers in the border zone cells also have intrinsic pacemaker properties, but depolarization is depressed by the surrounding atrial tissue.

Once the center nodal cells depolarize, the impulse is conducted through the nodal border zone toward the atrium. Atrial depolarization occurs both cell to cell and also through four specialized conduction pathways that exit the SA node (Figure 13-7, *A*). These conduction pathways are Bachmann's bundle, which is directed to the left atrium, and three internodal pathways that are directed to the AV node.

The atrioventricular node. The atrioventricular (AV) node is located posteriorly on the right side of the interatrial septum. Because the atria and ventricles are separated by nonconductive tissue, all electrical impulses initiated in the atria are conducted to the ventricles solely via the AV node. Although the AV node also possesses pacemaker cells, the intrinsic rate is less than that of the SA node (see Table 13-2). So, as an impulse from the SA node arrives at the AV node, the AV node is depolarized (Figure 13-7, *B*), resetting its own pacemaker potential. This prevents the AV node from initiating its own pacemaker impulse that would compete with the SA node.

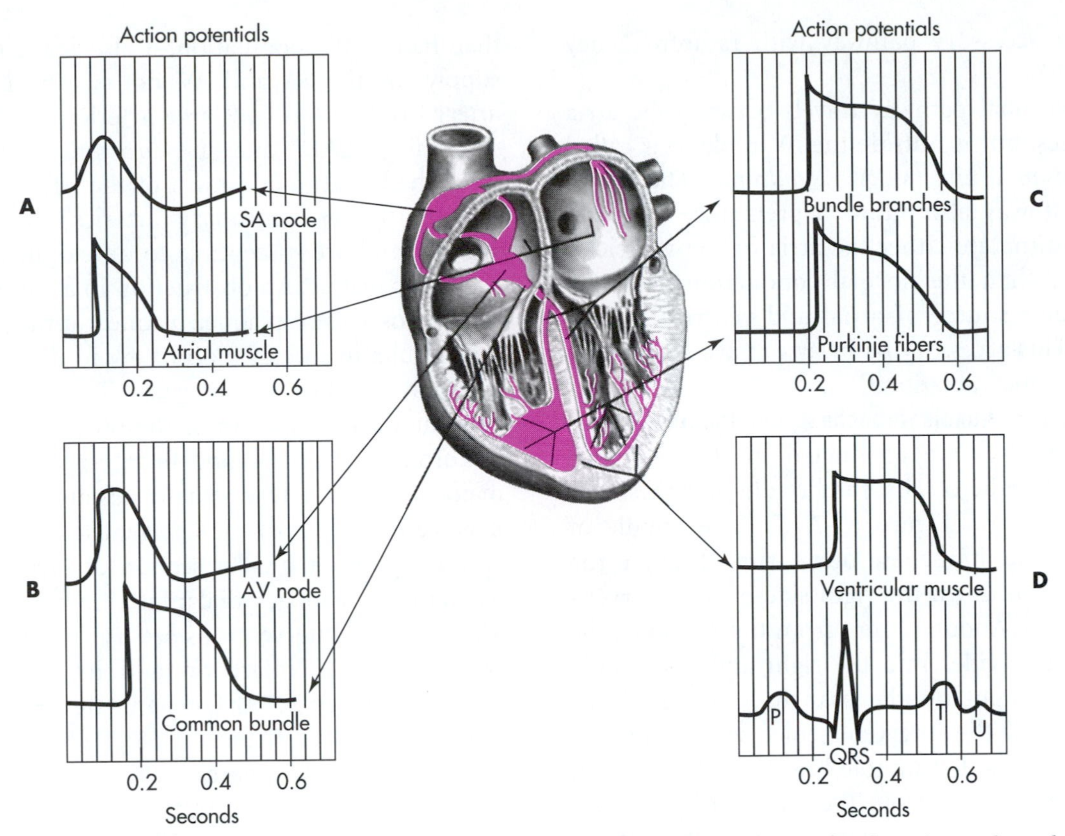

FIGURE 13-7. Heart with normal conduction pathways and transmembrane action potentials of **A,** SA node and atrial muscle; **B,** A-V node and common bundle; **C,** bundle branches; and **D,** ventricular muscle. (From Thompson JM and others: *Mosby's clinical nursing,* ed 4, St Louis, 1997, Mosby.)

As the depolarization impulse from the SA node arrives at the AV node, a slight conduction delay occurs through the AV node. This delay is a result of the inherent properties of the nodal structures that cause a slowing of conduction velocity. The purpose of this delay is to allow adequate time for optimal ventricular filling from atrial contraction. If no electrical delay occurred, the mechanical event of atrial contraction would not have sufficient time to add to ventricular filling. This would lower end-diastolic ventricular volume and potentially lead to lowered cardiac output. The AV nodal delay also provides a protective mechanism for the ventricles. As a result of the slowed conduction velocity through the AV node, the contraction frequency of the ventricles is limited. For example, when an abnormal number of electrical impulses bombard the AV node during atrial flutter or atrial fibrillation, the AV nodal delay limits the number of impulses that move through to the ventricles. Without this delay, the ventricles would receive each atrial impulse and the heart would quickly decompensate.[7]

Another property in the AV node is that of retrograde (backward) conduction. This means that an electrical impulse that is initiated in or below the AV node can be conducted in a backward fashion. When this happens, the propagation time is generally longer than that of antegrade (forward) conduction. This may manifest itself in a variety of heart and conduction disease conditions, as well as in the postoperative recovery period after certain cardiac surgical procedures. In this instance, the coordinated efforts of the atria and ventricles are diminished or lost, resulting in lack of atrial kick to ventricular filling. Detection of this condition is made by the electrocardiogram (ECG).[8]

The normal AV node contains only one pathway to conduct impulses from the atria to the ventricle. If more than one pathway—often called an *accessory pathway*—through the node is present, this allows the electrical impulse to use the second pathway to take a short cut and reenter the atrial circuit. This causes rapid atrial dysrhythmias and overrides normal sinus node firing. The dysrhythmias can be eliminated by ablating the accessory pathway with radiofrequency ablation (RFA).[9,10]

If an additional pathway travels between the atria and ventricles, but is outside the AV node, it is called *Wolff-Parkinson-White (WPW) syndrome.* The WPW accessory pathway also allows a premature electrical impulse to stimulate either the atria or the ventricles much earlier than the normal conduction pathways and is a major source of atrial and ventricular dysrhythmias. This accessory pathway can also be ablated by radiofrequency ablation.[11]

Bundle of His, bundle branches, and Purkinje fibers. Electrical impulses are conducted in the ventricles through the bundle of His, the bundle branches, and the Purkinje fibers (Figure 13-7, *C*). The bundle of His, the bundle branches, fibers run through the subendocardium down the right side of the interventricular septum. About 12 mm from the AV node, the bundle of His divides into the right and left bundle branches. The right bundle branch continues down the right side of the interventricular septum toward the right apex. The left bundle branch is thicker than the right and takes off from the bundle of His at almost a right angle. It then traverses the septum to the subendocardial surface of the left interventricular wall, where it divides into a thin anterior and a thick posterior branch. Functionally, when one of the left branches is blocked, it is referred to as a *hemiblock.* All of the bundle branches are subject to conduction defects (bundle branch blocks) and give rise to characteristic changes in the 12-lead ECG.

The right bundle branch and the two divisions of the left bundle branch eventually divide into the Purkinje fibers. These divide many times, terminating in the subendocardial surface of both ventricles. The Purkinje fibers have the fastest conduction velocity of all heart tissue. Ventricular muscle depolarization follows (Figure 13-7, *D*).

Coronary blood supply. The coronary circulation consists of those vessels that supply the heart structures with oxygenated blood (coronary arteries) and then return the blood to the general circulation (coronary veins). The right and left coronary arteries arise at the base of the aorta immediately above the aortic valve (Figure 13-8). After leaving the base of the aorta, the coronary arteries traverse along the outside of the heart in the natural grooves (sulci). To perfuse the thick heart muscle, branches from these main arteries arise at acute angles, penetrating the muscular wall and eventually feeding the endocardium (Figure 13-9).

The *right coronary artery* (RCA) serves the right atrium and the right ventricle in most people. In more than half of the population, it also is the usual blood supply for the SA and AV nodes. The *left coronary artery* divides into two large arteries, the *left anterior descending* (LAD) and the *circumflex.* These vessels serve the left atria and most of the left ventricle (Figure 13-10). The coronary arteries are small end-arteries, and are susceptible to development of atherosclerotic plaque. An obstruction in a coronary artery, by atherosclerotic plaque, plaque rupture, or thrombus, results in loss of blood flow to the myocardium normally supplied by that artery. This can be fatal, depending on the location of the obstruction. Blockage of coronary arterial blood flow, especially in the left main coronary artery usually results in death from massive infarction of the left ventricle. If the blocked artery supplies a smaller section of myocardium, the result may be a myocardial infarction but not death.[12,13] Many clinical interventions are used to limit and prevent myocardial infarction and its sequelae. (∞Myocardial Infarction, p. 490; Coronary Artery Bypass Surgery, p. 541; Thrombolytic Therapy, p. 561; Catheter Interventions for Coronary Artery Disease, p. 552.)

There is a huge spectrum of variation in the disposition of coronary arteries. The term *dominant* coronary artery describes the artery that traverses the posterior interventricular sulcus and supplies the posterior part of the ventricular septum and often part of the posterolateral wall of the left ventricle.

After blood passes through the coronary capillaries, the majority of it is returned to the right atrium via the coronary veins, exiting via the coronary sinus. In addition, the *Thebesian vessels* are small veins that connect capillary beds directly with the cardiac chambers and also communicate with cardiac veins and other Thebesian veins.[14] However, some of the blood returns directly to the chambers via vascular communications of irregular endothelium-lined sinuses within the muscular structure. These veins that drain into the left ventricle would therefore add unoxygenated blood to the freshly oxygenated blood. When unoxygenated blood mixes with freshly oxygenated blood in the left ventricle, it is called a *physiologic shunt.* An example of a normal shunt is the previously mentioned situation in which unoxygenated blood from the myocardium drains into the left ventricle. An example of an abnormal shunt is an opening in the ventricular septum, called a *ventricular septal defect (VSD),* which allows large amounts of venous blood from the right ventricle to mix with the freshly oxygenated blood in the left ventricle.[15]

Several clinical situations merit a brief discussion here. During ventricular contraction, no blood flows

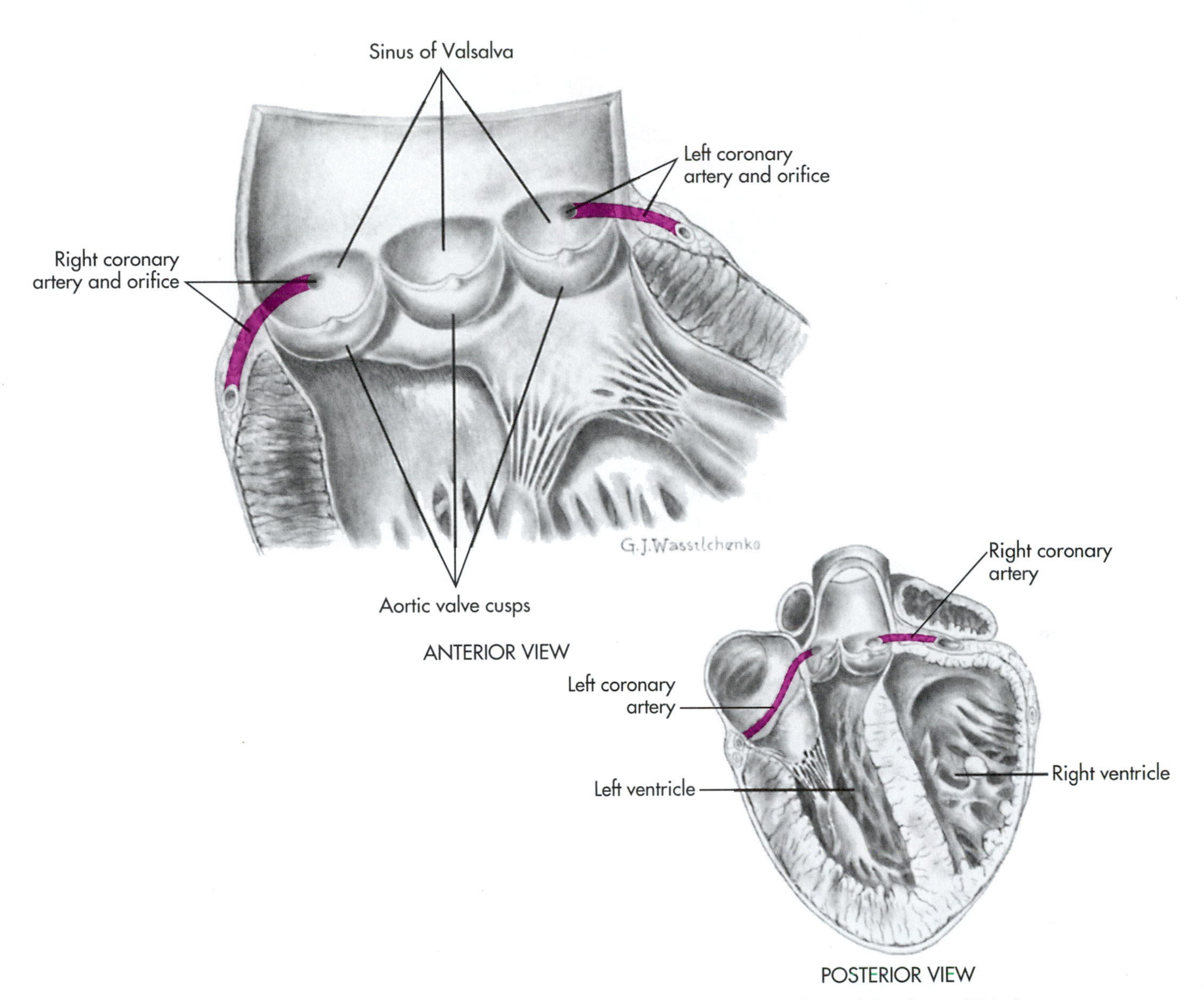

FIGURE 13-8. Proximity of the right and left coronary arteries to the aortic valve and the sinus of Valsalva.

to the cardiac tissue because of the contracted state of the cardiac muscle and resulting occlusion of arteries within the musculature. Coronary artery circulation is highest during early diastole, after the aortic valve has closed. During an episode of tachycardia, diastolic time is greatly diminished; hence coronary perfusion time is diminished. This offers a possible explanation for compromised coronary blood flow and fall in blood pressure during times of rapid heart rate.[16]

The systemic circulation. If the purpose of the heart is to generate enough pressure to pump the blood, it is the function of the vascular structures to act as conduits to carry vital oxygen and nutrients to each cell and also to carry away waste products. Also of primary importance is the ability to exchange those nutrients and waste products at the cellular level. The vascular system acts not only as a conducting system for the blood, but as a control mechanism for the pressure in the heart and vessels. So, it is actually the complex interplay between the heart and the blood vessels that maintains adequate pressure and velocity within this system for optimal functioning.

The arterial system. Arteries are constructed of three layers (Figure 13-11). The innermost layer, or the *intima,* is a thin lining of endothelium and a small amount of elastic tissue. This smooth lining decreases resistance to blood flow and minimizes the chance for platelet aggregation. The *media,* or middle layer, is made up of smooth muscle and elastic tissue. This muscular layer changes the lumen diameter when

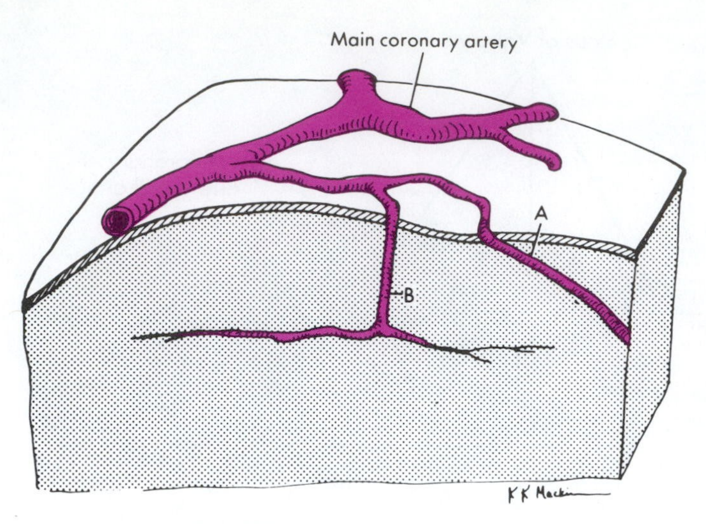

FIGURE 13-9. Intramyocardial distribution of coronary arteries. **A,** Epicardial arteries rise at acute angles from main coronary vessels to supply epicardial surface of the heart. **B,** Smaller vessels branch at oblique angles from main coronary vessels that penetrate deeper into the myocardium and endocardium (intramural arteries). (From Quaal S: *Comprehensive intraaortic balloon pumping,* St Louis, 1984, Mosby.)

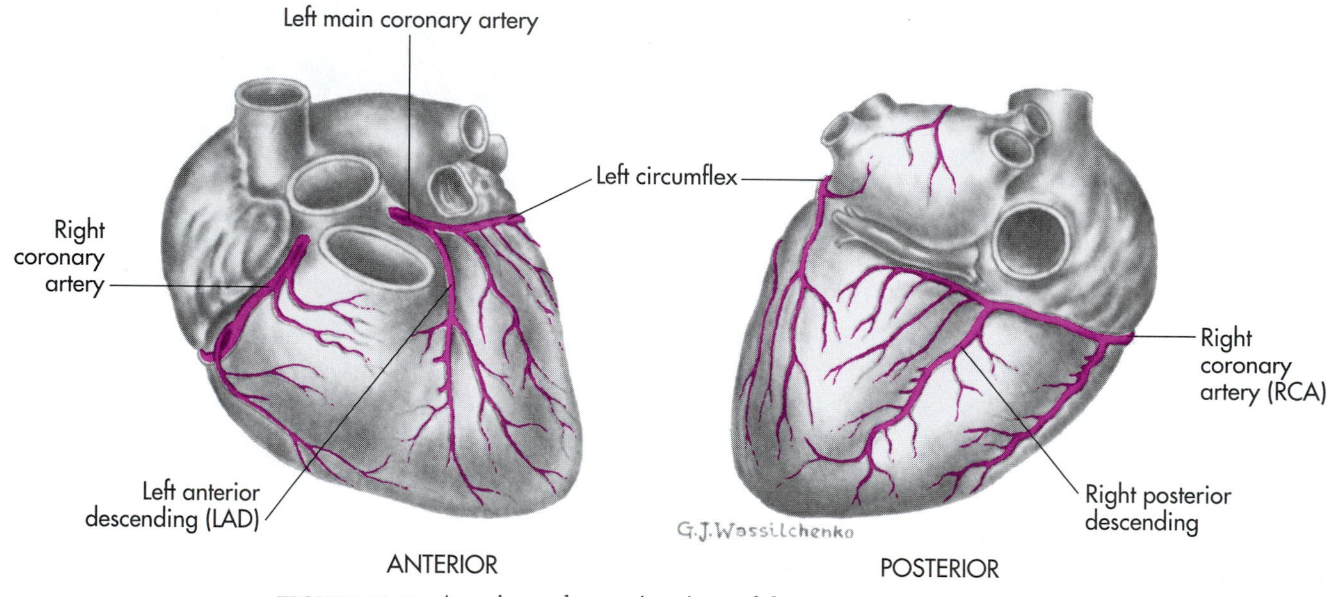

FIGURE 13-10. Anterior and posterior views of the coronary artery circulation.

necessary. The *adventitia,* which is the outermost layer, is largely a connective tissue coat that helps strengthen and shape the vessels.

The intima and the adventitia layers remain relatively constant in the vascular system, whereas the elastin and smooth muscle in the media change proportions, depending on the type of vessel. The aorta contains the greatest amount of elastic tissue. This is necessary because of the sudden shifts in pressure created by the left ventricle. The arterioles, or smaller arteries, and precapillary sphincters have more smooth muscle than do the larger arteries and aorta, because they function to change the luminal diameter when regulating blood pressure and blood flow to the tissues (Figure 13-12).

Blood flow and blood pressure. The pulsatile nature of arterial flow is caused by intermittent cardiac ejection and the stretch of the ascending aorta. The pressure wave initiated by left ventricular ejection (Figure 13-13) travels considerably faster than does the blood itself. Thus when an examiner palpates a pulse, it is this propagation of the pressure wave that is perceived.

In the normal arterial system, the blood flow is called *laminar,* or *streamlined,* because the fluid

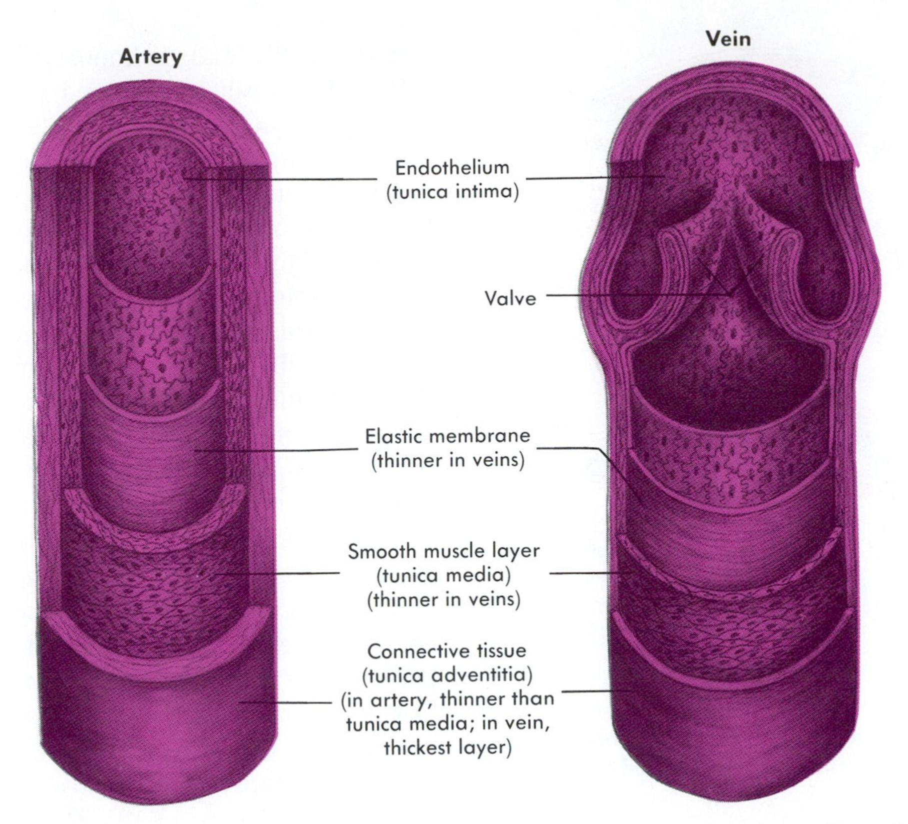

FIGURE 13-11. Cross-section of an artery and vein showing the three layers: tunica intima, tunica media, and tunica adventitia. Note the difference in wall thickness between the artery and the vein and the lack of valves within the artery. (From Thompson JM and others: *Mosby's clinical nursing,* ed 4, St Louis, 1997, Mosby.)

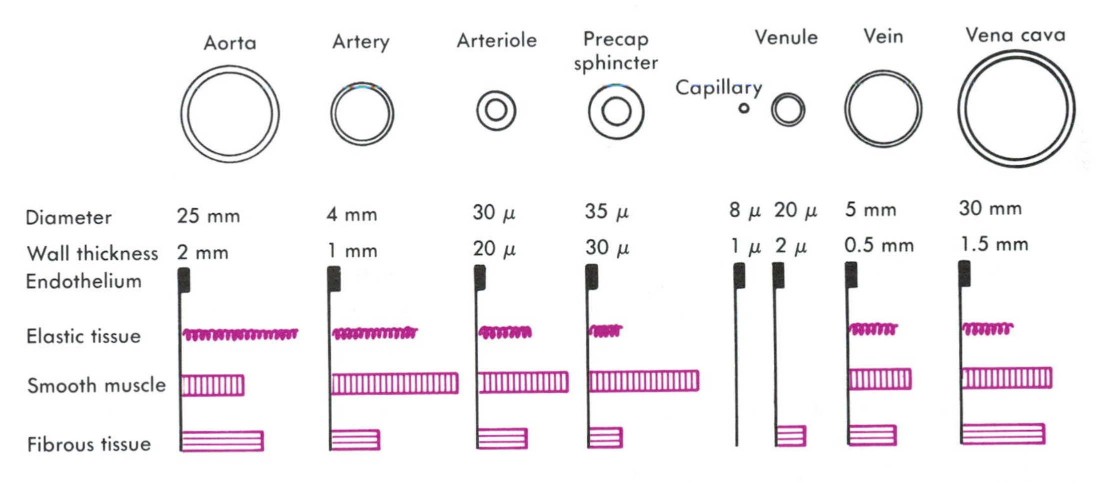

FIGURE 13-12. Internal diameter, wall thickness, and relative amounts of the principal components of the vessel circulatory system. Cross-sections of the vessels are not drawn to scale because of the huge range from aorta to vena cava to capillaries. (From Berne RM, Levy MN: *Cardiovascular physiology,* ed 6, St Louis, 1992, Mosby.)

moves in one direction. However, there are small differences in the linear velocities within a blood vessel. The layer of blood immediately adjacent to the vessel wall moves relatively slowly, because of the friction caused as it comes in contact with the motionless blood vessel wall. In contrast, the fluid more central in the lumen travels more rapidly. The most central blood travels at the highest velocity (Figure 13-14). Clinical implications include conditions in which the vessel wall has an abnormality, such as a small clot or plaque deposit. This disruption in the streamlined flow can set up eddy currents that may predispose the area to platelet aggregation and thus enlargement of the abnormality.[17,18]

Blood pressure (BP) measurement has several components. The systolic blood pressure (SBP) represents the ventricular volume ejection and the response of the arterial system to that ejection. The diastolic value

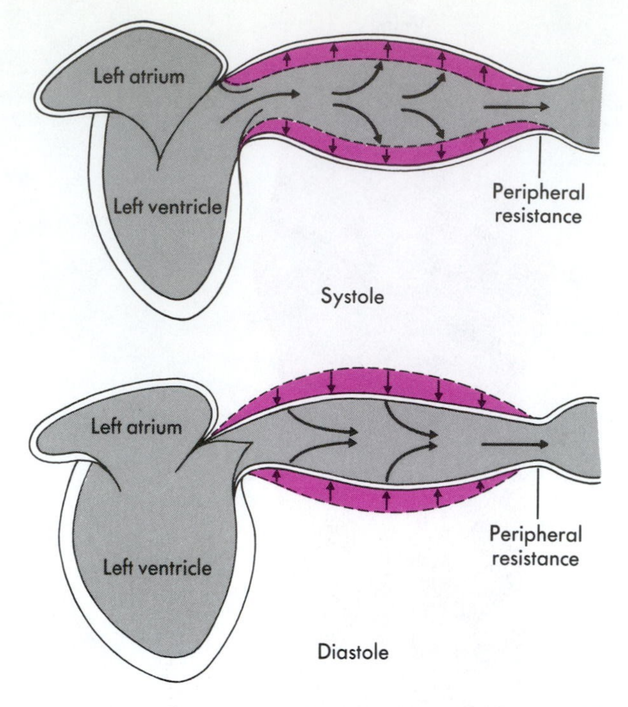

FIGURE 13-13. Elastic and recoil properties of the aorta. (From Berne RM, Levy MN: *Cardiovascular physiology,* ed 6, St Louis, 1992, Mosby.)

(DBP) indicates the ventricular resting state of the arterial system. The pulse pressure is the difference between the SBP and DBP. The mean arterial pressure (MAP) is the mean value of the area under the BP curve (Figure 13-15). BP may be measured several ways. Direct measurement is accomplished by means of a catheter inserted into an artery.[19] The most common indirect method is by means of a stethoscope and sphygmomanometer[20] (Figure 13-16). Figure 13-17 graphically summarizes blood pressures in various portions of the systemic circulatory system.

Vascular resistance is a reflection of arteriolar tone. The large amount of smooth muscle in the arterioles allows for relaxation or contraction of these vessels and causes changes in resistance and redistribution of blood flow. *Resistance* is the opposition to flow caused by the blood vessels. Most changes in resistance are caused by alterations in the tone of the arterial vessel walls, especially in the arterioles. The purpose of this mechanism is to maintain a constant blood pressure in the arterial system. The clinician can never assume that blood flow and blood pressure are identical. For example, poor blood flow to the tissues because of vasoconstricted peripheral arterioles causes the blood to back up and increases blood pressure. A higher blood pressure is a compensatory mechanism but does not necessarily mean there is adequate tissue perfusion.[19] Resistance values are measured by systemic vascular resistance (SVR) and pulmonary vascular resistance (PVR). These values are based on calculations from other hemodynamic parameters (see Appendix D).

Precapillary sphincters and the microcirculation. Where present, the precapillary sphincters are small cuffs of smooth muscle that control blood flow at the junction of the arterioles and the capillaries. The precapillary sphincters allow selective blood flow into capillary beds, depending on their contractile state. The precapillary sphincters are not innervated by the autonomic nervous system as are the arterioles; rather, they respond to local or circulating vasoactive agents. This means that they do not have direct nervous connection to sympathetic input but respond to circulating epinephrine released by the adrenal gland.

As the blood reaches the capillary level, the pulsatile nature of arterial flow is dampened (see Figure 13-17). Even though the diameter of a capillary is less than that of the arteriole, the pressure and flow velocity in the capillary bed is relatively low as a result of the branching nature and large cross-sectional area of the capillary bed (Figure 13-18). The capillary consists of a single cell layer of endothelium and is devoid of muscle or elastin (see Figure 13-12). Hence diffusion of solutes into and out of the capillary is not impeded by mechanical barriers. Thus the capillaries normally retain large structures, such as red blood cells, but are permeable to smaller solutes, such as electrolytes. Although true capillaries do not contain smooth muscle, there is evidence that the endothelium can change its shape and may even secrete substances that influence smooth muscle in other vessels.

The venous system. As the blood leaves the capillary system, it passes through the venules and into the veins. Both venules and veins contain elastic tissue, smooth muscle, and fibrous tissue (Figure 13-12). The veins, however, contain a greater percentage of smooth muscle and fibrous tissue to accommodate the large venous volume and demands for reserve capacity. The majority of circulating blood is contained in the veins that are referred to as *capacitance vessels* (Figure 13-19). Approximately 60% of the total blood volume is found in the veins and is hemodynamically "inactive," meaning that this blood volume does not directly contribute to blood pressure and other hemodynamic parameters. This enables the body to tap into a ready reserve during times of need. For example, when a person changes from a supine to a sitting position, approximately 7 to 10 ml blood/kg of body weight is pooled in the legs. Cardiac output decreases by approximately 20% and stroke volume by 20% to 50%.[21] Arterial BP is maintained by reflex vasoconstriction. Thus

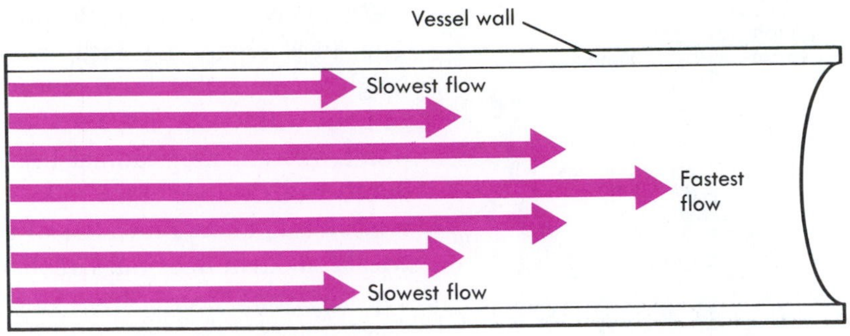

FIGURE 13-14. Laminar flow in an artery.

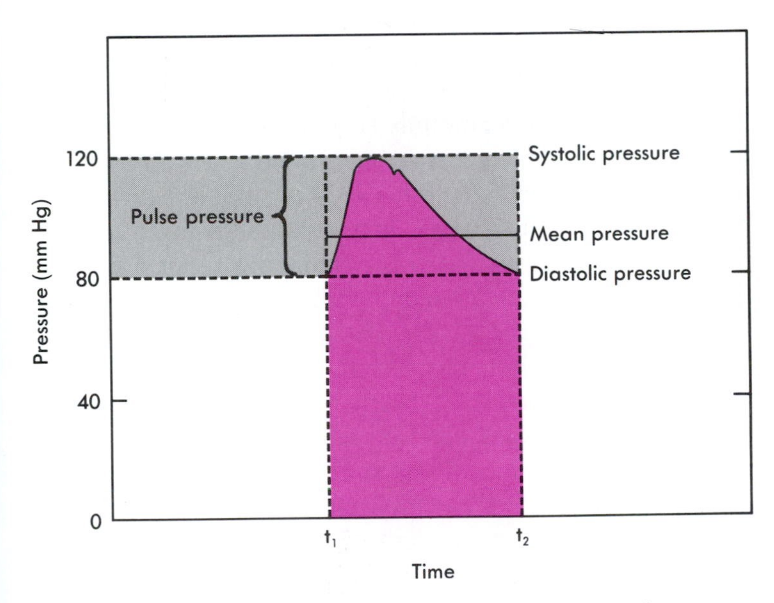

FIGURE 13-15. Arterial systolic, diastolic, pulse, and mean pressures. (From Berne RM, Levy MN: *Cardiovascular physiology,* ed 6, St Louis, 1992, Mosby.)

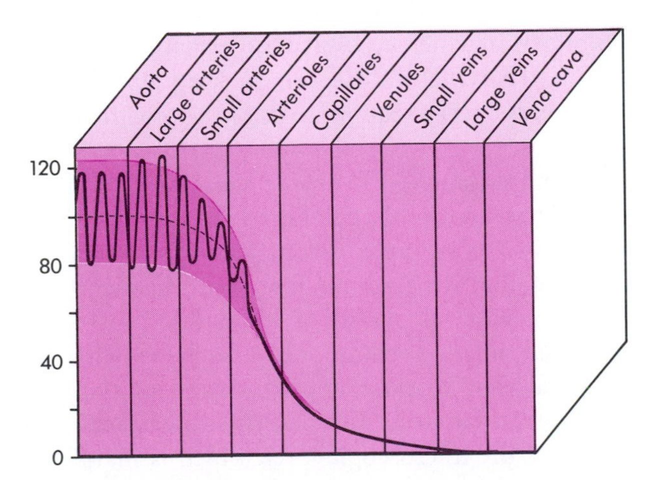

FIGURE 13-17. Blood pressures in the different portions of the systemic circulatory system.

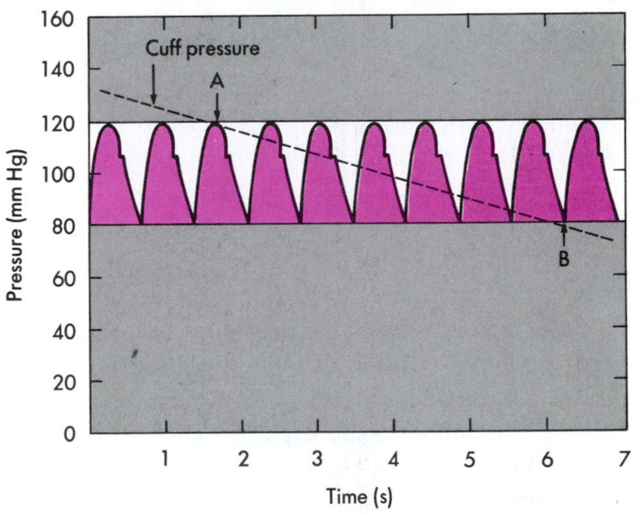

FIGURE 13-16. Principles of blood pressure measurements with a sphygmomanometer. The oblique line represents pressure in the inflatable bag in the cuff. At cuff pressures greater than the systolic pressure (*to the left of* **A**), no blood progresses beyond the cuff and no sounds can be detected below the cuff with the stethoscope. At cuff pressures between the systolic and diastolic levels (*between* **A** *and* **B**), spurts of blood traverse the arteries under the cuff and produce Korotkoff's sounds. At cuff pressures below the diastolic pressure (*to the right of* **B**), arterial flow past the region of the cuff is continuous and no sounds are audible. (From Berne RM, Levy MN: *Cardiovascular physiology,* ed 6, St Louis, 1992, Mosby.)

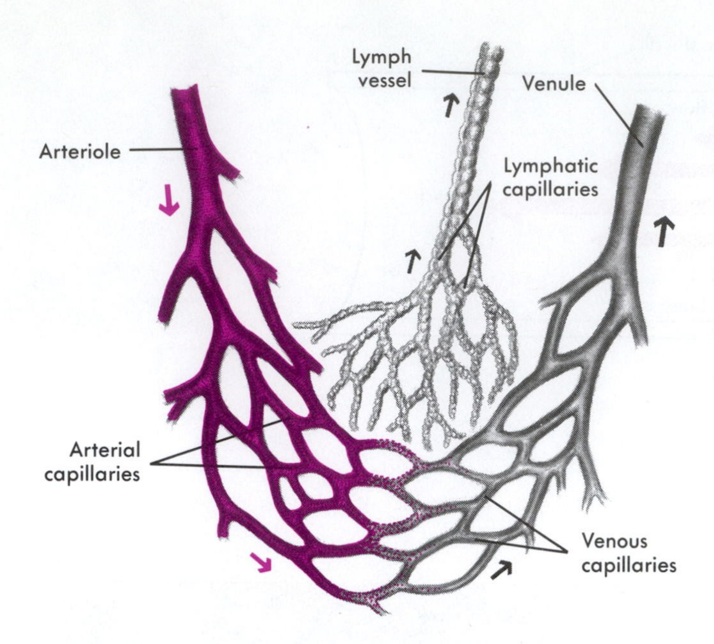

FIGURE 13-18. Microcirculation. Note the branching nature and large cross-sectional area of the capillary bed. (From Thompson JM and others: *Mosby's clinical nursing,* ed 3, St Louis, 1993, Mosby.)

the primary function of capacitance vessels under reflex control is to redistribute the blood to or from the heart to maintain optimal cardiac filling pressures. In humans, these reservoirs are greatest in the splanchnic bed (liver and intestines). Thus patients with decreased blood reserves, such as occurs in a dehydrated or hypovolemic individual, require special caution during position changes, especially from supine to standing. Before helping such a patient to stand, one must allow him or her to "dangle" (sit on the side of the bed) to check for adequate venous reserves.[21]

Microscopic Structure

To understand and appreciate the unique pumping ability of the heart, one must have knowledge of cardiac cell structure and function. This section reviews the anatomic mechanisms responsible for the contractile process in cardiac muscle cells.

Cardiac fibers. Cardiac muscle fibers are typically found in a latticework arrangement. The fiber cells (myofibrils) divide, rejoin, and then separate again, but they retain distinct cellular walls and possess a single nucleus. This differs greatly from skeletal muscle, in which the cells have fused together to form a fiber and have many nuclei.

In general, cardiac myofibrils run on a longitudinal axis, and the fibers appear striped, or striated. When viewed under an electron microscope, these striations are actually the contractile proteins (Figure 13-20). The areas separating each myocardial cell from its neighbor are called *intercalated discs,* which are continuous with the *sarcolemma,* or cell membrane. The point where a longitudinal branch of the cell meets another cell branch is the tight junction (or *gap junction*), which offers much less of an impedance to electrical flow than does the sarcolemma. Because of this, depolarization occurs from one cell to another with relative ease. Also, the cardiac muscle is a *functional syncytium,* in which depolarization started in any cardiac cell quickly is spread to all of the heart.

Cardiac cells. Each cardiac cell contains two types of intracellular contractile proteins, *actin* and *myosin.* These proteins abound in the cell in organized longitudinal arrangements. When visualized by electron microscopy, the myosin filaments appear thick, whereas the almost double amounts of actin filaments appear thin. The actin filaments are connected to the Z bands on one end, leaving the other end free to interact with the myosin cross-bridges. In the resting muscle cell, the actin and myosin partially overlap. The ends of the myosin filament that overlap with the actin have tiny projections (Figure 13-21). For contraction to occur, these projections interact with the actin to form cross-bridges (see Figure 13-21). The portion of the muscle fiber between two Z bands is called a *sarcomere.* In a normal resting state, the sarcomere is about 2.0 to 2.2 μm. Another extremely important intracellular structure necessary for successful contraction is the *sarcoplasmic reticulum* (SR). Calcium ions are stored in the SR and released for use after depolarization (Figure 13-22). Deep invaginations into the sarcomere are called *transverse tubules,* or T tubules. The T tubules are essentially an extension of the cell membrane and thus function to conduct depolarization to structures deep within the cytoplasm, such as the SR. The cardiac cells abound with *mitochondria,* which contain respiratory enzymes necessary for oxidative phosphorylation. This enables the cell to keep up with the tremendous energy requirements of the repetitive contraction.

The importance of these precise and complex anatomic structures is evidenced in several clinical conditions. For example, chronic cardiomyopathy is a disease of the myocardium that most frequently results from viral, alcoholic, or idiopathic causes. The ventricular dilation commonly associated with this condition leads to poor approximation of the actin and myosin filaments. This results in decreased contraction at the microscopic level, which is manifested by impaired myocardial contractility, low cardiac

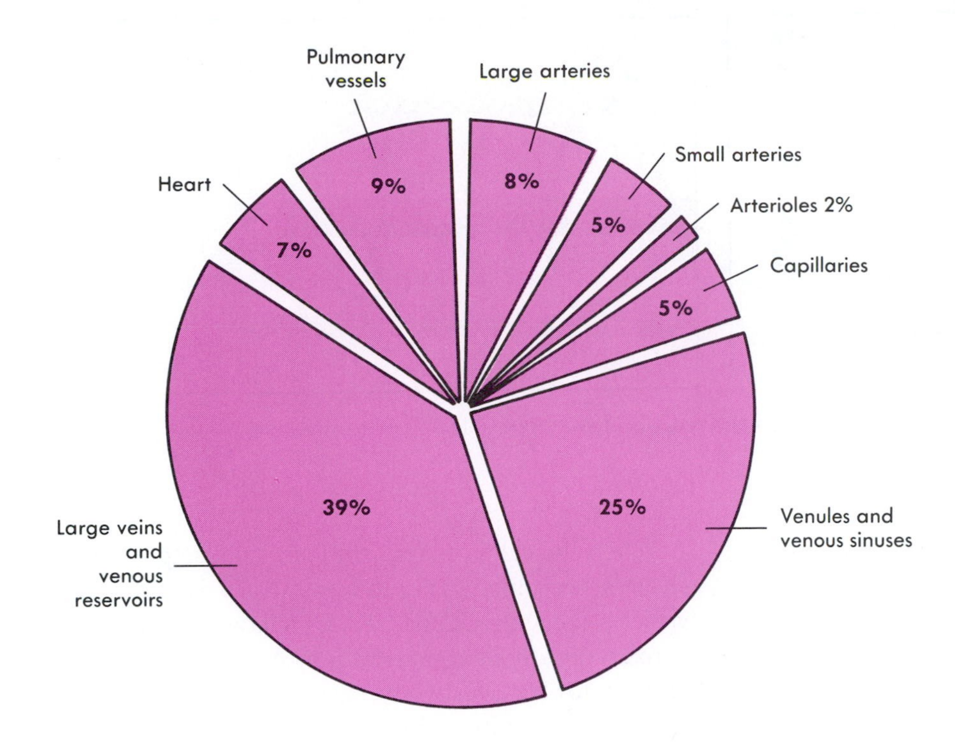

FIGURE 13-19. Percentage of the total blood volume in each portion of the circulation system.

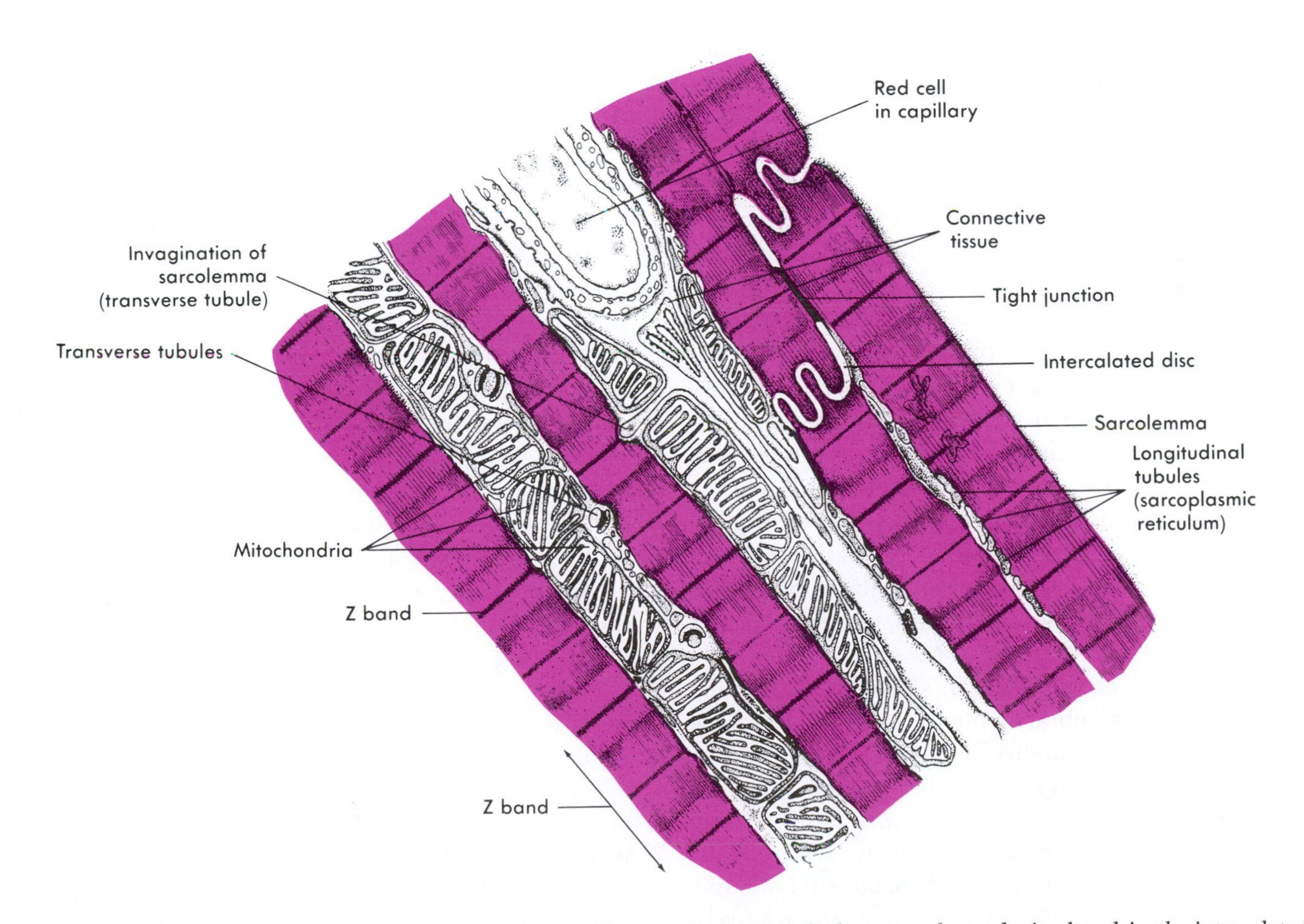

FIGURE 13-20. Diagram of an electron micrograph of cardiac muscle showing the large numbers of mitochondria, the intercalated discs with tight junctions, the transverse tubules, and the longitudinal tubules (also known as the sarcoplasmic reticulum) (approximately ×30,000). (From Berne RM, Levy MN: *Cardiovascular physiology,* ed 6, St Louis, 1992, Mosby.)

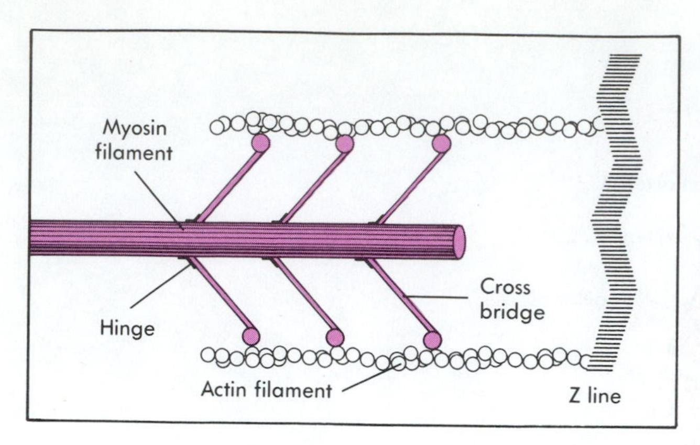

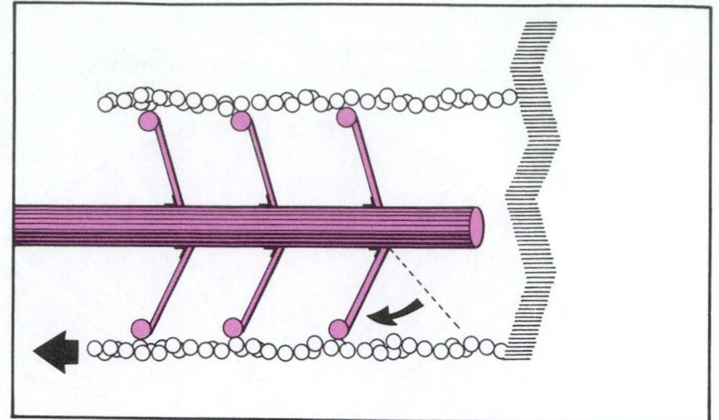

FIGURE 13-21. Actin and myosin filaments and cross-bridges responsible for cell contraction.

output, and increased diastolic volume. Eventually, biventricular heart failure may result.[4,5]

PHYSIOLOGY

The study of the electrical and mechanical properties of cardiac tissue has fascinated scientists for more than 100 years. These properties include excitability, conductivity, automaticity, rhythmicity, contractility, and refractoriness. The following section relates these concepts specifically to cardiac cells (Table 13-3).

Electrical Activity

Transmembrane potentials. Electrical potentials across cell membranes are present in essentially all cells of the body. Some cells, such as nerve and muscle cells, are specialized for conduction of electrical impulses along their membranes. This electrical potential, or transmembrane potential, refers to the relative electrical difference between the interior of a cell and that of the fluid surrounding the cell. Ionic channels are pores in cell membranes that allow for passage of specific ions at specific times or signals. Transmembrane potentials and ionic channels are extremely important in myocardial cells because they form the basis for electrical impulse conduction and muscular contraction.

Resting membrane potential. In a myocardial cell, the normal resting membrane potential (RMP) is approximately −80 to −90 millivolts (mV). This means that the interior of the cell is relatively negative compared with the exterior medium when the cell is at rest. The relative negativity of the cell interior is created by an uneven distribution of positively charged ions and negatively charged ions. Hence there are relatively more of the positively charged ions outside of the cell than there are inside.

When the cell is at rest, the intracellular potassium (K^+) is very high, and sodium (Na^+) is low. Conversely, the extracellular K^+ is relatively low, compared with a high concentration of Na^+ (Table 13-4). Similar to Na^+, calcium (Ca^{++}) also has a much higher concentration outside the cell. These large differences in individual ion concentrations are responsible for the *chemical gradients,* that is, the tendency of a ion to move from the area of higher concentration to the area of lower concentration. However, there is also an *electrical gradient,* in which the positively charged ions move to an area of relative negativity. For example, the chemical gradient of K^+ is to move out of the cell, because the intracellular concentration is so much higher than the outside medium. But, as a result of the relative negativity inside the cell, the electrical gradient works to retain the positively charged K^+ ion. An important factor influencing both gradients is *membrane permeability,* or the selectivity of the membrane to ionic movements. Even at rest, there is some slight movement of ions across the cell membrane. For example, the cell membrane is approximately 50 times more permeable to K^+ than it is to Na^+. Because K^+ movement out of the cell creates more negativity inside the cell, K^+ is therefore the most important ion for maintaining the negative RMP.

Phases of the action potential. In a myocardial cell, when a sudden increase in the permeability of the membrane to Na^+ occurs, a rapid sequence of events follows that lasts a fraction of a second. This sequence of events is termed *depolarization.* The graphic representation of depolarization is the *action potential* (AP) (Figure 13-23). As the membrane is depolarized, Na^+ begins to enter the cell, thus causing the interior of the cell to become more positive. At approximately −65 mV, the membrane reaches *threshold,* the point

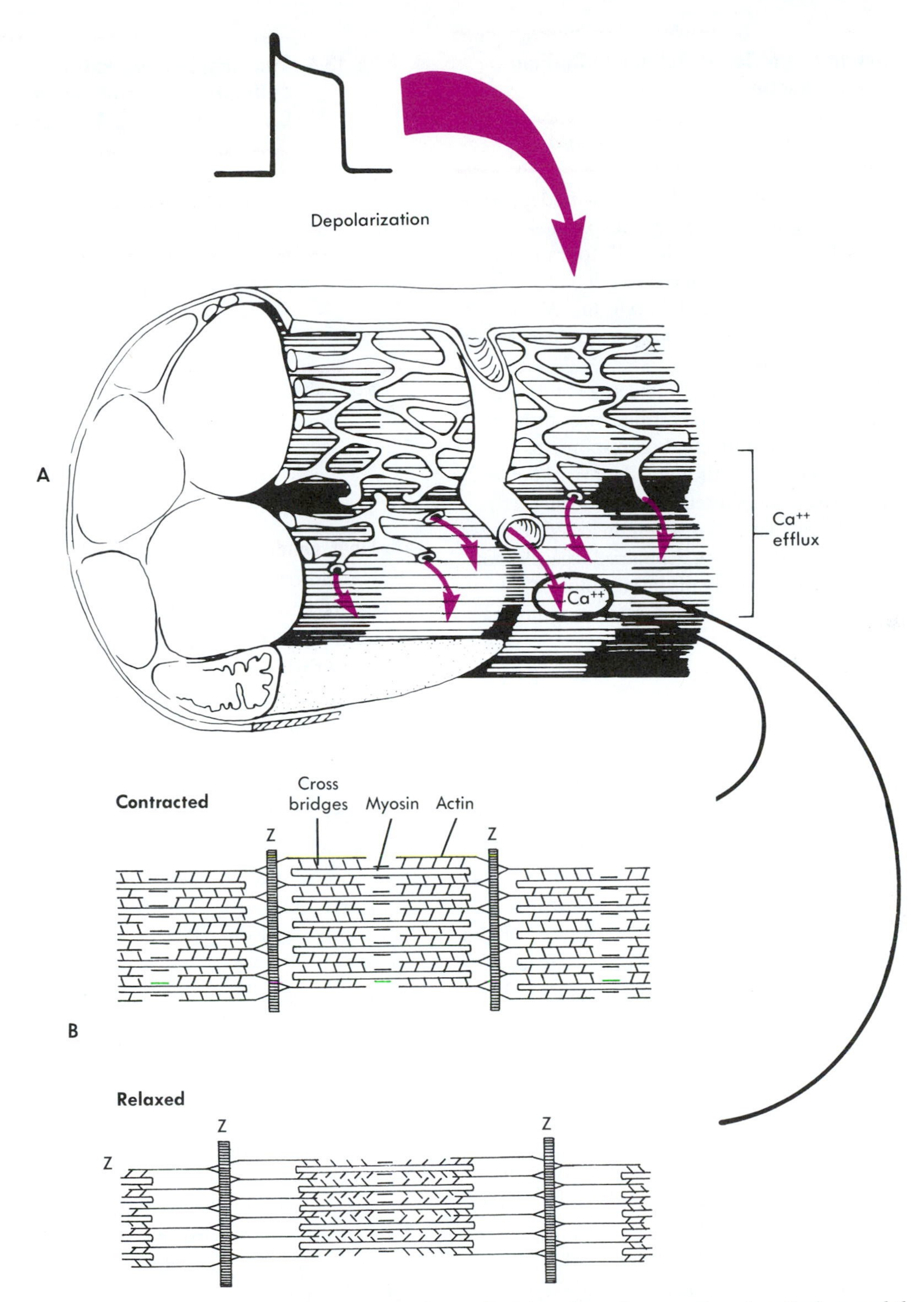

FIGURE 13-22. A, Depolarization of a myocardial cell causes release of calcium from the sarcoplasmic reticulum and the transverse tubules. **B,** Calcium release allows for the cross-bridges on the myosin filaments to attach to the actin filaments to effect cell contraction. (From Quaal S: *Comprehensive intraaortic balloon pumping,* St Louis, 1984, Mosby.)

at which the inward Na^+ current overcomes the efflux of K^+. This is accomplished by means of the fast Na^+ channels. With the fast Na^+ channels open, the inward rush of Na^+ is extremely rapid and briefly causes the inside of the cell to become slightly more positive than the outside of the cell. This is known as *phase 0 of the AP* and is reflected in the overshoot of the AP where the charge is +20 to +30 mV.

When the rapid influx of Na^+ is terminated, a brief period of partial repolarization occurs (phase 1 of

TABLE 13-3 Definitions of Terms Related to Cardiac Tissue Function

Term	Definition
Excitability	The ability of a cell or tissue to depolarize in response to a given stimulus
Conductivity	The ability of cardiac cells to transmit a stimulus from cell to cell
Automaticity	The ability of certain cells to spontaneously depolarize ("pacemaker potential")
Rhythmicity	Automaticity generated at a regular rate
Contractility	The ability of the cardiac myofibrils to shorten in length in response to an electrical stimulus (depolarization)
Refractoriness	The state of a cell or tissue during repolarization when the cell or tissue either cannot depolarize regardless of the intensity of the stimulus or requires a much greater stimulus than is normally required

TABLE 13-4 The Approximate Extracellular and Intracellular Concentrations of K^+, Na^+, and Ca^{++} in a Resting Myocardial Cell

Ion	Extracellular Concentration (mM/L)	Intracellular Concentration (mM/L)
K^+	4	135
Na^+	145	10
Ca^{++}	2	0.0001

From Berne RM, Levy MN: *Cardiovascular physiology,* ed 7, St Louis, 1997, Mosby.

the AP). This is followed by phase 2, or the plateau. During this phase, another set of channels—the slow Na^+ and Ca^{++} channels—open and allow the influx of Ca^{++} and Na^+. Also during phase 2, K^+ tends to diffuse out of the cell, balancing the slow inward flux of Na^+ and Ca^{++}, thereby maintaining the plateau of the AP. The Ca^{++} entering the cell at this phase causes cardiac contraction, which is described later in this chapter. The inward flux of Ca^{++} during this phase can be influenced by many factors. For example, agents such as verapamil, nifedipine, and diltiazem inhibit the inward Ca^{++} current and thus are known as *calcium channel blockers.*[22]

Phase 3 of the AP is the final repolarization phase and depends on two processes. The first is the inactivation of the slow channels, thereby preventing further influx of Ca^{++} and Na^+. The other is the continued efflux of K^+ out of the cell. Both of these processes cause the intracellular environment to become more negative, thereby reestablishing the RMP. Phase 4 of the AP is the return to RMP. The excess Na^+ that entered the cell during depolarization is now removed from the cell in exchange for K^+ by means of the Na^+/K^+ pump. This mechanism returns the intracellular concentrations of Na^+ and K^+ to the levels before depolarization and is essential for normal ionic balance (Table 13-5).

Fiber conduction and excitability. Different parts of the conduction system require different electrical currents and create individual transmembrane action potentials, as shown in Figure 13-7. In addition ionic shifts within the endocardium, myocardium, and epicardium are not uniform, although the clinical significance of this finding is not clear at this time.[23,24] Propagation of an AP along a cardiac fiber occurs as a result of ionic shifts discussed previously. As a local section of the cell becomes depolarized, reaches threshold, and completely depolarizes, it affects the adjacent area of the cell and begins depolarization in that area. Thus the AP propagates down the fiber in a wavelike fashion (Figure 13-24). This is somewhat analogous to a trail of gunpowder. When the gunpowder is lit at one end, a small area ignites, burns, and then ignites the area of gunpowder immediately adjacent, and so on.

The time from the beginning of the AP until the time when the fiber can accept another AP is called the *effective* or *absolute refractory period.* During this period, the cell cannot be depolarized regardless of the amount or intensity of the stimulus. This period lasts from the beginning of depolarization to approximately −50 mV during phase 3. Immediately after the absolute refractory period is the *relative refractory period.* At this time, the cell is not fully repolarized, but could depolarize with a strong enough stimulus (Figure 13-25). This period lasts from approximately −50 mV during phase 3 to when the cell returns to RMP. At phase 4, the cell is fully repolarized and is again at RMP, ready to respond to the next stimulus.

Pacemaker versus nonpacemaker action potentials. The action potential as just discussed is representa-

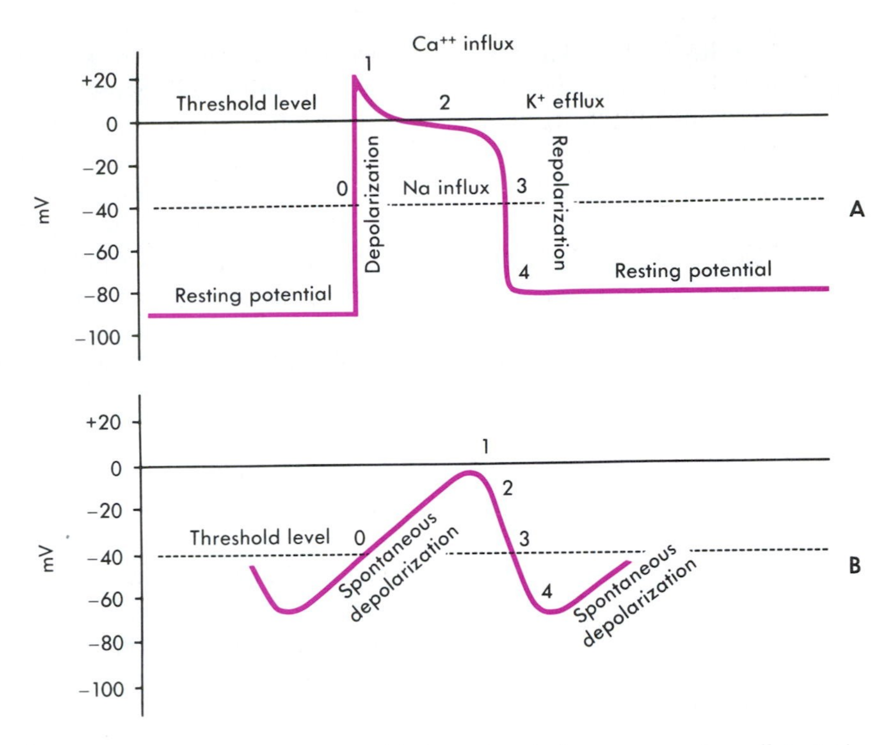

FIGURE 13-23. Cardiac action potentials. **A,** Action potential phases 0 to 4 of a nonpacemaker cell. **B,** Action potential of a pacemaker cell. (From Thompson JM and others: *Mosby's clinical nursing,* ed 4, St Louis, 1997, Mosby.)

TABLE 13-5 Summary of Phases 0 Through 4 of a Cardiac Cell Action Potential (AP)

Phase	Description	Ionic Movement	Mechanisms
0	Upstroke	Na^+ into cell	Fast channels open
1	Overshoot		Fast channels close
2	Plateau	Na^+, Ca^{++} into cell, K^+ out	Slow channels open
3	Repolarization	K^+ out of cell	Slow channels close
4	RMP	Na^+ out, K^+ in	Na^+/K^+ pump

tive of the depolarization of nonpacemaker myocardial cells. The AP generated by a Purkinje fiber is similar to that of a ventricular myocardial cell, except that phase 2 is usually more prolonged in the Purkinje fiber. Atrial myocardial cells exhibit a shortened plateau (phase 2) as compared with ventricular cells.

The pacemaker cells of the SA node have an AP that is very different from that of a myocardial or Purkinje cell. In the SA node, the RMP is approximately

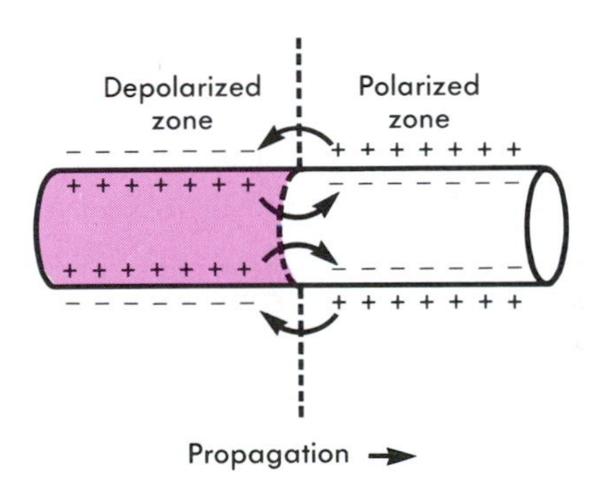

FIGURE 13-24. Schematic representation of the propagation of an action potential along a cell membrane.

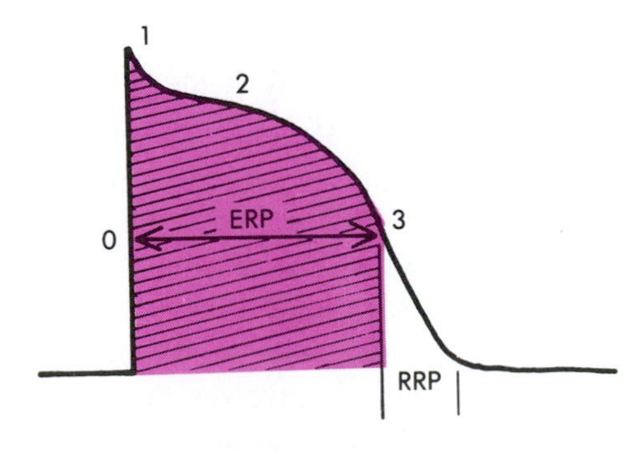

FIGURE 13-25. The two parts of the refractory period. The effective (absolute) refractory period (ERP) extends from phase 0 to approximately −50 m V in phase 3. The remainder of the action potential is the relative refractory period (RRP). (From Conover MB: *Understanding electrocardiography,* ed 6, St Louis, 1992, Mosby.)

−65 mV. And, rather than an RMP that remains constant, the cells slowly depolarize at a steady rate until threshold is reached (see Figure 13-23, *B*). Because there are no fast Na^+ channels in the pacemaker cells, the SA node AP has a different configuration from that of a myocardial cell and is referred to as the *slow response.* The lack of a true RMP is largely the result of a steady Na^+ influx through the slow channels. This mechanism explains how the cells can spontaneously depolarize (automaticity). It also provides the basis for understanding alterations in the pacemaker cells. The frequency of the pacemaker cell discharge may be altered by changing the rate of depolarization (changing the slope of phase 4), changing the level of the threshold, or raising or lowering the RMP.

Mechanical Activity

Excitation-contraction coupling. The electrical activity discussed in the previous section is the basis for mechanical contraction. As the myocardial cell is depolarized, specifically during phase 2 of the AP, some Ca^{++} enters the cytoplasm through the cell membrane via special Ca^{++} channels. The majority of Ca^{++} enters the cytoplasm from stores in the sarcoplasmic reticulum (SR). The cytoplasmic Ca^{++} then binds with troponin and tropomyosin, molecules that are present on the actin filaments, resulting in contraction. Occurring throughout the myocardium, the result is myocardial contraction. Once contraction has occurred, Ca^{++} is taken back up into the SR and the cytoplasmic concentration of Ca^{++} falls, leading to muscular relaxation. Both contraction and relaxation are active processes, because they require adenosine triphosphate (ATP) and because the Ca^{++} is removed from the cell by way of a Na^+/Ca^{++} pump. The role of this pump is not fully established, but it clearly contributes to intracellular Ca^{++} regulation during diastole. The question of increased contractility is also not completely elucidated. Variations in strength of contraction may involve recruitment of more or fewer cross-bridges or a change in the Ca^{++}-binding properties of the contractile proteins. There is also probably an increase in Ca^{++} sensitivity as the muscle fiber is stretched. However, the role of Ca^{++} is much more complex than is presented here, because it involves not only the mechanical events in the cell, but also several metabolic and regulatory processes.

The Cardiac Cycle

The cardiac cycle refers to one complete mechanical cycle of the heartbeat, beginning with ventricular contraction and ending with ventricular relaxation.

Ventricular systole. As the ventricles are depolarized, the septum and papillary muscles tense first. This provides a stable outflow tract and competent AV valves. The ventricles begin to tense (endocardium to epicardium), causing a rise in pressure. When the intraventricular pressure exceeds that of the intraatrial pressure, the mitral and tricuspid valves close. This stage is known as *isovolumic contraction* because, even though the ventricular muscle is tensing, the ventricular volume does not change. As the ventricular tension increases, the intraventricular pressures exceed those of the aorta and pulmonary arteries, causing the aortic and pulmonic valves to open. The blood ejected from the ventricles is called the *stroke volume.* Usually more than half of the total ventricular blood volume is ejected; the blood that remains in the ventricles is the *residual* or *end-systolic volume.*

The *ejection fraction* (EF) is the ratio of the stroke volume ejected from the left ventricle per beat to the volume of blood remaining in the left ventricle at the end of diastole (left ventricular end-diastolic volume, or LVEDV). EF is expressed as a percent, normal being at least greater than 50%. An ejection fraction of 30% could indicate either poor ventricular function (as in cardiomyopathy), poor ventricular filling, obstruction to outflow (as in some valve stenosis conditions), or a combination of these. Both ejection fraction and LVEDV are widely used clinically as indexes of contractility and cardiac function.

Ventricular diastole. After ventricular systole is ventricular diastole. The first phase is *isovolumic relaxation,* which occurs between closure of the semilunar (aortic and pulmonic) valves and the opening of the AV (mitral and tricuspid) valves. Immediately after is the rapid filling phase, in which the AV valves open and the majority of the ventricular filling occurs. The next phase is a reduced ventricular filling period. This is passive flow of blood from the periphery and pulmonary vasculature into the ventricles. The last part of ventricular diastole, known as *atrial kick,* provides approximately 30% of total ventricular filling.[25] With this, the cycle is complete and begins once again with systole (Figure 13-26).

Interplay of the Heart and Vessels: Cardiac Output

Cardiac output (CO) is defined as the volume of blood ejected from the heart over 1 minute. Therefore the determinants of CO are heart rate (HR) in beats per minute and stroke volume (SV) in milliliters per beat. The equation is as follows:

$$CO = HR \times SV$$

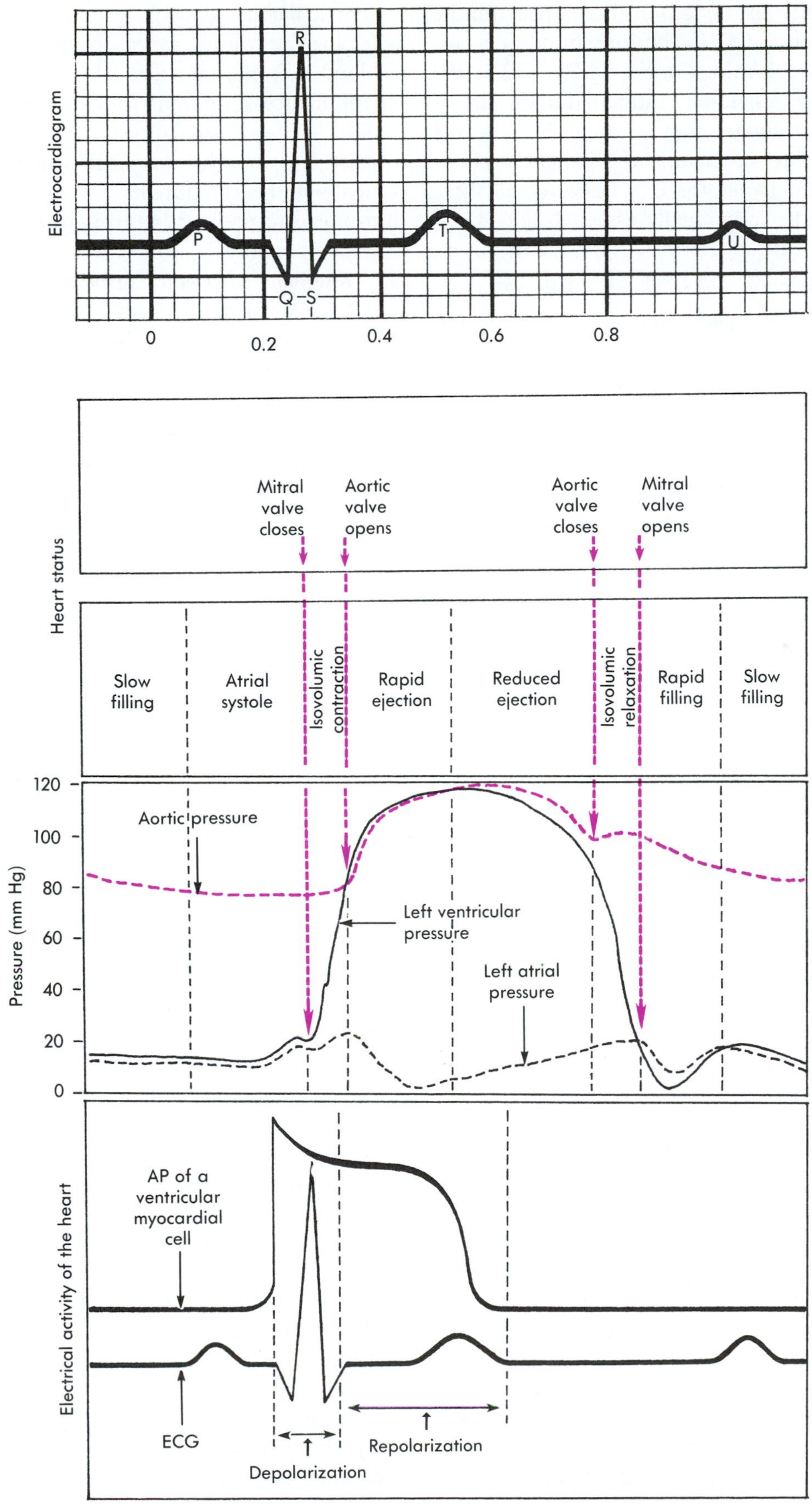

FIGURE 13-26. The cardiac cycle.

CO is normally expressed in liters per minute (L/min). The normal CO in the human adult is approximately 4 to 6 L/min. *Cardiac index* (CI) is the CO divided by the individual's estimated body surface area, expressed in square meters (m^2). The normal range for CI is 2.5 to 4.5 L/min/m^2. Changes in either the SV or HR can change the CO. However, all three parameters must be individually assessed. For example, for a person with an HR of 72 and SV of 70 ml:

$$CO = 72 \text{ (beats/min)} \times 70 \text{ (ml/beat)} = 5.04 \text{ L/min}$$

If, however, the parameters change to an HR of 140 and SV of 40 ml:

$$CO = 140 \text{ (beats/min)} \times 40 \text{ (ml/beat)} = 5.6 \text{ L/min}$$

Clearly, although the latter CO is greater, it does not reflect improved cardiac status. Rather, it could mean that cardiac decompensation is imminent. Although HR is influenced by many neurochemical factors, as discussed in the next section, this section focuses on the components of the SV (Figure 13-27). These are preload, afterload, and contractility.

Preload. The concept of preload was introduced in the early 1900s when Ernest Starling described his findings in an isolated dog heart preparation. Starling found that as he increased the volume infused into a denervated heart, the cardiac output increased, until it reached a point at which further infusion actually caused the CO to decrease. This is now known as *Starling's law of the heart,* and it is graphically described as the Starling curve (Figure 13-28). It can best be described on a molecular basis, using as a foundation the discussion of the actin and myosin cross-bridges in the myofibril. As the diastolic volume increases, it stretches the actin and myosin molecules in their resting state. As contraction occurs, the contractility increases as a result of the increased stretch. However, if the stretch is excessive and causes the actin and myosin to be stretched beyond their cross-bridging limits (i.e., greater than 2.2 μm), contractility decreases. This is the basis for Starling's curve. With the advent of critical care units and sophisticated monitoring, this principle has grown to great significance in clinical practice. For example, after a myocardial infarction (MI), the ability of the left ventricle to pump may be impaired. It is desirable to optimize the contractility of the remaining viable heart muscle by "stretching" it with added volume. But if the intravascular volume exceeds the stretch limit, CO diminishes.

Preload, then, is a function of the volume of blood presented to the left ventricle and also the compliance (the ability of the ventricle to stretch) of the ventricles at the end of diastole. It has been described as left ventricular end-diastolic pressure (LVEDP). Factors affecting the volume aspect include venous return, total blood volume, and atrial kick. Factors affecting the compliance of the ventricles are the stiffness and thickness of the muscular wall. For example, the hypovolemic patient has too little preload, whereas the patient with heart failure has too much preload. One way to measure preload is through the pulmonary artery wedge pressure.

Afterload. *Afterload* can be defined as the ventricular wall tension or stress during systolic ejection. An increase in afterload usually means an increase in the work of the heart. Afterload is increased by factors that oppose ejection. Examples of increased afterload include aortic impedance (high diastolic aortic pressure, aortic stenosis), septal hypertrophy (obstruction in the outflow tract), vasoconstriction (increased systemic vascular resistance), and increased blood volume or viscosity. Therapeutic management to decrease afterload is aimed at decreasing the work of the heart through the use of vasodilators to decrease the myocardial oxygen demand.

An increase in afterload can evoke a type of autoregulation in which the ventricle adapts to changes in filling pressure without a continued increase in resting fiber length (the Anrep effect). For example, when peripheral vascular resistance increases abruptly during vasoconstriction, ventricular diastolic pressure rises temporarily until the ventricle reaches a new equilibrium level of pressure.

Contractility. Contractility refers to the heart's contractile force. It is also referred to as *inotropy* (literally, *ino,* strength; *tropy,* enhancing), which can be positive (stronger contraction) or negative (weaker contraction). As discussed, contractility can be increased by Starling's mechanism and by the sympathetic nervous system. It can be greatly affected by pharmacologic agents, particularly those that mimic the sympathetic nervous system (sympathomimetics, adrenergics).

Contractility may also be altered by a variety of other physiologic phenomena. One such mechanism is the staircase—or treppe—phenomenon, which occurs when cardiac muscle contracts rapidly after a period of normal rate. During this tachycardia, the force of contraction progressively increases until a new steady state is reached. In addition, situations that cause an increase in the cytoplasmic Ca^{++} may result in positive inotropy. An example of this is the drug *digoxin.* Digoxin inhibits the Na^+/K^+ pump, which causes a slight rise in the intracellular Na^+. This rise in turn slows the Na^+/Ca^{++} pump that is responsible for removing the cytoplasmic Ca^{++} during diastole.

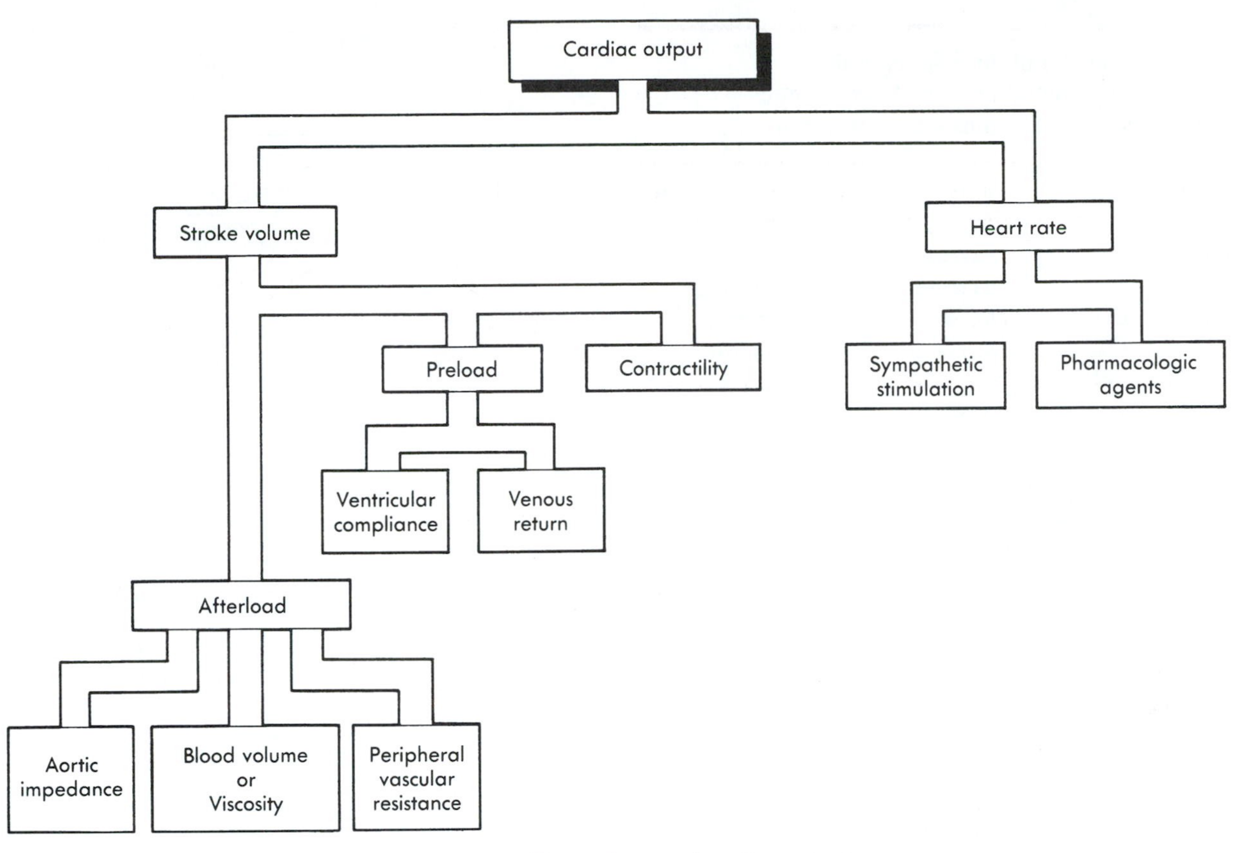

FIGURE 13-27. Determinants of cardiac output.

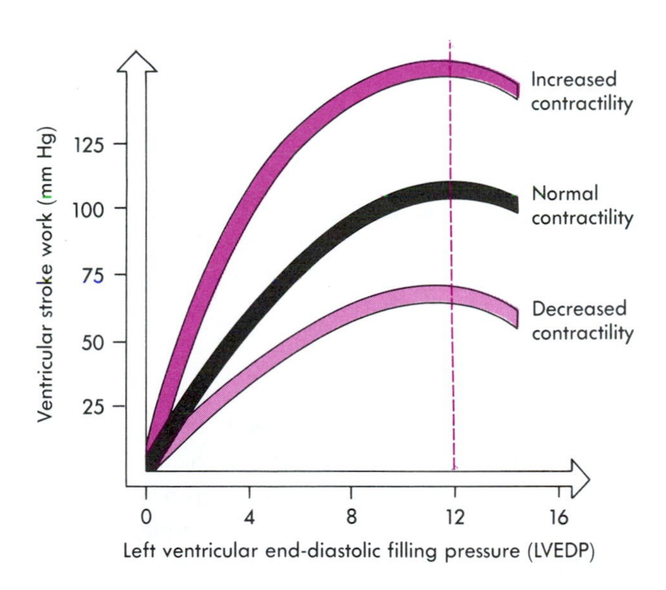

FIGURE 13-28. Starling curve. As the left ventricular end diastolic pressure (LVEDP) increases, so does ventricular stroke work or contractility. When left ventricular filling pressure exceeds a maximal point, contractility and cardiac output diminish.

The impaired Na^+/Ca^{++} pump causes a slight increase in cytoplasmic Ca^{++}, which is the basis for the increased inotropic properties of digoxin.

Regulation of the Heartbeat

Nervous control. Both the parasympathetic nervous system (PNS) and the sympathetic nervous system (SNS) are normally active to create a balance between maintenance and fight-or-flight cardiovascular functions, respectively. Table 13-6 summarizes the effects these divisions of the autonomic nervous system have on the heart.

Parasympathetic fibers are concentrated mostly near the SA and AV conduction tissue. Specifically, this involves the right and left vagus nerves (Figure 13-29). Stimulation of the vagus nerve produces bradycardia as a result of hyperpolarization of phase 4 of the AP, which causes the slope to take a longer time to reach threshold. There is also a concomitant decrease in sympathetic tone. Thus adjustments can be made by changes in both the PNS and the SNS or, under certain conditions, selective changes in one.

Sympathetic nerve fibers parallel the coronary circulation to some degree before the fibers penetrate the myocardium. The right and left sympathetic chains

TABLE 13-6 Summary of the Effects of the Parasympathetic and Sympathetic Nervous Systems on the Heart

Function	Parasympathetic	Sympathetic
Automaticity	Decrease	Increase
Contractility	Decrease	Increase
Conduction velocity	Decrease	Increase
Chronotropy (rate)	Decrease	Increase

probably have slightly different effects on the myocardium. It appears that the right chain has more effect on acceleration properties, whereas the left chain has a greater influence on contractility.

Intrinsic regulation. Supplementing the nervous control are several reflexes that serve as feedback mechanisms to the brain. These reflexes work to maintain even blood flow and perfusion.

The *baroreceptors,* or pressure sensors, are located in the aortic arch and the carotid sinuses. They are more sensitive to wall changes (wall strain) in these areas than to the absolute pressure. As the receptors sense a change in wall conformation, usually as a result of a decrease or increase in pressure, the autonomic nervous system is activated to either raise or lower the heart rate, respectively. For example, a drop in blood pressure alters the baroreceptor input to the vasomotor center in the medulla, causing a reflex tachycardia. Evidence also suggests that the baroreflex initiates changes in vascular capacity to alter CO according to need. Clinically, this is evidenced not only by a reflex tachycardia in response to a decreased BP, but also by venoconstriction to increase blood return to the heart and augment stroke volume. In the opposite situation, an elevated arterial pressure causes the baroreceptors to reset their sensitivity in a way that increases the threshold pressure necessary for baroreceptor activation. This helps to explain why hypertension is not controlled by the baroreceptor response.[26]

The arterial *chemoreceptors,* or aortic bodies, are located in the bifurcation of the aortic arch. They possess a rich capillary blood supply and extensive innervation of the PNS. Their main function is to signal changes in oxygen tension (usually less than 80 mm Hg), a drop in the pH level below 7.40, or a carbon dioxide tension ($PaCO_2$) of greater than 40 mm Hg. Stimulation of the chemoreceptors normally causes an increase in respiratory rate and depth.

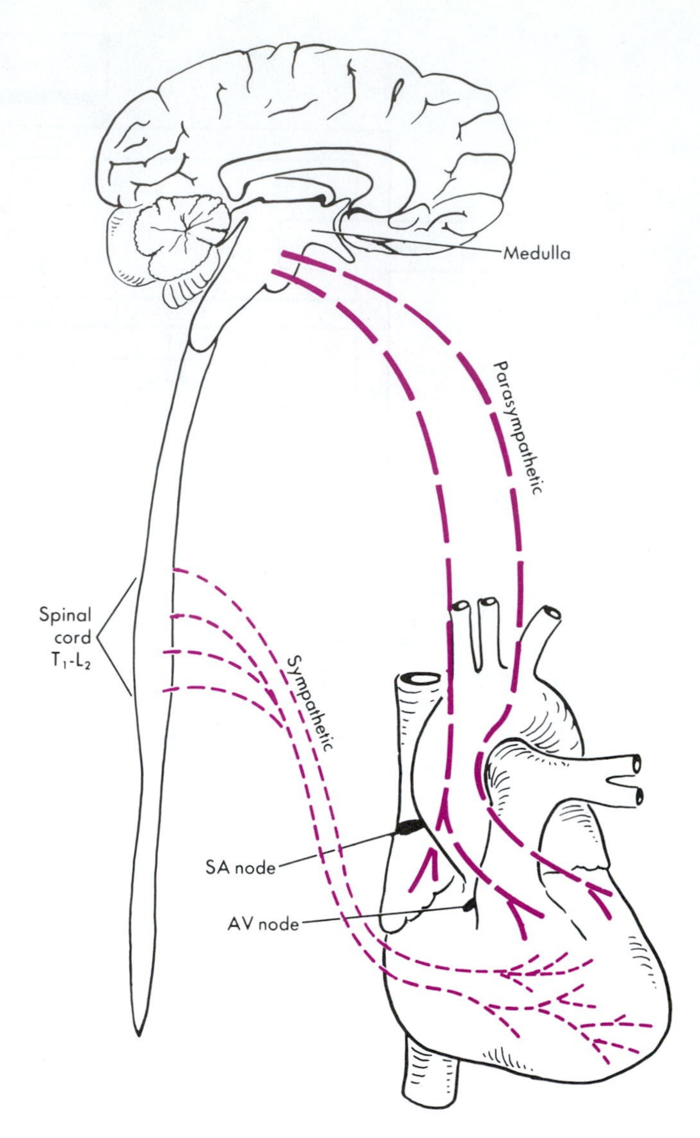

FIGURE 13-29. Autonomic nervous system innervation of nodal tissue and myocardium by parasympathetic vagus nerve fibers and sympathetic chains. (From Quaal S: *Comprehensive intraaortic balloon pumping,* St Louis, 1984, Mosby.)

The *Bainbridge reflex* is attributed to receptors in the right atrium. When the pressure in the right atrium rises sufficiently to stimulate these receptors, it causes a reflex tachycardia. The purpose of this reflex is probably to protect the right side of the heart from an overload state and to quickly equalize filling pressures of the right and left sides of the heart.

Another control mechanism involves *atrial natriuretic factor* (ANF).[27] It is a hormone secreted by the atria in response to increases in atrial pressure. This hormone causes Na^+ and water to be excreted by the kidneys and is also a potent vasodilator. Thus the body rids itself of excess extracellular volume and increases

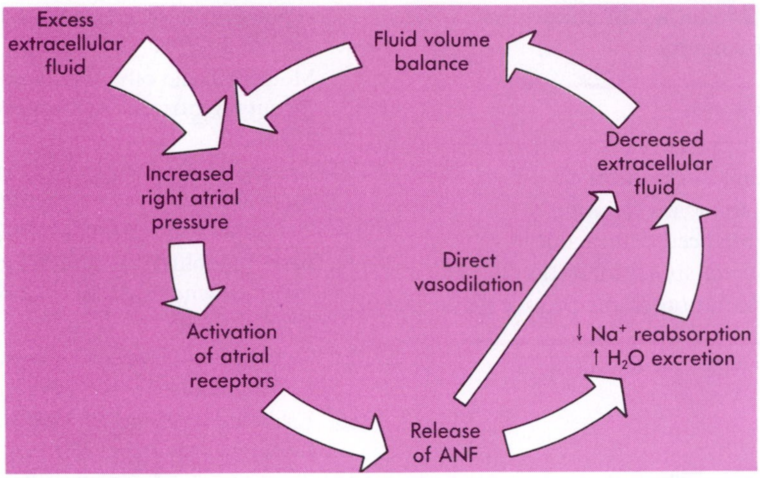

FIGURE 13-30. The atrial natriuretic factor system.

the capacity of the veins to restore total body blood volume. It is possible that ANF is the opposite regulatory mechanism countering the renin-angiotensin system, because the renin-angiotensin system works to conserve Na^+ and water and raise blood pressure (Figure 13-30).

Other reflexes involve the respiratory cycle and its effect on heart rate and stroke volume. Normally the heart rate varies slightly with the respiratory cycle. The heart usually accelerates on inspiration and decelerates with exhalation. Also, left ventricular stroke volume decreases during normal inspiration. There may be so many contributing factors to these phenomena that a single explanation would be inadequate. Possible contributors may include normal fluctuations in sympathetic and vagal tone during respiration, changes in intrathoracic pressure involving increased venous return and the Bainbridge reflex, stretch receptors in the lungs, interactions between the respiratory and cardiac centers in the medulla, increased capacity of the pulmonary vessels during lung inflation, decreased left ventricular compliance resulting from increased right ventricular return, increased impedance to left ventricular outflow related to the pleural pressure changes, or neural reflex mechanisms that are independent of mechanical influences. Thus many complex hemodynamic changes occur throughout the respiratory cycle. Consideration must also be given to underlying lung and cardiac disease, intravascular volume status, respiratory rate, and added effects of mechanical ventilation.

Control of Peripheral Circulation

Intrinsic control. Intrinsic or local control of the peripheral circulation is most influential at the arteriolar level.[26] The arterioles are the major *resistance vessels* because of the amount of smooth muscle in the vessel walls (see Figure 13-12). Although the vascular smooth muscle differs in arrangement and amount in different organ beds, it is still subject to many influences. Because the smooth muscle is normally under dual influence between the vasodilator and vasoconstrictor mechanisms, the arteriole has the potential for either increasing or decreasing its lumen substantially. Several local factors influence this balance. One is pharmacologic stimuli, such as locally released catecholamines, histamine, acetylcholine, serotonin, angiotensin, adenosine, and prostaglandins. These can be initiated by a variety of mechanisms, such as tissue injury, hypoxemia, or hormones. Other factors that influence circulation locally are temperature and carbon dioxide.

Extrinsic control. Extrinsic control is mediated by several mechanisms of the central nervous system. The first is that of the autonomic nervous system and the second that of the vascular reflexes, as discussed.

The autonomic nervous system exerts dual antagonistic control over most organ systems via the sympathetic and parasympathetic fibers. The vasoconstrictor region in the medulla is normally tonically active. Experimentally, the neuronal activity of this region is essential for maintenance of arterial BP and heart rate. Stimulation causes increases in mean

TABLE 13-7 Regions in the Medulla Affecting Cardiovascular Activity

Region	Activity
Dorsal lateral medulla (pressor region)	Vasoconstriction Cardiac acceleration Enhanced contractility
Ventromedial medulla (depressor region)	Direct spinal inhibition Inhibition of the pressor region

arterial pressure and heart rate by enhancing sympathetic outflow and possibly inhibiting PNS outflow. The sympathetic outflow targets the resistance vessels, causing vasoconstriction. Inhibition of these areas causes the opposite effect—vasodilation. Sympathetic fibers causing vasoconstriction supply the arteries, arterioles, and veins. However, the capacitance vessels (veins) are probably more responsive to sympathetic stimulation, but the effects are not as readily observed as are those on the arterial side. Table 13-7 summarizes the sympathetic receptors, including location and effects of stimulation.

Control of peripheral circulation is a combination of intrinsic and extrinsic mechanisms. Additional influences include emotions, temperature, and humoral substances.

REFERENCES

1. Pierce CD: Acute post-MI pericarditis, *J Cardiovasc Nurs* 6(4):46-56, 1992.
2. Ryan TJ and others: ACC/AHA guidelines for the management of patients with acute myocardial infarction: executive summary, *Circulation* 194: 2341-2350, 1996
3. Bayer AS: Infective endocarditis, *Clin Infect Dis* 19(2):368-370, 1994.
4. O'Connell JB, Moore CK, Waterer HC: Treatment of end-stage dilated cardiomyopathy, *Br Heart J* 72(suppl 6):S52-S56, 1994.
5. ACC/AHA Task Force Report: Guidelines for early management of patients with acute myocardial infarction, *J Am Coll Cardiol* 16(2):249-292, 1990.
6. Ling LH and others: Clinical outcome of mitral regurgitation due to flail leaflet, *New Engl J Med* 335(19):1417-1423, 1996.
7. Botteron GW, Smith JM: Quantitative assessment of the spatial organization of atrial fibrillation in the intact human heart, *Circulation* 93(3):513-518, 1996.
8. Wood K: Mechanisms and clinical manifestations of supraventricular tachycardias, *Prog Cardiovasc Nurs* 10(2):3-14, 1995.
9. Moulton L and others: Radiofrequency catheter ablation for supraventricular tachycardia, *Heart Lung* 22(1):3-14, 1995.
10. Craney JM: Radiofrequency catheter ablation of supraventricular tachyarrhythmias: clinical consideration and nursing care, *J Cardiovasc Nurs* 7(3):26-39, 1993
11. Berry V: Wolff-Parkinson-White syndrome and the use of radiofrequency catheter ablation, *Heart Lung* 22(1):15-25, 1995.
12. Cairns JA and others: Coronary thrombolysis, *Chest* 104(suppl 4):401S-423S, 1995.
13. Fishbein MC, Siegel RJ: How big are coronary plaques that rupture? *Circulation* 94(10):2662-2666, 1996.
14. Kar S, Nordlander R: Coronary veins: an alternate route to ischemic myocardium, *Heart Lung* 21(2):148-157, 1992.
15. Molchany CA: Ventricular septal and free wall rupture complicating acute MI, *J Cardiovasc Nurs* 6(4):38-45, 1992.
16. Robinson AW: Common varieties of supraventricular tachycardia: differentiation and dangers, *Heart Lung* 25(5):373-383, 1996.
17. McPherson DD: Three-dimensional arterial imaging, *Scientific American: Science and Medicine* March/April: 22-31, 1996.
18. Schwartz SM, Murry CE, O'Brien ER: Vessel wall response to injury, *Sci Am* March/April:12-21, 1996.
19. Hand HL: Direct and indirect blood pressure measurement for open heart surgery patients: an algorithm, *Crit Care Nurse* 12(6):52-60, 1992.
20. Anderson FD, Cunningham SG, Maloney JP: Indirect blood pressure measurement: a need to reassess, *Am J Crit Care* 2(4):272-277:1993.
21. Winslow EH, Lane LD, Woods RJ: Dangling: a review of relevant physiology, research and practice, *Heart Lung* 24(4):263-272, 1995.
22. Frishman WH, Somnenblick EH: Cardiovascular uses of calcium antagonists. In Messerli FH, editor: *Cardiovascular drug therapy,* ed 2, Philadelphia, 1996, WB Saunders.
23. Näbauer M and others: Regional differences in current density and rate-dependent properties of the transient outward current in subepicardial and subendocardial myocytes of the human left ventricle, *Circulation* 93(2):168-177, 1996.
24. Gan-Xin Y, Antzelevitch C: Cellular basis for the electrocardiographic J wave, *Circulation* 93(2):372-379, 1996.
25. Cash LA: Heart failure from diastolic dysfunction, *DCCN* 15(4):170-177, 1996.
26. Persson PB: Modulation of cardiovascular control mechanisms and their interaction, *Physiol Rev* 76(1):193-244, 1996.
27. Perreault T, Gutkowska J: Role of atrial natriuretic factor in lung physiology and pathology, *Am J Respir Crit Care Med* 151:226-242, 1995.

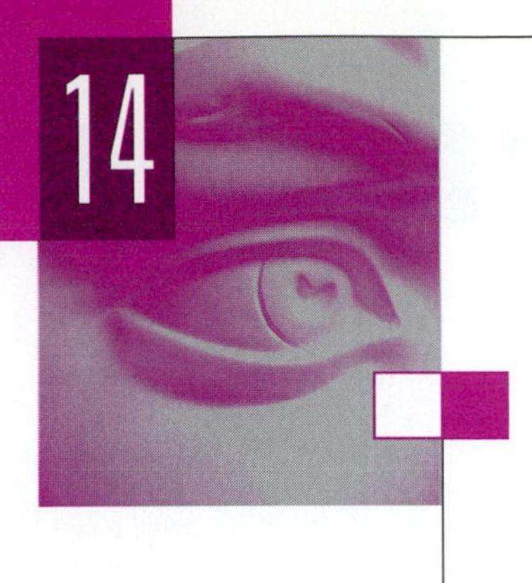

Cardiovascular Clinical Assessment

NOTHING IS MORE valuable to a patient in the critical care unit than a nurse who is proficient in physical assessment, who knows "normal" from "abnormal" appearances or behavior, and who recognizes subtle physical or behavioral changes. The cardiovascular abnormal signs can quickly develop, accelerate, and prove fatal without skilled nursing observation and intervention.

The purpose of this chapter is to demonstrate how the techniques of inspection, palpation, percussion, and auscultation are implemented in the monitoring of cardiovascular patients. Noninvasive assessment of the cardiovascular system provides easily attainable and valuable data on cardiac and vascular status and on any immediate localized or systemic response to treatment. This information, combined with the cardiovascular history and the data from any hemodynamic monitoring equipment, guides patient treatment and preserves the "excellence of care" reputation that critical care units have established.

What this chapter cannot so readily convey is the professional challenge offered by—and commensurate personal satisfaction derived from—becoming proficient with these techniques. The reward is the patient who does not succumb to acute cardiac failure, because new jugular venous distention (JVD) was observed early in his or her course; or the patient whose thrombophlebitis was discovered on a routine midshift vascular examination and treated appropriately, reducing his or her risk for pulmonary embolism.

HISTORY

The patient history is important for providing data that contribute to the cardiovascular diagnosis and the treatment plan, as shown in Box 14-1. It also provides an opportunity to assess baseline cognitive functioning. In the acute care setting, patients with cardiovascular diseases are at risk for changes in cognition caused by both diseases and treatments.[1]

The patient's presenting symptoms or complaints direct the history-taking part of the assessment. Each symptom is further explored with the questions detailed in Table 14-1. For example, the vague complaint of *chest pain* can become "classic angina" when the patient is more specific (e.g., ". . . a midsubsternal pressure that radiates into my jaw and makes me short of breath when I walk more than a block. If I sit down, it goes away in about 5 minutes"). Other symptoms that may be indicative of cardiovascular problems are listed in Box 14-1 under "common cardiovascular symptoms" and must be inquired about, even if the patient does not complain of them.

Box 14-1 also lists the other parts of the patient history, with specific cardiovascular information that must be solicited in each category. Obtaining information about the medical history, current medication usage, and cardiac studies that may have been performed in the past is useful in determining health/illness patterns and treatment of the current medical problem. Taking the time to obtain this information may prevent repetitive tests or ineffective therapy. Cardiac education and rehabilitation is focused on risk factor variables and personal life-style choices (patient profile) that place the patient at continued risk for cardiovascular disease.

PHYSICAL EXAMINATION

Inspection

The degree to which the body proclaims its condition is surprisingly explicit. To the educated observer,

BOX 14-1

COMMON CARDIOVASCULAR SYMPTOMS

Chest pains
Palpitations
Dyspnea
Cough
Nocturia
Edema
Dizziness/syncope/visual changes
Claudication/extremity pain or parasthesis
Fatigue

PATIENT PROFILE

Baseline cognitive functioning
Personal habits
 Use of tea, coffee, alcohol, recreational drugs; over-the-counter drug use; smoking; exercise; dietary habits
Life-style pattern
 Working, relaxing, coping, cultural habits
Recent life changes
 Within the past 12 months
Emotional state
 Evidence of psychologic stress, anger, anxiety, depression
Perception of illness and its meaning for the future

RISK FACTORS

Gender/age
Family history of premature CHD
Smoking history
Hypertension
Lipid disorders
Sedentary life-style
Diabetes mellitus
Obesity

FAMILY HISTORY

Coronary artery disease at < age 55 yrs
Myocardial infarction
Hypertension
Stroke
Diabetes mellitus
Lipid disorders
Collagen vascular disease

CARDIAC STUDIES OR INTERVENTIONS IN PAST

Cardiac catheterization
Cardiac ultrasound
ECG
Exercise tolerance test
Myocardial imaging with radiographic isotopes
Percutaneous transluminal coronary angioplasty
Atherectomy
Stent placement
Valvuloplasty

MEDICAL HISTORY

Childhood
 Murmurs, cyanosis, streptococcal infections, rheumatic fever
Adult
 Heart failure, coronary artery disease, heart valve disease, mitral valve prolapse, myocardial infarction, peripheral vascular disease, diabetes mellitus, hypertension, hyperlipidemia, dysrhythmias, murmurs, endocarditis, psychiatric illnesses, thrombophlebitis, deep vein thrombosis, systemic or pulmonary emboli
Allergies
 Especially to radiographic contrast agents or iodine
 Surgical history
 Coronary artery bypass grafting, valve replacement, peripheral vascular bypasses or repairs, pacemaker, defibrillator implants
 Recent dental work or infection

CURRENT MEDICATION USAGE

Anticoagulants
Antidysrhythmics
Antihypertensives
Antiplatelets
Beta-blockers
Calcium channel blockers
Cholesterol lowering agents
Digitalis
Diuretics
Hormones
Nitrates
Oral contraceptives
Potassium

CHD, Congestive heart disease.

skin color, body posture, and facial expression speak volumes in the absence of a single word from the patient. Inspection of the cardiovascular system focuses on the patient's general appearance—face, extremities, neck, thorax, and abdomen. Although experience eventually allows one to inspect the patient in a more spontaneous, less compartmentalized fashion, attending to each area suggested ensures the comprehensiveness of the inspection.

General appearance and face. The weight in proportion to the height is assessed to determine whether the patient is obese (a cardiac risk factor) or cachectic (which can indicate chronic heart failure). The face is observed for the color of the skin (cyanotic,

TABLE 14-1 Clarification of Symptoms by Asking Specific Questions

Determine	Typical Question
Location, radiation	Where is it? Does it move or stay in one place?
Quality	What's it like?
Quantity	How severe is it? How frequent? How long does it last?
Chronology	When did it begin? How has it progressed?
Aggravating and alleviating factors	What are you doing when it occurs? What do you do to get rid of it?
Associated findings	Are there any other symptoms you feel at the same time?
Treatment sought and effect	Have you seen a physician in the past for this same problem? What was the treatment?

pale, or jaundiced) and expressions of apprehension or pain. Body posture can indicate the amount of effort it takes to breathe or the position of comfort the patient chooses (e.g., sitting upright to breathe may be necessary with acute heart failure or leaning forward may be the least painful position for the patient with pericarditis).[2] The patient is observed for diaphoresis, confusion, or lethargy, each of which could indicate hypotension or low cardiac output. It is important to systematically inspect the skin, lips, tongue, mucous membranes, and conjunctiva for hydration, pallor, or cyanosis. Central cyanosis is a bluish discoloration of these areas and the nailbeds. It indicates circulation of a significant amount of "reduced" (unsaturated with oxygen) arterial hemoglobin as a result of right-to-left intracardiac shunting, impaired pulmonary function, or hypoxia from any cause.[2] It must be recognized and treated as a medical emergency. Pulse oximetry, arterial blood gas analysis, and treatment with 100% oxygen must be instituted immediately.[3] Multiracial studies indicate that the tongue is the most sensitive site for observation of cyanosis.[3] Box 14-2 summarizes the necessary information to obtain from the initial inspection of the patient.

BOX 14-2 Inspection of the Cardiovascular System
General appearance and face

GENERAL APPEARANCE

Weight
Nutritional status
Position of comfort
Color of skin

FACE

Expression
Emotional state
Presence of diaphoresis
Color of lips
Color of mucous membranes/tongue
Color of conjunctiva

Extremities. The nailbeds are inspected for clubbing and also for cyanosis. Peripheral cyanosis indicates reduction of peripheral blood flow as a result of vascular disease or decreased cardiac output and is usually seen in the nailbeds or the tip of the nose.[2]

Clubbing of the nailbeds is associated with central cyanosis as a sign of chronic oxygen deficiency. Clubbing is evaluated by assessing the angle between the nail and the nail base, which is normally less than 180 degrees. A flattened angle (180 degrees) with a springy or spongy nail base is "early" clubbing, and an angle greater than 180 degrees with a swollen nail base is "late" clubbing.

The extremities yield multiple signs of vascular disease. The parameters to be assessed are hair loss (sparse or lacking), skin texture (shiny, dry, cracked, or ulcerated), temperature (cool or warm), color (pale, dusky, or hyperpigmented), and the presence of edema. With arterial insufficiency, pallor is present when the legs are elevated. With venous thrombosis, the color of the extremity may be dusky and the circumference of the affected calf or thigh may be slightly larger compared with the other extremity.[4] The lower extremities are specifically inspected for varicosities that may predispose a patient to thrombophlebitis and/or require the patient to undergo special venous radiographic studies if coronary artery bypass grafting were needed. Table 14-2 lists the specific information to be obtained through inspection of the extremities and separates the abnormal findings into arterial or venous disease etiologies.

Neck. The jugular veins of the neck are inspected for a noninvasive estimate of intravascular volume

TABLE 14-2 Inspection and Palpation of Extremities: Comparison of Arterial and Venous Disease

Characteristics	Arterial Disease	Venous Disease
Hair loss	Present	Absent
Skin texture	Thin, shiny, dry	Flaking, stasis, dermatitis, mottled
Ulceration	Located at pressure points; painful, pale, dry with little drainage; well-demarcated with eschar or dried; surrounded by fibrous tissue; granulation tissue scant and pale	Usually at the ankle; painless, pinkish, moist with large drainage; irregular, dry and scaly; surrounded by dermatitis; granulation tissue healthy
Skin color	Elevational pallor, dependent rubor	Brawny, brown, cyanotic when down
Nails	Thick, brittle	Normal
Varicose veins	Absent	Present
Temperature	Cool	Warm
Capillary refill	> 3 seconds	< 3 seconds
Edema	None or mild, usually unilateral	Usually present foot to calf, unilateral or bilateral
Pulses	Weak or absent (0 to 1+)	Normal, strong and symmetrical

Modified from Krenzer ME: *AACN Clin Issues* 6(4):631, 1995.

and/or pressure. The bilateral external jugular veins are observed for the presence or absence of jugular vein distention (JVD). The right internal jugular vein pulsation is used to estimate jugular venous pressure (JVP), which can be extrapolated to estimate central venous pressure (CVP).

External jugular vein. Normally, at a trunk elevation higher than 30 degrees, the external jugular veins are nondistended. Jugular venous distention occurs when central venous pressure is elevated, as it is with right ventricular failure. To assess for JVD with the patient sitting up, first identify the external jugular veins bilaterally (Figure 14-1). Once identified, release the pressure and observe for true fullness (distention). Because inhalation decreases venous pressure, JVD is assessed at the end of exhalation. In the recumbent position (Figure 14-2), the external jugular veins are always distended, and the examiner simply elevates the trunk of the patient to determine the degree of elevation required to eliminate their visibility.[5] Generally, the higher the sitting angle of the patient with JVD, the higher the central venous pressure. This finding is reported by including the angle of the head of the bed at the time JVD was appreciated (e.g., "presence of JVD with head of bed elevated to 45 degrees").

Finding JVD during inspection of the neck veins can contribute to a cardiac failure diagnosis and help explain other findings of the physical examination, like shortness of breath, diaphoresis, or confusion. If JVD appears acutely, prompt treatment to reduce volume

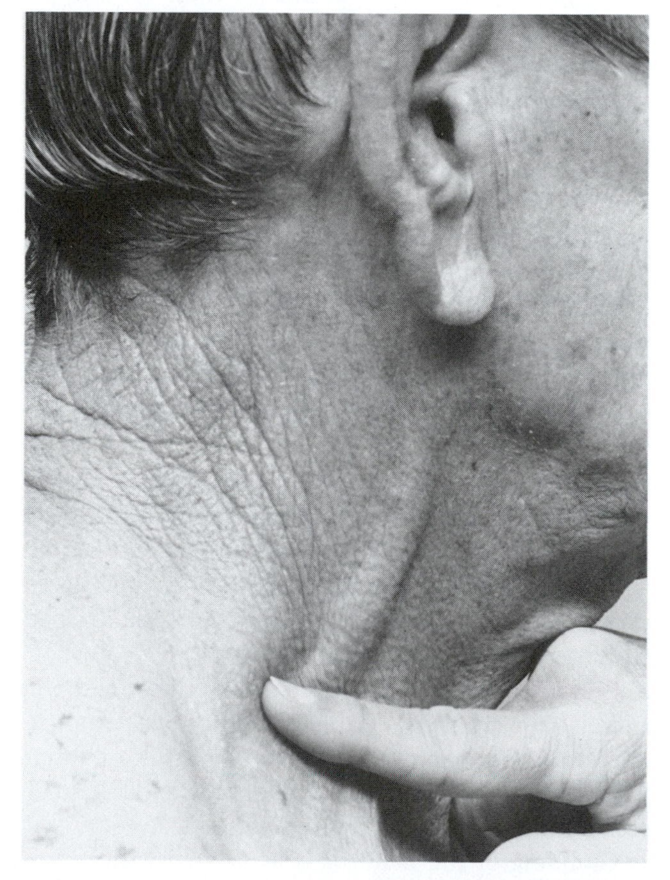

FIGURE 14-1. Assessment of jugular vein distention (JVD). Applying light finger pressure over the sternocleidomastoid muscle, parallel to the clavicle, helps identify the external jugular vein by occluding flow and distending it. Release the finger pressure and observe for true distention. *If the patient's trunk is elevated to 30 degrees or more JVD should not be present.*

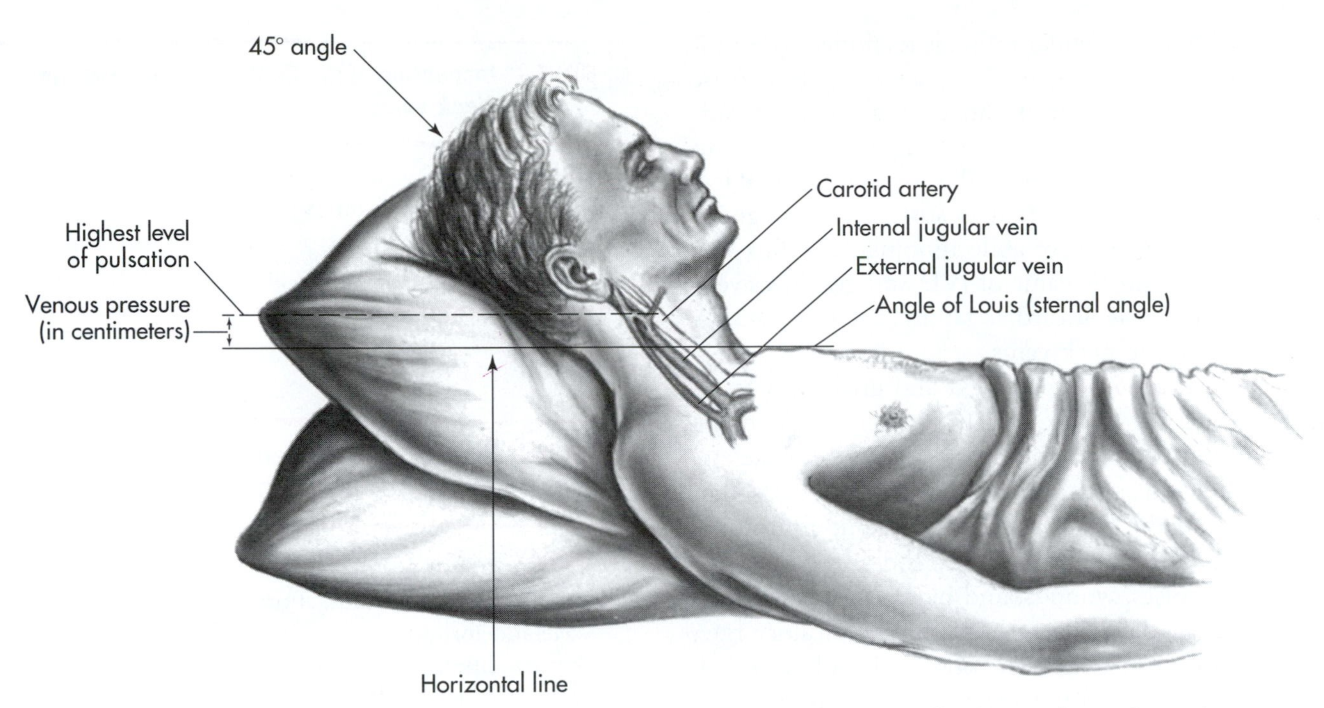

FIGURE 14-2. Position of internal and external jugular veins. Pulsation in the internal jugular vein can be used to estimate central venous pressure. (Modified from Thompson JM and others: *Mosby's clinical nursing,* ed 4, St Louis, 1997, Mosby.)

or pressure overload may prevent deterioration into acute ventricular failure.

Internal jugular vein. The pulsation of the internal jugular vein can be used to evaluate jugular venous pressure. This vein lies anterior to the external jugular at the level of the clavicle and follows a parallel path with the carotid artery and the trachea (see Figure 14-2). On the right side, it is directly in line with the right atrium and reflects the mean right arterial pressure or central venous pressure, thus giving a good indication of the patient's intravascular volume status.[6]

The procedure for examining the internal jugular vein pulsation and evaluating the JVP is as follows: examine the patient in a well-lit room, stand on the patient's right side, and turn the patient's head slightly toward the left. The head must be supported to relax the neck muscles. The patient's trunk must be elevated as high as necessary to visualize the top of the column of blood in the internal jugular vein (30 to 40 degrees above the horizontal position for patients with normal pressures). The highest point of pulsation in the internal jugular vein is observed during exhalation. The vertical distance between this pulsation, which is at the top of the fluid level, and the sternal angle (angle of Louis) is estimated in centimeters (see Figure 14-2). The normal level of the JVP is 4 cm or less. Elevated JVP (more than 4 cm) reflects an increased CVP.[6] The degree of elevation of the patient's trunk is included when reporting this finding (e.g., "JVP estimated at 8 cm with the head of the bed elevated 45 degrees").

It is clinically understood that to convert JVP to an estimated CVP, the examiner would add 5 cm to account for the distance of the sternal angle above the level of the midright atrium. The upper limit of normal for estimated CVP is 9 cm (JVP of 4 cm plus 5 cm). The right internal jugular vein pulsation wave can also be used (an advanced skill) to provide additional information about right-sided cardiac conduction, function, and tricuspid valve status.

Abdominojugular reflux. Right-sided cardiac failure is one cause of elevated central venous pressure. Noninvasive confirmation of cardiac failure can be achieved by performing a bedside test called the *abdominojugular reflux test.* It consists of observing the JVP in the right internal jugular vein before, during, and after midabdominal compression for 15 to 30 seconds. The patient is asked to relax and breathe normally through an open mouth. Firm pressure of approximately 20 to 35 mm Hg, if a blood pressure cuff bladder is placed between the examiner's hand and the abdomen, is applied to the midabdomen. Pressure on the abdomen causes increased venous return to the right atrium. If the heart is failing, it cannot pump away the extra volume of blood.[5] If the patient tenses or holds his or her breath, there is an increased venous return to the heart and the test may be falsely positive. A positive abdominojugular reflux is identified when abdominal compression causes a sustained JVP increase of 4 cm or more.[6] The negative or normal abdominojugular reflux includes no rise in JVP, a transient (less than 10 seconds) rise in JVP, or a rise in JVP less than or equal to 3 cm that is sustained throughout compression.[6] A positive abdominojugular reflux improves the diagnostic value of JVD and, noninvasively, aides the diagnosis of cardiac failure. See Box 14-3 for inspection of the neck veins.

Thorax and abdomen. The next and final areas of inspection are the thorax and the abdomen. Both the anterior and posterior thorax are assessed for skeletal deformities (e.g., pectus excavatum, straight back) that may displace the heart and cause systolic murmurs.[2] The skin on the chest wall and the abdomen is checked for scars, bruises, wounds, and bulges associated with pacemaker or defibrillator implants. Respiratory rate, pattern, and effort are also observed and recorded. Refer to Box 14-4 for inspection of the thorax and abdomen.

Thoracic reference points. The thoracic cage is divided with imaginary vertical lines (sternal, midclavicular, axillary, vertebral, and scapular), and the intercostal spaces (ICSs) are divided with horizontal lines to serve as reference points in locating or describing cardiac findings (Figure 14-3). The ribs are numbered from 1 (the first rib below the clavicle) to 12. The intercostal space between each rib is numbered the same as the rib that lies above it. The second rib is the easiest to locate, because it is attached to the sternum at the angle of Louis. This angle (also called the *sternal angle*) is the bony ridge on the sternum that lies approximately 2 inches below the sternal notch (see Figure 14-3, *A*). Once the second rib has been located, it can be used as a reference point to count off the other ribs and intercostal spaces.

Apical impulse. The anterior thorax must also be inspected for the apical impulse, sometimes referred to as the *point of maximal impulse (PMI)*. The apical impulse occurs as the left ventricle contracts during systole and rotates forward, causing the left ventricular apex to hit the chest wall. The impulse is a quick, localized (2×2 cm), outward movement normally located just lateral to the left midclavicular line at the 5th intercostal space in the adult patient (Figure 14-4). The apical impulse is the only normal pulsation visualized on the chest wall, and—if visible—the location, size, and character are noted. The rest of the anterior thorax is inspected for abnormal pulsations that can indicate cardiac enlargement (e.g., a visible pulsation in the left parasternal region suggests right ventricular enlargement). The abdomen is also inspected for normal pulsations of the aorta, commonly seen in the epigastric area (see Figure 14-4). For a summary of the thoracic and abdominal areas of inspection, see Box 14-4.

BOX 14-3 Inspection of the Cardiovascular System
Neck veins

External jugular vein for JVD
Internal jugular vein for JVP
Abdominojugular reflux test for confirmation of right-sided ventricular failure

BOX 14-4 Inspection of the Cardiovascular System
Thorax and abdomen

THORAX

Respiratory rate, rhythm, effort
Skeletal deformities
Skin condition (scars, bruises, wounds)
Presence of pacemaker generator
Apical impulse
Abnormal pulsations

ABDOMEN

Skin conditions (scars, bruises, wounds)
Abdominal aortic pulsation
Presence of implantable cardioverter defibrillator (ICD)

Palpation

Palpation is a technique that uses the sense of touch. The fingertips are sensitive to pressure, the backs of the fingers are sensitive to temperature, and the base of the fingers on the palmar side—as well as the lateral edge of the palm—are sensitive to pressure and vibrations. Palpation is done with a light touch and an unhurried, relaxed approach. Palpation is used to assess pulsations in the extremities, neck, thorax, and abdomen. Palpation is also used to assess the presence and amount of edema, the temperature of the skin, and capillary refill. The information obtained with palpation reinforces data collected with inspection and is especially important for the assessment of the vascular system (see Table 14-2).

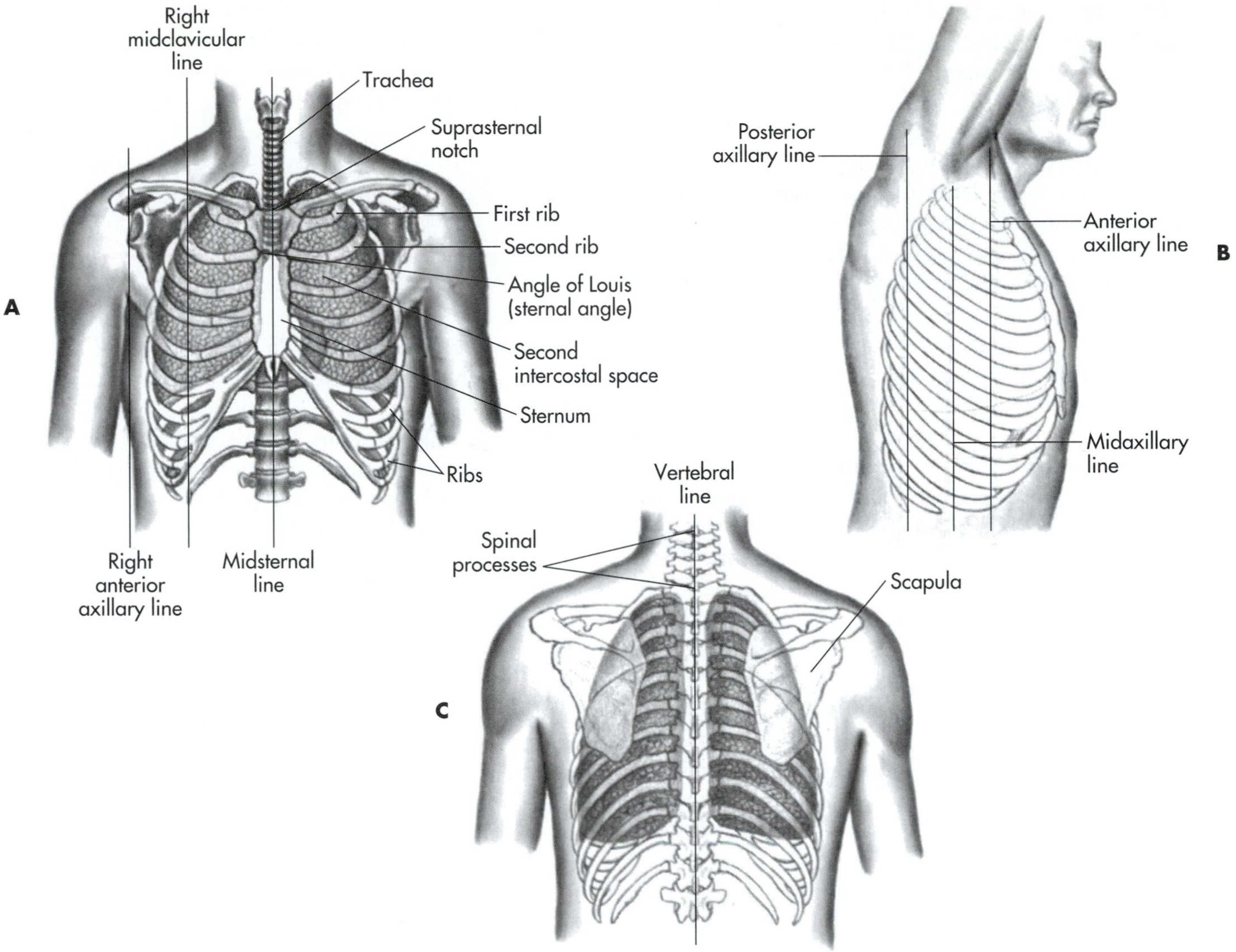

Right
midclavicular
line
Trachea
Suprasternal
notch
First rib
Second rib
Angle of Louis
(sternal angle)
Second
intercostal space
Sternum
Ribs
Right
anterior
axillary line
Midsternal
line
A
Posterior
axillary line
Anterior
axillary line
B
Midaxillary
line
Vertebral
line
Spinal
processes
Scapula
C

FIGURE 14-3. Thoracic landmarks. **A,** Anterior thorax. **B,** Right lateral thorax. **C,** Posterior thorax.

Pulmonic area
Aortic area
Erb's point
Parasternal areas
Right and left
sternal borders
Apical impulse
Mitral area
G.J.Wassilchenko
Epigastric area
Tricuspid area

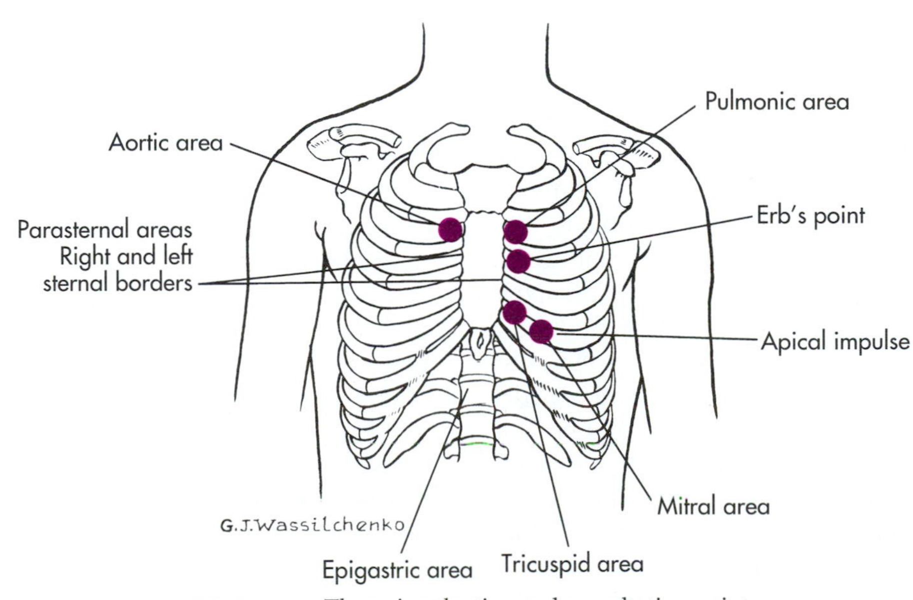

FIGURE 14-4. Thoracic palpation and auscultation points.

Arterial pulsations. Seven major arterial areas are assessed for pulse palpation. The examination incorporates bilateral assessment of the carotid, brachial, radial, ulnar, popliteal, dorsalis pedis, and posterior tibial arteries. The extremity pulses are assessed separately and compared bilaterally to check for consistency. Pulse volume is graded on a pulse assessment scale. An example of such a scale, which ranges from 0 to 3+ , is shown in Box 14-5. A diminished or absent pulse may indicate the presence of arterial stenosis or occlusion proximal to the site of the examination. An abnormally strong or bounding pulse suggests the presence of an aneurysm or an occlusion distal to the examination site.[4]

Upper extremities. The radial and the brachial arteries are palpated for pulse quality in the upper extremities. These same arteries also are often punctured or cannulated for arterial blood gas specimens. It is imperative to assess the pulse quality frequently when the artery is cannulated, as well as assessing the color, temperature, and pulse quality distal to the cannulated site. Occlusion of arterial blood flow is reflected by the absence of a pulse and/or coolness and pallor of the distal extremity.

Allen test. Before a radial artery is punctured or cannulated, the Allen test is done to assess adequate blood flow to the hand through the ulnar artery. If the patient is alert and cooperative, the procedure is as follows:

1. The patient is requested to make a tight fist to squeeze the blood out of his or her hand.
2. The radial artery is compressed with firm thumb pressure by the examiner.
3. The patient is requested to open the hand, palm side up, while the radial artery is still occluded.
4. The time it takes for the color to return to the hand is noted.

If the ulnar artery is patent, the color will return within 3 seconds. Delayed color return (a "failed" Allen test) implies that the ulnar artery is occluded; therefore the radial artery is the only source of blood flow to the hand and must not be punctured or cannulated.

If the patient is unable to cooperate, an alternative approach is to use a pulse oximeter that displays a pulse waveform.[7] With the photodetector of the pulse oximeter attached to the middle finger and an adequate pulse amplitude displayed on the monitor, simultaneously compress the radial and ulnar arteries until the waveform clearly decreases or vanishes. Release pressure off the ulnar artery only. If the ulnar artery is patent, the pulse amplitude recovers its normal appearance (a slightly lower amplitude can also be considered normal) and indicates adequate blood supply to the hand; therefore arterial catheterization of the radial artery can be accomplished safely.[7]

BOX 14-5 Pulse Palpation Scale

SCALE	DESCRIPTION
0	Not palpable
1+	Faintly palpable (weak and thready)
2+	Palpable (normal pulse)
3+	Bounding (hyperdynamic pulse)

Capillary refill. Capillary refill assessment is a maneuver done on the nailbeds to evaluate arterial circulation to the extremity. The nailbed is compressed to produce blanching, and release of the pressure should result in a return of blood flow and nail color in less than 3 seconds. The severity of arterial insufficiency is directly proportional to the amount of time necessary to reestablish flow and color.

Lower extremities. The lower extremity pulses are the most difficult to locate—the popliteal pulses perhaps the most elusive. The popliteal pulses are found behind the knee, deep in the popliteal fossa, just lateral of the midline. The knee can be bent slightly to gain easier access to this area. The knee can be bent slightly to gain easier access to this area. The posterior tibial pulses are located behind the medial malleolus, and the dorsalis pedis pulses are located on the dorsal areas of the feet, usually just lateral to the extensor tendon of the great toe. The lightest touch, with at least three fingertips, and systematic movement across the top of the foot help to locate the dorsalis pedis. The dorsalis pedis and the posterior tibial pulses may be congenitally absent, but their presence is not entirely ruled out until they are checked with the patient's extremity in the dependent position. Box 14-6 lists the important points of palpation for both the upper and lower extremities.

Edema. Edema is fluid accumulated in the extravascular spaces of the body, such as the abdomen and the dependent tissues of the legs and sacrum. One must note whether the edema is dependent, unilateral or bilateral, and pitting or nonpitting. The amount of edema is quantified by measuring the circumference of the limb or by pressing the skin of the feet, ankles, and shins against the underlying bone. If an impression is left in the tissue when the thumb is removed, it is called *pitting edema.* A patient with ventricular failure may gain 10 pounds or

BOX 14-6 Palpation of the Cardiovascular System
Upper and lower extremities

UPPER EXTREMITIES

Brachial pulses
Radial pulses
Temperature
Capillary refill

LOWER EXTREMITIES

Popliteal pulses
Posterior tibial pulses
Dorsalis pedis pulses
Edema of feet, ankles, shins
Presence of phlebitis

BOX 14-7 Pitting Edema Scale

SCALE	DESCRIPTION	DEPTH OF INDENTATION	TIME TO RETURN TO BASELINE
0	None present	0	—
1+	Trace	0-1/4″ (< 6.4 mm)	Rapid
2+	Mild	1/4-1/2″ (6.4-12.8 mm)	10-15 sec
3+	Moderate	1/2-1″ (12.8 mm-2.5 cm)	1-2 min
4+	Severe	> 1″ (> 2.5 cm)	2-5 min

more of excess fluid before pitting is noted. Liver or renal failure and venous insufficiency with venous stasis can also cause pitting edema in the lower extremities. There is no universally agreed upon scale for pitting edema. An example of one scale is shown in Box 14-7.

Thrombophlebitis and deep vein thrombosis. The veins of the lower extremities are assessed with palpation, specifically for thrombophlebitis, which is an inflammation of the vein with thrombus formation. Squeezing or pressing the calves against the tibia may elicit pain, tenderness, increased firmness, or tension in the muscle. These signs suggest phlebitis and should alert the examiner to check other parameters that may aid in diagnosis, such as comparing leg circumferences and checking for increased heat in the extremity, unexplained fever, or tachycardia. Also, Homan's sign, in the presence of the other signs, can assist in the diagnosis of phlebitis.[5] To elicit Homan's sign, the examiner flexes the patient's knee and forcefully and abruptly dorsiflexes the patient's foot. The sign is positive when pain is reported in the popliteal region and the calf.

Deep vein phlebitis or deep vein thrombosis (DVT) predisposes a patient to pulmonary emboli and chronic venous insufficiency. Although fewer than 50% of patients with DVT have signs or symptoms, nearly 1 in 10 patients with DVT develops pulmonary embolus; therefore detection of DVT is important.[4] Symptoms that may indicate DVT include intermittent or constant pain, tenderness, and a tight or heavy sensation in the affected extremity. Patients considered at risk for DVT include those hospitalized with heart disease, those with a history of DVT, and those older than 40 years who have had major surgery or myocardial infarction.[8]

Carotid pulses. The carotid pulses are assessed by palpation for cardiac rate and rhythm and also for the amplitude and contour of the pulsation. Normally there is a swift upstroke to this pulse, with a slight rounded plateau at its peak and a gradual descent (Figure 14-5). With an increased pulse pressure (the difference between the systolic and diastolic blood pressure readings), the carotid pulse is large and "bounding" and the descending portion of the wave is as rapid as the upstroke. Hyperdynamic states such as fever, anxiety, hyperthyroidism, anemia, and exercise can cause this type of waveform. Aortic insufficiency, because of the rapid runoff of blood through the incompetent valve, also can create a bounding carotid pulse. Conditions causing decreased cardiac output (aortic stenosis, ventricular failure, or hypotension) create a small wave with an upstroke as gradual as the descent. If the carotid pulse is regular and alternates between large and small waves with every other wave being small, it is called *pulsus alternans.* Pulsus alternans is evidence of left-ventricular failure[2] (see Figure 14-5).

If blood flow through the carotid arteries is compromised at all by arteriosclerosis or plaque, palpation could easily cause total occlusion; thus only one carotid artery at a time is palpated. Also, the carotid arteries are palpated in the lower half of the neck, well below the level of the carotid bodies, which—when stimulated—cause a decrease in heart rate.

Thorax. The chest wall is palpated for the apical impulse described previously. Its location, size, amplitude, and duration are recorded. An enlarged left ventricle

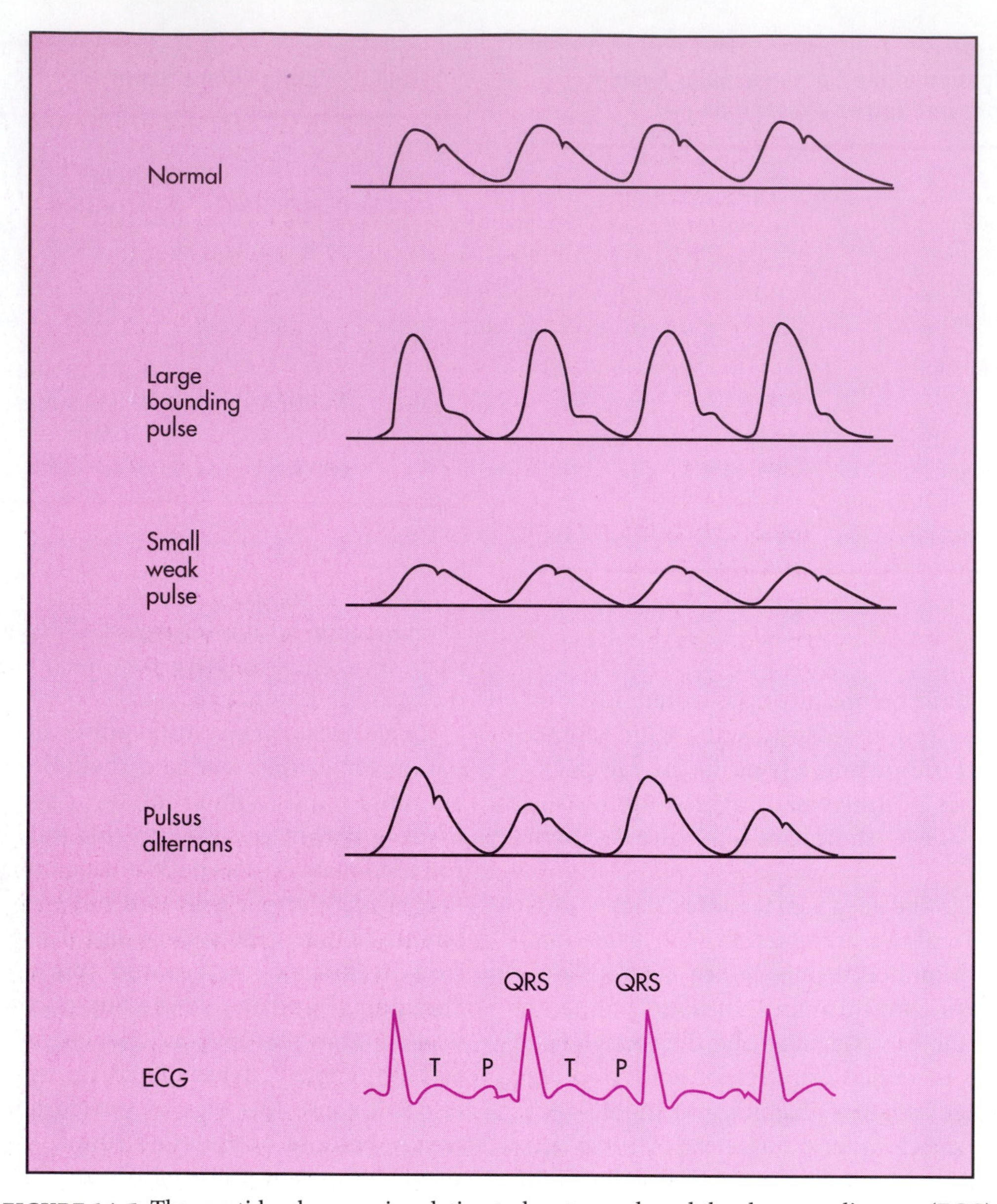

FIGURE 14-5. The carotid pulse wave in relation to heart sounds and the electrocardiogram (ECG).

(left ventricular hypertrophy secondary to ventricular failure or hypertension) is suspected when the apical impulse is enlarged (greater than 2 cm) and is displaced laterally. When the apical impulse is difficult to locate, the patient can be turned to the left lateral decubitus position. This facilitates palpation of the impulse, because the left ventricle is against the chest wall in the left lateral position. Although this makes palpation of the apical impulse easier, it may also distort the placement and size of the impulse—limitations the examiner must consider.[9] Once the apical impulse has been examined, the entire precordium (the chest area overlying the heart and great vessels) must be assessed for other pulsations. The precordial areas are labeled primarily for auscultation, and the locations are situated where the sounds originating from the valves are best heard (see Figures 14-4 and 14-6): the primary and secondary (Erb's point) aortic areas at the 2nd right intercostal space and 3rd left ICS adjacent to the sternum, respectively; the pulmonic area in the 2nd left ICS; the tricuspid area in the 4th and 5th ICSs adjacent to the left sternal border; and the mitral area, at the 4th and 5th ICSs midclavicular line, where the apical impulse occurs. Each area is palpated in a systematic fashion.

The terminology used to communicate palpatory findings must describe as accurately as possible the sensation the examiner feels. Generally, accepted ter-

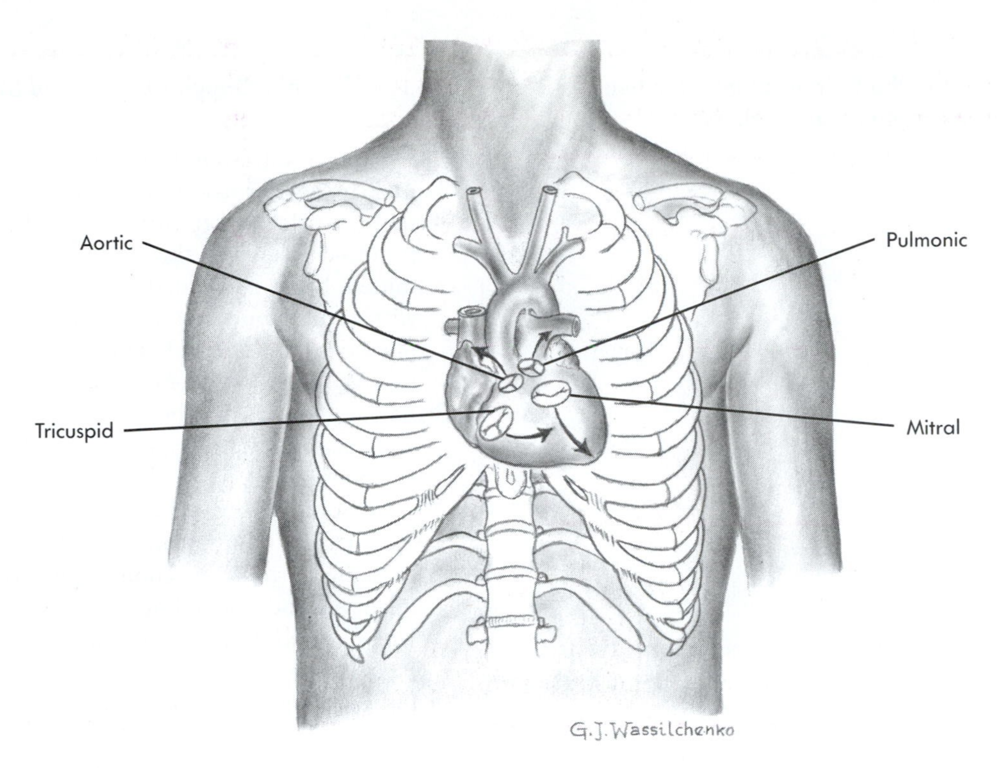

FIGURE 14-6. Transmission of heart sounds to the thorax and their relationship to the anatomic position of the heart valves.

minology refers to "thrusts" as localized and "heaves" or "lifts" as more diffuse movements. For example, right ventricular enlargement can cause a left parasternal "heave," and cor pulmonale—with both right atrial and right ventricular enlargement—can cause a sternal "lift." Left ventricular hypertrophy usually causes an apical "thrust." The paradoxical movement, or "heave," associated with ventricular aneurysm at the apex is often first detected by palpation. "Thrills" are vibrations that feel similar to a cat's purr and are associated with loud murmurs. Palpation of a thrill in the aortic area may indicate aortic stenosis or hypertension.[9] Description of location, amplitude, duration, direction (inward or outward), distribution (localized or diffuse), and timing in the cardiac cycle (systole or diastole) are helpful for determining the cause of a pulsation.

Abdomen. The abdomen is palpated for the pulsations of the femoral arteries and the abdominal aortic artery. The femoral arteries are palpated by pressing deeply into the groin beneath the inguinal ligament, approximately midway between the anterior superior iliac spine and the symphysis pubis on both the right and left sides.

The aortic pulsation is normally located in the epigastric area (see Figure 14-4) and can be felt as a forward movement by using firm fingertip pressure above the umbilicus. If the pulsation is prominent or diffuse, it may indicate an abdominal aneurysm. The normal width of the aorta is approximately the width of the patient's own thumb. To estimate aortic width, lay two to three fingers on one side of the aorta and the thumb, of the same hand, on the other side. Compare that width to the patient's thumb. A widened aorta also may indicate an aortic aneurysm.[4] Refer to Box 14-8 for specifics of palpation of the neck, precordium, and abdomen.

Percussion

Percussion may be used in the cardiac physical examination to outline the left cardiac border. The apical impulse, however, located by inspection and palpation, is more reliable in determining the size of the left ventricle and is more quickly assessed.

Auscultation

Auscultation is used for blood pressure measurement, detection of carotid and femoral bruits, and assessment of normal and abnormal heart sounds and murmurs. Many good references are available for detailed study of heart sounds and murmurs.[2,5,10-13] The following information introduces the normal heart sounds and the ventricular filling sounds that are abnormal when associated with cardiac dysfunction,

BOX 14-8 Palpation of the Cardiovascular System
Neck, precordium, and abdomen

NECK

Carotid pulses

PRECORDIUM

Apical impulse
Other chest pulsations (lifts, thrusts, heaves, thrills)

ABDOMEN

Femoral pulses
Abdominal aortic pulse

BOX 14-9 Use of a Doppler Ultrasound Stethoscope

The Doppler ultrasound stethoscope is a valuable tool in vascular assessment. Doppler ultrasonography, a velocity detector, detects the shift in ultrasound frequency that results when the transmitted beam is reflected off moving particles within the blood vessels. Doppler ultrasonography can detect arterial signals in a vessel with a pressure as low as 20 mm Hg.

Signals are generated by both arteries and veins, each with distinct characteristic patterns. Normal peripheral arteries have a biphasic or triphasic pulsatile sound. With a partially obstructed sound, one or more components are lost, but it remains pulsatile. A normal venous signal is a low frequency sound resembling a windstorm that varies with respiration. Venous signals can be absent during Valsalva maneuver. A positive Doppler signal indicates presence of blood flow but not adequacy of perfusion.

To use the Doppler ultrasound stethoscope, liberally apply ultrasound gel to the pulse point. Insert the tip of the probe into the gel at a 45-60 degree angle to the blood vessel, applying light pressure. Ultrasound waves do not pass through air, so use adequate gel to exclude air. Water soluble lubricating gel can be substituted, but never use electrocardiograph electrode gel, because it will damage the probe. Activate the stethoscope by turning it on or pressing the activation button.

From Krenzer ME: *AACN Clin Issues Crit Care Nurs* 6(4):631, 1995.

reduced compliance, or valvular disease. Murmurs are presented in the broad categories of systolic and diastolic occurrence. The murmurs most commonly occurring subsequent to a myocardial infarction are discussed in more detail. The extracardiac murmur of the pericardial friction rub is also discussed, because it often occurs in the critical care setting and can be easily treated when properly identified.

Vasculature. Using a stethoscope and sphygmomanometer or Doppler ultrasound stethoscope (Box 14-9), a blood pressure measurement is performed on the brachial arteries bilaterally. The inflatable bag of the sphygmomanometer cuff needs to be 20% wider than the diameter of the limb being measured and long enough to encircle the limb.

Cuffs that are too small can give falsely high readings, and cuffs that are too large can give falsely low readings. Normally the blood pressure between both arms varies only 5 to 10 mm Hg. A difference of 20 mm Hg or more suggests arterial compression or obstruction on the side with the lower pressure. Clearly document asymmetry, so that all subsequent measurements are made on the arm with the higher pressure.[4] *Pulsus alternans,* an alternating pulse amplitude previously discussed in the carotid artery section (see also Figure 14-5), can also be auscultated. The pulse sounds alternate between loud and soft. If the variation is slight, auscultation may be the only method of detection.

Pulsus paradoxus is another abnormality of the arterial pulse that is frequently only detected by sphygmomanometry. Pulsus paradoxus is a greater than 10 mm Hg difference in the systolic blood pressure heard during expiration that is heard during both inspiration and expiration. The pulse normally diminishes 5 to 10 mm Hg during inspiration because the increased negative intrathoracic pressure delays pulmonary venous return to the left side of the heart and stroke volume is reduced. Any restrictive pulmonary or cardiac disease, like pulmonary emboli or acute cardiac tamponade, can exaggerate this normal response to respiration and cause pulsus paradoxus. To auscultate for pulsus paradoxus, have the patient breathe normally (quietly) and inflate the cuff above the systolic pressure. Lower the cuff pressure slowly toward the systolic level and note the pressure reading when the first sound is heard during expiration. Continue to drop the pressure very slowly until sound can be heard throughout the respiratory cycle. Again note the pressure reading. If the readings are greater than 10 mm Hg apart, a pulsus paradoxus is present. This is a subtle, but early sign of cardiac tamponade and is assessed when the patient exhibits dyspnea, orthopnea (discomfort in breathing when lying flat), or a positive JVD after a myocardial infarction or cardiac surgery.

The carotid and femoral arteries are auscultated for *bruits.* A bruit is an extracardiac vascular sound resulting from either (1) blood flow through a tortuous or a partially occluded vessel or (2) increased blood flow through a normal vessel. The sound is a high-pitched "sh-sh" sound that vacillates in volume with systole and diastole. Because the diaphragm of the stethoscope is usually too big to auscultate the carotid or femoral areas comfortably, the bell—pressed firmly enough into the skin to create a seal—acts as a good substitute. The skin, then, becomes a diaphragm and transmits the high-pitched sound of the bruit. Light but firm pressure is the key when using the bell of the stethoscope to create a diaphragm. The auscultation of a bruit can expedite the diagnosis of arterial obstruction suspected with inspection and palpation of the lower extremities.

Heart. Auscultation of the heart can be the most challenging part of the cardiac physical examination. To summarize the advice given by most authors, the examiner must (1) discipline himself or herself to auscultate systematically across the precordium; (2) visualize the cardiac anatomy under each point of auscultation, expecting to hear the physiologically associated sounds; (3) memorize the cardiac cycle to enhance the ability to hear abnormal sounds; and (4) practice, practice, practice. Normal heart sounds are referred to as *sound one (S_1)* and *sound two (S_2)*. S_1 is produced by the rapid deceleration of blood flow when the atrioventricular (mitral and tricuspid) valves close at the beginning of systole. S_2 is heard at the end of systole when the semilunar (aortic and pulmonic) valves reach closure. The actual sounds are caused not by the valve leaflets touching each other when they close, but by the vibrations created by the abrupt interruption of retrograde blood flow against the closed, tensed valve leaflets.[2,12] Both sounds are high-pitched and heard best with the diaphragm of the stethoscope. Each sound is loudest in an auscultation area located "downstream" from the actual valvular component of the sound (see Figure 14-6). For example, S_2—which is associated with aortic and pulmonary valve closure—can be heard best at the base of the heart, at the second ICS to the right and left of the sternum, and in the areas labeled aortic and pulmonic. This is true because these areas overlie a section of vasculature "downstream" from the valves in the same direction that sound travels. S_1, associated with closure of the mitral and tricuspid valves, is heard best in the mitral and tricuspid areas. S_1 occurs immediately before the carotid upstroke. To identify it, if the heart rate is over 80 bpm, it may be helpful to simultaneously palpate the carotid artery pulsation while auscultating in the tricuspid or mitral area.

Both S_1 and S_2 are split sounds (Figure 14-7) because of asynchronous left and right ventricular contraction. When there are no ventricular conduction blocks, the left side of the heart contracts milliseconds before the right. The left-sided heart valves, mitral and aortic, are the first heard components of each sound and are usually the loudest. The splits are best heard in the areas overlying the quieter components, the tricuspid and pulmonic valves. The S_2 is more obviously split, and the audible distance between the aortic and pulmonary components is increased with inhalation. This respiratory variation is called physiologic splitting and occurs because inspiration causes changes in pulmonary vascular impedance and in systemic and pulmonary venous return. These changes result in a lengthening of right ventricular ejection time and a corresponding shortening of left ventricular ejection time.[2,5,10,12] All the components of the split sounds are high-pitched and best heard with the diaphragm of the stethoscope. This information helps to differentiate the normal split sound from the ventricular filling sounds that may indicate pathology. See Table 14-3 for detailed characteristics of the normal heart sounds.

An advanced skill in auscultation is determining whether the S_1 and S_2 are louder or softer than normal. The intensity of the sounds vary with dysrhythmias, hyperdynamic cardiac states, and the physical condition of the valves. Independent study, as well as practice and experience, prepare the novice to detect abnormal intensities and splits of S_1 and S_2.

Third and fourth heart sounds (S_3 and S_4). The usually abnormal heart sounds are labeled *sound three (S_3)*and *sound* four (S_4) and are referred to as *gallops* when auscultated during tachycardia. They are ventricular filling sounds, occurring during diastole, and are low-pitched. One can differentiate between right and left ventricular gallops by location. Left ventricular S_3 and S_4 are heard best with the bell of the stethoscope positioned lightly over the apical impulse and with the patient in the left lateral decubitus position; right ventricular gallops are heard best at the left lower sternal border (LLSB). S_3 and S_4 are rhythmic (sounding similar to horses cantering) and have mimetic sounds, as listed in Box 14-10. The sound of S_3 is similar to that of a stone dropping into water at the bottom of a well—dull and "thuddy." S_4 occurs at the end of diastole when the ventricle is full and is associated with the atrial contraction (kick). It is a hollow, snappy sound, as if the noncompliant ventricle cannot accept

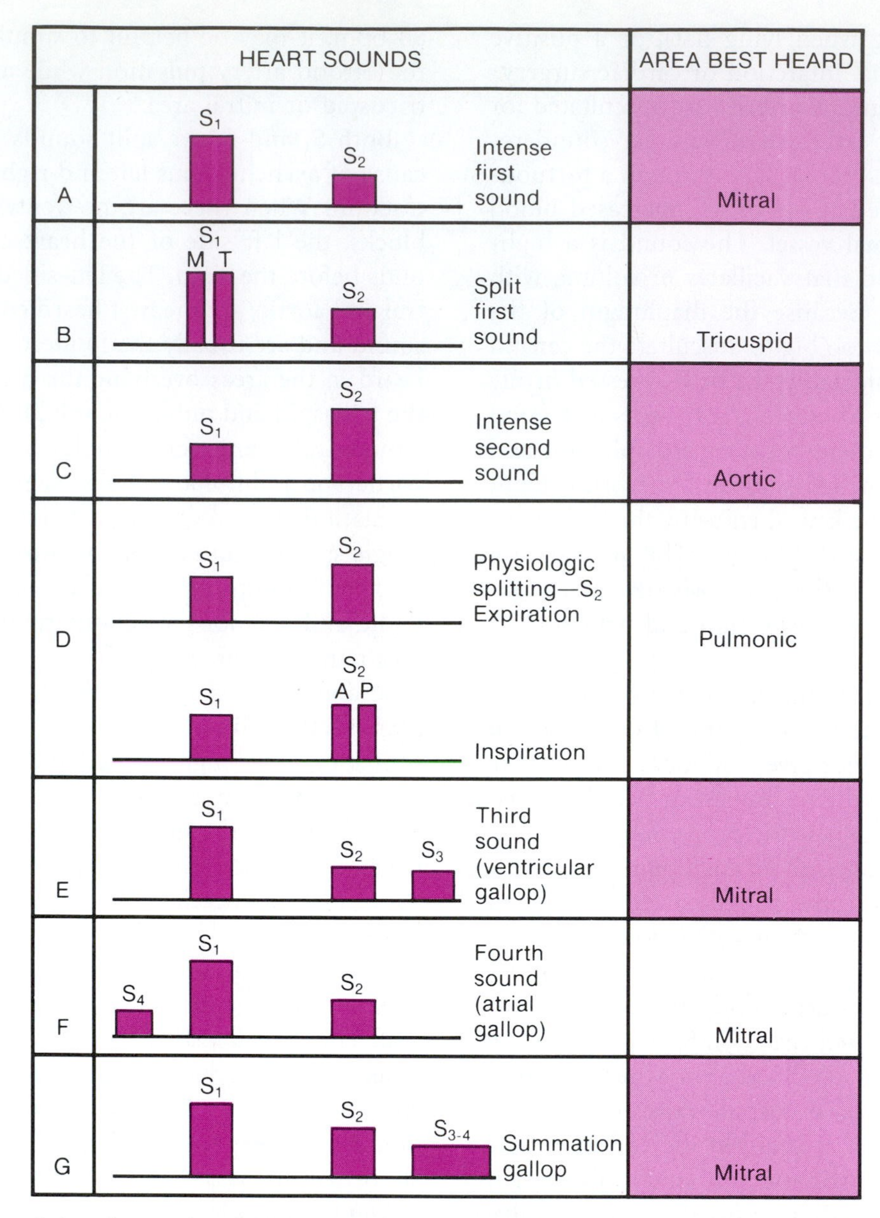

HEART SOUNDS
AREA BEST HEARD
A
S1
S2
Intense first sound
Mitral
B
S1
M T
S2
Split first sound
Tricuspid
C
S1
S2
Intense second sound
Aortic
D
S1
S2
Physiologic splitting—S2 Expiration
Pulmonic
S1
S2
A P
Inspiration
E
S1
S2
S3
Third sound (ventricular gallop)
Mitral
F
S4
S1
S2
Fourth sound (atrial gallop)
Mitral
G
S1
S2
S3-4
Summation gallop
Mitral

FIGURE 14-7. Characteristics of normal and abnormal heart sounds and the auscultatory area where each is best heard.

anymore volume unless it flows in hard and fast. The presence of S_3 is normal in persons younger than age 40 years because of rapid filling of the ventricle and the motion it causes in the young, healthy heart.[2,5,10]

It is important to remember that both S_3 and S_4 are diastolic sounds. If extra sounds are heard, they can best be labeled as systolic or diastolic by using the "inching technique."[5] This means the aortic area, where S_2 is loudest, is auscultated first; then the stethoscope is "inched" across the pericardium toward the mitral area, where S_1 is loudest. It can then be determined whether the extra sound(s) is coming before S_2 (systolic event) or after S_2 (diastolic event). Once the timing is ascertained, the pitch is assessed (high-pitched is a split S_1 or S_2, low-pitched is an S_3 or S_4). A useful test to differentiate between splits and ventricular fill-

TABLE 14-3 Characteristics of Heart Sounds One (S_1) and Two (S_2)

S_1	S_2
High-pitched	High-pitched
Loudest in mitral area (apex)	Loudest in aortic area (base)
Normal split <20 msec	Normal split <30 msec
Split heard best in tricuspid area	Split heard best in pulmonic area
Important to differentiate between split S_1 and S_4	↑ Split with inhalation
Occurs immediately before carotid upstroke	↓ Split with exhalation

↑, Increased; ↓, decreased.

BOX 14-10 Characteristics of Heart Sounds Three (S_3) and Four (S_4)

S_3	S_4
PHYSIOLOGIC CAUSES	
Related to diastolic motion and rapid filling of ventricles in early diastole	Related to diastolic motion and ventricular dilation with atrial contraction in late diastole
Can be normal in children and young adults (<40 yr)	May occur with or without cardiac decompensation
PATHOLOGIC CAUSES	
Ventricular dysfunction with an increase in end systolic volume (MI, heart failure, valvular disease, systemic or pulmonary hypertension)	Ventricular hypertrophy with a decrease in ventricular compliance (CAD, systemic hypertension, cardiomyopathy, aortic or pulmonary stenosis, ↑ in intensity with acute MI or angina)
Hyperdynamic states (anemia, thyrotoxicosis, mitral or tricuspid regurgitation)	Hyperkinetic states (anemia, thyrotoxicosis, arteriovenous fistula)
	Acute valvular regurgitation
RHYTHMIC WORD ASSOCIATION	
Kentucky	Tennessee
S_1 S_2 S_3	S_4 S_1 S_2
SYNONYMS	
Ventricular gallop	Atrial gallop
Protodiastolic gallop	Presystolic gallop

CAD, Coronary artery disease; ↑, increases.

ing sounds is to listen with the bell of the stethoscope. The examiner must press the bell down during auscultation, turning it into a diaphragm that accentuates only high-pitched sounds. If the extra sounds disappear, they may have been low-pitched S_3 or S_4. Detecting an S_3, S_4, or both during auscultation can contribute to the diagnoses of acute or chronic heart failure, chronic hypertension, or valvular disease.

Murmurs. Heart murmurs are prolonged extra sounds that occur during systole or diastole. The sounds are vibrations caused by turbulent blood flow through the cardiac chambers. As indicated in Box 14-11, not all murmurs are caused by cardiac valvular disease. Some murmurs are caused by a high rate of blood flow through the ventricle, as occurs with fever, anemia, and exercise (high output states); other murmurs may be caused by structural defects such as patent foramen ovale (opening in the septum between the right and left atria).[11] Murmurs are characterized by their timing (systolic/diastolic), location and radiation, quality (blowing, grating, harsh), pitch (high or low), and intensity (loudness graded on a scale of I to VI—the higher the number, the louder the murmur, as shown in Box 14-12. Table 14-4 describes the most common murmurs and usual characteristics heard on auscultation.

BOX 14-11 Causes of Cardiac Murmurs

- An increased rate of flow through cardiac structures
- Blood flow across a partial obstruction or irregularity
- Shunting of blood through an abnormal passage from high to low pressure
- Backflow across an incompetent valve

BOX 14-12 Grading of Cardiac Murmurs

GRADE	DESCRIPTION
I/VI	Very faint, may be heard only in a quiet environment
II/VI	Quiet, but clearly audible
III/VI	Moderately loud
IV/VI	Loud: may be associated with a thrill
V/VI	Very loud; thrill easily palpable
VI/VI	Very loud; may be heard with stethoscope off the chest. Thrill palpable and visible

TABLE 14-4 Characteristics of Some Murmurs

Defect	Timing in the Cardiac Cycle	Pitch, Intensity, Quality	Location, Radiation
SYSTOLIC MURMURS			
Mitral regurgitation	S_1 S_2	High Harsh Blowing	Mitral area May radiate to axilla
Tricuspid regurgitation	S_1 S_2	High Often faint, but varies Blowing	Tricuspid RLSB, apex, LLSB, epigastric areas Little radiation
Ventricular septal defect	S_1 S_2	High Loud Blowing	Left sternal border
Aortic stenosis	S_1 S_2	Chhhh hh Medium Rough, harsh	Aortic area to suprasternal notch, right side of neck, apex
Pulmonary stenosis	S_1 S_2	Low to medium Loud Harsh, grinding	Pulmonic area No radiation
DIASTOLIC MURMURS			
Mitral stenosis	Atrial kick S_2 S_1	Low Quiet to loud with thrill Rough rumble	Mitral area Usually no radiation
Tricuspid stenosis	Atrial kick S_2 S_1	Medium Quiet; louder with inspiration Rumble	Tricuspid area or epigastrium Little radiation
Aortic regurgitation	S_2 S_1	High Faint to medium Blowing	Aortic area to LLSB and aorta Erb's point
Pulmonic regurgitation	S_2 S_1	Medium Faint Blowing	Pulmonic area No radiation

RLSB, Right lower sternal border; *LLSB,* left lower sternal border.

BOX 14-13 Auscultation of the Cardiovascular System Precordium

AORTIC AREA

S_2 loud
Aortic systolic murmur

PULMONIC AREA

S_2 loud and split with inhalation
Pulmonic valve murmurs

ERB'S POINT

S_2 split with inhalation
Aortic diastolic murmur
Pericardial friction rub

TRICUSPID AREA

S_1 split
Right ventricular S_3 and S_4
Tricuspid valve murmurs
Murmur of ventricular septal defect

MITRAL AREA

S_1 loud
Left ventricular S_3 and S_4
Mitral valve murmurs

In children or adolescents, systolic "high flow" murmurs are common and are a result of vigorous ventricular contraction. These murmurs have a low-to-medium pitch (heard best with the bell of the stethoscope), grade I to II intensity, and a blowing quality. They are often heard best in the tricuspid area and do not radiate.

When auscultating murmurs, the examiner visualizes the cardiac anatomy, specifically the location of the heart valves and the direction of sound transmission with valve closure and murmur. Generally the systolic valvular murmurs radiate downstream from the valve that is narrowed (stenotic), and the diastolic valvular murmurs—indicating a backflow of blood through an incompetent valve—are auscultated best directly over the area of the valve (see Figure 14-6). Box 14-13 reviews where sounds are best heard on the specific areas of the precordium.

Murmurs associated with myocardial infarction. At the bedside, the nurse is often the first person to auscultate a murmur. The holosystolic or pansystolic murmurs that can occur acutely with myocardial infarction are good examples. The auscultation of a new, high-pitched, holosystolic, blowing murmur at the cardiac apex heralds mitral valve regurgitation secondary to papillary muscle dysfunction. This murmur may be soft (I/VI or II/VI) and occur only during ischemic episodes when the papillary muscle contractility is impaired, but its presence is associated with persistent pain, ventricular failure, and higher mortality.[12,14] If the murmur is loud (V/VI or VI/VI), harsh, and radiating in all directions from the apex, the papillary muscle or chordae tendineae may have ruptured.[15] This is an emergency situation necessitating immediate medical and, often, surgical intervention.

Ventricular septal defect, or rupture, is another emergency situation. It creates the same type of harsh, holosystolic murmur and is loudest along the left sternal border.[14,16] The clinical picture associated with both the papillary muscle rupture and the ventricular septal defect is that of acute ventricular failure and cardiogenic shock. Immediate diagnosis and treatment are necessary to prevent death. (∞Postinfarction Structural Complications, p. 497.)

Pericardial friction rub. A pericardial friction rub is a sound that can occur within 2 to 7 days of a myocardial infarction and/or cardiac surgery and is secondary to pericardial inflammation or pericarditis. Its appearance with other conditions such as congestive heart failure may indicate a pericardial effusion and warrants a cardiac ultrasound study.[17] Classically, it is a three-phase grating or scratching sound that is both systolic and diastolic, corresponding with cardiac motion within the pericardial sac (i.e., ventricular systole, ventricular diastole, and atrial systole). It is high-pitched, often transient, and best auscultated during inhalation at Erb's point (the 3rd ICS to the left of the sternum; see Figure 14-4). It is often associated with chest pain, which can be aggravated by deep inspiration, coughing, swallowing, and changing position. It is important to differentiate pericarditis from myocardial ischemia, and the detection of the pericardial friction rub through auscultation can assist in this differentiation, leading to the proper diagnosis and treatment.

Physical assessment of the cardiovascular patient is a skill that must not be lost in the technology of the critical care setting. Data collected from a thorough, thoughtful examination contributes to the nursing, as well as the medical, diagnoses and guides the decisions for invasive technology. Table 14-5 presents the cardiovascular assessment data for common cardiac diagnoses, using the techniques of inspection, palpation, and auscultation presented in this chapter.

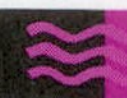

RESEARCH ABSTRACT

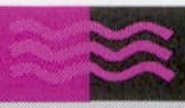

Factors associated with cognitive recovery after cardiopulmonary resuscitation.

Sauve M and others: *Am J Crit Care* 5(2):127, 1996.

PURPOSE

The purpose of this study was to determine to what extent factors associated with cardiopulmonary resuscitation, left ventricular function, and mood state are related to five cognitive outcomes: orientation, attention, memory, reasoning, and motor performances.

DESIGN

Repeated measures, longitudinal design

SAMPLE

The sample consisted of 45 subjects from the cardiac dysrythmia population of five hospitals who were at least 30 years old, had no history of brain pathology or psychiatric illness requiring medications, and had sustained a cardiac arrest within 3 weeks of enrollment in the study.

PROCEDURE

Neuropsychologic tests were used to assess cognitive outcomes and psychologic status over time. Baseline measures were done within 3 weeks of the initial arrest and administered again at 6 to 9 weeks, 12 to 15 weeks, and 22 to 25 weeks after the arrest. The relationship of the cardiopulmonary resuscitation, left ventricular function, and psychologic variables to cognitive outcomes were assessed at each data point. Testing completed in the hospital was finished before any major surgical intervention. Follow-up procedures, including interviews, were conducted in the subjects' homes.

RESULTS

During hospitalization, 84% of the survivors had mild to severe deficits in one or more cognitive area; 50% continued to be impaired in one or more cognitive area at 6 months. Of these, all had mild to severe deficits in at least one area of memory, with delayed recall the most common deficit. The time that it took the patients to awaken after surgery accounted for a portion of the variance in orientation and memory outcomes over time. The left ventricular function variables accounted for a significant portion of the variance in motor speed. There were significant decreases in tension and depression, but not anger, over time. Female subjects reported higher levels of tension and depression than the male subjects.

DISCUSSION/IMPLICATIONS

Findings from this study indicate that half of the long-term survivors of cardiopulmonary resuscitation are cognitively intact 6 months after resuscitation, and that 25% have moderate to severe impairment in memory. Although this study used a small sample, there are obvious implications that can be incorporated into practice. It is important to assess and document the time it takes patients to awaken after surgery, since those subjects who woke up in fewer than 24 hours had more positive outcomes, despite the confusion or combativeness that may have occurred during that time. This information is important to share with family members, who need reassurance and support after cardiopulmonary resuscitation of their loved ones. It is equally important to discuss the implications of the longer wakening period with family members and to consider implications for discharge and long-term follow-up care that may be needed by this population of patients.

TABLE 14-5 Possible Clinical Findings with the Cardiovascular Diagnoses of Heart Failure, Myocardial Infarction, Acute Cardiac Tamponade, Thrombophlebitis, Deep Vein Thrombosis, Pulmonary Emboli, and Pericarditis

Cardiovascular Clinical Assessment	Possible Abnormal Findings Associated with **Heart Failure**	Possible Abnormal Findings Associated with **Myocardial Ischemia** or **Infarction**	Possible Abnormal Findings Associated with **Tamponade**	Possible Abnormal Findings Associated with **Thrombophlebitis** (T), **Deep Vein Thrombosis** (DVT), and **Pulmonary Emboli** (PE)	Possible Abnormal Findings Associated with **Pericarditis**
Inspection: General appearance and face	Lethargy; confusion; anxiousness; cachexia; sitting upright to breathe; shortness of breath; cough; diaphoresis; yellow or pale face and conjunctiva; cyanotic lips, tongue, mucous membranes	Expression of pain, anxiousness, denial, anger, diaphoresis, gray or pale face, tachypnea, nausea and/or vomiting, weakness	Weakness; exhaustion; dyspnea on exertion; orthopnea; cold, clammy skin	Feverish (T); moderate malaise (T or DVT); anxiousness, shortness of breath, tachypnea, or diaphoresis (PE)	Expression of pain with deep inspiration, cough, change in position, and/or swallowing; sitting up and leaning forward as position of comfort; feverish
Inspection: External jugular vein; Internal jugular vein pulsation; Abdominojugular reflux. Palpation: Carotid artery. Auscultation: Carotid artery	Increased JVD, increased JVP, positive abdominojugular reflux, small carotid pulsation, pulsus alternans		Increased JVD, increased JVP		
Inspection: Chest and abdomen. Palpation: Chest and abdomen. Auscultation: Chest and abdomen	Increased respiratory rate and effort, apical impulse enlarged and displaced laterally, sternal lift or heave, S_3 present, mitral regurgitation murmur, ascites	Thrill over sternum, S_4 present (normally not heard), S_3 present, mitral regurgitation murmur, murmur of ventricular septal rupture	Quiet or muffled heart sounds, tachycardia		Pericardial friction rub
Inspection: Upper extremities. Palpation: Upper extremities	Nailbeds cyanotic and/or clubbed, decreased BP	Increased or decreased BP	Decreased BP, narrow pulse pressure, pulsus paradoxus	Pulsus paradoxus	

Continued

TABLE 14-5 **Possible Clinical Findings with the Cardiovascular Diagnoses of Heart Failure, Myocardial Infarction, Acute Cardiac Tamponade, Thrombophlebitis, Deep Vein Thrombosis, Pulmonary Emboli, and Pericarditis—*cont'd***

Cardiovascular Clinical Assessment	Possible Abnormal Findings Associated with **Heart Failure**	Possible Abnormal Findings Associated with **Myocardial Ischemia** or **Infarction**	Possible Abnormal Findings Associated with **Tamponade**	Possible Abnormal Findings Associated with **Thrombophlebitis** (T), **Deep Vein Thrombosis** (DVT), and **Pulmonary Emboli** (PE)	Possible Abnormal Findings Associated with **Pericarditis**
Inspection: Upper extremities Palpation: Upper extremities Inspection: Lower extremities Palpation: Lower extremities	Bilateral edema			Tenderness, increased firmness, tension in calf muscle with squeezing or pressing against tibia (T), increased warmth and/or redness of overlying skin (T), unequal leg circumference (T or DVT), positive Homan's sign (T or DVT), edema (T or DVT)	

REFERENCES

1. Minarik PA: Cognitive assessment of the cardiovascular patient in the acute care setting, *J Cardiovasc Nurs* 9(4):36, 1995.
2. Braunwald E: The physical examination. In Braunwald E, editor: *Heart disease: a textbook of cardiovascular medicine,* ed 4, Philadelphia, 1992, WB Saunders.
3. Carpenter KD: A comprehensive review of cyanosis, *Crit Care Nurse* 13(4):66, 1993.
4. Krenzer ME: Peripheral vascular assessment: finding your way through arteries and veins, *AACN Clin Issues Crit Care Nurs* 6(4):631, 1995.
5. Hurst JW: *Cardiovascular diagnosis: the initial examination,* St. Louis, 1993, Mosby.
6. Cook DJ, Simel DL: Does this patient have abnormal central venous pressure? *JAMA* 275(8):630, 1996.
7. Castella X: A practical way of performing Allen's test to assess palmar collateral circulation, *Anesth Analg* 77(5):1085, 1993, (letter).
8. Ecklund MM: Optimizing the flow of care for prevention and treatment of deep vein thrombosis and pulmonary emboli, *AACN Clin Issues Crit Care Nurs* 6(4):588, 1995.
9. O'Rourke RA, Silverman ME, Schlant RC: General examination of the patient. In RC Schlant and RW Alexander, editors: *Hurst's the heart, arteries, and veins,* ed 8, New York, 1994, McGraw-Hill.
10. Adolph RJ: The value of bedside examination in an era of high technology. III. *Heart Disease and Stroke* 3:236, 1994.
11. Adolph RJ: The value of bedside examination in an era of high technology. IV. *Heart Disease and Stroke* 3:312, 1994.
12. Shaver JA, Salerni R: Auscultation of the heart. In RC Schlant and RW Alexander, editors: *Hurst's the heart, arteries, and veins,* ed 8, New York, 1994, McGraw-Hill.
13. Adolph RJ: The value of bedside examination in an era of high technology. II. *Heart Disease and Stroke* 3:188, 1994.
14. Tawa CB, Raizner AE: Recognition and treatment of myocardial rupture, *Heart Disease and Stroke,* 3:143, 1994.
15. O'Sullivan CK: Mitral regurgitation as a complication of MI: pathophysiology and nursing implications, *J Cardiovas Nurs* 6(4):26, 1992.
16. Molchany CA: Ventricular septal and free wall rupture complicating acute MI, *J Cardiovasc Nurs* 6(4):38, 1992.
17. Pierce CO: Acute post-MI pericarditis, *J Cardiovasc Nurs* 6(4):46, 1992.

15 Cardiovascular Diagnostic Procedures

LABORATORY ASSESSMENT

INFORMATION NEEDED FOR assessment of the cardiovascular patient's status can be obtained through laboratory studies of blood serum. Accurate interpretation of these laboratory studies, along with the clinical picture, enables the critical care team to diagnose, treat, and assess the response to therapeutic interventions.

Laboratory studies of blood serum are performed to assess (1) electrolyte levels that directly affect cardiac function, (2) other organ systems that reflect or secondarily affect cardiac status, (3) enzyme levels that may reflect myocardial infarction, (4) hematologic status for determination of anemia or infection that may be a cause of cardiac disease, (5) coagulation levels, and (6) serum lipid levels for treatment of a coronary artery disease risk factor.

Electrolytes

Potassium. During depolarization and repolarization of nerve and muscle fiber, potassium and sodium exchange occurs intracellularly and extracellularly. The potassium gradient across the cell membrane determines conduction velocity and helps confine pacing activity to the sinus node.[1] Thus either an excess or a deficiency of potassium can alter cardiac muscle function.

Hyperkalemia. Too much potassium (hyperkalemia) decreases the rate of ventricular depolarization, shortens repolarization, and also depresses atrioventricular (AV) conduction. As the serum levels of potassium rise from normal levels (3.5 to 5.5 mEq/L), evidence of these phenomena can be seen on the electrocardiogram (ECG) (Figure 15-1, *A*). Tall, peaked T waves are usually, although not uniquely, associated with early hyperkalemia and are followed by widening of the QRS complex and prolongation of the P wave and PR interval. With severe hyperkalemia (greater than 8 mEq/L), depressed AV conduction (Figure 15-1, *B*) leads to cardiac standstill or ventricular fibrillation. This life-threatening condition can be acutely managed with an intravenous insulin/glucose infusion, and permanently managed with Kayexalate or dialysis. Coexisting low serum sodium, calcium, or pH levels potentiate the cardiac effects of hyperkalemia.

Hypokalemia. A low serum potassium level, called *hypokalemia* (less than 3.5 mEq/L), is commonly caused by gastrointestinal losses, diuretic therapy with insufficient replacement, or chronic steroid therapy and is also reflected by the ECG (Figure 15-2). Myocardial conduction is impaired, and ventricular repolarization is prolonged, as evidenced by a prominent U wave. The U wave is not totally unique to hypokalemia, but its presence is a signal for the nurse to check the serum potassium level. The occurrence of or increase in numbers of premature ventricular contractions (PVCs) can also be a result of decreased potassium levels. Supposedly normal potassium levels (less than 4.9 mEq/L), even in the healthy population, are associated with higher prevalence rates of various ventricular dysrhythmias.[2] In the critical care unit where patients are receiving diuretics and/or have nasogastric tubes to suction, the serum potassium is checked frequently by the critical care nurse and replaced intravenously to normal levels to prevent dysrhythmias. Other ECG indicators of hypokalemia are the occurrence of bradycardia, AV block, atrial flutter, and an exaggeration of toxic effects of digitalis.[1] All of these dysrhythmias are usually reversible with

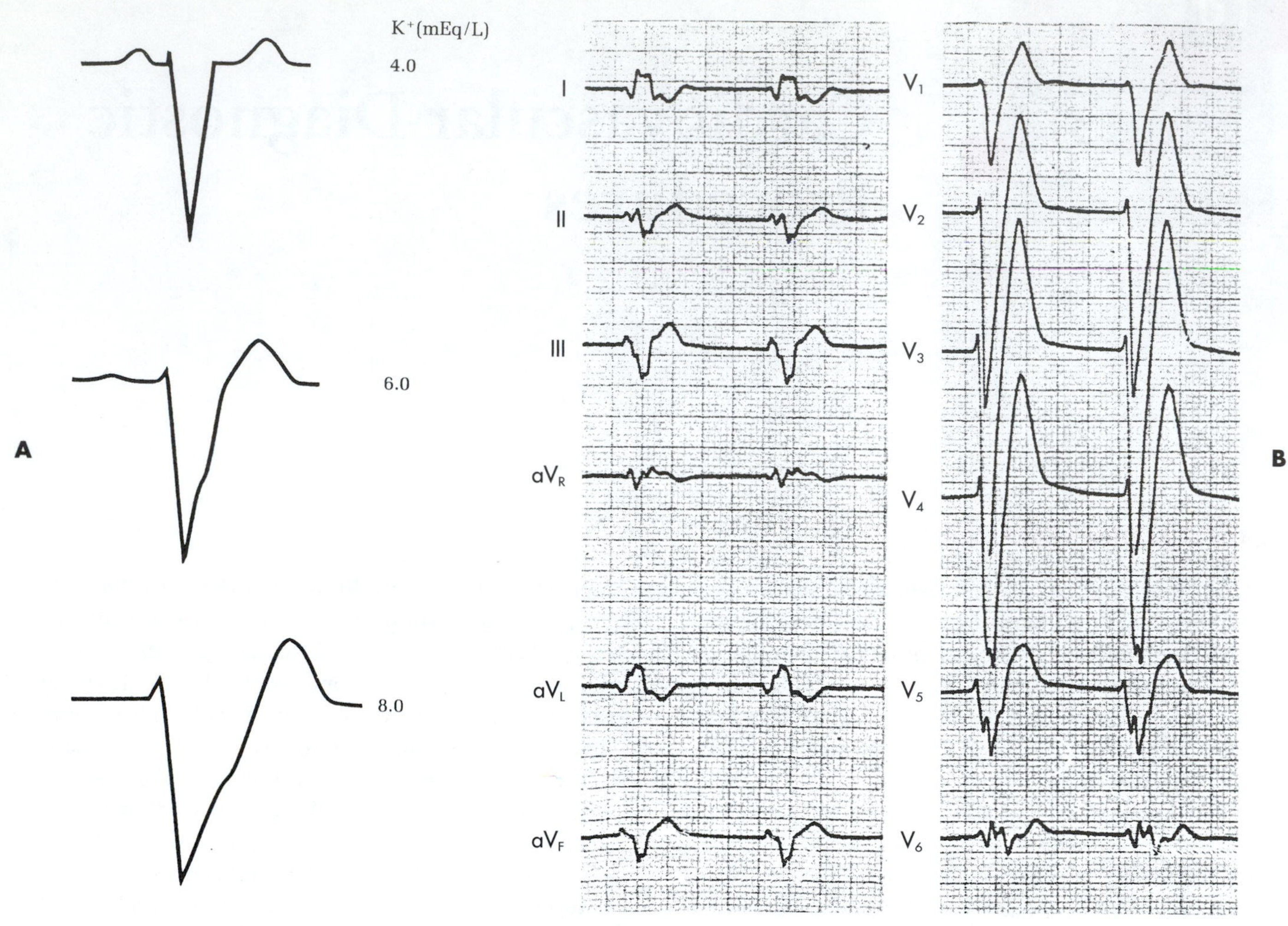

FIGURE 15-1. Effects of hyperkalemia. **A,** Stages in hyperkalemia from normal potassium levels to plasma levels of 8 mEq/L. At 6 mEq/L the P wave flattens, the QRS broadens, and the ST segment disappears, with the S wave flowing into the tall, tented T wave. **B,** Life-threatening hyperkalemia. Note the absence of P waves, lack of ST segment (in V_1 to V_5) and peaked T waves. These changes do not necessarily occur with a specific serum potassium level. For example, some patients can have a normal ECG with a potassium level of 7 mEq/L (patients with chronic renal failure), whereas other patients with an *acute* rise in serum potassium to a similar level will have ventricular fibrillation. (From Conover MB: *Understanding electrocardiography,* ed 7, 1996, Mosby-Year Book.)

potassium replacement. If concomitant hypomagnesemia exists, successful replenishment of potassium deficit cannot be accomplished until the hypomagnesemia is reversed. See Box 15-1 for electrolyte values that affect cardiac contractility.

Calcium. Calcium (Ca^{++}) is an important mediator of many cardiovascular functions because of its effect on vascular tone, myocardial contractility, and cardiac excitability. Although the most commonly performed blood test for calcium levels is total serum calcium (8.5 to 10.5 mg/dL), the portion of the total calcium called *ionized* or "free" calcium is what is biologically active. The inactive forms of plasma calcium are bound to protein (primarily albumin) and complexed to anions such as chloride and phosphate. Ionized calcium is primarily responsible for the pathophysiologic effects of hypercalcemia and hypocalcemia. The serum concentration of ionized calcium is maintained within very narrow limits (4 to 5 mg/dL), and direct measurement is considered to be the most accurate method for assessing calcium status.[3] If this laboratory service is unavailable, then total calcium levels (along with other blood tests, such as albumin, pH, phosphate, and serum osmolarity, that reflect calcium-protein binding prop-

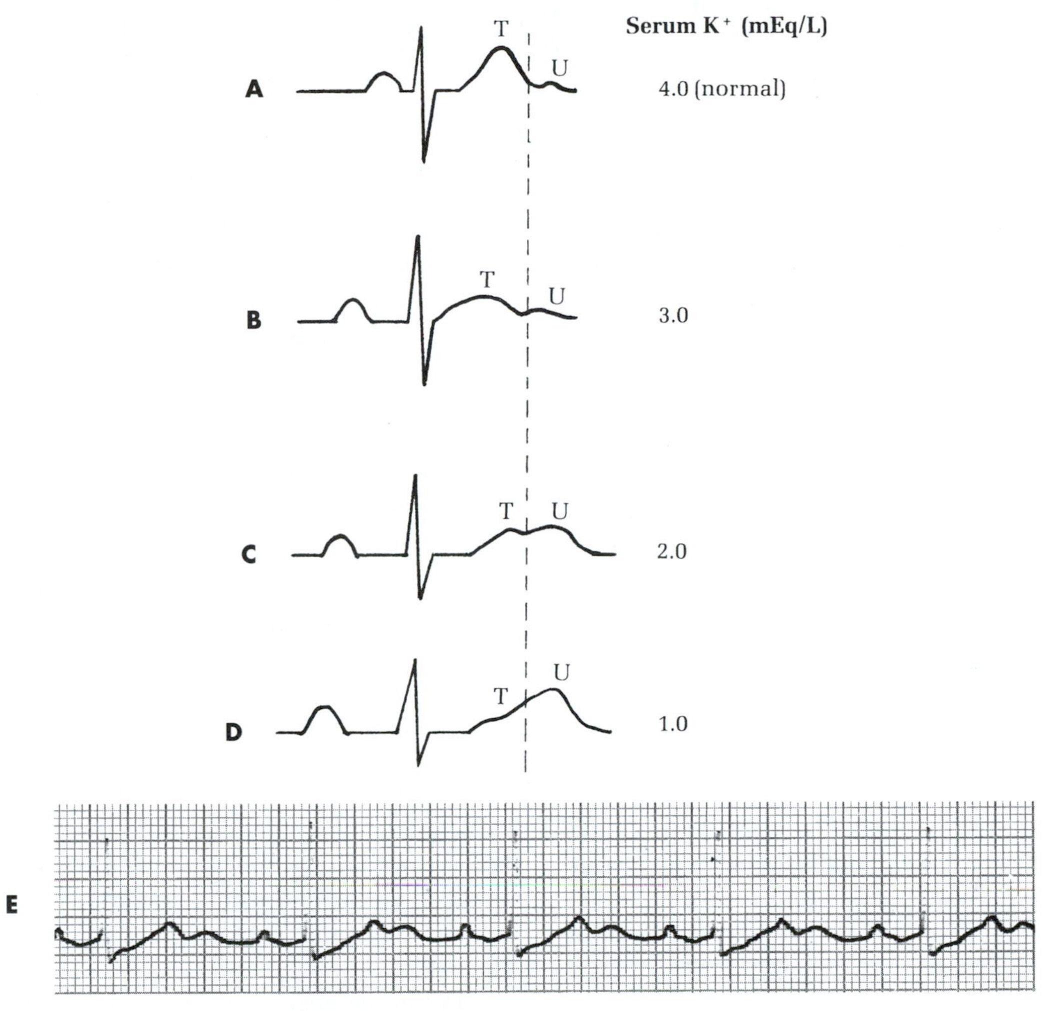

FIGURE 15-2. Hypokalemia. **A,** At a normal serum concentration of 4-5.5 mEq/L the amplitude of the T wave is appreciably greater than that of the U wave. **B,** By the time the serum potassium level has dropped to 3 mEq/L, the amplitude of the T and U waves are approaching each other. **C** and **D,** With a further drop in the level of potassium the U wave begins to tower over and fuse with the T wave. **E,** Tracing from a patient with hypokalemia (serum K + level 2.5 mEq/L). The ST depression typical of hypokalemia and the prominent U wave are evident. (From Conover MB: *Understanding electrocardiography,* ed 7, 1996, Mosby.)

erties and affect the level of available ionized calcium) are used to assess for hypercalcemia or hypocalcemia. The critical care team monitors the serum levels of calcium, potassium, and magnesium on an ongoing basis to prevent the clinical manifestations that occur with abnormal levels of any of these electrolytes.

Calcium levels are disrupted by tumors of the bone and lung, endocrine disorders, hypomagnesemia or hypermagnesemia, excessive intake or deficiency of vitamin D, intestinal malabsorption of calcium, kidney failure, and pancreatitis.

BOX 15-1 Chemistry Values That Affect Cardiac Contractility and Conduction

	NORMAL RANGE
Potassium (K)	3.5-5.5 mEq/L
Ionized Calcium (Ca)	4-5 mg/dL
Total Calcium (Ca)	8.5-10.5 mg/dL
Magnesium (Mg)	1.8-2.4 mg/dL
(may be reported in mg/dL or mEq/L)	1.5-2.0 mEq/L

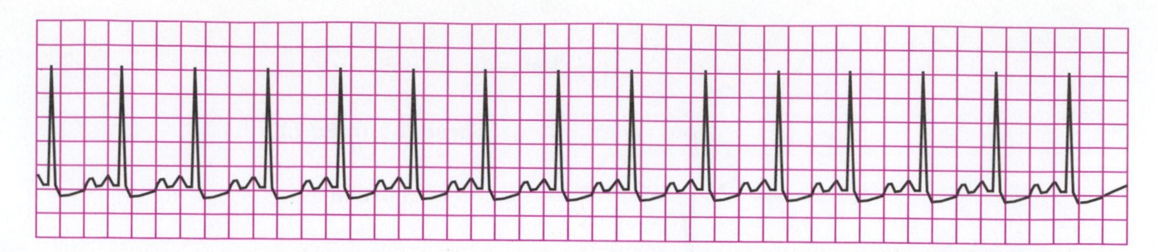

FIGURE 15-3. Abnormal QT prolongation in a hypocalcemic patient. The patient is a 50-year-old female admitted to the critical care unit with alcoholic liver disease and malnourishment. Total calcium is 5.1 mg/dL, and albumin is 1.3 mg/dL. The QT interval (0.55 second) is markedly prolonged for the heart rate (100/min). The QT interval varies with the heart rate and can be "corrected" using the formula $\frac{QT}{RR} = QT_C$ (corrected QT). The corrected QT (QT_C) should be < 0.44 second. The QT_c in the ECG tracing pictured is 0.55 second. Hypocalcemia lengthens ventricular repolarization. A quick method of assessing the QT interval is that it is less than half of the RR interval. If it is more than half of the RR interval, it is prolonged. (From Yucha CB, Toto KH: Calcium and phosphorus derangements, *Crit Care Clin North Am* 6(4):747, 1994.)

Hypercalcemia. *Hypercalcemia* is increased amounts of ionized calcium (greater than 4.8 mg/dL) or increased amounts of total serum calcium (greater than 10.5 mg/dL). This condition has a cardiovascular effect of strengthening contractility and shortening ventricular repolarization. The ECG demonstrates the shortened repolarization with a shortened QT interval. Rhythm disturbances may include bradycardia; first-, second-, and third-degree heart block; and bundle branch block. Hypercalcemia can potentiate the effects of digitalis, precipitate digitalis toxicity, and cause hypertension.[3]

Hypocalcemia. Ionized calcium levels greater than 4.0 mg/dL or total serum calcium levels less than 8.5 mg/dL (with a concurrent normal albumin level and normal or acidotic serum pH) is hypocalcemia. Hypocalcemia is common in critically ill and postsurgical patients because of blood transfusions, magnesium imbalances, shock, or alkalosis.[3] The cardiovascular effects of hypocalcemia include decreased myocardial contractility, reduced cardiac output, decreased cardiac responsiveness to digitalis, and hypotension. Rhythm disturbances range from bradycardia to ventricular tachycardia and asystole. When the ionized calcium is less than 3.2 mg/dL, the ECG commonly demonstrates a prolonged QT interval (Figure 15-3). This predisposes a patient to the life-threatening ventricular dysrhythmia *torsades de pointes*. An ionized calcium level this low is considered a medical emergency and requires immediate reversal with an intravenous infusion of calcium.[1] (∞Calcium, p. 378; Intervals Between Waveforms, p. 392.)

Magnesium. Magnesium (Mg^{++}) is essential for many enzyme, protein, lipid, and carbohydrate functions in the body and is critical for the production and use of energy.[4] In the blood stream, it is found predominantly within the cells, although an adequate serum level (extracellular) is essential to normal cardiac and skeletal muscle function. The normal serum range is from 1.5 to 2.0 mEq/L or 1.8 to 2.4 mg/dL. The incidence of hypermagnesemia is rare in comparison with hypomagnesemia and occurs secondary to renal insufficiency or iatrogenic overtreatment.[4] Hypomagnesemia can be caused by insufficient intake in the diet or in total parental nutrition (TPN); chronic alcohol abuse; diuresis; diarrhea; or rapid administration of citrated blood products, causing citrate-chelation.

Hypomagnesemia. A serum magnesium concentration less than 1.5 mEq/L is called hypomagnesemia. It is commonly associated with other electrolyte imbalances, most notably alterations in potassium, sodium, calcium, and phosphorous. Both hypokalemia and hypocalcemia are likely to be unresponsive to replacement therapy until the hypomagnesemia is corrected.[4] Cardiac-related changes with hypomagnesemia are hypertension and vasospasm, including coronary artery spasm. Several studies have linked magnesium depletion to sudden cardiac death, to an increased incidence of acute myocardial infarction,[4] and to the occurrence of ventricular dysrythmias.[2]

The ECG changes are similar to those seen with hypokalemia (see Figure 15-2) and hypocalcemia (see Figure 15-3)—prolonged PR and QT intervals, presence of U waves, T wave flattening, and a widened QRS complex. Cardiac dysrythmias may be supraventricular or ventricular and include torsades de pointes. Dysrhythmias associated with hypomagnesemia may not respond to usual antidysrhythmic treatment, but they often respond well to magnesium infusions. The American Heart Association is currently recommending intravenous magnesium as the treatment of choice for torsades de pointes.[1] It is important to evaluate renal function when administering magnesium to avoid hypermagnesium states. (∞Magnesium, p. 380; Torsades De Pointes, p. 418.)

General Chemistry Studies

The chemistry studies most helpful in the diagnosis of cardiovascular abnormalities give information about glucose metabolism, thyroid function, kidney function, liver function, and electrolyte concentrations. The presence of increased serum glucose (more than 115 mg/dL) during a fasting state (serum drawn 12 hours after most recent ingestion of food or drink) may indicate diabetes mellitus. Patients with diabetes, insulin or non–insulin dependent, are at increased risk of developing all manifestations of atherosclerotic vascular disease. Eighty percent of all deaths occurring in non–insulin-dependent diabetes mellitus (NIDDM) patients is a result of complications of atherosclerosis.[5]

Thyroid hormone levels are not routinely ordered but are often helpful diagnostically. Elevated levels of the thyroid hormones T_3 and T_4 may result in thyrotoxicosis and a resultant hyperdynamic cardiovascular picture (palpitations, tachycardia, bounding pulses). Decreased levels of the thyroid hormones (hypothyroidism) may be an explanation for fatigue, dyspnea on exertion, decreased cardiac output, and heart failure.[6] (∞Thyroid Gland, p. 983.)

Blood urea nitrogen (BUN) and creatinine are blood chemistries that reflect renal function. With renal failure, BUN and creatinine levels are increased. Renal failure may cause electrolyte imbalances of potassium and calcium, which affect cardiac conduction and contractility.

Liver function indexes seen on the chemistry report include alkaline phosphatase, bilirubin, aspartate aminotransferase (AST), and alanine aminotransferase (ALT). Abnormal liver function tests may alert the medical team to liver dysfunction caused by failure of the right side of the heart. "Normal" laboratory values vary from institution to institution but must be readily available to the critical care nurse. (∞Laboratory Assessment, p. 377.)

Cardiac enzymes. Cardiac enzymes are proteins that are released from irreversibly damaged myocardial tissue cells. The traditional "gold standard" for diagnosing myocardial infarction (MI) is the rise and fall of the serum MB fraction of the enzyme creatine phosphokinase (CK) within 24 hours after the onset of symptoms.[7] The CK-MB serum levels elevate 4 to 8 hours after MI, peak at 15 to 24 hours, and remain elevated for 2 to 3 days (Table 15-1). Serial samples are drawn routinely every 6 to 12 hours, and three samples are usually sufficient to support or rule out the diagnosis of MI. Newer methods of detection include evaluating myoglobin, troponin T, and troponin I levels.

Current treatment of acute MI is to open the coronary artery obstructed by a thrombus and reperfuse the injured area within 3 to 4 hours of injury. Reperfusion treatments include thrombolytic agents ("clotbusters"), cardiac catheterization with percutaneous transluminal coronary angioplasty (PTCA), and surgery to provide coronary artery bypass grafting (CABG). If successful, these treatments may totally abort the MI or limit the amount of cardiac muscle damage. After reperfusion, the serum CK-MB level rises dramatically (doubles within 90 minutes) and peaks early (6 to 10 hours). Blood samples are drawn at admission; at time of thrombolytic therapy; and then at 3, 6, 12, 18, and 24 hours to detect the rise and assess the return of effective myocardial reperfusion.[8]

Reperfusion must be performed early in the course of the MI to save cardiac tissue, because the rise of CK-MB occurs 4 to 6 hours after the MI. It is current clinical practice to diagnose an acute MI by ECG and clinical symptoms, without the aid of elevated cardiac enzymes. Serologic tests that are more sensitive than CK-MB (i.e., those that detect damaged myocardium earlier) are being actively researched. When the methodology becomes widely available, levels of protein markers such as MB_1 and MB_2 (CK-MB isoforms), myoglobin, cardiac troponin T (cTnT), and cardiac troponin I (cTnI) may markedly improve the rapidity with which acute MI can be diagnosed.[7] See Table 15-1 for a summary of this information.

Lactate dehydrogenase (LDH, or LD) is another cardiac enzyme that is almost always elevated after MI. Its levels are useful for late diagnosis of MI, when CK-MB levels have returned to normal. LDH levels begin to increase 10 to 12 hours after injury, peak at 48 to 72 hours, and remain elevated for 10 to 14 days. LDH isoenzymes, LDH_1 and LDH_2, delineate the tissue source (increase the cardiac specificity) of the elevated LDH. Normally, serum levels of LDH_1 are less than those of LDH_2 (LDH_1/LDH_2 less than or equal to 1.0), and with MI, both levels rise, but LDH_1

TABLE 15-1 Summary of Increased Serum Markers After Acute MI

Serum Marker	Earliest Increase (hours)*	Peak (hours)*	Return to Normal (days)*	Amplitude of Increase
Total CK	3-6	24-36	3	6-12
CK-MB	4-8	15-24	3-4	16
CK-MB_2/MB_1	2	4-6	2	
Total LD	10-12	48-72	11	3
LD_1	8-12	72-144	8-14	
LD_1/LD_2	>6		>3	
Myoglobin	2-3	6-9	Often 12 hours	10
Troponin T	4-6	10-24	10-15	
Troponin I	4-6	10-24	10-15	

(Adapted from Wallach J: *Interpretation of diagnostic tests,* ed 6, Boston, 1996, Little, Brown.)
*Time periods represent average reported values.
NOTE: There is a range of reported values because different studies used different time periods after onset of symptoms, different benchmarks for establishing the diagnosis, and different patient populations, etc.
CK, creatine phosphokinase; *LD,* lactate dehydrogenase.

levels become greater than LDH_2 levels. This is called a "flipped" LDH_1-to-LDH_2 ratio (LDH_1/LDH_2 greater than 1.0). The flipped ratio usually appears in 12 to 24 hours after injury and never appears before CK-MB elevation. It may flip back and forth, making it important to collect serial specimens, and it may remain flipped for longer than the total LDH stays elevated (see Table 15-1).[8]

Hematologic Studies

Hematologic laboratory studies that are routinely ordered for the management of patients with altered cardiovascular status are red blood cell (RBC, or erythrocyte) level; hemoglobin (Hgb) level; hematocrit (Hct) level; erythrocyte sedimentation rate (ESR), white blood cell (WBC, or leukocyte) level; and coagulation tests.

Red blood cells. The normal amount of RBCs varies with age, gender, environmental temperature, altitude, and exercise. Males produce 4.5 million to 6 million RBCs per cubic millimeter, whereas the normal level for females is 4 million to 5.5 million per cubic millimeter.

RBCs are composed of Hgb, which transports and releases oxygen to the tissues of the body. Hgb levels range from 14 to 18 g/dL in males and from 12 to 16 g/dL in females. Hct is the volume percentage of RBCs in whole blood—40% to 54% for males and 38% to 48% for females. When the serum level of total RBCs falls, it is logical to also see a fall in Hgb and Hct levels. Anemia, a hematologic disorder of insufficient amounts of RBCs (and concurrently, decreased Hgb and Hct levels), can cause an increase in cardiac workload and cardiac dilation and eventually cardiac failure. An increase in the number of RBCs (polycythemia) also results in increased levels of hemoglobin and hematocrit and often occurs as a response to tissue hypoxia.

Erythrocyte sedimentation rate. The ESR is a measurement of how quickly RBCs separate from plasma in 1 hour. With injury (e.g., myocardial infarction), inflammation (e.g., endocarditis), or pregnancy, RBCs have higher globulin and fibrinogen levels, which cause faster precipitation and increase the sedimentation rate. Heart failure can decrease the ESR because of the associated decrease in levels of serum fibrinogen.

White blood cells. Most inflammatory processes such as rheumatic fever, endocarditis, and myocardial infarction that produce necrotic tissue within the heart muscle increase the WBC level. The normal level of serum leukocytes for both genders is 5000 to 10,000 per cubic millimeter.

Blood coagulation studies. Coagulation studies are ordered to determine serum clotting effectiveness. Anticoagulants, most notably heparin, warfarin, and platelet inhibitory agents (e.g., aspirin) are adminis-

BOX 15-2 Normal and Therapeutic Adult Coagulation Values

TEST	NORMAL VALUE	THERAPEUTIC VALUE	
PT	11-16 sec*	1.5-2.5 times normal	
INR	< 2.0	Chronic atrial fibrillation	2.0-3.0
		(if patient > 70 yrs)	< 2.5
		Treatment of DVT/PE	2.0-3.0
		Tissue heart valve	2.0-3.0
		Survivor of acute MI	2.5-3.5
		Mechanical heart valve(s)	2.5-3.5
APTT	28-38 sec	1.5-2.5 times normal	
PTT	60-90 sec	1.5-2.0 times normal	
ACT†	70-120 sec	150-190 sec	
		> 300 sec post PTCA/stent	

*PT normal value may vary by 2 sec between different laboratories.
†ACT normal, therapeutic, and post PTCA/stent values may vary with type of activator used.[10]
PT, Prothrombin time; *INR,* international normalized ratio; *APPT,* activated partial thromboplastin time; *PTT,* partial thromboplastin time; *ACT,* activated coagulation time; *DVT,* deep vein thrombosis; *PE,* pulmonary embolism.

tered to reduce the incidence of reocclusion after successful reperfusion and to decrease myocardial infarct extension.[7] Patients who have stasis of blood (e.g., with atrial fibrillation or prolonged bed rest), valvular heart disease, or a history of thrombosis are at risk for developing a thrombus and usually require anticoagulation. Coagulation studies are ordered to guide dosage of these anticoagulating drugs.

Most coagulation study results are reported as the length of time *in seconds* it takes for blood to form a clot in the laboratory test tube. The *prothrombin time* (PT) is used to determine the therapeutic dosage of warfarin necessary to achieve anticoagulation. The PT is also reported as an *international normalized ratio* (INR). The INR was developed by the World Health Organization (WHO) in an attempt to standardize PT results between clinical laboratories worldwide. Box 15-2 illustrates target INR ranges for different cardiovascular conditions that require anticoagulation.[9] The *partial thromboplastin time* (PTT) and *activated partial thromboplastin time* (APTT) are used to measure the effectiveness of intravenous or subcutaneous heparin administration. An additional test of heparin effect is the *activated coagulation time* (ACT). The ACT can be performed outside of the laboratory setting in areas such as the cardiac catheterization laboratory, the operating room, or specialized critical care units.[11] Normal and therapeutic values for all of these coagulation studies are shown in Box 15-2.

Serum Lipid Studies

Four primary blood lipid levels are important in evaluating an individual's risk of developing and/or progressing coronary artery disease: total cholesterol; low density lipoprotein–cholesterol (LDLC); triglycerides; and high density lipoprotein-cholesterol (HDLC). When levels of cholesterol, LDLs, and triglycerides are elevated or the level of HDLs is low, the patient is considered "at risk" for developing or progressing coronary heart disease (CHD) and is offered intensive interventions in diet therapy, exercise prescription, and/or drug therapy.

Total cholesterol. Cholesterol is a fatlike substance (lipid) that is present in cell membranes and is a precursor of bile acids and steroid hormones. It is produced by the liver. The cholesterol level in the blood is determined partly by genetics and partly by acquired factors such as diet, calorie balance, and level of physical activity. Cholesterol in excess amounts (more than 200 mg/dL) in the serum forces the progression of atherosclerosis (athrogenesis). See Table 15-2 for normal lipid levels.

Low-density lipoproteins. About 60% to 70% of the total serum cholesterol is found in *low density lipoproteins-cholesterol* (LDL-C). Both the LDL-C and total serum cholesterol levels are directly correlated with risk for CHD, and high levels of each are significant predictors of future myocardial infarctions in patients with established coronary artery atherosclerosis.[11] LDL-C is

TABLE 15-2 **Desirable Lipid Levels to Lower the Risk of Coronary Heart Disease (CHD) and to Reduce Morbidity and Mortality in Patients with Established CHD**

Lipid	Desirable Level
Total cholesterol	< 200 mg/dL
LDL-C	< 130 mg/dL without CHD < 100 mg/dL with CHD
Triglycerides	< 200 mg/dL
HDL-C	> 35 mg/dL

(Adapted from the National Cholesterol Education Program: *Second report from the expert panel on detection, evaluation, and treatment of high blood cholesterol in adults (adult treatment panel II)*, NIH Pub. No. 93-3095, 1993, US Dept of Health and Human Services.)
LDL-C, Low density lipoprotein-cholesterol; *HDL-C*, high density lipoprotein-cholesterol.

TABLE 15-3 **X-ray Densities of Intrathoracic Structures**

Metal or Bone (White)	Fluid (Gray)	Air (Black)
Ribs, clavicle, sternum, spine	Blood	Lung
Calcium deposits	Heart	
Surgical wires or clips	Veins	
Prosthetic valves	Arteries	
Pacemaker wires	Edema	

the major atherogenic lipoprotein and thus is the primary target for cholesterol-lowering efforts.

Very low density lipoproteins and triglycerides. The *very low density lipoproteins* (VLDL) contain 10% to 15% of the total serum cholesterol along with most of the triglycerides in fasting serum; VLDLs are precursors of LDL-C, and some forms of VLDL (phenotype B) appear to be atherogenic.[11] Elevated triglyceride levels are often associated with reduced HDL-C levels and directly correlate with the phenotype B of LDL-C.

High density lipoproteins. *High density lipoproteins-cholesterol* (HDL-C) are particles that carry 20% to 30% of the total serum cholesterol. A low HDL-C level (less than 35 mg/dL) is another independent, significant risk factor for CHD. Several studies,[11] however, also support a protective role of HDL-C against atherogenesis, and a level greater than 60 mg/dL may act as a "shield" against the risk of CHD.

DIAGNOSTIC PROCEDURES

Chest Radiography

Basic principles and technique. Chest radiography is the oldest noninvasive method for visualizing images of the heart, yet it remains a frequently used and valuable diagnostic tool. Information about cardiac anatomy and physiology can be obtained with ease and safety at a relatively low cost. In the critical care unit, the nurse may be the first person to view the chest radiograph of an acutely ill patient. Nurses also have an important role in influencing the quality of the film through proper positioning and instruction of the patient. For these reasons, it is vital that critical care nurses gain a basic understanding of chest x-ray techniques and interpretation as they apply to the cardiovascular system.

Tissue densities. As x-rays travel through the chest from the emitting tube to the film plate, they are absorbed to a varying degree by the tissues through which they pass (Table 15-3). Very dense tissue, such as bone, absorbs almost all the x-rays, leaving the film unexposed, or white. The heart, aorta, pulmonary vessels, and the blood they contain are moderately dense structures, appearing as gray areas on the x-ray film. These vascular structures are surrounded by air-filled lung that allows the greatest penetration of x-rays, resulting in fully exposed (black) areas on the film. Thoracic structures can be studied best by examining their borders. Two structures with the same density, when located next to each other, have no visible border. If a structure is located next to a contrasting density (e.g., vascular structures next to an air-filled lung), even subtle changes in size and shape can be seen.

Standard positions. In most institutions, a standard radiographic examination of the heart and lungs consists of posteroanterior (PA) and lateral films. Fluoroscopy is a simple and inexpensive tool for examination of the dynamics of cardiac contraction, but it has been replaced at the bedside by two-dimensional echocardiography, which is noninvasive and just as accurate. The major use of fluoroscopy currently is for guidance during right catheterization and other instrumentation of the heart.

Ideally, the chest radiograph is taken in the x-ray department with the patient in an upright position; the film exposed during a deep, sustained inhalation; and the x-ray tube aimed horizontally 6 feet from the film. This is a PA film, because the beam traverses the patient from posterior to anterior.

Because most patients in critical care units are too ill to go to the x-ray department, chest radiographs are routinely obtained by using portable x-ray machines, with the patient either sitting upright or lying supine, depending on the patient's clinical condition and the judgment of the nurse. In both cases, the film plate is placed behind the patient's back and an anteroposterior (AP) projection is used, in which the x-ray beam enters from the front of the chest. In the supine film the x-ray tube can be only approximately 36 inches from the patient's chest because of ceiling height and x-ray equipment construction, resulting in an inferior quality film from a diagnostic standpoint, because the images of the heart and great vessels are somewhat magnified and not as sharply defined. Whenever possible, the upright (AP) film is preferred to the supine because it provides more accurate hemodynamic data; it shows more of the lung, since the diaphragm is lower; and the images are sharper and less magnified. With an upright film, the x-ray tube must be 50 inches from the film plate.[12] It is important to remove extrinsic tubing and other objects when possible from the patient's chest to avoid opacities resulting from artifact.

A deep, sustained inhalation is important. During exhalation, the lungs appear to cloud and the heart appears larger, possibly leading to an erroneous diagnosis of congestive heart failure, diffuse atelectasis, or consolidation. Alert patients are encouraged by the radiology technician to take in a deep breath and hold it while the exposure is taken. With patients receiving mechanical ventilatory support, the exposure must be timed to coincide with maximal inhalation. Some patients are simply unable to maintain a sustained inhalation on command, resulting in a distorted cardiac shadow and poor visualization of the lung fields. For this reason it is important to be able to compare and contrast serial chest films before determining that progress or deterioration has occurred.

Indications. In the past it was common practice for most patients in a critical care unit to have a daily chest x-ray performed. Recently the cost-effectiveness of this practice has been questioned. Indeed, the value of a chest x-ray is difficult to measure, because it is only one piece of data that must be evaluated with the patient's clinical situation and other test results in mind. It is difficult to weigh how much the chest film results alone may have affected the patient's diagnosis or management. Initial admission films are important because they provide a baseline from which deviations can be more clearly seen. Chest radiographs have high diagnostic accuracy in identifying the malposition of tubes or lines in the critically ill; they can be quite confusing in a patient who has several abnormalities at once, such as pneumonia and acute heart failure. The American College of Radiology (ACR) has published the following general recommendations based on review of the current literature: (1) a daily chest x-ray is indicated for patients with acute cardiopulmonary problems and those receiving mechanical ventilation, (2) patients who require cardiac monitoring but are otherwise stable need only an admission film, and (3) a chest x-ray is performed whenever a new device is placed or whenever there is a specific question about the patient's cardiopulmonary status that the chest x-ray could address.[12]

Cardiac radiographic film analysis. Evaluation of a chest film is a systematic process. All invasive tubes and lines must be located and identified. This discussion is limited to cardiovascular devices, although there are other tubes commonly used in critical care patients that require x-ray verification, including endotracheal, tracheostomy, chest, nasogastric, and enteral feeding tubes. Major thoracic structures including the lungs, pleural space, mediastinum, diaphragm, and vascular structures are assessed and compared with previous films, if available. Variations from previous films can alert the clinician to possible complications and provide information about the patient's hemodynamic status.

Cardiovascular tubes, lines, and devices. Multiple devices are routinely used in the care of cardiovascular patients for monitoring and support. Recognizing these devices and being able to identify deviations from normal is essential, since improper positioning can be life-threatening. A chest x-ray is indicated immediately after initial placement and after any invasive manipulation of a tube or catheter to evaluate its position and to assess for complications related to the procedure. Table 15-4 summarizes the most common cardiovascular appliances and their correct position on the chest radiograph.

Central venous catheters are used to monitor central venous pressure (CVP) and to provide reliable venous access. On the chest film, they are seen as moderately radiopaque tubes extending centrally from a subclavian, internal jugular, or femoral vein insertion site. The ideal location of the catheter tip is within the superior vena cava (SVC), so that it is close to the right atrium, yet beyond the most proximal venous valves.

TABLE 15-4 Cardiovascular Appliances

Appliance	Function	Position
Swan-Ganz catheter	Measures PAWP and right heart pressures	Tip in right or left pulmonary artery
CVP catheter	CVP measurement, venous access	Superior vena cava
LA catheter	Left atrial pressure	Left atrium
Mediastinal drains	Mediastinal fluid evacuation	Anterior mediastinum, posterior pericardium
Pacemaker leads	Cardiac pacing	Over right heart
IABP	Assists LV function	Tip just below top of aortic arch

PAWP, Pulmonary artery wedge pressure; *CVP,* central venous pressure; *LA,* left atrium; *IABP,* intraaortic balloon pump; *LV,* left ventricle.

Placement of the catheter tip beyond venous valves is important for accurate CVP measurement. Examples of malposition include placement into the wrong vein, intracardiac placement, or arterial cannulation. Placement into a vein other than the vena cava would not preclude use of the catheter for venous infusion, but would result in inaccurate CVP measurements. Placement into the right atrium or right ventricle could cause dysrhythmias, endocardial damage, or cardiac perforation and pericardial tamponade. Arterial cannulation would result in an inaccurate CVP measurement and would be unsafe for fluid infusion. Other potential complications of central line placement include pneumothorax, ectopic placement in the pleural space, infection, and catheter knotting or fragmentation. Since air rises, a pneumothorax can usually be seen in the apicolateral region of the affected side on an upright film. Supine films are more difficult to interpret, but a pleural air collection may be seen at the anteromedial aspect of the thorax. Sometimes the appearance of the pneumothorax on the chest film is delayed, because of very slow leakage of air into the pleural space. For this reason, at least one follow-up film several hours after catheter insertion is necessary to be certain that a pneumothorax has not occurred.[13] Ectopic placement in the pleural space can lead to infusion of fluid into the pleural space if not detected on the initial chest film. The result would appear as a large pleural effusion on the affected side only, developing suddenly after central line placement and fluid infusion through that line. Knotting and/or catheter fragmentation are rare but serious complications that may result in thrombosis, dysrhythmias, vascular injury, or embolization. Frontal as well as lateral views are necessary for accurate localization of catheter fragments.[13]

Pulmonary artery catheters, also known as Swan-Ganz catheters, are commonly used to obtain more specific hemodynamic data. The insertion site is generally a subclavian or internal jugular vein. The catheter progresses from the superior vena cava to the right atrium, to the right ventricle, to the pulmonary outflow tract, and finally into the right or left main pulmonary artery. If the tip of the catheter is too peripheral, blood flow may be obstructed and result in pulmonary infarction. If the catheter tip can be seen on the chest film more than 2 cm lateral to the pulmonary hilum, it is too peripheral. If the tip of the catheter is located too proximal (in the right ventricle or pulmonary outflow tract), dysrhythmias, endothelial damage, or perforation may occur. In addition, the catheter must not be directed toward an upper lobe, since upper lobe pulmonary blood vessels may be somewhat compressed by surrounding alveoli, rendering measurements less accurate.[14] Since pulmonary artery catheters are placed via central venous access, all of the other aforementioned potential complications of central venous line insertion are also risks of these catheters, and they must be kept in mind when viewing postplacement films.

A *left atrial catheter* is sometimes placed during open heart surgery to measure left atrial pressures directly. It is also radiopaque, and is seen in the left atria on the chest film.

Two or three *mediastinal drainage tubes* are also commonly inserted during cardiac surgery. They are inserted in the midline incision; one is directed superiorly to drain the anterior mediastinum, and the other is left of the incision site and is directed inferiorly to drain the posterolateral pericardial space.[14]

An *intraaortic balloon pump (IABP)* provides mechanical support for the failing heart. It is a 26 to 28 mm inflatable balloon that surrounds a catheter that is inserted into the descending aorta, either percutaneously via the femoral artery or operatively into the thoracic aorta. A chest x-ray must be obtained immediately after insertion to evaluate the position of the IABP. The distal tip of the catheter contains a small radiopaque rectangle that is helpful in determining its position on the chest film. This rectangle must be just distal to the origin of the left subclavian artery in the descending thoracic aorta, just below the top of the aortic arch. If it is not inserted far enough, counterpulsation is less effective and occlusion of the intraabdominal vessels could occur, resulting in renal or mesenteric ischemia. If the catheter is advanced too far, it may enter or obstruct the left subclavian or carotid artery, causing ischemia. Even when inserted properly, there is a risk of aortic dissection, especially when there is preexisting aortic disease. Aortic dissection can be seen on the chest x-ray as a loss of sharpness of the borders of the descending thoracic aorta.[13]

A *pacemaker* is another cardiovascular device that can be visualized and evaluated on a chest film. Used in the treatment of bradydysrhythmias and heart block, a pacemaker consists of a pulse generator, atrial and/or ventricular lead wires, and terminal electrodes. If the pacemaker is permanently implanted, the entire system is seen on the chest film. If it is only a temporary pacemaker, the pulse generator is external to the body and is not seen on the chest film. The electrodes are usually placed transvenously into the right side of the heart; even when placed epicardially, they are usually sutured onto the right atrium or right ventricle. On the frontal chest x-ray, the transvenous ventricular electrode must project slightly to the left of the midline and over the apex. Ideally, there is a slight bend in the catheter just before its tip. Complications that can occur and that can be seen radiographically include malposition of the electrode, myocardial perforation, lead-wire fracture, and infection. All of these complications, although possibly identifiable on a very good quality radiograph, are actually very subtle, and may require multiple views or even fluoroscopy for accurate diagnosis. Malposition is identified by comparing serial films and examining the position of the terminal electrodes. Even subtle changes in electrode position can cause serious pacemaker failure. Myocardial perforation is identified on the chest film if the tip of the electrode is seen projecting beyond the border of the heart. Clinical and radiographic signs of pericardial tamponade, such as progressive enlargement of the cardiac silhouette, may be present. Sharp angulation, fixation, or flexion of the lead wire increases the risk of fracture. Fractures commonly occur in three locations—the tip, near the pulse generator, and at the venous entry site. Radiographic evidence of infection, such as soft tissue swelling, gas accumulation, and air-fluid levels, may accompany clinical signs of infection.[13]

Hemodynamic assessment. A wealth of physiologic data can be gleaned from a chest x-ray. To be valid, this information needs to be interpreted in the context of a thorough physical examination. Keeping that in mind, the following parameters can be evaluated on a standard chest x-ray: systemic blood volume, pulmonary blood volume, central venous pressure, pulmonary artery pressure, and pulmonary artery wedge pressure (PAWP).

Systemic blood volume can be estimated by examining the vascular pedicle—that portion of the superior mediastinum that contains the great vessels (Figure 15-4, *arrows*). The right margin of the vascular pedicle is the lateral border of the superior vena cava, and the left margin is the lateral border of the left subclavian artery. These vessels are easily distensible; therefore they change in diameter with changes in circulating blood volume. To properly evaluate this, serial chest x-rays with consistent patient positioning are essential. Comparison of the cardiothoracic (CT) ratio (see Figure 15-4) from one day to the next can be used to assess this parameter also, but it is not as sensitive—a 66% increase in systemic blood volume is necessary to cause a visible change.[15]

Pulmonary blood volume is determined by examining the diameter of the pulmonary blood vessels. If blood flow through the lungs is increased, the diameter of the vessels throughout the lungs also are increased. In a low-flow state, the vessels appear constricted.

Central venous pressure can be estimated by noting the relative width of the azygous vein. This vein can be seen just above the right main bronchus overlying the outline of the superior vena cava, and it responds directly to right atrial pressure rather than circulating blood volume as a whole.

Pulmonary artery pressure is reflected in the relative diameter of central (hilar) pulmonary blood vessels compared with peripheral pulmonary vessels. Large hilar vessels with small or nonexistent peripheral vessels are indicative of chronic pulmonary hypertension, often seen in patients with chronic pulmonary disease. The lack of peripheral vessels is sometimes referred to as "pruning" because it looks like the pulmonary vessels have been cut off, similar to the pruning of a tree. The extent to which these changes are present is a fairly accurate indication of the severity of the chronic pulmonary hypertension. However, it does not accurately reflect acute changes in pulmonary artery pressure.[15]

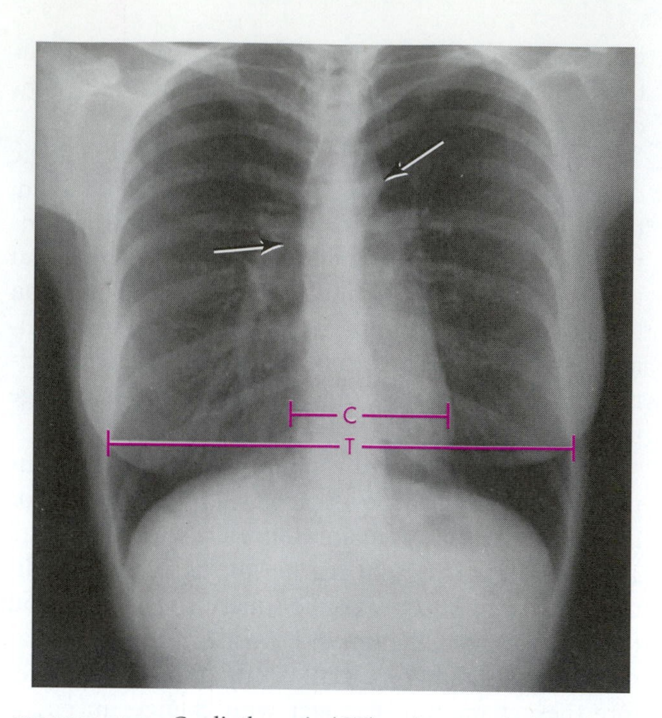

FIGURE 15-4. Cardiothoracic (CT) ratio—a technique for estimating heart size on a PA chest film. Normally the cardiac diameter is 50% or less of the thoracic diameter when measured during full inhalation. *C*, Maximal cardiac diameter; *T*, maximal thoracic diameter measured to the inside of the ribs. The width of the vascular pedicle *(arrows)* is a more accurate indicator of systemic blood volume.

TABLE 15-5 Chest X-ray Estimation of Pulmonary Artery Wedge Pressure (PAWP)*

Pulmonary Artery Wedge Pressure (mm Hg)	Chest X-ray Findings
5-12	Normal
12-15	Equal perfusion of upper and lower lung fields
15-20	Upper lung perfusion > lower lung perfusion
20-25	Interstitial edema in lower lobes; Kerley B lines; perivascular cuffing and peribronchial cuffing
> 25	Perihilar haze; diffuse perihilar infiltrates

*These PAWP values are guidelines. PAWP values may vary in individual patients; see text for further discussion.

The final hemodynamic variable that can be assessed on a portable chest film is *pulmonary artery wedge pressure* (Table 15-5). Considerable controversy exists surrounding the accuracy of PAWP estimates based solely on a chest film. However, the information obtained radiographically is still clinically useful if it is placed in a clinical perspective and potential sources of error are understood. On a normal, high-quality, upright chest x-ray, the diameter of the blood vessels in the lower lobes is greater than the diameter of the blood vessels in the upper lobes. This is because blood flows preferentially to the lung bases as a result of gravitational forces in the upright position. The vessel margins are normally sharply defined. When the PAWP rises above 12 mm Hg, the diameter of upper and lower blood vessels begins to equalize. Eventually, as the PAWP nears 20 mm Hg, the diameter of upper lobe blood vessels becomes greater than that of the lower lobe vessels. This is referred to as "cephalization" of blood flow. As the PAWP increases to between 20 and 25 mm Hg, blurring of the blood vessel margins occurs. Known as "perivascular cuffing," the blurring is a result of fluid surrounding the pulmonary vessels. The pressure within the vessels has exceeded the colloid osmotic pressure of the blood, causing a transudate of fluid into the interstitium. This fluid also accumulates around the bronchi, causing "peribronchial cuffing." Fluid gathers as well along the interlobar septae, resulting in linear opacities on the chest x-ray that extend to the pleural surface, especially near the costophrenic angles. These are called "Kerley B lines." When the PAWP exceeds 25 mm Hg, the transudate collects in large amounts in the interstitial and alveolar compartments. This development of alveolar pulmonary edema is seen on the chest film as hazy, fluffy opacification of the lungs, particularly in the hilar regions.[15]

Discrepancies between the degree of pulmonary congestion in acute heart failure identified on the chest x-ray and the actual measurement of PAWP are common. There are three main reasons for this. Other lung problems—emphysema, interstitial lung disease, or pneumonia—or even the inability of the patient to take a deep breath for the x-ray, cloud the picture and make subtle changes difficult to see. Time is another important variable; whereas hemodynamic measurements reflect a specific instance in time, movement of water in or out of the extravascular compartment may take hours or even days. Finally, many critically ill patients cannot tolerate an upright position and must therefore have their portable chest film taken in the supine position. When the patient is supine, hydrostatic differences occur from the anterior to the posterior aspects of the lung, rather than from bases to apices. Even in a normal supine patient, vessel diameter appears equalized from base to apex. Distribution of edema can also change.

Future trends. Digital radiography systems are being widely implemented in hospitals, although few use them for portable films at present. In a digital radiograph, the image is divided into discrete elements (pixels) that are assigned a specific value and stored for later display, either on a computer screen or by means of a laser printer. Pixel sizes vary; the smaller the pixel, the better the resolution. Currently, the resolution of a digital radiograph is not quite as good as that of a standard chest film, although it is considered adequate.[16] This will certainly improve as technology progresses. Digital systems have many advantages. No film development is necessary, so the image can be displayed rapidly on a video display in the clinical area. The image can be expanded or compressed. This system also lends itself to computer-assisted diagnosis, which involves computer analysis of the image to detect and quantify pathologic findings. If a baseline film has been digitally recorded, the baseline film can be "subtracted" from the current film, highlighting any areas of change, such as increased heart size or new pulmonary infiltrates. There are still technical difficulties to overcome with this technique, but it has the potential to greatly increase the value of chest radiography as a cardiovascular diagnostic technique.

Electrocardiography

Electrocardiography is a complex subject about which much literature has been written and to which entire books have been devoted—and justifiably so. A detailed evaluation of a 12-lead ECG can provide a wealth of cardiac diagnostic information and often provides the basis on which other definitive diagnostic tests are selected. This section provides a comprehensive discussion of the many clinical factors that the critical care nurse considers when monitoring a patient for dysrhythmias. Specific dysrhythmias commonly encountered in clinical practice are discussed in the section on dysrhythmia interpretation later in the chapter. The beginning section covers 12-lead ECG analysis and describes the skills needed to evaluate lead placement, left ventricular axis, and changes in the 12-lead ECG caused by ischemia or infarction. The intent is to provide a sound basis for understanding the value of the many clinical applications of electrocardiography. (∞Dysrhythmia Interpretation, p. 406.)

Basic principles. The ECG records electrical changes in heart muscle. It does not record mechanical contraction, which usually immediately follows electrical depolarization. However, a condition known as *pulseless electrical activity (PEA)* occasionally occurs, in which the heart is mechanically at a standstill while rhythmic electrical impulses continue to be generated and then recorded on the ECG.

A review of the cardiac action potential illustrates electrical changes that occur (Figure 15-5). During phase 0 (*depolarization*), the electrical potential changes rapidly from a baseline of − 90 mV to + 20 mV and stabilizes at about 0 mV. Because this is a significant electrical change, it appears on the ECG. Phases 1 and 2 represent an electrical plateau, during which time mechanical contraction occurs. Because there is no significant electrical change at this time, nothing shows on the ECG. During phase 3 (*repolarization*), the electrical potential again changes, this time a little more slowly, from 0 mV back to − 90 mV. This is another major electrical event, and it is reflected on the ECG. Phase 4 represents a resting period, during which chemical balance is restored by the sodium pump, but since positively charged ions are exchanged on a one-for-one basis, there is no electrical activity and no visible change occurs on the ECG tracing. (∞Electrical Activity, p. 344).

Electrocardiographic leads. All electrocardiographs use a system of one or more *leads.* A lead consists of three electrodes: a positive electrode, a negative electrode, and a ground electrode. The function of the ground electrode is to prevent the display of background electrical interference on the ECG tracing. Leads do not transmit any electricity to the patient—they just sense and record it.

The positive electrode on the skin acts as a camera. If the wave of depolarization travels toward the positive electrode, an upward stroke, or *positive deflection,* is written on the ECG paper (Figure 15-6, *A*). If the wave of depolarization travels away from the positive electrode, a downward line, or *negative deflection,* is recorded on the ECG (Figure 15-6, *B*). When depolarization moves perpendicularly to the positive electrode, a biphasic complex occurs. Sometimes the complex may even appear almost flat or isoelectric if the electrical forces traveling in opposite directions are equal and have the effect of canceling out each other (Figure 15-6, *C*). The size of the muscle mass being depolarized also has an effect, with the larger muscle mass having a greater influence on the tracing.

The wave of ventricular depolarization in the healthy heart travels from right to left and head to toe. The appearance of the waveforms in different ECG leads will vary, depending on the location of the positive electrode. The standard 12-lead ECG provides a picture of electrical activity in the heart from the 12 different positions of the positive electrodes.

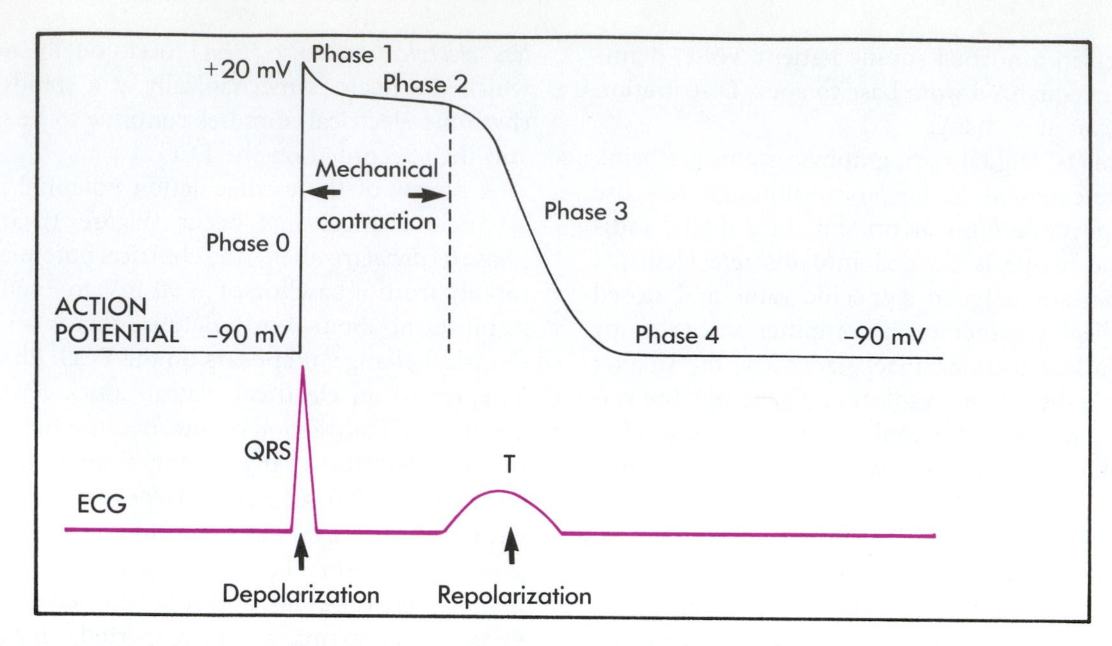

FIGURE 15-5. Correlation of the action potential of a ventricular myocardial cell with the electrical events recorded on the surface ECG. Note that the ECG is "silent" during phase 2 of the action potential. Mechanical contraction is occurring, but there is no significant electrical activity.

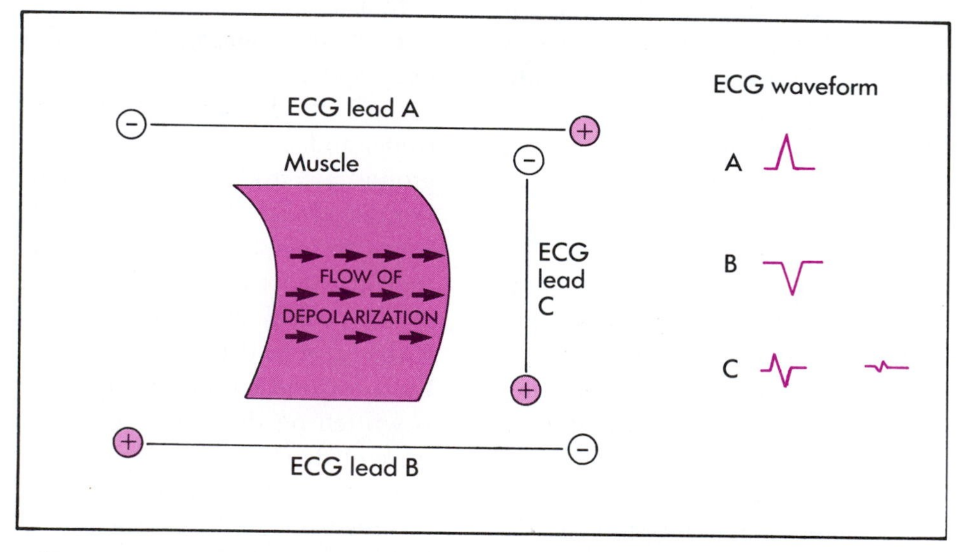

FIGURE 15-6. Effect of lead position on the ECG tracing. **A,** Flow of depolarization toward the positive electrode results in a positive deflection on the ECG. **B,** Flow of depolarization away from the positive electrode results in a negative deflection on the ECG. **C,** Flow of depolarization perpendicular to the positive electrode results in a biphasic or nearly isoelectric deflection on the ECG. This basic principle applies to both the P wave and the QRS complex.

A standard 12-lead ECG consists of six limb leads and six chest leads. The limb leads are obtained by placing electrodes on all four extremities. The exact location on the extremities does not matter, as long as skin contact is good and bone is avoided. The machine interprets all extremity signals as coming from the connection of the extremity to the torso, (i.e., from the shoulder or groin).

Leads I, II, and III are bipolar limb leads in that they consist of a positive and a negative electrode. The other three limb leads are labeled aV_R, aV_L, and aV_F, representing augmented vector right, left, and foot (Figure 15-7, *A*). These unipolar leads consist only of a positive electrode, with the negative electrode calculated within the machine at roughly the center of the heart. Under these circumstances the ECG tracing

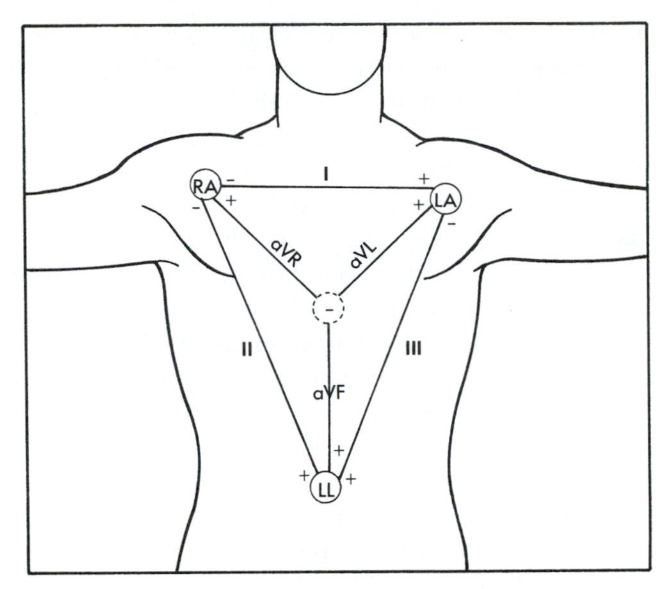

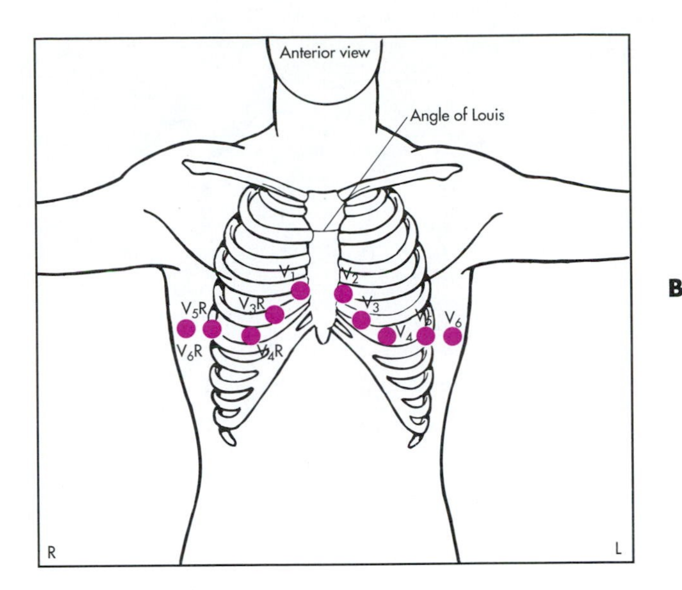

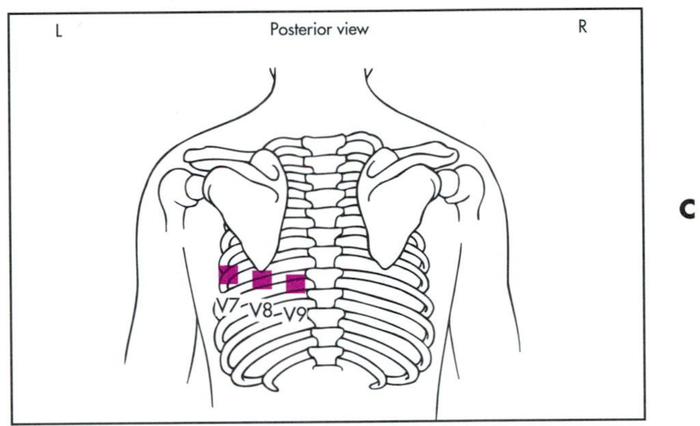

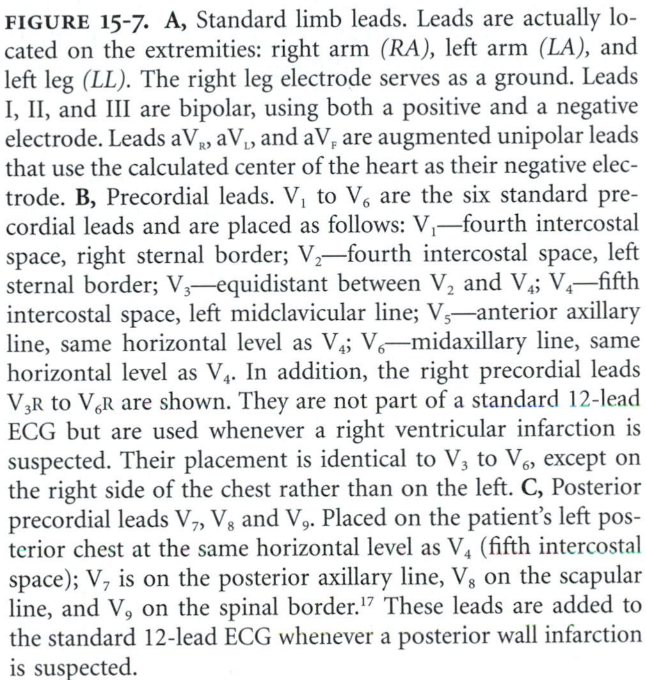

FIGURE 15-7. A, Standard limb leads. Leads are actually located on the extremities: right arm *(RA)*, left arm *(LA)*, and left leg *(LL)*. The right leg electrode serves as a ground. Leads I, II, and III are bipolar, using both a positive and a negative electrode. Leads aV_R, aV_L, and aV_F are augmented unipolar leads that use the calculated center of the heart as their negative electrode. **B,** Precordial leads. V_1 to V_6 are the six standard precordial leads and are placed as follows: V_1—fourth intercostal space, right sternal border; V_2—fourth intercostal space, left sternal border; V_3—equidistant between V_2 and V_4; V_4—fifth intercostal space, left midclavicular line; V_5—anterior axillary line, same horizontal level as V_4; V_6—midaxillary line, same horizontal level as V_4. In addition, the right precordial leads V_3R to V_6R are shown. They are not part of a standard 12-lead ECG but are used whenever a right ventricular infarction is suspected. Their placement is identical to V_3 to V_6, except on the right side of the chest rather than on the left. **C,** Posterior precordial leads V_7, V_8 and V_9. Placed on the patient's left posterior chest at the same horizontal level as V_4 (fifth intercostal space); V_7 is on the posterior axillary line, V_8 on the scapular line, and V_9 on the spinal border.[17] These leads are added to the standard 12-lead ECG whenever a posterior wall infarction is suspected.

would ordinarily be very small, so the machine enhances, or *augments,* it. The term *vector* refers to directional force.

The six standard precordial chest leads are labeled "V" leads and are distributed in an arch around the left side of the chest. They are useful for viewing electrical forces traveling from right to left or front to back but are not helpful in evaluating vertical forces in the heart. For an accurate interpretation, all 12 leads must be considered (Figure 15-7, *B*).

At times, additional leads are helpful in evaluating the extent of myocardium involved in an acute myocardial infarction. Both the right ventricle and the posterior wall of the left ventricle are areas of the heart that are not well-represented on a standard 12-lead ECG. The right ventricle can be assessed by adding right-sided chest leads (Figure 15-7, *B*). Labeled V_3R, V_4R, and V_6R, they are added to the standard 12-lead ECG whenever right ventricular infarction is suspected. A right ventricular infarction is most commonly associated with an inferior or posterior left ventricular infarction. The posterior wall of the left ventricle can be assessed using posterior chest leads (Figure 15-7, *C*). These leads are labeled V_7, V_8 and V_9. Although posterior lead placement can be somewhat technically challenging, the information obtained is very useful clinically and may influence decisions regarding clinical management.[17]

Baseline distortion. It is important that the tracing have a flat baseline, which is that portion of the tracing that is between the various waveforms. Two forms of artifact can distort the baseline: 60-cycle interference and muscular movement. Sixty-cycle interference (Figure 15-8, *A*) results from leakage of electrical current somewhere within the system and appears as a generalized thickening of the baseline. It can usually

A

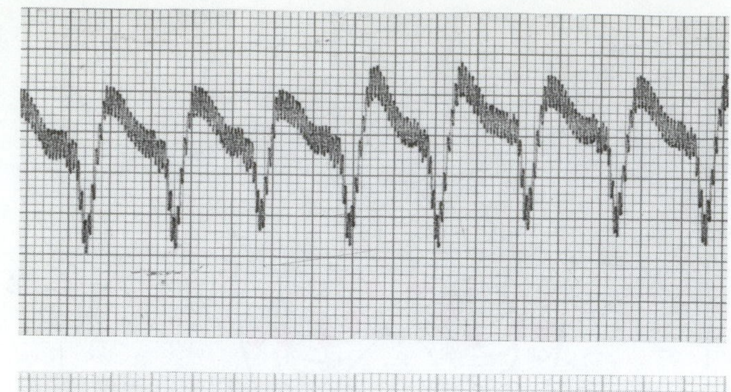

B

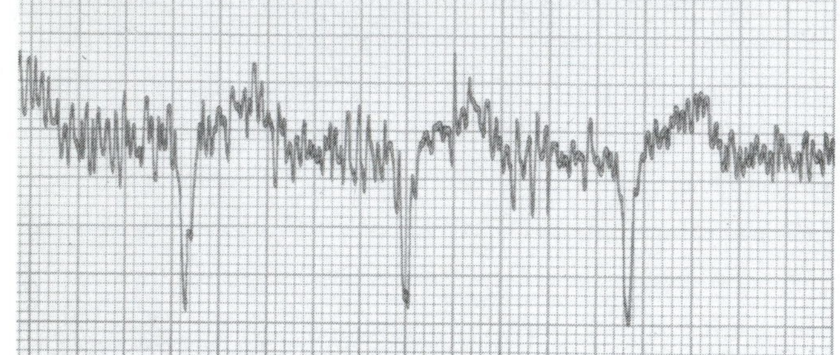

FIGURE 15-8. **A,** Artifact—60-cycle interference. **B,** Artifact—muscular movement.

be resolved by ensuring that all electrical equipment at the bedside is well-grounded. Occasionally, it may be necessary to unplug one piece of equipment at a time until the offending device is found. Muscular movement (Figure 15-8, *B*) is displayed as a coarse, erratic disturbance of the baseline. In most cases, asking the patient to lie quietly while the ECG is being run is sufficient. If movement is caused by shivering or seizure activity, it is best to wait until the activity subsides before obtaining the 12-lead ECG. If tremor is caused by Parkinson's disease or other neuromuscular disorders, a resolution may not be possible. It must be remembered that the artifact has an adverse effect on the accurate interpretation of the tracing.

Twelve-lead ECG analysis

Specialized ECG paper. ECG paper records the speed and magnitude of electrical impulses on a grid composed of small and large boxes (Figure 15-9). There are five small boxes in every large box. At a standard paper speed of 25 mm/second, one small box (1 mm) is equivalent to 0.04 second, and one large box (5 mm) represents 0.20 second. Distances along the horizontal axis represent speed and are stated in seconds rather than in millimeters or number of boxes. The vertical axis represents magnitude or strength of force.

Calibration. At standard calibration, one small box equals 0.1 mV, and one large box equals 0.5 mV. It is important to look for the standardization mark, which is usually located at the beginning of the tracing (Figure 15-10, *A*). The mark indicates 1 mV and at standard calibration goes up two large boxes. Twelve-lead ECGs are sometimes run at different calibrations. If, at standard calibration, some complexes are so tall they run off the paper, the tracing is repeated at half standard (Figure 15-10, *B*), and the calibration mark rises only one large box. If all of the complexes on a standard tracing are very small, it may be repeated at double standard, with the calibration mark going up four large boxes (Figure 15-10, *C*). In any case, the calibration must be clearly marked on the tracing, because some diagnostic conclusions are based on the magnitude of specific portions of the ECG complex.

Waveforms. The analysis of waveforms and intervals provide the basis for ECG interpretation (Figure 15-11). The P wave represents atrial depolarization. The QRS complex represents ventricular depolarization, corresponding to phase 0 of the ventricular action potential. It is referred to as a *complex* because it can actually consist of several different waves, depending on the placement of the positive electrode and the direction of the spread of electrical activity in the heart. Basically, the letter Q is used to describe an *initial* negative deflection; in other words, only if the first deflection from the baseline is negative will it be labeled a Q wave. The letter R applies to any positive deflection. If there are two positive deflections in one QRS complex, the second is labeled R′ (read "R prime") and is commonly seen in lead V_1 in right bundle branch block. The letter S refers to any subsequent negative deflections. Any combination of these deflections can occur and is collectively called the *QRS complex* (Figure 15-12). The QRS duration is normally 0.10 second (2 1/2 small boxes) or less.

The T wave represents ventricular repolarization, corresponding to phase 3 of the ventricular action potential. The onset of the QRS to approximately the midpoint or peak of the T wave represents an absolute refractory period, during which the heart muscle cannot respond to another stimulus no matter how strong that stimulus might be (Figure 15-13). From the midpoint to the end of the T wave, the heart muscle is in the relative refractory period. The heart muscle has not yet fully recovered, but it could be depolarized again if a strong enough stimulus were received. This can be a particularly dangerous time for ectopy to occur, especially if any portion of the myocardium is ischemic, because the ischemic muscle takes even longer to fully repolarize. This sets the stage for the disorganized, self-perpetuating depolarizations of various sections of the myocardium that is known as *ventricular fibrillation.*

Intervals between waveforms. Intervals between waveforms are also evaluated (see Figure 15-11). The

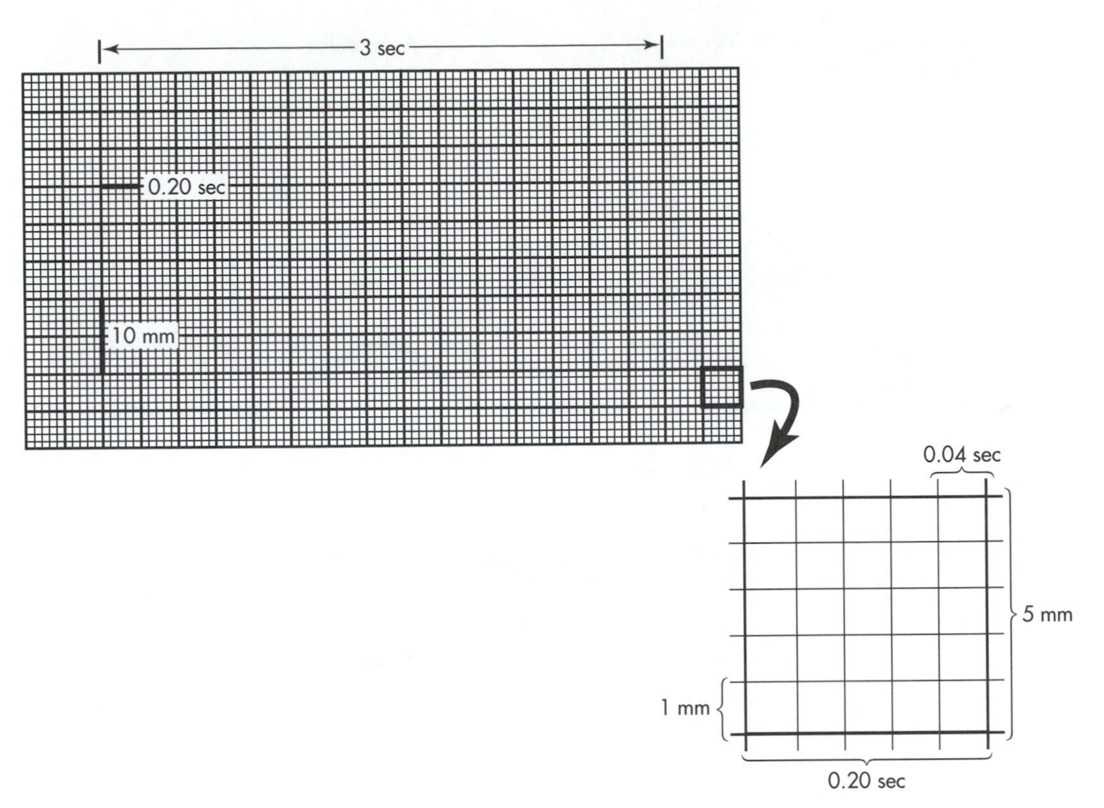

FIGURE 15-9. ECG graph paper. The horizontal axis represents time, and the vertical axis represents magnitude of voltage. Horizontally, each small box is 0.04 second and each large box is 0.20 second. Vertically, each large box is 5 mm. Markings are present every 3 seconds at the top of the paper for ease in calculating heart rate.

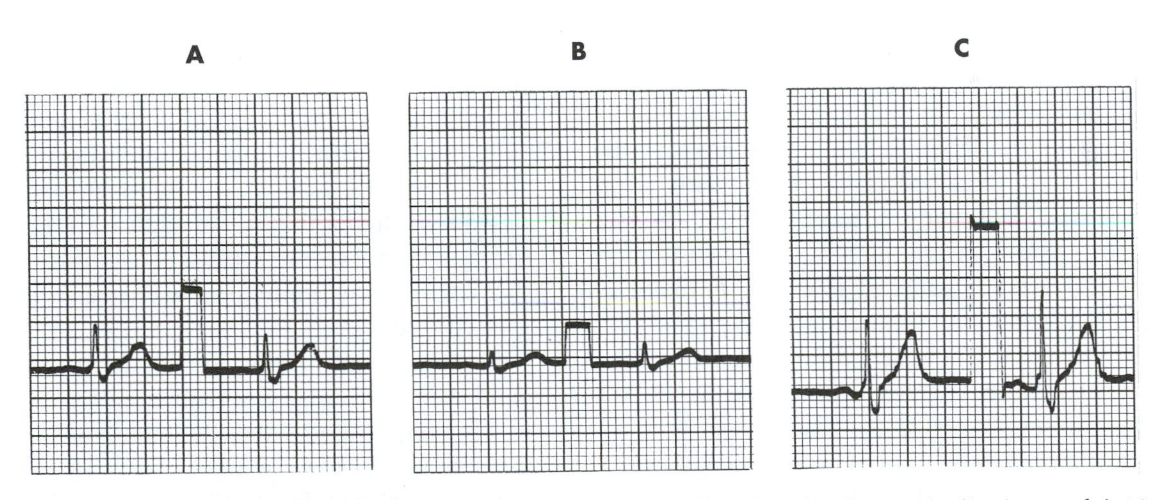

FIGURE 15-10. A, Normal standardization mark, in which the machine is calibrated so that the standardization mark is 10 mm tall. **B,** Half standardization, used whenever QRS complexes are too tall to fit on the paper. **C,** Twice normal standardization, used whenever QRS complexes are too small to be adequately analyzed.

PR interval is measured from the beginning of the P wave to the beginning of the QRS complex. Normally, the PR interval is 0.12 to 0.20 second in length and represents the time between sinus node discharge and the beginning of ventricular depolarization. Because most of this time period results from delay of the impulse in the AV node, the PR interval is an indicator of AV nodal function.

The portion of the wave that extends from the end of the QRS to the beginning of the T wave is labeled the *ST segment.* Its duration is not measured. Instead, its shape and location are evaluated. The ST segment is normally flat and at the same level as the isoelectric baseline. Elevation or depression is expressed in millimeters and may indicate ischemia. The QT interval is measured from the beginning of the QRS complex

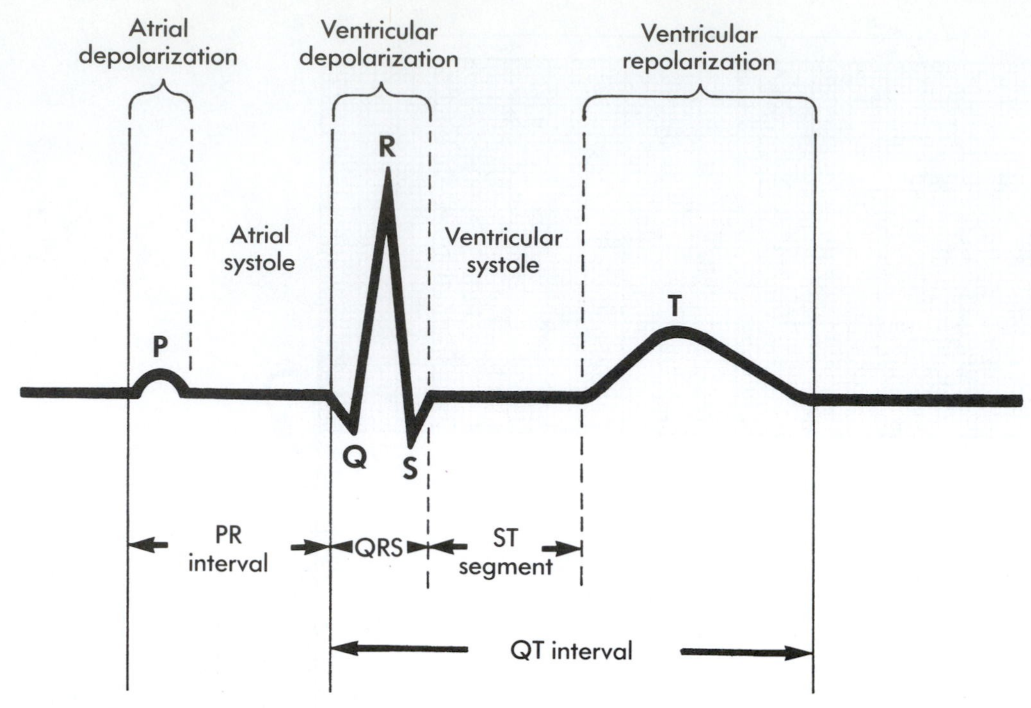

FIGURE 15-11. Normal ECG waveforms, intervals, and correlation with events of the cardiac cycle. The P wave represents atrial depolarization, followed immediately by atrial systole. The QRS represents ventricular depolarization, followed immediately by ventricular systole. The ST segment corresponds to phase 2 of the action potential, during which time the heart muscle is completely depolarized and contraction normally occurs. The T wave represents ventricular repolarization. The PR interval, measured from the beginning of the P wave to the beginning of the QRS, corresponds to atrial depolarization and impulse delay in the AV node. The QT interval, measured from the beginning of the QRS complex to the end of the T wave, represents the time from initial depolarization of the ventricles to the end of ventricular repolarization.

to the end of the T wave and indicates the total time interval from the onset of depolarization to the completion of repolarization. At normal heart rates, the QT interval is less than half of the RR interval (measured from one QRS complex to the next). However, the normal value of a QT interval is dependent on heart rate and must be adjusted according to the heart rate to be evaluated in a meaningful way. The corrected QT interval (QTc) can be calculated by dividing the measured QT interval, in seconds, by the RR cycle length[18] (see Figure 15-3). The normal QTc interval is less than 0.44 second. A prolonged QT interval is significant because it can predispose the patient to the development of polymorphic ventricular tachycardia, known also as *torsades de pointes.* A long QT interval can be congenital (adrenergic dependent) or it can be acquired (pause dependent) as a result of electrolyte imbalance or antidysrhythmic drug therapy. Quinidine is the antidysrhythmic drug most commonly responsible for the acquired form of prolonged QT interval, although any Class Ia drug (quinidine, procainamide, and disopyramide); Class III drug (amiodarone or sotalol); or Class IV drug (bepridil) can prolong the QT interval and initiate an episode of torsades de pointes. The prodysrhythmic effect of these drugs is not related to serum drug levels or the duration of treatment.[18] It is an idiosyncratic response, which can be intensified by hypokalemia, hypomagnesemia, or hypocalcemia. In addition, it is much more likely to occur in the setting of significant bradycardia, either sinus bradycardia or second- or third-degree AV block.

Both forms of prolonged QT interval may produce similar dysrhythmias, but there are distinct differences in their response to sympathetic nervous system stimulation and in their management. The acquired, or pause-dependent, long QT syndrome is thought to arise from prolongation of the ventricular refractory period. Acute therapy is directed at increasing the heart rate, which will shorten the QT interval. This may include placement of a temporary pacemaker; careful infusion of isoproterenol; and intravenous (IV) magnesium supplementation, especially if serum levels of magnesium are low. Long-term management includes correction of electrolyte abnormalities or removal of the responsible drug. In the congenital, or adrenergic-dependent, long QT syndrome an autonomic imbalance exists, resulting in an enhanced response to

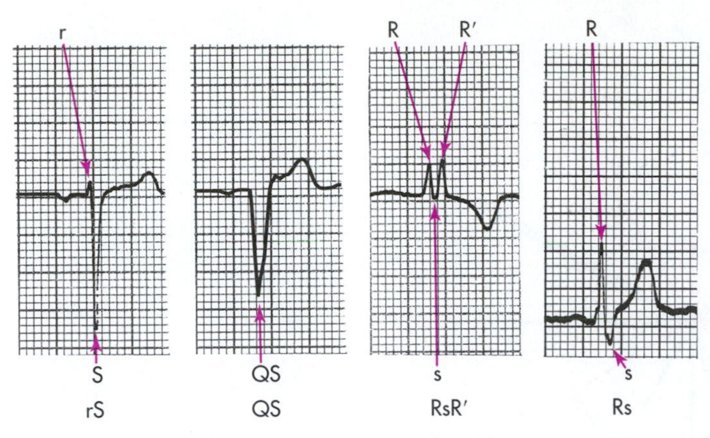

FIGURE 15-12. Examples of QRS complexes. Small deflections are labeled with lowercase letters, whereas uppercase letters are used for larger deflections. A second upward deflection is labeled R′ ("R prime").

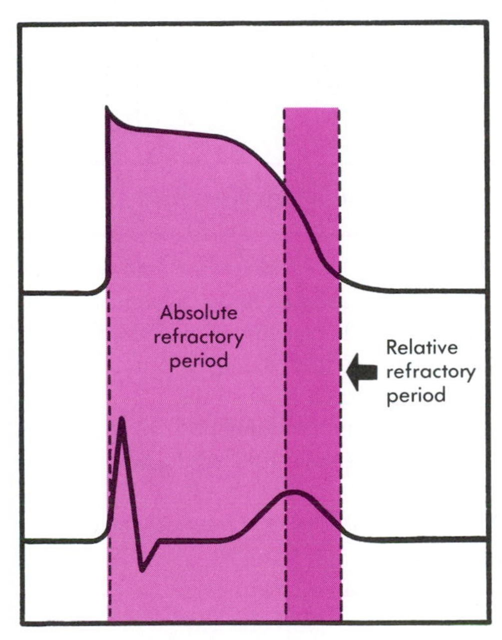

FIGURE 15-13. Absolute and relative refractory periods correlated with the cardiac muscle's action potential and with an ECG tracing.

sympathetic stimulation. Torsades de pointes usually occurs after some form of sympathetic discharge, such as sudden exertion, fright, emotional stress, delirium tremens, or cocaine use. Management in that case is aimed at blocking beta-adrenergic receptors with either medication (beta-blockers) or surgery (left sympathectomy). Sometimes pacemaker therapy is necessary to allow adequate doses of beta-blockers to be tolerated without causing symptomatic bradycardia. Only 1% of patients with congenital long QT syndrome require placement of an implantable cardioverter defibrillator.[18]

Although the ECG records only electrical events, it is helpful to understand the correlation of these intervals to the physiologic events of the cardiac cycle. Immediately after the P wave and during the PR interval, atrial systole occurs. Similarly, ventricular systole begins immediately after the QRS complex and continues until approximately the midpoint of the T wave (Figure 15-11).

Ventricular axis. Electrical impulses spread through cardiac muscle tissue in many directions at once when the ventricular muscle is depolarized. Using the 12-lead ECG, all of these individual forces can be averaged to describe the overall direction that current is traveling, which is called the *mean vector.* The mean vector can be plotted on a circular graph known as the *hexaxial reference system* (Figure 15-14), and a degree can be assigned to it. This degree represents the ventricular axis.

Normal range for ventricular axis varies slightly, but it is approximately −30 to +110 degrees. Right-axis deviation is present if the axis falls between +110 and +180 degrees. Left-axis deviation is present if the axis falls between −30 and −90 degrees. If the axis plots in the upper left portion of the circle, it is called an *indeterminate axis* and can occur only if the wave of depolarization starts in the bottom of the ventricle and spreads upward toward the atria. Clinically, this can be seen in beats of ventricular origin, such as premature ventricular contractions (PVCs) and some pacemaker-initiated beats. To determine the frontal plane ventricular axis, the six limb leads are examined to find the lead with the smallest QRS complex, or the most equiphasic (equal portions above and below the baseline) if no complex is clearly the smallest. In Figure 15-15, lead aV_F is the smallest. Next, using the

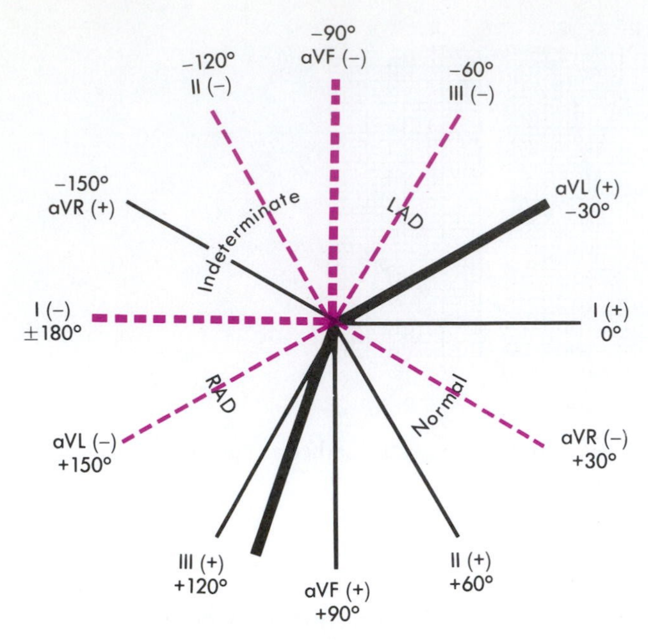

FIGURE 15-14. Hexaxial reference system. *RAD,* right axis deviation; *LAD,* left axis deviation.

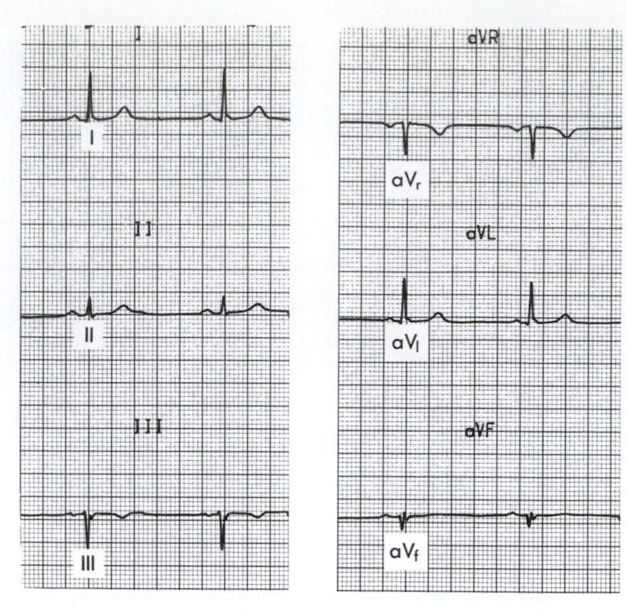

FIGURE 15-15. Limb leads of normal ECG illustrating normal axis of 0 degrees.

hexaxial reference system (see Figure 15-14), the lead is found that is perpendicular to the one that had the smallest complex. For example, perpendicular to lead aV_F is lead I, so the mean vector lies parallel with lead I. The third step is to determine whether the QRS complex is positive or negative in the lead parallel to the mean vector (in this case, I). If the QRS is positive, the mean vector is directed toward the positive electrode. If the QRS is negative, the mean vector is directed away from the positive electrode. In Figure 15-15, the QRS in lead I is upright, or positive. The positive pole of lead I is at the right midpoint of the hexaxial reference system and corresponds to a numeric degree of zero, which is normal (Box 15-3).

BOX 15-3 Steps in Determining Axis

1. Find the most isoelectric limb lead.
2. Using the hexaxial reference system, find the lead that is perpendicular to the one identified in step 1.
3. Determine whether the QRS is positive or negative in the perpendicular lead.
4. Look at the corresponding positive or negative pole of the perpendicular lead on the hexaxial reference system.
5. The degree listed on the hexaxial reference system is the axis.

Cardiac monitor lead analysis. During continuous cardiac monitoring, adhesive, pre-gelled electrodes are used to obtain an ECG tracing that is similar to one lead of a 12-lead ECG. At a minimum, this requires three electrodes: one positive, one negative, and one ground. In many clinical areas, five electrodes are used, either to monitor two leads simultaneously or to allow selection of several different leads at any time through a lead selector switch on the monitor. Typical placement of the five electrodes in a multilead system is illustrated in Figure 15-16. Three leads—II, MCL_1, and MCL_6—are commonly used for continuous monitoring, although others may also be used. Accurate lead placement is essential for accurate cardiac monitoring. Lead placement must be verified at the beginning of each shift. Once a transient dysrhythmia has occurred, it is too late to change lead placement so that an accurate analysis can be performed.

Lead II. On a standard 12-lead ECG, lead II is formed by a positive electrode attached to the left leg, a negative electrode attached to the right arm, and a ground electrode on the right leg. It is not practical to connect electrodes to the arms and legs during continuous monitoring, but the general placement remains the same. The positive electrode is placed on the lower left torso, at least below the level of the sixth rib and preferably below the rib cage completely. The negative electrode is placed on the right shoulder, and the ground electrode is usually placed on the left shoulder (Figure 15-17). The location of the ground is not

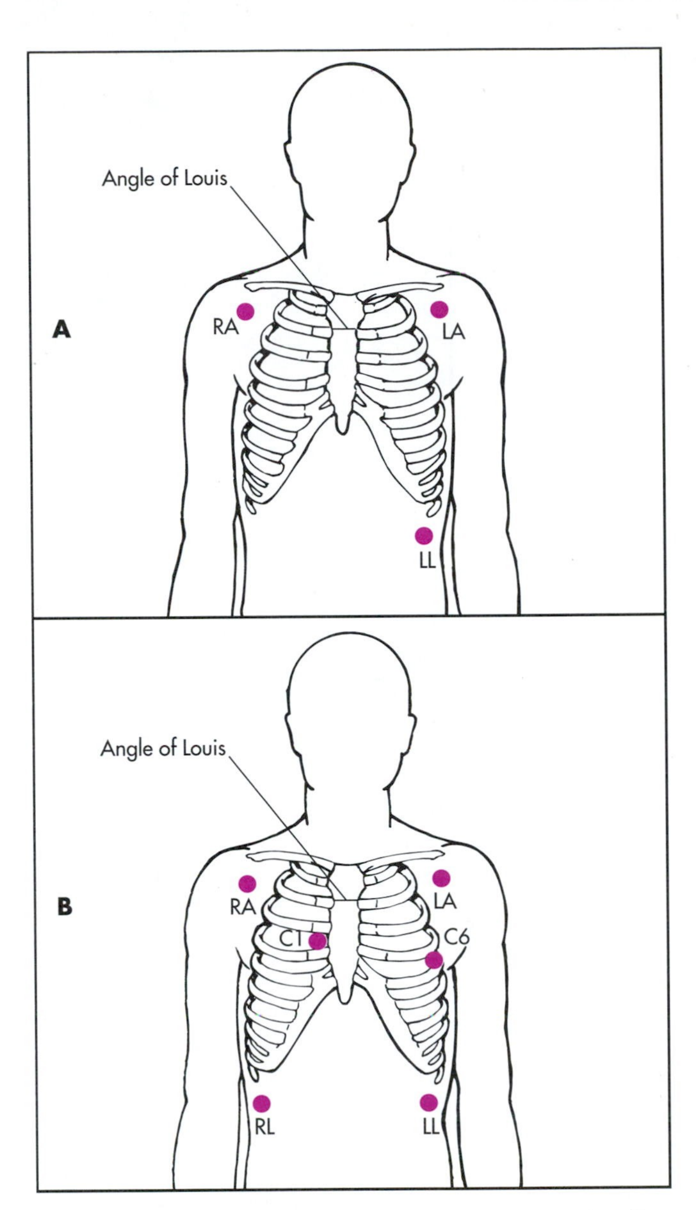

FIGURE 15-16. **A,** Three electrodes and lead-wire cables allow monitoring of three of the limb leads (I, II, and III) and can also be rearranged to monitor MCL_1 and MCL_6 (see Figure 15-18, *A*). **B,** Multilead monitoring system: Five electrodes and lead-wire cables allow monitoring of any of the six standard limb leads (I, II, III, aV_R, aV_L, or aV_F) and any one precordial lead, either V_1 or V_6. C_1 indicates the proper position of the chest electrode for monitoring lead V_1, and C_6 indicates the proper position of the chest electrode for monitoring V_6. The cable attachments are color-coded for quick identification and placement. Accurate electrode placement is essential.

significant. In patients with a normal electrical axis, this lead displays a waveform that is predominantly upright, has the greatest amplitude, and thus has the best signal-to-noise ratio. For this reason it is a popular monitoring lead and one that is often recommended by manufacturers of monitoring equipment.[19] P waves are usually easy to identify in lead II. However, it is difficult to identify right bundle branch block (RBBB) and left bundle branch block (LBBB) in this lead, because this is a vertical lead that does not clearly display horizontal interventricular conduction changes. This lead is also nondiagnostic in differentiating ventricular tachycardia from supraventricular tachycardia with aberrant conduction.

Lead MCL_1. Identification of an RBBB pattern is important in continuous cardiac monitoring, not only for diagnosing a new conduction defect, but also for verifying placement of a pacemaker wire, differentiating between ventricular tachycardia and supraventricular tachycardia with aberrant conduction, and determining whether PVCs are originating in the right or left ventricle. Lead MCL_1 is a good selection for this purpose.

"MCL_1" stands for "modified chest lead one." It is equivalent to a V_1 lead on a 12-lead ECG. The tracings are similar but not identical. In both, the positive electrode is at the 4th intercostal space just to the right of the sternum (Figure 15-18, *A*). It is extremely important for this electrode to be placed accurately. If placement is incorrect by even one intercostal space, the diagnostic value of this lead is completely lost.[20]

With V_1 the ECG machine calculates the negative electrode at the center of the heart, whereas with MCL_1 the negative electrode is located just below the left shoulder. In MCL_1 the ground electrode is placed on the right shoulder.

Because the positive electrode is to the right of the heart and most of the electrical activity in the heart is directed toward the left ventricle, the QRS complex in lead MCL_1 normally is negative (Figure 15-18, *B*). Any abnormal activity directed toward the right ventricle, such as in RBBB, results in an upright QRS complex, often in an RSR′ pattern.

Lead MCL_6. An alternative to lead MCL_1 is lead MCL_6. This is a modified V_6, with the positive electrode located in the V_6 position (left 5th intercostal space, midaxillary line). The negative electrode is placed below the left shoulder, and the ground can be placed below the right shoulder. Lead MCL_6 is also an adequate lead for monitoring interventricular conduction changes (see Figure 15-18, *A* and *C*).

Lead selection for optimal bedside monitoring. In the early years of critical care nursing, the primary goals of cardiac monitoring were heart rate surveillance, detection of "warning" dysrhythmias (mostly PVCs), and early detection of lethal dysrhythmias (ventricular fibrillation or asystole). Although these are still goals of ECG monitoring in the critical care unit today, several more complex issues are now of concern. It is now known that not all wide QRS complex tachycardias are

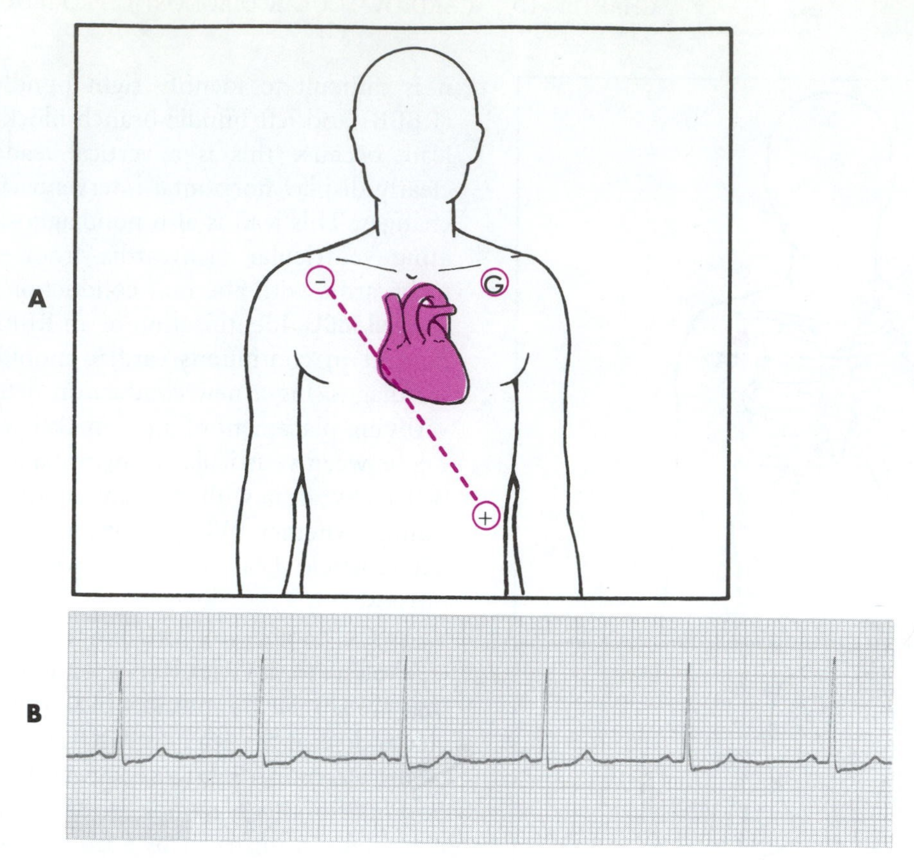

FIGURE 15-17. Monitoring lead II. **A,** Electrode placement. The negative electrode is placed below the right shoulder; the positive electrode is placed on the lower left torso (preferably below the rib cage); the ground electrode is placed on the left shoulder. **B,** Typical ECG tracing in Lead II.

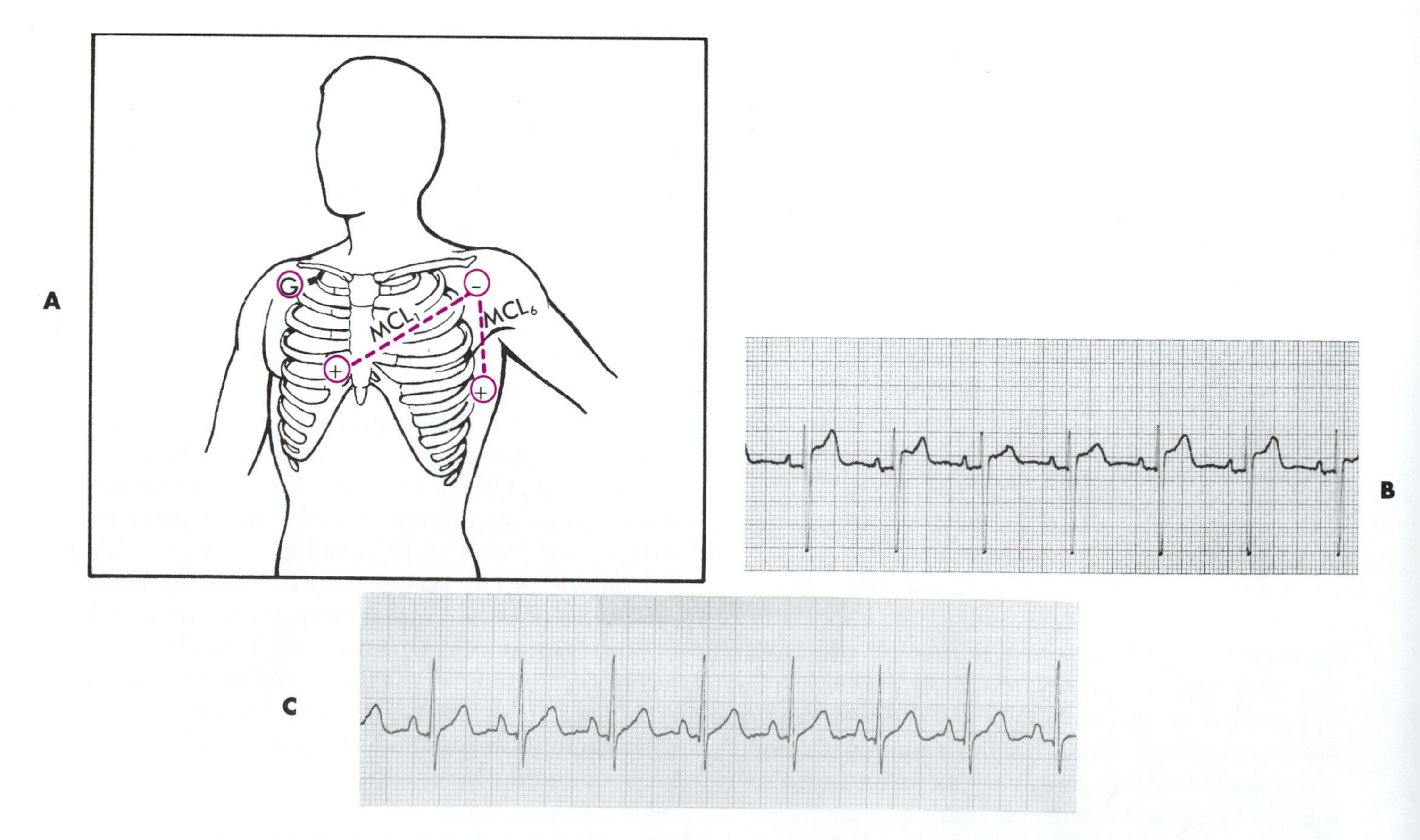

FIGURE 15-18. **A,** Monitoring lead placement in MCL_1 and MCL_6. **B,** Typical ECG tracing in MCL_1. **C,** Typical ECG tracing in MCL_6.

ventricular in origin; sometimes they are supraventricular with aberrant ventricular conduction. Many patients are now undergoing reperfusion therapy involving balloon angioplasty or thrombolysis, and these patients require continuous monitoring for ST-segment changes that may represent ischemia even in the absence of clinical symptoms. It is now important that the nurse admitting a patient to the critical care unit or telemetry unit make a well-planned choice of monitoring lead(s) that is tailored to the clinical needs of that particular patient. In addition, accuracy of lead placement is extremely important if these leads are to be used for specialized diagnostic purposes. Limb electrodes need to be placed close to where the limb joins the torso. Diagnostic accuracy is lost if these electrodes are moved closer to the heart.[20]

Dysrhythmia monitoring. Patients with serious cardiac diseases such as acute myocardial infarction, heart failure, and cardiomyopathy are at risk for the development of bundle branch blocks, complex ectopy, and wide complex tachycardias. These patients need to be monitored with a precordial lead that documents interventricular conduction changes. This is lead MCL_1 or MCL_6 in a three lead–wire system or V_1 or V_6 in a five lead–wire system. Current five lead–wire systems usually offer the clinician the choice of MCL_1 or V_1. The tracings in these two leads are not identical, and V_1 must be chosen over MCL_1 because it has a higher diagnostic accuracy.[20] If only a single lead can be displayed, lead MCL_1 or V_1 is the best choice, with MCL_6 a good second choice if for some reason an electrode cannot be placed in the V_1 position (e.g., in patients with a sternal incision).

V_1 is preferred over V_6 because both RBBB and ventricular tachycardia can be diagnosed with slightly greater accuracy in V_1 than in V_6. If a second lead can be displayed simultaneously, lead MCL_6 or V_6 would be the best choice, but this is not practical with many five lead–wire systems, because they include only one designated chest electrode.

Instead, any one of the six standard limb leads will do as a second lead, and selection is based on the patient's other monitoring needs, such as the need for ST-segment monitoring for ischemia. From a dysrhythmia standpoint, lead I or aV_F is also a good second choice, because either can be used to identify a QRS axis diagnostic of ventricular dysrhythmias. (Both lead aV_F and lead I are required for this, but in a five lead–wire system the critical care nurse can rapidly scroll through all six limb leads to obtain this information.) If three leads can be displayed simultaneously, lead V_1 plus lead aV_F and lead I are the best choices. It is no longer recommended to monitor lead II alone, since it is not helpful in diagnosing wide-complex tachycardias, and if they are not sustained there may not be time to document the dysrhythmia in a more helpful lead. Lead II can still be chosen as a second choice if two or more leads can be monitored simultaneously.

ST-segment monitoring. In this era of thrombolytic therapy and percutaneous transluminal coronary angioplasty (PTCA), one of the major new responsibilities of the critical care nurse is monitoring for myocardial ischemia. Myocardial ischemia may be accompanied by classic symptoms such as chest pain, or it may be "silent," without any clinical symptoms being recognized. Patients at risk for the development of silent ischemia include all patients experiencing an acute myocardial infarction (AMI), including those treated with thrombolytics, nitrates, or anticoagulation therapy. In addition, PTCA patients are at risk for coronary artery spasm or reocclusion, which may or may not be symptomatic, but which is reflected by ST-segment changes very similar to those seen during balloon inflation at the time of the procedure.[21] Any patient admitted to the critical care unit with a history of a previous MI, angina, or diabetes mellitus is likely to experience silent ischemia. Elderly patients undergoing surgical procedures can be assumed to have coronary artery disease and are monitored for silent ischemia intraoperatively. It is estimated that 60% to 90% of patients with known coronary artery disease experience episodes of silent ischemia.[22] Patients can have both symptomatic and asymptomatic (silent) episodes of transient myocardial ischemia, although in these patients symptoms generally indicate a more severe ischemic episode.

ST-segment monitoring identifies high risk patients in whom additional interventions or therapy may be indicated. It also can provide evidence that reperfusion has occurred after thrombolytic therapy or acute angioplasty.

Myocardial ischemia is represented on the cardiac monitor as a change in the level of the ST segment in relation to the isoelectric line. Many cardiac monitoring systems are now equipped with an ST-segment monitoring option that allows parameters to be set and alarms to be triggered when ST deviation is noted. Under normal (nonischemic) conditions the ST segment is at the same level as the TP segment (Figure 15-19). If the TP segment cannot be identified because of tachycardia, the PR segment can be used as a reference point to identify the isoelectric line (see Figure 15-19), although the PR segment can be altered

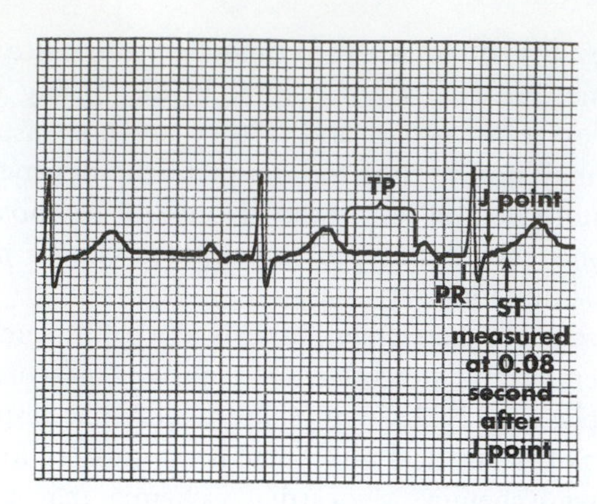

FIGURE 15-19. The TP interval is used as the reference point for the isoelectric line if the heart rate is slow enough for the TP interval to be clearly seen. If not, the PR interval can be used.

because of pericarditis or atrial enlargement.[22] Ischemia can cause either ST-segment depression or ST-segment elevation. ST elevation represents more severe, usually transmural, ischemia.[22] ST depression may indicate less severe (subendocardial) ischemia or may be a reciprocal, "mirror-image," pattern seen from a location directly opposite from the actual area of ischemic myocardium. Clinically, ST depression is more commonly seen with transient silent ischemia.[21]

ST-segment deviation can also occur in the absence of myocardial ischemia. Hyperkalemia may cause ST elevation, whereas hypokalemia and hypomagnesemia cause ST depression. Other nonischemic causes of ST-segment changes include hyperventilation, pericarditis, hypothermia, ventricular aneurysm, hypothyroidism, and pulmonary infarction.[14,21] Poor electrode contact with the skin can cause false ST-segment changes, emphasizing the need for adequate skin preparation before electrode placement. Certain drugs, especially digitalis and quinidine, can cause ST depression. Controversy exists regarding the accuracy of ST-segment monitoring in patients with preexisting LBBB. ST-segment changes still occur, although the ST-segment "baseline" is not at the isoelectric line, and monitoring parameters must be adjusted accordingly.[21]

ST-segment deviation is measured as the number of millimeters of ST-segment displacement from the isoelectric line, or from the patient's baseline, measured 60 to 80 msec from the J-point (Figure 15-20). Measurement at 60 msec from the J-point may be a more sensitive indicator of ischemia, but also results in more false-positive alarms. The 80 msec measurement point is more specific. ST elevation is displayed as a positive number, whereas ST depression is indicated by a negative number (Figure 15-20). To be clinically significant, the ST-segment change must be at least 1 mm and last at least 60 seconds.

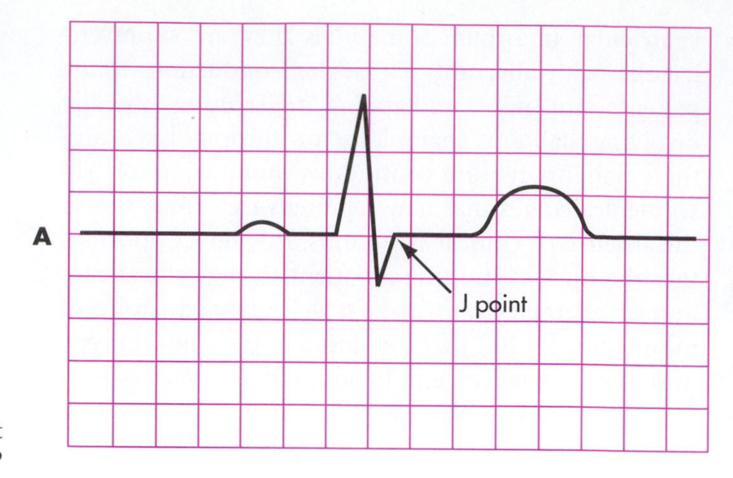

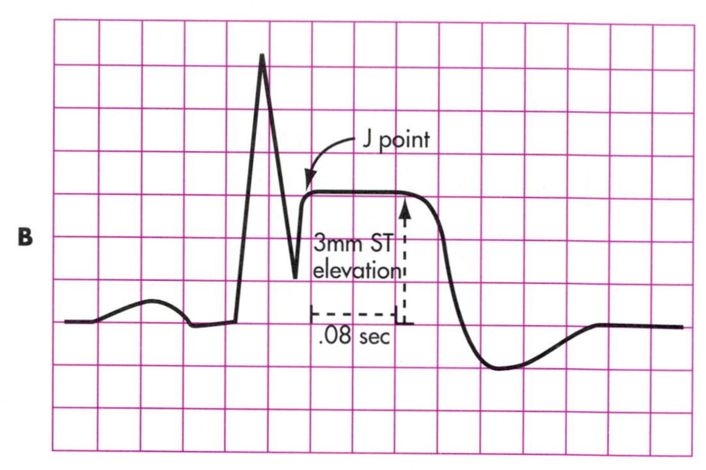

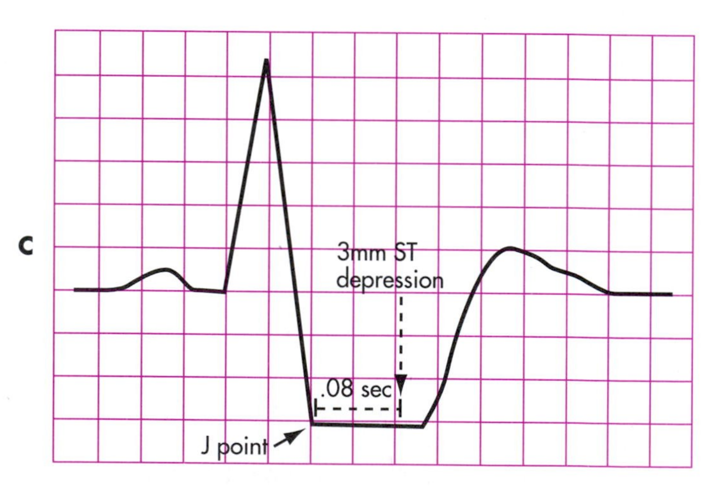

FIGURE 15-20. A, Normal position of the J-point. B, 3 mm ST elevation. C, 3 mm ST depression. ST changes are measured 0.08 msec after the J-point.

It must be remembered that the gain (calibration) on a bedside monitor is adjusted to maximize visibility of the tracing at a distance; as a result, the magnitude of ST-segment deviation is not accurate and must always be confirmed with a 12-lead ECG. In addition, ST-segment changes can sometimes occur as a result of position changes and be falsely interpreted as ischemia.[21] A 12-lead ECG is needed to confirm or refute the existence of true ischemic changes.

The effectiveness of ST-segment monitoring in identifying episodes of myocardial ischemia depends on appropriate lead selection. Myocardial ischemia is localized, not diffuse, and is different for each patient, depending on the location and extent of his or her coronary artery disease. As discussed previously, lead V_1 is chosen first for monitoring, since it is the most diagnostic lead for analyzing dysrhythmias and identifying the new development of a bundle branch block.[19] It is not a very valuable lead for ST-segment monitoring. The best way to choose a lead for monitoring ST segments for ischemia is to look at the patient's 12-lead ECG during an episode of ischemia, if available. The standard 12-lead ECG obtained in an acute MI before thrombolytic therapy would reveal the leads that best demonstrated ischemia in that patient. Leads that showed ST-segment deviation during balloon inflation at the time of PTCA are the best leads to monitor after the procedure. If this information is not available, lead III or aV_F is the best choice for a second monitoring lead.[19] Currently, a system for continuous monitoring of a derived 12-lead ECG is being developed and tested, which shows great promise for more accurate ST-segment monitoring in the future.[23] (∞Myocardial Infarction, p. 490.)

Hypertrophy. Cardiac chamber enlargement can be suspected or diagnosed using the 12-lead ECG because muscle size influences the ECG tracing. Atrial hypertrophy is identified by the size and shape of the P waves and is usually seen best in lead II. Wide m-shaped P waves are seen in left atrial hypertrophy and are called P-*mitrale,* because left atrial hypertrophy is often caused by mitral stenosis (Figure 15-21, *A*). Tall, peaked P waves occur in right atrial hypertrophy and are referred to as P-*pulmonale,* because this condition is often the result of chronic pulmonary disease (Figure 15-21, *B*).

Ventricular hypertrophy is basically an increase in the size and muscle mass of one or both ventricles. Because a larger muscle is being depolarized, a greater amount of electrical activity is recorded on the ECG during depolarization. In ventricular hypertrophy, specific changes occur in the QRS complex. Upright QRS complexes become taller, and negative QRS complexes become even more negative. Often the QRS becomes slightly wider, because it takes longer to depolarize a larger muscle. The QRS axis often shifts toward the enlarged ventricle, because a greater portion of the total electrical activity of the heart occurs there.

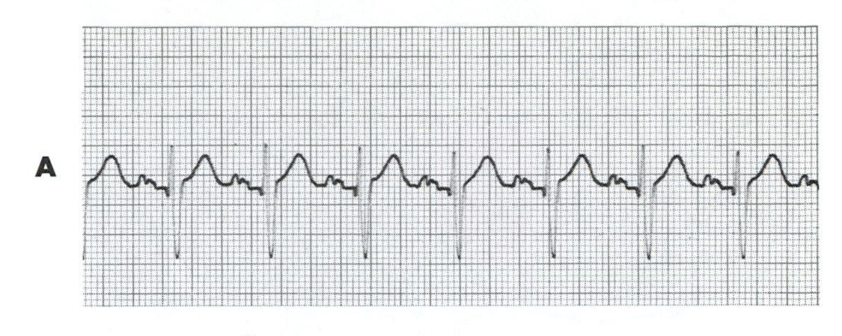

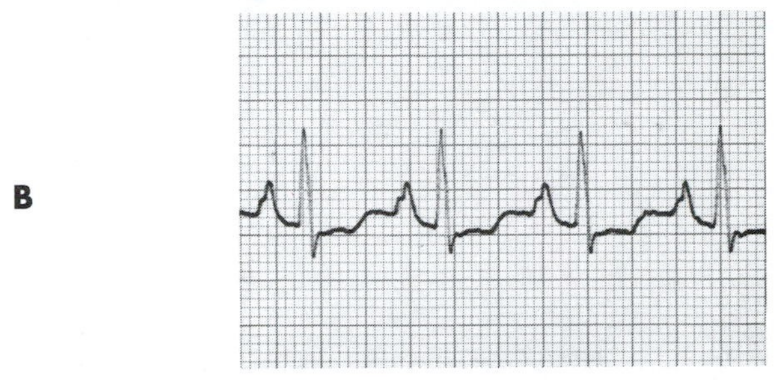

FIGURE 15-21. Atrial hypertrophy. **A,** In left atrial hypertrophy the P wave is broad and notched and is sometimes called "P-mitrale," because it is often associated with mitral valve disease. **B,** In right atrial hypertrophy the P wave is tall and peaked and is sometimes called "P-pulmonale," because it is often associated with pulmonary disease.

Ischemia and infarction. Ischemia occurs when the delivery of oxygen to the tissues is insufficient to meet metabolic demand. Cardiac ischemia can be the result of a sudden decrease in supply, such as when coronary artery spasm occurs, or can be the result of a sudden increase in demand, such as exercise. Ischemia is by nature a transient process. Either the balance of supply and demand is restored and the muscle tissue recovers or the imbalance becomes so great that the tissue can no longer survive and it becomes necrotic. Many nursing and medical interventions are directed toward saving as much ischemic tissue as possible. Infarction refers to the actual death and disintegration of muscle cells and their eventual replacement by scar tissue. Once infarction has occurred, that process cannot be reversed.

ECG changes. Both ischemia and infarction cause changes in the way cardiac muscle cells respond to electrical stimuli, and these changes can usually be seen in a 12-lead ECG tracing. The ECG changes that result from myocardial ischemia involve transient ST-segment and T wave abnormalities. ST-segment elevation is seen when the positive electrode lies directly over an area of transmural ischemia (Figure 15-22, *A*).

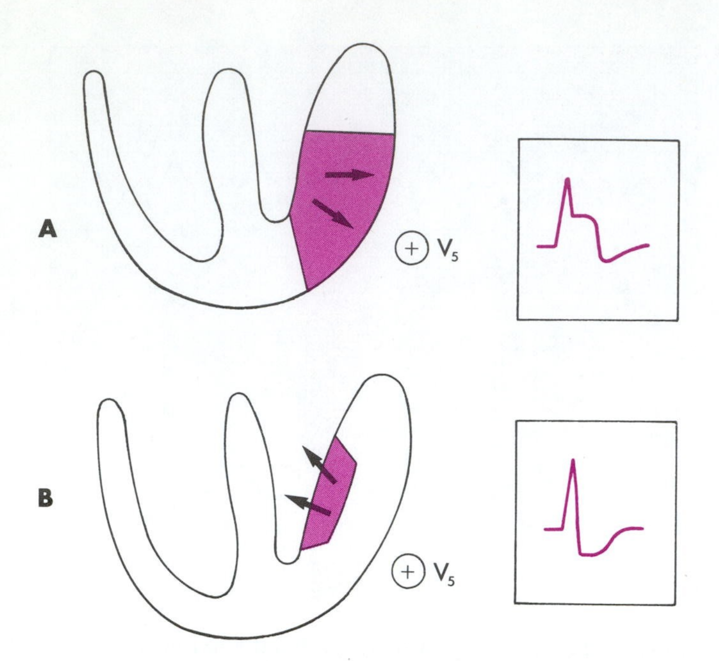

FIGURE 15-22. **A,** Acute transmural ischemia. The electrical forces *(arrows)* responsible for the ST segment are directed outward through the entire thickness of the heart muscle wall, causing ST elevation in leads directly over the ischemic area. **B,** Acute subendocardial ischemia. The electrical forces responsible for the ST segment are deviated toward the inner layer of the heart, resulting in ST depression in leads directly over that area of the heart muscle wall.

If the reduction of blood flow is limited to the endocardium and some normal muscle tissue remains between the ischemic area and the positive electrode, ST-segment depression is recorded.[20] In subendocardial ischemia, the ischemic area is closest to the inner cavity wall of the heart, and there is a layer of normal muscle tissue left surrounding it (Figure 15-22, *B*). ST-segment depression would result, because the positive electrode is separated from the ischemic area by normal tissue. T waves most commonly flatten or become inverted, in part because of the influence of the depressed ST segment "dragging" them down. Occasionally, T waves that were inverted on a normal 12-lead ECG become suddenly upright on a tracing obtained during an ischemic episode. Essentially, a baseline ECG must be available for comparison, and any change in ST segment or T waves from that baseline is significant.

Infarction involves actual necrosis (death) of muscle cells with eventual formation of scar tissue. These cells can no longer be depolarized when an impulse reaches them. If the infarction involves the epicardial (outer) layer of the heart muscle or the entire thickness of the heart wall (transmural), the QRS complex changes. Abnormal Q waves will develop in the leads overlying the affected area. Occasionally, the entire QRS complex just becomes smaller, without actual development of Q waves.

If only the subendocardial layer of the heart muscle is infarcted, abnormal Q waves do not develop. In fact, there may be no change in the QRS complex. The diagnosis then depends on CK-MB or LDH_1 isoenzyme results and the clinical presentation. Non-Q wave infarctions account for 25% to 40% of all acute myocardial infarctions. As a group, they are smaller and result in fewer short-term complications than Q wave (transmural) MIs. However, non-Q wave MIs are associated with higher rates of reinfarction and unstable angina.[24]

The location of the infarction can be roughly determined by noting the specific leads in which the ST-segment and T wave changes are seen on the 12-lead ECG. See Table 15-6 for a summary of the anticipated changes. Right ventricular infarction and posterior wall infarction are particularly difficult to identify on a standard 12-lead ECG, because none of the standard leads directly view these areas. A right ventricular infarction can be suspected in the setting of an acute inferior wall MI when the ST-segment elevation in lead III is greater than in lead II. To avoid missing this diagnosis, right-sided precordial leads (Figure 15-7, *B*) should be placed and a tracing obtained on any patient with a suspected inferior wall MI. It is estimated that right ventricular infarction occurs in as many as 52% of patients with an inferior wall MI involving the proximal right coronary artery.[25] A posterior wall MI can be suspected in a patient with an acute inferior wall MI when there is ST-segment depression in leads V_1, V_2, and V_3 on the standard 12-lead ECG. Posterior wall involvement can be verified by adding posterior precordial leads V_7, V_8, and V_9 (Figure 15-7, *C*).[17]

Infarct age. The relative age of the infarction can also be estimated. When blood flow in a coronary artery is occluded, the entire area of heart muscle normally perfused by that artery becomes ischemic. Collateral arterioles exist, which overlap and supply the perimeter of this area, and may prevent necrosis of some of the affected tissue. At the center of the ischemic area, collateral blood flow is minimal or does not exist at all. Within a few hours, this tissue begins to necrose, or die. On the ECG tracing, this process is illustrated as follows. Within minutes of the onset of infarction, ST-segment elevation occurs in the leads directly overlying the affected heart wall. This ST-segment elevation persists for several days, gradually becoming less

TABLE 15-6 Location of ECG Changes During Myocardial Infarction

Location of Infarction	Artery Involved	Leads Involved; EGG Changes
Anterior wall	LAD	V_{2-4}; Q waves, ST↑, T↓
Inferior wall	RCA or LCx	II, III, aV_F; Q waves, ST↑, T↓
Ventricular septum	LAD	V_{1-2}; Q waves, ST↑, T↓
Lateral wall	LCx or LAD	V_{5-6}, I, aV_L; Q waves, ST↑, T↓
True posterior wall	RCA or LCx	V_{1-3}; tall, upright R; ST↓; ST↑ V_{7-9}
Right ventricle	Proximal RCA	V_4R-V_6R; ST↑

LAD, Left anterior descending; ↑, elevated; ↓, depressed; *RCA*, right coronary artery; *LCx*, left circumflex.

severe. Within the first few hours, T waves may become tall and symmetric. These are known as "hyperacute" T waves and also indicate acute ischemia. Meanwhile, usually within 4 to 24 hours from the onset of the infarction, abnormal Q waves begin to develop in the affected leads, and T waves begin to invert. Sometimes, instead of actual Q waves developing, the R waves just become smaller. This still indicates necrosis of muscle tissue. The ST segments become isoelectric again in several days or weeks, and the T wave becomes symmetric and deeply inverted in the affected leads. Occasionally, these T wave changes do not ever resolve. Usually, however, the T waves return to normal within several months. The Q waves usually persist for the remainder of the patient's life. Table 15-7 summarizes the timing of these changes.

TABLE 15-7 Timing of ECG Changes During Myocardial Infarction

Timing	Change
Immediate	ST-segment elevation in leads over the area of infarction
Within a few hours	Giant upright T waves
Several hours to 2 weeks	ST segment normalizes; T waves invert symmetrically
Several hours to days; usually remain for life	Q waves or reduced R-wave voltage

Ventricular conduction defects. Intraventricular conduction defects are the result of an abnormal pathway of conduction through the ventricles. Normally, conduction spreads from the AV node to the bundle of His and from there down the right and left bundle branches. The right bundle branch is long and thin and terminates in a mass of Purkinje fibers, which spread the wave of depolarization to the surrounding right ventricular muscle. The left bundle branch divides after only a short distance into the left anterior fascicle, the left posterior fascicle, and the left septal fibers (Figure 15-23). Each of these fascicles causes depolarization of separate areas of the left ventricle. If any part of the conduction system fails, the muscle cells in that area are still depolarized, but not as quickly. Depolarization must then spread from cell to cell, a slower process than activation through specialized conduction pathways.

On the ECG, intraventricular conduction defects cause a widening of the QRS because of the slower spread of depolarization. The affected muscle tissue begins the slower cell-to-cell depolarization just as the other areas in the ventricle are almost finished. This later depolarization is then tacked onto the end of the normal QRS, making it prolonged and altering its shape.

Any part of the conduction system can be affected. The term *bundle branch block* refers to complete interruption of conduction through either the right bundle or the entire left bundle branch. In complete right or left bundle branch block, the QRS is always 0.12 second or longer in duration. When only one fascicle of the left bundle branch is blocked, the QRS duration is within normal limits, although usually more prolonged than before the conduction disturbance occurred.

Right and left bundle branch block. The chest leads are the most useful in identifying complete right and left bundle branch blocks. Specifically, V_1 and V_6 are the best leads from which to identify forces traveling in a horizontal direction, because they are located on the right and left sides of the heart, respectively. Figure

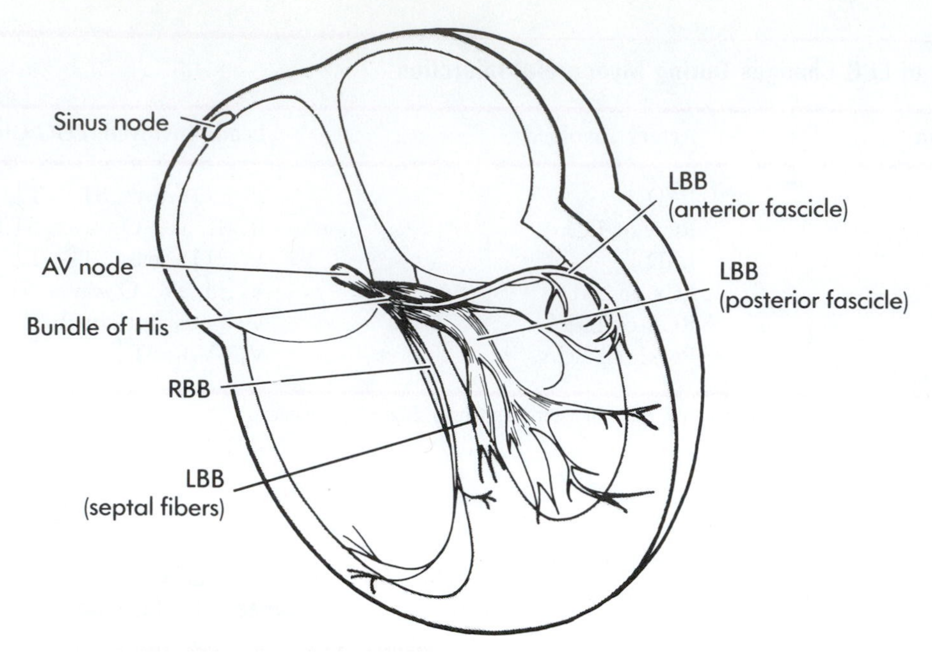

FIGURE 15-23. Cardiac conduction system. (Modified from Conover MB: *Understanding electrocardiography: arrhythmias and the 12-lead ECG,* ed 6, St Louis, 1992, Mosby.)

15-24, *A* illustrates the normal sequence of ventricular activation and the usual shape of the QRS complex in V_1 and V_6.

In complete right bundle branch block (Figure 15-24, *B*), the right ventricle is not activated through the rapid conduction system. Rather, it must be activated slowly, from one cell to the next. Electrical forces, not counterbalanced by opposing forces on the left, travel toward the right at the end of the ventricular activation. The septum is depolarized first, in a normal manner from left to right. Next the wave of depolarization spreads through the left ventricle and is recorded in lead V_1 as a negative deflection. The final portion of the QRS complex is upright, indicating final forces traveling toward the right. This represents right ventricular depolarization that occurs after left ventricular depolarization is nearly complete. In lead V_6, the positive electrode is on the left side of the chest, so the waveforms are reversed. The final forces of the QRS are negative, because they are traveling toward the right and away from the positive electrode of V_6. Note that the final negative deflection in V_6 is smaller than the final upright deflection in lead V_1, because the positive electrode in V_6 is at a greater distance from the right ventricle.

In complete left bundle branch block (Figure 15-24, *C*), the conduction through the left ventricle must spread from cell to cell. Because a portion of the common left bundle normally initiates depolarization of the septum, the septum also is depolarized in an abnormal direction, from right to left. In lead V_1 this is recorded as an initial negative deflection. Next, the right ventricle is depolarized, seen as a small upright notch in the QRS as the forces travel briefly toward the positive electrode of V_1. Sometimes this notch is absent. The sequence of events has not changed, but the left ventricle is already beginning to be depolarized cell to cell and may offset the rightward forces of right ventricular depolarization. The final forces travel toward the left as the left ventricle is being depolarized. The left ventricle is a very large muscle mass, so these final forces are large and wide. In lead V_1 the final deflection is a deep negative deflection (S wave), whereas in lead V_6 these final forces inscribe a tall, upright deflection (R wave).

Bundle branch blocks can easily be diagnosed at the bedside if the patient is being monitored with lead MCL_1 or MCL_6, because these correlate closely with the precordial leads V_1 and V_6, respectively. A bundle branch block exists when the QRS complex is wider than 0.12 second (and when the complex did not originate in the ventricles such as does a PVC or paced beat). To determine which bundle branch is blocked, examine the last part of the QRS just before it returns to the baseline in leads V_1 and V_6. If upright in V_1 and negative in V_6, a right bundle branch block exists. If negative in V_1 and upright in V_6, a left bundle branch block is present.

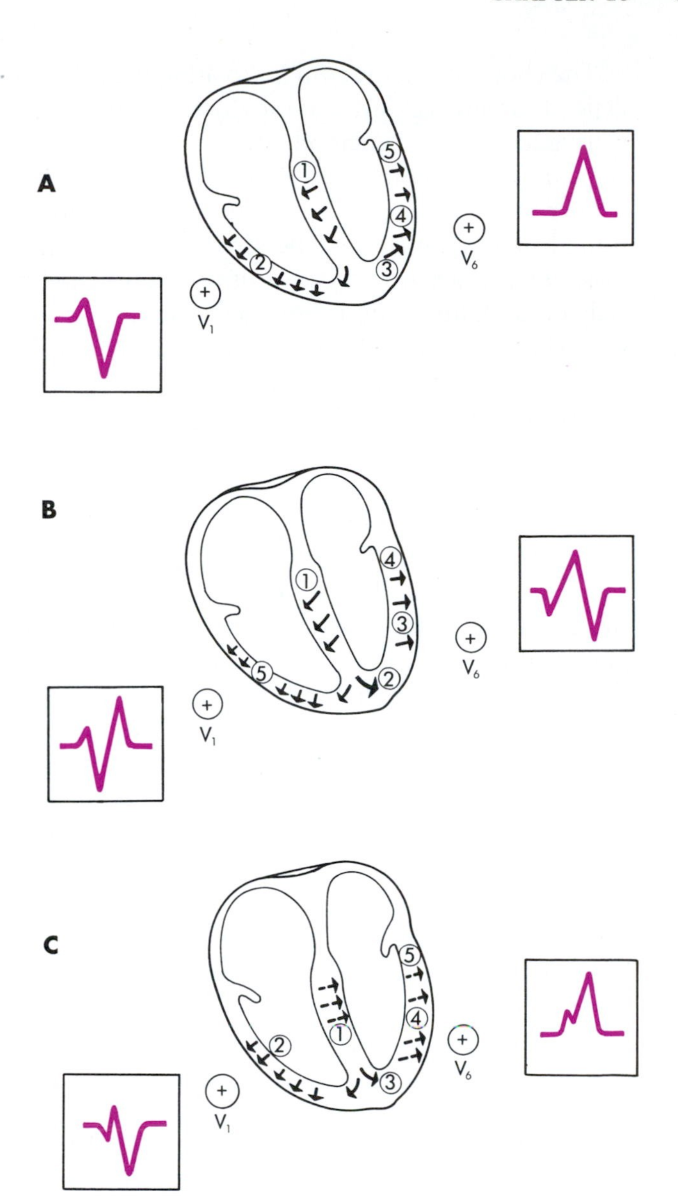

FIGURE 15-24. **A,** Sequence of ventricular depolarization and resulting QRS complex, as seen in leads V_1 and V_6. **B,** Sequence of ventricular depolarization when right bundle branch block is present and resulting QRS complex, as seen in leads V_1 and V_6. **C,** Sequence of ventricular depolarization when left bundle branch block is present and resulting QRS complex, as seen in leads V_1 and V_6.

Hemiblocks. Hemiblocks involve conduction failure of only part of the left bundle branch. In left anterior fascicular block (also called *left anterior hemiblock*), left ventricular depolarization begins in the left posterior fascicle and spreads anteriorly through Purkinje fibers distal to the block. The QRS is only slightly prolonged, up to 0.02 second longer than the patient's previous QRS. However, the axis changes dramatically and becomes more negative than − 30 degrees (left-axis deviation). Other causes of left-axis deviation must be ruled out before a clinical diagnosis of left anterior hemiblock can be made (Boxes 15-4 and 15-5). In left posterior fascicular block (also called *left posterior hemiblock*), the anterior portion of the left ventricle is depolarized first. Conduction then spreads slowly to the right, inferiorly and posteriorly. Once again the QRS is slightly prolonged. The axis then swings entirely the other direction and becomes greater than + 110 degrees (right-axis deviation). Other causes of right-axis deviation must be ruled out before a clinical diagnosis of left posterior hemiblock can be made (see Box 15-5).

Bifascicular block. Blockage of any two branches of the ventricular conduction system constitutes bifascicular block. Any combination of these conduction disturbances can occur and can evolve into complete heart block. Development of right bundle branch block with left anterior fascicular block occurs in approximately 5% of patients with acute myocardial infarction, as does left bundle branch block. Right bundle branch block in combination with left posterior fascicular block is rare, probably because the left posterior fascicle is short and thick and has a dual blood supply from the left anterior descending and right posterior descending coronary arteries.

BOX 15-4 Causes of Left-Axis Deviation

- Normal variation
- Mechanical shifts: exhalation; high diaphragm caused by pregnancy, ascites, or abdominal tumor
- Left anterior hemiblock
- Left ventricular hypertrophy
- Pulmonary emphysema (uncommon)
- Wolff-Parkinson-White syndrome
- Hyperkalemia
- Cardiomyopathy

BOX 15-5 Causes of Right-Axis Deviation

- Normal variation
- Mechanical shifts: inhalation, emphysema
- Left posterior hemiblock
- Right ventricular hypertrophy
- Lateral wall myocardial infarction
- Right bundle branch block
- Dextrocardia

Bifascicular block that develops during an acute myocardial infarction warrants placement of a temporary pacemaker prophylactically in case complete heart block develops. When bifascicular block occurs in other patient populations, use of a pacemaker can be avoided if the patient is asymptomatic. However, in most cases, bifascicular block eventually progresses to complete heart block.

Dysrhythmia interpretation. In clinical practice the terms *dysrhythmia* and *arrhythmia* often are used interchangeably. There may be discussion over which word is the most accurate. Both are correct, and either may be used in practice. In this textbook, dysrhythmia is the more commonly used term. A dysrhythmia is any disturbance in the normal cardiac conduction pathway. Dysrhythmias can be detected on a 12-lead ECG, but very often they occur only sporadically. For this reason patients in a critical care unit are monitored continuously, using a single or dual lead system, and rhythm strips are recorded routinely, as well as any time there is a change in the patient's rhythm. A systematic approach to evaluation of a rhythm strip is introduced first in this section, followed by specific criteria for common dysrhythmias encountered in clinical practice. (Cardiac Care IVD.)

Heart rate determination. The first thing to assess when evaluating a rhythm strip is the ventricular rate. Regardless of the dysrhythmia involved, the ventricular rate holds the key to whether the patient is able to tolerate the dysrhythmia (i.e., maintain adequate blood pressure, cardiac output, and mentation). If the ventricular rate is consistently greater than 200 or less than 30, emergency measures must be started to correct the rate. A detailed analysis of the underlying rhythm disturbance can proceed later when the immediate crisis is over. There are three methods for calculating rate (Figure 15-25, *A*):

1. Number of RR intervals in 6 seconds times 10 (NOTE: ECG paper is usually marked at the top in 3-second increments, making a 6-second interval easy to identify.)
2. Number of large boxes between QRS complexes divided into 300
3. Number of small boxes between QRS complexes divided into 1500

In the healthy heart, the atrial rate and the ventricular rate are the same. However, in many dysrhythmias the atrial and ventricular rates are different; thus both must be calculated. To find the atrial rate, the PP interval, instead of the RR interval, is used in one of the three methods listed for determining rate.

The choice of method for calculating the heart rate depends on the regularity of the rhythm. If the rhythm is irregular, the first method (RRs in 6 seconds × 10) is the only method that can be used (Figure 15-25, *A*). If the rhythm is regular, it is more accurate to use the second or third method. The second method can be easier to use when two consecutive R waves fall exactly on dark lines, and it provides a rapid estimate of rate. The third method is recommended when both R waves do not fall exactly on dark lines.

Rhythm determination. The term *rhythm* refers to the regularity with which the P waves or R waves occur. Calipers assist in determining rhythm. One point of the calipers is placed on the beginning of one R wave, while the other point is placed on the very next R wave. Leaving the calipers "set" at this interval, each succeeding RR interval is checked to be sure it is the same width.

In describing the rhythm, three terms are used. If the rhythm is *regular,* the RR intervals are the same, ± 10%. For example, if there are 20 small boxes in an RR interval, an R wave could be off by two small boxes, but the rhythm would still be considered regular.

If the rhythm is *regularly irregular,* the RR intervals are not the same, but some sort of pattern is involved, which could be grouping, rhythmic speeding up and slowing down, or any other consistent pattern (Figure 15-26, *A*).

If the rhythm is *irregularly irregular,* the RR intervals are not the same, and no pattern can be found (Figure 15-26, *B*).

P wave evaluation. The P wave is analyzed by answering the following questions. First, is the P wave present or absent? Second, is it related to the QRS? It is hoped that one P wave will be in front of every QRS. Sometimes there may be two, three, or four P waves in front of every QRS. If this pattern is consistent, the P wave and QRS are still related, although not on a 1:1 basis.

PR interval evaluation. The duration of the PR interval, which normally is 0.12 to 0.20 second, is measured first. This is done by measuring from the start of a P wave to the beginning of the following QRS (Figure 15-27). Next, all PR intervals on the strip are checked to be sure they are the same duration as the original interval.

QRS evaluation. The entire ECG strip must be evaluated to ascertain that the QRS complexes are consistently the same shape and width. The normal QRS duration is 0.06 to 0.10 second. If more than one QRS shape is on the strip, each QRS must be measured. The QRS is measured from where it leaves the

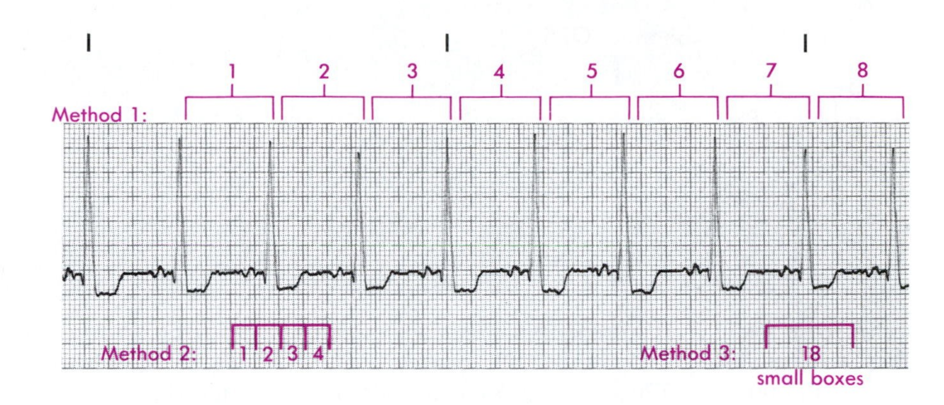

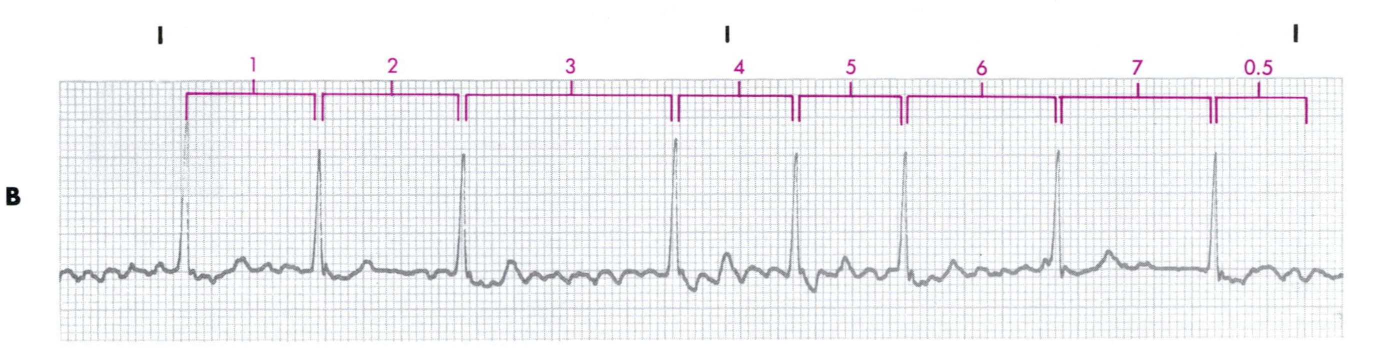

FIGURE 15-25. **A,** Calculation of heart rate. Method 1: number of RR intervals in 6 seconds multiplied by 10 (e.g., 8 × 10 = 80/min). Method 2: number of large boxes between QRS complexes divided into 300 (e.g., 300 ÷ 4 = 75/min). Method 3: number of small boxes between QRS complexes divided into 1500 (e.g., 1500 ÷ 18 = 84/min). **B,** Rate calculation if the rhythm is irregular. Only method 1 can be used (e.g., 7.5 intervals × 10 = 75/min).

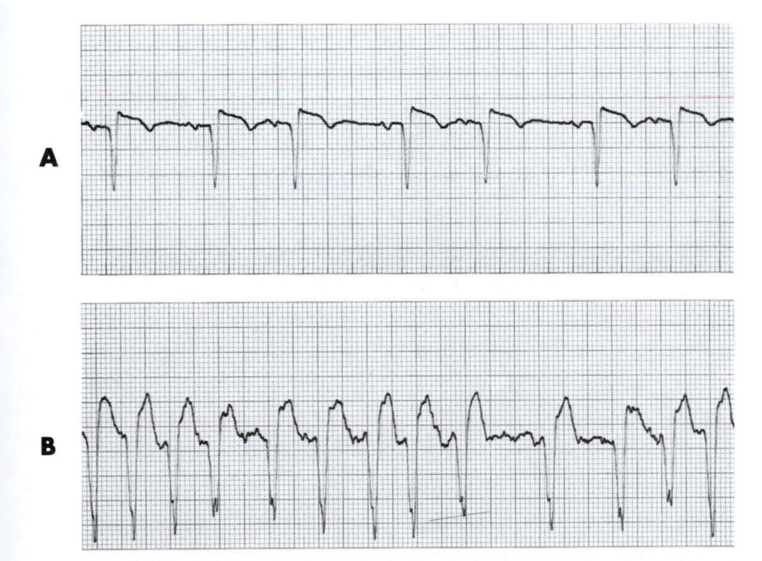

FIGURE 15-26. **A,** Regularly irregular rhythm—irregular but with a consistent pattern, in that every other beat is premature. **B,** Irregularly irregular rhythm—irregular with no consistent pattern.

baseline to where it returns to the baseline (see Figure 15-27).

Sinus rhythms. The cardiac cycle begins when an impulse originates in the sinus node. As the wave of depolarization spreads through the atria, a P wave is inscribed on the ECG. The impulse is delayed briefly in the AV node, which corresponds to the PR interval on the ECG. After leaving the AV node, the wave of depolarization spreads rapidly through the bundle of His and the bundle branches and causes ventricular depolarization, which is recorded as a QRS complex by the ECG. Contraction immediately follows depolarization. Contraction is terminated by repolarization, which is demonstrated as a T wave on the ECG.

Normal sinus rhythm. If all of the events just discussed occur in their normal sequence with normal rates and intervals, the patient is in normal sinus rhythm. Specifically, the following are the criteria for normal sinus rhythm:

1. Rate. The intrinsic rate of the sinus node is 60 to 100 beats per minute. *Intrinsic rate* is the normal rate at which a pacemaker site in the heart

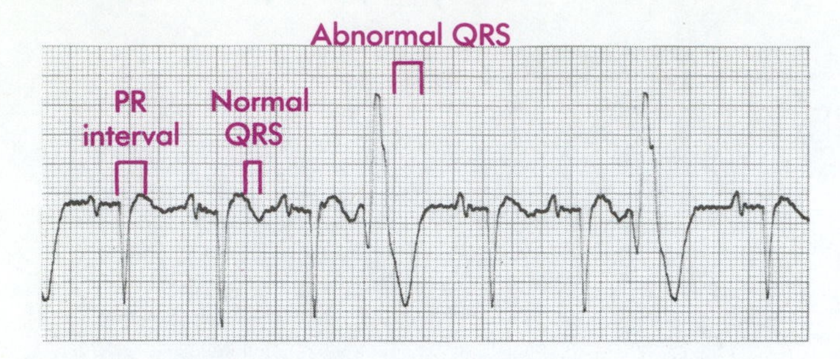

FIGURE 15-27. PR interval measurement, from the beginning of the P wave to the beginning of the QRS complex. The PR interval on this tracing is 0.20 second. QRS duration illustrating both normal and abnormal intervals. The narrow QRS complexes measure 0.08 second, which is normal. The wide QRS complexes measure 0.20 second and are caused by ventricular ectopy.

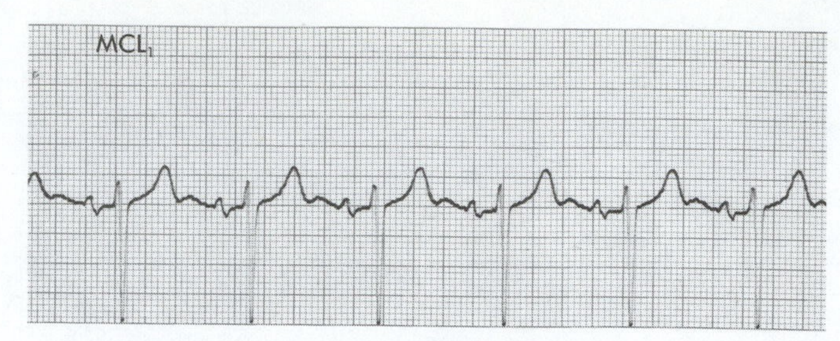

FIGURE 15-28. Normal sinus rhythm. The rate is 70; the rhythm is regular. One P wave is present before each QRS complex. The PR interval is 0.18 second and does not vary throughout the strip. The QRS duration is 0.08 second. All evaluation criteria are within normal limits.

TABLE 15-8 Sinus Rhythms

Parameters	Normal Sinus Rhythm	Sinus Bradycardia	Sinus Tachycardia	Sinus Dysrhythmia
Rate	60-100/min	60/min	100/min	Variable
Rhythm	Regular	Regular	Regular	Irregular; respiratory variation
P wave	Present, with one per QRS	Present, with one per QRS	Present, with one per QRS	Present, with one per QRS
PR interval	0.12-0.20 sec and constant	0.12-0.20 sec and constant	0.12-0.20 sec and constant	0.12-0.20 sec and constant
QRS	0.06-0.10 sec	0.06-0.10 sec	0.06-0.10 sec	0.06-0.10 sec

depolarizes automatically with no outside influences, such as drugs, fever, or exercise. In normal sinus rhythm, the rate must be whatever is "normal" for the sinus node, (i.e., 60 to 100 beats per minute).

2. Rhythm. The rhythm must be regular, ± 10%.
3. P wave. P waves must be present, and one and only one must precede every QRS complex.
4. PR interval. This interval represents delay in the AV node. In normal sinus rhythm the PR interval is 0.12 to 0.20 second.
5. QRS. Size and shape does not matter in this complex, because it depends on lead placement and gain adjustments on the monitor. However, all QRS complexes must look alike. If conduction through the ventricles is normal, the QRS duration is 0.06 to 0.10 second. Figure 15-28 is an example of normal sinus rhythm in MCL_1.

Sinus bradycardia. Sinus bradycardia meets all of the criteria for normal sinus rhythm except that the rate is less than 60 (Table 15-8). It is normally seen in well-trained athletes at rest or in many other individuals during sleep. Other conditions in which sinus bradycardia occurs include vagal stimulation, increased intracranial pressure, drug therapy with digoxin or beta-blockers, and ischemia of the sinus node caused by an acute inferior wall myocardial infarction. Sinus bradycardia is generally not treated unless the patient displays symptoms of hypoperfusion, such as hypotension, dizziness, chest pain, or changes in level of consciousness.

Sinus tachycardia. Sinus tachycardia meets all the criteria for normal sinus rhythym except that the rate is greater than 100 beats per minute (see Table 15-8). Rates may be as high as 180 to 200 beats per minute in healthy, young adults with strenuous exercise. However, in the critical care setting, bedrest has been prescribed for most patients. It is wise to be skeptical of any "sinus tachycardia" with a rate greater than 150 and to search for a triggering focus other than the sinus node. For example, atrial flutter waves might be difficult to see at first glance because of baseline distortion caused by the high ventricular rate (Figure 15-29).

Sinus tachycardia can be caused by a wide variety of factors, such as exercise, emotion, pain, fever, hemorrhage, shock, and congestive heart failure. Many drugs used in critical care can also cause sinus tachycardia, and common culprits are aminophylline, dopamine, hydralazine, beta stimulants such as epinephrine, and overzealous use of atropine. Tachycardia is detrimental to anyone with ischemic heart disease because it decreases time for ventricular filling, decreases stroke volume, and thus compromises cardiac output. In addition, tachycardia increases heart work and myocardial oxygen demand while decreasing oxygen supply by decreasing coronary artery filling time.

If the cause of the tachycardia can be determined (e.g., fever or pain), the cause is treated rather than trying to treat the heart rate directly. Several drugs are available to decrease the heart rate, and both calcium channel blockers and beta-blockers are widely used for this purpose. However, a word of caution is warranted here. Cardiac output (CO) is determined by heart rate and stroke volume. If an injured heart can no longer maintain an adequate stroke volume, heart rate can be increased to maintain CO and supply an adequate blood flow to vital body tissues. If a drug is administered to force the sinus node to slow, severe and relatively immediate heart failure can result. The sinus node is controlled by many neural and humoral influences in the body, and the rate is set to try to meet the perceived demands; thus a close examination of the reason for the tachycardia is mandatory before treatment decisions are made.

Sinus dysrhythmia. Sinus dysrhythmia meets all of the criteria for normal sinus rhythm except that the rhythm is irregular (see Table 15-8). Usually this irregularity coincides with the respiratory pattern; heart rate increases with inhalation and decreases with exhalation (Figure 15-30). Sinus dysrhythmia frequently occurs in children, and the incidence decreases with age. No treatment is required. To avoid being misled by other rhythm disturbances, one must examine all P waves closely to be sure that they are all the same shape and that the PR intervals are all constant.

Atrial dysrhythmias. Atrial dysrhythmias originate from an ectopic focus in the atria, somewhere other than the sinus node. The ectopic impulse occurs prematurely before the normal sinus impulse is due to occur. Usually, the premature P wave initiates a normal QRS complex. However, some exceptions do occur. The early P wave usually looks different than the sinus P wave and often is inverted. The PR interval may be longer, shorter, or the same as the PR interval of a sinus beat.

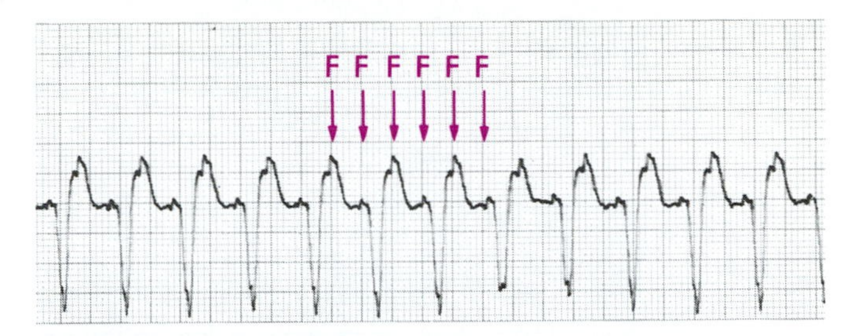

FIGURE 15-29. Sinus tachycardia? In fact, this is atrial flutter with 2:1 conduction. Note how difficult it is to see the extra flutter waves (F) that are hidden in the QRS complexes.

Premature atrial contractions. Premature atrial contractions (PACs) are isolated, early beats from an ectopic focus in the atria. The underlying rhythm is usually sinus. The regular sinus rhythm is interrupted by an early, abnormally shaped P wave. If the impulse arrives in the AV node after the AV node is fully repolarized, it is conducted to the ventricles. If the ventricles are also fully repolarized, conduction through them is normal and a normal QRS is recorded on the ECG (Figure 15-31, *A*).

Sometimes, the ectopic P wave arrives so early that the AV node is still in its absolute refractory period. In this case, the wave of depolarization does not move past the AV node and no QRS follows. All that is seen on the ECG is an early, abnormal P wave followed by a pause until the next sinus P wave occurs (Figure 15-31, *B*). This is called a *nonconducted PAC.* Usually these P waves are so early that they are superimposed on the T wave of the previous beat, making them somewhat difficult to find. The pause that follows is still clearly seen. Whenever an unexpected pause occurs in a rhythm, the T wave preceding the pause must be examined very carefully and compared with other T waves on the same strip to locate distortions that may reveal a hidden, early P wave.

Occasionally, the early ectopic P wave can be conducted through the AV node, but part of this conduction pathway through the ventricles is blocked. Because the right bundle branch normally has the longest refractory period, it is usually the right bundle branch that is still blocked when the early impulse arrives. On

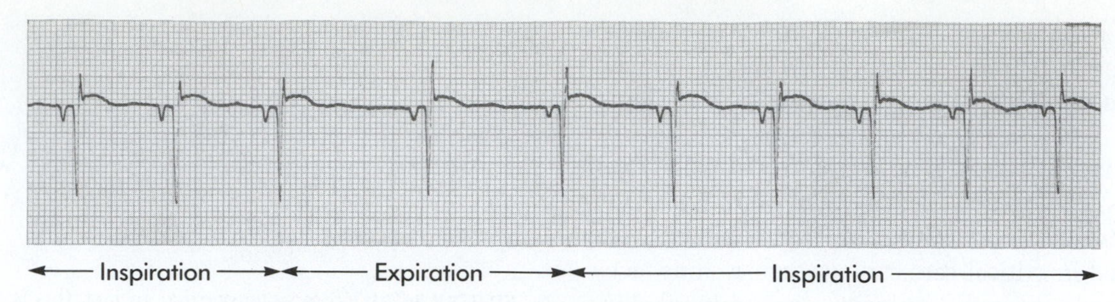

FIGURE 15-30. Sinus dysrhythmia. Note the increase in heart rate during inspiration and decrease in heart rate during expiration.

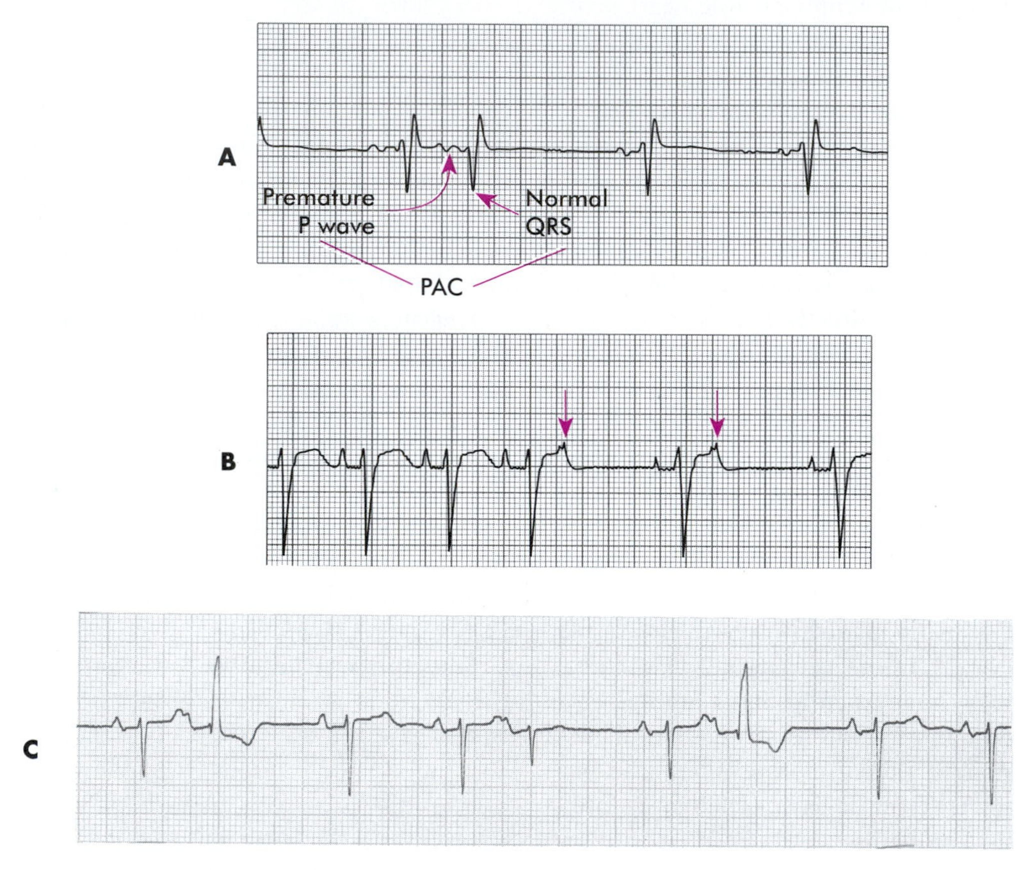

FIGURE 15-31. Premature atrial contractions (PACs). **A,** Normally conducted PAC. The early P wave is indicated by the *arrow,* and the QRS that follows is of normal shape and duration. **B,** Nonconducted (blocked) PACs. The early P waves are indicated by *arrows.* Note how they distort the T waves, making them appear peaked, compared with the normal T waves seen after the third and fourth QRS complexes. **C,** Right bundle branch block aberration after a PAC.

the ECG, this appears as an early, abnormal P wave, followed by an abnormally wide QRS, usually with a shape consistent with right bundle branch block (Figure 15-31, *C*). Conduction through the ventricles that is different from normal is referred to as *aberrant.* Consequently, these early, abnormally conducted PACs are called aberrantly conducted PACs.

PACs can occur in normal individuals. They are accentuated by emotional disturbances, nicotine, tea, caffeine, and digitalis. Mitral valve prolapse is associated with an increased frequency of atrial dysrhythmias. Heart failure can also cause PACs because of increased pressure within the atria. As atrial pressure begins to rise, the atrial walls are stretched, causing irritability of atrial cells and the occurrence of PACs.

Paroxysmal supraventricular tachycardia. "Paroxysmal" means starting and stopping abruptly. Paroxysmal supraventricular tachycardia (PSVT) refers to

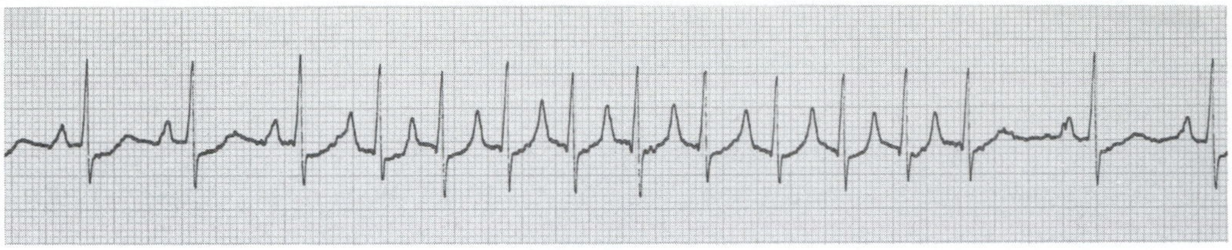

FIGURE 15-32. Paroxysmal supraventricular tachycardia (PSVT). Note that the atrial rate during the tachycardia is 158 beats per minute. The run starts and stops abruptly.

the sudden interruption of sinus rhythm by an atrial ectopic focus that fires repetitively at a rate of 150 to 250 beats per minute and eventually stops as suddenly as it began (Figure 15-32). The rhythm of PSVT is perfectly regular, because the reentry loop has a specific length; each circuit through the loop requires exactly the same amount of time to complete. Reentry, either within the atria itself or involving the AV node, is the mechanism responsible for most supraventricular tachycardias, including PSVT.[26] Other common underlying mechanisms include abnormal automaticity and triggered activity. P waves are present and abnormally shaped, although they may be difficult to identify because they often blend in with the previous T wave because of the rapid rate. It is most helpful if the beginning of the PSVT run is captured and recorded on ECG paper, because the early, abnormal P wave is often easiest to identify in front of the first beat of the run. The PR interval should be the same for each cycle in the run, but it will probably be different from the PR interval of the patient's own normal sinus rhythm. Just as with PACs, the QRS complex is usually normal, because once the impulse passes through the AV node, conduction through the ventricles follows the usual pathway (Table 15-9). However, aberrant conduction, often in the form of right bundle branch block, can occur. It causes a wide QRS complex, leading to difficulty in differentiating this relatively benign dysrhythmia from its more serious counterpart, ventricular tachycardia. Sometimes, because of refractoriness in the AV node, not all of the ectopic P waves are conducted to the ventricles. Usually, at least every other P wave conducts a QRS, but occasionally the conduction ratio may drop to three P waves for every QRS.

PSVT has essentially the same causal factors as PACs. PSVT has greater clinical significance, because it may be sustained for long periods and because it occurs at such a rapid rate. As stressed in the discussion of sinus tachycardia, rapid rates decrease ventricular filling time, increase myocardial oxygen consumption, and decrease oxygen supply. Heart failure, angina, or even myocardial infarction can result.[27] PSVT usually responds rapidly to medical management, which may include the use of direct or indirect vagal maneuvers, intravenous calcium channel blocking agents, or electrical cardioversion. Intravenous adenosine is the drug of choice to briefly block conduction through the AV node.[26] Often, adenosine alone restores normal sinus rhythm, but if not, it will unmask the ectopic P waves and confirm the diagnosis of the dysrhythmia.

Multifocal atrial tachycardia. Multifocal atrial tachycardia, sometimes referred to as *chaotic atrial tachycardia,* occurs when there are numerous irritable atrial foci that intermittently fire and generate an impulse (Figure 15-33). The atrial rate is greater than 100 beats per minute but generally does not exceed 160. The distinguishing feature on the ECG is that there are at least three different P wave shapes, indicating at least three different irritable foci. This is most commonly seen in elderly patients with chronic obstructive pulmonary disease (COPD). COPD causes chronic pulmonary hypertension, which in turn causes chronically elevated right atrial and right ventricular pressures. The abnormally high right atrial pressure causes stretching of the right atrial muscle cells and chronic irritability. Because the underlying cause cannot be resolved, this dysrhythmia usually is refractory to any treatment.

Atrial flutter. Atrial flutter (AF) is believed to be caused by a steady circular pathway through which the wave of depolarization is continually moving. The loop is sufficiently large (or conduction through it sufficiently slow) that the current always finds the cells in front of it to be repolarized and ready to receive another stimulus. As a consequence, the current

TABLE 15-9 Atrial Dysrhythmias

Parameter	Paroxysmal Supraventricular Tachycardia	Multifocal Atrial Tachycardia	Atrial Flutter	Atrial Fibrillation
Rate				
Atrial	150-250/min	100-160/min	250-350/min	>350/min (unable to count it)
Ventricular	Same or less	Same	Half or less	100-180/min (uncontrolled); <100/min (controlled)
Rhythm	Regular	Irregular	Atrial—regular; ventricular—may or may not be regular	Irregularly irregular
P wave	Present; abnormally shaped	Present; three or more different shapes	F waves	F waves
PR interval	May be normal or prolonged	Variable	Conduction ratio: flutter waves per QRS	Absent
QRS	0.06-0.10 sec	0.06-0.10 sec	0.06-0.10 sec	0.06-0.10 sec

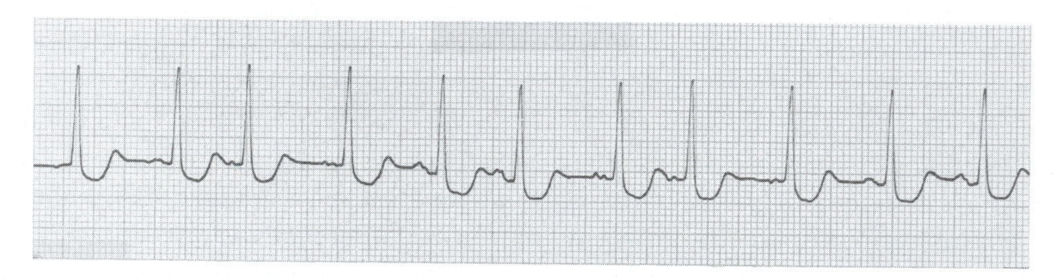

FIGURE 15-33. Multifocal atrial tachycardia (MAT). Note that there are several differently shaped P waves and that the PR intervals vary.

continually perpetuates itself. The atrial rate in atrial flutter is 250 to 350 beats per minute and is most often at 300 (see Table 15-9). At this rate, separate distinction of individual P waves is lost, and they blend together in a saw-tooth pattern (Figure 15-34). In this state, P waves are more appropriately called *F waves* (flutter waves). Fortunately, the AV node does not allow conduction of all these impulses to the ventricles. When evaluating the rate of atrial flutter, one must calculate both atrial and ventricular rates.

The atrial rhythm is always regular, because the circuit is always the same length and therefore always requires the same time to complete. The ventricular rhythm is regular if the same number of flutter waves occurs between each QRS complex—in other words, if the degree of block at the AV node remains constant. Sometimes the refractoriness in the AV node changes from beat to beat, resulting in an irregular ventricular response. When describing atrial flutter, "PR interval" no longer applies; instead, it is a "conduction ratio," such as 3:1 or 4:1, that is used. In normal sinus rhythm, measuring the PR interval allows evaluation of the speed of conduction through the AV node; in atrial flutter, the number of flutter waves that bombard the AV node before one is allowed to pass through to the ventricles is a measure of AV nodal conduction. Once the impulse has passed the AV node, conduction through the ventricles is unaltered. The QRS duration remains normal or at least the same as it was in normal sinus rhythm.

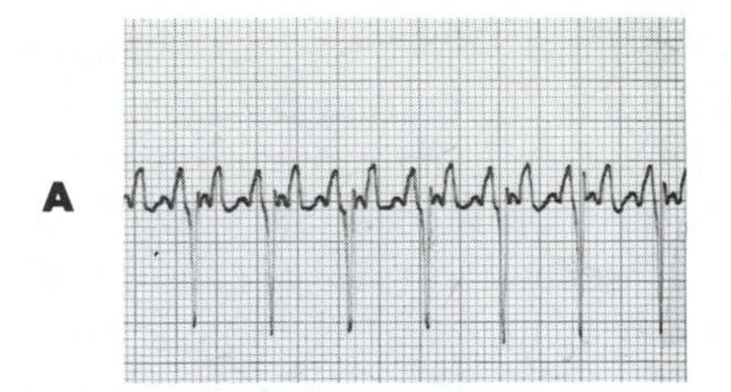

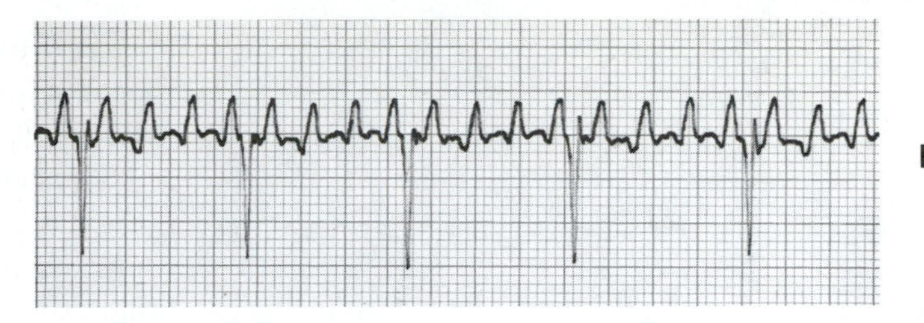

FIGURE 15-34. **A,** Initial strip shows atrial flutter with 2:1 conduction through the AV node. **B,** During carotid sinus massage, the AV conduction rate is decreased, more clearly revealing the flutter waves.

The major key to the clinical significance of atrial flutter is the ventricular response rate. If the atrial rate is 300 and the AV conduction ratio is 4:1, the ventricular response rate is 75 beats per minute and should be well-tolerated. If, on the other hand, the atrial rate is 300 but the AV conduction ratio is 2:1, the corresponding ventricular rate of 150 may cause angina, acute heart failure, or other signs of cardiac decompensation. An atrial rate of 250 with a 1:1 AV conduction ratio yields a ventricular response rate of 250, and emergency measures are needed to decrease the ventricular rate.

Sometimes it is difficult to identify the flutter waves, especially if the conduction ratio is 2:1. Intravenous adenosine or vagal maneuvers can be useful diagnostic tools to increase briefly the refractory period of the AV node and allow better visualization of the F waves (see Figure 15-34). Vagal maneuvers or IV adenosine terminate atrial flutter. Electrical or pharmacologic cardioversion is usually required to restore sinus rhythm. Type I antidysrhythmic drugs, such as quinidine, procainamide, or disopyramide, cause the flutter waves to become slower but may result in an increase in the ventricular response rate, which may not be well-tolerated.[26] A new class III IV antidysrhythmic agent, Ibutilide, has also shown promise in pharmacologic cardioversion of atrial flutter and atrial fibrillation.[28] If cardioversion is unsuccessful, ventricular rate control can be achieved using digoxin, calcium channel blockers, or beta-adrenergic blockers. (∞Antidysrythmic Drugs, p. 578.)

Atrial fibrillation. When numerous sites in the atria fire spontaneously and rapidly, an organized spread of depolarization can no longer take place, and atrial fibrillation results (Figure 15-35). Small sections of atrial muscle are activated individually, resulting in quivering of the atrial muscle without effective contraction. The ECG tracing in atrial fibrillation is characterized by an uneven baseline without clearly defined P waves and an irregularly irregular ventricular rhythm. Sometimes rapid atrial fibrillation appears as a regular rhythm at first glance. However, if examined closely, the ventricular response always is irregular.[29] If on careful examination the RR intervals are truly regular, there are only two possible explanations. Either the rhythm is not atrial fibrillation but some other form of SVT, or the patient has atrial fibrillation but has also developed complete heart block with a regular "default" pacemaker at or below the level of the AV node. In atrial fibrillation, the QRS complex is usually normal, because the pathway through the ventricles is unchanged once the impulse leaves the AV node. The AV node acts as a filter to protect the ventricles from the 350 to 600 sporadic atrial impulses that are occurring each minute (see Table 15-9). In addition, the AV node itself does not receive all of the atrial impulses. When the atrial muscle tissue immediately surrounding the AV node is in a refractory state, impulses generated in other areas of the atria cannot reach the AV node, helping to explain the wide variation in RR intervals during atrial fibrillation.

A normal AV node conducts impulses to the ventricles at a rate of 100 to 180 times per minute. This rapid rate is not desirable, and a major therapeutic goal is to reduce the ventricular response rate to 60 to 90 beats per minute at rest and fewer than 110 beats per minute during exertion.[29] There are two ways to approach this goal: (1) convert the atrial fibrillation back to sinus rhythm using electrical cardioversion or chemical cardioversion with pharmacologic agents or (2) allow the atrial fibrillation to exist and use pharmacologic measures to control the ventricular response rate.

Electrical cardioversion may be successful in converting the rhythm to sinus if attempted within a few days or weeks of the onset of atrial fibrillation. Its success is less likely if the atrial fibrillation has existed for a long time. Cardioversion also carries with it the threat of precipitating emboli. During atrial

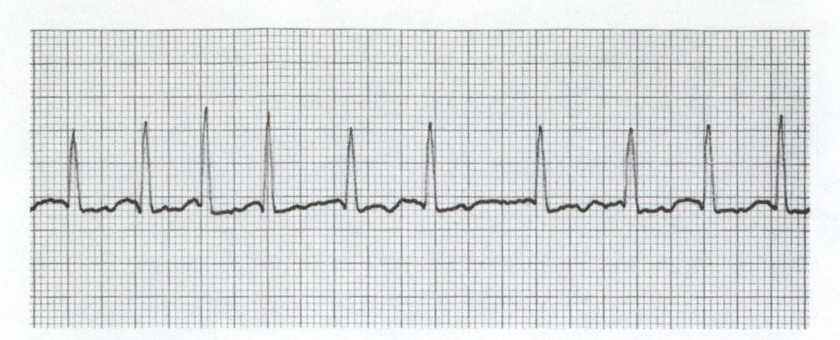

FIGURE 15-35. Atrial fibrillation. Note the irregularly irregular ventricular rhythm.

fibrillation the atria do not contract; hence blood may pool in areas of the atrial walls. This pooling can promote thrombus formation (mural thrombi) within the atria. If cardioversion is successful and normal sinus rhythm is restored, the atria again contracts forcibly and, if thrombus formation has occurred, may send clots traveling through the pulmonary or systemic circulation. To prevent this, it is recommended that patients who have been in atrial fibrillation for 3 or more days be anticoagulated for 3 weeks before elective cardioversion.[29] Transesophageal echocardiography (TEE) may be helpful in identifying the presence of thrombi in the atria, and is sometimes used as a screening tool before elective cardioversion. However, thrombi may be missed or may be transient. Inability to visualize thrombi on the echocardiogram does not negate the need for anticoagulation.

Sometimes patients are in a rapid atrial fibrillation for only a few hours or days at a time and then convert back to sinus rhythm spontaneously. This is called *paroxysmal atrial fibrillation.* If it occurs often, these patients are also at risk for development of mural thrombi and subsequent emboli and must receive long-term anticoagulation therapy unless it is contraindicated. (∞Transesophageal Echocardiography, p. 433.)

The three most common causes of atrial fibrillation are rheumatic heart disease, ischemic heart disease, and hyperthyroidism. Of these, hyperthyroidism is the most correctable, and atrial fibrillation can be effectively reversed in 60% of these cases by correcting the thyrotoxic condition. Often atrial fibrillation is the presenting symptom in patients with previously undiagnosed hyperthyroidism, and nurses have a key role in identifying these patients through careful history-taking and physical assessment. If not recognized and treated, excess thyroid hormone makes rate control difficult, increases risk of a thromboembolic event, and causes higher morbidity and mortality.[30]

Calcium channel blockers, beta-blockers, and digoxin are the most commonly used drugs to control ventricular response rate in atrial fibrillation.

Supraventricular tachycardia (SVT). Any tachycardia originating above the ventricles is considered to be a supraventricular tachycardia. The rate is rapid (more than 100 beats per minute), and it is not ventricular tachycardia. The distinction between ventricular tachycardia (VT) and SVT is important, because treatment is very different. However, "SVT" is not a very specific term. SVT includes sinus tachycardia, atrial tachycardia, atrial flutter, atrial fibrillation, and junctional tachycardia. Each of these entities has a distinct pathophysiology, specific long-term therapy, and expected outcome. In an acute situation, a rapid dysrhythmia may be difficult to identify precisely. Tachycardia alone can cause hemodynamic instability. It is important to at least differentiate VT from SVT; then the focus can be directed to rate control until the acute situation is resolved and hemodynamic stability is restored. At that point, a more careful analysis is needed to determine the specific dysrhythmia responsible for the SVT.

SVT is a common dysrhythmia in critical care, occurring in 15% to 40% of patients in the first few days after coronary artery bypass graft (CABG) surgery,[31] as well as in other critically ill patients with or without coronary artery disease. These patients may already be hemodynamically compromised; thus prompt and effective treatment is essential. Conversion to sinus rhythm is ideal; failing that, slowing of the ventricular response (e.g. heart rate) is essential. New therapies that are showing promise in this regard are intravenous (IV) magnesium and IV amiodarone. Moran and others[32] reported conversion from SVT to sinus rhythm within 24 hours in 74% of patients given IV magnesium and in 50% of patients in whom IV amiodarone was used. In the remainder of the patients, both drugs were about equally effective in slowing the ventricular response rate. For long-term therapy, the newest development has been radiofrequency catheter ablation (RFA). Radiofrequency energy is delivered to a very specific, localized area of heart muscle to cause necrosis of that exact area. This therapy is especially effective if reentry is the mechanism involved in causing the SVT, since RFA can interrupt the reentry path. Success rates of up to 99% have been reported.[33] (∞Antidysrhythmic Drugs, p 578.)

Junctional dysrhythmias. Only certain areas of the AV node have the property of automaticity. The entire area around the AV node is collectively called the *junction;* hence impulses generated there are called *junctional.*

TABLE 15-10 **Junctional Rhythms**

Parameter	Junctional Escape Rhythm	Accelerated Junctional Rhythm	Junctional Tachycardia
Rate	40-60/min	60-100/min	>100/min
Rhythm	Regular	Regular	Regular
P waves	May be present or absent; inverted in lead II	May be present or absent; inverted in lead II	May be present or absent; inverted in lead II
PR interval	<0.12 sec	<0.12 sec	<0.12 sec
QRS	0.06-0.10 sec	0.06-0.10 sec	0.06-0.10 sec

After an ectopic impulse arises in the junction, it spreads in two directions at once. One wave of depolarization spreads upward into the atria and depolarizes them, causing the recording of a P wave on the ECG. At the same time, another wave of depolarization spreads downward into the ventricles through the normal conduction pathway, resulting in a normal QRS complex. Depending on timing, the P wave may be seen in front of the QRS, but with a short PR interval, the P wave may be obscured entirely by the QRS, or the P wave may immediately follow the QRS. When atrial depolarization begins in the junction, the wave of depolarization spreads from the bottom of the atria upward, causing inversion of the P wave in lead II.

Premature junctional contraction. If only a single ectopic impulse originates in the junction, it is simply called a *premature junctional contraction.* On the ECG, the rhythm is regular from the sinus node except for one early QRS complex of normal shape and duration. The P wave can be entirely absent. If a P wave can be found, it very closely precedes or follows the QRS. In lead II, the P wave appears inverted (having a negative deflection), because the atria are being depolarized from the AV node upward, which is the opposite direction from the wave of depolarization that occurs when triggered by the sinus node. If the P wave appears before the QRS, the PR interval is less than 0.12 second. Premature junctional contractions have virtually the same clinical significance as do PACs. However, if the patient is receiving digoxin, digitalis toxicity is suspected. Although digoxin slows conduction through the AV node, it also increases automaticity in the junction.

Junctional escape rhythm. Sometimes the junction becomes the dominant pacemaker of the heart (Table 15-10). Normally the intrinsic rate of the junction is 40 to 60 beats per minute. The intrinsic rate of the sinus node is 60 to 100 beats per minute. Under normal conditions the junction never has a chance to "escape" and depolarize the heart because it is overridden by the sinus node. However, if the sinus node fails, the junctional impulses can depolarize completely and pace the heart. This is called a *junctional escape rhythm* and is a protective mechanism to prevent asystole in the event of sinus node failure. Generally, a junctional escape rhythm (Figure 15-36) is well-tolerated, although efforts must be directed toward restoring sinus rhythm. Sometimes a pacemaker is inserted as a protective measure because of concern that the junction may also fail.

Junctional tachycardia and accelerated junctional rhythm. A junctional rhythm can also occur at a faster rate (see Table 15-10). As with sinus rhythm, the term *tachycardia* is reserved for rates greater than 100 per minute; thus junctional tachycardia is a junctional rhythm, usually regular, at a rate greater than 100. But what if the junctional rate is greater than 60 and less than 100 (faster than the intrinsic rate of the junction, yet not fast enough to be considered a tachycardia)? The phrase *accelerated junctional rhythm* applies to this situation. Accelerated junctional rhythm is usually well-tolerated by the patient, mainly because the heart rate is within a reasonable range. Junctional tachycardia may not be tolerated as well, depending on the rate and the patient's underlying cardiac reserve. Once again, digitalis toxicity is strongly suspected, because digoxin enhances automaticity of the AV node. If digitalis toxicity is present, the only treatment is to withhold digoxin until the dysrhythmia resolves.

Ventricular dysrhythmias. Ventricular dysrhythmias result from an ectopic focus in any portion of the ventricular myocardium. The usual conduction pathway through the ventricles is not used, and the wave of depolarization must spread from cell to cell. As a result, the QRS complex is prolonged and is always greater than 0.12 second. It is the width of the QRS,

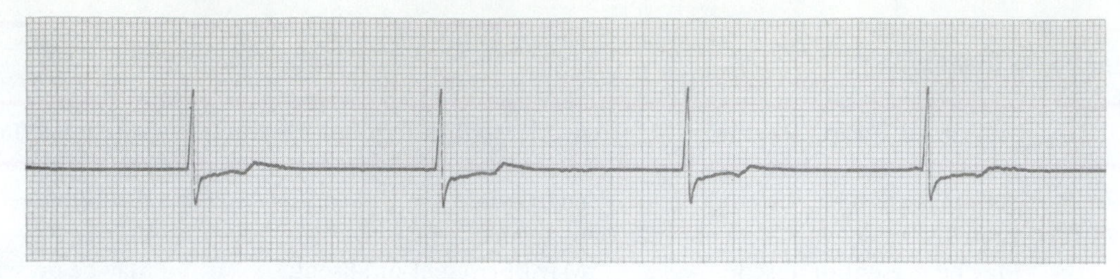

FIGURE 15-36. Junctional escape rhythm. The ventricular rate is 38. P waves are absent, and the QRS is normal width.

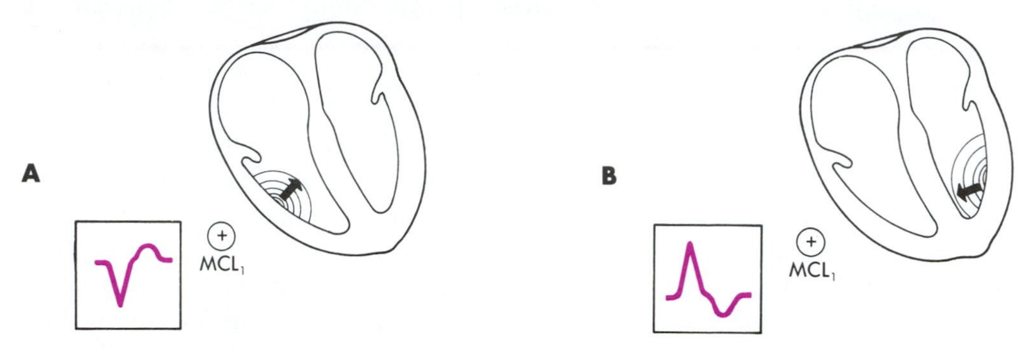

FIGURE 15-37. **A,** Right ventricular premature ventricular contraction (PVC). The spread of depolarization is from right to left, away from the positive electrode in lead MCL_1, resulting in a wide, negative QRS complex. **B,** Left ventricular PVC. The spread of depolarization is from left to right, toward the positive electrode in lead MCL_1. The QRS complex is wide and upright.

not the height, that is important in diagnosing ventricular ectopy.

Premature ventricular contractions. A single ectopic impulse originating in the ventricles is called a *premature ventricular contraction (PVC).* Some PVCs are very small in height but remain wider than 0.12 second. If in doubt, a different lead is evaluated. The shape of the QRS varies, depending on the location of the ectopic focus. If the ectopic focus is in the right ventricle, the impulse spreads from right to left and the QRS resembles a left bundle branch block pattern, because the left ventricle is the last to be depolarized. In MCL_1, this is a wide, negative QRS (Figure 15-37, *A*). If the ectopic focus is in the left ventricular free wall, the wave of depolarization spreads from left to right (Figure 15-37, *B*).

Because the ectopic focus could be any cell in the ventricle, the QRS might take an unlimited number of shapes or patterns. If all of the ventricular ectopic beats look the same in a particular lead, they are called *unifocal,* which means that they probably all result from the same irritable focus (Figure 15-38, *A*). Conversely, if the ventricular ectopics are of various shapes in the same lead, they are called *multifocal* (Figure 15-38, *B*). Multifocal ventricular ectopics are more serious than unifocal ventricular ectopics, because they indicate a greater area of irritable myocardial tissue and are more likely to deteriorate into ventricular tachycardia or fibrillation. In general, ventricular dysrhythmias have more serious implications than do atrial or junctional dysrhythmias and occur only rarely in healthy individuals.

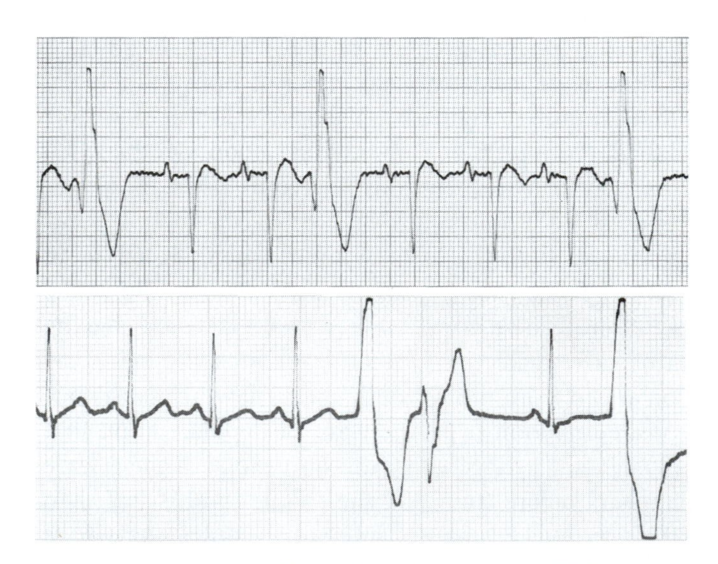

FIGURE 15-38. **A,** Unifocal PVCs. **B,** Multifocal PVCs.

A PVC originates in a ventricular cell that has become abnormally permeable to sodium, usually as a result of damage of one kind or another. Because of this new permeability to sodium, the cell reaches depolarization threshold before an impulse is received from the sinus node. Once depolarization threshold is reached, the cell automatically depolarizes, thus beginning total ventricular depolarization. Ordinarily, the ventricular impulse does not conduct back through the AV node; hence the sinus node is not disturbed and continues to depolarize the atria, resulting in a normal P wave. Conduction from the sinus node will not proceed into the ventricles if they are in a refractory state. The next sinus beat, assuming there is no further ventricular ectopy, conducts normally through the AV node and into the ventricles.

Compensatory pause. If the interval from the last normal QRS preceding the PVC to the one following it is exactly equal to two complete cardiac cycles (Figure 15-39, *A*), a compensatory pause is present. It does not usually occur in PACs or premature junctional contraction, so when present it is somewhat diagnostic of ventricular ectopy. If the normal sinus P wave that occurs immediately after the PVC finds the ventricles sufficiently recovered to accept another impulse, a normal QRS results and the PVC is sandwiched between two normal beats (Figure 15-39, *B*). This PVC is referred to as *interpolated,* meaning "between." Interpolated PVCs usually occur when either the PVC is very early or the normal sinus rate is relatively slow.

Occasionally, the ventricular impulse spreads backward across the AV node to depolarize the atria. When this occurs, the sinus node is reset, and there is not a full compensatory pause.

Describing ventricular ectopy. PVCs can develop concurrently with any supraventricular dysrhythmia. Therefore it is not sufficient to describe a patient's rhythm as "frequent PVCs" or even "frequent unifocal PVCs." The underlying rhythm must always be described first (e.g., "sinus bradycardia with frequent unifocal PVCs" or "atrial fibrillation with occasional multifocal PVCs"). Timing of PVCs can also be described. When a PVC follows each normal beat, *ventricular bigeminy* is present (Figure 15-40). If a PVC follows every two normal beats, it is called *ventricular trigeminy.*

The timing of PVCs can be important, especially if myocardial ischemia is present. The relative refractory period, represented on the ECG by the last half of the T wave, is a particularly vulnerable time for ectopy to occur because repolarization is not yet complete. Repolarization is even more delayed in ischemic tissue so that various portions of the ventricular muscle are not repolarized simultaneously. If a PVC occurs at this critical point when only a part of the muscle is repolarized, individual segments of muscle can depolarize separately from each other, resulting in ventricular fibrillation. This is called the *R-on-T phenomenon* (Figure 15-41).

Two consecutive PVCs are described as a *couplet,* and three consecutive PVCs are called either a *triplet* or a *three-beat run of ventricular tachycardia.* More than three consecutive PVCs are considered ventricular tachycardia, but it is still useful to state how many beats of ventricular tachycardia occurred if the run was short, (i.e., fewer than 20 beats).

Causes of PVCs. There are many causes of PVCs. They have been known to occur, although rarely, in healthy individuals with no evidence of heart disease. The critical care nurse has an important role in identifying factors that may be causing or at least contributing to the occurrence of PVCs. Acute ischemia is the most dangerous cause of ventricular ectopy. Ischemia causes cell membrane permeability to change, giving rise to early depolarization and the initiation of ectopic impulses. Ventricular ectopy that occurs during an acute ischemic event may require treatment with intravenous lidocaine or other antidysrhythmic drugs.

Metabolic abnormalities are common causes of the development of PVCs. Hypokalemia, hypoxemia, and acidosis predispose the cell membrane to instability and may cause ventricular ectopy. Treatment is directed toward identifying the metabolic disturbance and correcting it. Arterial blood gas values and serum potassium and magnesium levels are obtained if no recent results are available. The ability of oxygen and potassium values to change very rapidly in a critically ill patient must not be underestimated. If PVCs develop during suctioning of an intubated patient, a few additional breaths of 100% oxygen usually are sufficient to restore adequate oxygenation and to eliminate the ventricular ectopy.

Any form of heart disease can lead to the development of ventricular ectopy. Patients with cardiomyopathy or ventricular aneurysms can have chronic, severe ventricular ectopy, which may prove to be refractory to any antidysrhythmic agent. Invasive procedures, such as insertion of a pulmonary artery catheter or cardiac catheterization, can cause PVCs by mechanically irritating the ventricular muscle. In these situations the ectopy resolves with removal or advancement of the catheter. As a temporary measure, a one-time bolus of lidocaine can be used as a precaution against the development of a life-threatening dysrhythmia during these procedures.

Certain drugs can cause ventricular ectopy. Digitalis toxicity is often accompanied by PVCs, which are somewhat resistant to conventional antidysrhythmic

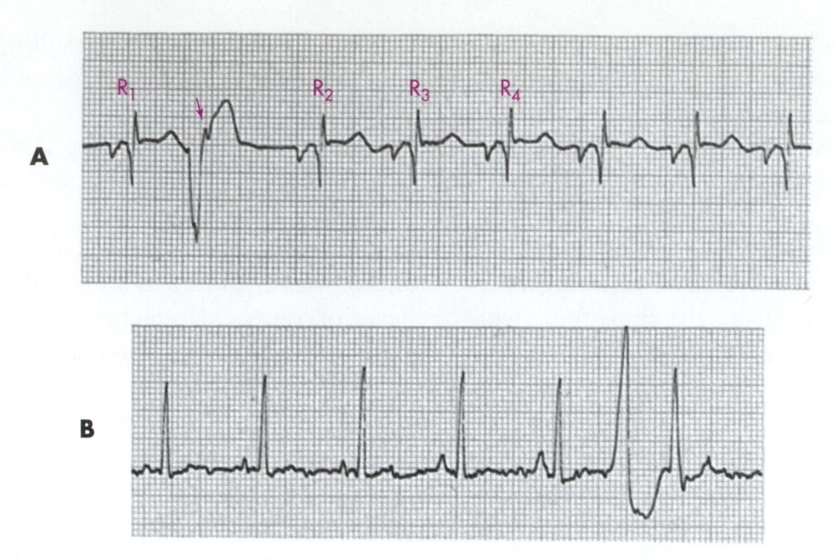

FIGURE 15-39. **A,** PVC with a fully compensatory pause. The interval between the two sinus beats that surround the PVC (R_1 and R_2) is exactly two times the normal interval between sinus beats (R_3 and R_4). The fully compensatory pause occurs because the sinus node continues to pace despite the PVC. Note the sinus P wave *(arrow)* hidden in the ST segment of the PVC. This P wave did not conduct through to the ventricles because they had just been depolarized and were still in the absolute refractory period. **B,** Interpolated PVC. The PVC falls between two normal QRS complexes without disturbing the rhythm. Note that the RR interval between sinus beats remains the same.

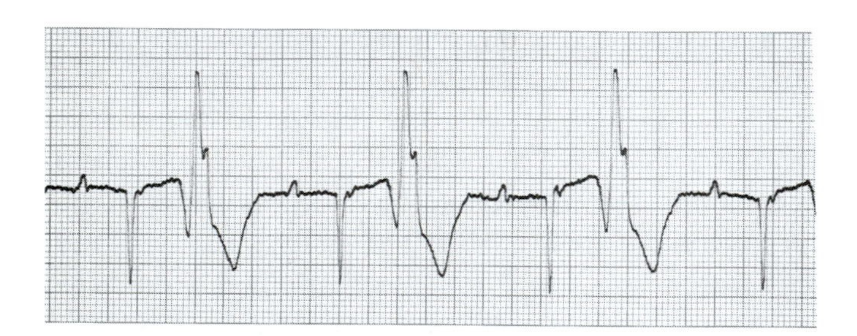

FIGURE 15-40. Ventricular bigeminy.

therapy. Some Class I antidysrhythmic drugs can actually cause more serious dysrhythmias than those they were intended to treat. This is called a *prodysrhythmic effect* and can sometimes be fatal. These drugs prolong the QT interval by lengthening the ventricular refractory period. This is a therapeutic effect, but when the QT prolongation becomes excessive, a characteristic form of polymorphic ventricular tachycardia called *torsades de pointes* develops (Figure 15-42). In this dysrhythmia the ventricular tachycardia is very rapid and the QRS complexes appear to twist in a spiral pattern around the baseline. Clinically, torsades de pointes is poorly tolerated because of the extremely rapid rate. If not terminated, death will result. Sometimes torsades de pointes stops spontaneously, although the patient may experience a syncopal episode or seizure at the time of the dysrhythmia.

Treatment of PVCs. Not all ventricular ectopy requires treatment. In individuals without significant underlying heart disease, PVCs do not represent an increased risk for sudden death and are considered benign. If the patient complains of palpitations, therapy initially includes reassurance and elimination of such factors as caffeine or alcohol ingestion, emotional stress, and sympathomimetic drugs that increase ventricular irritability. If symptoms continue, mild tranquilizers can be administered, followed by beta-blockers to reduce the response to sympathetic stimulation. Antidysrhythmic drugs are used only as a last resort.

In patients with underlying heart disease, PVCs and/or episodes of nonsustained ventricular tachycardia are potentially malignant. Nonsustained ventricular tachycardia is defined as three or more consecutive premature ventricular beats at a rate faster than 110 per minute, lasting less than 30 seconds.[34]

Because the occurrence of ventricular dysrhythmias in patients with heart disease has been shown to increase the risk of both sudden and nonsudden cardiac death,[35] these dysrhythmias have been treated aggressively with antidysrhythmic drugs for many years. However, until recently no well-controlled clinical trials had been performed to demonstrate that reduction of ventricular ectopics with antidysrhythmic drugs really improved morbidity and mortality statistics. In 1987 the National Institutes of Health began a randomized,

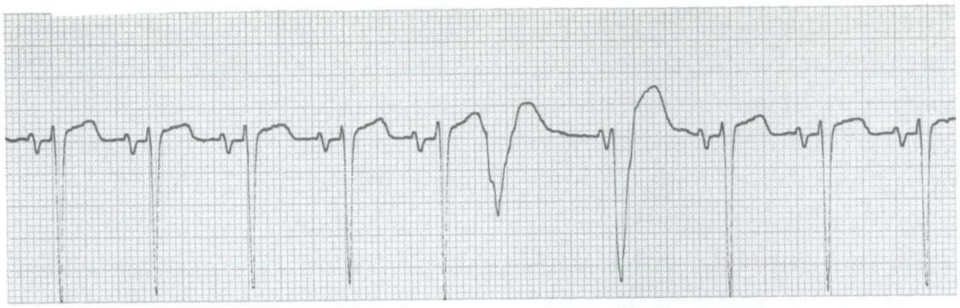

FIGURE 15-41. R-on-T phenomenon.

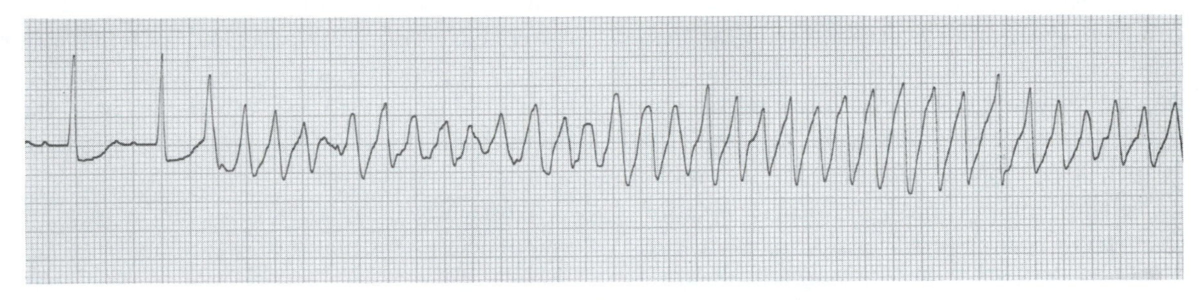

FIGURE 15-42. Torsades de pointes.

double-blind study known as the *Cardiac Arrhythmia Suppression Trial (CAST)* to test the assumption that the treatment of ventricular dysrhythmias prolongs life. Patients with potentially malignant ventricular dysrhythmias were randomized into one of four groups: treatment with (1) encainide, (2) flecainide, (3) moricizine, and (4) placebo. These three drugs were chosen because they were the most effective in suppressing ventricular ectopics, as documented by Holter monitor recordings, and had the lowest incidence of side effects. They are classified as class IC antidysrythmics. The study was aborted, and interim results were released in 1989, when it was found that patients treated with encainide and flecainide had a significantly increased mortality over the placebo group, despite excellent suppression of ventricular ectopics and episodes of nonsustained ventricular tachycardia. The study was continued briefly with moricizine (CAST II), but it was also found to result in higher mortality rates than placebo.[35] Although the results of this study cannot be generalized to other groups of antidysrhythmic drugs, or to patients with episodes of symptomatic sustained ventricular tachycardia (VT), they have cast serious doubts on the efficacy of antidysrhythmic drug therapy in general. The final recommendation of the CAST investigators was that post-MI patients with asymptomatic or only mildly symptomatic ventricular ectopic must not receive antidysrhythmic drugs until improved survival can be documented in a clinical trial.[35] Amiodarone has shown promise in this regard, and several large clinical trials are currently in progress. Beta-blockers have been shown to significantly decrease mortality after a myocardial infarction, and although they are only moderately effective in suppressing ventricular ectopic activity, they are safer than conventional antidysrhythmic drugs. Calcium channel blockers are associated with increased mortality post-MI and are used only when there are convincing clinical reasons to do so. (∞Antidysrythmic Drugs, p. 578.)

Patients who have already experienced sustained ventricular tachycardia or cardiac arrest are at risk for sudden death. Additional risk factors for sudden cardiac death include poor left ventricular function, ongoing myocardial ischemia, and cardiac conduction or rhythm disturbances.[35] An extensive clinical evaluation of these patients is warranted, including cardiac catheterization and electrophysiologic testing with programmed ventricular stimulation. Therapy is aimed at eliminating malignant ventricular ectopy and preventing recurrence of sustained ventricular tachycardia or ventricular fibrillation. It may include treating the underlying cause, administering antidysrhythmic drugs, performing ablation of the reentrant pathway within the ventricle, or implanting an implantable cardioverter defibrillator (ICD). Many new ICDs have "tiered therapy" available, which may include several bursts of overdrive pacing in an attempt to terminate the VT before cardioversion. This has the advantage of being more comfortable for the patient, since it prevents the discomfort of an internal shock if the overdrive pacing is successful. Antitachycardia pacing is a good treatment if combined with defibrillation backup. It is risky without defibrillator support, since one of the complications of antitachycardiac pacing is acceleration of the ventricular tachycardia being treated to a faster VT, polymorphic VT, or even ventricular fibrillation (VF).[36] (∞Implantable Cardioverter defibrillator, p. 550.)

Radiofrequency ablation for ventricular tachycardia requires the presence of an inducible, hemodynamically stable ventricular tachycardia, allowing time to localize the critical area via endocardial mapping. If a bundle branch is part of the reentrant circuit (which it is in 6% of all monomorphic VT), catheter ablation of the right bundle branch provides a permanent cure. Controlled trials are currently in progress comparing drug therapy, ICD implantation, and ablation in these high risk patients.[36]

Idioventricular rhythm. At times an ectopic focus in the ventricle can become the dominant pacemaker of the heart (Table 15-11). If both the sinus node and the AV junction fail, the ventricles depolarize at their own intrinsic rate of 20 to 40 times per minute. This is called an *idioventricular rhythm* and is protective in nature. Rather than trying to abolish the ventricular beats, the aim of treatment is to increase the effective heart rate and reestablish a higher pacing site, such as the sinus node or AV junction. The heart rate may be increased pharmacologically with an infusion of isoproterenol (Isuprel). Or more commonly a temporary pacemaker is used to increase heart rate until the underlying problems that caused failure of the other pacing sites can be resolved.

An *accelerated idioventricular rhythm* occurs when a ventricular focus assumes control of the heart at a rate greater than its intrinsic rate of 40 per minute but less than 100 per minute (Figure 15-43). Although relatively benign in and of itself, this rhythm must be closely observed for any increase in rate, or hemodynamic deterioration. Usually it is not treated pharmacologically if well-tolerated, although a transvenous temporary pacemaker should be inserted electively as a precaution against sudden hemodynamic deterioration. Intravenous lidocaine must never be administered to a patient with an idioventricular rhythm, because it suppresses the ventricular pacemaker and converts the rhythm to asystole.

Ventricular tachycardia. Ventricular tachycardia is caused by a ventricular pacing site firing at a rate of 100 times or more per minute (Figure 15-44). The complexes are wide, and the rhythm may be slightly irregular, often accelerating as the tachycardia continues (see Table 15-11). In most cases the sinus node is not affected, and it continues to depolarize the atria on schedule. P waves can sometimes be seen on the ECG tracing. They are not related to the QRS and may even conduct a normal impulse to the ventricles if their timing is just right. If the sinus impulse and the ventricular ectopic impulse meet in the middle of the ventricles, a fusion beat results. Fusion beats are narrower than ventricular beats and look like a cross between the patient's sinus QRS and the ventricular ectopic QRS (Figure 15-45). When present, P waves and fusion beats are helpful in verifying the diagnosis of ventricular tachycardia.

Ventricular tachycardia can occur acutely in a variety of clinical situations, including myocardial ischemia, digitalis toxicity, and electrolyte disturbances and as an adverse reaction of certain antidysrhythmic drugs. Patients with chronic, severe heart disease, such as cardiomyopathy or ventricular aneurysm, may experience frequent episodes of ventricular tachycardia. Ventricular tachycardia is a serious dysrhythmia and must be treated quickly. Its rapid rate alone makes this dysrhythmia poorly tolerated. The benefit of the proper timing of atrial contraction, which would add volume to the ventricles just before contraction and enhance the force of contraction, is lost, thus greatly reducing cardiac output (CO). The fall in CO may cause the patient to lose consciousness. Finally, if not terminated quickly, ventricular tachycardia is very likely to degenerate into ventricular fibrillation and death.

Ventricular fibrillation. Ventricular fibrillation is the result of chaotic electrical activity in the ventricles from either repetitive small areas of reentry or a series of rapid discharges from various foci within the ventricular myocardium.[34] This causes the ventricles to be unable to contract completely and effectively. The ventricles merely quiver, and there is no forward flow of blood. Without forward flow, there is no palpable pulse or audible apical heart tones. Clinically, ventricular fibrillation is indistinguishable from asystole (absence of electrical activity). On the ECG, ventricular fibrillation appears as a continuous, undulating pattern without clear P, QRS, or T waves (Figure 15-46). When VF occurs in the setting of an acute ischemic event and is not accompanied by a significant amount of myocardial damage, it is referred to as *primary VF.* If primary VF is treated immediately the survival rate is excellent. In contrast, *secondary VF* occurs in the setting of severe left ventricular dysfunction,

TABLE 15-11 Ventricular Rhythms

Parameter	Idioventricular Rhythm	Accelerated Idioventricular Rhythm	Ventricular Tachycardia	Ventricular Fibrillation
Rate	20-40/min	40-100/min	>100/min	None
Rhythm	Usually regular	Usually regular	Usually regular	Irregular
P waves	Absent or retrograde	Absent or retrograde	Absent or retrograde	None
PR interval	None	None	None	None
QRS	>0.12 sec	>0.12 sec	>0.12 sec	Fibrillatory waves

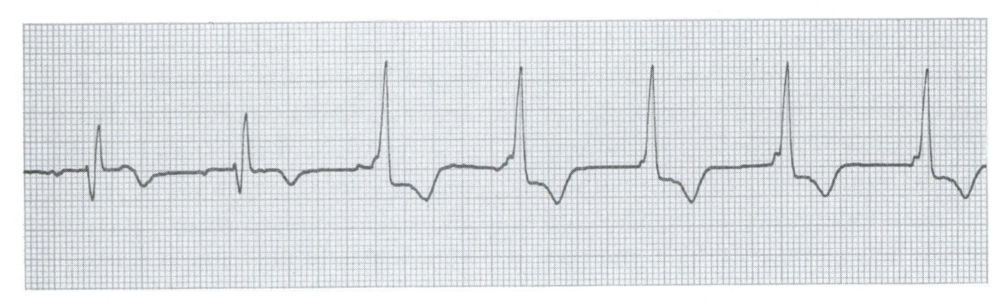

FIGURE 15-43. Accelerated idioventricular rhythm (AIVR). The QRS duration is 0.14 second, and the ventricular rate is 65.

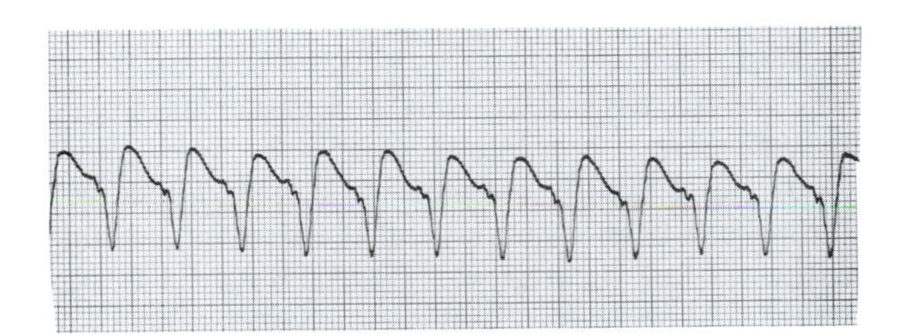

FIGURE 15-44. Ventricular tachycardia.

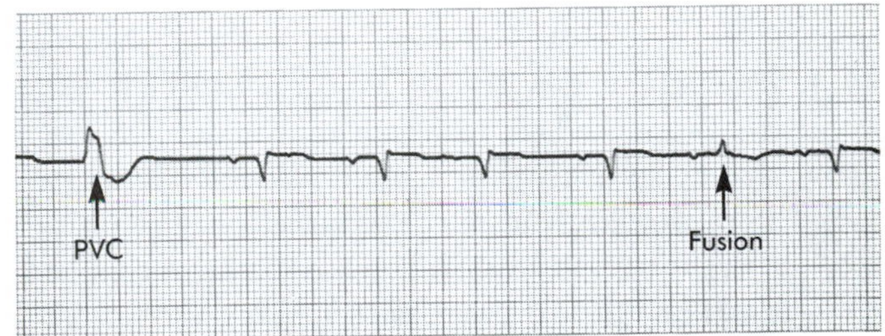

FIGURE 15-45. Ventricular fusion beat *(arrows)*. The QRS duration is only 0.08 second, and the shape represents both the normal QRS and the previous PVC.

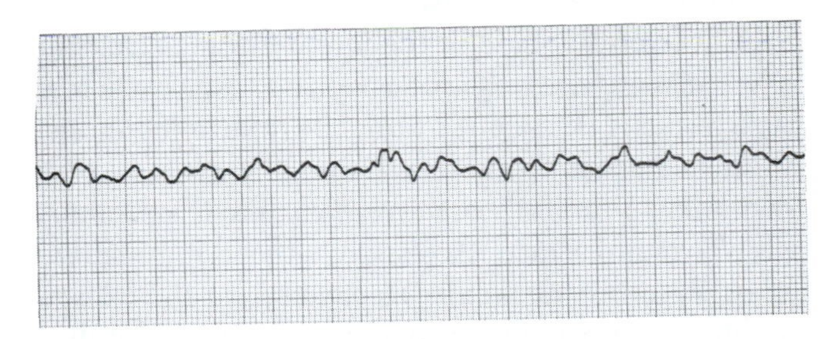

FIGURE 15-46. Ventricular fibrillation.

cardiogenic shock, and deteriorating hemodynamics. Resuscitation is often unsuccessful, recurrence rates are high in those who are resuscitated, and there is a 70% to 80% mortality rate.[34]

Ventricular fibrillation is sometimes further described as "coarse" or "fine." Coarse ventricular fibrillation is seen on the ECG as large, erratic undulations of the baseline. This usually indicates recent onset of ventricular fibrillation and is usually more easily defibrillated. In fine ventricular fibrillation the ECG baseline exhibits only a mild tremor, with waveforms greater than 0.2 mV.[34] In either case, the patient does not have a pulse, no blood is being pumped forward, and defibrillation is the only definitive therapy. Generally, coarse ventricular fibrillation is more likely to be successfully defibrillated. Epinephrine can be used to try to change fine ventricular fibrillation to coarse ventricular fibrillation to facilitate defibrillation attempts. Antidysrhythmic drugs, such as intravenous lidocaine and bretylium, are also given if initial attempts at defibrillation fail. As with any cardiac arrest situation, supportive measures, such as CPR, intubation, and correction of metabolic abnormalities, are performed concurrently with definitive therapy. (See Appendix C, Advanced Cardiac Life Support [ACLS] Guidelines.)

Differential diagnosis of a wide QRS complex tachycardia. Tachycardias that are triggered by an ectopic atrial or junctional focus are called *supraventricular,* meaning that they come from an irritable site above the ventricles. Typical supraventricular tachycardia (SVT) has a narrow QRS complex (less than 0.12 second), because the electrical impulse enters the ventricle through the AV node and still follows the normal conduction pathway via the bundle branches through the ventricles. Ventricular tachycardia (VT) always has a wide QRS complex (greater than 0.12 second), because the impulse begins somewhere within the ventricles and must spread slowly—cell to cell—without the benefit of the usual conduction system. Therefore it is easy to distinguish between typical SVT and ventricular tachycardia by QRS width alone.

Unfortunately, not all SVTs result in a narrow QRS complex. There are three situations in which a supraventricular tachycardia has a wide QRS complex.[37]

1. The patient may already have a right or left bundle branch block, resulting in a wide QRS even during sinus rhythm. Understandably, if that patient develops an atrial or junctional tachycardia, the bundle branch block remains unchanged and the QRS complex is still wide.
2. A supraventricular impulse may arrive in the ventricles so early that only part of the conduction system is repolarized. One of the bundle branches is still refractory, causing the wave of depolarization to spread abnormally *(aberrantly)* through the ventricles and resulting in a wide QRS complex.
3. Occasionally an anatomic variant occurs in which the patient has a small strip of muscle tissue connecting the atria with the ventricles and bypassing the AV node. This is called an *accessory pathway,* or *bypass tract,* the most common of which is *Wolff-Parkinson-White syndrome,* or WPW. This is not a problem in normal sinus rhythm, although it sometimes causes subtle ECG changes that allow it to be detected. However, when rapid atrial dysrhythmias occur, they can be conducted directly to a portion of the ventricular myocardium without normal AV delay. Depolarization through the ventricles then proceeds from cell to cell rather than through the normal pathway of the conduction system, resulting in a wide QRS complex tachycardia that closely resembles ventricular tachycardia.

Significance. Standard treatment for ventricular tachycardia includes administration of intravenous lidocaine, whereas supraventricular tachycardia is typically managed with intravenous diltiazem or verapamil. If the diagnosis is incorrect and a supraventricular tachycardia is treated with lidocaine, the treatment is ineffective. If a ventricular tachycardia is mistakenly diagnosed as SVT and verapamil is given, the consequences can be acute, severe hypotension or loss of consciousness requiring immediate cardioversion. Therefore it is important in patients who are relatively hemodynamically stable to be sure of the etiology of the tachycardia before treatment is initiated.

Regardless of the site of origin, a wide QRS complex tachycardia may not be well-tolerated, mainly because of the rapid heart rate that prevents adequate ventricular filling during diastole, as well as increasing myocardial oxygen demand while decreasing time for coronary artery filling. Hemodynamic deterioration is evidenced by syncope, severe hypotension, or symptoms of ischemia. In this case, emergency cardioversion needs to be performed regardless of whether the tachycardia is of ventricular or supraventricular origin.

Correct diagnosis of a wide QRS complex tachycardia may have an impact on the long-term management of a patient as well. If atrial flutter or fibrillation is determined to be the underlying mechanism, long-term treatment probably involves digoxin or a calcium channel blocker to reduce the heart rate response when these dysrhythmias occur. These drugs have little or no value in the long-term management of recurrent ventricular tachycardia. If ventricular tachycardia is determined to be the underlying mechanism in a patient without a history of ventricular dysrhythmias, a careful search for the cause (hypoxemia, electrolyte imbalance, excess sympathetic stimulation, or ischemia) is warranted. Depending on the clinical situation, the patient may require long-term antidysrhythmic therapy. If there is a history of ventricular tachycardia or "sudden death" and the patient is already on antidysrhythmic therapy, a recurrent episode of ventricular tachycardia indicates that the current treatment regimen is not effective and the therapy needs to be changed.

Clinical differentiation. Contrary to popular belief, hemodynamic stability or instability does not help to differentiate between ventricular tachycardia and SVT with a wide QRS complex.[37] In theory, a supraventricular tachycardia is better tolerated, especially if atrial contraction is still occurring before each ventricular contraction (AV synchrony). However, clinically this is often untrue. Ventricular tachycardia may be well-tolerated, especially if the rate is less than 150 per minute. Some patients can be in sustained VT for hours without significant hemodynamic compromise. Conversely, AV synchrony is still lost in atrial fibrillation or atrial flutter, and the ventricular response rate may be very rapid, compromising ventricular filling and, in turn, cardiac output.

Careful physical examination can be of value in determining the source of the tachycardia. The jugular venous pulse can be assessed for the presence of *cannon "a" waves.* When the atria contract at the same time as ventricular systole, the AV valves are closed and the blood in the atria is forced to regurgitate into the venous system. This is seen as a very large pulsation in the jugular vein. If it occurs sporadically (i.e., not with every beat), it is a sign of *AV dissociation,* or independent beating of the atria and ventricles. Heart sounds provide another diagnostic clue. Variation of the intensity of the first heart sound (S_1) from beat to beat favors ventricular tachycardia, because this is also indicative of AV dissociation.

By far the most reliable means of diagnosing a wide QRS complex tachycardia is through careful analysis of the ECG. Heart rate and rhythm are evaluated first, although they are not diagnostic by themselves. Rates of 130 to 170 per minute favor ventricular tachycardia. Rates greater than 170 per minute favor SVT with aberrant conduction, because healthy hearts can usually conduct impulses at rates less than 170 without altering the normal conduction pathway through the ventricles. Ventricular tachycardia is not always perfectly regular, but a grossly irregular rhythm is more likely to be atrial fibrillation with aberrant conduction through the ventricles.[37] Rates greater than 220 per minute, especially if accompanied by an irregular rhythm, favor atrial fibrillation with conduction around the AV node via a bypass tract.

The QRS width is measured in more than one lead, because the lead with the widest QRS complex is the most reliable indicator of true QRS duration. (It is assumed that some portion of the QRS complex is isoelectric in leads where the QRS appears to be more narrow.) QRS widths of less than 0.14 second favor SVT with aberrant conduction, whereas widths of greater than 0.14 second in a RBBB pattern or of greater than 0.16 second in an LBBB pattern favor ventricular tachycardia.[34]

The tracing is examined closely for the presence of P waves. If P waves can be identified and they do not correlate on a 1:1 basis with the QRS complexes, AV dissociation exists and strongly suggests ventricular tachycardia.[34]

Although P waves may be found in any lead, they are most likely to be visible in V_1 or MCL_1. If the sinus node remains in control of the atria and a ventricular ectopic focus is in control of the ventricles, it is likely that at some point the timing will be just right for the sinus impulse to conduct through the AV node and begin to depolarize the ventricles just as the ventricular ectopic focus fires. The resulting QRS complex is a fusion beat (see Figure 15-45), which looks like a blend of the patient's normal QRS and the wide QRS complex of the ventricular dysrhythmia. Fusion beats also strongly suggest ventricular tachycardia.[34]

Another helpful diagnostic criterion for ventricular tachycardia is a QRS axis in the northwest quadrant of -90 degrees to ± 180 degrees (see Figure 15-14). An axis in this quadrant means that the wave of depolarization is directed upward and to the right, exactly the opposite of normal ventricular depolarization. Even when ventricular conduction is abnormal, as in bundle branch blocks, ventricular depolarization begins at the level of the AV junction and spreads downward toward the apex, although conduction disturbances direct the current flow more to the right or left than normal. Although not all ventricular tachycardias have an axis in the northwest quadrant, about one fourth of them do, and when present, an axis in the northwest quadrant confirms the diagnosis of ventricular tachycardia. Figure 15-47 illustrates how this abnormal axis can be rapidly identified from a five lead–wire bedside monitor by noting the shape of the QRS in leads I and aV_F.

Finally, the shape of the QRS complex in the right precordial lead MCL_1 or V_1 and the left precordial lead MCL_6 or V_6 can be diagnostic of ventricular tachycardia or of SVT with aberrant conduction. Figure 15-48 summarizes these QRS patterns. In addition, if the QRS complex is either entirely positive from V_1 through V_6 or entirely negative, the diagnosis is ventricular tachycardia.[34,37]

This phenomenon is known as *precordial concordance* and is also valid when only V_1 and V_6 are analyzed without the benefit of V_{2-5} as well.

Implications for critical care nursing management. Proper electrode placement and appropriate lead selection have already been discussed but cannot be overemphasized. In addition to correct lead placement and selection, every effort must be made to record the wide QRS complex tachycardia on a standard 12-lead ECG. Certainly emergency treatment must not be

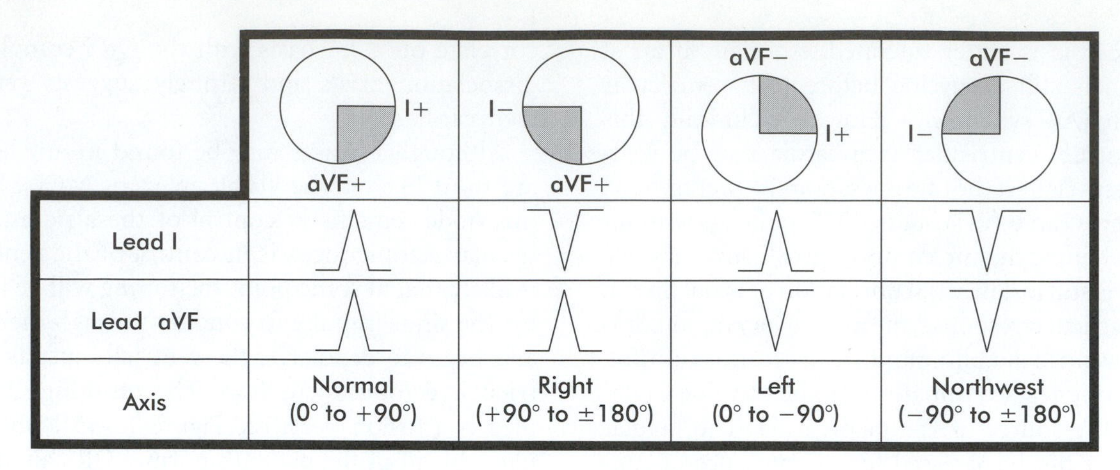

FIGURE 15-47. Determination of QRS axis quadrant by noting predominant QRS polarity in leads I and aV_F. If QRS during tachycardia is primarily positive in both I and aV_F, the axis falls within the normal quadrant from 0 to 90 degrees. If the QRS complex is primarily negative in I and positive in aV_F, right axis deviation is present. If the QRS complex is predominantly positive in I and negative in aV_F, left axis deviation is present. Finally, if QRS is primarily negative in both I and aV_F, markedly abnormal "northwest" axis is present that is diagnostic of ventricular tachycardia. (From Drew B: *Heart Lung* 20(6):615, 1991.)

delayed if the patient is hemodynamically unstable, but documenting the dysrhythmia by recording a "stat" 12-lead ECG must be given a high priority if time permits. Ventricular tachycardia and SVT are often nonsustained, and waiting for a physician's order or a technician to perform the test could result in failure to document the dysrhythmia at all, leaving the cause and subsequent therapy a mystery. Finally, if in doubt as to the origin of the wide QRS complex tachycardia, verapamil must be avoided because it has been known to cause rapid hemodynamic deterioration.

Atrioventricular conduction disturbance. Normally, the sinoatrial (SA) node triggers electrical depolarization in the heart. From there, the impulse travels through internodal tracts to the atrioventricular (AV) node. The impulse is delayed in the AV node to allow the atria to contract before the impulse is conducted to the bundle of His, bundle branches, and Purkinje fibers.

Clinically, the ability of the AV node to conduct is evaluated by measuring the PR interval and the relationship of P waves to QRS complexes (Table 15-12). The normal PR interval, measured from the beginning of the P wave to the beginning of the QRS complex, ranges from 0.12 to 0.20 second.

First-degree AV block. When all atrial impulses are conducted to the ventricles but the PR interval is greater than 0.20 second, a condition known as *first-degree AV block* exists (Figure 15-49). First-degree AV block is not clinically significant by itself, but in a patient with an acute myocardial infarction, it may be a forerunner of more severe conduction disturbances and deserves close monitoring.

Second-degree AV block. Second-degree AV block can be broadly defined as a condition in which one or more (but not all) atrial impulses that are conducted fail to reach the ventricles. This very general description covers a wide variety of patterns with markedly variable clinical significance. Second-degree AV block can be divided into Mobitz Type I (also known as Wenckebach) and Mobitz Type II.

Mobitz Type I. In Mobitz Type I block, the AV conduction time progressively lengthens until a P wave is not conducted. Mobitz I is caused by an abnormally long relative refractory period. The rate of conduction depends on the moment of impulse arrival: the earlier the impulse arrives in the AV node, the longer it takes to conduct; the later it arrives, the shorter the conduction time. Mobitz I second-degree AV block develops because each successive sinus impulse arrives earlier and earlier in the relative refractory period of the AV node until one sinus impulse finally arrives during the absolute refractory period and fails to conduct.

On the ECG, Mobitz Type I AV block can be distinguished by PR intervals that progressively lengthen until a P wave finally is not conducted and is therefore not followed by a QRS (Figure 15-50). If four P waves are conducted to the ventricles and the fifth one is not, a 5:4 conduction ratio is present (five P waves to four QRS complexes). The PR interval lengthening is usually greatest with the second beat of the cycle. The RR intervals become progressively shorter until the sinus P wave is not conducted. After that pause, the cycle repeats itself. It is useful to look at the RP

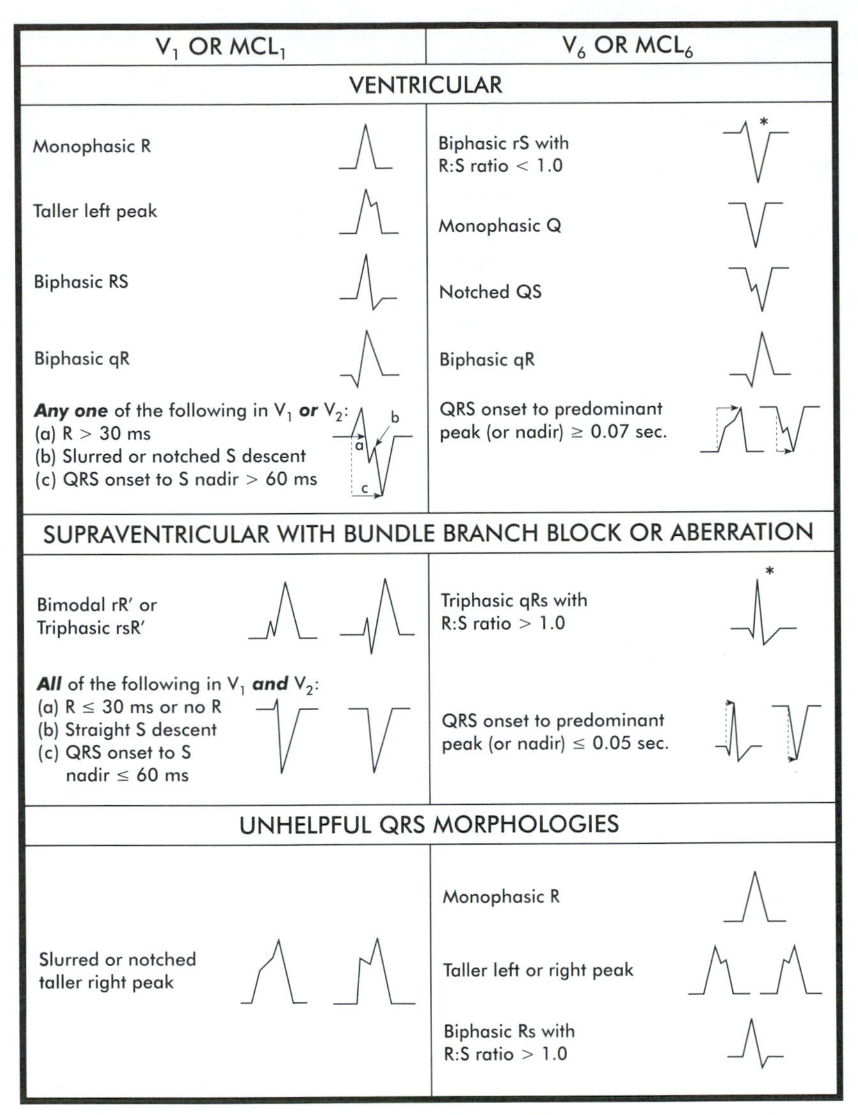

V1 OR MCL1
V6 OR MCL6
VENTRICULAR
Monophasic R
Taller left peak
Biphasic RS
Biphasic qR
Any one of the following in V1 or V2:
(a) R > 30 ms
(b) Slurred or notched S descent
(c) QRS onset to S nadir > 60 ms
Biphasic rS with
R:S ratio < 1.0
Monophasic Q
Notched QS
Biphasic qR
QRS onset to predominant
peak (or nadir) ≥ 0.07 sec.
SUPRAVENTRICULAR WITH BUNDLE BRANCH BLOCK OR ABERRATION
Bimodal rR′ or
Triphasic rsR′
All of the following in V1 and V2:
(a) R ≤ 30 ms or no R
(b) Straight S descent
(c) QRS onset to S
nadir ≤ 60 ms
Triphasic qRs with
R:S ratio > 1.0
QRS onset to predominant
peak (or nadir) ≤ 0.05 sec.
UNHELPFUL QRS MORPHOLOGIES
Slurred or notched
taller right peak
Monophasic R
Taller left or right peak
Biphasic Rs with
R:S ratio > 1.0
* Tachycardias with a right bundle branch block pattern in V1 only

FIGURE 15-48. Summary of morphologic clues in V_1 or MCL_1 (left column) and in V_6 or MCL_6 (right column) that are valuable in distinguishing supraventricular tachycardia with bundle branch block or aberration from ventricular tachycardia. If wide complex tachycardia with taller right peak pattern (i.e., unhelpful morphology) develops in a patient monitored with a single MCL_1 lead, the nurse changes leads to determine whether the wide complex falls into one of the diagnostic patterns in MCL_6. (From Drew B: *Heart Lung* 20(6):614, 1991.)

interval to determine the earliness of the sinus impulse arrival in the AV node. The RP interval is measured from the beginning of the QRS to the beginning of the following P wave. As the RP interval decreases, the PR interval increases, and vice versa. This phenomenon is known as *RP-PR reciprocity* and always indicates Mobitz Type I block.

In Mobitz Type I block the actual anatomic site of the block is at the level of the AV node itself. Usually, with an acute inferior wall infarction, the block is caused by ischemia and is transient. Still, the possibility of progression to a more serious conduction disturbance exists, warranting close observation and, occasionally, placement of a temporary pacemaker as a precautionary measure.

Mobitz Type II. Mobitz Type II block occurs in the presence of a long absolute refractory period with virtually no relative refractory period. This results in an "all or nothing" situation. Sinus P waves either will or will not be conducted. When conduction does occur, all PR intervals are the same. There is no RP-PR reciprocity. Usually, Mobitz II indicates block below the AV node, either in the His bundle or in both bundle branches. Most often, it occurs when one bundle

TABLE 15-12 Atrioventricular (AV) Block

Parameter	First Degree	Second-Degree Mobitz I (Wenckebach)	Second-Degree Mobitz II	Third Degree (Complete)
PR interval	>0.20 sec and constant	Increases with each consecutively conducted P wave	Constant	Varies randomly
P waves	1 P wave for each QRS	Intermittently not conducted, yielding more P waves than QRS complexes	Intermittently not conducted, yielding more P waves than QRS complexes	P waves independent and not related to QRS complexes
QRS	0.06-0.10 sec	0.06-0.10 sec	May be normal, but usually co-exists with bundle branch block (>0.12)	0.06-0.10 sec if junctional escape pacemaker activates the ventricles >0.12 if ventricular escape pacemaker activates the ventricles

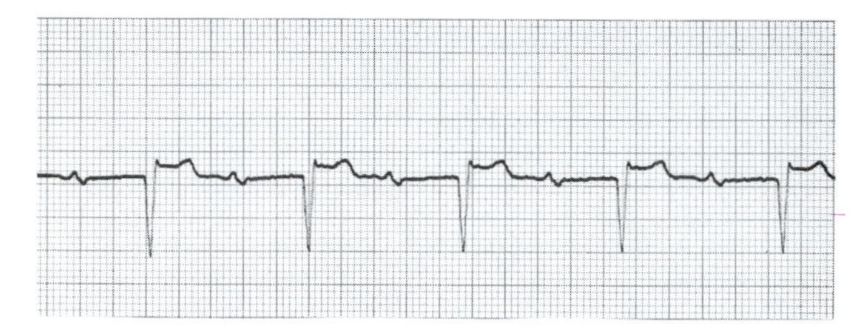

FIGURE 15-49. First-degree AV block. The PR interval is prolonged to 0.44 second.

branch is blocked and the other one is ischemic. Mobitz II block is more ominous clinically than is Mobitz I and often progresses to complete AV block. On the ECG the PR interval is constant (Figure 15-51). If consecutive P waves are conducted, the difference between Mobitz I and Mobitz II second-degree AV block is apparent: in Mobitz I the PR interval gradually lengthens until finally a P wave is not conducted or is missed; in Mobitz II the PR intervals remain exactly the same, but suddenly a normal P wave (not premature) fails to conduct.

Occasionally, only every other P wave is conducted through the AV node (Figure 15-52). This pattern could indicate either Mobitz I or II, because consecutive conduction of P waves—which would reveal either a lengthening or constant PR—does not occur. In Mobitz I the conduction ratios may have decreased from 4:3 to 3:2 to 2:1, yet the site and type of block have not changed. The change in conduction ratio may be caused by an increase in atrial rate, or it may change spontaneously.

In 2:1 conduction it is impossible to be certain whether the block is Mobitz Type I or II from the surface ECG. If it occurs along with other Mobitz I ratios, it is probably still Mobitz I, and vice versa. If it is an isolated occurrence with no other strips for comparison, the QRS width and the PR interval offer valuable clues to the site of the block. In Mobitz I the QRS is usually normal and the PR interval is usually prolonged. In Mobitz II the QRS is usually wide and the PR interval is usually normal. Also, during an acute inferior myocardial infarction, Mobitz Type I AV block with 2:1 conduction is much more common than is Type II.

Third-degree AV block. Third-degree, or complete, AV block is a condition in which no atrial impulses can conduct through the AV node to cause ventricular depolarization. The opportunity for conduction is optimal, yet none occurs. It is hoped that a junctional or ventricular focus will depolarize spontaneously at its intrinsic rate of 20 to 40 beats per minute and ventricular contraction will continue. If not, asystole occurs; there is no pulse, and death will result if intervention is not immediate.

On the ECG, P waves are present and usually occur at regular intervals. If a junctional focus is pacing the heart, normal QRSs are present but occur at a rate and timing interval totally independent of the P waves. The PR intervals vary widely, because the P wave and QRS are not related to each other. If a ventricular focus

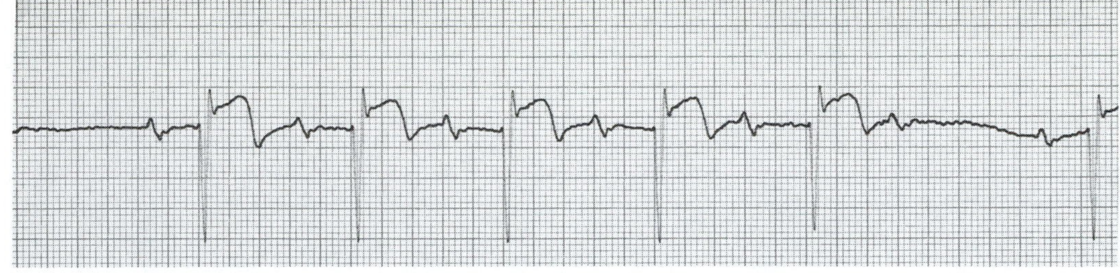

FIGURE 15-50. Mobitz Type I (Wenckebach) second-degree AV block. Note that the PR intervals gradually increase from 0.36 to 0.46 second until, finally, a P wave is not conducted to the ventricles.

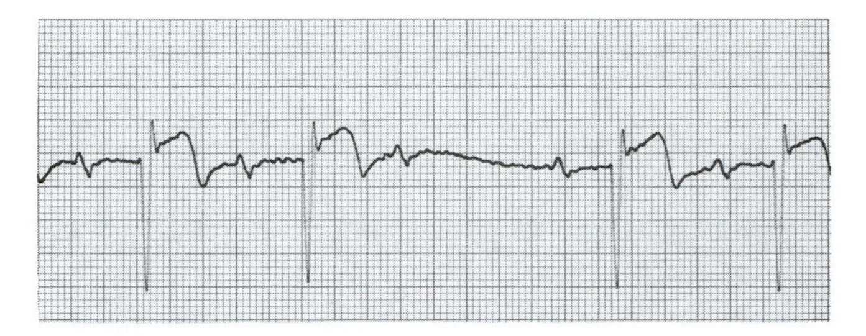

FIGURE 15-51. Mobitz Type II second-degree AV block. Note that the PR intervals remain constant.

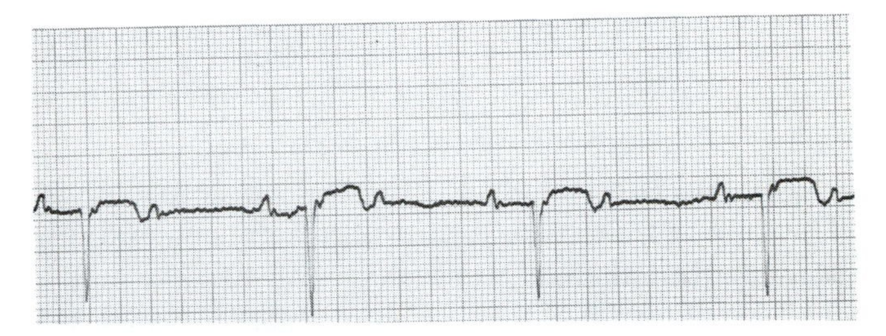

FIGURE 15-52. 2:1 AV block. Because no two consecutive P waves are conducted, it is not possible to determine with certainty whether this is Mobitz I or Mobitz II second-degree AV block.

is pacing the heart, the QRS complex is wide and unrelated to the P waves (Figure 15-53).

Medical management of AV block. Clinically, the consequences of AV block range from benign to life-threatening. First-degree AV block is seldom of immediate concern but bears close observation for progression of the conduction disturbance. Second degree Mobitz I (Wenckebach) is usually benign, especially during an acute ischemic episode. If hemodynamic compromise is present or deemed likely, a temporary pacemaker can be inserted prophylactically until the situation stabilizes or normal conduction is restored. Second-degree Mobitz II is more serious and often precedes complete AV block. Use of a temporary pacemaker is usually necessary, but its insertion can be elective if the patient remains hemodynamically stable. Complete heart block almost always requires use of a pacemaker. If the patient is hemodynamically unstable, an external pacemaker can be used to maintain an adequate ventricular rate until a temporary pacemaker can be inserted.

Ambulatory electrocardiography

Definition and purpose. Ambulatory electrocardiography is a technique that records the ECG of patients while they perform their usual activities. It was designed to document abnormal cardiac electrical activity that occurs at random during spontaneous activity or is induced by specific circumstances such as sleep, emotional stress, or physical activity. Clinical indications include palpitations, dizziness, syncope, and pacemaker evaluation.

Procedure. Two types of recording systems are available: continuous and intermittent. Although different in design, advantages, and limitations, each type can be used by ambulatory patients within or outside the hospital setting.

Continuous recording systems. Holter monitors are the most widely used continuous recording system. The patient wears skin electrodes and carries a small box that contains an analog tape recorder, either with a shoulder strap or clipped to his or her belt or pocket. Usually the monitor is left on for 24 hours and then is returned to the hospital or clinic for reading. This is a totally noninvasive procedure with no adverse effects.

All Holter monitors record at least two leads, primarily to minimize inaccurate interpretation caused by artifact. Usually five electrodes are placed. Two of them are positive electrodes, corresponding approximately to the V_1 and V_5 positions on a standard 12-lead ECG. There are also two negative electrodes and one ground. Occasionally, additional electrodes are used to improve diagnostic capabilities. For example, a separate lead can be used to detect pacemaker spikes if the patient is being monitored for pacemaker dysfunction. The skin electrodes are disposable, pregelled,

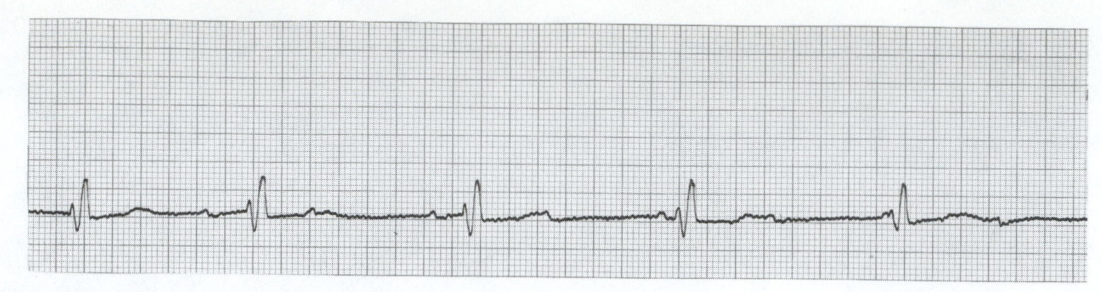

FIGURE 15-53. Third-degree (complete) heart block.

and self-adhering. They should be kept dry—not because of any electrical danger, but to prevent their falling off before the recording is completed.

The tape saves all of the ECG tracings for 24 hours. The tape can correlate time with the tracing and display the time that an event occurred when the tape is decoded. Most also have an event marker, which the patient can press to indicate the onset of symptoms or another event that may be important. The patient is asked to keep a diary of his or her activities, symptoms, and any medications that are taken.

Continuous recording systems are the most thorough form of ambulatory electrocardiography, because they record every heartbeat for 24 hours. They do not require the active participation of the patient (although a detailed patient log is helpful) and therefore do not miss asymptomatic ECG changes or dysrhythmias that may be accompanied by a loss of consciousness. When dysrhythmias occur that correlate with symptoms or symptoms occur in the absence of dysrhythmias, one of the primary goals of Holter monitoring has been achieved. Unfortunately, most patients do not have typical symptoms daily. If no significant dysrhythmias or symptoms occur during the 24-hour monitoring period, the test is completely useless. If dysrhythmias occur in the absence of symptoms, very little is gained, because people normally have asymptomatic dysrhythmias quite frequently and the dysrhythmias documented may or may not be the ones responsible for the patient's presenting symptoms. Holter monitoring is quite expensive because of the sophisticated equipment required, especially for analysis of the recording, and the technician time involved. In this era of increasing health care costs, the expense of this test must be weighed against its potential benefits in individual cases.

Ambulatory monitoring is most useful in evaluating the effectiveness of antidysrhythmic therapy.[38] For instance, transient ST-segment elevation after acute MI can be detected through Holter monitoring.[39] This is important because ST-segment elevation after an acute MI is associated with a higher 5-year mortality rate in patients with a large MI than in post-MI patients without ST-segment elevation.[39]

Intermittent recording systems. A device similar to a Holter monitor that does not record the ECG continuously can be attached to the patient. When the patient is having symptoms, he or she presses a button to initiate the recording manually. Advantages of this mode center around the ability to leave the recorder on the patient for longer periods. With the intermittent recorder mode, the device can be worn for up to 96 hours and the patient can trigger active recording at the appropriate times. The disadvantage of this approach is that the ECG tracing just before the onset of symptoms is not recorded, leaving the precipitating factors a mystery. Also, the patient must be able to trigger the device; if loss of consciousness occurs rapidly, this is not possible and the dysrhythmia is not recorded.

Transtelephonic systems. Transtelephonic monitors are not attached to the patient all the time. These monitors consist of a small box, about 4" × 2½" with four metal plates on the bottom. The box is issued to the patient for a specific time, often 1 month. The patient carries the box at all times. Whenever symptoms are experienced, the patient places the recording box in the center of the chest and places the four metal plates (electrodes) in firm contact with the skin. An alternative method, often preferred by patients, is to use two arm bracelets rather than direct chest placement. A button is then depressed to activate the recording, which lasts 1 to 2 minutes. The recording is stored until it is convenient for the patient to call in the recording to a central analysis facility. At that time, the receiver of the patient's telephone is placed over a transmitter on the box and the recording is transmitted to the analysis facility, where it is printed out as a readable ECG tracing. A copy of the tracing is sent to the patient's physician, and the patient is advised if urgent medical attention is necessary. The center can contact the patient's physician or emergency medical personnel if the dysrhythmia is life-threatening. This system can be quite cost-effective, because it is less expensive than a continuous 24-hour Holter monitor and provides for a longer monitoring time, thereby increasing the chance that a recording will occur during symptoms. However, if symptoms are incapacitating, the patient may not be able to activate the system. Dysrhythmias that are asymptomatic are missed because the patient has no reason to activate the system.

Nursing management. Some cardiac telemetry units have added a transtelephonic telephone to the unit so that patients recently discharged home can immediately transmit a signal if they have unexpected symptoms. It is the responsibility of the nurse to interpret the rhythm and provide instructions over the telephone. If it is an emergency, the patient is instructed to dial 911 and alert emergency personnel.

A well-informed patient can greatly enhance the quality of the recording. Many patients' symptoms do not occur every day and may be missed during a random 24-hour recording. Often symptoms tend to occur in association with specific activities. The nurse needs to inquire about the types of activities that tend to provoke symptoms for a specific patient and encourage the patient to pursue those activities while wearing the monitor. In general, the patient is encouraged to be as active as possible. Keeping an accurate diary of activities is important, because it allows correlation of an identified dysrhythmia with a specific activity or symptom. Examples of items that the patient must record include medications, meals, exercise, emotional stress, arguments, smoking, bowel movements, urination, sexual intercourse, and sleep periods. In addition, any symptoms such as palpitations, lightheadedness, or chest pressure are recorded.

The only activities that are restricted while wearing a Holter monitor are those that would get the chest electrodes or monitor wet, eliminating swimming and taking a shower or tub bath. Sponge baths are permitted as long as the chest electrodes are avoided. No activities are restricted when using a transtelephonic monitor, because it is not worn all the time.

Exercise electrocardiography

Definition. Exercise electrocardiography consists of the recording of an ECG tracing during a period of stress on the heart muscle and its blood supply reserves to uncover and diagnose ischemia, which is not apparent at rest. Exercise places unique demands on the cardiovascular system. Systemic oxygen consumption increases markedly, requiring the heart to increase cardiac output (CO) to meet these demands. Myocardial contractility increases, resulting in greater stroke volume and systolic blood pressure. Heart rate is increased also as a result of circulating catecholamines. Normally, as heart rate and stroke volume rise, CO is increased dramatically and the tissue needs for oxygen are met. This enhanced myocardial performance is not without its price. Even at rest, the heart muscle extracts 70% of the oxygen available in the circulating blood. When the myocardial demand for oxygen increases during exercise, coronary blood flow must increase to maintain an adequate oxygen supply. In patients with coronary artery disease, coronary blood flow is not able to increase sufficiently to meet the high metabolic needs of the myocardium during exercise, and ischemia results.[40]

Indications. Exercise tolerance testing, or stress testing, is clinically useful in several settings. It helps evaluate the presence, absence, or severity of coronary artery disease, both in patients with known coronary heart disease and those initially seen with chest pain of unclear origin. Stress testing can evaluate the functional capacity of patients with or without heart disease and can be done serially to evaluate the effectiveness of medical or surgical therapy.

In this era of cost-containment, treadmill testing is being incorporated in various protocols to reduce the cost of caring for patients with known or suspected coronary artery disease. One such study, the *Rapid Rule-Out of Myocardial Ischemia Observation (ROMIO)*, used stress testing for high risk patients who went to an emergency room with chest pain and who had negative initial ECGs and cardiac enzymes. These patients underwent either a symptom-limited exercise test or a dobutamine stress echo within 12 hours of admission, and were discharged home if the results were negative. The study found that stress testing was useful in significantly reducing both the length of the hospital stay and total cost in this patient population.[41] Other studies have looked at exercise testing as a major factor in deciding which patients with stable coronary artery disease are to undergo additional invasive procedures and which patients are to be managed medically.[42]

Procedure. Originally exercise tests were conducted using a two-step platform that the patient climbed up and down repeatedly. This is called a *Master's two-step exercise test* and is still used in a few places because the cost of the equipment is minimal. The majority of exercise tests in the United States, however, are now performed using a treadmill on which both speed and slope can be varied or using a bicycle ergometer. A number of protocols have been developed using a treadmill. All reach virtually the same end point, but they vary the speed with which they approach that end point. Two popular ones are the Bruce protocol, in which both grade and speed are varied every 3 minutes, and the Balke protocol, in which speed remains constant and grade is gradually increased every minute.

Regardless of the protocol used, the ECG is printed at 1-minute intervals, as well as during any symptoms, visible ECG changes, or dysrhythmias. Blood pressure is also measured and recorded every minute.

The treadmill test is terminated when a desirable level, based on the patient's heart rate, is reached. A maximal stress test is one in which the predicted maximal heart rate for that patient is achieved. The maximal predicted heart rate can be estimated using the formula of 220 minus the patient's age. A goal of 85% to 90% of the predicted maximal heart rate is set for a submaximal test, and in most patients this level of exercise is sufficient to unmask any significant coronary artery disease. The test can also be aborted before that point if symptoms occur. Blood pressure is expected to rise during exercise, but a systolic blood pressure greater than 220 mm Hg or a diastolic blood pressure greater than 110 mm Hg is considered high enough to stop the test.

A low-level stress test is sometimes performed before discharge from the hospital on patients who have had an acute myocardial infarction. In this case the heart rate is raised only to 120 or 130 beats per minute. ST-segment depression or elevation that occurs during the predischarge low-level stress test is a reliable indicator of additional myocardium at risk. However, exercise-induced angina or abnormal blood pressure responses to exercise often do not appear during a low-level stress test, so a "normal" predischarge stress test must be followed later by a test closer to maximal level.

Nursing management. During the exercise test the patient is encouraged to continue as long as possible. However, the test is stopped if the patient requests, because of symptoms such as fatigue, shortness of breath, or leg cramps. In addition, the nurse stops the test for significant ECG changes, blood pressure changes, or development of angina. The diagnostic value of the test is based on the maximal heart rate achieved, not on the length of time that the patient remains on the treadmill. A well-trained athlete might be able to stay on the treadmill for 15 minutes, whereas an elderly or sedentary person may tolerate it for only 3 to 5 minutes; yet if 85% of the predicted maximal heart rate is achieved, both tests are equally diagnostic.

After the exercise test is completed, the patient is assisted into a supine position. The ECG, pulse rate, and blood pressure are monitored for at least 10 more minutes to detect dysrhythmias or signs of ischemia. The patient is instructed to rest for the next 30 to 60 minutes after release from the exercise laboratory. Hot showers are to be avoided for 3 to 4 hours to prevent development of orthostatic hypotension.

The nurse performing the test must be certain that emergency medications and a defibrillator are available in the test area and be familiar with their use. (See Appendix C, ACLS Guidelines.)

Patient education. Many patients are anxious about undergoing exercise testing, and the anxiety is often multifactorial. Patients without known heart disease may be afraid that they will "fail" the test, find they have heart disease, and perhaps need open heart surgery. If the patient generally follows a sedentary lifestyle, anxiety may be caused by the fear of "collapsing" on the treadmill or spending several days recovering from exhaustion. Some are afraid that they will be forced to go beyond their endurance. Often, low-level exercise testing is performed before discharge on patients who have been hospitalized for an acute myocardial infarction. These patients may be afraid that the strain on their heart is too great or that they will die during the test.

Patient teaching can do much to allay these fears. In addition to describing the procedure itself, the nurse instructs the patient to fast for 3 hours before the test, refrain from smoking for at least 2 hours before the test, and wear comfortable shoes and loose-fitting clothes. The patient is reassured that his or her heart will be monitored closely during the test and a physician will be standing by.

Echocardiography

Definition. Echocardiography uses waves of ultrasound to obtain and display images of cardiac structures. Normal human hearing occurs at a sound frequency of 20 to 20,000 cycles per second (hertz). Ultrasound uses sound frequencies greater than 20,000 hertz (Hz). When used to image cardiac structures, the best results are achieved using 1.5 megahertz to 10 megahertz (mHz). Usually 2.25 mHz are used with adults to allow optimal depth penetration, whereas 3 mHz to 5 mHz are used in pediatric patients to provide a clearer image of the smaller structures.

Indications. Echocardiography is used to detect cardiac abnormalities such as mitral valve stenosis and regurgitation, prolapse of mitral valve leaflets, aortic stenosis and insufficiency, hypertrophic cardiomyopathy, atrial septal defects, and pericardial effusions. Standard transthoracic echocardiography is capable of providing all of the information needed for decision-making in 90% to 95% of all cardiac patients.[43] For another 5% of patients in whom the transthoracic image is inadequate, transesophageal echocardiography (TEE) is a new technique that eliminates the interference of the thoracic structures and provides an excellent image of the heart and great vessels from a posterior view. Recent developments also allow detection of wall-motion abnormalities, estimation of ejection fraction and pulmonary artery pressures, and identification of intracardiac myomas. In the future, intracoronary echocardiography may routinely be able to detect and quantify coronary artery disease.[44]

Procedure. While a transthoracic echocardiogram is performed, the patient is in either a supine, left lateral, or semi-Fowler's position. Which position is used depends on the patient's clinical condition and on which position provides the best view of the structures examined. A transducer is placed on the skin, with lubricant between the transducer and the skin to improve contact and reduce artifact. The active element in the transducer is a piezoelectric crystal. *Piezoelectric* refers to the ability to transform electrical energy into mechanical (in this case, sound) energy, and vice versa. The transducer emits ultrasound waves and receives a signal from the reflected sound waves. Periods of sound transmission alternate with periods of sound reception.

Ultrasonic waves do not travel through air very well, and they are unable to penetrate very dense structures, such as bone; hence, in adults, the transducer is usually placed in the 3rd or 4th intercostal space to the left of the sternum, because at that point the pericardium is in direct contact with the chest wall and the ultrasonic waves are not obstructed by either air or bone. Other positions are sometimes used if the standard location does not provide adequate visualization of the cardiac structures.

Ultrasound is reflected best at interfaces between tissues that have different densities. In the heart these are the blood, cardiac valves, myocardium, and pericardium. Because all these structures differ in density, their borders can be seen on the echocardiogram. In one type of echocardiography, a thin beam of ultrasound is directed through the heart (Figure 15-54, *A*). Each interface is represented by a dot, and when recorded over time (like an ECG), each dot becomes a line on an oscilloscope. A strip-chart recording can be made of this tracing as the heart beats. Because this is a recording of heart motion over time, this technique is called an *M-mode* (motion-mode) echocardiogram. A typical M-mode echo is shown in Figure 15-54, *B*.

M-mode echocardiogram. The M-mode echocardiogram is particularly useful for measuring cardiac wall thickness and chamber size, evaluating valve motion, and assessing contractile motion of certain portions of the heart wall. It provides a good view of the anterior interventricular septum, the left ventricular posterior wall from the base to the midportion, the aortic and mitral valves, and the left atrium. Areas that cannot be studied include the apex, lateral or free wall segments, and the true posterior and inferior wall of the left ventricle. Because all portions of the ventricular wall cannot be examined, it is difficult to determine the size of dyskinetic areas using this technique. Aneurysms are also hard to diagnose, depending on their location. If the heart muscle is contracting uniformly throughout, estimates of left ventricular function are quite accurate. However, if wall-motion abnormalities exist, this estimate of cardiac contractility is unreliable. Estimates of left ventricular size and function are also unreliable if significant aortic regurgitation is present. M-mode echocardiograms are particularly useful in detecting small pericardial effusions and cardiac tamponade.

Two-dimensional echocardiogram. Two-dimensional (2-D) echocardiograms use numerous crystals in the transducer to create a cross-sectional imaging plane. Sections of the heart are then viewed from a number of different angles (Figure 15-55). The picture is displayed on an oscilloscope, and photographs are taken to serve as a permanent record. In many ways it is superior to the M-mode echocardiogram. The 2-D echocardiogram provides better quantification of valvular stenosis and a greater ability to detect ventricular aneurysms. Because a whole "slice" of the heart is seen at once, the location of various structures in relationship to the rest of the heart is better appreciated, and the size of dyskinetic wall segments can be determined. Wall-motion abnormalities can be detected in nearly all patients within 4 hours after an acute myocardial infarction, and the extent of muscle dysfunction is predictive of later complications. Performing an echocardiogram on all patients

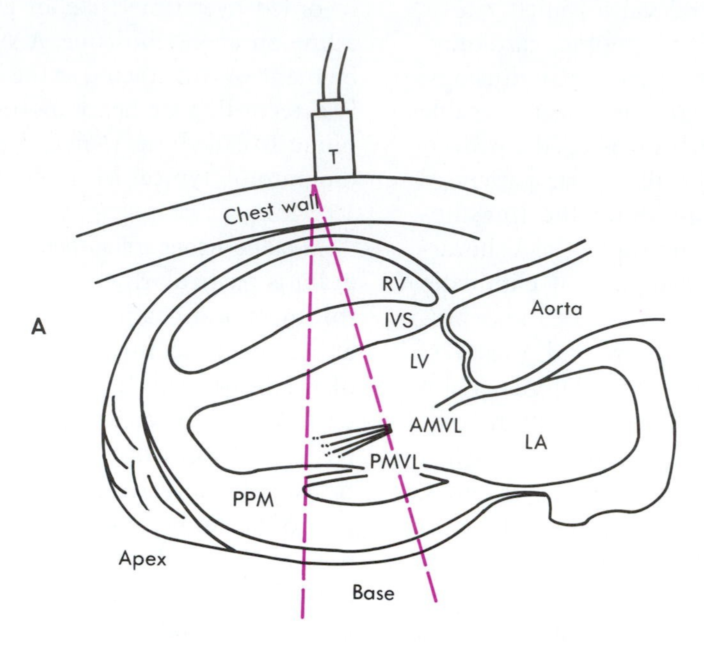

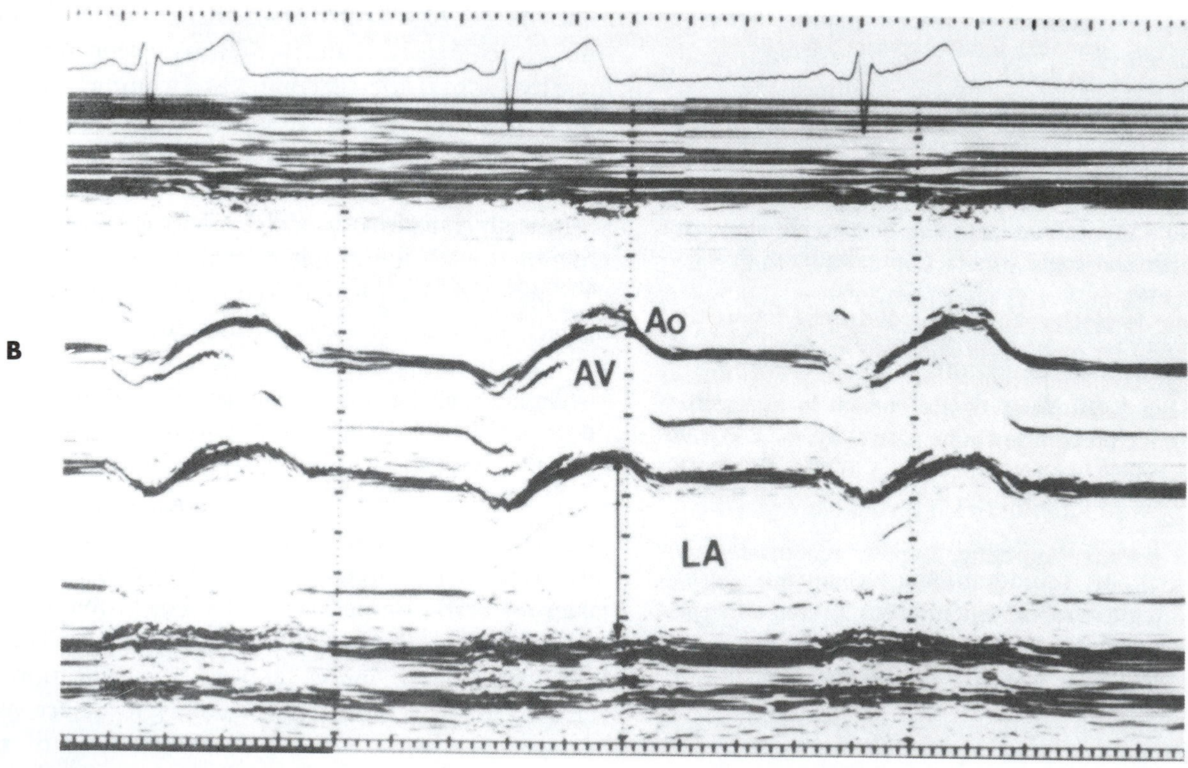

FIGURE 15-54. **A,** Schematic presentation of cardiac structures transversed by two echobeams. **B,** Normal, M-mode echocardiogram at the level of the aorta, aortic valve leaflets, and left atrium. RV, right ventricle; *LV,* left ventricle; *IVS,* interventricular septum; *AMVL,* anterior mitral valve leaflet; *PMVL,* posterior mitral valve leaflet; *PPM,* posterior papillary muscle; *LA,* left atrium; *T,* transducer; *Ao,* aorta; *AV,* aortic valve. (**A** from Urden L, Davie J, Thelan L: *Essentials of critical care nursing,* St Louis, 1992, Mosby; **B** from Kinney M and others: *Comprehensive cardiac care,* ed 7, St Louis, 1991, Mosby)

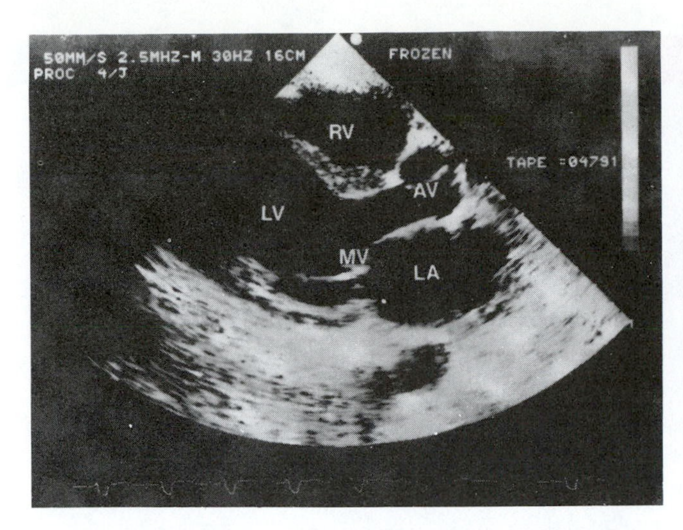

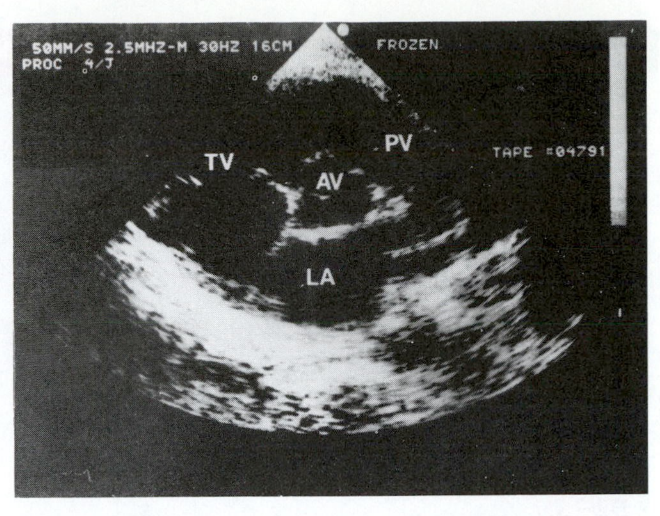

FIGURE 15-55. Two-dimensional echocardiogram. Note that several sections of the heart can be viewed at one time, and it is easier to see the relationship of the chambers to one another. Abbreviations are as in Figure 15-54, plus *TV*, tricuspid valve. (From Kinney M and others: *Comprehensive cardiac care*, ed 7, St. Louis, 1991, Mosby.)

being evaluated for chest pain could help identify those patients who are likely to have had a myocardial infarction or who are at risk for complications and could benefit from admission to a coronary care unit.

Phonocardiogram. Phonocardiography is frequently combined with echocardiography to evaluate valvular dysfunction. It provides a graphic display of the sounds that occur in the heart and great vessels. The transducer placed on the chest wall records heart sounds that correspond to auscultation with a stethoscope. (∞Heart Sounds, p. 367.)

Color-flow Doppler echocardiography. Doppler echocardiography provides a special kind of echocardiogram that assesses blood flow. It uses a pulsed or continuous wave of ultrasound that records frequency shifts of reflected sound waves, showing velocity and direction of blood flow relative to the transducer. Doppler signals are usually displayed in color. Known as color-flow mapping or imaging, this technique analyzes Doppler signals from multiple intracardiac sites simultaneously. The Doppler tracing for each site is displayed in a color-coded format superimposed on a real-time 2-D echocardiographic image. Flow toward the transducer is displayed in one color, whereas flow away from the transducer is displayed in a contrasting color. The brightness of the color is varied to signify varying flow velocities. Doppler echocardiography is especially useful in patients with valvular heart disease. Both regurgitation and stenosis can be detected and estimates made of their severity. When multiple valves are involved, the Doppler technique can clarify the extent of damage to the individual valves. Other uses for Doppler echocardiography include evaluation of congenital shunts and atresias, measurement of volume flow, and assessment of cardiac output. By measuring flow velocity in the right ventricular outflow tract, mean pulmonary artery pressure can be estimated.

Transesophageal echocardiography. This is a relatively new technique in which the transducer (either single-plane, bi-plane, or multi-plane) is mounted on a flexible shaft similar to a gastroscope and advanced to various locations in the esophagus where images are examined. The multi-plane transducer has a single array of crystals that can be rotated in a 180-degree arc, requiring less manipulation of the probe within the esophagus.[45] Because of the close anatomic relationship between the heart and the esophagus, transesophageal echocardiography (TEE) produces high-quality images of intracardiac structures and the thoracic aorta without the interference of the chest wall, bone, or air-filled lung.

The procedure is similar to an upper GI endoscopy. The patient is asked to fast for a minimum of 6 hours before the procedure to prevent nausea and vomiting.[45] Medication is usually given to inhibit salivary secretions, reducing the risk of aspiration.[43] Sedation agents are also given to reduce fear and anxiety and to provide retrograde amnesia. Routine antibiotic prophylaxis against bacteremia and endocarditis is not necessary, although it is still considered for high risk patients, such as those with prosthetic valves, previous endocarditis,[46] or very poor dentition.[43] The pharyngeal region is

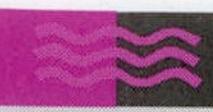

RESEARCH ABSTRACT

Reducing time in bed after cardiac catheterization (TIBS II).

Keeling A and others: *Am J Crit Care* 5(4):277, 1996.

PURPOSE

The purpose of this study was to determine whether there would be a significant difference in the incidence of bleeding from femoral artery insertion sites among cardiac catheterization patients who remained in bed for 4 hours and those who remained in bed for 6 hours after sheath removal.

DESIGN

Experimental, control group.

SAMPLE

The convenience sample consisted of 86 adult patients undergoing diagnostic coronary angioplasty. Subjects were suspected of having or were diagnosed with coronary artery disease and were not receiving heparin or other anticoagulant or thrombolytic agents after the procedure. The mean age of the control group subjects was 58 years, with an average of 61 years for the experimental group. There was no significant difference between the two groups regarding the amount of time spent in the procedure.

PROCEDURE

Subjects were randomly assigned to remain in bed for 4 hours (experimental) or 6 hours (control) after arterial sheath removal. All subjects received heparin before the procedure and protamine upon conclusion of the procedure. Pressure was applied to the groin area for 20 minutes after removal of the sheath. Sterile 4 × 4 gauze pads were applied over the catheter site and secured with Elastoplast tape or clear tape. A 5-pound sandbag was placed over the dressing. Patients were instructed to keep their affected leg extended during their time in bed; the head of the bed could be elevated 30 degrees during this time.

RESULTS

There was no significant difference in the incidence of bleeding or hematoma formation related to getting out of bed between the two groups. Five patients in the experimental group bled at sometime after the procedure; however, only one incident was related to getting out of bed.

DISCUSSION/IMPLICATIONS

Findings from this study indicate that reduced time in bed for coronary angioplasty patients from 6 to 4 hours did not produce an increase in femoral insertion site bleeding. The standard of 6 hours of bedrest after the procedure can be reduced with no untoward effects. The change in practice can lead to greater patient satisfaction, reduced length of stay, and more efficient use of staff time. It is important to evaluate traditional practices such as the one in this study so that cost-effective quality of care and services can be implemented.

anesthetized with 2% viscous lidocaine (Xylocaine) and 10% (Xylocaine) spray to lessen the gag reflex and prevent retching and laryngospasm. The patient is usually placed in the left lateral decubitus position, although the supine position can be used in the critical care or operative setting if necessary. A soft bite block is inserted between the teeth to prevent damage to the echoscope. As the echoscope is inserted, the patient is asked to swallow. The echoscope is advanced to 25 cm from the mouth, and imaging is begun. Advancement to additional locations permits additional views (Figure 15-56). TEE is also used intraoperatively, in which case sedation and local anesthetics are not required.

TEE is useful whenever the transthoracic approach is unsatisfactory, as in COPD and obesity and when chest wall changes caused by aging create obstacles to clear image visualization. In addition, TEE is superior to transthoracic echocardiography in a variety of situations. The entire thoracic aorta can be visualized clearly, and TEE is rapidly becoming the diagnostic procedure of choice in suspected dissecting aortic aneurysm, even surpassing aortic angiography. Angiograms require the use of intravenous contrast agents (dye), which can cause further renal damage in patients who already have compromised renal function. TEE carries no such risk.

Both atrial chambers are well-imaged with TEE, and the left atrial appendage is particularly well-observed, making TEE the procedure of choice for detection of left atrial thrombus. Diagnosis and quantification of atrial septal defects can also be done with this method, and the addition of Doppler capabilities allows assessment of atrial shunting after percutaneous mitral

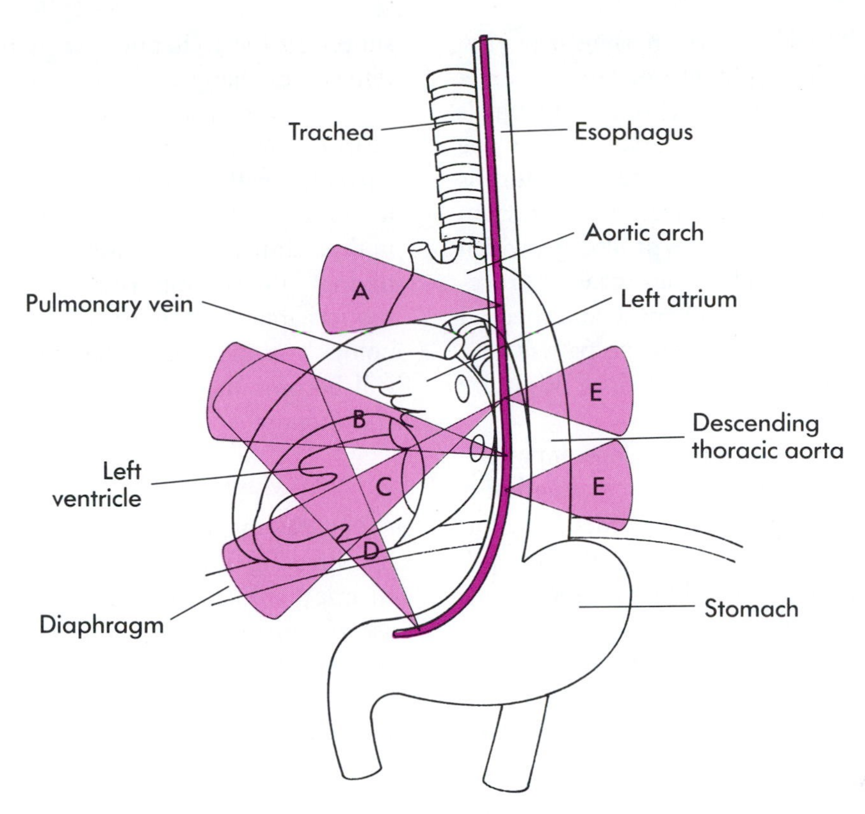

FIGURE 15-56. Diagram of common scan planes during a transesophageal two-dimensional echocardiogram. **A,** Horizontal scan plane of aortic arch and distal portion of aorta. **B,** Basal short-axis (transverse), long-axis (sagittal) views, and short-axis views of both atria. **C,** Four-chamber and left atrioventricular long-axis views. Sagittal scan plane can image a cross section of the left ventricle. **D,** Transgastric short-axis view of left and right ventricles. **E,** Transverse and sagittal scan sections of descending aorta.

valvuloplasty. Because of the ability to use higher-frequency ultrasonic waves than those used with transthoracic echocardiography, TEE is useful in evaluating patients with infective endocarditis to investigate the source of emboli, assess valve regurgitation, and identify valvular vegetations.[45] Both native and prosthetic mitral valves can be assessed for regurgitation or stenosis. Proximal coronary arteries and large pulmonary veins can also be imaged, although the value of this in relation to coronary angiography must be investigated further.

One other advantage of TEE over transthoracic echocardiography is that it is a convenient way to monitor cardiac function during open heart and general surgery. Transthoracic echocardiography is rarely used for this purpose, because it requires manual placement of the transducer on the chest at all times. The transesophageal probe can be placed and left in position during the operative procedure. Global myocardial function can be monitored, new areas of dyskinesis (indicating ischemia) detected, and intracardiac air detected if present.

The risks involved in TEE are surprisingly low, even in unstable critically ill patients. The overall incidence of complications is less than 1%. Respiratory depression and aspiration secondary to sedation can occur. Manipulation of the probe within the esophagus can cause a vasovagal response, resulting in severe bradycardia and hypotension. The most serious risk of the procedure is esophageal bleeding. This can occur during intraoperative use because of the large doses of heparin that are often administered during surgery. Patients with liver cirrhosis and/or esophageal varices are also at risk for esophageal bleeding. The procedure must always be performed under constant monitoring, and if esophageal entry is difficult, it cannot be forced.

Nursing management. In the critical care unit, the echocardiograph is usually brought to the bedside. The lighting in the room can be dimmed to improve the visual clarity of the images displayed on the screen. For transthoracic echocardiography, lubricant is placed on the patient's chest, and a transducer is placed in various positions to visualize cardiac and valvular structures. The nursing care consists of monitoring the patient during the procedure, which is usually performed by an echocardiography technician.

Patient education. Transthoracic echocardiography is completely noninvasive, and the nurse explains the purpose to the patient and family. The procedure is not uncomfortable, but it may be tiresome for certain patients because of the length of the procedure, which is usually 30 to 60 minutes. TEE is an invasive procedure, and the nurse explains the purpose and method to the patient. The nurse also assures the patient that sedation agents will be given, as needed, to minimize discomfort.

TEE is somewhat more uncomfortable, comparable to an upper GI endoscopy. It is important to administer appropriate sedation agents, if needed. Suction equipment must be available in the event that the patient vomits or has difficulty handling oral secretions.

Future trends in echocardiography. Stress echocardiography was first developed in the 1970s, and is currently being evaluated as a less-expensive alternative to nuclear perfusion imaging. Stress causes an imbalance of myocardial oxygen supply and demand, which causes ischemia and eventually results in wall-motion abnormalities, which are detectable with an echocardiogram. A 30% reduction in blood supply can be detected with nuclear perfusion imaging, whereas an approximately 70% reduction is necessary to cause wall-motion abnormalities detectable on an echocardiogram.[47] Although less expensive, stress echocardiography is also a less-sensitive measure of myocardial perfusion.

Stress can be applied to the heart by both physical and pharmacologic means. Exercise is one of the most reliable sources of stress, but is the least practical because of patient movement, hyperventilation, and tachycardia.[48] Pharmacologic sources of stress include dobutamine infusion, dobutamine plus atropine, dipyridamole (Persantine), and adenosine. Dobutamine most closely resembles exercise, because it causes myocardial ischemia through a dramatic increase in myocardial oxygen demand as a result of an increase in heart rate, contractility, and systemic blood pressure.[48] Potential side effects include hypotension, hypertension, dysrhythmias, nausea, headache, anxiety, and tremor.[45] Atropine is sometimes given if dobutamine alone does not cause an adequate increase in heart rate. Persantine and adenosine can both cause ischemia by causing coronary vasodilation and maldistribution of blood flow. Normal coronary arteries will dilate, using more of the blood available and will "steal" blood from diseased, stenotic vessels. Blood supply to the ischemic area is reduced, but demand remains unchanged.

Three-dimensional echocardiography allows the heart to be viewed as a reconstructed model.[49] Though currently in the experimental phase, commercial systems are rapidly becoming available. Viewing the heart in three dimensions greatly improves accuracy in identifying valvular abnormalities, cardiac masses, wall-motion abnormalities, and regurgitant jets.[49] As technology improves, three-dimensional echocardiography will become more useful in cardiovascular diagnosis and therapy.

Nuclear Magnetic Resonance

Nuclear magnetic resonance (NMR) is a noninvasive imaging technique that can obtain specific biochemical information from body tissue without the use of ionizing radiation. The procedure does not present any known hazard to living cells. In many respects, the image created is superior to both x-ray film and ultrasonography because bone does not interfere with magnetic resonance imaging (MRI). NMR application is limited in critical care because patients have to leave the unit, and many patients are too unstable to be transported to the MRI lab.

Indications. Currently, cardiac magnetic resonance imaging can provide information about tissue integrity, wall-motion abnormalities and aneurysms, ejection fraction, cardiac output, patency of proximal coronary arteries, and flow rates through coronary artery bypass grafts.[50] NMR is useful in diagnosing complications of myocardial infarction, such as pericarditis or pericardial effusion, valvular dysfunction, ventricular septal defects, aneurysm, and intracardiac thrombus.[51]

Blood that is actively flowing does not emit a magnetic resonance signal; thus it provides a natural dark contrast material in the lumen of proximal coronary arteries. As a result, abnormalities of lumen size such as narrowing—which may provide evidence of obstruction—can be visualized. For this reason, NMR has replaced computed tomography (CT) scanning and angiography for evaluating aortic disease and for assessing veins in the chest, abdomen, and pelvis.[51]

Procedure. The method by which NMR scanning is performed is quite complex, but the basic concept is fairly simple. Certain atoms within molecules act as tiny bar magnets with north and south poles. The nuclei spin around this axis like a spinning top. Under normal conditions these small atomic magnets are arranged at random. If a patient is placed within a strong magnetic field, many of the nuclei line up in the same direction as the magnetic force. When a radio frequency wave is sent, some of the nuclei absorb this energy, causing them to fall out of alignment and wobble like a gyroscope that is winding down. This "wobbling" out of alignment is termed *resonance.* The process of returning to alignment with the magnetic field after the radio frequency signal is turned off is called *relaxation.* These energy changes can be detected and recorded by the scanner.

Each type of atom has its own unique resonance and relaxation pattern. The easiest one to record at present is the hydrogen ion, although other atoms such as phosphorus, sodium, and carbon are also being studied. Because there are two hydrogen ions per molecule of water, magnetic resonance imaging is especially sensitive to changes in tissue water content. Myocardial ischemic injury results in predictable increases in regional myocardial water content, allowing differentiation between normal and ischemic tissue. Infarction leading to myocardial scarring results in tissue with a decreased water content, which can be identified on a magnetic resonance scan as an area of decreased signal intensity.

Magnetic resonance imaging works well for structures that have little or no motion, such as the brain. Cardiac applications have been limited because of the constant motion of the heart. In an attempt to overcome this limitation, various gating or slicing techniques have been used to time the images at exact phases of the cardiac cycle. The gating can be timed from the R wave of the ECG or from the arterial pulse tracing. Either method is satisfactory as long as the patient is in normal sinus rhythm. With any irregularity of the rhythm, the gating technique becomes much less helpful.[51]

Nursing management. Magnetic resonance imaging is actually a very safe procedure. The main hazard is related to the presence of other metal substances in the environment. Because the magnetism used is approximately 40,000 times stronger than the magnetic field of the earth, metal objects such as IV poles or oxygen tanks can become projectiles if they come close enough to the magnet's pull. There are significant limitations of NMR in the critical care setting. The narrow size of the magnet bore requires that the patient be able to lie flat. The patient must also be able to lie motionless for up to 7 minutes at a time. The close quarters inside the magnet bore tend to provoke claustrophobia in anyone already predisposed to it, and sedation may be required. Standard ventilators, monitoring equipment, and infusion pumps cannot be used. Special pneumatically driven ventilators with nonmagnetic accessories are available, as well as special ECG and pulse oximetry devices. IV infusions need to be hand regulated by plastic drip controllers.

TABLE 15-13 Metallic Implants and Nuclear Magnetic Resonance Imaging

Safe	Unsafe
Nonferromagnetic aneurysm clips	Cardiac pacemaker
Hemostatic vascular slips	Implanted cardioverter defibrillator (ICD)
Staples	Thermodilution
Carotid artery clamps*	Swan-Ganz catheter
Cochlear implants	Implanted drug infusion pump
Wire sutures	Detectable metal in the eye
Vascular access ports	Intracranial aneurysm clips
Plastic endotracheal tubes	Bullets†
Chest tubes	
Catheters	
Orthopedic devices and prostheses	
Prosthetic heart valves‡	
Intravascular coils, stents, and filters§	

*Exceptions: Poppen-Blalock carotid artery clamp and clips made of 17-7PH stainless steel

†Most are nonferromagnetic and therefore safe. However, steel shotgun pellets are replacing lead and are ferromagnetic, as are foreign-made ballistic material and shrapnel. Bullets are less likely to move if imbedded in scar tissue. The risk/benefit ratio must be considered.

‡Exception: Starr-Edwards Pre-6000 valve.

§Safe if they have been in place several weeks.

Many patients have implanted metallic devices that may cause concern. Table 15-13 lists some guidelines about which implants are safe and which are not.[51] Implanted drug infusion pumps may stop working during the procedure, but should resume normal function without reprogramming when the patient is removed from the magnetic field.

Neither a cardiac pacemaker nor an implantable cardioverter defibrillator (ICD) is safe because they may turn off or switch modes when exposed to a strong external magnetic field. Aneurysm clips are composed of ferromagnetic materials and could experience significant torque when exposed to the magnetic field.

Patient education. The patient who is claustrophobic needs considerable reassurance and education before lying supine and motionless inside the MRI tube. Careful assessment for presence of a pacemaker, ICD, or other metallic devices is important so that the nurse can explain why these devices cannot be exposed to the MRI magnetic field. Table 15-13 shows which metallic implants are safe and which are unsafe in nuclear resonance imaging.

Radionuclide Study: Thallium Scan

Indications. The purpose of a thallium scan is to determine whether there is a perfusion defect in cardiac muscle. The study was developed as an adjunct to the exercise ECG stress test. A thallium scan is indicated for the patient with chest pain and known or suspected coronary artery disease and for the patient with a left bundle branch block (LBBB) or a permanent pacemaker in whom an ECG stress test may be difficult to interpret because of distortion of the QRS complex.

A thallium scan combines the techniques of both cardiology and radiology. In cardiology, coronary artery anatomy is important because regional myocardial blood supply is from specific coronary arteries and any blockage of an artery can lead to a discrete myocardial perfusion defect, meaning that the blood supply to this area is either decreased or absent. Although coronary arteriography defines the anatomy of the coronary arteries, it does not show whether the arteries perfuse the cardiac muscle. The radiology component involves the use of thallium-201 and a specialized perfusion-scanning camera. Thallium-201 is a low-energy radioactive isotope. It is an analog of potassium and acts like potassium when injected into the blood stream. Because thallium is similar to potassium, it is absorbed from the blood stream by cardiac muscle cells as part of the sodium-potassium adenosine triphosphatase (ATPase) pump. Thallium uptake depends on two factors: (1) the patency of the coronary arteries and (2) the amount of healthy myocardium with a functional sodium-potassium ATPase pump. If an area of myocardium is infarcted (dead), it will not take up thallium. Once thallium has been injected, a specialized scintillation camera and computer system can detect the areas of thallium concentration (uptake).

Procedure. Before the thallium scan the procedure is fully explained, including a description of the equipment, since it may be overwhelming to some patients. The thallium test takes place in a specialized laboratory that contains ECG monitoring equipment, cardiovascular exercise equipment (treadmill or stationary bicycle), and an Anger gamma scintillation camera. The patient is usually fasting, because a thallium scan involves vigorous exercise. A patent IV line is inserted before the test. Once in the laboratory the patient is asked to exercise vigorously for up to 1 minute or longer or until angina or fatigue develops. At this point the thallium (or other isotope) is injected into the blood stream. After the injection the patient is asked to exercise vigorously for another minute to stress the heart and circulate the thallium. As soon as possible after exercise (within 10 minutes), the patient is asked to lie on the examination table for the first perfusion scan by the scintillation camera. The camera examines the heart from three angles—anterior, left anterior oblique, and left lateral oblique—to increase accuracy. On the camera screen the heart image looks like a circle with a hole. The myocardium appears, but the fluid-filled center does not.

Significance. If no perfusion defect is seen, the test is complete for that patient. If a perfusion defect is noted, the patient is asked to return for a repeat scan in 4 hours. If a perfusion defect is present 4 hours later, this means the area is infarcted. If the perfusion defect has taken up thallium since the first test (redistribution), the area is ischemic.

Occasionally, a patient who cannot tolerate a thallium/ECG stress test will have a pharmacologic thallium test. In this case the patient is given dipyridamole (Persantine) to increase coronary artery blood flow, and the thallium test is then performed.

Cardiac Catheterization and Coronary Arteriography

Indications. Cardiac catheterization and coronary arteriography are routine diagnostic procedures for patients with known or suspected heart disease. Clinical indications for cardiac catheterization include myocardial ischemia, unstable angina, evolving myocardial infarction, heart failure with a history that suggests coronary artery disease or cardiac valvular disease, and congenital heart disease. Cardiac catheterization is used both to confirm physical findings and to provide a baseline for medical or surgical therapy.

During catheterization of the left side of the heart, hemodynamic pressure measurements are taken in the aortic root, the left ventricle, and the left atrium. Radiopaque contrast (dye) is used to visualize the left side of the heart (angiogram) and the coronary arteries (arteriogram). Catheterization of the right side of the heart is performed using a thermodilution pulmonary artery catheter. Information obtained includes hemodynamic pressure measurements in the right atrium, right ventricle, pulmonary artery, and pulmonary capillary wedge position, as well as the measurement of cardiac output, calculated hemodynamic values, oxygen saturations, and an angiogram of the right-heart chambers using radiopaque contrast. If an arteriogram (visualization) of the coronary arteries is undertaken, that is a separate procedure.

Procedure. Before the catheterization the patient meets with the cardiologist to discuss the purpose, benefit, and risks of the study. For many patients, cardiac catheterization is the first major invasive procedure after a diagnosis of possible cardiac disease. The patient is often very anxious and has many questions. It is important that both nursing and medical staff fully answer patients' questions about the catheterization experience.

The morning of the procedure the patient fasts except for ingesting prescribed cardiac medications. Light premedication is given before the patient goes to the catheterization laboratory. If there is a history of allergy, an antihistamine or corticosteroid may be administered to prevent an anaphylactic reaction to the radiopaque contrast. Throughout the cardiac catheterization the patient remains awake and alert. He or she is positioned on a hard table with a C- or U-shaped camera arm overhead or to the side. This arm can be moved to view the heart from several different angles. Cardiac catheterization catheters, available in a variety of designs and sizes, are placed in the groin area after the patient receives a local anesthetic. The choice of catheters is based on the cardiologist's experience and the diagnostic study required. The femoral artery is used to catheterize the left side of the heart, including the coronary arteries. The femoral vein is used to pass catheters to the right side of the heart. During the study the patient receives heparin systemically to reduce the risk of emboli. Many patients also receive nitroglycerin to control chest pain, particularly when the coronary arteries are full of contrast material during the coronary arteriographic procedure. At this time the patient may also experience bradycardia or hypotension. To move the contrast dye more quickly and minimize the vagal effect on heart rate and blood pressure, the patient may be asked to cough. If the bradycardia persists, atropine or—occasionally—a transvenous pacemaker may be used. If hypotension continues, IV fluids are administered as a bolus. At the end of the study the femoral catheters are removed from the vessels. After the catheterization, once the patient is stable, the cardiologist meets with the patient and family to discuss the findings and plan of care.

Nursing management

Femoral artery site care. After the catheters are removed from the femoral artery and vein, pressure is applied to the groin area until bleeding has stopped. After catheterization the patient remains flat for 6 hours to allow the femoral arterial puncture site to form a stable clot. Most bleeding occurs within the first 2 to 3 hours after the procedure.[52-54] During this time the groin site is checked frequently for evidence of bleeding or hematoma. There has been considerable nursing research focused on the most appropriate method of controlling bleeding at the femoral arterial puncture site. Methods used include manual pressure, sandbag, elastic pressure dressing, and mechanical compression devices. The patient is asked to lie still and not to bend at the hip. It usually takes about 40 minutes for a stable clot to form, but can take longer in some patients, including those with a large body surface area.[52-54]

Most patients lie flat for up to 6 hours after a cardiac catheterization procedure. This time period is to allow a stable clot to form at the femoral arterial puncture site. Some institutions' protocols call for gradually increasing the height of the head of the bed over time while carefully monitoring the groin site for bleeding or hematoma formation.[55]

Sometimes when the patient needs to void urine this movement can dislodge the clot. If the patient is unable to void in the supine position, a urinary catheter is usually inserted.

Peripheral pulses. Pedal and posterior tibial pulses are assessed every 15 minutes for the first hour after the catheterization and every 30 minutes to 1 hour thereafter. The affected limb is assessed for changes in color, temperature, pain, or parasthesia to detect early evidence of acute arterial occlusion.

Rehydration. The patient is encouraged to drink large amounts of clear liquids, and the IV fluid rate is increased to 100 ml/hour. Fluid is given for rehydration because the radiopaque contrast acts as an osmotic diuretic. Patients who have elevated blood urea nitrogen (BUN) or creatinine levels before catheterization are at risk for acute renal failure from the dye.[56] For these patients the quantity of contrast material is consciously limited and fluid boluses given to preserve kidney function.

Angina. The patient is assessed for chest pain after the procedure. Usually, sublingual nitroglycerin is sufficient to relieve the pain, discomfort, or pressure.

Not all patients describe their angina as "pain," and many other descriptors may be used. A 1 to 10 pain scale can be used to quantify the angina. A 12-lead ECG must be obtained immediately to identify the coronary arteries involved, and the cardiologist is notified. If the chest pain persists, this may indicate that a clot has formed in a coronary artery, and the patient may need to return to the cardiac catheterization laboratory for an interventional cardiology procedure. (∞Angina, p. 486; Catheter Interventions for Coronary Artery Disease, p. 552.)

Dysrhythmias. Dysrhythmias are always a concern after an invasive cardiovascular diagnostic procedure. They occur secondary to the underlying cardiac disease and low potassium levels that can occur secondary to excessive diuresis.

Patient education. Because of the invasive nature of cardiac catheterization, many patients express considerable anxiety.[57,58] Relevant information concerns the sensory details of the procedure, such as lying flat and motionless on a hard table for many hours and sometimes experiencing a feeling of warmth when the dye is injected. Pain is uncommon because narcotic analgesics and sedative medications are always provided. Information about possible outcomes—both positive and negative—and possible complications must be provided.[57-60] Also, postcatheterization requirements such as lying still and the need to drink large quantities of fluids are explained. The basic information can be provided using written material and videotapes, but it is vital to individualize the content and answer any specific concerns or questions. Patients are also asked to report any other unusual symptoms, such as chest pain or nausea.

Electrophysiology Study

Indications. The electrophysiology study (EPS) is an invasive diagnostic tool used to record intracardiac electrical activity. A person may have an EPS performed because of a history of a syncopal episode (loss of consciousness), rapid wide complex tachycardia, or other cardiac electrical problems not diagnosed by the noninvasive diagnostic studies, such as the 12-lead ECG, treadmill stress test, signal-averaged ECG, or Holter monitoring. The EPS is performed in a specially equipped cardiac catheterization laboratory.

Before the electrophysiology study, written and verbal education is given to the patient and family to increase their sense of security and to decrease stress and anxiety. All antidysrhythmic medications are discontinued several days before the study so that any ventricular dysrhythmias may be readily induced during the EPS. Premedication is administered before the study to induce a relaxed state, and during the procedure the patient is conscious but receives sedation agents at regular intervals. The patient fasts 6 hours before the EPS, and during the procedure, lies supine on a hard table with a C- or U-shaped camera arm to the side or overhead to verify the position of the EPS catheters in the heart.

Electrophysiology equipment for stimulation of dysrhythmias and monitoring is usually nearby. A peripheral IV, radial arterial line, and surface ECG leads are placed. Then, electrophysiology catheters are inserted into the femoral vein and advanced to the right side of the heart under fluoroscopy. These catheters, similar to pacing catheters, are placed at specific anatomic sites within the heart to record the earliest electrical activity. These sites include the sinoatrial (SA) node, the atrioventricular (AV) node, the coronary sinus, the bundle of His, the bundle branches, and other selected areas of myocardium. Once the catheters are in position, a pacing technique known as *programmed electrical stimulation* is used to trigger the dysrhythmia. This technique delivers pulses of two to four early ventricular pacing beats, via the catheter, to the selected area of myocardium. Once the dysrhythmia is induced, it can be converted to normal sinus rhythm spontaneously or be converted by rapid atrial pacing, cardioversion/defibrillation, or IV antidysrhythmic medications. During the EPS the electrophysiologist looks for a site of early electrical activation that stimulates the myocardium before the SA node. At the end of the study, all of the electrophysiology catheters are removed before the patient returns to the nursing unit.

Medical management. After the EPS diagnosis, depending on the findings, the options for treatment are discussed with the patient and family. Many of the possible interventions necessitate a return to the electrophysiology (EP) laboratory to monitor the effectiveness of the treatment. For example, if the diagnosis is Wolff-Parkinson-White (WPW) syndrome, the solution may be a radiofrequency catheter ablation of the accessory tract. If it is a bradydysrhythmia, a permanent pacemaker may be inserted. If the diagnosis is reentry ventricular tachycardia, the treatment may be antidysrhythmic drugs or an implantable cardioverter defibrillator (ICD). When an electrophysiology study is required for a patient with an ICD, the device can substitute for the EP catheters. In the latest generation of ICD generators, known as *tiered therapy devices* because of their three therapeutic components (pace termination, back-up bradycardia pacing, and cardioversion/defibrillation), it is not necessary for the patient to have EP catheters placed in the femoral vein. The EPS can be performed via the external ICD programmer in the EP laboratory. The ICD generator and leads perform programmed electrical stimulation in a similar manner to a full EPS. (∞Implantable Cardioverter Defibrillator, p. 550.)

In summary the electrophysiology study can provide valuable information about intracardiac electrical abnormalities and reveal specialized diagnostic clues that can be used to guide medical and nursing management of the patient with significant cardiac dysrhythmias.

Nursing management. The nursing care of the patient after removal of the EPS catheter is similar to the care provided for the cardiac catheterization patient. The nursing interventions focus on achieving hemostasis at the femoral puncture site, assessing pedal pulses and perfusion in the affected limb, monitoring for chest pain and dysrhythmias, and providing comprehensive patient education. (∞Cardiac Catheterization Nursing Management, p. 439.)

Signal-Averaged ECG

The signal-averaged ECG is used to identify individuals at risk for sudden cardiac death from ventricular dysrhythmias. It is different from the 12-lead ECG, Holter monitoring, and stress test, and it is used in the subset of patients predisposed to lethal ventricular dysrhythmias. This is a noninvasive test. The patient lies in a supine position and is asked to keep muscle movement to a minimum. Electrode leads are applied to the anterior and posterior chest walls, and the leads are connected to a signal-averaged ECG computer. This computer produces a high-resolution, high-magnification ECG signal. This "noise-free" ECG is then analyzed for both QRS duration and for the presence, duration, and measurement of late myopotentials. After computer analysis, the signal-averaged ECG is described as either negative (normal) or positive (abnormal). A positive signal-averaged ECG is a predictor of increased risk for sudden cardiac death.

Myocardium that is damaged, either by myocardial infarction or by cardiomyopathy, produces late-activating myopotentials that may cause reentry ventricular dysrhythmias. The 12-lead ECG is not sufficiently sensitive to detect these low-amplitude, late potentials—hence the need for a high-resolution signal.

Many patients with a positive signal-averaged ECG (abnormal) display a normal signal-averaged ECG when placed on antidysrhythmic medications. The signal-averaged ECG is not analyzed in isolation. It is used in conjunction with other cardiac diagnostic tests, including the electrophysiology study. It is a helpful adjunct to the electrophysiology study but does not replace it.

Head Up–Tilt Table Test

A patient who is being evaluated for unexplained transient loss of consciousness (syncope) may undergo a head up–tilt table test (HUTT) in addition to EPS and neurologic examination. Etiology of syncope is divided into cardiac and noncardiac causes. Noncardiac-related syncope has a mortality rate of 5% at 1 year. Syncope that occurs as a result of a cardiac condition, such as cardiomyopathy or valvular stenosis, carries a 1 year mortality rate that ranges from 20% to 30%.[61]

If the neurologic examination is normal and the EPS is negative for dysrhythmias, the cause of loss of consciousness may be vasovagal related. This condition is also called vasodepressor syncope (VDS), or neurocardiogenic syncope (NCS).[61] The syncopal episodes are evaluated by a HUTT. Vasovagal-related syncope describes transient loss of consciousness caused by hypotension secondary to parasympathetic vasodilation and venous pooling, which reduces cerebral perfusion and creates the syncopal episode.

The HUTT is usually conducted in the radiology department. The patient lies supine on a table and is connected to an ECG monitor. A noninvasive blood pressure cuff is applied, and an IV line is established. The table head is elevated to between 40 and 80 degrees, following a standard protocol. Blood pressure and heart rate measurements are determined frequently. A positive vasovagal response occurs if the patient loses consciousness as the head of the table is raised. However, not all susceptible individuals experience syncope under resting conditions. In this situation, isoproterenol (Isuprel) 1 to 8 μg/min may be infused to increase heart rate and circulating catecholamines. If the patient has a HUTT-induced syncopal episode, secondary ventricular dysrhythmias may also occur. Therefore antidysrhythmic medications and a defibrillator must always be nearby.

Treatment of vasovagal syncope varies according to the cause. If increased circulating catecholamine levels are the problem, beta-blockers are used to decrease catecholamine effect. If increased vagal tone is the cause, atropine-like drugs that block the parasympathetic nervous system may be prescribed. After treatment with appropriate medications, the HUTT is repeated. For the patient who has experienced syncope of unknown cause, the HUTT is a highly effective test if the EPS and neurologic examination are negative.

Bedside Hemodynamic Monitoring

Invasive hemodynamic monitoring is one of the major competencies required for the critical care nurse. Using invasive catheters and sophisticated monitors, the nurse evaluates a patient's cardiac function, circulating blood volume, and physiologic response to treatment. Knowledge of the theoretic base that underlies hemodynamic monitoring assists the clinician in developing decision-making skills to interpret and analyze trends and to formulate a nursing management plan appropriate for each individual patient. Critical care nurses and physicians who frequently manage patients with invasive hemodynamic lines more accurately assess hemodynamic waveforms than clinicians who infrequently work in critical care.[62-64]

Indications. The range of medical diagnoses for which hemodynamic monitoring can be used is enormous. Most of these medical diagnoses are linked by three nursing diagnoses: (1) Alteration in Cardiac Output, (2) Alteration in Fluid Volume, and (3) Alteration in Tissue Perfusion. These nursing diagnoses are based on pathophysiologic processes that alter one of the four hemodynamic mechanisms that support normal cardiovascular function: preload, afterload, heart rate, and contractility. Treatment of alterations in cardiac output, fluid volume, and tissue perfusion vary, based on the precipitating cause and medical diagnosis, as discussed later in this chapter in the section on pulmonary artery catheters. (∞Cardiac Output, p. 460; Pulmonary Artery Pressure Monitoring, p. 459.)

There are different levels of hemodynamic monitoring intensity, depending on the clinical needs of the patient. The simplest level includes monitoring heart rhythm, central venous pressure (CVP), and arterial blood pressure—a combination that is commonly used after uncomplicated general surgery. If the patient has a low cardiac output (CO), such as might occur subsequent to an acute myocardial infarction, a more intense level of surveillance may be necessary. It might involve use of a thermodilution pulmonary artery catheter, which provides hemodynamic information that includes intracardiac pressures, direct measurement of CO, and—if necessary—continuous measurement of pulmonary arterial oxygen saturation (SvO_2). Another catheter used in critical care is the left atrial pressure line, which may be used in selected patients after cardiac surgery. (Hemodynamic Pressure Monitoring: Nursing Management; Cardiac Care IVD)

Overview of hemodynamic monitoring

Equipment. A hemodynamic monitoring system has four component parts as shown in Figure 15-57 and described in the following list:

A. The invasive catheter in the patient and the and high pressure tubing connecting the patient and the transducer.

B. The transducer, which receives the physiologic signal from the catheter and tubing and converts it into electrical energy.

C. The flush system, which maintains catheter patency of the fluid-filled system.

D. The bedside monitor contains the amplifier/recorder, which increases the volume of the electrical signal and displays it on an oscilloscope and on a digital scale in millimeters of mercury (mm Hg).

Although many different invasive catheters are inserted to monitor hemodynamic pressures, all catheters are connected to similar equipment (see Figure 15-57). This consists of a bag of 0.9% normal saline solution, which will usually contain 1 unit of heparin (range 0.25 to 2 units per milliliter of saline depending on the institutional protocol). A 300 mm Hg pressure infusion cuff, IV tubing, three-way stopcocks, and an in-line flow device for both continuous fluid infusion and manual flush are also attached. The high pressure tubing connects the invasive catheter to the transducer to prevent damping (flattening) of the waveform. The most commonly used transducers are disposable, use a silicon chip, and are highly accurate.[65]

Heparin. Heparin is added to the infusion/flush setup to maintain catheter patency. Arterial monitoring lines maintained with a heparin flush solution have a greater probability of remaining patent than do lines maintained with nonheparinized solutions, such as normal saline.[66,67] A recent study reported that the distal port of the pulmonary artery (PA) may not require anticoagulation to maintain catheter patency.[67] However, most critical care units empirically anticoagulate PA catheters to decrease the risk of clot in the catheter lumen.

Calibration of equipment. To ensure accuracy of hemodynamic pressure readings, two baseline measurements are necessary: (1) calibration of the system to atmospheric pressure, also known as "zeroing" the transducer, and (2) determination of the phlebostatic axis for transducer height placement; this is sometimes called "leveling" the transducer.

Zeroing the transducer. To calibrate the equipment to atmospheric pressure, also called *zeroing the transducer,* the three-way stopcock nearest to the transducer is turned simultaneously to open the transducer to air (atmospheric pressure) and to close it to the patient and the flush system. The monitor is adjusted so that "0" is displayed, which equals atmospheric pressure. Atmospheric pressure is not actually

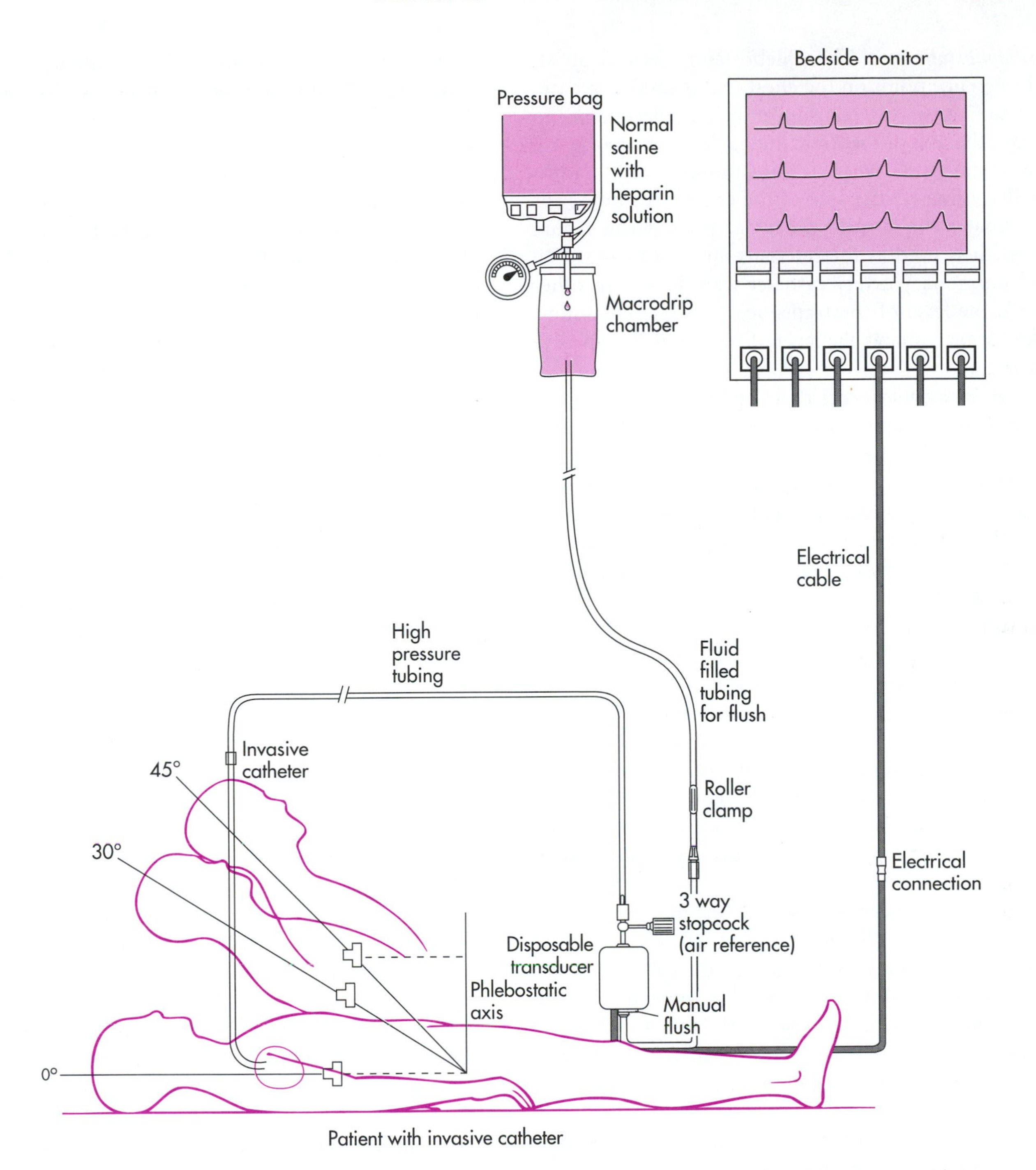

FIGURE 15-57. The four parts of a hemodynamic monitoring include invasive catheter attached to high pressure tubing to connect to the transducer; transducer; flush system, including a manual flush; and bedside monitor

"0"—it is 760 mm Hg at sea level. Using "0" to represent current atmospheric pressure provides a convenient baseline for hemodynamic measurement purposes.[68]

Some monitors also require calibration of the upper scale limit while the system remains open to air. At the end of the calibration procedure, the stopcock is returned to the closed position and a closed cap is placed over the open port. At this point the patient's waveform and hemodynamic pressures are displayed.

Disposable transducers are now so accurate that once they are calibrated to atmospheric pressure, drift from the zero baseline is minimal.[68] While in theory this means that repeated calibration is unnecessary, clinical protocols in most units require the nurse to calibrate the transducer at the beginning of each shift.

Phlebostatic axis. The phlebostatic axis is a physical reference point on the chest that is used as a baseline for consistent transducer height placement. To obtain the axis, a theoretic line is drawn from the 4th intercostal space, where it joins the sternum, to a midaxillary line on the side of the chest. This point approximates the level of the atria, as shown in Figure 15-57. It is used as the reference mark for both CVP and pulmonary artery catheter transducers. In other words the level of the transducer "air reference stopcock" approximates the level of the tip of the invasive catheter.

Leveling the transducer. Leveling the transducer is different from zeroing. This process aligns the disposable transducer with the tip of the invasive catheter. Some critical care units use a carpenter's level for this purpose. If the transducer air-reference stopcock is level with the phlebostatic axis reference point, accurate hemodynamic pressure measurements can be obtained for most patients.

Error in measurement can occur if the transducer is placed *below* the phlebostatic axis, because the fluid in the system will weigh on the transducer (hydrostatic pressure) and produce a false high reading. For every inch the transducer is below the tip of the catheter, the fluid pressure in the system increases the measurement by 1.87 mm Hg.[68] For example, if the transducer is positioned 6 inches below the tip of the catheter, this falsely elevates the displayed pressure by 11 mm Hg.[68]

If the transducer is placed *above* this atrial level, gravity and lack of fluid pressure will give an erroneously low reading. Once again, for every inch the transducer is positioned above the catheter tip, the measurement is 1.87 mm Hg less than the true value.[68] If several clinicians are taking measurements, the reference point can be marked on the side of the patient's chest to ensure accurate measurements. See Box 15-6 for a description of other nursing activities associated with hemodynamic monitoring.

Patient position. Patient position in the hemodynamically monitored patient would not be an issue if critical care patients always lay flat and supine in bed. However, this is not always a comfortable position, especially if the patient is alert, or if the head of the bed needs to be elevated to decrease work of breathing.

Nurse researchers have determined that the CVP, PAP, and PAWP can be reliably measured at head-of-bed positions from 0 (flat) to 60 degrees if the patient is lying on his or her back.[69-72] In general, if the patient is normovolemic and hemodynamically stable, raising the head of the bed does not affect hemodynamic pressure measurements. If the patient is so hemodynamically unstable or hypovolemic that raising the head of the bed negatively affects intravascular volume distribution, correcting the hemodynamic instability and leaving the patient in a supine position is the first priority. In summary, the majority of patients *do not* need the head of the bed to be lowered to "0" to obtain accurate CVP, PAP, or PAWP readings. However, there is no such agreement if patients are turned to the side in the lateral position. This is mainly because it is difficult to identify the true phlebostatic axis in this position, and also because of the position of the heart in the left chest. Currently, measurements taken in the lateral position are not considered as accurate as measurements taken when the patient is lying on his or her back.[69,72]

Intraarterial Blood Pressure Monitoring

Indications. Intraarterial blood pressure monitoring is indicated for any major medical or surgical condition that compromises cardiac output, tissue perfusion, or fluid volume status. The system is designed for continuous measurement of three blood pressure parameters—systole, diastole, and mean arterial blood pressure (MAP). In addition, the direct arterial access is helpful in the management of patients with acute respiratory failure who require frequent arterial blood gas (ABG) measurements.

Catheters. The size of the catheter used is proportionate to the diameter of the cannulated artery. In small arteries—such as the radial and dorsalis pedis—a 20-gauge, 3.8 to 5.1 cm, nontapered Teflon catheter is most often used. If the larger femoral or axillary arteries are used, a 19- or 20-gauge, 16 cm, Teflon catheter is used. Teflon catheters are preferred because of their lower risk of causing thrombosis.

The catheter insertion is usually percutaneous, although the technique varies with vessel size. Cannulas are most often inserted in the smaller arteries, using a "catheter-over-needle" unit in which the needle is used as a temporary guide for catheter placement. With this method, once the unit has been inserted into the artery, the needle is withdrawn, leaving the supple plastic cannula in place. Insertion of a cannula into a larger artery usually necessitates use of the Seldinger technique. This procedure involves (1) entry into the artery using a needle, (2) passage of a supple guidewire through the needle into the artery, (3) removal of the needle, (4) passage of the catheter over the guidewire, and (5) removal of the guidewire, leaving the cannula in the artery. If a cannula cannot be inserted into the artery using percutaneous methods, an arterial cut-

NURSING INTERVENTION CLASSIFICATIONS

BOX 15-6 Invasive Hemodynamic Monitoring

DEFINITION: Measurement and interpretation of invasive hemodynamic parameters to determine cardiovascular function and regulate therapy as appropriate

ACTIVITIES:

Assist with insertion and removal of invasive hemodynamic lines
Assist with Allen test for evaluation of collateral ulnar circulation before radial artery cannulation, if appropriate
Assist with chest x-ray examination after insertion of pulmonary artery catheter
Monitor heart rate and rhythm
Zero and calibrate equipment per hospital protocol, with transducer at the level of the right atrium
Monitor blood pressure (systolic, diastolic, and mean), central venous/right atrial pressure, pulmonary artery pressure (systolic, diastolic, and mean), and pulmonary capillary/artery wedge pressure
Monitor hemodynamic waveforms for changes in cardiovascular function
Compare hemodynamic parameters with other clinical signs and symptoms
Use closed-system cardiac output setup
Obtain cardiac output by administering cardiac output injectate within 4 sec and average three injections that are within less than 1 L of each other
Monitor pulmonary artery and systemic arterial waveforms; if dampening occurs, check tubing for kinks or air bubbles, check connections, aspirate clot from tip of catheter, gently flush system, or assist with repositioning of catheter
Document pulmonary artery and systemic arterial waveforms
Monitor peripheral perfusion distal to catheter insertion site every 4 hr or as appropriate
Monitor for dyspnea, fatigue, tachypnea, and orthopnea
Monitor for forward progression of pulmonary catheter resulting in spontaneous wedge, and notify physician if it occurs
Refrain from inflating balloon more frequently than per hospital protocol
Monitor for balloon rupture (e.g., assess for resistance when inflating balloon and allow balloon to passively deflate after obtaining pulmonary capillary/artery wedge pressure)
Prevent air emboli (e.g., remove air bubbles from tubing; if balloon rupture is suspected, refrain from attempts to reinflate balloon and clamp balloon port)
Maintain sterility of ports
Maintain closed-pressure system to ports, as appropriate
Perform sterile dressing changes and site care, as appropriate
Inspect insertion site for signs of bleeding or infection
Change IV solution and tubing every 24 to 72 hr, based on protocol
Monitor laboratory results to detect possible catheter-induced infection
Administer fluid and/or volume expanders to maintain hemodynamic parameters within specified range
Administer pharmacological agents to maintain hemodynamic parameters within specified range
Instruct patient and family on therapeutic use of hemodynamic monitoring catheters
Instruct patient on activity restriction while catheters remain in place

Modified from McCloskey JC, Bulechek GM: *Nursing intervention classifications,* ed 2, St Louis, 1996, Mosby.

down may be performed. This procedure is avoided if possible, because it involves a skin incision to expose the artery directly and is associated with a higher risk of infection.

Insertion. Several major peripheral arteries are suitable for receiving a cannula and for long-term hemodynamic monitoring. The most frequently used site is the radial artery. If this artery is not available, the femoral, dorsalis-pedis, axillary, or brachial arteries may be used.

Allen test. The major advantage of the radial artery is that collateral circulation to the hand is provided by the ulnar artery and palmar arch in most of the population; thus there are other avenues of circulation if the radial artery becomes blocked after catheter placement. Before radial artery cannulation, collateral circulation must be assessed, either by using the Doppler flowmeter or by the Allen test. In the Allen test the radial and ulnar arteries are compressed simultaneously. The patient is asked to clench and unclench the hand until it blanches. One of the arteries is then released, and the hand should immediately flush from that side. The same procedure is repeated for the remaining artery.

Nursing management. Intraarterial blood pressure monitoring is designed for continuous assessment of arterial perfusion to the major organ systems of the body. Mean arterial pressure (MAP) is the clinical parameter most frequently used to assess perfusion, because MAP represents perfusion pressure throughout the cardiac cycle. Because one third of the cardiac cycle is spent in systole and two thirds in diastole, the MAP calculation must reflect the greater amount of time spent in diastole. The MAP formula when calculated by hand is as follows:

$$[(\text{Diastole} \times 2) + (\text{systole} \times 1)] \div 3$$

Thus a blood pressure of 120/60 mm Hg produces a MAP of 80 mm Hg. However, the bedside hemodynamic monitor may show a slightly different digital number because most computers calculate the area under the curve of the arterial line tracing (Table 15-14).

Perfusion pressure. A MAP greater than 60 mm Hg is necessary to perfuse the coronary arteries, brain, and kidneys. A MAP between 70 and 90 mm Hg is ideal for the cardiac patient to decrease LV work load. After a carotid endarterectomy or neurologic surgery, a MAP of 90 to 110 mm Hg may be more appropriate to increase cerebral perfusion pressure. Systolic and diastolic pressures are monitored in conjunction with the MAP as a further guide to the accuracy of perfusion. Should cardiac output decrease, the body compensates by constricting peripheral vessels to maintain the blood pressure. In this situation the MAP may remain constant, but the pulse pressure (difference between systolic and diastolic pressures) narrows. The following examples explain this point:

Mr. A: BP, 90/70 mm Hg; MAP, 76 mm Hg

Mr. B: BP, 150/40 mm Hg; MAP, 76 mm Hg

Both of these patients have a perfusion pressure of 76 mm Hg, but clinically they are very different. Mr. A is peripherally vasoconstricted, as is demonstrated by the narrow pulse pressure (90/70 mm Hg). His skin is cool to touch, and he has weak peripheral pulses. Mr. B has a wide pulse pressure (150/40 mm Hg), warm skin, and normally palpable peripheral pulses. Thus nursing assessment of the patient with an arterial line includes comparison of clinical findings with arterial line readings, including perfusion pressure and MAP.

Pulse pressure. Another clinical example of hemodynamic nursing assessment is seen in patient JW 1 day after his coronary artery bypass graft (CABG) surgery. JW has recently been weaned from low-dose dopamine (Intropin) and sodium nitroprusside (Nipride) and has received a diuretic (20 mg of furosemide IV). He has voided 800 ml of urine via the Foley catheter during the last 2 hours. JW's MAP remains at 80 mm Hg, but his pulse pressure has narrowed by 30 mm Hg from 120/60 to 100/70 mm Hg. His heart rate has increased from 90 to 110 beats per minute (bpm). This clinical situation is not uncommon after furosemide (Lasix) administration, but the narrowed pulse pressure and increased heart rate may indicate hypovolemia. The nurse caring for JW will monitor the trend of the MAP. If the MAP begins to decrease and JW shows signs of a low cardiac output, his physician will be notified. In most nonemergency situations, following the *trend* of the arterial pressure is more valuable than an isolated measurement.

Cuff blood pressure. If the arterial line becomes unreliable or dislodged, a cuff pressure can be used as a reserve system. In the normovolemic patient, little difference exists between the cuff blood pressure and arterial pressure.

Pressure differences are to be expected because the arterial catheter measures flow within the artery, whereas the mercury sphygmomanometer and stethoscope measure pressure from the outside. In the normovolemic patient, differences of 5 to 10 mm Hg do not affect clinical management. If the patient has a low CO or is in shock, the cuff pressure is unreliable because of vasoconstriction, and an arterial line is inserted. If there is ever any doubt about the accuracy of the arterial waveform or pressure reading, a cuff blood pressure reading is always taken.

Arterial pressure waveform interpretation. As the aortic valve opens, blood is ejected from the left ventricle and is recorded as an increase of pressure in the arterial system. The highest point recorded is called *systole.* After peak ejection (systole), force is decreased and pressure drops. A notch (the dicrotic notch) may be visible on the downstroke of this arterial waveform, representing closure of the aortic valve. The dicrotic notch signifies the beginning of diastole. The remainder of the downstroke represents diastolic runoff of blood flow into the arterial tree. The lowest point recorded is called *diastole.* A normal arterial pressure tracing is described in Figure 15-58. Note that electrical stimulation (QRS) is always first and that the ar-

TABLE 15-14 Hemodynamic Pressures and Calculated Hemodynamic Values

Hemodynamic Pressure	Definition and Explanation	Normal Range*
Mean arterial pressure (**MAP**)	Average perfusion pressure created by arterial blood pressure during the cardiac cycle. The normal cardiac cycle is one third systole and two thirds diastole. These three components are divided by 3 to obtain the average perfusion pressure for the whole cardiac cycle.	70-100 mm Hg
Central venous pressure (**CVP**)	Pressure created by volume in the right side of the heart. When the tricuspid valve is open, the CVP reflects filling pressures in the right ventricle. Clinically, the CVP is often used as a guide to overall fluid balance.	2-5 mm Hg 3-8 cm water (H_2O)
Left atrial pressure (**LAP**)	Pressure created by volume in the left side of the heart. When the mitral valve is open, the LAP reflects filling pressures in the left ventricle. Clinically, the LAP is used after cardiac surgery to determine how well the left ventricle is ejecting its volume. In general, the higher the LAP, the lower the ejection fraction from the left ventricle.	5-12 mm Hg
Pulmonary artery pressure (**PAP**) (systolic, diastolic, mean) (**PA systolic [PAS], PA diastolic [PAD], PAP mean [PAPm]**)	Pulsatile pressure in the pulmonary artery, measured by an indwelling catheter.	PAS 20-30 mm Hg PAD 5-10 mm Hg PAP_M 10-15 mm Hg
Pulmonary capillary wedge pressure, or pulmonary artery wedge pressure (**PCW,** or **PCWP** or **PAWP**)	Pressure created by volume in the left side of the heart. When the mitral valve is open, the PAWP reflects filling pressures in the pulmonary vasculature, and pressures in the left side of the heart are transmitted back to the catheter "wedged" into a small pulmonary arteriole.	5-12 mm Hg
Cardiac output (**CO**)	The amount of blood pumped out by a ventricle. Clinically, it can be measured using the thermodilution CO method, which calculates CO in liters per minute (L/min).	4-6 L/min (at rest)
Cardiac index (**CI**)	CO divided by body surface area (BSA), tailoring the CO to individual body size. A BSA conversion chart is necessary to calculate CI, which is considered more accurate than CO because it is individualized to height and weight. CI is measured in liters per minute per square meter BSA ($L/min/m^2$).	2.2-4.0 $L/min/m^2$
Stroke volume (**SV**)	Amount of blood ejected by the ventricle with each heartbeat. Hemodynamic monitoring systems calculate SV by dividing cardiac output (CO in L/min) by the heart rate (HR) then multiplying the answer by 1000 to change liters to milliliters (ml).	60-70 ml
Stroke volume index (**SI**)	SV indexed to BSA.	40-50 ml/m^2
Systemic vascular resistance (**SVR**)	Mean pressure difference across the systemic vascular bed, divided by blood flow. Clinically, SVR represents the resistance against which the left ventricle must pump to eject its volume. This resistance is created by the systemic arteries and arterioles. As SVR increases, CO falls. SVR is measured in either units or $dynes/sec/cm^{-5}$. If the number of units is multiplied by 80, the value is converted to $dynes/sec/cm^{-5}$.	10-18 units or 800-1400 $dynes/sec/cm^{-5}$
Systemic vascular resistance index (**SVRI**)	SVR indexed to BSA.	2000-2400 $dynes/sec/cm^{-5}/m^2$

*The formulas for these hemodynamic values are listed in Appendix D.

Continued

TABLE 15-14 Hemodynamic Pressures and Calculated Hemodynamic Values—cont'd

Hemodynamic Pressure	Definition and Explanation	Normal Range*
Pulmonary vascular resistance (**PVR**)	Mean pressure difference across pulmonary vascular bed, divided by blood flow. Clinically, PVR represents the resistance against which the right ventricle must pump to eject its volume. This resistance is created by the pulmonary arteries and arterioles. As PVR increases, the output from the right ventricle decreases. PVR is measured in either units or dynes/sec/cm^{-5}. PVR is normally one sixth of SVR.	1.2-3.0 units or 100-250 dynes/sec/cm^{-5}
Pulmonary vascular resistance index (**PVRI**)	PVR indexed to BSA.	225-315 dynes/sec/cm^{-5}/m^2
Left cardiac work index (**LCWI**)	Amount of work the left ventricle does *each minute* when ejecting blood. The hemodynamic formula represents pressure generated (MAP) multiplied by volume pumped (CO). A conversion factor is used to change mm Hg to kilogram-meter (kg-m). LCWI is always represented as an indexed volume (BSA chart). LCWI increases or decreases because of changes in either pressure (MAP) or volume pumped (CO).	3.4-4.2 kg-m/m^2
Left ventricular stroke work index (**LVSWI**)	Amount of work the left ventricle performs with *each heartbeat.* The hemodynamic formula represents pressure generated (MAP) multiplied by volume pumped (SV). A conversion factor is used to change ml/mm Hg to gram-meter (g-m). LVSWI is always represented as an indexed volume. LVSWI increases or decreases because of changes in either pressure (MAP) or volume pumped (SV).	50-62 g-m/m^2
Right cardiac work index (**RCWI**)	Amount of work the right ventricle performs *each minute* when ejecting blood. The hemodynamic formula represents pressure generated (PAP mean) multiplied by volume pumped (CO). A conversion factor is used to change mm Hg to kilogram-meter (kg-m). RCWI is always represented as an indexed value (BSA chart). Similar to LCWI, the RCWI increases or decreases because of changes in either pressure (PAP mean) or volume pumped (CO).	0.54-0.66 kg-m/m^2
Right ventricular stroke work index (**RVSWI**)	Amount of work the right ventricle does *each heartbeat.* The hemodynamic formula represents pressure generated (PAP mean) multiplied by volume pumped (SV). A conversion factor is used to change mm Hg to gram-meter (g-m). RVSWI is always represented as an indexed value (BSA chart). Similar to LVSWI, the RVSWI increases or decreases because of changes in either pressure (PAP mean) or volume pumped (SV).	7.9-9.7 g-m/m^2

terial pressure tracing follows the initiating QRS. The relationship of the arterial pressure waveform to the ejection phase of left ventricular systole is shown in Figure 13-26. (∞Cardiac Cycle, p. 348.)

Decreased arterial perfusion. Specific problems with heart rhythm can translate into poor arterial perfusion if cardiac output decreases. Poor perfusion may be seen as a single, nonperfused beat after a premature ventricular contraction (PVC) (Figure 15-59) or as multiple, nonperfused beats (Figure 15-60). In ventricular bigeminy, every second beat is poorly perfused (Figure 15-61). A disorganized atrial baseline resulting from atrial fibrillation creates a variable arterial pulse because of the differences in stroke volume between each beat (Figure 15-62). All of these examples illustrate that when two beats are close together, the left ventricle does not have time to fill adequately and the second beat is poorly perfused or is not perfused at all.

Pulse deficit. A pulse deficit occurs when the apical heart rate and the peripheral pulse are not equal. In the critical care unit this can be seen on the bedside

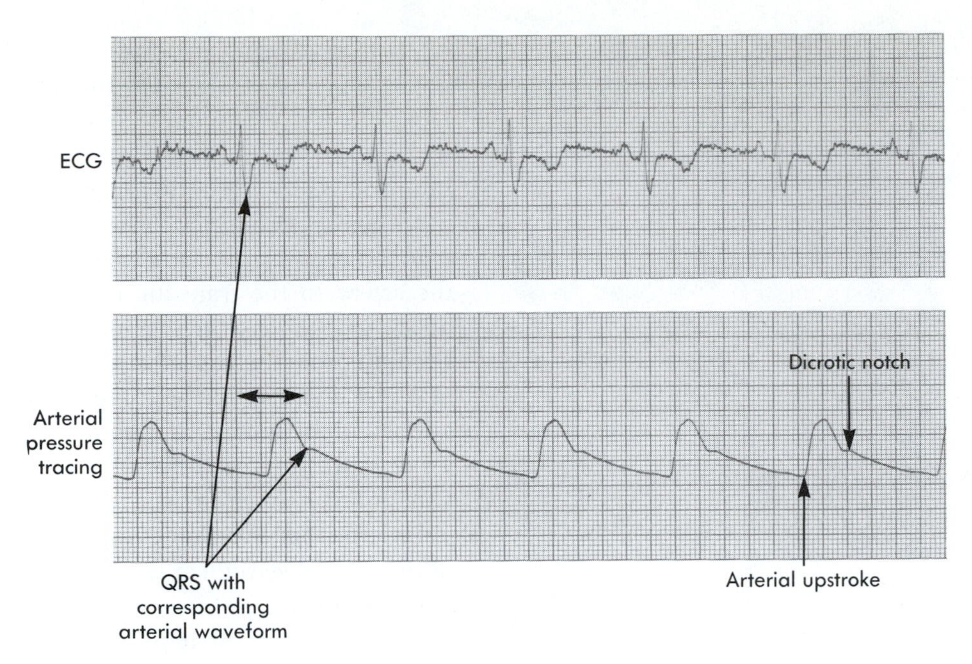

FIGURE 15-58. Simultaneous ECG and normal arterial pressure tracing.

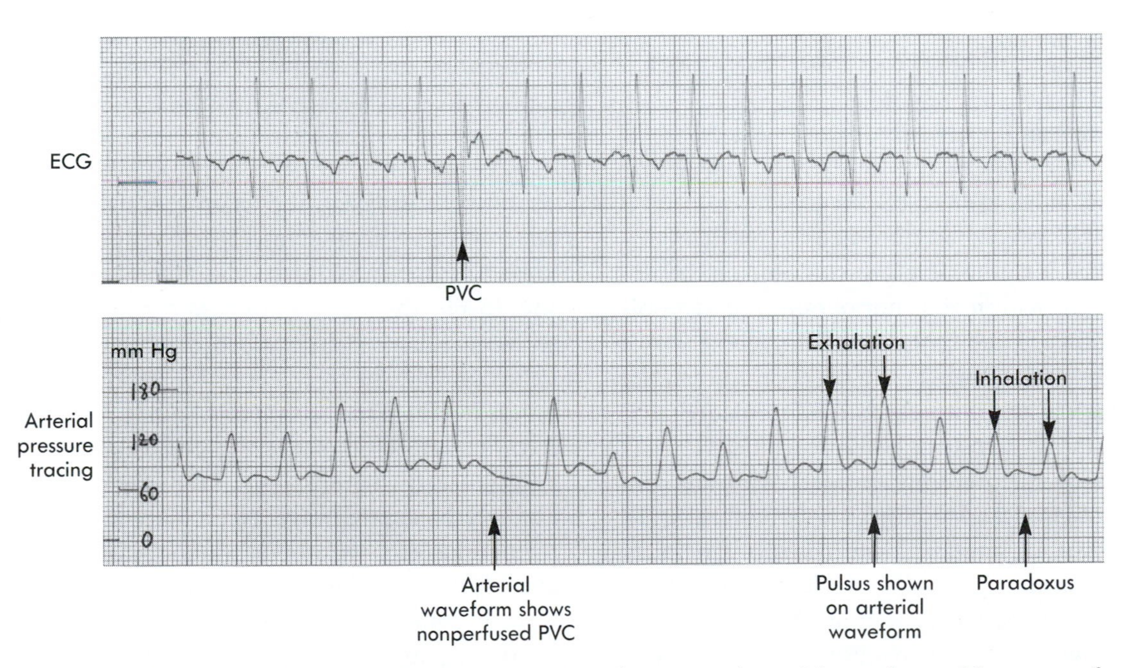

FIGURE 15-59. Simultaneous ECG and arterial pressure tracings show normal arterial waveform with a nonperfused premature ventricular contraction (PVC). Arterial waveform also shows evidence of pulsus paradoxus in a patient who is mechanically ventilated.

monitor. Normally there is one arterial upstroke for each QRS, and if there are more QRS complexes than arterial upstrokes, a pulse deficit is present, as shown in Figures 15-59 and 15-62. To identify a pulse deficit in an unmonitored patient, a stethoscope is placed over the apex of the heart. The heartbeat can be heard, but it cannot be felt as a radial pulse. To determine whether a pulse deficit is significant, it is necessary to evaluate the clinical impact on the patient and whether there is any change in MAP or pulse pressure.

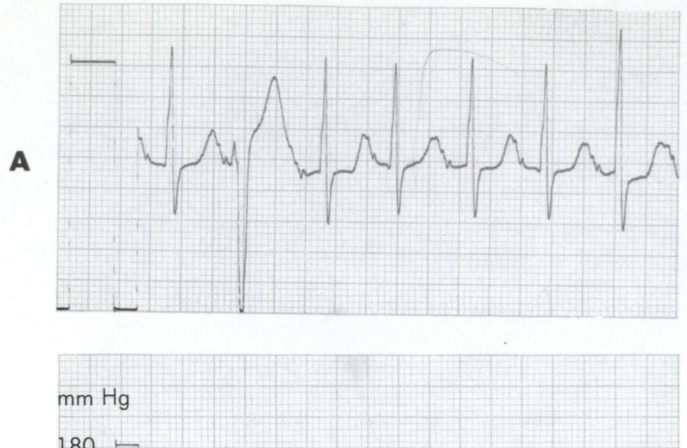

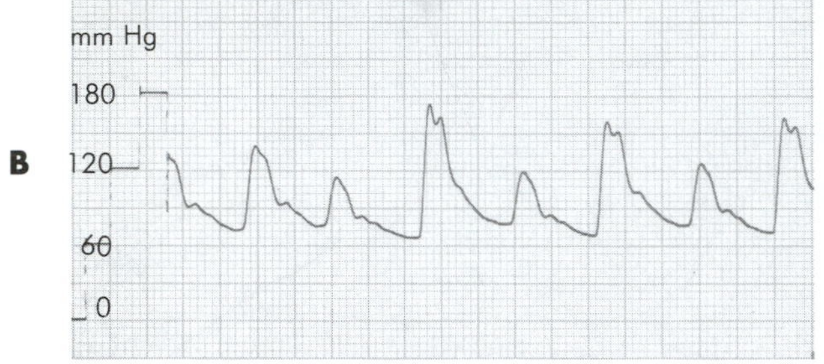

FIGURE 15-60. Simultaneous **A,** ECG and **B,** arterial pressure tracings show pulsus alternans. A nonperfused PVC is also present.

Generally, the more nonperfused beats, the more serious the problem.

Pulsus paradoxus. Pulsus paradoxus is a decrease of more than 10 mm Hg in the arterial waveform that occurs during inhalation (see Figure 15-59). It is caused by a fall in cardiac output as a result of increased negative intrathoracic pressure during inhalation. As pressure within the thorax falls, blood pools in the large veins of the lungs and thorax and stroke volume is decreased. This can be seen on an arterial waveform in a patient with cardiac tamponade, pericardial effusion, or constrictive pericarditis. It commonly occurs in hypovolemic patients who are mechanically ventilated and use large tidal volumes (12 to 15 ml/kg), or in patients who are spontaneously breathing very deeply.

In pulsus alternans, every other arterial pulsation is weak. This sometimes occurs in patients with advanced left ventricular failure.

Damped waveform. If the arterial monitor shows a low blood pressure, it is the responsibility of the nurse to determine whether it is a true patient problem or a problem with the equipment, as described in Table 15-15. A low arterial blood pressure waveform is shown in Figure 15-63. In this case the digital readout correlated well with the patient's own cuff pressure, confirming that the patient was hypotensive. This arterial waveform is more rounded, without a dicrotic notch, when compared with the normal waveform in Figure 15-58. A damped (flattened) arterial waveform is shown in Figure 15-64. In this case the patient's cuff pressure was significantly higher than the digital readout, thus representing a problem with equipment. A damped waveform occurs when communication from the artery to the transducer is interrupted and produces false values on the monitor and oscilloscope. Damping may be caused by a clot at the end of the catheter, by kinks in the catheter or tubing, or by air bubbles in the system. Troubleshooting techniques (see Table 15-15) are used to find the origin of the problem and to remove the cause of damping.

Underdamped waveform. Another cause of distortion of the arterial waveform is underdamping, often called *overshoot* or *fling.* This is recognized by a narrow upward systolic peak that produces a false high systolic reading when compared with the patient's cuff blood pressure as shown in Figure 15-65. The overshoot is caused by increased dynamic response or oscillations within the system.

Fast-flush square wave test. The monitoring system dynamic response can be checked at the bedside by performing the "fast-flush square wave," or "frequency response," test. This test involves use of the manual flush system on the transducer. Normally the flush device allows only 3 ml of fluid/hour. With the normal waveform displayed, the manual fast-flush is used to generate a rapid increase in pressure, which is displayed on the monitor oscilloscope. As shown in Figure 15-66, the normal dynamic response waveform shows a square pattern with one or two oscillations before the return of the arterial waveform. If the system is overdamped, a sloped—rather than square-pattern is seen. If the system is underdamped, there are additional oscillations—or vibrations—seen on the "fast-flush square wave test." This test can be performed for any hemodynamic monitoring system.[73] If air bubbles, clots, or kinks are in the system, the waveform becomes damped, or flattened, and this is seen in the square wave test. At this point, the troubleshooting methods described in Table 15-15 can be implemented.

The nurse caring for the patient with an arterial line must be able to assess whether a low MAP or narrowed perfusion pressure represents decreased arterial perfusion or equipment malfunction. Assessment of the arterial waveform on the oscilloscope, in combination with clinical assessment, will yield the answer.

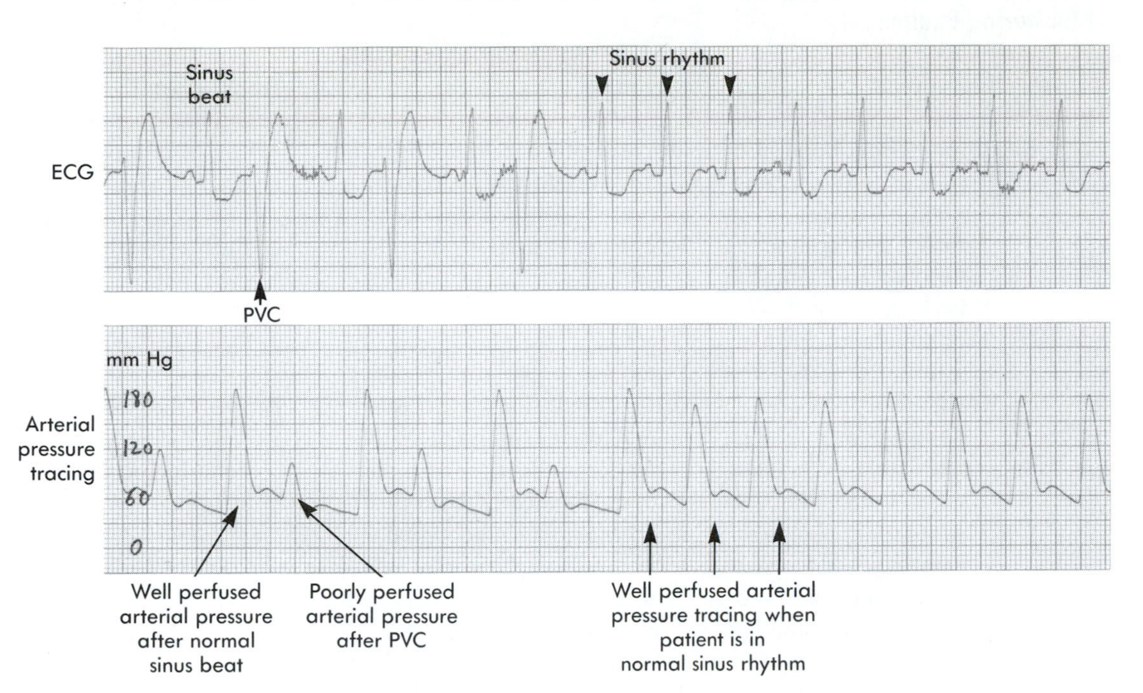

FIGURE 15-61. Simultaneous ECG and arterial pressure tracings show ventricular bigeminy in which every other ventricular beat is poorly perfused on the arterial pressure waveform in the first part of the tracing. In the second half of the tracing, there is a well-perfused arterial pressure tracing as the patient converts to normal sinus rhythm.

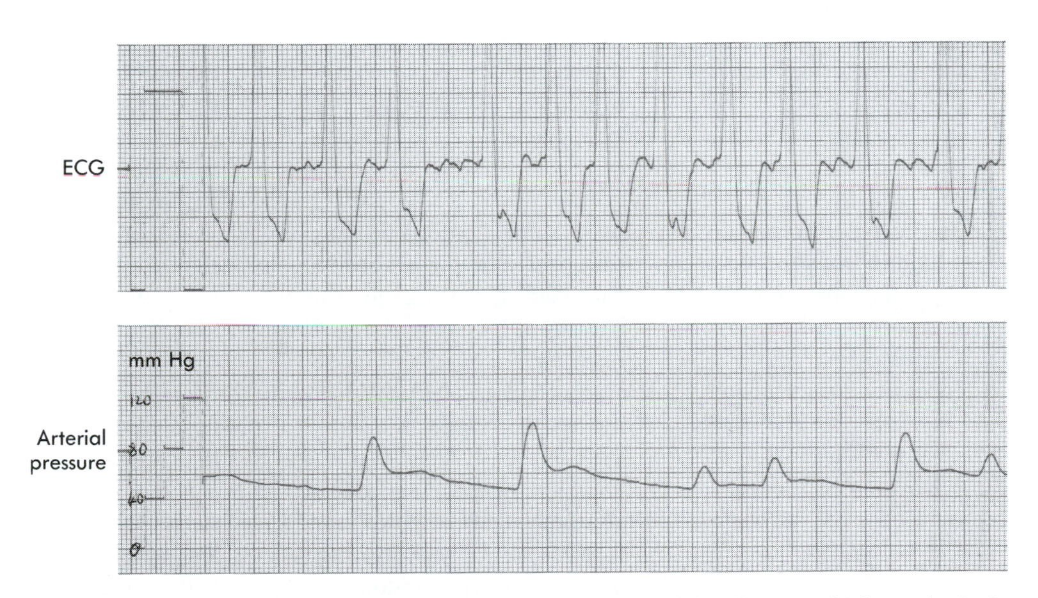

FIGURE 15-62. Simultaneous ECG and arterial pressure tracings show atrial fibrillation, which results in irregular atrial pulsations. They create differences in beat-to-beat ventricular upstroke volume, resulting in diminished or absent ventricular output, as seen on the arterial waveform.

Central Venous Pressure Monitoring

Indications. Central venous pressure (CVP) monitoring is indicated whenever a patient has significant alteration in fluid volume (see Table 15-14). The CVP can be used as a guide in fluid volume replacement in hypovolemia and to assess the impact of diuresis after diuretic administration in the case of fluid overload. In addition, when a major IV line is required for volume replacement, a central venous line is a good choice because large volumes of fluid can easily be delivered.

Catheters. CVP catheters are available as single-, double-, or triple-lumen infusion catheters, depending

TABLE 15-15 **Nursing Measures to Ensure Patient Safety and to Troubleshoot Problems with Hemodynamic Monitoring Equipment**

Problem	Prevention	Rationale	Troubleshooting
Overdamping of waveform	Provide continuous infusion of solution containing heparin through an in-line flush device (1 unit of heparin for each millimeter of flush solution).	To ensure that recorded pressures and waveform are accurate because a damped waveform gives inaccurate readings.	Before insertion, completely flush the line and/or catheter. In a line attached to a patient, back flush through the system to clear bubbles from tubing or transducer.
Underdamping, ("overshoot" or "fling")	Use short lengths of noncompliant tubing. Use "fast-flush square wave" test to demonstrate optimal system damping. Verify arterial waveform accuracy with the cuff blood pressure.	If the monitoring system is underdamped, both the systolic and diastolic values will be overestimated by both the waveform and the digital values. False high systolic values may lead to clinical decisions based on erroneous data.	Perform the "fast-flush square wave" test to verify optimal damping of the monitoring system.
Clot formation at end of catheter	Provide continuous infusion of solution containing heparin through an in-line flush device (1 unit of heparin for each millimeter of flush solution).	Any foreign object placed in the body can cause local activation of the patient's coagulation system as a normal defense mechanism. The clots that are formed may be dangerous if they break off and travel to other parts of the body.	If a clot in the catheter is suspected because of a damped waveform or resistance to forward flush of the system, gently aspirate the line using a small syringe inserted into the proximal stopcock. Then flush the line again once the clot is removed and inspect the waveform. It should return to a normal pattern.
Hemorrhage	Use Luer-Lok (screw) connections in line setup. Close and cap stopcocks when not in use.	A loose connection or open stopcock creates a low-pressure sump effect, causing blood to back into the line and into the open air.	Once a blood leak is recognized, tighten all connections, flush the line, and estimate blood loss.
	Ensure that the catheter is either sutured or securely taped in position.	If a catheter is accidentally removed, the vessel can bleed profusely, especially with an arterial line or if the patient has abnormal coagulation factors (resulting from heparin in the line) or has hypertension.	If the catheter has been inadvertently removed, put pressure on the cannulation site. When bleeding has stopped, apply a sterile dressing, estimate blood loss, and inform the physician. If the patient is restless, an armboard may protect lines inserted in the arm.
Air emboli	Ensure that all air bubbles are purged from a new line setup before attachment to an indwelling catheter.	Air can be introduced at several times, including when central venous pressure (CVP) tubing comes apart, when a new line setup is attached, or when a new CVP or pulmonary artery (PA) line is inserted. During insertion of a CVP or PA line, the patient may be asked to hold his or her breath at specific times to prevent drawing air into the chest during inhalation.	Because it is impossible to get the air back once it has been introduced into the blood stream, prevention is the best cure.

TABLE 15-15 Nursing Measures to Ensure Patient Safety and to Troubleshoot Problems with Hemodynamic Monitoring Equipment—cont'd

Problem	Prevention	Rationale	Troubleshooting
Air emboli—cont'd	Ensure that the drip chamber from the bag of flush solution is more than half full before using the in-line, fast-flush system.	The in-line, fast-flush devices are designed to permit clearing of blood from the line after withdrawal of blood samples.	If any air bubbles are noted, they must be vented through the in-line stopcocks and the drip chamber must be filled.
	Some sources recommend removing all air from the bag of flush solution before assembling the system.	If the chamber of the IV tubing is too low or empty, the rapid flow of fluid will create turbulence and cause flushing of air bubbles into the system and into the blood stream.	The left atrial pressure (LAP) line setup is the only system that includes an air filter specifically to prevent air emboli.
Normal waveform with *low* digital pressure	Ensure that the system is calibrated to atmospheric pressure.	To provide a 0 baseline relative to atmospheric pressure.	Recalibrate the equipment if transducer drift has occurred.
	Ensure that the transducer is placed at the level of the phlebostatic axis.	If the transducer has been placed *higher* than the phlebostatic level, gravity and the lack of hydrostatic pressure will produce a false *low* reading.	Reposition the transducer at the level of the phlebostatic axis. Misplacement can occur if the patient moves from the bed to the chair or if the bed is placed in a Trendelenburg position.
Normal waveform with *high* digital pressure	Ensure that the system is calibrated to atmospheric pressure.	To provide a 0 baseline relative to atmospheric pressure.	Recalibrate the equipment if transducer drift has occurred.
	Ensure that the transducer is placed at the level of the phlebostatic axis.	If the transducer has been placed *lower* than the phlebostatic level, the weight of hydrostatic pressure on the transducer will produce a false *high* reading.	Reposition the transducer at the level of the phlebostatic axis. This situation can occur if the head of the bed was raised and the transducer was not repositioned. Some centers require attachment of the transducer to the patient's chest to avoid this problem.
Loss of waveform	Always have the hemodynamic waveform monitored so that changes or loss can be quickly noted.	The catheter may be kinked, or a stopcock may be turned off.	Check the line setup to ensure that all stopcocks are turned in the correct position and that the tubing is not kinked. Sometimes the catheter migrates against a vessel wall, and having the patient change position restores the waveform.

on the specific needs of the patient. They are made from polyvinyl chloride and are very soft and flexible.

Insertion. The large veins of the upper thorax (subclavian [SC] or internal jugular [IJ]) are most commonly used for percutaneous CVP line insertion. During insertion using the SC or IJ veins, the patient may be placed in a Trendelenburg position. Placing the head in a dependent position causes the internal jugular veins in the neck to become more prominent, facilitating line placement. To minimize the risk of air

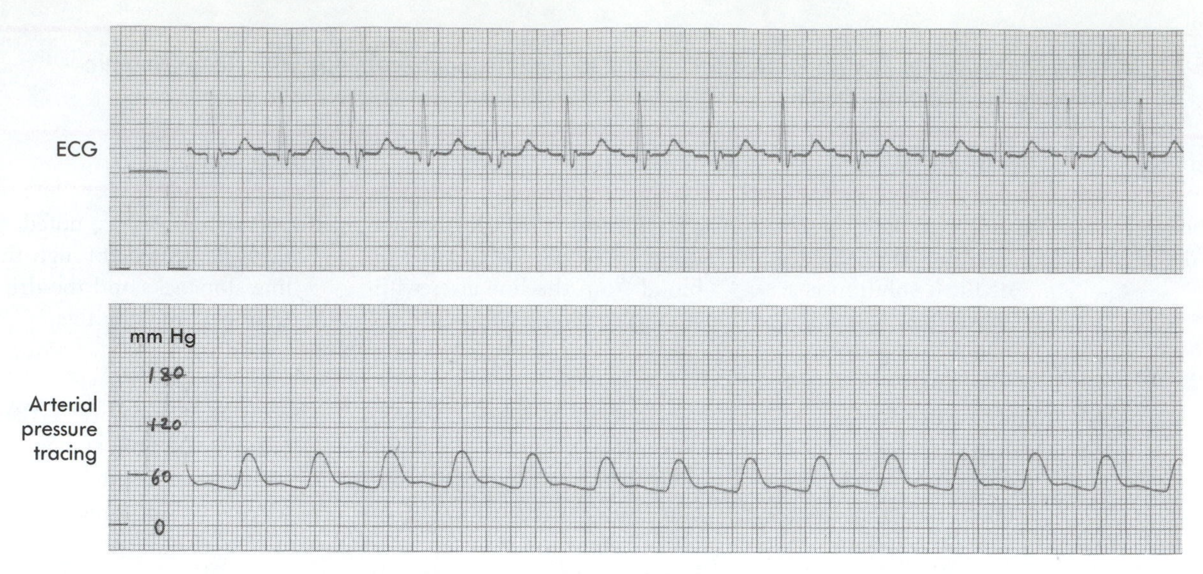

FIGURE 15-63. Simultaneous ECG and arterial pressure tracings show a low arterial pressure waveform.

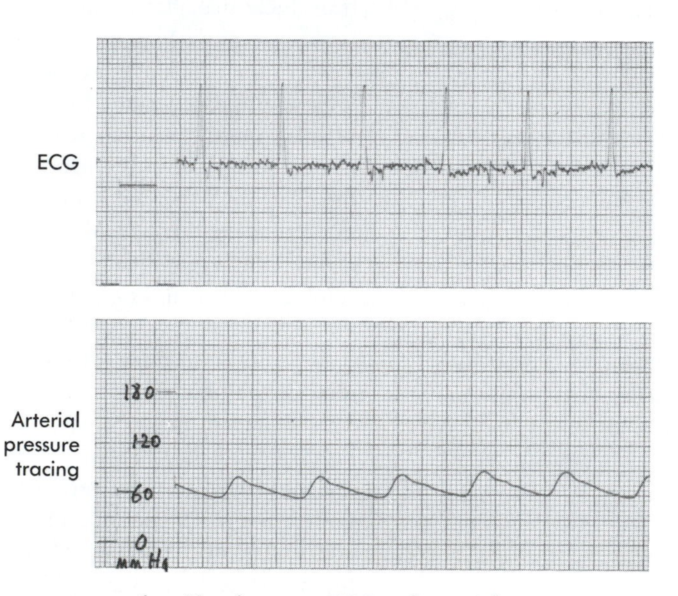

FIGURE 15-64. Simultaneous ECG and arterial pressure tracings show a damped arterial pressure waveform.

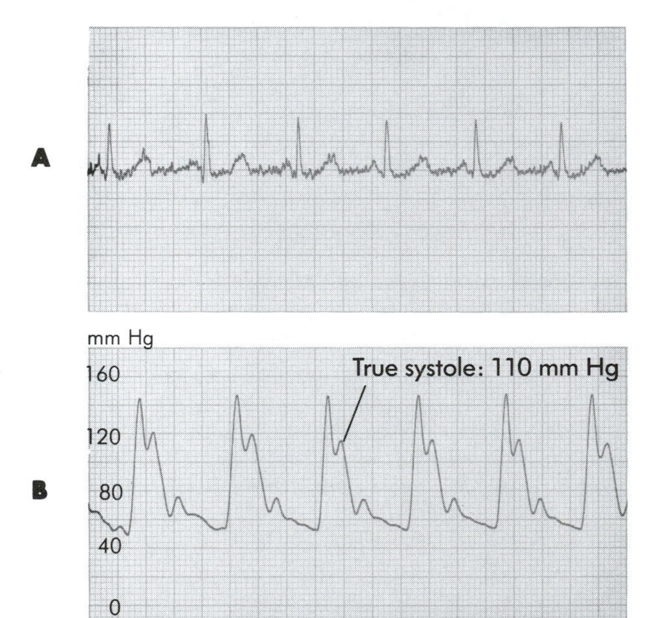

FIGURE 15-65. Simultaneous **A,** ECG and **B,** arterial pressure tracings showing "overshoot" or "fling" caused by a heightened dynamic response in the monitoring system. The monitor recorded an arterial line blood pressure of 141/51 mm Hg. The patient's true blood pressure with cuff was 110/54 mm Hg. The 110 mm Hg cuff systolic is consistent with the arterial line tracing without "overshoot."

embolus during the procedure, the patient may be asked to "take a deep breath and hold it" any time the needle or catheter is open to air. The tip of the catheter is designed to remain in the vena cava and should not migrate into the right atrium. If the IJ or SC veins are not available, the femoral veins can be used for CVP access. The femoral veins are further away from the heart, so for accurate measurements the tip of the catheter must be advanced into the inferior vena cava near the right atrium.[74]

Because many patients are awake and alert when a CVP catheter is inserted, a brief explanation about the procedure will minimize patient anxiety and result in

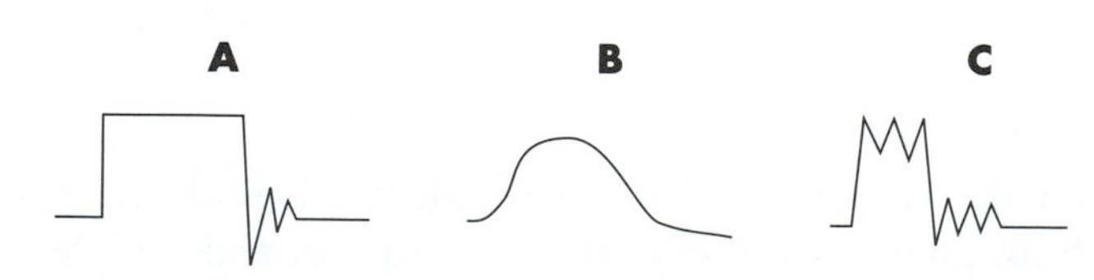

FIGURE 15-66. Fast-flush square wave test. **A,** Normal system dynamic response. **B,** System overdamped. **C,** System underdamped.

cooperation during the insertion. This cooperation is important, because insertion is a sterile procedure and because the supine or Trendelenburg position may not be comfortable for many patients.

CVP catheters are designed for placement by percutaneous injection after skin preparation and administration of a local anesthetic. Usually, a prepackaged CVP kit is used for the procedure. The standard CVP kit contains sterile towels, a needle introducer, syringe, guidewire, and catheter. The Seldinger technique, in which the vein is located by using a needle and syringe, is the preferred method of placement. A guidewire is passed through the needle, the needle is removed, and the catheter is passed over the guidewire. Once the catheter is correctly placed in the vena cava, the guidewire is removed. Finally, an IV setup is attached and the catheter is sutured in place.

After CVP catheter placement, a chest radiograph is obtained to verify placement and the absence of an iatrogenic hemothorax or pneumothorax. Other suitable insertion sites include the femoral and antecubital fossae veins. In the rare case that it is not possible to insert a CVP catheter percutaneously, a surgical cutdown may be performed.

Nursing management. The CVP catheter is used to measure the filling pressures of the right side of the heart. During diastole, when the tricuspid valve is open and blood is flowing from the right atrium to the right ventricle, the CVP accurately reflects right ventricular end-diastolic pressure (RVEDP). The normal CVP is 2 to 5 mm Hg (3 to 8 cm H_2O).

Low CVP. A low CVP often occurs in the hypovolemic patient and suggests there is insufficient blood volume in the ventricle at end-diastole to produce an adequate stroke volume. Thus to maintain normal cardiac output, the heart rate must increase. This increase produces the tachycardia often observed in hypovolemic states and increases myocardial oxygen demand.

The CVP is used in combination with the mean arterial pressure (MAP) and other clinical parameters to assess hemodynamic stability. In the hypovolemic patient, the CVP falls before there is a significant fall in MAP, because peripheral vasoconstriction keeps the MAP normal. Thus the CVP is an excellent early warning system for the patient who is bleeding, vasodilating, receiving diuretics, or rewarming after cardiac surgery.

High CVP. An elevated CVP occurs in cases of fluid overload. To circulate the excess blood volume, the heart must greatly increase its contractile force to move the large volume of blood. This increases the cardiac workload and increases myocardial oxygen consumption. The critical care nurse follows the trend of the CVP measurements to determine subsequent interventions for optimal fluid volume management.

CVP limitations. The CVP is not a reliable indicator of left ventricular dysfunction. Left ventricular dysfunction, which can occur after an acute myocardial infarction, increases filling pressures on the left side of the heart. The CVP, because it measures RVEDP, remains normal until the increase in pressure from the left side of the heart is reflected back through the pulmonary vasculature to the right ventricle. In this situation a pulmonary artery catheter that measures pressures on the left side of the heart is the monitoring method of choice. (∞Pulmonary Artery Pressure Monitoring, p. 459.)

Water versus mercury CVP. To take CVP measurements the clinician can choose from two methods: either a mercury (mm Hg) system, using a transducer and a hemodynamic monitor, or a water (cm H_2O) manometer system. If a patient changes from one system to the other, the CVP value will also change because mercury is heavier than water and 1 mm Hg is equal to 1.36 cm H_2O. To convert water to mercury, the water value is divided by 1.36 ($H_2O \div 1.36$). To convert mercury to water, the mercury value is multiplied by 1.36 (mm Hg $\times$ 1.36).

Patient position. To achieve accurate CVP measurements, the phlebostatic axis is used as a reference point on the body, and the transducer or water manometer zero must be level with this point. If the phlebostatic axis is used and the transducer or water manometer is correctly aligned, any head-of-bed position of up to 60 degrees may be accurately used for CVP readings for most patients. Elevating the head of the bed is especially helpful for the patient with respiratory or cardiac problems who will not tolerate a flat position.[71]

Air embolus. The risk of air embolus, although uncommon, is always present for the patient with a central venous line in place. Air can enter during insertion, through a disconnected or broken catheter, or along the path of a removed CVP catheter. This is more likely if the patient is in an upright position, because air can be pulled into the venous system with the increase in negative intrathoracic pressure during inhalation. If a large volume of air (200 to 300 ml) is infused rapidly, it may become trapped in the right ventricular outflow tract, stopping blood flow from the right side of the heart to the lungs. The patient may experience respiratory distress and cardiovascular collapse. Treatment involves administering 100% oxygen and placing the patient on the left side with the head downward (left lateral Trendelenburg position). This position displaces the air from the right ventricular outflow tract to the apex of the heart, where it can be either resorbed or aspirated. Precautions to prevent an air embolism in a CVP line include using only Luer-Lok connections, avoiding long loops of IV tubing, and using screw caps on three-way stopcocks.

Infection. Infection related to the use of CVP catheters is a major problem. It is estimated that more than 50,000 infections related to catheter use occur annually in the United States with a 10% to 20% associated mortality.[75] Risk factors include extremes of age, impaired host defense mechanisms, severe illness, malnutrition, and presence of other invasive lines. Generalized manifestations of infection are often present, however, inflammation at the catheter site is often absent.[75] To determine whether the catheter is contaminated, after removal, the tip is placed in a sterile container and cultured. The CVP catheter is left in place until there is evidence of infection. No decrease in infections was found when catheters were routinely changed every 3 days.[75] Catheters changed over guidewires usually have a higher rate of infection.[76] Prevention is the best defense against complications resulting from infections. Most infections are transmitted via the skin. Therefore current recommendations include that the physician use optimal sterile technique during catheter insertion, including maximal barrier precautions and chlorhexidine site preparation.

Nurses are to follow aseptic procedures in site care and any time they enter the system to withdraw blood, give medications, or change tubing. There is a higher incidence of infection with transparent occlusive dressings that do not allow removal of moisture. Therefore nonocclusive dressings such as cotton gauze or other moisture-permeable dressings are recommended.[75] Site dressings that have antimicrobial properties are now being developed to try to lower infection rates. New developments in catheter design may also help to reduce central line infection. Catheters are available that are impregnated with an antimicrobial substance or have a silver-impregnated, tissue-barrier cuff attached to the catheter. These catheters are designed to lower the rate of central line infection.[75]

CVP waveform interpretation. The normal right atrial (CVP) waveform has three positive deflections—called *a, c,* and *v waves*—that correspond to specific atrial events in the cardiac cycle[77] (Figure 15-67). The *a wave* reflects atrial contraction and follows the P wave seen on the ECG. The downslope of this wave is called the *x descent* and represents atrial relaxation. The *c wave* reflects the bulging of the closed tricuspid valve into the right atrium during ventricular contraction. The *c wave* is small and not always visible but corresponds to the QRS-T interval on the ECG. The *v wave* represents atrial filling and increased pressure against the closed tricuspid valve in early diastole. The downslope of the *v wave* is named the *y descent* and represents the fall in pressure as the tricuspid valve opens and blood flows from the right atrium to the right ventricle.

Cannon waves. Dysrhythmias can change the pattern of the CVP waveform. In a junctional rhythm or after a premature ventricular contraction (PVC), the atria are depolarized after the ventricles if there is retrograde conduction to the atria. This may be seen as a retrograde P wave on the ECG and as a large combined *ac wave* or *cannon wave* on the CVP waveform (Figure 15-68). These cannon waves can be easily detected as large "pulses" in the jugular veins.[77] Other pathologic conditions, such as advanced right ventricular failure or tricuspid valve insufficiency, allow regurgitant backflow of blood from the right ventricle to the right atrium during ventricular contraction, producing large *v waves* on the right atrial waveform. In atrial fibrillation the CVP waveform has no recognizable pattern because of the disorganization of the atria.

Left Atrial Pressure Monitoring

Indications. Left atrial pressure (LAP) monitoring is used in selected cases after major cardiac surgery. Until the advent of the pulmonary artery catheter in the 1970s, LAP monitoring was used to assess hemodynamics on the left side of the heart. Today it is not used for routine monitoring. It is a clinical choice on rare occasions in the postoperative management of the cardiac surgery patient who has significant pulmonary hypertension. In this situation, accurate left atrial pressures may be difficult to obtain with a pulmonary artery catheter.

Insertion. The LAP catheter is inserted into the left atrium during open heart surgery. The single-lumen catheter exits through the chest wall and is attached to a routine hemodynamic monitoring setup that contains an in-line air filter.

Nursing management. The placement of the LAP catheter directly into the left atrium places the patient at particular risk for air or tissue emboli. Nursing care is planned to reduce these equipment-related risks. An in-line air filter is added to the flush system that contains heparin to reduce the risk of air emboli. If the waveform becomes damped, noninvasive methods of troubleshooting—such as repositioning the patient—are performed. The catheter is not manually flushed, because to do so may increase the risk of emboli, resulting from clot formation at the tip of the catheter. Pericardial tamponade is a potential complication of LAP catheter removal. Therefore mediastinal chest

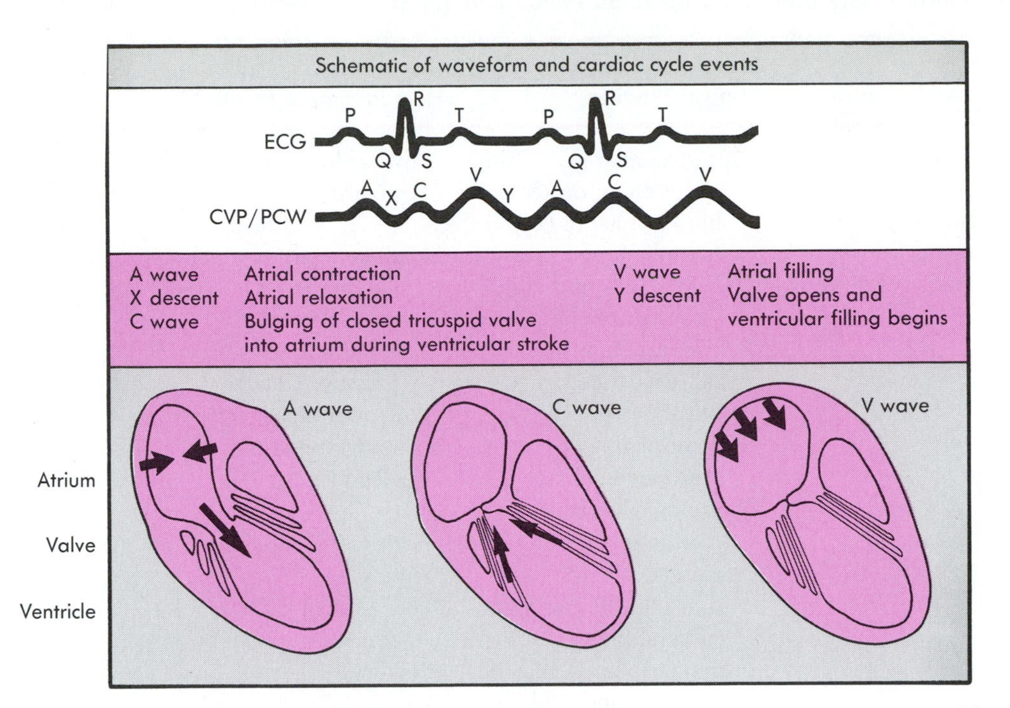

FIGURE 15-67. Cardiac events that produce the CVP waveform with a, c, and v waves. A wave represents atrial contraction. X descent represents atrial relaxation. C wave represents the bulging of the closed tricuspid valve into the right atrium during ventricular systole. V wave represents atrial filling. Y descent represents opening of the tricuspid valve and filling of the ventricle.

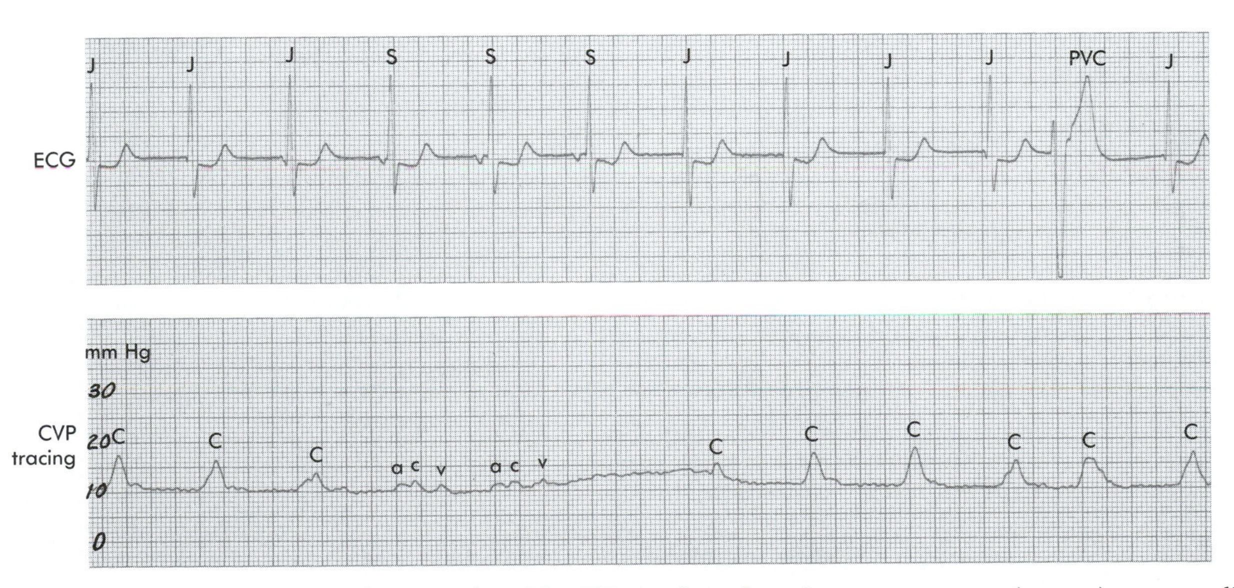

FIGURE 15-68. Simultaneous ECG and CVP tracings. The CVP waveform shows large cannon waves (c waves) corresponding to the junctional beats or premature ventricular contractions *(strip above)*. As the patient converts to sinus rhythm, the CVP waveform has a normal configuration. J, Junctional rhythm followed by cannon waves on CVP waveform; *PVC,* premature ventricular contraction followed by cannon wave on CVP; S, sinus rhythm followed by normal CVP tracing with a, c, and v waves; *C,* cannon waves on CVP tracing; *ac,* normal right atrial pressure tracing.

tubes are left in position until after the catheter is removed. Because of these risks, the LAP catheter is rarely left in place for more than 48 hours.

LAP waveform interpretation. The LAP waveform consists of two positive deflections, which are termed the *a* and *v waves.* The *a wave* represents atrial contraction, and the *v wave* represents filling of the left atrium against a closed mitral valve. Normal LAP pressure ranges from 5 to 12 mm Hg and is elevated with mitral valve disease or severe heart failure on the left side.

TABLE 15-16 **Pulmonary Artery Catheters: Selected Indications for Use and Response to Treatment**

Diagnostic Indications*	Possible Cause	Associated Clinical Findings	Hemodynamic Profile†	Treatment and Expected Response
Hypovolemic shock	Trauma Surgery Bleeding Burns Excessive diuresis	Cardiovascular (CV): sinus tachycardia, decreased blood pressure (BP) (systolic blood pressure [SBP] <90 mm Hg), weak peripheral pulses Pulmonary: lungs clear Renal: decreased urinary output Skin: normal skin temperature, no edema Neurologic: variable	Low cardiac output (CO) Low cardiac index (CI) (<2.2 L/min/m^2) High systemic vascular resistance (SVR) (>1600 dynes/sec/cm^{-5}) Low pulmonary artery pressure (PAP) Low pulmonary artery wedge pressure (PAWP)	Treatment: fluid challenge Expected hemodynamic response: Decreased heart rate (HR) Increased BP Increased PAP Increased PAWP Increased central venous pressure (CVP) Increased CO/CI Decreased SVR
Early septic shock	Sepsis	CV: sinus tachycardia, decreased BP (SBP <90 mm Hg), bounding peripheral pulses Pulmonary: lungs may be clear *or* congested, depending on the origin of the sepsis Renal: decreased urinary output Skin: warm and flushed Neurologic: variable	High CO (>8 L/min) High CI Low SVR (<600 dynes/sec/cm^{-5}) Low PAP Low PAWP Low CVP	Treatment: IV fluid to maintain hemodynamic function Peripheral vasoconstricting agent (alpha) to increase SVR Antibiotics and laboratory cultures to find site of infection Expected hemodynamic response: Decreased HR Increased BP Increased PAP Increased PAWP Increased CVP Increased CO/CI Increased SVR
Advanced septic shock or multisystem failure shock	Sepsis Multiple Organ Dysfunction Syndrome (MODS)	CV: normal sinus rhythm or sinus tachycardia, decreased BP, weak peripheral pulses Pulmonary: lungs may be clear *or* congested, depending on the site of sepsis; acidosis based on arterial blood gas (ABG) values, may require mechanical ventilation Renal: decreased urinary output, may have increased blood urea nitrogen (BUN) and increased creatinine levels Skin: cool and mottled Neurologic: variable, depending on fluid status and drugs used in treatment	Low CO Low CI (<2.2 L/min/m^2) High SVR (>1600 dynes/sec/cm^{-5}) High or low PAP High or low PAWP High or low CVP	Treatment: Vasodilators to decrease SVR Antibiotics Support of body systems as necessary (e.g., mechanical ventilation or hemodialysis) Expected hemodynamic response: Decreased HR Increased BP Normal PAP/PAWP/CVP Decreased SVR, decreased pulmonary vascular resistance Increased CO/CI

*Patients undergoing major vascular or cardiac surgery may also have a PA catheter in situ to follow the trend of CO/CI, SVR/PVR, and fluid status during the first 24 hours after surgery.

†See Table 15-14 for definitions and Appendix D for normal values of hemodynamic parameters listed in this table.

TABLE 15-16 Pulmonary Artery Catheters: Selected Indications for Use and Response to Treatment—cont'd

Diagnostic Indications*	Possible Cause	Associated Clinical Findings	Hemodynamic Profile†	Treatment and Expected Response
Cardiogenic shock	Left ventricular pump failure caused by acute myocardial infarction or severe mitral or aortic valve disease	CV: sinus tachycardia, possibly dysrhythmias, systolic BP <90 mm Hg, S_3 or S_4, weak peripheral pulses Pulmonary: lungs may have crackles or pulmonary edema Renal: decreased urinary output Skin: cool, pale, and moist Neurologic: may have decreased mentation caused by low BP and CO	Low CO Low CI (<2.2 L/min/m²) High SVR (>1600 dynes/sec/cm⁻⁵) High PAP High PAWP (>15 mm Hg) High CVP Low stroke volume index (SI) Low left cardiac work index (LCWI) Low left ventricular stroke work index (LVSWI)	Treatment: Inotropic drugs to increase left ventricular contractility Vasodilators or intraaortic balloon pump (IABP) to decrease afterload Diuretics to decrease preload Optimization of heart rate and control of dysrhythmias Expected hemodynamic response: Decreased HR Increased BP Decreased PAP Decreased PAWP Decreased CVP Decreased SVR Decreased PVR Increased CO/CI Increased SI Increased LCWI Increased LVSWI
Acute respiratory distress syndrome (ARDS) *or* noncardiogenic pulmonary edema	Trauma Sepsis Shock Inhaled toxins (smoke, chemicals, 100% oxygen) Aspiration of gastric contents Metabolic disorders	CV: sinus tachycardia, high or low BP, normal peripheral pulses Pulmonary: poor oxygenation and pulmonary edema, increased respiratory rate, or need for mechanical ventilation Renal: increased or decreased urinary output Skin: normal temperature Neurologic: anxiety or confusion associated with respiratory distress and poor oxygenation	Normal CO Normal CI Normal SVR Normal PAWP High PAP High PVR (>250 dynes/sec/cm⁻⁵) Low right cardiac work index (RCWI) Low right ventricular stroke work index (RVSWI)	Treatment: Eliminate cause of ARDS Support pulmonary function as necessary Expected hemodynamic response: Decreased HR Normal BP Decreased PAP Decreased PVR Increased RCWI Increased RVSWI Normal CO/CI Normal SVR

Pulmonary Artery Pressure Monitoring

Indications. When specific hemodynamic and intracardiac data are required for diagnostic and treatment purposes, a thermodilution pulmonary artery (PA) catheter may be inserted. This catheter is used for diagnosis and evaluation of heart disease, shock states, and medical conditions that compromise cardiac output or fluid volume. In addition, the PA catheter is used to evaluate patient response to treatment, as described in Table 15-16.

A significant advantage of the PA catheter over the previously described methods of monitoring is that it simultaneously assesses several hemodynamic parameters—including pulmonary artery systolic and diastolic pressures, the pulmonary artery mean pressure, and the pulmonary artery wedge pressure (PAWP)—and includes the capability of measuring cardiac output and of calculating additional hemodynamic parameters.[78]

Cardiac output determinants. Cardiac output is the product of heart rate multiplied by stroke volume.* *Stroke volume* (SV) is the volume of blood ejected by the heart each beat in milliliters. The normal adult SV is 50 to 70 ml. The clinical factors that contribute to the heart's stroke volume are preload, afterload, and contractility (Figure 15-69). All three of these can be measured by the pulmonary artery catheter. Another factor of CO is heart rate, which is recorded by the ECG leads or by clinical assessment.

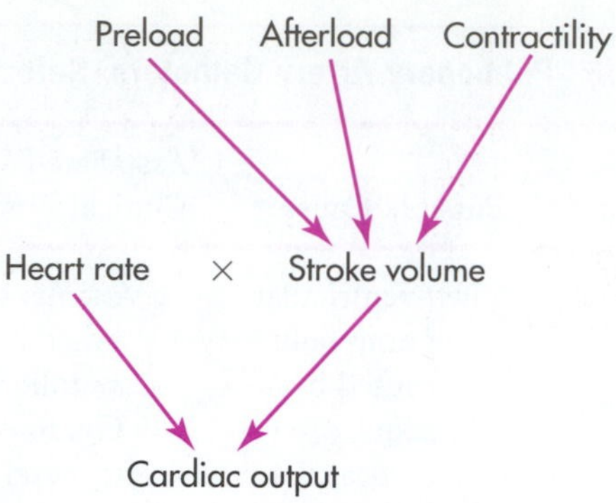

FIGURE 15-69. Preload, afterload, and contractility all contribute to the heart's stroke volume. Stroke volume × heart rate = cardiac output.

Oxygen supply and demand. In the healthy heart when the peripheral tissues need more oxygen—for example during exercise or fever—the normal heart can augment both heart rate and stroke volume and greatly increase cardiac output. In the critically ill patient when the tissues require more oxygen these normal mechanisms are often nonfunctional, and it is the critical care nurse who assesses the need for and optimizes hemodynamic function. The following discussion provides a basic understanding of the clinical factors that determine cardiac output and the role of the critical care nurse in caring for the patient with an alteration in any of these factors. (Hemodynamic Pressure Monitoring: Concepts)

Preload. Clinicians commonly describe the hemodynamic numbers related to preload as "filling pressures." These numbers include pulmonary artery diastolic (PAD) pressure, left atrial pressure (LAP), and pulmonary artery wedge pressure (PAWP), which measure preload in the left side of the heart; and CVP, which measures preload in the right side of the heart.

Preload is the *volume* in the ventricle at end-diastole. Because diastole is the filling stage of the cardiac cycle, the volume in the ventricle at end-diastole represents the presystolic volume available for ejection for that cardiac cycle. It is not possible to measure left ventricular volume directly in the critical care unit. However, the presence of blood within the ventricle creates pressures that can be measured by the PA catheter and transducer, and can be displayed on the bedside monitor.

Measurement of preload. When the PA catheter is correctly positioned, with the tip in one of the large branches of the pulmonary artery, the only valve between the PA catheter tip and the left ventricle is the mitral valve. During diastole, when the mitral valve is open, there is no obstruction between the tip of the PA catheter and the left ventricle (Figure 15-70). The left ventricular preload volume creates *left ventricular end-diastolic pressure (LVEDP)*. This is measured clinically by the *left atrial pressure (LAP)* or the *pulmonary artery wedge pressure (PAWP)*. The PAWP and PAD are the values most frequently referred to in this chapter, because they are the values most often used in clinical practice. Normal LAP or PAWP is 5 to 12 mm Hg.

Starlings's law of the heart. Clinically the PAWP has significance because a change in left ventricular volume (preload) is reflected by a change in the measured PAWP. Change in preload relies on a concept known as *Starling's law of the heart*. This concept states that the force of ventricular ejection is directly related to two elements: (1) the volume in the ventricle at end-diastole (preload) and (2) the amount of myocardial stretch placed on the ventricle as a result. If the volume in the left ventricle is low, CO is also suboptimal. If intravenous fluids (volume) are infused, CO increases as LV volume and myocardial fiber stretch increase. This is true up to a point. Past this point, more fluid volume overdistends the ventricle and stretches the myocardial fibers so much that cardiac output actually decreases. This scenario is seen clinically in the setting of acute heart failure with pulmonary edema. The impact of preload on CO is represented in Figures 15-71 and 15-72, using the Starling curve as a model. (∞Preload, p. 350.)

Ejection fraction. The relationship of preload to the cardiac output is complex. This is because not all preload volume is ejected with every heartbeat. The percentage of preload volume ejected from the left ven-

*Heart rate × stroke volume = cardiac output

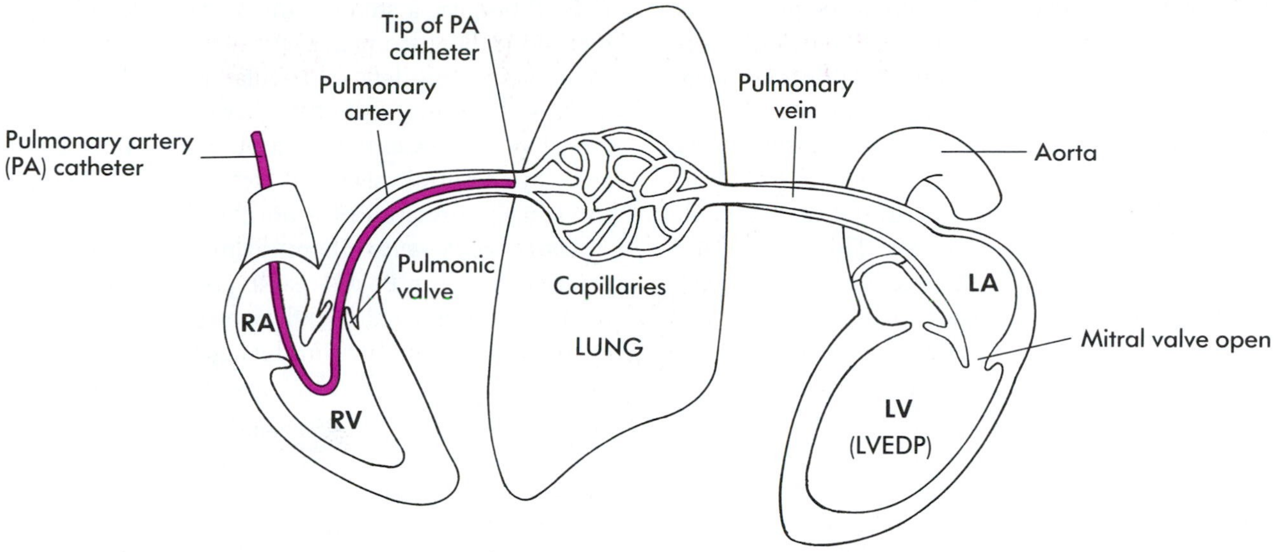

Tip of PA catheter
Pulmonary artery
Pulmonary artery (PA) catheter
Pulmonary vein
Aorta
Pulmonic valve
Capillaries
LUNG
LA
RA
RV
Mitral valve open
LV (LVEDP)

FIGURE 15-70. Relationship of PAWP to LVEDP/preload. This diagram illustrates why, in the majority of clinical situations, the PAWP accurately reflects LVEDP, or preload. During diastole, when the mitral valve is open, there are no other valves or other obstructions between the tip of the catheter and the left ventricle. Thus the pressure exerted by the volume in the LV is reflected back through the left atrium through the pulmonary veins and to the pulmonary capillaries.

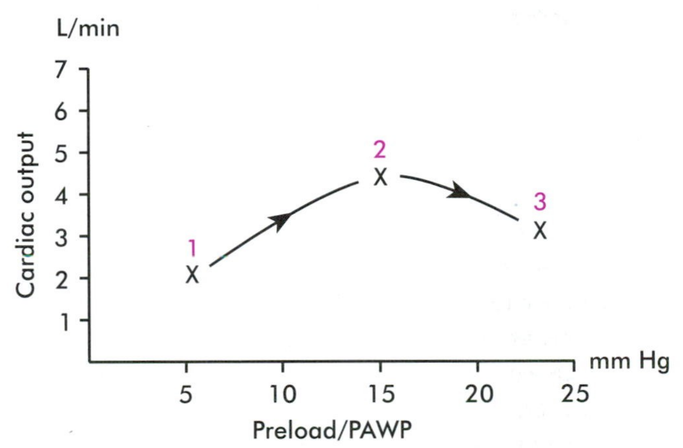

FIGURE 15-71. Impact of preload on cardiac output. *1,* Poor CO with low preload as a result of hypovolemia. *2,* Hypovolemia is corrected after the administration of 2 L of intravenous (IV) fluid. The preload volume in the ventricle is increased, and PAWP has risen. Because of the increased fiber stretch secondary to the increase in preload, CO has also risen. *3,* After the infusion of 2 more liters of IV solution, the myocardial fibers are overdistended, preload (PAWP) has increased, and CO has fallen as the volume in the left ventricle rises.

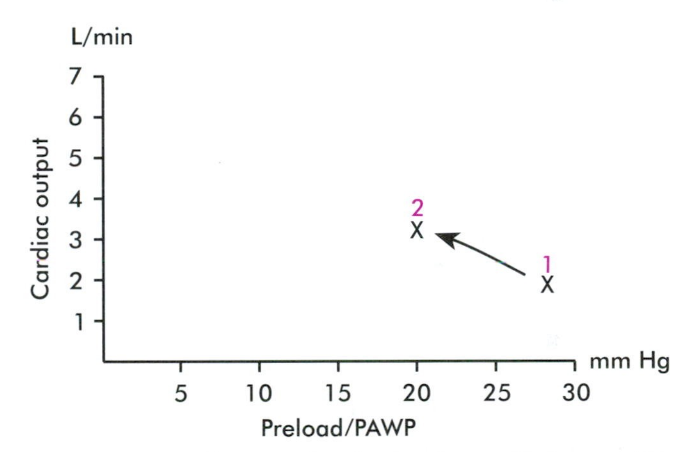

FIGURE 15-72. Impact of preload and venodilation on CO. *1,* After an acute anterior wall myocardial infarction that has created significant left ventricular dysfunction, this patient has LV pump failure with low CO and elevated filling pressures (↑ PAWP). One of the clinical problems faced by this patient is too much preload. *2,* After administration of diuretics to remove volume and nitroglycerin to dilate the venous system, preload is reduced and CO rises.

tricle per beat is measured during cardiac catheterization and is described as the *ejection fraction (EF).* A normal ejection fraction in a healthy heart is 70%. The volume ejected from the left ventricle with each beat is known as the *stroke volume (SV)* and can be calculated at the bedside by dividing the CO by the heart rate per minute.

Myocardial dysfunction. A significant relationship exists between LVEDP and myocardial dysfunction. As a general rule, the higher the LVEDP, the greater is the degree of myocardial dysfunction, because the compromised ventricle is unable to eject all of the preload blood volume. The greater the degree of myocardial dysfunction, the lower is the ejection fraction and the higher the preload and LVEDP. Hemodynamically this translates into elevated PAWP and PAD pressures.

In a patient with dilated cardiomyopathy, the preload volume might be 100 ml. However, the stroke volume ejected may be only 30 ml. The ejection fraction in this patient is 30% (normal EF is 70%). The remaining preload volume (70 ml in this example) will significantly elevate PAWP. When the mitral valve opens at the beginning of diastole, the pressure in the left atrium (LA) needs to be slightly higher than pressures in the LV to allow filling. The 70 ml remaining in the ventricle will produce high LV diastolic pressures. This will elevate the LA filling pressure and consequently elevate PAWP. In this example the left ventricle is overstretched by excessive preload, and therefore CO will be below normal. A plan of care for this patient would include decreasing LV preload through restriction of IV/PO fluids, venodilation, and diuresis.

PAD/PAWP relationship. LVEDP can be measured by two methods using a PA catheter. The most accurate is the PAWP. The second method involves using pulmonary artery diastolic (PAD) pressure, because during diastole in most patients, the PAD is equal to or 1 to 3 mm Hg higher than the mean PAWP and LVEDP.

It is physiologically impossible for the PAWP to ever be higher than the PAD pressure. The nurse must recalibrate and troubleshoot the monitoring system if this appears to occur (see Table 15-15).

Pulmonary hypertension. It is important to be aware that specific clinical conditions can alter the normal PAD/PAWP relationship. If the patient has vascular lung disease that has elevated the PA pressures independently from the cardiac pressures, the PAD pressure will not accurately reflect function of the left side of the heart. The clinical conditions that cause PA pressures to rise but PAWP to remain normal are primary pulmonary hypertension and acute respiratory distress syndrome (ARDS). The numerical difference between the PAD and the PAWP values is called a *gradient.* If there is a large gradient between the PAWP and PAD pressure when the PA catheter is inserted, the patient has pulmonary hypertension (Table 15-17, *C*).

Heart failure. In failure of the left side of the heart, both the PAWP and the PAD pressure are elevated and approximately equal (Table 15-17, *B*). The heart failure may cause secondary pulmonary hypertension. In other words, over time, the damage to the lung vasculature occurs because of exposure to high cardiac pressures.

Mitral stenosis. Pathology of the mitral valve, either stenosis or regurgitation, alters the accuracy of PAWP and PAD pressures as parameters of left ventricular function. In mitral valve stenosis, left atrial pressure and PAWP are increased and cause pulmonary congestion; however, these values are *not* reflective of LVEDP because a stenotic mitral valve decreases normal blood flow from the left atrium to the left ventricle, decreasing left ventricular preload and consequently lowering LVEDP. Therefore a nonstenotic mitral valve is essential for accurate readings because a narrowed mitral valve increases PAWP and PAD pressures in the presence of a normal LVEDP.

Mitral regurgitation. If mitral regurgitation (MR) is present, the mean PAWP reading is artificially elevated because of abnormal backflow of blood from the left ventricle to the left atrium during systole. This PAWP reading is distinguished by very large v waves on the PAWP tracing and may not be reflective of true LVEDP (Table 15-17, *F*).

The v waves can be dramatic in some patients. However, the size of the v wave is not related to the amount of mitral regurgitation, but to the compliance of the left atrium. If the mitral regurgitation is chronic and the left atrium is compliant, v waves may not be large. By contrast, in the setting of acute mitral regurgitation after infarction of a papillary muscle, the noncompliant atrium contributes to the large v waves. Reading the PAWP tracing in the presence of mitral regurgitation is difficult. It has been suggested that if there are large v waves (acute MR), the trough of the x descent is the best predictor of LVEDP. If the v wave is small (chronic MR), the mean PAWP or LAP pressure can still estimate LV preload (LVEDP).

Afterload. *Afterload* is defined as the pressure the ventricle has to generate to overcome the resistance to ejection created by the arteries and arterioles. It is a calculated measurement derived from information obtained from the PA catheter. As a response to increased afterload, ventricular wall tension rises. After a decrease in afterload, wall tension is lowered. The technical name for afterload is *systemic vascular resistance.*

Systemic vascular resistance. Resistance to ejection from the left side of the heart is measured by the systemic vascular resistance (SVR). The SVR formula, normally calculated by the bedside computer, is as follows:

$$\frac{\text{MAP} - \text{CVP}}{\text{CO}} \times 80 = \text{SVR}$$

The normal value is 800 to 1200 dynes/sec/cm^{-5}. To index this value to the patient's body surface area, the cardiac index (CI) is placed in the formula in the same position as the CO. The critical care nurse frequently manipulates prescribed vasoactive drugs to therapeutically alter afterload. In general, the lower the SVR, the higher the cardiac output.

Pulmonary vascular resistance. Resistance to ejection from the right side of the heart is measured by the

TABLE 15-17 Clinical Interpretation of Pulmonary Artery (PA) Waveforms

PA Pressure	Clinical Interpretation	mm Hg	Waveform Interpretation
Pulmonary artery systolic (PAS) pressure	PAS pressure reflects the systolic pressure in the pulmonary vasculature. See waveform A for normal waveform. It is elevated in pulmonary hypertension because of idiopathic causes, in some congenital heart defects, and in lung disease.	20, 10	A: Normal (PAS; Dicrotic notch; PAD)
Pulmonary artery diastolic (PAD) pressure	In the patient with healthy lung vasculature, PAD pressure reflects left ventricular end-diastolic pressure (LVEDP), as shown in waveform B. Even if the patient experiences heart failure, the PAWP and PAD increase together.	30, 20, 10	B: PAD/PAWP Correlation in a Patient with Normal Lungs (PAD; PAWP)
	In the presence of ARDS or pulmonary hypertension, PAD pressure is *not* an accurate reflection of pulmonary artery wedge pressure (PAWP), as shown in waveform C.	60, 40, 20, 0	C: Poor PAD/PAWP Correlation in a Patient With Pulmonary Hypertension (PAD; PAWP)
Mean pulmonary artery pressure (PAP mean or PAP_M)	PAP mean pressure is used in the calculation of pulmonary vascular resistance (PVR) and pulmonary vascular resistance index (PVRI), as described in Table 15-14. High mean pressures can be reflective of either cardiac or pulmonary disease. Low mean pressures are reflective of hypovolemia. See waveform D for PAP mean placement.	20, 10, 0	D: Placement of PAP Mean Value (PAS; PAP mean; PAD)
Pulmonary artery wedge pressure (PAWP) or pulmonary capillary wedge pressure (PCWP)	In the healthy patient, PAWP reflects blood in the left ventricle at end-diastole (LVEDP). The normal PAWP waveform is a left atrial waveform, as shown in waveform E.	13, 10	E: Normal PAWP Tracing with a and v Waves (a; v)
	If a patient has mitral valve regurgitation, the v waves are larger than normal, increasing PAWP and possibly not reflecting true LVEDP, as shown in waveform F. PAWP is elevated in many cardiac disease states in which left ventricular function is compromised. PAWP is low in hypovolemic states.	20, 15, 10	F: PAWP Tracing with Elevated v Waves Caused by Mitral Valve Regurgitation (a; v)

pulmonary vascular resistance (PVR). The PVR value is normally one sixth of the SVR. Normal PVR is 50 to 250 dynes/sec/cm^{-5}. The formula for PVR is listed in Appendix D.

Afterload reduction. Pharmacologic manipulation of afterload to improve cardiac performance is commonly used with the critically ill patient. Many drugs, with different modes of action, are available. Drugs that vasodilate the arterial system and reduce SVR when given as a continuous infusion include sodium nitroprusside (Nipride) and high dose nitroglycerin (NTG). Other vasodilators commonly used include IV hydralazine and oral ACE inhibitor drugs. (∞Cardiac Drugs, p. 574.)

If the SVR is extremely low (less than 500 dynes/sec/cm^{-5}) the cardiac output will be elevated and can induce cardiac failure because of the extreme work requirements. In this situation medications may be used to "tighten up" the SVR. If the patient is refractory to dopamine or dobutamine, norepinephrine (Levophed) is used as a vasopressor to vasoconstrict the peripheral vasculature.[79] The critical care nurse evaluates the effectiveness of the medication by the increase in SVR into the therapeutic range. Frequent assessment of the peripheral circulation is required when drugs that increase SVR are used, since excessive vasoconstriction can negatively affect tissue perfusion. (∞Septic Shock, p. 1111.)

Vasodilation of the pulmonary arterial vasculature is achieved by either a nitroglycerin drip (at doses that do not lower the systemic blood pressure) or prostaglandin E_1.

CASE STUDY

Mr. T had a large anterior wall myocardial infarction (MI) 2 days ago. As a result, he has symptoms of acute heart failure, an elevated SVR of 1840 dynes/sec/cm^{-5}, and a low cardiac output of 2.8 L/min. In a heart with decreased contractility after an MI, an afterload measurement above the normal range lowers cardiac output. To optimize Mr. T's cardiac function, systemic vasodilators or "afterload-reducing drugs" are prescribed to lower SVR into the normal range. After the administration of sodium nitroprusside 1 to 4 μg/kg/min, Mr. T's SVR decreased to 970 dynes/sec/cm^{-5} and his cardiac output increased to 4.1 L/min. In this situation, decreasing the systemic resistance to ejection greatly increased the amount of blood ejected from the left ventricle.

In contrast, for the person with a normal heart without cardiac dysfunction, an elevated SVR may have minimal impact on CO. In summary, the importance of afterload on CO is related to the functional quality of the myocardium. Whether the heart muscle is globally damaged (cardiomyopathy) or regionally damaged (MI), small changes in SVR can produce significant changes in cardiac output. (∞Afterload, p. 462.)

Contractility. Many factors have an impact on contractility, including preload volume as measured by PAWP, afterload (SVR), myocardial oxygenation, electrolyte balance, positive and negative inotropic drugs, and the amount of functional myocardium available to contribute to contraction. These factors can have either a positive inotropic effect and enhance contractility or a negative inotropic effect and decrease contractility. Significant factors related to contractility that can be measured by the PA catheter include preload filling pressures, afterload, and cardiac output. Additional contractility numbers can be calculated and are displayed in the hemodynamic profile on the bedside monitor. These include left and right stroke work index values (LVSWI and RVSWI).[80] These values estimate the force of cardiac contraction (see Table 15-14).

Preload has an impact on contractility by Starling's mechanism. As volume in the ventricle rises, contractility increases. If the ventricle is overdistended with volume, contractility falls (see Figures 15-71 and 15-72). Afterload alters contractility by changes in resistance to ventricular ejection. If afterload is high, contractility is decreased. If afterload is low, contractility is augmented. Hypoxemia is known to act as a negative inotrope. The myocardium must have oxygen available to the cells to contract efficiently. Some cardiac drugs can also alter contractility. Calcium channel blocking agents may have a negative inotropic effect. In this case if the cardiac depression is severe, calcium is the antidote, because it is a positive inotrope.

Optimizing contractility. Intravenous drugs such as dopamine and dobutamine are prescribed for their positive inotropic effect, whereas beta-blockers such as propranolol (Inderal) have a negative inotropic effect and lower CO. The nurse considers the impact of these pharmacologic agents on contractility when following the trend of the patient's hemodynamic profile. There is no single hemodynamic number that reflects contractility. However, if LV contractility is increased in response to treatment, this is reflected by changes in PAWP and by an increase in cardiac output and LVSWI.[80] (∞Contractility, p. 350.)

Pulmonary artery catheters. The traditional pulmonary artery (PA) catheter, invented by Swan and Ganz, has four lumens for measurement of right atrial pressure (RAP or CVP), PA pressures, PAWP, and CO[79] (Figure 15-73, *A*). Multifunction catheters may have additional lumens, which can be used for IV infusion (Figure 15-73, *B*), to measure continuous mixed venous oxygen saturation (Svo_2), right ventricular volume (Figure 15-73, *C*), continuous cardiac output (Figure 15-73, *D*), or to pace the heart using transvenous pacing electrodes.[81]

The PA catheter is 110 cm in length, and it is made of polyvinyl chloride. This supple material is ideal for flow-directional catheters. The most commonly used size is 7.5 or 8.0 Fr, although 5.0 and 7.0 Fr sizes are available. Each of the four lumens exits into the heart at a different point along the catheter length (see Figure 15-73, *A*).

Right atrial lumen. The proximal lumen is situated in the right atrium and is used for IV infusion, CVP measurement, withdrawal of venous blood samples, and injection of fluid for CO determinations. This port is often described as the right atrial port (RAP), also called the CVP port.

Pulmonary artery lumen. The distal (PA) lumen is located at the tip of the PA catheter and is situated in the pulmonary artery. It is used to record PA pressures and can be used for withdrawal of blood samples to measure Svo_2.

Balloon lumen. The third lumen opens into a latex balloon at the end of the catheter that can be inflated with 0.8 (7 Fr) to 1.5 (7.5 Fr) ml of air. The balloon is inflated during catheter insertion once the catheter reaches the right atrium to assist in forward flow of the catheter and to minimize right ventricular ectopy from the catheter tip. It is also inflated to obtain PAWP measurements when the PA catheter is correctly positioned in the pulmonary artery.

Thermistor lumen. The fourth lumen is a thermistor used to measure changes in blood temperature. It is located 4 cm from the catheter tip and is used to measure thermodilution CO. The connector end of the lumen is attached directly to the CO computer.

Additional features. If continuous Svo_2 is measured, the catheter has an additional fiberoptic lumen that exits at the tip of the catheter (see Figure 15-73, *C*). If cardiac pacing is used, two PA catheter methods are available. One type of catheter has three atrial (A) and two ventricular (V) pacing electrodes attached to the catheter so that when it is properly positioned, the patient can be connected to a pacemaker and be AV-paced. The other catheter method uses a specific transvenous pacing wire that passes through an additional catheter lumen and exits in the right ventricle if ventricular pacing is required. In addition, a right ventricular volumetric PA catheter is available that measures stroke volume in the RV, as illustrated in Figure 15-73, *C*.

Insertion. If a PA catheter is to be inserted into a patient who is awake, some brief explanations about the procedure are helpful to ensure that the patient understands what is going to happen. The initial insertion techniques used for placement of a PA catheter are similar to those described in the section on CVP line insertion. In addition, because the PA catheter is positioned within the heart chambers and pulmonary artery on the right side of the heart, catheter passage is monitored, using either fluoroscopy or waveform analysis on the bedside monitor (Figure 15-74).

Before inserting the catheter into the vein, the physician—using sterile technique—tests the balloon for inflation and flushes the catheter with normal saline solution to remove any air. The PA catheter is then attached to the bedside hemodynamic line setup and monitor, so that the waveforms can be visualized while the catheter is advanced through the right side of the heart (see Figure 15-74). A larger introducer sheath (8.5 Fr)—which has the tip positioned in the vena cava and an additional IV side-port lumen—is often used to cannulate the vein first. This remains in place, and the supple PA catheter is threaded through the introducer.

Pulmonary artery waveform interpretation.

Right atrial waveform. As the PA catheter is advanced into the right atrium during insertion, a right atrial waveform must be visible on the monitor, with recognizable a, c, and v waves (see Figure 15-74). The normal mean pressure in the right atrium is 2 to 5 mm Hg. Before passage through the tricuspid valve, the balloon at the tip of the catheter is inflated for two reasons. First, it cushions the pointed tip of the PA catheter so that if the tip comes into contact with the right ventricular wall, it will cause less myocardial irritability and consequently fewer ventricular dysrhythmias. Second, inflation of the balloon assists the catheter to float with the flow of blood from the right ventricle into the pulmonary artery. It is because of these features and the balloon that PA catheters are described as flow-directional catheters.

Right ventricular waveform. The right ventricular waveform is pulsatile, with distinct systolic and diastolic pressures. Normal RV pressures are 20 to 30 mm Hg systolic and 0 to 5 mm Hg diastolic. Even with the balloon inflated, it is not uncommon for some ventricular ectopy to occur during passage through the RV. All patients who have a PA catheter inserted must

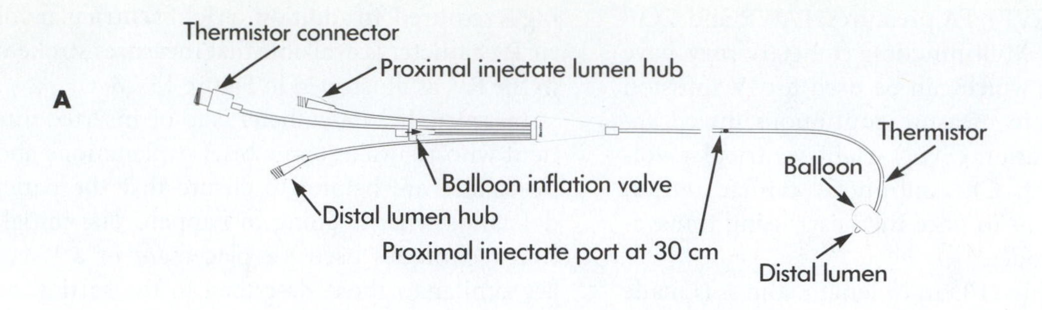

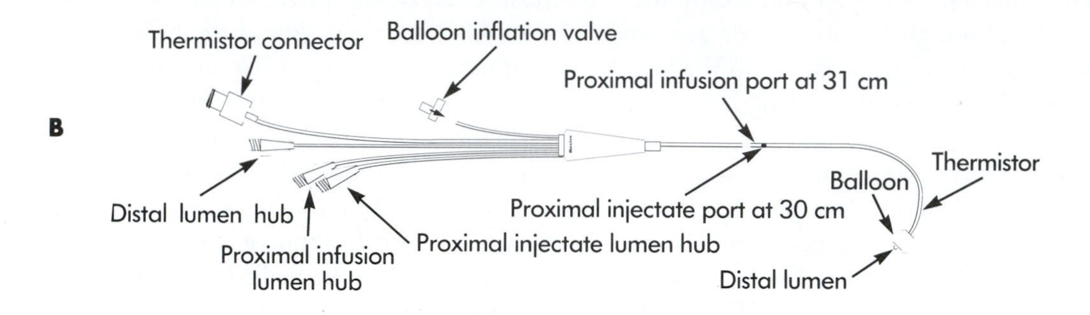

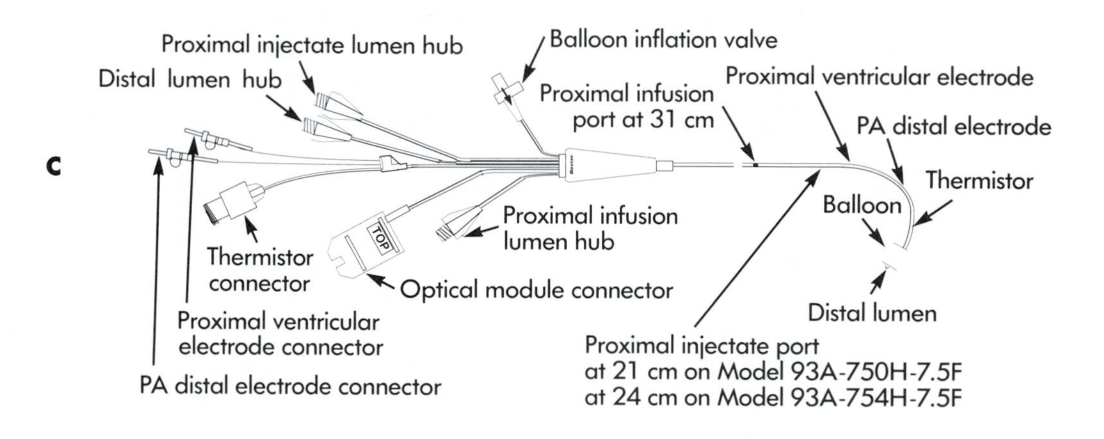

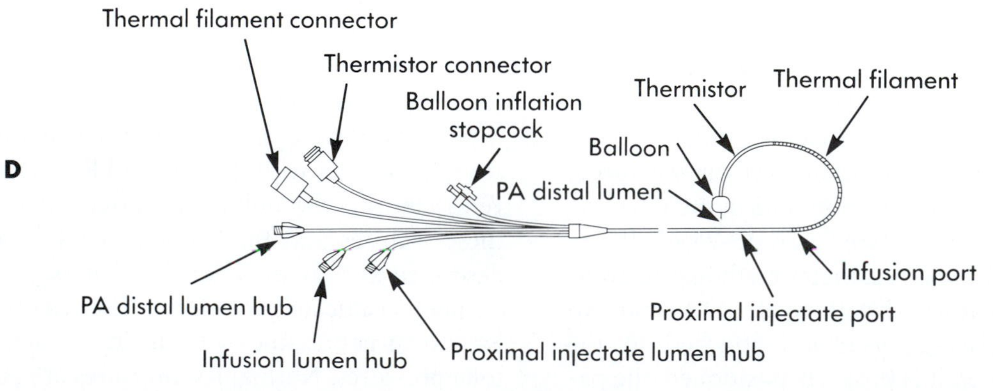

FIGURE 15-73. Types of pulmonary artery catheters available for clinical use. **A,** Four-lumen catheter. **B,** Five-lumen catheter that includes an additional infusion lumen in the right atrium. **C,** Multifunction six-lumen catheter that combines an additional infusion lumen, right ventricular volume measurement, and continuous $S\bar{v}O_2$ monitoring. **D,** Six-lumen catheter with continuous cardiac output capability. (Courtesy Baxter Healthcare Corporation, Edwards Critical Care Division.)

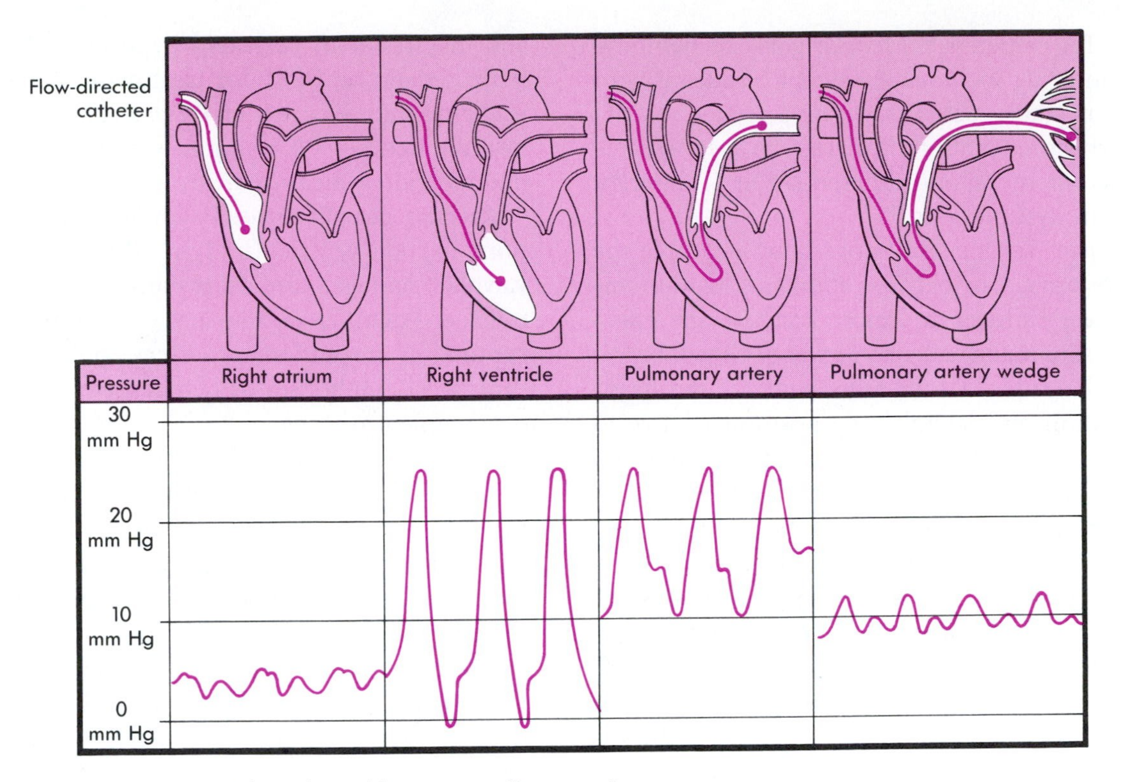

FIGURE 15-74. PA insertion with corresponding waveforms.

have simultaneous electrocardiographic monitoring, with defibrillator and emergency resuscitation equipment nearby.

Pulmonary artery waveform. As the catheter enters the pulmonary artery, the waveform again changes. The diastolic pressure rises. Normal PA pressures range from 20 to 30 mm Hg systolic over 10 mm Hg diastolic. A dicrotic notch, visible on the downslope of the waveform, represents closure of the pulmonic valve.

Pulmonary artery wedge waveform. While the balloon remains inflated, the catheter is advanced into the wedge position. Here, the waveform decreases in size and is pulsatile—reflective of a normal left atrial tracing with *a* and *v wave* deflections. This is described as a *wedge tracing,* because the balloon is "wedged" into a small pulmonary vessel (see Figure 15-74). The balloon occludes the pulmonary vessel so that the PA lumen is exposed only to left atrial pressure and is protected from the pulsatile influence of the PA. When the balloon is deflated, the catheter should spontaneously float back into the PA. When the balloon is reinflated, the wedge tracing should be visible. The normal PAWP ranges from 5 to 12 mm Hg.

After insertion, the catheter is sutured to the skin, and a chest radiograph is taken to verify placement. If the catheter is advanced too far into the pulmonary bed, the patient is at risk for pulmonary infarction. If the catheter is not sufficiently advanced into the PA, it will not be useful for PAWP readings. However, in many critical care units, if the patient's PAD and PAWP values approximate (within 0 to 3 mm Hg), the PAD is reliably used to follow the trend of LV filling pressure (preload). This prevents possible trauma from frequent balloon inflation; in such a situation the PA catheter would be consciously pulled back into a nonwedging position in the pulmonary artery.

After insertion, a chest radiograph or fluoroscopy is used to verify PA catheter position to make sure that it is not looped or knotted in the RV and to rule out pneumothorax or hemorrhagic complications. A thin plastic cuff can be placed on the outside of the catheter when it is inserted to maintain sterility of that part of the PA catheter that exits from the patient. Then, if the catheter is not in the desired position or if it migrates out of position, the PA catheter can be repositioned. The plastic cuff is designed to keep the external catheter sterile for a short period after insertion.

Medical management. There is considerable controversy in the medical community over the routine use of pulmonary artery catheters. Some physicians believe the complication rates associated with PA catheters are too high and discourage their use.[82-84] Others firmly advocate their use and clinical benefit.[85,86] Practice guidelines are available for physicians who routinely work with PA catheters.[87] Medical goals of hemodynamic monitoring include assessment of adequacy of perfusion in stable patients, early detection of decreased perfusion, titration of therapy to meet specific therapeutic outcomes, and differentiation of different organ system dysfunctions.[78]

Nursing management. The more knowledgeable the critical care nurse can become about use of the pulmonary artery catheter, the more accurate and effective the nursing management interventions will be.[63,64]

Factors that affect PA measurement are the head-of-bed position and lateral body position relative to transducer height placement, respiratory variation, and positive end-expiratory pressure (PEEP).

Patient position. In the supine position, if the transducer is placed at the level of the phlebostatic axis, a head-of-bed position from flat up to 60 degrees is appropriate for most patients. PA and PAWP measurements in the lateral position may be significantly different from those taken when the patient is lying supine. At this point, if there is concern over the validity of pressure readings in a particular patient, it is more reliable to take measurements with the patient on his or her back, with the head-of-bed elevated up to 60 degrees. A stabilization period of only 5 minutes is required before taking pressure readings after a patient changes position.[88]

Respiratory variation. All PAD and PAWP tracings are subject to respiratory interference, especially if the patient is on a positive-pressure, volume-cycled ventilator. During inhalation the ventilator "pushes up" the PA tracing, which produces an artificially high reading (Figure 15-75, *A*). During spontaneous respiration, negative intrathoracic pressure "pulls down" the waveform and can produce an erroneously low measurement (Figure 15-75, *B*). To minimize the impact of respiratory variation, the PAD is read at end-expiration, which is the most stable point in the respiratory cycle. If the digital number fluctuates with respiration, a paper readout can be obtained to verify true PAD. In some clinical settings, airway pressure and flow are recorded simultaneously with the PAD/PAWP tracing to identify end-expiration.[70,89]

PEEP. Some clinical diagnoses, such as acute respiratory distress syndrome (ARDS), require the use of high levels of PEEP to treat refractory hypoxemia. If a PEEP of greater than 10 cm H_2O is used, PAWP and PA pressures will be artificially elevated. Because of this impact of PEEP, in the past, patients in some critical care units were taken off the ventilator to record PA pressure measurements. It has since been shown that this practice decreases the patient's oxygenation and may result in persistent hypoxemia. Because patients remain on PEEP for treatment, they remain on it during measurement of PA pressures. In this situation the trend of PA readings is more important than one individual measurement.

Avoiding complications. Potential cardiac complications include ventricular dysrhythmias, endocarditis, valvular damage, cardiac rupture, and cardiac tamponade. Potential pulmonary complications include rupture of a pulmonary artery, pulmonary artery thrombosis, embolism or hemorrhage, and infarction of a segment of lung.

The PA tracing is continuously monitored. This is to ensure that the catheter does not migrate forward into a spontaneous wedge position. A segment of lung can be infarcted if the wedged catheter occludes an arteriole for a prolonged period. If the catheter is wedged the critical care nurse can pull the catheter back out of the wedge position, if the institutional policy allows.[90]

Infection is always a risk with a PA catheter. The risks are similar to those discussed in the section on central venous catheters. (∞Infection, p. 456.)

PA catheter removal. PA catheters are routinely removed by the critical care nurse without major complications.[90,91] The most common incidents are premature ventricular contractions (PVC) as the catheter is pulled through the RV.

Cardiac output. The PA catheter measures cardiac output (CO) using the bolus thermodilution method. This technique can be performed at the bedside and results in CO calculated in liters per minute. Generally, three cardiac outputs that are within a 10% mean range are obtained at one time and are averaged to calculate CO.[92]

Cardiac output method. A known amount (5 ml or 10 ml bolus) of iced or room temperature normal saline solution is injected into the proximal lumen of the catheter. The injectate exits into the right atrium (RA) and travels with the flow of blood past the thermistor (temperature sensor) at the distal end of the catheter in the pulmonary artery. The injectate can be delivered by hand injection via individual syringes of saline or, as done more commonly, by a closed in-line system attached to a 500 ml bag of normal saline.

Sometimes the right atrial (proximal) port is clotted off and not usable. If another right atrial port is available, this can be substituted.[93] However, if a usable port is not available, to ensure accurate cardiac output data, a new pulmonary artery catheter is inserted.

Cardiac output curve. The thermodilution CO method uses the indicator-dilution principle, in which a known temperature is the indicator. It is based on

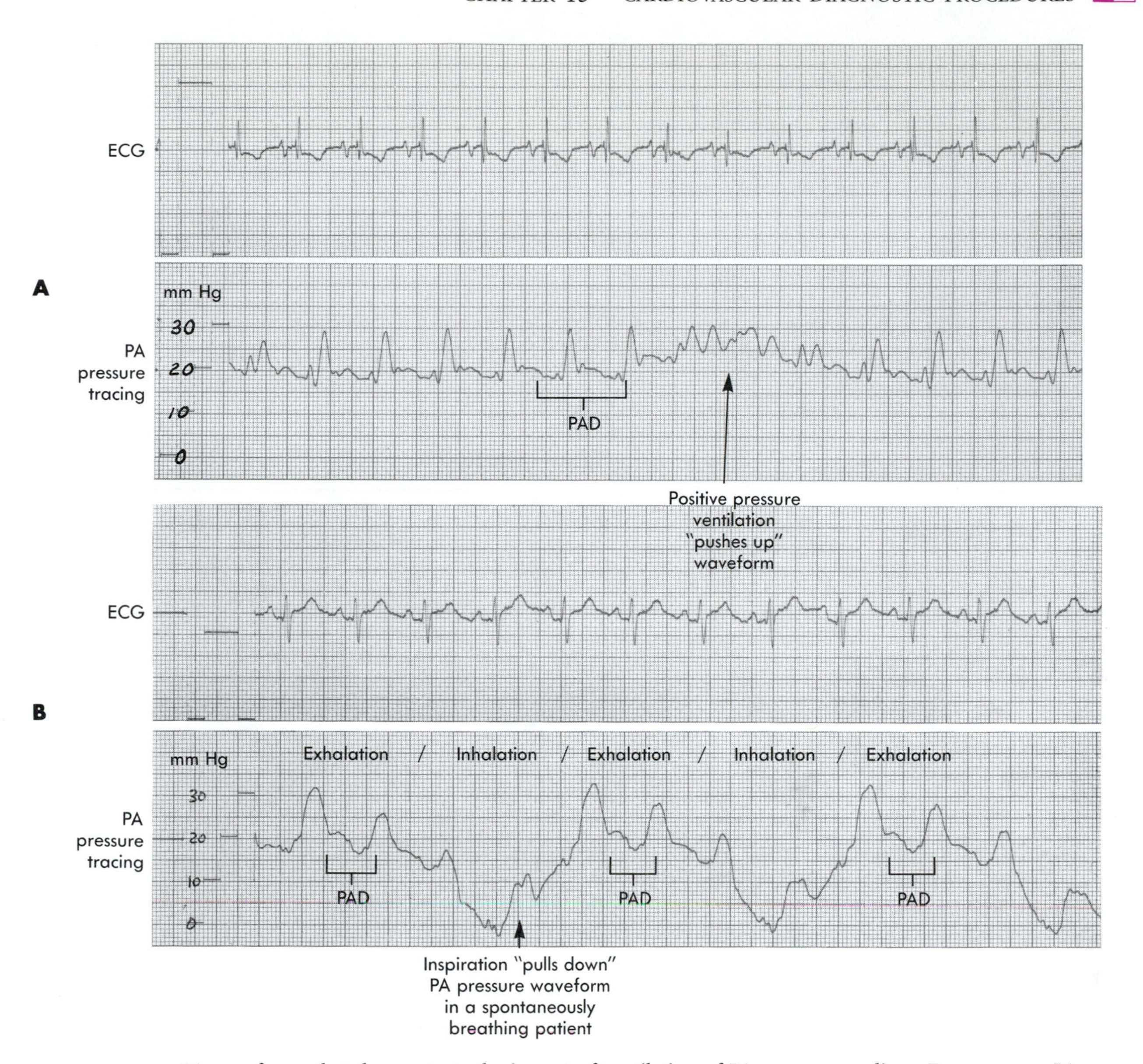

FIGURE 15-75. PA waveforms that demonstrate the impact of ventilation of PA pressure readings. For accuracy, PA pressures are read at end-exhalation. **A,** Positive pressure ventilation: the increase in intrathoracic pressure during inhalation "pushes up" the PA pressure waveform, creating a false high reading. **B,** Spontaneous breathing: the decrease in intrathoracic pressure during normal inhalation "pulls down" the PA waveform, creating a false low reading.

the principle that the change in temperature over time is inversely proportional to blood flow. Blood flow can be diagrammatically represented as a cardiac output curve, on which temperature is plotted against time (Figure 15-76, *A*). Most hemodynamic monitors display this CO curve, which must then be interpreted to determine whether the CO injection is valid. The normal curve has a smooth upstroke, with a rounded peak and a gradually tapering downslope. If the curve has an uneven pattern, it may indicate faulty injection technique, and the CO measurement is repeated. Patient movement or coughing also alters the CO (Figure 15-76, *B*).

Injectate temperature. If the cardiac output is within the normal range it is equally accurate, whether iced or room temperature injectate is used. However, if the cardiac outputs are extremely high or very low, iced injectate may be more accurate.[94] To ensure accurate readings, the difference between injectate temperature and body temperature must be at least 10° C, and the injectate must be delivered within 4 seconds, with minimal handling of the syringe to prevent warming of the solution. This is particularly important if iced injectate is used. With all delivery systems, the injectate is delivered at the same point in the respiratory cycle, usually end-exhalation.

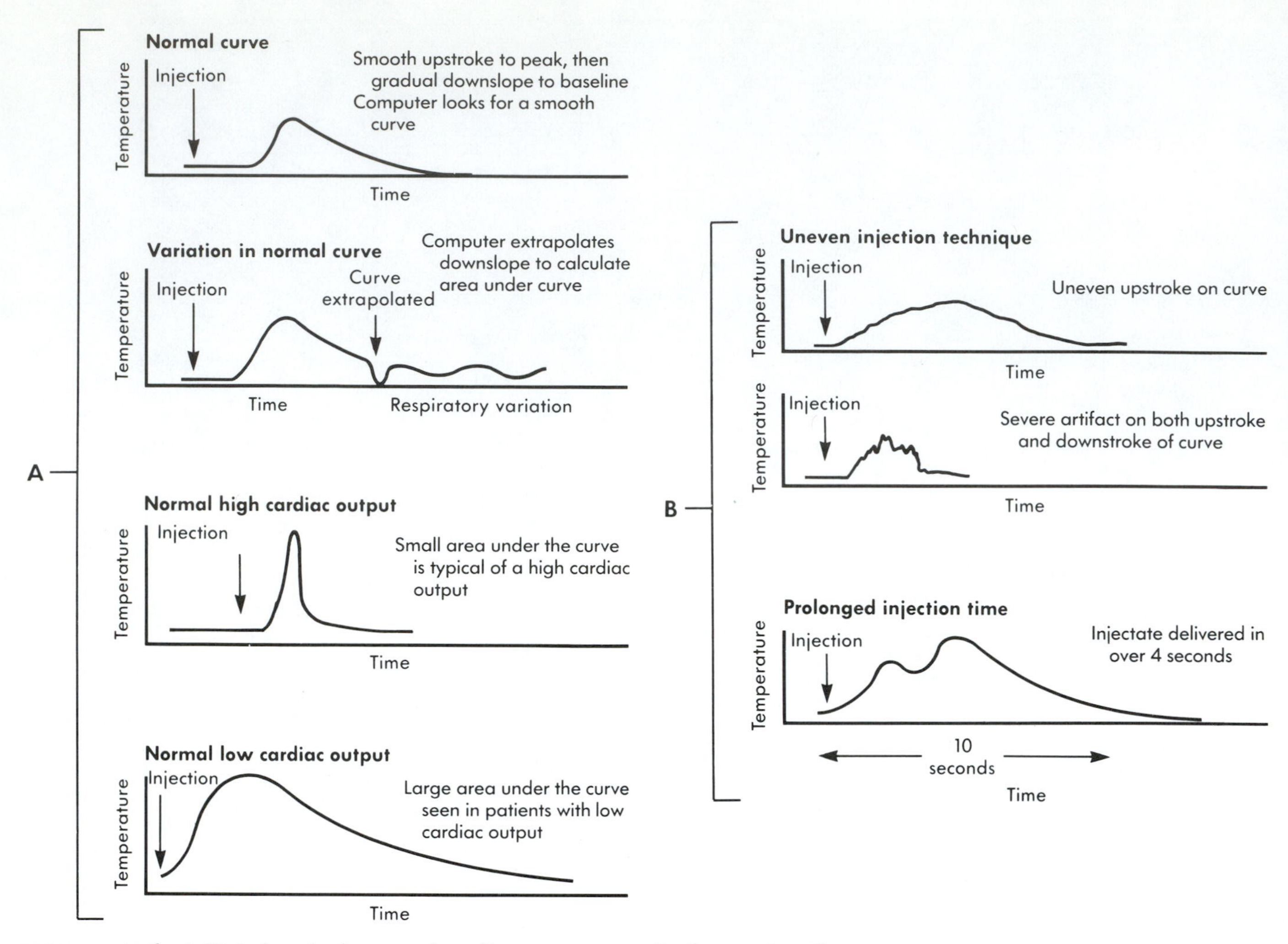

FIGURE 15-76. **A,** Variations in the normal cardiac output curve. **B,** Abnormal cardiac output curves produce an erroneous cardiac output value.

Patient position. In the normovolemic stable patient, reliable CO measurements can be obtained in a supine position with the head of the bed elevated up to 60 degrees.[69,72] If the patient is hypovolemic or unstable, leaving the head of the bed in a flat position, or only slightly elevated, is the most clinically appropriate choice. Cardiac output measurements performed when the patient is turned to the side are not considered as accurate as those performed with the patient in the supine position.

Clinical errors. Two clinical conditions produce errors in the thermodilution CO measurement: tricuspid valve regurgitation and ventricular septal defect (VSD). If the patient has tricuspid valve regurgitation, the expected flow of blood from the right atrium to the pulmonary artery is disrupted by backflow from the right ventricle to the right atrium. This creates a lower CO measurement than the patient's actual output. If the person has an intracardiac left-to-right shunt, such as occurs with a VSD, the thermodilution CO measures the large pulmonary volume and records a higher CO than the patient's true systemic output.

Continuous cardiac output measurement. The bolus thermodilution method is reliable but performed intermittently. Researchers are investigating continuous methods of monitoring cardiac output. At present no one method has come to the fore to replace current practice, but several are under active investigation.

One method of continuous cardiac output measurement is impedance cardiography.[95] Impedance cardiography works by emitting a low-voltage, high-frequency, alternating electrical current through the thorax via spot or band electrodes. The electrical impedance changes within the thorax are detected by the sensing electrodes. Because blood flow through the thoracic aorta causes shifts in impedance this information can be used to calculate stroke volume, and from this continuous cardiac output can be measured.[95] Another method of continuous cardiac output uses heat as the thermodilution indicator.[96,97]

Calculated hemodynamic profiles. For the patient with a thermodilution PA catheter in place, additional hemodynamic information can be calculated using routine vital signs, CO, and body surface area (BSA). These measurements are calculated using specific formulas that are indexed to a patient's body size, using either the DuBois body area surface chart or the computer program associated with the new generation of hemodynamic monitors. (See Appendix D.)

The calculated hemodynamic profiles are described in Table 15-14. Clinical use of these profiles is described in two case studies. In Box 15-7, the case study is a step-by-step interpretation of the hemodynamic profile to familiarize the reader with use of calculated values. In Box 15-8, the case study uses only values indexed to body weight and illustrates the impact of treatment on these values over time.

Continuous Monitoring of Mixed Venous Oxygen Saturation

Indications. Continuous monitoring of mixed venous oxygen saturation (SvO_2) is indicated for the patient who has the potential to develop an imbalance between oxygen supply and metabolic tissue demand. This includes the patient in shock and the patient with severe respiratory compromise, such as acute respiratory distress syndrome (ARDS).[98]

Continuous SvO_2 monitoring measures the balance achieved between arterial oxygen supply (SaO_2) and oxygen demand at the tissue level by sampling desaturated venous mixed blood from the pulmonary artery (SvO_2). It is called *mixed venous blood,* because it is a mixture of all of the venous blood saturations from many body tissues. Under normal conditions the cardiopulmonary system achieves a balance between oxygen supply and demand. The four factors that contribute to this balance include cardiac output (CO), hemoglobin (Hgb), arterial oxygen saturation (SaO_2), and tissue metabolism (VO_2). Three of these factors (CO, Hgb, and SaO_2) contribute to the supply of oxygen to the tissues. Tissue metabolism (VO_2) determines the quantity of oxygen extracted at tissue level, or oxygen consumption, and creates the demand for oxygen. The relationship of all these factors is illustrated in Figure 15-77. (∞Cardiac Output Determinants, p. 460.)

In addition to interpreting SvO_2, it is possible to calculate the quantity of oxygen that is provided by the cardiopulmonary system and the amount of oxygen consumed by the body tissues. These calculations are based on the principles of oxygen transport physiology and are the basis for calculation of SvO_2. These formulas are explained in greater detail in Table 15-18 and are listed in Appendix D.

Catheters. The SvO_2 catheter contains the traditional four lumens plus a lumen containing two or three optical fibers. The fiberoptics are attached to an optical module that is connected to a small bedside computer. The optical module transmits a narrow band of light down one optical fiber. This light is reflected off the hemoglobin in the blood, and returns to the optical module through the receiving fiberoptic. The SvO_2 signal is recorded on a continuous display.

SvO_2 calibration. The catheter is calibrated before insertion into the patient through a standard color reference system, which is part of the catheter package. Insertion technique and sites are identical to those used for placement of a conventional PA catheter. Waveform analysis and/or SvO_2 can be used for accurate placement. Once the catheter is inserted, recalibration is unnecessary unless the catheter becomes disconnected from the optical module. To calibrate when the catheter is inserted in a patient, a mixed venous blood sample must be withdrawn from the PA lumen and sent to the laboratory for oxygen saturation (SvO_2) analysis.

Nursing management. SvO_2 monitoring provides a continuous assessment of the balance between oxygen supply and demand for an individual patient. Nursing assessment includes evaluation of the SvO_2 value and evaluation of the four factors (SaO_2, CO, Hgb, and VO_2) that maintain the oxygen supply-demand balance.

Normal SvO_2 is 75%. For most critically ill patients, an SvO_2 value between 60% and 80% is evidence of adequate balance between oxygen supply and demand. If the SvO_2 value changes by more than 10% and this change is maintained for more than 10 minutes, the nurse must determine which of the four factors is affecting SvO_2.

SvO_2 and arterial oxygen saturation. A change in SvO_2 may be caused by a change in arterial oxygen saturation (SaO_2). If the SaO_2 is increased because supplemental oxygen is being given, the SvO_2 also rises. If the SaO_2 is decreased, SvO_2 falls. Decreased SaO_2 can be caused by any action or disease that reduces oxygen supply, including ARDS, endotracheal suctioning, removing a patient from the ventilator, or removal of an oxygen mask. Figure 15-78 demonstrates a fall in SvO_2 during suctioning in a patient with ARDS. Transient decreases in SvO_2 related to a nursing action such as endotracheal suctioning are not usually a cause for concern. Some patients may be slow to resaturate up to the presuction level of SvO_2. In this case an appropriate nursing intervention

BOX 15-7 Hemodynamic Profile: Case Study 1

Mr. SR has a medical history of cardiomyopathy and chronic obstructive pulmonary disease (COPD). He is admitted to a coronary care unit because of an exacerbation of his biventricular heart failure. He has been complaining of anginal pain and shortness of breath. His nursing diagnoses are Decreased Cardiac Output and Impaired Gas Exchange.

Height	163 cm	PAD	27 mm Hg	PVR	322 dynes/sec/cm^{-5}
Weight	79 kg	PAPM	36 mm Hg	PVRI	612 dynes/sec/cm^{-5}/m^2
Body surface area (BSA)		PAWP	26 mm Hg	LCW	2.1 kg-m
	1.9 m^2	CVP	24 mm Hg	LCWI	1.1 kg-m/m^2
HR	104 bpm	CO	2.48 L/min	LVSW	2.4 g-m
ABP		CI	1.31 L/min/m^2	LVSWI	10.7 g-m/m^2
Systolic	88 mm Hg	SV	23.8 ml	RCW	1.21 kg-m
Diastolic	51 mm Hg	SI	12.5 ml/m^2	RCWI	0.64 kg-m/m^2
MAP	63 mm Hg	SVR	1257 dynes/sec/cm^{-5}	RVSW	11.7 g-m
PAS	55 mm Hg	SVRI	2388 dynes/sec/cm^{-5}/m^2	RVSWI	6.2 g-m/m^2

ANALYSIS OF HEMODYNAMIC PROFILE*

PROFILE	ANALYSIS
HR	Heart rate of 104 beats per minute (bpm) is above normal limits (normal, 60-100 bpm).
ABP (arterial blood pressure)	Narrow pulse pressure of 88/51 mm Hg with a low mean arterial pressure (MAP) of 63 mm Hg (normal MAP, 65-90 mm Hg).
Pulmonary artery pressure	Pulmonary artery pressures are elevated (55/27 mm Hg), consistent with diagnosis of cardiomyopathy, failure of left side of heart, and COPD (normal PAP, 25/10 mm Hg).
PAWP (pulmonary artery wedge pressure)	Elevated PAWP (26 mm Hg), consistent with diagnosis of cardiomyopathy and failure of left side of heart (normal PAWP, 5-12 mm Hg).
CVP (central venous pressure)	Elevated CVP (24 mm Hg), consistent with diagnosis of cardiomyopathy, failure of right side of heart, and COPD (normal CVP, 4-6 mm Hg).
CO (cardiac output) and CI (cardiac index)	Poor CO and CI (CO, 2.48 L/min; CI, 1.31 L/min/m^2). Both values are below normal (normal CO, 4-6 L/min; normal CI, 2.2-4 L/min/m^2).
SV (stroke volume) and SI (stroke volume index)	SV and SI are low (SV, 23.8 ml; SI, 12.5 ml/m^2). These results would be anticipated from the low cardiac output (normal SV, 60-70 ml; normal SI, 40-50 ml/min/m^2).
SVR (systemic vascular resistance) and SVRI (systemic vascular resistance index)	SVR and SVRI are at the upper normal range (SVR, 1257 dynes/sec/cm^{-5}, SVRI, 2388 dynes/sec/cm^{-5}/m^2). These values are not contributing to the low cardiac output at this time (normal SVR, 800-1400 dynes/sec/cm^{-5}; normal SVRI, 2000-2400 dynes/sec/cm^{-5}/m^2).
PVR (pulmonary vascular resistance) and PVRI (pulmonary vascular resistance index)	PVR and PVRI are elevated (PVR, 322 dynes/sec/cm^{-5}; PVRI 612 dynes/sec/cm^{-5}/m^2). High pulmonary vascular resistance may be contributing to the low cardiac output (normal PVR, 100-250 dynes/sec/cm^{-5}; normal PVRI, 225-315 dynes/sec/cm^{-5}/m^2).
LCWI (left cardiac work index) and LVSWI (left ventricular stroke work index)	Both LCWI and LVSWI are below normal (LCWI, 1.1 kg-m/m^2; LVSWI, 10.7 g-m/m^2), indicating that left ventricular myocardial damage may be present. This is consistent with SR's diagnosis of cardiomyopathy (normal LCWI, 3.4-4.2 kg-m/m^2; normal LVSWI, 50-62 g-m/m^2).
RCWI (right cardiac work index) and RVSWI (right ventricular stroke work index)	RCWI is normal, but RVSWI is below normal (RCWI, 0.64 kg-m/m^2; RVSWI, 6.2 g-m/m^2), indicating that right ventricular myocardial damage may be present. This is consistent with SR's diagnosis of cardiomyopathy and history of COPD (normal RCWI, 0.54-0.66 kg-m/m^2, normal RVSWI, 7.9-9.7 g-m/m^2).
Nursing impression	The hemodynamic data confirm the nursing clinical diagnosis of poor CO. The goal is to improve CO within the limits of SR's myocardial dysfunction and COPD. As CO improves and PA pressures decrease, the patient will have less pulmonary congestion, which will improve alveolar gas exchange.

*Formulas and normal values for the hemodynamic values are in Table 15-14 and Appendix D.

BOX 15-8 Hemodynamic Profile: Case Study 2

1. ADMISSION

Mrs. JL has been admitted to the critical care unit with pulmonary edema. She has a history of anterior wall myocardial infarction and severe chronic obstructive pulmonary disease (COPD).

Height	159 cm	MAP	106 mm Hg	SI	9.9 ml/m^2
Weight	45.8 kg	PAS	53 mm Hg	SVRI	5351 dynes/sec/cm^{-5}/m^2
Body surface area (BSA)		PAD	27 mm Hg	PVRI	1046 dynes/sec/cm^{-5}/m^2
	1.40 m^2	PAPM	44 mm Hg	LCWI	1.9 kg-m/m^2
HR	131 bpm	PAWP	27 mm Hg	LVSWI	14.3 g-m/m^2
ABP		CVP	19 mm Hg	RCWI	0.78 kg-m^2/m^2
Systolic	160 mm Hg	CO	1.82 L/min	RVSWI	5.9 g-m/m^2
Diastolic	80 mm Hg	CI	1.3 L/min/m^2		

*Analysis of hemodynamic profile 1**

In the above hemodynamic profile, note the fast heart rate; high MAP; high PA and CVP filling pressures; low CI, SI, LVSWI, and RVSWI; and high SVRI and PVRI. These values are consistent with a diagnosis of failure of the left side of the heart, causing pulmonary edema, which may lead to cardiogenic shock. Treatment is focused on increasing the cardiac index by lowering SVRI and PVRI and using IV sodium nitroprusside and IV nitroglycerin in continuous infusion.

2. 3 HOURS LATER

Height	159 cm	MAP	83 mm Hg	SI	16.5 ml/m^2
Weight	45.8 kg	PAS	41 mm Hg	SVRI	3088 dynes/sec/cm^{-5}/m^2
Body surface area (BSA)		PAD	26 mm Hg	PVRI	300 dynes/sec/cm^{-5}/m^2
	1.40 m^2	PAPM	33 mm Hg	LCWI	2.1 kg-m/m^2
HR	113 bpm	PAWP	26 mm Hg	LVSWI	18.6 g-m/m^2
ABP		CVP	11 mm Hg	RCWI	0.84 kg-m/m^2
Systolic	104 mm Hg	CO	2.61 L/min	RVSWI	7.4 g-m/m^2
Diastolic	69 mm Hg	CI	1.86 L/min/m^2		

Analysis of hemodynamic profile 2

Results 3 hours later after sodium nitroprusside administration: note improving hemodynamics shown above as normal MAP and lower intracardiac filling pressures (PA and CVP). However, CI and SI remain low, and SVRI is above normal. Mrs JL remains in severe left ventricular failure because of her low CI.

3. THE NEXT DAY

Height	159 cm	MAP	77 mm Hg	SI	22.5 ml/m^2
Weight	45.8 kg	PAS	31 mm Hg	SVRI	2423 dynes/sec/cm^{-5}/m^2
Body surface area (BSA)		PAD	15 mm Hg	PVRI	273 dynes/sec/cm^{-5}/m^2
	1.40 m^2	PAPM	23 mm Hg	LCWI	2.4 kg-m/m^2
HR	104 bpm	PAWP	15 mm Hg	LVSWI	22.9 g-m/m^2
ABP		CVP	4 mm Hg	RCWI	0.74 kg-m/m^2
Systolic	111 mm Hg	CO	3.28 L/min	RVSWI	7.1 g-m/m^2
Diastolic	60 mm Hg	CI	2.34 L/min/m^2		

Analysis of hemodynamic profile 3

The following day Mrs. JL's hemodynamics have improved with continued use of sodium nitroprusside and nitroglycerin. CI is in the low-normal range, and SVRI and PVRI are in the high-normal range. LVSWI remains low, reflecting the patient's compromised left ventricle from the previous anterior wall myocardial infarction.

*See Box 15-7 for explanation of abbreviations, and see Table 15-14 and Appendix D for explanation of hemodynamic values.

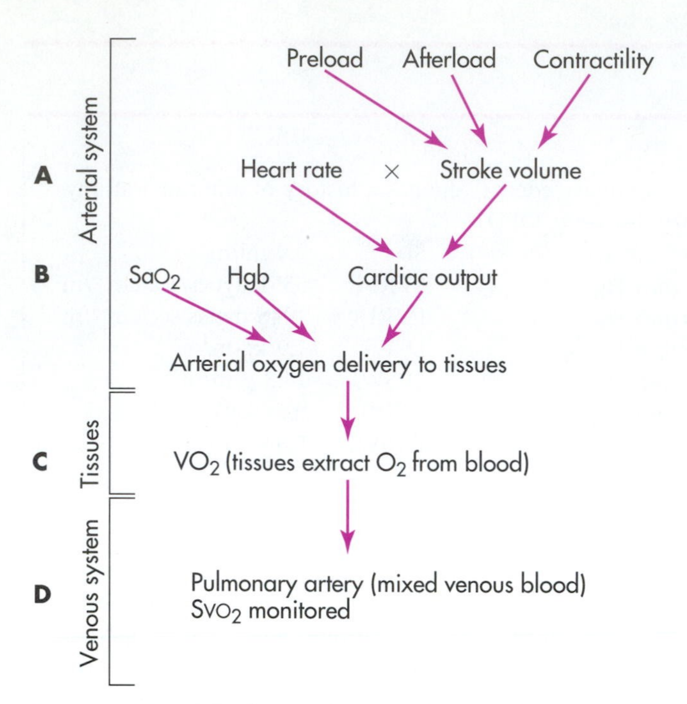

FIGURE 15-77. The factors that contribute to the SvO_2 value. **A,** Cardiac output (CO) is determined by HR × SV. **B,** The SaO_2, Hgb, and CO all contribute to arterial oxygen delivery at the tissue level. **C,** Tissues extract and use the oxygen carried in the blood. This process of cellular oxygen consumption is termed VO_2. **D,** Blood returns to the pulmonary artery where the mixed venous blood is recorded as SvO_2.

is to wait until SvO_2 has again returned to baseline before initiating other nursing activities. (Oxygenation: Clinical Assessment and Evaluation)

SvO_2 and cardiac output. A change in SvO_2 may also be caused by an alteration in cardiac output (CO). Four hemodynamic factors affect CO—preload, afterload, contractility, and heart rate, as shown in Figure 15-77. Changes in one or more of these individual factors affects CO. Figure 15-79 shows an improvement in a patient's SvO_2 from 70% to 80% after volume administration that increased preload *(point A)*. Later this patient's CO fell abruptly during a short run of ventricular tachycardia *(point B)*. Any major loss of heart rate causes a decrease in CO. Alterations in contractility and afterload (systemic vascular resistance) also have the potential to alter CO. Because CO is an important component of the continuous SvO_2 value, several researchers questioned whether SvO_2 could be substituted for thermodilution CO as a monitoring tool. Studies of adult patients after cardiac surgery and myocardial infarction indicate that a sustained change in the SvO_2 value does not automatically mean there has been a change in CO. There was not a consistent or reliable correlation between SvO_2 and CO in these clinical studies. Rather, SvO_2 changes indicate a need to check a thermodilution CO at the bedside to determine the cause of the change in SvO_2. The SvO_2 measurement is very sensitive and serves as an early warning for changes in patient condition, whether or not the change is the result of an alteration in CO. Therefore SvO_2 monitoring is an additional level of hemodynamic monitoring but does not replace thermodilution CO.[99-101]

This principle is clearly illustrated in the SvO_2 case study in Box 15-9 where an increase in SvO_2 is not associated with a significant rise in CO. The rationale and explanation for this finding are also discussed in the section on assessment of oxygen consumption.

SvO_2 and hemoglobin. Hemoglobin (Hgb) is the transport mechanism for oxygen in the blood. If the Hgb level falls as a result of bleeding or red cell destruction, the body maintains oxygen transport by increasing cardiac output and using oxygen reserves in the venous blood return. Therefore the body can compensate efficiently for anemia. In the healthy person, Hgb must be extremely low before SvO_2 falls. However, in an anemic patient with a compromised cardiovascular system who cannot adequately increase CO, SvO_2 declines as venous oxygen reserves are consumed by the body.

SvO_2 and oxygen consumption. Oxygen consumption (VO_2) describes the amount of oxygen the body tissues consume for normal function in 1 minute. If the body's metabolic demands increase because of exercise or increased metabolic rate, the body increases cardiac output to augment oxygen supply and also uses reserve oxygen in the venous system. Normal oxygen delivery to the tissues is 1000 ml of oxygen per minute. At rest a person might consume one quarter of available oxygen or 250 ml of oxygen per minute. This leaves a venous oxygen reserve of 750 ml of oxygen per minute (see Table 15-18). Thus for the normal individual, the combination of increased CO and use of considerable venous oxygen reserve provides adequate compensation for increased metabolic needs. However, for the critically ill patient with either cardiac or respiratory dysfunction, an increase in activity leading to increased oxygen consumption may overwhelm the cardiopulmonary system and oxygen reserves.[101-103]

In the critically ill patient, routine nursing procedures can increase VO_2 by 10% to 36% (Table 15-19). The critical care nurse can observe the effect of increased VO_2 during routine nursing care and in conditions that increase metabolic rate. Activities such as turning, giving a backrub, or getting a patient out of bed are often accompanied by a sudden, temporary decrease in the patient's continuous SvO_2 reading. Once

TABLE 15-18 Calculations and Explanation of Oxygen Transport Physiology

Name	Formula	Normal Value	Explanation
Arterial oxygen saturation (SaO_2)	$\frac{HgbO_2}{(Hgb + HgbO_2)} \times 100$	>96%	Hgb, hemoglobin; $HgbO_2$, oxyhemoglobin. The arterial oxygen saturation represents the amount of oxyhemoglobin (oxygen bound to hemoglobin) divided by the total hemoglobin. Normally 96% of oxygen is bound to hemoglobin.
Blood oxygen content CaO_2 (arterial) CvO_2 (venous)	(O_2 dissolved) + (O_2 saturation) $(PO_2 \times 0.0031) + (1.34 \times Hgb \times SO_2)$	19-20 ml/dL 12-15 ml/dL	Blood oxygen (O_2) content represents the amount of oxygen dissolved in 100 ml of blood. It can be calculated for both arterial blood (CaO_2) and for venous blood (CvO_2). It is measured in ml/dL. It is the combination of both dissolved O_2 (PaO_2) and O_2 saturation (SaO_2).
Blood oxygen transport (also called "oxygen delivery")	$CO \times CaO_2 \times 10$ (arterial) $CO \times CvO_2 \times 10$ (venous)	1000 ml/min 750 ml/min	Oxygen transport represents the amount of oxygen transported to or from the tissues each minute in milliliters (ml/min). Arterial O_2 transport is a measure of the O_2 delivered to the tissues. Venous O_2 transport reflects the venous return to the right side of the heart. Oxygen transport is calculated by multiplying the cardiac output (CO) by the oxygen content (CaO_2 or CvO_2) and by the number 10. The difference between normal arterial and normal venous O_2 return represents oxygen consumption by the tissues.
Tissue oxygen consumption (VO_2)	Arterial O_2 transport minus venous O_2 transport $(CO \times CaO_2 \times 10) - (CO \times CvO_2 \times 10)$	250 ml/min	Oxygen consumption represents the amount of oxygen consumed by the tissues in 1 minute. To calculate VO_2, it is necessary to know both arterial oxygen transport and venous oxygen transport values, which are calculated in ml/min. The difference represents oxygen consumption.
Arterial venous oxygen difference (A-VO_2 difference)	Arterial O_2 content minus venous O_2 content $CaO_2 - CvO_2$	3.0-5.5 ml/dL	The arterial venous oxygen difference represents the difference between the arterial oxygen content (CaO_2) and the venous oxygen content (CvO_2). Because CaO_2 and CvO_2 are measured ml/dL, A-VO_2 difference is also measured in ml/dL.
Mixed venous oxygen saturation (SvO_2)	Arterial O_2 transport minus tissue consumption equals venous return $(CO \times CaO_2 \times 10) - VO_2$	60%-80%	Mixed venous oxygen saturation (SvO_2) represents the venous oxygen return that is bound (saturated) with hemoglobin. Saturation is measured in percent (%). The SvO_2 value is a function of the amount of oxygen delivered to the tissues minus the amount of oxygen consumed by the tissues (VO_2) in milliliters per minute. The higher the amount (ml) of oxygen in the venous return, the greater the hemoglobin saturation will be.

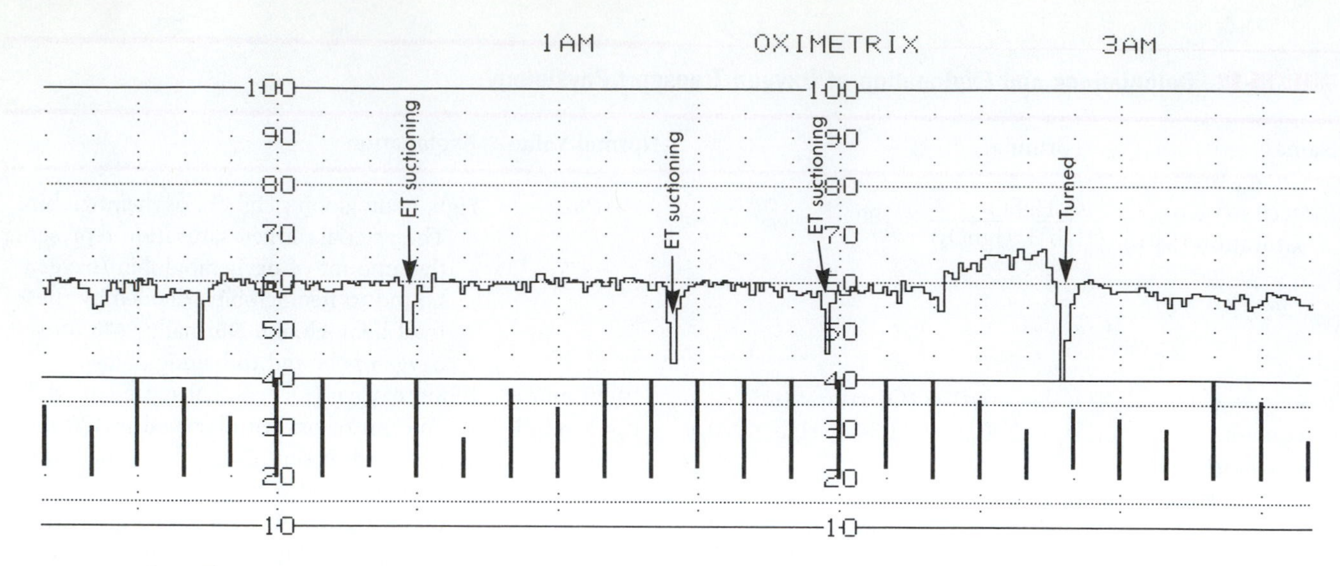

FIGURE 15-78. Fall in $S\bar{v}O_2$ during endotracheal (ET) suctioning. The ET suction decreases SaO_2. The baseline $S\bar{v}O_2$ is low (60%) because the patient has ARDS and is hypoxemic.

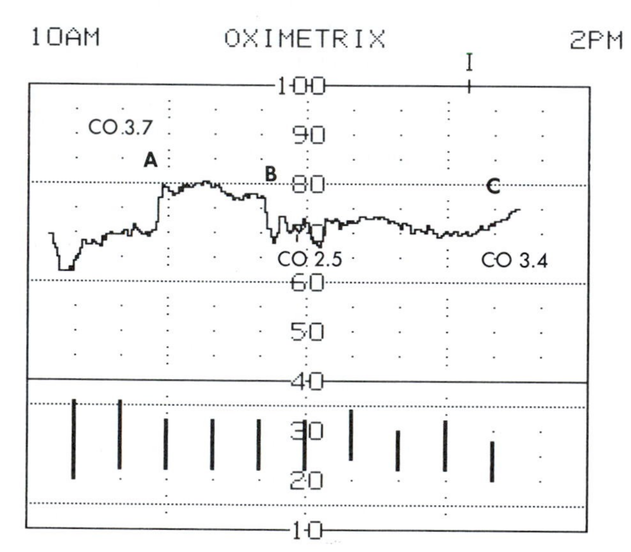

FIGURE 15-79. Impact of changes in cardiac output (CO) on $S\bar{v}O_2$ values. Point *A:* Just before point A, $S\bar{v}O_2$ readings are low because CO and pulmonary artery pressures were low as a result of excessive diuresis. Infusion of 500 ml of colloid solution and 1000 ml of lactated Ringer's solution crystalloid increased the $S\bar{v}O_2$ and improved the CO, which rose to 3.7 L/min. Point *B:* A short run of ventricular tachycardia caused the CO to fall abruptly to 2.5 L/min and decreased the $S\bar{v}O_2$ value. Point *C:* The beginning of an upward trend in $S\bar{v}O_2$ is related to administration of fluids and to improvement in CO and in filling pressures. CO is now 3.4 L/min. The graph represents a 4-hour printout; the space between each dotted line represents 20 minutes.

the movement is finished, most patients resaturate up to their preactivity $S\bar{v}O_2$ level within 4 to 5 minutes. In critically ill patients it may take up to a full 5 minutes for resaturation (rise in $S\bar{v}O_2$) to occur. In this situation the appropriate nursing action is to observe the patient clinically, in conjunction with monitoring $S\bar{v}O_2$, and to postpone additional maneuvers until the $S\bar{v}O_2$ has returned to baseline.[101]

Many clinical conditions that dramatically increase $\dot{V}O_2$ are frequently seen in critical care units. Conditions such as sepsis, multiple organ dysfunction syndrome (MODS), burns, head injury, and shivering can more than double normal oxygen tissue requirements (see Table 15-19). Such dramatic increases in $\dot{V}O_2$ translates into a low $S\bar{v}O_2$, even if the CO is normal, as discussed in the following case study.

$S\bar{v}O_2$ Case Study

An example of the impact of increased oxygen consumption and low cardiac output on $S\bar{v}O_2$ is shown in the case study in Box 15-9. Patient EH has just been admitted to the critical care unit and is cold and shivering after cardiopulmonary bypass and cardiac surgery.

At *point A* (see figure on p. 478), $S\bar{v}O_2$ is low at 40%. The low $S\bar{v}O_2$ is caused by postoperative shivering, which has greatly increased EH's oxygen consumption. The oxygen consumption ($\dot{V}O_2$) is high at 322 ml/min. An additional factor is that EH has a low cardiac output. The CO is 3.0 L/min, which provides below normal flow to the tissues. The oxygen delivery is low at only 505 ml/min. The increased $\dot{V}O_2$ and the low CO both contribute to the low $S\bar{v}O_2$.

BOX 15-9 Hemodynamic Profile: Case Study 3

Mr. EH has just been admitted to the cardiovascular critical care unit after open heart surgery. At *point A* (see figure on p. 477) he has an extremely low mixed venous oxygen saturation (Svo_2) of 40%. An Svo_2 below 40% indicates that the oxygen supply is not adequate to meet the demands of the body tissues, resulting in metabolic acidosis. To determine the reason for the low Svo_2, one must know the hemoglobin (Hgb), the arterial oxygen saturation (Sao_2), the cardiac output (CO), and the tissue oxygen consumption (Vo_2). EH's Hgb value is 11.6 g/dL (normal male Hgb, 13.5-18.0 g/dL), which is acceptable after major surgery; the Sao_2 is 99.6% (normal, 97%), which is high because this patient is receiving mechanical ventilation with 70% oxygen immediately after surgery; and the CO is low at 3.15 L/min (normal, 4-6 L/min). EH is receiving dopamine 5 μg/kg/min for his low CO. He is shivering and cold because his body temperature is only 35.2° C after the surgery. Using the values described above—Hgb 11.6 g/dL; Sao_2, 99.6%; and CO 3.15 L/min—it is possible to calculate the tissue oxygen consumption (Vo_2) for EH.

ARTERIAL SUPPLY	VENOUS RETURN
CO ($Pao_2 \times 0.0031$) + ($1.34 \times$ Hgb $\times Sao_2$)10 −	CO ($Pvo_2 \times 0.0031$) + ($1.34 \times$ Hgb $\times Svo_2$)10 = Vo_2

(To calculate arterial oxygen supply, the oxygen in the venous return, Vo_2, and the difference between the arterial and venous oxygen content [A-Vo_2 difference], insert EH's values [in bold] into the above formula.)

ARTERIAL SUPPLY	VENOUS RETURN	*Vo2*	*A-Vo2 Difference*
3.15(354 × 0.0031) + (1.34 × 11.6 × 0.99)10 −	3.15(20 × 0.0031) + 1.34 × 11.6 × 0.38)10		
3.15(1.0 + 15.3)10	3.15(0.06 + 5.90)10		
3.15(16.3)10	3.15(5.90)10		
505 ml/min (see figure)	183 ml/min	= 322 ml/min	10.4 ml/dL

At *point A* (see figure) the arterial oxygen supply to the tissues is 505 ml/min (normal, 1000 ml/min), whereas the oxygen returned in the venous blood is only 183 ml/min (normal, 750 ml/min). EH's Vo_2 is elevated at 322 ml/min (normal, 250 ml/min). The clinical goals for this patient would be to (1) increase the CO and (2) use sedation or muscle relaxants to decrease oxygen consumption by controlling the shivering. The difference between the oxygen content in the arterial and the venous blood (A-Vo_2 difference) is very large at 10.4 ml/dL (normal, 3.5-5.0 ml/dL). These calculated values confirm the nursing diagnosis of Altered Tissue Perfusion with a decreased cardiac output.

Two hours later, at *point B* (see figure), EH's Svo_2 has improved to a low-normal value of 60%. Additional inotropic drugs have been administered. At this time the Hgb is 10.8 g/dL, Sao_2 is 99.6%, and CO remains low at 3.3 L/min. Thus the improvement in Svo_2 has not been caused by a dramatic increase in CO. When EH's oxygen consumption is calculated at *point B*, it becomes evident that the decrease in physical activity after sedation with morphine to reduce shivering has improved the Svo_2. EH's values are emphasized in bold.

ARTERIAL SUPPLY	VENOUS RETURN
CO ($Pao_2 \times 0.0031$) + ($1.34 \times$ Hgb $\times Sao_2$)10 −	CO ($Pvo_2 \times 0.0031$) + ($1.34 \times$ Hgb $\times Svo_2$)10 = Vo_2

ARTERIAL SUPPLY	VENOUS RETURN	*Vo_2*	*A-Vo_2 Difference*
3.3(266 × 0.0031) + (1.34 × 10.8 × 0.99)10 −	3.3(28 × 0.0031) + (1.34 × 10.8 × 0.60)10		
3.3(0.82 + 14.32)10	3.3(0.86 + 8.6)10		
3.3(15.1)10	3.3(9.4)10		
498 ml/min	300 ml/min	198 ml/min	5.7 ml/dL

At *point B* (see figure), EH's arterial oxygen supply is still low at 498 ml/min, and the oxygen in his mixed venous blood return remains low at 300 ml/min. Vo_2 is now lower than normal (typical after sedation)—198 ml/min. At this time the A-Vo_2 difference is almost within normal limits at 5.7 ml/dL. These findings are confirmed by the low-normal Svo_2 value of 60% at *point B*. This case study illustrates the point that tissue oxygen consumption (O_2 demand) can be as important as cardiac output (CO) and oxygenation (O_2 supply) in determining mixed venous oxygen saturation (Svo_2) in the patient with a compromised cardiovascular system.

*See Box 15-7 for explanation of abbreviations, and see Table 15-14 and Appendix D for explanation of hemodynamic values.

Continued

BOX 15-9 Hemodynamic Profile—cont'd

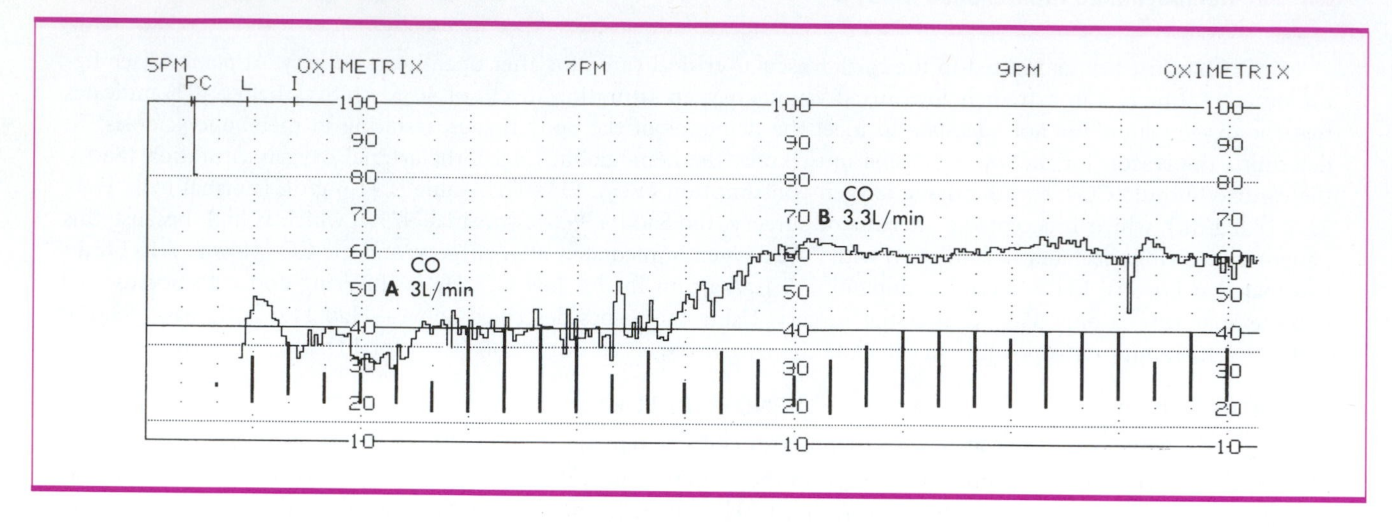

TABLE 15-19 Conditions and Activities That Alter Oxygen Consumption (Vo_2)

Condition or Activity	% Increase Over Resting Vo_2	% Decrease Under Resting Vo_2
CLINICAL CONDITIONS THAT INCREASE Vo_2		
Fever	10% (for each 1° C over normal)	
Skeletal injuries	10%-30%	
Work of breathing	40%	
Severe infection	60%	
Shivering	50%-100%	
Burns	100%	
Routine postoperative procedures	7%	
Nasal intubation	25%-40%	
Endotracheal tube suctioning	27%	
Chest trauma	60%	
Multiple organ dysfunction syndrome	20%-80%	
Sepsis	50%-100%	
Head injury, with patient sedated	89%	
Head injury, with patient not sedated	138%	
Critical illness in emergency department	60%	
NURSING ACTIVITIES THAT INCREASE Vo_2		
Dressing change	10%	
Electrocardiogram	16%	
Agitation	18%	
Physical examination	20%	
Visitor	22%	
Bath	23%	
Chest x-ray examination	25%	
Position change	31%	
Chest physiotherapy	35%	
Weighing on sling scale	36%	
CONDITIONS THAT DECREASE Vo_2		
Anesthesia		25%
Anesthesia in burned patients		50%

From White KM and others: *Heart Lung* 19(5):550, 1990.

TABLE 15-20 Clinical Interpretation of Svo_2 Measurements

Svo_2 Measurement	Physiologic Basis for Change in Svo_2	Clinical Diagnosis and Rationale
High Svo_2 (80%-95%)	Increased oxygen supply	Patient receiving more oxygen than required by clinical condition
	Decreased oxygen demand	Anesthesia, which causes sedation and decreased muscle movement
		Hypothermia, which lowers metabolic demand (e.g., with cardiopulmonary bypass)
		Sepsis caused by decreased ability of tissues to use oxygen at a cellular level
		False high positive because PA catheter is wedged in a pulmonary capillary
Normal Svo_2 (60%-80%)	Normal oxygen supply and metabolic demand	Balanced oxygen supply and demand
Low Svo_2 (less than 60%)	Decreased oxygen supply caused by:	
	Low hemoglobin (Hgb)	Anemia or bleeding with compromised cardiopulmonary system
	Low arterial saturation (Sao_2)	Hypoxemia resulting from decreased oxygen supply or lung disease
	Low cardiac output (CO)	Cardiogenic shock caused by left ventricular pump failure
	Increased oxygen consumption (Vo_2)	Metabolic demand exceeds oxygen supply in conditions that increase muscle movement and increase metabolic rate, including physiologic states such as shivering, seizures, and hyperthermia and nursing interventions such as obtaining bedscale weight and turning

At *point B* (see figure on p. 477.), the shivering has stopped after sedation; consequently, his tissue oxygen consumption (Vo_2) has decreased to 198 ml/min, which is within normal range. As a result, his Svo_2 has risen to 60%. However, EH's cardiac output remains low. Thus the very low Svo_2 at *point A* was caused by increased oxygen consumption caused by shivering, and was not related to the low cardiac output. However, since an Svo_2 of 60% is considered a "low-normal value," nursing interventions would now focus on improving the cardiac output to increase the Svo_2 value.

Normal Svo_2. If Svo_2 is within the normal range of 60% to 80% and the patient is not clinically compromised, one can assume that oxygen supply and demand are balanced for that individual. The situation becomes out of balance when there is either a decrease in oxygen delivery because of changes in (Sao_2), CO, or Hgb or an increase in oxygen demand (increased Vo).

Low Svo_2. If Svo_2 falls below 60% and is sustained, the clinician must assume that oxygen supply is not equal to demand (Table 15-20). It is helpful to assess the cause of decreased Svo_2 in a logical sequence that reflects knowledge of the meaning of the Svo_2 value. The following is one such assessment sequence:

1. Clinically assess the patient.
2. Assess whether the decreased Svo_2 is caused by low oxygen supply. Verify the effectiveness of the ventilator or oxygen mask or check arterial oxygen saturation (Sao_2) by transcutaneous oximetry or from arterial blood gas values.
3. Assess cardiac function by performing a CO measurement.
4. Assess Hgb value by checking recent laboratory results or by withdrawing a blood sample for laboratory analysis.
5. Assess whether the decreased Svo_2 is the result of a recent patient movement or nursing action that may have temporarily increased Vo.

If Svo_2 falls below 40%, the balance of oxygen supply and demand may not be adequate to meet tissue needs at the cellular level. The cells change from an aerobic to anaerobic mode of metabolism, which results in the production of lactic acid and is representative of a shock state in which cellular injury or cell death may result. At this point every attempt must be made to determine the cause of the low SvO_2 and to correct the oxygen supply-demand imbalance.

High SvO_2. In certain clinical conditions, SvO_2 may increase to an above normal level (greater than 80%). This occurs during times of low oxygen demand (decreased VO_2) such as during anesthesia. In certain cases of septic shock, the tissue cells cannot use the oxygen supplied to them and, as a consequence, the oxygen is not extracted from the blood at the tissue level. In this situation the venous oxygen reserve remains elevated and SvO_2 is higher than normal (see Table 15-20). Finally if the SvO_2 catheter drifts into a wedged position, the SvO_2 increases because the fiberoptics are in contact with newly oxygenated blood.

The range of diagnostic tools available to the bedside critical care nurse will continue to expand. As critical care patient needs become more complex and nursing responsibilities augment, incorporation of appropriate diagnostic information into the nursing management plan will only increase in importance.

REFERENCES

1. Conover MB: *Understanding electrocardiography,* ed 7, St Louis, 1996, Mosby.
2. Tsuji H and others: The association of levels of serum potassium and magnesium with ventricular premature complexes (the Framingham Heart Study), *Am J Cardiol* 74:232, 1994.
3. Yucha CB, Toto KH: Calcium and phosphorus derangements, *Crit Care Clin North Am* 6(4):747, 1994.
4. Toto KH, Yucha CB: Magnesium homostasis, intolerances, and therapeutic uses, *Crit Care Clin North Am* 6(4):767, 1994.
5. Wilson PWF, Kannel WB: Epidemiology of hyperglycemia and atherosclerosis. In Ruderman N, Williamson J, Brownlee M, editors: *Hyperglycemia, diabetes, and vascular disease,* New York, 1992, Oxford University Press.
6. Coffland FI: Endocrine disorders affecting the cardiovascular system, *Crit Care Clin North Am* 6(4):735, 1994.
7. Williams K, Morton PG: Diagnosis and treatment of acute myocardial infarction, *AACN Clin Issues in Crit Care Nurs* 6(3):375, 1995.
8. Wallach JW: *Interpretation of diagnostic tests,* ed 6, Boston, 1996, Little, Brown.
9. Hirsh J and others: Oral anticoagulants: mechanism of action, clinical effectiveness, and optimal therapeutic range, *Chest,* 108(4)suppl:231S, 1995.
10. Popma JJ and others: Antithrombic therapy in patients undergoing coronary angioplasty, *Chest,* 108(4)supp:486S, 1995.
11. National Cholesterol Education Program: *Second report of the expert panel on detection, evaluation, and treatment of high blood cholesterol in adults (adult treatment panel II),* NIH Pub. No. 93-3095, 1993, U.S. Department of Health and Human Services.
12. Henschke CI and others: Accuracy and efficacy of chest radiography in the intensive care unit, *Radiol Clin North Am* 34(1):21-31, 1996.
13. Zarshenas Z, Sparschu RA: Catheter placement and misplacement, *Crit Care Clin* 10(2):417-436, 1994.
14. Henry DA: Radiologic evaluation of the patient after cardiac surgery, *Radiol Clin North Am* 34(1):119-135, 1996.
15. Cascade PN, Kazerooni EA: Aspects of chest imaging in the intensive care unit, *Crit Care Clin* 10(2):247-265, 1994.
16. MacMahon H, Giger M: Portable chest radiography techniques and teleradiology, *Radiol Clin North Am* 34(1):1-20, 1996.
17. Stewart S, Haste M: Prediction of right ventricular and posterior wall ST elevation by coronary care nurses: the 12-lead electrocardiograph versus the 18-lead electrocardiograph, *Heart Lung* 25(1):14-23, 1996.
18. Futterman LG, Lemberg L: The long QT syndrome: when syncope is common to the young and the elderly, *Am J Crit Care* 4(5):405-412, 1995.
19. Hebra JD: The nurse's role in continuous dysrhythmia monitoring, *AACN Clin Issues in Crit Care Nurs* 5(2):178-185, 1994.
20. Drew BJ: Bedside electrocardiogram monitoring, *AACN Clin Issues in Crit Care Nurs* 4(1):25-33, 1993.
21. Tisdale LA, Drew BJ: ST segment monitoring for myocardial ischemia, *AACN Clin Issues in Crit Care Nurs* 4(1):34-43, 1993.
22. Creel CA: Silent myocardial ischemia and nursing implications, *Heart Lung* 23(3):218-227, 1994.
23. Drew BJ and others: ST segment monitoring with a derived 12-lead electrocardiogram is superior to routine cardiac care unit monitoring, *Am J Crit Care* 5(3):198-206, 1996.
24. Williams K, Morton PG: Diagnosis and treatment of acute myocardial infarction, *AACN Clin Issues in Crit Care Nurs* 6(3):375-386, 1995.
25. Turner DM, Turner LA: Right ventricular myocardial infarction: detection, treatment and nursing implications, *Crit Care Nurse,* 15(1):22-27, 1995.
26. Chun HM, Sung RJ: Supraventricular tachyarrhythmias: pharmacologic versus nonpharmacologic approaches, *Med Clin North Am* 79(5):1121-1133, 1995.
27. Califf RM: Acute ischemic syndromes, *Med Clin North Am* 79(5):999-1023, 1995.
28. Stambler BS: Efficacy and safety of repeated intravenous doses of Ibutilide for rapid conversion of atrial flutter on fibrillation, *Circulation* 94:1613-1621, 1996.

29. Ukani ZA, Ezekowitz MD: Contemporary management of atrial fibrillation, *Med Clin North Am* 79(5):1135-1152, 1995.
30. Tregear K, McCauley K: Thyrotoxic atrial fibrillation: pathophysiology, detection, and management, *J Cardiovasc Nurs* 7(3):1-7, 1993.
31. Nally BR and others: Supraventricular tachycardia after coronary artery bypass grafting surgery and fluid and electrolyte variables, *Heart Lung* 25(1):31-36, 1996.
32. Moran JL and others: Parenteral magnesium sulfate versus amiodarone in the therapy of atrial tachyarrhythmias: a prospective, randomized study, *Crit Care Med* 23(11):1816-1824, November 1995.
33. Craney JM: Radiofrequency catheter ablation of supraventricular tachycardias: clinical consideration and nursing care, *J Cardiovasc Nurs* 7(3):26-39, 1993.
34. Nicolai C: Ventricular dysrhythmias in ischemic heart disease, *AACN Clin Issues in Crit Care Nurs* 6(3):452-463, 1995.
35. Kellen JC and others: The cardiac arrhythmia suppression trial: implications for nursing practice, *Am J Crit Care* 5(1):19-25, 1996.
36. Hamdan M, Scheinman M: Current approaches in patients with ventricular tachyarrhythmias, *Med Clin North Am* 79(5):1097-1119, 1995.
37. Fabius DB: Diagnosing and treating ventricular tachycardia, *J Cardiovasc Nurs* 7(3):8-25, 1993.
38. Kessler DK, Kessler KM, Myerburg RJ: Ambulatory electrocardiography: a cost per management decision analysis, *Arch Intern Med* 155:165-169, 1995.
39. Mickley H and others: Characteristics and prognostic importance of ST-segment elevation on Holter monitoring early after acute myocardial infarction, *Am J Cardiol* 76:537-542, 1995.
40. Crawford MH: Approach to cardiac disease diagnosis. In Crawford MH, editor: *Current diagnosis & treatment in cardiology*, Norwalk, Conn, 1995, Appleton & Lange.
41. Gomez MA and others: An emergency department-based protocol for rapidly ruling out myocardial ischemia reduces hospital time and expense: results of a randomized study (ROMIO), *J Am Coll Cardiol* 28(1):25-33, 1996.
42. Marcus R and others: The exercise test as gatekeeper: limiting access or appropriately directing resources? *Chest* 107(5):1442-1446, 1995.
43. Khandheria BK, Tajik AJ, Seward JB: Multiplane transesophageal echocardiography: examination technique, anatomic correlations, and image orientation, *Crit Care Clin* 12(2):203-233, 1996.
44. McPherson D: Three dimensional arterial imaging, *Sci Am: Science and Medicine* 3(2):22-31, 1996.
45. Laurienzo JM: Transesophageal dobutamine stress echocardiography: the nurse's role, *J Cardiovasc Nurs* 9(4):24-35, 1995.
46. Khandheria BK, Seward JB, Tajik AJ: Critical appraisal of transesophageal echocardiography: limitations and pitfalls, *Crit Care Clin* 12(2):235-251, 1996.
47. Botvinick EH: Stress imaging: current clinical options for the diagnosis, localization, and evaluation of coronary artery disease, *Med Clin North Am* 79(5):1025-1061, 1995.
48. Aronson S, Han LK: Stress echocardiography, contrast echocardiography, and tissue characterization, *Crit Care Clin* 12(2):429-450, 1996.
49. Legget ME, Bashein G: Automatic border detection and three-dimensional reconstruction with echocardiography, *Crit Care Clin* 12(2):478-496, 1996.
50. Steffens JC and others: Magnetic resonance imaging in ischemic heart disease, *Am Heart J* 132(1):156-173, 1996.
51. Soulen RL, Duman RJ, Hoeffner E: Magnetic resonance imaging in the critical care setting, *Crit Care Clin* 10(2):401-415, 1994.
52. Simon AW: Use of a mechanical pressure device for hemostasis following cardiac catheterization, *Am J Crit Care* 3(1):62-64, 1994.
53. Hogan-Miller E and others: Effects of three methods of femoral site immobilization on bleeding and comfort after coronary angiogram, *Am J Crit Care* 4(2):143-148, 1995.
54. Bogart MA: Time to hemostasis: a comparison of manual versus mechanical compression of the femoral artery, *Am J Crit Care* 4(2):149-156, 1995.
55. Rein A and others: Positioning post-outpatient cardiac catheterization, *Prog Cardiovasc Nurs* 10(4):4-10, 1995.
56. Soloman R and others: Effects of saline, manitol, and furosemide on acute decreases in renal function induced by radiocontrast agents, *N Engl J Med* 331(21):1416-1420, 1994.
57. Davis TM and others: Preparing adult patients for cardiac catheterization: informational treatment and coping style interactions: *Heart Lung* 23(2):130-139, 1994.
58. Davis TM and others: Undergoing cardiac catheterization: the effects of informational preparation and coping style on patient anxiety during the procedure, *Heart Lung* 23(2):140-150, 1994.
59. Weld L: Developing a cardiac catheterization program, *J Cardiovasc Nurs* 11(2):47-57, 1997.
60. Beckerman A, Grossman D: Cardiac catheterization, *Heart Lung* 24(3):213-219, 1995.
61. Futterman LG, Lemberg L: Unexplained syncope: diagnostic value of tilt-table testing, *Am J Crit Care* 3(4):322-325, 1994.
62. Iberti TJ and others: A multicenter study of physicians' knowledge of the pulmonary artery catheter, *JAMA* 264(22):2928-2932, 1990.
63. Iberti TJ and others: Assessment of critical care nurses' knowledge of the pulmonary artery catheter, *Crit Care Med* 22(10):1674-1678, 1994.
64. Burns D and others: Critical care nurses' knowledge of pulmonary artery catheters, *Am J Crit Care* 5(1):49-54, 1996.
65. Gardner RM: Accuracy and reliability of disposable pressure transducers coupled with modern pressure monitors, *Crit Care Med* 24(5):879-882, 1996.

66. American Association of Critical Care Nurses: Evaluation of the effects of heparinized and nonheparinized flush solutions on the patency of arterial pressure monitoring line: the AACN Thunder Project, *Am J Crit Care* 2(1):3-15, 1993.
67. Zevola DR, Dioso J, Moggio R: Comparison of heparinized and nonherarinized solutions for maintaining patency of arterial and pulmonary artery catheters, *Am J Crit Care* 6(1):52-55, 1997.
68. Ahrens T, Penick JC, Tucker MK: Frequency requirements for zeroing transducers in hemodynamic monitoring, *Am J Crit Care* 4(6):466-471, 1995.
69. Doering LV: The effect of position change on hemodynamics and gas exchange in the critically ill: a review, *Am J Crit Care* 2(3):208-216, 1993.
70. Dobbin K and others: Pulmonary artery mean pressure measurement in patients with elevated pressures: effect of backrest elevation and methods of measurement, *Am J Crit Care* 1(2):61-69, 1992.
71. Potger KC, Elliott D: Reproducibility of central venous pressures in supine and lateral positions: a pilot evaluation of the phlebostatic axis in critically ill patients, *Heart Lung* 23(4):285-299, 1994.
72. Emerson RJ, Banasik JL: Effect of position on selected hemodynamic parameters in postoperative cardiac surgery patients, *Am J Crit Care* 3(4):289-299, 1994.
73. Quaal SJ: Quality assurance in hemodynamic monitoring, *AACN Clin Issues in Crit Care Nurs* 4(1):197-206, 1993.
74. Joynt GM and others: Comparison of intrathoracic and intraabdominal measurements of central venous pressure, *Lancet* 347:1155-1157, 1996.
75. Hoppe B: Central venous catheter-related infections: pathogenesis, predictors, and prevention, *Heart Lung* 24(4):333-339, 1995.
76. Bradley AD and others: Infectious rates of central venous pressure catheters: comparison between newly placed catheters and those that have been changed, *Mayo Clin Proc* 71(9):838-846, 1996.
77. Cook DJ, Simel DL: Does this patient have abnormal central venous pressure? *JAMA* 275(8):630-634, 1996.
78. Ginosak Y, Sprung CL: The Swan-Ganz catheter: twenty-five years of monitoring, *Crit Care Clin* 12(4):771-776, 1996.
79. Wiessner WH, Casey LC, Zbilut JP: Treatment of sepsis and septic shock: a review, *Heart Lung* 24(5):380-392, 1995.
80. Ramsey JD, Tisdale LA: Use of ventricular stroke work index and ventricular function curves in assessing myocardial contractility, *Crit Care Nurse* 15(1):61-67, 1995.
81. Nelson LD: The new pulmonary arterial catheters, *Crit Care Clin* 12(4): 795-818, 1996.
82. Conners AF Jr and others: The effectiveness of right heart catheterization in the initial care of critically ill patients, *JAMA* 276(11):889-897, 1996.
83. Pulmonary Artery Catheter Consensus Conference Participants: Pulmonary artery catheter consensus conference: consensus statement, *Crit Care Med* 25(6):910-925, 1997.
84. Liebowitz AB: Do pulmonary artery catheters improve patient outcomes? No, *Crit Care Clin* 12(3):559-568, 1996.
85. DelGuerico LRM: Does pulmonary artery catheter use change outcome? Yes, *Crit Care Clin* 12(3):553-557, 1996.
86. Hoyt JW: *Society of Critical Care Medicine,* letter to membership, Sept 16, 1996.
87. American Society of Anesthesiologists Task Force on Pulmonary Artery Catheterization: Practice guidelines for pulmonary artery catheterization, *Anesthesiology* 78:380-394, 1993.
88. Shinners PA, Pease MO: A stabilization period of 5 minutes is adequate when measuring pulmonary artery pressures after turning, *Heart Lung* 2(6):474-477, 1993.
89. Booker KJ, Arnold JS: Respiratory-induced changes on the pulmonary capillary wedge pressure tracing, *Crit Care Nurs* 13(3):80-88, 1993.
90. Hitchens M, Stotts JR: The RN's role in manipulation of pulmonary artery catheters, *Crit Care Nurse* 15(1):30-35, 1995.
91. Wades TA: Pulmonary artery catheter removal, *Crit Care Nurs* 14(3):62-72, 1994.
92. Smith MA: Noninvasive hemodynamic monitoring with thoracic electrical bioimpedance, *Crit Care Nurse* 14(5):56-59, 1994.
93. Pesola GR, Plante L: Room temperature thermodilution cardiac output: proximal injectate lumen vs proximal infusion lumen, *Am J Crit Care* 2(2):132-133, 1993.
94. Wallace DC, Winslow EH: Effects of iced and room temperature injectate on cardiac output measurements in critically ill patients with both low and high cardiac outputs, *Heart Lung* 22(1):55-63, 1993.
95. Jensen L, Yakimets J, Teo KK: A review of impedance cardiography, *Heart Lung* 24(3):194-206, 1995.
96. Guilbeau JR, Applegate AR: Thermodilution: an advanced technique for measuring continuous cardiac output, *DCCN* 15(1):25-30, 1996.
97. Ditmyer CE and others: Comparison of continuous with intermittent bolus thermodilution cardiac output measurements, *Am J Crit Care* 4(6):460-465, 1995.
98. White KM: Using continuous Svo_2 to assess oxygen supply/demand balance in the critically ill patient, *AACN Clin Issues in Crit Care Nurs* 4(1):134-147, 1993.
99. Headley JM: Strategies to optimize the cardiorespiratory status of the critically ill, *AACN Clin Issues in Crit Care Nurs* 6(1):1231-1234, 1995.
100. Noll ML, Byers JF: Comparison of Svo_2, Spo_2 and clinical parameters with arterial blood gases during ventilatory weaning after cardiac surgery, *Am J Crit Care* 3(5):353-355, 1994.
101. Epstein CD, Henning RJ: Oxygen transport variables in the identification and treatment of tissue hypoxia, *Heart Lung* 22(4):328-345, 1993.
102. Bearden EF: The costs and benefits of monitoring perfusion in the critically ill, *Crit Care Nurs Clin North Am* 7(2):239-248, 1996.
103. Gawlinski A: Effect of positioning on mixed venous oxygen saturation, *J Cardiovasc Nurs* 7(4):71-81, 1993.

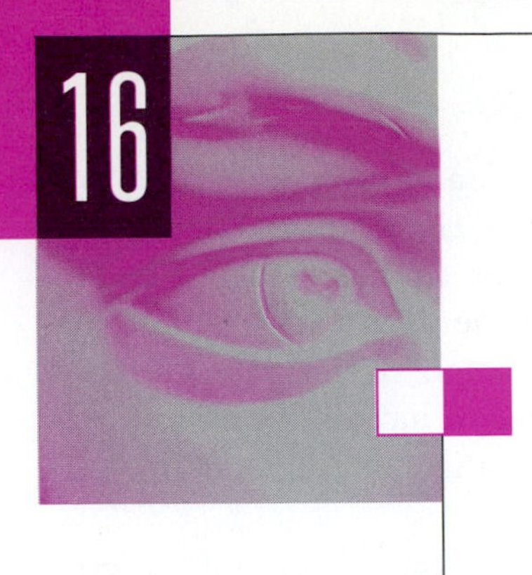

Cardiovascular Disorders

CARDIOVASCULAR DISEASE REMAINS the leading cause of mortality in the United States. It claims more than 950,000 lives annually and places a heavy emotional and financial burden on society.[1] An understanding of the pathology of cardiovascular disease processes, the areas of assessment on which to focus, and current medical and nursing management allow the critical care nurse to accurately anticipate and plan interventions. This chapter focuses on cardiac disorders commonly seen in the critical care environment.

BOX 16-1 Etiology of Coronary Artery Disease

- Atherosclerosis
- Thrombosis
- Spasm
- Coronary dissection
- Aneurysm formation

CORONARY ARTERY DISEASE

Description

Coronary artery disease (CAD) is an insidious, progressive disease of the coronary arteries that results in their narrowing or complete occlusion. There are multiple causes of coronary artery narrowing (Box 16-1), but atherosclerosis is the most prevalent. Atherosclerosis affects not only the coronary arteries but also arterial vessels in the brain, kidneys, and peripheral arteries.

Etiology

CAD has a long latent period.[2] Fatty streaks can appear within the aorta during childhood, but symptoms occur only when the atherosclerotic plaque occludes 75% of the vessel lumen, usually in late middle age.[3]

Epidemiologic data collected during the past 40 years has demonstrated an association between specific risk factors and the development of CAD. One of the most important epidemiologic studies is the Framingham Heart Study, which began in 1948 and continues today with a third and fourth generation of subjects. Blood cholesterol, smoking, activity level, blood pressure, and electrocardiographic results are checked on a regular basis for participants in this study. As a result, specific CAD risk factors that are associated with an increased probability of CAD development have been identified. These life-style habits are referred to as *CAD risk factors.*[4]

Risk Factors for Coronary Artery Disease

Public awareness of the risk factors that contribute to the development of coronary artery disease is increasing. However, because people are living longer than ever before and cardiovascular disease is most prevalent in elderly persons, CAD continues to be a worldwide public health problem.[5]

Factors that increase risk for development of CAD include age, gender, race, genetic inheritance (family history), elevated serum cholesterol, hypertension, cigarette smoking, glucose intolerance, sedentary life-style, stress, and a type A behavior pattern. These factors are further delineated into nonmodifiable and modifiable CAD risk factors (Box 16-2).

Age. The symptoms of CAD occur as a person ages. In general CAD is a disease of middle and old age.[2-4]

BOX 16-2 Coronary Artery Disease Risk Factors

NONMODIFIABLE

Age
Gender
Family history
Race

MODIFIABLE

Major

Elevated serum lipids
Hypertension
Cigarette smoking
Impaired glucose tolerance
Diet high in saturated fat, cholesterol, and calories
Physical inactivity

Minor

Psychologic stress
Personality type

Gender. CAD occurs approximately 10 years later in women than it does in men. After menopause, rates are the same for both genders.[4-6]

Family history. A positive family history is one in which a close blood relative had a myocardial infarction or stroke before the age of 60 years. This family history suggests a genetic predisposition to the development of coronary artery disease.[4]

Race. Nonwhite populations of both genders have higher CAD mortality rates than do white populations.

Cholesterol. Hyperlipidemia is a leading factor responsible for severe atherosclerosis and the development of CAD.[7] Total serum cholesterol levels more than 200 mg/dL are associated with a higher risk of CAD, and levels greater than 270 mg/dL carry a fourfold increase in risk.[7] Total cholesterol is subdivided into the following specific lipoproteins:

1. High density lipoprotein-cholesterol (HDL-C).
2. Low density lipoprotein-cholesterol (LDL-C).
3. Very low density lipoprotein-cholesterol (VLDL-C).
4. Triglycerides.

Low density refers to a low protein content. Elevated LDL-C, VLDL-C, and triglyceride levels are associated with an increased incidence of CAD. *High density* implies a high protein content. Low HDL-C levels also increase CAD risk.[7,8] Very low density lipoproteins-cholesterol (VLDL-C) transport mainly triglycerides. Low density lipoproteins-cholesterol (LDLs-C) are metabolized from VLDL-C and carry 60% to 75% of the total plasma cholesterol. High density lipoproteins-cholesterol (HDLs-C) clear cholesterol from the tissues and transport it to the liver. Children and premenopausal women have high HDL-C levels. HDL-C levels increase in response to increased physical exercise, weight loss, and cessation of cigarette smoking. (∞Serum Lipids, p. 383.)

Homocystine. Homocystinuria is a rare inborn error of metabolism. It has received attention recently because patients with high levels of plasma homocystine have a very high incidence of atherosclerotic coronary artery and vascular disease.[9,10] As with other risk factors, the chance for CAD to develop increases if the person also smokes cigarettes, has hyperlipidemia, is overweight, or is physically inactive.

Hypertension. Hypertension is the elevation of either systolic blood pressure (SBP) or diastolic blood pressure (DBP). The higher the BP, the greater is the risk of coronary artery disease. Hypertension is a risk factor because of the damage it causes to the endothelium of the vessel. The risk of developing CAD is reduced when the SBP and DBP are less than 140/90 mm Hg.[11] Hypertension has many predisposing factors that overlap with CAD risk factors including older age, high dietary sodium intake, obesity, sedentary life-style, excessive alcohol consumption, cocaine abuse, the use of oral contraceptives, and being of African-American descent. Other risk factors include medications and medical problems that influence intrinsic mediators of blood pressure, such as the renin-angiotensin-aldosterone system and the sympathetic nervous system. Management of hypertension is initially directed toward life-style modifications such as weight loss, decrease of dietary sodium chloride, increase in physical activity, reduced alcohol consumption, stress management, and if these are not successful, by pharmacologic therapy.[11,12] Hypertensive emergencies are managed by intravenous (IV) antihypertensive agents and vasodilators.

Cigarette smoking. The greater the number of cigarettes smoked per day, the greater the CAD risk. Cigarette smoking unfavorably alters serum lipid levels, decreasing HDL-C levels and increasing LDL-C and triglyceride levels. Smoking results in cardiac electrical instability within cell membranes and impairs oxygen transport and use while increasing myocardial oxygen demand. Smoking also is thought to alter intimal endothelial permeability and to foster platelet agglutination. Fortunately, the damage from smoking is not unalterable, and after cessation the coronary risk falls rapidly, with a decrease of approximately 50% within 1 year.[6]

Diabetes mellitus. Individuals with diabetes mellitus have a higher incidence of coronary artery disease than does the general population. In fact, diabetes triples or quadruples the risk of developing CAD.[13] Premenopausal women with diabetes are at increased risk of developing CAD, compared with nondiabetic women of the same age, because diabetes negates the protective effect of estrogen. CAD risk from diabetes also rises in the presence of increased serum cholesterol, hypertension, and cigarette smoking.[13]

Oral contraceptives. Oral contraceptives increase a woman's risk of developing CAD, especially after age 35 years, because they (1) alter blood coagulation, (2) alter platelet function, (3) alter fibrinolytic activity, and (4) may inversely affect the integrity of vascular endothelium. The risk is increased more if the woman also smokes cigarettes.

Obesity. Obesity is often associated with a sedentary life-style. It also increases susceptibility to the development of other risk factors, such as hypertension, impaired glucose tolerance, and hyperlipidemia, with increased LDL-C and decreased HDL-C levels.

Physical inactivity. Evidence continues to accumulate that a sedentary life-style increases the risk for CAD. Physical inactivity is also associated with lower HDL-C levels, higher LDL-C levels, hypertension, obesity, increased glucose intolerance, and hyperlipidemia.[4]

Stress and anxiety. Type A behavior patterns that include time-urgency, hostility, anger, and anxiety have also been associated with the development of CAD.[14,15] How stress and behavior influences the development of CAD is not well-understood, but stress is associated with increased circulating catecholamines, which may precipitate hypertension, alteration in platelet function, increased fatty acid mobilization, and a resultant elevation of free fatty acids.

Multifactorial risk. At present, researchers are uncertain why a risk factor in one individual may result in serious consequences but may not cause problems for another individual. Studies show that CAD is a multifactorial disease and as the number of known risk factors increase, the risk of developing the disease increases in an exponential, rather than additive, manner.

Pathophysiology

CAD is a progressive disorder of the coronary arteries that results in narrowing or complete occlusion. There are multiple causes for coronary artery narrowing, but *atherosclerosis* is the most prevalent. Atherosclerosis affects the medium-sized arteries perfusing the heart, brain, and kidneys and the large arteries branching off the aorta. Atherosclerotic lesions may take different forms, depending on their anatomic location; the individual's age, genetic makeup, physiologic status; and the number of risk factors present. Normal arterial walls are composed of three cellular layers: the intima, or innermost endothelial layer; the media, or middle muscular layer; and the adventitia, or outermost connective tissue layer. (∞The Arterial System, p. 337.)

Three major elements are associated with atherosclerotic plaque development and luminal narrowing[16-18]: (1) smooth muscle proliferation; (2) formation of a connective tissue matrix composed of collagen, elastic fibers, and proteoglycans; and (3) accumulation of lipids (Figure 16-1).

Stages of plaque development. Specific stages of atherosclerotic plaque development have been identified.[2,16-18] The first stage is the development of fatty streaks. These are broad-based lesions composed of lipid-laden macrophages and smooth muscle cells. During the second stage, streaks develop into fatty plaques. Subsequently, collagen and dense connective tissue create atherosclerotic fibrous plaques. Finally, the third stage—the advanced or complicated lesion phase—is when the fibrous plaque becomes vascularized, the core calcifies, and the surface ulcerates, resulting in hemorrhage and thromboembolic episodes. Furthermore, the media may develop aneurysmal changes resulting from the decrease in smooth muscle cells (see Figure 16-1).

CAD hemodynamic effects. The major hemodynamic effect of CAD is the disturbance of the delicate balance between myocardial oxygen supply and demand. Atherosclerosis alters the normal coronary artery's response to increased demand in two ways: (1) lesions that result in a 75% or more vessel-lumen occlusion restrict flow under resting conditions and (2) vessels become stiff and lose the ability to dilate. The result is decreased driving pressure beyond the site of the lesion and less oxygenated blood available to the myocardial cells perfused by that vessel. During periods of ischemia—felt as angina by the patient—the myocardium is forced to shift from aerobic metabolism to anaerobic metabolism, the consequences of which are (1) less-efficient energy production, (2) lactic acid build-up, (3) intracellular hypokalemia, (4) intracellular acidosis, (5) intracellular hypernatremia, and (6) interference with the release of calcium from its storage sites in the sarcoplasmic reticulum. Tissue hypoxia or ischemia is the end result of this process.

Plaque rupture. Superficial tears in vessel wall atherosclerotic plaque are found—on autopsy—in about 17% of patients who die from noncardiac causes.[19] This suggests that damage to atherosclerotic plaque is a routine event. In individuals who die from a known coronary event, the vessel luminal diameter is more

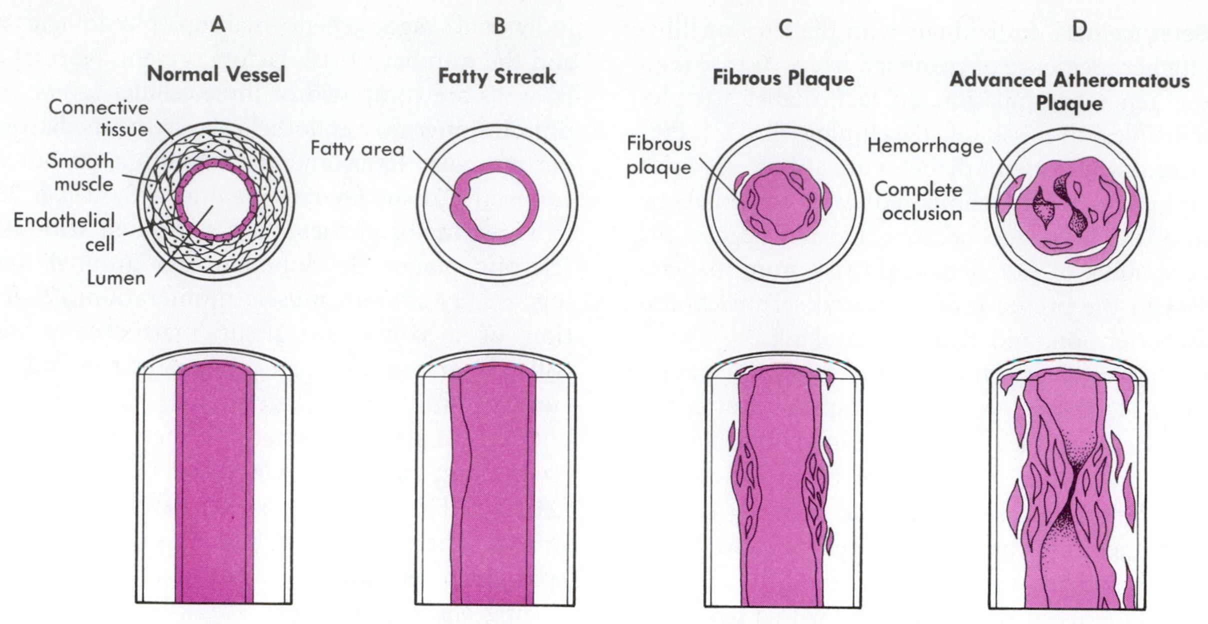

FIGURE 16-1. The progression of atherosclerosis shown in both the longitudinal and the cross-sectional views. **A,** Normal vessel. **B,** First stage, fatty streaks. **C,** Second stage, fibrous plaque development. **D,** Third stage, advanced (complicated) lesions.

than 75% occluded by plaque.[18,19] In individuals with more lumen than not occluded by plaque, there is a greater risk of plaque rupture from the damaged plaque surface. It is believed that unstable angina, acute myocardial infarction, and ischemic sudden cardiac death are the result of ruptured plaque and a rapidly evolving thrombus.[20] Deep fissures in the fibrous cap expose procoagulant factors within the plaque core to the blood plasma. When platelets in the blood are exposed to collagen, necrotic debris, von Willebrand factor, and thromboxane, a clot is formed that can occlude the coronary artery.[20] Highly fibrotic plaques do not rupture. The type of atherosclerotic plaque that is prone to rupture has a weak fibrous cap and a large amount of cholesterol within the core.[20] For this reason it is thought that reducing the plasma cholesterol, and ultimately the cholesterol within the plaque, will decrease the risk of an acute coronary event.[21,22]

Plaque regression. Reduction of blood cholesterol decreases the plaque size by decreasing the amount of cholesterol within the plaque core. It will not change the dimensions of the fibrous or calcified portions of the plaque. If diet is not effective in lowering blood cholesterol levels, lipid-lowering drugs are used to lower the LDL-C level to less than 100 mg/dL, the HDL-C level to less than 50 mg/dL, and triglycerides to less than 140 mg/dL.[7,21]

Angina

Angina pectoris, or chest pain caused by myocardial ischemia, is not a separate disease, but rather a symptom of CAD. It is caused by a blockage or spasm of a coronary artery, leading to diminished blood supply to the myocardium. The lack of oxygen causes ischemia, which is felt as pain. Angina may occur anywhere in the chest, neck, arms, or back, but the most commonly described location is behind the sternum. The pain often radiates to the left arm but can also radiate to both arms, the mandible, and/or the neck (Figure 16-2). Angina has other characteristics in addition to pain (Box 16-3). It is classified as stable, unstable, and variant.[23,24]

The patient who comes to the emergency department with a recent history of unstable angina is usually admitted to the critical care unit as a patient with "rule out MI."[25] Factors to consider when assessing chest pain are listed in Box 16-4. If the patient is having unrelenting chest pain, obviously this is more than angina, and all interventions will focus on clearing the blocked coronary artery. Angina pectoris is covered under diagnosis-related group (DRG) 140 and has an anticipated length of stay of 3.8 days.[26]

Stable angina. *Stable angina* is predictable and caused by similar precipitating factors each time, such as exercise, emotional upset, and tachycardia. Patients become used to the pattern of this type of angina and may describe it as "my usual chest pain." Control of pain is achieved by rest and administration of a coronary artery vasodilator such as sublingual nitroglycerin. Stable angina is the result of fixed lesions (blockages) of more than 75%. Ischemia and chest pain occur when myocardial demand exceeds blood

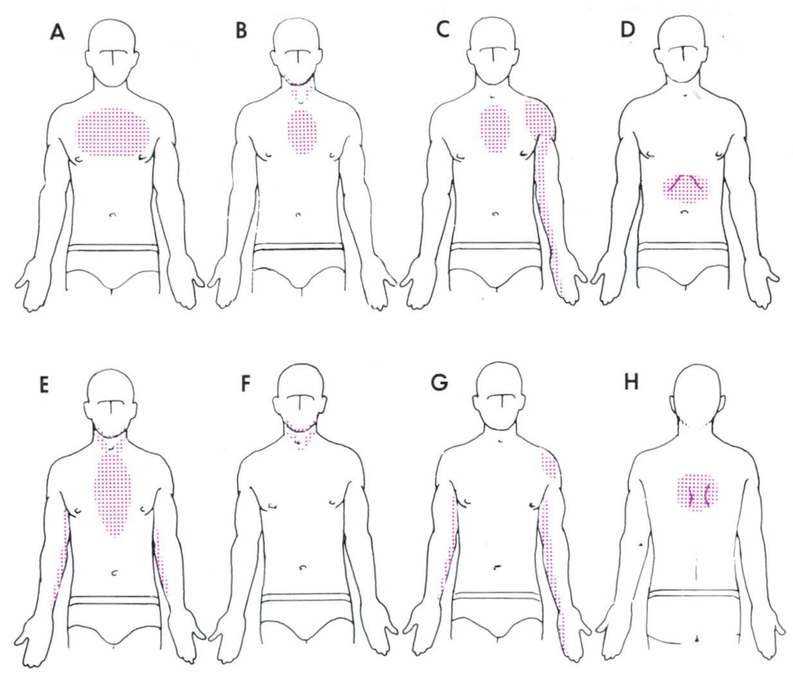

FIGURE 16-2. Common sites for anginal pain. **A,** Upper part of chest. **B,** Beneath sternum, radiating to neck and jaw. **C,** Beneath sternum, radiating down left arm. **D,** Epigastric. **E,** Epigastric, radiating to neck, jaw, and arms. **F,** Neck and jaw. **G,** Left shoulder. **H,** Intrascapular.

oxygen supply. It can be managed medically for long periods.

Unstable angina. *Unstable angina* is defined as a change in a previously established stable pattern of angina or a new onset of severe angina. It usually is more intense than stable angina, may awaken the person from sleep, or may necessitate more than nitrates for pain relief. A change in the level or frequency of symptoms requires immediate medical evaluation.[24] Severe angina that persists for more than 20 minutes and is not relieved by three nitroglycerin tablets is called *preinfarction,* or *crescendo, angina.* This is a medical emergency, and the person must be taken to a hospital emergency room immediately.[25] The pathology underlying the change from stable to unstable angina may be plaque hemorrhage or fissure that causes an increase in localized platelet agglutination and acute thrombosis.[20]

Variant angina. *Variant,* or *Prinzmetal's, angina* is caused by coronary artery spasm. It is believed to result from spasm, with or without atherosclerotic lesions. Variant angina commonly occurs when the individual is at rest and also can be cyclic, occurring at the same time every day. It usually is associated with ST-segment elevation and occasionally with transient abnormal Q waves. Smoking tobacco and ingesting alcohol and cocaine also may precipitate spasm. Drugs of choice for the treatment of spasm are agents that vasodilate the coronary arteries, such as nitroglycerin or calcium channel blockers (e.g., nifedipine and diltiazem).

Silent ischemia. *Silent ischemia* is defined as objective ECG evidence of myocardial ischemia (ST-segment changes) without the patient experiencing any symptoms of angina.[27] It is classified into three clinical types (Box 16-5). Patients with Type I ischemia are asymptomatic, without manifestations of cardiovascular disease, yet continuous monitoring or stress testing demonstrates myocardial ischemia. Often, these patients are found to have multivessel CAD when tested later using coronary arteriography. Type II patients are those who have had an acute myocardial infarction and demonstrate active ischemia but have no anginal symptoms. Patients with Type III ischemia have some ischemic episodes that are accompanied by chest pain and other episodes without chest discomfort. Type III patients may or may not have had a prior infarction. Once identified, silent ischemia usually is treated in the same manner as classic angina—with nitrates, beta-blockers, calcium channel blockers, and life-style changes.[27,28]

Medical Management

The major goals of medical therapy for coronary artery disease and angina are to (1) increase coronary artery perfusion, (2) decrease myocardial workload,

BOX 16-3 Characteristics of Angina Pectoris

LOCATION

Beneath sternum, radiating to neck and jaw
Upper chest
Beneath sternum, radiating down left arm
Epigastric
Epigastric, radiating to neck, jaw, and arms
Neck and jaw
Left shoulder, inner aspect of both arms
Intrascapular

DURATION

0.5 to 30 minutes (stable)
Duration of longer than 30 minutes, without relief from rest or medication, indicates unstable or preinfarction symptoms

QUALITY

Sensation of pressure or heavy weight on the chest
Feeling of tightness, like a vise
Visceral quality (deep, heavy, squeezing, aching)
Burning sensation
Shortness of breath, with feeling of suffocation
Most severe pain ever experienced

RADIATION

Medial aspect of left arm
Jaw
Left shoulder
Right arm

PRECIPITATING FACTORS

Exertion/exercise
Cold weather
Exercising after a large, heavy meal
Walking against the wind
Emotional upset
Fright, anger
Coitus

MEDICATION RELIEF

Usually within 45 seconds to 5 minutes of sublingual nitroglycerin administration

BOX 16-4 Factors to Consider When Assessing Chest Pain

Onset (either sudden or gradual)
Precipitating factors (did visitors come or leave; was the patient up moving around?)
Location (was it substernal; was it located in same area as previous pain?)
Radiation (did it radiate to the jaw, neck, arm, or shoulder?)
Quality (was it similar to previous anginal pain; was it less or worse?)
Intensity (on a scale of 1 to 10, where would the patient rate it?)
Duration (did it last seconds or minutes; how soon after onset did the patient call for help?)
Relieving factors (what made it better—changing position, nitroglycerin, oxygen, the presence of the nurse?)
Aggravating factors (did the environment, telephone calls, waiting for help worsen the pain?)
Associated symptoms (was the pain accompanied by nausea, vomiting, diaphoresis, or dyspnea?)
Emotional response (how did the patient feel about the pain; anxious, fearful, angry?)

BOX 16-5 Silent Ischemia

TYPE	CLINICAL CHARACTERISTICS
I	Objective evidence of myocardial ischemia without chest pain/symptoms
II	No anginal symptoms after a previous MI, but objective evidence of myocardial ischemia continues
III	Symptoms of angina with some episodes of ischemia, and asymptomatic with other ischemic events; may or may not have had a previous MI

MI, myocardial infarction.
Objective evidence of myocardial ischemia: ST-segment changes seen on ECG monitoring.

(3) prevent myocardial infarction (MI) disability or death, and (4) intervene in cases of unstable angina. Specific medical management depends on the frequency, severity, duration, and hemodynamic consequences of the angina.

Myocardial supply/demand balance. Pharmacologic therapy such as oxygen, nitrates, and vasodilators[23] are used to increase coronary artery perfusion and myocardial oxygen supply. Lytic therapy may be used to restore blood flow to the coronary artery if the patient arrives at the emergency department within 6 hours of the onset of chest pain. Bedrest, beta-blockers, ACE (angiotensin-converting enzyme) inhibitors, and calcium channel blockers are used to decrease myocardial oxygen demand. Analgesics such as morphine are used to relieve anginal pain.[23,29,30] (∞Cardiac Drugs, p. 574.)

MI prevention. CAD risk factors, such as hypertension or hyperlipidemia, are treated aggressively. A low-sodium, low-cholesterol diet may be recommended. Activity is restricted until episodes of angina are controlled.

Angina management. The change from stable to unstable angina represents a serious problem. The patient is admitted to a hospital, and bedrest is prescribed. It is important that any identified precipitating problems be treated. If the anginal pain continues, cardiac catheterization, intraaortic balloon support, thrombolytic therapy, interventional cardiology procedure, or coronary artery bypass graft (CABG) surgery may be indicated.[29,30] (∞Cardiac Catheterization, p. 438; Intraaortic Balloon Pump, p. 567; Thrombolytic Therapy, p. 561; CABG, p. 541.)

BOX 16-6 NURSING DIAGNOSIS AND MANAGEMENT

CORONARY ARTERY DISEASE/ANGINA

- Acute Pain related to transmission and perception of cutaneous, visceral, muscular, or ischemic impulses, secondary to myocardial ischemia p. 197
- Altered Myocardial Tissue Perfusion related to acute myocardial ischemia p. 595
- Activity Intolerance related to cardiopulmonary dysfunction, p. 596
- Powerlessness related to lack of control over current situation, p. 89
- Anxiety related to threat to biologic, psychologic, and/or social integrity, p. 99
- Knowledge Deficit: Discharge Regimen related to lack of previous exposure to information, p. 61 (see Patient Education Box 16-7)

Nursing Management

Nursing management of the patient with CAD and angina incorporates a variety of nursing diagnoses (Box 16-6). Nursing interventions focus on early identification of chest pain, pain control, maintaining a calm environment, and patient education.

Assessment of chest pain. Complaints of chest discomfort are evaluated quickly. Chest pain in the patient with known or suspected coronary disease may represent myocardial ischemia, which must be treated while it is still reversible. The patient is asked to rate the intensity of the chest discomfort on a scale of 1 to 10. The words "chest pain" are not to be used exclusively, since some patients describe their angina as "pressure" or "heaviness." It is also important to document the characteristics of the pain, the patient's heart rate and rhythm, the presence of ectopic beats or conduction defects, the patient's mentation, and overall tissue perfusion. This includes skin color, temperature, peripheral pulses, and urine output. A 12-lead electrocardiogram (ECG) is used to identify the area of ischemic myocardium.[31] The major concern is that the chest pain may represent preinfarction angina, and early identification is essential so that the patient can be immediately transported to the cardiac catheterization laboratory for diagnosis and possibly treatment. If the hospital does not have a cardiac catheterization laboratory, thrombolytics may be prescribed to prevent the development of an acute myocardial infarction.

Relieve chest pain. In the critical care unit, control of angina is achieved by a combination of supplemental oxygen, nitrates, and analgesia.

1. *Oxygen:* all patients with acute ischemic pain are administered supplemental oxygen to increase myocardial oxygenation. Those patients who develop symptoms of acute heart failure may require emergency intubation and mechanical ventilation to correct significant hypoxemia.[23,30]
2. *Nitrates:* a combination of intravenous and sublingual nitroglycerin is used to vasodilate the coronary arteries and control pain. After nitrate administration, the nurse closely observes the patient for relief of chest pain, return of the ST segment to baseline, and for the development of unwanted side effects such as hypotension and headache.[23,30]
3. *Analgesia:* morphine is the analgesic of choice for preinfarction angina; it both relieves pain and decreases fear and anxiety. After administration the critical care nurse assesses the patient for pain relief and the development of unwanted side effects such as hypotension and respiratory depression.[23,30]

Maintaining a calm environment. Patients admitted to a critical care unit with acute angina experience extreme anxiety and fear of death. The critical care nurse is met with the challenge of combining the elements of a calm environment that alleviate fear and anxiety, while at the same time always being ready to respond to an acute patient emergency such as a cardiac arrest or to assist with emergency intubation or insertion of hemodynamic monitoring catheters.

Coronary precautions. Nursing research studies have shown that many of the "coronary precautions" previously practiced to decrease energy expenditure by the patient do not have a scientific basis.[32] These precautions included withholding iced oral fluids and caffeine, feeding patients, avoiding rectal temperatures, providing full bed baths, having patients use bedpans rather than bedside commodes, and avoiding vigorous backrubs.[32] One precaution that has proved valid is teaching patients to avoid the Valsalva maneuver.[32]

Acute MI patients who are stable and pain free can feed themselves and do not need to be fed by the nurse, although most acute MI patients do not have a large appetite. If patients are accustomed to drinking coffee at home, withholding it in the hospital can cause symptoms of acute caffeine withdrawal. Therefore coffee drinkers may have one to four cups of coffee a day during hospitalization.[32] There is no reason to withhold iced fluids, because they do not have any clinical effect on dysrhythmias.

Vigorous backrubs are not contraindicated and do not increase angina. In addition, full bed baths are no longer considered necessary for the stable patient who can assist with the bath. In the past many MI patients were given full bed baths to conserve their energy, even when the patients were pain free and stable. Most stable patients are also able, and prefer, to use the bedside commode, rather than a bedpan. Finally, the issue of obtaining rectal temperatures (not contraindicated) has largely been resolved by the increasing use of less-invasive tympanic membrane thermometers that use the ear canal as the route.

A coronary precaution that must always be taught in the acute period is the importance of avoiding the *Valsalva maneuver,* defined as forced expiration against a closed glottis. This can be explained as "bearing down" when going to the bathroom or breath holding when repositioning in bed. The Valsalva maneuver has been associated with changes in blood pressure and heart rate, because the increase in intrathoracic pressure decreases venous return to the right side of the heart.[32]

Patient education. In the critical care unit, the patient's ability to retain educational information is severely affected by stress and pain. However, it is imperative to teach the importance of avoiding the Valsalva maneuver as previously described. Once the ischemic pain is controlled, patient and family education can begin. Points to cover include risk factor modification, signs and symptoms of angina, when to call the physician, medications, and dealing with emotions and stress.[33] However, since the acute hospital length of stay for uncomplicated angina is usually less than 4 days, referral to a cardiac rehabilitation program for a controlled exercise program and risk factor modification after discharge is perhaps the most helpful teaching intervention a critical care nurse can provide (Box 16-7).

MYOCARDIAL INFARCTION

Description

Myocardial infarction is the term used to describe irreversible myocardial necrosis (cell death) that results from an abrupt decrease or total cessation of coronary blood flow to a specific area of the myocardium.[30] Acute MI is covered under DRGs 121, 122, and 123, depending on the clinical presentation (Box 16-8). The anticipated length of stay ranges from 4.9 to 8.4 days.[26]

Etiology

Atherosclerosis is responsible for most myocardial infarctions, because it causes luminal narrowing and reduced blood flow, resulting in decreased oxygen delivery to the myocardium. The three mechanisms that are primarily responsible for the acute reduction in oxygen delivery to the myocardium are (1) coronary artery thrombosis, (2) plaque fissure or hemorrhage, and (3) coronary artery spasm. Infarction is more prevalent in the left ventricle, with multivessel occlusions, and in myocardium distal to vessels that have not developed collateral flow.

Coronary artery thrombi. Thrombi are now known to be present in almost all acute coronary artery occlusions. These thrombi, usually composed of platelets, fibrin, erythrocytes, and leukocytes, may be superimposed on a plaque or may be aligned adjacent to a plaque. They release thromboxane A_2, serotonin, and thrombin—all vasoconstricting substances that compound vessel narrowing and set up a vicious cycle of recurrent occlusion. Scientists have not determined the cause of thrombus formation, but plaque fissure or hemorrhage, or both, are thought to be predisposing events.[16-19]

Atherosclerotic plaques. Plaques are classified according to their composition. Hard plaques are heavily calcified and fibrotic, whereas soft plaques are composed of cholesterol esters and lipids. Coronary artery thrombosis has been associated with rupture, or cracks, of the plaques and release of the plaque material into the vascular lumen. Plaque rupture can induce thrombosis by (1) forming a platelet plug, (2) releasing tissue thromboplastin from the plaque material that activates the clotting cascade, and (3) obstructing the vessel lumen with plaque components. Coronary artery spasm is often present in acute occlusions. How-

BOX 16-7 PATIENT EDUCATION

ANGINA

- Angina: describe signs and symptoms such as pain, pressure, and heaviness in chest, arms, or jaw
- Preinfarction or unstable angina: any chest pain that is not relieved by 2-3 sublingual nitroglycerin (NTG) tablets provides reason to call 911 (Emergency Services) or to be driven to the nearest hospital emergency department
- Use of the pain scale from 1 to 10: notify critical care nurse or emergency personnel of any changes in pain intensity
- Use of sublingual NTG for angina: pain intensity should decrease on the pain scale after NTG administration; at home, NTG must be kept in a dark, airtight container or it loses its potency; to ensure potency, the NTG supply is replaced about every 6 months; active NTG has a slight burning sensation when placed under the tongue
- Avoidance of the Valsalva maneuver
- Risk factor modification tailored to the patient's individual risk factor profile: decrease fat intake to <30% of total calories a day; stop smoking; reduce salt intake; control hypertension; treat diabetes, if patient is diabetic; increase physical activity; achieve ideal body weight
- Refer to cardiac rehabilitation program
- Medication teaching: indications, side effects
- Follow-up care
- Symptoms to report to a health care professional
- How to handle emotional stress and anger

ever, it is not known whether this results from hyperactive smooth muscle or whether it is a secondary response related to a plaque rupture and the release of vasoactive substances.[16-19]

Pathophysiology

Infarction. The area of cellular death and muscle necrosis in the myocardium is known as the *zone of infarction* (Figure 16-3). On the ECG, evidence of this zone is seen by pathologic Q waves, which reflect a lack of depolarization from the cardiac surface involved in the myocardial infarction (Figure 16-4, *D*). As healing takes place, the cells in this area are replaced by scar tissue.

Injury. The infarcted zone is surrounded by injured but still potentially viable tissue in an area known as the *zone of injury* (see Figure 16-3). Cells in this area do not fully repolarize because of the deficient blood supply. This is recorded as elevation of the ST segment (Figure 16-4, *C*).

Ischemia. The outer region of the myocardium is the *zone of ischemia,* as illustrated in Figure 16-3, and is composed of viable cells. Repolarization in this zone is impaired but eventually is restored to normal. Repolarization of the cells in this area manifests as T wave inversion (Figure 16-4, *B*).

MI Evolution. During the first 6 weeks after an infarction, the damaged myocardium undergoes many changes. Approximately 6 hours after the infarction, the muscle becomes distended, pale, and cyanotic. Over the next 2 days the myocardium becomes reddish purple, and an exudate may form on the epicardium. Leukocyte scavenger cells begin to infiltrate the muscle and carry away the necrotic debris, thereby thinning the necrotic wall. Approximately 3 to 4 weeks after the infarction, scar tissue begins to form and the affected wall becomes whiter and thicker.

Transmural MI. Myocardial infarctions are classified according to their location on the myocardial surface and the muscle layers affected. A transmural MI involves all three muscle layers—the endocardium, the myocardium, and the epicardium (Figure 16-5)—and involves significant ECG changes.

Non-Q wave MI. Nontransmural infarctions are classified as either *subendocardial,* involving the endocardium, or *subepicardial,* involving the epicardium. Some myocardium may be involved in a nontransmural MI, but it is not a full thickness MI. Generally, abnormal Q waves are not seen, so a nontransmural MI is commonly called a *non-Q wave MI.* A 12-lead ECG of a non-Q wave MI is shown in Figure 16-6.

BOX 16-8 Myocardial Infarction *Diagnosis-Related Groups (DRGs)*[26]

DRG NUMBER		LENGTH OF STAY
121	Circulatory disorders with acute myocardial infarction and cardiovascular complication, discharged alive.	8.4 days
122	Circulatory disorders with acute myocardial infarction without cardiovascular complication, discharged alive.	5.8 days
123	Circulatory disorders with acute myocardial infarction, discharged alive.	4.9 days

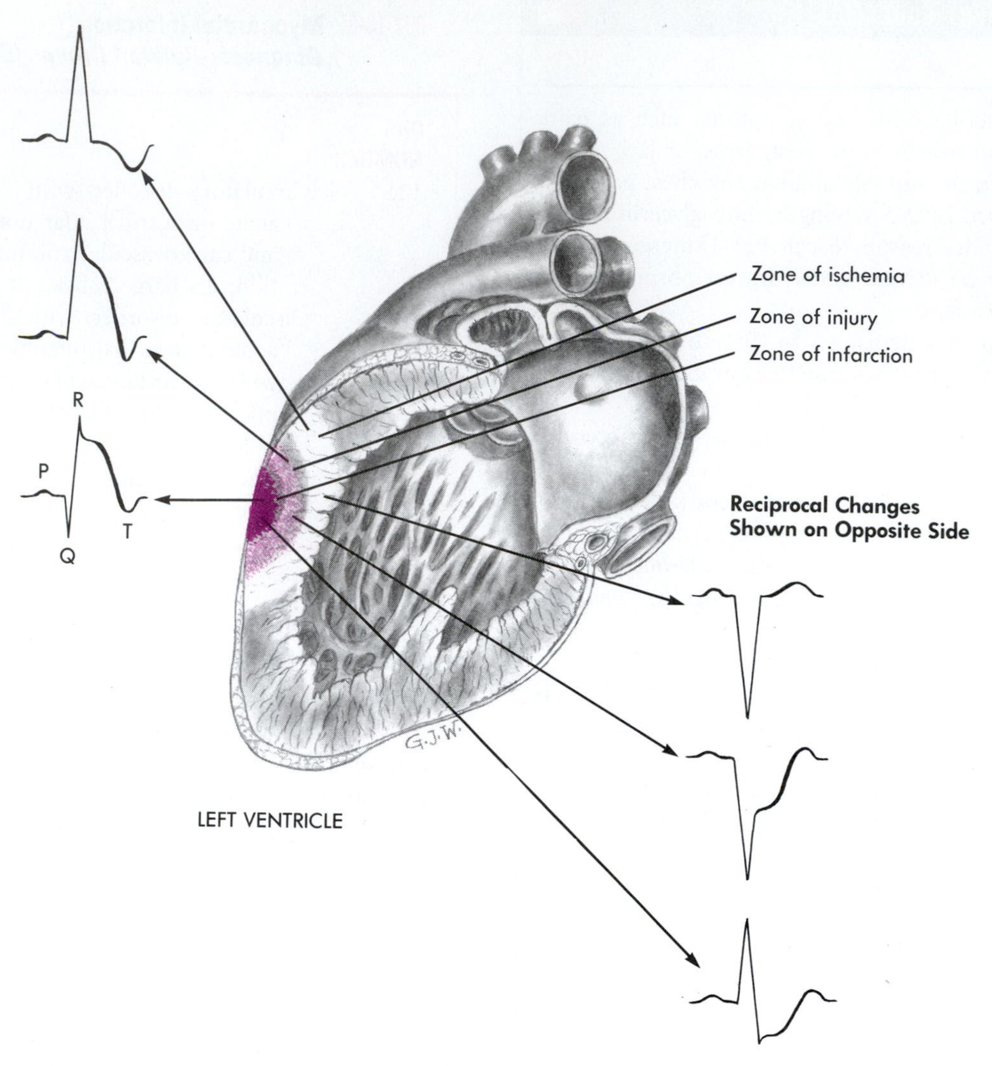

FIGURE 16-3. Zone of ischemia, zone of injury, and zone of infarction, shown through ECG waveforms and reciprocal waveforms corresponding to each zone.

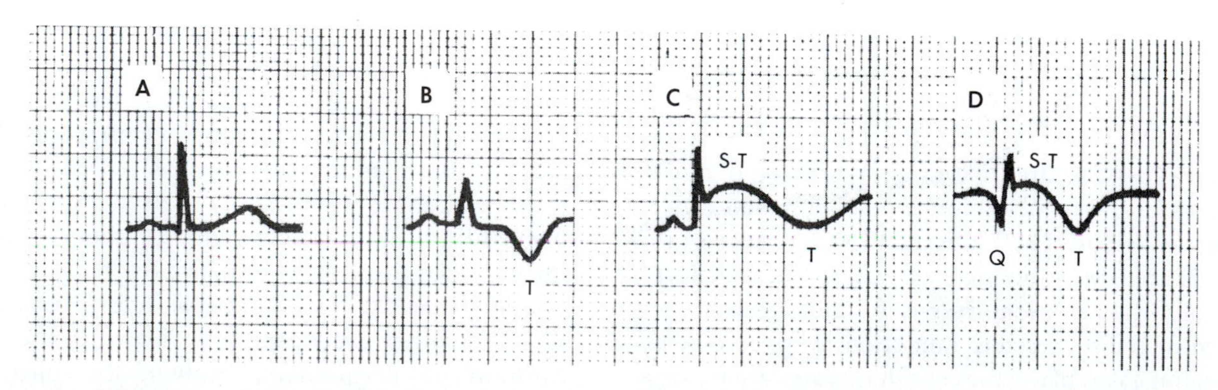

FIGURE 16-4. ECG changes indicative of ischemia, injury, and infarction (necrosis) of the myocardium. **A,** Normal ECG. **B,** Ischemia indicated by inversion of the T wave. **C,** Ischemia and current of injury indicated by T wave inversion and ST-segment elevation. The ST segment may be elevated above or depressed below the baseline, depending on whether the tracing is from a lead facing toward or away from the infarcted area and depending on whether epicardial or endocardial injury occurs. Epicardial injury causes ST elevation in leads facing the epicardium. **D,** Ischemia, injury, and myocardial necrosis. The Q wave indicates necrosis of the myocardium. (From Kinney M and others: *Comprehensive cardiac care,* ed 8, St Louis, 1996, Mosby.)

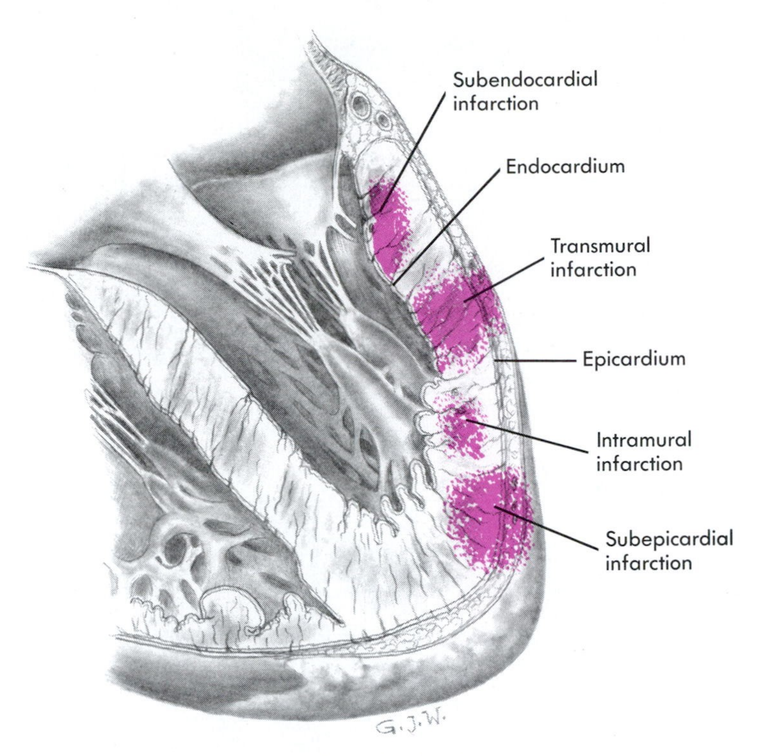

FIGURE 16-5. Location of infarctions in myocardium.

12-lead ECG changes. The ECG changes produced by a transmural infarction demonstrate alteration in both myocardial depolarization (QRS complex) and repolarization (ST segment). The changes in repolarization are seen by the presence of new Q waves. These Q waves are deeper (more than one third the height of the corresponding R wave) and wider than normal (more than 0.04 seconds).[31]

MI location. The location of infarction is determined by correlating the ECG leads with Q waves and the ST segment T wave abnormalities (Table 16-1). Infarction most commonly occurs in the left ventricle and the interventricular septum; however, almost 25% of patients who sustain an inferior myocardial infarction have some right ventricular damage.[30] The ECG manifestations that are used to diagnose an MI and pinpoint the area of damaged ventricle include inverted T waves, ST-segment elevation, and pathologic Q waves.[31]

Anterior wall infarction. Anterior wall infarction results from occlusion of the proximal left anterior descending (LAD) artery and may involve the left main artery. ST-segment elevation is expected in leads V_1 through V_4, and T wave inversion may occur in leads I, aV_L, and V_2 through V_5 (Figure 16-7). There is a loss of positive R wave progression in leads V_1 through V_6. A large anterior wall MI may be associated with left ventricular (LV) pump failure, cardiogenic shock, or death. Because the anterior wall is so large, it is commonly described in sections, as in the following discussion.

Anteroseptal infarctions. Anteroseptal infarction results from an occlusion of the LAD artery. Leads V_1 through V_4 on the 12-lead ECG reflect the electrical activity of the anterior wall. There is a loss of R wave progression in V_1 and V_2, leaving a QS complex. Q waves are seen in leads V_2 through V_4. If the infarct involves only the septum this will appear only in the V_1 lead. Reciprocal changes usually are not seen with an anteroseptal myocardial infarction.

Anterolateral infarction. Anterolateral infarction occurs as a result of occlusion of the circumflex coronary artery. On a 12-lead ECG, Q waves and ST-T wave changes are seen in leads I, aV_L, V_4, V_5, and V_6. Reciprocal changes occur in the inferior leads II, III, and aV_F.

Inferior wall infarction. Inferior wall infarction occurs with occlusion of the right coronary artery (RCA). This infarction is manifested by ECG changes in leads II, III, and aV_F. Reciprocal changes occur in leads I and aV_L (Figure 16-8). Because the RCA perfuses the sinoatrial (SA) node, the proximal bundle of His, and the atrioventricular (AV) node, conduction disturbances may be seen with an inferior wall MI.

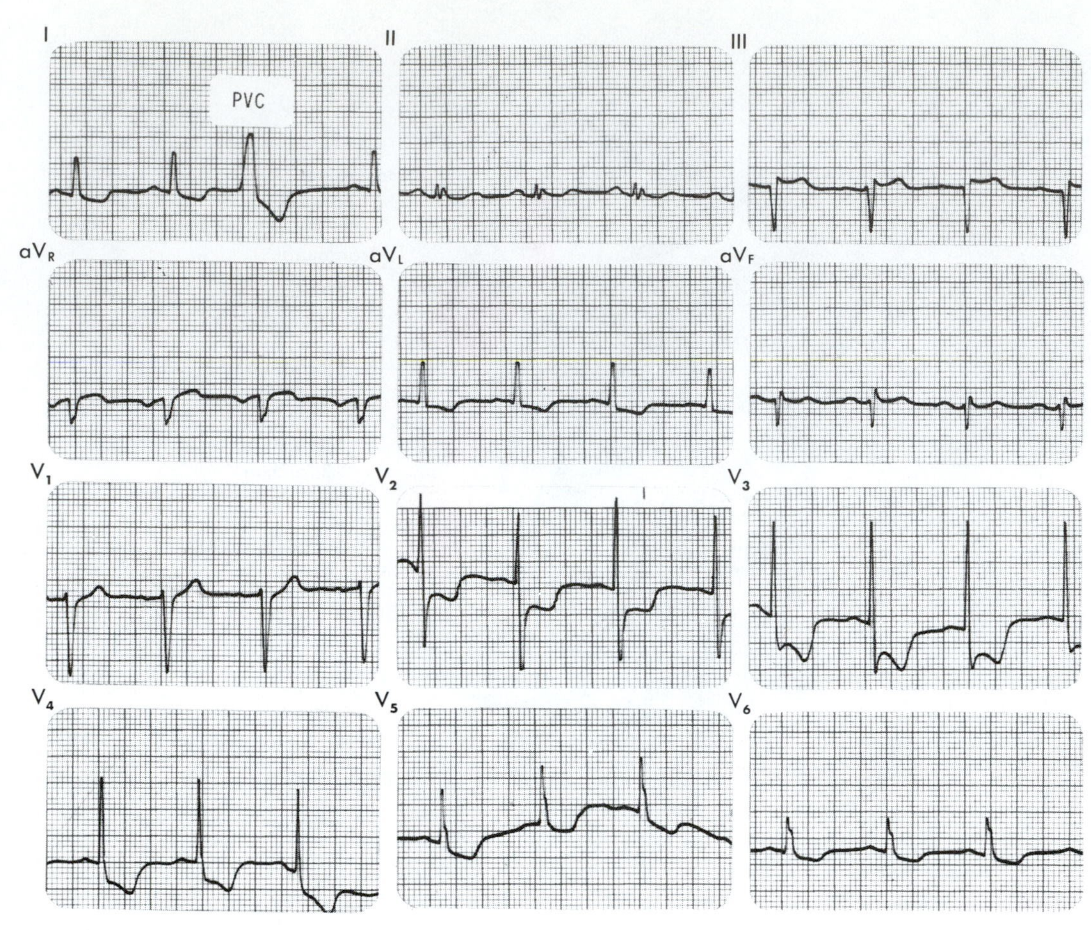

FIGURE 16-6. Subendocardial myocardial infarction, also known as a non-Q wave MI. Note the marked ST-segment depressions, best seen in chest leads V_2 to V_5, consistent with a subendocardial infarction. Slight ST-segment elevations are seen in reciprocal leads a V_F and III. (From Goldberger AL, Goldberger E: *Clinical electrocardiography: a simplified approach,* ed 5, St. Louis, 1994, Mosby.)

TABLE 16-1 Correlation Between Ventricular Surfaces, ECG Leads, and Coronary Arteries

Surface of Left Ventricle	ECG Leads	Coronary Artery Usually Involved
Inferior	II, III, aV_F	Right coronary
Lateral	V_5-V_6, I, aV_L	Left circumflex
Anterior	V_2-V_4	Left anterior descending
Septal	V_1-V_2	Left anterior descending
Posterior	V_1-V_2 (reciprocal changes)	Left circumflex

Right ventricular infarction. Infarction of the right ventricle occurs when there is a blockage in a proximal section of the right coronary artery. This places all of the right ventricle and the inferior wall at risk.[30]

Posterior wall infarction. Posterior wall infarction occurs with occlusion of the circumflex branch of the left coronary artery. Because the standard 12-lead ECG does not directly record activity on the posterior surface of the myocardium, a posterior wall myocardial infarction is documented by reciprocal changes, seen as tall R waves and ST-segment depression in leads V_1 and V_2.[31]

MI diagnosis. The definitive diagnosis of myocardial infarction is based on a combination of the patient's clinical symptoms, 12-lead ECG changes, and cardiac enzyme levels.[30] MI location can help predict risk of mortality. Anterior and anteroseptal infarctions are associated with twice the mortality of inferior wall infarctions.

Chest pain during MI. The most common clinical manifestation of infarction is prolonged severe chest pain, which often is associated with nausea, vomiting, and diaphoresis. This pain generally lasts 30 or more minutes and usually is located in the substernal or left precordial area. Unlike angina, which often is described

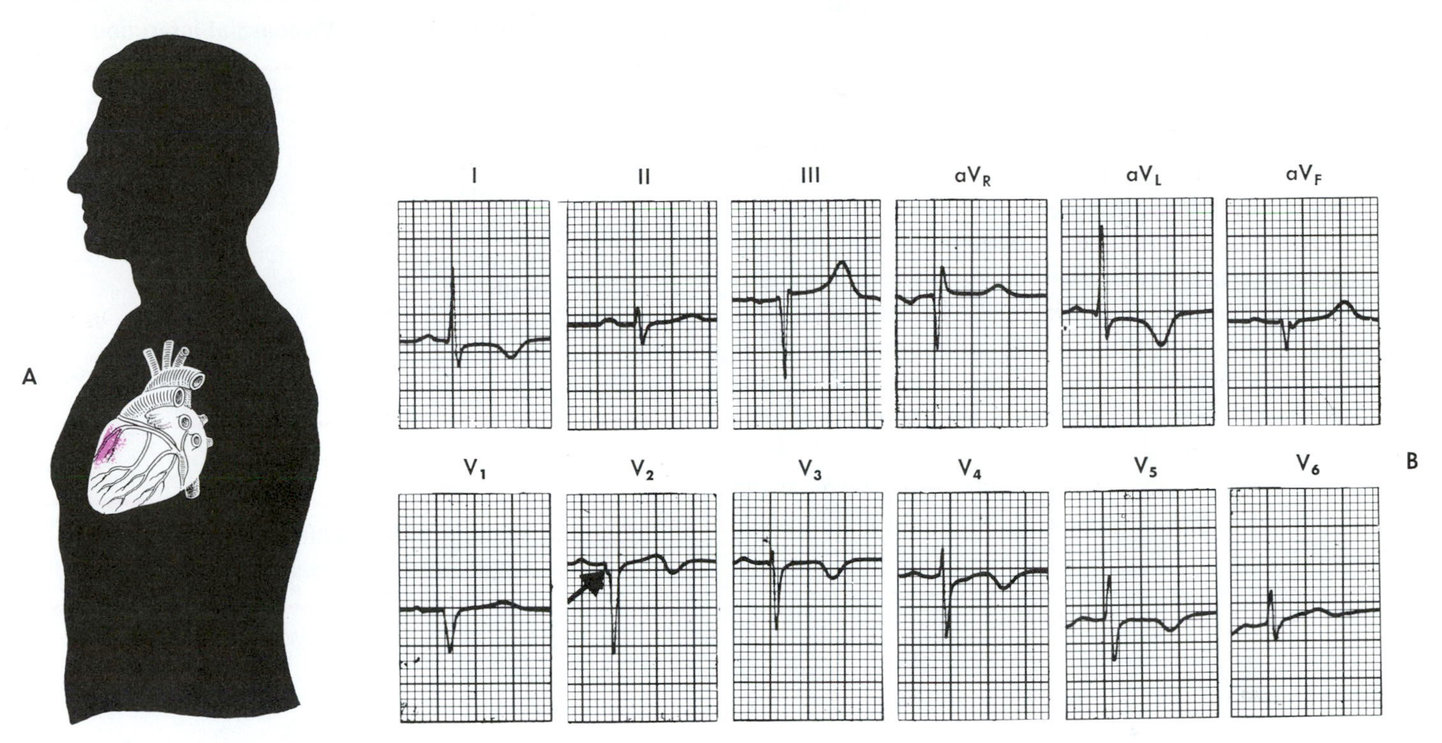

FIGURE 16-7. A, Position of an anterior wall infarction. **B,** Anterior wall infarction. Note the QS complexes in leads V_1 and V_2, indicating anteroseptal infarction. There is also a characteristic notching (*arrow,* V_2) of the QS complex, often seen in infarctions. In addition, note the diffuse ischemic T wave inversions in leads I, aV_L, and V_2 through V_5, indicating generalized anterior wall ischemia. (From Goldberger AL, Goldberger E: *Clinical electrocardiography: a simplified approach,* ed 5, St Louis, 1994, Mosby.)

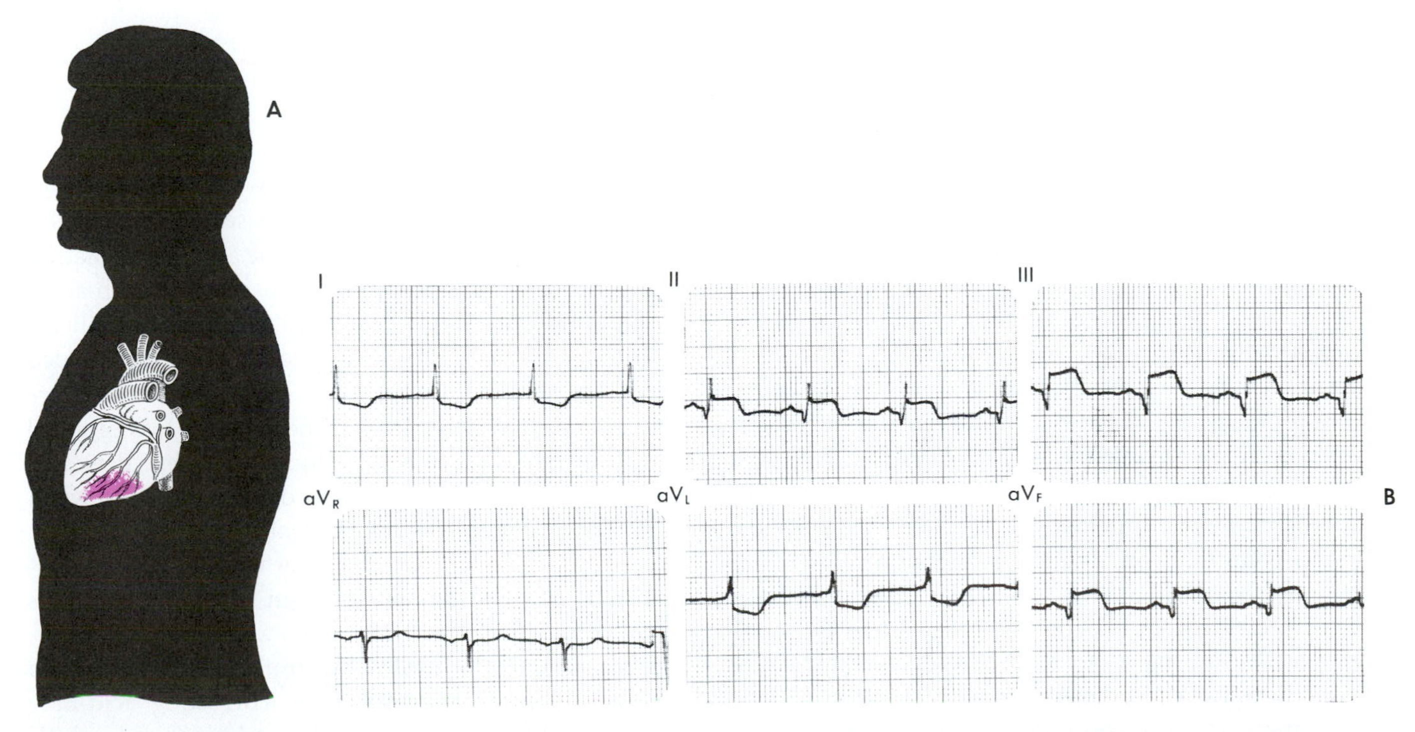

FIGURE 16-8. A, Position of an inferior wall infarction. **B,** Acute inferior wall infarction. Note the ST elevations in leads II, III, and aV_R, with reciprocal ST depressions in leads I and aV_L. Abnormal Q waves also are seen in leads II, III, and aV_F. Changes are not seen in leads V_4-V_6, so these leads are not shown. (From Goldberger AL, Goldberger E: *Clinical electrocardiography: a simplified approach,* ed 5, St Louis, 1994, Mosby.)

as discomfort, the pain of infarction may be described as the most severe pain the individual has ever experienced. Descriptions used are "like an elephant sitting on my chest" or a viselike tightness. The pain may radiate to the back, neck, jaw, or left arm, particularly down the ulnar aspect (see Figure 16-2). Neither rest nor nitrates relieves the pain.

Cardiac enzymes during MI. Specific cardiac enzymes and isoenzymes are released in the presence of damaged or infarcted myocardial cells. To confirm the diagnosis of MI, serum CK-MB isoenzymes are measured at 6-hour intervals for the first 24 hours and then daily.[30] With a large anterior MI the CK-MB level can rise to more than 150 U/L with a total CK level of more than 1,000 U/L. Troponin levels also can be used for early detection of acute MI. (∞Cardiac Enzymes, p. 381.)

Dysrhythmias and Acute MI

Many patients experience complications, occurring either early or late in the postinfarction course (Box 16-9). These complications may result from a pump problem or an electrical dysfunction. Pumping complications cause heart failure (HF), pulmonary edema, and cardiogenic shock. Electrical dysfunctions include bradycardia, bundle branch blocks, and varying degrees of heart block.[30] Almost 95% of patients who experience a MI will have dysrhythmias. There are many potential causes (Box 16-10). The major goal of treatment of any dysrhythmia is preservation, or return, of adequate cardiac output.

Sinus rhythms during MI. Sinus bradycardia (heart rate less than 60 beats/minute) occurs in approximately 40% of patients who sustain an acute myocardial infarction and is more prevalent with an inferior wall infarction. It is seen most frequently in the immediate postinfarction period. Symptomatic bradycardia with hypotension and low cardiac output is treated with atropine 0.5 mg IV push, repeated every 5 minutes to a maximum dose of 2 mg.[30] Sinus tachycardia (heart rate more than 100 beats/minute) most often occurs with anterior wall myocardial infarctions. Anterior infarctions impair left ventricular pumping ability, thereby reducing the ejection fraction and stroke volume. In an attempt to maintain cardiac output, the heart rate increases. Sinus tachycardia must be corrected, not only because it greatly increases myocardial oxygen consumption, but because it shortens diastolic filling time, thereby decreasing stroke volume, systemic perfusion, and coronary artery filling.

Atrial dysrhythmias during MI. Premature atrial contractions (PAC) occur frequently in patients who sustain an acute infarction. PACs most commonly are caused by cell irritability, resulting from distention of the left atrium secondary to increased left ventricular end-diastolic pressure and volume. Atrial fibrillation is a common atrial dysrhythmia associated with acute MI and is more prevalent with an anterior wall infarction. It may occur spontaneously or be preceded by PACs or atrial flutter. With atrial fibrillation there is loss of atrial contraction, and hence a loss of atrial kick and the extra stroke volume it carries. It is estimated that cardiac output can decrease by 30% when atrial kick is lost. (∞Atrial Dysrhythmias, p. 408.)

Ventricular dysrhythmias during MI. Premature ventricular contractions are seen in almost all patients within the first few hours after a myocardial infarction. They are controlled by administering oxygen to reduce myocardial hypoxia, by correcting acid-base or electrolyte imbalances, and by administering an IV lidocaine bolus and infusion. In the setting of an acute MI, PVCs are treated if they are (1) frequent (more than 6/minute), (2) closely coupled (R-on-T

BOX 16-9 Complications of Myocardial Infarction

Dysrhythmias
Ventricular aneurysm
Ventricular septal defect
Papillary muscle rupture
Pericarditis
Cardiac rupture
Sudden death
Heart failure
Pulmonary edema
Cardiogenic shock

BOX 16-10 Etiology of Dysrhythmias in Myocardial Infarction

Tissue ischemia
Hypoxemia
Autonomic nervous system influences
Metabolic derangements
  Acid-base imbalances
Hemodynamic abnormalities
Drugs (especially digoxin toxicity)
Electrolyte imbalances (e.g., hypokalemia, hypomagnesemia)
Fiber stretch
  Chamber dilation
  Cardiomyopathy

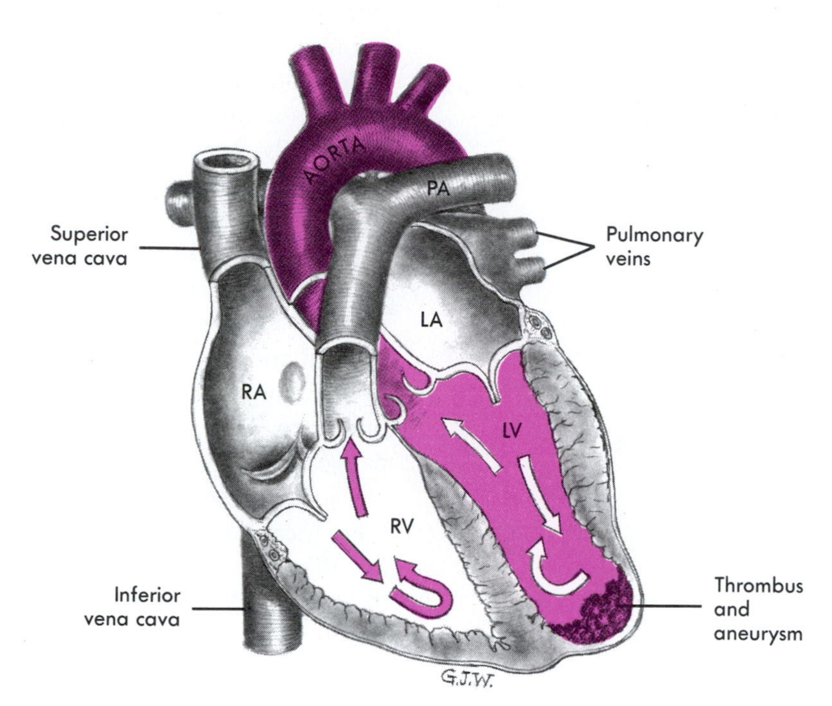

FIGURE 16-9. Ventricular aneurysm after acute MI. *PA*, pulmonary artery; *LA*, left atrium; *RA*, right atrium; *LV*, left ventricle; *RV*, right ventricle.

phenomenon), (3) multiform in shape, and (4) occur in bursts of 3 or more.[30] PVCs and ventricular tachycardia (VT) occurring within the first few hours postinfarction usually are transient. When, however, these same dysrhythmias occur late in the course, they tend to be associated with high in-hospital mortality, because they usually are related to the cumulative loss of myocardium. Ventricular fibrillation (VF) is a life-threatening dysrhythmia associated with high mortality in acute MI. (∞Ventricular Dysrhythmias, p. 415.)

AV heart block during MI. AV heart block during MI most frequently follows an inferior wall MI. Because the right coronary artery perfuses the AV node in 90% of the population, RCA occlusion leads to ischemia and infarction of the AV node cells. Symptomatic AV block with hemodynamic compromise is treated with IV atropine or by insertion of a temporary pacemaker.[30] (∞AV Conduction Disturbances, p. 424; Temporary Pacemaker, p. 529.)

Structural Complications After Acute MI

Ventricular aneurysm after MI. A ventricular aneurysm (Figure 16-9) is a noncontractile, thinned left ventricular wall, which results in a reduction of the stroke volume. It occurs in approximately 12% to 15% of patients who survive acute transmural infarction. The most common complications of a ventricular aneurysm are acute heart failure, systemic emboli, and VT. Treatment is directed toward management of these complications and surgical repair by left ventricular aneurysmectomy. The prognosis depends on the size of the aneurysm, overall left ventricular function, and the severity of coexisting CAD. Rupture of the aneurysm is rare, but nonetheless life-threatening, and usually occurs only if there is reinfarction of the border of the aneurysm.

Ventricular septal defect after MI. Rupture of the ventricular septal wall (Figure 16-10) affects approximately 1% to 2% of patients who sustain acute transmural MI and usually occurs in the first week after MI.[34] However, acute ventricular septal defect (VSD) patients make up 5% to 20% of acute MI associated deaths. The rupture often is followed by acute heart failure, shock, and death. Ventricular septal defect manifests as severe chest pain, syncope, hypotension, and sudden hemodynamic deterioration caused by shunting of blood from the high-pressure left ventricle into the low-pressure right ventricle through the new septal opening. A holosystolic murmur (accompanied by a thrill) can be auscultated and is best heard

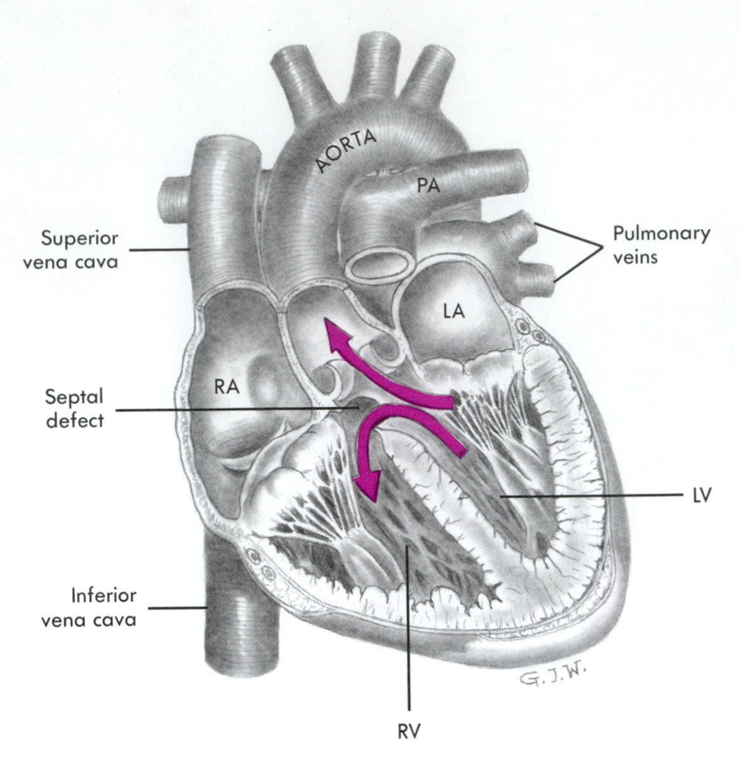

FIGURE 16-10. Ventricular septal defect after acute MI. See Figure 16-9 for explanation of abbreviations.

along the left sternal border. A diagnosis of postinfarction VSD can be made at the bedside with use of a pulmonary artery catheter or by transesophageal echocardiography (TEE). Rupture of the septum is a medical and surgical emergency. The patient's condition is stabilized with vasodilators and an intraaortic balloon pump (IABP) to decrease afterload. The goal of afterload reduction in these patients is to decrease the amount of blood being shunted to the right side of the heart and to increase the forward flow of blood to the systemic circulation. Mortality is very high with medical therapy alone; therefore most patients need emergency surgery to close the ventricular septum.[34]

Papillary muscle rupture after MI. Papillary muscle rupture can occur when the infarct involves the area around the mitral valve. It is rare but accounts for 1% to 5% of acute MI related deaths.[11] Infarction of the papillary muscles results in ineffective mitral valve closure, and blood is forced back into the low-pressure left atrium during ventricular systole.[35] The rupture may be partial or complete. Complete rupture is catastrophic and precipitates severe acute mitral regurgitation, shock, and death. Partial rupture (Figure 16-11) also results in mitral regurgitation, but usually the condition can be stabilized with aggressive medical management using the intraaortic balloon pump and vasodilators. Urgent surgical intervention is required to replace the mitral valve.[34]

Cardiac wall rupture after MI. Of the deaths that occur after myocardial infarction, 3% to 4% can be attributed to cardiac rupture, which often occurs in older patients who have systemic hypertension during the acute phase of their infarction.[34,36] Rupture commonly occurs around the fifth postinfarction day when leukocyte scavenger cells are removing necrotic debris, thus thinning the myocardial wall. The onset is sudden and usually catastrophic. Bleeding into the pericardial sac results in cardiac tamponade, cardiogenic shock, electromechanical dissociation, and death. Survival is rare. If rupture occurs in the hospital, emergency pericardiocentesis is required to relieve the tamponade until a surgical repair can be attempted.[34,36]

Pericarditis after MI. Pericarditis is inflammation of the pericardial sac. It can occur during a transmural MI after an acute MI when the damage extends into the epicardial surface of the heart. The damaged epicardium then becomes rough and tends to irritate and inflame the pericardium lying adjacent to it, precipitating pericarditis.[37] Pain is the most common symptom of pericarditis, and a pericardial friction rub is the most common sign. The friction rub is best heard at the sternal border and is described as a grating, scraping, or leathery scratching. Pericarditis may result in a pericardial effusion. Once the effusion (fluid) occurs, the friction rub may disappear. Pericarditis is treated with either aspirin or nonsteroidal antiinflammatory drugs.[37]

Medical Management

The goals of medical management during myocardial infarction include preservation of myocardium, pain control, management of complications, and pharmacologic therapy.

Preservation of myocardium. The first 6 hours after the onset of chest pain constitute the crucial period for salvaging the myocardium. During this period it may be possible to achieve reperfusion of the infarcting myocardium with either one or a combination of the following interventions:[30] (1) intravenous or intracoronary thrombolysis, (2) emergency percutaneous transluminal coronary angioplasty (PTCA) or coronary atherectomy, or (3) emergency coronary artery bypass surgery. Myocardial tissue can be salvaged for at least 4 hours after the onset of anginal symptoms, but in some patients this period may extend to 6 hours. Unfortunately, many persons do not seek treatment until this phase has passed.

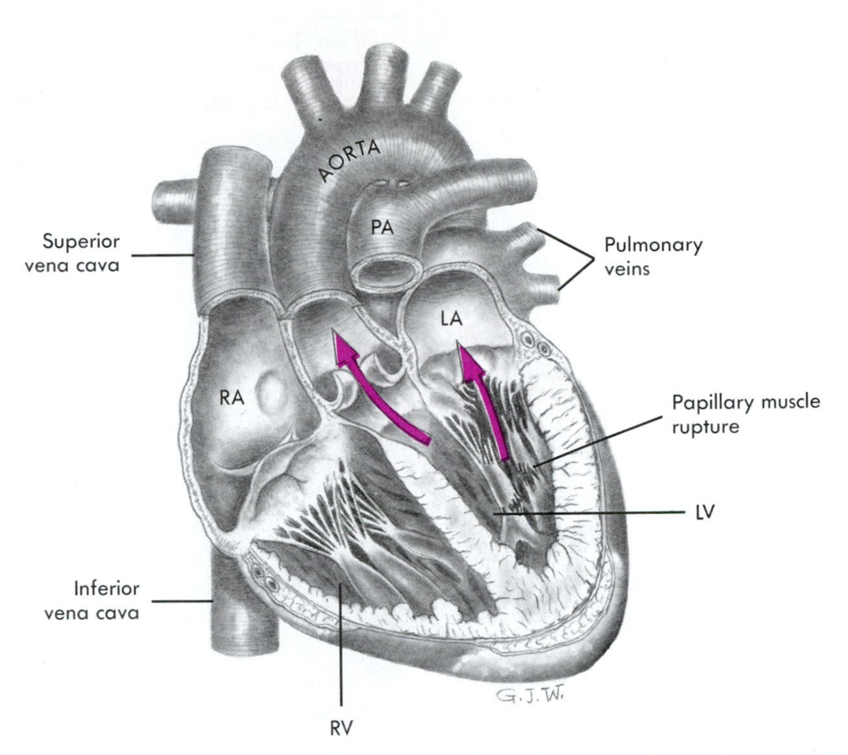

FIGURE 16-11. Papillary muscle rupture after acute MI. See Figure 16-9 for explanation of abbreviations.

Pain control. Pain control is a priority because continued pain is a symptom of ongoing ischemia, which places additional risk on noninfarcted myocardial tissue. Morphine remains the analgesic agent of choice; it decreases anxiety, restlessness, autonomic nervous system activity, and preload, thereby decreasing myocardial oxygen demands. Oxygen is used for a minimum of 24 to 48 hours after infarction to prevent tissue hypoxia.

Management of complications. Many times a pulmonary artery catheter is inserted.[30] This allows for correlation of chamber pressures to heart rate, blood pressure, cardiac output, and the patient's clinical condition. Thus pharmacologic and fluid replacement decisions can be based on concrete parameters of ventricular function. The goal is to manage acute heart failure more effectively. Heart failure is responsible for one third of the deaths of patients with an acute MI.[30] (∞Pulmonary Artery Pressure Monitoring, p. 459.)

Pharmacologic therapy. The major goals of drug therapy are anticoagulation, reduction in myocardial workload, and analgesia.

Anticoagulation is divided into three therapeutic sections: antiplatelet, anticoagulant, and lytic. Antiplatelet agents act against the initial "white clot" that forms the platelet plug. Low-dose aspirin is used for many patients. Aspirin decreases platelet release of thromboxane A_2, which reduces vasoconstriction and further platelet aggregation.[38] This therapy may be continued for an indefinite period, and studies have documented the beneficial antiplatelet effect of low-dose prophylactic aspirin.[38] If a patient cannot tolerate aspirin, the antiplatelet agent ticlopidine (Ticlid) may be prescribed.[39]

Anticoagulants are used to decrease the incidence of embolic complications (e.g., deep vein thrombosis and left ventricular thrombi), especially while bedrest is prescribed. Anticoagulants include heparin, as an IV infusion or by subcutaneous injection, or oral warfarin (Coumadin). The effectiveness of these agents is determined by measurement of blood coagulation times.[30,40,41] (∞Blood Coagulation Studies, p. 382.)

The third level of coagulation-related drugs that may be used are the lytic agents. If an acute MI is diagnosed within 6 hours, lytic agents may be used to dissolve the clot and restore blood flow in the occluded artery. (∞Thrombolytic Therapy, p.561.)

Beta-blocking agents are used to reduce infarct size by decreasing myocardial oxygen demand during the first few hours of infarction. However, beta-blockers are contraindicated if there is LV failure, because they depress cardiac contractility.[30] Beta blockade is also used after the completed infarction to lower the risks of reinfarction or death. Calcium channel blockers are a diverse group of drugs that are used in conjunction with the other agents previously described to decrease coronary artery spasm and as antihypertensives.[30] (∞Cardiac Drugs, p. 574.)

Nursing Management

Nursing management of the patient with an acute myocardial infarction incorporates a variety of nursing diagnoses (Box 16-11). Acute nursing interventions are directed toward continuous patient assessment, control of anginal pain, achievement of myocardial oxygen supply/demand balance and optimal cardiac output, prevention of complications, and provision of patient education.

Patient assessment. The clinical manifestations of an acute MI are shown in Box 16-12 and provide a baseline of expected findings. A considerable portion of time will be spent monitoring the patient for dysrhythmias; assessing vital signs for hemodynamic deterioration, breath sounds for signs of pulmonary congestion, heart sounds for abnormalities, such as development of a new murmur—S_3, S_4, or the murmur of a VSD or of mitral regurgitation; and evaluating side effects from the medication regimen. If left ventricular pump failure is present, hemodynamic assessment using a pulmonary artery catheter is required.[30] (∞Heart Sounds, p. 367.)

Pain control. Continued ischemic pain represents myocardium at risk. While pain can be controlled by nitroglycerin and morphine, if the patient is within the 4-hour window in which the myocardium can be salvaged by thrombolytic therapy or emergency PTCA, these are the interventions of choice.[29,30]

Myocardial oxygen supply/demand balance. In the acute period, if there is severe myocardial damage, myocardial oxygen supply is increased by the use of positive inotropic drugs such as dobutamine and dopamine and by avoiding negative inotropic agents such as beta-blockers. Supplemental oxygen is administered to prevent tissue hypoxia. To decrease cardiac work and myocardial oxygen consumption, bedrest with bedside commode privileges is usually prescribed during the first 24 to 48 hours.

Preventing complications. For the first 24 hours the acute MI patient may receive a light diet because appetite is often poor. It is no longer considered necessary to restrict iced fluids or caffeine.[32] While the patient is in bed, an upright position is preferable to foster better lung expansion. Deep breathing decreases the risk of atelectasis. An upright position also decreases venous return, lowers preload, and decreases cardiac work.

BOX 16-11 NURSING DIAGNOSIS AND MANAGEMENT

MYOCARDIAL INFARCTION AND COMPLICATIONS

- Acute Pain related to transmission and perception of cutaneous, visceral, muscular, or ischemic impulses, p. 197
- Decreased Cardiac Output related to alterations in preload, p. 590
- Decreased Cardiac Output related to alterations in afterload, p. 592
- Decreased Cardiac Output related to alterations in contractility, p. 592
- Decreased Cardiac Output related to alterations in heart rate, p. 593
- Activity Intolerance related to cardiopulmonary dysfunction, p. 596
- Altered Myocardial Tissue Perfusion related to acute myocardial ischemia, p. 595
- Sleep Pattern Disturbance related to fragmented sleep, p. 118
- Anxiety related to threat to biologic, psychologic, and/or social integrity, p. 99
- Ineffective Individual Coping related to situational crisis and personal vulnerability, p. 95
- Powerlessness related to lack of control over current situation or disease progression, p. 89
- Knowledge Deficit: Discharge Regimen related to lack of previous exposure to information, p. 61 (see Patient Education Box 16-13)

The patient is taught to avoid increasing intraabdominal pressure (Valsalva maneuver). Also, stool softeners are used to lessen the risk of constipation from analgesics and bedrest and to decrease the risk of straining. The nurse controls the critical care unit environment by decreasing noise, diminishing sensory overload, and allowing adequate rest periods.

Patient Education

The patient who comes into the emergency room within 6 hours of onset of chest pain immediately receives education about possible therapies to salvage the threatened myocardium, such as thrombolytic therapy or emergency PTCA. If the patient is admitted to the hospital outside the window of time when the myocardium can be saved, he or she is admitted to the critical care unit and will have lost myocardial tissue. In the acute period the patient receives education about the reasons he or she is in the critical care unit and the importance of avoiding straining when coughing, moving, or using the commode or bathroom.

BOX 16-12 Clinical Manifestations of Acute Myocardial Infarction

Tachycardia *with* or *without* ectopy
Bradycardia
Normotension or hypotension
Tachypnea
Diminished heart sounds, especially S_1
If left ventricular dysfunction present, may have S_3 and/or S_4
Systolic murmur
Pulmonary crackles
Pulmonary edema
Air hunger
Orthopnea
Frothy sputum
Decreased cardiac output
 Decreased urine output
 Decreased peripheral pulses
 Slow capillary refill
Restlessness
Confusion
Anxiety
Agitation
Denial
Anger

Once the acute phase has passed, education for the patient and family is focused on risk factor reduction, manifestations of angina, when to call a physician or emergency services, medications, and resumption of physical and sexual activity.[42] If possible, a referral is made to a cardiac rehabilitation program so that this education can be reinforced outside the acute care hospital environment[33] (Box 16-13).

BOX 16-13 PATIENT EDUCATION

MYOCARDIAL INFARCTION

- Pathophysiology of coronary artery disease, angina, and acute MI
- Angina: describe signs and symptoms, such as pain, pressure, or heaviness in chest, arms, or jaw
- Use of the pain scale from 1 to 10: notify critical care nurse or emergency personnel of any changes in chest pain intensity
- Avoid the Valsalva maneuver
- Risk factor modification tailored to the patient's individual risk factor profile: decrease fat intake to < 30% of total calories a day and total cholesterol to <200 mg/dL; stop smoking; reduce salt intake; control hypertension; treat diabetes, if patient is diabetic; increase physical activity; achieve ideal body weight
- Refer to cardiac rehabilitation program
- Medication teaching: indications, side effects
- Follow-up care
- Symptoms to report to a health care professional
- How to handle emotional stress and anger

SUDDEN CARDIAC DEATH

Description

About 500,000 cardiac deaths occur each year. Two thirds, or about 350,000 deaths, occur within 1 hour of symptom onset.[43] The most likely mechanism is ventricular tachycardia, which degenerates into ventricular fibrillation. This syndrome is called *sudden cardiac death (SCD)*. In spite of aggressive cardiopulmonary resuscitation (CPR) initiated outside the hospital, few who sustain an out-of-the-hospital cardiac arrest survive to hospital discharge.[43] In general, the longer the time period the patient was unconscious, the poorer the prognosis.

Etiology

Most incidents of SCD occur in patients with preexisting ventricular dysfunction secondary to multivessel cardiac disease with or without a history of myocardial infarction. The sudden death episode usually begins as VT, which deteriorates into VF. Other SCD risk factors include dilated or hypertrophic cardiomyopathy, aortic stenosis, AV block, ventricular preexcitation (Wolff-Parkinson-White [WPW] syndrome), and prolonged QT syndrome. Extensive atherosclerosis (more than 75% blockage) is the most common pathologic finding in the arteries of victims of SCD (Box 16-14). An ejection fraction less than 30% and a history of ventricular dysrhythmias are powerful predictors for sudden cardiac death.[44] Most victims of SCD are male and between the ages of 45 and 69 years.

Medical Management

Depending on the length of time the patient was unconscious as a result of the cardiac arrest, cognitive defects may be present because of the lack of cerebral blood flow.[43] The cardiac arrest may also have damaged the myocardium and other tissue. Therapy is tailored to the needs of the patient. Survivors usually receive antidysrhythmic agents and have an internal cardioverter defibrillator (ICD) unit implanted.[45] Prevention focuses on identification and treatment of

BOX 16-14 Causes of Sudden Cardiac Death (SCD)

MOST COMMON DYSRHYTHMIAS

Ventricular tachycardia → Ventricular fibrillation

UNDERLYING CARDIAC CONDITIONS

Heart failure
Hypertrophic cardiomyopathy (HCM)
Dilated cardiomyopathy
Coronary artery disease
Myocardial infarction (MI)
Severe aortic stenosis
Wolff-Parkinson-White (WPW) syndrome
Long QT syndrome

high risk cardiac patients. (∞Implantable Cardioverter Defibrillator, p. 550; Antidysrhythmic Medications, p. 574.)

HEART FAILURE

Description

The National Heart, Lung, and Blood Institute estimates that more than 2 million Americans have heart failure (HF) and that about 400,000 new cases are diagnosed each year.[46] The heart failure rate is higher in men than in women for all age-groups. The 5-year mortality rate in men is about 60%, whereas in women it is about 45%.[47] Heart failure is the most common cause of in-hospital mortality for patients with cardiac disease and is responsible for one third of the deaths of patients with an acute MI. Heart failure is covered under DRG 127, with an anticipated length of stay of 6.7 days.[26]

Pathophysiology

Heart failure is a response to cardiac dysfunction, a condition in which the heart cannot pump blood at a volume required to meet the body's needs.[46] For many years heart failure was known as *congestive heart failure (CHF)*. However, because the patient in heart failure does not always have pulmonary congestion, the terms *acute heart failure* and *chronic heart failure* are increasingly being used. The function of the heart is to transfer blood coming into the ventricles from the venous system into the arterial system. Impaired cardiac function results in failure to empty the venous system and reduced delivery of blood to the pulmonary and arterial circulations—hence, heart failure. Many precipitating causes of heart failure are listed in Box 16-15.

BOX 16-15 Precipitating Causes of Heart Failure

Reduction or cessation of medication
Dysrhythmias
Systemic infection
Pulmonary embolism
Physical, environmental, and emotional stress
Pericarditis, myocarditis, and endocarditis
High ventricular output states
Development of serious systemic illness
Administration of a cardiac depressant or salt-retaining drug
Development of a second form of heart disease

TABLE 16-2 New York Heart Association Functional Classification of Heart Failure

Class	Definition
I	Normal daily activity does not initiate symptoms
II	Normal daily activities initiate onset of symptoms, but symptoms subside with rest
III	Minimal activity initiates symptoms; patients are usually symptom free at rest
IV	Any type of activity initiates symptoms, and symptoms are present at rest

Assessment and Diagnosis

Heart failure is described in many ways, including (1) using the New York Heart Association (NYHA) classification, (2) as primary ventricular involvement—right or left, (3) as progressing forward or backward, or (4) as primarily systolic or diastolic LV dysfunction. However heart failure is classified, it is important to remember that the ventricles do not function in isolation. They have a common septal wall and are encircled and bound together by continuous muscle fibers. Thus any interruption or damage to one chamber eventually affects all the chambers.

NYHA classification. A commonly used method is the New York Heart Association functional classification of heart failure, which is based on patient symptoms (Table 16-2).

Right heart failure. Failure of the right side of the heart is defined as *ineffective right ventricular contractile function*. Pure failure of the right side of the heart may result from an acute condition such as a pulmonary embolus or a right ventricular infarction, but it is most commonly caused by failure of the left side

TABLE 16-3 **Clinical Manifestations of Failure of Right and Left Sides of Heart**

Left Ventricular Failure		Right Ventricular Failure	
Signs	**Symptoms**	**Signs**	**Symptoms**
Tachypnea Tachycardia Cough Bibasilar crackles Gallop rhythms (S_3 and S_4) Increased pulmonary artery pressures Hemoptysis Cyanosis Pulmonary edema	Fatigue Dyspnea Orthopnea Paroxysmal nocturnal dyspnea Nocturia	Peripheral edema Hepatomegaly Splenomegaly Hepatojugular reflux Ascites Jugular venous distention Increased central venous pressure Pulmonary hypertension	Weakness Anorexia Indigestion Weight gain Mental changes

of the heart or the backing up of blood behind the left ventricle. Its common manifestations are weakness, peripheral or sacral edema, jugular venous distention, hepatomegaly, jaundice, liver tenderness, and elevated central venous pressure (CVP). If peripheral perfusion is greatly compromised, cyanosis may be present. Gastrointestinal symptoms include anorexia, nausea, and a feeling of fullness (Table 16-3).

Left heart failure. Failure of the left side of the heart is defined as a *disturbance of the contractile function of the left ventricle,* resulting in pulmonary congestion and edema or decreased cardiac output, or both.[45] Most frequently it occurs in patients with left ventricular infarctions, hypertension, and aortic and/or mitral valve disease. Classic clinical manifestations include decreased peripheral perfusion, such as weak or diminished pulses; cool, pale extremities; and peripheral cyanosis (see Table 16-3). Over time with progression of the disease state, the fluid accumulation behind the dysfunctional left ventricle produces dysfunction of the right ventricle, resulting in failure of the right side of the heart and its manifestations.

Forward heart failure. Forward heart failure is defined as *inadequate delivery of blood into the arterial system.* It occurs when systemic vascular resistance (afterload) is increased, producing decreased flow of blood out of the ventricles. This decrease results in a reduced cardiac output and hypoperfusion of vital organs. Forward failure often occurs with aortic stenosis or systemic hypertension.

Backward heart failure. Backward heart failure is defined as *failure of the ventricle to empty.* This is usually a result of left ventricular systolic dysfunction caused by myocardial infarction or cardiomyopathy. Backward heart failure results in a decreased systolic ejection fraction (EF), usually less than 30%, that causes an accumulation of fluid and elevation of pressure in all the chambers and in the venous system behind the ventricle. When the left ventricle pumps ineffectively, blood pools within the LV and left ventricular end-diastolic pressure (LVEDP) increases. As the mitral valve opens, the increased LVEDP results in increased atrial pressure, which is transmitted back into the pulmonary circuit, increasing pulmonary pressures.[46,47]

Acute versus chronic heart failure. Acute versus chronic heart failure refers to the rapidity with which the syndrome develops, the presence and activation of compensatory mechanisms, and the presence or absence of fluid accumulation in the interstitial space. Acute heart failure has a sudden onset, with no compensatory mechanisms. The patient may experience acute pulmonary edema, low cardiac output, or even cardiogenic shock. Patients with chronic heart failure are hypervolemic, have sodium and water retention, and have structural heart chamber changes such as dilation or hypertrophy. Chronic failure is ongoing, with symptoms that may be made tolerable by medication, diet, and a low activity level. A change to acute failure, however, can be precipitated by the onset of dysrhythmias, acute ischemia, sudden illness, or cessation of medications. This may necessitate admission to a critical care unit.

Compensatory mechanisms in heart failure. When the heart begins to fail and the cardiac output is no longer sufficient to meet the metabolic needs of the tissues, the body activates major compensatory mechanisms such as the adrenergic system, the renin-angiotensin-aldosterone system, sinus tachycardia, and the development of ventricular hypertrophy, as described in the following:

1. *Adrenergic system:* the adrenergic compensatory mechanism raises blood pressure. As a result of increased sympathetic activity, levels of circulating catecholamines are increased, resulting in peripheral vasoconstriction. This leads to shunting of blood from nonvital organs, such as the skin, to vital organs, such as the heart and brain.
2. *Renin-angiotensin-aldosterone system:* activation of the renin-angiotensin-aldosterone system promotes fluid retention. It causes constriction of the renal arterioles, decreased glomerular filtration, and increased reabsorption of sodium from the proximal and distal tubules. In addition, diminished hepatic metabolism of aldosterone increases the antidiuretic hormone (ADH) level and enhances water retention.
3. *Sinus tachycardia:* initially helpful, sinus tachycardia eventually may become a negative factor because it increases myocardial oxygen demand while shortening the amount of time for coronary artery perfusion. This imbalance can lead to myocardial ischemia, which may decrease ventricular contraction, reduce ventricular filling, and necessitate a higher filling pressure. If heart failure progresses to the point at which tissue perfusion is inadequate to meet the body's needs, the patient will be in cardiogenic shock. (∞Cardiogenic Shock, p. 1102.)
4. *Ventricular hypertrophy:* ventricular hypertrophy is the final compensatory mechanism. Because myocardial hypertrophy increases the force of contraction, hypertrophy helps the ventricle overcome an increase in afterload.[48]

Complications of Heart Failure

The clinical manifestations of acute heart failure result from tissue hypoperfusion and organ congestion (see Table 16-3). The severity of clinical manifestations progresses as heart failure worsens. Initially, manifestations appear only with exertion but eventually occur at rest (see Table 16-2).

Shortness of breath in heart failure. The patient experiences the feeling of shortness of breath first with exertion, but as heart failure worsens, symptoms are present at rest. Breathlessness in heart failure is described by the following terms:

1. *Dyspnea:* the patient's sensation of shortness of breath; it results from pulmonary vascular congestion and decreased lung compliance
2. *Orthopnea:* describes difficulty in breathing when lying flat because of an increase in venous return that occurs in the supine position
3. *Paroxysmal nocturnal dyspnea:* a severe form of orthopnea in which the patient awakens from sleep gasping for air
4. *Cardiac asthma:* dyspnea with wheezing, a nonproductive cough, and pulmonary crackles that progress to the gurgling sounds of pulmonary edema

Pulmonary edema in heart failure. Pulmonary edema, or fluid in the alveoli (Figure 16-12), inhibits gas exchange by impairing the diffusion pathway between the alveolus and the capillary. It is caused by increased left atrial and ventricular pressures and results in an excessive accumulation of serous or serosanguineous fluid in the interstitial spaces and alveoli of the lungs. This may be coughed up as a frothy, pink sputum. Two stages mark the formation of pulmonary edema. Stage I is characterized by interstitial edema, engorgement of the perivascular and peribronchial spaces, and increased lymphatic flow. Stage II is characterized by alveolar edema resulting from fluid moving into the alveoli from the interstitium. Eventually, blood plasma moves into the alveoli faster than the lymphatic system can clear it, interfering with diffusion of oxygen, depressing the arterial partial pressure of oxygen (PaO_2), and leading to tissue hypoxia.

Symptoms of pulmonary edema. With acute onset, patients are extremely breathless and anxious with a sensation of suffocation. They expectorate pink, frothy liquid and feel as if they are drowning. They may sit bolt upright, gasp for breath, or thrash about. The respiratory rate is elevated, and accessory muscles of ventilation are used, with nasal flaring and bulging neck muscles. Respirations are characterized by loud inspiratory and expiratory gurgling sounds. Diaphoresis is profuse; and the skin is cold, ashen, and cyanotic, reflecting low cardiac output, increased sympathetic stimulation, peripheral vasoconstriction, and desaturation of arterial blood.

Arterial blood gases in pulmonary edema. Arterial blood gas (ABG) values are variable. In the early stage of pulmonary edema, respiratory alkalosis may be present because of hyperventilation, which eliminates CO_2. As the pulmonary edema progresses and as gas exchange becomes impaired, acidosis (pH less than 7.35) and hypoxemia ensue. A chest x-ray usually confirms an enlarged cardiac silhouette, pulmonary venous congestion, and interstitial edema. (∞Arterial Blood Gas Interpretation, p. 641.)

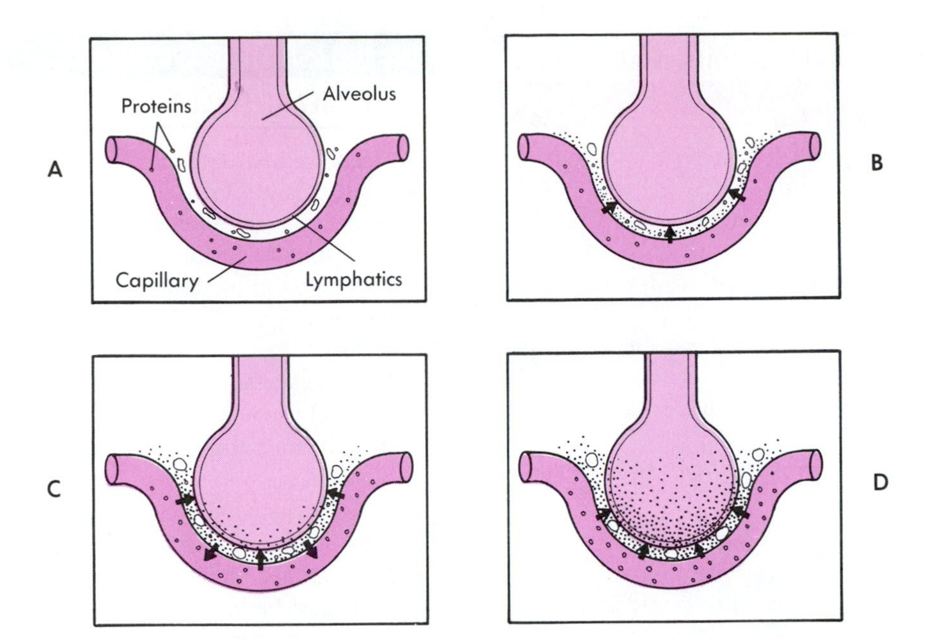

FIGURE 16-12. As pulmonary edema progresses, it inhibits oxygen and carbon dioxide exchange at the alveolar capillary interface. **A,** Normal relationship. **B,** Increased pulmonary capillary hydrostatic pressure causes fluid to move from the vascular space into the pulmonary interstitial space. **C,** Lymphatic flow increases in an attempt to pull fluid back into the vascular or lymphatic space. **D,** Failure of lymphatic flow and worsening of left-sided heart failure results in further movement of fluid into the interstitial space and the alveoli.

Medical Management

The goals of medical management of heart failure are to relieve heart failure symptoms, enhance cardiac performance, and identify and correct the precipitating causes of acute heart failure.

Relieve symptoms and enhance cardiac performance. In the acute phase the patient usually has a pulmonary artery catheter in place so that LV function can be followed closely. Control of symptoms involves management of fluid overload, improvement of cardiac output by decreasing systemic vascular resistance, and increasing contractility. Diuretics are administered to decrease preload and to eliminate fluid from the body. If pulmonary edema develops, additional diuretics are used. Morphine is given to facilitate peripheral dilatation and decrease anxiety. Afterload is decreased by vasodilators, such as sodium nitroprusside and nitroglycerin. Nitrates are used to decrease preload and vasodilate the coronary arteries if CAD is an underlying cause of the acute heart failure.[49] For some patients an IABP is also required. Contractility is increased by digitalis and positive inotropic agents, such as dopamine or dobutamine. Angiotensin-converting enzyme (ACE) inhibitors may alter chamber remodeling and slow the decline in contractility.[50]

Correct precipitating causes. Once symptoms of heart failure are controlled, diagnostic studies such as cardiac catheterization, echocardiogram, and thallium scan are undertaken to uncover the cause of the heart failure and tailor long-term management to treat the cause. Some structural problems such as valvular disease may require surgical correction.

Nursing Management

Nursing management of the patient with heart failure incorporates a variety of nursing diagnoses (Box 16-16). Nursing management goals are to optimize cardiopulmonary function, ensure rest, monitor the effectiveness of pharmacologic therapy, provide adequate nutrition, maintain skin integrity, and educate the patient and family about heart failure.

Optimize cardiopulmonary function. The patient's ECG is evaluated for any dysrhythmias that may be present or may develop as a result of drug toxicity or electrolyte imbalance. Patients experiencing heart failure are prone to digoxin toxicity secondary to decreased renal perfusion, as well as to electrolyte imbalances. Breath sounds are auscultated frequently to determine adequacy of respiratory effort and to assess for onset or worsening of congestion. Oxygen through a nasal cannula is administered to relieve dyspnea. Diuretics or vasodilators are used to decrease excessive preload and afterload. If the patient is not hypotensive, morphine may be administered to

BOX 16-16 NURSING DIAGNOSIS AND MANAGEMENT

ACUTE HEART FAILURE

- Impaired Gas Exchange related to ventilation/perfusion mismatching or intrapulmonary shunting, p. 725
- Decreased Cardiac Output related to alterations in preload, p. 590
- Decreased Cardiac Output related to alterations in contractility, p. 592
- Decreased Cardiac Output related to alterations in heart rate, p. 593
- Activity Intolerance related to cardiopulmonary dysfunction, p. 596
- Anxiety related to threat to biologic, psychologic, and/or social integrity, p. 99
- Ineffective Individual Coping related to situational crisis and personal vulnerability, p. 95
- Sleep Pattern Disturbance related to circadian desynchronization, p. 119
- Knowledge Deficit: Medications related to lack of previous exposure to information, p. 61 (see Patient Education Box 16-17)

BOX 16-17 PATIENT EDUCATION

ACUTE HEART FAILURE

- Heart Failure: pathophysiology of heart failure
- Fluid Balance: low-salt diet to reduce fluid retention; intake and output measurement; signs of fluid overload, such as peripheral edema
- Daily weight: increase or loss of 1-2 pounds in a few days is a sign of fluid gain or loss, not true weight gain or loss
- Breathlessness: increasing shortness of breath, wheezing, and sleeping upright on pillows are symptoms that must be monitored and reported to a health care professional
- Activity: activity conservation with rest periods as heart failure progresses
- Medications: medications are complex, and information must be in writing, as well as oral
  - Preload: purpose of diuretics, increased urine output, and control of fluid volume
  - Afterload: purpose of vasodilators or ACE inhibitors in decreasing the workload of the heart
  - Heart rate: purpose of digoxin to control atrial fibrillation—a frequent dysrhythmia in heart failure
  - Contractility: with the exception of digoxin, there are no oral contractility drugs that are approved by the FDA
  - Anticoagulation: patients with distended atria, enlarged ventricles, or with atrial fibrillation may be prescribed anticoagulants (warfarin [Coumadin]); risks of bleeding, importance of correct dosages, prothrombin times (INR), and nutritional-pharmacologic interactions are emphasized
- Follow-up care
- Symptoms to report to a health care professional

decrease hyperventilation and anxiety. If the patient's ventilatory status worsens, the nurse must be prepared for endotracheal intubation and mechanical ventilation. Obtaining daily weights is important until the weight stabilizes at a "dry" weight. Generally, the daily weight is used in fluid management, and a weekly weight is used for tracking body weight (muscle, fat).

Promote rest. During periods of breathlessness, activity must be restricted; bedrest usually is prescribed for the patient, who is positioned with the head of the bed elevated to allow for maximal lung expansion. The arms can be supported on pillows so that there is no undue stress placed on the shoulder muscles. The legs may be placed in a dependent position to encourage venous pooling, thereby decreasing venous return. Rest periods must be carefully planned and adhered to, while independence within the patient's activity prescription is fostered.[51] Vital signs are recorded before an activity is begun and after it is completed. Signs of activity intolerance, such as dyspnea, fatigue, sustained increase in pulse, and onset of dysrhythmias are documented and reported to the physician. Activity is gradually increased according to patient tolerance.

Pharmacologic therapy. Patients experiencing acute heart failure require aggressive pharmacologic therapy.[52,53] The nurse must know the action, side effects, therapeutic levels, and toxic effects of the diuretics; the positive inotropic agents used to increase ventricular contractility; and the vasodilators used to decrease preload. The patient's hemodynamic response to these agents, as well as to diuretic therapy and fluid restrictions, is closely monitored.

Provide nutrition. Patients experiencing heart failure frequently experience decreased appetite and nausea; therefore small, frequent meals may be more appropriate than the standard three large meals. Food must be as tasty as possible; favorite foods, as well as food from home, may be worked into the diet as long as the foods are compatible with nutritional restrictions.

Skin integrity. Skin breakdown is a risk because of immobility, bedrest, inadequate nutrition, edema, and decreased perfusion to the skin and subcutaneous tissue. Frequent position changes are helpful to prevent this complication.

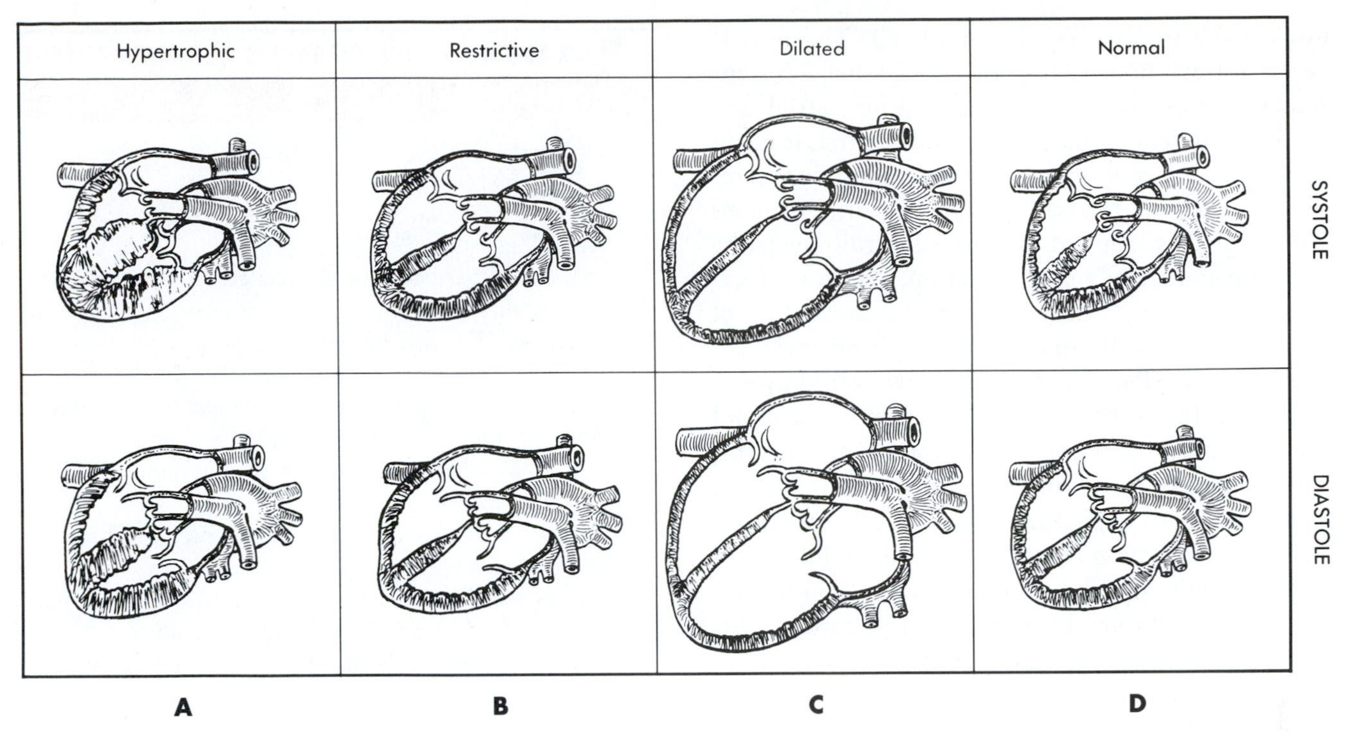

FIGURE 16-13. Types of cardiomyopathies and the differences in ventricular diameter during systole and diastole, compared with a normal heart. **A,** Hypertrophic. **B,** Restrictive. **C,** Dilated. **D,** Normal.

Patient Education

The nurse assesses the patient's understanding of conservation of energy in planning activities and collaborates with the patient in organizing the day's schedule. Other topics to cover include the importance of a low-salt diet and the multiple medications used to control the symptoms of heart failure (Box 16-17).

CARDIOMYOPATHY

Description

Cardiomyopathy is a disease of the heart muscle: *cardio = heart, myo = muscle,* and *pathy = pathology.* Cardiomyopathies are described as primary or secondary and further classified on the basis of associated structural abnormalities. These categories are hypertrophic, restrictive, and dilated cardiomyopathy (Figure 16-13).

Cardiomyopathies are covered under DRGs 124 and 125; anticipated length of stay ranges from 3.2 to 5.3 days.[26] The longer length of stay is for patients with associated complications.

Etiology

Primary cardiomyopathy. *Primary,* or *idiopathic, cardiomyopathy* is defined as a heart muscle disease of unknown cause, although both viral infections and autoimmune disorders have been implicated.

Secondary cardiomyopathy. Secondary cardiomyopathy is defined as heart muscle disease resulting from some other systemic disease, such as coronary artery disease, valvular heart disease, severe hypertension, alcohol abuse, or known autoimmune disease.

Hypertrophic cardiomyopathy. Hypertrophic cardiomyopathy (HCM) is characterized by stiff, noncompliant myocardial muscle with left ventricular hypertrophy and bizarre cellular hypertrophy of the upper ventricular septum. This septal hypertrophy results in obstruction of the aortic valve outflow tract (Figure 16-13, *A*). It also pulls the papillary muscle out of alignment, causing mitral regurgitation. This disorder used to be known as *idiopathic hypertrophic subaortic stenosis (IHSS);* however, because IHSS described only 25% of affected patients, the more general term of HCM is now used.[54,55] Symptoms include exertional dyspnea, myocardial ischemia, supraventricular tachycardia (SVT), VT, syncope, and heart failure. Sudden cardiac death occurs in 2% to 3% of adults with HCM per year.[56] Medical management includes limitation of physical activity, beta-blockers, calcium channel blockers, antidysrhythmic therapy, treatment of heart failure, and for some patients an implantable cardioverter defibrillator (ICD), surgical myectomy, or mitral valve replacement.[54]

Dilated cardiomyopathy. Dilated cardiomyopathy is characterized by grossly dilated ventricles without muscle hypertrophy (Figure 16-13, *C*). The muscle fibers contract poorly, resulting in global left ventricular dysfunction, low cardiac output, atrial and ventricular dysrhythmias, blood pooling that leads to ventricular clots and embolic episodes, and finally, refractory heart failure and premature death. The goals of medical management of dilated cardiomyopathy are improvement of pump function, removal of excess fluid, control of heart failure, and prevention of sudden cardiac death and other complications.[57]

Restrictive cardiomyopathy. Restrictive cardiomyopathy (Figure 16-13, *B*) is the least common form and is characterized by abnormal diastolic function. This cardiomyopathy results in ventricular wall rigidity as a consequence of myocardial fibrosis. The overall effect is the obstruction of ventricular filling. Restrictive cardiomyopathy may be misdiagnosed as constrictive pericarditis. Backward heart failure, low cardiac output, dyspnea, orthopnea, and liver engorgement are the most common clinical manifestations of restrictive cardiomyopathy. Medical management is directed toward the improvement of pump function, removal of excess fluid, and a low-sodium diet.

BOX 16-18 NURSING DIAGNOSIS AND MANAGEMENT

CARDIOMYOPATHY

- Decreased Cardiac Output related to alterations in preload, p. 590
- Decreased Cardiac Output related to alterations in afterload, p. 592
- Decreased Cardiac Output related to alterations in contractility, p. 592
- Decreased Cardiac Output related to alterations in heart rate, p. 593
- Impaired Gas Exchange related to ventilation/perfusion mismatching or intrapulmonary shunting, p. 725
- Activity Intolerance related to cardiopulmonary dysfunction, p. 596
- Anxiety related to threat to biologic, psychologic, and/or social integrity, p. 99
- Powerlessness related to lack of control over current situation and/or disease progression, p. 89
- Knowledge Deficit: Discharge Regimen related to lack of previous exposure to information, p. 61 (see Patient Education Box 16-19)

Nursing Management

Nursing management of the patient with cardiomyopathy incorporates a variety of nursing diagnoses (Box 16-18). Nursing interventions are individualized according to the type of cardiomyopathy and are focused on achievement of a therapeutic fluid balance, effective pharmacologic therapy, mobility, and patient and family education about cardiomyopathy.

Fluid balance. Patients are monitored for clinical manifestations of worsening heart failure, such as tissue edema, increased ventricular filling pressures, neck vein engorgement, pulmonary congestion, weight gain, increased fatigue, and onset of gallop rhythms. Daily weight and strict fluid restriction with accurate intake and output records are required.

Pharmacologic therapy. The patient with cardiomyopathy usually takes a wide range of medications that includes diuretics, calcium channel blockers, beta-blockers, vasodilators, anticoagulant or antiplatelet agents, and antidysrhythmics. Often the transition from IV to oral administration is supervised by the critical care nurse, and knowledge of appropriate and unwanted side effects is essential. For example, patients with cardiomyopathy are prone to digoxin toxicity related to decreased excretion of the drug secondary to a decreased glomerular filtration rate.

Mobility. Nursing interventions are directed at maintaining the patient's current level of conditioning and toward collaborating with the physical therapist to maintain or improve current functional level. Activity plans need to reflect energy conservation; therefore activities are clustered and include frequent rest periods.

Patient Education

Topics of education include all of those applicable to acute heart failure. Also, assessment of the patient's understanding of this illness, adaptive coping mechanisms, and support systems must be incorporated into the teaching plan. Patients and families need to know what support services are available. Most cardiomyopathies have only palliative treatments, and patients may need to be educated for several possible outcomes, including heart transplantation, cardiac disability, or sudden cardiac death (Box 16-19).

ENDOCARDITIS

Description

Infection by a microorganism of a platelet-fibrin vegetation on the endothelial surface of the heart results in infective endocarditis. Acute and subacute endocarditis is covered under DRG 126, with an anticipated length of stay of 16.3 days.[26]

Etiology

Development of endocarditis depends on two factors: (1) a susceptible lesion in the vascular endothelium and (2) an organism to establish the infection.[58]

BOX 16-19 PATIENT EDUCATION

CARDIOMYOPATHY

Cardiomyopathy produces symptoms of heart failure; patient education covers many of the same issues.

- Cardiomyopathy: explain pathophysiology of cardiomyopathy and heart failure
- Fluid balance: low-salt diet to reduce fluid retention; intake and output measurement; signs of fluid overload, such as peripheral edema
- Daily weight: increase or loss of 1-2 pounds in a few days is a sign of fluid gain or loss, not true weight gain or loss
- Breathlessness: increasing shortness of breath, wheezing, and sleeping upright on pillows are symptoms that must be monitored and reported to a healthcare professional
- Activity: activity conservation with rest periods as heart failure progresses
- Medications: medications are complex, and information must be in writing, as well as oral
  - Preload: purpose of diuretics, increased urine output, and control of fluid volume
  - Afterload: purpose of vasodilators or ACE inhibitors in decreasing the workload of the heart
  - Heart rate: purpose of digoxin to control atrial fibrillation—a frequent dysrhythmia in heart failure
  - Contractility: with the exception of digoxin, there are no oral contractility drugs that are approved by the FDA
  - Anticoagulation: patients with distended atria, enlarged ventricles, or atrial fibrillation may be prescribed anticoagulants (Coumadin); risk of bleeding, importance of correct dosages, prothrombin times (INR), and nutritional-pharmacologic interactions are emphasized
- Follow-up care
- Symptoms to report to a health care professional

BOX 16-20 Predisposing Factors in Endocarditis

Rheumatic heart disease
Congenital heart disease
Mitral valve prolapse
Marfan's syndrome
Peripheral arteriovenous fistulas
Indwelling intravenous or intraarterial catheters
Cardiac and prosthetic valve surgery
Prosthetic aortic grafts
Degenerative heart disease
Alcoholism
Chronic hemodialysis
Intravenous drug abuse
Syphilitic aortic disease
Immunosuppression
Severe burns

BOX 16-21 Endocarditis/Myocarditis: Most Common Causative Organisms in United States

RNA VIRUSES

Coxsackie viruses A and B
ECHO virus
Influenza A and B
Mumps

DNA VIRUSES

Varicella zoster
Cytomegalovirus
Epstein-Barr

The source of the organism may be unknown, or it may be traced to an invasive procedure, such as a biopsy; cannulation of the veins or arteries; urogenital procedures; dental work; or intravenous drug use[59] (Box 16-20). Almost any bacterium or fungus can infect a susceptible site. In Western Europe and North America, streptococci and staphylococci account for 75% to 85% of all endocarditis cases (Box 16-21). For this reason aggressive treatment of all streptococcal pharyngitis cases is encouraged.[60]

Pathophysiology

Endocarditis begins after the onset of bacteremia and the colonization of thrombotic vegetation. The bacteria is then encased in a platelet and fibrin shell, which protects it from destruction by phagocytic neutrophils, leading to a zone of localized agranulocytosis. It is because of this extensive protective mechanism, which restricts the body's normal response to infection, that antibiotic therapy must be so intensive and prolonged.

Assessment and Diagnosis

Endocarditis may be described as either acute or subacute. Acute infection develops on normal valves, progresses rapidly, causes severe destruction, and may be fatal if the patient is not treated. Subacute infection occurs on damaged heart valves and progresses much more slowly. The term *subacute bacterial endocarditis (SBE)* is not always accurate because, although

BOX 16-22 Clinical Manifestations of Endocarditis

Fever
Splenomegaly
Hematuria
Petechiae
Cardiac murmurs
Easy fatigability
Osler's nodes (small, raised, tender areas most commonly found in pads of fingers and toes)
Splenic hemorrhages
Roth's spots (round or oval spots consisting of coagulated fibrin; seen in the retina and leads to hemorrhage)

most infections are bacterial, some are caused by yeast or fungus. It is much more useful to classify the disease according to the causative microorganism. In cases of prosthetic valve endocarditis, antibiotics are usually not a sufficient treatment, and surgical replacement of the valve is required.[61] Clinical manifestations of endocarditis are listed in Box 16-22.

Medical Management

Treatment requires prolonged parenteral therapy with adequate doses of bactericidal antibiotics. An increasing number of patients are being discharged home earlier than in the past and continuing the parenteral therapy via a surgically implanted line, such as a Port-A-Cath, at home.

Nursing Management

Nursing management of the patient with endocarditis incorporates a variety of nursing diagnoses (Box 16-23). Nursing management supports resolution of the infectious process, prevention of complications, increased activity as tolerated, and patient and family education about endocarditis.

Resolution of infection. Endocarditis requires a long course of intravenous antibiotics, usually 6 weeks. This is begun in the hospital and continued at home with an indwelling central catheter. Nursing assessment includes monitoring for signs of worsening infection, such as temperature elevation, malaise, weakness, easy fatigability, and night sweats.

Prevention of complications. A patient with infective endocarditis is at risk for embolic events, either cerebral or pulmonary. Therefore level of consciousness, visual changes, and headache are assessed. As valvular dysfunction accelerates, acute heart failure develops. Cardiac assessment includes auscultation of heart sounds

BOX 16-23 NURSING DIAGNOSIS AND MANAGEMENT

ENDOCARDITIS

- Decreased Cardiac Output related to alterations in preload, p. 590
- Decreased Cardiac Output related to alterations in afterload, p. 592
- Decreased Cardiac Output related to alterations in contractility, p. 592
- Decreased Cardiac Output related to alterations in heart rate, p. 593
- Activity Intolerance related to cardiopulmonary dysfunction, p. 596
- Acute Pain related to transmission and perception of cutaneous, visceral, muscular, or ischemic impulses, p. 197
- Risk for Infection risk factor: invasive monitoring devices, p. 598
- Anxiety related to threat to biologic, psychologic, and/or social integrity, p. 99
- Knowledge Deficit (Specify) related to lack of previous exposure to information, p. 61 (see Patient Education Box 16-24)

to detect the presence or change in a cardiac murmur. Shortness of breath or chest pain with hemoptysis must be reported. This could be caused either by worsening heart failure or by pulmonary emboli.

Activity. During the most critical period, bedrest is prescribed for the patient. Mobility is addressed by range-of-motion exercises to maintain muscle tone and by frequent turning and repositioning to prevent skin breakdown. Support and diversional activity are important at this time if the patient is hemodynamically unstable and the hospital stay is prolonged. If the patient is active, discharge to home with an indwelling vascular access for IV antibiotics is encouraged.

Patient Education

The patient needs to know the manifestations of infection, how to take an oral temperature, activities that increase risk of a recurrence of the endocarditis, the necessity of providing other health care professionals such as the dentist or podiatrist with the endocarditis history, and information on how to obtain Medic Alert bracelets and cards if required (Box 16-24).

VALVULAR HEART DISEASE

Description

Valvular heart disease describes structural and/or functional abnormalities of single or multiple cardiac valves. The result is alteration in blood flow across the

BOX 16-24 PATIENT EDUCATION

ENDOCARDITIS

- Pathophysiology of endocarditis
- Medications: importance of long-term intravenous antibiotics
- Temperature: daily temperature
- Infection control: prophylactic antibiotics related to dental work or other invasive procedures, when current medical crisis controlled
- Activity tolerance: increase activity as tolerated; rest periods as needed
- Heart failure: if symptoms of heart failure are present, education is given on fluid and sodium restriction, fluid balance, diuretic management, daily weight, and controlling breathlessness

valve. There are two types of valvular lesions—stenotic and regurgitant. These are described in this section of the chapter, with reference to the specific cardiac valves involved.

Medical management of valve disease does not have a septate DRG. Usually, if a person is admitted to the critical care unit with valve disease, they either have acute heart failure (DRG 127) or are admitted for cardiac surgical valvular procedure (DRGs 104 or 105). The anticipated length of stay is 3.2 to 5.3 days for medical management (circulatory disorders excluding acute MI, DRG 124 and 125).[26] The longer time period (DRG 124, 5.3 days) is for patients who also undergo cardiac catheterization.

Etiology

In the past in the United States, most valvular lesions were rheumatic in origin; that is, damage was a direct result of group A beta-hemolytic streptococcal pharyngitis. Today, with the aging population, degenerative valve changes are equally important (Box 16-25).

BOX 16-25 Etiology of Valvular Heart Disease

Rheumatic fever
Infective endocarditis
Inborn defects of connective tissue
Dysfunction or ruptures of the papillary muscles
Congenital malformations
Aging valve tissue

Pathophysiology

Mitral valve stenosis. Mitral stenosis describes a progressive narrowing of the mitral valve orifice from the normal size of 4 to 6 cm to less than 1.5 cm. This narrowing is usually caused by aging valve tissue or by acute rheumatic valvulitis (Table 16-4, *A*). The diffuse valve leaflet fibrosis and fusion of one or both commissures reduces leaflet mobility. Also the chordae tendineae may be thickened, shortened, and fused—further contributing to the stenotic mitral orifice. As a result, the mitral valve no longer can open and close passively in response to chamber pressure changes, and blood flow across the valve is impeded.[62,63]

Mitral valve regurgitation. Mitral regurgitation may occur secondary to rheumatic disease or aging of the valve, or it can be caused by endocarditis, papillary muscle dysfunction, or a number of other events (Table 16-4, *B*). In mitral valve regurgitation the valve annulus, leaflets, commissures, chordae tendineae, and papillary muscles may all be dysfunctional or the dysfunction may be isolated to just one component of the valve. Mitral valve regurgitation results in retrograde flow of blood into the left atrium with each ventricular contraction. The left atrium dilates to accommodate this additional volume, whereas the left ventricle hypertrophies as it tries to maintain forward flow and an adequate stroke volume. Acute mitral valve regurgitation caused by papillary muscle rupture secondary to acute MI is a medical emergency. This condition is not tolerated without aggressive medical therapy to stabilize the patient's condition, which frequently includes the use of an intraaortic balloon pump. Once the patient's condition has stabilized, surgical replacement of the incompetent valve is performed.[64] (∞AV Valves, p. 333.)

Aortic valve stenosis. Aortic stenosis can result from aging, calcification of a congenital bicuspid valve, or rheumatic valvulitis (Table 16-4, *C*). Irrespective of its cause, the effect is the impedance of ejection of blood from the left ventricle into the aorta, resulting in increased left ventricular systolic pressure, left ventricular hypertrophy, and eventually, at end-stage disease, left ventricular dilation. In addition, when the increase in volume and pressure are communicated back to the atrial and pulmonary vasculature, the result is an increase in left atrial pressure and volume, elevated pulmonary venous pressure, and pulmonary congestion. The goal of medical and surgical management is to prevent left ventricular damage from occurring.[65]

Aortic valve regurgitation. Aortic regurgitation or insufficiency can occur as a result of rheumatic fever, systemic hypertension, Marfan's syndrome, syphilis, rheumatoid arthritis, aging valve tissue, or discrete subaortic stenosis (Table 16-4, *D*). Aortic valve incompetence

TABLE 16-4 Valvular Dysfunction

	Pathophysiology	Clinical Manifestations	Physical Signs
A 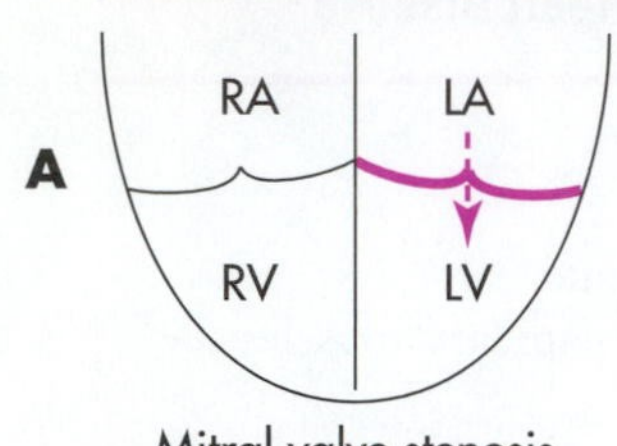 Mitral valve stenosis 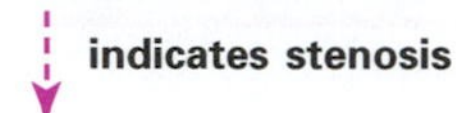 indicates stenosis	**MITRAL VALVE STENOSIS** Left atrium must generate more pressure to propel blood beyond the lesion Rise in left atrial pressure and volume reflected retrograde into pulmonary vessels Right ventricular hypertrophy Right ventricular failure	Dyspnea on exertion Fatigue and weakness Pronounced respiratory symptoms—orthopnea, paroxysmal nocturnal dyspnea Mild hemoptysis with bronchial capillary rupture Susceptibility to pulmonary infections	Chest radiograph—pulmonary congestion, redistribution of blood flow to upper lobes ECG—atrial fibrillation and other atrial dysrhythmias Auscultation—diastolic murmur, accentuated S_1, opening snap Catheterization—elevated pressure gradient across valve; increased left atrial pressure, pulmonary artery wedge pressure, and pulmonary artery pressure; low cardiac output
B 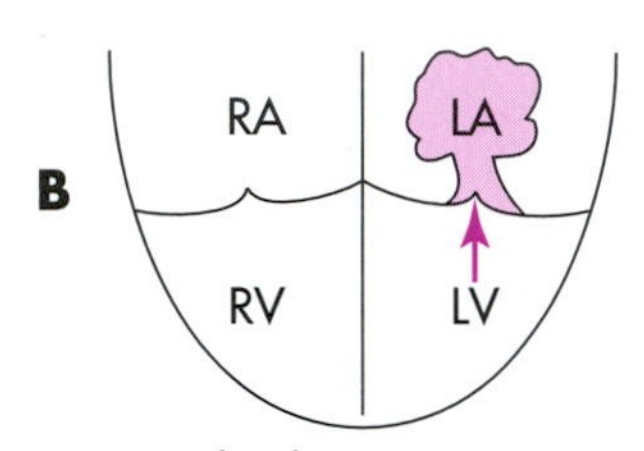 Mitral valve regurgitation 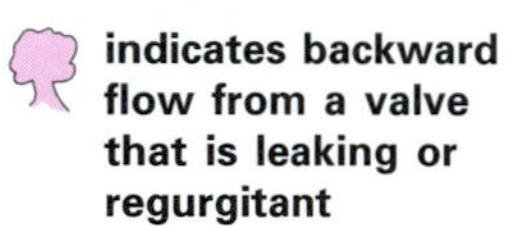 indicates stenosis of the valve indicates backward flow from a valve that is leaking or regurgitant	**MITRAL VALVE REGURGITATION** Left ventricular dilation and hypertrophy Left atrial dilation and hypertrophy	Weakness and fatigue Exertional dyspnea Palpitations Severe symptoms precipitated by left ventricular failure, with consequent low output and pulmonary congestion	Chest radiograph—left atrial and left ventricular enlargement, variable pulmonary congestion ECG—P-mitrale, left ventricular hypertrophy, atrial fibrillation Auscultation—murmur throughout systole Catheterization—opacification of left atrium during left ventricular injection, V waves, increased left atrial and left ventricular pressures Variable elevations of pulmonary pressures
C 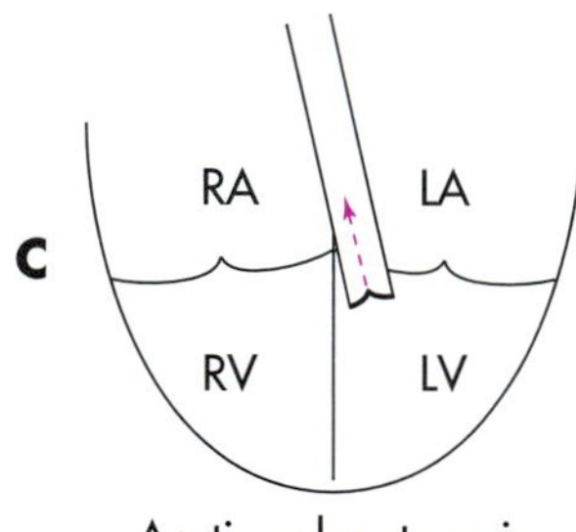 Aortic valve stenosis 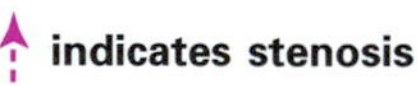 indicates stenosis	**AORTIC VALVE STENOSIS** Left ventricular hypertrophy Progressive failure of ventricular emptying Pulmonary congestion Failure of right side of heart, with systemic venous congestion Sudden cardiac death	Exertional dyspnea Exercise intolerance Syncope Angina Heart failure (left ventricular failure)	Chest radiograph—poststenotic aortic dilation, calcification ECG—left ventricular hypertrophy Auscultation—systolic ejection murmur Catheterization—significant pressure gradient, increased left ventricular end-diastolic pressure
D 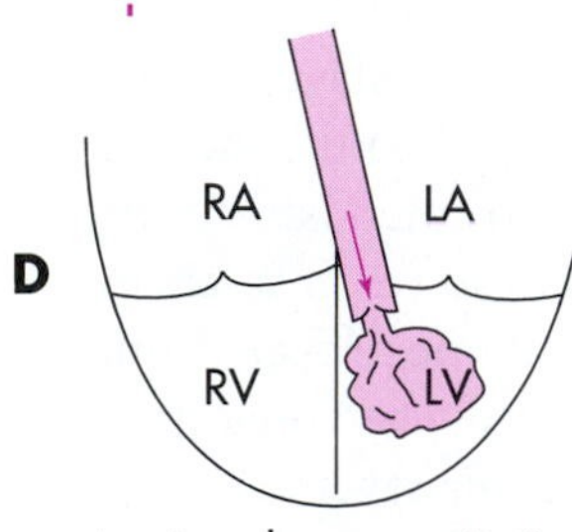 Aortic valve regurgitation indicates stenosis of the valve 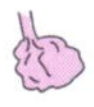 indicates backward flow from a valve that is leaking or regurgitant	**AORTIC VALVE REGURGITATION** Increased volume load imposed on left ventricle Left ventricular dilation and hypertrophy	Fatigue Dyspnea on exertion Palpitations	Chest radiograph—boot-shaped elongation of cardiac apex ECG—left ventricular hypertrophy Auscultation—diastolic murmur Catheterization—opacification of left ventricle during aortic injection Peripheral signs—hyperdynamic myocardial action and low peripheral resistance

TABLE 16-4 Valvular Dysfunction—cont'd

	Pathophysiology	Clinical Manifestations	Physical Signs
E RA LA RV LV Tricuspid valve stenosis (arrow) **indicates stenosis**	**TRICUSPID VALVE STENOSIS** Right atrium must generate higher pressure to eject blood beyond the lesion Right atrial dilation Systemic venous engorgement Increased venous pressures	Venous distention Peripheral edema Ascites Hepatic engorgement Anorexia	Chest radiograph—right atrial enlargement ECG—right atrial enlargement (P-pulmonale) Auscultation—diastolic murmur Catheterization—elevated right atrial pressure with large a waves; pressure gradient across the tricuspid valve
F RA LA RV LV Tricuspid valve regurgitation (arrow) **indicates stenosis of the valve** (cloud) **indicates backward flow from a valve that is leaking or regurgitant**	**TRICUSPID VALVE REGURGITATION** Right ventricular hypertrophy and dilation	Decreased cardiac output Neck vein distention Hepatic engorgement Ascites Edema Pleural effusions	Chest radiograph—right atrial and ventricular enlargement ECG—right ventricular hypertrophy and right atrial enlargement, atrial fibrillation Auscultation—murmur throughout systole Catheterization—elevated right atrial pressure and V waves

results in reflux of blood back into the left ventricle during ventricular diastole. To accommodate this extra volume, the left ventricle initially dilates and then hypertrophies in an attempt to empty more completely and to meet the needs of the peripheral circulation. Recent research indicates that women, because of their smaller left ventricular size, may benefit from aortic valve repair surgery earlier than do men.[66] (∞Semilunal Valves, p. 334.)

Tricuspid valve stenosis. Tricuspid stenosis is rarely an isolated lesion; it frequently occurs in conjunction with mitral or aortic disease, or both. Its origin most often is rheumatic fever (Table 16-4, *E*). Tricuspid stenosis increases the pressure work of the usually low-pressure right atrium, resulting in right atrial hypertrophy. In addition, the right atrium dilates in an attempt to accommodate the residual right atrial volume and the incoming venous return. As a result, systemic venous congestion occurs—the consequences of which include jugular venous congestion, liver failure, hepatomegaly, ascites, and peripheral edema.[67,68]

Tricuspid valve regurgitation. Tricuspid regurgitation usually results from advanced failure of the left side of the heart that eventually affects the right side of the heart (backward heart failure), or severe pulmonary hypertension[67,68] (Table 16-4, *F*).

Pulmonic valve disease. Pulmonary valve disease is not a common disorder in adults. It is most often related to congenital anomalies and produces failure of the right side of the heart.

Mixed valvular lesions. Many persons have mixed lesions (i.e., an element of both stenosis and regurgitation). Mixed lesions can accentuate the severity of a condition. For example, when combined, aortic stenosis and aortic regurgitation increase left ventricular volume and pressure and thereby multiply the degree of left ventricular work.

Medical Management

Management of valvular disorders includes pharmacologic therapy to control symptoms of heart failure, balloon dilatation, or cardiac surgical repair or replacement. (∞Valvular Surgery, p. 542.)

Nursing Management

Nursing management of the patient with valvular disease incorporates a variety of nursing diagnoses (Box 16-26). Nursing interventions are directed toward maintenance of adequate cardiac output, optimizing fluid balance, and patient and family education.

BOX 16-26 NURSING DIAGNOSIS AND MANAGEMENT

VALVULAR HEART DISEASE

- Decreased Cardiac Output related to alterations in preload, p. 590
- Decreased Cardiac Output related to alterations in afterload, p. 592
- Decreased Cardiac Output related to alterations in contractility, p. 592
- Decreased Cardiac Output related to alterations in heart rate, p. 593
- Activity Intolerance related to cardiopulmonary dysfunction, p. 596
- Knowledge Deficit: Discharge Regimen related to lack of previous exposure to information, p. 61 (see Patient Education Box 16-27)

BOX 16-27 PATIENT EDUCATION

VALVULAR HEART DISEASE

- Pathophysiology of the valvular disease
- Infection control: prophylactic antibiotics related to dental work or other invasive procedures
- Heart failure: if symptoms of heart failure are present, education is provided on fluid and sodium restriction, fluid balance, diuretic management, daily weight, and controlling breathlessness
- Medications: medications may be complex, and information must be in writing, as well as oral
  - Preload: purpose of diuretics, increased urine output, and control of fluid volume
  - Afterload: purpose of vasodilators or ACE inhibitors in decreasing the workload of the heart
  - Heart rate: purpose of digoxin to control atrial fibrillation—a frequent dysrhythmia in heart failure
  - Contractility: with the exception of digoxin, there are no oral contractility drugs that are approved by the FDA
  - Anticoagulation: patients with distended atria, enlarged ventricles, or atrial fibrillation may be prescribed anticoagulants (Coumadin); risks of bleeding, importance of correct dosages, prothrombin times (INR), and nutritional-pharmacologic interactions are emphasized
- Follow-up care
- Symptoms to report to a health care professional

Assessing cardiac output. Low cardiac output is a common finding in patients with valvular heart disease. It can occur because of decreased forward flow through a stenotic valve or because of bi-directional flow across an incompetent valve. Vital signs and the effect of positive inotropic and afterload-reducing agents are assessed and documented. If the patient has hemodynamic catheters, cardiac output and hemodynamic parameters are measured and evaluated. Patient care activities are carefully planned to provide adequate rest periods to prevent fatigue.

Managing fluid balance. Fluid status is assessed by auscultating breath and heart sounds. The appearance of pulmonary crackles or an S_3 may indicate volume overload. The jugular vein may be assessed for signs of increased distention. Diuretics and vasodilators are administered, if required. The patient is weighed daily, and fluid intake and output is monitored and recorded.

Patient Education

Patient education includes information related to diet and/or fluid restrictions, actions and side effects of heart failure medications, the need for prophylactic antibiotics before undergoing any invasive procedures such as dental work,[58] and when to call the health care provider to report a change in cardiac symptoms (Box 16-27).

ATHEROSCLEROTIC DISEASES OF THE AORTA

Description

Two atherosclerotic aortic conditions are described—aortic aneurysm and aortic dissection. An *aortic aneurysm* is a localized dilation of the arterial wall that results in an alteration in vessel shape and blood flow. Figure 16-14 displays the four types of aneurysms. An *aortic dissection* occurs when a column of blood separates the vascular layers. This creates a false lumen, which communicates with the true lumen through a tear in the intima.[69]

The incidence of aortic aneurysm is higher in men than in women, and it is diagnosed most commonly after the fifth decade of life. Abdominal aortic aneurysm is four times more common than is thoracic aneurysm. Aortic aneurysm and aortic dissection are covered under the same diagnosis-related groups as the peripheral vascular diseases: DRG 130 and 131. Length of stay ranges from 5.5 to 7.2 days.[26] The longer length of stay (DRG 130) is for patients with additional complications.

Etiology

Most patients with an aortic aneurysm (90%) have a history of systemic hypertension. Other causes of aortic aneurysm include (1) atherosclerotic changes in

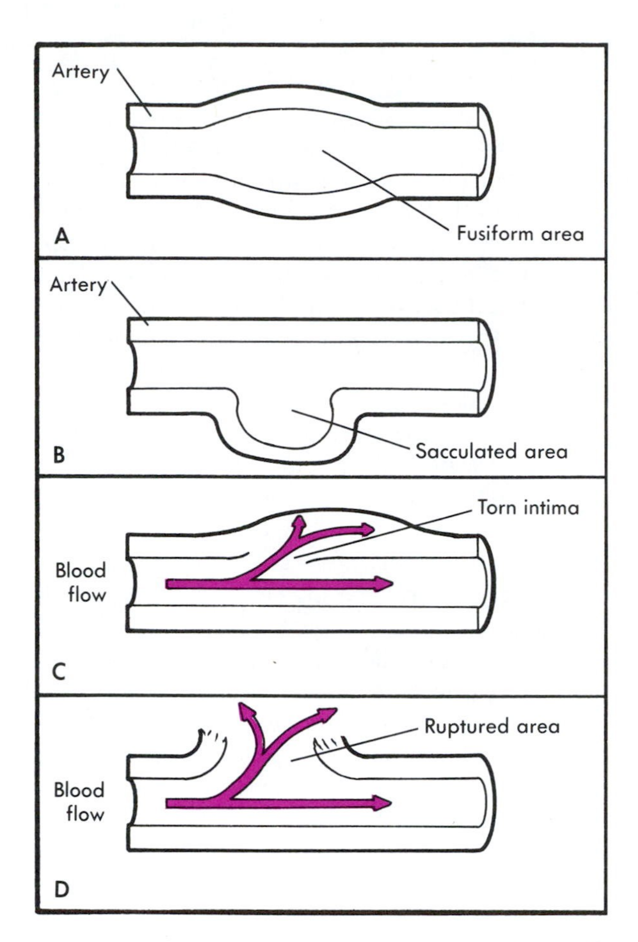

FIGURE 16-14. Four types of aneurysms. **A,** Fusiform aneurysm, in which an entire segment of an artery is dilated, thus taking on a spindle or bulbous shape. Fusiform aneurysms occur most often in the abdominal aorta secondary to atherosclerosis. **B,** Sacculated aneurysm, which involves only one side of an artery and usually is located in the ascending aorta. **C,** Dissecting aneurysm, which occurs because of a tear in the intima, resulting in the shunting of blood between the intima and media of a vessel. **D,** Pseudoaneurysm, which results from a ruptured artery.

the thoracic and abdominal aorta, (2) blunt trauma, (3) Marfan's syndrome, (4) pregnancy, and (5) iatrogenic injury or dissection.[69]

Assessment and Diagnosis

An aortic aneurysm does not always have symptoms. It may be detected during routine abdominal examination as a palpable, pulsatile mass located in the umbilical region of the abdomen to the left of the midline. A thoracic aneurysm may be identified on a routine chest x-ray film. An aortic dissection is usually identified emergently by the onset of acute pain as described in the following.

Aortic aneurysm. An aneurysm less than 4 cm in diameter can be managed on an outpatient basis with frequent blood pressure monitoring and ultrasound testing to document any changes in the aneurysm's size. The patient is encouraged to lose weight if obesity is a factor, and hypertension is treated to decrease hemodynamic stress on the site. An aneurysm greater than 5 cm usually requires surgical intervention (Box 16-28). After surgical repair, a patient generally is admitted to the critical care unit.

BOX 16-28 Indications for Aortic Aneurysm Repair

- Aneurysm greater than 5 cm
- Aneurysm progressively increasing in size
- Impending rupture
- Symptoms resulting from cerebral or coronary ischemia
- Pericardial tamponade
- Uncontrollable pain
- Aortic insufficiency

Aortic dissection. Aortic dissections are classified according to site of the tear. There are two classification systems used in clinical practice. These use either the letters A and B or numerals I, II, or III, as shown in Figure 16-15. The classic clinical manifestation is the sudden onset of intense, severe, tearing pain, which may be localized initially in the chest, abdomen, or back. As dissection extends, pain radiates to the back or distally toward the lower extremities. Cardiovascular signs may include severe hypertension, acute neurologic deficits, fleeting peripheral pulses, or a new murmur indicative of aortic regurgitation. The location of the dissection may be established by the site of pain. A descending aortic dissection usually is accompanied by pain that radiates to the back, abdomen, or legs. An ascending aortic dissection produces central chest pain. Invasive diagnostic procedures that may be performed include an aortogram (aortic angiogram with radiopaque contrast), magnetic resonance imaging (MRI), and a computed tomographic (CT) scan using contrast.[70]

Medical Management

Medical management of an aortic aneurysm involves controlling hypertension and educating the patient about the need for corrective surgery if the aneurysm is more than 5 cm. Medical management of acute aortic dissection involves control of hypertension with intravenous agents and control of pain with narcotics such as morphine. Progression of the

LEGAL REVIEW 

Products Liability

There are three theories of recovery for harm or injury suffered from defective medical products (drugs, diagnostic and treatment devices and equipment, and blood and blood components): (1) strict liability, (2) negligence, and (3) warranty.

Most states have adopted and codified the Restatement (Second) of Torts, Section 402A, definition of strict liability: One who sells a defective product that is unreasonably dangerous to the consumer is liable for harm to the consumer, even if the seller has exercised all possible care in the preparation and sale of the product and the consumer has not bought the product from the seller. The underlying public policy in this law is that consumers should be protected from the inevitable risks of harm brought about by mass production and marketing of products.

To prevail under this theory, the plaintiff must prove the defendant sold the product, the product was defective, the defect rendered the product unreasonably dangerous when used in a reasonably foreseeable manner, the defendant was in the business of selling the product and the defect existed at the time of the sale, the defect was the proximate cause of the damages, and the plaintiff suffered damages. However, under many state statutes, "sellers" may be immune from liability if the seller is not engaged in the assembly, design, or manufacture of the product and the defect originated in one of these areas of production.

There are three types of product defects: (1) defective manufacture, (2) defective design, and (3) inadequate or absent warnings (which are usually litigated under a negligence theory).

Under the negligence theory, the duty of reasonable care applies to the design, manufacture, and testing of the product to ensure safety. There is also a duty to provide adequate information and warnings to the consumer about the product. In strict liability the plaintiff's proof focuses on the condition of the product that is designed or manufactured in a certain way, whereas in negligence the proof focuses on the reasonableness of the defendant's conduct in designing, manufacturing, or selling the product and in providing product information and warnings.

Under the warranty liability theory, statements or representations about the character, fitness, condition, or quality of the product are at issue. Product warranties may be express or they may be presumed—that is, implied.

A hospital may be liable for negligence under corporate and respondeat superior theories for failure to monitor and maintain equipment safety and for failure to provide adequately trained staff to operate medical equipment and devices. Critical care nurses may be held personally liable for negligence or malpractice for using defective products or devices, for failure to properly monitor or use equipment, and for failure to comply with printed instructions for use.

Hospitals, doctors, and nurses frequently reuse medical devices (particularly heart catheters) for cost containment reasons. In the event the reused device proves or becomes defective and causes injury, the hospital and staff—as well as the manufacturer and seller—may be liable under all three products liability doctrines.

In the Hawaii and Texas cases cited below, both states have "blood shield" statutes that bar certain claims against hospitals arising from a patient's contraction of acquired immunodeficiency syndrome from transfusion of contaminated blood. In *Gibson v. Methodist Hosp.*, the court held that blood was not a product for purposes of product liability and breach of warranty claims. In Hawaii, entities are statutorily exempt from strict liability for preparing or transfusing blood or blood components but are not exempt from liability for negligence. In *Smith v. Cutter Biological, Inc.*, the court held that the Hawaii blood shield statute did not preclude negligence claims against four manufacturers of Factor VIII (antihemophilic factor concentrate) by a hemophiliac who became exposed to human immunodeficiency virus through Factor VIII injections, despite his inability to positively identify the actual tortfeasor (wrongdoer).

See Geddes A: Free movement of pharmaceuticals within the community: the remaining barriers, *Eur L Rev* 16:295, 1991; *Gibson v Methodist Hosp.*, 822 S.W.2d 95 (Tex. App. 1991); *Grubb v Albert Einstein Med. Center,* 387 A.2d 480 (Pa. 1978); Lynn JSR: Implantable medical devices: a survey of products liability case law, *Med Trial Tech Q* 38:44, 1991; *May v Broun,* 492 P.2d 776 (Or. 1972); *Phelps v Sherwood Med. Indus.,* 836 F.2d 296 (7th Cir. 1987); *Phillips v Medtronic, Inc:,* No. 86-4231-R (D. Kan. Feb. 23, 1990); Prosser WL and others: *Prosser and Keeton on the law of torts,* ed 5, St Paul, 1988, West; *Restatement (Second) of Torts* Sec. 402A; Shimm DS, Spece RG: Conflict of interest and informed consent in industry-sponsored clinical trials, *J Legal Med* 12:477, 1991; *Smith v Cutter Biological, Inc.,* 823 P.2d 717 (Haw. 1991).

dissection is evaluated by the patient's report of worsening or new pain. Surgery is usually performed for dissections that involve the ascending aorta to prevent death from cardiac tamponade. This includes Type A, or Type I and II, dissections. The surgical procedure includes resection of the affected area, followed by graft placement and restoration of blood flow to major branches of the aorta. Replacement of the aortic valve may be performed if the dissection involves the valve.[70] Dissections that involve the de-

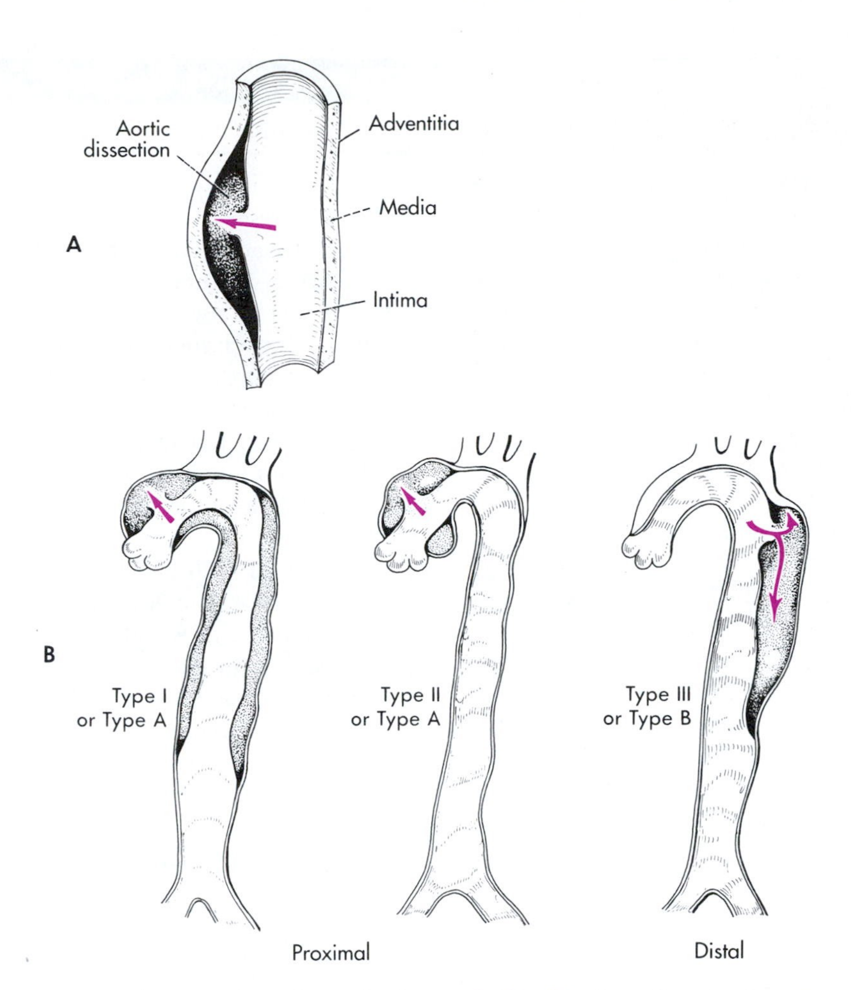

FIGURE 16-15. Aortic dissection. **A,** Separation of vascular layers. **B,** Classification of aortic dissection. (Modified from Price SA, Wilson LM: *Pathophysiology: clinical concepts of disease processes,* ed 4, St Louis, 1992, Mosby.)

scending aorta (Type B, or Type III) do not always require surgery.

Nursing Management

Nursing management of the patient with aortic aneurysm or aortic dissection incorporates a variety of nursing diagnoses (Box 16-29). Nursing interventions are directed toward control of hypertension, pain control, and education of the patient and family.

Hypertension management. The cardiovascular status is assessed hourly, including monitoring blood pressure in both arms, checking peripheral pulses bilaterally, auscultating for an aortic murmur, and monitoring the ECG for ischemic changes or dysrhythmias. Patients usually require an arterial line and receive potent vasodilators such as labetalol or sodium nitroprusside.

Pain control. Acute pain is a classic sign of aortic dissection. Analgesics are given to control pain, decrease anxiety, and increase comfort. Because analgesics can mask the pain of further dissection, they are administered judiciously. The patient's neurovascular status is assessed hourly. Documentation includes the presence and distribution of pain, pallor, paresthesia, paralysis, and pulselessness.

Patient Education

In the acute period education is limited to an explanation of the critical care environment and the importance of blood pressure control. If additional procedures such as an aortogram, CT scan, or surgery are to be performed, the critical care nurse assists with the explanations (Box 16-30).

PERIPHERAL VASCULAR DISEASE

Description

Peripheral vascular disease (PVD) is divided into arterial and venous disease of the peripheral vessels. *Venous disease* is a chronic condition that is managed on an outpatient basis and does not require admission to a critical care unit. By contrast, *arterial PVD* may require critical care admission for an acute thrombotic occlusion. PVD can occur in any

BOX 16-29 NURSING DIAGNOSIS AND MANAGEMENT

AORTIC ANEURYSM AND AORTIC DISSECTION

- Decreased Cardiac Output related to alterations in preload, p. 590
- Acute Pain related to transmission and perception of cutaneous, visceral, muscular, or ischemic impulses, p. 197
- Altered Peripheral Tissue Perfusion related to decreased peripheral blood flow, p. 596
- Altered Myocardial Tissue Perfusion related to acute myocardial ischemia, p. 595
- Risk for Infection risk factor: invasive monitoring devices, p. 598
- Anxiety related to threat to biologic, psychologic, and/or social integrity, p. 99
- Altered Renal Tissue Perfusion related to decreased renal blood flow, p. 916
- Activity Intolerance related to cardiopulmonary dysfunction, p. 596
- Knowledge Deficit: Discharge Regimen related to lack of previous exposure to information, p. 61 (see Patient Education Box 16-30)

BOX 16-30 PATIENT EDUCATION

AORTIC ANEURYSM AND AORTIC DISSECTION

- Pathophysiology of atherosclerotic aortic disease: aortic aneurysm or aortic dissection
- Hypertension control: hypertension increases risk of aneurysm rupture or increasing the aortic dissection
- Pain control: use of 1-10 pain scale; provide information about availability of pain medications for acute pain
- Preprocedure teaching for aortic angiogram, CT scan, or TEE
- Preoperative teaching for aortic surgical repair
- Risk factor modification: after the acute episode, if the cause of the aortic aneurysm or aortic dissection is atherosclerosis, an individual risk factor profile is developed for each patient; topics include: decrease fat intake to less than 30% of total calories a day, achieve total blood cholesterol of less than 200 mg/dL, stop smoking, reduce salt intake, control hypertension, treat diabetes if patient is diabetic, increase physical activity, achieve ideal body weight
- Symptoms to report to a health care professional: pain, signs and symptoms of infection
- Follow-up care

CT, Computed tomography; TEE, transoephageal echocardiogram.

peripheral vessel, but is most frequently seen in the lower extremities. The following descriptions relate to arterial PVD.

Peripheral vascular disorders are covered under DRG 130 and DRG 131; length of stay ranges from 5.5 to 7.2 days.[26]

Etiology

Atherosclerosis is the most common cause of chronic arterial occlusion. Up to 5% of men and 2.5% of women 60 years or older have symptoms of intermittent claudication.[71] Risk factors are the same as those for CAD. In addition to atherosclerosis, diabetes, smoking, hypertension, hyperlipidemia, and male gender all increase the risk of developing PVD.

Pathophysiology

The most commonly affected vessels are the superficial femoral artery and the popliteal artery in the legs, followed by the distal aorta and iliac arteries.[71]

Assessment and Diagnosis

Intermittent claudication. Arterial occlusion obstructs blood flow to the distal extremity. The lack of blood flow produces ischemic muscle pain, or intermittent claudication. This cramping, aching pain while walking usually is the first symptom of peripheral occlusive disease. The pain is relieved by rest and may remain stable in occurrence and intensity for many years. Symptoms do not occur until more than 75% of the vessel lumen is occluded. Arterial pulses are diminished, transiently present (vessel spasm), or absent distal to the site of occlusion. Diabetic patients have a much higher incidence of peripheral vascular disease than does the general population. Cardiovascular disease, in general, causes 80% of the mortality in diabetic patients.[72]

Rest pain. As PVD progresses, 20% to 30% of patients develop pain during rest. Pain at rest threatens the viability of the limb and requires immediate catheter or surgical intervention to relieve the blockage and restore circulation to the extremity.[73,74]

Acute occlusion. The symptoms of acute occlusion from thrombosis are sudden onset of severe pain, loss of pulses, collapse of superficial veins, coldness, pallor, and impaired motor and sensory function. As with rest pain, acute occlusion requires immediate intervention to open the artery.[74]

Atrophic tissue changes. Skin changes include thickening of the nails and drying of the skin. Hair loss is common on the lower leg, dorsum of the feet, and toes. A temperature gradient usually is present as a line of demarcation between areas that are well-perfused and those that are poorly perfused. There also may be wasting of muscle or soft tissue. As the disease progresses, ulcerations and gangrene may result.

Medical Management

Medical therapy is geared toward controlling or eliminating risk factors, providing good foot care, and suggesting alterations in life-style to promote rest and pain relief. Pharmacologic management may include the use of anticoagulants, vasodilators, or antiplatelet agents.[73] If these therapies do not produce positive results, the patient may be a candidate for percutaneous transluminal angioplasty (PTA), stent placement, or surgery. PTA or stent placement is effective if the lesion (blockage) is discrete and localized.[74] However, if the arterial disease is diffuse, then bypass surgery is usually performed. If gangrene (cell death) is present, limb or partial limb amputation is required.

Nursing Management

Nursing management of the patient with peripheral arterial insufficiency incorporates a variety of nursing diagnoses (Box 16-31). Nurses assess the quality of the peripheral arterial pulses, intervene to maintain skin integrity, control pain, and educate the patient and family about peripheral vascular disease.

Arterial pulses. Assessment of peripheral pulses, limb color, and temperature are all critical in the evaluation of an ischemic limb. Many hospitals use a standard scale to improve documentation of pulses. If the pulse cannot be palpated, a Doppler may be used to assess blood flow. (∞Arterial Pulsations, p. 362.)

Skin integrity. Care is taken to protect the limb from injury, such as pressure sores. Healing is often impaired because of poor blood flow or diabetes. Feet may be protected from injury by cotton or lamb's wool placed between the toes or by a bed cradle. However, for an acute ischemic limb, removal of the thrombus is the only treatment that will salvage ischemic tissue.

Pain control. Intermittent claudication is managed by rest. However, the pain of an acute ischemic limb is extreme, and morphine is used for pain control.[73]

Patient Education

Education topics include risk factor modification similar to that taught for coronary artery disease, smoking cessation, promoting exercise, inspection of the feet and legs, foot care, avoidance of foot trauma, and medications.[75,76] Walking is good exercise to increase blood flow to the lower extremities and is highly recommended for the individual with PVD.[71]

If a surgically implanted prosthetic bypass graft is in place, teaching must include information about bacterial endocarditis precautions.[58] If the patient is diabetic, education about diabetes management is also included in the teaching plan. Box 16-32 lists the salient points to include when teaching patients and families about peripheral vascular disease.

BOX 16-31 NURSING DIAGNOSIS AND MANAGEMENT

PERIPHERAL VASCULAR DISEASE

- Acute Pain related to transmission and perception of cutaneous, visceral, muscular, or ischemic impulses, p. 197
- Altered Peripheral Tissue Perfusion related to decreased peripheral blood flow, p. 596
- Altered Myocardial Tissue Perfusion related to acute myocardial ischemia, p. 595
- Activity Intolerance related to prolonged immobility or deconditioning, p. 597
- Anxiety related to threat of biologic, psychologic, and/or social integrity, p. 99
- Powerlessness related to lack of control over current situation and/or disease progression, p. 89
- Knowledge Deficit: Discharge Regimen related to lack of previous exposure to information, p. 61 (see Patient Education Box 16-32)

CAROTID ARTERY DISEASE

Description

The bifurcation of the carotid arteries is a common site of atherosclerotic plaque development (Figure 16-16). Because these arteries carry the blood supply to the brain, when they are obstructed, the symptoms are neurologic. Carotid artery disorders are covered under DRG 15 TIA (transient ischemic attack) and precerebral occlusion. Anticipated length of stay is 4.2 days.[26]

Carotid artery disease is the most readily treatable type of lesion leading to stroke. The blood supply to the brain is provided by the vertebral arteries and the internal carotid arteries, branches of which anastomose to form the cerebral arterial circle of Willis. An abrupt interruption in circulation for 4 to 8 minutes produces permanent brain damage. When circulation to an area is impaired gradually, collateral circulation is often able to develop and maintain an adequate supply of blood to that area of the brain. With an abrupt interruption in blood supply, an acute stroke will occur.

Etiology

The most common cause of cerebrovascular disease in the United States is atherosclerosis, which accounts for 90% of all cases. Other causes include fibromuscular dysplasia, irradiation, carotid dissection, and

BOX 16-32 PATIENT EDUCATION

PERIPHERAL VASCULAR DISEASE

- Pathophysiology of peripheral vascular disease
- Daily inspection and care of feet and legs
- Avoidance of trauma to feet or legs
- Increase walking distance gradually
- Risk factor modification: after the acute episode, if the cause of the aortic aneurysm or aortic dissection is atherosclerosis, an individual risk factor profile is developed for each patient; topics include: decrease fat intake to less than 30% of total calories a day, achieve total blood cholesterol of less than 200 mg/dL, stop smoking, reduce salt intake, control hypertension, control diabetes if patient is diabetic, increase physical activity, achieve and maintain ideal body weight
- Preprocedure teaching for angiogram, percutaneous angioplasty, or stent placement in the lower extremities
- Risks and benefits of thrombolytic therapy for acute peripheral arterial occlusion
- Presurgery teaching for revascularization surgery
- Rehabilitation education if amputation is indicated
- Medications
  Antithrombotic therapy: usually asprin to decrease platelet adhesiveness
  Lipid-lowering agents: HMG-CoA reductase inhibitors and other agents
  Antihypertensive agents: antihypertensive medications and how to self-monitor own blood pressure
- Symptoms to report to a health care professional: pain (chest or legs), leg or foot trauma
- Follow-up care

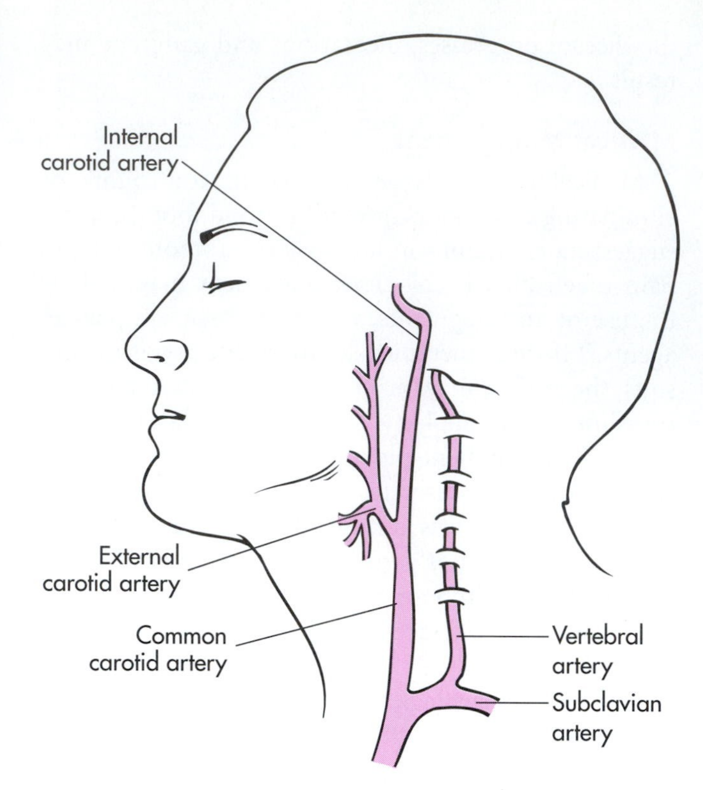

FIGURE 16-16. Carotid arteries (common, internal, and external). Atherosclerotic plaque develops in the common carotid artery at the bifurcation into the internal and external carotid arteries. Plaque also develops in the common, internal, and external carotid arteries.

arteritis. The major mechanisms by which atherosclerosis causes ischemic symptoms are embolization and thrombosis. Ulcerated lesions frequently accumulate platelet thrombi which, along with cholesterol deposits, may travel in the blood stream to become emboli to the brain. Stenotic areas of more than 75% in the carotid arteries are prone to thrombosis because of sluggish flow across the lesion. The carotid arteries can be studied noninvasively by Doppler.[77]

Manifestations of carotid artery disease vary, depending on which vessel is involved. Common neurologic manifestations include hemiparesis, monoparesis, dysphasia, dysarthria, global aphasia, diplopia, vertigo, syncope confusion, and monocular blindness. The duration of symptoms is the most common means of classifying events; symptoms lasting fewer than 24 hours are classified as transient ischemic attacks (TIAs). Symptoms lasting longer than 24 hours but less than 72 hours are classified as reversible ischemic neurologic deficit (RIND), and symptoms lasting longer than 72 hours are considered completed stroke. (∞Cerebrovascular Accident, p. 798.)

Medical Management

Medical management is focused on lowering the atherosclerotic risk factors over which the patient has control. This includes regulation of hypertension, smoking cessation, seeking medical attention for treatable cardiac abnormalities such as atrial fibrillation, reducing weight, and reducing the cholesterol level to less than 200 mg/dL. The symptomatic patient with carotid stenosis greater than 75% will benefit from carotid surgical endarterectomy.

Asymptomatic patients who have carotid stenosis pose a quandary. In these patients the risk of stroke needs to be weighed against the risks of surgery—specifically stroke. Clinical studies suggest that carotid endarterectomy combined with aspirin and risk factor reduction is superior to aspirin and risk factor reduction alone in preventing stroke in asymptomatic patients with significant stenosis; however, not all clinicians interpret the findings in this way. Asymptomatic patients needs to be informed of the risks involved with the procedure, along with their risk for future cerebral vascular events.[78-80]

Nursing Management

Nursing management is focused on assessment of cerebral perfusion; vital signs; respiratory pattern; level of consciousness; pupil reaction; pupil size; and possible cranial nerve deficits such as difficulty in swallowing, loss of gag reflex, changes in speech, and loss of facial symmetry. The nurse educates the patient and family about the causes of the current event and provides information on preventing further cerebrovascular events. Several nursing diagnoses are associated with management of the patient with carotid artery disease (Box 16-33).

Neurologic assessment. Neurologic assessment in the patient with carotid artery disease is divided into two parts: (1) level of consciousness, mental alertness, and cerebral perfusion; and (2) cranial artery function.

A neurologic assessment is performed to make sure that the patient has not suffered a TIA or stroke. Thus questions to ascertain level of conscious relate to time and place and reason for hospital admission. Mental alertness is assessed by the ability with which the patient responds to these and other questions. In addition, the person is asked to move all four limbs on command. To assess the cranial nerves the patient is asked to make a grimace, which should demonstrate bilateral facial symmetry; to stick out the tongue to ensure it is midline; and to swallow and speak, which should be done without difficulty. (∞Pupillary Function and Eye Movement, p. 769; Rapid Neurologic Examination, p. 774.)

Patient Education

If the patient is admitted to a critical care unit, a severe cerebrovascular accident or stroke may have already occurred. If however, the patient has known carotid artery disease and has not had a cerebrovascular event, preventative education is essential. Since there are many causes of stroke, it is important to discuss the mechanism of stroke in carotid artery disease. It is usually embolic to a specific area of the brain. It may also occur secondary to a thrombus that develops across the narrowed carotid artery lumen, causing widespread cerebral hypoperfusion. Many patients who have atherosclerotic carotid artery disease also have coronary artery disease (CAD) or peripheral vascular disease (PVD) and are diabetic or hypertensive. The major areas of education are listed in Box 16-34. (∞Risk Factors for Coronary Artery Disease, p. 483; Pathophysiology of Coronary Artery Disease, p. 485; Peripheral Vascular Disease, p. 517.)

BOX 16-33 NURSING DIAGNOSIS AND MANAGEMENT

CAROTID ARTERY DISEASE

- Altered Cerebral Tissue Perfusion, p. 842
- Anxiety related to threat to biologic, psychologic, and/or social integrity, p. 99
- Knowledge Deficit: Discharge Regimen related to lack of previous exposure to information, p. 61 (see Patient Education Box 16-34)

DEEP VEIN THROMBOSIS

Description

Deep vein thrombosis (DVT) describes a clot accompanied by inflammation, pain, tenderness, and redness at the site that forms in a deep vein of the leg, pelvis, and less commonly, the arm. The concern over DVT is that it may migrate, via the venous circulation, to the pulmonary vascular bed, causing a fatal pulmonary embolus. Thrombophlebitis, or injury and inflammation of the vein, is often the precursor of a DVT. The most commonly affected vessels are the saphenous, femoral, and popliteal veins in the leg.[81-83]

Etiology

Thrombophlebitis and DVT occur when there is an alteration in the integrity of veins, resulting in decreased venous return or thrombosis. Stasis of blood, endothelial injury, and hypercoagulability of blood are referred to as *Virchow's triad;* usually two of these three conditions must be present for thrombosis to occur. DVT markedly increases the patient's risk of pulmonary embolism and long-term disability, which result from chronic venous insufficiency. The incidence of DVT increases with age. At 65 years the incidence is 1.8 per 1000 person years. At age 85 the incidence is 3.1 per 1000 person years.[81] The most common risk factors are age older than 40 years, followed by obesity and major surgery.[81] Inherited coagulation disorders and hypercoagulability create a higher propensity for clotting and increase the DVT risk profile. (∞Pulmonary Embolus, p. 668.)

Assessment and Diagnosis

Development of deep vein thrombosis may be insidious. It occurs as a result of immobility or edema—causes of which include increased intravascular volume

BOX 16-34 PATIENT EDUCATION

CAROTID ARTERY DISEASE

- Pathophysiology of atherosclerotic carotid artery disease
- Pathophysiology of embolic stroke (emboli from carotid artery)
- Warning signs of impending stroke
- Risk factor modification: after the acute episode, if the cause of the carotid artery disease is atherosclerosis, an individual risk factor profile is developed for each patient; topics include: decrease fat intake to less than 30% of total calories a day, achieve total blood cholesterol of less than 200 mg/dL, stop smoking, reduce salt intake, control hypertension, control diabetes if patient is diabetic, increase physical activity, achieve and maintain ideal body weight
- Signs and symptoms to report to a health care professional
- Follow-up care

and increased intravascular pooling of blood. Pain is described as an aching or throbbing sensation, which worsens with ambulation. As many as half of the patients with DVT are asymptomatic.[81] A positive Homans' sign, which is pain on dorsiflexion of the foot, heightens the suspicion of a deep vein thrombosis. If DVT is present in the upper extremity, the entire arm swells.[81] Other manifestations include redness with swelling, increased skin temperature, dilation of superficial veins, and mottling and cyanosis caused by stagnant blood flow.

Medical Management

Major therapeutic emphasis is placed on prophylaxis. The patient is confined to bedrest, along with elevation of the limb, and anticoagulation therapy. Analgesics are prescribed to reduce discomfort. Anticoagulants are prescribed to reduce further clotting.

The risks and benefits of anticoagulation are discussed with the patient before therapy begins. In the acute phase, the DVT can be treated with either intravenous or subcutaneous heparin. Subsequently, oral warfarin (Coumadin) may be used. Antiplatelet therapy with aspirin is added to prevent DVT from occurring again and to reduce the incidence of pulmonary embolism.[81] None of the aforementioned antithrombotics dissolve the existing clot, but they will prevent new thrombi from forming. If a DVT is identified in the formation phase, thrombolytic agents may be used to dissolve the clot. Lytic therapy is most effective if performed within 48 hours of clot formation. Because of the risks associated with thrombolytics, this therapy is generally reserved for limb ischemia with DVT.[81] Patients receiving anticoagulation therapy require careful assessment for bleeding tendencies, including obtaining frequent bleeding studies (activated partial prothoplastin time [aPTT], international normalized ratio [INR], or prothrombin time [PT]), testing stool and urine for occult blood, and inspecting gums for bleeding. Once the patient begins to ambulate, full-length, custom-fitted elastic stockings are ordered. Complaints of or observation of dyspnea or chest pain must be quickly evaluated to assess the risk of pulmonary embolism.[82,83]

Medical management with anticoagulants is adequate for most patients; however, those at risk for pulmonary embolism (i.e., patients with cancer, bleeding disorders, or spinal cord injury or patients who are comatose) may require surgical intervention for protection. Possible procedures include venous embolectomy, femoral vein interruption, inferior vena cava interruption, and insertion of filtering devices into the inferior vena cava.

Nursing Management

The focus of management for the patient with venous disease is to rest the affected extremity, prevent complications resulting from deep vein thrombosis, and monitor anticoagulant therapy. Several nursing diagnoses are used in the management of the patient with DVT (Box 16-35).

Activity. During the acute phase, self-care activities are limited and bedrest is maintained. The affected limb may be elevated above the level of the right atrium to decrease edema and venous stasis. Range-of-motion exercises can be performed with the unaffected leg. The patient is instructed to avoid bending at the knees or hips, because this impedes venous return. Thigh-high antiembolism stockings that have been custom-fitted can also be used. It is not clear when it is "safe" to resume normal activity, such as walking, after DVT. Normally it is after study results of the extremity are negative and after symptoms have abated.[81] Prevention strategies again become important since the patient remains at risk for a recurrence. In general, early ambulation after surgery or other procedures and avoidance of bedrest are the most effective prevention strategies.

Risk of pulmonary embolism. The patient with a deep vein thrombosis is closely monitored for signs of pulmonary embolism and instructed to report immediately any chest pain, dyspnea, hemoptysis, or tachypnea. Risk factors for DVT are nearly identical to those of pulmonary embolism; almost 90% of the 50,000 to

BOX 16-35 NURSING DIAGNOSIS AND MANAGEMENT

DEEP VEIN THROMBOSIS

- Altered Peripheral Tissue Perfusion, p. 596
- Activity Intolerance related to prolonged immobility or deconditioning, p. 597
- Acute Pain related to transmission and perception of cutaneous, visceral, muscular, or ischemic impulses, p. 197
- Powerlessness related to lack of control over current situation and/or disease progression, p. 89
- Anxiety related to threat to biologic, psychologic, and/or social integrity, p. 99
- Knowledge Deficit: Discharge Regimen related to lack of previous exposure to information, p. 61 (see Patient Education Box 16-36)

BOX 16-36 PATIENT EDUCATION

DEEP VEIN THROMBOSIS

- Pathophysiology of deep vein thrombosis
- Discuss risk of pulmonary embolus, need for antiembolism stockings, or pneumatic compression devices on legs; avoid trauma legs and report any chest pain, breathlessness, or increased respiratory rate
- Medications: anticoagulants (heparin or Coumadin) to prevent formation of new thrombus at the site; asprin to decrease platelet aggregation

200,000 pulmonary emboli each year originate from a DVT.[81] For patients who must remain immobile because of their clinical condition, external pneumatic compression devices, antiembolism stockings, or low-dose heparin are commonly used.

Anticoagulation. Anticoagulant therapy is monitored by obtaining daily coagulation values—aPTT, INR, or PT. Signs of bleeding are monitored and treated promptly. Stools are checked for occult blood. Mechanical trauma is avoided by asking the patient to use a soft toothbrush and an electric razor.

Patient Education

Patient education emphasizes DVT prevention for all patients who are immobile in the critical care unit for any length of time. This includes explanations about activity prophylaxis such as early ambulation after major surgery, external pneumatic compression boots, and low-dose heparin.

For patients who have a diagnosed DVT, education is focused on immobilization of the limb, avoidance of trauma to the limb, and elevation of the limb to decrease venous pooling and increase blood flow. If the patient is anticoagulated, the risks and benefits of this therapy are discussed, as well as the risk of pulmonary embolus. The patient is instructed to report any chest pain, shortness of breath, or respiratory distress (Box 16-36).

HYPERTENSIVE CRISIS

Description

Hypertensive crises are relatively uncommon, but when they do occur they are life threatening and demand early recognition and management to minimize morbidity and mortality. There are two types of hypertensive crises: (1) hypertensive emergencies, which develop rapidly over hours to days and place the patient at risk for end-organ damage; and (2) hypertensive urgencies, which develop over days to weeks and are characterized by a serious elevation in blood pressure but do not put the patient at risk for end-organ damage. Hypertensive crisis is characterized by a rise in diastolic blood pressure to greater than 120 to 130 mm Hg (Table 16-5).[84]

Etiology

Hypertensive crisis may occur in patients with no history of the condition or can be precipitated by noncompliance with medical therapy or diet, or both, or by inadequate treatment.

In patients with no known history of hypertension, common causes of crisis include (1) acute renal failure, (2) acute central nervous system (CNS) events, (3) drug-induced hypertension, (4) ingestion of tyramine-containing foods or beverages (beer or cheese) during treatment with a monoamine oxidase inhibitor (MAOI), and (5) pregnancy-induced eclampsia.

Pathophysiology

The exact mechanism of hypertensive crisis is not known, but it is characterized by fibrinoid necrosis of the arterioles.

Assessment and Diagnosis

Hypertensive crisis is manifested by CNS compromise (headache, papilledema, coma); cardiovascular compromise (angina, myocardial infarction); acute renal failure; and a history consistent with catecholamine excess. Other symptoms include nausea and vomiting, confusion, lethargy, altered mental status, and blurring of vision. Worsening of such symptoms may indicate

TABLE 16-5 Classification of Blood Pressure (BP)

Category	Systolic mm Hg	Diastolic mm Hg
NORMAL BP		
Normal	<130	<85
High-Normal	130-139	85-89
HYPERTENSION		
Stage 1	140-159	90-99
Stage 2	160-179	100-109
Stage 3	180-209	110-119
Stage 4	>210	>120

Data from Expert Panel on Detection, Evaluation and Treatment of High Blood Cholesterol in Adults: JAMA 269:3015-3022, 1993.

TABLE 16-6 Hypertensive Emergencies

Emergency	Examples of Causes
CARDIOVASCULAR COMPROMISE	
Chest pain	Unstable angina, myocardial infarction, aortic dissection
Acute heart failure	Myocardial infarction, severe hypertension
Hypertension after vascular surgery	Aortic aneurysmectomy, carotid endarterectomy, coronary artery bypass grafting
CENTRAL NERVOUS SYSTEM (CNS) COMPROMISE	
Papilledema	Increased intracranial pressure—mass lesion Malignant hypertension—any cause
Headache, agitation, lethargy, confusion	Hypertensive encephalopathy—any cause, subarachnoid hemorrhage, cerebrovascular accident (CVA)
Coma	CVA, advanced hypertensive encephalopathy, trauma, tumor
Seizures	Advanced hypertensive encephalopathy, CNS tumor, eclampsia, CVA (less common)
Focal neurologic deficit	CVA, CNS tumor, hypertensive encephalopathy
ACUTE RENAL FAILURE	Malignant hypertension, vasculitis, scleroderma, glomerulonephritis
CATECHOLAMINE EXCESS	Pheochromocytomas, monoamine oxidase inhibitor (MAOI) in combination with certain drugs and foods, clonidine and guanabenz withdrawal

hypertensive encephalopathy. Table 16-6 lists symptoms and clinical findings associated with hypertensive emergencies.

Diagnostic studies include blood pressure measurement in both arms and placement of an intraarterial line for close monitoring of blood pressure. A 12-lead ECG is taken to evaluate for evidence of acute MI or left ventricular hypertrophy. Other pathologic diseases associated with acute hypertension include aortic dissection, stroke, acute heart failure, and acute renal failure.

Medical Management

Hypertensive emergencies necessitate admission of the patient to the critical care unit, where antihypertensive therapy can be administered parenterally and blood pressure monitored continuously by means of an arterial line. Several intravenous medications, in several different drug classes, are available for acute reduction of blood pressure. Medications include vasodilators such as sodium nitroprusside (SNP), nitroglycerin (NTG), hydralazine, and diazoxide. Short-acting beta-blockers that are effective are labetalol and esmolol. Beta-blockers are especially effective if aortic dissection is present. The intravenous ACE inhibitor enalaprilat will also lower blood pressure. Sometimes, combinations of the aforementioned agents are used to more effectively bring the hypertension under control.[84,85] An intravenous diuretic (furosemide) is used if fluid retention is present. It is important to be aware that cerebral hypoperfusion can occur if mean blood pressure is lowered too rapidly. During the first 24 hours of treatment, it is recommended that mean arterial pressure be decreased by no more than 20 to 30 mm Hg. Once the blood pressure is stabilized, oral antihypertensive therapy is initiated to achieve blood pressure values of less than 140/90 mm Hg.[7] (∞Vasodilator Drugs, p. 579.)

Hypertensive urgencies may not necessitate admission to a critical care unit, because they can be treated with rapid-acting oral antihypertensive agents. The agent of choice is the calcium channel blocker

BOX 16-37 NURSING DIAGNOSIS AND MANAGEMENT

HYPERTENSIVE CRISIS

- Altered Cerebral Tissue Perfusion related to vasospasm or hemorrhage, p. 842
- Altered Myocardial Tissue Perfusion related to acute myocardial ischemia, p. 595
- Anxiety related to threat to biologic, psychologic, and/or social integrity, p. 99
- Knowledge Deficit: Discharge Regimen related to lack of previous exposure to information, p. 61 (see Patient Education Box 16-38)

nifedipine. A single 5 or 10 mg dose, when the capsule is bitten and then swallowed, will reduce blood pressure within 20 to 30 minutes. Captopril (25 mg), an ACE inhibitor, is also highly effective at lowering blood pressure. The beta-blocker labetalol can also be prescribed in oral doses. Other oral drugs that may be used include clonidine, guanabenz, prazosin, and minoxidil. A loop diuretic (furosemide) is generally prescribed in addition to the antihypertensive agents.[84]

Hypertensive crisis with current therapy is associated with a 25% mortality 1 year after the event and 50% 5 years after the event. The most common causes of death are uremia, myocardial infarction, heart failure, and cerebrovascular accident.

BOX 16-38 PATIENT EDUCATION

HYPERTENSIVE CRISIS

- Pathophysiology of hypertensive crisis
- Normal and abnormal blood pressure values
- Self-monitoring of blood pressure at home
- Connection between hypertension and other atherosclerotic diseases such as CAD, PVD, and cerebrovascular disease
- Warning signs of a "heart attack," or MI
- Warning signs of a "brain attack," or stroke
- Warning signs of intermittent claudication or PVD
- Risk factor modification: after the acute episode, if the cause of the carotid artery disease is atherosclerosis, an individual risk factor profile is developed for each patient; topics include: decrease fat intake to less than 30% of total calories a day, achieve total blood cholesterol of less than 200 mg/dL, stop smoking, reduce salt intake, control hypertension, control diabetes if patient is diabetic, increase physical activity, achieve and maintain ideal body weight
- Medications: antihypertensive medications, rationale, and side effects
- Signs and symptoms to report to a health care professional
- Follow-up care

CAD, Coronary artery disease; *PVD,* peripheral vascular disease; *MI,* myocardial infarction.

Nursing Management

The focus of nursing management for the patient with hypertensive crisis is to return the blood pressure to the desired range without introducing other complications as a result of the therapy. Then, once the hypertension is controlled, identify the factors that resulted in this life-threatening condition. Several nursing diagnoses are associated with hypertensive crisis (Box 16-37).

During the acute phase the patient is closely observed for clinical manifestations in other organ systems, including the neurologic, cardiac, and renal systems. Neurologic compromise may be manifested by mental confusion, stupor, seizures, coma, or stroke. Cardiac compromise may be exhibited by aortic dissection, myocardial ischemia, or dysrhythmias. Acute renal failure may not be evident immediately, but urine output, blood urea nitrogen (BUN), and serum creatinine values are evaluated over several days to determine whether the kidneys were affected by the hypertensive episode. When short-acting intravenous antihypertensive agents are administered, the blood pressure is closely monitored. If potent antihypertensive drugs such as sodium nitroprusside or labetalol are being used, an arterial line must be inserted and the drugs infused through an infusion pump.

Patient Education

Patient education during the acute phase is limited to an explanation of the need to control blood pressure and the purpose of the equipment used in the critical care unit. Once the hypertensive crisis is resolved, the focus of education is on life-style changes related to risk factor modification. Hypertension is emphasized as a risk factor for CAD, PVD, and cerebrovascular disease. The major points to discuss are listed in Box 16-38.

REFERENCES

1. Kelly DT: Our future society: a global challenge, *Circulation* 95(11): 2459-2464, 1997.
2. Teplitz L, Siwik DA: Cellular signals in atherosclerosis, *J Cardiovasc Nurs* 8(3):28-52, 1994.
3. Effat MA: Pathophysiology of ischemic heart disease: an overview, *AACN Clin Issues in Crit Care Nurs* 6(3):369-374, 1995.
4. Hunink MG and others: The recent decline in mortality from coronary heart disease, 1980-1990, *JAMA* 277(7): 535-542, 1997.
5. Tunstall-Pedoc H and others: Myocardial infarction and coronary deaths in the World Health Organization MONICA project: WHO Monica project, *Circulation* 90(1):583-612, 1994.
6. Njølstad I, Arnesen E, Lund-Larsen PG: Smoking, serum lipids, blood pressure, and sex differences in myocardial infarction: a 12 year follow-up of the Finnmark study, *Circulation* 93(3):450-456, 1996.
7. Expert Panel on Detection, Evaluation and Treatment of High Blood Cholesterol in Adults: *Summary of the second report of the National Cholesterol Education Program* (Adult treatment panel II), *JAMA* 269:3015-3022, 1993.
8. Dietary Guidelines For Healthy American Adults: A statement for health professionals from the Nutrition Committee, American Heart Association, *Circulation* 94(7):1795-1800, 1996.
9. Boushey CJ and others: A quantitative assessment of plasma homocystine as a risk factor for vascular disease, *JAMA* 274(13):1049-1057, 1995.
10. Nygård O and others: Total plasma homocystine and cardiovascular risk profile: the Hordaland Homocystine Study, *JAMA* 274:1526-1533, 1995.
11. Joint National Committee on Detection, Evaluation and Treatment of High Blood Pressure: The fifth report of the joint national committee on detection, evaluation and treatment of high blood pressure, *Arch Intern Med* 153:154-183, 1993.
12. Sytkowski PA and others: Secular trends in long-term sustained hypertension, long-term treatment, and cardiovascular mortality: the Framingham Heart Study 1950 to 1990, *Circulation* 93(4):697-703, 1996.
13. Stamler J and others: MRFIT 12 year follow-up: diabetes and mortality, *Diabetes Care* 16:434-444, 1993.
14. Kawachi I and others: Symptoms of anxiety and risk of coronary heart disease: the normative aging study, *Circulation* 90(5):2225-2229, 1994.
15. Allison TG: Identification and treatment of psychosocial risk factors for coronary artery disease, *Mayo Clin Proc* 71(1):817-819, 1996.
16. Fuster V and others: The pathogenesis of coronary artery disease and the acute coronary syndromes. II. *N Engl J Med* 326(5):310-318, 1992.
17. Fuster V and others: The pathogenesis of coronary artery disease and the acute coronary syndromes. I. *N Engl J Med* 326(4):242-250, 1992.
18. Fuster V: Elucidation of the role of plaque instability and rupture in acute coronary events, *Am J Cardiol* 76(9):24C-33C, 1995.
19. Fishbein MC, Siegel RJ: How big are coronary atherosclerotic plaques that rupture? *Circulation* 94(10):2662-2666, 1996
20. Waters D: Plaque stabilization: a mechanism for the beneficial effect of lipid-lowering therapies in angiography studies, *Prog Cardiovasc Dis* 27(3):107-120, 1994.
21. Superko HR, Krauss RM: Coronary artery disease regression: convincing evidence of the benefit of aggressive lipoprotein management, *Circulation* 90:1056-1069, 1994.
22. Lamarche B and others: Apolipoprotein A-I and B levels and risk of ischemic heart disease during a five-year follow-up of men in the Québec Cardiovascular Study, *Circulation* 94:273-278, 1996.
23. Braunwald E and others: *Unstable angina: diagnosis and management,* Clinical practice guideline No 10, AHCPR Publ No 94-0602, Rockville, Md, 1994, Agency for Health Care Policy and Research and the National Heart, Lung, and Blood Institute, Public Health Service, US Department of Health and Human Services.
24. Catherwood E, O'Rourke DJ: Critical pathway management of unstable angina, *Prog Cardiovasc Dis* 27(3):121-148, 1994.
25. Bankwala Z, Swenson LJ: Unstable angina pectoris: what is the likelihood of further cardiac events? *Postgrad Med* 98(6):155-158, 1995.
26. *St. Anthony's DRG guidebook,* Reston, Va, 1996, St. Anthony.
27. Cohn P: Silent ischemia. In Fuster V, Ross R, Topol EJ, editors: *Atherosclerosis and coronary artery disease,* vol 2, New York, 1996, Lippincott-Raven.
28. Pepine CJ: Prognostic implications of silent myocardial ischemia, *N Engl J Med* 334(2):113-114, 1996.
29. Pilote L and others: Regional variation across the United States in the management of acute myocardial infarction, *N Engl J Med* 333(9):565-572, 1995.
30. Ryan TJ and others: ACC/AHA guidelines for the management of patients with acute myocardial infarction: a report of the American College of Cardiology/American Heart Association Task Force on practice guidelines (Committee on Management of Acute Myocardial Infarction), *J Am Coll Cardiol* 28(5):1328-1428, 1996.
31. Hearns PA: Differentiating ischemia, injury, infarction: expanding the 12-lead electrocardiogram, *DCCN,* 13(4):172-183, 1994.
32. Riegel B and others: Are nurses still practicing coronary precautions? A national survey of nursing care of acute myocardial infarction patients, *Am J Crit Care* 5(2):91-98, 1996.
33. Wang WWT: The educational needs of myocardial infarction patients, *Prog Cardiovasc Nurs* 9(4):28-36, 1994.
34. Kuhn FE, Gersh BJ: Mechanical complications of acute myocardial infarction. In Fuster V, Ross R, Topol EJ, editors: *Atherosclerosis and coronary artery disease* vol 2, New York, 1996, Lippincott-Raven.
35. Van Dantzig JM and others: Pathogenesis of mitral regurgitation in acute myocardial infarction: importance of changes in left ventricular shape and regional function, *Am Heart J,* 131(5):865-871, 1996.

36. Becker RC and others: A composite view of cardiac wall rupture in the United States National Registry of Myocardial Infarction, *J Am Coll Cardiol* 27(6):1321-1326, 1996.
37. Pierce CD: Acute post-MI pericarditis, *J Cardiovasc Nurs* 6(4):46-56, 1992.
38. Antiplatelet Trialist's Collaboration: Collaborative overview of randomized trials of antiplatelet therapy: prevention of death, myocardial infarction and stroke by prolonged antiplatelet therapy in various categories of patients, *Br Med J* 308:81-106, 1994.
39. Schühlen H and others: Major benefit from antiplatelet therapy for patients at high risk for adverse cardiac events after coronary Palmaz-Schatz stent placement, *Circulation* 95:2015-2021, 1996.
40. Azar AJ and others: Optimal intensity of oral anticoagulant therapy after myocardial infarction, *J Am Coll Cardiol* 27(6):1349-1355, 1996.
41. Cairns JA and others: Antithrombotic agents in coronary artery disease, *Chest* 108(Suppl 4):380S-400S, 1995.
42. Steinke EE, Patterson P: Sexual counselling of MI patients, *J Cardiovasc Nurs* 10(1):81-87, 1995.
43. Sauve MJ and others: Patterns of cognitive recovery in sudden cardiac arrest survivors: the pilot study, *Heart Lung* 25(3):172-181, 1996.
44. Gilman JK, Sohail J, Narccarelli GV: Predicting and preventing sudden death from cardiac causes, *Circulation* 90:1083-1092, 1994.
45. Moss AJ and others: Improved survival with an implanted defibrillator in patients with coronary disease at high risk for ventricular arrhythmia, *New Engl J Med* 335(26):1933-1940, 1996.
46. Konstam M and others: *Heart failure: evaluation and care of patients with left-ventricular systolic dysfunction*, Clinical practice guideline No 11, AHCPR Publ No 94-0612, Rockville, Md, 1994, Agency for Health Care Policy and Research and the National Heart, Lung, and Blood Institute, Public Health Service, US Department of Health and Human Services.
47. Funk M: Epidemiology of heart failure, *Crit Care Nurs Clin North Am* 5(4):569-573, 1993.
48. Piano MR: Cellular and signaling mechanisms of cardiac hypertrophy, *J Cardiovasc Nurs* 8(4):1-26, 1994.
49. Elkayam U: Nitrates in the treatment of congestive heart failure, *Am J Cardiol* 77(13):41C-51C, 1996.
50. The SOLVD Investigators: Effect of enalapril on survival in patients with reduced left ventricular ejection fraction and congestive heart failure, *N Engl J Med* 325(5):293-302, 1991.
51. Schaefer KM, Polylycki MJS: Fatigue associated with congestive heart failure: use of Levine's Conservation model, *J Adv Nurs,* 18(2):260-268, 1993.
52. Whalen DA, Izzi G: Pharmacologic treatment of acute congestive heart failure resulting from left ventricular systolic and diastolic dysfunction, *Crit Care Nurs Clin North Am* 5(2):261-269, 1993.
53. Col NF and others: The impact of clinical trials on the use of medications for acute myocardial infarction, *Arch Intern Med,* 156:54-60, 1996.
54. Louie EK, Edwards LC: Hypertrophic cardiomyopathy, *Prog Cardiovasc Dis* 36(4):275-308, 1994.
55. Uszenski HJ and others: Hypertrophic cardiomyopathy: medical, surgical and nursing management, *J Cardiovasc Nurs* 7(2):13-22, 1993.
56. Chang AC, McAreavery D, Fananapazir L: Identification of patients with hypertrophic cardiomyopathy at high risk for sudden death, *Curr Opin Cardiol* 10(1):9-15, 1995.
57. Larsen L, Markham J, Haffajee CI: Sudden death in idiopathic dilated cardiomyopathy: role of ventricular arrhythmias. I. *Pacing Clin Electrophysiol* 16(5):1051-1059, 1995.
58. Dajac AS and others: Prevention of bacterial endocarditis: recommendations by the American Heart Association, *Circulation* 96(1):358-366, 1997.
59. Steckelberg JM, Wilson WR: Risk factors for infective endocarditis, *Infect Dis Clin North Am* 7(1):9-19, 1993.
60. Dajani A and others: Treatment of acute streptococcal pharyngitis and prevention of rheumatic fever: a statement for health professionals, *Pediatrics* 96(4):758-764, 1995.
61. Wolff M and others: Prosthetic valve endocarditis in the ICU, *Chest* 108(3):688-694, 1995.
62. Walter BF, Howard J, Fes S: Pathology of mitral valve stenosis and pure mitral regurgitation. I. *Clin Cardiol* 17(6):330-336, 1994.
63. Walter BF, Howard J, Fess S: Pathology of mitral valve stenosis and pure mitral regurgitation. II. *Clin Cardiol* 17(7):395-402, 1994.
64. Ling LH and others: Clinical outcome of mitral regurgitation due to flail leaflet, *N Engl J Med* 335(19):1417-1423, 1996.
65. Carabello BA: Indications for valve surgery in asymptomatic patients with aortic and mitral stenosis, *Chest* 108(6):1678-1682, 1995.
66. Klodas E and others: Surgery for aortic regurgitation in women: contrasting indications and outcomes compared with men, *Circulation* 94(10):2472-2478, 1996.
67. Walter BF, Howard J, Fess S: Pathology of tricuspid valve stenosis and pure tricuspid regurgitation. I. *Clin Cardiol* 18(2):97-102, 1995.
68. Walter BF, Howard J, Fess S: Pathology of tricuspid valve stenosis and pure tricuspid regurgitation. II. *Clin Cardiol* 18(3):167-174, 1995.
69. House-Fancher MA: Aortic dissection: pathophysiology, diagnosis, and acute care management, *AACN Clin Issues in Crit Care Nurs* 6(4):602-613, 1995.
70. Guilmet D and others: Aortic dissection: anatomic types and surgical approaches, *J Cardiovasc Surg* 34(1):23-32, 1993.
71. Weitz JI and others: Diagnosis and treatment of chronic arterial insufficiency of the lower extremities: a critical review, *Circulation* 94(11):3026-3049, 1996.
72. Dowdell HR: Diabetes and vascular disease: a common association, *AACN Clin Issues in Crit Care Nurs* 6(4):526-535, 1995.

73. Karch AM: Pain, pills and possibilities: drug therapy in peripheral vascular disease, *AACN Clin Issues in Crit Care Nurs* 6(4):614-630, 1995.
74. Poskus DB: Revascularization in peripheral vascular disease: stents, atherectomies, lasers and thrombolytics, *AACN Clin Issues in Crit Care Nurs* 6(4):536-546, 1995.
75. Calligaro KD and others: Impact of clinical pathways on hospital costs and early outcome after major vascular surgery, *J Vasc Surg* 22(6):649-660, 1996.
76. Cookingham A: Peripheral vascular disease: educational concerns for patients with a chronic disease in a changing health care environment, *AACN Clin Issues in Crit Care Nurs* 6(4):670-676, 1995.
77. Blakeley DD and others: Noninvasive carotid artery testing: a meta-analytic review, *Am J Intern Med* 122:360-367, 1995.
78. Brott T, Toole JF: Medical compared with surgical treatment of asymptomatic carotid artery stenosis, *Ann Intern Med,* 123(9):720-722, 1995.
79. Chervu A: Recurrent carotid artery stenosis: diagnosis, management, and prevention *Semin Vasc Surg* 8(1):70-76, 1995.
80. The European Carotid Surgery Trialist's Collaborative Group: Risk of stroke in the distribution of an asymptomatic carotid artery, *Lancet* 345:209-312, 1995.
81. Ecklund MM: Optimizing the flow of care for prevention and treatment of deep vein thrombosis and pulmonary embolism, *AACN Clin Issues in Crit Care Nurs* 6(4):588-601, 1995.
82. Ginsberg JS: Management of venous thromboembolism, *N Engl J Med* 335(24):1816-1821, 1996.
83. Hirsh J, Hoak J: Management of deep vein thrombosis and pulmonary embolism: a statement for healthcare professionals from the Council on Thrombosis (in consultation with the Council on Cardiovascular Radiology), American Heart Association, *Circulation* 93(12):2212-2235, 1996.
84. Porsche R: Hypertension: diagnosis, acute anti-hypertensive therapy, and long-term management, *AACN Clin Issues in Crit Care Nurs* 6(4):515-525, 1995
85. Ram CV: Immediate management of severe hypertension, *Cardiol Clin* 13(4):579-591, 1995.

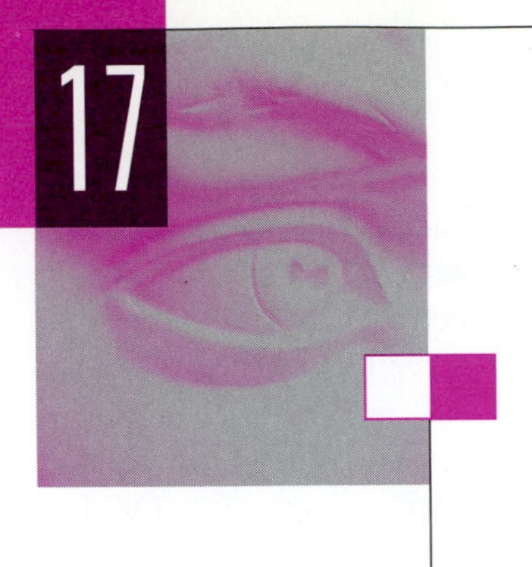

Cardiovascular Therapeutic Management

TEMPORARY PACEMAKERS

PACEMAKERS ARE ELECTRONIC devices that can be used to initiate the heartbeat when the heart's intrinsic electrical system is unable to effectively generate a rate adequate to support cardiac output. Pacemakers can be used temporarily, either supportively or prophylactically, until the condition responsible for the rate or conduction disturbance resolves. Pacemakers also can be used on a permanent basis if the patient's condition persists despite adequate therapy. The use of temporary pacemakers as a diagnostic tool is gaining popularity.

This section emphasizes temporary pacemakers, because the critical care nurse is responsible for preventing, assessing, and managing pacemaker malfunctions when these devices are used in the clinical setting. A brief discussion of permanent pacemakers is provided, and similarities between implanted and temporary pacemakers are presented, where appropriate.

Indications

The clinical indications for instituting temporary pacemaker therapy are similar regardless of the cause of the rhythm disturbance that necessitates the placement of a pacemaker (Box 17-1). Such causes range from drug toxicities and electrolyte imbalances to sequelae related to acute myocardial infarction or cardiac surgery. (∞AV Conduction Disturbances, p. 424.)

BOX 17-1 Indications for Temporary Pacing

- Bradydysrhythmias
  - Sinus bradycardia and arrest
  - Sick sinus syndrome
  - Heart blocks
- Tachydysrhymias
  - Supraventricular
  - Ventricular
- Permanent pacemaker failure
- Support cardiac output after cardiac surgery
- Diagnostic studies
  - Electrophysiology studies (EPS)
  - Atrial electrograms (AEG)

Therapeutic indications. Dysrhythmias that are unresponsive to drug therapy and result in compromised hemodynamic status are a definite indication for pacemaker therapy. The goal of therapy in the case of bradydysrhythmia is to increase the ventricular rate and thus enhance cardiac output. Alternately, "overdrive" pacing can be used to decrease the rate of a rapid supraventricular or ventricular rhythm. This rapid pacing of the heart, or overdrive pacing, functions either to prevent the "breakthrough" ectopy that can result from a slow rate or to "capture" an ectopic focus and allow the natural pacemaker to regain control.

Temporary pacing may be used in the treatment of symptomatic bradycardia or progressive heart block that occurs secondary to myocardial ischemia or drug toxicity. After cardiac surgery, temporary pacing can be used to improve a transiently depressed, rate-dependent cardiac output. In addition, conduction disturbances that can occur after valvular surgery can be managed effectively with temporary pacing.

Diagnostic indications. Several diagnostic uses for temporary pacing have evolved during the past several years. Electrophysiology studies (EPS) are now performed in cardiac catheterization laboratories equipped with specialized pacing equipment. During an electrophysiology study special pacing electrodes are used to diagnose the patient's potential for dysrhythmias.[1] These electrodes are used to induce dysrhythmias in patients with recurrent symptomatic tachydysrhythmias. This allows the physician to closely evaluate the particular dysrhythmia and to determine appropriate therapy. For those patients whose tachydysrhythmia is found to be refractory to conventional antidysrhythmic therapy, *radiofrequency (RF) current catheter ablation* of the responsible tissue can be done safely and effectively in the electrophysiology laboratory. After a mapping procedure localizes the site of dysrhythmia formation, short bursts of radiofrequency current are delivered through the catheter, destroying the offending tissue with heat. Radiofrequency ablation is more effective than its predecessor, direct current (DC) ablation, because it delivers a more precise localized ablation current that lowers the incidence of complications and does not require general anesthesia.[2,3]

The atrial electrogram (AEG) is simply an amplified recording of atrial activity that can be obtained through the use of atrial pacing wires and a standard electrocardiogram (ECG) machine. It often is used after cardiac surgery to facilitate the diagnosis of supraventricular dysrhythmias in patients with temporary atrial epicardial electrodes already in place.[4]

The Pacemaker System

A pacemaker system is a simple electrical circuit consisting of a pulse generator and a pacing lead (an insulated electrical wire) with either one or two electrodes.

Pacing pulse generator. The pulse generator is designed to generate an electrical current that travels through the pacing lead and exits through an electrode (exposed portion of the wire) that is in direct contact with the heart. This electrical current initiates a myocardial depolarization. The current then seeks to return by one of several ways to the pulse generator to complete the circuit.

The power source for a temporary external pulse generator is the standard 9-volt alkaline battery inserted into the generator. Implanted permanent pacemaker batteries are generally long-lived lithium cells.

Pacing lead systems. The pacing lead used for temporary pacing may be *bipolar* or *unipolar.* In a bipolar system, two electrodes (positive and negative) are located within the heart, whereas in a unipolar system only one electrode (negative) is in direct contact with the myocardium. In both unipolar and bipolar systems the current flows from the negative terminal of the pulse generator, down the pacing lead to the negative electrode, and into the heart. The current is then picked up by the positive electrode (*ground*) and flows back up the lead to the positive terminal of the pulse generator.

The bipolar lead used in transvenous pacing has two electrodes on one catheter (Figure 17-1, *D*). The distal, or negative, electrode is at the tip of the pacing lead and is in direct contact with the heart, usually inside the right atrium or ventricle. Approximately 1 cm from the negative electrode is a positive electrode. The negative electrode is attached to the negative terminal, and the positive electrode is attached to the positive terminal of the pulse generator, either directly or via a bridging cable (Figure 17-1).

An epicardial lead system is frequently used for temporary pacing after cardiac surgery. The bipolar epicardial lead system has two separate insulated wires (one negative and one positive electrode) that are loosely secured with sutures to the cardiac chamber to be paced. Both leads are in contact with the myocardial tissue, so either wire may be used as the negative, or pacing, electrode. The remaining wire is then used as the positive, or ground, electrode.

A unipolar pacing system (epicardial or transvenous) has only one electrode (the negative electrode) making contact with the heart. In the case of a permanent pacemaker, the positive electrode can be created by the metallic casing of the subcutaneously implanted pulse generator (Figure 17-2). Or as is the case with a unipolar epicardial lead system, the positive electrode can be formed by a piece of surgical steel wire sewn into the subcutaneous tissue of the chest or the metal portion of a surface ECG electrode.

There are advantages and disadvantages to both systems. Because the unipolar pacing system has a wide sensing area as a result of the relatively large distance between the negative and positive electrodes, it has better sensing capabilities than does a bipolar system. This feature, however, makes the unipolar system more susceptible to sensing extraneous signals, such as the electrical artifact created by normal muscle movements (myopotentials) or external electromagnetic interference (EMI), that may result in inappropriate inhibition of the pacing stimulus. This problem is generally of more concern in permanent pacing systems, in which the "can" of the pacemaker generator may be used as a part of the pacing circuit. Because the "can" is located near a large muscle mass, upper body movement can result in the inappropriate sensing of myopotentials.[5]

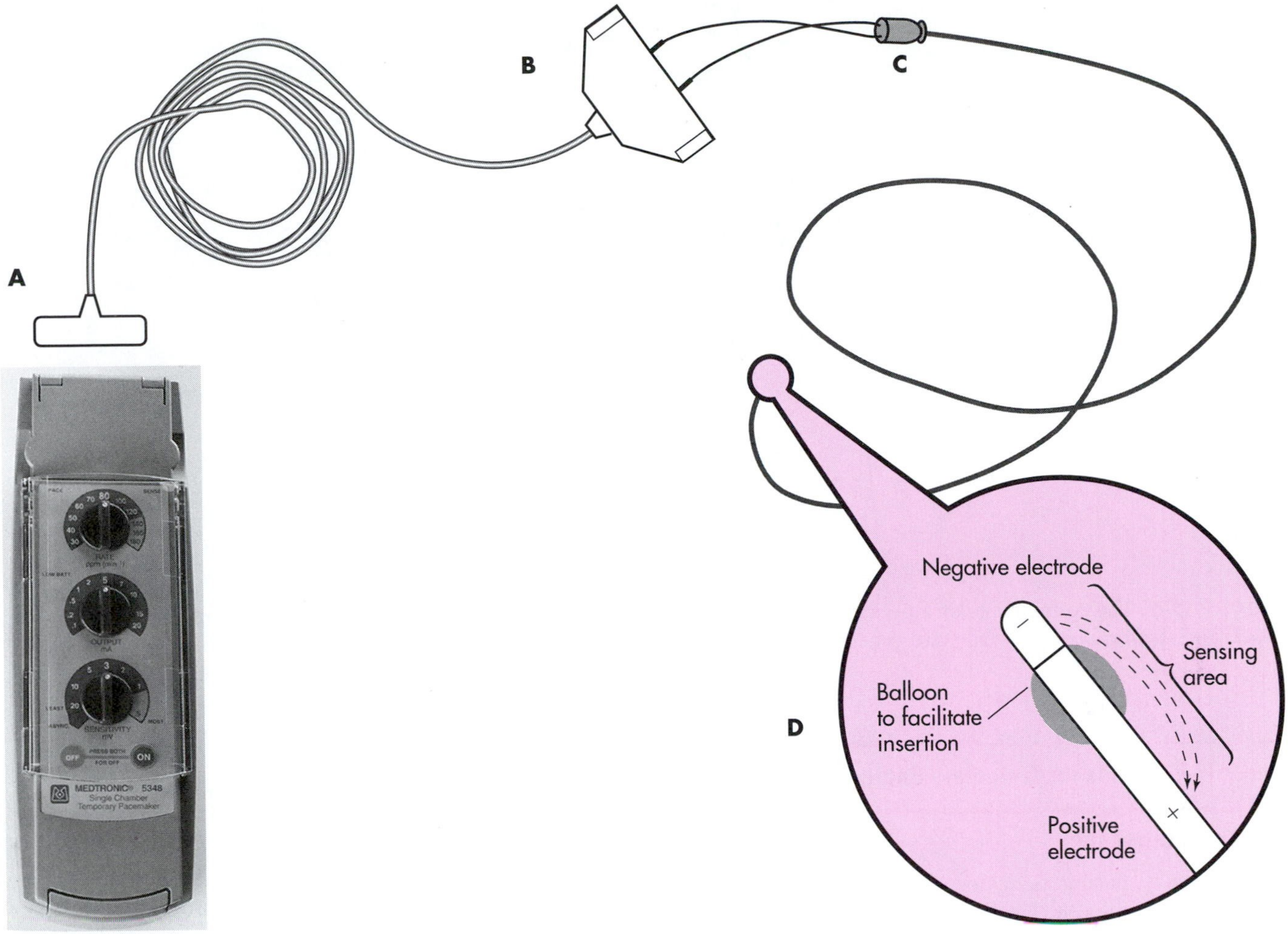

FIGURE 17-1. The components of a temporary bipolar transvenous system. A, Single-chamber temporary (external) pulse generator. B, Bridging cable. C, Pacing lead. D, Enlarged view of the pacing lead tip.

Pacing Routes

Several routes are available for temporary cardiac pacing (Box 17-2). Permanent pacing usually is accomplished transvenously; although in situations in which a thoracotomy is otherwise indicated, such as cardiac surgery, the physician may elect to insert permanent epicardial pacing wires.

Transcutaneous cardiac pacing involves the use of two large skin electrodes, one placed anteriorly and the other posteriorly on the chest, connected to an external pulse generator. It is a rapid, noninvasive procedure that nurses can perform in the emergency setting and is recommended as a primary intervention in the Advanced Cardiac Life Support (ACLS) algorithm for the treatment of bradycardia.[6] Improved technology related to stimulus delivery and the development of large electrode pads that help disperse the energy have helped reduce the pain associated with cutaneous nerve and muscle stimulation.[5] Discomfort may still be an issue in some patients, particularly when higher energy levels are required to achieve capture. This route is generally used as a short-term therapy until the situation resolves or another route of pacing can be established. (See ACLS algorithms in Appendix C.)

The insertion of temporary epicardial pacing wires has become a routine procedure during most cardiac surgical cases. Ventricular, and in many cases atrial, pacing wires are loosely sewn to the epicardium. The terminal pins of these wires are pulled through the skin before the chest is closed. If both chambers have pacing wires attached, the atrial wires exit subcostally to the right of the sternum and the ventricular wires exit in the same region but to the left of the sternum.[7] These wires can be removed several days after surgery by gentle traction at the skin surface with minimal risk of bleeding.

Temporary transvenous endocardial pacing is accomplished by advancing a pacing electrode wire

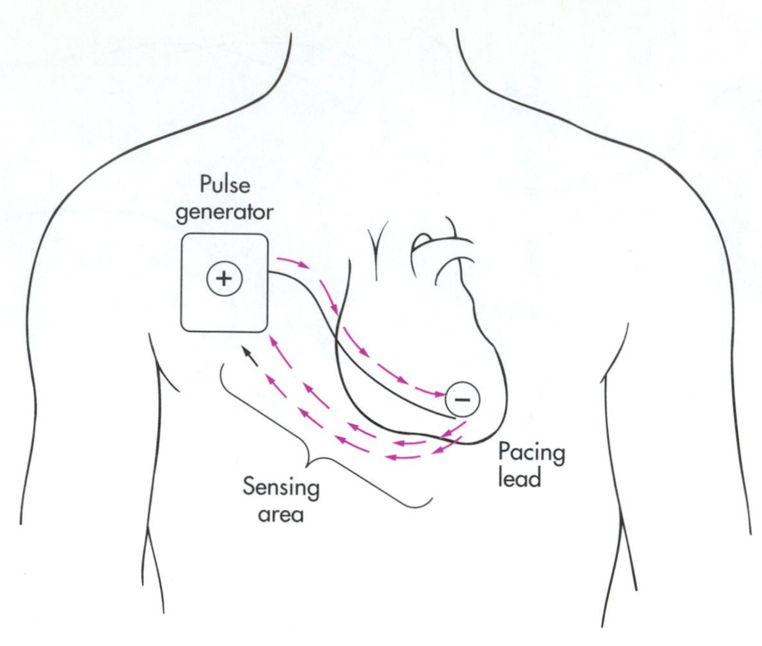

FIGURE 17-2. The components of a permanent unipolar transvenous pacing system. The pacing lead contains the negative electrode, and the metal case of the pulse generator acts as the positive terminal.

BOX 17-2 Routes for Temporary Pacing

TRANSCUTANEOUS

Emergency pacing is achieved by depolarizing the heart through the chest by means of two large skin electrodes.

TRANSTHORACIC

A pacing wire is inserted emergently by threading it through a transthoracic needle into the right ventricle.

EPICARDIAL

Pacing electrodes are sewn to the epicardium during cardiac surgery.

TRANSVENOUS (ENDOCARDIAL)

The pacing electrode is advanced through a vein into the right atrium or right ventricle, or both.

through a vein, often the subclavian or internal jugular, and into the right atrium or right ventricle. Insertion can be facilitated either through direct visualization with fluoroscopy or by the use of the standard ECG. In some cases the pacing wire is inserted through a special pulmonary artery catheter via a port that exits in the right ventricle.

Five-Letter Pacemaker Codes

In the 1960s, pacemaker terminology was limited to "fixed-rate" and "demand" pacing, followed by the introduction of "AV sequential" pacing in the early 1970s. Although these terms are still useful today for understanding pacemaker function (Box 17-3), the continued expansion of functional capabilities of pulse generators made it necessary to develop a more precise classification system. Therefore in 1974 the Inter-Society Commission for Heart Disease (ICHD) adopted a three-letter code for describing the various pacing modalities available. The code has since undergone several revisions, including the addition of two more letters representing programming characteristics and antitachycardia functions, to accommodate the development of newer devices that are rate-responsive or that combine pacing and cardioversion/defibrillation capabilities (see Table 17-1 for a description of the five-letter code).[8] The original three-letter code, however, remains adequate to describe temporary pacemaker function.

The original code is based on three categories, each represented by a letter. The first letter refers to the cardiac chamber that is paced. The second letter designates which chamber is sensed, and the third letter indicates the pacemaker's response to the sensed event. These three letters are used to describe the mode of pacing. For example, a VVI pacemaker paces the ventricle when the pacemaker fails to sense an intrinsic

BOX 17-3 Pacemaker Terminology

FIXED-RATE (ASYNCHRONOUS)

Delivers a pacing stimulus at a set (fixed) rate regardless of the occurrence of spontaneous myocardial depolarizations; occurs in nonsensing modes

DEMAND (SYNCHRONOUS)

Delivers a pacing stimulus only when the heart's intrinsic pacemaker fails to function at a predetermined rate; the pacing stimulus is either inhibited or triggered by the sensing of intrinsic activity

ATRIOVENTRICULAR (AV) SEQUENTIAL (DUAL-CHAMBER)

Delivers a pacing stimulus to both the atrium and ventricle in physiologic sequence with sufficient AV delay to permit adequate ventricular filling

ventricular depolarization. Sensing of a spontaneous ventricular depolarization, however, inhibits ventricular pacing. On the other hand, a VOO pacemaker paces the ventricle at a fixed rate and has no sensing capabilities (see Table 17-2 for a description of temporary pacing modes).

Physiologic pacing modes are those in which the normal physiologic, or sequential, relationship between atrial and ventricular stimulation and contraction is maintained. Atrioventricular (AV) synchrony increases the volume in the ventricle before contraction and thus helps to improve cardiac output. This may be achieved with atrial pacing in patients who have an intact conduction system, where each atrial pacing stimuli depolarizes the atria and is then conducted through to the ventricles. When atrial-to-ventricular conduction is impaired (i.e., during heart block), AV synchrony may be maintained via dual-chamber (i.e, both atrial and ventricular) pacing modes. The newest of these is the DDD mode, which is sometimes referred to as the "universal mode" because of its flexibility.[9] In DDD pacing, atrial and ventricular leads are used for both pacing and sensing. In response to sensed activity the pacemaker inhibits the pacing stimulus so that a sensed P wave in the atria will inhibit the atrial spike and a sensed R wave in the ventricle will inhibit the ventricular pacing spike. In addition, a sensed P wave may also be used to "trigger" a ventricular pacing stimulus when normal conduction through the AV node is impaired. Although the DDD mode is more complicated to program and interpret than earlier modes, it offers the most options for maintaining physiologic pacing.

Pacemaker Settings

The controls on all external temporary pulse generators are similar, and their function must be thoroughly understood so that pacing can be initiated quickly in an emergency situation and troubleshooting can be facilitated should problems with the pacemaker arise.

The *rate control* (Figure 17-3) regulates the number of impulses that can be delivered to the heart per minute. The rate setting depends on the physiologic needs of the patient, but in general it is maintained between 60 and 80 beats per minute. Pacing rates for overdrive suppression of tachydysrhythmias may greatly exceed these values. Some generators have special controls for overdrive pacing that allow for rates of up to 800 stimuli per minute. If the pacemaker is operating in a dual-chamber mode, the ventricular rate control also regulates the atrial rate.

The *output dial* regulates the amount of electrical current (measured in milliamperes [mA]) that is delivered to the heart to initiate depolarization. The point at which depolarization occurs is termed *threshold* and is indicated by a myocardial response to the pacing stimulus (capture). Threshold can be determined by gradually decreasing the output setting until 1:1 capture is lost. The output setting is then slowly increased until 1:1 capture is reestablished; this threshold to pace is less than 1.0 mA with a properly positioned pacing electrode. The output, however, is set two to three times higher than threshold because thresholds tend to fluctuate over time. Separate output controls for both the atrium and the ventricle are used with a dual-chamber pulse generator.

The *sensitivity control* regulates the ability of the pacemaker to detect the heart's intrinsic electrical activity. Sensitivity is measured in millivolts (mV) and determines the size of the intracardiac signal that the generator will recognize. If the sensitivity is adjusted to its most sensitive setting—a setting of 1 mV—the pacemaker can respond even to low-amplitude electrical signals coming from the heart. On the other hand, turning the sensitivity to its least sensitive setting (adjusting the dial to a setting of 20 mV or to the area labeled *async*) will result in the inability of the pacemaker to sense *any* intrinsic electrical activity and cause the pacemaker to function at a fixed rate. A sense indicator (often a light) on the pulse generator signals each time intrinsic cardiac electrical activity is sensed.

TABLE 17-1 NASPE/BPEG Generic (NBG) Code

Position	I	II	III	IV	V
	Chamber(s) paced	Chamber(s) sensed	Response to sensing	Programmability	Antitachydysrhythmia function(s)
	0 = None A = Atrium	0 = None A = Atrium	0 = None T = Triggered	0 = None P = Simple programmability (rate, output, sensitivity)	0 = None P = Pacing (antitachydysrhythmia)
	V = Ventricle	V = Ventricle	I = Inhibited	M = Multiprogrammability	S = Shock
	D = Dual (A + V) S* = Single (A or V)	D = Dual (A + V) S = Single (A or V)	D = Dual (T + I)	C = Communicating R = Rate modulation (rate responsive)	D = Dual (P + S)

Modified from Bernstein AD and others: The NASPE/BPEG generic pacemaker code for antibradycardia and adaptive rate pacing and antitachyarrhythmia devices, PACE 10:794, 1987.
*Used by manufacturer only.
NOTE: Positions I through III are used exclusively for antibradydysrhythmia function.
NASPE, North American Society of Pacing and Electrophysiology; BPEG, British Pacing and Electrophysiology Group; NBG, North American British Generic.

TABLE 17-2 Examples of Temporary Pacing Modes

Pacing Mode	Description
FIXED RATE:	
AOO	Atrial pacing, no sensing
VOO	Ventricular pacing, no sensing
DOO	Atrial and ventricular pacing, no sensing
DEMAND:	
AAI	Atrial pacing, atrial sensing, inhibited response to sensed P waves
VVI	Ventricular pacing, ventricular sensing, inhibited response to sensed QRS complexes
DVI	Atrial and ventricular pacing, ventricular sensing; both atrial and ventricular pacing are inhibited if a spontaneous ventricular depolarization is sensed
UNIVERSAL:	
DDD	Both chambers are paced and sensed; inhibited response of the pacing stimuli to sensed events in their respective chamber; triggered response to sensed atrial activity to allow for rate-responsive ventricular pacing

A pulse generator may be designed to sense atrial or ventricular activity, or both (see Box 17-4 for the procedure for measuring sensitivity). The sensitivity is set at half the value of the sensitivity threshold, to ensure that all appropriate intrinsic cardiac signals are sensed. For example, if the measured sensitivity threshold is 3 mV, the generator is set at 1.5 mV. The pacemaker's sensing ability can be quickly evaluated by observing for a change in pacing rhythm in response to spontaneous depolarizations.

The *AV interval* control (available only on dual-chamber generators) regulates the time interval between the atrial and ventricular pacing stimuli. This interval is analogous to the PR interval that occurs in

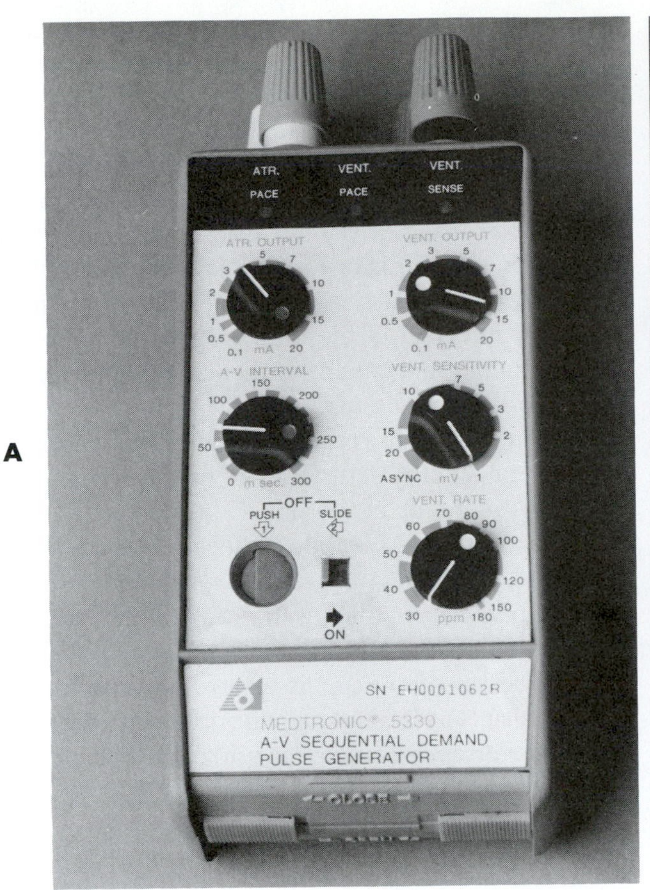

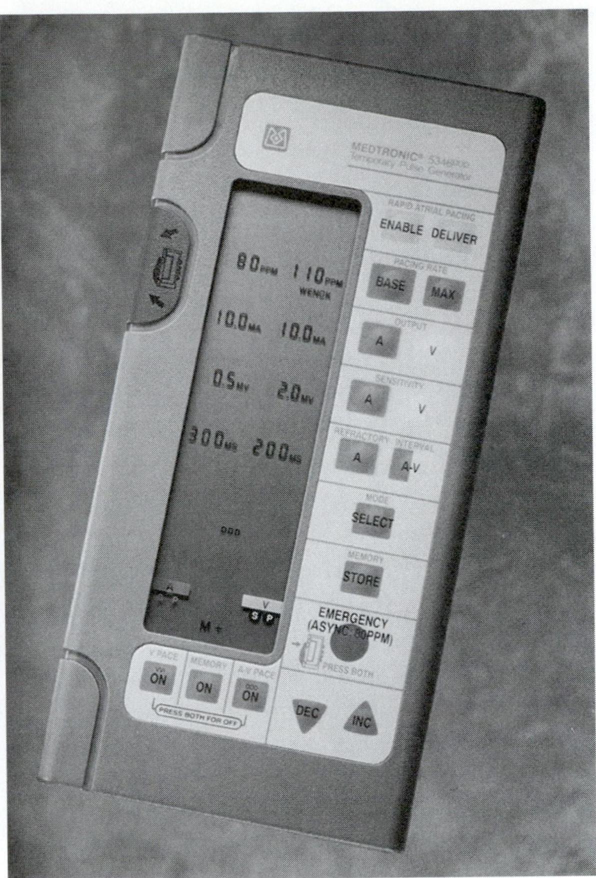

FIGURE 17-3. Temporary dual-chamber pulse generators (external). (An example of a temporary single-chamber pulse generator is shown in Figure 17-1.) **A,** An older model AV sequential demand pulse generator. **B,** A newer model DDD pulse generator. (Courtesy Medtronic Inc., Minneapolis.)

BOX 17-4 Temporary Pacemaker Sensitivity Thresholds

- Set the sensitivity control to its most sensitive setting
- Adjust the pulse generator rate to 10 beats/min less than the patient's intrinsic rate (the flash indicator should flash regularly)
- Reduce the generator output to the minimal value to prevent the risk of competing with the intrinsic rhythm
- Gradually increase the sensitivity value until the sense indicator stops flashing and the pace indicator starts flashing
- Decrease sensitivity until the sense indicator begins to flash again; this is the sensitivity threshold
- Adjust the sensitivity setting on the generator to half the threshold value; restore generator output and rate to their original values

the intrinsic ECG. Proper adjustment of this interval to between 150 to 250 msec preserves AV synchrony and permits maximal ventricular stroke volume and enhanced cardiac output.

Temporary DDD pacemakers have several other digital controls that are unique to this newer type of temporary pulse generator (Figure 17-3, *B*). The lower rate, or *base rate,* determines the rate at which the generator will pace when intrinsic activity falls below the set rate of the pacemaker. The *upper rate* determines the fastest ventricular rate the pacemaker will deliver in response to sensed atrial activity. This setting is needed to protect the patient's heart from being paced in response to rapid atrial dysrhythmias.[10] The *pulse width,* which can be adjusted from 0.05 to 2.0 msec, controls the length of time that the pacing stimulus is delivered to the heart. There also is an *atrial refractory period,* programmable from 150 to 500 msec, which regulates the length of time after either a sensed or paced ventricular event during which the pacemaker cannot respond to another atrial stimulus. An emergency button is also available on some models to allow for rapid initiation of asynchronous (DOO) pacing during an emergency.

Finally, on all temporary pacemakers, an *on/off* switch is provided with a safety feature that prevents the accidental termination of pacing.

Pacing Artifacts

All patients with temporary pacemakers require continuous ECG monitoring. The pacing artifact is the spike that is seen on the ECG tracing as the pacing stimulus is delivered to the heart. A *P wave* is visible after the pacing artifact if the atrium is being paced (Figure 17-4, *A*). Similarly, a QRS complex follows a ventricular pacing artifact (Figure 17-4, *B*). With dual-chamber pacing a pacing artifact precedes both the P wave and the QRS complex (Figure 17-4, *C*).

Not all paced beats look alike. For example, the artifact (spike) produced by a unipolar pacing electrode is larger than that produced by a bipolar lead (Figure 17-5). Furthermore, the QRS complex of paced beats appears different, depending on the location of the pacing electrode. If the pacing electrode is positioned in the right ventricle, a left bundle branch block (LBBB) pattern is displayed on the ECG. On the other hand, a right bundle branch block (RBBB) pattern is visible if the pacing stimulus originates from the left ventricle.

Pacemaker Malfunctions

Most pacemaker malfunctions can be categorized as abnormalities of either pacing or sensing.

Problems with pacing can involve the failure of the pacemaker to deliver the pacing stimulus, a pacing stimulus that depolarizes the heart, or the correct number of pacing stimuli per minute.

Pacing abnormalities. Failure of the pacemaker to deliver the pacing stimulus results in the disappearance of the pacing artifact, even though the patient's intrinsic rate is less than the set rate on the pacer (Figure 17-6). This can occur either intermittently or continuously and can be attributed to failure of the pulse generator or its battery, a loose connection between the various components of the pacemaker system, broken lead wires, or stimulus inhibition as a result of EMI. Tightening connections, replacing the batteries or the pulse generator itself, or removing the source of EMI may restore pacemaker function.

If the pacing stimulus fires but fails to initiate a myocardial depolarization, a pacing artifact will be present but will not be followed by the expected P wave or QRS complex, depending on the chamber being paced (Figure 17-7). This "loss of capture" most often can be attributed either to displacement of the pacing electrode or to an increase in threshold (electrical stimulus necessary to elicit a myocardial depolarization) as a result of drugs, metabolic disorders, electrolyte imbalances, or fibrosis or myocardial ischemia at the site of electrode placement. In many cases, increasing the output (mA) may elicit capture. For transvenous leads, repositioning the patient to the left side may improve lead contact and restore capture.

Pacing also can occur at inappropriate rates. For example, impending battery failure in a permanent pacemaker can result in a gradual decrease in the paced rate, or "rate drift." Another phenomenon, commonly referred to as *runaway pacemaker,* results in the firing of the pacemaker stimulus at rates greater than the set rate. This malfunction, which is caused by failure of the pulse generator's circuitry, necessitates replacement.

Sensing abnormalities. Sensing abnormalities include both undersensing and oversensing. *Undersensing* is the inability of the pacemaker to sense spontaneous myocardial depolarizations. This results in competition between paced complexes and the heart's intrinsic rhythm. This malfunction can be demonstrated on the ECG by pacing artifacts that occur *after* or unrelated to spontaneous complexes (Figure 17-8). Undersensing can result in the delivery of pacing stimuli into a relative refractory period of the cardiac depolarization cycle. Ventricular pacing stimuli delivered into the downslope of the T wave (R-on-T phenomenon) is a real danger with this type of pacer aberration, since it may precipitate a lethal dysrhythmia. The nurse must act quickly to determine the cause and initiate appropriate interventions. Often the cause can be attributed to inadequate wave amplitude (or height of the P or R wave). If this is the case, the situation can be promptly remedied by increasing the sensitivity (moving the sensitivity dial toward its lowest setting). Other possible causes include inappropriate (i.e., asynchronous) mode selection, lead displacement or fracture, loose cable connections, and pulse generator failure.

Oversensing results from the inappropriate sensing of extraneous electrical signals, leading to unnecessary triggering or inhibiting of stimulus output, depending on the pacer mode. The source of these electrical signals can range from the presence of tall, peaked T waves to EMI in the critical care environment. Because most temporary pulse generators are programmed in demand modes, oversensing results in unexplained pauses in the ECG tracing as the extraneous signals

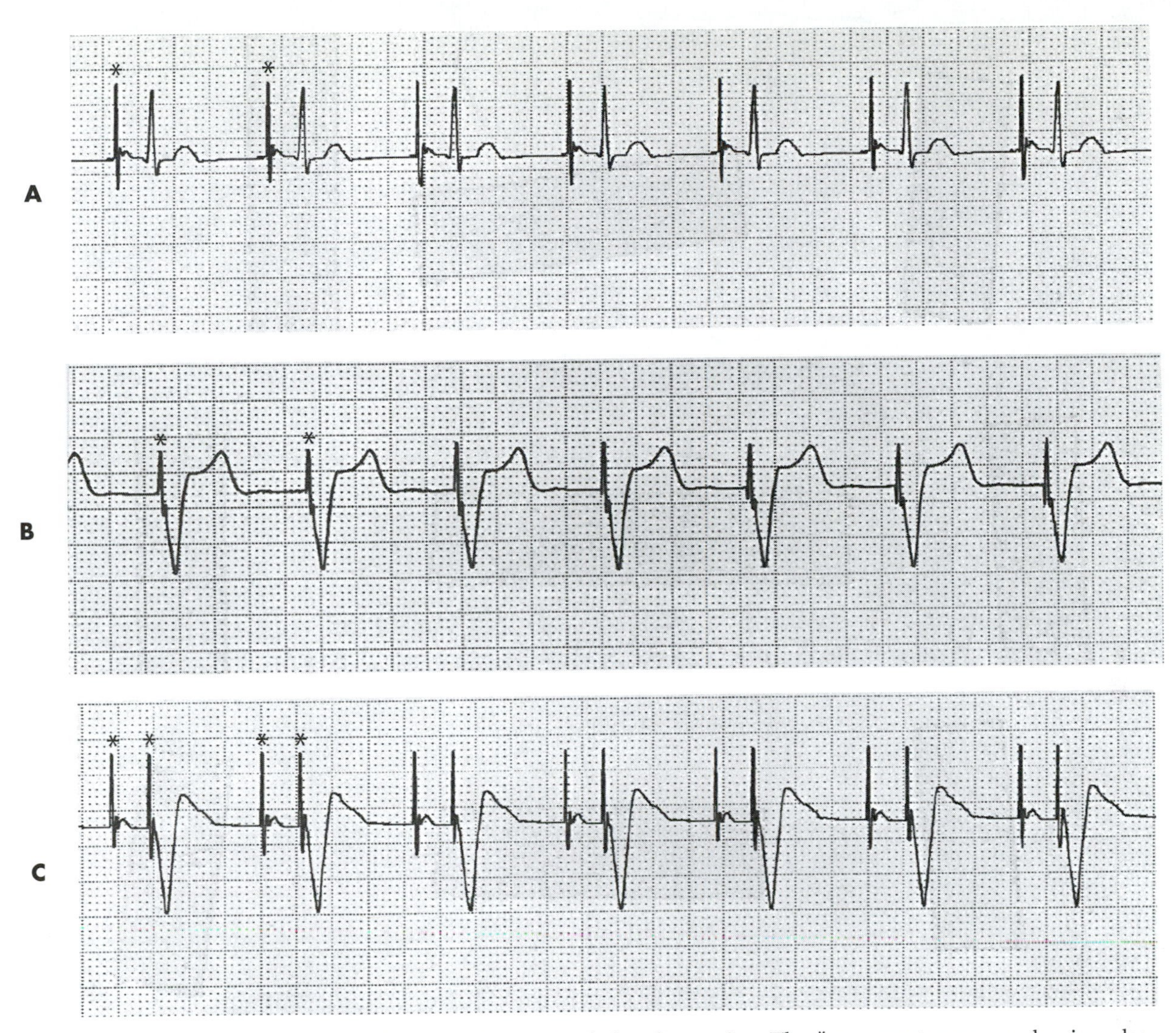

FIGURE 17-4. **A,** Atrial pacing. **B,** Ventricular pacing. **C,** Dual-chamber pacing. The * represents a pacemaker impulse.

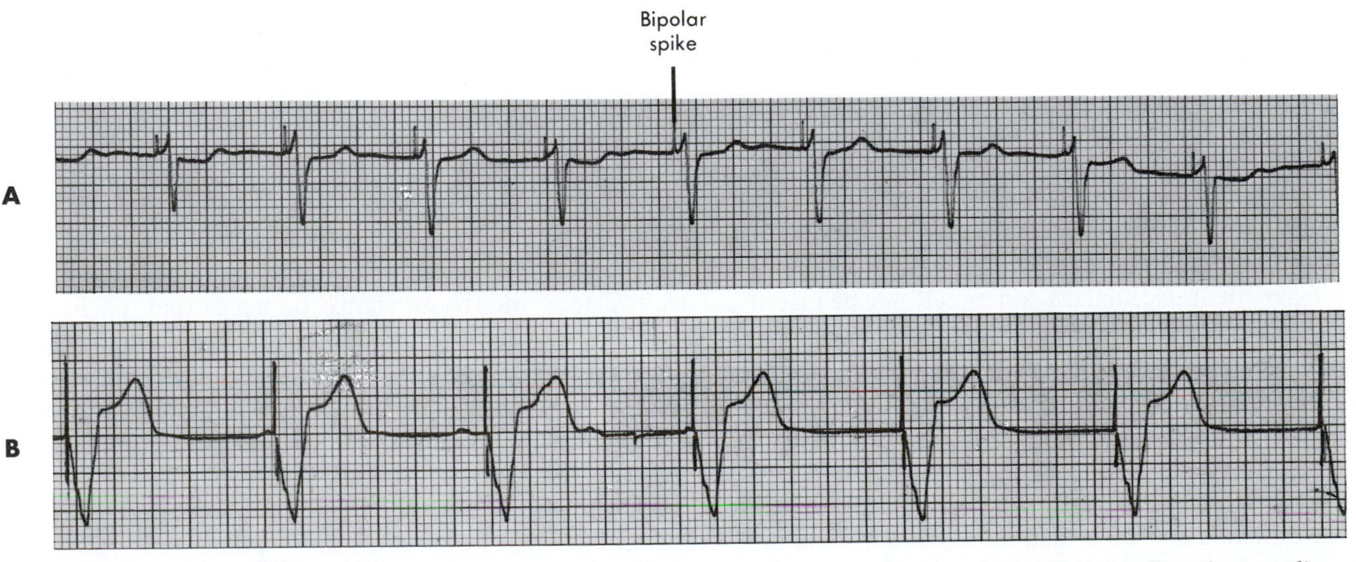

FIGURE 17-5. **A,** Bipolar pacing artifact. **B,** Unipolar pacing artifact. (From Conover MB: *Understanding electrocardiography: arrhythmias and the 12-lead ECG,* ed 6, St Louis, 1992, Mosby.)

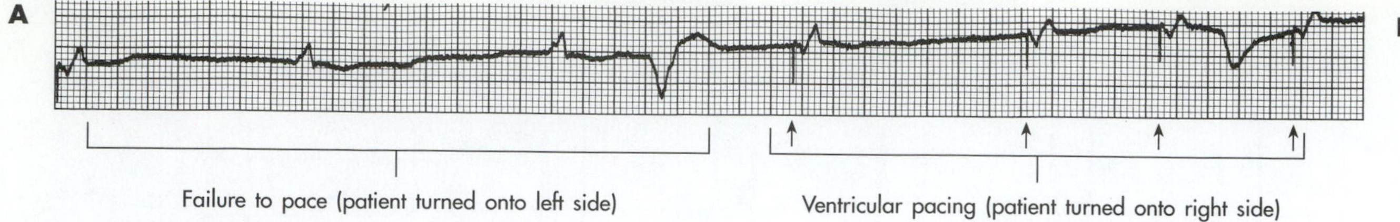

FIGURE 17-6. Pacemaker malfunction: failure to pace. **A,** Patient with a transvenous pacemaker is turned onto the left side. Immediately there is a failure to pace (loss of pacer artifacts on ECG). The patient's heart rate is extremely low without pacemaker support. **B,** The nurse turns the patient onto the right side, the transvenous electrode floats into contact with the right ventricular wall, and pacing is resumed. (From Kesten KS, Norton CK: *Pacemakers: patient care, troubleshooting, rhythm analysis,* Baltimore, 1985, Resource Applications, Inc.)

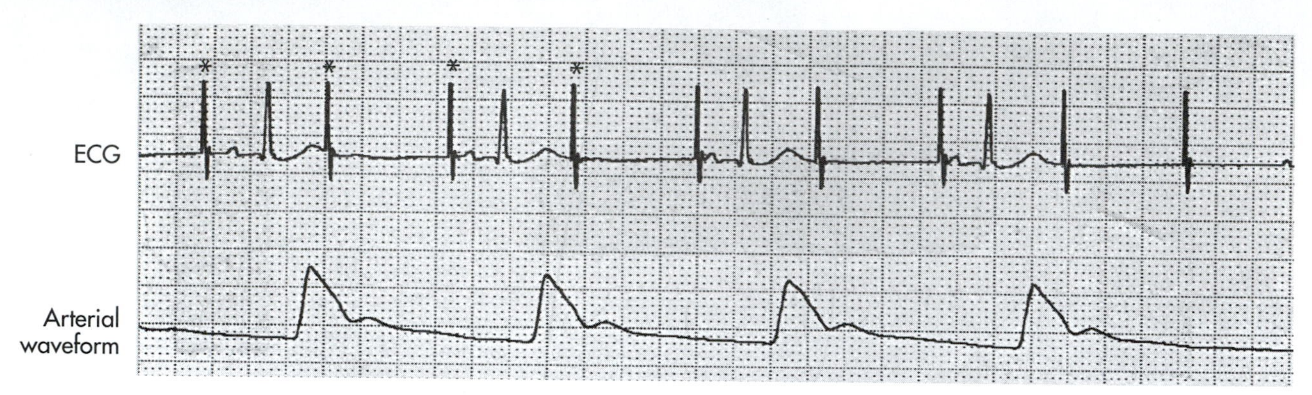

FIGURE 17-7. Pacemaker malfunction: failure to capture. Atrial pacing and capture occur after pacer spikes(s) 1, 3, 5, and 7. The remaining pacer spikes fail to capture the tissue, resulting in loss of the P wave, no conduction to the ventricles, and no arterial waveform. The * represents a pacemaker impulse.

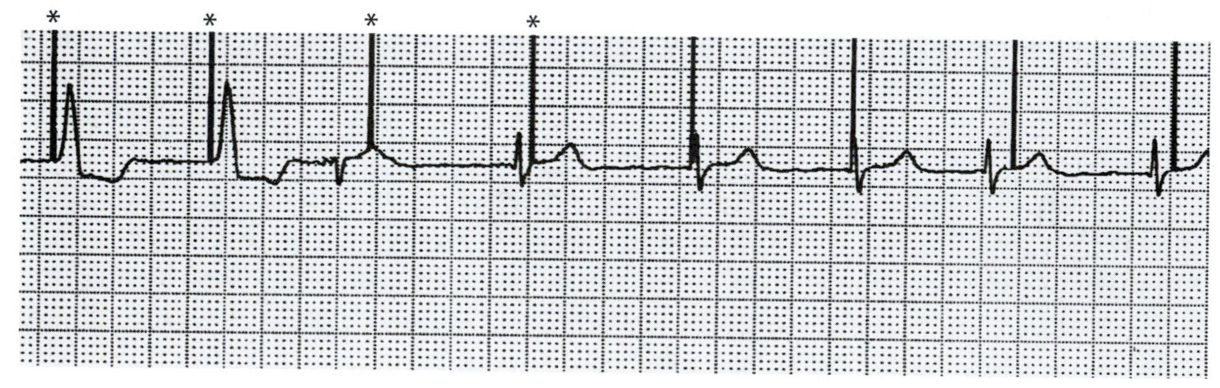

FIGURE 17-8. Pacemaker malfunction: undersensing. Notice that after the first two paced beats there is a series of intrinsic beats. Failure of the pacemaker unit to sense these intrinsic QRS complexes leads to inappropriate pacemaker spikes(s), which fall on top of or after the intrinsic QRS complexes. These spikes do not capture the ventricle because they occur during the refractory period of the cardiac cycle. The * represents a pacemaker impulse.

are sensed and inhibit pacing. Often, simply moving the sensitivity dial toward 20 mV stops the pauses. With permanent pacemakers, a magnet may be placed over the generator to restore pacing in an asynchronous mode until appropriate changes in the generator settings can be programmed.

Medical Management

The physician determines the pacing route, based on the patient's clinical situation. Generally transcutaneous pacing is used in emergent situations, until a transvenous lead can be secured. If the patient is undergoing heart surgery, epicardial leads may be electively placed at the end of the operation. The physician places the transvenous or epicardial pacing lead(s), repositioning as needed to obtain adequate pacing and sensing thresholds. Decisions regarding lead placement may later limit the pacing modes available to the clinician. For example, to perform dual-chamber pacing, both atrial and ventricular leads must be placed. In emergent situations, however, interventions are focused on establishing ventricular pacing, and atrial lead placement may not be feasible. After lead placement, the initial settings for output and sensitivity are determined, the pacing rate and mode are selected, and the patient's response to pacing is evaluated.

Nursing Management

Nursing responsibilities associated with the care of a patient with a temporary pacemaker are associated with several nursing diagnoses (Box 17-5) and can be combined into four primary areas: assessment and prevention of pacemaker malfunction, protection against microshock, surveillance for complications such as infection, and patient education.

Prevention of pacemaker malfunction. Continuous ECG monitoring is essential to facilitate prompt recognition of and appropriate intervention for pacemaker malfunction. In addition, proper care of the pacing system can do a great deal to prevent pacing abnormalities.

The temporary pacing lead and bridging cable must be properly secured to the body with tape to prevent the accidental displacement of the electrode, which can result in failure to pace or sense. The external pulse generator can be secured to the patient's waist with a strap or placed in a telemetry bag for the mobile patient. For the patient on a regimen of bedrest, the pulse generator can be suspended with twill tape from an intravenous (IV) pole mounted overhead on the ceiling, which not only will prevent tension on the lead while the patient is moved (given adequate length of bridging cable) but also will alleviate the possibility of accidental dropping of the pulse generator.

The nurse inspects for loose connections between the lead(s) and pulse generator on a regular basis. In addition, replacement batteries and pulse generators must always be available on the unit. Although the battery has an anticipated life span of 1 month, it probably is sound practice to change the battery if the pacemaker has been operating continually for several days. Newer generators provide a low battery signal 24 hours before complete loss of battery function to prevent inadvertent interruptions in pacing. The pulse generator must always be labeled with the date that the battery was replaced.

Microshock protection. It is important to be aware of all sources of EMI, which, within the critical care environment, could interfere with the pacemaker's function. Sources of EMI in the clinical area include electrocautery, defibrillation current, radiation therapy, magnetic resonance imaging devices, and transcutaneous electrical nerve stimulation (TENS) units. In most cases, if EMI is suspected of precipitating pacemaker malfunction, converting to the asynchronous mode (fixed rate) will maintain pacing until the cause of the EMI is removed.

BOX 17-5 NURSING DIAGNOSIS AND MANAGEMENT
TEMPORARY PACEMAKER

- Decreased Cardiac Output related to alterations in heart rate, p. 593
- Altered Myocardial Tissue Perfusion related to acute myocardial ischemia, p. 595
- Risk for Infection risk factor: invasive monitoring devices, p. 598
- Anxiety related to threat to biologic, psychologic, and/or social integrity p. 99
- Body Image Disturbance related to functional dependence on life sustaining technology, p. 86
- Knowledge Deficit: Discharge Regimen related to lack of previous exposure to information, p. 61 (see Patient Education Box 17-6)

Because the pacing electrode provides a direct, low-resistance path to the heart, the nurse takes special care while handling the external components of the pacing system to avoid conducting stray electrical current from other equipment. Even a small amount of stray current transmitted via the pacing lead could precipitate a lethal dysrhythmia. The possibility of "microshock" can be minimized by the wearing of rubber gloves when handling the pacing wires and by proper insulation of terminal pins of pacing wires when they are not in use. The latter can be accomplished either by using caps provided by the manufacturer or by improvising with a needle cover or section of disposable rubber glove. The wires are to be taped securely to the patient's chest to prevent accidental electrode displacement. Additional safety measures include using a nonelectric or a properly grounded electric bed, keeping all electrical equipment away from the bed, and permitting the use of only rechargeable electric razors.

Infection risk. Infection at the lead insertion site is a rare but serious complication associated with temporary pacemakers. The site(s) is carefully inspected for purulent drainage, erythema, and edema, and the patient is observed for signs of systemic infection. Site care is performed according to the institution's policy and procedure. Although most infections remain localized, endocarditis can occur in patients with endocardial pacing leads. A less common complication associated with transvenous pacing is myocardial perforation, which can result in rhythmic hiccoughs or cardiac tamponade.

Patient Education

Patient teaching for the person with a temporary pacemaker emphasizes prevention of complications (Box 17-6). The patient is instructed not to handle any exposed portion of the lead wire and to notify the nurse if the dressing over the insertion site becomes soiled, wet, or dislodged. The patient also is advised not to use any electrical devices brought in from home that could interfere with pacemaker functioning. Furthermore, patients with temporary transvenous pacemakers need to be taught to restrict movement of the affected extremity to prevent lead displacement.

BOX 17-6 PATIENT EDUCATION

TEMPORARY PACEMAKERS

- Description of pacemaker therapy
- Care of the pacemaker system:
  - Minimize handling of leads or cables
  - Notify nurse if dressing becomes wet or loose
- Activity restrictions (minimize upper extremity movement with transvenous leads)
- Electrical safety precautions (no electric razors)
- Symptoms to report (dizziness)

Permanent Pacemakers

About 110,000 permanent pacemakers are implanted annually in the United States, and critical care nurses are likely to encounter these devices in their clinical practice.[11] Originally designed to provide an adequate ventricular rate in patients with symptomatic bradycardia, the goal of pacemaker therapy today is to simulate, as much as possible, normal physiologic cardiac depolarization and conduction. Sophisticated generators now permit rate-responsive pacing, either in response to sensed atrial activity (DDD) or in response to a variety of physiologic sensors (body motion, blood temperature, and minute ventilation).[10] Table 17-3 describes the types of rate-responsive pacing generators currently in clinical use.

The patient who has a permanent pacemaker implanted is covered under two diagnosis-related groups: DRG 115 and 116, depending on the presence of complications. The anticipated length of stay ranges from 5.9 to 11.2 days. The longer length of stay is for patients with serious complications such as myocardial infarction or shock (DRG 115).[12]

Recent technologic advances in the computer industry have had a major impact on today's permanent pacemakers. Microprocessors have allowed for the development of increasingly smaller generators despite the incorporation of more complex features. Today's generators are not only smaller, but also more energy efficient and more reliable than previous models.[5] An example of a modern pacemaker is shown in Figure 17-9.

Medical Management

Permanent pacemakers may be implanted with the patient under local anesthesia in either the operating room or the cardiac catheterization laboratory. Generally, transvenous leads are inserted via the cephalic or subclavian vein and positioned in the right atrium and/or the right ventricle, under fluoroscopy. Satisfactory lead placement is determined by testing stimulation and sensitivity thresholds with a pacing system analyzer. The lead(s) is then attached to the generator, which is inserted into a surgically created "pocket" in the subcutaneous tissue below the clavicle.

Nursing Management

Nursing management for patients after permanent pacemaker implant includes monitoring for complications related to insertion, as well as for pacemaker malfunction. Postoperative complications are rare but include pneumothorax, hematoma, lead displacement, and infection.[13]

Identification of pacemaker malfunction is the same as that described previously for temporary pacemakers. To evaluate pacemaker function the nurse must minimally know the pacemaker's programmed mode of pacing and the lower rate setting. With permanent pacemakers, settings are adjusted noninvasively through a specialized programmer that uses pulsed magnetic fields or a radiofrequency signal. If a pacemaker problem is suspected, ECG strips are obtained and the physician notified so that the pacemaker settings can be reprogrammed as needed. If the patient experiences symptoms of decreased cardiac output, they may require support with temporary transcutaneous pacing until the problem is corrected.

The foregoing discussion has provided an introduction to the basic concepts of pacemaker therapy. It is essential, however, that the nurse who cares for patients with either permanent or temporary pacemakers be familiar with even the most sophisticated modes of pacemaker function. Only by keeping "pace" with current technology can the nurse accurately interpret pacer function and thereby safely and effectively care for patients with pacemakers.

TABLE 17-3 Permanent Pacemaker Rate-Responsive Pacing Modes

Pulse Generator	Description
AAIR	AAI features, plus rate-responsive pacing. It is used for patients with a symptomatic bradycardia with a paceable atrium and intact atrioventricular (AV) conduction.
VVIR	VVI features, plus rate-responsive pacing. It is used for patients with an unpaceable atrium caused by chronic atrial fibrillation or other atrial dysrhythmia.
DDDR	DDD features, plus rate-responsive pacing. It is used for patients with a symptomatic bradycardia in which the atrium is paceable but AV conduction is, or may become, unreliable.

Because these generators are rate-responsive (R), they can increase (modulate) heart rate in response to a sensed physiologic variable, usually upper body movement.

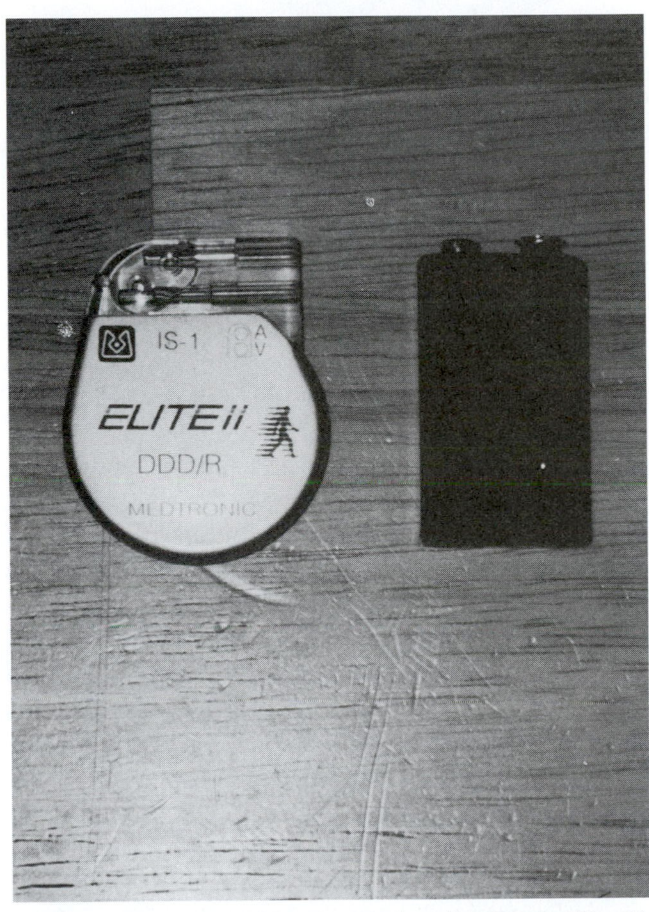

FIGURE 17-9. A permanent pacemaker (Medtronic Elite II) placed next to a 9-volt battery for comparison of size. This dual-chamber generator is 7.5 mm thick and weights only 26 g.

CARDIAC SURGERY

The nursing management of the patient undergoing cardiac surgery is demanding yet exciting work that requires the talents of an experienced team of critical care nurses. The following discussion introduces basic cardiac surgical techniques and principles of cardiopulmonary bypass and highlights the key points about postoperative care of the adult patient who requires either valve replacement or coronary artery revascularization.

Coronary Artery Bypass Surgery

Since its introduction more than 2 decades ago, coronary artery bypass surgery has been proved both safe and effective in relieving medically uncontrolled angina pectoris in most patients. With improved medical management of coronary artery disease (CAD), however, much debate has been generated regarding the efficacy of medical versus surgical therapy for CAD. (∞Coronary Artery Disease, Medical Management, p. 487; Catheter Interventions for Coronary Artery Disease, p. 552.)

The combined results of three major randomized trials continue to support the view that coronary artery bypass grafting (CABG) affords dramatic symptomatic improvement and an improved quality of life.[14] CABG is more effective than medical therapy for improving survival in patients with left main–vessel or triple-vessel disease or with double-vessel disease involving the left anterior descending artery (LAD), as well as for relieving exercise-induced ischemia or chronic ischemia leading to left ventricular (LV) dysfunction. Medical therapy is recommended when ischemia is prevented by antianginal drugs that are well-tolerated by the patient.[14]

Coronary artery bypass surgery is covered under two DRGs: DRG 106 and 107. The anticipated length of stay ranges from 9.8 to 12.7 days. The longer length of stay is for patients who undergo cardiac catheterization and CABG surgery (DRG 106).[12]

Myocardial revascularization involves the use of a conduit, or channel, designed to bypass an occluded coronary artery. Currently, the two most common conduits are the saphenous vein graft and the internal mammary artery (IMA). Saphenous vein graft (SVG) involves the anastomosis of an excised portion of the saphenous vein proximal to the aorta and distal to the

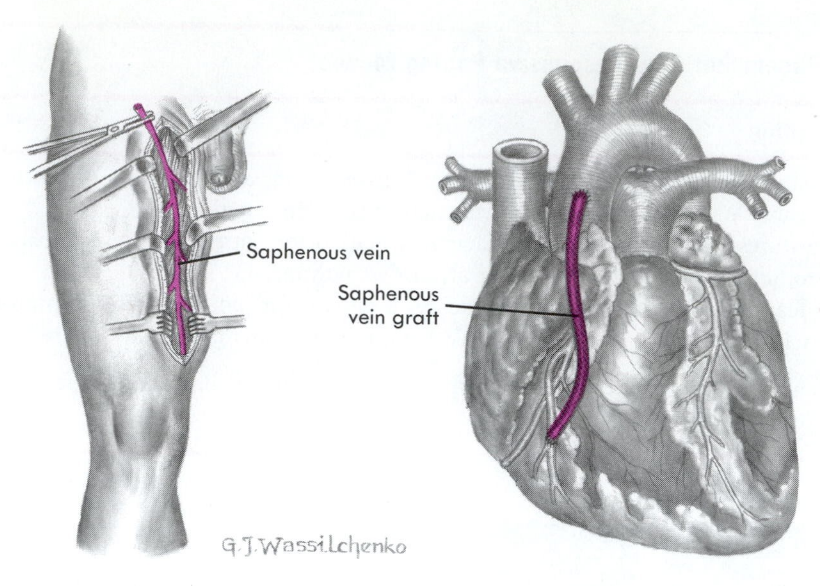

FIGURE 17-10. Saphenous vein graft.

coronary artery below the obstruction (Figure 17-10). The IMA, which usually remains attached to its origin at the subclavian artery, is swung down and anastomosed distal to the coronary artery (Figure 17-11).

Both the right IMA (RIMA) and the left IMA (LIMA) may be used as conduits. Of note, urgent coronary artery bypass surgery may preclude the use of the IMA because of the extra time required to mobilize the artery, as well as the inability to effect cardioplegia through this conduit. The current trend, however, is to use arterial conduits such as the IMA when possible, because their long-term patency rates are superior to those of the SVG.[15]

The right gastroepiploic artery (GEA) has recently been introduced as an alternate conduit for CABG. The GEA, which is a branch of the gastroduodenal artery, is pulled up to the pericardial cavity and anastomosed to a distal portion of the coronary artery (Figure 17-12). Although it is a little smaller in diameter than the IMA, studies indicate that patency rates are excellent.[16,17] Because of its size and anatomic location, the GEA is well-suited for bypassing the right coronary artery and the posterior descending artery.[18] The technical aspects of obtaining this conduit, however, may limit its widespread use.

The potential benefit of long-term patency associated with arterial conduits has recently led to revived interest in the use of radial artery (RA) grafts. First introduced as a potential conduit for myocardial revascularization in the 1970s, RA grafts were abandoned secondary to a high incidence of early graft occlusion and vasospasm. Current early patency rates of 90% or better have been attributed to improved harvesting techniques and the use of postoperative calcium channel blockers to minimize vasospasm.[19] A comparison of conduits used for myocardial revascularization is provided in Table 17-4.

Valvular Surgery

Valvular disease results in various hemodynamic dysfunctions that usually can be managed medically as long as the patient remains symptom free. There is reluctance to intervene surgically early in the course of this disease because of the surgical risks and long-term complications associated with prosthetic valve replacement. These consequences, however, must be weighed against the possibility of irreversible deterioration in left ventricular function that may develop during the compensated asymptomatic phase. (∞Valvular Heart Disease, p. 510.)

Surgical therapy for aortic valve disease is limited at this time to aortic valve replacement (AVR). Three surgical procedures, however, are available to treat mitral valve disease: commissurotomy, valve repair, and valve replacement. Commissurotomy is performed for mitral stenosis and involves incising fused leaflets and debriding calcium deposits to increase valve mobility. In the setting of mitral regurgitation, valve repair may be attempted, often with the use of a ring to reduce the size of the dilated mitral annulus, thus enhancing leaflet coaptation (annuloplasty). Both forms of valve reconstruction avoid the complications inherent with a prosthetic valve and may obviate the need for long-term anticoagulation.[20] If reconstruction of the mitral

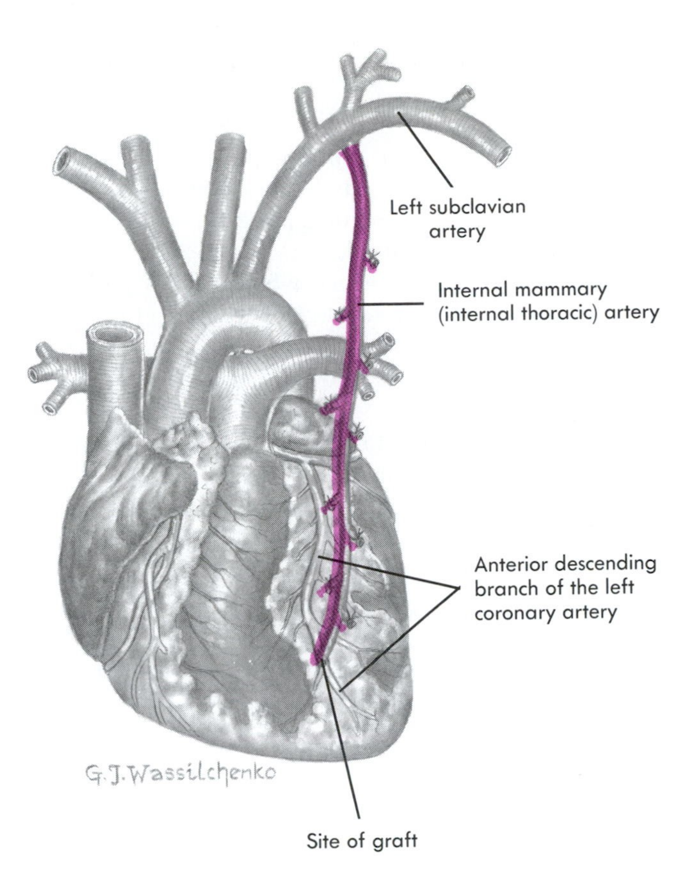

FIGURE 17-11. Internal mammary artery graft.

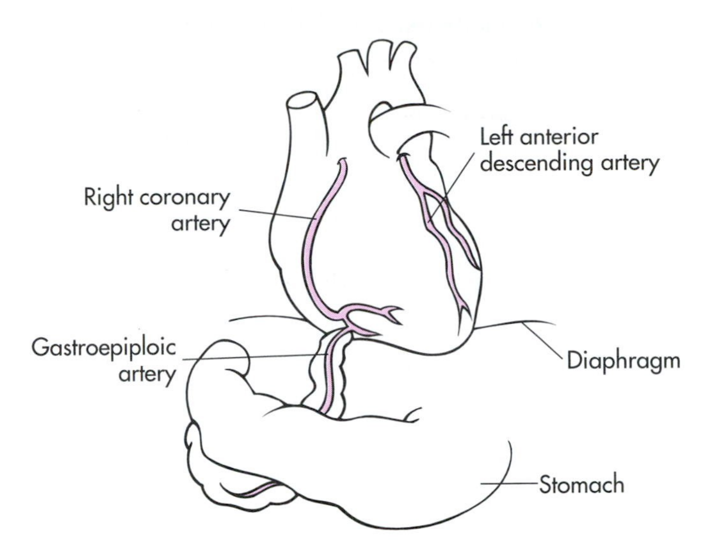

FIGURE 17-12. Gastroepiploic artery graft.

valve is not possible, it is replaced (mitral valve replacement [MVR]).

Valvular surgery is covered under two DRGs: DRG 104 and 105. The anticipated length of stay ranges from 12.0 to 16.0 days. The longer length of stay is for patients who undergo cardiac catheterization in addition to valvular surgery (DRG 104).[12]

There are two categories of prosthetic valves: mechanical and biologic, or tissue, valves. Mechanical valves are made from combinations of metal alloys, pyrolite carbon, Dacron, and Teflon (Figure 17-13). Their construction renders them highly durable, but all patients with mechanical valves require anticoagulation to reduce the incidence of thromboembolism. On the other hand, biologic, or tissue valves, because of their low thrombogenicity, offer the patient freedom from therapeutic anticoagulation. Their durability, however, is limited by their tendency toward early calcification (see Box 17-7 for a description of various valvular prostheses). Biologic valves are usually constructed from animal or human cardiac tissue.

The choice of a valvular prosthesis depends on many factors. Because mechanical valves are more durable, for example, they may be chosen over a tissue valve for a young person who is anticipated to have a relatively long life span ahead. Similarly, a bioprosthesis (tissue valve) may be chosen for an older patient (older than 65 years); even though the valve has a reduced longevity, the patient has a decreased life expectancy.[21] For patients with medical contraindications to anticoagulation or for patients whose past compliance with drug therapy has been questionable, a tissue valve is selected. Technical considerations, such as the size of the annulus (or anatomic ring in which the valve sits), also can influence the choice of valve (a bioprosthesis may be too big for a small aortic root).

Cardiopulmonary Bypass

Cardiopulmonary bypass (CPB) is a mechanical means of circulating and oxygenating a patient's blood while diverting most of the circulation from the heart and lungs during cardiac surgical procedures. The extracorporeal circuit consists of cannulas that drain off venous blood, an oxygenator that oxygenates the blood by one of several methods, and a pump head that pumps the arterialized blood back to the aorta through a single cannula. The patient is systemically heparinized before initiation of bypass to prevent clotting within the bypass circuit.

Systemic hypothermia during bypass can reduce tissue oxygen requirements to 50% of normal, which affords the major organs additional protection from ischemic injury. Lowering the body temperature to about 28° C (82.4° F) is accomplished through a heat exchanger incorporated into the pump. The blood is warmed back up to normal body temperature before bypass is discontinued.

TABLE 17-4 Conduits Used for Coronary Artery Bypass Grafts

Type of Graft	Advantages	Disadvantages
Saphenous vein	Easily harvested Length allows for multiple grafts No anatomic limitations to graft sites	Long-term patency is not as good as arterial grafts Requires at least two anastomosis sites Associated with leg edema postoperatively
Internal mammary artery	Improved patency over venous grafts Only requires one anastomosis	Requires extensive dissection Not accessible for emergency bypass Associated with increased chest-wall discomfort postoperatively Anatomic limitations to bypassing some areas of the heart
Gastroepiploic artery	Improved patency over venous grafts Only requires one anastomosis Associated with increased gastrointestinal complications postoperatively	Technically difficult to harvest Not accessible for emergency bypass Anatomic limitations to bypassing some areas of the heart
Radial artery	Suspected improved patency rates Easily harvested	Requires adequate collateral flow to hand via ulnar artery May be associated with higher rates of vasospasm Requires two anastomosis sites

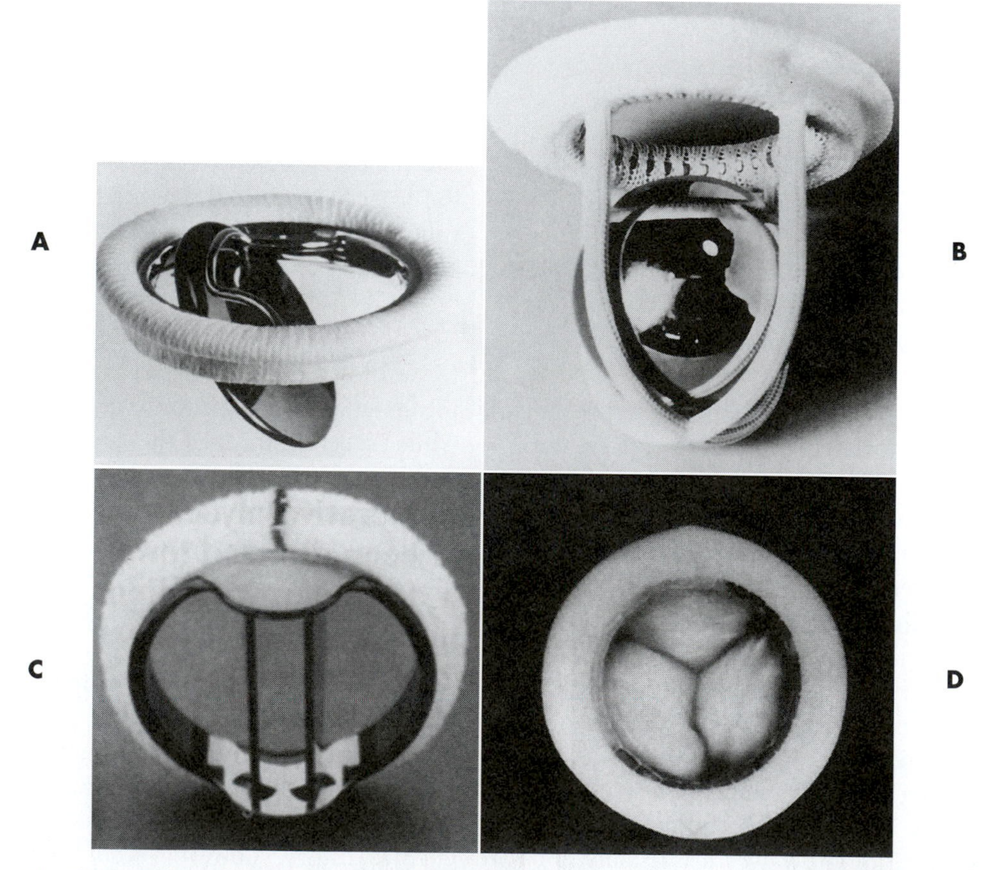

FIGURE 17-13. A, The Björk-Shiley tilting-disk valve with pyrolytic-carbon disk, Stellite cage, and Teflon cloth sewing ring. The valve opens to 60 degrees. **B,** The Starr-Edwards caged-ball valve model 6320 with completely cloth-covered Stellite cage and hollow Stellite ball, with specific gravity close to that of blood. **C,** The St. Jude Medical mechanical heart valve, a mechanical central flow disk. **D,** The Hancock II porcine aortic valve. The flexible Derlin stent and sewing ring are covered in Dacron cloth. (**A, B,** and **D** from Eagle K and others: *The practice of cardiology,* ed 2, Boston, 1989, Little, Brown; **C** courtesy St. Jude Medical, Inc, Copyright 1993, St Paul, Minn.)

BOX 17-7 Classification of Prosthetic Cardiac Valves

MECHANICAL VALVES

Tilting-disk: a free-floating, lens-shaped disk mounted on a circular sewing ring
- Björk-Shiley
- Omniscience (Lillehei-Kaster)
- Medtronic-Hall (Hall-Kaster)

Caged-ball: a ball moves freely within a three- or four-sided metallic cage mounted on a circular sewing ring
- Starr-Edwards

Bileaflet: two semicircular leaflets, mounted on a circular sewing ring, that open centrally
- St. Jude Medical

BIOLOGIC (TISSUE) VALVES (BIOPROSTHESES)

Porcine heterograft: a porcine aortic valve mounted on a semiflexible stent and preserved with glutaraldehyde
- Hancock
- Carpentier-Edwards

Bovine pericardial heterograft: bovine pericardium fashioned into three identical cusps that are then mounted on a cloth-covered frame
- Ionescu-Shiley

Homograft: a human heart valve (aortic or pulmonic) harvested from a donated heart and cryopreserved; may or may not be mounted on a support ring

The technique of hemodilution also is used to enhance tissue oxygenation by improving blood flow through the systemic and pulmonary microcirculation during bypass. *Hemodilution* refers to the dilution of autologous (patient's own) blood with the isotonic crystalloid solution used to prime the pump. Capillary perfusion is enhanced by hemodilution, because the reduced viscosity (stickiness) of the blood decreases both resistance to flow through the capillaries and the possibility of microthrombi formation. At the completion of CPB, the large quantities of "pump blood" that remain in the bypass circuit can be collected and used for initial postoperative volume replacement.

In response to findings that the low cardiac output syndrome often seen postoperatively might be a result of intraoperative myocardial ischemia or necrosis, efforts have been directed toward providing additional protection to the myocardium during bypass. Rapidly stopping the heart in diastole by perfusing the coronary arteries with a cold potassium cardioplegic ("heart-paralyzing") agent has been the method of choice for intraoperative myocardial protection. Continued research in this area has resulted in the emergence of blood as a vehicle for the cardioplegic components to enhance the supply of oxygen and nutrients to the arrested myocardial cells.[22] Warm (normothermic) cardioplegia is also being investigated and is believed by some to result in less ventricular dysfunction postoperatively.[23] Regardless of the type of cardioplegic solution used, it must be reinfused at regular intervals during bypass to keep the heart in an arrested state and to minimize myocardial oxygen requirements.

Numerous clinical sequelae can result from CPB (Table 17-5). Knowledge of these physiologic effects allows the nurse to anticipate problems and intervene effectively.

Postoperative Management

Medical and nursing management of the postoperative cardiac surgery patient are often overlapping. The physician prescribes therapeutic interventions and identifies specific hemodynamic endpoints that are individualized for each patient. The nurse is then responsible for applying these therapies to maintain the patient's hemodynamic parameters within the desired range. For example, orders may be written to maintain the patient's blood pressure, filling pressures, cardiac output, and systemic vascular resistance within a desired range, using a combination of volume, vasodilator, and inotropic infusions. In most institutions, standard protocols are used to facilitate the postoperative nursing diagnoses and management of cardiac surgical patients (Box 17-8).

Cardiovascular support. Postoperative cardiovascular support often is indicated because of a low output state resulting from preexisting heart disease, a prolonged CPB pump run, and/or inadequate myocardial protection. Cardiac output can be maximized by adjustments in heart rate, preload, afterload, and contractility.

Heart rate. In the presence of low cardiac output, the heart rate can be appropriately regulated by means of temporary pacing or drug therapy. Temporary epicardial pacing usually is instituted when the heart rate of the adult patient who has had cardiac surgery drops to less than 80 beats per minute. In the case of tachycardia, intravenous beta-blockers (esmolol) or calcium channel blockers (diltiazem) may be used to slow supraventricular rhythms with a ventricular response that exceeds 110 beats per minute. Because ventricular ectopy can result from hypokalemia, serum potas-

TABLE 17-5 Physiologic Effects of Cardiopulmonary Bypass (CPB)

Effects	Causes
Intravascular fluid deficit (hypotension)	Third spacing Postoperative diuresis Sudden vasodilation (drugs, rewarming)
Third spacing (weight gain, edema)	Decreased plasma protein concentration Increased capillary permeability
Myocardial depression (decreased cardiac output)	Hypothermia Increased systemic vascular resistance Prolonged CPB pump run Preexisting heart disease Inadequate myocardial protection
Coagulopathy (bleeding)	Systemic heparinization Mechanical trauma to platelets Depressed release of clotting factors from liver as a result of hypothermia
Pulmonary dysfunction (decreased lung mechanics and impaired gas exchange)	Decreased surfactant production Pulmonary microemboli Interstitial fluid accumulation in lungs
Hemolysis (hemoglobinuria)	Red blood cells damaged in pump circuit
Hyperglycemia (rise in serum glucose)	Decreased insulin release Stimulation of glycogenolysis
Hypokalemia (low serum potassium) and	Intracellular shifts during bypass
Hypomagnesemia (low serum magnesium)	Postoperative diuresis secondary to hemodilution
Neurologic dysfunction (decreased level of consciousness, motor/sensory deficits)	Inadequate cerebral perfusion Microemboli to brain (air, plaque fragments, fat globules)
Hypertension (transient rise in blood pressure)	Catecholamine release and systemic hypothermia causing vasoconstriction

sium levels are maintained in the high-normal range (4.5 to 5.0 mEq/L) to provide some margin for error. Maintaining serum magnesium in a therapeutic range (2.0 mEq/L) has also been shown to reduce the incidence of dysrhythmias in the postoperative period.[24,25]

BOX 17-8 NURSING DIAGNOSIS AND MANAGEMENT

STATUS POST OPEN HEART SURGERY

- Decreased Cardiac Output related to alterations in preload, p. 590
- Decreased Cardiac Output related to alterations in afterload, p. 592
- Decreased Cardiac Output related to alterations in contractility, p. 592
- Decreased Cardiac Output related to alterations in heart rate, p. 593
- Impaired Gas Exchange related to ventilation/perfusion mismatching or intrapulmonary shunting, p. 725
- Ineffective Airway Clearance related to excessive secretions of abnormal viscosity of mucus, p. 722
- Activity Intolerance related to cardiopulmonary dysfunction, p. 596
- Fluid Volume Deficit related to absolute loss, p. 914
- Risk for Infection risk factor: invasive monitoring devices, p. 598
- Acute Pain related to transmission and perception of cutaneous, visceral, muscular, or ischemic impulses, p. 197
- Anxiety related to threat to biologic, psychologic, and/or social integrity, p. 99
- Sleep Pattern Disturbance related to fragmented sleep, p. 118
- Knowledge Deficit: Discharge Regimen related to lack of previous exposure to information, p. 61 (see Patient Education Box 17-10)

Preload. In most patients, reduced preload is the cause of low postoperative cardiac output. If a pulmonary artery catheter has been inserted during surgery, monitoring pulmonary artery wedge pressure (PAWP) can provide a more convenient and accurate guide to left ventricular preload than can monitoring central venous pressure (CVP) alone. To enhance preload, volume may be administered in the form of crystalloid, colloid, or packed red cells. It is not uncommon to achieve the greatest hemodynamic stability in cardiac surgery patients when filling pressures (pulmonary artery diastolic or PAWP) are in the range of 18 to 20 mm Hg (normally 5 to 12 mm Hg).

Afterload. Partly as a result of the peripheral vasoconstrictive effects of hypothermia, many patients who have had cardiac surgery demonstrate postoperative hypertension. Although transient, postoperative hypertension can precipitate or exacerbate bleeding from the mediastinal chest tubes. In addition, the high systemic vascular resistance (afterload) resulting from the intense vasoconstriction can increase left ventricular workload. Therefore vasodilator therapy with intravenous sodium nitroprusside often is used to reduce afterload and thus control hypertension and improve cardiac output.

The use of warm cardioplegia may alter the traditional hemodynamic picture of postoperative cardiac surgery patients. These patients may have peripheral vasodilation, associated with hypotension and a low systemic vascular resistance. Therapy for these patients usually includes volume loading and vasopressors such as phenylephrine or dopamine to tighten the peripheral vasculature and maintain an adequate mean arterial pressure.[26]

Contractility. If these adjustments in heart rate, preload, and afterload fail to produce significant improvement in cardiac output, contractility can be enhanced with positive inotropic support or intraaortic balloon pumping (IABP), thus augmenting circulation. (∞IABP, p. 567; Inotropic Drugs, p. 577.)

Temperature regulation. Hypothermia can contribute to depressed myocardial contractility in the patient who has had cardiac surgery. To prevent subsequent excessive temperature elevations while hyperthermia blankets are used to warm the patient, care must be taken to remove the blankets promptly when the temperature reaches 98.4° F (36.9° C).

Control of bleeding. Postoperative bleeding from the mediastinal chest tubes can be caused by inadequate hemostasis, disruption of suture lines, or coagulopathy associated with CPB. Bleeding is more likely to occur with IMA grafts as a result of the extensive chest-wall dissection required to free the IMA. If bleeding in excess of 150 ml/hour occurs early in the postoperative period, clotting factors (fresh-frozen plasma and platelets) and additional protamine (used to reverse the effects of heparin) may be administered, along with prompt blood replacement.

In some institutions, autotransfusion devices, which facilitate the collection and reinfusion of shed mediastinal blood, may be used to replace red cell loss.[27] A number of chest drainage systems are configured for either intermittent or continuous autotransfusion. These systems contain a special reservoir section where blood is collected directly from the chest tubes (Figure 17-14). The accumulated blood is then passed through a microaggregate filter before reinfusion into the patient. Once bleeding slows and autotransfusion is no longer required, the chest tubes are connected directly to the chest tube drainage system (Box 17-9).

The use of prophylactic positive end-expiratory pressure (PEEP) in conjunction with mechanical ventilation may be helpful in controlling bleeding in some cases by increasing intrathoracic pressure enough to effect tamponade of oozing mediastinal blood vessels. Rewarming the patient reverses the depressed manufacture and release of clotting factors that result from hypothermia. Persistent mediastinal bleeding, however—usually in excess of 500 ml in 1 hour or 400 ml/hour for 2 consecutive hours despite normalization of clotting studies—is an indication for reexploration of the surgical site.

Chest tube patency. Chest tube stripping to maintain patency of the tubes is controversial because of the high negative pressure generated by routine methods of stripping. It is believed to result in tissue damage that can actually contribute to bleeding. This risk, however, must be carefully weighed against the very real danger of cardiac tamponade if blood is not effectively drained from around the heart. Therefore chest tube stripping frequently is advocated in instances of excessive postoperative bleeding. The technique of "milking" the chest tubes, however, may be advisable for routine postoperative care, because this technique generates less negative pressure and decreases the risk of bleeding.[28]

Pulmonary care. Until recently, overnight intubation to facilitate lung expansion and optimize gas exchange was common in patients who had cardiac surgery. Newer protocols that facilitate early extubation (within the first 4 to 8 hours) have now been implemented in many institutions.[29,30] Early extubation requires a multidisciplinary approach that incorporates anesthesiologists, surgeons, nurses, and respiratory therapists. Potential candidates must be identified preoperatively so that the anesthetic regimen can be modified to support early extubation. Generally, short-acting anesthetic agents such as propofol (Diprivan) are used at the end of the surgery, and narcotics are minimized. Postoperatively, patients are evaluated for hemodynamic stability, adequate control of bleeding, and normothermia. Once these criteria are met, the patient is weaned off propofol and ventilator weaning can begin. If needed, narcotics are given in small increments to manage pain and anxiety. Patients who exhibit hemodynamic instability or intraoperative complications or who have underlying pulmonary disease related to long-term valvular dysfunction may require longer periods of mechanical ventilation. After extubation, supplemental oxygen is administered, and patients are medicated for incisional pain to facilitate adequate coughing and deep breathing.

Neurologic complications. The transient neurologic dysfunction often seen in patients who have had cardiac surgery probably can be attributed to decreased

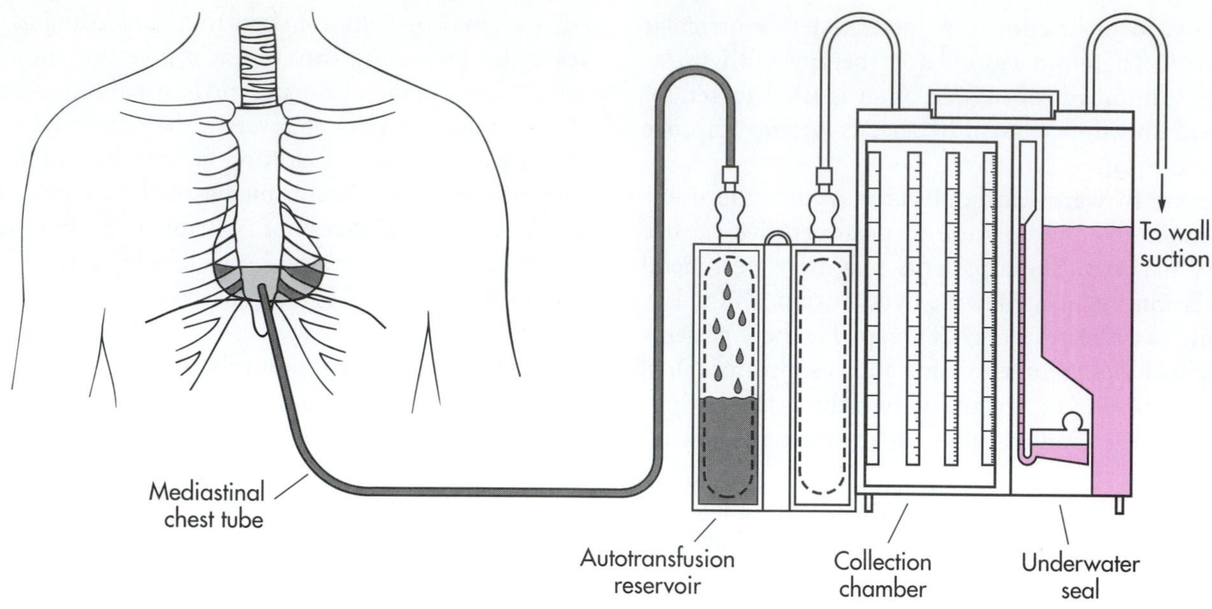

FIGURE 17-14. Components of an autotransfusion system.

NURSING INTERVENTION CLASSIFICATIONS

BOX 17-9 Autotransfusion

DEFINITION: Collecting and reinfusing blood which has been lost intraoperatively or postoperatively from clean wounds

ACTIVITIES:

Screen for appropriateness of salvage (contraindications include sepsis or infection or tumor at the site, blood containing an irrigant that is not injectable, hemostatic agents, or microcrystalline collagen)
Determine the risk/benefit ratio
Obtain patient's informed consent
Instruct patient regarding procedure
Use appropriate blood retrieval system
Label collection device with the patient's name, hospital number, date, and time that collection was begun
Monitor patient and system frequently during retrieval
Maintain integrity of the system before, during, and after blood retrieval
Screen blood for appropriateness of reinfusion
Maintain integrity of blood between salvage and reinfusion
Prepare blood for reinfusion
Document time of initiation of collecting, condition of blood, type and amount of anticoagulants, and retrieval volume
Reinfuse transfusion within 6 hr of retrieval
Maintain universal precautions

From McCloskey JC, Bulechek GM: *Nursing interventions classification,* ed 2, St Louis, 1996, Mosby.

cerebral perfusion and to cerebral microemboli, both related to the CPB pump run. Compounding these are environmental factors, such as sensory deprivation and sensory overload associated with being in a critical care unit. The term *postcardiotomy psychosis* has been used to describe this postoperative syndrome that initially may be seen as only a mild impairment of orientation but that may progress to agitation, hallucinations, and paranoid delusions.[31]

Patients and family members need to be reassured that postcardiotomy psychosis is a temporary phenomenon that will resolve quickly. Meanwhile, every effort must be made to keep the patient informed of all that is going on in the surroundings so that unfamiliar sights, sounds, and smells are not overwhelming and confusing. Painful stimuli are kept to a minimum, and meaningful stimuli, such as touching, is encouraged. Nursing management is organized to maximize optimal sleep patterns whenever possible. (∞Sleep Deprivation, p. 109.)

Infection. Postoperative fever is fairly common after CPB. However, persistent temperature elevation to more than 101° F (37.8° C) must be investigated. Sternal wound infections and infective endocarditis are the most devastating infectious complications, but leg wound infection, pneumonia, and urinary tract infection also can occur.[32]

Renal involvement. Hemolysis caused by trauma to the red blood cells in the extracorporeal circuit results in hemoglobinuria, which can damage renal tubules. Therefore small amounts of furosemide (Lasix) usually are given to promote urine flow if the urine output is low (less than 25 to 30 ml/hour) and "pink-tinged."

Patient Education

Patient education includes information related to the surgical procedure, as well as content related to risk factor management for the prevention of atherosclerosis. Patients who have undergone valve surgery may also require information regarding the need for antibiotic prophylaxis before invasive procedures, as well as specifics pertaining to their anticoagulation regimen (Box 17-10).

BOX 17-10 PATIENT EDUCATION

STATUS POST OPEN HEART SURGERY

- Pathophysiology of disease (either coronary artery or valvular disease)
- Risk factor modification to prevent CAD (smoking cessation, regular exercise, weight loss)
- Postoperative incisional care
- Activity limitations (no lifting, pushing, or pulling of anything >10 lb for 6-8 weeks; no driving for 6-8 weeks)
- Recommended exercise progression after surgery
- Recommended diet after surgery
- Information regarding prescribed medications (including prescribed pain medication)
- Anticipated mood changes after surgery
- Follow-up appointments for clinic or primary physician
- Additional information for valve patients:
  - Symptoms of endocarditis
  - Antibiotic prophylaxis before invasive procedures
  - Information regarding anticoagulant therapy and follow-up

Recent Advances

Surgical treatment of cardiac dysrhythmias. The increasing success of radiofrequency ablation has limited the use of surgery for intractable supraventricular and ventricular tachydysrhythmias. If catheter ablation of the dysrhythmia is not feasible or has proved ineffective, the patient may be evaluated for surgical treatment. During surgery the origin of the dysrhythmia first is localized with specialized pacing electrodes (referred to as *intraoperative mapping*). The offending area of myocardium is then either excised or eliminated by cryosurgery (freezing) or laser. This procedure is most successful in patients who have an organized type of tachydysrhythmia originating from a defined area, such as a scar or aneurysm.[33]

The *maze procedure* is a new surgical intervention for patients with atrial fibrillation or atrial flutter that has not responded to medical therapy.[34] A series of cuts are made in the atrial tissue to create an electrical maze that disrupts the reentrant pathways and directs the sinus impulse through the AV node.[35] The goal of treatment is not only to prevent the recurrence of atrial tachydysrhythmias, but to restore sinus rhythm and AV synchrony, if possible. If the sinus node is no longer functioning, a pacemaker may be implanted to restore an AV sequential rhythm. Initial success rates for this procedure have been promising, and research is now focused on the development of specialized ablation catheters to facilitate a nonsurgical version of the maze procedure.

Surgical treatment of cardiomyopathy. *Cardiomyoplasty* is an investigational alternative treatment to heart transplant for patients with ischemic or dilated cardiomyopathy. The patient's latissimus dorsi muscle is wrapped around the ventricle to augment ventricular function. The muscle is not stimulated for the first 2 weeks after surgery to allow time for adhesions to form between the muscle and the heart. Once the muscle has begun to adhere to the myocardium, the graft is stimulated to contract during cardiac systole by a special pacemaker (cardiostimulator).[36,37] Cardiomyoplasty is not a substitute for cardiac transplant, but it may be an option for patients who don't meet transplant criteria because of associated noncardiac diseases, age, or other reasons.[38]

Minimally invasive bypass surgery. An alternative method of revascularizing coronary arteries without the use of cardiopulmonary bypass is now being investigated by several researchers.[39,40] A small thoracotomy or laparotomy incision is made and a thoracope is introduced to allow the surgeon to visualize the vessels. The arterial conduit (LIMA, RIMA, or GEA) is harvested and attached to the myocardium without opening the sternum. Although the research is preliminary, this procedure may prove to be an option for patients who are unable to tolerate CPB.

Although future trends in the surgical management of cardiac disease are difficult to predict, the critical care nurse must continue to be prepared to meet the challenge of providing a high level of nursing management at the bedside. A solid knowledge base and keen assessment skills are prerequisites for the accurate anticipation of problems and prompt intervention necessary to stabilize the patient and prevent the occurrence of life-threatening complications.

IMPLANTABLE CARDIOVERTER DEFIBRILLATOR

If a ventricular tachydysrhythmia is not amenable to surgical or radiofrequency ablation or to antidysrhythmic drugs, an implantable cardioverter defibrillator (ICD) may be inserted. The ICD is capable of identifying and terminating life-threatening ventricular dysrhythmias. A recent clinical trial suggests that ICD therapy may be the preferred treatment for patients at increased risk for sudden cardiac death. Researchers found that patients who received an ICD had a decreased mortality when compared with those who received antidysrhythmic therapy with amiodarone.[41] (∞Sudden Cardiac Death, p. 501; Ventricular Tachycardia and Ventricular Fibrillation, p. 420.)

ICD System

The ICD system contains sensing electrodes to recognize the dysrhythmia and defibrillation electrodes or patches that are in contact with the heart and can deliver a "shock." These electrodes are connected to a generator that is surgically placed in the subcutaneous tissue in the upper left abdominal quadrant (Figure 17-15). The early model generators could defibrillate or cardiovert only lethal dysrhythmias. Recent improvements in ICD treatment include the use of "tiered" therapy generators that incorporate antitachycardia pacing, bradycardia back-up pacing, low-energy cardioversion, and high-energy defibrillation options. With tiered therapy, antitachycardia pacing is used as the first line of treatment in some cases of ventricular tachycardia (VT). If the VT can be pace-terminated successfully, the patient will not receive a "shock" from the generator and may not even realize that the ICD terminated the dysrhythmia. If programmed bursts of pacing do not terminate the VT, the ICD will "cardiovert" the rhythm. If the dysrhythmia deteriorates into ventricular fibrillation (VF), the ICD is programmed to defibrillate at a higher energy. If the dysrhythmia terminates spontaneously, the device will not discharge (Figure 17-15). Occasionally, the electrical rhythm may deteriorate to asystole or a slow idioventricular rhythm. In such cases the bradycardia back-up pacing function is activated.

ICD Insertion

The ICD has progressed not only in the area of programmable functions but also in the insertion design. Initially, all ICDs were implanted surgically either during open heart surgery, with electrode patches sewn directly onto the epicardium, or by means of a thoracotomy incision, with the electrode patches attached to the outside of the pericardium. Recently, several new devices have become available that obviate the need for a thoracic surgical intervention. Transvenous electrode leads are inserted into the subclavian vein and advanced into the right side of the heart where contact with the endocardium is achieved. To improve defibrillation efficacy, an additional subcutaneous patch may be placed with some models. The endocardial leads are used for sensing, pacing, and cardioversion/defibrillation. They are connected to the generator by tunneling through the subcutaneous tissue; thus thoracotomy is avoided. The endocardial lead system offers several advantages: it is less invasive, requires shorter hospitalization, and is associated with significantly lower implantation mortality.[42] Technical advances and the development of smaller ICDs have made it feasible to implant these devices in the pectoral position, similar to that used for permanent pacemakers.[43]

Medical Management

Medical management of the ICD patient begins before implantation, with a thorough evaluation of the patient's dysrhythmia and underlying cardiac function. A number of noninvasive studies are available to help identify patients at risk for sudden cardiac death (SCD). These include signal averaged electrocardiography, echocardiography, baroreceptor sensitivity testing, and heart rate variability studies. Generally, patients identified at risk for SCD undergo an electrophysiology study to identify the origin of the dysrhythmia and to determine the effect of antidysrhythmic agents in suppressing or altering the rate of the dysrhythmia. Further assessment of cardiac status is made to determine whether additional interventions (cardiac surgery, angioplasty)

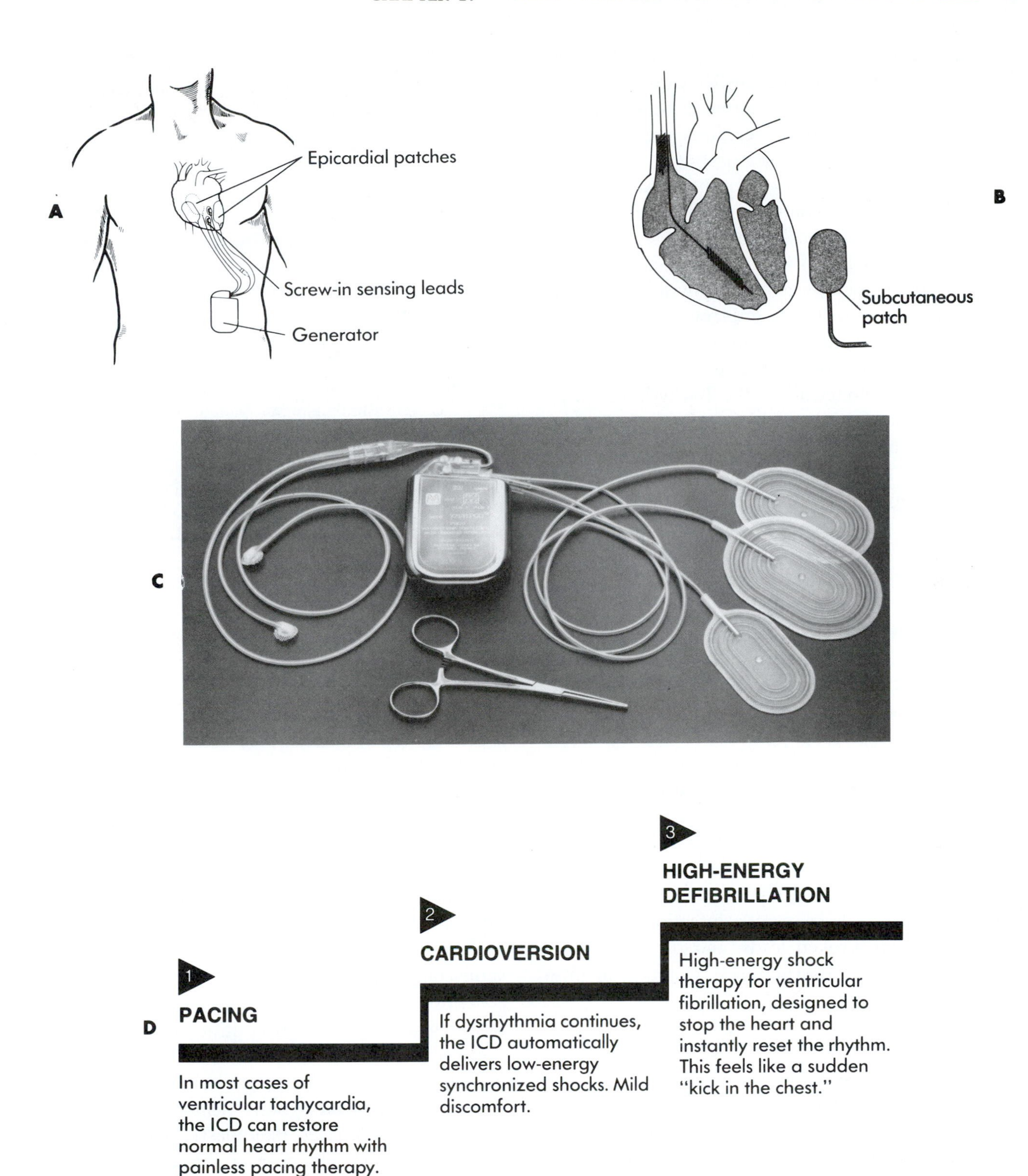

FIGURE 17-15. **A,** Placement of an implantable cardioverter defibrillator (ICD) and epicardial lead system. The generator is placed in a subcutaneous "pocket" in the left upper abdominal quadrant. The epicardial screw-in sensing leads monitor the heart rhythm and connect to the generator. If a life-threatening dysrhythmia is sensed, the generator can pace-terminate the dysrhythmia or deliver electrical cardioversion or defibrillation through the epicardial patches. With this system, the leads/patches must be placed during open-chest (sternal or thoracotomy) surgery. **B,** In the transvenous lead system, open-chest surgery is not required. The pacing/cardioversion/defibrillation functions are all contained in a lead (or leads) inserted into the right atrium and ventricle. A subcutaneous patch may be placed under the skin. **C,** An example of an ICD tiered therapy generator (Medtronic PCD) with epicardial screw-in sensing leads and patches. **D,** Tiered therapy is designed to use increasing levels of intensity to terminate ventricular dysrhythmias. (Courtesy Medtronic Inc., Minneapolis.)

are indicated to improve cardiac function. This part of the work up may include cardiac catheterization, stress testing, and echocardiography. Based on the aforementioned evaluation, decisions are made regarding the implantation approach (i.e., thoracotomy at the time of surgery or nonthoracotomy) as well as the type of therapy required (antitachypacing, cardioversion, defibrillation).

ICD programming. Initial programming of the device is generally performed by an electrophysiologist at the time of implantation. During implantation, defibrillation threshold measurements are obtained. This involves inducing the dysrhythmia and then evaluating the device's ability to terminate the dysrhythmia. Once it is determined that the ICD functions adequately, further follow-up is conducted on an outpatient basis to monitor the number of discharges and the battery life of the device.

Nursing Management

If the ICD system was implanted during open heart surgery, the postoperative nursing management is similar to that for any patient undergoing cardiac surgery. If an endocardial lead system is implanted, the nursing management is less intense and the hospital stay is shorter. The nursing diagnoses and management of the patient with an ICD are listed in Box 17-11. In the case of a ventricular dysrhythmia, it is important to know the type of ICD implanted, how the device functions, and whether it is activated (i.e., *on*). Most patients will continue to take some antidysrhythmic medications to decrease the number of "shocks" required.[44] Complications associated with the ICD include infection from the implanted system, broken leads, and the sensing of supraventricular tachydysrhythmias resulting in unneeded discharges.[45]

Patient Education

To facilitate a positive psychologic adjustment to the ICD, education of the patient and family about the device is vital (Box 17-12). Preoperative teaching for the ICD patient includes information about how the device works and what to expect during the implantation procedure. After implantation, education is focused on aspects of living with an ICD. Patients need information pertaining to scheduled device follow-up and instructions about what to do if they experience a "shock." Many institutions also have successfully used family support groups for this patient population.

BOX 17-11 NURSING DIAGNOSIS AND MANAGEMENT

IMPLANTABLE CARDIOVERTER DEFIBRILLATOR

- Decreased Cardiac Output related to alterations in heart rate, p. 593
- Altered Myocardial Tissue Perfusion related to acute myocardial ischemia, p. 595
- Activity Intolerance related to cardiopulmonary dysfunction, p. 596
- Acute Pain related to transmission and perception of cutaneous, visceral, muscular, or ischemic impulses, p. 197
- Body Image Disturbance related to actual change in body structure, function, or appearance, p. 87
- Ineffective Family Coping related to critically ill family member, p. 97
- Knowledge Deficit: Discharge Regimen related to lack of previous exposure to information, p. 61 (see Patient Education Box 17-12)

CATHETER INTERVENTIONS FOR CORONARY ARTERY DISEASE

During the last 2 decades there has been a growing trend toward catheter-based interventions for the treatment of coronary artery disease. Percutaneous transluminal coronary angioplasty (PTCA) was first introduced in 1977 as an alternative to coronary artery bypass surgery.[46] The advantages of PTCA included avoiding the risks involved with cardiac surgery (general anesthesia, thoracotomy, extracorporeal circulation, and mechanical ventilation) and significantly decreasing convalescence time. Disadvantages included acute complications related to the procedure itself, late restenosis, and difficulty in accessing certain lesions. Research in this area has continued, and a growing number of interventional devices have been developed to address the limitations of conventional angioplasty. Today catheter-based options include not only PTCA, but atherectomy; laser angioplasty; and stent placement, used either alone or in conjunction with angioplasty. Percutaneous catheter-based interventions are covered under DRG 112, with an anticipated length of stay of 5.0 days.[12]

Indications for Catheter-Based Interventions

Indications for catheter-based interventions have been considerably broadened since the initial application of balloon angioplasty (Box 17-13). Whereas once

BOX 17-12 PATIENT EDUCATION

POST IMPLANTABLE CARDIOVERTER DEFIBRILLATOR

- Pathophysiology of underlying disease process, including sudden cardiac death and ventricular dysrythmias
- Information regarding how the ICD is programmed to function
- Actions to take if a shock occurs
- Importance of continuing antidysrhythmic medications
- Activity limitations related to driving and avoiding strong magnetic fields
- Signs and symptoms of device failure
- Follow-up schedule with health care professional
- Cardiopulmonary resuscitation (CPR) training for family members

BOX 17-13 Traditional Eligibility Criteria for PTCA

Single-vessel disease exclusive of left main lesions
Characteristics of the lesion
- Concentric
- Noncalcified
- Proximal
- Discrete (less than 1 cm length)
- No total occlusions

History of disease
- Short history of angina (less than 1 year)
- Inadequate control on medications

Normal ventricular function
Not in the setting of acute myocardial infarction
Must be a candidate for CABG

only patients with single-vessel coronary artery disease were considered for PTCA, now patients with multivessel disease, even those who have previously undergone SVG and IMA grafting or thrombolytic therapy for acute myocardial infarction may be candidates for catheter intervention.[46]

Earlier restrictions regarding the characteristics and location of the atherosclerotic lesion have also changed with improved technology. Left main coronary lesions have been successfully dilated under certain conditions. Also, no longer is the presence of an eccentric (uneven distribution of plaque), moderately calcified, or nonproximal lesion an absolute contraindication. Furthermore, it is now sometimes possible to traverse and dilate a totally occluded vessel. Lesion morphology related to shape, size, location, and amount of calcification has been more clearly defined through clinical experience and is now used to guide the selection of specific catheter-based interventions.[47] (∞Coronary Artery Disease, p. 485.)

Surgical backup. Initially, most institutions required that patients preparing to undergo PTCA be candidates for coronary artery bypass surgery. Complications such as abrupt closure may arise during the procedure, which necessitates immediate aortocoronary bypass grafting. Because urgent bypass surgery is required in only 1% to 3% of cases, a more selective surgical backup plan is appropriate. Thus only those patients undergoing high-risk interventions, who are otherwise ideal surgical candidates, require formal surgical backup support. Nevertheless, the availability of cardiac surgical services on site remains mandatory for all patients.[46]

Percutaneous Transluminal Coronary Angioplasty

PTCA involves the use of a balloon-tipped catheter that, when advanced through an atherosclerotic lesion (atheroma), can be inflated intermittently for the purpose of dilating the stenotic area and improving blood flow through it (Figure 17-16). The high balloon-inflation pressure stretches the vessel wall, fractures the plaque, and enlarges the vessel lumen. A successful angioplasty procedure is one in which the stenosis is reduced to less than 50% of the vessel lumen diameter, although most clinicians aim for less than 30% final diameter stenosis.[46] Procedural success is influenced by patient variables such as age, cardiac function, and comorbidities such as diabetes as well as by characteristics of the lesion itself. Lesions that are discrete (less than 1 cm in length), concentric, easily accessible, and have little or no calcification are most likely to be treated successfully with PTCA.[46] PTCA is also a valuable adjunct to thrombolytic therapy in terms of reducing a severe stenosis that persists after thrombolysis.[48]

Procedure

PTCA is performed in the cardiac catheterization laboratory under fluoroscopy. Introducer catheters or "sheaths" are inserted percutaneously into the femoral artery and vein. The venous sheath can be used to perform a right heart catheterization with a pulmonary artery (PA) catheter or to insert a pacing catheter, or both. A catheter with pacing capabilities may be indicated if dilation of the right coronary artery or circumflex artery is anticipated because the

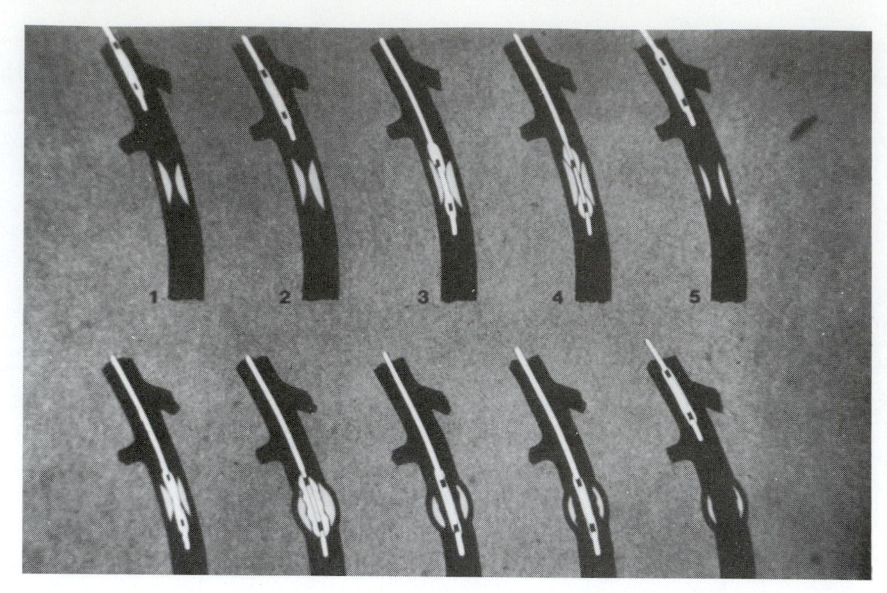

FIGURE 17-16. Balloon compression of an atherosclerotic lesion. (From Kinney M and others: *Comprehensive cardiac care,* ed 8, St Louis, 1996, Mosby.)

blood supply to the conduction system of the heart may be interrupted, requiring emergency pacing. The pacing catheter also serves as an anatomic landmark for locating the lesions to be dilated. The patient is systemically heparinized to prevent clots from forming on or in any of the catheters. A special guiding catheter designed to engage the coronary ostia is inserted through the arterial sheath and advanced in a retrograde manner through the aorta. Nitroglycerin or calcium channel blockers may be given at this time to prevent coronary artery spasm and to maximize coronary vasodilation during the procedure. A guidewire is then advanced down the coronary artery and negotiated across the occluding atheroma. The balloon catheter is advanced over this guidewire and positioned across the lesion. The balloon is inflated and deflated repetitively (each inflation not to exceed 90 seconds) until evidence of dilation is demonstrated on an angiogram (Figure 17-17). In cases that require prolonged balloon inflations, however, an autoperfusion angioplasty catheter is available with side holes that allow passive blood flow through the central lumen to the distal coronary artery if adequate systemic blood pressure is present.

The patient is transferred to the coronary care or angioplasty unit for overnight care and observation. The introducer sheaths are left in place for several reasons. First, the intravenous infusion of heparin is continued for 6 to 24 hours after PTCA to prevent clot formation on the roughened endothelium at the site of dilation.[49] Therefore removal of the sheaths during this time causes a predisposition to bleeding. Second, it allows for rapid vascular access should redilation become necessary. The arterial sheath must be attached to a continuous heparinized saline flush, however, and intravenous fluids must be infused through the venous sheath to maintain luminal patency. If the patient's postangioplasty course is uneventful, the heparin infusion is discontinued and the sheaths are removed within 24 hours of the procedure. After sheath removal the patient may be discharged home 6 to 12 hours later.

Complications

As stated earlier, serious complications can result from angioplasty that necessitate emergency CABG surgery. These complications include persistent coronary artery spasm, myocardial infarction, and acute coronary occlusion. Abciximab (Reopro) has recently been approved by the Food and Drug Administration (FDA) as an adjunct to PTCA for the prevention of abrupt closure of arteries in high risk patients. Reopro is a human-mouse monocolonal antibody that inhibits platelet aggregation. In a large-scale clinical trial, Reopro, administered as a bolus and followed with a continuous infusion for 12 hours after angioplasty, was found to decrease the risk of reocclusion.[50] The major complication of Reopro is bleeding, and nursing management requires careful assessment of all potential bleeding sites, especially at the femoral sheath site. Extra precautions are used to immobilize the sheath in-

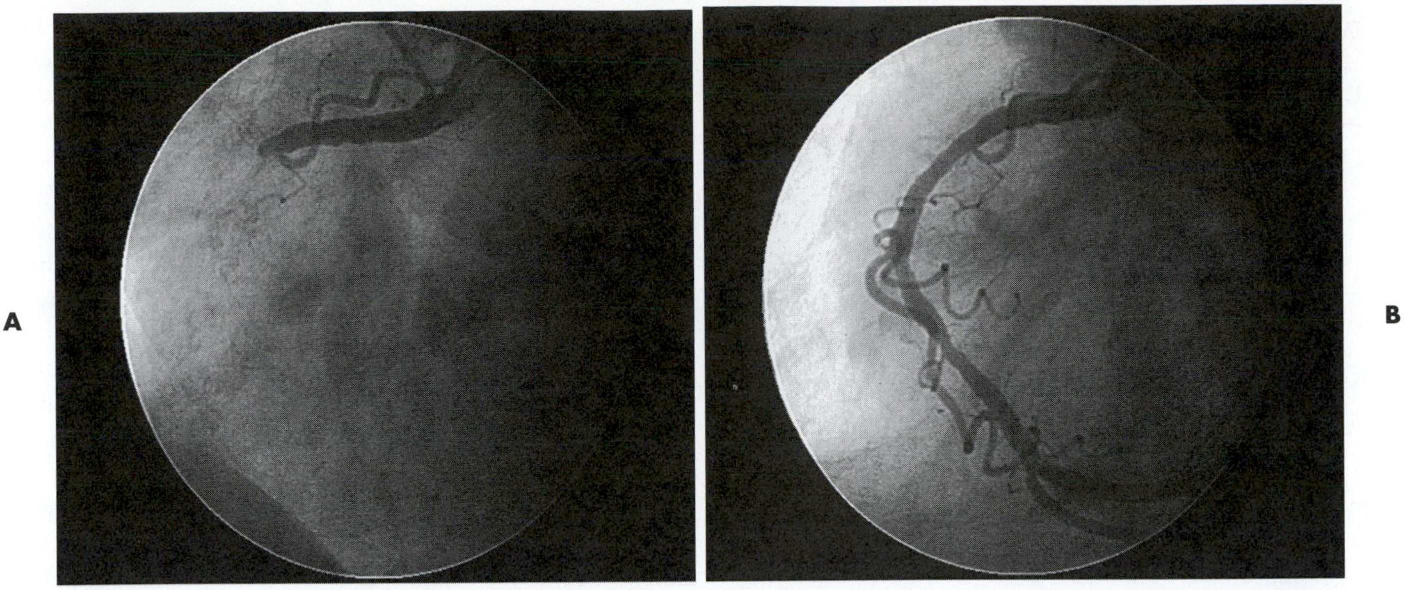

A

B

FIGURE 17-17. **A,** Coronary arteriogram of an acute proximal total occlusion of the right coronary artery (RCA). Patient had sudden onset of chest pain at home and was emergently admitted to the cardiac catherization laboratory. **B,** The same vessel (RCA) shown in **A** after successful coronary atherectomy and intracoronary thrombolytic therapy to open the occluded artery. Symptoms of chest pain resolved after the procedure.

sertion site, either with a sheet tuck to the affected leg or a leg restraint.[51]

Other complications that can occur in the period immediately after angioplasty include bleeding and hematoma formation at the site of vascular cannulation; compromised blood flow to the involved extremity; allergic reaction to radiopaque contrast dye; dysrhythmias; and vasovagal response (hypotension, bradycardia, and diaphoresis) during manipulation or removal of introducer sheaths. Restenosis can occur up to 6 months after angioplasty; however, this late complication typically is amenable to repeat angioplasty. The mechanism involved in restenosis remains unclear, but it is thought to be related to intimal hyperplasia, as well as to platelet deposition and thrombus formation. For this reason, patients are started on a regimen of antiplatelet drugs (e.g., a combination of aspirin and dipyridamole or ticlopidine).

Although PTCA has relatively high success rates in initially opening occluded vessels, this technique has major limitations, including a high frequency of restenosis and abrupt vessel closure. The fact that angioplasty does not remove the occlusive material but rather compresses it to widen the vessel lumen is thought to contribute to the rate of restenosis. Coronary atherectomy, laser angioplasty, and placement of endovascular prostheses (stents) are interventional technologies developed to address the problems of acute closure and restenosis associated with PTCA.[46]

Atherectomy

Atherectomy is the excision and removal of the atherosclerotic plaque by cutting, shaving, or grinding; specialized coronary catheters are used to achieve a more controlled mechanism of injury, with the hope of fewer complications.[52]

Three atherectomy devices are described in Table 17-6: directional coronary atherectomy (DCA), rotational ablation (Rotablator), and transluminal extraction catheter. All three devices are FDA-approved for use in coronary as well as peripheral arteries. Because these devices use different mechanisms, they may offer special advantages for different types of lesions. The current trend is to use a "lesion-specific" approach in the selection of a device for catheter intervention.

Directional coronary atherectomy. The mechanism of action of the DCA catheter is shown in Figure 17-18. The DCA catheter has presented a significant research advantage for understanding the pathogenesis of CAD and also the restenosis process after catheter interventions. Because DCA extracts pieces of atheroma that can be studied microscopically (rather like a biopsy specimen), progress has been made in the

TABLE 17-6 Atherectomy Devices

Device	Design	Uses
Directional atherectomy (Simpson Atherocath)	Rotating cup-shaped cutter within a windowed cylindric housing; plaque that protrudes into window is shaved off and collected within nose cone of cutter housing (Figure 17-18)	Ostial lesions SVG Eccentric lesions in large vessels Proximal, discrete lesions
Rotational ablation (Rotablator)	A high-speed rotating diamond-studded bur; "sanding effect"; generates microparticles that pass distally into microcirculation	Distal lesions Long, diffuse lesions Tortuous vessels Calcified lesions Eccentric lesions Ostial lesions Small vessels
Transluminal extraction catheter (TEC)	Motorized cutting head with triangular blades; excised plaque removed by suction	Diffuse disease SVG

SVG, Saphenous venous graft.

understanding of both CAD and the restenosis process caused by intimal hyperplasia. This device is well-suited for lesions that are located in the proximal or midportion of the coronary artery, as well as eccentric lesions and those occurring in saphenous vein grafts.[52]

Rotablator. The Rotablator device has a diamond-coated burr that drills through the plaque, creating tiny particles. This particulate matter is carried through the blood stream and disposed of by the reticuloendothelial system. This device is the preferred treatment for heavily calcified lesions, since the burr drill preferentially ablates calcified plaque and is deflected by the elastic elements of the vessel wall.[53] The Rotablator has also proved effective in removing lesions from tortuous vessels. Improved lumen diameter may be achieved when angioplasty is used after the Rotablator procedure (adjunctive angioplasty).[47]

Transluminal extraction catheter. The transluminal extraction catheter (TEC) consists of a motorized cutting head with triangular blades that rotate at 700 revolutions per minute to shave atherosclerotic lesions. As the plaque is excised, a suction device incorporated into the catheter is used to remove the plaque from the vessel. This device has been successful in the treatment of long, diffuse lesions as well as stenosis that occurs in bypass grafts. Unlike PTCA and DCA, the TEC catheter may also be used to establish reperfusion through total occlusions.[54] TEC atherectomy may

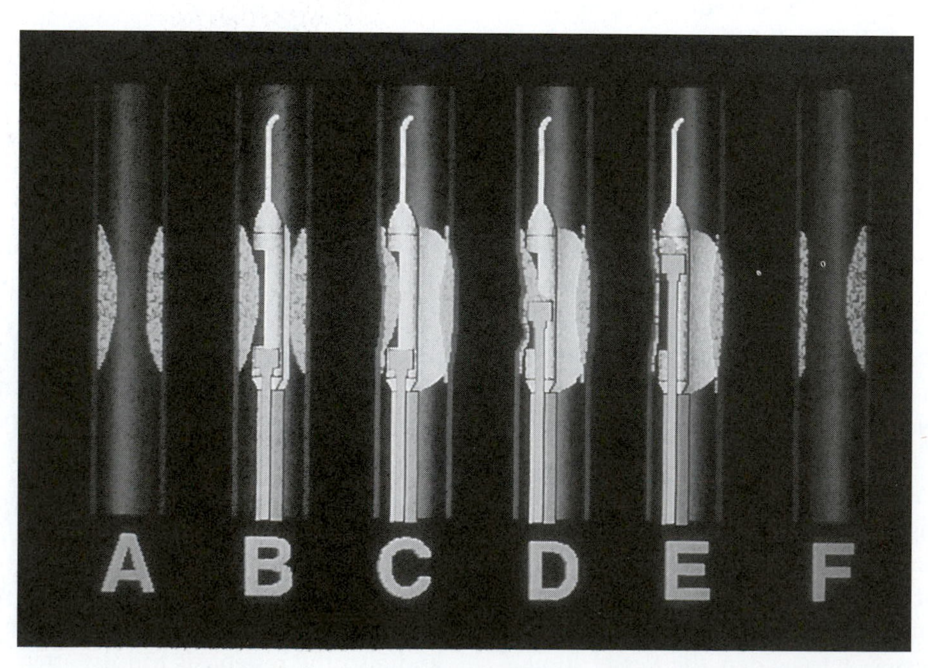

FIGURE 17-18. Directional coronary atherectomy: **A,** atheroma (plaque) in vessel lumen; **B,** DCA device in position; **C,** inflation of low-pressure support balloon that pushes the plaque into the "window" of the device (the ability to turn the atherocath in different directions within the artery explains the name of the DCA device); **D,** the cutter begins to shear away plaque; **E,** the plaque is pushed into the nose cone (collection chamber) of the atherocath; **F,** vessel lumen shows decreased plaque after removal of catheter.

be performed first to debulk the lesion, and then is followed by angioplasty to further decrease the amount of residual stenosis.

Procedure. The procedure for atherectomy is similar to that described for PTCA. The sheaths required are larger to facilitate passage of the larger atherectomy catheters. As a result, postprocedure complications related to the sheaths may be increased. Patients undergoing Rotablator procedures may also have an increased need for continued nitroglycerin in the postprocedure period to treat vasospasm.[49,55]

Laser Angioplasty

Laser is an acronym for *l*ight *a*mplification by *s*timulated *e*mission of *r*adiation. Laser plaque ablation in coronary arteries, using the excimer laser, is currently being studied in clinical trials. The excimer laser is a contact cutter, meaning that it only ablates tissue that it touches. The catheter is advanced by a guidewire system similar to that used in angioplasty. The excimer laser, which uses high-energy pulsed ultraviolet light—so-called cold laser—to vaporize plaque, is particularly suited for distal disease and occluded SVGs.[56]

Coronary Stents

Another major coronary technology is the coronary stent prosthesis. This is a self-expanding or balloon-expandable stent that is introduced into the coronary artery over a guidewire in a region that has been previously dilated with PTCA to prevent acute closure and restenosis, as well as to obtain a larger vascular lumen diameter.[56,57]

Procedure. The procedure for stent placement is similar to that used in other catheter interventions. Access to the coronary arteries is obtained via a femoral sheath, which allows for placement of a catheter over a guidewire. A stent is positioned at the target side, is expanded, and the catheter is removed, leaving the stent in place. Several types of stents are now available. As shown by the examples in Figure 17-19, stents have either thermal memory (Figure 17-19, *A*), are self-expanding (Figure 17-19, *B*), or are balloon-expandable (Figure 17-19, *C*).[57] At present, approved indications for stents include threatened or abrupt vessel closure ("failed" angioplasty or atherectomy) and primary stenting as an alternative to angioplasty or bypass surgery.[58]

Because the stent is a foreign object (generally made of stainless steel) in the blood stream, the stent's presence in the coronary artery activates the coagulation cascade. To prevent acute thrombosis of the stent, intense anticoagulation and antiplatelet therapy was initially used during and after stent placement. This consisted of preprocedure aspirin and dypyridamole and the administration of IV heparin both during and after the procedure to prevent acute thrombosis of the stent. Consequently, bleeding was a major complication of stent placement. Recent studies have indicated that reduced anticoagulation may be sufficient to maintain stent patency. Many physicians now use heparin only during the procedure and remove access sheaths as soon as the activated clotting time (ACT) returns to normal.[58] Aspirin is continued indefinitely, and ticlopidine and/or low molecular weight heparin are commonly prescribed after stent placement. Conventional medications for treatment of coronary artery disease, such as IV nitroglycerin and calcium channel blockers, may also be prescribed.

Ongoing development in both stent design and stenting procedures may expand clinical indications for these devices. Research is currently being conducted on stents coated with heparin that may allow for favorable outcomes with the use of only postprocedural antiplatelet agents such as ticlopidine and aspirin.[58] Intravascular ultrasound is being used by some clinicians to evaluate the vessel lumen diameter after stent deployment.[59] Information obtained from ultrasound may provide a better estimate of residual plaque than that provided by angiography, since contrast material may surround the lattice-work of the stent, giving the appearance of a large lumen even when the stent is not fully open.[58] Multiple stents have also been implanted sequentially within a vessel to fully cover the area of the lesion.[60]

Despite the rapid expansion of research in the area of interventional cardiology, no one device has emerged as the preferred methodology for all patients. It is likely that stents will continue to be an adjunct to angioplasty, atherectomy, and thrombolytic drugs as part of an increasing number of interventional cardiology devices used to treat acute manifestations of coronary artery disease.

Nursing Management

Nursing management and diagnoses after angioplasty, atherectomy, or stent insertion focuses on accurate assessment of the patient's condition and prompt intervention (Box 17-14). The nurse at the bedside is in the unique position to continuously monitor for clinical manifestations of potential problems and take quick and appropriate action to minimize the deleterious effects of complications related to the interventional catheter procedure.

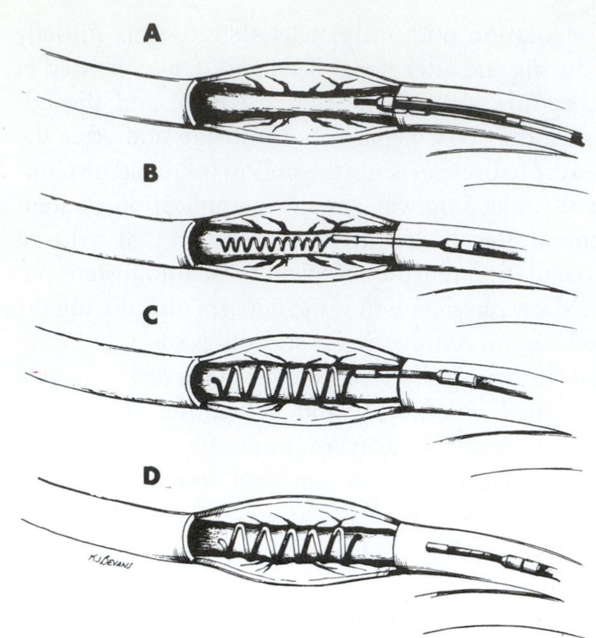

A. Stent is cooled with ice and straightened in catheter for placement.
B. Exposed to blood temperature, coil begins to expand.
C. Coil expands to full size in coronary artery.
D. Stent is released from delivery device and supports vessel. Catheter is removed from coronary artery.

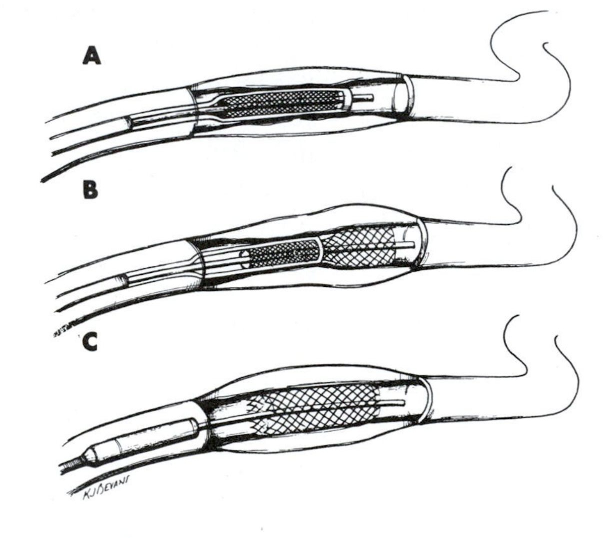

A. Stent is constricted in constraining catheter.
B. Stent is released from catheter.
C. Stent is fully expanded to support vessel. Catheter is removed from coronary artery.

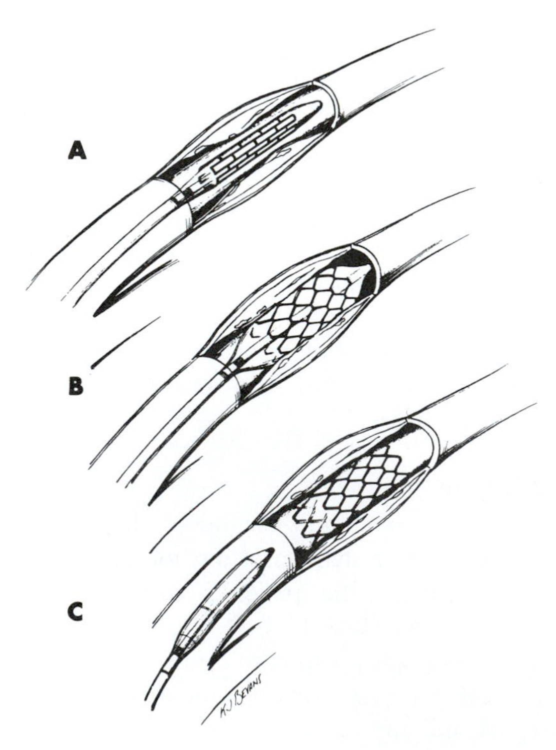

A. Stent is crimped onto balloon catheter for placement.
B. Stent is expanded against vessel wall.
C. Stent is supporting the vessel wall. Balloon catheter is withdrawn from coronary artery.

FIGURE 17-19. Intracoronary stents. **Top,** nitinol stent (heat-sensitive). **Middle,** Medinvent stent (self-expanding). **Bottom,** Palmaz-Schatz stent (balloon-expandable). (From Bevans M, McLimore E: *J Cardiovasc Nurs* 7(1):34, 1992.)

BOX 17-14 NURSING DIAGNOSIS AND MANAGEMENT

POST PTCA, CORONARY ATHERECTOMY, AND STENT

- Altered Myocardial Tissue Perfusion related to acute myocardial ischemia, p. 595
- Altered Peripheral Tissue Perfusion related to decreased peripheral blood flow, p. 596
- Activity Intolerance related to prolonged immobility or deconditioning, p. 597
- Acute Pain related to transmission and perception of cutaneous, visceral, muscular, or ischemic impulses, p. 197
- Anxiety related to threat to biologic, psychologic, and/or social integrity, p. 99
- Knowledge Deficit: Discharge Regimen related to lack of previous exposure to information, p. 61 (see Patient Education Box 17-15)

Angina. It is essential that the nurse observe the patient for recurrent angina, a clinical indication of myocardial ischemia. Angina may be accompanied by elevated ST segments on the bedside monitor or the 12-lead ECG. Angina during interventional cardiology procedures is an expected occurrence at the time of balloon inflation or manipulation within the coronary artery. Intraprocedure angina is caused by the temporary interruption of blood flow through the involved artery, which should subside with deflation or removal of the balloon or nitroglycerin administration, or both. Angina after a coronary interventional procedure may be a result of transient coronary vasospasm, or it may signal a more serious complication. In any case the nurse must act quickly to assess for manifestations of myocardial ischemia and initiate clinical interventions, as indicated. The physician usually orders intravenous nitroglycerin to be titrated to alleviate chest pain. Continued angina despite maximal vasodilator therapy generally rules out transient coronary vasospasm as the source of ischemic pain, and redilation or emergency coronary artery bypass surgery must be considered. The risk is that a clot in the coronary artery, usually occurring at a site where the intimal wall has been dissected, will cause an acute occlusion. (∞Acute Myocardial Infarction, p. 490.)

Femoral site care. While the sheath is in place or after its removal, bleeding or hematoma at the sheath insertion site may occur as a result of the effects of heparin. The nurse observes the patient for bleeding or swelling at the puncture site and frequently assesses adequacy of circulation to the involved extremity. The nurse also assesses the patient for back pain, which can indicate retroperitoneal bleeding from the internal arterial puncture site. The patient is instructed to keep the involved leg straight and not to elevate the head of the bed any more than 30 degrees while the sheath is in place (to prevent dislodgment) and for several hours after its removal (to prevent bleeding). Use of an eggcrate mattress may help alleviate the lower back pain many patients experience while immobile after an interventional catheter procedure. After sheath removal, direct pressure is applied to the puncture site for 15 to 30 minutes; a sandbag may be ordered if direct pressure is inadequate for hemostasis. For stents or atherectomy, which require a larger sheath size, a C-clamp or fem-stop may be used to apply continued pressure for 1 to 2 hours to ensure adequate hemostasis. A surgical approach to the problem of controlling femoral bleeding after percutaneous interventional cardiology procedures has recently been developed. The percutaneous vascular surgical device is inserted into the femoral artery in the same position as a conventional introducer sheath (Figure 17-20, *A*). The device contains needles and sutures that are used to suture the artery closed after the interventional procedure (Figure 17-20, *B*). At the end of the procedure, when the artery is sealed, the needles are removed by the cardiologist and the sutures are knotted firmly (Figure 17-20, *C*). This device is used in Europe and recently received approval from the Food and Drug Administration in the United States. If devices such as this are successful, bleeding complications in patients undergoing percutaneous catheter interventions will be greatly reduced.

Patients usually are allowed to resume ambulation 6 to 8 hours later, depending on institutional protocol. Excessive bleeding or hematoma formation can become a serious problem because it may result in hypotension or compromised blood flow to the involved extremity. For this reason, pulses are usually monitored every 15 minutes for the first couple of hours immediately after the procedure, and then every 1 to 2 hours until the sheaths are removed. After sheath removal, pulses are again monitored at 15-minute intervals for a brief period.

Patient Education

Typically, patients undergoing elective angioplasty, atherectomy, or laser procedures are hospitalized for approximately 24 hours. Stent procedures may require a slightly longer hospital stay. All patients require education about their medication regimen and about

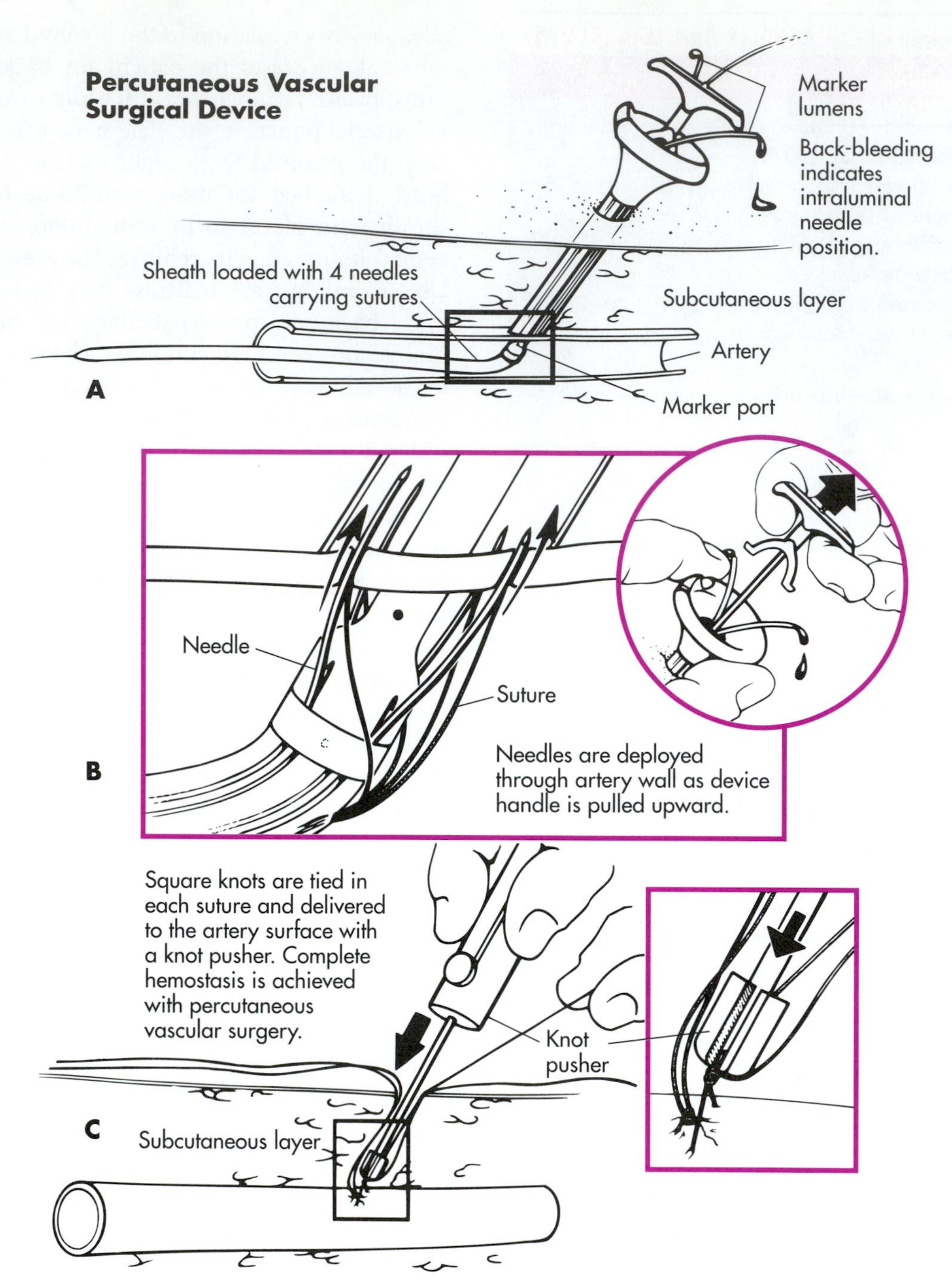

Percutaneous Vascular Surgical Device
Marker lumens
Back-bleeding indicates intraluminal needle position.
Sheath loaded with 4 needles carrying sutures
Subcutaneous layer
Artery
A
Marker port
Needle
Suture
Needles are deployed through artery wall as device handle is pulled upward.
B
Square knots are tied in each suture and delivered to the artery surface with a knot pusher. Complete hemostasis is achieved with percutaneous vascular surgery.
Knot pusher
C
Subcutaneous layer

FIGURE 17-20. Example of a percutaneous vascular surgical device used to close the femoral artery after catheter interventions for coronary artery disease. **A,** Insertion of device into femoral artery. **B,** After the interventional procedure, the device is removed by pulling upward to allow needles—in the device—to close the artery. **C,** The sutured artery is secured with a knot pusher. (Courtesy Perclose Inc., Menlo Park, Calif.)

risk-factor modification. (Box 17-15). Because of the abbreviated hospital stay, the nurse often has insufficient time to do more than identify the offending risk factors and initiate basic instruction. Patients are referred to local cardiac rehabilitation centers for more extensive teaching and follow-up to facilitate understanding and compliance with risk factor modification.

Another point of instruction that must be addressed is the patient's knowledge deficit related to discharge medications. Patients frequently are sent home on a regimen of antiplatelet drugs, as well as a nitrate such

BOX 17-15 PATIENT EDUCATION

POST PTCA, CORONARY ATHERECTOMY, AND STENT

- Pathophysiology of atherosclerosis
- Risk factor modification (diet, exercise, smoking cessation, weight loss)
- Information about prescribed medications (antiplatelet agents, nitrates, calcium channel blockers, etc.)
- Symptoms to report to the health care professional (chest pain, shortness of breath, bleeding)
- Follow-up appointments

as isosorbide to promote vasodilation. In addition, if the patient has demonstrated evidence of a vasospastic component to the disease, calcium channel blockers are prescribed. It is essential that the patient clearly understand the rationale for therapy, as well as potential side effects of each drug. It is important that patients be provided with written information as well as a number to call if problems occur.[61]

BALLOON VALVULOPLASTY

After the development of percutaneous balloon angioplasty for coronary artery disease, it became reasonable to consider adaptation of this technique as a nonsurgical intervention for stenotic cardiac valves. Although long-term results are not promising at this point, especially for aortic valvuloplasty, balloon valvuloplasty can provide palliation and short-term symptomatic relief in selected patient populations[62] (Box 17-16).

Balloon valvuloplasty is performed in the cardiac catheterization laboratory. The procedure is similar to a routine cardiac catheterization, including cannulation of the femoral artery and vein with percutaneous introducer sheaths. The balloon dilation catheter is then threaded over a guidewire across the stenotic valvular orifice. The valves may be approached either retrograde via the aorta or antegrade across the interatrial septum. In the antegrade transseptal approach, the balloon catheter is passed across the interatrial septum, which results in the creation of a small atrial septal defect.[63] Subsequent inflations of the balloon increase the valve opening by separating fused commissures, cracking calcified leaflets, and stretching valve structures. Inflations are continued until the balloon "waist" disappears which indicates full inflation.[64] Regurgitant flow can result, particularly after mitral valvuloplasty. The risks of balloon valvuloplasty, which are similar to those inherent in most catheterization procedures, include, but are not limited to, cardiac perforation, thromboembolic events, dysrhythmias, hypotension, and bleeding.[63] The postprocedure nursing management is similar to that for other percutaneous cardiac catheter procedures. (∞Catheter Interventions For CAD: Nursing Management, p. 552.)

BOX 17-16 Indications for Balloon Valvuloplasty

AORTIC

Nonsurgical candidates with incapacitating symptoms

Patients with aortic stenosis who require urgent noncardiac surgery

Patients with severe heart failure or cardiogenic shock because of aortic stenosis whose conditions need to be stabilized until valve replacement is deemed safer

Patients with poor left ventricular function, low cardiac output, and small gradient across a stenotic aortic valve whose need for aortic valve replacement requires assessment

MITRAL

As an alternative to open mitral commissurotomy

THROMBOLYTIC THERAPY

Thrombolytic therapy is an important clinical intervention for the patient experiencing acute myocardial infarction (AMI). Before the introduction of thrombolytic agents, the medical management of AMI was focused on decreasing myocardial oxygen demands to minimize myocardial necrosis and thus preserve ventricular function. Recently, however, efforts to limit the size of infarction have been directed toward the timely reperfusion of the jeopardized myocardium. The use of thrombolytic therapy to accomplish this objective is predicated on the prevailing theory that the significant event in most transmural infarctions is the rupture of an atherosclerotic plaque with thrombus formation. The thrombus occludes the coronary artery, depriving the myocardium of oxygen previously supplied by that artery. The administration of a thrombolytic agent results in the lysis of the acute thrombus, thus recanalizing, or opening, the obstructed coronary artery and restoring blood flow to the affected tissue. Once perfusion is restored, adjunctive measures are taken to prevent further clot formation and reocclusion. Thrombolytic therapy does not have a specific DRG. The DRGs are the same as those used for acute myocardial infarction (DRGs 121, 122, and 123).

Eligibility Criteria

Certain criteria have been developed, based on research findings, to determine the patient population that would most likely benefit from the administration of thrombolytic therapy. In general, patients with recent onset of chest pain (less than 6 hours' duration) are candidates. Research suggests that the earlier the treatment is instituted, the higher the likelihood of successful reperfusion. (∞Angina, p. 486.)

Patients with persistent ST-segment elevation despite sublingual nitroglycerin or nifedipine, a sign of impending transmural infarction, are considered candidates for therapy. Patients with abnormal Q waves are not excluded from therapy because this finding is not necessarily evidence of a completed infarction. (∞Acute Myocardial Infarction, p. 490.)

Exclusion criteria is usually based on the increased risk of bleeding incurred by the use of thrombolytics. Patients who have stable clots that might be disrupted by thrombolytic therapy (secondary to recent surgery or a recent cerebrovascular accident) are generally not considered candidates for thrombolytic therapy. Other common criteria for the use of thrombolytic therapy are included in Box 17-17.

BOX 17-17 Thrombolytic Therapy Selection Criteria

No more than 6 hours from onset of chest pain, and less if possible
ST-segment elevation on ECG
Ischemic chest pain of 30 minutes' duration
Chest pain unresponsive to sublingual nitroglycerin or nifedipine
No conditions that might cause a predisposition to hemorrhage

Thrombolytic Agents

Five thrombolytic agents are currently available for either intracoronary or intravenous treatment of acute myocardial infarction. Although these agents differ in their mechanism of clot lysis, all have been found effective in lysing clots and restoring perfusion. A comparison of these agents is provided in Table 17-7. Because patients with an area of plaque disruption are still at risk for clot formation and reocclusion, intravenous heparin and oral aspirin are prescribed either during or immediately after thrombolytic therapy. The timing of these interventions may vary, based on the specific thrombolytic agent used and institutional protocols. Heparin therapy is usually continued for 24 to 72 hours, whereas daily aspirin is continued indefinitely.

Streptokinase. Streptokinase (SK) is a thrombolytic agent derived from beta-hemolytic streptococci, which when combined with plasminogen, catalyzes the conversion of plasminogen to *plasmin*—the enzyme responsible for clot dissolution in the body.

SK can be administered either intravenously or by an intracoronary approach, which necessitates cardiac catheterization. The efficacy of both routes has been established, and both have been used in clinical practice. Intravenously administered SK, although not as effective in terms of recanalizaton as intracoronary streptokinase, has the advantage of being more practical in that it can be administered more rapidly after the onset of symptoms. SK is considerably more effective in thrombi that are less than 3 hours old, compared with older thrombi.[65]

Side effects. The three major problems associated with the use of SK are its systemic lytic effects coupled with a long half-life, potential antigenic effects if readministered, and hypotension. Because the anticoagulant action of SK is systemic (nonclot-specific) and prolonged (half-life 20 to 25 minutes), bleeding is the most common complication; thus the patient requires careful observation during the 12 hours immediately after administration (Box 17-18). In addition, because SK is a bacterial protein, it can produce a variety of allergic reactions, including anaphylaxis, especially when administered to a patient who either has received SK therapy previously or has had a recent streptococcal infection. It is necessary to be familiar with the possible allergic manifestations (see Box 17-19), as well as cognizant of the fact that as a result of delayed antibody formation, symptoms may develop several days after infusion. Diphenhydramine (Benadryl) or steroids are often prescribed before streptokinase administration to blunt this unwanted effect. Hypotension is sometimes associated with the rapid administration of SK. This fall in blood pressure usually responds to volume replacement but occasionally requires vasopressor support.

Urokinase. Urokinase (UK) is an enzymatic protein secreted by the parenchyma of the human kidney. Its thrombolytic effect results from the direct activation of plasminogen to form plasmin. This differs from SK,

TABLE 17-7 Thrombolytic Agents Approved by the FDA for use in Acute Myocardial Infarction

Drug	Dosage	Actions	Special Considerations
Anistreplase (APSAC)	30 mg via slow IV bolus over 2-5 min	A molecular combination of streptokinase and plasminogen with actions similar to streptokinase Has systemic lytic effects	May cause allergic reactions and hypotension Long half-life, so heparin is usually started 4-6 hr after APSAC Aspirin begun with treatment and continued q day
rPA (reptelase)	IV: 10 million U given as a bolus, repeated in 30 min	Binds to fibrin at the clot and promotes activation of plasminogen to plasmin	Heparin started with administration of the drug and continued for 24 hr Aspirin begun with treatment and continued q day
Streptokinase	IV: 1.5 million U given over 60 min	Catalyzes the conversion of plasminogen to plasmin, which causes lysis of fibrin Has systemic lytic effects	May cause allergic reactions and hypotension Heparin may be administered IV or SQ Aspirin begun with treatment and continued q day May be administered intracoronary
t-PA (alteplase)	Conventional IV: 100 mg over 3 hr, with the first 10 mg given as a bolus, followed by 40 mg the first hour and 20 mg/hr for the second and third hr Front-loaded IV: 100 mg over 1.5 hr, with the first 15 mg given as a bolus Accelerated-dose IV: 100 mg over 90 min with the first 15 mg given as a bolus	Binds to fibrin at the clot (clot-specific) and promotes activation of plasminogen to plasmin	Short half-life, so heparin is usually started with the t-PA as a bolus and then followed with an infusion Aspirin begun with treatment and continued q day
Urokinase	IV: 2 million U over 1 hr IC: 4000-6000 U/min, average dose 500,000 U	Non-selective thrombolysis when given IV	No allergic side effects (nonantigenic) May be administered intracoronary Aspirin begun with treatment and continued q day

BOX 17-18 Signs of Inadequate Hemostasis Related to Thrombolytic Therapy

Bleeding or hematoma at puncture sites
Hematuria, hematemesis, hemoptysis, melena, epistaxis
Bruising or petechiae (pinpoint hemorrhages)
Flank ecchymoses with complaints of low back pain (suggestive of retroperitoneal bleeding)
Gingival bleeding
Change in neurologic status (intracranial bleeding)
Deterioration in vital signs, decreased hematocrit values (internal bleeding)

BOX 17-19 Possible Allergic Manifestations Related to Streptokinase Therapy

Anaphylaxis
Urticaria
Itching
Nausea
Flushing
Fever
Chills

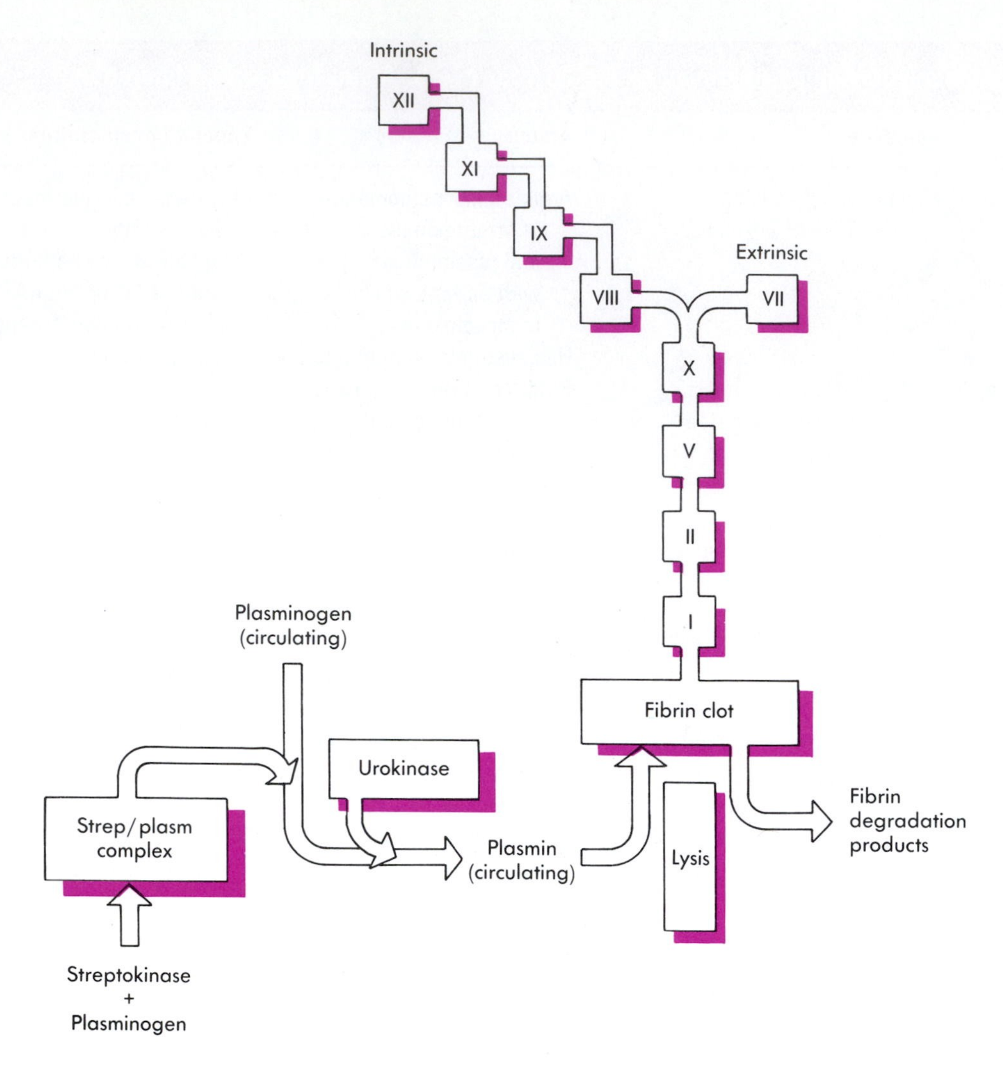

FIGURE 17-21. Site of action of streptokinase and urokinase.

which first must form a complex with plasminogen that will activate plasmin to dissolve the clot (Figure 17-21). UK also is nonclot-specific (activates circulating, nonclot-bound plasminogen, as well as clot-bound plasminogen) but has a shorter half-life than does SK. Because UK is produced by the kidney, it is nonantigenic and thus well-suited for use if subsequent thrombolytic therapy is indicated. Currently, however, it is difficult and expensive to produce, precluding extensive clinical use. It is used in the cardiac catheterization laboratory during PTCA, stent placement, or atherectomy for acute ischemic syndromes, in which the use of adjunctive intracoronary UK to treat thrombus accumulation often results in maintained vessel patency.[66] Urokinase is also the preferred thrombolytic agent for treatment of acute peripheral arterial inclusion because of its nonantigenic properties and a lower incidence of bleeding complications.[67]

Tissue plasminogen activator. Another mode of thrombolytic therapy is tissue plasminogen activator (t-PA or alteplase). Marketed under the name Activase, t-PA is a naturally occurring enzyme (thus nonantigenic) that is clot-specific and has a very short half-life (5 to 10 minutes). It converts plasminogen to plasmin after binding to the fibrin-containing clot. This clot specificity results in an increased concentration and activity of plasmin at the site of the clot where it is needed (Figure 17-22). It was hoped that this characteristic of t-PA would prevent the induction of a systemic lytic state that occurs with SK therapy. The results of studies comparing the adverse effects of SK and t-PA, however, show similar incidences of bleeding after administration.[68] Tissue plasminogen activator was approved specifically for intravenous administration. Several different dosing regimens have been proposed and tested in the clinical setting (see Table

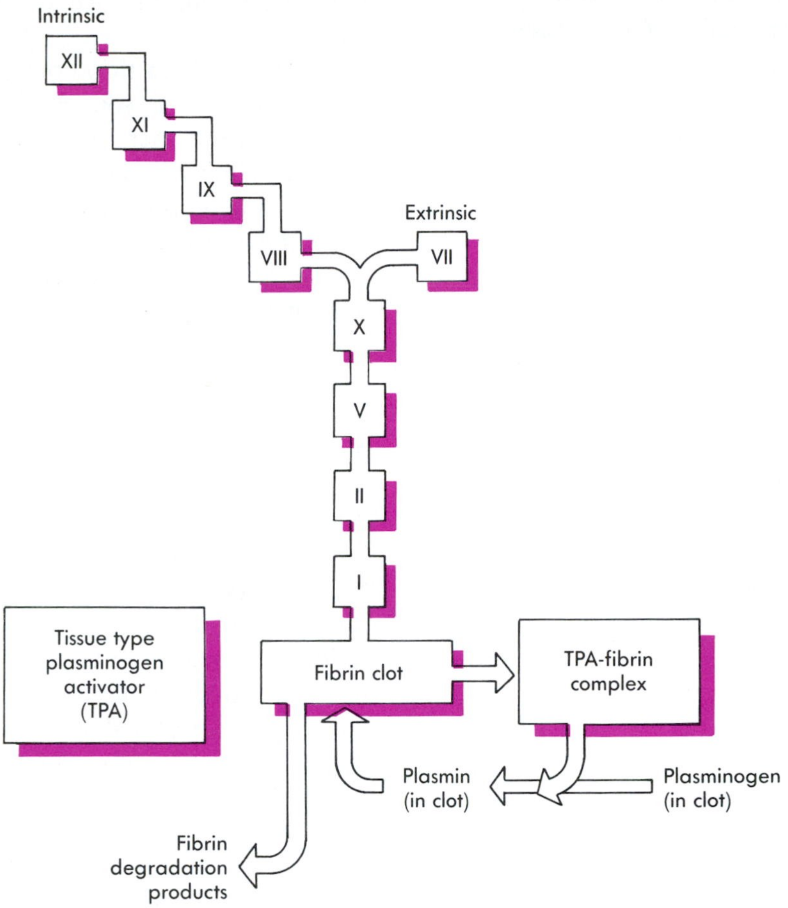

FIGURE 17-22. Site of action of tissue plasminogen activator.

17-7). Front-loaded or accelerated-dose t-PA has proved effective in recent clinical trials, in which the 100 mg dose is administered over 90 minutes, with the first 10 to 15 mg given as a bolus.[68]

Anistreplase. Anistreplase, also known as anisoylated plasminogen-streptokinase activator complex (APSAC; Eminase), was approved by the FDA in 1990 for use in the treatment of AMI. Often referred to as a second-generation streptokinase, it has certain advantages over SK that are related specifically to duration of action and ease of administration. Because it is inactive on administration, APSAC can be given rapidly as a bolus injection. The half-life of APSAC is markedly increased (90 minutes), so concomitant heparin therapy, if employed, should begin 4 to 6 hours after administration to decrease the risk of bleeding associated with the prolonged fibrinolytic activity (see Table 17-7).[65]

Disadvantages, which are similar to those of SK, include the potential for allergic reactions and hypotension. Evidence suggests, however, that the lytic state produced by APSAC and the other nonclot-specific agents (UK, SK) may account for the reduced tendency for thrombosis to recur after thrombolytic therapy.[69] APSAC has similar efficacy to streptokinase in terms of clot lysis, but is much more expensive.

Recombinant plasminogen activator (rPA, or reteplase) is the newest of the thrombolytic agents. This new generation plasminogen activator is given as a double bolus, and then followed with a heparin infusion. Studies have shown that reteplase is as effective as other thrombolytic agents in the treatment of AMI, without an increased risk of complications.[70]

The area of thrombolytic therapy is rapidly evolving, and drug dose ranges and regimens are subject to change when research findings are updated. For example, the results of a large, randomized thrombolytic study recently demonstrated a significant reduction in mortality, even when t-PA therapy was begun between 6 and 12 hours after onset of chest pain.[71] A similar trial evaluating the administration of streptokinase showed no significant reduction in mortality for patients treated 7 to 12 hours after the onset of symptoms.[72] This

BOX 17-20 Noninvasive Evidence of Reperfusion

Cessation of chest pain
Reperfusion dysrhythmias, primarily ventricular
Return of elevated ST segments to baseline
Early and marked peaking of creatine kinase (CK)

suggests that if therapy is begun after the recommended 6 hour timeframe, t-PA may be the preferred thrombolytic agent.

Evidence of Reperfusion

Several phenomena may be observed after the reperfusion of an artery that has been completely occluded by a thrombus (Box 17-20). Recognition of these noninvasive markers of recanalization is essential for documenting the patient's response to thrombolytic therapy.

Pain and reperfusion dysrhythmias. Initially, when there is reperfusion there is an abrupt cessation of ischemic chest pain as blood flow is restored. Another reliable indicator of reperfusion is the appearance of various "reperfusion" dysrhythmias. Premature ventricular contractions, bradycardias, heart block, ventricular tachycardia, and, rarely, ventricular fibrillation may occur. The reason for the occurrence of these dysrhythmias remains unclear, but is thought to be the result of restored flow to ischemic tissue. Generally, reperfusion dysrhythmias are self-limiting or nonsustained, and aggressive antidysrhythmic therapy is not required. Vigilant monitoring of the patient's ECG is essential, however, because a stable condition may deteriorate rapidly and the dysrhythmias may require emergency treatment.

ST segment. Another noninvasive marker of recanalization is the rapid resolution of the previously elevated ST segments, which indicates restoration of blood flow to previously ischemic myocardial tissue. For this reason a monitoring lead should be chosen that clearly demonstrates ST elevation before initiation of therapy.[73] (∞ST-Segment Monitoring, p. 399.)

Creatine kinase. The serum concentration of creatine kinase (formerly known as creatine phosphokinase) rises rapidly and markedly after reperfusion of the ischemic myocardium. This phenomenon is termed *washout,* because it is thought to result from the rapid readmission of creatine kinase—an enzyme released by damaged myocardial cells—into the circulation after restoration of blood flow to previously unperfused areas of the heart. (∞Cardiac Enzymes, p. 381.)

When the three thrombolytic agents approved for intravenous use are compared in terms of reperfusion, t-PA achieves higher, early patency rates. By 24 hours, however, all three agents have uniformly high patency rates.[68] In addition, the administration of heparin extends the anticoagulant effect of therapy beyond that of the thrombolytic agents and often is used 1 to 3 days or more after lytic therapy.[74] Also, the combined effects of aspirin's antiplatelet therapy have been shown to decrease mortality.

Residual coronary stenosis. In most cases, thrombolytic therapy has been determined to be successful in reopening occluded coronary arteries in the setting of acute myocardial infarction. This results in the salvage of myocardium by limiting infarct size, thus preserving left ventricular function and significantly reducing morbidity and mortality. However, residual coronary stenosis resulting from the atherosclerotic process remains even after successful thrombolysis. This residual coronary stenosis can cause rethrombosis. Therefore thrombolytic therapy is recognized as an emergency procedure to restore patency until more definitive therapy can be initiated to effectively reduce the degree of stenosis (interventional catheter procedure) or to bypass the offending occlusion (coronary artery bypass surgery). The optimal timing of these interventions is yet to be determined.

Nursing Management

Nursing management of the patient undergoing thrombolytic therapy begins with identifying potential candidates. In many institutions, checklists are used to facilitate rapid identification of patients who are candidates for thrombolytics. The nurse prepares the patient for thrombolytic therapy by starting intravenous lines and obtaining baseline laboratory values and vital signs. Assessment of the patient continues throughout administration of the thrombolytic agent for clinical indicators of reperfusion as well as complications related to therapy. There are several nursing diagnoses linked to the management of the patient receiving thrombolytic therapy (Box 17-21). The most common complication related to thrombolysis is bleeding, not only as a result of the thrombolytic therapy itself but also because the patients routinely receive anticoagulation therapy for several days to minimize the possibility of rethrombosis. Therefore the nurse must continually monitor for clinical manifestations of bleeding (see Box 17-18).

BOX 17-21 NURSING DIAGNOSIS AND MANAGEMENT

POST THROMBOLYTIC THERAPY

- Altered Myocardial Tissue Perfusion related to acute myocardial ischemia, p. 595
- Acute Pain related to transmission and perception of cutaneous, visceral, muscular, or ischemic impulses, p. 197
- Anxiety related to threat of biologic, psychologic, and/or social integrity, p. 99
- Fluid Volume Deficit related to absolute loss, p. 914
- Knowledge Deficit: Discharge Regimen related to lack of previous exposure to information, p. 61 (see Patient Education Box 17-22)

BOX 17-22 PATIENT EDUCATION

POST THROMBOLYTIC THERAPY

- Pathophysiology of atherosclerosis
- Risk factor management
- Description of thrombolytic agent and how it works
- Measures to minimize bleeding and bruising associated with thrombolytic therapy
- Recognition and actions to take for recurrent ischemic symptoms
- Information regarding prescribed medications (antiplatelet agents, anticoagulants)

BOX 17-23 Indications for the Use of Intraaortic Balloon Pump

Left ventricular failure after cardiac surgery
Unstable angina refractory to medications
Recurrent angina after AMI
Complications of AMI
  Cardiogenic shock
  Papillary muscle dysfunction/rupture with mitral regurgitation
  Ventricular septal defect
  Refractory ventricular dysrhythmias

Mild gingival bleeding and oozing around venipuncture sites are common and not a cause of concern. Should serious bleeding occur, such as intracranial or internal bleeding, all fibrinolytic and heparin therapies are discontinued, and volume expanders or coagulation factors, or both, are administered. In addition to accurate assessment of the patient for evidence of bleeding, nursing management includes preventative measures to minimize the potential for bleeding. For example, patient handling is limited, injections are avoided if at all possible, and additional pressure is provided to ensure hemostasis at venipuncture and arterial puncture sites. Intravenous lines are placed before administering lytic therapy, and a heparin lock may be used for obtaining laboratory specimens during treatment. Antacids can be given prophylactically, especially if the patient complains of gastric discomfort.

Patient Education

Education for the patient receiving thrombolytic therapy includes information regarding the actions of thrombolytic agents, with emphasis on precautions to minimize bleeding (Box 17-22). For example, the patient is cautioned against vigorous toothbrushing and told to refrain from using straight-edge razors. In addition information is provided regarding ongoing risk factor management in the prevention of atherosclerotic coronary artery disease.

MECHANICAL CIRCULATORY ASSIST DEVICES

Mechanical circulatory assist devices are used in the treatment of heart failure when conventional pharmacologic therapy has proved ineffective. The primary goals of mechanical assist devices are to decrease myocardial workload and maintain adequate perfusion to vital organs. There is no specific DRG for mechanical assist devices. The DRG refers only to the primary medical diagnosis. Therefore the DRGs associated with acute MI, acute heart failure, and shock can all be used. If the cardiac failure is reversible, a short duration of ventricular assistance is used to allow the myocardium time to recover. If the condition is irreversible, a mechanical assist device may be used as a bridge for transplant for qualified candidates. (∞Heart Transplantation, p. 1179.)

Intraaortic Balloon Pump

The intraaortic balloon pump (IABP) currently is the most widely used temporary mechanical circulatory assist device to support failing circulation (Box 17-23). Its therapeutic effects are based on the hemodynamic principles of diastolic augmentation and afterload reduction.

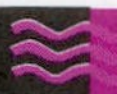
RESEARCH ABSTRACT
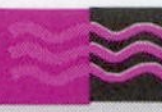

Spouse stressors while awaiting heart transplantation.

Collins E, White-Williams C, Jalowiec A: *Heart Lung* 25(1):4, 1996.

PURPOSE

The purpose of this study was threefold: (1) to identify common stressors experienced by spouses of heart transplantation (HT) candidates; (2) to identify differences in stressors among spouses of HT candidates based on selected demographic variables; and (3) to report preliminary psychometric data on the newly developed Spouse Transplant Stressor Scale.

DESIGN

Comparative, cross-sectional survey.

SAMPLE

The nonrandom sample consisted of 85 spouses of patients awaiting HT at three sites. The mean age of the study subjects was 51.5 years; the average age of the HT candidate was 53.9 years. The spouse sample was primarily female (90.5%) and white (94.1%), and the participants had been married an average of 26.2 years. The majority were educated at the college level, were in their first marriage, and had three children. Patients waited for a donor heart an average of 222 days (range, 1 day to 3.7 years).

PROCEDURE

Subjects were administered five instruments in the overall study: (1) the Spouse Transplant Stressor Scale (STSS), which was developed by one of the investigators of this study; (2) Family Inventory of Resources for Management; (3) the Jalowiec Coping Scale; (4) the Quality of Life Index (Ferrans and Powers); and (5) a six-item rating form that assessed the impact of the HT experience. The newly developed STSS had been tested and refined in a pilot study before this investigation. Four subscales were identified: transplantation stressors, socioeconomic stressors, responsibility stressors, and stressors related to self.

RESULTS

Spouses of HT candidates reported high levels of stress during the waiting period. Factors directly related to the transplantation experience were rated as the most stressful. Fear that the patient would die before a donor heart became available was rated as the top stressor for the spouses. Working spouses perceived more stressors related to responsibility, socioeconomics, and self. Stressors associated with the transplantation process itself were equally stressful for those spouses who worked and those who did not work. Alpha coefficients for the STSS subscales range from .79-.92.

DISCUSSION/IMPLICATIONS

The alpha coefficients for the STSS demonstrate initial reliability for the newly developed tool. Additional testing for reliability is needed. Findings from this study indicate multiple nursing implications. The high levels of stress reported by the spouses may lead them to be more prone to stress-related illnesses. Information regarding this link can be given by nurses, with an emphasis on self-care and stress-reduction strategies. Since not knowing when or whether the transplant would take place was highly stressful for spouses, additional support and interventions may be necessary during this time. Study results also illustrate that working spouses have special needs and concerns that need to be assessed, addressed, and supported during the process.

The most commonly used intraaortic balloon consists of a single sausage-shaped polyurethane balloon that is wrapped around the distal end of a vascular catheter and positioned in the descending thoracic aorta just distal to the takeoff of the left subclavian artery. The second generation of intraaortic balloon catheters is more flexible and can be wrapped to a smaller diameter than its predecessors and therefore can be inserted into the femoral artery percutaneously rather than surgically. When attached to a bedside pumping console and properly synchronized to the patient's cardiac cycle, the intraaortic balloon inflates during diastole and deflates just before systole.

Initially, as the balloon is inflated in diastole concurrent with aortic valve closure, the blood in the aortic arch above the level of the balloon is displaced retrograde (backward) toward the aortic root, augmenting diastolic coronary arterial blood flow and increasing myocardial oxygen supply (Figure 17-23, *A*). The blood volume in the aorta below the level of the balloon is propelled forward toward the peripheral vascular system, which may enhance renal perfusion. Subsequently, the deflation of the balloon just before the opening of the aortic valve creates a potential space or vacuum in the aorta, toward which blood flows unimpeded during ventricular ejection

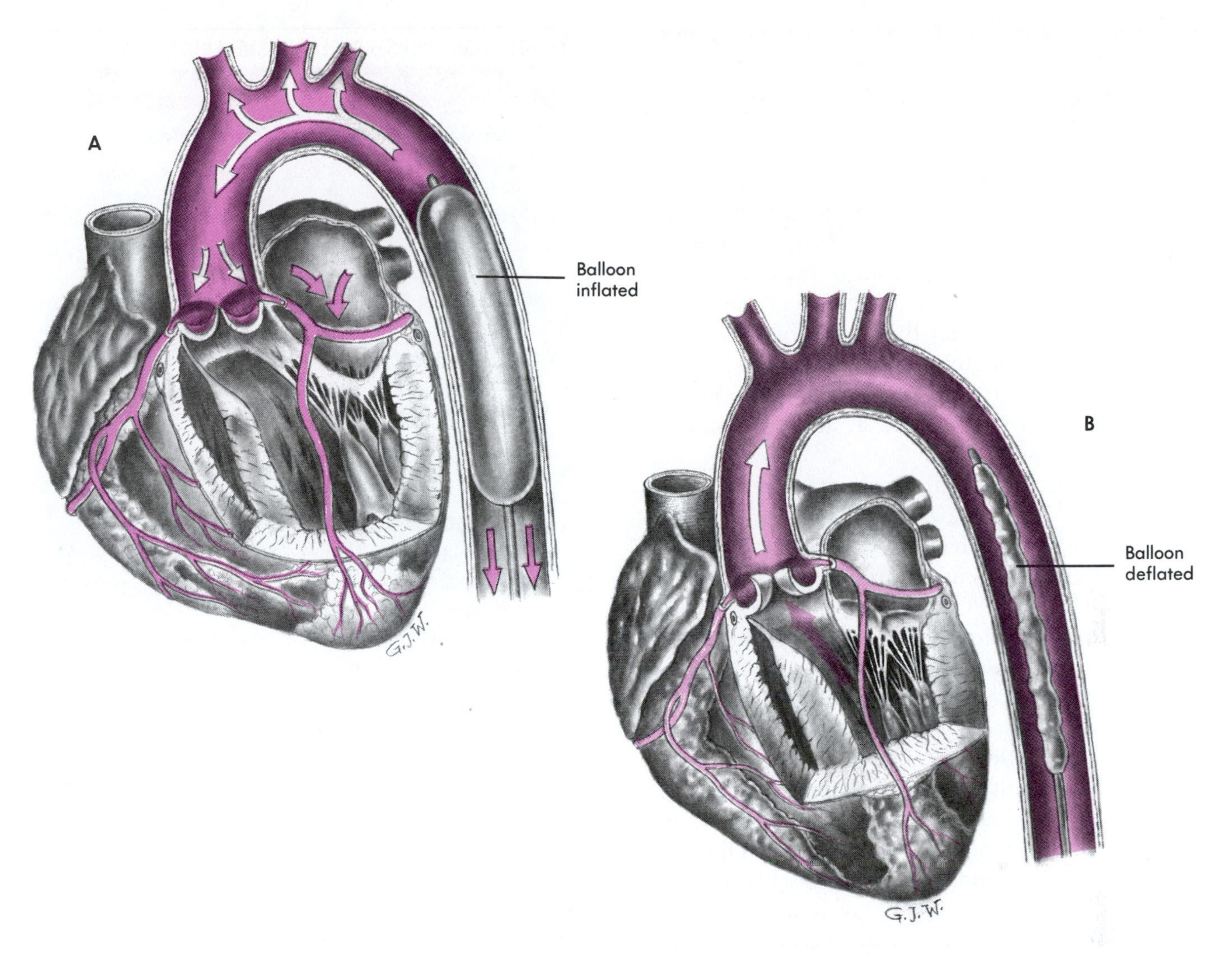

FIGURE 17-23. Mechanisms of action of intraaortic balloon pump. **A,** Diastolic balloon inflation augments coronary blood flow. **B,** Systolic balloon deflation decreases afterload.

(Figure 17-23, *B*). This decreased resistance to left ventricular ejection, or decreased afterload, facilitates ventricular emptying and reduces myocardial oxygen demands. The overall physiologic effect of IABP therapy is an improvement in the balance between myocardial oxygen supply and demand.[75] Contraindications to balloon pumping include aortic aneurysm, aortic valve insufficiency, and severe peripheral vascular disease.

Medical management. The intraaortic balloon may be inserted in the operating room, the cardiac catheterization laboratory, or the critical care unit. The IAB is usually inserted percutaneously through the femoral artery and advanced to the correct position in the descending thoracic aorta. The physician may insert the balloon through an introducer sheath, or perform a sheathless insertion to minimize the degree of vessel occlusion created by the catheter. If percutaneous catheter placement is not feasible, the catheter may be placed via surgical cutdown or a direct thoracic approach. After insertion, the balloon is attached to the console and filled with the prescribed volume of helium, and pumping is initiated. If the balloon fails to unwrap completely during filling, the physician may rapidly inflate and deflate the balloon manually, using a syringe.

Nursing management. Although the actual management of the pumping console and its timing functions may be delegated to specially trained personnel on the unit, several important nursing diagnosis and management responsibilities relate to the management of the patient receiving IABP therapy (Box 17-24).

Dysrythmias. The ECG and arterial pressure tracing are constantly monitored to verify the timing and effect of balloon counterpulsations (Figure 17-24). For counterpulsation to occur, the pump must receive a trigger signal to identify the beginning of a new cardiac cycle. The trigger can be the R wave of the ECG, the upstroke of the arterial pressure waveform, or a pacemaker spike.[76] Dysrhythmias can adversely affect the timing of balloon inflation and deflation; thus rhythm disturbances must be detected and treated promptly. Mean arterial pressure is ideally maintained at about 80 mm Hg with adequate pumping.

Peripheral ischemia. The most common complication of IABP is lower extremity ischemia secondary to occlusion of the femoral artery, either by the catheter itself or by emboli from thrombus formation on the balloon.[77] Consequently, the presence and quality of peripheral pulses distal to the catheter insertion site are assessed frequently, along with color, temperature, and capillary refill of the involved extremity. Doppler localization of peripheral pulses may be required if pulses are difficult to palpate on the cannulated extremity. Signs of diminished perfusion must be reported immediately. Anticoagulation, such as a heparin infusion, may be prescribed to decrease the incidence of thrombosis. Other vascular complications of IABP include acute aortic dissection and the development of pseudoaneurysms at the catheter insertion site.

Balloon perforation. Another potential complication of IAB therapy is balloon perforation. Perforation occurs secondary to repeated contact of the balloon membrane with calcified plaque in the aorta as the balloon inflates and deflates. The patient is monitored for evidence of a balloon leak, such as a gas leak alarm from the pump console and the presence of blood in the IAB tubing. If a balloon leak is detected, pumping is stopped and the physician immediately notified so that the balloon can be removed. If the balloon isn't promptly removed or pumping is attempted after the perforation, the IAB may become entrapped as the blood hardens within the catheter, creating a mass. If this occurs, the balloon must be surgically removed.

Balloon catheter position. The balloon catheter must be maintained in proper position to optimize its effectiveness and minimize complications. The balloon may migrate proximally and occlude the left subclavian artery, or it may move distally, compromising renal circulation. Therefore careful assessment of the left radial pulse and urinary output is essential. Measures to prevent accidental displacement of the balloon catheter include ensuring that the patient observes complete bedrest, with the head of the bed elevated no more than 30 degrees, and avoiding any flexion of the involved hip.

Preventing complications. Log rolling, in which the patient is moved from side to side every 2 hours, is used to maintain skin integrity and to prevent pulmonary atelectasis. Some institutional protocols call for implementation of continuous lateral rotation therapy to help facilitate pulmonary toilet in the IAB patient. Since thrombocytopenia may occur as a result of mechanical destruction of the platelets by the pumping action of the balloon, platelet counts are closely monitored and the patient is observed for evidence of bleeding. Because infection of the insertion site is a potential complication, the IAB dressing is changed in accordance with the hospital policy for other invasive lines.

Psychologic needs. Finally, the psychologic needs of the patient must not be overlooked. Sleep deprivation

BOX 17-24 NURSING DIAGNOSIS AND MANAGEMENT

INTRAAORTIC BALLOON PUMP

- Decreased Cardiac Output related to alterations in preload, p. 590
- Decreased Cardiac Output related to alterations in afterload, p. 592
- Decreased Cardiac Output related to alterations in contractility, p. 592
- Decreased Cardiac Output related to alterations in heart rate, p. 593
- Activity Intolerance related to cardiopulmonary dysfunction, p. 596
- Altered Myocardial Tissue Perfusion related to acute myocardial ischemia, p. 595
- Altered Peripheral Tissue Perfusion related to decreased peripheral blood flow, p. 596
- Risk for Infection risk factor: invasive monitoring devices, p. 598
- Sleep Pattern Disturbance related to circadian desynchronization, p. 119
- Body Image Disturbance related to functional dependence on life-sustaining technology, p. 86
- Knowledge Deficit: Discharge Regimen related to lack of previous exposure to information, p. 61 (see Patient Education Box 17-25)

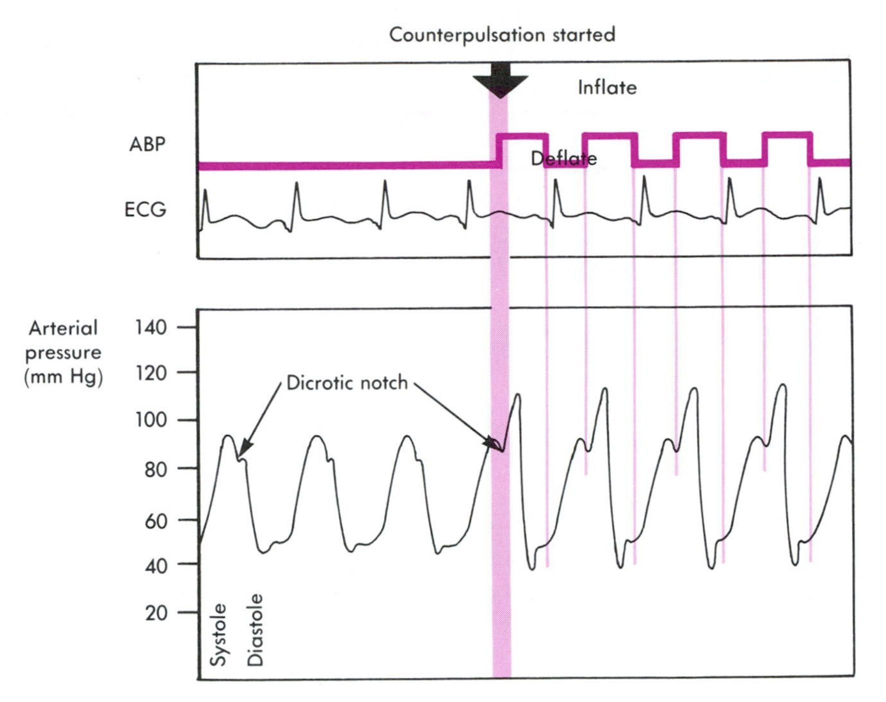

FIGURE 17-24. The timing and effect of balloon counterpulsations. Timing is adjusted by synchronizing balloon inflation with the dicrotic notch on the arterial waveform, resulting in an elevated diastolic pressure. Inflation is maintained throughout diastole, to augment coronary perfusion. Deflation occurs just before the next systole, resulting in a reduced systolic pressure and decreased afterload. (From Guzzetta CE, Dossey BM: *Cardiovascular nursing: holistic practice,* St Louis, 1992, Mosby.)

is not at all uncommon, partly caused by the continuous nursing management requirements of the patient but also related to the noise level in the unit, including the sounds made by the balloon pumping device. In addition, anxiety related to fear of not recovering and loss of control because of forced immobility are common occurrences. Pharmacologic agents such as midazolam (Versed) may be used to decrease patient anxiety and promote rest.

IABP weaning. Weaning from the balloon pump is considered when hemodynamic stability has been achieved with no, or only minimal, pharmacologic support. One weaning procedure consists of slowly decreasing the pumping frequency from every beat to every eighth beat, as tolerated. Decreasing balloon volume is another method of weaning.[77] To prevent thrombus formation on the balloon surface, the IABP must remain at a minimal pumping ratio (or volume) until its removal. Dependence on the balloon for more than 48 hours, indicative of severe cardiac dysfunction, usually is associated with a poor prognosis.

Patient education. Patient education for the IAB patient is presented in Box 17-25. Many of the IABP manufacturers provide helpful educational booklets designed for patients and families.

BOX 17-25 PATIENT EDUCATION

INTRAAORTIC BALLOON PUMP

- Description of the IABP and how it works
- Activity restrictions (minimize leg movement)
- Symptoms to report to the health care professional (pain in the back, leg, chest)

Ventricular Assist Devices

The ventricular assist device (VAD) is designed to support a failing natural heart with flow assistance. Diversion of varying amounts of systemic blood flow around a failing ventricle by means of an extracorporeal pump reduces cardiac workload while maintaining the circulation. VADs also can maintain adequate perfusion during periods of cardiac arrest.[78] Device selection is based on individual VAD capabilities and institutional preference (Table 17-8).

The VAD currently is indicated for two types of clinical applications. The first category of patients includes those who, despite aggressive medical therapy, continue to demonstrate persistent cardiac failure but who have the potential for regaining normal heart function if the heart is given time to rest. This category, termed

TABLE 17-8 Ventricular Assist Devices

Type	Example	Use	Description	Insertion
Centrifugal	Biomedicus	Univentricular or biventricular support	Blood is diverted to a cone-shaped pump head where blades rotate and propel blood back through return cannula via continuous (nonpulsatile) flow	Cannulate LA or femoral artery to aorta for LVAD Cannulate RA and PA for RVAD
Rotary	Hemopump	LV support	A propeller housed in the LV cannula draws blood from the LV and propels it into the aorta	Via femoral artery, across aortic valve, and into LV
Pneumatic	Thoratec	Univentricular or biventricular support	External pulsatile pump that uses a pressurized air sac to eject blood through outflow cannula	Cannulate LA and aorta for LVAD Cannulate RA and PA for RVAD Inflow through ventricular apex when cardiotomy is expected
	Abiomed BVS 5000	Univentricular or biventricular support	A two-chamber external pump with bladders that fill by gravity; blood pumps are positioned at a level relative to the patient	Cannulate LA and aorta for LVAD Cannulate RA and PA for RVAD
	TCI Heartmate	LVAD	A pneumatically driven, totally implantable pump with external drive console	Inflow from LV apex with outflow to aorta via graft
Electric	Novacor	LVAD	An electrically driven pulsatile pump that is implanted in an upper abdominal quadrant	Via LV apex and ascending aorta
	TCI Heartmate Vented Electric	LVAD	Totally implantable pump, powered by two 12-volt batteries or a direct power source	LV to aorta
Cardiopulmonary support	Bard CPS	Emergency resuscitation (e.g., supported angioplasty)	Femoral-femoral bypass; venous blood delivered to centrifugal pump that passes through normothermic heat exchanger to membrane oxygenator and back to patient	Percutaneous or cutdown insertion of catheters into femoral vein and femoral artery

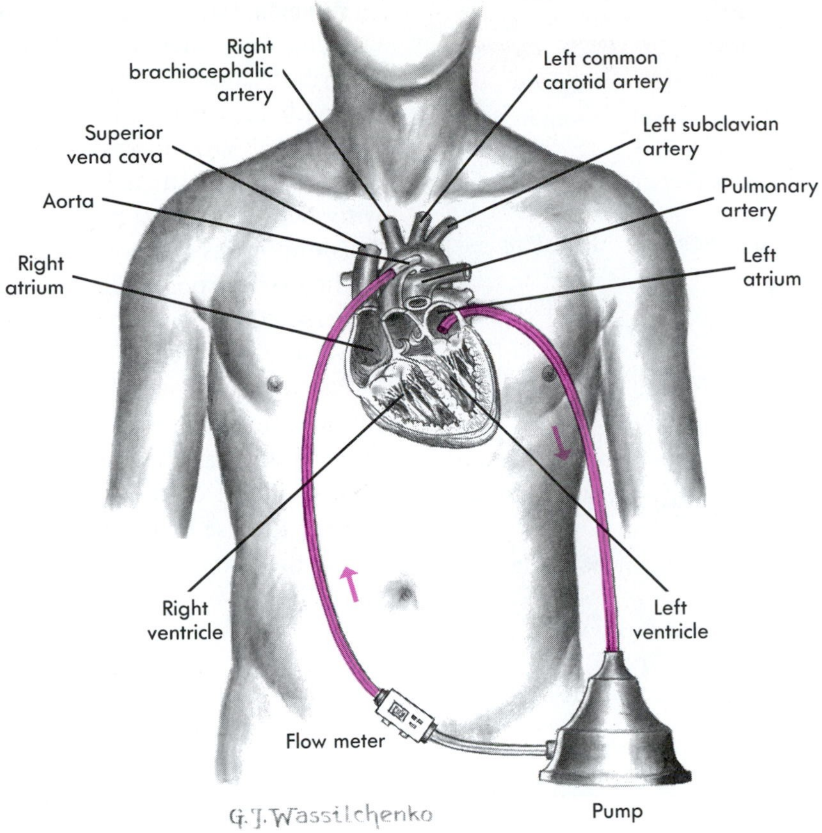

FIGURE 17-25. Conceptual diagram of a left centrifugal ventricular assist device (LVAD).

pending recovery, consists of patients who either cannot be weaned from cardiopulmonary bypass or are in refractory cardiogenic shock after AMI. The second category, termed *bridge to transplant,* includes those patients who need circulatory support until heart transplantation can be performed.[79]

The left ventricular assist device (LVAD) is used most commonly because left ventricular (LV) failure occurs more often than does right ventricular (RV) failure. Use of biventricular support (bi-VAD) is becoming more common because RV failure often follows LV failure.[80] Outflow cannulas that divert blood from the heart to the LVAD for LV support are surgically placed in either the left atrium or LV apex depending on the indication for the device. For example, if the patient is "pending recovery" of the natural heart, preservation of LV function mandates left atrial cannulation. The right atrium is cannulated for outflow for right ventricular support. Inflow back to the heart from the pump is accomplished by cannulation of the aorta or femoral artery for the LVAD and pulmonary artery for the right ventricular assist device (RVAD). (See Figure 17-25 for cannula placement in LVAD configuration of the centrifugal pump.) Flow rates between 1 and 6 L/minute are used to maintain adequate cardiac output while decreasing ventricular workload.

Nursing management. Nursing diagnosis and management for a patient with a ventricular assist device includes monitoring for hemodynamic changes as well as for complications related to the device (Box 17-26). The same interventions to optimize cardiac output by manipulation of heart rate, preload, afterload, and contractility that are used with cardiac surgery patients apply to patients with a VAD. Adequate filling volumes are required to maintain pump flow. Afterload reduction may be needed to improve output from the unassisted ventricle when univentricular support is used.

Device failure. Because of the life-saving nature of this therapy, device failure is a life-threatening event. Since VAD designs vary considerably, troubleshooting methods for device failure are unique to each device.

Anticoagulation. The requirement for anticoagulation varies with the type of VAD, the flow rate, and institutional protocol. If patients are anticoagulated with heparin, nurses are responsible for maintaining

BOX 17-26 NURSING DIAGNOSIS AND MANAGEMENT

VENTRICULAR ASSIST DEVICE

- Decreased Cardiac Output related to alterations in preload, p. 590
- Decreased Cardiac Output related to alterations in afterload, p. 592
- Decreased Cardiac Output related to alterations in contractility, p. 592
- Decreased Cardiac Output related to alterations in heart rate, p. 593
- Activity Intolerance related to cardiopulmonary dysfunction, p. 596
- Altered Myocardial Tissue Perfusion related to acute myocardial ischemia, p. 595
- Risk for Infection risk factor: invasive monitoring devices, p. 598
- Sleep Pattern Disturbance related to circadian desynchronization, p. 119
- Body Image Disturbance related to functional dependence on life-sustaining technology, p. 86
- Knowledge Deficit: Discharge Regimen related to lack of previous exposure to information, p. 61 (see Patient Education Box 17-27)

the activated clotting time (ACT) within a therapeutic range and monitoring for complications of bleeding. If bleeding occurs, additional coagulation studies, such as partial thromboplastin time (PTT), prothrombin time (PT), and fibrinogen and platelet counts, may be performed. Continued bleeding may necessitate holding the heparin infusion and administering fresh frozen plasma and platelets. If patients are not anticoagulated, the risk of thrombi obstructing a VAD cannula increases, as does the risk of an embolic event.

Infection. Patients with a VAD are at considerable risk for infection. The most common infection is pneumonia secondary to immobility and the need for ventilatory support. Other infectious risks are posed by the presence of invasive catheters and the surgically implanted VAD. Infection is prevented by using strict aseptic technique with all invasive tubing and dressing changes. Site care varies, depending on institutional protocols and the type of ventricular assist device that is used. Nurses monitor patients for infection by obtaining temperatures, inspecting insertion sites and incisions, and following daily leukocyte counts. If an infection is suspected, pan-cultures (blood, urine, and sputum) are taken to guide appropriate antibiotic therapy.

Weaning. Weaning is accomplished by gradually decreasing flow rates to allow the patient's ventricle to contribute more to total blood flow. Controversy exists with regard to anticoagulation; however, during weaning of VAD flow rates to less than 2 L/minute, ACTs are maintained between 160 and 480 seconds with heparin, depending on institutional protocols. This minimizes the potential for thrombus formation in the extracorporeal circuit during weaning but also increases the risk of bleeding and therefore necessitates close monitoring.

Patient education. The rapid and acute nature of cardiogenic shock limits the nurse's ability to prepare patients and families for VAD insertion. Despite the critical nature of the illness, nurses explain the reason for the use of the VAD and provide information about the critical care environment and equipment (Box 17-27).

EFFECTS OF CARDIOVASCULAR DRUGS

Multiple medications are used in the treatment of critically ill cardiovascular patients. The critical care nurse is responsible for preparation and administration of these drugs and often is required to titrate the dose on the basis of the patient's hemodynamic response. The medications used to treat cardiovascular disease are rapidly changing and expanding as more is learned about the pathophysiology of cardiac disease and as improved formulas are developed by pharmaceutical companies. The critical care nurse who has a general understanding of the mechanisms of action of the various drug classifications can readily apply this knowledge to new drugs within the same classification. The following discussion provides a concise review of drugs commonly administered to support cardiovascular function in the critical care setting. The emphasis is on intravenously administered medications that are used for the acute, rather than the chronic, management of cardiovascular conditions.

Antidysrhythmic Drugs

Antidysrhythmic drugs comprise a diverse category of pharmacologic agents used to terminate or prevent an array of abnormal cardiac rhythms. These drugs commonly are classified according to their primary effect on the action potential of cardiac cells (Figure 17-26). The classification scheme shown in Table 17-9 is the most commonly used system. Classification of newer agents becomes more difficult because some of these agents have characteristics of more than one class

BOX 17-27 PATIENT EDUCATION

VENTRICULAR ASSIST DEVICE

- Description of the ventricular assist device and how it works (VAD specific)
- Activity restrictions during VAD therapy
- Symptoms to report to the health care professional

and others have no characteristics of the current system. (∞Cardiac Action Potential, p. 344.)

Class I drugs. Class I agents are sodium channel blockers that decrease the influx of sodium ions through "fast" channels during phase 0 depolarization. This prolongs the absolute (effective) refractory period, thus decreasing the risk of premature impulses from ectopic foci. In addition, these drugs depress automaticity by slowing the rate of spontaneous depolarizations of pacemaker cells during the resting phase (phase 4).

Class I drugs can be further subdivided into three groups, according to their potency as sodium channel inhibitors and their effect on phase 3 repolarization.[81] Class IA agents—quinidine, procainamide, and disopyramide—block not only the fast sodium channels but also phase 3 repolarization and thereby prolong the action potential duration. Clinically, this may result in measurable increases in the QRS duration and the QT interval. All class IA agents may depress myocardial contractility, with disopyramide having the most potent negative inotropic effect.[82] Drugs in class IB have only a moderate effect on sodium channels and actually accelerate phase 3 repolarization to shorten the action potential duration; lidocaine, mexiletine, and tocainide belong in this group. Class IC agents are the most potent sodium channel blockers, with little effect on repolarization. Class IC drugs increase both the PR and the QRS intervals. Included in this group are encainide, flecainide, and propafenone. The results of the Cardiac Arrhythmia Suppression Trial (CAST) indicated that treatment with encainide and flecainide may be associated with increased mortality and have thus decreased the use of these agents in clinical practice.[83]

Class II drugs. Class II drugs are beta-adrenergic blockers (beta-blockers). These agents inhibit dysrhythmias mediated by the sympathetic nervous system by competing with endogenous catecholamines for available receptor sites. As a result, spontaneous depolarization during the resting phase (phase 4) is depressed and atrioventricular conduction is slowed.

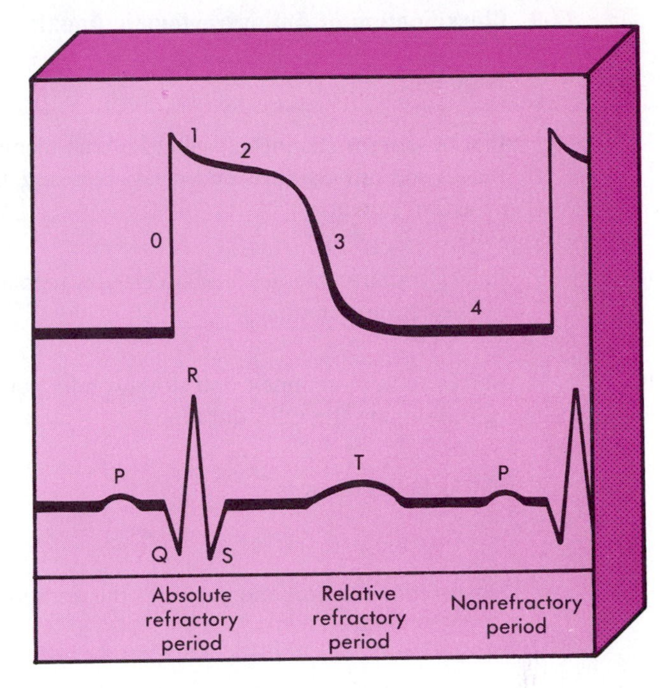

FIGURE 17-26. The phases of the cardiac action potential and their relationship to the heart's refractory periods. *Phase 0,* Depolarization—rapid influx of sodium. *Phase 1,* Rapid repolarization—rapid eflux of potassium ions and decreased sodium conductance. *Phase 2,* Plateau—slow influx of sodium and calcium ions. *Phase 3,* Repolarization—continued eflux of potassium ions. *Phase 4,* Resting phase—restoration of ionic balance by sodium and potassium pumps.

Drugs in this class can be further subdivided into cardioselective (those that block only $beta_1$ receptors) and noncardioselective (those that block both $beta_1$ and $beta_2$ receptors). Knowledge of the effects of adrenergic-receptor stimulation allows for anticipation of not only the therapeutic responses brought about by beta-blockade but also the potential adverse effects of these agents (Table 17-10). For example, bronchospasm can be precipitated by noncardioselective beta-blockers in a patient with chronic obstructive pulmonary disease (COPD) secondary to blocking the effects of $beta_2$ receptors in the lungs. Beta-blockers also are negative inotropes and must be used cautiously in patients with left ventricular dysfunction. Although numerous beta-blockers are available, only esmolol, metoprolol, and propranolol are available as intravenous agents for the treatment of acute dysrhythmias. Of these, esmolol (Brevibloc) offers significant advantages in the critically ill patient because of its short half-life (approximately 9 minutes). It is used in the treatment of supraventricular tachycardias, such as atrial fibrillation and atrial flutter.

TABLE 17-9 Classification of Antidysrhythgmic Agents

Class	Action	Drugs
I	Blocks sodium channels ("stabilizes" cell membrane)	
IA	Blocks sodium channels and delays repolarization, thus lengthening the duration of the action potential	Quinidine Procainamide Disopyramide
IB	Blocks sodium channels and accelerates repolarization, thus shortening the duration of the action potential	Lidocaine Mexiletine Tocainide
IC	Blocks sodium channels and slows conduction through the His-Purkinje system, thus prolonging the QRS duration	Flecainide Encainide Propafenone
II	Blocks beta receptors	Esmolol Metoprolol Propranolol
III	Slows repolarization and prolongs the duration of the action potential	Amiodarone Ibutilide Sotalol
IV	Blocks calcium channels	Diltiazem Verapamil

Class III drugs. Class III agents include amiodarone, bretylium, ibutilide, and sotalol. These agents markedly slow the rate of phase 3 repolarization, increasing the effective refractory period and the action potential duration. Although their effect on the action potential is similar, these drugs differ greatly in their mechanism of action and their side effects. At this time, sotalol is approved only for oral use. Intravenous bretylium is used in the treatment of life-threatening ventricular dysrhythmias that are refractory to other antidysrhythmic agents, such as lidocaine and procainamide.[6] Amiodarone has only recently been approved for intravenous use in the United States. It is considered a second-line therapy for serious ventricular dysrhythmias that are refractory to other medications.[84] Ibutilide (Covert) is a short-term antidysrhythmic agent used for the rapid conversion of acute atrial fibrillation or atrial flutter to sinus rhythm. The drug is administered as a 10-minute infusion in a carefully monitored clinical setting. The most serious side effect of ibutilide is its potential for inducing life-threatening dysrhythmias, especially torsades de pointes.[85]

Class IV drugs. Class IV agents are calcium channel blockers that inhibit the influx of calcium through slow calcium channels during the plateau phase (phase 2). This effect occurs primarily in tissue in which slow calcium channels predominate, primarily in the sinus and atrioventricular (AV) nodes and the atrial tissue. Verapamil was the first drug in this category available as an intravenous antidysrhythmic. It depresses sinus and AV node conduction and is effective in terminating supraventricular tachycardias caused by AV nodal reentry.[81] Recently, diltiazem (Cardizem) has become available in IV form. Studies suggest that diltiazem may be as effective as verapamil in treating supraventricular dysrhythmias, with fewer hypotensive side effects.[86] Because accessory pathways are not affected by calcium channel blockade, both of these agents must be avoided in the treatment of atrial fibrillation for patients with Wolff-Parkinson-White syndrome.[87]

Unclassified antidysrhythmics. Adenosine (Adenocard) is a newer antidysrhythmic agent that remains unclassified under the current system. Adenosine occurs endogenously in the body as a building block of adenosine triphosphate (ATP). Given in intravenous boluses, adenosine slows conduction through the AV node, causing transient AV block. It is used clinically to convert supraventricular tachycardias and to facilitate differential diagnosis of rapid dysrhythmias. Be-

TABLE 17-10 Effects of Adrenergic Receptors

Receptor	Location	Response to Stimulation
alpha	Vessels of skin, muscles, kidneys, and intestines	Vasoconstriction of peripheral arterioles
$beta_1$	Cardiac tissue	Increased heart rate Increased conduction Increased contractility
$beta_2$	Vascular and bronchial smooth muscle	Vasodilation of peripheral arterioles Bronchodilation

cause of its short half-life, the drug is administered intravenously as a rapid bolus, followed by a saline flush. The bolus is delivered as centrally as possible, so that the drug reaches the heart before it is metabolized.[88] Side effects are transient because the drug is rapidly taken up by the cells and is cleared from the body within 10 seconds.

Magnesium is also unclassified under the present system. Though its action as an antidysrhythmic agent is not entirely understood, clinical studies suggest that it may reduce the incidence of both ventricular and supraventricular dysrhythmias in selected patient populations. It is considered the treatment of choice in patients with torsades de pointes. For acute treatment 1 to 2 g of magnesium is administered over 1 to 2 minutes. In patients with confirmed hypomagnesemia, this bolus may be followed with a 24-hour infusion.[89]

Side effects. Antidysrhythmic drugs carry the risk of serious side effects, some of which may be life threatening. The major side effects of the intravenous antidysrhythmic agents are listed in Table 17-11. The most severe complication is the potential for a "prodysrhythmic" effect. This may result in a worsening of the underlying dysrhythmia, the occurrence of a new dysrhythmia, or the development of a bradydysrhythmia. Torsades de pointes is a prodysrhythmia caused by Class IA agents.[89] The development of a prodysrhythmia is unpredictable; thus the nurse plays an important role in evaluating ECG changes, monitoring drug levels, and assessing patient symptoms. Antidysrhythmic agents may also alter the amount of energy required for defibrillation and pacing. For example, increases in an antidysrhythmic dose may increase the amount of output (mA) required to depolarize the myocardium.

Inotropic Drugs

Critically ill patients with compromised cardiac function frequently require the use of medications to enhance myocardial contractility (positive inotropes). Clinically available inotropes include cardiac glycosides, sympathomimetics, and phosphodiesterase inhibitors. These agents increase myocardial contractility, resulting in improved cardiac output, more complete emptying of the ventricles, and decreased filling pressures.

Cardiac glycosides include digitalis and its derivatives. Although these drugs have been used for centuries, their slow onset of action and risk of toxicity make them more appropriate for the management of chronic heart failure. Because digoxin also causes slowing of the sinus rate and a decrease in AV conduction, it may be administered intravenously in the acute care setting to control supraventricular dysrhythmias.

Sympathomimetic agents stimulate adrenergic receptors, thereby simulating the effects of sympathetic nerve stimulation. Included in this category are naturally occurring catecholamines (epinephrine, dopamine, and norepinephrine), as well as synthetic catecholamines (dobutamine and isoproterenol). The cardiovascular effects of these drugs, which vary according to their selectivity for specific receptor sites, are often dose-dependent as well.[90] Table 17-12 describes the cardiovascular effects of sympathomimetic drugs at various dosages.

Dopamine. Dopamine (Intropin) is one of the most widely used drugs in the critical care setting. It is a chemical precursor of norepinephrine, which, in addition to both alpha- and beta-receptor stimulation, can activate dopaminergic receptors in the renal and mesenteric blood vessels. The actions of this drug are entirely dose-related.[6] At low dosages of 1 to 2 μg/kg/min, dopamine stimulates dopaminergic receptors, causing renal and mesenteric vasodilation. The resultant increase in renal perfusion increases urinary output. Moderate dosages result in stimulation of $beta_1$ receptors to increase myocardial contractility and improve cardiac output. At dosages greater than 10 μg/kg/min, dopamine predominantly stimulates alpha receptors, resulting in vasoconstriction that often negates both the beta-adrenergic and dopaminergic effects.

Dobutamine. Dobutamine (Dobutrex) is a synthetic catecholamine with predominantly $beta_1$ effects. It also produces some $beta_2$ stimulation, resulting in a mild vasodilation. Dobutamine is as effective as dopamine in increasing myocardial contractility, but it lacks the dopaminergic effects of that drug. Dobutamine is useful in the treatment of heart failure,

TABLE 17-11 Pharmacology of Selected Antidysrhythmic Agents

Drug/Site of Action	Indications	Dosage	Major Side Effects
SINUS NODE, ATRIA, OR AV NODE			
Adenosine	SVT, PSVT	6.0 mg IV rapid push, repeat with 12 mg over 1-2 sec; follow with IV fluid (NS or D5W)	Transient: flushing, dyspnea, hypotension
Digoxin	AFib, AF, PSVT	0.5-1.0 mg loading dose in divided doses; maintenance dose of 0.125-0.375 mg q day	Bradycardia, heart block Toxicity: CNS and GI symptoms
Diltiazem	SVT, AFib, AF	Bolus dose of 0.25 mg/kg IV over 2 min, followed by an infusion of 5.0-15 mg/h	Bradycardia, hypotension, AV block
Esmolol	ST, SVT	Loading dose of 500 μg/kg/min over 1 min, followed by an infusion of 50 μg/kg/min for 4 min; repeat procedure q 5 min, increasing infusion by 25-50 μg/kg/min to maximum of 200 μg/kg/min	Hypotension, bradycardia, heart failure
Ibutilide	AFib, AF	0.010-0.025 mg/kg infused over 10 min (may repeat once)	Minimal side effects except for polymorphic VT (torsades de pointes)
Propranolol	SVT	1.0-3.0 mg IV q 5 min not to exceed 0.1 mg/kg	Bradycardia, heart block, heart failure
Verapamil	AF, PSVT	5.0-10 mg IV, may repeat in 15-30 min	Hypotension, bradycardia, heart failure
VENTRICLE			
Bretylium	Refractory VF VT	5.0 mg/kg IV bolus, followed by 10 mg/kg dosages repeated at 15-30 min intervals for total of 30 mg/kg; or 500 mg in 50 ml D5W to infuse over 8-10 min, then continuous infusions at 1.0-2.0 mg/min	Initially: hypertension, tachycardia, PVCs Subsequently: hypotension, bradycardia, nausea and vomiting
Lidocaine	PVCs, VT, VF	1.0-1.5 mg/kg bolus, followed by continuous infusion of 1.0-4.0 mg/min	CNS toxicity, nausea, vomiting with repeated doses
ATRIA AND VENTRICLE			
Amiodarone	Refractory VT (effective in AFib and AF)	5.0-10 mg/kg slowly IV, followed by an infusion of 10 mg/kg/day for 3-5 days	Hypotension, abnormal liver function tests
Procainamide	AF, SVT, PVCs, VT	Loading dose of 12-17 mg/kg at a rate of 50 mg/min, followed by infusion of 1.0-4.0 mg/min	Hypotension, GI effects Widening of QRS and QT

SVT, Supraventricular tachycardia; PSVT, paroxysmal supraventricular tachycardia; AFib, atrial fibrillation; AF, atrial flutter; CNS, central nervous system; VT, ventricular tachycardia; VF, ventricular fibrillation; PVC, premature ventricular contraction.

especially in hypotensive patients who cannot tolerate vasodilator therapy. The usual dosage range is 2.5 to 20 μg/kg/min, titrated on the basis of hemodynamic parameters.

Epinephrine. Epinephrine (Adrenalin) is produced by the adrenal gland as part of the body's response to stress. This agent has the ability to stimulate both alpha and beta receptors, depending on the dose administered (see Table 17-12). At doses of 1 to 2 μg/min, epinephrine binds with beta receptors to increase heart rate, cardiac conduction, contractility, and vasodilation, thereby increasing cardiac output. As the dosage is increased, alpha receptors are stimulated, resulting in increased vascular resistance and blood pressure. At these doses epinephrine's impact on cardiac output depends on the heart's ability to pump against the in-

TABLE 17-12 Physiologic Effects of Sympathomimetic Agents

		Receptor Activated				Cardiovascular Effects		
Drug	Dosage	Alpha	Beta$_1$	Beta$_2$	Dopa	CO	HR	SVR
Dobutamine	<5 μg/kg/min	0	↑↑↑	↑	0	↑↑	↑	0/↓
	5-20 μg/kg/min	0	↑↑↑	↑↑	0	↑↑↑	↑↑	↓
	>20 μg/kg/min	0	↑↑↑	↑↑	0	↑↑↑	↑↑↑	↓↓
Dopamine	<3 μg/kg/min	0	↑	↑	↑↑↑	0/↑	0/↑	0
	3-10 μg/kg/min	↑	↑↑↑	↑	↑↑↑	↑↑↑	↑	↑
	11-20 μg/kg/min	↑↑	↑↑↑	↑	↑↑	↑↑	↑↑	↑↑↑
	>20 μg/kg/min	↑↑↑↑	↑↑	↑	↑	↑	↑	↑↑↑↑
Epinephrine	<2 μg/min	0	↑	↑↑	0	0/↑	0/↑	↓
	2-8 μg/min	↑↑	↑↑↑	↑↑	0	↑↑↑	↑	↑
	9-20 μg/min	↑↑↑	↑↑	↑↑	0	↑↑	↑↑	↑↑
Isoproterenol	1-7 μg/min	0	↑↑↑	↑↑↑	0	↑↑↑	↑↑↑	↓↓↓
Norepinephrine	<2 μg/min	↑↑↑	↑↑	0	0	↑	0/↓	↑↑↑
	2-16 μg/min	↑↑↑↑	↑↑	0	0	↓	↓	↑↑↑↑
Phenylephrine	10-100 μg/min	↑↑↑↑	0	0	0	0/↓	↓	↑↑↑

NOTE: Refer to Table 17-10, p. 577, for actions of receptors.
CO, Cardiac output; HR, heart rate; SVR, systemic vascular resistance; 0, no effect; ↑, increased; ↓, decreased (the number of arrows indicates the degree of effect [e.g., ↑ = mild and ↑↑↑↑ = strong effect.]).

creased afterload. Epinephrine accelerates the sinus rate and may precipitate ventricular dysrhythmias in the ischemic heart. Other side effects include restlessness, angina, and headache.

Norepinephrine. Norepinephrine (Levophed) is similar to epinephrine in its ability to stimulate beta$_1$ and alpha receptors, but it lacks the beta$_2$ effects. At low infusion rates, beta$_1$ receptors are activated to produce increased contractility and thus augment cardiac output. At higher doses the inotropic effects are limited by marked vasoconstriction mediated by alpha receptors. Clinically, norepinephrine is used most often as a vasopressor to elevate blood pressure in shock states.

Isoproterenol. Isoproterenol (Isuprel) is a pure beta-receptor stimulant with no alpha effects. It produces dramatic increases in heart rate, conduction, and contractility via beta$_1$ stimulation and vasodilation via beta$_2$ stimulation. Isoproterenol also produces vasodilation of the pulmonary arteries and bronchodilation. It greatly increases the automaticity of cardiac cells and frequently precipitates dysrhythmias, such as premature ventricular contractions and even ventricular tachycardia. These effects limit its usefulness in the compromised heart. Its most common use is as a temporary treatment for symptomatic bradycardia until a pacemaker is available.

Phosphodiesterase inhibitors. Phosphodiesterase inhibitors are a new group of inotropic agents that also are potent vasodilators. Drugs in this classification inhibit the enzyme phosphodiesterase, resulting in increased levels of cyclic adenosine monophosphate (AMP) and intracellular calcium. *Amrinone* (Inocor) and *milrinone* (Primacor) were the first of these agents approved for use in the United States. Increases in cardiac output occur as a result of increased contractility (inotropic effects) and decreased afterload (vasodilative effects). Filling pressures tend to decrease, whereas the heart rate and blood pressure remain fairly constant. Amrinone may cause thrombocytopenia, so platelet counts are monitored and patients observed for hemorrhagic complications.[89] Milrinone is associated with a lower rate of thrombocytopenia but can induce ventricular dysrhythmias (premature ventricular complexes, ventricular tachycardia) in a significant number of patients.

Vasodilator Drugs

Vasodilators are pharmacologic agents that improve cardiac performance by various degrees of arterial or venous dilation, or both. The goal of vasodilator therapy may be a reduction of preload or afterload, or both. Afterload reduction is accomplished by vasodilation of arterial vessels. This results in decreased resistance to left ventricular ejection and may improve cardiac output without increasing myocardial oxygen demands. Reduction of preload is accomplished by dilating venous vessels to increase capacitance. This results in decreased filling pressures for a failing heart. These drugs may be classified into four groups on the basis of mechanism of action (Table 17-13).

Direct smooth muscle relaxants. Direct-acting vasodilators include sodium nitroprusside (Nipride), nitroglycerin (Tridil), and hydralazine (Apresoline). These drugs produce relaxation of vascular smooth muscle, resulting in decreased peripheral vascular resistance. Hypotension may occur as a result of peripheral vasodilation, and headaches may be caused by cerebral vasodilation. Compensatory mechanisms can occur in response to the drop in blood pressure. These include baroreceptor activation that causes reflex tachycardia and activation of the renin-angiotensin-aldosterone system, with resultant sodium and water retention.[91]

Sodium nitroprusside (Nipride) is a potent, rapidly acting venous and arterial vasodilator, particularly suitable for rapid reduction of blood pressure in hypertensive emergencies and perioperatively. It also is effective for afterload reduction in the setting of severe heart failure. The drug is administered by continuous intravenous infusion, with the dosage titrated to maintain the desired blood pressure and systemic vascular resistance (SVR). Prolonged administration can result in thiocyanate toxicity, manifested by nausea, confusion, and tinnitus.[90]

Intravenous nitroglycerin (Tridil) causes both arterial and venous vasodilation, but its venous effect is more pronounced. It is used in the critical care setting for the treatment of acute heart failure (HF) because it reduces cardiac filling pressures, relieves pulmonary congestion, and decreases cardiac workload and oxygen consumption. In addition, nitroglycerin dilates the coronary arteries and is a useful adjunct in the treatment of unstable angina and acute myocardial infarction. The initial dosage is 10 μg/minute, and the infusion is titrated upward to achieve the desired clinical effect: a reduction or elimination of chest pain, decreased pulmonary artery wedge pressure (PAWP), or a decrease in blood pressure. Nitroglycerin also is administered prophylactically to prevent coronary vasospasm after coronary angioplasty, atherectomy, stent insertion, or thrombolytic therapy. The most common side effects of this drug include hypotension, flushing, and headache.[92] *Hydralazine* (Apresoline) is a potent arterial vasodilator. It seldom is given as a continuous infusion, but rather in intravenously administered dosages of 5 to 10 mg every 4 to 8 hours. Occasionally, hydralazine is given as an intermediate drug in the transition between the weaning of a continuous infusion and the initiation of oral antihypertensive medications. The major side effect is reflex tachycardia mediated by the sympathetic nervous system. This may be diminished by the concomitant administration of beta-blockers.

Calcium channel blockers. Calcium channel blockers are a chemically diverse group of drugs with differing pharmacologic effects (Table 17-14).

Nifedipine (Procardia) and *nicardipine* (Cardene) are dihydropyridines. This group of calcium channel blockers (with the suffix "pine") is used primarily as arterial vasodilators. These drugs reduce the influx of calcium in the arterial resistance vessels. Both coronary and peripheral arteries are affected. They are used in the critical care setting to treat hypertension. Nifedipine is available in an oral form only but often is prescribed sublingually. Although controversy exists over the absorption of sublingual nifedipine, studies indicate that if the drug is bitten before swallowing, the drug is absorbed more quickly.[93] Nicardipine recently became available as an intravenous calcium channel blocker, and as such it offers more accurate titration for effective control of hypertension.[94]

Side effects of nifedipine and nicardipine are related to vasodilation and include hypotension, reflex tachycardia, flushing, headache, and ankle edema.

Verapamil (Calan, Isoptin) and *diltiazem* (Cardizem) are part of another group of calcium channel blockers with differing functions. These drugs dilate coronary arteries but have little effect on the peripheral vasculature. They are used in the treatment of angina, especially that which has a vasospastic component, and as antidysrhythmics in the treatment of supraventricular tachycardias.

ACE inhibitors. Angiotensin-converting enzyme (ACE) inhibitors produce vasodilation by blocking the conversion of angiotensin I to angiotensin II. Because angiotensin is a potent vasoconstrictor, limiting its production decreases peripheral vascular resistance. In contrast to the direct vasodilators and nifedipine, ACE inhibitors do not cause reflex tachycardia nor induce sodium and water retention. However, these drugs may cause a profound fall in blood pressure, especially in patients who are volume-depleted. Blood pressure must be monitored carefully, especially during initiation of therapy.[95]

Captopril (Capoten) and *enalapril* (Vasotec) are used in patients with heart failure to decrease SVR (afterload) and pulmonary artery wedge pressure (pre-

TABLE 17-13 Characteristics of Selected Vasodilators

Drug Classification	Dosage	Preload	Afterload	Side Effects
DIRECT SMOOTH MUSCLE RELAXANTS				
Sodium nitroprusside (Nipride)	0.25-6.0 μg/kg/min IV infusion	Moderate	Strong	Hypotension, thiocyanate toxicity, reflex tachycardia
Nitroglycerin (Tridil)	5.0-300 μg/min IV infusion	Strong	Mild	Headache, reflex tachycardia, hypotension
CALCIUM CHANNEL BLOCKERS				
Nicardipine (Cardene)	5.0 mg/hr IV, titrated to 15 mg/hr	None	Strong	Hypotension, headache, reflex tachycardia
Nifedipine (Procardia)	10-30 mg SL	None	Strong	Hypotension, headache, reflex tachycardia
ACE INHIBITORS				
Captopril (Capoten)	6.25-100 mg PO q 8-12 hr	Moderate	Moderate	Hypotension, chronic cough, neutropenia
Enalapril (Vasotec)	0.625 mg IV over 5 min, then q 6 hr	Moderate	Moderate	Hypotension, elevation of liver enzymes
ALPHA-ADRENERGIC BLOCKERS				
Labetalol (Normodyne)	20-80 mg IV bolus q 10 min, then 1.0-2.0 mg/min infusion	Moderate	Moderate	Orthostatic hypotension, bronchospasm, AV block
Phentolamine (Regitine)	1.0-2.0 mg/min infusion	Moderate	Moderate	Hypotension, tachycardia

ACE, Angiotensin-converting enzyme; *SL,* sublingual; *PO,* by mouth.

TABLE 17-14 Characteristics of Calcium Channel Blockers

Drug	Actions	Dosage	Special Considerations
DIHYDROPYRIDINES			
Nicardipine (Cardene)	Short-term control of hypertension	5.0 mg/hr IV, titrated to 15 mg/hr	Hypotension, headache, nausea
Nifedipine (Procardia)	Hypertension	10-30 mg SL	Hypotension, headache, reflex tachycardia
BENZOTHIAZEPINES			
Diltiazem (Cardizem)	SVT, AFib, AF, angina	Bolus dose of 0.25 mg/kg IV over 2 min, followed by an infusion of 5.0-15 mg/hr	Bradycardia, hypotension, AV block
PHENYLALKYLAMINES			
Verapamil (Calan, Isoptin)	AF, PSVT	5.0-10 mg IV, may repeat in 15-30 min	Hypotension, bradycardia, heart failure

SVT, Supraventricular tachycardia; *AFib,* atrial fibrillation; *AF,* atrial flutter; *AV,* atrioventricular; *PSVT,* paroxysmal supraventricular tachycardia.

load). Captopril is available in an oral form only but has a relatively rapid onset of action (approximately 1 hour). Enalapril is available in an intravenous form and may be used to decrease afterload in more emergent situations.

Alpha-adrenergic blockers. Peripheral adrenergic blockers block alpha receptors and veins, resulting in vasodilation. Orthostatic hypotension is a common side effect and may result in syncope. Long-term therapy also may be complicated by fluid and water retention.[91]

Labetalol (Normodyne), a combined alpha- and beta-blocker, is used in the treatment of hypertensive emergencies. Because the blockade of $beta_1$ receptors permits the decrease of blood pressure without the risk of reflexive tachycardia and increased cardiac output, this drug also is useful in the treatment of acute aortic dissection.

Phentolamine (Regitine) is a peripheral alpha-blocker that causes decreased afterload via arterial vasodilation. It is given as a continuous infusion at a rate of 1 to 2 mg/minute and is titrated to achieve the required reduction in blood pressure and SVR.[90] This drug also is used to treat the extravasation of dopamine. If this occurs, 5 to 10 mg is diluted in 10 ml normal saline and administered intradermally into the infiltrated area.

Vasopressors. Vasopressors are sympathomimetic agents that mediate peripheral vasoconstriction through stimulation of alpha-receptors (see Table 17-12). This results in increased systemic vascular resistance and thus elevates blood pressure. Some of these drugs (epinephrine and norepinephrine) also have the ability to stimulate beta receptors. Vasopressors are not widely used in the treatment of critically ill cardiac patients, because the dramatic increase in afterload is taxing to a damaged heart. Occasionally, vasopressors may be used to maintain organ perfusion in shock states. For example, *phenylephrine* (Neo-Synephrine) or *norepinephrine* (Levophed) may be administered as a continuous intravenous infusion to maintain organ perfusion by increasing peripheral vascular resistance in the warm phase of septic shock.

REFERENCES

1. Darling EJ: Overview of cardiac electrophysiologic testing, *Crit Care Clinics North Am* 6(1):1, 1994.
2. Zipes DP and others: Guidelines for clinical intracardiac electrophysiological and catheter ablation procedures (ACC/AHA task force report), *J Am Coll Cardiol* 26(2):555, 1995.
3. Fischer JD and others: Catheter ablation for cardiac arrhythmias: clinical applications, personnel and facilities (ACC position statement), *J Am Coll Cardiol* 24(3):828, 1994.
4. Bumgarner LI: Diagnostic uses of epicardial electrodes after cardiac surgery, *Prog Cardiovasc Nurs* 7(4):21, 1992.
5. Moses HW and others: *A practical guide to cardiac pacing,* ed 4, Boston, 1995, Little, Brown.
6. American Heart Association: *Textbook of advanced cardiac life support,* Dallas, 1994, The Association.
7. Manion PA: Temporary epicardial pacing in the postoperative cardiac surgical patient, *Crit Care Nurs* April:30, 1993.
8. Bernstein AD and others: The NASPE/BPEG generic pacemaker code for antibradycardia and adaptive rate pacing and antitachyarrhythmia devices, *Pacing Clin Electrophysiol* 10:794, 1987.
9. Vlay SC: *A practical approach to cardiac arrhythmias,* ed 4, Boston, 1995, Little, Brown.
10. Witherell CL: Cardiac rhythm control devices, *Crit Care Nurs Clin* 6(1):85, 1994.
11. Das G, Carlblom D: Artificial cardiac pacemakers, *Int J Clin Pharmacol Ther* 28:5, 1990.
12. St. Anthony's DRG guidebook, Reston, Va, 1996, St. Anthony.
13. Chauhan A and others: Early complications after dual chamber vs. single chamber pacemaker implantation. II. *Pacing Clin Electrophysiol* 17(11):2012, 1994.
14. Kirklin JW and others: ACC/AHA guidelines and indications for CABG surgery, *Circulation* 83:1125, 1991.
15. Alfieri O, Lorusso R: Developments in surgical techniques for coronary revascularization, *Curr Opin Cardiol* 10(6):556, 1995.
16. Jegaden O and others: Technical aspects and late functional results of gastroepiploic bypass grafting (400 cases), *Eur J Cardiothorac Surg* 9(10):575, 1995.
17. Pym J and others: Right gastroepiploic-to-coronary artery bypass: the first decade of use, *Circulation* 92(suppl 9):II45, 1995.
18. Dietl CA and others: Which is the graft of choice for the right coronary and posterior descending arteries? Comparison of the right internal mammary artery and the right gastroepiploic artery, *Circulation* 92(suppl 9):II92, 1995.
19. Brodman RF and others: Routine use of unilateral and bilateral radial arteries for coronary artery bypass graft surgery, *J Am Coll Cardiol* 28(40):959, 1996.
20. Atunes MJ: Mitral valve repair in the 1990s, *Eur J Cardiothorac Surg* 6(suppl 1):S13, 1992.
21. Jamieson WR: Modern cardiac valve devices—bioprotheses and mechanical prostheses: state of the art, *J Card Surg* 8(1):89, 1993.
22. Brown KK: Surgical therapy of chronic heart failure and severe ventricular dysfunction, *Crit Care Nurs Q* 18(1):45, 1995.
23. Buckberg GD: Update on current techniques of myocardial protection, *Ann Thorac Surg* 60:805, 1995.
24. Colquhoun IW and others: Arrhythmia prophylaxis after coronary artery surgery: a randomized controlled trial of intravenous magnesium chloride, *Eur J Cardiothorac Surg* 7(10):520, 1993.
25. Casthely PA and others: Magnesium and arrhythmias after coronary artery bypass surgery, *J Cardiothorac Vasc Anesth* 8(2):188, 1994.
26. Barden C, Hansen M: Cold versus warm cardioplegia: recognizing hemodynamic variations, *DCCN* 14(3):114, 1995.
27. Ley SJ: Intraoperative and postoperative blood salvage, *AACN Clin Issues Crit Care Nurs* 7(2):238, 1996.

28. Gross SB: Current challenges, concepts and controversies in chest tube management, *AACN Clin Issues Crit Care Nurs* 4(2):260, 1993.
29. Gross SB: Early extubation: preliminary experience in the cardiothoracic patient population, *Am J Crit Care* 4(4):262, 1995.
30. Maxam-Moore VA, Goedecke RS: The development of an early extubation algorithm for patients after cardiac surgery, *Heart Lung* 25(1):61, 1996.
31. Leahy NM: Neurologic complications after open heart surgery, *J Cardiovasc Nurs* 7(2):41, 1993.
32. Vaska PL: Sternal wound infections, *AACN Clin Issues Crit Care Nurs* 4(3):475, 1993.
33. Geha AS and others: Strategies in the surgical treatment of malignant ventricular arrhythmias: an 8 year experience, *Ann Surg,* 216(3):309, 1992.
34. Cox JL and others: Modification of the maze procedure for atrial flutter and atrial fibrillation. I. Rationale and surgical results, *J Thorac Cardiovasc Surg* 110(2):473, 1995.
35. Futterman LG, Lemberg L: An alternative to pharmacologic management of atrial fibrillation: the maze procedure, *Am J Crit Care* 3(3):238, 1994.
36. Bove LA and others: Nursing care of patients undergoing dynamic cardiomyoplasty, *Crit Care Nurs* June:96, 1995.
37. Vollman MW: Dynamic cardiomyoplasty: perspectives on nursing care and collaborative management, *Prog Cardiovasc Nurs* 10(2):15, 1995.
38. Futterman LG, Lemberg L: Cardiomyoplasty: a potential alternative to cardiac transplantation, *Am J Crit Care,* 5(1):80, 1996.
39. Benetti FJ: Video assisted coronary bypass surgery, *J Card Surg* 10(6):620, 1995.
40. Acuff TE and others: Minimally invasive coronary artery bypass grafting, *Ann Thorac Surg* 61(1):135, 1996.
41. Moss AJ and others: Improved survival with an implanted defibrillator in patients with coronary disease at high risk for ventricular arrhythmia, *N Engl J Med* 335(26):1933-1940, 1996.
42. Jordaens L and others: A new transvenous internal cardioverter defibrillator: implantation technique, complications and short-term follow-up, *Am Heart J,* 129(2):251, 1995.
43. Akhtar M and others: Role of implantable cardioverter defibrillator therapy in the management of high-risk patients, *Circulation* 85(suppl 1):I131, 1992.
44. Collins MA: When your patient has an implantable cardioverter defibrillator, *Am J Nurs* March:34, 1994.
45. Burke LR, Rodgers BL, Jenkins LS: Living with recurrent ventricular dysrhythmias, *Focus Crit Care* 19(1):60, 1992.
46. Ryan TJ and others: Guidelines for percutaneous transluminal coronary angioplasty, *J Am Coll Cardiol* 22(7):2033, 1993.
47. Safian RD and others: Do excimer laser angioplasty and rotational atherectomy facilitate balloon angioplasty? Implications for lesion-specific coronary intervention, *J Am Coll Cardiol* 27(3):552, 1996.
48. Holmes DR and others: Emergency "rescue" percutaneous transluminal coronary angioplasty after failed thrombolysis with streptokinase: early and late results, *Circulation* 81(suppl 3):51, 1990.
49. Murphy MC and others: Differences in symptoms during post PTCA versus rotational ablation, *Prog Cardiovasc Nurs* 9(2):4, 1994.
50. EPIC investigators: Use of monoclonal antibody directed against platelet glycoprotein IIb/IIIa receptor in high risk coronary angioplasty, *N Engl J Med* 330:956, 1994.
51. Brezina K and others: Care of the patient receiving Reopro™ following angioplasty, *J Invas Cardiology* 6(suppl A):38A, 1994.
52. Perra BM: Managing coronary atherectomy patients in a special procedure unit, *Crit Care Nurs* 15(3):57, 1995.
53. Dussaillant GR and others: Effect of rotational atherectomy in noncalcified atherosclerotic plaque: a volumetric intravascular ultrasound study, *J Am Coll Cardiol* 28(4):856, 1996.
54. Fogarty and others: Atherectomy: a review of current devices and methods. In Kerstein MD, White JV, editors: *Alternatives to open vascular surgery,* Philadelphia, 1995, Lippincott.
55. Deelstra MH: Coronary rotational ablation: an overview with related nursing interventions, *Am J Crit Care* 2(1):16, 1993.
56. Albert NM: Laser angioplasty and intracoronary stents: going beyond the balloon, *AACN Clin Issues Crit Care Nurs* 5(1):15, 1994.
57. Bevans M, McLimore E: Intracoronary stents: a new approach to coronary artery dilation, *J Cardiovasc Nurs* 7(1):34, 1992.
58. Pepine CJ and others: Coronary artery stents (ACC Expert Concensus Document), *J Am Coll Cardiol* 28(3):782, 1996.
59. Columbo A and others: Intracoronary stenting without anticoagulation accomplished with ultrasound guidance, *Circulation* 91:1676, 1995.
60. Columbo A and others: Results of coronary stenting for restenosis, *J Am Coll Cardiol* 28(4):830, 1996.
61. Gardner E and others: Intracoronary stent update: focus on patient education, *Crit Care Nurse* 16(2):65, 1995.
62. Oakley CM: Management of valvular stenosis, *Curr Opin Cardiol* 10(2):117, 1995.
63. Kawaniski DT, Rahimtoola SH: Catheter balloon commissurotomy for mitral stenosis: complications and results, *J Am Coll Cardiol* 19(1):192, 1992.
64. Barden C and others: Balloon aortic valvuloplasty: nursing care implications, *Crit Care Nurse* 10(6):22, 1990.
65. Majoros KA: Comparisons and controverises in clot buster drugs, *Crit Care Nurs Q* 16(2):46, 1993.
66. Schieman G and others: Intracoronary urokinase for intracoronary thrombus accumulation complicating PTCA in acute ischemic syndromes, *Circulation* 82(6):2052, 1990.
67. Coen SD, Silverman E: Peripheral intra-arterial thrombolytic therapy for acute arterial occlusion, *Crit Care Nurs,* 14(5):23, 1994.

68. Habib GB: Current status of thrombolysis in acute myocardial infarction. I. Optimal drug selection and delivery of a thrombolytic drug, *Chest* 107(1):225, 1995.
69. Sherry S: Pharmacology of anistreplase, *Clin Cardiol* 13(3)(suppl V):V3, 1990.
70. Smalling RW and others: More rapid, complete, and stable coronary thrombolysis with bolus administration of reteplase compared with ateplase infusion in acute myocardial infarction, *Circulation* 91(11):2725, 1995.
71. LATE Study Group: Late assessment of thrombolytic efficacy (LATE) study with ateplase after acute oneset of acute myocardial infarction, *Lancet* 342:767, 1993.
72. EMERAS Collaborative Group: Randomized trial of late thrombolysis in patients with suspected acute myocardial infarction, *Lancet* 342:767, 1993.
73. Drew BJ, Tisdale LA: ST segment monitoring for coronary artery reocclusion following thrombolytic therapy and coronary angioplasty: identification of optimal bedside monitoring leads, *Am J Crit Care* 2(4):280, 1993.
74. Habib GB: Current status of thrombolysis in acute myocardial infarction. III. Optimalization of adjunctive therapy after thrombolytic therapy, *Chest* 107(3):809, 1995.
75. Wojner AJ: Assessing the five points of intra-aortic balloon pump waveform, *Crit Care Nurs* 14(3):48, 1994.
76. Cadwell CA, Quaal SJ: Intra-aortic balloon counterpulsation timing, *Am J Crit Care* 5(4):254, 1996.
77. Shinn AE, Joseph D: Concepts on intraaortic balloon pulsation, *J Cardiovasc Nurs* 8(2):45, 1994.
78. Moroney DA, Reedy JE: Understanding ventricular assist devices: a self study guide, *J Cardiovasc Nurs* 8(2):1, 1994.
79. Vaca KJ, Lohmann DP, Moroney DA: Current status and future trends of mechanical circulatory support, *Crit Care Nurs Clin North Amer* 7(2):249, 1995.
80. Emery RW, Joyce LD: Directions in cardiac assistance, *J Cardiac Surg* 6(3):400, 1991.
81. Stier F: Antidysrhythmic agents, *AACN Clin Issues Crit Care Nurs* 3(2):483, 1992.
82. Weiner B: Hemodynamic effects of antidysrhythmic drugs, *J Cardiovasc Nurs* 5(4):39, 1991.
83. Bennett B, Singh S: Management of ventricular arrhythmias: then and now, *Am J Crit Care* 1(3):107, 1992.
84. Levine JH and others: Intravenous amiodarone for recurrent sustained hypotensive ventricular tachyarrhythmias, *J Am Coll Cardiol* 27(1):67, 1996.
85. Ellenbogen KA and others: Efficacy of intravenous ibutilide for rapid termination of atrial fibrillation and flutter: a dose response study, *J Am Coll Cardiol* 28:130, 1996.
86. Peitz TJ: Intravenous diltiazem hydrochloride rather than verapamil for resistant paroxysmal supraventricular tachycardia, *West J Med* 19(5):598, 1993.
87. Paul SC: New pharmacologic agents for emergency management of supraventricular tachydysrhythmias, *Crit Care Nurs Q* 16(2):35, 1993.
88. Morton PG: Update on new antiarrhythmic drugs, *Crit Care Nurs Clin North Am* 6(1):69, 1994.
89. Lefor N, Cardello FP, Felicetta JV: Recognizing and treating torsades de pointes, *Crit Care Nurs* 12(6):23, 1992.
90. Clements JV: Sympathomimetics, inotropics, and vasodilators, *AACN Clin Issues Crit Care Nurs* 3(2):395, 1992.
91. Deglin JH, Deglin S: Hypertension: current trends and choices in pharmacotherapeutics, *AACN Clin Issues Crit Care Nurs* 3(2):507, 1992.
92. Kuhn M: Nitrates, *AACN Clin Issues Crit Care Nurs* 3(2):409, 1992.
93. Schumann D: Sublingual nifedipine controversy in drug delivery, *DCCN* 10(6):314, 1991.
94. Halpern NA and others: Postoperative hypertension: a multicenter, prospective, randomized comparison between intravenous nicardipine and sodum nitroprusside, *Crit Care Med* 20(12):1637, 1992.
95. Kuhn M: Angiotensin-converting enzyme inhibitors, *AACN Clin Issues Crit Care Nurs* 3(2):461, 1992.

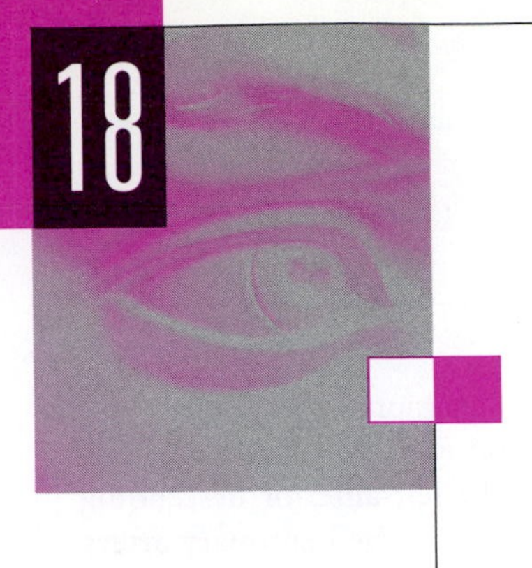

Cardiovascular Nursing Diagnosis and Management

THIS CHAPTER IS designed to supplement the preceding chapters in the *Cardiovascular Alterations* unit by integrating theoretic content into clinically applicable case studies and nursing management plans.

The case study is designed to illustrate clinical problem solving and patient care management occurring in actual patients. The case, reviewed retrospectively, demonstrates how medical and nursing diagnoses may be effectively used in critical care. The case study also demonstrates revisions to the plan of care and the nursing and medical management outcomes that are apt to occur during the course of a complicated hospitalization as the patient responds physiologically to treatment. Often in a short case anecdote, such as presented in this chapter, the clinical answer may appear to be obvious from the day of admission. In practice, however, critical care patient management is sometimes investigative and the "correct" diagnosis for an individual patient may not become apparent until midway in the hospitalization. Or a patient with an apparently straightforward diagnosis may develop an unexected complication, and the plan of care and potential outcomes will then require revision. Many of the case studies demonstrate this principle.

The nursing management plans, which—unlike the case study—are not patient-specific, provide a basis nurses can use to individualize care for their patients. In the previous *Cardiovascular Alterations* chapters, each medical diagnosis is assigned a Nursing Diagnosis and Management box. Using this box as a page guide, the reader can access relevant nursing management plans for each medical diagnosis. For example, nursing management of *endocarditis,* described on p. 508, may involve several nursing diagnoses and management plans outlined in this chapter and in other Nursing Diagnosis and Management chapters. Specific examples are (1) *Risk for Infection risk factor: invasive monitoring devices,* p. 598; and (2) *Knowledge Deficit: Home Intravenous Medication Regimen related to lack of previous exposure to information,* on p. 61. These examples highlight the interrelationship of the various physiologic systems in the body and the fact that pathology often has a multisystem impact on the critically ill.

Use of the case study and management plans can enhance the understanding and application of the *Cardiovascular* content in clinical practice.

CASE STUDY 1

CARDIOVASCULAR

CLINICAL HISTORY

Mrs. C is a 68-year-old white woman with history of coronary artery disease and hypertension. She has an 8-year history of exertional angina, which became unstable 3 weeks ago. A myocardial infarction (MI) was ruled out, and a cardiac catheterization procedure was performed, revealing significant obstruction in the left anterior descending (LAD) artery and in the right coronary artery (RCA) with an ejection fraction of 35%. She received coronary artery bypass grafting (CABG) to the LAD and RCA. Her postoperative course was uneventful until postoperative day 4.

She returned to the critical care unit from the medical/surgical ward, with acute shortness of breath and a rapid pulse, reported to be 124 beats per minute.

CURRENT PROBLEMS

Mrs. C was lying in bed with the head of bed (HOB) elevated. Her expression was anxious, her color was pale, and she was diaphoretic. She stated that she felt extremely weak and in the past 12 hours became short of breath (SOB) with only mild exertion.

Clinical data were as follows: Ht., 5′8″; Wt., 160 lb (10 lb more than preoperative weight according to medical record); BP, 104/70; HR, 115/irreg; respiratory rate (RR), 28/min; assessment with HOB elevated to 30 degrees revealed jugular venous distention (JVD) and an estimated jugular venous pressure (JVP) of 7 cm H_2O by internal jugular venous pulsation.

Bilateral lower extremity edema was present. There was a surgical wound on the left leg, groin to ankle.

Lung sounds were decreased in the right lower lobe (RLL) and absent in the left lower lobe (LLL). There were no crackles and no production with coughing. Room air O_2 saturation was 90%.

Heart sounds S_1 and S_2 were normal; there was no S_3. No murmurs were heard; pericardial friction rub was present.

Laboratory data included the following: hemoglobin (Hgb), 10.8 g/dL; hematocrit (Hct), 31.3%; sodium, 149 mEq/L; potassium, 4.4 mEq/L; chloride, 105 mEq/L; bicarbonate, 26 mEq/L; urea nitrogen, 17 mg/dL; creatinine, 1.2 mg/dL; and glucose, 98 mg/dL. Room air arterial blood gas (ABG) values were pH, 7.48; Po_2, 62 mm Hg; Pco_2, 47 mm Hg; bicarbonate, 25 mEq. The 12-lead electrocardiogram (ECG) showed atrial fibrillation with ventricular response of 128 beats per minute. Chest X-ray examination demonstrated new pulmonary vascular congestion and large left pleural effusion since CABG.

MEDICAL DIAGNOSES

Heart failure
Atrial fibrillation

NURSING DIAGNOSES

Decreased Cardiac Output related to alterations in preload and afterload
Impaired Gas Exchange related to ventilation/perfusion mismatching
Activity Intolerance related to decreased cardiac output and/or myocardial tissue perfusion alterations
Anxiety related to threat to biologic, psychologic, and/or social integrity

PLAN OF CARE

1. In collaboration with MD, administer diuretics to decrease preload and fluid volume excess and digoxin to decrease ventricular response rate to atrial fibrillation.
2. Decrease fluid intake; maintain strict I&O record.
3. Monitor vital signs and physical examination for response to treatment or continued deterioration.
4. Provide oxygen therapy with O_2 saturation monitoring to improve oxygenation without suppressing respiratory drive.
5. See that patient maintains strict bedrest in position of comfort to decrease energy expenditure.
6. Explain symptoms and management of care to reduce anxiety.

CASE STUDY 1—CONT'D

CARDIOVASCULAR

MEDICAL AND NURSING MANAGEMENT AND PATIENT OUTCOME

After 40 mg furosemide was given intravenously, the patient urinated 300 ml in the next hour. The atrial fibrillation converted to sinus tachycardia 110/min.

The physical examination revealed the following: BP, 80/60; HR, 110/regular; RR, 28/min.

Patient continued to be diaphoretic with a change in mental status. Her lips and tongue appeared cyanotic.

She complained of SOB at rest and requested HOB to be elevated more.

JVD was present with HOB elevated to 45 degrees.

Hepatojugular reflux was present.

JVP was estimated at 13 cm H_2O using the internal jugular vein pulsation with the HOB elevated to 45 degrees.

Auscultation of breath sounds revealed crackles in lower one third of right lung.

O_2 saturation was 88% on 2 L O_2 via nasal prongs.

Heart sounds S_1 and S_2 were normal; S_3 was present; no murmurs were heard. A pericardial friction rub was present.

MEDICAL DIAGNOSIS

Heart failure

NURSING DIAGNOSIS

Decreased Cardiac Output related to excessive preload and afterload

REVISED PLAN OF CARE

Insert pulmonary artery (PA) catheter.

MEDICAL AND NURSING MANAGEMENT AND PATIENT OUTCOME

Pulmonary artery catheter readings were as follows: RA, 8; PA, 30/15; PAWP, 15 mm Hg. The catheter monitor readout showed good waveform for all pressures, but the pressures did not correlate with the physical assessment of JVD, estimated CVP of 18 cm H_2O, JVP, 13 cm, and 5 cm hepatojugular reflux, + S_3, and subjective symptoms. The height of the transducer was found to be higher than phlebostatic axis level. Once the transducer was lowered, the PA catheter readings were the following: RA, 13 mm Hg; PA, 60/26 mm Hg; PAWP, 25 mm Hg.

Dopamine IV at 2 μg/kg/min and dobutamine IV at 5 μg/kg/min were started. Urine output increased to 2500 ml over the next 8 hours, and the PA catheter readings were RA, 8; PA, 40/15; PAWP, 15 mm Hg. The patient's JVD disappeared, and subjectively she felt less SOB. Her ABGs with 2 L O_2 via nasal prongs were the following: pH, 7.44; Po_2, 86 mm Hg; Pco_2, 42 mm Hg; and bicarbonate, 26 mEq/L. Her cardiac rhythm remained in sinus with a ventricular rate of 96 beats per minute. The dobutamine was discontinued after 10 hours, and the patient was able to be weaned from the dopamine and oxygen within 24 hours. She left the critical care unit and continued postoperative CABG cardiac rehabilitation in preparation for discharge.

CASE STUDY 2

CARDIOVASCULAR

CLINICAL HISTORY

Mr. H is a 70-year-old white man. He has a long history of coronary artery disease with associated ventricular dysrhythmias as described as follows:

1. Inferior wall myocardial infarction (MI) in 1985
2. Coronary artery bypass grafting (CABG) using vein grafts in 1995
3. Atherectomy to unblock one vein graft in 1997
4. Recurrent ventricular tachycardia (VT) at rate of 160/min in 1997; patient's VT poorly controlled on multiple antidysrhythmic medications

Continued

CASE STUDY 2—CONT'D

CARDIOVASCULAR

CLINICAL HISTORY—cont'd

5. Development of first-degree heart block in 1997
6. Placement of implantable cardioverter defibrillator (ICD) in 1997 as protection against sudden cardiac death; the ICD device has antitachycardia capability in addition to cardioversion/defibrillation functions.

CURRENT PROBLEMS

Recently Mr. H developed unstable angina. He underwent a cardiac catheterization. This showed severe coronary artery disease in three native vessels, with progressive disease in the vein grafts and a posterior basilar aneurysm at the site of the old inferior MI. Because of his continued episodes of VT, Mr. H also underwent an electrophysiology study (EPS). The EPS included an endocardial catheter map of the ventricle to locate the focus of the VT. The EPS showed atypical left bundle branch VT arising from an area adjacent to the site of the inferior MI. The ICD also was tested and was functioning correctly.

MEDICAL DIAGNOSES

Coronary artery disease
Ventricular tachycardia

NURSING DIAGNOSES

Decreased Cardiac Output related to alterations in heart rate
Acute Pain related to transmission and perception of cutaneous, visceral, muscular, or ischemic impulse
Anxiety related to threat to biologic, psychologic, and/or social integrity

PLAN OF CARE

Mr. and Mrs. H discussed with the cardiologist, surgeon, and electrophysiologist that Mr. H should be admitted to the hospital for a redo coronary artery bypass graft operation with a plan to use the internal mammary arteries. Because of the recurrent ventricular tachycardia and poorly controlled VT despite antidysrhythmic medications and ICD, Mr. H would also undergo ventricular cryoablation of the focus of his VT during the open heart surgery procedure.

MEDICAL AND NURSING MANAGEMENT AND PATIENT OUTCOME

Mr. H underwent open heart surgery with cardiopulmonary bypass (CPB) that involved CABG using both right and left internal mammary arteries and cryoablation of VT foci. Mr. H returned from the operating room to the critical care unit in stable condition after surgery. The nursing assessment revealed the following:

Neuro: Mr. H remained sedated and nonresponsive postanesthesia.

Resp: He was intubated and ventilated. Lungs were clear to auscultation, with bilateral breath sounds.

CV: Heart rate of 120, sinus tachycardia with occasional PVCs. Atrial and ventricular epicardial pacing wires were present. The wires were connected to a temporary pacemaker generator, which was turned off. (Temporary epicardial pacing wires are routinely inserted at the time of cardiac surgery). The ICD was programmed "on." The ICD either paces, cardioverts, or defibrillates, depending on the specific dysrhythmia. There was a pulmonary artery catheter with side-port, a radial arterial line, and a peripheral IV in situ. His hemodynamics were stable: MAP, 60 mm Hg; CVP, 6 mm Hg; pulmonary artery wedge pressure (PAWP), 10 mm Hg; cardiac output (CO), 2.9 L/min; cardiac index (CI), 1.87 L/min/m^2; systemic vascular resistance (SVR), 1659 dynes/sec/cm^{-5}.

Mr. H was bleeding via the mediastinal chest tubes (200 ml/hr).

Integument/Temp: Skin was cool and dry with palpable peripheral pulses. Initial core temperature was 35.3° C. (The low temperature was expected after CPB, and Mr. H was expected to rewarm and vasodilate in the next 6 to 8 hours.)

Medications: IV drips were dopamine at 3.0 μg/kg/min; sodium nitroprusside (SNP) at 0.6 μg/kg/min; and nitroglycerin at 66 μg/min.

GI: Nasogastric tube was in place to decompress stomach; there was minimal bile-colored drainage. No bowel sounds were present.

CASE STUDY 2—CONT'D

CARDIOVASCULAR

MEDICAL AND NURSING MANAGEMENT AND PATIENT OUTCOME—cont'd

GU: A large volume of dilute urine drained via the urinary catheter (400 ml/hr). This was secondary to diuretics given at the end of the CPB.

Lab: Hematocrit (Hct), 28.9%; platelets, 98,000; glucose, 146 mg/dL; K^+, 3.2 mEq/L (replaced); magnesium, 1.9 mEq/L; prothombin time (PT), 15.9 secs or 47%; partial thromboplastin time (PTT), 38 seconds; and fibrinogen, 129 mg/dL.

MEDICAL DIAGNOSES

CABG and ventricular cryoablation
ICD (previous surgery)

NURSING DIAGNOSES

Hypothermia related to exposure to cold environment
Fluid Volume Deficit related to absolute loss: blood
Decreased Cardiac Output related to alterations in afterload
Decreased Cardiac Output related to alterations in preload

REVISED PLAN OF CARE

1. Increase body temperature by using warm blankets.

2a. (first intervention) Replace fluid lost as a result of bleeding, urine output, and rewarming, by CPB cell-saver, and Plasmanate (blood not given at this time because Hct is greater than 25%).

2b. (second intervention) Slow bleeding by correcting prolonged coagulation times by administration of IV coagulation products: fresh frozen plasma, cryoprecipitate, and platelets.

3. Increase cardiac output by correcting the fluid volume deficit and decreasing SVR.

4. Continue to monitor for dysrhythmias.

MEDICAL AND NURSING MANAGEMENT AND PATIENT OUTCOME

Eight hours after returning from surgery Mr. H was awake and had been medicated for incisional pain. His core temperature had risen to 38.3° C, and his periphery (hands and feet) was warm. Fluid volume replacement had been effective, and hemodynamic filling pressures had increased: MAP, 75-80 mm Hg; CVP, 18 mm Hg; PAWP, 22 mm Hg. (In a patient with a previously damaged heart from an MI, higher filling pressures are often necessary to optimize contractility [Starling's law]).

Four hours after surgery mediastinal bleeding had slowed to 50 ml/hr after administration of the IV coagulation products. Because of the clinical improvement, coagulation factors were not retested.

The cardiac output had increased to 5.12 L/min; cardiac index, 3.3 L/min/m^2; and SVR, 732 dynes/sec/cm^{-5}. The nurse had maintained the dopamine drip at a constant rate, but had increased the SNP to 1.2 µg/kg/min. The increased SNP combined with rewarming had decreased SVR and raised CO effectively.

One hour after his return from surgery Mr. H's heart rate slowed to a sinus rhythm (79 bpm) with demonstration of his chronic first-degree heart block and bundle branch block. Because his cardiac output and peripheral perfusion remained stable, the nurse continued to monitor the situation. No treatment was given at that time. Two hours later Mr. H had a short burst of VT (6 beats). The VT was self-terminating. The nurse informed the MD and continued to monitor the rhythm. No treatment was given at that time. Six hours later the heart rhythm deteriorated into a second-degree heart block, Mobitz Type II. The nurse immediately turned on the temporary pacemaker generator that was connected to the epicardial pacing wires, and Mr. H was successfully AV-paced at a rate of 88 paced-bpm.

MEDICAL DIAGNOSES

CABG
Second-degree heart block
Ventricular dysrhythmias

NURSING DIAGNOSIS

Decreased Cardiac Output related to alterations in heart rate

Continued

CASE STUDY 2—CONT'D

CARDIOVASCULAR

REVISED PLAN OF CARE

1. Maintain AV-paced rhythm while second-degree heart block is evaluated.
2. Continue to monitor cardiac rhythm while ventricular dysrhythmias are evaluated.

MEDICAL AND NURSING MANAGEMENT AND PATIENT OUTCOME

The remainder of Mr. H's stay in the critical care unit was uneventful. On the first postoperative day the endotracheal tube was removed without difficulty. His hemodynamics remained stable. He was weaned off the IV drips, which were replaced by oral afterload-reducing medications. On the second postoperative day chest tubes were removed without problems and Mr. H was transferred out of the critical care unit to the telemetry cardiac surveillance unit.

Because Mr. H's second-degree heart block persisted, he remained on the telemetry unit, AV-paced with a temporary generator. To protect Mr. H from the consequences of further deterioration in his conduction system, the cardiologist implanted a permanent, dual-chamber (DDD) pacemaker before Mr. H was discharged from the hospital.

MEDICAL DIAGNOSES

CABG
Ventricular dysrhythmias
Second-degree heart block
Permanent pacemaker

NURSING DIAGNOSIS

Knowledge Deficit: Discharge for CABG, Permanent Pacemaker, and Antidysrhythmic Drugs related to lack of previous exposure to information

REVISED PLAN OF CARE

Provide discharge teaching to Mr. H and his wife for his home care. Topics include CABG surgery and cardiac risk factor modification, instructions on his pacemaker, and information on the effects of the antidysrhythmic drugs.

MEDICAL AND NURSING MANAGEMENT AND PATIENT OUTCOME

Mr. H received discharge teaching from both the CV nurse specialist and staff nurses in the days before his discharge from the hospital. The CABG was successful in eliminating Mr. H's angina. The ventricular dysrhythmias were more effectively controlled after the cryoablation. In addition, with the combination of the permanent pacemaker, the implantable cardioverter defibrillator, and adjusted antidysrhythmic medications, Mr. H's risk of sudden death caused by dysrhythmias was significantly decreased.

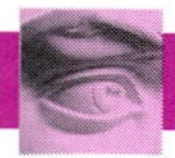

NURSING MANAGEMENT PLAN

DECREASED CARDIAC OUTPUT

DEFINITION:

The state in which the blood pumped by an individual's heart is sufficiently reduced to the extent that it is inadequate to meet the needs of the body's tissues.

Decreased Cardiac Output Related to Alterations in Preload

EXCESSIVE PRELOAD RISK FACTORS

- Acute heart failure/cardiomyopathy
- Decreased cardiogenic shock
- Acute renal failure

PRELOAD RISK FACTORS

- Bleeding
- Coagulopathy
- Surgery
- Sepsis with vasodilation
- Hypovolemic shock

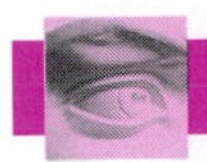

NURSING MANAGEMENT PLAN—CONT'D

Decreased Cardiac Output Related to Alterations in Preload

DEFINING CHARACTERISTICS

- Systolic blood pressure (SBP) <90 mm Hg
- Mean arterial pressure (MAP) <60 mm Hg
- Cardiac index (CI) <2.2 L/min/m^2
- Urine output <0.5 ml/kg/hr or <30 ml/hr

Excessive preload

- Pulmonary artery wedge pressure (PAWP) >15 mm Hg
- Pulmonary artery diastolic pressure (PAD) >15 mm Hg

Decreased preload

- PAWP <6 mm Hg and PAD <6 mm Hg or significantly below patient's baseline
- Bibasilar fluid crackles
- Faint peripheral pulses
- Ventricular gallop rhythm (S_3)
- Skin cool, pale, moist
- Activity intolerance

OUTCOME CRITERIA

- Cardiac index is 2.2-4.0 L/min/m^2.
- Heart rate is <100 bpm.
- SBP is >90 mm Hg.
- MAP is >60 mm Hg.
- PAWP, PAD, and CVP are >6 mm Hg to <15 mm Hg.

NURSING INTERVENTIONS AND *RATIONALE*

The following interventions *reduce* preload:

1. Monitor the assessment parameters listed under "Defining Characteristics - Excessive Preload," and with physician collaboration, administer diuretics.
2. Titrate venous vasodilators and inotropic drips, per protocol, to desired SBP, MAP, PAWP, and/or PAD. Withhold and/or change drip rate when SBP, MAP, PAWP, PAD, and CVP begin to normalize.
3. Implement fluid restriction.
4. Double concentrate intravenous drug drips when possible ***to decrease the amount of volume infused to the patient.***
5. Monitor intake and output balance.
6. Monitor daily weight.

The following interventions *increase* preload:

1. Monitor assessment parameters listed under "Defining Characteristics - Decreased Preload."
2. Assess reason for low preload and reverse process or stop patient bleeding.
3. Calculate the patient's 24-hour fluid requirements per body surface area (BSA), and replace with the appropriate electrolyte solution.
4. Administer solutions using the fluid challenge technique: infuse precise amounts of fluid (usually 5 to 20 ml/min) over 10-minute periods and monitor cardiac loading pressure serially to determine successful challenging. If the PAWP or PAD elevates more than 7 mm Hg above beginning level, the infusion is stopped. If the PAWP or PAD rises only to 3 mm Hg above baseline or falls, another fluid challenge is given.
5. If the patient is bleeding, assess whether this is from a coagulopathy or represents loss of blood volume from trauma or GI bleeding, or at an arterial cannulation site. If from coagulopathy, fresh frozen plasma, platelets, and other clotting factors are infused. If from bleeding, surgical or other procedures may be required.
6. If Hgb is <9 g/dL or Hct is <25%, in collaboration with physician, infuse red blood cells (RBCs).
7. Assess for signs and symptoms of fluid overload once fluid replacement has begun. These may include elevations of PAP or CVP to above normal levels, pulmonary crackles, or dyspnea.
8. Monitor intake and output balance.
9. Monitor daily weight.

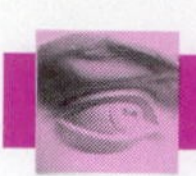

NURSING MANAGEMENT PLAN

Decreased Cardiac Output Related to Alterations in Afterload

RISK FACTORS

- Multiple organ dysfunction syndrome (MODS)
- Acute myocardial infarction (MI)
- Sepsis
- Cardiac surgery

DEFINING CHARACTERISTICS

High afterload

- Cardiac output (CO) <4.0 L/min
- Cardiac index (CI) <2.2 L/min/m^2
- Systemic vascular resistance (SVR) >1400 dynes/sec/cm^{-5}
- Systolic blood pressure (BP) <90 mm Hg
- Cool, pale, mottled extremities

Low afterload

- Cardiac output >6.0 L/min
- Cardiac index >4.4 L/min/m^2
- SVR <600 dynes/sec/cm^{-5}
- Systolic BP <90 mm Hg
- Pink, warm, vasodilated extremities

OUTCOME CRITERIA

- CI is >2.2.
- SVR is >600 and <1400 dynes/sec/cm^{-5}
- Systolic BP is >90 mm Hg.

NURSING INTERVENTIONS AND *RATIONALE*

The following interventions *reduce* afterload:

1. Monitor the assessment parameters listed under "Defining Characteristics - High Afterload."
2. With physician collaboration, administer vasodilator drugs, such as sodium nitroprusside (SNP), high dose nitroglycerin, and angiotensin-converting enzyme (ACE) inhibitors. Monitor the effect of the vasodilator drugs or the SVR/CI, and adjust accordingly.

The following interventions *increase* afterload:

1. Monitor the assessment parameters listed under "Defining Characteristics - Low Afterload."
2. With physician collaboration, administer vasopressor drugs to support BP and increase SVR (phenylephrine, epinephrine, high-dose dopamine).
3. Monitor peripheral perfusion closely while administering vasopressor drugs.
4. If BP drops suddenly, the patient may be placed in a Trendelenburg (head downward) position until BP stabilizes. This action is contraindicated if there is head injury.
5. Fluid volume resuscitation may be required if the systemic vasodilation causes a relative decrease in preload.

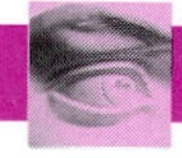

NURSING MANAGEMENT PLAN

Decreased Cardiac Output Related to Alterations in Contractility

RISK FACTORS FOR LOW CONTRACTILITY

- Acute myocardial infarction
- Cardiomyopathy
- Cardiogenic shock

DEFINING CHARACTERISTICS

- Systolic blood pressure (SBP) <90 mm Hg
- Mean arterial blood pressure (MAP) <60 mm Hg
- Cardiac index (CI) < 2.2L/min/m^2
- Pulmonary artery wedge pressure (PAWP) >15 mm Hg
- Pulmonary artery diastolic (PAD) pressure >15 mm Hg
- Urine output <0.5 ml/kg/hr or <30 ml/hr.
- Decreased mentation

OUTCOME CRITERIA

- Systolic blood pressure is >90 mm Hg.
- Mean arterial blood pressure is >60 mm Hg.
- Cardiac index is >2.2 L/min/m^2.
- Pulmonary artery wedge pressure and pulmonary artery diastolic pressure are >15 mm Hg.
- Urine output is >0.5 ml/kg/hr or >30 ml/hr.

NURSING INTERVENTIONS AND *RATIONALE*

The following interventions *increase* contractility

1. Monitor the assessment parameters outlined under "Defining Characteristics."
2. Using the "Starling Curve" concept, optimize preload for the patient with impaired contractility—use of diuretics, venous dilators (nitroglycerin) lower cardiac filling pressures (PAWP, CVP [central venous pressure]).
3. In collaboration with physician, optimize cardiac output with inotropic drugs to increase contractility—dopamine, dobutamine, amrinone, digoxin.
4. In collaboration with physician, use arterial vasodilation (sodium nitroprusside, hydralazine, angiotensin-converting enzyme [ACE] inhibitors) to lower afterload and enhance contractility.

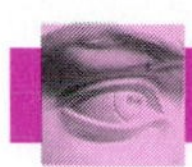

NURSING MANAGEMENT PLAN

Decreased Cardiac Output Related to Alterations in Heart Rate

DEFINING CHARACTERISTICS

- Systolic blood pressure (SBP) <90 mm Hg
- Mean arterial pressure (MAP) <60 mm Hg
- Ventricular rate <60 bpm
- Decreased mentation or syncope
- Decreased urine output

OUTCOME CRITERIA

- Systolic blood pressure is >90 mm Hg.
- Mean arterial pressure is >60 mm Hg.
- Ventricular rate is >60 bpm.
- The patient is awake and responsive.
- Urine output is >30 ml/hr.

NURSING INTERVENTIONS AND *RATIONALE*

First-degree AV block

1. Monitor the assessment parameters listed under "Defining Characteristics."
2. Monitor closely, measuring PR intervals ***to determine further prolongation, which would suggest progression of heart block.*** Often, no specific intervention is required.
3. With physician collaboration, consider withholding supraventricular antidysrhythmic agents such as digitalis, quinidine, beta-blocking agents, and calcium channel blockers.

Second-degree AV block—Mobitz I (Wenckebach pattern)

1. Monitor the assessment parameters listed under "Defining Characteristics."
2. Monitor for symptomatic decompensation resulting from slow ventricular rate (rare).
3. While symptomatic, position patient supine ***to increase preload and therefore cardiac output.***
4. Monitor for progression to complete heart block.
5. With physician collaboration, consider withholding digitalis.
6. Eliminate sources of vagal stimulation. ***Vagal stimulation increases the delay in conduction at the AV node.***

Second-degree AV block—Mobitz II

1. Monitor the assessment parameters listed under "Defining Characteristics."
2. Monitor closely for symptomatic decompensation as a result of slow ventricular rate (common).
3. While symptomatic, position patient supine ***to increase preload and therefore cardiac output.***
4. Monitor for progression of existing block, such as 2:1, 3:1, 4:1 conduction, and for progression to complete heart block.
5. Follow critical care emergency standing orders regarding the administration of positive chronotropic agents, such as atropine, or isoproterenol.
6. Anticipate possibility of temporary transvenous pacemaker insertion or use of external pacemaker.

Third-degree (complete) AV block

1. Monitor the assessment parameters listed under "Defining Characteristics."
2. Monitor closely for symptomatic decompensation resulting from slow ventricular rate (common).
3. While symptomatic, position patient supine ***to increase preload and therefore cardiac output.***
4. Follow critical care emergency standing orders regarding the administration of isoproterenol.
5. Anticipate the necessity of pacemaker insertion or use of external pacemaker.

Sinus bradycardia

1. Monitor the assessment parameters listed under "Defining Characteristics."
2. Monitor for symptomatic decompensation resulting from slow ventricular rate.
3. Anticipate the necessity of pacemaker insertion or use of external pacemaker.

Supraventricular tachycardias

1. Monitor the assessment parameters listed under "Defining Characteristics."
2. Distinguish supraventricular tachycardia from ventricular tachycardia. Monitoring the patient in lead V_1 or MCL_1 ***may assist in distinguishing ventricular ectopy from aberrancy.***
3. Follow critical care emergency standing orders regarding the administration of supraventricular antidysrhythmic agents, such as verapamil, quinidine, procainamide, propranolol, digoxin, and adenosine.
4. Consider positioning patient supine ***to increase preload.***
5. Identify precipitating factors when possible, such as emotional stress, caffeine, nicotine, and sympathomimetic drugs, and intervene to reduce or eliminate their effect.
6. Assess apical-radial pulse ***to identify deficits indicating nonperfused beats.*** Monitor amplitude of peripheral pulses ***to ascertain perfusion to extremities.***
7. Monitor arterial blood pressure ***to determine symptomatic decompensation.***
8. With physician collaboration, consider carotid sinus massage or Valsalva maneuver, ***thereby increasing vagal tone.***

Continued

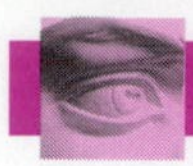

NURSING MANAGEMENT PLAN—CONT'D

Decreased Cardiac Output Related to Alterations in Heart Rate

Supraventricular tachycardias—cont'd

9. Anticipate possibility of synchronized cardioversion or overdrive pacing.
10. For atrial fibrillation that is either spontaneously, pharmacologically, or electrically converted, monitor for signs of cerebral, pulmonary, and/or peripheral thromboembolization as a result of liberation of mural thrombi.
11. If patient is hypoxemic or if dysrhythmia is suspected to be a result of or exacerbated by ischemia, administer oxygen observing the following principles:

    Without physician collaboration, liter flow must be no greater than 2 L/min via nasal prongs in patients whose pulmonary history either is unknown or reveals a pattern of chronic CO_2 retention. ***Administration of oxygen at concentrations higher than 2 L/min via nasal prongs may induce CO_2 narcosis in patients who chronically retain CO_2.***

    Oxygen is administered with the goal of achieving ***an oxygen saturation (Sao_2) above 92% when measured by pulse oximetry or arterial blood gases (ABGs).***

    Observe caution when administering oxygen at an FIO_2 greater than 40% ***in view of the higher risk for oxygen toxicity.***
12. Assess serum electrolyte levels, especially potassium and calcium, ***because increased or decreased electrolyte levels may exacerbate the dysrhythmia or may impair treatment of the dysrhythmia.***

Ventricular tachycardia

1. Monitor the assessment parameters listed under "Defining Characteristics," plus for the possibility of syncope and loss of consciousness.
2. Carefully distinguish ventricular tachycardia from supraventricular tachycardia. Monitoring the patient in lead V_1 or MCL_1 ***may assist in distinguishing ventricular ectopy from aberrancy.***
3. Monitor and treat the "warning dysrhythmias" (i.e., > 6 premature ventricular contractions [PVCs] per minute, multifocal PVCs, R-on-T phenomenon, couplets, bursts of ventricular tachycardia, bigeminy, trigeminy).
4. Assess serum electrolyte levels (potassium/magnesium) and ABGs, ***because altered electrolytes, acid-base imbalance, and hypoxemia may exacerbate the dysrhythmia or may impair effectiveness of treatment.***
5. Follow critical care emergency standing orders regarding the administration of ventricular antidysrhythmic agents, such as lidocaine, bretylium, and procainamide.
6. For asymptomatic ventricular tachycardia, treat with lidocaine. For symptomatic ventricular tachycardia, treat with synchronized cardioversion. For pulseless ventricular tachycardia, treat as ventricular fibrillation and defibrillate.
7. Position patient supine ***to increase preload.***
8. Anticipate possibility that sporadic ventricular dysrhythmias may progress to ventricular tachycardia or ventricular fibrillation, and be prepared to treat with implementation of synchronized cardioversion and defibrillation, respectively.
9. Anticipate possibility of cardiac standstill and activation of resuscitation protocol.
10. When safe rhythm is reestablished, carefully assess for femoral and carotid pulsations ***to rule out pulseless electrical activity (PEA).***
11. Identify precipitating factors when possible, such as hypoxia, electrolyte abnormalities, drug toxicity (especially amrinone, digitalis, quinidine, disopyramide, procainamide, phenothiazines, tricyclic and tetracyclic antidepressants), or recent MI, and intervene to reduce or eliminate their effect.

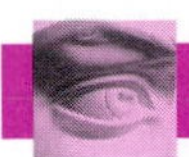

NURSING MANAGEMENT PLAN

ALTERED MYOCARDIAL TISSUE PERFUSION

DEFINITION:

The state in which an individual experiences a decrease in nutrition and oxygenation at the myocardial cellular level due to a deficit in capillary blood supply

Altered Myocardial Tissue Perfusion Related to Acute Myocardial Ischemia

DEFINING CHARACTERISTICS

- Angina for more than 30 min
- ST-segment elevation on 12-lead electrocardiogram (ECG)
- Elevation of CK and CK-MB enzymes
- Apprehension

OUTCOME CRITERIA

- Systolic blood pressure (SBP) is >90 mm Hg.
- Mean arterial pressure (MAP) is >60 mm Hg.
- Ventricular heart rate is <100 bpm.
- Pulmonary artery (PA) pressures are within normal limits or back to baseline.
- Cardiac index (CI) is >2.2 L/min/m^2
- Urine output is >0.5 ml/kg/hr or >30 ml/hr.
- 12-lead ECG is normalized without new Q waves.
- Angina is absent.
- CK and CK-MB enzymes are within normal range.
- Patient and family are educated about coronary artery disease (CAD) risk factor modification.

NURSING INTERVENTIONS AND *RATIONALE*

Monitor the assessment parameters listed under "Defining Characteristics."

The following interventions control pain:

1. Evaluate 12-lead ECG for signs of myocardial ischemia.
2. In collaboration with the physician, administer sublingual nitroglycerin (NTG) and start an intravenous (IV) NTG infusion. Titrate IV NTG ***to control pain.*** Maintain SBP >90 mm Hg.
3. Administer morphine IV.

The following interventions decrease myocardial oxygen demand:

1. Administer oxygen 2 L/min to achieve Spo_2 >92%.
2. Promote bedrest, with head of bed at 45 degrees.

The following interventions are to lyse clot in coronary artery:

1. Administer low dose aspirin (80 mg to 325 mg) PO.

OR

2. In collaboration with physician, if appropriate for patient, infuse thrombolytic agent of choice ***to lyse clot in coronary artery.*** Maintain SBP at >90 mm Hg.
3. Infuse IV heparin and assess coagulation studies (activated clotting time or partial thromboplastin time) per hospital protocol ***to prevent recurrent thrombosis.***
4. Prepare for cardiac catheterization and emergency angioplasty/atherectomy to remove coronary thrombus.

Monitor hemodynamic/cardiac ryhthm status.

1. Monitor cardiac rhythm for presence of dysrhythmias. Assess serum electrolytes (potassium and magnesium) and arterial blood gases (AGBs). Correct any imbalance. Administer lidocaine IV (1 mg/kg body weight) if premature ventricular contractions (PVCs) are >6/min.
2. In case of cardiac/respiratory arrest, follow ACLS/hospital protocols. Have cardioversion/defibrillation equipment nearby.
3. Monitor SBP ***because many conditions (drugs, dysrhythmias, myocardial ischemia) may cause hypotension (SBP <90 mm Hg).***
4. If clinical condition deteriorates, a pulmonary artery (PA) catheter may be required. Be prepared to assist with insertion of PA catheter and to assess hemodynamic profile (PA pressures, pulmonary artery wedge pressure [PAWP], cardiac output [CO], and CI).
5. In collaboration with the physician, if appropriate for the patient, titrate additional vasodilator medications (sodium nitroprusside) or inotropic medications (dopamine, dobutamine) to maintain SBP > 90 mm Hg and CI >2.2 L/min/m^2.

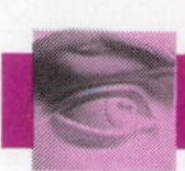

NURSING MANAGEMENT PLAN

Altered Peripheral Tissue Perfusion Related to Decreased Peripheral Blood Flow

RISK FACTORS

- Femoral artery cannulation for interventional cardiology or vascular procedures, intraaortic balloon pump (IABP), or hemodynamic monitoring catheters
- Radial artery cannulation or puncture
- Acute arterial thrombus
- Orthopedic trauma to an extremity

DEFINING CHARACTERISTICS

- Weak and/or unequal peripheral pulses
- Delayed capillary refill
- Ischemic pain from extremity
- Cool skin on extremity
- Pale extremity
- Paresthesias from extremity

OUTCOME CRITERIA

- Peripheral pulses are full and equal bilaterally.
- Capillary refill is equal bilaterally.
- There is no ischemic pain.
- There is equal skin temperature in both extremities.
- The skin is pink and warm in both extremities.
- Paresthesias are absent.

NURSING INTERVENTIONS AND *RATIONALE*

Monitor the assessment parameters listed under "Defining Characteristics" frequently.

Observe cannulation/injury site to prevent hematoma formation or bleeding.

Do not bend limb at cannulation/injury site.

Notify physician of any changes in peripheral pulses, pallor, paresthesias, or pain in the extremity.

Prepare for return to surgery, peripheral arterial embolectomy, or peripheral lytic therapy.

In consultation with physician, medicate for pain from limb ischemia.

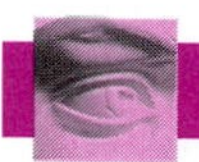

NURSING MANAGEMENT PLAN

ACTIVITY INTOLERANCE

DEFINITION:

The state in which an individual has insufficient physiological or psychological energy to endure or complete required or desired daily activities.

Activity Intolerance Related to Cardiopulmonary Dysfunction

DEFINING CHARACTERISTICS

- Chest pain on activity
- Electrocardiographic changes on activity
- Heart rate elevations 30 beats/minute (bpm) above baseline on activity; heart rate elevations 15 bpm above baseline on activity for patients on beta-blockers or calcium channel blockers
- Heart rate elevations above baseline 5 minutes after activity
- Breathlessness on activity
- $SpO_2 < 92\%$ on activity
- Postural hypotension when moving from supine to upright position
- Subjective fatigue on activity

OUTCOME CRITERIA

- Heart rate elevations are < 20 bpm above baseline on activity and are < 10 bpm above baseline on activity for patients on beta-blockers or calcium channel blockers.
- Heart rate returns to baseline 5 minutes after activity.
- Chest pain is absent on activity.
- The patient has subjective tolerance to activity.

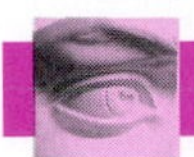

NURSING MANAGEMENT PLAN—CONT'D

Activity Intolerance Related to Cardiopulmonary Dysfunction

NURSING INTERVENTIONS AND *RATIONALE*

1. Monitor the assessment parameters listed under "Defining Characteristics."
2. Encourage active or passive range-of-motion exercises while the patient is in bed ***to keep joints flexible and muscles stretched.*** Teach patient to refrain from holding breath while performing exercises. ***Avoid the Valsalva maneuver.***
3. Encourage performance of muscle-toning exercises at least 3 times daily, ***because a toned muscle uses less oxygen when performing work than an untoned muscle.***
4. Progress ambulation.
5. Teach patient to take pulse ***to determine activity tolerance:*** take pulse for full minute before exercise, then for 10 seconds and multiply by 6 at exercise peak.

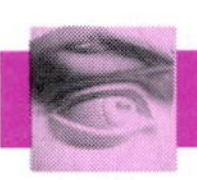

NURSING MANAGEMENT PLAN

Activity Intolerance Related to Prolonged Immobility or Deconditioning

DEFINING CHARACTERISTICS

- Systolic blood pressure (SBP) drop >20 mm Hg; heart rate increase >20 bpm on postural change
- Vertigo on postural change
- Syncope on postural change

OUTCOME CRITERIA

- SBP drop is <10 mm Hg; heart rate increase is < 10 bpm on postural change.
- Vertigo or syncope is absent on postural change.

NURSING INTERVENTIONS AND *RATIONALE*

1. Monitor the assessment parameters listed under "Defining Characteristics."
2. ***To increase muscular and vascular tone,*** instruct and assist in the following bed exercises: straight leg raises, dorsiflexion/plantar flexion, and quadriceps setting and gluteal setting exercises.
3. Determine that the patient is hydrated to 24-hour fluid requirements per body surface area (BSA) ***to increase preload and thus stroke volume and cardiac output.*** Hydrate accordingly if not contraindicated by cardiac or renal disorders.
4. Assist with postural changes accomplished in increments:
   Head of bed to 45 degrees and hold until symptom free
   Head of bed to 90 degrees and hold until symptom free
   Dangle until symptom free
   Stand until symptom free and ambulate
5. As soon as it is medically safe, assist patient to sit at bedside for meals.
6. When treating pain with narcotic analgesics, plan ambulation to occur well before peak action of drug.

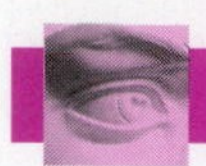

NURSING MANAGEMENT PLAN

RISK FOR INFECTION

DEFINITION:

The state in which an individual is at increased risk for being invaded by pathogenic organisms.

Risk for Infection Risk Factor: Invasive Monitoring Devices

RISK FACTOR

- Invasive monitoring devices

DEFINING CHARACTERISTICS

- Fever of undetermined origin
- Tachycardia
- Elevated white blood cell count
- Reddened, inflamed catheter insertion sites
- Drainage from catheter insertion sites

OUTCOME CRITERIA

- Patient is afebrile.
- Heart rate is within range of baseline.
- Catheter insertion sites are clear and dry.

NURSING INTERVENTIONS AND *RATIONALE*

NOTE: *The rationale for each of the following interventions is the avoidance of contamination and colonization of invasive lines and is based on national standards and supported with research.*

1. Monitor the assessment parameters listed under "Defining Characteristics."
2. Practice handwashing—consisting of 10 seconds using mechanical friction and soap and water—before drawing blood or any line manipulation in which the closed system is interrupted.
3. Secure catheters to prevent piston movement (in and out).
4. Maintain an occlusive, sterile dressing. Gauze dressings over arterial lines are recommended.
5. Eliminate all nonessential stopcocks.
6. A different anatomic site is selected for each catheter inserted.
7. Use uniform, prepackaged, sterile transducer/pressure monitoring and flush assembly.
8. A sterile gown is worn when inserting central lines. For skin preparation, clean the skin with iodophor. Wear gloves, mask, and cap and use sterile drapes.
9. Use sterile normal saline as the flush solution.
10. To the extent possible, limit blood drawing by obtaining all specimens at the same time.
11. After obtaining a sample of blood, the stopcock is flushed with saline to clear. All ports are capped when not in use.
12. Transparent, occlusive dressings are changed every 72 hours or when integrity is disrupted. Gauze dressings are changed every 24 hours or sooner if soiled, saturated, or disrupted. Change IV tubing every 72 hours and IV fluids every 24 hours, or as required by institutional policy.
13. Catheters inserted in an emergency, without proper asepsis, are removed and, if necessary, replaced under aseptic conditions.
14. At any sign of infection (localized pain, inflammation, sepsis, fever of undetermined origin), catheters are removed and cultured.

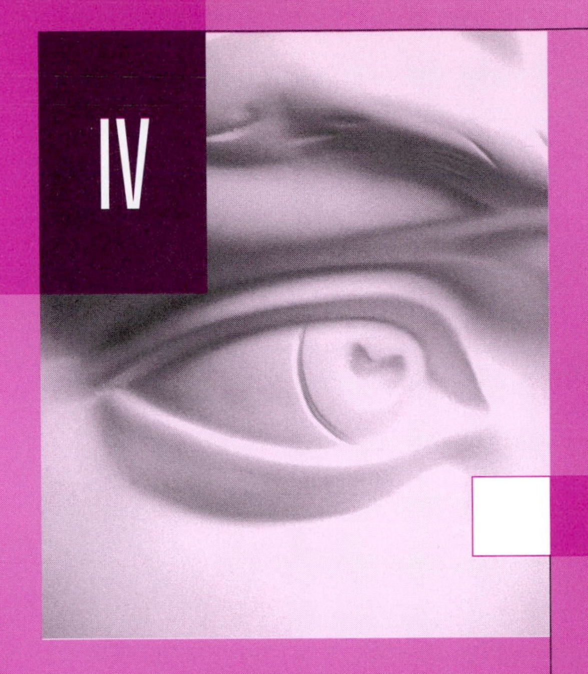

PULMONARY ALTERATIONS

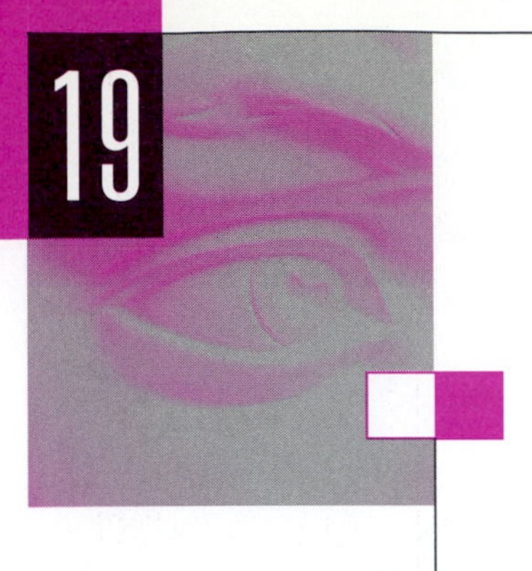

Pulmonary Anatomy and Physiology

THE PULMONARY SYSTEM consists of the thorax, conducting airways, respiratory airways, and pulmonary blood and lymph supply. The primary functions of the pulmonary system are ventilation and respiration. *Ventilation* is the movement of air in and out of the lungs. *Respiration* is the process of gas exchange (i.e., the movement of oxygen from the atmosphere into the blood stream and the movement of carbon dioxide from the blood stream into the atmosphere). The anatomic structures that constitute the pulmonary system are intimately related to function, and structural abnormalities can readily translate into pulmonary disorders; thus an applicable knowledge of anatomy and physiology is imperative in caring for the patient with pulmonary dysfunction.

THORAX

The thorax contains the major organs of respiration. It consists of the thoracic cage, lungs, pleura, and muscles of ventilation. Together these structures form the ventilatory pump, which performs the work of breathing.

Thoracic Cage

The thoracic cage is a cone-shaped structure that is rigid but flexible. It must be somewhat rigid to protect the underlying structures, yet it also must be flexible to accommodate inhalation and exhalation. The cage consists of 12 thoracic vertebrae, each with a pair of ribs. Posteriorly, each rib is attached to its own vertebra, but anteriorly, attachment varies (Figure 19-1). The first seven pairs of ribs are attached directly to the sternum. The eighth, ninth, and tenth pairs are attached by cartilage to the ribs above. The eleventh and twelfth ribs have no anterior attachment, and for this reason they sometimes are referred to as *floating ribs.* The second rib is attached to the sternum at the angle of Louis, which is the raised ridge that can be felt just below the suprasternal notch.[1]

Lungs

The lungs are cone-shaped organs that have a total volume of approximately 3.5 to 8.5 L. The superior portion is known as the *apex,* and the inferior portion is known as the *base.* The apical portion of each lung rises a few centimeters above the clavicle (See Figure 19-1). Each lung is firmly attached to the thoracic cavity at the hilum and at the pulmonary ligament.[2]

Lobes and segments. The lungs are divided into lobes and segments (Figure 19-2), with the lobes being separated by pleural membrane–covered fissures. The right lung, which is larger and heavier than the left, is divided into upper, middle, and lower lobes. The left lung is divided into only an upper and a lower lobe.[2] A portion of the left lung, the lingula, corresponds anatomically with the right middle lobe. The horizontal fissure divides the right upper lobe from the right middle lobe. The oblique fissure divides the right upper and middle lobes from the lower lobe and the left upper lobe from the lower lobe. The lobes are divided into 18 segments, each of which has its own bronchus branching immediately off a lobar bronchus. Ten segments are located in the right lung and eight in the left lung.[1]

Mediastinum. The area between the two lungs, the mediastinum, contains the heart, great vessels, lymphatics, and esophagus. A portion of the mediastinal area contains the root of the lungs, also known as the hilum, in which the visceral and parietal pleura form a sheath around the main-stem bronchi, the

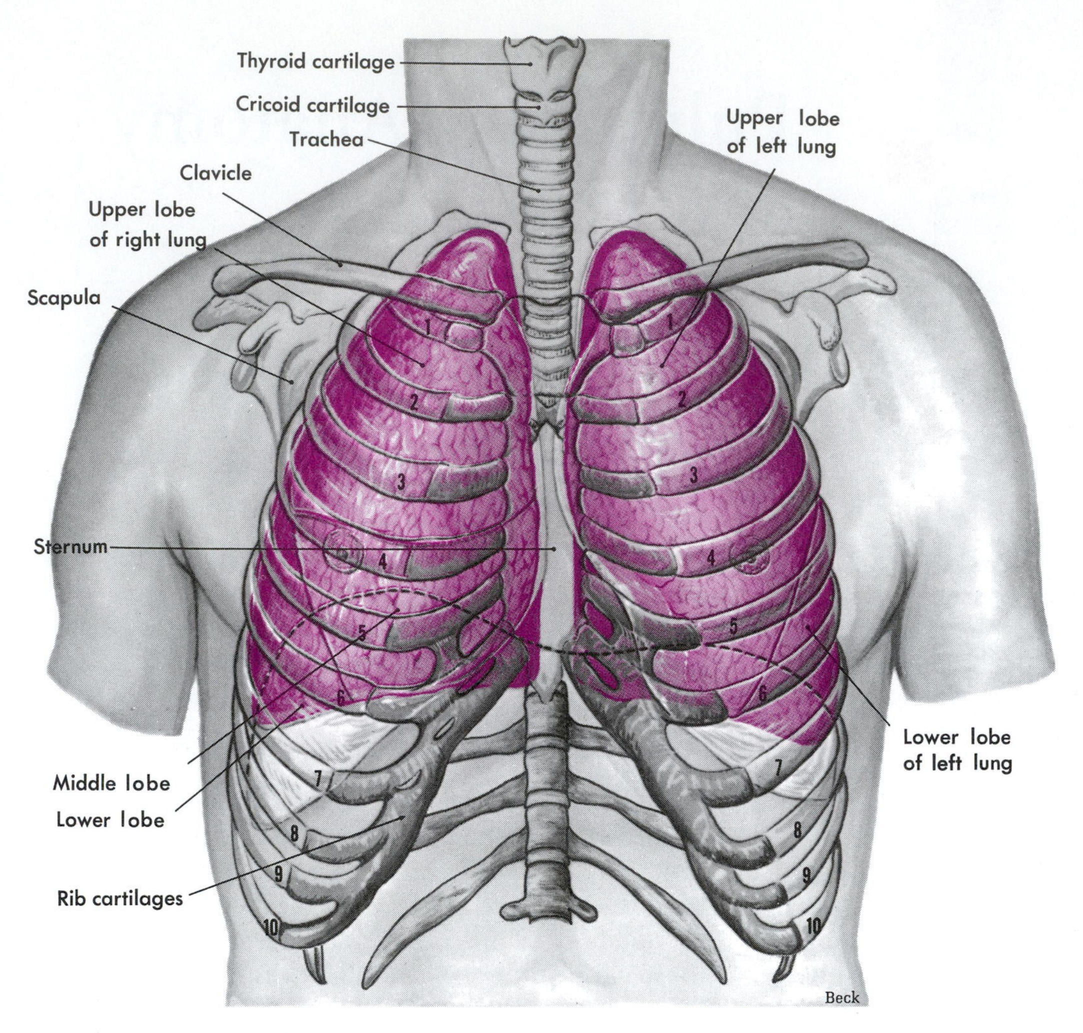

FIGURE 19-1. Ventilatory structures of the chest wall and lungs, showing ribs (numbered) and lobes of the lungs. Each intercostal space takes the number of the rib above it. The dotted line indicates the location of the diaphragm at inhalation and exhalation. Note the apex of each lung rising above the clavicle. (From Thibodeau GA: *Anthony's textbook of anatomy and physiology,* ed 13, St Louis, 1990, Mosby.)

major blood vessels, and the nerves that enter and exit the lungs.[2]

Pleura

The pleura is a thin membrane that lines the outside of the lungs and the inside of the chest wall. The visceral pleura adheres to the lungs, extending onto the hilar bronchi and into the major fissures. The parietal pleura lines the inner surface of the chest wall and mediastinum.[2] The two pleural surfaces are separated by an airtight space, which contains a thin layer of lubricating fluid. Pleural fluid allows the visceral and parietal pleural membranes to glide against each other during inhalation and exhalation.[1,3] The pleural space has the capacity to hold much more fluid than its normal volume of a few milliliters.[1]

Intrapleural pressure. The pleural space has a pressure within it termed the *intrapleural pressure,* which differs from the intraalveolar (pressure within the alveoli) and atmospheric pressure.[4] Under normal conditions intrapleural pressure is less than the intraalveolar and atmospheric pressure, with a normal range of −4 cm H_2O to −10 cm H_2O during exhalation and inhalation, respectively.[3] A deep inhalation can generate intrapleural pressures of −12 to −18 cm H_2O. This negative intrapleural pressure results from forces within the chest wall that exert pressure to pull the parietal pleura outward and away from the visceral pleura while the elastic fibers within the lungs exert pressure to pull the visceral pleura inward away from the parietal pleura. The constant "pull" of the two pleural membranes in opposite directions

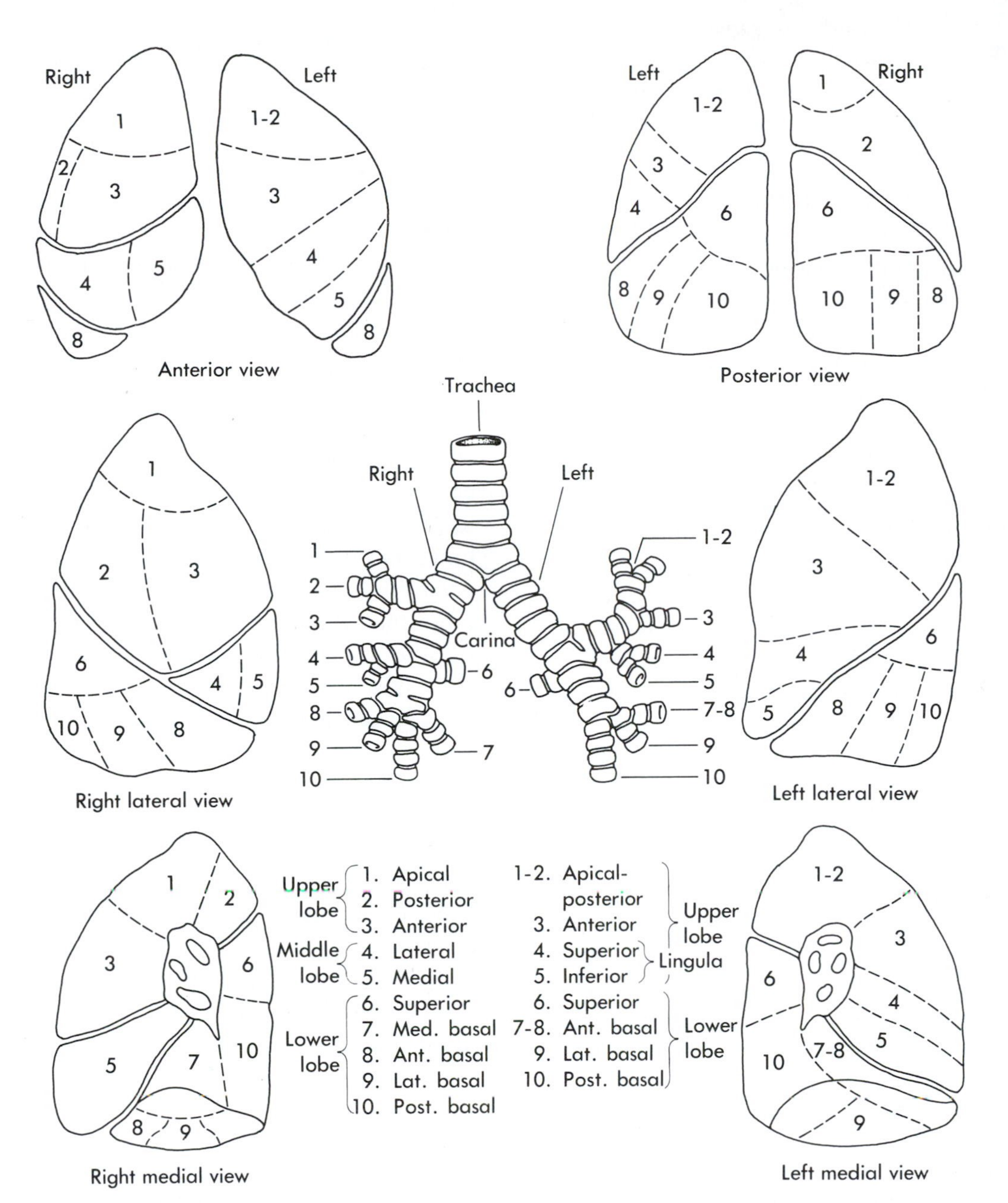

FIGURE 19-2. Lungs divided into lobes and segments. Note the differences between the right and left lungs. (From Ruppel GL, Tesoriero J: Functional anatomy of the respiratory system. In Scanlan CL, Spearman CB, Sheldon RL: *Egan's fundamentals of respiratory care,* ed 6, St Louis, 1995, Mosby.)

from each other causes the pressure within the space to be subatmospheric.[4] It is the negative pressure in the pleural space that keeps the lungs inflated (Box 19-1). If atmospheric pressure enters the pleural space, all or part of a lung will collapse, producing a pneumothorax.[1]

Muscles of Ventilation

The muscles of ventilation (Figure 19-3) are governed by the regulatory activity of the central nervous system, which sends messages to the muscles to stimulate contraction and relaxation. This muscular activity controls inhalation and exhalation. Muscles that increase the size of the chest are termed *muscles of inhalation;* those that decrease the size of the chest are termed *muscles of exhalation.*[5]

Inhalation. The main muscle of inhalation is the diaphragm. The diaphragm is a dome-shaped fibromuscular septum that separates the thoracic and abdominal cavities. It is connected to the sternum,

BOX 19-1 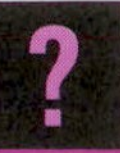 **Why The Lungs Stay Inflated**

The lungs stay inflated because the pressure surrounding them (intrapleural) is always less than the pressure within them (intrapulmonary).

WHY IS THE INTRAPLEURAL PRESSURE LESS THAN THE INTRAPULMONARY PRESSURE?

The intrapleural pressure is always (1) less than intrapulmonary pressure, (2) less than atmospheric pressure, and (3) considered negative because of the "pull" of the two pleural membranes in opposite directions. The parietal pleura is pulled outward by forces within the chest wall while the visceral pleura is pulled inward by the force of the elastic fibers within the lungs.

WHY DO THE TWO PLEURAL MEMBRANES "PULL" IN OPPOSITE DIRECTIONS?

The parietal pleura, attached to the chest, is pulled outward because the elastic fibers within the intercostal muscles exert outward pressure on the ribs. These fibers are in a relaxed state when the rib cage is fully expanded, such as during a deep inhalation. The visceral pleura, attached to the lungs, is pulled inward because the elastic fibers within the lungs, responsible for elastic recoil, exert pressure to make the lungs smaller. Elastic fibers in the lungs are in a relaxed position only when the lung is at its smallest configuration, such as occurs with a pneumothorax. Hence, because of the opposite pull of the chest wall and the lung and because the pleural membranes are attached to these structures, there is a constant pull of the two membranes in opposite directions. The subatmospheric pressure, which results within the pleural space, plus the greater than atmospheric intrapulmonary pressure within the lungs allow the lungs to remain inflated. Anything that causes the pressure within the pleural space to rise to atmospheric pressure or above will cause the lung(s) to collapse—a pneumothorax.

ribs, and vertebrae. During normal, quiet breathing the diaphragm does approximately 80% of the work of breathing. On inhalation the diaphragm contracts and flattens, pushes down on the viscera, and displaces the abdomen outward. Diaphragmatic contraction also lifts and expands the rib cage to some extent.[1,5,6]

The action of the diaphragm is governed by the medulla, which sends its impulses through the phrenic nerve. The phrenic nerve arises from the cervical plexus through the fourth cervical nerve, with secondary contributions by the third and fifth cervical nerves. For this reason and because the diaphragm does most of the work of inhalation, trauma involving C3 to C5 levels causes ventilatory dysfunction.[5]

Other muscles of inhalation include those that lift the rib cage. The most important of these are the external intercostal muscles, which elevate the ribs and expand the chest cage outward. In addition, the scalene, serratus anterior, and sternocleidomastoid muscles also participate in the elevation of the first two ribs and sternum.[1,5,6]

Exhalation. Exhalation in the healthy lung is a passive event requiring very little energy. Exhalation occurs when the diaphragm relaxes and moves back up toward the lungs. The intrinsic elastic recoil of the lungs assists with exhalation. Because exhalation is a passive act, there are no true muscles of exhalation other than the internal intercostal muscles, which assist the inward movement of the ribs. During exercise, however, exhalation becomes a more active event, requiring some participation of the accessory muscles of ventilation. Several muscles of the abdomen have long been thought to contribute to active exhalation.[4,5]

Accessory muscles. The accessory muscles of ventilation usually are considered those muscles that enhance chest expansion during exercise but that are not active during normal, quiet breathing. These muscles include the scalene; sternocleidomastoid; and other chest and back muscles, such as the trapezius and pectoralis major.[1,5,6]

CONDUCTING AIRWAYS

The conducting airways consist of the upper airways, trachea, and bronchial tree (Figure 19-4). The purpose of the conducting airways is threefold: to warm and humidify the inhaled air, to act as a protective mechanism that prevents the entrance of foreign matter into the gas exchange areas, and to serve as a passageway for air entering and leaving the gas exchange regions of the lungs.[1-3]

Upper Airways

The upper airways consist of the nasal and oral cavities, pharynx, and larynx (see Figure 19-4). Their main contribution to ventilation is the conditioning of inspired air. *Conditioned air* is air that has been warmed, humidified, and cleansed of some irritants. Warming and humidifying, which are essential to achieving a

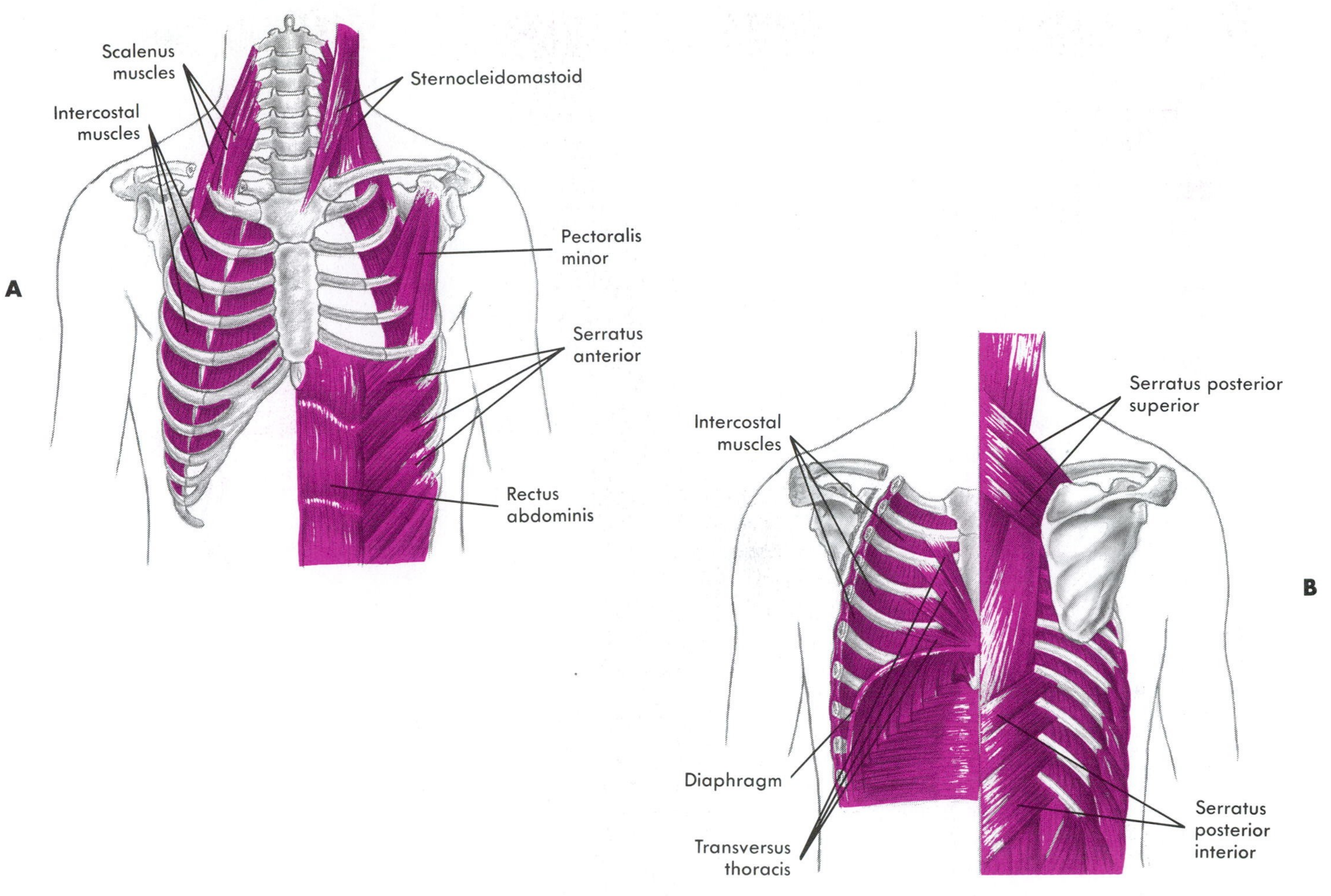

FIGURE 19-3. Muscles of ventilation. **A,** Anterior view. **B,** Posterior view.

nonirritant effect on the lower airways, occur mainly within the nose through a dense vascular network that lines the nasal passages. The air is cleansed by the coarse hairs that line the nasal passages by filtering large inhaled particles.[1,3]

Epiglottis. Also located in the upper airways is the epiglottis. It protects the lower airways by closing the opening to the trachea during swallowing, so that food passes into the esophagus and not the trachea. The epiglottis is a thin, leaf-shaped, elastic cartilage located directly posterior to the root of the tongue (i.e., attached to the thyroid cartilage [Figure 19-4]). It opens widely during inhalation, permitting air to pass through the trachea into the lower airways.[1,7]

Trachea

The trachea is a hollow tube approximately 11 cm (4.5 inches) in length and 2.5 cm (1 inch) in diameter (Figure 19-5). It begins at the cricoid cartilage and ends at the bifurcation (the major carina) from which the two main-stem bronchi arise. The carina is approximately at the level of the aortic arch, the fifth thoracic vertebra,[8] or just below the level of the angle of Louis.[1] The trachea consists of smooth muscle supported anteriorly by 16 to 20 C-shaped, cartilaginous rings. These prevent tracheal collapse during bronchoconstriction and strong coughing. The posterior wall of the trachea lies contiguous with the anterior wall of the esophagus. Having no cartilaginous support, this wall is composed only of muscle tissue, which is separated from the anterior esophageal wall by loose connective tissue (see Figure 19-5).[1]

Bronchial Tree

The two main-stem bronchi are structurally different (see Figure 19-5). The left bronchus is slightly narrower than the right, and because of its position above the heart, the left bronchus angles directly toward the left lung at approximately 45 to 55 degrees from the midline. The right bronchus is wider and angles at 20 to 30 degrees from the midline. Because of this angulation and the forces of gravity, the most common site of aspiration of

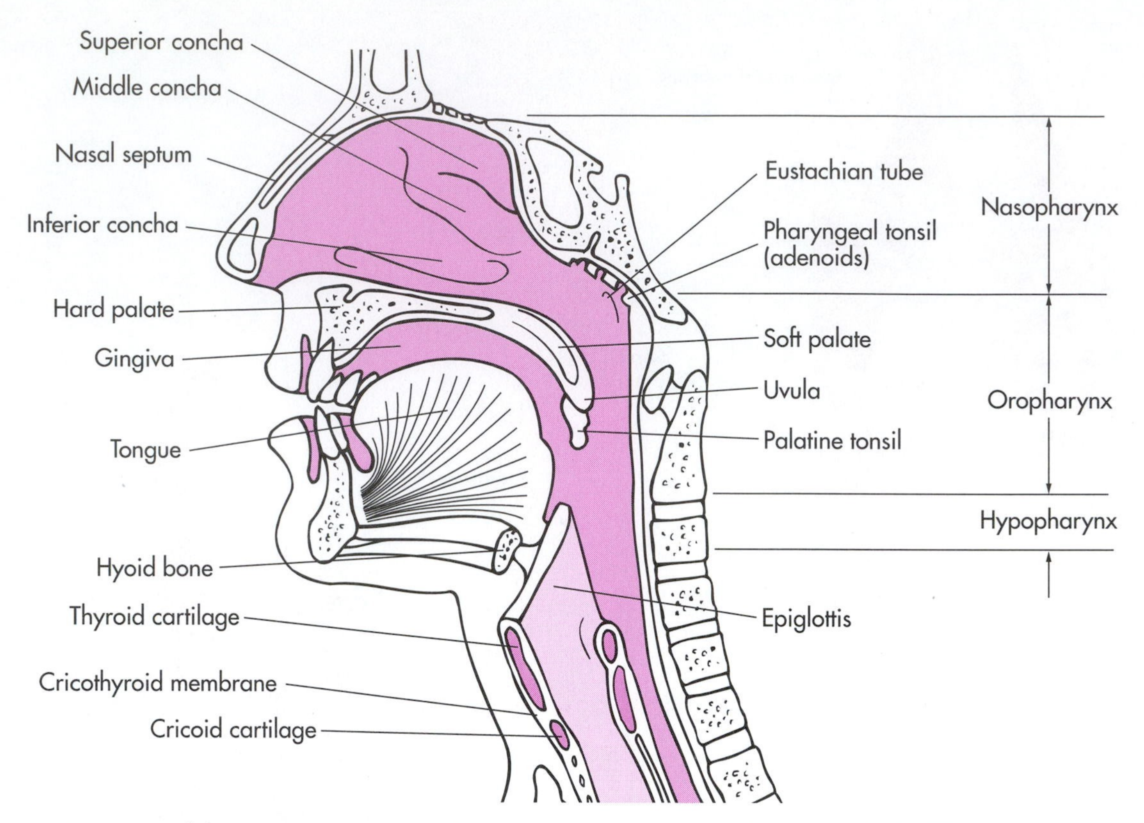

FIGURE 19-4. Structures of the upper airways. Note the placement of the epiglottis. (From Ellis PD, Billings DM: *Cardiopulmonary resuscitation: procedures for basic and advanced life support,* St Louis, 1980, Mosby.)

foreign objects is through the right main-stem bronchus into the lower lobe of the right lung.[2,3]

Bronchi. Each branching of the tracheobronchial tree produces a new generation of tubes (Figure 19-6). The main-stem bronchi are the first generation; the next branch, the five lobar bronchi, is the second generation. The third generation includes the 18 segmental bronchi. The fourth through approximately ninth generations are referred to as the *small bronchi,* beginning with the subsegmental bronchi. In these bronchi, diameters decrease; however, because the number of bronchi increases with each generation, the total cross-sectional area increases with each generation. This great increase in the cross-sectional area of the lung is extremely significant in that it allows easy ventilation despite the decreasing airway lumens.[1]

Bronchioles. The final subdivision of the conducting airways is the bronchioles. These are tubes with a diameter less than 1 mm and without connective tissue and cartilage within their walls. Their walls do, however, contain smooth muscle.[2] When smooth-muscle constriction occurs, these airways may close completely from lack of structural support. The terminal bronchioles form the last branch of the conducting airways, after which the gas exchange areas of the lungs begin. There are more than 32,000 terminal bronchioles.[1]

Defense system. The main defense system within the airways is the mucociliary escalator, or mucous blanket, a combination of mucus and cilia. The mucus, which floats atop the cilia (Figure 19-7), traps foreign particles. Ciliary movement then propels the entire mucous blanket and any trapped particles upward toward the pharynx at an average speed of 1 mm/minute in the smaller bronchioles and 12 mm/minute in the larger airways and trachea.[9] The mucus is either swallowed or cleared once it reaches the pharynx. The submucous glands of the airways produce approximately 100 ml of mucus per day, with all but about 10 ml reabsorbed through the bronchial lining.[8] The mucociliary escalator is so efficient that almost no particles larger than the size of 3 μm reach the alveoli. The cough reflex is another protective mechanism present in the lungs. Excessive amounts of foreign particles in the trachea and bronchi can initiate the cough reflex. Once initiated, the rapid expulsion of air carries any foreign particles with it.[9]

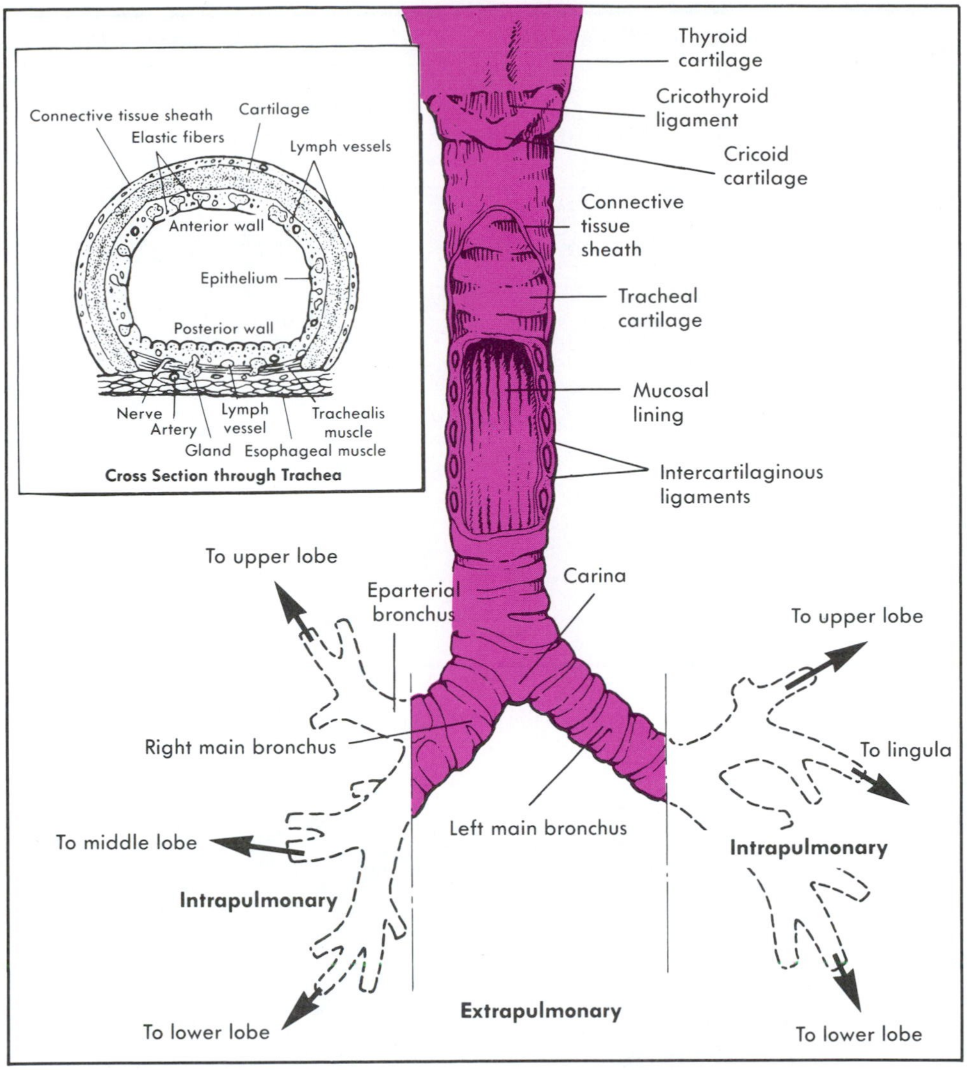

FIGURE 19-5. Anterior view of the trachea and primary bronchi and a cross-section through a part of the trachea, including a C-shaped cartilaginous element. (From Martin DE: *Respiratory anatomy and physiology,* St Louis, 1988, Mosby.)

RESPIRATORY AIRWAYS

The respiratory airways consist of the respiratory bronchioles and the alveoli. The respiratory airways also are known as the *terminal respiratory units,* or the *acini.* It is in these areas of the lungs that gas exchange takes place.

Respiratory Bronchioles

Each terminal bronchiole gives rise to two respiratory bronchioles, each branching two to four more times.[2] The respiratory bronchioles form the transition zone of the lungs, acting as both conducting airways and gas exchange units. While air is moving through the respiratory bronchioles, alveolar outpouchings on their surfaces allow gas exchange to take place.[1]

Alveoli

Each respiratory bronchiole gives rise to several alveolar ducts, which terminate in clusters of 10 to 16 alveoli. Thus each terminal respiratory unit contains approximately 100 alveolar ducts and 2000 alveoli.[10] The alveolus is the primary site of gas exchange and the end point in the respiratory tract. Within the two lungs there are approximately 300 million alveoli. The alveoli are composed of several types of cells, including Type I and Type II alveolar epithelial cells and alveolar macrophages.[1,3]

Type I alveolar epithelial cells. Type I alveolar epithelial cells comprise approximately 90% of the total alveolar surface within the lungs (Figure 19-8). They are the chief structural cells of the alveolar wall and play a major role in the maintenance of the gas-blood

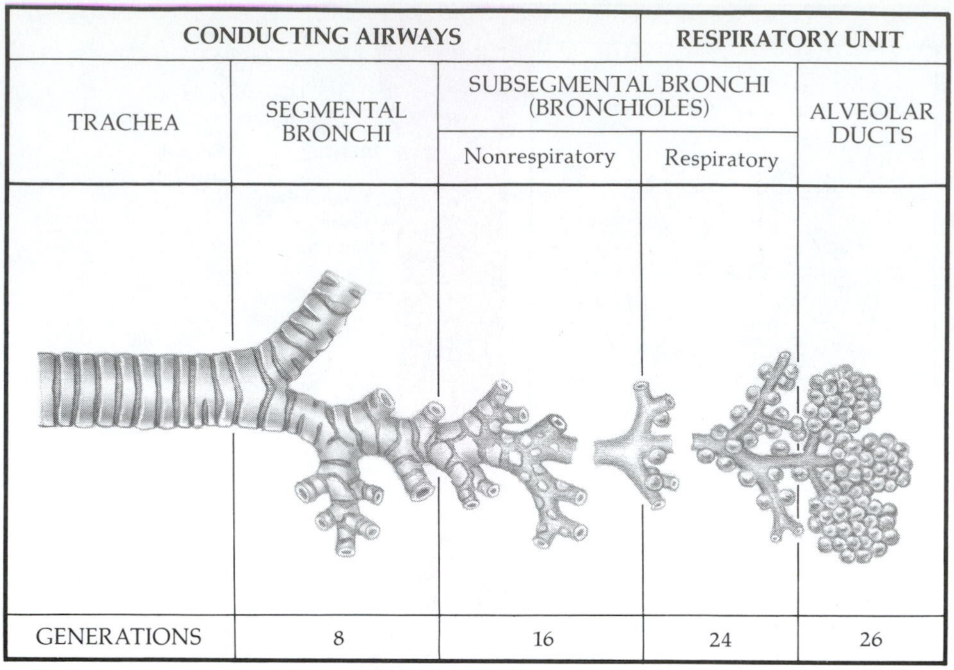

CONDUCTING AIRWAYS			RESPIRATORY UNIT	
TRACHEA	SEGMENTAL BRONCHI	SUBSEGMENTAL BRONCHI (BRONCHIOLES)		ALVEOLAR DUCTS
		Nonrespiratory	Respiratory	
GENERATIONS	8	16	24	26

FIGURE 19-6. Conducting and respiratory airways. Note the branching with increasing generations. (From Thompson JM and others: *Mosby's clinical nursing,* ed 4, St Louis, 1997, Mosby.)

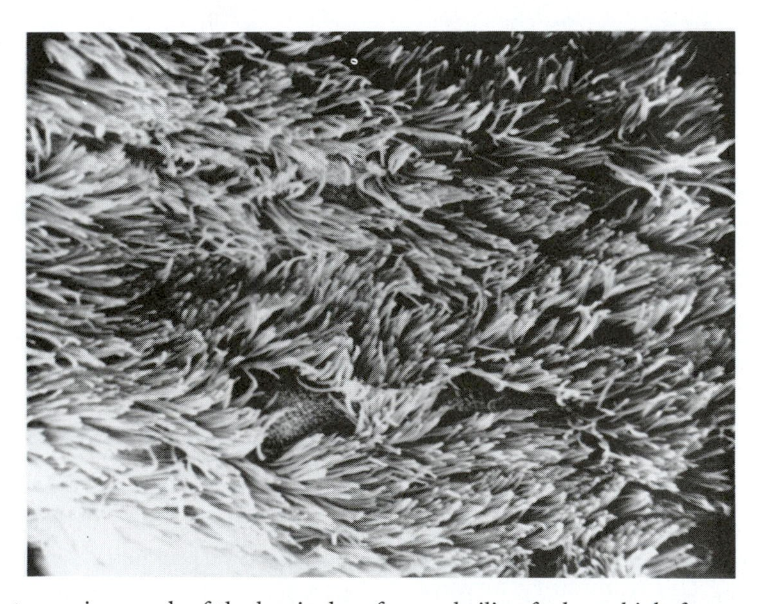

FIGURE 19-7. Scanning electron micrograph of the luminal surface and cilia of a bronchiole from a normal adult male (× 2000). (From Ebert RV, Terracio MJ: Observation of the secretion on the surface of the bronchioles with the scanning electron microscope, *Am Rev Respir Dis* 112:491, 1975.)

barrier and gas exchange. Type I cells are extremely susceptible to injury and become inflamed when exposed to inhaled toxins.[1,9]

Collateral air passages. There are a variety of collateral air passages located within the lower regions of the lungs. Within the walls of the Type I cells are the pores of Kohn (Figure 19-9), which allow collateral movement of air between alveoli. The canals of Lambert are collateral air pathways that exist between the alveoli and the respiratory and terminal bronchioles.[9] They are of particular benefit when a respiratory bronchiole is blocked or collapsed, because they allow gas to pass into alveoli distal to the blockage. Thus collateral air passages are of significant benefit in any pathologic condition of the lung that results in obstruction of airflow into a portion of the lungs.

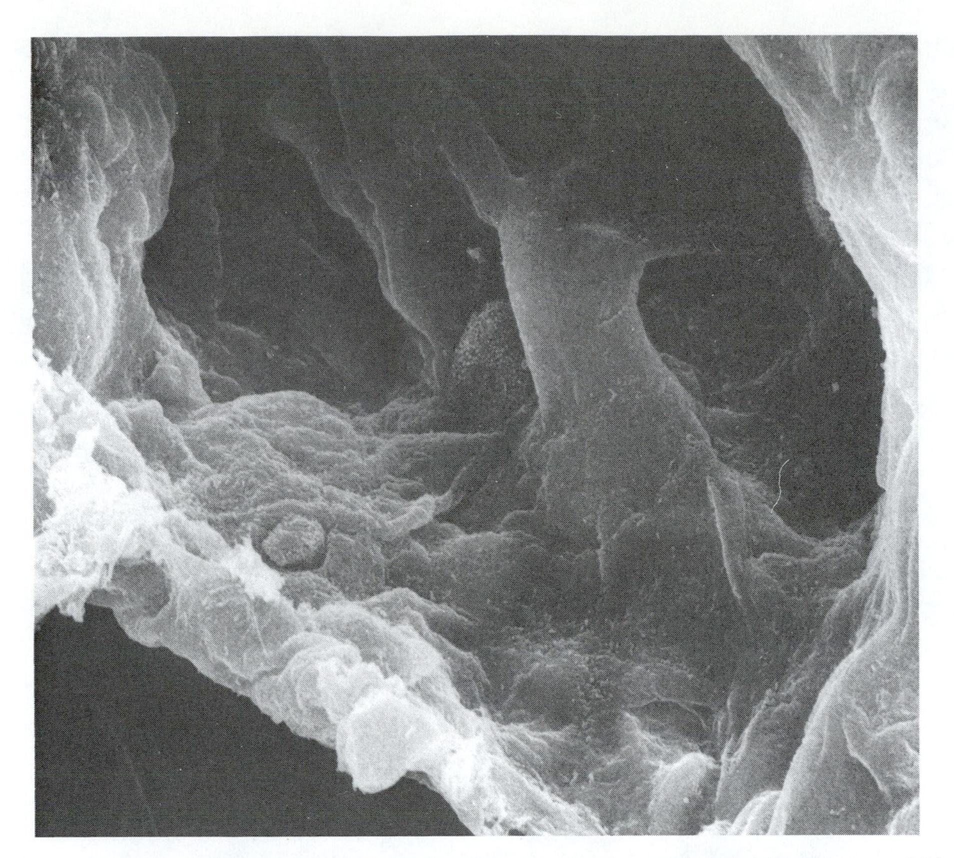

FIGURE 19-8. Detail of an alveolar surface composed chiefly of Type I alveolar epithelial cells. (Picture width—1 cm equals 3.46 μm). (From Martin DE: *Respiratory anatomy and physiology,* St Louis, 1988, Mosby.)

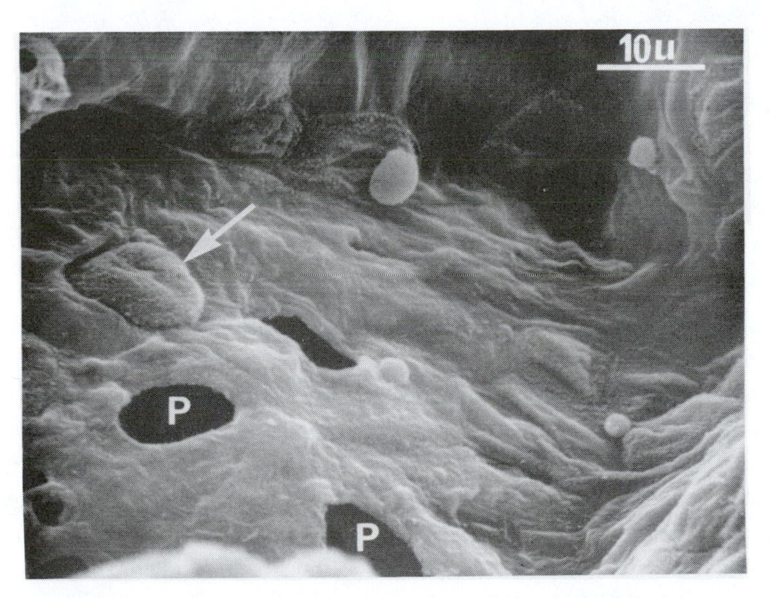

FIGURE 19-9. Scanning electron micrograph of the surface of a human alveolus, showing pores of Kohn *(P)* and a macrophage *(arrow)* (× 1500). (Courtesy Dr MS Wang.)

In contrast, however, these pores and canals also allow the movement of microorganisms through lung tissue.[1,2]

Type II alveolar epithelial cells. Type II alveolar epithelial cells occur in much greater numbers than Type I cells, but because of their minute size, they comprise a smaller portion of the total alveolar wall. After injury to the alveolar wall, Type II cells rapidly divide to line the surface; later they transform into Type I cells. The most important function of Type II

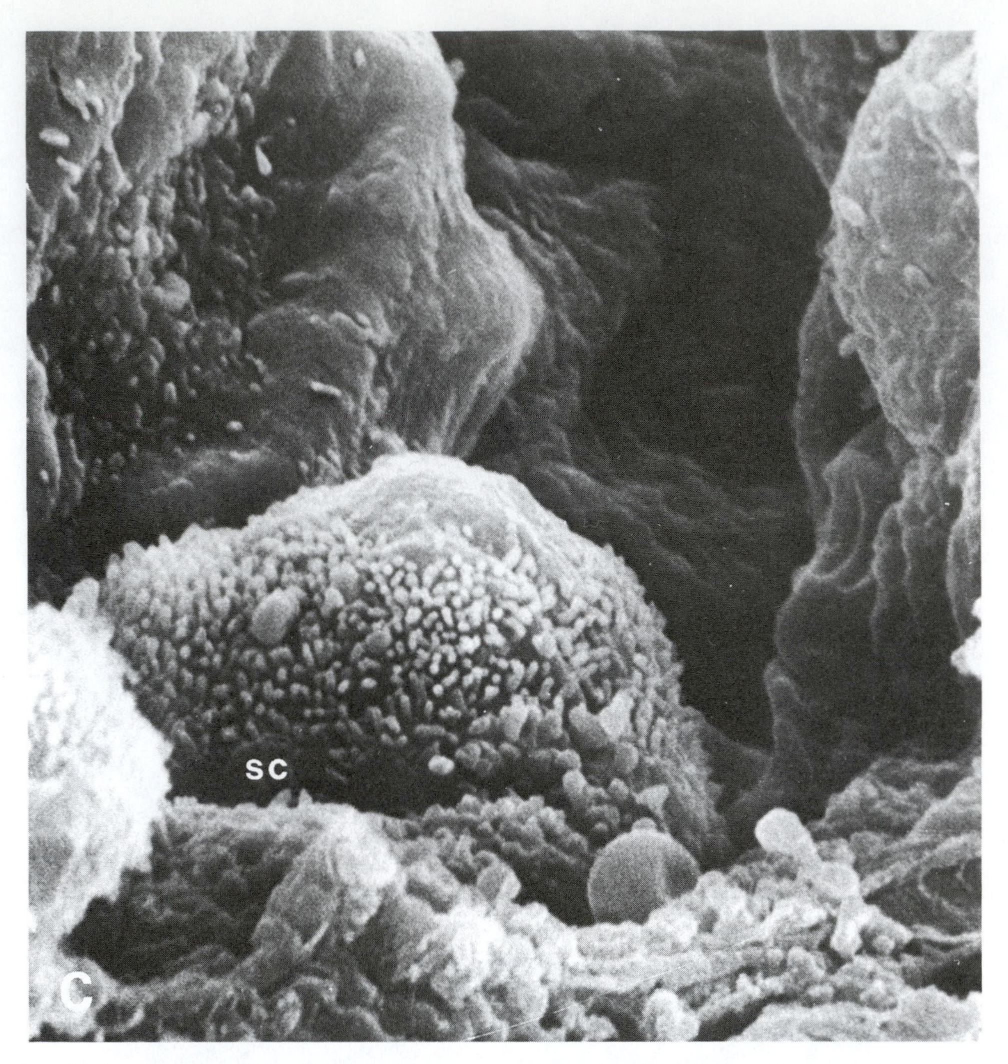

FIGURE 19-10. Type II alveolar epithelial cell. Note the presence of brush microvilli on all except the bald top of the round luminal surface. Type II cells produce surfactant. (Picture width—1 cm equals 0.85 μm). (From Martin DE: *Respiratory anatomy and physiology,* St Louis, 1988, Mosby.)

cells is their ability to produce, store, and secrete pulmonary surfactant (Figure 19-10).[1,3,9]

Surfactant. Surfactant is a phospholipid composed of fatty acids bound to lecithin. Like other surfactants, such as detergents and soaps, pulmonary surfactant functions to lower surface tension of the alveoli. Whereas with detergents and soaps this decrease in surface tension cleans clothes, within the lungs it stabilizes the alveoli, increases lung compliance, and eases the work of breathing. When pulmonary disease disrupts the normal synthesis and storage of surfactant, the lungs become less compliant and the work of breathing increases. Severe loss of surfactant results in alveolar instability and collapse and impairment of gas exchange.[11]

Defense system. Alveolar macrophages are monocytes that originate in the bone marrow and are released into the blood stream (Figure 19-11).[1-3] Upon entering the pulmonary capillary circulation, they move through the capillary membrane wall into the interstitial space and the alveoli. Once in the alveoli, the monocytes transform into macrophages and assume a phagocytic role. They move from alveolus to alveolus through the pores of Kohn, keeping the alveoli clean and sterile through phagocytosis and microbial killing activity, which includes the secretion of hydrogen peroxide, lysozyme, and other substances that kill microorganisms.[2,3]

PULMONARY BLOOD AND LYMPH SUPPLY

Two vascular systems and one lymphatic system make up the pulmonary blood and lymph supply. The pulmonary circulation is the vascular system that

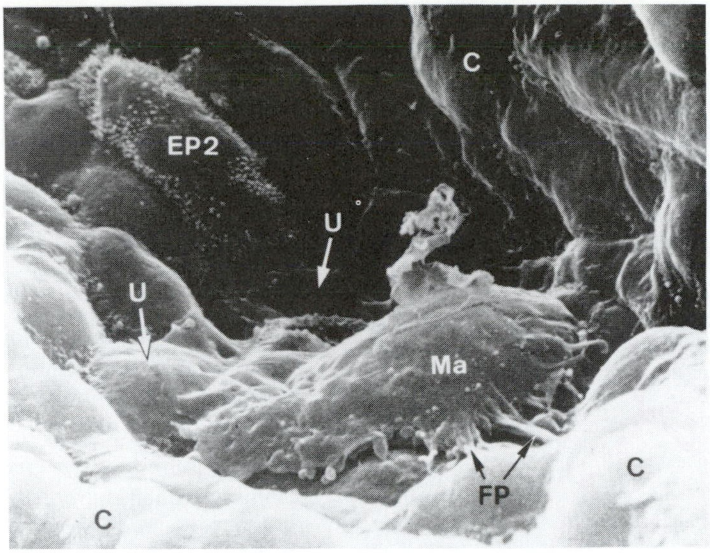

FIGURE 19-11. Scanning electron micrograph of a healthy human lung, showing an alveolar macrophage *(Ma)* attached to the epithelium partly by filopodia *(FP)* and forming an undulating membrane *(U)* in the direction of forward movement to the left. Several capillaries *(C)* are evident, and a Type II alveolar epithelial cell *(EP2)* can be seen in the background. (Original magnification × 3700.) (From Gehr P, Bachofen M, Weibel ER: The normal human lung: ultrastructure and morphometric estimation of diffusion capacity, *Respir Physiol* 32[2]:121, 1978.)

forms the gas exchange network surrounding the alveoli. The bronchial circulation is the vascular system that perfuses the tracheobronchial tree.

Pulmonary Circulation

The pulmonary circulatory system begins at the pulmonary artery, which receives venous blood from the right side of the heart. The pulmonary artery then divides into main-stem left and right branches and continues to branch until it forms the capillaries that surround the alveoli (see Figure 19-12). After gas exchange takes place, the blood is returned to the left side of the heart through the pulmonary veins.[2,12]

Pulmonary artery pressures. The pulmonary circulation is by far the largest vascular bed within the body and is the only one that receives the entire cardiac output. Just as the systemic circulation has a systolic and a diastolic blood pressure, so does the pulmonary circulation. Because of the relative lack of smooth muscle within the vessels of the pulmonary circulation, however, the pressures are vastly lower than within the systemic circulation.[1,13] Pulmonary artery systolic (PAS) pressure averages 25 mm Hg, pulmonary artery diastolic (PAD) pressure averages 10 mm Hg, and pulmonary artery mean (PAM) pressure is 15 mm Hg.[12] Because of the low pulmonary artery pressures, right ventricular wall thickness needs to be only approximately one third of left ventricular wall thickness. However, just as hypertension can occur within the systemic circulation, it also can occur within the pulmonary circulation (Box 19-2).[14]

Alveolar-Capillary Membrane

The vessels of the alveolar-capillary membrane form a network around each alveolus that is so dense it forms an almost continuous sheet of blood covering the alveoli.[2] The interior diameter of each capillary segment is just large enough to allow red blood cells to squeeze by in single file so that their cell membranes touch the capillary walls (Figure 19-13).[4] In this way, oxygen and carbon dioxide need not pass through significant amounts of plasma when diffusing into and out of the alveoli, making a highly efficient vehicle for gas exchange. Each red blood cell spends approximately three fourths of a second in the alveolar-capillary network and is exposed to the alveolar gas of two or three alveoli.[1] In that short time hemoglobin is brought from its normal venous blood saturation level of 75% to its arterial saturation level of more than 96%.[4] Actually, hemoglobin levels have been shown to reach normal within only a 0.25 second exposure to alveolar gas; thus under conditions such as tachycardia in which the red blood cells spend less time within the pulmonary capillary network, normal oxygenation can still occur.[3]

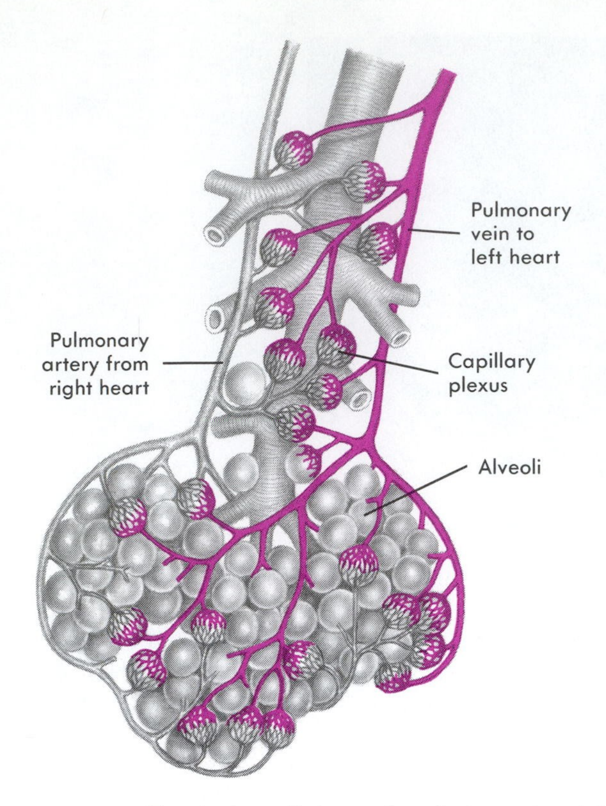

FIGURE 19-12. Terminal ventilation and perfusion units of the lung. Pulmonary arterial blood is venous *(dark gray)*, and pulmonary venous blood is oxygenated *(purple)*. (From Thompson JM and others: *Mosby's clinical nursing,* ed 4, St Louis, 1997, Mosby.)

BOX 19-2 Pulmonary Hypertension

Pulmonary hypertension is defined as increased pressure (PAS greater than 30 mm Hg and PAM greater than 18 mm Hg) within the pulmonary arterial system. It occurs when the cross-sectional area of the pulmonary bed decreases as a result of vasoconstriction and/or structural changes in the vascular bed. These changes may be a result of a variety of pathophysiologic conditions, including impedance to pulmonary venous drainage (e.g., mitral stenosis); increased pulmonary blood flow (e.g., septal defect); impedance to flow through large pulmonary arteries (e.g., pulmonary embolus) or small pulmonary blood vessels (e.g., collagen vascular diseases); and impedance to flow from hypoxic vasoconstriction.

The pulmonary hypertension resulting from hypoxic vasoconstriction, although caused in part by vasospasm, is largely a result of alterations in the structure of the blood vessels of the pulmonary circulation, which results in an increase in the medial thickness and a reduction in the size of the vascular lumen. Pulmonary hypertension increases the afterload of the right ventricle and, when chronic, can result in right ventricular hypertrophy (cor pulmonale) and failure.

Membrane layers. The alveolar-capillary membrane is less than 0.5 μm thick[15] and is composed of several layers of cells: the alveolar epithelium, the alveolar basement membrane, the interstitial space, the capillary basement membrane, and the capillary endothelium (Figure 19-14). Oxygen and carbon dioxide traverse easily across these layers, which present no barrier to diffusion because the membrane is very thin.[3]

Bronchial Circulation

The bronchial circulation, also known as the systemic blood supply to the lungs, is the system that perfuses the tracheobronchial tree, visceral pleura, interstitial and connective tissue, some arteries and veins, lymph nodes, and the nerves within the thoracic cavity. The bronchial arteries that perfuse structures in the left side of the thorax branch off the aorta, and those that perfuse the right-sided structures branch from the intercostal, subclavian, or internal mammary artery. After perfusing the specific lung structures, most of the venous blood returns to the right side of the heart; however, some venous blood from the bronchial circulation returns directly into the pulmonary veins and the left atrium.[16]

Physiologic shunting. The left atrium normally contains pure oxygenated blood, with a hemoglobin saturation at 100%. The mixing of venous blood from the bronchial circulation with the oxygenated blood in the left atrium decreases the saturation of left atrial blood to a range between 96% and 99%. For this reason, while a person is breathing room air, the oxygen saturation of arterial blood is less than 100%. The dumping of venous blood into the left atrium is known as an *anatomic shunt.* The thebesian veins, which drain blood from the myocardium, are also responsible for the addition of venous blood to the left atrium. These two systems constitute the normal anatomic shunt, which comprises approximately 3% to 5% of the total cardiac output.[17]

Lymphatic Circulation

The lungs are more richly supplied with lymphatic tissue than any other organ, perhaps because of their

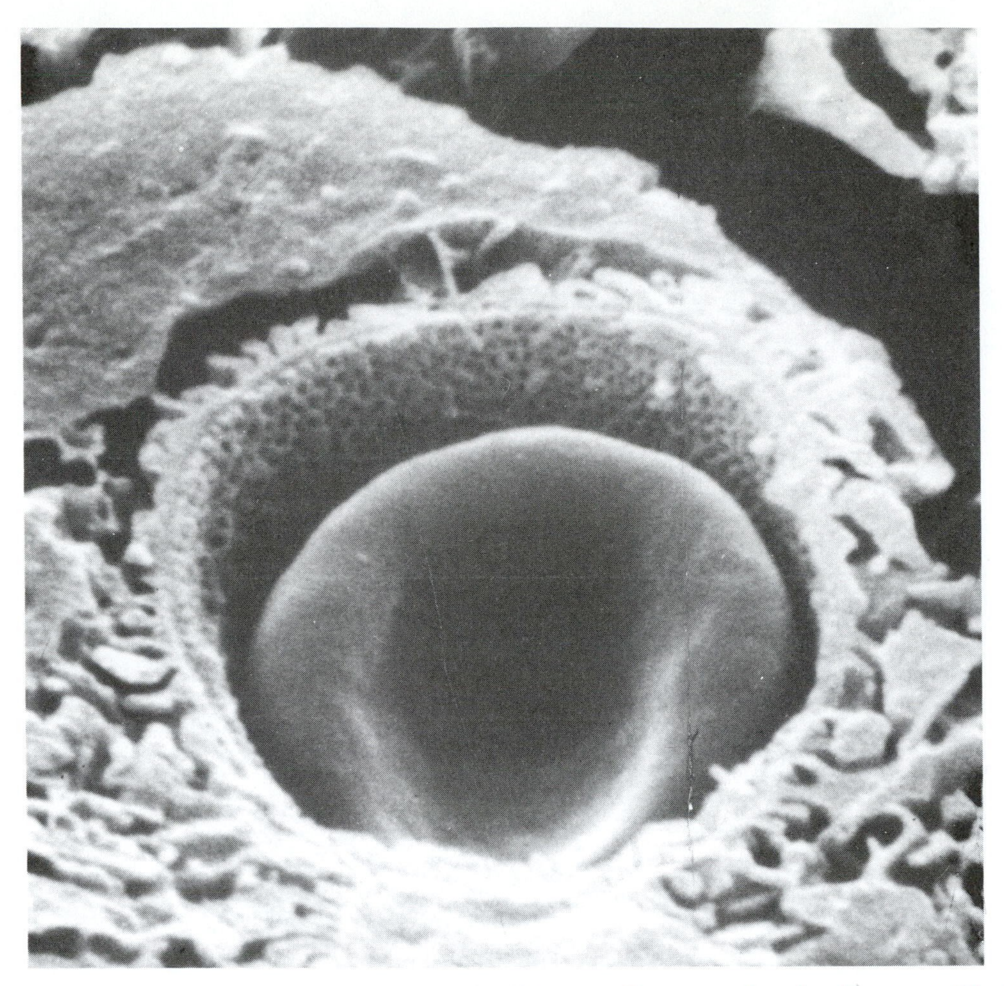

FIGURE 19-13. Scanning electron micrograph of a red blood cell in a capillary. Note that the diameters of both are similar. In many instances the red blood cells course through even smaller capillaries, often through capillaries that are one half the diameter of the red blood cell. This is possible because the cells are pliable, mainly as a result of their biconcave disk shape. (From Martin DE: *Respiratory anatomy and physiology,* St Louis, 1988, Mosby.)

constant exposure to the external environment. The lymphatic vessels parallel much of the pulmonary vasculature and the tracheobronchial tree to the level of the terminal and respiratory bronchioles. Lymphatic vessels also are located within the connective tissue of lung parenchyma and within the pleural membranes. These vessels eventually drain into the primary lymph nodes located at the hila of the lungs. The lymphatic system in the lungs serves two purposes: as part of the immune system, it is responsible for removing foreign particles and cell debris from the lungs and for producing both antibody and cell-mediated immune responses; it also is responsible for removing fluid from the lungs and for keeping the alveoli clear.[1-3]

VENTILATION

Air moves into and out of the lungs because of the difference between intrapulmonary pressure (pressure inside the lungs) and atmospheric pressure (Figure 19-15). The movement of air into the lungs is known as *inhalation,* whereas the movement of air out of the lungs is known as *exhalation.* At the command of the central nervous system, the muscles of ventilation contract, the thorax and lungs expand, and intrapulmonary pressure falls. When the pressure falls below atmospheric pressure, air enters the lungs and inhalation occurs. At the end of inhalation, the muscles of ventilation relax, the thorax contracts and the lungs are compressed, and intrapulmonary pressure rises. When the pressure rises above atmospheric pressure, air exits the lungs and exhalation occurs.[4,18]

Work of Breathing

The work of breathing is the amount of work that must be performed to overcome the elastic and resistive properties of the lungs. The elastic properties are determined by lung recoil, chest-wall recoil, and

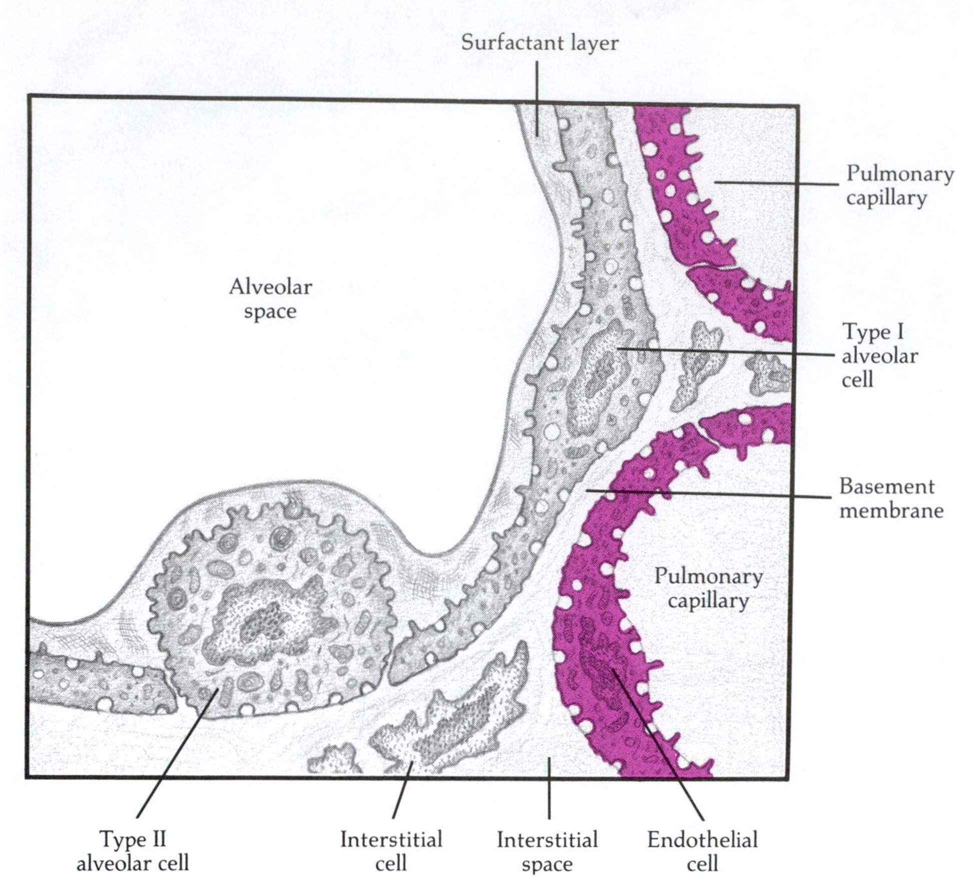

FIGURE 19-14. Layers of the alveolar-capillary membrane. (From Thompson JM and others: *Mosby's clinical nursing,* ed 4, St Louis, 1997, Mosby.)

the surface tension of the alveoli. The resistive properties are determined by airway resistance.[1,18,19] Normally the work of breathing occurs during inhalation. Even exhalation, however, can be a strain when lung recoil, chest-wall recoil, and/or airway resistance is/are abnormal.[4,18]

During normal, quiet ventilation only 1% to 2% of basal oxygen consumption is required by the pulmonary system.[19] During heavy exercise the amount of energy required by the pulmonary system can become progressively greater; thus the work of breathing can limit exercise in the patient with pulmonary disease. Pathologic conditions of the pulmonary system can drastically change the energy requirement for ventilation. Pulmonary diseases that decrease lung compliance (e.g., atelectasis, pulmonary edema); decrease chest wall compliance (e.g., kyphoscoliosis); increase airway resistance (e.g., bronchitis, chronic obstructive pulmonary disease); or decrease lung recoil (i.e., emphysema) can increase the work of breathing so much that one third or more of the total body energy is used for ventilation (Box 19-3).[4,18]

Pulmonary Volumes and Capacities

Pulmonary ventilation can be described in terms of volumes and capacities (Figure 19-16). Tidal volume (V_T) is the amount of air inhaled and exhaled with each breath. Inspiratory reserve volume (IRV) is the maximum amount of air that can be inhaled over and above the normal tidal volume. Expiratory reserve volume (ERV) is the maximum amount of air that can be exhaled beyond the normal tidal volume. The residual volume (RV) is the amount of air left in the lungs after a complete exhalation. Inspiratory capacity (IC) is the sum of the tidal volume and the inspiratory reserve volume. Functional residual capacity (FRC) is the sum of the expiratory reserve volume and the residual volume. Vital capacity (VC) is the sum of the inspiratory reserve volume, the tidal volume, and the expiratory reserve volume. Total lung capacity (TLC) is the sum of all four volumes and represents the maximal amount of air that can be inhaled.[3,18]

Physiologic dead space. The portion of total ventilation that participates in gas exchange is known as *alveolar ventilation.* The portion of ventilation that

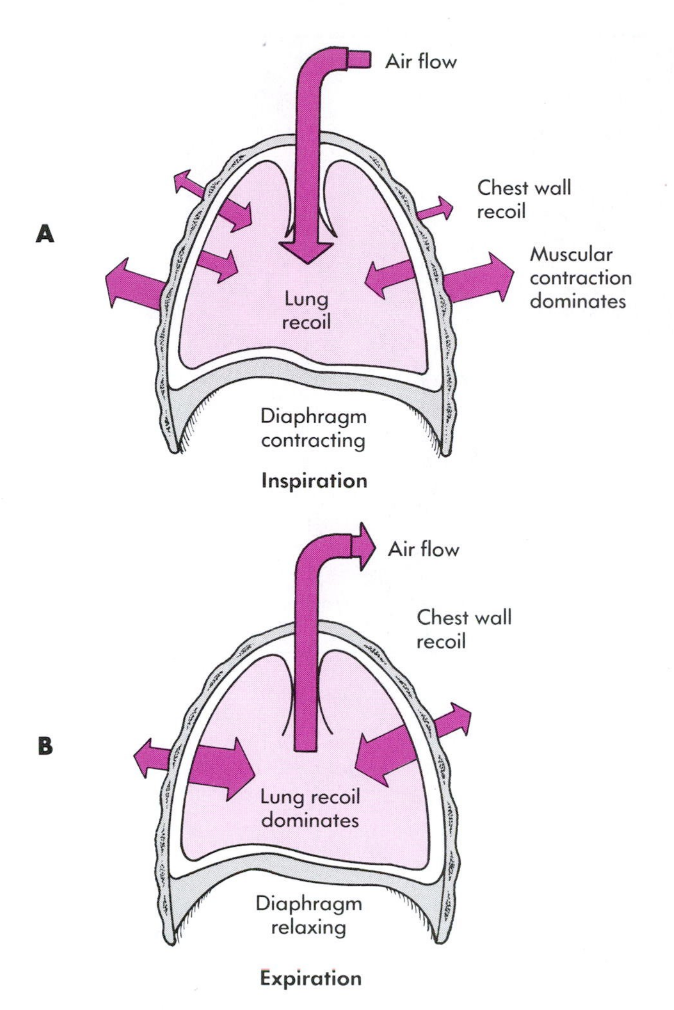

FIGURE 19-15. The process of inhalation and exhalation. **A,** During inhalation, the muscles of ventilation contract, the thorax and lungs expand, and air enters the lungs. **B,** During exhalation, the muscles of ventilation relax, the thorax and lungs are compressed, and air exits the lungs. (Modified from Davey SS, Huether SE, Budd M: Structure and function of the pulmonary system. In McCance KL, Huether SE, editors: *Pathophysiology: the biologic basis for disease in adults and children,* ed 2, St Louis, 1994, Mosby.)

does not take part in gas exchange is known as *wasted ventilation.* The areas in the lungs that are ventilated but in which no gas exchange occurs are known as *dead space regions.* The conducting airways are referred to as *anatomic dead space,* because they are ventilated but not perfused; thus they are not able to participate in gas exchange. In addition, some ventilation goes to unperfused alveoli. Without perfusion, gas exchange cannot take place, and thus the ventilation is wasted. These unperfused alveoli are known as *alveolar dead space.* Anatomic dead space plus alveolar dead space is termed *physiologic dead space.*[3,17,18]

BOX 19-3 ? How Lung Disease Can Alter Ventilation

Normal muscular action of the diaphragm, flexibility of the rib cage, elasticity of the lungs, and airway diameter are instrumental in allowing easy inhalation and exhalation. Any interference with these actions impairs normal ventilation. Pulmonary diseases can be categorized into obstructive or restrictive diseases, depending on how the underlying cause affects normal ventilation.

Restrictive diseases "restrict" lung or chest-wall movement and include diffuse interstitial lung fibrosis, atelectasis, kyphoscoliosis, and severe chest-wall pain. These conditions can be either acute or chronic, and because they restrict lung or chest-wall expansion, or both, patients have smaller tidal volumes but an increased ventilatory rate to maintain minute ventilation.

Obstructive diseases result in obstruction to normal airflow. The classic examples are emphysema, in which airflow is decreased because of a decrease in lung recoil, and asthma, in which airflow is decreased because of diffuse airway narrowing. Emphysema results in lungs that inflate easily but, lacking the normal elastic recoil, do not compress to assist with exhalation. Patients with emphysema may have little difficulty inhaling but struggle to exhale.

Regulation of Ventilation

Regulation of ventilation by the brain is complex and not completely understood. Ventilation is regulated by a triad comprising a controller (located within the central nervous system), a group of effectors (muscles of ventilation), and a variety of sensors that include chemoreceptors (central and peripheral) and mechanoreceptors (located in the chest wall and lungs).[7] Efferent nerve fibers convey impulses from the controller to the effectors, whereas afferent nerve fibers carry impulses from some of the sensors to the controller (Figure 19-17).[20]

Controller. The central nervous system houses what is known as the controller of ventilation. Actually, the controller is not located in one specific area; rather, it is in several areas that work together to provide coordinated ventilation. The brainstem regulates automatic ventilation; the cerebral cortex allows voluntary ventilation; and neurons housed in the spinal cord process information from the brain and from the peripheral receptors, allowing them to send final information to the muscles of ventilation.[7,21]

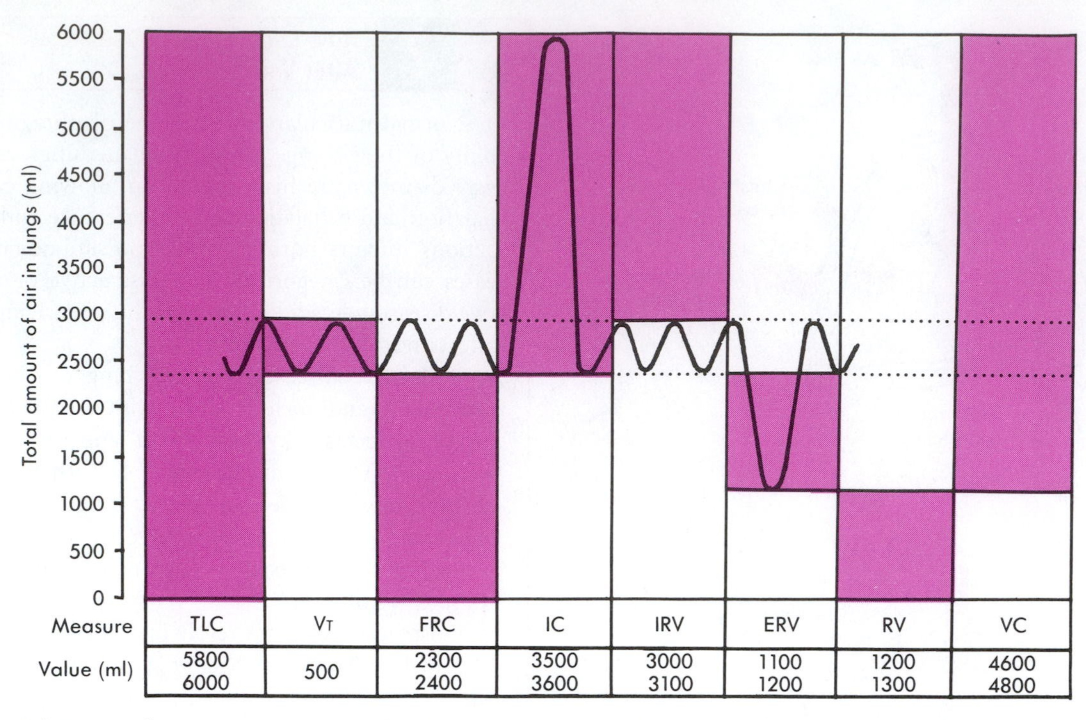

FIGURE 19-16. Lung volume measurements. All values are approximately 25% less in women. *TLC,* Total lung capacity; *Vt,* tidal volume; *FRC,* functional residual capacity; *IC,* inspiratory capacity; *IRV,* inspiratory reserve volume; *ERV,* expiratory reserve volume; *RV,* residual volume; *VC,* vital capacity.

Brainstem. In the brainstem, both the medulla oblongata and the pons are involved in ventilation. Four different groups of neurons are thought to participate in the regulation of inhalation and exhalation. The dorsal respiratory group, located in the medulla, is responsible for the basic rhythm of ventilation. Cells in this area are believed to automatically fire and trigger inhalation. The pneumotaxic center in the pons is responsible for limiting inhalation and thus triggering exhalation. This response also facilitates control of the rate and pattern of respiration. The ventral respiratory group, located in the medulla, is responsible for both inspiration and expiration during periods of increased ventilation. The apneustic center in the lower pons is thought to work with the pneumotaxic center to regulate the depth of inspiration.[6]

Cerebral cortex. The cerebral cortex functions by allowing voluntary ventilation to override the automatic controls of the medulla and pons. Voluntary ventilatory control is most important during behavioral states such as crying, laughing, singing, and talking. During these states, voluntary control may override the automatic control, which responds chiefly to chemical stimuli and changes in lung inflation.[3,21]

Effectors. The effectors of ventilation are the muscles of ventilation (see Figure 19-3). In considering their function in the control of ventilation, however, the most important issue is that they function in a coordinated fashion. The central nervous system regulates this function.[7]

Sensors. The main sensors for the regulation of ventilation are the central and peripheral chemoreceptors (see Figure 19-17). These chemoreceptors respond to changes in the chemical composition of the blood or other fluid around them. Other sensors that are found in the lung include the irritant receptors, stretch receptors, and the juxtacapillary (J) receptors.[3,7,21]

Central chemoreceptors. The central chemoreceptors are located near the ventral surface of the medulla in the chemosensitive area (see Figure 19-17). These chemoreceptors are surrounded by cerebral extracellular fluid and respond primarily to changes in the hydrogen ion concentration of that fluid. Ventilation increases when the hydrogen ion concentration rises and decreases when the hydrogen ion concentration falls. A rise in the partial pressure of carbon dioxide (Pa_{CO_2}) causes the movement of carbon dioxide across the blood-brain barrier into the cerebrospinal fluid, stimulating the movement of hydrogen ions into the brain's extracellular fluid. These hydrogen ions then stimulate the chemoreceptors, and ventilation is increased. Consequently, the increase in ventilation causes exhalation

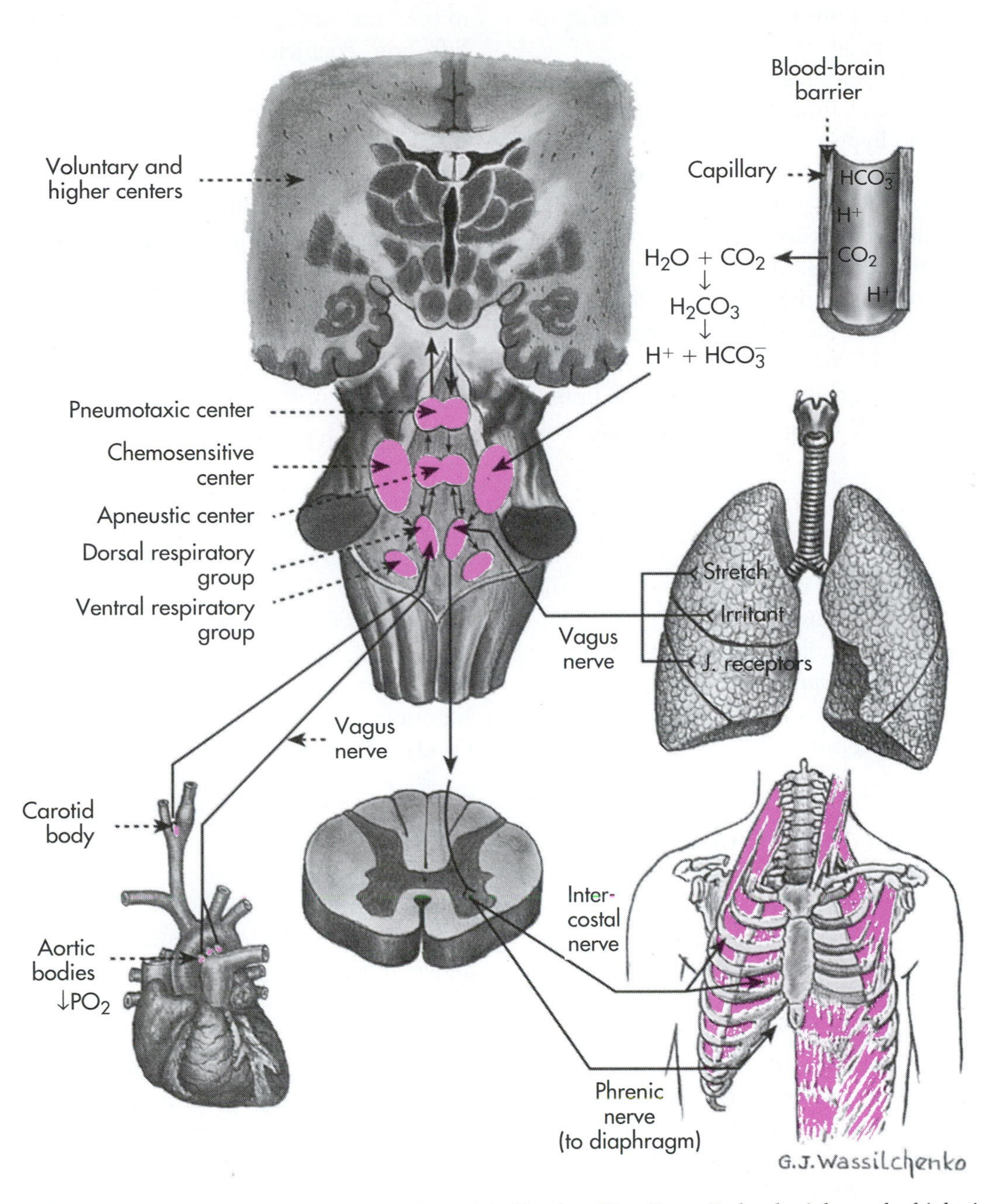

FIGURE 19-17. Respiratory control system. (From McCance KL, Huether SE, editors: Pathophysiology: the biologic basis for disease in adults and children, ed 2, St Louis.)

of excess carbon dioxide, a fall in Pa_{CO_2}, and the return of normal ventilation. Central chemoreceptors are not affected by changes in the partial pressure of oxygen (Pa_{O_2}).[4,7,21]

Peripheral chemoreceptors. The peripheral chemoreceptors are located above and below the aortic arch and at the bifurcation of the common carotid arteries (see Figure 19-17). The most important action of the peripheral chemoreceptors is their response to changes in the Pa_{O_2}, because they are the primary receptors that increase ventilation in response to arterial hypoxemia. Thus immediate hyperventilation, one of the principal compensatory mechanisms in response to hypoxemia, is governed by these chemoreceptors. The peripheral chemoreceptors also respond to changes in Pa_{CO_2} and hydrogen ion concentration. An increase in either results in an increase in ventilation. Studies indicate that the peripheral chemoreceptors probably are more involved with short-term response to carbon dioxide, whereas the central chemoreceptors are responsible for the long-term response to carbon dioxide.[7,21]

Other receptors. Irritant receptors lie between airway epithelial cells and function to stimulate bronchoconstriction and hyperpnea in response to inhaled irritants. Stretch receptors, which are located in the airways, are stimulated by changes in lung volume. They inhibit inhalation and are thought to protect the lung from overinflation (Hering-Breuer reflex). Juxtacapillary receptors lie in the alveolar walls close to the capillaries. They are stimulated by engorgement of the pulmonary capillaries and an increase in the interstitial fluid volume of the alveolar wall. Stimulation of the J receptors is thought to cause rapid, shallow breathing.[21]

RESPIRATION

Respiration refers to the movement of oxygen and carbon dioxide. Gas exchange that takes place at the lung level through the alveolar-capillary membrane is referred to as *external respiration.* The diffusion of gases in and out of the cells at the tissue level is referred to as *internal respiration.*[3]

Diffusion

Oxygen and carbon dioxide move throughout the body by diffusion. Diffusion moves molecules from an area of high concentration to an area of low concentration. The difference in the concentrations of the gases is referred to as the *driving pressure.* The greater the driving pressure of the gas through the membrane, the greater the diffusion.[3] Within the lungs, diffusion occurs because of the difference in the driving pressure between the pulmonary capillaries and the alveoli. Oxygen is in high concentration within the alveoli and thus exerts a higher driving pressure as compared with the pulmonary capillaries; therefore oxygen moves by diffusion from the alveoli into the pulmonary capillaries. On the other hand, carbon dioxide is in higher concentration and thus has a higher driving pressure within the pulmonary capillaries as compared with the alveoli; therefore carbon dioxide diffuses out of the capillaries into the alveoli, where it is exhaled (Figure 19-18).[4,22] The driving pressure of oxygen is lower at higher altitudes because the effects of gravity on the gases are lessened[20] and is higher when supplemental oxygen is administered.[23]

In addition to the driving pressure of the gases, several other factors affect the rate of diffusion. These include the thickness of the alveolar-capillary membrane,[3] the surface area of the membrane,[24] and the diffusion coefficient of the gas.[23] An increase in the thickness of the alveolar-capillary membrane (e.g., pulmonary edema, fibrosis)[14] or a decrease in the surface area of the membrane (e.g., pneumonectomy, lobectomy, pulmonary embolus, emphysema)[24] will decrease the rate of diffusion. The diffusion coefficient of each gas is determined by its solubility. The higher the diffusion coefficient, the faster the gas diffuses. Carbon dioxide has a much higher diffusion coefficient than oxygen; thus carbon dioxide diffuses 20 times more rapidly than does oxygen.[23]

VENTILATION/PERFUSION RELATIONSHIPS

Ventilation (V) and perfusion (Q) should be equally matched at the alveolar-capillary membrane level for optimal gas exchange to take place, but because of normal regional variations in the distribution of ventilation and perfusion, this is not the case. Normally alveolar ventilation is approximately 4 L/minute and pulmonary capillary perfusion is approximately 5 L/minute. Thus the normal ventilation to perfusion (V/Q) ratio is 4:5, or 0.8.[17,23]

Distribution of Ventilation

The distribution of ventilation throughout the lungs is not even. This is the result of a variety of factors, including the configuration of the thorax and the effects of gravity on intrapleural pressure. The thorax allows more lung expansion at the base than at the apex, which permits more ventilation to the base and limits ventilation to the apex. Gravity also produces regional variations in intrapleural pressure. At rest the negative intrapleural pressure at the apex is greater than at the base, thus alveoli in the apexes are larger and have more air left in them at the end of expiration. Because the alveoli are larger, they are less compliant and more difficult to inflate. On inhalation the alveoli at the base expand more because they have less pressure to overcome.[3,17,18] In the upright person the base of the lung receives about four times more ventilation than does the apex.[18] In the supine person, gravity produces the same effects in the dependent zones of the lungs (posterior regions).[3,17,18]

Distribution of Perfusion

The distribution of perfusion through the lungs is related to gravity and intraalveolar pressures. Because of the effects of gravity, the pressure in the capillaries in the lungs is higher in the bases than in the

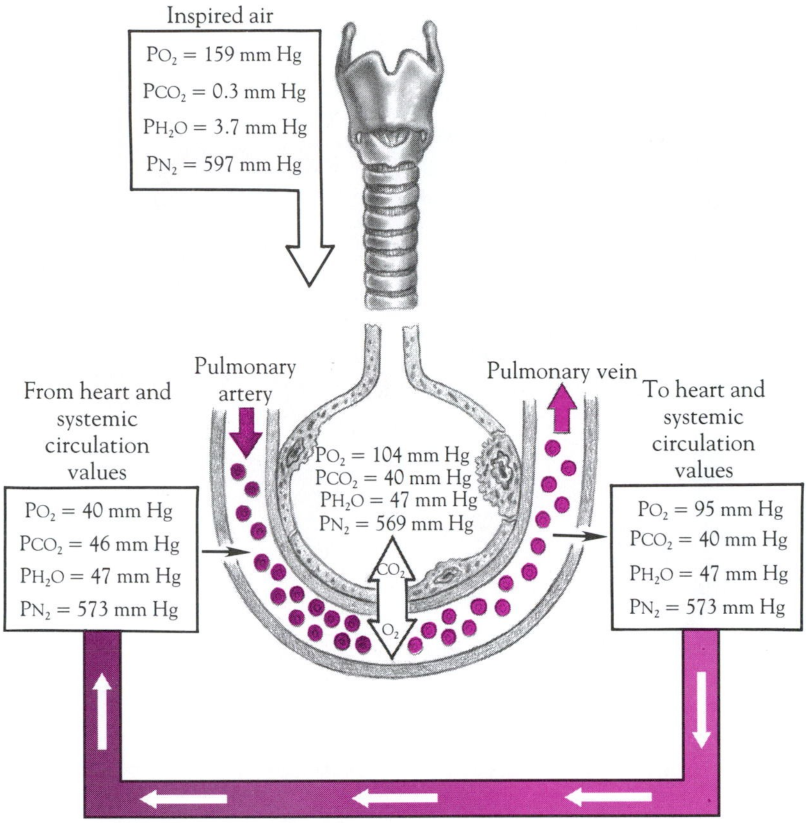

FIGURE 19-18. Process of respiration. (From Thompson JM and others: *Mosby's clinical nursing,* ed 4, St Louis, 1997, Mosby.)

apexes. This promotes preferential blood flow to the gravity-dependent areas of the lungs. Intraalveolar pressures also vary throughout the different regions of the lungs, with the highest pressure in the apexes and the lowest pressure in the bases. Thus in some areas of the lungs the intraalveolar pressure has the potential of exceeding capillary hydrostatic pressure, resulting in an absence of blood flow to these areas. On the basis of this concept the lung can be divided into three zones. Zone 1 is the nondependent portion of the lung, which has the potential of no perfusion. Zone 2 is the middle portion of the lung, which receives varying blood flow. Zone 3 is the gravity-dependent area of the lung, which receives a constant blood flow (Figure 19-19).[3,17]

Ventilation/Perfusion Mismatching

A variety of factors can affect the matching of ventilation to perfusion in the lungs, and their relationship can be considered as a continuum (Figure 19-20). At one end of the continuum there is the alveolus that is receiving ventilation but is not receiving any perfusion, thus unable to participate in gas exchange. This situation is referred to as *alveolar dead space.* On the other end of the continuum there is the alveolus that is receiving perfusion but is not receiving any ventilation, thus unable to participate in gas exchange. This situation is referred to as *intrapulmonary shunting.* In this case the blood is returned to the left side of the heart unoxygenated.[24] Between these two extremes exist an infinite number of ventilation/perfusion mismatches. Situations in which ventilation exceeds perfusion (V/Q greater than 0.8) are considered *dead space producing,* whereas situations in which perfusion exceeds ventilation (V/Q less than 0.8) are considered *shunt producing.* Although minor mismatching of ventilation may not significantly affect gas exchange, significant alterations in the relationship result in hypoxemia.[17,24]

Hypoxic vasoconstriction. The distribution of perfusion is also affected by the amount of oxygen in the

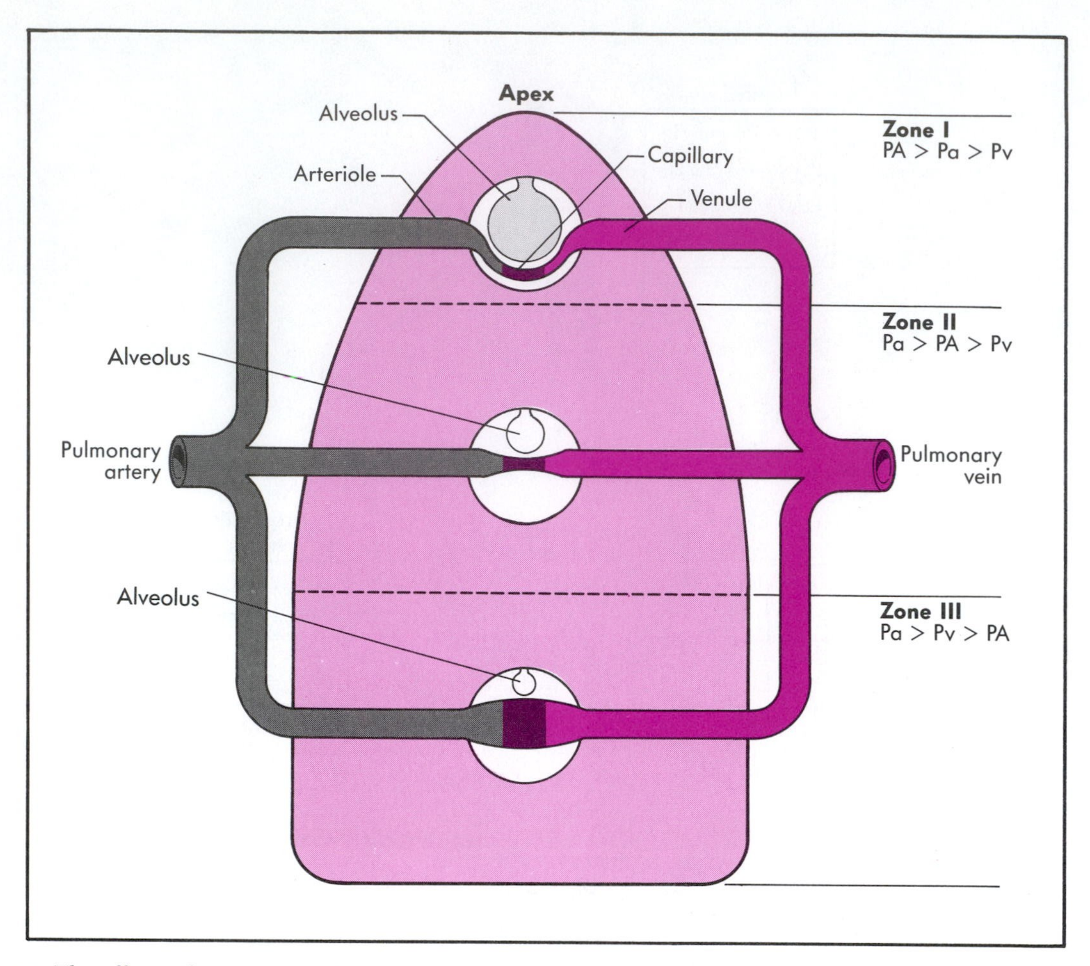

FIGURE 19-19. The effects of gravity and alveolar pressure on pulmonary blood flow. Note the three different lung zones. (From Davey SS, Huether SE, Budd M: Structure and function of the pulmonary system. In McCance KL, Huether SE, editors: *Pathophysiology: the biologic basis for disease in adults and children,* ed 2, St Louis, 1994, Mosby.)

alveoli. Although most blood vessels in the body dilate in response to hypoxia, the pulmonary vessels constrict when the PaO_2 is less than 60 mm Hg. This event is known as *hypoxic vasoconstriction,* and it generally occurs when a portion of the pulmonary capillaries perfuses unventilated or underventilated alveoli. It is thought to be a compensatory response used to limit the returning of unoxygenated blood to the left side of the heart. If the response is prolonged and generalized throughout the lungs, pulmonary hypertension will result.[25]

GAS TRANSPORT

Gas transport refers to the movement of oxygen and carbon dioxide to and from the tissue cells. The transportation vehicle is the blood stream, which is moved by the pumping action of the heart (cardiac output). At the tissue level, both oxygen and carbon dioxide move into and out of the cell by diffusion. Oxygen diffuses into the cell because of the pressure gradient that exists between oxygen in the capillary and oxygen in the cell (Figure 19-21, *A*). Carbon dioxide diffuses into the capillary because of the pressure gradient that exists between carbon dioxide in the cell and carbon dioxide in the capillary (Figure 19-21, *B*).[3]

Oxygen Content

Oxygen is transported to the tissues by the blood in two ways. It is either dissolved in plasma (PaO_2) or bound to hemoglobin molecules (oxygen saturation [SaO_2]). Most of the oxygen is transported by hemoglobin, with the portion of oxygen dissolved in plasma equal to approximately 3% of the total oxygen within

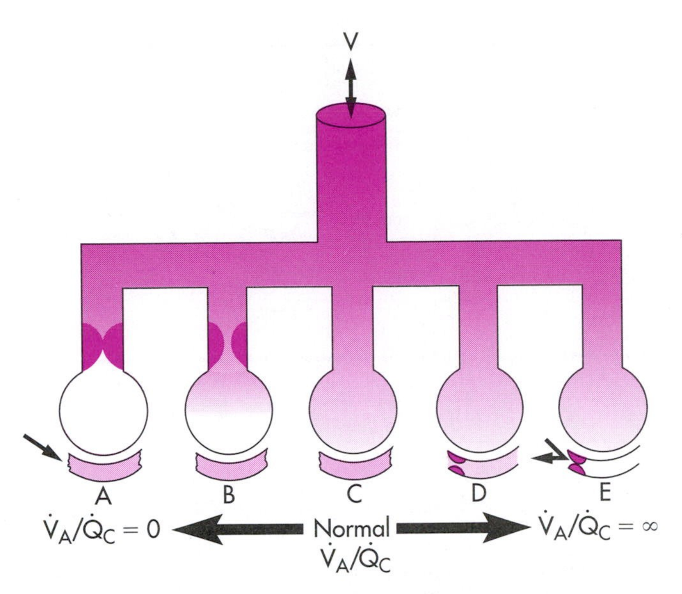

FIGURE 19-20. Continuum of ventilation/perfusion relationships. **A,** Intrapulmonary shunting. **B,** V/Q mismatching—shunt-producing situation. **C,** Normal V/Q ratio. **D,** V/Q mismatching—dead space–producing situation. **E,** Alveolar dead space. (From Misasi RS, Keyes JL: Matching and mismatching ventilation and perfusion in the lung, *Crit Care Nurse* 16(3):23, 1996.)

the blood.[26] The pressure exerted by the oxygen dissolved in plasma is important because this oxygen diffuses across the capillary membrane into the cells first and serves as the vehicle for unloading the oxygen from the hemoglobin molecule. As molecules of dissolved oxygen leave the plasma and diffuse into the cells, the molecules of oxygen move off the hemoglobin, dissolve into the plasma and, in turn, diffuse into the cells.[20] For this process to begin, a pressure gradient must exist between the oxygen level in the capillary and the oxygen level in the cell.

Oxygen content formula. The amount of oxygen in the arterial blood can be calculated using the arterial oxygen content (CaO_2) formula. The amount of oxygen in the venous blood can be calculated using the venous oxygen content (CvO_2) formula (see Appendix D).[27]

Oxyhemoglobin dissociation curve. The relationship between dissolved oxygen and hemoglobin-bound oxygen is illustrated graphically as the oxyhemoglobin dissociation curve (Figure 19-22). The sigmoid shape of the oxyhemoglobin dissociation curve illustrates several essential points about the relationship between the two ways oxygen is carried. The steep lower portion of the curve, at PaO_2 levels of 10 to 60 mm Hg, shows that the peripheral tissues can withdraw large amounts of oxygen from the hemoglobin molecule with only a small change in PaO_2, thus preserving the gradient for the continued unloading of hemoglobin.[20,26] The area at PaO_2 levels of 60 to 100 mm Hg is called the *flat upper portion* of the curve. This portion shows that the saturation of hemoglobin remains high, even as the PaO_2 declines. For example, in a healthy person, a PaO_2 of 60 mm Hg yields a saturation of 89%, whereas a PaO_2 of 100 mm Hg yields a saturation of 98%. The great drop in PaO_2 (from 100 to 60 mm Hg) causes only a small drop in oxygen saturation (from 98% to 89%).[23,26]

Shifting of the oxyhemoglobin dissociation curve. Under normal circumstances, hemoglobin has a steady and predictable affinity for oxygen. The combination of oxygen and hemoglobin based on this affinity is responsible for the position of the oxyhemoglobin dissociation curve, wherein a given PaO_2 yields a predictable oxygen saturation.[20,26,27] Occasionally, events occur that alter the affinity hemoglobin has for oxygen. These events include changes in pH, $PaCO_2$, temperature, and 2,3-diphosphoglycerate (2,3-DPG) (Box 19-4).[23] Any time this affinity is altered, the position of the oxyhemoglobin dissociation curve shifts (see Figure 19-22). Shifts in the position of the curve mean there is a change in the way oxygen is taken up by the hemoglobin molecule at the alveolar level, as well as a change in the way oxygen is delivered at the tissue level.[23,26,27]

Shift to the right. When the curve is shifted to the right (see Figure 19-22, *curve C*), there is a lower oxygen saturation for any given PaO_2; in other words, hemoglobin has less affinity for oxygen. Although the saturation is lower than expected, a right shift enhances

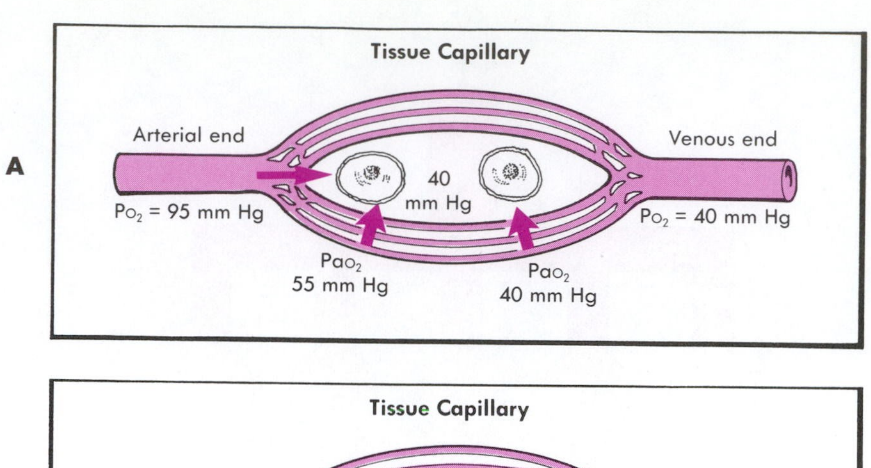

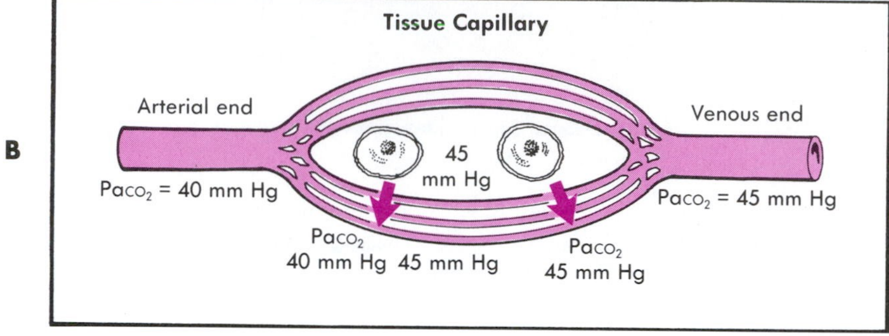

FIGURE 19-21. Internal respiration. **A,** Diffusion of oxygen from a tissue capillary into a tissue cell. **B,** Diffusion of carbon dioxide from a tissue cell into a tissue capillary.

oxygen delivery at the tissue level, because hemoglobin unloads more readily. Factors that cause this change in oxygen-hemoglobin affinity and shift the curve to the right include fever, increased $Paco_2$, acidosis, and an increase in 2,3-DPG.[23,26,27]

Shift to the left. When the curve is shifted to the left (see Figure 19-22, *curve A*), quite the reverse occurs; there is a higher arterial saturation for any given Pao_2, because hemoglobin has an increased affinity for oxygen. Although the saturation is higher, oxygen delivery to the tissues is impaired because hemoglobin does not unload as easily. Factors that contribute to the effect include hypothermia, alkalemia, decreased $Paco_2$, and decreased 2,3-DPG.[23,26,27]

Abnormalities of hemoglobin. Hemoglobin carries approximately 97% of the total amount of oxygen held within the blood stream. This great carrying capacity depends on hemoglobin that is normal in amount and molecular structure.[20] Most hemoglobin abnormalities affect the oxygen-carrying capability of this molecule.[23] The most common abnormality involving hemoglobin is a decrease in amount. This can be an acute or a chronic situation (anemia). Abnormal hemoglobin structure also can pose problems, such as hemoglobin S, which is responsible for sickle cell anemia.[22,28] Hemoglobin S has less affinity for oxygen than does normal hemoglobin. Normal hemoglobin can become abnormal hemoglobin under certain conditions. Methemoglobin and carboxyhemoglobin are two such examples. Methemoglobin occurs when the iron atoms within the hemoglobin molecule are oxidized from the ferrous state to the ferric state. Methemoglobin does not carry oxygen. Carboxyhemoglobin occurs when carbon monoxide combines with hemoglobin. Carbon monoxide uses the same binding site as does oxygen and has a much greater affinity for hemoglobin.[24,28]

Carbon Dioxide Content

Carbon dioxide, one of the end products of aerobic cellular metabolism, is produced continuously within the cells. On its way from the cells to the lungs, carbon dioxide is transported within the plasma and the erythrocytes. Carbon dioxide is transported; physically dissolved as the $Paco_2$ (5%); bound to blood proteins (including hemoglobin) in the form of carbaminohemoglobin compounds (5% to 10%); and combined with water to form carbonic acid (80% to 90%), some of which dissociates into hydrogen ions and bicarbonate.[4] In the lungs these methods of carbon dioxide carriage are reversed as the carbon dioxide leaves the plasma and erythrocytes for exhalation.[23]

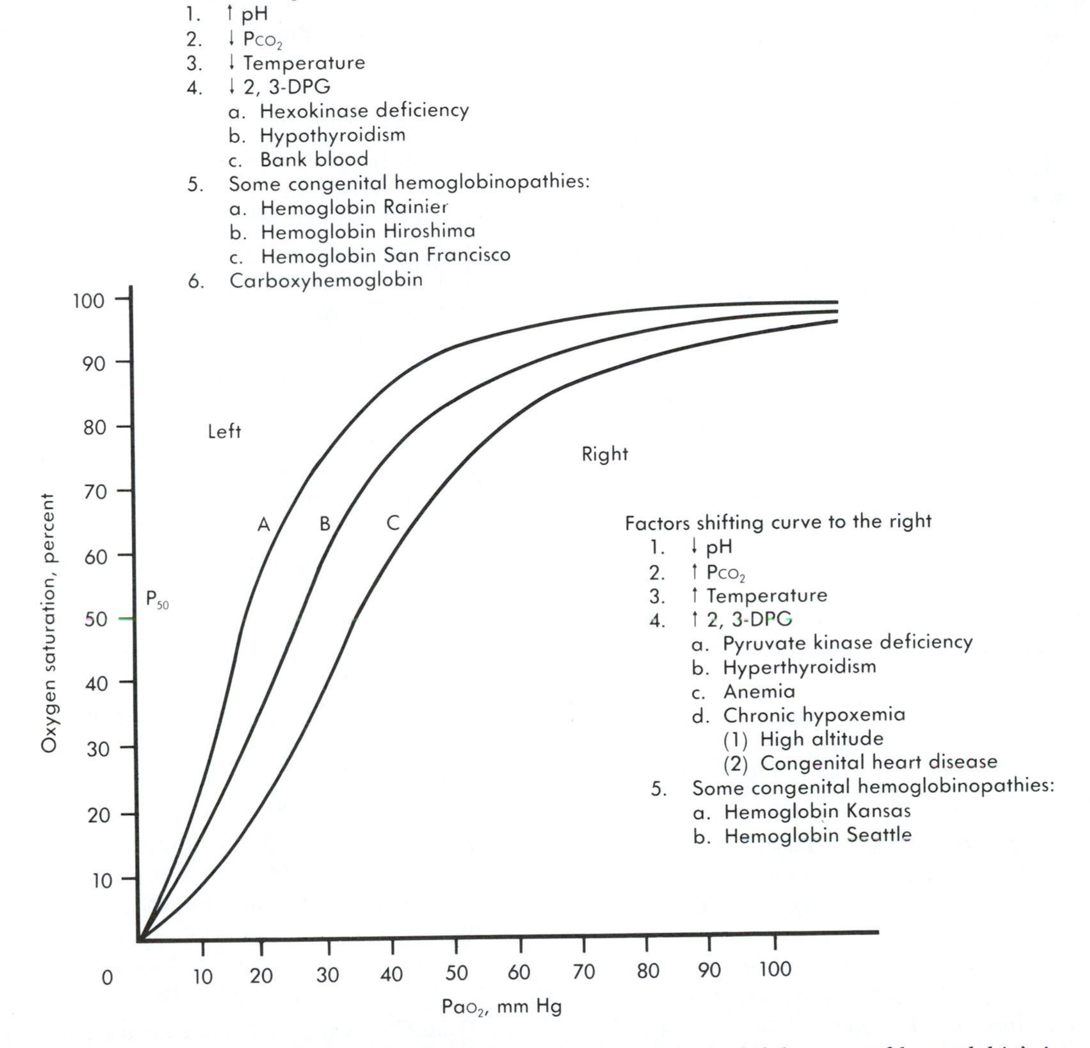

FIGURE 19-22. Oxyhemoglobin dissociation curve. **A,** The curve is shifted to the left because of hemoglobin's increased affinity for oxygen. **B,** The standard oxyhemoglobin dissociation curve. **C,** The curve is shifted to the right because of hemoglobin's decreased affinity for oxygen. (Modified from Ahrens TS, Nelson G: Pulmonary anatomy and physiology. In Kinney MR, Packa DR, Dunbar SB, editors: *AACN's clinical reference for critical-care nursing,* ed 3, St Louis, 1993, Mosby.)

BOX 19-4 ? What is 2,3-DPG?

2,3-Diphosphoglycerate (2,3-DPG), an organic phosphate found primarily in red blood cells, has the ability to alter the affinity of hemoglobin for oxygen. When the level of 2,3-DPG increases within the red blood cells, hemoglobin's affinity for oxygen is decreased (a shift in the oxyhemoglobin curve to the right), thus making more oxygen available to the tissues. Increased synthesis of 2,3-DPG apparently is an important component of the adaptive responses in healthy persons to an acute need for more tissue oxygen. Tissue hypoxia acts as the stimulus for production of 2,3-DPG, and increased amounts have been found in patients with anemia, right-to-left shunts, and congestive heart failure and in persons residing at high altitudes.

A decrease in the amount of 2,3-DPG is detrimental to tissue oxygenation because this decrease causes hemoglobin's affinity for oxygen to increase (a shift in the oxyhemoglobin curve to the left). Situations resulting in decreased 2,3-DPG levels include hypophosphatemia, septic shock, and the use of banked blood. Blood preserved with acid citrate dextrose loses most of its red cell 2,3-DPG within several days. Blood preserved with citrate phosphate dextrose maintains its 2,3-DPG levels for several weeks. Transfusion of blood with low 2,3-DPG will not be beneficial for tissue oxygenation until the 2,3-DPG level is restored, which may take 18 to 24 hours.

REFERENCES

1. Ruppel GL, Tesoriero JV: Functional anatomy of the respiratory system. In Scanlan CL, Spearman CB, Sheldon RL, editors: *Egan's fundamentals of respiratory care,* ed 6, St Louis, 1995, Mosby.
2. Sobonya RE: Normal anatomy and development of the lung. In Baum GL, Wolinsky E, editors: *Textbook of pulmonary diseases,* ed 5, Boston, 1994, Little, Brown.
3. Davey SS, Huether SE, Budd M: Structure and function of the pulmonary system. In McCance KL, Huether SE, editors: *Pathophysiology: the biologic basis for disease in adults and children,* ed 2, St Louis, 1994, Mosby.
4. Guyton AC: *Textbook of medical physiology,* ed 9, Philadelphia, 1996, WB Saunders.
5. Epstein SK: An overview of respiratory muscle function, *Clin Chest Med* 15:619, 1995.
6. Rochester DF, Esau SA: The respiratory muscles. In Baum GL, Wolinsky E, editors: *Textbook of pulmonary diseases,* ed 5, Boston, 1994, Little, Brown.
7. Johnson DC, Kazam H: Central control of ventilation in neuromuscular disease, *Clin Chest Med* 15:607, 1994.
8. Cosenza JL, Norton LC: Secretion clearance: state-of-the-art from a nursing perspective, *Crit Care Nurse* 6(4):23, 1986.
9. Romberger D and others: Respiratory tract defense mechanisms. In Baum GL, Wolinsky E, editors: *Textbook of pulmonary diseases,* ed 5, Boston, 1994, Little, Brown.
10. Staub NC, Albertine KH: Anatomy of the lungs. In Murray JF, Nadel JA, editors: *Textbook of respiratory medicine,* ed 2, Philadelphia, 1994, WB Saunders.
11. Haas CF, Weg JG: Exogenous surfactant therapy: an update, *Respir Care* 41:397, 1996.
12. Malik AB, Feustel PJ: Pulmonary circulation and lung fluid and solute exchange. In Murray JF, Nadel JA, editors: *Textbook of respiratory medicine,* ed 2, Philadelphia, 1994, WB Saunders.
13. Gil J: The normal lung circulation: state of the art, *Chest* 93(suppl 3):80S, 1988.
14. Murray JF: General principles and diagnostic approach. In Murray JF, Nadel JA, editors: *Textbook of respiratory medicine,* ed 2, Philadelphia, 1994, WB Saunders.
15. Grant BJB, Saltzman AR: Respiratory functions of the lung. In Baum GL, Wolinsky E, editors: *Textbook of pulmonary diseases,* ed 5, Boston, 1994, Little, Brown.
16. Charan NB, Carvalho PG: Anatomy of the normal bronchial circulatory system in humans and animals. In Butler J, editor: *The bronchial circulation,* New York, 1992, Marcel Dekker.
17. Misasi RS, Keyes JL: Matching and mismatching ventilation and perfusion in the lung, *Crit Care Nurse* 16(3):23, 1996.
18. Scanlan CL, Ruppel GL: Ventilation. In Scanlan CL, Spearman CB, Sheldon RL, editors: *Egan's fundamentals of respiratory care,* ed 6, St Louis, 1995, Mosby.
19. Ward ME, Roussos C, Macklem PT: Respiratory mechanics. In Murray JF, Nadel JA, editors: *Textbook of respiratory medicine,* ed 2, Philadelphia, 1994, WB Saunders.
20. Carpenter KD: Oxygen transport in the blood, *Crit Care Nurse* 11(9):20, 1991.
21. Kelsen SG, Cherniack NS: Control of ventilation. In Baum GL, Wolinsky E, editors: *Textbook of pulmonary diseases,* ed 5, Boston, 1994, Little, Brown.
22. West JB: Ventilation, blood flow, and gas exchange. In Murray JF, Nadel JA, editors: *Textbook of respiratory medicine,* ed 2, Philadelphia, 1994, WB Saunders.
23. Gross GW, Scanlan CL: Gas exchange and transport. In Scanlan CL, Spearman CB, Sheldon RL, editors: *Egan's fundamentals of respiratory care,* ed 6, St Louis, 1995, Mosby.
24. Misasi RS, Keyes JL: The pathophysiology of hypoxia, *Crit Care Nurse* 14(8):55, 1994.
25. Vender RL: Chronic hypoxic pulmonary hypertension, *Chest* 106:236, 1994.
26. Dickson SL: Understanding the oxyhemoglobin dissociation curve, *Crit Care Nurse* 15(5):54, 1995.
27. Hayden RA: What keeps oxygenation on track? *Am J Nurs* 92(12):32, 1992.
28. Ahrens TS: Concepts in the assessment of oxygenation, *Focus Crit Care* 14(1):36, 1987.

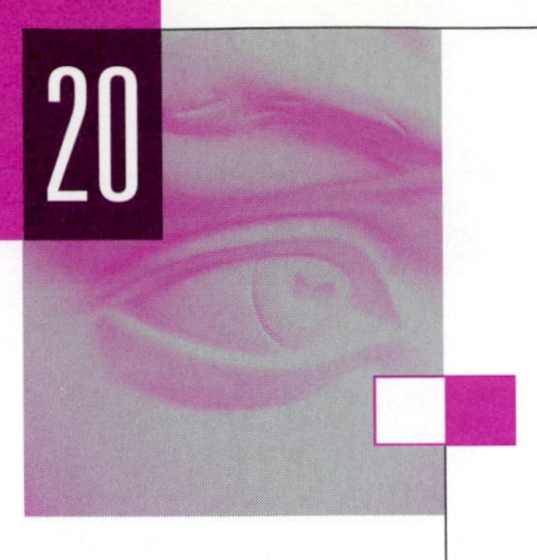

Pulmonary Clinical Assessment

Assessment of the patient with pulmonary dysfunction is a systematic process that incorporates both an inquiry into the chronology of the present illness (better known as a history) and an investigation of the current physical manifestations (better known as a physical examination). The purpose of the assessment is twofold: first, to recognize changes in the patient's pulmonary status that would necessitate nursing or medical intervention; and second, to determine the ways in which the patient's pulmonary dysfunction is interfering with his or her self-care activities.[1] Once completed, the assessment serves as the foundation for developing the management plan for the patient. The assessment process can be brief or can involve a detailed history and examination, depending on the nature and immediacy of the patient's situation. Whatever the setting, the nurse must develop and practice a sequential pattern of assessment to avoid omitting portions of the examination.[1]

BOX 20-1 Manifestations of Respiratory Decompensation

INADEQUATE AIRWAY

Stridor
Noisy respirations
Supraclavicular and intercostal retractions
Flaring of nares
Labored breathing with use of accessory muscles

INADEQUATE VENTILATION

Absence of air exchange at nose and mouth (breathlessness)
Minimal/absent chest-wall motion
Manifestations of obstructed airway
Central cyanosis
Decreased or absent breath sounds (bilateral, unilateral)
Restlessness, anxiety, confusion
Paradoxical motion involving significant portion of chest wall
Decreased $Pa{O_2}$, increased $Pa{CO_2}$, decreased pH

INADEQUATE GAS EXCHANGE

Tachypnea
Decreased $Pa{O_2}$
Increased dead space
Central cyanosis
Chest infiltrates on x-ray evaluation

HISTORY

Taking a thorough and accurate history is extremely important to the assessment process. The patient's history provides the foundation and direction for the rest of the assessment. The overall goal of the patient interview is to expose key clinical manifestations that will facilitate the identification of the underlying cause of the illness. This information will then assist in the development of an appropriate management plan.[2]

The initial presentation of the patient determines the rapidity and direction of the interview. For a patient in acute distress (Box 20-1), the history is curtailed to just a few questions about the patient's chief complaint and precipitating events. For a patient in no obvious distress, the history focuses on five different areas: (1) review of the patient's present illness, (2) overview of the patient's general respiratory status, (3) examination of the patient's general health

BOX 20-2 DATA COLLECTION FOR PULMONARY HISTORY

CHIEF COMPLAINT

Cough

- Onset and duration
  - Sudden or gradual
  - Episodic or continuous
- Characteristics
  - Dry or wet
  - Hacking, hoarse, barking, or congested
  - Productive or nonproductive
- Sputum
  - Present or absent
  - Frequency of production
  - Appearance—color (clear, mucoid, purulent, blood-tinged, mostly bloody), foul odor, frothy
  - Amount
- Pattern
  - Paroxysmal
  - Related to time of day, weather, activities, talking, or deep breathing
  - Change over time
- Severity
  - Causes fatigue
  - Disrupts sleep or conversation
  - Produces chest pain
- Associated symptoms
  - Shortness of breath
  - Chest pain or tightness with breathing
  - Fever
  - Upper respiratory tract signs (sore throat, congestion, increased mucus production)
  - Noisy respirations or hoarseness
  - Gagging or choking
  - Anxiety, stress, or panic reactions
- Efforts to treat
  - Prescription or nonprescription drugs
  - Vaporizers
  - Effective or ineffective

Shortness of breath (SOB) or dyspnea on exertion (DOE)

- Onset and duration
  - Sudden or gradual
  - Gagging or choking episode a few days before onset
- Pattern
  - Related to position—improves when sitting up or with head elevated; number of pillows used to alleviate problems
  - Related to activity—exercise or eating; extent of activity that produces dyspnea
  - Related to other factors—time of day, season, or exposure to something in the environment
  - Harder to inhale or harder to exhale
- Severity
  - Extent activity is limited
  - Breathing itself causes fatigue
  - Anxiety about getting enough air
- Associated symptoms
  - Pain or discomfort—exact location in trespiratory tree
  - Cough, diaphoresis, swelling of ankles, or cyanosis
- Efforts to treat
  - Prescription or nonprescription drugs
  - Oxygen
  - Effective or ineffective

Chest pain

- Onset and duration
  - Gradual or sudden
  - Associated with trauma, coughing, or lower respiratory tract infection
- Associated symptoms
  - Shallow breathing
  - Uneven chest expansion
  - Fever
  - Cough
  - Radiation of pain to neck or arms
  - Anxiety about getting enough air
- Efforts to treat
  - Heat, splinting, or pain medication
  - Effective or ineffective

Patient's perception of the problem

- Degree of concern about the symptoms
- Opinion of its cause

Patient history: factors relating to respiratory disorders (causes or aggravating factors)

- Tobacco use—both present and past
  - Type of tobacco—cigarettes, cigars, pipes, or smokeless
  - Duration and amount—age started, inhale when smoking, amount used in the past and present
  - Pack years—number of packs per day multiplied by number of years patient has smoked
  - Efforts to quit—previous attempts and current interest
- Work environment
  - Nature of work
  - Environmental hazards: chemicals, vapors, dust, pulmonary irritants, or allergens
  - Use of protective devices
- Home environment
  - Location
  - Possible allergens: pets, house plants, plants and trees outside the home, or other environmental hazards
  - Type of heating
  - Use of air conditioning or humidifier
  - Ventilation
  - Stairs to climb

BOX 20-2 DATA COLLECTION FOR PULMONARY HISTORY—cont'd

CHIEF COMPLAINT—cont'd

Medical history

Infectious respiratory diseases
- Strep throat
- Mumps
- Tonsillitis

Thoracic trauma or surgery

Previous diagnosis of pulmonary disorders—dates of hospitalization

Chronic pulmonary diseases—date, treatment, and compliance with therapy
- Tuberculosis
- Bronchitis
- Emphysema
- Bronchiectasis
- Asthma
- Cystic fibrosis
- Sinus infection

Other chronic disorders—cardiovascular, cancer, musculoskeletal, neurologic
- Nasal surgery or injury
- Obstruction of one or both nares
- Mouth breathing often necessary (especially at night)
- History of nasal discharge

Nosebleeds
- Affects one or both nostrils
- Aggravated by crusting

Previous tests
- Allergy testing
- Pulmonary function tests
- Tuberculin and fungal skin tests
- Chest x-rays

Family history

Tuberculosis
Cystic fibrosis
Emphysema
Allergies
Asthma
Atopic dermatitis
Smoking by household members
Malignancy

From Wilson SF, Thompson JM: *Respiratory disorders,* St Louis, 1990, Mosby

status, (4) survey of the patient's family and social background, and (5) description of the patient's current symptoms.[1-4] Specific items regarding each of these areas are outlined in Box 20-2.[1,3]

A description of the patient's current symptoms is also obtained. Symptoms that are common in the pulmonary patient include dyspnea, cough, wheezing, edema, palpitations, fatigue, chest pain,[4] hemoptysis, and sputum.[5] Information is elicited regarding the location, onset and duration, characteristics, setting, aggravating and alleviating factors, associated symptoms,[4] and efforts to treat the symptoms.[6] If the cough is productive, the patient is asked questions about the color, amount, odor, and consistency of the sputum.[7]

PHYSICAL EXAMINATION

Four techniques are used in physical assessment: inspection, palpation, percussion, and auscultation. Inspection is the process of looking intently at the patient. Palpation is the process of touching the patient to judge the size, shape, texture, and temperature of the body surface or underlying structures. Percussion is the process of creating sound waves on the surface of the body to determine abnormal density of any underlying areas. Auscultation is the process of concentrated listening with a stethoscope to determine characteristics of body functions.[8]

Inspection

Inspection of the patient focuses on three areas: (1) observation of the tongue and sublingual area, (2) assessment of chest-wall configuration, and (3) evaluation of respiratory effort. If possible, patients are positioned upright, with their arms resting at their sides.[3] Inspection generally begins during the interview process.[1]

Tongue and sublingual area. The tongue and sublingual area are observed for a blue, gray, or dark purple tint or discoloration, indicating the presence of central cyanosis. Central cyanosis is a sign of hypoxemia, or inadequate oxygenation of the blood, and is considered to be life threatening. It occurs when the amount of reduced hemoglobin (unsaturated hemoglobin) exceeds 5 g/dL. The fingers and toes may also appear discolored, an indication of the presence of peripheral cyanosis.[9]

CULTURAL INSIGHTS 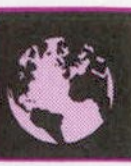

The Family Perspective

The ability to communicate effectively with the family of the critical care patient is a most important psychosocial element for the critical care nurse. To succeed at this task, the nurse must understand the structure of the family and who its leaders and members are.

In contrast to traditional Anglo-American families that consist of comparatively few important members, immigrant families are generally *extended units* in which aunts, uncles, cousins, and grandparents are closely bound and have a central importance in each other's eyes. Many families extend even beyond blood relatives to include *fictive kin*—individuals who are loved and regarded as family members but who are not related by biology or marriage—especially within the African-American culture, as well as within the *compadres* and *comadres* (godparents) tradition of the Hispanic culture.

The implication for critical care nurses of the extended and fictive family lies primarily in the importance of respecting the wishes of the patient concerning visiting rights. Hospital rules must also be respected, but the nurse should make no rash judgments about who really matters to the patient, who is capable of rendering valuable support, and who is not. In addition, the nurse must not believe that she or he has been lied to if a patient refers to a non-blood "relative" as "brother," "sister," "aunt," or "uncle." These designations are merely affectionate terms and are not meant to manipulate the nurse into allowing a nonfamily member to visit the patient.

With respect to visitation, the importance of family support to the critically ill immigrant patient cannot be overemphasized. In Gypsy culture—to cite an extreme—the presence of the family is believed to bring healing energy to the patient. Among those from the Middle East, the family brings very tangible hope to the critically ill patient. In short, the family functions not just as a support system but as a central component in the healing process.

Because of the central role played by the extended family in the care of the immigrant patient, the nurse must know how to address the family to ensure mutual respect and cooperation. Above all else, the nurse must use last names, proceed slowly, and generally respect the more formal social rules of immigrant cultures. The nurse must also be able to determine who is the family's spokesperson and decision maker. Only in this way will the professional be able to establish rapport, maintain respect, and ensure good communication.

Within Middle Eastern families, for example, the spokesperson is likely to be the father or eldest brother, although the eldest female is likely to hold a great deal of power within the home. This distinction between public power and private control is an important one and must be honored by the health care worker. In Hispanic culture, the public head of the household is very likely the father, but within the home, it is the woman who controls many of the decisions. A similar situation occurs within the Italian household. Despite this covert power of the woman, the nurse must respect the male in public and address him with respect and formality.

The issue of whom to address becomes even more complicated when considering the existence of tribal systems within certain immigrant cultures. The Samoans, Laotians, and Gypsies, for example, each practice a form of tribal culture that has as one of its components a tribal leader who functions as the spokesperson and decision maker for the community. By showing respect for the family and the tribal structure of the group, the nurse can dramatically improve patient and family cooperation.

Chest-wall configuration. Assessment of chest-wall configuration incorporates observations about the size and shape of the patient's chest. Normally, the ratio of anteroposterior (AP) diameter to lateral diameter ranges from 1:2 to 5:7 (Figure 20-1, *A*).[1,10,11] An increase in the AP diameter is suggestive of chronic obstructive pulmonary disease (COPD).[1] The shape of the chest is inspected for any structural deviations. Some of the more commonly seen abnormalities are pectus excavatum, pectus carinatum, barrel chest, and spinal deformities. In pectus excavatum (funnel chest), the sternum and lower ribs are displaced posteriorly, creating a funnel or pit-shaped depression in the chest. This causes a decrease in the AP diameter of the chest and may interfere with respiratory function. In pectus carinatum (pigeon breast), the sternum projects forward, causing an increase in the AP diameter of the chest. The barrel chest also results in an increase in AP diameter of the chest and is characterized by displacement of the sternum forward and the ribs outward (Figure 20-1, *B*). Spinal deformities such as kyphosis, lordosis, and scoliosis may also be present and can interfere with respiratory function.[10-12]

Respiratory effort. Evaluation of respiratory effort incorporates observations on the rate, rhythm, symmetry, and quality of ventilatory movements.[1] Normal breathing at rest is effortless and regular and occurs at a rate of 12 to 20 breaths per minute.[3] There are a number of abnormal respiratory patterns (Table 20-1). Some of the more commonly seen patterns in

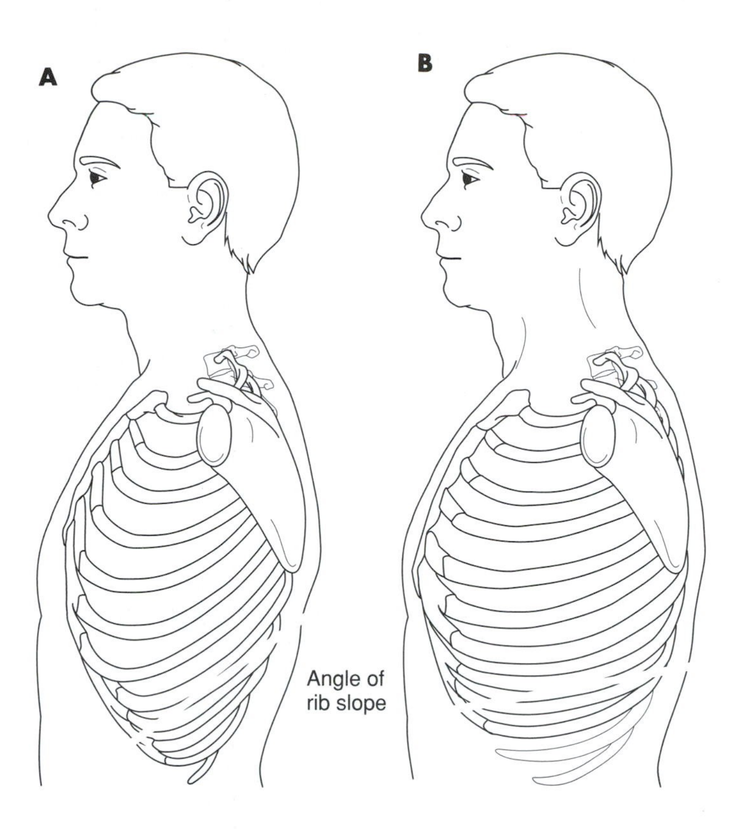

FIGURE 20-1. Chest-wall configuration. **A,** Normal configuration. **B,** Increased anteroposterior diameter. (From Barkauskas V and others: *Health and physical assessment,* St Louis, 1994, Mosby.)

patients with pulmonary dysfunction are tachypnea, hyperventilation, and air trapping. Tachypnea is manifested by an increase in the rate and decrease in the depth of ventilation. Hyperventilation is manifested by an increase in both the rate and depth of ventilation. Patients with COPD often experience obstructive breathing, or air trapping. As the patient breathes, air becomes trapped in the lungs and ventilations become progressively shallower until the patient actively and forcefully exhales.[13]

Additional assessment areas. Other areas assessed are patient position, active effort to breathe, use of accessory muscles, presence of intercostal retractions, unequal movement of the chest wall, flaring of nares, and pausing midsentence to take a breath.[1,11] The presence of other iatrogenic features, such as chest tubes, central venous lines, artificial airways, and nasogastric tubes, are noted, because they may affect assessment findings.

Palpation

Palpation of the patient focuses on three areas: (1) confirmation of the position of the trachea, (2) assessment of respiratory excursion, and (3) evaluation of fremitus. In addition, the thorax is assessed for any areas of tenderness, lumps, or bony deformities. The anterior, posterior, and lateral areas of the chest are evaluated in a systematic fashion.[10,12]

Position of trachea. Confirmation of the position of the trachea is performed to verify that the trachea is midline. It is assessed by placing the fingers in the suprasternal notch and moving upward.[13] Deviation of the trachea to either side can indicate pneumothorax, unilateral pneumonia, diffuse pulmonary fibrosis, a large pleural effusion, or severe atelectasis. With atelectasis the trachea shifts to the same side as the problem, and with pneumothorax the trachea shifts to the opposite side of the problem.[12]

Respiratory excursion. Assessment of respiratory excursion involves measuring the degree and symmetry of respiratory movement. It is assessed by placing the hands on the anterolateral chest with the thumbs extended along the costal margin, pointing to the xiphoid process, or by placing the hands on the posterolateral chest with the thumbs on either side of the spine at the level of the tenth rib (Figure 20-2). The patient is instructed to take a few normal breaths, then a few deep breaths. Chest movement is assessed for equality, which signifies symmetry of thoracic expansion.[3,11,12] Asymmetry is an abnormal finding that can occur with pneumothorax, pneumonia, or other disorders that interfere with lung inflation. The degree of chest movement is felt to ascertain the extent of lung expansion. The thumbs should separate 3 to 5 cm during deep inspiration.[12] Lung expansion of a hyperinflated chest is less than that of a normal one.[4,10]

Tactile fremitus. Assessment of tactile fremitus is performed to identify, describe, and localize any areas of increased or decreased fremitus. *Fremitus* refers to the palpable vibrations felt through the chest wall when the patient speaks. It is assessed by placing the palmar surface of the hands against opposite sides of the chest wall and having the patient repeat the word "ninety-nine" (Figure 20-3). The hands are moved systematically around the thorax until the anterior, posterior, and both lateral areas have been assessed.[11,12] If only one hand is used, it is moved from one side of the chest to the corresponding area on the other side of the chest until all areas have been assessed.[12]

Fremitus varies from patient to patient and depends on the pitch and intensity of the voice. Fremitus is described as normal, decreased, or increased. With normal fremitus, vibrations can be felt over the trachea but are barely palpable over the periphery. With decreased fremitus, there is interference with the transmission of vibrations. Examples of disorders that

TABLE 20-1 Abnormal Patterns of Respiration

Pattern	Description	Associated conditions
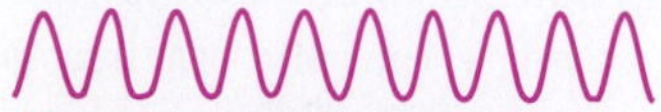	**Normal:** smooth and even at a rate of 12-20 per minute	
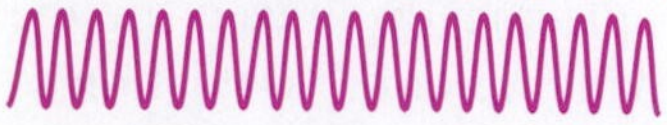	**Tachypnea:** shallow breathing at a rate of > 20 per minute	Anxiety, pain, massive liver enlargement, abdominal ascites
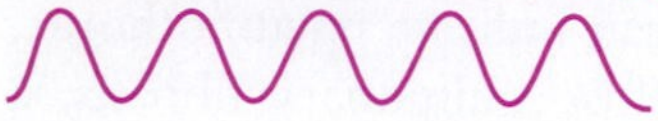	**Bradypnea:** < 12 per minute	Neurogenic disorders, electrolyte imbalance, infection, protective response to pain or pleurisy or other discomfort aggravated by breathing
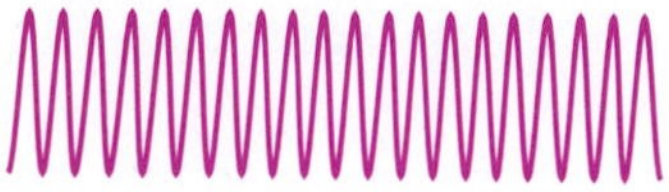	**Hyperpnea** or hyperventilation: deep breathing at a rate of > 20 per minute	Exercise, acute anxiety, panic reactions, metabolic disorders
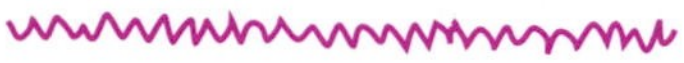	**Central neurogenic hyperventilation:** hyperpnea over a sustained period	Lesions in lower midbrain or upper pons, often from transtentorial herniation
	Air trapping: normal breathing pattern interspersed with forced expirations	Obstructive lung disease
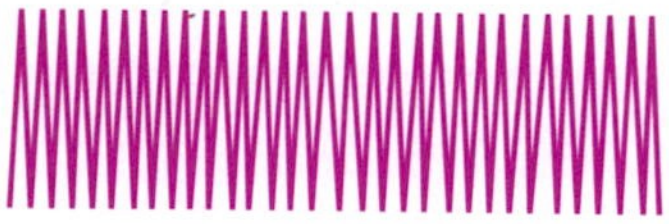	**Kussmaul:** fast (> 20 per min), deep, sighing breaths without pauses; labored breathing	Renal failure, metabolic acidosis
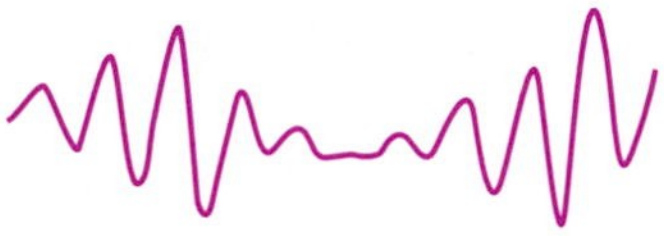	**Cheyne-Stokes:** alternating hyperpnea and apnea	In adults, bilateral lesions in cerebral hemisphere, basal ganglia, midbrain, pons, or cerebellum. In infants this pattern is normal Injury to mid or lower pons
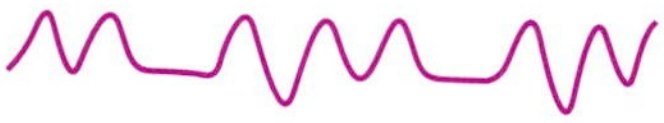	**Apneustic:** end-inspiratory phase, often followed by expiratory phase	Lesions of lower pons or upper medulla
	Biot's or cluster: disorganized sequence of breaths with irregular periods of apnea	Lesions of medulla
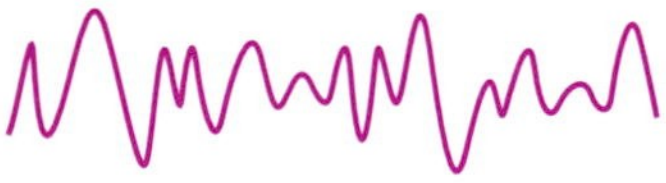	**Ataxic breathing:** irregular breathing patterns with both deep and shallow breaths occurring randomly	

From Wilson SF, Thompson JM: *Respiratory disorders,* St Louis, 1990, Mosby.

decrease fremitus include pleural effusion, pneumothorax, bronchial obstruction, pleural thickening, and emphysema. With increased fremitus, there is an increase in the transmission of vibrations. Examples of disorders that increase fremitus include pneumonia, lung cancer, and pulmonary fibrosis.[3]

Percussion

Percussion of the patient focuses on two areas: (1) evaluation of the underlying lung structure and (2) assessment of diaphragmatic excursion. Although not an often-used technique, percussion is useful for confirming suspected abnormalities.

Underlying lung structure. Evaluation of the underlying lung structure is performed to estimate the amounts of air, liquid, or solid material present. It is performed by placing the middle finger of the nondominant hand on the chest wall. The distal portion, between the last joint and the nailbed, is then struck with the middle finger of the dominant hand. The hands are moved side-to-side, systematically around the thorax, to compare similar areas, until the anterior, posterior, and both lateral areas have been assessed (Figure 20-4). Five different tones can be elicited: resonance, hyperresonance, tympany, dullness, and flatness. These tones are distinguished by differences in intensity, pitch, duration, and quality. Table 20-2 describes the different percussion tones and their associated conditions.[1,10,13]

Diaphragmatic excursion. Assessment of diaphragmatic excursion is accomplished by measuring the difference in the level of the diaphragm on inspiration and expiration. It is performed by instructing

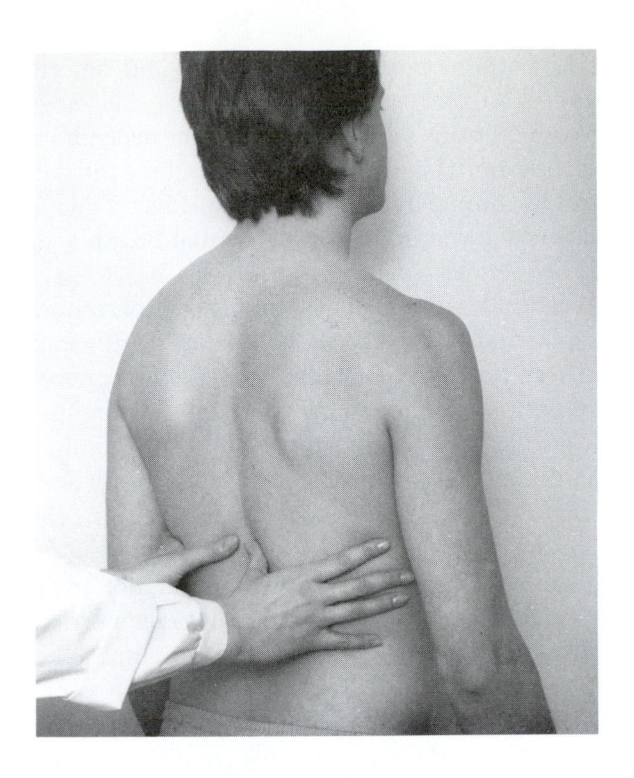

FIGURE 20-2. Assessment of respiratory excursion. (From Malasanos L, Barkauskas V, Stoltenberg-Allen K: *Health assessment,* St Louis, 1990, Mosby.)

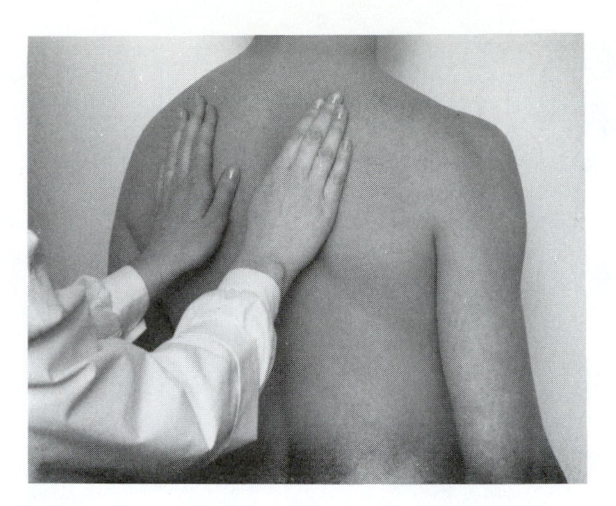

FIGURE 20-3. Assessment of tactile fremitus, showing simultaneous application of the fingertips of both hands to compare sides. (From Malasanos L, Barkauskas V, Stoltenberg-Allen K: *Health assessment,* St Louis, 1990, Mosby.)

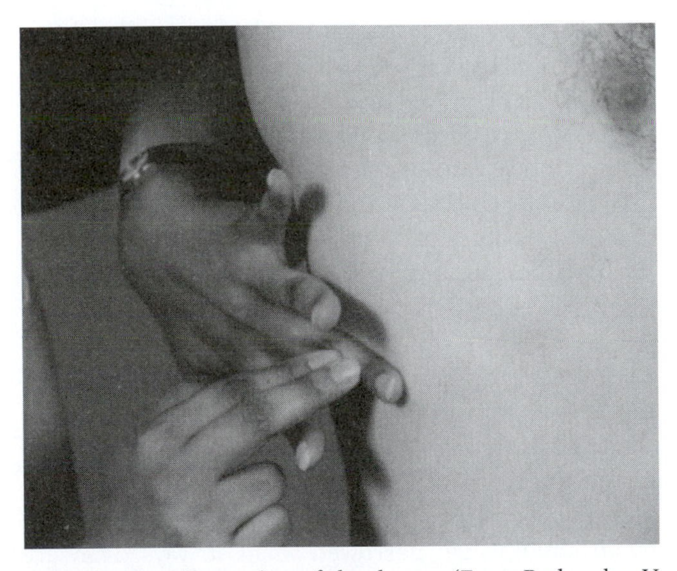

FIGURE 20-4. Percussion of the thorax. (From Barkauskas V and others: *Health and physical assessment,* St Louis, 1994, Mosby.)

TABLE 20-2 Percussion Tones and Their Associated Conditions

Tone	Description	Condition
Resonance	Intensity—loud Pitch—low Duration—long Quality—hollow	Normal lung Bronchitis
Hyperresonance	Intensity—very loud Pitch—very low Duration—long Quality—booming	Asthma Emphysema Pneumothorax
Tympany	Intensity—loud Pitch—musical Duration—medium Quality—drumlike	Large pneumothorax Emphysematous blebs
Dullness	Intensity—medium Pitch—medium-high Duration—medium Quality—thudlike	Atelectasis Pleural effusion Pulmonary edema Pneumonia Lung mass
Flatness	Intensity—soft Pitch—high Duration—short Quality—extremely dull	Massive atelectasis Pneumonectomy

the patient to inhale and hold the breath. The posterior chest is percussed downward, over the intercostal spaces, until the dull sound produced by the diaphragm is heard. The spot is marked. The patient is then instructed to take a few breaths in and out, exhale completely, and then hold his or her breath. The posterior chest is percussed again, and the new area of dullness over the diaphragm is then located and marked. The difference between the two spots is noted and measured (Figure 20-5). Normal diaphragmatic excursion is 3 to 5 cm.[10,12] It is decreased in disorders or conditions such as ascites, pregnancy,

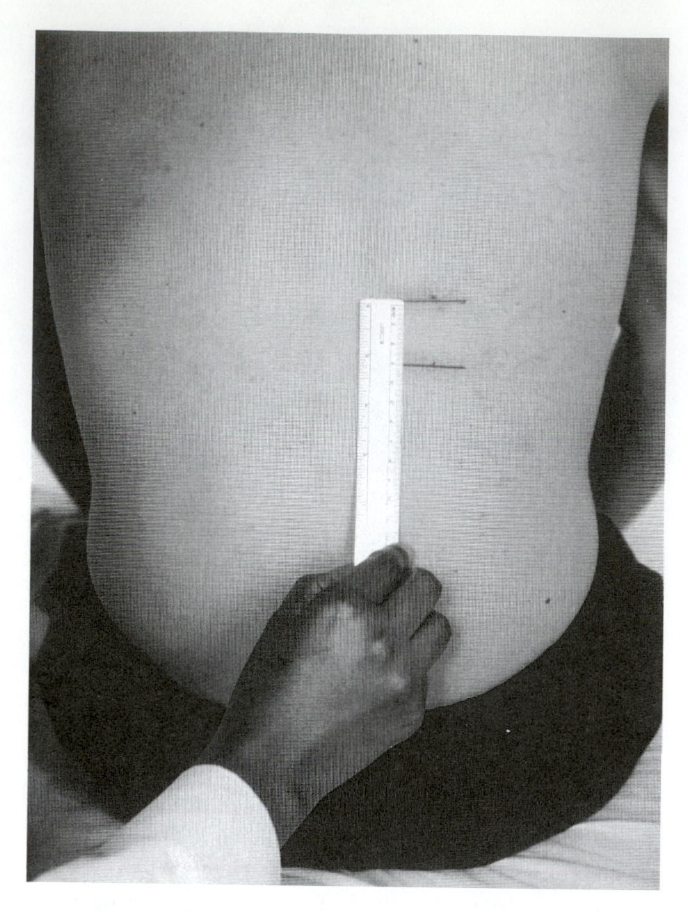

FIGURE 20-5. Assessment of diaphragmatic excursion. (From Barkauskas V and others: *Health and physical assessment,* St Louis, 1994, Mosby.)

hepatomegaly, and emphysema. It is increased in pleural effusion or disorders that elevate the diaphragm, such as atelectasis or paralysis.

Auscultation

Auscultation of the patient focuses on three areas: (1) evaluation of normal breath sounds, (2) identification of abnormal breath sounds, and (3) assessment of voice sounds. Auscultation requires a quiet environment, proper positioning of the patient, and a bare chest.[14] Breath sounds are best heard with the patient in the upright position.[5]

Normal breath sounds. Evaluation of normal breath sounds is performed to assess air movement through the pulmonary system and to identify the presence of abnormal sounds. It is performed by placing the diaphragm of the stethoscope against the chest wall and instructing the patient to breathe in and out slowly with his or her mouth open. Both the inspiratory and expiratory phases are assessed. Auscultation is done in a systematic sequence—side to side, top to bottom, posteriorly, laterally, and anteriorly (Figure 20-6).[5,10,12]

Normal breath sounds are different, depending on their location. They are classified into three categories: bronchial, bronchovesicular, and vesicular. Table 20-3 describes the characteristics of normal breath sounds and their associated conditions.[3,10,13,14]

Abnormal breath sounds. Identification of abnormal breath sounds occurs once the normal breath sounds have been clearly delineated. There are three categories of abnormal breath sounds: absent or diminished breath sounds, displaced bronchial breath sounds, and adventitious breath sounds. Table 20-4 describes the various abnormal breath sounds and their associated conditions.[3,7,14]

An absent or diminished breath sound indicates that there is little or no airflow to a particular portion of the lung (either a small segment or an entire lung).[14] Displaced bronchial breath sounds are normal bronchial sounds heard in the peripheral lung fields instead of over the trachea. This condition is usually indicative of fluid or exudate present in the alveoli.[14] Adventitious breath sounds are extra or added sounds heard in addition to the other sounds already discussed. They are classified as crackles, rhonchi, wheezes, and friction rubs. Crackles (also called rales) are short, discrete, popping or crackling sounds produced by fluid in the small airways or alveoli or by the snapping open of collapsed airways during inspiration. They can be heard on inspiration and expiration and may clear with coughing.[5,14] Crackles can be further classified as fine, medium, or coarse, depending on pitch.[3] Rhonchi are coarse, rumbling, low-pitched sounds produced by airflow over secretions in the larger airways or by narrowing of the large airways. They are mainly heard on expiration and sometimes can be cleared with coughing. Rhonchi can be further classified as bubbling, gurgling, or sonorous, depending on the characteristics of the sound.[14] Wheezes are high-pitched, squeaking, whistling sounds produced by airflow through narrowed small airways. They are mainly heard on expiration but may be heard throughout the ventilatory cycle. Depending on their severity, wheezes can be further classified as mild, moderate, or severe.[14] A pleural friction rub is a creaking, leathery, loud, dry, coarse sound produced by irritated pleural surfaces rubbing together. It is usually heard best in the lower anterolateral chest area during both inspiration and expiration. Pleural friction rubs are caused by inflammation of the pleura.[3,7,11,12]

Voice sounds. Assessment of voice sounds is particularly useful in detecting lung consolidation or lung

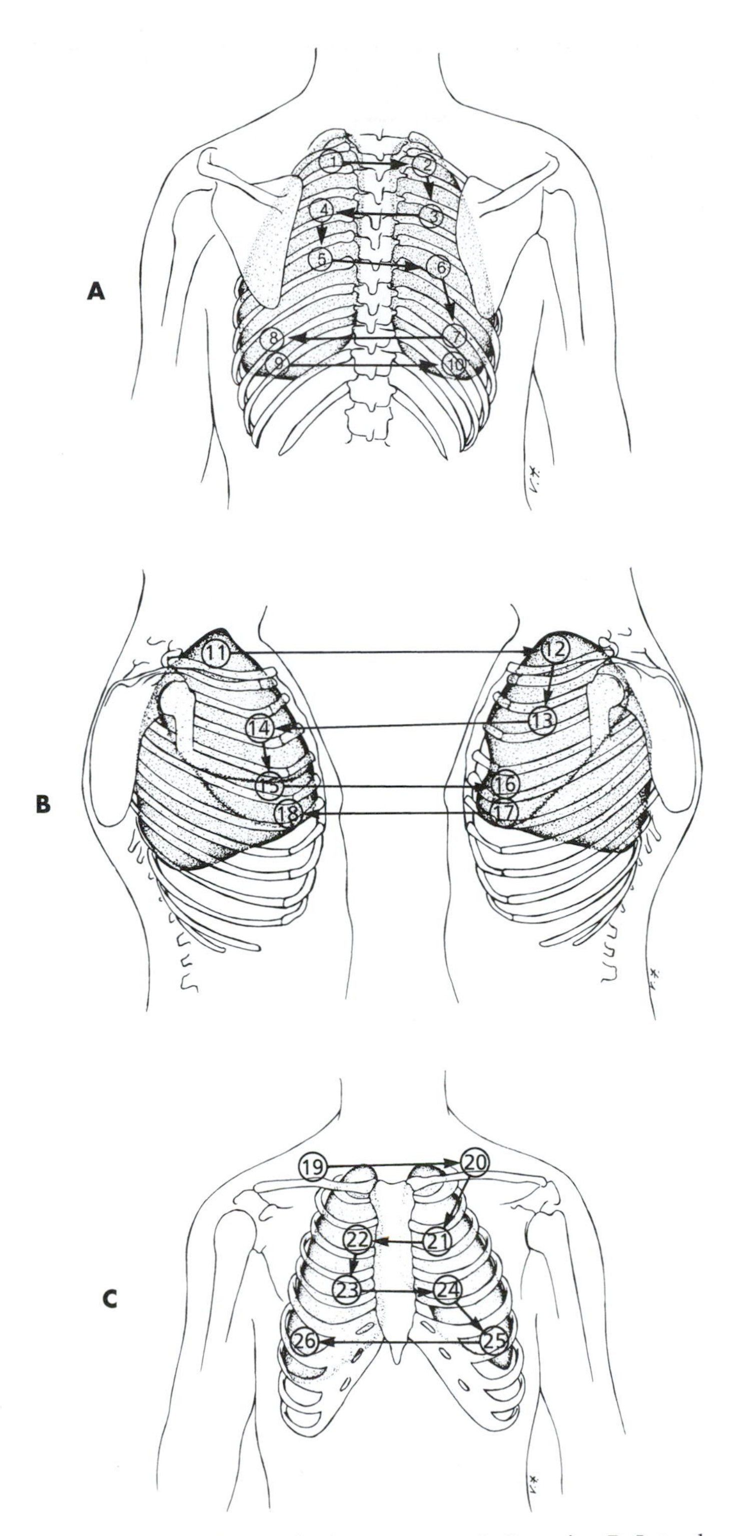

FIGURE 20-6. Auscultation sequence. **A,** Posterior. **B,** Lateral. **C,** Anterior. (From Perry AG, Potter PA: *Clinical nursing skills and techniques,* ed 3, St Louis, 1994, Mosby.)

TABLE 20-3 Characteristics of Normal Breath Sounds

Sound	Characteristics
Vesicular	Heard over most of lung field; low pitch; soft and short exhalation and long inhalation
Bronchovesicular	Heard over main bronchus area and over upper right posterior lung field; medium pitch; exhalation equals inhalation
Bronchial	Heard only over trachea; high pitch; loud and long exhalation

Adapted from Thomspon JM and others: *Mosby's clinical nursing,* ed 3, St Louis, 1993, Mosby.

compression. Three abnormal types of voice sounds are bronchophony, whispering pectoriloquy, and egophony. Bronchophony describes a condition in which the spoken voice is heard on auscultation with higher intensity and clarity than usual. Normally the spoken word is muffled when heard through the stethoscope. It is assessed by placing the diaphragm of the stethoscope against the posterior side of the patient's chest and instructing the patient to say "ninety-nine." Bronchophony is present when the sound heard is clear, distinct, and loud. Whispering pectoriloquy describes a condition of unusually clear transmission of the whispered voice on auscultation. Normally the whispered word is unintelligible when heard through the stethoscope. It is assessed by placing the stethoscope against the posterior side of the patient's chest and instructing the patient to whisper "one, two, three." Whispering pectoriloquy is present when the sound heard is clear and distinct. Egophony describes a condition in which the voice sounds increase in intensity and develop a nasal bleating quality on auscultation. It is assessed by placing the stethoscope against the posterior side of the patient's chest and instructing the patient to say "e-e-e." Egophony is present when the "e" sound changes to an "a" sound.[12,14]

ASSESSMENT FINDINGS OF COMMON DISORDERS

Table 20-5 presents a variety of common pulmonary disorders and their associated assessment findings.

TABLE 20-4 Abnormal Breath Sounds and Their Associated Conditions

Abnormal Sound	Description	Condition
Absent breath sounds	No airflow to particular portion of lung	Pneumothorax Pneumonectomy Emphysematous blebs Pleural effusion Lung mass Massive atelectasis Complete airway obstruction
Diminished breath sounds	Little airflow to particular portion of lung	Emphysema Pleural effusion Pleurisy Atelectasis Pulmonary fibrosis
Displaced bronchial sounds	Bronchial sounds heard in peripheral lung fields	Atelectasis with secretions Lung mass with exudate Pneumonia Pleural effusion Pulmonary edema
Crackles (rales)	Short, discrete, popping or crackling sounds	Pulmonary edema Pneumonia Pulmonary fibrosis Atelectasis Bronchiectasis
Rhonchi	Coarse, rumbling, low-pitched sounds	Pneumonia Asthma Bronchitis Bronchospasm
Wheezes	High-pitched, squeaking, whistling sounds	Asthma Bronchospasm
Pleural friction rub	Creaking, leathery, loud, dry, coarse sounds	Pleural effusion Pleurisy

TABLE 20-5 Assessment Findings Frequently Associated With Common Lung Conditions

Condition*	Breath Sound†	Description	Inspection	Palpation	Percussion	Auscultation
Healthy lung		Tracheobronchial tree and alveoli are clear; pleurae are thin and close together; chest wall is mobile.	Symmetric rib and diaphragmatic movement—absence of accessory muscle activity Regular respiratory rhythm	Trachea—midline Expansion—equal bilaterally Tactile fremitus—present Diaphragmatic excursion—3 to 5 cm	Resonant	Breath sounds—vesicular over periphery areas Voice sounds—normal Adventitious sounds—none except for a few transient crackles at the bases that clear with deep breathing
Asthma Bronchospasm Normal bronchial lumen		Asthma is characterized by intermittent episodes of airway obstruction caused by bronchospasm, excessive bronchial secretion, or edema of bronchial mucosa.	Central cyanosis Tachypnea with audible wheezing Use of accessory muscles of ventilation	Tactile fremitus—decreased	Hyperresonant	Breath sounds—distant, decreased Voice sounds—decreased Adventitious sounds—wheezes

From Malasanos L and others: *Health assessment,* ed 4, St Louis, 1990, Mosby.

*Although some disease conditions are bilateral, one diseased lung and one healthy lung are illustrated for each condition to provide contrast. Pathologic condition is illustrated on the left side, and the normal lung is on the right side.

† •••• denotes auscultation of crackles; ᴡᴡ denotes auscultation of wheezes; ||||| denotes auscultation of pleural friction rub.

Continued

TABLE 20-5 Assessment Findings Frequently Associated With Common Lung Conditions—cont'd

Condition*	Breath Sound†	Description	Inspection	Palpation	Percussion	Auscultation
Atelectasis 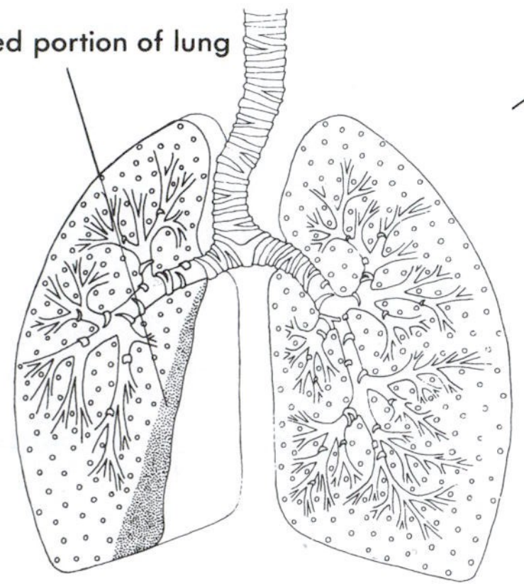 Collapsed portion of lung	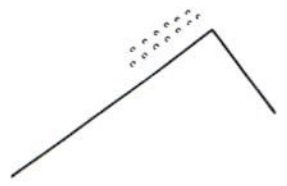	Atelectasis is the collapse of alveolar lung tissue, and findings reflect the presence of a small, airless lung; this condition is caused by complete obstruction of a draining bronchus by a tumor, thick secretions, or an aspirated foreign body, by persistent hypoventilation, and by lack of sighing.	Decreased chest motion on affected side Affected side retracted, with ribs appearing close together Cough may or may not be present Intercostal retraction on affected side during inhalation and bulging during exhalation	Trachea—shifted to affected side Expansion—decreased on affected side Tactile fremitus—decreased or absent over atelectasis	Dull to flat over affected area	Breath sounds—decreased or absent over affected area; high-pitched bronchial sounds when partial obstruction present Adventitious sounds—high-pitched; possible crackles during terminal portion of inspiration
Bronchiectasis 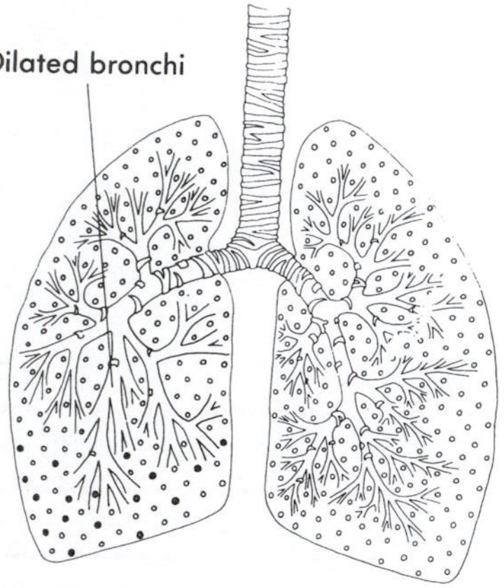 Dilated bronchi	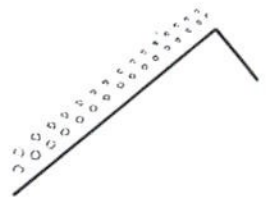	Bronchiectasis is abnormal dilation of the bronchi or bronchioles, or both. It results in copious amounts of thick mucus.	If mild, normal respirations; if severe, tachypnea Less expansion on affected side Cough with purulent sputum	Expansion—decreased on affected side Tactile fremitus—increased	Resonant or dull	Breath sounds—usually vesicular Voice sounds—usually normal Adventitious sounds—crackles

TABLE 20-5 Assessment Findings Frequently Associated With Common Lung Conditions—cont'd

Condition*	Breath Sound†	Description	Inspection	Palpation	Percussion	Auscultation
Bronchitis—chronic Bronchial inflammation with abnormal secretion		Chronic bronchitis is an inflammation of the bronchial tree characterized by partial airway obstruction or constrictions; it results in abnormal amounts of mucus, which—if not expectorated—cause abnormal ventilation/perfusion inequalities.	Rasping cough with mucoid sputum Central cyanosis Dependent edema	Tactile fremitus—normal or increased	Resonant or dull	Breath sounds—vesicular Adventitious sounds—localized crackles Wheezes Possibly decreased breath sounds if airways obstructed
Emphysema Abnormally distended alveoli		Emphysema is a permanent hyperinflation of the lung beyond the terminal bronchioles, with destruction of alveolar walls.	Dyspnea with exertion Barrel chest Tachypnea Use of accessory muscles of respiration Pursed-lip breathing High-Fowler's position, forward leaning shoulders, hunched position Possible clubbing of fingers	Expansion—diminished Tactile fremitus—decreased	Resonant to hyper-resonant Diaphragmatic excursion—decreased	Breath sounds—decreased intensity; often prolonged exhalation Adventitious sounds—occasional wheeze, fine crackles during late inhalation

Continued

TABLE 20-5 Assessment Findings Frequently Associated With Common Lung Conditions—cont'd

Condition*	Breath Sound†	Description	Inspection	Palpation	Percussion	Auscultation
Pleural effusion with thickening 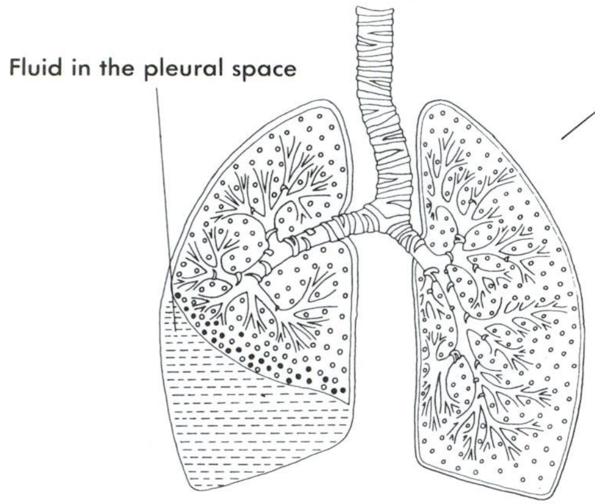 Fluid in the pleural space	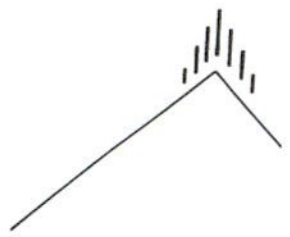	Pleural effusion is a collection of fluid in the pleural space; if pleural effusion is prolonged, fibrous tissue may also accumulate in the pleural space. The clinical picture depends on the amount of fluid or fibrosis present and the rapidity of development; fluid tends to gravitate to the most dependent areas of the thorax, and the adjacent lung is compressed.	Tachypnea Decreased chest expansion on the affected side (expansion may be normal when effusion is small)	Trachea—no deviation in small effusions; deviation toward normal side with large effusion Expansion—decreased on affected side with large effusions Tactile fremitus—decreased or absent	Dull to flat over effusion area	Breath sounds—decreased or absent over area involved in the effusion Adventitious sounds—sometimes pleural friction rub; possible crackles in thoracic area overlying effusion/normal lung interface
Pneumonia with consolidation 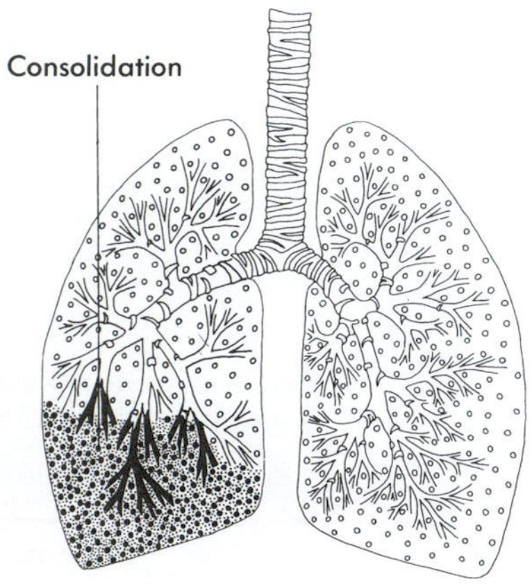 Consolidation	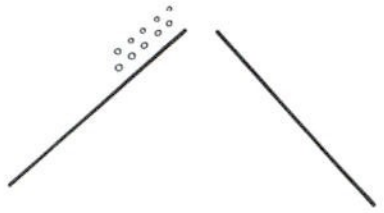	Pneumonia with consolidation occurs when alveolar air is replaced by fluid or tissue; physical findings depend on the amount of parenchymal tissue involved.	Tachypnea Guarding and less motion on the affected side or on both sides when bilateral pneumonia present Cough Possible sputum production	Expansion—limited on the affected side or bilaterally Tactile fremitus—usually increased but may be decreased if a bronchus leading to the affected area is plugged Trachea—no deviation or deviation to unaffected side in unilateral pneumonias	Dull to flat	Breath sounds—increased in intensity; bronchovesicular or bronchial breath sounds over affected area Voice sounds—increased bronchophony, egophony, whisper pectoriloquy Adventitious sounds—crackles when consolidation is small Changes may be minimal or absent

TABLE 20-5 Assessment Findings Frequently Associated With Common Lung Conditions—cont'd

Condition*	Breath Sound†	Description	Inspection	Palpation	Percussion	Auscultation
Pneumothorax Air in the pleural space		Pneumothorax implies air in the pleural space. There are three types of pneumothorax: (1) closed—air in the pleural space does not communicate with the air in the lung; (2) open—air in the pleural space freely communicates with the air in the lung, and air in the pleural space is atmospheric; and (3) tension—air in the pleural space communicates with air in the lungs only during inhalation; air pressure in the pleural space is greater than atmospheric pressure. Physical signs depend on the degree of lung collapse and the presence or absence of pleural effusion.	Decreased chest-wall motion If large, tachypnea and dyspnea Bulging of intercostal spaces on the affected side during exhalation Central cyanosis	Trachea—deviated toward normal side Expansion—decreased on affected side Tactile fremitus—absent over affected area Possible subcutaneous emphysema (crepitus)	Hyperresonant over affected area	Breath sounds—usually decreased or absent; if open pneumothorax, have an amorphic quality Voice sounds—decreased or absent Adventitious sounds—none Possible Hamman's sign (mediastinal crepitus)
Pulmonary fibrosis—diffuse Fibrotic portion of lung		Pulmonary fibrosis is the presence of an excessive amount of connective tissue in the lungs; consequently, the lungs are smaller than normal and less compliant; the lower lobes are usually the most affected.	Dyspnea on exertion Tachypnea Diminished thoracic expansion Central cyanosis	Trachea—deviated to most affected side	Resonant to dull	Breath sounds—reduced or absent, bronchovesicular or bronchial Vocal fremitus—increased; possible whisper pectoriloquy Adventitious sounds—crackles during inhalation and exhalation

REFERENCES

1. Rokosky JS: Assessment of the individual with altered respiratory function, *Nurs Clin North Am* 16:195, 1981.
2. Gehring PE: Physical assessment begins with a history, *RN* 54(11):26, 1991.
3. Brenner M, Welliver J: Pulmonary and acid-base assessment, *Nurs Clin North Am* 25:761, 1990.
4. Dettenmeier PA: *Pulmonary nursing care,* St Louis, 1992, Mosby.
5. Wilkins RL: Bedside assessment of the patient. In Scanlan CL, Spearman CB, Sheldon RL, editors: *Egan's fundamentals of respiratory care,* ed 6, St Louis, 1995, Mosby.
6. Wilson SF, Thompson JM: *Respiratory disorders,* St Louis, 1990, Mosby.
7. Stiesmeyer JK: A four-step approach to pulmonary assessment, *Am J Nurs* 93(8):22, 1993.
8. Fitzgerald MA: The physical exam, *RN* 54(11):34, 1991.
9. Carpenter KD: A comprehensive review of cyanosis, *Crit Care Nurse* 13(4):66, 1993.
10. King C: Examining the thorax and respiratory system, *RN* 45(8):55, 1982.
11. Kuhn KW, McGovern M: Respiratory assessment of the elderly, *J Gerontol Nurs* 18(5):40, 1992.
12. Malasanos L, Barkauskas V, Stoltenberg-Allen K: *Health assessment,* ed 4, St Louis, 1990, Mosby.
13. Seidel HM and others: *Mosby's guide to physical examination,* ed 2, St Louis, 1991, Mosby.
14. Boyda EK and others: *Pulmonary auscultation,* St Paul, 1987, 3M Health Care Group.

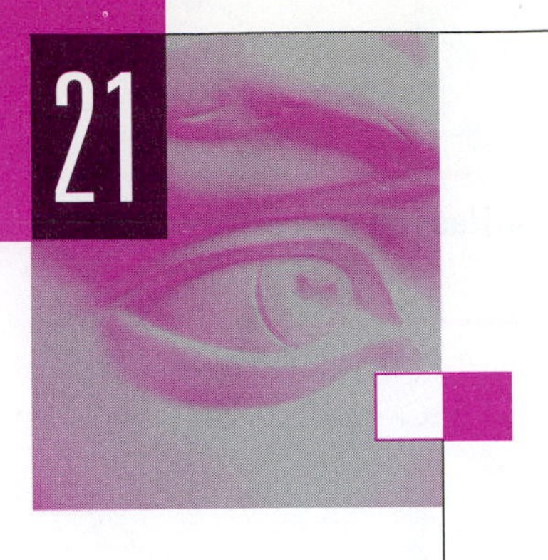

Pulmonary Diagnostic Procedures

To complete the assessment of the critically ill pulmonary patient, a review of the patient's laboratory studies and diagnostic tests is performed. Although many procedures exist for diagnosing pulmonary disease, their application in the critically ill patient is limited. Only those studies and tests that are currently used in the critical care setting are presented here. Bedside monitoring devices are also discussed.

LABORATORY STUDIES

Arterial Blood Gases

Interpretation of arterial blood gas (ABG) levels can be difficult, especially if one is under pressure to do it quickly and accurately. One method that can help ensure accuracy when analyzing arterial blood gas levels is to follow the same steps of interpretation each time. A specific method to be used each time that blood gas values must be interpreted is presented here (Box 21-1).

Step 1: Look at the Pao_2 level and answer the question, "Does the Pao_2 show hypoxemia?" The Pao_2 is a measure of the partial pressure of oxygen dissolved in arterial blood plasma, with "P" standing for "partial pressure" and "a" standing for "arterial." Sometimes Pao_2 is shortened to Po_2. It is reported in millimeters of mercury (mm Hg). Pao_2 reflects 3% of total oxygen in the blood.[1]

The normal range in Pao_2 for persons breathing room air at sea level is 80 to 100 mm Hg. However, the normal range is age-dependent in two groups: infants and persons 60 years and older. The normal level for infants breathing room air is 40 to 70 mm Hg.[2] The normal level for persons 60 years and older decreases with age as changes occur in the ventilation/perfusion (V/Q) matching in the aging lung.[1] The correct Pao_2 for older persons can be ascertained as follows: 80 mm Hg (the lowest normal value) minus 1 mm Hg for every year that a person is over the age of 60. Using this formula, a 65-year-old individual can have a Pao_2 as low as 75 mm Hg and still be within the normal range (formula for 5 years over 60 years of age: 80 mm Hg −5 mm Hg = 75 mm Hg). An acceptable range for an 80-year-old person is 60 mm Hg (formula for 20 years over the age of 60: 80 mm

BOX 21-1 Steps for Interpretation of Blood Gas Levels

STEP 1

Look at the Pao_2 level and answer the question, *"Does the Pao_2 level show hypoxemia?"*

STEP 2

Look at the pH level and answer the question, *"Is the pH level on the acid or alkaline side of 7.40?"*

STEP 3

Look at the $Paco_2$ level and answer the question, *"Does the $Paco_2$ level show respiratory acidosis, alkalosis, or normalcy?"*

STEP 4

Look at the Hco_3 level and answer the question, *"Does the Hco_3 level show metabolic acidosis, alkalosis, or normalcy?"*

STEP 5

Look back at the pH level and answer the question, *"Does the pH show a compensated or an uncompensated condition?"*

Hg − 20 mm Hg = 60 mm Hg). At any age, a $Pa{O_2}$ lower than 40 mm Hg represents a life-threatening situation that requires immediate action.[1] In addition, a $Pa{O_2}$ less than the predicted lowest value indicates hypoxemia, which means that a lower-than-normal amount of oxygen is dissolved in plasma.

Several reasons support analysis of the $Pa{O_2}$ level before analysis of other blood gas components. First, a $Pa{O_2}$ of less than 40 mm Hg severely compromises tissue oxygenation and calls for the immediate administration of supplemental oxygen and/or mechanical ventilation. Second, the test results for the $Pa{O_2}$ level can be quickly analyzed. If the $Pa{O_2}$ level is more than the lowest value for the patient's age, it is normal.

Step 2: Look at the pH level and answer the question, "Is the pH on the acid or alkaline side of 7.40?" The pH is the hydrogen ion (H^+) concentration of plasma. Calculation of pH is accomplished by using the partial pressure of carbon dioxide ($Pa{CO_2}$) and the plasma bicarbonate level (HCO_3^-). The formula used is the Henderson-Hasselbalch equation (Box 21-2).[3]

BOX 21-2 The Henderson-Hasselbalch Equation for Blood pH

The blood pH depends on the ratio of bicarbonate to dissolved carbon dioxide. As long as the ratio is 20:1, the pH will be 7.4.

$$pH = pK^* + \log \frac{base}{acid}$$

$$pH = pK + \log \frac{HCO_3^-}{Co_2}$$

$$pH = 6.1 + \log \frac{24 \text{ mEq/L}}{40 \times .03 \text{ mEq/L}}$$

$$pH = 6.1 + \log 20$$

$$pH = 6.1 + 1.3$$

$$pH = 7.4$$

*pK is the pH at which the substance is half dissociated and half undissociated—value here is 6.1; HCO_3^- normal is 24 mEq/L; CO_2 normal for arterial blood is 40 mm Hg and must be converted to mEq/L to be used in this equation. Therefore the 40 mm Hg is multiplied by .03 to convert to mEq/L.

The normal pH of arterial blood is 7.35 to 7.45, with the mean being 7.40. If the pH level is less than 7.40, it is on the acid side of the mean. A pH level less than 7.35 is known as *acidemia,* and the overall condition is called *acidosis.* If the pH level is greater than 7.40, it is on the alkaline side of the mean. A pH level greater than 7.45 is known as *alkalemia,* and the overall condition is called *alkalosis.*[1]

Step 3: Look at the $Pa{CO_2}$ level and answer the question, "Does the $Pa{CO_2}$ show respiratory acidosis, alkalosis, or normalcy?" The $Pa{CO_2}$ is a measure of the partial pressure of carbon dioxide dissolved in arterial blood plasma, and it is reported in mm Hg. It is the acid-base component that reflects the effectiveness of ventilation in relation to the metabolic rate.[1] In other words, the $Pa{CO_2}$ value indicates whether the patient can ventilate well enough to rid the body of the carbon dioxide produced as a consequence of metabolism.

The normal range for $Pa{CO_2}$ is 35 to 45 mm Hg. This range does not change as a person ages. A $Pa{CO_2}$ value of greater than 45 mm Hg defines *respiratory acidosis,* which is caused by alveolar hypoventilation. Hypoventilation can result from chronic obstructive pulmonary disease (COPD), oversedation, head trauma, anesthesia, drug overdose, neuromuscular disease, or hypoventilation with mechanical ventilation.[4]

Ventilatory failure results whenever the $Pa{CO_2}$ level exceeds 50 mm Hg. Acute ventilatory failure occurs when the $Pa{CO_2}$ level is greater than 50 mm Hg and the pH level is less than 7.30. It is referred to as *acute* because the pH is abnormal, thereby not allowing enough time for the body to compensate by returning the pH to the normal range. *Chronic ventilatory failure* is defined as a $Pa{CO_2}$ value of greater than 50 mm Hg, with a pH level of greater than 7.30.[1,5]

A $Pa{CO_2}$ value that is less than 35 mm Hg defines *respiratory alkalosis,* which is caused by alveolar hyperventilation. Hyperventilation can result from hypoxia, anxiety, pulmonary embolism, pregnancy, and hyperventilation with mechanical ventilation or as a compensatory mechanism to metabolic acidosis.[4]

Step 4: Look at the HCO_3^- level and answer the question, "Does the HCO_3^- show metabolic acidosis, alkalosis, or normalcy?" The bicarbonate (HCO_3^-) is the acid-base component that reflects kidney function. The bicarbonate is reduced or increased in the plasma by renal mechanisms. The normal range is 22 to 26 mEq/L.[6] A bicarbonate level of less than 22 mEq/L defines *metabolic acidosis,* which can result from ketoacidosis, lactic acidosis, renal failure, or diarrhea. The cumulative effect is a gain of acids or a loss of base. A bicarbonate level that is greater than 26 mEq/L defines *metabolic alkalosis,* which can result from fluid loss from the upper gastrointestinal tract (vomiting or nasogastric suction), diuretic therapy, severe hypokalemia, alkali administration, or steroid therapy.[3,4]

Step 5: Look back at the pH level and answer the question, "Does the pH show a compensated or an uncompensated condition?" If the pH level is abnormal (less than 7.35 or greater than 7.45), the $Pa{CO_2}$ value or the HCO_3^- level, or both, will also be abnormal. This is an uncompensated condition because there has not been enough time for the body to return the pH to its normal range.[1,3] See Box 21-3 for two examples of uncompensated ABGs. If the pH level is within normal limits and both the $Paco_2$ value and the HCO_3^- level are abnormal, the condition is compensated because there has been enough time for the body to restore the pH to within its normal range.[3] Differentiating the primary disorder from the compensatory response can be difficult. The primary disorder is the abnormality that caused the pH level to shift initially; thus, on whichever side of 7.40 the pH level occurs is considered the primary disorder.[1] See Box 21-4 for two examples of compensated ABGs. Partial compensation may also be present and is evidenced by abnormal pH, $Paco_2$, and HCO_3^- levels, indications that the body is attempting to return the pH to its normal range.[4]

Table 21-1 summarizes the changes in the acid-base components that accompany various acid-base disorders.[1,4] In addition to the parameters previously discussed, other factors must be considered when reviewing a patient's ABGs, including oxygen saturation, oxygen content, expected Pao_2, base excess and deficit, and anion gap analysis.

Oxygen saturation. Oxygen saturation is a measure of the amount of oxygen bound to hemoglobin, compared with hemoglobin's maximal capability for binding oxygen. It can be assessed as a component of the ABG (Sao_2) or can be measured noninvasively using a pulse oximeter (Spo_2).[7] Oxygen saturation is reported as a percentage or as a decimal, with normal being greater than 95% on room air. Normally, the saturation level cannot reach 100% (on room air) because of the physiologic shunting.[1] However, when supplemental oxygen is administered, oxygen saturation may approach 100% so closely that it is reported as 100%.

Proper evaluation of the oxygen saturation level is vital. For example, an Sao_2 of 97% means that 97% of the available hemoglobin is bound with oxygen. The word "available" is essential to evaluating the Sao_2 level, because the hemoglobin level is not always within normal limits and oxygen can bind only with what is available. A 97% saturation level associated with 10 g of hemoglobin does not deliver as much oxygen to the tissues as does a 97% saturation associated with 15 g of hemoglobin. Thus assessing only the Sao_2 level and finding it within normal limits must not lead one to believe that the patient's oxygenation status is normal. The hemoglobin level must also be evaluated before a decision on oxygenation status can be made.[6]

Oxygen content. Oxygen content (Cao_2) is a measure of the total amount of oxygen carried in the blood, including the amount dissolved in plasma (measured by the Pao_2) and the amount bound to the hemoglobin molecule (measured by the Sao_2). Cao_2 is reported in milliliters (ml) of oxygen carried per 100 ml of

BOX 21-3 Uncompensated ABGs

EXAMPLE 1:

Pao_2: 90 mm Hg
pH: 7.25
$Paco_2$: 50 mm Hg
HCO_3^-: 22 mEq/L
Interpretation: Uncompensated respiratory acidosis

EXAMPLE 2

Pao_2: 90 mm Hg
pH: 7.25
$Paco_2$: 40 mm Hg
HCO_3^-: 17 mEq/L
Interpretation: Uncompensated metabolic acidosis

BOX 21-4 Compensated ABGs

EXAMPLE 1:

Pao_2: 90 mm Hg
pH: 7.37
$Paco_2$: 60 mm Hg
HCO_3^-: 38 mEq/L
Interpretation: Compensated respiratory acidosis with metabolic alkalosis. (The acidosis is considered the main disorder and the alkalosis the compensatory response, because the pH is on the acid side of 7.40.)

EXAMPLE 2

Pao_2: 90 mm Hg
pH: 7.42
$Paco_2$: 48 mm Hg
HCO_3^-: 35 mEq/L
Interpretation: Compensated metabolic alkalosis with respiratory acidosis. (The alkalosis is considered the main disorder and the acidosis the compensatory response, because the pH is on the alkaline side of 7.40.)

TABLE 21-1 Summary of Arterial Blood Gas Assessment

Disorder	pH	$PaCO_2$	HCO_3^-
Respiratory Acidosis			
Uncompensated	<7.35	>45 mm Hg	22-26 mEq/L
Partially compensated	<7.35	>45 mm Hg	26 mEq/L
Compensated	7.35-7.39	>45 mm Hg	26 mEq/L
Respiratory Alkalosis			
Uncompensated	>7.45	<35 mm Hg	22-26 mEq/L
Partially compensated	>7.45	<35 mm Hg	22 mEq/L
Compensated	7.41-7.45	<35 mm Hg	22 mEq/L
Metabolic Acidosis			
Uncompensated	<7.35	35-45 mm Hg	22 mEq/L
Partially compensated	<7.35	<35 mm Hg	22 mEq/L
Compensated	7.35-7.39	35 mm Hg	22 mEq/L
Metabolic Alkalosis			
Uncompensated	>7.45	35-45 mm Hg	26 mEq/L
Partially compensated	>7.45	45 mm Hg	26 mEq/L
Compensated	7.41-7.45	45 mm Hg	26 mEq/L
Combined Respiratory and Metabolic Acidosis	<7.35	45 mm Hg	22 mEq/L
Combined Respiratory and Metabolic Alkalosis	>7.45	35 mm Hg	26 mEq/L

blood. The normal value is 20 ml of oxygen per 100 ml of blood. To calculate the oxygen content, the PaO_2, the SaO_2, and the hemoglobin level are used (see Appendix D). A change in any one of these parameters will affect the CaO_2.[1,8]

The value of assessing the CaO_2 is best illustrated by the examples in Table 21-2. Here, the ABG parameters that are most commonly used to evaluate oxygenation status (PaO_2 and SaO_2) are both normal. Assessing only the PaO_2 and the SaO_2 would lead to the invalid conclusion that Patient B's oxygenation status is normal. However, consideration of the hemoglobin and the CaO_2 reveals that the oxygenation of Patient B's blood is significantly abnormal.

Expected PaO_2. When a patient receives supplemental oxygen, the PaO_2 level is expected to rise. Knowing the level to which the PaO_2 should rise in normal subjects on a given FIO_2 and comparing that with the level to which the PaO_2 actually does rise in patients with pulmonary disease has value, because it illustrates how well the lung is functioning. Calculating the expected PaO_2 is accomplished by multiplying the FIO_2 value by 5.[1] Thus the expected PaO_2 on an FIO_2 of 30% is at least 150 mm Hg (30 × 5), whereas the expected PaO_2 on an FIO_2 of 50% is 250 mm Hg (50 × 5). These expected PaO_2 values represent the oxygen level achievable with healthy lungs. Pulmonary disease can radically decrease the expected PaO_2 level. It is impossible to apply the "FIO_2 value × 5" rule to achieve the expected PaO_2 value when the patient is on a system that delivers oxygen by liters per minute. For these situations, Table 21-3 shows the FIO_2 levels that correspond to various oxygen delivery systems.

TABLE 21-2 Assessing Oxygenation Status

Patient	PaO_2 Level (mm Hg)	SaO_2 Level (%)	Hgb Level (g%)	CaO_2 Level (vol%)
A	100	97	15	19.8
B	100	97	10	13.3

Table 21-4 illustrates three examples of what can occur when the expected PaO_2 level does not reach normal. Patient A shows a normal expected PaO_2; thus it is assumed that his or her lungs are performing normally. The fact that the expected PaO_2 has been reached means that he or she may not require supplemental

TABLE 21-3 Guidelines for Estimating FIO_2 With Low-flow Oxygen Devices

100% O_2 Flow Rate (L)	FIO_2 (%)
NASAL CANNULA OR CATHETER	
1	24
2	28
3	32
4	36
5	40
6	44
OXYGEN MASK	
5-6	40
6-7	50
7-8	60
MASK WITH RESERVOIR BAG	
6	60
7	70
8	80
9	90
10	99+

From Shapiro BA, Peruzzi WT, Kozelowski-Templin R: *Clinical application of blood gases,* ed 5, St Louis, 1994, Mosby. NOTE: Normal ventilatory pattern assumed.

TABLE 21-4 The Expected PaO_2 Compared with the Actual PaO_2

Patient*	FIO_2 level(%)	Expected PaO_2 Level (mm Hg)	Actual PaO_2 Level (mm Hg)
A	30	150	160
B	50	250	85
C	50	250	60

*Patients are all younger than 60 years.

oxygen. Patient B has not reached the expected PaO_2, but at least he or she is not hypoxemic. The administration of supplemental oxygen should bring the PaO_2 level above 80 mm Hg. However, because the expected PaO_2 level has not been achieved, it must be assumed that removal of oxygen will result in hypoxemia.[1] Patient C has not reached the expected PaO_2, and is therefore having trouble with oxygenation.

Base excess and base deficit. Base excess and base deficit reflect the nonrespiratory contribution to acid-base balance and are reported in milliequivalents per liter above or below the normal range of −2 mEq/L to +2 mEq/L. A negative base level is reported as a base deficit, which correlates with metabolic acidosis, whereas a positive base level is reported as a base excess, which correlates with metabolic alkalosis.[1]

BOX 21-5 Anion Gap

Formula: Extracellular fluid cations minus extracellular fluid anions plus measured bicarbonate level

OR

Sodium (Na^+) − (chloride [Cl^-] + bicarbonate [HCO_3^-]) = 8-16 mEq/L

EXAMPLE

Na^+ 145 Cl^- 105 HCO_3^- 15

145 − 105 + 15 = 145 − 120 = 25

Interpretation: High anion-gap metabolic acidosis

Anion gap. Calculation of the anion gap can give a more complete analysis of metabolic disturbances that occur in the critically ill patient. The anion gap is computed by subtracting the major plasma anions—chloride and bicarbonate—from the major plasma cation—sodium (Box 21-5).[1] The remainder is made up of minor plasma anions such as organic ions, phosphates, and negatively charged proteins. The normal anion gap is 8 to 16 mEq/L.[1] Any process that significantly increases the minor plasma anions creates a high anion-gap metabolic acidosis. Elevation of the anion gap is seen with processes such as diabetic or alcoholic ketoacidosis, lactic acidosis, renal failure, rhabdomyolysis, and toxins such as salicylates and methanol.[1,4] A nonanion-gap metabolic acidosis can occur through the loss of bicarbonate and the retention of the chloride ion (hyperchloremic metabolic acidosis).[3] Clinically, a nonanion-gap acidosis is associated with diarrhea, renal failure, and ureterosigmoidoscopy. Therefore, anion-gap calculation is helpful in the classification of metabolic acidosis.

Classic Shunt Equation and Oxygen Tension Indices

The efficiency of oxygenation can be assessed by measuring the degree of intrapulmonary shunting that occurs in a patient at any one time, using the classic shunt equation and oxygen tension indices.

Intrapulmonary shunting (QS/QT [the portion of cardiac output not exchanging with alveolar blood divided by the total cardiac output]) refers to venous blood that flows to the lungs without being oxygenated because of nonfunctioning alveoli.[1,7] Other names for this condition include shunt effect, low V/Q, wasted blood flow, and venous admixture.[2] Direct determination of intrapulmonary shunting requires the use of the classic shunt equation (see Appendix D), which is both invasive and cumbersome. A shunt greater than 10% is considered abnormal and indicative of a shunt producing disorder.[1]

Often times, intrapulmonary shunting is estimated by using the oxygen tension indices. One advantage to these methods is the ease of performance, though they have been found to be unreliable in critically ill patients.[1] An estimate of intrapulmonary shunting can be determined by computing the difference between the alveolar and arterial oxygen concentrations. Normally, alveolar and arterial PO_2 values are approximately equal.[7] When they are not, it indicates that venous blood is passing malfunctioning alveoli and returning unoxygenated to the left side of the heart.[8] The most common oxygen tension indices used to estimate intrapulmonary shunting are the PaO_2/FIO_2 ratio, the PaO_2/PAO_2 ratio, and the A-a gradient ($P[A\text{-}a]O_2$)

PaO_2/FIO_2 ratio. The PaO_2/FIO_2 ratio is clinically the easiest formula to calculate because it does not call for the computation of the alveolar PO_2. Normally, the PaO_2/FIO_2 ratio is greater than 286, with the lower the value the worse the lung function.[7]

PaO_2/PAO_2 ratio. The PaO_2/PAO_2 ratio (arterial/alveolar O_2 ratio) is normally greater than 60%. The disadvantage to using this formula is that it calls for the computation of the alveolar PO_2 (see Appendix D), but the advantage is that it is unaffected by changes in the FIO_2, as long as the underlying lung condition is stable.[1]

Alveolar-arterial gradient. The A-a gradient ($P[A\text{-}a]O_2$) is normally less than 20 mm Hg on room air for patients younger than 61 years old. This estimate of intrapulmonary shunting is the least reliable clinically, but is frequently used in clinical decision making. One of the major disadvantages to using this formula is that it is greatly influenced by the amount of oxygen the patient is receiving.[1,7]

Serial determinations of the estimates of intrapulmonary shunting provide the practitioner with objective data on which to base clinical decisions.[1,7] Table 21-5 illustrates the change in intrapulmonary shunting in the hypoxemic patient using the previously described oxygen tension indices to estimate severity of shunting.

Dead Space Equation

The efficiency of ventilation can be measured using the clinical dead space (V_D/V_T) equation (see Appendix D). The formula measures the fraction of tidal volume not participating in gas exchange. Dead space greater than 0.6 indicates a dead space–producing disorder and is considered abnormal. The major limitations to using this formula are that it requires the measurement of exhaled carbon dioxide to complete and that the work of breathing by patients must remain stable during the collection.[1] (∞Ventilation/Perfusion Relationships, p. 618.)

Sputum Studies

Careful analysis of sputum specimens is crucial for the rapid identification and treatment of pulmonary infections. The most difficult aspect of sputum examination is proper collection of the specimen. In general, collection of a good sputum sample requires a conscious, cooperative, sufficiently hydrated patient.[9] When the patient has difficulty producing sputum, heated, nebulized saline may help to loosen secretions for expectoration.[10] Chest physiotherapy combined with nebulization improve the success rate. Collection of a sputum specimen is best done in the morning, because there is a greater volume of secretions as a result of nighttime pooling.[11]

Many critically ill patients cannot cough effectively, and thus sputum collection by other means is required. These methods include tracheobronchial aspiration, transtracheal aspiration, and the use of a fiberoptic bronchoscopy with a protected brush catheter. Because each method has its own benefits and risks, the patient's clinical condition determines the appropriate technique.[12]

Many critically ill patients have endotracheal or tracheostomy tubes already in place. Collecting sputum specimens from these patients requires special attention to technique (Box 21-6). Deep specimens are obtained to avoid collecting specimens that contain resident upper airway flora that may have migrated down the tube. Colonization of the lower airways with upper airway flora can occur within 48 hours of intubation.[13]

Once a sputum specimen is obtained, it is examined for volume, physical properties, mucopurulence, and color. Next, a microscopic examination is done to identify the source of the specimen. If a bacterial infection is suspected, a Gram stain

TABLE 21-5 Calculation of Intrapulmonary Shunting in a Hypoxemic Patient

FIO_2	PaO_2 Level (mm Hg)	PAO_2 Level (mm Hg)	PaO_2/FIO_2	a/A Ratio (%)	A-a Gradient (mm Hg)
.21	40	97	190	.41	57
.50	80	300	160	.27	220
1.0	150	610	60	.25	460

Data from Murray JF, Nadel JA: *Textbook of respiratory medicine,* Philadelphia, 1988, WB Saunders.

BOX 21-6 Procedure for Collection of Tracheal or Endotracheal Specimen

1. Clear the endotracheal or tracheostomy tube of all local secretions, avoiding deep airway penetration.
2. Attach a sputum trap to a sterile suction catheter, and advance the catheter into the trachea while trying to avoid contact with the endotracheal tube or tracheostomy tube.
3. After the catheter is fully advanced, apply suction until secretions return to the sputum trap. When enough secretions are collected, discontinue suctioning and remove the catheter.
4. Do not apply suction while the catheter is being withdrawn, because this can contaminate the sample with sputum from the upper airway. Do not flush the catheter with sterile water, because this dilutes the sample.
5. If the catheter becomes plugged with secretions, place it in a sterile container and send it to the laboratory. The specimen must be transported immediately or refrigerated if a delay is necessary.

followed by a culture and sensitivity (C&S) is performed.

DIAGNOSTIC PROCEDURES

Bronchoscopy

Fiberoptic bronchoscopy is a relatively safe procedure, done at the bedside, and is most often used as both a diagnostic and therapeutic tool. Diagnostic indications include hemoptysis, infectious pneumonia, difficult intubation, pulmonary injury after chest trauma, acute burn inhalation injury, aspiration lung injuries, and acute upper airway obstruction. Therapeutic indications include the aspiration of foreign bodies; removal of obstructing secretions; atelectasis; difficult intubation; and resection of small, benign growths from the airway.[14,15]

Before the bronchoscopy, a complete patient history and examination, including a chest x-ray examination, are performed.[15] Preprocedure evaluation of the patient also includes clotting studies (prothrombin time [PT], partial thromboplastin time [PTT], and platelet count) and evaluation of the arterial blood gas levels.[11,15] Hypoxemic patients need supplemental oxygen during the procedure. The patient must have nothing by mouth for 6 to 8 hours before the bronchoscopy to reduce the risk of aspiration.[15,16]

Although a topical anesthetic can be used alone, it is generally supplemented by an intravenous sedative and/or analgesic. A benzodiazepine for sedative effects and/or a narcotic analgesic are administered intravenously during the procedure.[15,16] Preprocedure medications for a diagnostic bronchoscopy may include atropine and intramuscular codeine. Atropine lessens the vasovagal response and reduces the secretions, whereas codeine decreases the cough reflex. When a bronchoscopy is performed therapeutically to remove secretions, decreased cough and gag reflexes are present, which may impair secretion clearance.[16] Maintenance of the airway is essential to prevent complications.

Complications of the procedure may be related to the procedure itself, the anesthetic, or an ancillary procedure. Minor complications include laryngospasm, bronchospasm, epistaxis, fever, vomiting, altered pulmonary mechanics, and hemodynamic instability. Major complications include anaphylaxis, infection, hypotension, cardiac dysrhythmias, pneumothorax, hemorrhage, respiratory failure, hypoxemia, and cardiopulmonary arrest.[14,15]

Thoracentesis

Thoracentesis is a simple, usually uncomplicated procedure done at the bedside for the removal of fluid or air from the pleural space. It is most frequently used as a diagnostic measure, or it may be performed therapeutically for the drainage of a pleural effusion or empyema.[17] No absolute contraindications to thoracentesis exist, although there are risks that generally contraindicate the procedure in all but emergency situations. These risk factors include unstable hemodynamics, coagulation defects, mechanical ventilation, the presence of an intraaortic balloon pump, or patients who are uncooperative. In most clinical situations, diagnostic thoracentesis can be delayed until these risk factors are eliminated.[18]

The patient is placed in a sitting position with legs over the side of the bed and hands and arms supported on a padded overbed table. If the patient's condition precludes sitting, the side-lying position with the back flush with the edge of the bed and the affected side down can be used.[18] The patient is cautioned not to move or cough during the procedure.[17] During the thoracentesis, the site of the needle insertion is usually determined by previous chest x-ray examination, computed tomography (CT) scan, or chest percussion. A local anesthetic is used to minimize patient discomfort during insertion of the thoracentesis needle.[18,19]

Complications associated with thoracentesis include pain, pneumothorax, and reexpansion pulmonary edema. Reexpansion pulmonary edema can occur when a large amount of effusion fluid (approximately 1000 to 1500 ml) is removed from the pleural space.[17,18] Removal of the fluid increases the negative intrapleural pressure, which can lead to edema when the lung does not reexpand to fill the space. The patient experiences severe coughing and shortness of breath. The onset of these symptoms is an indication to discontinue the thoracentesis. If the physician is measuring the negative pressure during the thoracentesis, withdrawal of fluid is stopped when pressure exceeds −20 cm of water pressure.[18,19] Although therapeutic thoracentesis may be associated with a decrease in dyspnea, removal of large pleural effusions is associated with a higher morbidity.[18]

Bedside Pulmonary Function Tests

Pulmonary function tests (PFTs) are designed to quantify respiratory function and are an essential component of a thorough pulmonary evaluation. PFTs are used for a variety of purposes, including preoperative assessment, evaluating lung mechanics, diagnosing and tracking pulmonary diseases, and monitoring therapy. Results are individualized according to age, gender, and body size.[20]

A complete pulmonary function test consists of four components: lung volumes, mechanics of breathing, diffusion, and arterial blood gases. PFTs may take as long as 2 hours to complete. Because of the severity of illness encountered in the critical care area, all four components are rarely completed. Most frequently, measurements of pulmonary function in the critically ill are limited to those areas that give the practitioner information about the patient's need for or ability to wean from mechanical ventilation. This section covers the areas most frequently tested at the bedside of critically ill individuals.

Measurement of lung volumes and capacities (Box 21-7) provides valuable information about the origin of a disease process. There are four lung volumes and four lung capacities that can be measured. Measurement of volumes at the bedside is limited to tidal volume and vital capacity. Generally, a vital capacity of 10 to 15 ml/kg is a minimally accepted value for weaning, with a respiratory rate of less than 24 breaths per minute.[11,20]

The assessment of the mechanics of breathing includes measurement of the flow of gas, lung and chest compliance, respiratory muscle strength, and tissue resistance. In the critical care area, dynamic and static compliance are measured at the bedside. Compliance is a measure of the distensibility of the lungs (how easily they are inflated). Dynamic compliance is measured during the breathing cycle. A value of 35 to 50 ml/cm H_2O is normal (see Appendix D). It should be noted that measurement of dynamic compliance does not separate resistance forces. Therefore conditions that increase resistance alter the dynamic compliance value. Dynamic compliance decreases with any decrease in lung compliance or increase in airway resistance, such as occurs with bronchospasm and retained secretions. Static compliance is measured under no-flow conditions so that resistance forces are removed. Static compliance decreases with any decrease in lung compliance, such as occurs with pneumothorax, atelectasis, pneumonia, pulmonary edema, and chest-wall restrictions. A normal value is 60 to 100 ml/cm of H_2O (see Appendix D).[11]

Assessment of inspiratory muscle strength can be evaluated through the measurement of maximal inspiratory pressure (MIP) and negative inspiratory pressure (NIP). Both should be more negative than −20 to −25 cm H_2O. Other names for these same tests are negative inspiratory effort (NIE), peak inspiratory pressure (PIP), and peak inspiratory force (PIF). Both the MIP and NIP require a cooperative patient and can provide useful information about spontaneous breathing ability.[11,20] Maximal expiratory pressure (MEP) can be measured to test the ability to cough in

BOX 21-7 Lung Volumes and Capacities

Tidal volume (VT): The volume of air exhaled after a normal resting inhalation. VT × respiratory rate = minute ventilation. Normal is 500 ml.

Inspiratory reserve volume (IRV): The amount of additional air that can be taken in after a normal inhalation. Normal is 3000-3100 ml.

Inspiratory capacity (IC): The maximal amount of air that can be inhaled after a normal exhalation. Normal is 3500-3600 ml.

Expiratory reserve volume (ERV): The additional amount of air that can be exhaled after a normal resting exhalation. Normal is 1100-1200 ml.

Vital capacity (VC): The maximal amount of air that can be exhaled after a maximal inhalation. Normal is 4600-4800 ml.

Residual volume (RV): The amount of air left in the lung after maximal exhalation. Normal is 1200-1300 ml.

Functional residual capacity (FRC): The amount of air left in the lung after a normal exhalation. The total of the ERV and RV. Normal is 2300-2400 ml.

Total lung capacity (TLC): The maximal volume of air in the lung after a maximal inspiration. The total of all lung volumes. Normal is 5800-6000 ml.

TABLE 21-6 Bedside Pulmonary Function Tests

Test	Description
Respiratory rate (f)	Number of breaths per minute
Tidal volume (VT)	Volume of air exhaled after a normal resting inhalation
Minute ventilation (VE)	Volume of air expired per minute (tidal volume respiratory rate = minute ventilation)
Maximal voluntary ventilation (MVV)	Maximal amount of air that can be moved into and out of the lungs in 1 minute
Forced vital capacity (FVC)	Maximal amount of air that can be forcefully exhaled from the lungs after maximal inhalation
Maximal inspiratory pressure (MIP)	Maximal negative pressure generated on inhalation
Maximal expiratory pressure (MEP)	Maximal positive pressure generated on exhalation
Peak expiratory flow rate (PEFR)	Maximal flow rate achieved during forced exhalation
Forced expiratory flow at midpoint of vital capacity ($FEF_{25\%-75\%}$)	Measure of the average flow rate during the middle 50% of exhalation
Forced expiratory flow at 1 second (FEV_1)	Volume of air exhaled in first second of forced exhalation

neuromuscular patient populations. Other common methods used to assess respiratory muscle strength are maximum voluntary ventilation (MVV), minute ventilation (VE), and breathing pattern.

Dynamic pulmonary function tests are designed to evaluate the function of the respiratory muscles, thorax, and lungs. These tests are timed breathing studies that evaluate the degree of respiratory impairment and include forced vital capacity (FVC), peak expiratory flow rate (PEFR), forced expiratory volume in 1 second (FEV_1), and forced expiratory volume divided by the forced vital capacity (FEV_1/FVC). Forced expiratory flow ($FEF_{25\%-75\%}$) is the mean rate of air flow over the middle half of the FVC and is a good index of airway resistance.[20] When these studies are performed at the bedside they require the use of spirometry for volume measurement.[20] The tests can be performed with intubated or nonintubated patients. In the intubated patient, the spirometer is attached to the end of the endotracheal tube. In the nonintubated patient, a nose clip is placed on the patient and the patient is instructed to breathe through a spirometer tube. The patient is seated on the side of the bed if possible.[20] Table 21-6 provides a description of each of these parameters.

Ventilation/Perfusion Scanning

Ventilation/perfusion scanning is indicated when a serious alteration of the normal ventilation/perfusion (V/Q) relationship is suspected. V/Q studies are most frequently ordered to diagnose and follow a suspected pulmonary embolus. V/Q scanning is approximately 90% accurate in determining this diagnosis. Comparing the perfusion scan with the results of a clinical examination may improve these percentages somewhat.

The V/Q scan consists of both a ventilation scan and a perfusion scan. The ventilation scan is performed by having the patient inhale a radiolabeled gas and air mixture through a mask. The perfusion scan is performed by intravenously injecting the patient with a radioisotope. Scintillation cameras record the gamma radiation images produced by the isotope as it is breathed or perfused into the lung. When an obstruction of the isotope's flow into an area of the lung occurs, the diminished radioactivity is reflected in the camera image of that zone.[21]

Because the results are less than 100% accurate in predicting pulmonary emboli, most V/Q scans are interpreted in one of four ways. The scan is interpreted as normal when the perfusion scan is normal and the probability of pulmonary embolism approaches zero. A low probability interpretation is given when there are small V/Q mismatches, focal V/Q matches with no corresponding radiographic abnormalities, or when the perfusion defects are considerably smaller than the radiographic abnormalities. An intermediate or indeterminant probability reading is used when there are severe diffuse airflow obstructions; perfusion defects corresponding in size and position to radiographic abnormalities; and a single, moderate V/Q mismatch without a corresponding radiographic abnormality. A high probability interpretation is used when the perfusion defects are substantially larger than the radiographic abnormalities or when there is one or more large or two or more moderate V/Q mismatches with no corresponding radiographic abnormalities. This finding is infrequently seen but has a predictive value of 97%.[22]

Chest Radiography

Chest radiography is an important diagnostic procedure for any critically ill patient. Chest x-ray examinations aid in the diagnosis of various disorders and complications and assist in the evaluation of treatment.[23]

When interpreting a chest x-ray film, a systematic method is used for viewing it (Box 21-8). Areas of the film that are assessed include bones, mediastinum, diaphragm, pleural space, and lung tissue. See Figure 21-1 for an example of a normal chest x-ray film.

Bones. The clavicles, ribs, thoracic and cervical spine, and scapulae are assessed. The clavicles should be symmetric, and the ribs should be an equal distance apart. At least eight to nine ribs should overlie lung tissue on an inspiratory film.[24] The thoracic and cervical spine should be straight without signs of curvature. The scapulae usually appear as areas of added density in the upper lung fields. There should be no evidence of fractures, calcification and lesions (increased density), or demineralization (decreased density).[24,25]

Mediastinum. The structures in the mediastinal area that are assessed are the cardiac silhouette and the trachea. The trachea should be midline with a slight deviation to the right as it approaches the carina.[25] Shifting of the mediastinal structures can occur with atelectasis and removal of all or a portion of a lung (toward the area of involvement), pneumothorax (away from the area of involvement), pleural effusion, and tumors.[24,26]

Diaphragm. The diaphragm should be clearly visible with sharp costophrenic angles (where the chest wall and the tapered edges of the diaphragm meet).[23,24] The level of the diaphragm (on deep inspiration) should appear at the tenth or eleventh rib,[24] with the right side 1 to 2 cm higher than the left side.[26] A gastric air bubble may be found under the left side of the diaphragm.[26] An elevated diaphragm may be seen in pregnancy, obesity, conditions that cause air or fluid to accumulate in the peritoneal space, and intestinal obstruction.[24] An elevated hemidiaphragm is associated with a number of conditions, including phrenic nerve injury, previous chest surgery, subphrenic abscess, trauma, stroke, tumor, pneumonia, and radiation therapy.[26] Flattening of the diaphragm can be a sign of increased air in the lungs, such as occurs with chronic obstructive pulmonary disease (COPD) or a pleural effusion.[24] Obliteration of

BOX 21-8 Steps for Interpretation of a Chest X-Ray Film

STEP 1

Look at the different densities (black, gray, and white), and answer the question, "*What is air, fluid, tissue, and bone?*"

STEP 2

Look at the shape or form of each density, and answer the question, "*What normal anatomic structure is this?*"

STEP 3

Look at both right and left sides, and answer the question, "*Are the findings the same on both sides or are there differences (both physiologic and pathophysiologic)?*"

STEP 4

Look at all the structures (bones, mediastinum, diaphragm, pleural space, and lung tissue), and answer the question, "*Are there any abnormalities present?*"

STEP 5

Look for all tubes, wires, and lines, and answer the question, "*Are the tubes, wires, and lines in the proper place?*"

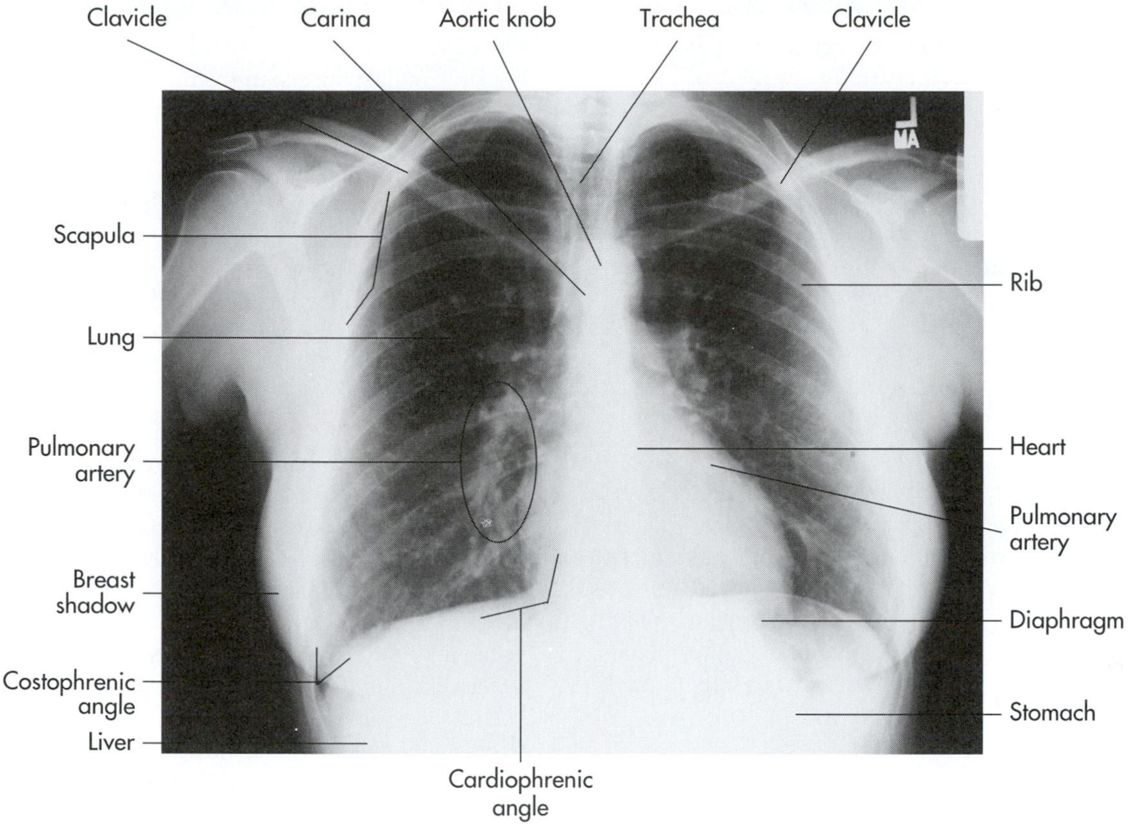

Clavicle
Carina
Aortic knob
Trachea
Clavicle
Scapula
Rib
Lung
Pulmonary artery
Heart
Pulmonary artery
Breast shadow
Diaphragm
Costophrenic angle
Stomach
Liver
Cardiophrenic angle

FIGURE 21-1. Location of structures on a normal chest x-ray. (From Dettenmeir PA: *Radiographic assessment for nurses,* St Louis, 1995, Mosby.)

"blunting" of the costophrenic angle can occur with pleural effusion, atelectasis, or pneumothorax.[24,26]

Pleural space. Identification of the pleural space on a chest x-ray film is an abnormal finding. The pleural space is not visible unless air (pneumothorax) or fluid (pleural effusion) enters it. As fluid accumulates in the pleural space, it surrounds the lung and eventually compresses it. With a pleural effusion, blunting of the costophrenic angle may be evident first, with flattening of the diaphragm and obscuring of the heart borders occurring as the effusion grows.[24] With a pneumothorax, the pleural edges become evident as one looks through and between the images of the ribs on the film. A thin line appears just parallel to the chest wall, indicating where the lung markings have pulled away from the chest wall.[26] In addition, the collapsed lung will be manifested as an area of increased density separated by an area of radiolucency (blackness).[26]

Lung tissue. The lung tissue is viewed for any areas of increased density or increased radiolucency that could indicate an abnormality. Increased density can be the result of accumulation of fluid in the lungs (e.g., water, pus, blood, edema fluid) or collapse of lung tissue (as occurs with atelectasis or pneumothorax). Increased radiolucency is caused by increased air in the lungs, as may occur with COPD.[24] In some patients a fine line may be present on the right side at about the level of the sixth rib in the midlung field. This is a normal finding and represents the horizontal fissure, which separates the right upper lobe from the right middle lobe.[26]

Tubes, wires, and lines. The chest x-ray film also is assessed for proper placement of all tubes, wires, and lines. When properly positioned, an endotracheal tube is 2 to 3 cm above the carina, and a nasogastric tube runs the length of the esophagus, with the tip in the stomach.[24] The origin of a central venous catheter is observed as a thin continuous radiopaque line at the level of the jaw, progressing toward the superior vena cava in an internal jugular approach, whereas a subclavian approach originates in the clavicular area. A pulmonary artery catheter is viewed running through

RESEARCH ABSTRACT

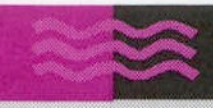

Stress in critical care nurses: actual and perceived.

Sawatzky JA: *Heart Lung* 25(5):409, 1996.

PURPOSE

The purpose of this study was twofold: to describe the stressful work environment experiences and the perception of stress in female critical care nurses and to explore possible relationships between these variables.

DESIGN

Descriptive, correlational, survey design.

SAMPLE

The convenience sample consisted of 96 female nurses with at least 1 year of critical care experience who were currently employed in adult critical care units in two large tertiary university-affiliated hospitals. Subjects ranged in age from 20 to 49 years, most (80%) were prepared at the diploma level, 41% worked full time, and 83% had completed a formal critical care program.

PROCEDURE

Subjects were administered the Critical Care Nursing Stress Scale (CCNSS), the Perceived Stress Scale, and a demographic questionnaire. Data collection took place over 3 weeks at each institution.

RESULTS

The top six work stressors were ranked on the basis of total scores for frequency, intensity, threat, and challenges. Unnecessary prolongation of life ranked high in the frequency, intensity, and threat categories. Management-related stressors, such as apathetic and incompetent nursing staff, ranked highest in the threat category. Noise and routine procedures ranked highest for frequency of occurrence. Inadequate knowledge and unfamiliar situations received high overall scores for perceived challenge. Lack of control was a common element among situations that ranked as the most stressful. There were significant correlations between perceived life stress and the perceived severity of work stressors ($p < .005$) and between actual (frequency) and perceived (intensity) stressful work events ($p < .001$).

DISCUSSION/IMPLICATIONS

Findings from this study provide information regarding stressors that are real or perceived by critical care nurses. It is important to identify specific stressors and analyze their impact on nursing care delivered, outcomes of care, organizational outcomes, and the personal well-being of critical care nurses. The CCNSS, which was developed by the investigator for this study, demonstrated initial reliability for examining stressors encountered by critical care nurses. Additional testing and potential refinement of the scale is needed. Several stressors were identified in the study, which differed among the various specialties. It is important to further explore these differences and design strategies to decrease the stressors. Staff nurses need to understand the impact of work stressors on their personal lives and take steps to find balance and an acceptable level of positive work stress. It is important that educators and administrators work collaboratively with bedside practitioners to identify and decrease work environment stressors so that positive outcomes can be maintained and enhanced.

the right atrium and right ventricle into the pulmonary artery.[24] Additional items that may be present include temporary or permanent pacing wires, a permanent pacing generator, an implantable cardioverter defibrillator (ICD), a peripherally inserted central catheter (PICC), chest tubes (pleural or mediastinal), electrocardiography (ECG) electrodes, and surgical markers and clips.

Nursing Management

Nursing management of a patient undergoing a diagnostic procedure involves a variety of interventions, which include preparing the patient psychologically and physically for the procedure, monitoring the patient's responses to the procedure, and assessing the patient after the procedure. Preparing the patient includes teaching the patient about the procedure, answering any questions, and positioning the patient for the procedure. Monitoring the patient's responses to the procedure includes observing the patient for signs of pain, anxiety, or respiratory distress (see Box 20-1) and monitoring vital signs, breath sounds, and oxygen saturation. Assessing the patient after the procedure includes observing for complications of the procedure and medicating the patient for any postprocedural discomfort. (∞Conscious Sedation, p. 193; Acute Respiratory Failure, p. 655.)

BEDSIDE MONITORING

Capnography

Capnography is the measurement of exhaled carbon dioxide gas and can be used to monitor a patient's ventilatory status. A capnograph is also known as an *end-tidal CO_2 monitor,* because the CO_2 is measured near the end of the exhalation.[11] Most often, the gas sample is analyzed through infrared gas analysis.[27] Frequently the CO_2 is measured via the exhalation port of the ventilator tubing; as the gas passes through the sensor, the data are transferred to the display unit. A display unit produces a waveform, called a capnogram (Figure 21-2), and a numeric recording approximating the $Paco_2$. The ability of the capnograph to approximate arterial $Paco_2$ is altered with abnormal cardiopulmonary function.[11,27] Clinical application of capnography can provide information in a number of areas, including estimation of $Paco_2$ levels, assessment of dead space (increased V/Q), assessment of pulmonary blood flow, and endotracheal tube placement.[7]

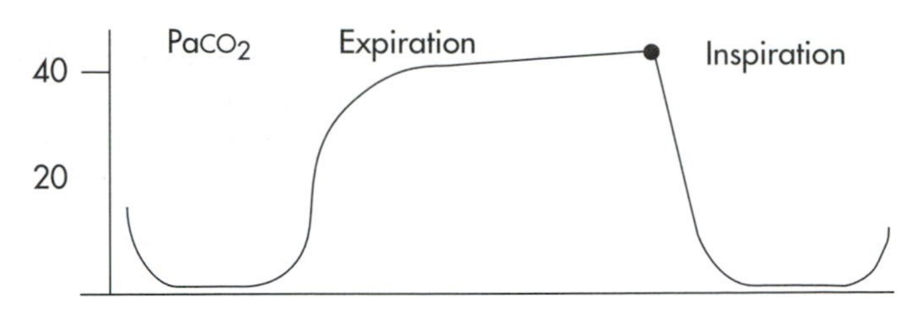

FIGURE 21-2. Normal capnographic waveform. (From Flynn JBM, Bruce NP: *Introduction to critical care skills,* St Louis, 1993, Mosby.)

Normally alveolar and arterial CO_2 concentrations are equal in the presence of normal ventilation/perfusion relationships. In a patient who is hemodynamically stable, the end-tidal CO_2 ($Petco_2$) can be used to estimate the $Paco_2$, with the $Petco_2$ levels 1 to 5 mm Hg less than $Paco_2$ levels.[7] The practitioner must determine first that a normal V/Q relationship exists before correlation of the $Petco_2$ and the $Paco_2$ can be assumed.[1,7]

Assessment of changes in physiologic dead space can be carried out with end-tidal CO_2 monitoring, based on the degree of difference between the $Paco_2$ and the $Petco_2$. As the severity of pulmonary impairment increases so does the disparity between the $Paco_2$ and the $Petco_2$, as indicated by an increased gradient. A gradient of greater than 5 mm Hg can be seen with underperfused alveolar-capillary units (dead space producing situations) and nonperfused alveolar-capillary units (alveolar dead space). Increased dead space ventilation is a result of decreased pulmonary blood flow/cardiac output and lung disease. This leads to an abnormality in the transfer of CO_2 from the blood to the lung. The result is a $Petco_2$ level that is lower than the $Paco_2$ because of the mixing of carbon dioxide between perfused and nonperfused units. The end result is an increased or widened $Paco_2$ to $Petco_2$ gradient.[1,7,11]

The noninvasive measurement of $Petco_2$ allows for the assessment of adequacy of cardiopulmonary resuscitation and endotracheal tube placement. Decreased pulmonary blood flow is associated with lower $Petco_2$ values, reflected clinically by decreased cardiac output, as in the case of cardiopulmonary resuscitation.[1,7] During endotracheal intubation, a low $Petco_2$ reading would indicate the tube is positioned in the stomach, because the amount of carbon dioxide in the esophagus is expected to be low.[1]

Capnography has also been used successfully to assist in the induction of cerebral vasoconstriction in patients with head injuries.[27] Capnography and $Petco_2$ analysis have many diverse applications in the critical care area, however, the practitioner must never assume the $Petco_2$ values reflect $Paco_2$ values.[7,27]

Pulse Oximetry

Pulse oximetry is a noninvasive method for monitoring oxygen saturation (Spo_2). It is indicated in any situation in which the patient's oxygenation status requires continuous observation. It consists of a microprocessor and a probe that attaches to the patient (finger, ear, toe, or nose). The probe consists of two light-emitting diodes and a photodetector (Figure 21-3). The diodes transmit red and infrared light wavelengths through the pulsating vascular bed to the photodetector on the other side. The photodetector converts the light signals into an electric signal, which is then sent to the microprocessor, which converts it to a digital reading. The pulse oximeter is considered very accurate, +4% to +5% at a saturation greater than 70%. However, several physiologic and technical factors limit the monitoring system.[27]

Physiologic limitations. Physiologic limitations include elevated levels of abnormal hemoglobins, presence of vascular dyes, and poor tissue perfusion. The pulse oximeter cannot differentiate between normal and abnormal hemoglobin. Elevated levels of abnormal hemoglobin falsely elevate the Spo_2. Vascular dyes, such as methylene blue, indigo carmine, indocyanine

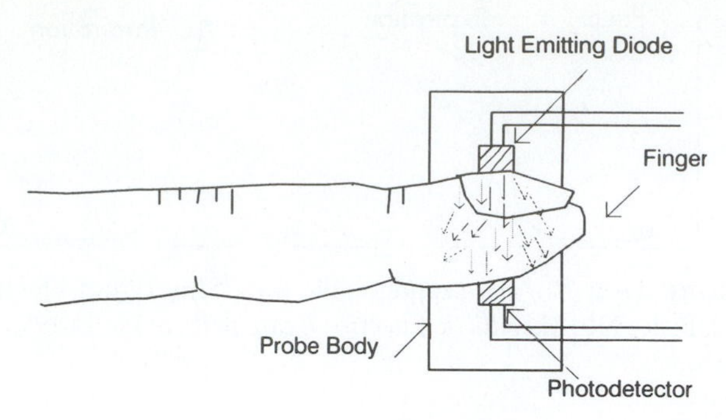

FIGURE 21-3. Pulse oximeter finger probe. (From Van Hooser T: Analysis of gas exchange. In Scanlan CL, Spearman CB, Sheldon RL, editors: *Egan's fundamentals of respiratory care,* ed 6, St Louis, 1995, Mosby.)

green, and fluorescein, also interfere with pulse oximetry and can lead to falsely low readings. Poor tissue perfusion to the area with the probe leads to loss of pulsatile flow and signal failure.[27]

Technical limitations. Technical limitations include bright lights, excessive motion, and incorrect placement of the probe. Bright lights may interfere with the photodetector and cause inaccurate results. The probe must be covered to limit optical interference. Excessive motion can mimic arterial pulsations and can lead to false readings. Incorrect placement of the probe can lead to inaccurate results, because part of the light can reach the photodetector without having passed through blood (optical shunting).[28] Interventions to limit these problems include using the proper probe in the appropriate spot (e.g., not using a finger probe on the ear), applying the probe according to the directions, and ensuring that the area being monitored has adequate perfusion.[29]

REFERENCES

1. Shapiro BA, Peruzzi WT, Kozelowski-Templin R: *Clinical application of blood gases,* St Louis, ed 5, 1994, Mosby.
2. Hazinski MF: *Nursing care of the critically ill child,* ed 2, St Louis, 1992, Mosby.
3. McCance KL, Huether SE: *Pathophysiology: the biologic basis for disease in adults and children,* ed 2, St Louis, 1994, Mosby.
4. Haber RJ: A practical approach to acid-base disorders, *West J Med* 155:146, 1991.
5. Des Jardins T, Burton GG: *Clinical manifestations and assessment of respiratory disease,* ed 3, St Louis, 1995, Mosby.
6. Ahern J: A guide to blood gases, *Nurs Stand* 9:50, 1995.
7. Ahrens T: Respiratory monitoring in critical care, *AACN Clin Issues Crit Care Nurs* 4:56, 1993.
8. Pier AF: Using mixed venous oxygen saturation to trend overall oxygenation in cardiothoracic surgical patients, *Crit Care Nurs Q* 16:72, 1993.
9. Smeltzer SC, Bare BG: *Brunner and Suddarth's textbook of medical-surgical nursing,* ed 7, Philadelphia, 1992, JB Lippincott.
10. Fink J: Humidity and aerosol therapy. In Scanlan CL, Spearman CB, Sheldon RL, editors: *Egan's fundamentals of respiratory care,* ed 6, St Louis, 1995, Mosby.
11. Boggs RL, Wooldridge-King M, editors: *AACN procedure manual for critical care,* ed 3, Philadelphia, 1993, WB Saunders.
12. MacLeod JA: Collecting specimens for laboratory analysis, *Nurs Stand* 5:36, 1992.
13. Estes RJ, Meduri GU: The pathogenesis of ventilator-associated pneumonia: mechanisms of bacterial transcolonization and airway inoculation, *Intensive Care Med* 21:365, 1995.
14. American Association of Respiratory Care: Clinical practice guidelines: fiberoptic bronchoscopy assisting, *Respir Care* 38:1173, 1993.
15. Pue CA, Pacht ER: Complications of fiberoptic bronchoscopy at a university hospital, *Chest* 107:430, 1993.
16. Reed AP: Preparation of the patient for awake flexible fiberoptic bronchoscopy, *Chest* 101:244, 1992.
17. Quigley RL: Thoracentesis and chest tube drainage, *Crit Care Clin* 11:111, 1995.
18. Quershi N, Zahir MA, Brandsetter RD: Thoracentesis in clinical practice, *Heart Lung* 23:376, 1994.
19. Barbers R, Patel P: Thoracentesis made safe and simple, *J Respir Dis* 15:841, 1994.
20. Douce FH: Basic pulmonary function measurements. In Scanlan CL, Spearman CB, Sheldon RL, editors: *Egan's fundamentals of respiratory care,* ed 6, St Louis, 1995, Mosby.
21. Ecklund MM: Optimizing the flow of care for the prevention and treatment of deep vein thrombosis and pulmonary embolism, *AACN Clin Issues Crit Care Nurs* 6:588, 1995.
22. Kersten RS, Jonas EA: New help with diagnostic and therapeutic dilemmas, *Consultant* 34:673, 1994.
23. Desai S: Interpretation of a normal chest x-ray, *Nurs Stand* 7:38, 1992.
24. Dettenmeir PA: *Radiographic assessment for nurses,* St Louis, 1995, Mosby.
25. Kelly-Heidenthal P, O'Connor M: Nursing assessment of portable chest x-rays, *DCCN* 13:127, 1994.
26. Sheldon RL: Systematic analysis of the chest x-ray. In Scanlan CL, Spearman CB, Sheldon RL, editors: *Egan's fundamentals of respiratory care,* ed 6, St Louis, 1995, Mosby.
27. Van Hooser T: Assessment of gas exchange. In Scanlan CL, Spearman CB, Sheldon RL, editors: *Egan's fundamentals of respiratory care,* ed 6, St Louis, 1995, Mosby.
28. Clark JS and others: Noninvasive assessment of blood gases, *Am Rev Respir Dis* 145:220, 1992.
29. Grossbach I: Case studies in pulse oximetry monitoring, *Crit Care Nurse* 13(4):63, 1993.

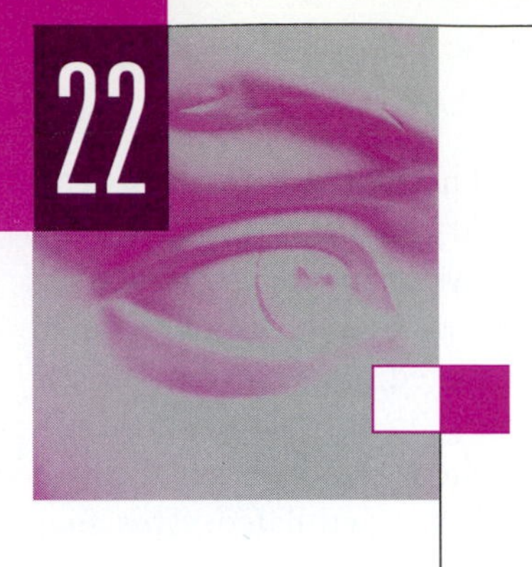

Pulmonary Disorders

UNDERSTANDING THE PATHOLOGY of a disease, the areas of assessment on which to focus, and the usual medical management allows the critical care nurse to more accurately anticipate and plan nursing interventions. This chapter focuses on pulmonary disorders commonly seen in the critical care environment.

ACUTE RESPIRATORY FAILURE

Description

Acute respiratory failure (ARF) is a clinical condition in which the pulmonary system fails to maintain adequate gas exchange.[1] It is probably the most prevalent problem seen in critical care today.[2] ARF can be classified as hypoxemic normocapnic respiratory failure (Type I) or hypoxemic hypercapnic respiratory failure (Type II), depending on the patient's arterial blood gases (ABGs). In Type I respiratory failure the patient has a low PaO_2 level and a normal $PaCO_2$ level, whereas in Type II respiratory failure, the PaO_2 level is low and the $PaCO_2$ level is high.[3]

Though any number of diagnosis-related groups (DRGs) may apply to the patient with ARF, depending on the underlying cause and subsequent treatment, DRG 475 (Respiratory system diagnosis with ventilator support), with an anticipated length of stay of 12.3 days, is normally used.[4]

Etiology

ARF results from a deficiency in the performance of the pulmonary system.[1-3] It usually occurs secondary to another disorder that has altered the normal function of the pulmonary system in such a way as to decrease the ventilatory drive, muscle strength, chest-wall elasticity, or the lung's capacity for gas exchange or to increase airway resistance or metabolic oxygen requirements.[5]

The etiologies of ARF may be classified as extrapulmonary or intrapulmonary, depending on the component of the respiratory system that is affected. Extrapulmonary causes include disorders that affect the brain, spinal cord, neuromuscular system, thorax, pleura, and upper airways. Intrapulmonary causes include disorders that affect the lower airways and alveoli, pulmonary circulation, and alveolar-capillary membrane.[6] Table 22-1 lists the etiologies of ARF and their associated disorders.[5]

Pathophysiology

Hypoxemia is the result of impaired gas exchange and is the hallmark of acute respiratory failure. Hypercapnia may be present, depending on the underlying cause of the problem. The main causes of hypoxemia are alveolar hypoventilation, ventilation/perfusion (V/Q) mismatching, and intrapulmonary shunting.[7] Type I respiratory failure usually results from V/Q mismatching and intrapulmonary shunting, whereas Type II respiratory failure usually results from alveolar hypoventilation, which may or may not be accompanied by V/Q mismatching and intrapulmonary shunting.[1] (∞Ventilation/Perfusion Relationships, p. 618.)

Alveolar hypoventilation. Alveolar hypoventilation occurs when the amount of oxygen being brought into the alveoli is insufficient to meet the metabolic needs of the body.[6] This can be the result of increasing metabolic oxygen needs or decreasing ventilations.[5] Hypoxemia caused by alveolar hypoventilation is often associated with hypercapnia and commonly results from extrapulmonary disorders.[1,7]

Ventilation/perfusion mismatching. V/Q mismatching occurs when ventilation and blood flow are mismatched

TABLE 22-1 Etiologies of Acute Respiratory Failure

Affected Area	Disorders*
EXTRAPULMONARY	
Brain	Drug overdose Central alveolar hypoventilation syndrome Brain trauma or lesion Postoperative anesthesia depression
Spinal cord	Guillain-Barré syndrome Poliomyelitis Amyotrophic lateral sclerosis Spinal cord trauma or lesion
Neuromuscular system	Myasthenia gravis Multiple sclerosis Neuromuscular-blocking antibiotics Organophosphate poisoning Muscular dystrophy
Thorax	Massive obesity Chest trauma
Pleura	Pleural effusion Pneumothorax
Upper airways	Sleep apnea Tracheal obstruction Epiglottitis
INTRAPULMONARY	
Lower airways and alveoli	Chronic obstructive pulmonary disease (COPD) Asthma Bronchiolitis Cystic fibrosis Pneumonia
Pulmonary circulation	Pulmonary emboli
Alveolar-capillary membrane	Pulmonary edema Acute respiratory distress syndrome (ARDS) Inhalation of toxic gases Near-drowning

*Not an inclusive list.

in various regions of the lung in excess of what is normal. Blood passes through alveoli that are underventilated for the given amount of perfusion, leaving these areas with a lower-than-normal amount of oxygen. V/Q mismatching is the most common cause of hypoxemia and is usually the result of alveoli that are partially collapsed or partially filled with fluid.[7,8]

Intrapulmonary shunting. The extreme form of V/Q mismatching—intrapulmonary shunting—occurs when blood reaches the arterial system without participating in gas exchange. The mixing of unoxygenated (shunted) blood and oxygenated blood lowers the average level of oxygen present in the blood. Intrapulmonary shunting occurs when blood passes through a portion of a lung that is not ventilated. This may be the result of alveolar collapse (e.g., atelectasis); alveolar consolidation (e.g., pneumonia); or excessive mucus accumulation (e.g., chronic bronchitis).[7,8]

Complications. If allowed to progress, hypoxemia can result in a deficit of oxygen at the cellular level. As the tissue demands for oxygen continue and the supply diminishes, an oxygen supply/demand imbalance occurs and tissue hypoxia develops. Decreased oxygen to the cells contributes to impaired tissue perfusion and the development of lactic acidosis and multiple organ dysfunction syndrome.[8] (∞Multiple Organ Dysfunction Syndrome, p. 1124.)

Assessment and Diagnosis

The patient with ARF may experience a variety of clinical manifestations, depending on the underlying cause and the extent of tissue hypoxia. The clinical manifestations commonly seen in the patient with ARF are usually related to the development of hypoxemia, hypercapnia, and acidosis (Table 22-2). Because the clinical symptoms are so varied, they are not considered reliable in predicting the degree of hypoxemia or hypercapnia.[8-10]

Diagnosing and following the course of respiratory failure is best accomplished by ABG analysis. ABG analysis confirms the level of $Pa{CO_2}$, $Pa{O_2}$, and blood pH. ARF is generally accepted as being present when the $Pa{O_2}$ level is less than 50 mm Hg and/or the $Pa{CO_2}$ level is greater than 50 mm Hg.[2,3] In patients with chronically elevated $Pa{CO_2}$ levels, these criteria must be broadened to include a pH level less than 7.35.[5]

Medical Management

Medical management of the patient with ARF is aimed at treating the underlying cause, promoting adequate gas exchange, correcting acidosis, and preventing complications.[5] Medical interventions to promote gas exchange are aimed at improving oxygenation and ventilation.

Oxygenation. Actions to improve oxygenation include supplemental oxygen administration and the use of positive airway pressure. The purpose of oxygen therapy is to correct hypoxemia, and although the absolute

TABLE 22-2 Clinical Manifestations of Acute Respiratory Failure

Organ System	Signs and Symptoms		
	Hypoxemia	Hypercapnia	Acidosis
Central nervous	Restlessness Agitation Irritability Confusion Personality changes Impaired judgment Memory loss Sleep disturbance Bizarre behavior Decreased level of consciousness	Headache Drowsiness Decreased level of consciousness Papilledema Blurred vision Confusion Seizures Sleep disturbances	Drowsiness Confusion Decreased level of consciousness
Cardiovascular	Tachycardia Bounding pulse Hypertension (systolic) Wide pulse pressure Dysrhythmias Palpitations Chest pain	Same as hypoxemia Flushing of the skin	Weak pulse Hypotension Dysrhythmias (bradycardia)
Pulmonary	Tachypnea Hyperventilation Dyspnea Shortness of breath Active accessory muscles (neck and shoulders) Active abdominal movement during respiration Ascites, edema, neck vein distention Intercostal retractions, tracheal tugging, flaring nares	Same as hypoxemia	Same as hypoxemia
Renal	Decreased urinary output Polycythemia Hypertension Edema	Decreased urinary output Hypochloremia Edema Hypertension	Hypochloremic metabolic alkalosis
Gastrointestinal	Decreased bowel sounds Abdominal distention Anorexia Nausea Vomiting Constipation Gastrointestinal bleeding	Same as hypoxemia	Same as hypoxemia
Skin	Pallor Cyanosis Clammy Cool Plethora	Flushed Clammy	Sympathetic nervous system responses (cool, clammy, pale)

Modified from Vaughan P: *Crit Care Nurse* 1(6):46, 1981.

level of hypoxemia varies in each patient, most treatment approaches aim to keep the oxygen saturation at 90% or more. The goal is to keep the tissues' needs satisfied but not produce hypercapnia or oxygen toxicity.[5] Supplemental oxygen administration is effective in treating hypoxemia related to alveolar hypoventilation and V/Q mismatching. When intrapulmonary shunting exists, supplemental oxygen alone is ineffective.[11] In this situation, positive pressure—in the form of constant positive airway pressure (CPAP) or positive end-expiratory pressure (PEEP)—is necessary to open collapsed alveoli and facilitate their participation in gas exchange. Positive pressure may be delivered noninvasively via a mask[12] or invasively via an endotracheal tube.[13] (∞Oxygen Therapy p. 689; Noninvasive Mechanical Ventilation, p. 710.)

Ventilation. Interventions to improve ventilation include intubation and mechanical ventilation. Intubation can be accomplished either orally or nasally. If prolonged intubation is required, a tracheostomy must be considered. Once intubated, the patient is placed on a positive-pressure ventilator. The selection of mode and settings depends on the patient's underlying condition, severity of respiratory failure, and body size. In the patient with chronic hypercapnia, the settings are adjusted to keep the pH level normal, but not the $Paco_2$ level.[14] (∞Invasive Mechanical Ventilation, p. 703.)

Pharmacology. Medications to facilitate removal of secretions and dilate airways may also be of benefit in the treatment of the patient with ARF. Mucolytics are administered to help liquefy secretions, which facilitates their removal. Bronchodilators, such as xanthines (e.g., theophylline and aminophylline); $beta_2$ agonists (e.g., albuterol, bitolterol, isoetharine, metaproterenol, and terbutaline); and anticholinergic agents (e.g., ipratropium), aid in smooth muscle relaxation and are of particular benefit to patients with airflow limitations. Steroids are also often administered to decrease airway inflammation and to enhance the effects of the $beta_2$ agonists.[5,14] (∞Bronchodilators and Adjuncts, p. 713.)

Sedation is necessary in many patients to assist with maintaining adequate ventilation. It can be used to comfort the patient and decrease the work of breathing, particularly if the patient is fighting the ventilator. Analgesics are administered for pain control.[14] In some patients, sedation does not decrease spontaneous respiratory efforts enough to allow adequate ventilation. Neuromuscular paralysis may be necessary to facilitate optimal ventilation. Paralysis also may be necessary to decrease oxygen consumption in the severely compromised patient. Three neuromuscular blocking agents commonly used are pancuronium (Pavulon), vecuronium (Norcuron), and atracurium (Tracrium).[15] (∞Neuromuscular Blocking Agents, p. 713.)

Acidosis. Acidosis may occur for a number of reasons. Hypoxemia causes impaired tissue perfusion, which leads to the production of lactic acid and the development of metabolic acidosis. Impaired ventilation leads to the accumulation of carbon dioxide and the development of respiratory acidosis. Once the patient is adequately oxygenated and ventilated, the acidosis should correct itself. Bicarbonate administration may be necessary if the acidosis persists or is severe (pH level less than 7.2).[5]

Complications. The patient with acute respiratory failure may experience a number of complications, including cardiac dysrhythmias, pulmonary embolism, gastrointestinal bleeding, and complications associated with mechanical ventilation. Dysrhythmias can be precipitated by hypoxemia, acidosis, electrolyte imbalances, and the administration of $beta_2$ agonists and xanthines. Maintaining oxygenation, normalizing electrolytes, and monitoring drug levels assist in the prevention of dysrhythmias. Symptomatic dysrhythmias are treated in the conventional manner. Pulmonary embolism can be prevented through the use of deep vein thrombosis prophylaxis with heparin. In addition, the patient receives stress ulcer prophylaxis, with a histamine blocker or sucralfate, to prevent gastrointestinal bleeding.[5]

Nursing Management

Nursing management of the patient with acute respiratory failure incorporates a variety of nursing diagnoses and interventions (Boxes 22-1 and 22-2). Nursing management is directed by the specific etiology of the respiratory failure, although some common interventions are used. The nurse has a significant role in optimizing oxygenation and ventilation, facilitating nutritional support, providing comfort and emotional support, and maintaining surveillance for complications. Nursing interventions to optimize oxygenation and ventilation include positioning, preventing desaturation, and promoting secretion clearance.

Positioning. Positioning of the patient with ARF depends on the type of lung injury. The goal is to facilitate or optimize V/Q matching and thus help alleviate hypoxemia. Patients with unilateral lung disease are positioned with the good lung down.[16-18] Patients with diffuse lung disease are positioned prone, with the right lung down, or are continuously turned. Some patients benefit from nonrecumbent positions, such as sitting or a semierect position.[18] Though not often used, the

BOX 22-1 NURSING DIAGNOSIS AND MANAGEMENT

ACUTE RESPIRATORY FAILURE

- Impaired Gas Exchange related to alveolar hypoventilation, p. 726
- Impaired Gas Exchange related to ventilation/perfusion mismatching or intrapulmonary shunting, p. 725
- Ineffective Breathing Pattern related to musculoskeletal fatigue or neuromuscular impairment, p. 724
- Risk for Aspiration, p. 727
- Altered Nutrition: Less than Body Requirements related to lack of exogenous nutrients or increased metabolic demand, p. 165
- Risk for Infection, p. 1119
- Inability to Sustain Spontaneous Ventilation related to respiratory muscle fatigue or metabolic factors, p. 724
- Acute Confusion related to sensory overload, sensory deprivation, and sleep pattern disturbance, p. 90
- Anxiety related to threat to biologic, psychologic, and/or social integrity, p. 99
- Body Image Disturbance related to functional dependence on life-sustaining technology, p. 86
- Ineffective Family Coping related to critically ill family member, p. 97
- Knowledge Deficit: Discharge Regimen related to lack of previous exposure to information, p. 61 (see Patient Education Box 22-2)

BOX 22-2 PATIENT EDUCATION

ACUTE RESPIRATORY FAILURE

- Pathophysiology of disease
- Specific etiology
- Precipitating factor modification
- Importance of taking medications
- Breathing techniques (e.g., pursed-lip breathing, diaphragmatic breathing)
- Energy conservation techniques
- Measures to prevent pulmonary infections (e.g., proper nutrition, handwashing, immunization against *Streptococcus pneumoniae* and influenza viruses)
- Signs and symptoms of pulmonary infection (e.g., sputum color change, shortness of breath, fever)
- Cough enhancement techniques (e.g., cascade cough, huff cough, end-expiratory cough, augmented cough)

prone position has also been shown to increase oxygenation in patients with severe respiratory failure.[16,17]

Preventing desaturation. A number of activities can prevent desaturation from occurring. These include performing procedures only as needed, hyperoxygenating the patient before suctioning, providing adequate rest and recovery time between various procedures,[18,19] and minimizing oxygen consumption.[20] Interventions to minimize oxygen consumption include limiting the patient's physical activity, administering sedation to control anxiety, and providing measures to control fever.[20] The patient is continuously monitored with a pulse oximeter for warning signs of desaturation.[19]

Promoting secretion clearance. Interventions to promote secretion clearance include those that prevent secretion retention and facilitate secretion removal. Actions to prevent secretion retention include providing adequate systemic hydration, humidifying supplemental oxygen, and preventing hypoventilation. Activities to facilitate secretion removal include suctioning (endotracheal or nasotracheal) and chest physical therapy (percussion, vibration, postural drainage, and coughing).[19] (∞Suctioning, p. 701.)

Preventing hypoventilation. To facilitate deep breathing the patient's thorax is maintained in alignment, and the head of the bed is elevated at least 30 degrees. This position best accommodates diaphragmatic descent and intercostal muscle action. Frequent repositioning (at least every 2 hours) or lateral rotation therapy is essential, because it results in a change in ventilatory pattern and V/Q matching.[19]

Once the patient is extubated, deep breathing and incentive spirometry are started as soon as possible. Deep breathing involves having the patient take a deep breath and hold it for approximately 3 seconds or longer. Incentive spirometry involves having the patient take at least 10 deep, effective breaths per hour using an incentive spirometer. These actions help prevent atelectasis and reexpand any collapsed lung tissue. The chest is auscultated during inflation to ensure that all dependent parts of the lung are well-ventilated and to help the patient understand the depth of breath necessary for optimal effect. Coughing is avoided unless secretions are present, because it promotes collapse of the smaller airways.[19]

Facilitating nutritional support. The initiation of nutritional support is of utmost importance in the management of the patient with ARF. The goals of nutritional support are to improve the patient's overall nutritional status, enhance the immune system, and promote respiratory muscle function. Because of the severity of the patient's illness, initially the patient may begin receiving parenteral nutrition (TPN), with the goal to change to enteral feedings as soon as the patient is able to tolerate them.[7,10] (∞Nutrition and Pulmonary Alterations, p. 133.)

Patient Education

Early in the patient's hospital stay, the patient and family are taught about acute respiratory failure, its etiologies, and its treatment. As the patient moves toward discharge, teaching focuses on the interventions necessary for preventing the reoccurrence of the precipitating disorder (see Box 22-2). If the patient smokes, he or she is encouraged to stop smoking and referred to a smoking cessation program. In addition, the importance of participating in a pulmonary rehabilitation program is stressed. (∞Patient Education, p. 659.)

ACUTE RESPIRATORY DISTRESS SYNDROME

Description

Acute (formerly called "adult") respiratory distress syndrome (ARDS)[20] is an inflammatory syndrome marked by disruption of the alveolar-capillary membrane.[21] A number of theories postulate that ARDS is part of the multisystem response to injury. Instead of multiple organ dysfunction syndrome (MODS) being the consequence of ARDS, newer theories indicate that ARDS starts from the same inflammatory-immune-mediated response as and is part of MODS. ARDS appears to occur first, because of the immediate nature of impaired gas exchange.[22] The mortality rate from ARDS has been declining over the last several years, but it still ranges from 23% to 57%, depending on the initiating event.[23] (∞Multiple Organ Dysfunction Syndrome, p. 1124.)

Though any number of DRGs may apply to the patient with ARDS, depending on the underlying cause and subsequent treatment, DRG 475 (Respiratory system diagnosis with ventilator support), with an anticipated length of stay of 12.8 days, is normally used.[4]

Etiology

A variety of clinical conditions are associated with the development of ARDS (Box 22-3).[20,24,25] They can be divided into direct and indirect injuries, depending on the primary event or site of injury.[20] Sepsis, aspiration of gastric contents, pulmonary contusion, pneumonia, and near-drowning were found to be major risk factors for the development of ARDS.[24]

BOX 22-3 Risk Factors for ARDS

DIRECT INJURY

Aspiration
Near-drowning
Toxic inhalation
Pulmonary contusion
Pneumonia
Oxygen toxicity
Transthoracic radiation

INDIRECT INJURY

Sepsis
Nonthoracic trauma
Hypertransfusion
Cardiopulmonary bypass
Severe pancreatitis
Embolism—air, fat, amniotic fluid
Disseminated intravascular coagulation (DIC)
Shock states

Pathophysiology. Though the exact cause of ARDS is unclear, it is generally believed that stimulation of the inflammatory-immune system initiates a systemic response that includes the sequestering of neutrophils in the lungs, activation of alveolar macrophages, and the release of endotoxin (Figure 22-1). Once stimulated these cellular systems release a variety of mediators, which result in increased capillary membrane permeability, changes in the diameter of the small airways, pulmonary vasoconstriction, injury to the pulmonary vasculature, and microemboli formation in the lungs. Several of the mediators implicated in this response are oxygen-free radicals, tumor necrosis factor, interleukin 1, proteases, platelet-activating factor, and eicosanoids.[26]

Permeability defect. Increased capillary membrane permeability results in a permeability defect, which allows leakage of fluid and protein into the pulmonary interstitium. As the fluid and protein accumulate in the interstitium, normal local controlling factors (e.g., oncotic pressure, capillary hydrostatic pressure, lymphatic drainage) are overwhelmed, and damage to the Type I alveolar epithelial cells occurs. Eventually, fluid and protein enter the alveoli and damage the Type II alveolar epithelial cells, resulting in impaired surfactant production. Injury to the cells and the loss of surfactant leads to alveoli collapse, resulting in intrapulmonary shunting, V/Q mismatching, decreased functional residual capacity (FRC), and decreased lung compliance.[22,26]

Bronchoconstriction. Changes in the diameter of the small airways lead to bronchoconstriction, which results in increased airway resistance, decreased lung

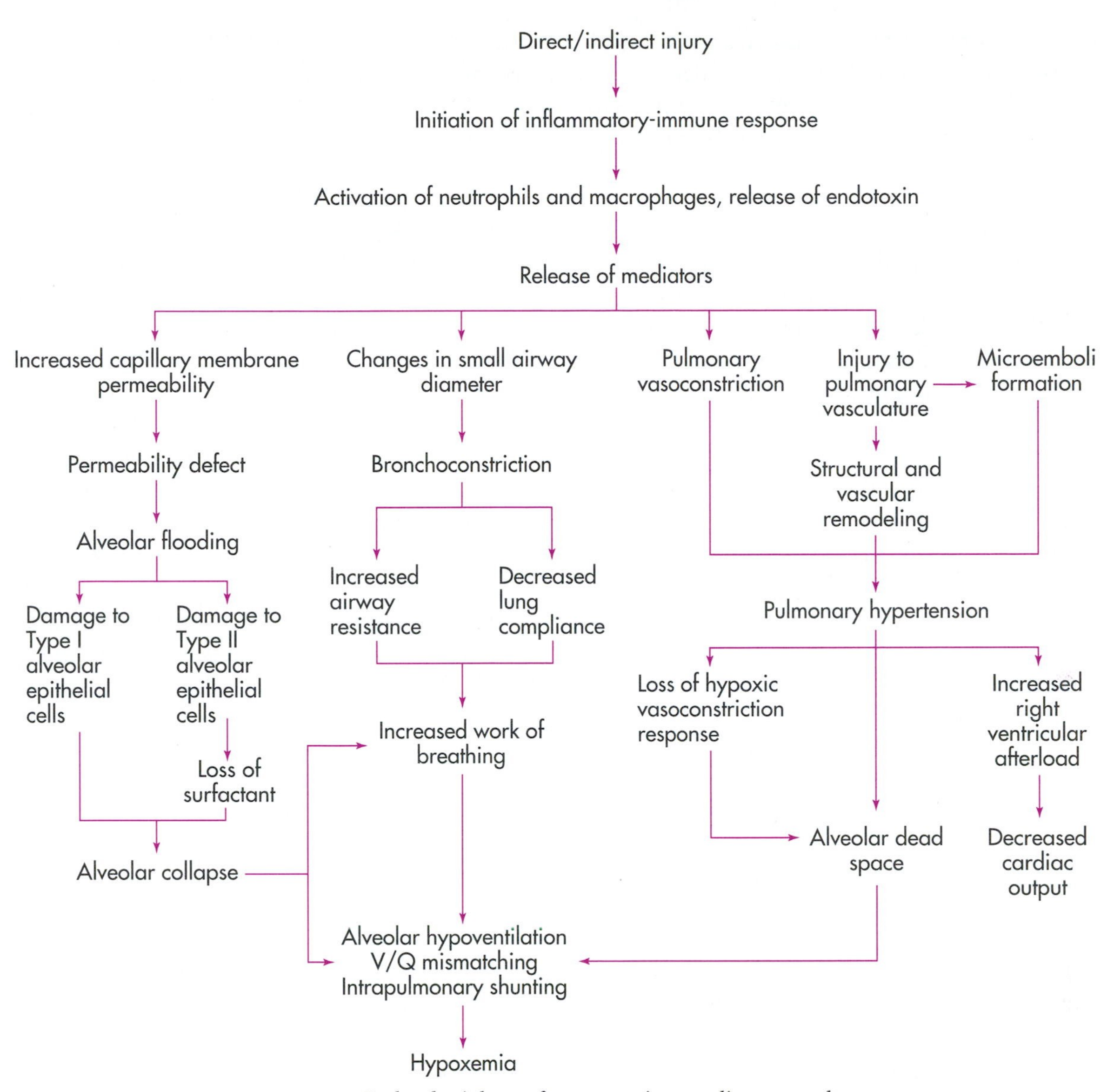

FIGURE 22-1. Pathophysiology of acute respiratory distress syndrome.

compliance, and increased V/Q mismatching. Hypoxemia and the work of breathing increases, which leads to fatigue and hypoventilation, which further heighten hypoxemia.[22,26]

Pulmonary hypertension. Injury to the pulmonary vasculature leads to structural abnormalities and vascular remodeling, which results in pulmonary hypertension. The formation of microemboli in the lungs and pulmonary artery vasoconstriction also contribute to the development of elevated pulmonary pressures. In addition, damage to the pulmonary circuit can lead to impairment of the compensatory response of hypoxic vasoconstriction. The end result is increased alveolar dead space, V/Q mismatching, and intrapulmonary shunting, which further increases hypoxemia and the work of breathing. Pulmonary hypertension also increases right ventricular afterload and can lead to right ventricular dysfunction and decreased cardiac output.[22,26]

The progression of ARDS can be described in phases. Phase 1 is the acute, or exudative, phase and occurs within 5 to 7 days of the onset of the disorder. During this phase the pulmonary capillaries leak and flood the alveoli, damaging the alveolar epithelial cells. Hyaline membranes start to develop along the alveoli. Phase 2 is the proliferative phase, and it occurs after 7 days of the onset of the disorder. During this phase fibroblasts and other inflammatory cells infiltrate the lungs in an attempt to repair the damage. This results in the structural abnormalities and vascular remodeling that precipitate development of pulmonary hypertension.

Phase 3 is the chronic, or fibrotic, phase and occurs after 2 to 3 weeks of the onset of the disorder. During this phase the remodeling of the lung is complete, with diffuse fibrotic scarring appearing in the alveoli and interstitial space.[26]

Assessment and Diagnosis

The patient with ARDS may exhibit a variety of clinical manifestations, depending on the precipitating event. Initially, the patient has tachypnea, restlessness, apprehension, and moderate accessory muscle use that progresses to agitation, dyspnea, fatigue, excessive accessory muscle use, and fine crackles as respiratory failure occurs.[26]

Arterial blood gas analysis reveals a low PaO_2 level, despite increases in supplemental oxygen administration (refractory hypoxemia).[25,26] Initially, the $PaCO_2$ level is low as a result of hyperventilation, but eventually the $PaCO_2$ level increases as the patient fatigues. The pH level is high initially but decreases as respiratory acidosis develops.[21,25]

Initially the chest x-ray may be normal, because changes in the lungs do not become evident for up to 24 hours. As the pulmonary edema becomes apparent, diffuse patchy interstitial and alveolar infiltrates appear. This progresses to multifocal consolidation of the lungs, which appears as a "white out" on the chest x-ray.[27]

Many criteria have been used to diagnose ARDS, which has led to confusion. In 1992, the American-European Consensus Committee on ARDS recommended defining ARDS as acute in onset, with a PaO_2/FIO_2 ratio less than or equal to 200 mm Hg (regardless of PEEP level), bilateral infiltrates on chest radiography, and a pulmonary artery wedge pressure less than or equal to 18 mm Hg or no clinical evidence of left atrial hypertension.[20]

Medical Management

Medical management of the patient with ARDS involves a multifaceted approach. This strategy includes treating the underlying cause, promoting gas exchange, supporting tissue oxygenation, and monitoring for complications.[25] Medical interventions to promote gas exchange include supplemental oxygen administration, PEEP, intubation, and mechanical ventilation.[20]

Oxygenation. Oxygen is administered at the lowest level possible to support tissue oxygenation. Continued exposure to high levels of oxygen can lead to oxygen toxicity, which further perpetuates the entire process. The goal of oxygen therapy is to maintain an SaO_2 of 90 mm Hg or greater using the lowest FIO_2. Because the hypoxemia that develops with ARDS is often refractory to oxygen therapy, it is usually necessary to facilitate oxygenation with PEEP.[25,27] (∞Oxygen Therapy, p. 689.)

The purpose of using PEEP in the patient with ARDS is to improve oxygenation while reducing FIO_2 to less toxic levels. PEEP has several positive effects on the lungs, including recruiting collapsed alveoli, increasing FRC, and redistributing fluid in the intraalveolar space to the interstitial space. Thus PEEP decreases intrapulmonary shunting and V/Q mismatching, increases compliance, and improves gas exchange. PEEP also has several negative effects, including decreased cardiac output (CO) because of decreased venous return, ventricular dysfunction as a result of increasing pulmonary vascular resistance, and barotrauma. The amount of PEEP a patient requires is determined by considering both SaO_2 and CO.[25,27] The goal of PEEP is to administer the least amount necessary to keep the SaO_2 level at 90 mm Hg or greater and the FIO_2 level at 60 mm Hg or less.[27]

Ventilation. Intubation and mechanical ventilation are usually required to facilitate ventilation, particularly as fatigue develops and ventilatory failure occurs. During the acute phase of ARDS the patient receives complete ventilatory support. This allows the ventilator to do the majority of the work of breathing and the patient to rest. Usually, the assist/control (also called continuous mandatory ventilation) mode and the synchronized intermittent mandatory ventilation (SIMV) mode are used. The assist/control mode allows the patient to rest completely, thus decreasing the work of breathing. The SIMV mode allows the patient to be ventilated with lower mean airway pressures, thus reducing the incidence of hemodynamic compromise and barotrauma.[27] (∞Invasive Mechanical Ventilation, p. 703.)

An alternative ventilatory modality that is also used in managing the patient with ARDS is inverse ratio ventilation (IRV), either pressure-controlled or volume-controlled. IRV prolongs the inspiratory (I) time and shortens the expiratory (E) time, thus reversing the normal I:E ratio. The effect is intentional air trapping, which increases FRC and alveolar recruitment while maintaining lower airway pressures. Disadvantages to IRV include the development of auto-PEEP, which can cause hemodynamic compromise and worsen gas exchange. In addition, patients receiving IRV usually require neuromuscular blockade and sedation to prevent them from fighting the ventilator.[25,27] (∞Neuromuscular Blocking Agents, p. 713.)

Tissue perfusion. Interventions to support tissue perfusion include cautious fluid management and maintenance of CO. Newer approaches to fluid management include maintaining a very low intravascular volume (pulmonary artery wedge pressure of 5 to 8 mm Hg) with fluid restriction and diuretics while supporting the CO with vasoactive and inotropic medications. The goal is to decrease the amount of fluid leakage into the lungs.[25,27]

Investigational therapies. A number of investigational studies of other therapies for the treatment of ARDS are under way. These therapies include drugs to block or neutralize the various mediators released as part of the inflammatory-immune response and methods to limit the damage to the lungs. A number of drugs are being tested, including nonsteroidal antiinflammatory agents, antioxidant agents, polyclonal and monoclonal antibodies, thromboxane synthetase inhibitors, and prostaglandin E_1. Methods to limit damage to the lungs include surfactant replacement, extracorporeal membrane oxygenation, and extracorporeal carbon dioxide removal. Inhaled nitric oxide is also being investigated to help reverse pulmonary vasoconstriction and improve perfusion of ventilated regions of the lungs.[25,27]

Nursing Management

Nursing management of the patient with ARDS incorporates a variety of nursing diagnoses (Box 22-4). Nursing interventions include optimizing oxygenation and ventilation, maximizing tissue perfusion, facilitating nutritional support, providing comfort and emotional support, and maintaining surveillance for complications.

Optimizing oxygenation and ventilation. Nursing interventions to optimize oxygenation and ventilation include positioning, preventing desaturation, and promoting secretion clearance. For further discussion on these interventions, see Nursing Management of Acute Respiratory Failure earlier in this chapter.

Maximizing tissue perfusion. Adequate tissue perfusion depends on an adequate supply of oxygen being transported to the tissues. An adequate CO and hemoglobin level are critical to oxygen transport. CO depends on heart rate, preload, afterload, and contractility. A variety of fluids and medications are used to manipulate this parameter. The types of fluids include both crystalloids and colloids. The types of medications include vasoconstrictors, vasodilators, positive inotropes, antidysrhythmics, and diuretics.[26] (∞Pulmonary Artery Pressure Monitoring, p. 456.)

Facilitating nutritional support. The initiation of nutritional support is of utmost importance in the management of the patient with ARDS. The goals of nutritional support are to improve the patient's overall nutritional status, enhance the immune system, and prevent the development of multiple organ dysfunction syndrome. Because of the severity of the patient's illness, initially the patient may begin receiving total parenteral nutrition (TPN), with the goal to change to enteral feedings as soon as the patient is able to tolerate them.[21] (∞Nutrition and Pulmonary Alterations, p. 133.)

BOX 22-4 NURSING DIAGNOSIS AND MANAGEMENT

ACUTE RESPIRATORY DISTRESS SYNDROME

- Impaired Gas Exchange related to ventilation/perfusion mismatching or intrapulmonary shunting, p. 725
- Decreased Cardiac Output related to alterations in preload, p. 590
- Altered Nutrition: Less than Body Requirements related to lack of exogenous nutrients or increased metabolic demand, p. 165
- Risk for Aspiration, p. 727
- Risk for Infection, p. 1119
- Anxiety related to threat to biologic, psychologic, and/or social integrity, p. 99
- Body Image Disturbance related to functional dependence on life-sustaining technology, p. 86
- Ineffective Family Coping related to critically ill family member, p. 97

PNEUMONIA

Description

Pneumonia is an acute inflammation of the lung parenchyma that is caused by an infectious agent that can lead to alveolar consolidation. Pneumonia can be classified as community-acquired (CAP) or hospital-acquired (nosocomial). Community-acquired pneumonia is acquired outside of the hospital and is usually less virulent than hospital-acquired pneumonia. CAP can be further classified as typical or atypical pneumonia. Typical pneumonia is an infection produced by bacterial organisms that normally inhabit the nasopharyngeal airway. Atypical pneumonia is an infection acquired from inhalation of organisms from the environment. Hospital-acquired pneumonia (HAP) is acquired inside the hospital and is usually much more serious than CAP, because many of the causative agents are resistant to conventional antibiotic therapy.[28] Ventilator-associated pneumonia (VAP) is a subgroup of HAP that refers to an infection that develops during mechanical ventilation more than 48 hours after intubation.[29]

Pneumonia falls under two different DRGs, depending on whether the patient develops complications or comorbid conditions (CC). DRG 79 (Respiratory infections and inflammation, age greater than 17 years with CC) and DRG 80 (Respiratory infections and inflammation, age greater than 17 years without CC) have average lengths of the stay of 9.3 days and 6.6 days, respectively.[4]

Etiology

The etiologies of pneumonia vary greatly with the type. Causes of typical CAP include *Streptococcus pneumoniae, Klebsiella pneumoniae, Moraxella catarrhalis,* group A streptococci, and *Haemophilus influenzae.* Causes of atypical CAP include *Mycoplasma pneumoniae,* influenza viruses, *Legionella pneumophila, Chlamydia pneumoniae,* and fungi.[30] *Pneumocystis carinii* is the predominate cause of pulmonary infection in patients with acquired immunodeficiency syndrome (AIDS) (Box 22-5).[31] Nosocomial pneumonia is usually caused by *Staphylococcus aureus, Klebsiella pneumoniae, Escherichia coli, Enterobacter* species, *Pseudomonas aeruginosa,* and *Serratia marcescens.*[32] Often, institutions have their own resident flora that predominates in nosocomial infection. Usually, the pathogens are the aerobic gram-negative bacilli[27] from the aquatic environment of the hospital.[30]

A number of conditions predispose a patient to developing pneumonia, including depressed gag and cough reflexes, decreased ciliary activity, increased secretions, decreased lymphatic flow, atelectasis, fluid in the alveoli, immunologic defect, and impaired alveolar macrophages.[33] Table 22-3 lists the precipitating conditions and their causes.

Risk factors for these conditions are host-related, device-related, and personnel/procedure-related. Host-related factors include age greater than 65 years, underlying illness (e.g., chronic obstructive pulmonary disease [COPD], immunosuppression, diabetes), alcoholism, smoking, depressed consciousness and malnutrition, and thoracic or abdominal surgery. Device-related factors include endotracheal intubation, mechanical ventilation, and gastric intubation with enteral feedings. Personnel/procedure-related factors include cross-contamination by hands, infected personnel, antibiotic therapy, and histamine blockers and antacid therapy.[32,34] Histamine blockers, antacid therapy, and enteral feedings elevate the pH level of the stomach and promote bacterial overgrowth. The nasogastric

BOX 22-5 Pneumocystis Carinii Pneumonia

Pneumocystis carinii pneumonia (PCP) is the most common pulmonary infection seen in the patient with acquired immunodeficiency syndrome (AIDS). PCP is a protozoan infection that commonly occurs in childhood. This opportunistic infection lies dormant until the immunocompromised state of the patient allows its recurrence.

The onset of the pneumonia may be sudden or gradual with the clinical manifestations becoming apparent over weeks. Clinical manifestations include a dry cough, dyspnea, fever, and malaise. As the pneumonia progresses, the patient develops hypoxemic normocapnic respiratory failure.

The two drugs used for the treatment of PCP are trimethoprim-sulfamethoxazole (TMP-SMX) and pentamidine isethionate. Both drugs are given intravenously and are very toxic. Pentamidine also can be administered via aerosol. Adverse reactions to these drugs include high fever, nausea and vomiting, liver and renal dysfunction, neutropenia, and thrombocytopenia.

TABLE 22-3 Precipitating Conditions of Pneumonia

Condition	Etiologies
Depressed epiglottal and cough reflexes	Unconsciousness, neurologic disease, endotracheal or tracheal tubes, anesthesia, aging
Decreased cilia activity	Smoke inhalation, smoking history, oxygen toxicity, hypoventilation, intubation, viral infections, aging, COPD
Increased secretion	COPD, viral infections, bronchiectasis, general anesthesia, endotracheal intubation, smoking
Atelectasis	Trauma, foreign body obstruction, tumor, splinting, shallow ventilations, general anesthesia
Decreased lymphatic flow	CHF, tumor
Fluid in alveoli	CHF, aspiration, trauma
Abnormal phagocytosis and humoral activity	Neutropenia, immunocompetent disorders, patients receiving chemotherapy
Impaired alveolar macrophages	Hypoxemia, metabolic acidosis, cigarette smoking history, hypoxia, alcohol use, viral infections, aging

COPD, Chronic obstructive pulmonary disease; *CHF,* congestive heart failure.

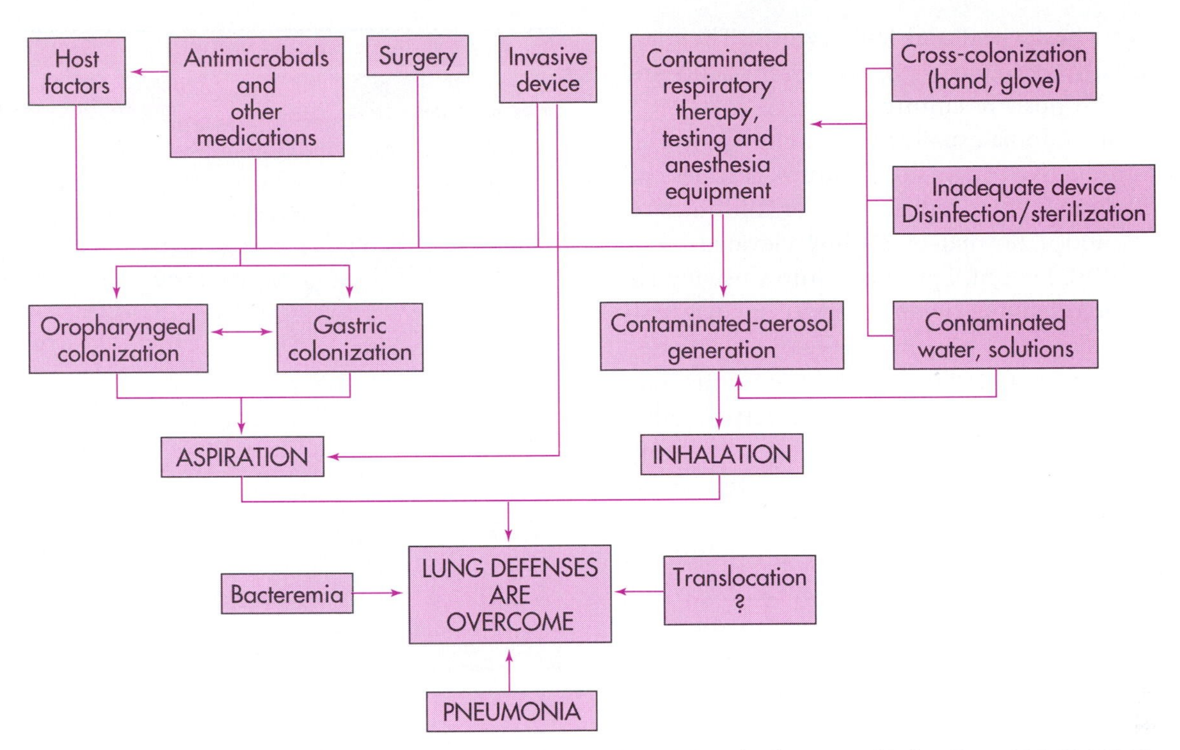

FIGURE 22-2. Pathophysiology of pneumonia. (From Tablan OC and others: *Am J Infect Contr* 22:247, 1994.)

tube acts as a wick, facilitating the movement of bacteria to the oropharynx, where it can be aspirated.[28]

Pathophysiology

Development of acute pneumonia implies a defect in host defenses, a particularly virulent organism, or an overwhelming inoculation event. Bacterial invasion of the lower respiratory tract can occur by inhalation, aspiration, migration from adjacent sites or colonization, direct inoculation, exogenous penetration from an infected site, and hematogenous seeding from another site. The most common method appears to be microaspiration of bacteria colonized in the upper airway (Figure 22-2).[34]

The oropharynx has a stable population of resident flora that may be anaerobic or aerobic. When stress occurs, such as with illness, surgery, or a viral infection, pathogenic organisms replace normal resident flora. Previous antibiotic therapy affects the resident flora population, making replacement by pathologic organisms more likely. The pathogens are then able to invade the sterile lower respiratory tract. Critically ill patients usually have gram-negative bacteria present in the oropharynx. Disruption of the gag and cough reflexes, altered consciousness, abnormal swallowing, and artificial airways all predispose the patient to aspiration and colonization of the lungs and subsequent infection. Histamine blockers, antacids, and enteral feedings also contribute to this problem, because they raise the pH level of the stomach and promote bacterial overgrowth. The nasogastric tube then acts as a wick facilitating the movement of bacteria from the stomach to the pharynx, where it too can be aspirated.[36]

Infection results in pulmonary inflammation with or without significant exudates. Increased capillary permeability occurs with increased interstitial and alveolar fluid. V/Q mismatching and intrapulmonary shunting occur, resulting in hypoxemia as lung consolidation progresses. Untreated pneumonia can result in ARF and initiation of the inflammatory-immune response. In addition, the patient may develop a pleural effusion. This is the result of the vascular response to inflammation, whereby capillary permeability is increased and fluid from the pulmonary capillaries diffuses into the pleural space.[33]

Assessment and Diagnosis

The clinical manifestations of pneumonia vary with the type of pneumonia. Typical pneumonia usually produces fever and chills, productive cough, purulent sputum, crackles on auscultation, localized alveolar infiltrates on chest x-ray, and leukocytosis. The diagnosis is usually based on a positive Gram stain and confirmed with positive cultures.[28]

Atypical pneumonia usually produces flu-like symptoms, nonproductive cough, little sputum, crackles and rhonchi on auscultation, diffuse alveolar infiltrates on chest x-ray, and a normal or slightly elevated white blood cell (WBC) count. Sputum cultures usually fail to identify the offending organism, thus the diagnosis is usually made with a positive serology test, though the test may take weeks to be diagnostic. Sputum Gram stains are usually negative, though a variety of other staining techniques (e.g., direct fluorescent antibody, acid-fast stain, potassium hydroxide preparation) may be more helpful.[28]

The clinical manifestations of HAP are similar to those of CAP but depend on the patient's underlying condition. Nosocomial pneumonia has an onset of more than 72 hours after hospitalization. Physical examination reveals rales, dullness on percussion, or an infiltrate on the chest x-ray and at least one of the following findings: purulent sputum, isolation of a pathogen from blood, transtracheal aspirate, biopsy specimen or a bronchial brush specimen, isolation of a virus in respiratory secretions, diagnostic antibody titers, or histopathologic evidence of pneumonia.[36]

BOX 22-6 NURSING DIAGNOSIS AND MANAGEMENT

PNEUMONIA

- Ineffective Airway Clearance related to excessive secretions or abnormal viscosity of mucus, p. 722
- Impaired Gas Exchange related to ventilation/perfusion mismatching or intrapulmonary shunting, p. 725
- Altered Nutrition: Less than Body Requirements related to lack of exogenous nutrients or increased metabolic demand, p. 165
- Risk for Aspiration, p. 727
- Risk for Infection Risk Factor: invasive monitoring devices, p. 598
- Anxiety related to threat to biologic, psychologic, and/or social integrity, p. 99
- Powerlessness related to lack of control over current situation or disease progression, p. 89
- Ineffective Family Coping related to critically ill family member, p. 97

Medical Management

Medical management of the patient with pneumonia includes antibiotic therapy, oxygen therapy for hypoxemia, mechanical ventilation if ARF develops, fluid management for hydration, nutritional support, and treatment of associated medical problems and complications. For patients having difficulty mobilizing secretions, mucolytics and therapeutic bronchoscopy may be necessary.

Antibiotic therapy. Although bacteria-specific antibiotic therapy is the goal, it may not always be possible because of difficulties in identifying the organism and the seriousness of the patient's condition. The time involved obtaining cultures must be balanced against the need to begin some treatment based on patient condition. Empirical therapy has become a generally acceptable approach. In this approach, choice of antibiotic treatment is based on the most likely etiologic organism while avoiding toxicity, superinfection, and unnecessary cost. If available, Gram stain results are used to guide antibiotic choices. Antibiotics chosen must offer broad coverage of the usual pathogens in the hospital or community. The patient's failure to respond to such therapy may indicate that the selected antibiotic regimen does not appropriately cover all of the etiologic pathogens, or it may indicate that a new source of infection has developed.[30]

Nursing Management

Nursing management of the patient with pneumonia incorporates a variety of nursing diagnoses (Box 22-6). Nursing interventions include optimizing oxygenation and ventilation, preventing the spread of infection, providing comfort and emotional support, and maintaining surveillance for complications. In addition, the patient's response to the antibiotic therapy is monitored for adverse effects.

Optimizing oxygenation and ventilation. Nursing interventions to optimize oxygenation and ventilation include positioning, preventing desaturation, and promoting secretion clearance. For further discussion on these interventions, see Nursing Management of Acute Respiratory Failure earlier in this chapter.

Preventing the spread of infection. Prevention is directed at eradicating pathogens from the environment and interrupting the spread of organisms from person to person. Significant progress has been made in removing contaminants from the patient environment through proper disinfection of respiratory equipment and increased use of disposable supplies. Other possible environmental sources of pathogens include suctioning equipment and indwelling lines. These invasive tools must be given proper aseptic care. Proper handwashing technique is the single most important measure available to prevent the spread of bacteria from person to person.[35] In addition, meticulous oral care is critical in decreasing the bacterial colonization of the oropharynx.

ASPIRATION LUNG DISORDER

Description

The presence of abnormal substances in the airways and alveoli as a result of aspiration is misleadingly called *aspiration pneumonia.* This term is misleading because the aspiration of toxic substances into the lung may or may not involve an infection. Aspiration lung disorder is a more accurate title, because injury to the lung can result from the chemical, mechanical, and/or bacterial characteristics of the aspirate.

Aspiration lung disorder falls under two DRGs, depending on whether the patient develops complications or comorbid conditions. DRG 101 (Other respiratory system diagnoses with CC) and DRG 102 (Other respiratory system diagnoses without CC) have average lengths of the stay of 5.2 days and 3.1 days, respectively.[4]

Etiology

A number of factors have been identified that place the patient at risk for aspiration (Box 22-7). Gastric contents and oropharyngeal bacteria (see Pneumonia) are the most common agents aspirated by the critically ill patient.[37] The effects of gastric contents on the lungs vary, based on the pH level of the liquid. If the pH level is less than 2.5, then the patient will develop severe chemical pneumonitis, resulting in hypoxemia.[38] If the pH level is greater than 2.5, the immediate damage to the lungs will be lessened[38] but the elevated pH level may have promoted bacterial overgrowth of the stomach.[28] Once the gastric contents are aspirated into the lungs, overwhelming bacterial pneumonia can develop.[35]

BOX 22-7 Risk Factors for Aspiration

- Altered level of consciousness
- Depressed gag, cough, or swallowing reflexes
- Presence of feeding tubes (all types)
- Presence of artificial airways
- Ileus or gastric distention
- History of gastrointestinal disorders
  - Dysphagia
  - Achalasia
  - Gastroesophageal reflux disease
  - Esophageal strictures

Pathophysiology

The type of lung injury that develops after aspiration is determined by a number of factors, including the quality of the aspirate and the status of the patient's respiratory defense mechanisms.

Acid liquid. The aspiration of acid (pH level less than 2.5) liquid gastric contents results in the development of bronchospasm and atelectasis almost immediately. Over the next 4 hours tracheal damage, bronchitis, bronchiolitis, alveolar-capillary breakdown, interstitial edema, and alveolar congestion and hemorrhage occur. Severe hypoxemia develops as a result of intrapulmonary shunting and V/Q mismatching. As the disorder progresses, necrotic debris and fibrin fill the alveoli, hyaline membranes form, and hypoxic vasoconstriction occurs, resulting in elevated pulmonary artery pressures.[39] The clinical course follows one of three patterns: (1) rapid improvement in 1 week, (2) initial improvement followed by deterioration and development of ARDS or pneumonia, or (3) rapid death from progressive ARF.[37,38]

Acid food particle. The aspiration of acid (pH level less than 2.5) nonobstructing food particles can produce the most severe pulmonary reaction because of extensive pulmonary damage. Severe hypoxemia, hypercapnia, and acidosis occur.[38]

Nonacid liquid. The effects of aspiration of nonacid (pH level greater than 2.5) liquid gastric contents are similar to those of acid liquid aspiration initially but with minimal structural damage occurring. Intrapulmonary shunting and V/Q mismatching usually start to reverse within 4 hours, and hypoxemia clears within 24 hours.[38]

Nonacid food particles. The effects of aspiration of nonacid (pH level greater than 2.5) nonobstructing food particles are similar to those of acid aspiration initially, with significant edema and hemorrhage occurring within 6 hours. After the initial reaction, the response changes to a reaction similar to that caused by a foreign body, with granuloma formation occurring around the food particles within 1 to 5 days. In addition to hypoxemia, hypercapnia and acidosis occur as a result of hypoventilation.[38]

Assessment and Diagnosis

Clinically, the patient demonstrates signs of acute respiratory distress,[37] and gastric contents may be present in the oropharynx.[38] The patient will have shortness of breath, coughing, wheezing, cyanosis, and signs of hypoxemia.[38] Tachypnea, tachycardia, hypotension, fever, and crackles also are present. Copious amounts of sputum are produced as alveolar edema develops.[37]

ABGs reflect severe hypoxemia. Chest x-ray changes appear 12 to 24 hours after the initial aspiration, with no one pattern being diagnostic of the event. Infiltrates will appear in a variety of distribution patterns, depending on the position of the patient during the aspiration event and the volume of the aspirate. If bacterial infection becomes established, leukocytosis and positive sputum cultures occur.[37]

Medical Management

Management of the patient with aspiration lung disorder includes both emergency and follow-up treatment. When aspiration is witnessed, emergency treatment is instituted to secure the airway and minimize pulmonary damage. The patient is placed in a slight (6 to 8 inches head-down) Trendelenburg position and turned to the right lateral decubitus position to aid drainage and avoid involvement of other lung areas. Oropharyngeal suctioning immediately follows.[38] Direct visualization by bronchoscopy is indicated for the removal of large particulate aspirate or to confirm an unwitnessed aspiration event. Bronchoalveolar lavage is not recommended, because this practice disseminates the aspirate in the lungs and increases damage. Prophylactic antibiotics are not recommended either.[38]

After airway clearance, attention is given to supporting oxygenation and hemodynamics. Hypoxemia is corrected with supplemental oxygen or mechanical ventilation with PEEP, if necessary. Hemodynamic changes result from fluid shifts that can occur after massive aspirations, causing noncardiogenic pulmonary edema. Monitoring intravascular volume is essential, and judicious amounts of replacement fluids are provided to maintain adequate urinary output and vital signs.[37,38]

Nursing Management

Nursing management of the patient with aspiration lung disorder incorporates a variety of nursing diagnoses (Box 22-8). Nursing interventions include optimizing oxygenation and ventilation, preventing further aspiration events, providing comfort and emotional support, and maintaining surveillance for complications.

Optimizing oxygenation and ventilation. Nursing interventions to optimize oxygenation and ventilation include positioning, preventing desaturation, and promoting secretion clearance. For further discussion on these interventions, see Nursing Management of Acute Respiratory Failure earlier in this chapter.

BOX 22-8 NURSING DIAGNOSIS AND MANAGEMENT

ASPIRATION LUNG DISORDER

- Impaired Gas Exchange related to ventilation/perfusion mismatching or intrapulmonary shunting, p. 725
- Ineffective Airway Clearance related to excessive secretions or abnormal viscosity of mucus, p. 722
- Risk for Aspiration, p. 727
- Risk for Infection, p. 1119
- Anxiety related to threat to biologic, psychologic, and/or social integrity, p. 99
- Ineffective Individual Coping related to situational crisis and personal vulnerability, p. 95
- Ineffective Family Coping related to critically ill family member, p. 97

Preventing aspiration. One of the most important interventions to prevent aspiration is identifying the patient at risk for aspiration. Actions to prevent aspiration include confirming feeding tube placement, checking for signs and symptoms of feeding intolerance and aspiration of gastric contents into the lungs, elevating the head of the bed at least 30 degrees or turning the patient on his or her right side if he or she must remain flat, ensuring proper inflation of artificial airway cuffs, and frequent suctioning of the oropharynx of intubated patients to prevent secretions from pooling above the cuff of the tube.[40]

PULMONARY EMBOLUS

Description

A pulmonary embolus (PE) occurs when clots (thrombotic emboli) or other matter (nonthrombotic emboli) lodge in the pulmonary arterial system, disrupting the blood flow to a region of the lungs. The majority of thrombotic emboli arise from the deep leg veins, particularly the iliac, femoral, and popliteal veins.[41] Other sources include the right ventricle, the upper extremities, and the pelvic veins. Nonthrombotic emboli arise from fat, tumors, amniotic fluid, air, and foreign bodies.[42] This section focuses on thrombotic emboli.

Pulmonary embolus falls under DRG 78 (Pulmonary embolism), with an average length of stay of 8.3 days.[4]

Etiology

A number of predisposing factors and precipitating conditions put a patient at risk for developing a PE (Box 22-9). Of the three predisposing factors (i.e., hy-

BOX 22-9 Risk Factors for Pulmonary Thromboembolism

PREDISPOSING FACTORS

- Venous stasis
  - Atrial fibrillation
  - Decreased cardiac output (CO)
  - Immobility
- Injury to vascular endothelium
  - Local vessel injury
  - Infection
  - Incision
  - Atherosclerosis
- Hypercoagulability
  - Polycythemia

PRECIPITATING CONDITIONS

- Previous pulmonary embolus
- Cardiovascular disease
  - Congestive heart failure
  - Right ventricular infarction
  - Cardiomyopathy
  - Cor pulmonale
- Surgery
  - Orthopedic
  - Vascular
  - Abdominal
- Cancer
  - Ovarian
  - Pancreatic
  - Stomach
  - Extrahepatic bile duct system
- Trauma (injury or burns)
  - Lower extremities
  - Pelvis
  - Hips
- Gynecologic status
  - Pregnancy
- Postpartum
- Birth control pills
- Estrogen replacement therapy

percoagulability, injury to vascular endothelium, and venous stasis [Virchow's triad]), venous stasis appears to be the most significant.[43]

Pathophysiology

A massive PE occurs with the blockage of a lobar or larger artery, resulting in occlusion of more than 40% of the pulmonary vascular bed. Blockage of the pulmonary arterial system has both pulmonary and hemodynamic consequences. The effects on the pulmonary system are increased alveolar dead space, bronchoconstriction, and compensatory shunting. The hemodynamic effects include an increase in pulmonary vascular resistance and right ventricular workload.[44] (∞Ventilation/Perfusion Relationships, p. 618.)

Increased dead space. An increase in alveolar dead space occurs because an area of the lung is receiving ventilation without being perfused. The ventilation to this area is known as *wasted ventilation,* because it does not participate in gas exchange. This effect leads to alveolar dead space ventilation and an increase in the work of breathing. To limit the amount of dead-space ventilation, localized bronchoconstriction occurs.[44]

Bronchoconstriction. Bronchoconstriction develops as a result of alveolar hypocarbia, hypoxia, and the release of mediators. Alveolar hypocarbia occurs as a consequence of decreased carbon dioxide in the affected area and leads to constriction of the local airways, increased airway resistance, and redistribution of ventilation to perfused areas of the lungs. A variety of mediators are released from the site of the injury, either from the clot or the surrounding lung tissue, which further causes constriction of the airways.[44] Bronchoconstriction promotes the development of atelectasis.[43]

Compensatory shunting. Compensatory shunting occurs as a result of the unaffected areas of the lungs having to accommodate the entire cardiac output. This creates a situation in which perfusion exceeding ventilation and blood is returned to the left side of the heart without participating in gas exchange. This leads to the development of hypoxemia.[44]

Hemodynamic consequences. The major hemodynamic consequence of a PE is the development of pulmonary hypertension, which is part of the effect of a mechanical obstruction when more than 50% of the vascular bed is occluded. In addition, the mediators released at the injury site and the development of hypoxia cause pulmonary vasoconstriction, which further exacerbates pulmonary hypertension. As the pulmonary vascular resistance increases, so does the workload of the right ventricle, as reflected by a rise in pulmonary artery (PA) pressures. Consequently, right ventricular failure occurs, which can lead to decreases in left ventricular preload, CO and blood pressure and shock.[44] (∞Heart Failure, p. 502.)

Assessment and Diagnosis

The patient with a PE may exhibit a number of clinical manifestations. Common symptoms include dyspnea, chest pain, cough, palpitations, apprehension, and diaphoresis. The chest pain is pleuritic in nature, with an abrupt onset and aggravated by deep breathing.[45,46] Syncope may be present if right ventricular failure occurs.[43]

Common signs include an increase in tachypnea, tachycardia, crackles, decreased breath sounds over the affected side, and a low-grade fever.[45] If right ventricular failure occurs, distended neck veins and a third heart sound (S_3) on auscultation may be present. Additional signs that indicate right ventricular decompensation are fixed splitting of the second heart sound (P_2), which results from delayed closure of the pulmonic valve, and a diastolic murmur, which is caused by pulmonic insufficiency.[46]

Initial laboratory studies that may be done are an ABG analysis, electrocardiogram (ECG), and chest radiography. ABGs may show a low Pao_2 level, indicating hypoxemia; a low $Paco_2$ level, indicating hypocarbia; and a high pH level, indicating respiratory alkalosis. The hypocarbia with resulting respiratory alkalosis is caused by tachypnea.[45] Common ECG findings are transient ST-segment depression and sinus tachycardia. The classic findings of P-pulmonale, S wave in lead I, and Q wave with inverted T wave in lead III, are seen in fewer than 15% of the patients with a PE.[45] Chest x-ray findings vary from normal to abnormal, with enlargement of the descending pulmonary artery, elevation of the diaphragm, and the presence of pleural effusion as the most common signs.[45]

Differentiating a PE from other illnesses can be difficult, because many of its clinical manifestations are found in a variety of other disorders.[45] Thus a variety of other tests may be necessary, including a V/Q scan and pulmonary angiogram and deep vein thrombosis (DVT) studies. A definitive diagnosis of a PE requires confirmation by a high probability V/Q scan, positive pulmonary angiogram, or strong clinical suspicion coupled with abnormal findings on lower extremity DVT studies.[44]

Medical Management

Prevention of PE is the first line of treatment for the disorder. Patients at risk for a thromboembolism are to receive prophylactic anticoagulation with adjusted-dose heparin, low molecular–weight heparin, or oral anticoagulants. In one study, the prophylactic use of low-dose subcutaneous heparin in surgical patients demonstrated a 60% to 70% decrease in the incidence of deep vein thrombosis. Risk patients are anticoagulated to maintain the activated partial thromboplastin time (aPTT) in the high-normal range or an international normalization ratio (INR) of 2.0 to 2.5.[47]

Medical management for the patient with a PE includes both prophylactic and definitive measures and the correction of the hypoxemia.

Prophylactic measures. Prophylactic interventions are focused on preventing the recurrence of a PE and include the administration of heparin and warfarin (Coumadin) and interruption of the inferior vena cava.

Heparin is administered to prevent further clots from forming and has no effect on the existing clot. Heparin may be administered by continuous drip, intermittent intravenous injection, or subcutaneous injection. The heparin is adjusted to maintain the aPTT at 1.5 to 2 times the control. Warfarin is started at the same time as the heparin, and when the INR reaches 2.0 to 3.0 the heparin is discontinued. The patient continues to receive warfarin for at least 3 months.[47]

Interruption of the inferior vena cava is reserved for patients in whom anticoagulation is contraindicated. The procedure involves placement of a percutaneous venous filter into the vena cava, usually below the renal arteries. The filter prevents further thrombotic emboli from migrating into the lungs.[44]

Definitive measures. Definitive actions are directed at treating the current PE and include the administration of thrombolytic agents and surgery to remove the clot. Measures to correct the hypoxemia include supplemental oxygen administration and intubation and mechanical ventilation.

The administration of thrombolytic agents in the treatment of PE has had limited success. Currently, thrombolytic therapy is reserved for the patient with a massive PE and concomitant hemodynamic instability,[43] though that criteria is broadening.[48] Either recombinant tissue-type plasminogen activator (rt-PA), streptokinase, or urokinase may be used. The therapeutic window for using thrombolytic therapy is 14 days of the onset of a PE.[48]

Surgical embolectomy is considered a last resort that involves the extraction of the embolus from the pulmonary arterial system. It is reserved for the patient with a massive PE that is refractory to all other measures. It is an extremely risky surgery with a high operative mortality.[44]

To reverse the hemodynamic effects of pulmonary hypertension, additional measures may be taken. These include the administration of inotropic agents and fluid. Fluids are administered to increase right ventricular preload, which would stretch the right ventricle and increase contractility, thus overcoming the elevated pulmonary arterial pressures. Inotropic agents also can be used to increase contractility to facilitate an increase in CO.[44]

Nursing Management

Prevention of PE is a major nursing focus, because the majority of critically ill patients are at risk for this disorder. Nursing actions are aimed at preventing the development of DVT, which is a major complication of immobility and a leading cause of PE. These measures include the use of antiembolic stockings and/or pneumatic compression stockings, elevation of the legs, active/passive range of motion, adequate hydration, and progressive ambulation. Patients at risk are routinely assessed for signs of a DVT—specifically, deep calf pain (Homan's sign), calf tenderness, or redness.[46]

Nursing management of the patient with a PE incorporates a variety of nursing diagnoses (Box 22-10). Nursing interventions focus on optimizing oxygenation and ventilation, monitoring for bleeding, providing comfort and emotional support, and maintaining surveillance for complications.

Optimizing oxygenation and ventilation. Nursing interventions to optimize oxygenation and ventilation include positioning, preventing desaturation, and promoting secretion clearance. For further discussion on these interventions, see Nursing Management of Acute Respiratory Failure earlier in this chapter.

Monitoring for bleeding. The patient receiving anticoagulant or thrombolytic therapy is observed for signs of bleeding. The patient's gums, skin, urine, stool, and emesis are screened for signs of overt or covert bleeding. In addition, following the patient's INR or aPTT is critical to managing the anticoagulation therapy.[46]

BOX 22-10 NURSING DIAGNOSIS AND MANAGEMENT

PULMONARY EMBOLUS

- Impaired Gas Exchange related to ventilation/perfusion mismatching or intrapulmonary shunting, p. 725
- Acute Pain related to transmission and perception of cutaneous, visceral, muscular, or ischemic impulses, p. 197
- Risk for Infection, p. 1119
- Anxiety related to threat to biologic, psychologic, and/or social integrity, p. 99
- Powerlessness related to lack of control over current situation or disease progression, p. 89
- Ineffective Family Coping related to critically ill family member, p. 97
- Knowledge Deficit: Discharge Regimen related to lack of previous exposure to information, p. 61 (see Patient Education Box 22-11.)

BOX 22-11 PATIENT EDUCATION

PULMONARY EMBOLUS

- Pathophysiology of disease
- Specific etiology
- Precipitating factor modification
- Measures to prevent deep vein thrombosis (e.g., avoid tight fitting clothes, crossing legs, and prolonged sitting or standing; elevate legs when sitting; exercise)
- Signs and symptoms of deep vein thrombosis (e.g., redness, swelling, sharp or deep leg pain)
- Importance of taking medications
- Signs and symptoms of anticoagulant complications (e.g., excessive bruising, discoloration of the skin, change in color of urine or stools)
- Measures to prevent bleeding (e.g., use soft-bristled toothbrush, caution when shaving)

Patient Education

Early in the patient's hospital stay, the patient and family are taught about pulmonary embolus, its etiologies, and its treatment. As the patient moves toward discharge, teaching focuses on the interventions necessary for preventing the reoccurrence of deep vein thrombosis and subsequent emboli, signs and symptoms of deep vein thrombosis and anticoagulant complications, and measures to prevent bleeding (Box 22-11). If the patient smokes, he or she is encouraged to stop smoking and referred to a smoking cessation program.

STATUS ASTHMATICUS

Description and Etiology

Asthma is a chronic obstructive pulmonary disease that is characterized by reversible airflow obstruction, airway inflammation, and hyperresponsiveness to a variety of stimuli.[49] Status asthmaticus is a severe asthma attack that fails to respond to conventional therapy with bronchodilators and may result in acute respiratory failure.[50] The precipitating cause of the attack is usually an upper respiratory infection, allergen exposure, or a decrease in antiinflammatory medications.[50] Other factors that have been implicated include overreliance on bronchodilators, environmental pollutants, lack of access to health care, failure to identify worsening airflow obstruction, and noncompliance with the health care regimen.[51]

Status asthmaticus falls under DRG 88 (Chronic obstructive pulmonary disease), with an average length of the stay of 6.1 days if the patient does not require intubation. If the patient does require intubation, DRG

475 (Respiratory system diagnosis with ventilator support) is then used, with an expected length of stay of 12.3 days.[4]

Pathophysiology

An asthma attack is initiated when exposure to an irritant or trigger occurs, resulting in the initiation of the inflammatory-immune response in the airways. Bronchospasm occurs along with increased vascular permeability and increased mucus production. Mucosal edema and thick tenacious mucus further increase airway responsiveness. The combination of bronchospasm, airway inflammation, and hyperresponsiveness results in narrowing of the airways and airflow obstruction.[49] These changes have significant effects on the pulmonary and cardiovascular systems.

Pulmonary effects. As the diameter of the airways decreases, airway resistance increases, resulting in increased residual volume, hyperinflation of the lungs, increased work of breathing, and abnormal distribution of ventilation. V/Q mismatching occurs, resulting in hypoxemia. Alveolar dead space also increases as hypoxic vasoconstriction occurs, resulting in hypercapnia.[50]

Cardiovascular effects. Inspiratory muscle force also increases in an attempt to ventilate the hyperinflated lungs. This results in a significant increase in negative intrapleural pressure, leading to an increase in venous return and pooling of blood in the right ventricle. The stretched right ventricle causes the intraventricular septum to shift, impinging on the left ventricle. In addition the left ventricle has to work harder to pump blood from the markedly negative pressure in the thorax to the elevated pressure in systemic circulation. This leads to a decrease in cardiac output and a fall in systolic blood pressure on inspiration (pulsus paradoxus).[50]

Assessment and Diagnosis

Initially, the patient may have a cough, wheezing, and dyspnea. As the attack continues tachypnea, tachycardia, diaphoresis, increased accessory muscle use, and pulsus paradoxus greater than or equal to 25 mm Hg develop.[50] Decreased level of consciousness, inability to speak, significantly diminished or absent breath sounds, central cyanosis,[51] and inability to lie supine[52] herald the onset of acute respiratory failure.

Initial ABG values indicate hypocapnia and respiratory alkalosis because of hyperventilation. As the attack continues and the patient starts to fatigue, hypoxemia and hypercapnia develop. Lactic acidosis may also occur because of lactate overproduction of the respiratory muscles. The end result is the development of respiratory and metabolic acidosis.[50,51]

Deterioration of pulmonary function tests despite aggressive bronchodilator therapy is diagnostic of status asthmaticus and indicates the potential need for intubation. FEV_1 (maximum volume of gas that the patient can exhale in 1 second) and/or PEFR (maximum flow rate that the patient can generate) less than 30% to 50% of predicted or patient's personal best indicates severe airflow obstruction, and the need for intubation with mechanical ventilation may be imminent.[52]

Medical Management

Medical management of the patient with status asthmaticus is directed toward supporting oxygenation and ventilation. Bronchodilators, corticosteroids, oxygen therapy, intubation, and mechanical ventilation are the mainstays of therapy.

Bronchodilators. Inhaled $beta_2$ agonists and anticholinergics are the bronchodilators of choice for status asthmaticus. $Beta_2$ agonists promote bronchodilation and can be administered by a nebulizer or a metered dose inhaler (MDI).[50-52] Usually, larger and more frequent doses are given,[52] and the drug is titrated to the patient's response.[50] Anticholinergics that inhibit bronchoconstriction are not very effective by themselves, but in conjunction with $beta_2$ agonists, they have a synergistic effect and produce a greater improvement in airflow. The routine use of xanthines is not recommended in the treatment of status asthmaticus, because they have been shown to have no therapeutic benefit.[50,51] (∞Bronchodilators and Adjuncts, p. 713.)

Corticosteroids. Systemic corticosteroids are also used in the treatment of status asthmaticus. Their antiinflammatory effects limit mucosal edema, decrease mucus production, and potentiate $beta_2$ agonists. Inhaled corticosteroids must also be continued or started, if the patient was not using them before the attack.[52] It usually takes 6 to 12 hours for the effects of the corticosteroids to become evident.[50,51]

Oxygen therapy. Supplemental oxygen is usually the initial treatment for hypoxemia. Low-flow oxygen therapy is administered to keep the patient's SaO_2 level greater than 92%.[50,52]

Intubation and mechanical ventilation. Indications for mechanical ventilation include cardiac or respiratory arrest,[51] disorientation,[52] failure to respond to bronchodilator therapy, and exhaustion.[50] A large endotracheal tube (greater than or equal to 8 mm) is used to decrease airway resistance and to facilitate suctioning of secretions.[51,52] Ventilating the patient with status asthmaticus can be very difficult. High inflation pressures must be avoided, because they can result in barotrauma. PEEP must also not be used, because the patient is prone to developing air trapping. Patient-ventilator asynchrony can also be a major problem. Sedation and neuromuscular paralysis may be necessary to allow for adequate ventilation of the patient.[50-52]

Investigation therapies. A number of therapies are currently under investigation for the treatment of status asthmaticus, including the use of general anesthesia, magnesium, and heliox (helium-oxygen mixture). General anesthetics are being studied because of their ability to reduce airflow obstruction. Agents that have been used include halothane, ketamine, and isoflurane.[51] A number of studies have focused on the bronchodilator abilities of magnesium. Though it has been demonstrated that magnesium is inferior to $beta_2$ agonists as a bronchodilator, magnesium may benefit patients whose conditions are refractory to conventional treatment. A bolus of 2 g of intravenous magnesium given over 20 minutes and followed by a continuous infusion of 2 g per hour has been reported to produce desirable effects.[50] Heliox is a gas that is fairly light and flows more easily through constricted areas. Studies have shown that it reduces air trapping and carbon dioxide and helps relieve respiratory acidosis.[52]

Nursing Management

Nursing management of the patient with status asthmaticus incorporates a variety of nursing diagnoses (Box 22-12). Nursing interventions focus on optimizing oxygenation and ventilation, providing comfort and emotional support, and maintaining surveillance for complications.

Optimizing oxygenation and ventilation. Nursing interventions to optimize oxygenation and ventilation include positioning, preventing desaturation, and promoting secretion clearance. For further discussion on these interventions, see Nursing Management of Acute Respiratory Failure earlier in this chapter.

Patient Education

Early in the patient's hospital stay, the patient and family are taught about asthma, its triggers, and its treatment. As the patient moves toward discharge, teaching focuses on the interventions necessary for preventing the reoccurrence of status asthmaticus, early warning signs of worsening airflow obstruction, correct use of an inhaler and a peak flow meter, measures to prevent pulmonary infections, and signs and symptoms of a pulmonary infection (Box 22-13). If the patient smokes, he or she is encouraged to stop smoking and referred to a smoking cessation program. In addition, the importance of participating in a pulmonary rehabilitation program must be stressed.

BOX 22-12 NURSING DIAGNOSIS AND MANAGEMENT

STATUS ASTHMATICUS

- Impaired Gas Exchange related to alveolar hypoventilation, p. 726
- Impaired Gas Exchange related to ventilation/perfusion mismatching or intrapulmonary shunting, p. 725
- Ineffective Breathing Pattern related to musculoskeletal fatigue or neuromuscular impairment, p. 724
- Ineffective Airway Clearance related to excessive secretions or abnormal viscosity of mucus, p. 722
- Risk for Infection, p. 1119
- Anxiety related to threat to biologic, psychologic, and/or social integrity, p. 99
- Body Image Disturbance related to actual change in body structures, function, or appearance, p. 87
- Ineffective Family Coping related to critically ill family member, p. 97
- Knowledge Deficit: Discharge Regimen related to lack of previous exposure to information, p. 61 (see Patient Education Box 22-13)

AIR LEAK DISORDERS

Description

Air leak disorders consist of conditions that result in extraalveolar air accumulation. These disorders are commonly classified into two categories: pneumothorax and barotrauma. A pneumothorax occurs as the result of the accumulation of air or another gas in the pleural space, whereas barotrauma occurs as the result of the accumulation of air in the interstitial space.[53] The individual disorders comprising these two categories are described in Table 22-4.

Air leak disorders fall under two DRGs, depending on whether the patient develops complications or comorbid conditions (CC): DRG 94 (Pneumothorax with CC) and DRG 95 (Pneumothorax without CC), which have average lengths of stay of 7.1 days and 4.1 days, respectively.[4]

Etiology

The three main causes of air leak disorders are disruption of the parietal or visceral pleura, allowing air to enter the pleural space; formation of gas within the pleural space from an infectious process; and rupture

BOX 22-13 PATIENT EDUCATION

STATUS ASTHMATICUS

- Pathophysiology of disease
- Specific etiology
- Early warning signs of worsening airflow obstruction (20% drop in PERF below predicted or personal best, increase in cough, shortness of breath, chest tightness, wheezing)
- Treatment of attacks
- Importance of taking prescribed medications and avoidance of over-the-counter asthma medications
- Correct use of an inhaler (with and without a spacer device)
- Correct use of a peak flow meter
- Removal or avoidance of environmental triggers (e.g., pollen; dust; mold spores; cat and dog dander; cold, dry air; strong odors; household aerosols; tobacco smoke; air pollution)
- Measures to prevent pulmonary infections (e.g., proper nutrition and handwashing, immunization against *Streptococcus pneumoniae* and influenza viruses)
- Signs and symptoms of pulmonary infection (e.g., sputum color change, shortness of breath, fever)
- Importance of participating in pulmonary rehabilitation program

of alveoli, allowing air to enter the interstitial space.[53] Disruption of the parietal pleura occurs as the result of penetrating trauma to the chest wall, allowing atmospheric air to enter the pleural space (traumatic open pneumothorax).[54] Disruption of the visceral pleura occurs as the result of air entering the pleural space from the lung. This may be a result of blunt chest-wall trauma (traumatic closed pneumothorax), diagnostic or therapeutic procedures (traumatic iatrogenic pneumothorax),[53] diseases of the pulmonary system (secondary spontaneous pneumothorax), or ruptured subpleural blebs (primary spontaneous pneumothorax).[52] Alveolar rupture occurs as the result of a change in the pressure gradient between the alveoli and the surrounding interstitial space. An increase in alveolar pressure or a decrease in interstitial pressure can lead to overdistention of the alveoli, rupture, and air leakage into the interstitial space. One of the most common causes of barotrauma is mechanical ventilation.[52]

Pathophysiology

The pathologic consequences of pneumothorax and barotrauma are different.

TABLE 22-4 Air Leak Disorders

Type	Description
PNEUMOTHORAX	
Spontaneous	
Primary	Disruption of the visceral pleura that allows air from the lung to enter the pleural space; occurs spontaneously in patients without underlying lung disease
Secondary	Disruption of the visceral pleura that allows air from the lung to enter the pleural space; occurs spontaneously in patients with underlying lung disease
Traumatic	
Open	Laceration in the parietal pleura that allows atmospheric air to enter the pleural space; occurs as a result of penetrating chest trauma
Closed	Laceration in the visceral pleura that allows air from the lung to enter the pleural space; occurs as a result of blunt chest trauma
Iatrogenic	Laceration in the visceral pleura that allows air from the lung to enter the pleural space; occurs as a result of therapeutic or diagnostic procedures, such as central line insertion, thoracentesis, and needle aspirations
Tension	Occurs when air is allowed to enter the pleural space but not exit it; as pressure increases inside the pleural space, the lung collapses and the mediastinum shifts to the unaffected side; may be a result of a spontaneous or traumatic pneumothorax
BAROTRAUMA	
Pulmonary interstitial emphysema	Air in the pulmonary interstitial space
Subcutaneous emphysema	Air in the subcutaneous tissues
Pneumomediastinum	Air in the mediastinal space
Pneumopericardium	Air in the pericardial space
Pneumoperitoneum	Air in the peritoneal space
Pneumoretroperitoneum	Air in the retroperitoneal space

Pneumothorax. Regardless of the etiology, once air or gas enters the pleural space, the affected lung becomes compressed. As the lung collapses, the alveoli become underventilated and unventilated, causing V/Q mismatching and intrapulmonary shunting. If the pneumothorax is large, hypoxemia ensues and acute respiratory failure quickly develops. In addition, increased pressure within the chest can lead to shifting of the mediastinum, compression of the great vessels, and decreased cardiac output.[54]

Barotrauma. Once air enters the interstitial space, it travels through the pulmonary interstitium (pulmonary interstitial emphysema) out through the hilum and into the mediastinum (pneumomediastinum), pleural space (pneumothorax), subcutaneous tissues (subcutaneous emphysema), pericardium (pneumopericardium), peritoneum (pneumoperitoneum), and retroperitoneum (pneumoretroperitoneum). Except for pneumothorax, the resultant disorders are usually fairly benign. Pneumomediastinum has been associated with decreased venous return and upper airway obstruction, and pneumopericardium has been associated with cardiac tamponade.[53,55]

Assessment and Diagnosis

The clinical manifestations of a pneumothorax depend on the degree of lung collapse. When a pneumothorax is large, decreased respiratory excursion on the affected side may be noticed, along with bulging intercostal muscles. The trachea may deviate away from the affected side. Percussion reveals hyperresonance with decreased or absent breath sounds over the affected area. ABG values will demonstrate hypoxemia and hypercapnia. A chest x-ray will confirm the pneumothorax, with increased translucency evident on the affected side (Figure 22-3).[54]

The clinical manifestations of barotrauma are much more subtle. Subcutaneous emphysema is manifested by crepitus, usually around the face, neck, and upper chest. Stabbing substernal pain with position changes and increased ventilation is the most commonly reported symptom of a pneumomediastinum. In addition, a clicking or crunching sound synchronous with the heart sounds may be heard over the apex of the heart (Hamman's sign). A friction rub may be heard with a pneumopericardium. Barotrauma is also confirmed with an x-ray. Extraalveolar air, as evidenced by increased translucency, will be present in the affected area (e.g., chest, abdomen).[53]

Medical Management

Medical management of the patient with air leak disorders varies depending on the severity of the specific disorder. Usually only a pneumothorax would require treatment, and that would depend on the size of the pneumothorax. A pneumothorax of less than 20% usually requires only supplemental oxygen administration, unless complications occur or underlying lung disease or injury is present.[54]

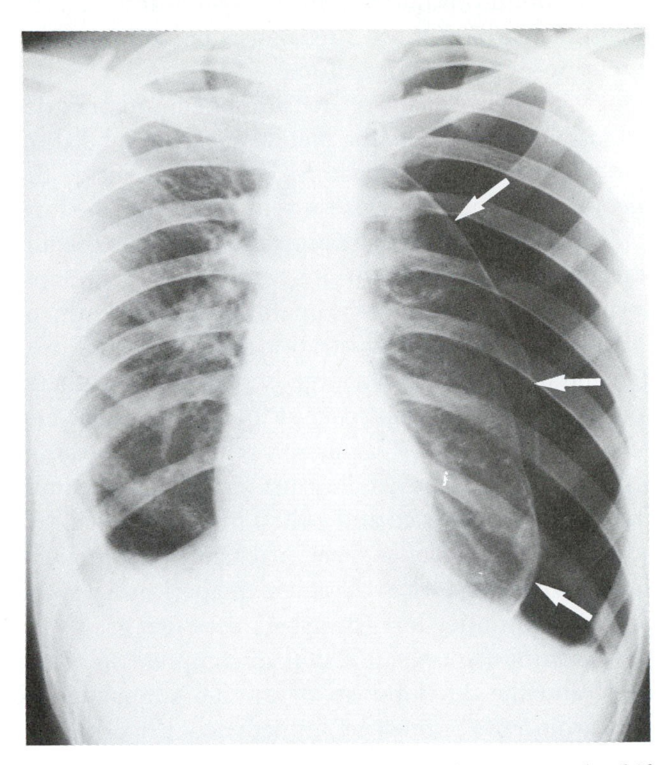

FIGURE 22-3. Left-sided tension pneumothorax. Note the shift of the heart and mediastinum to the right. (From Des Jardins T, Burton GC: *Clinical manifestations and assessment of respiratory disease,* ed 3, St Louis, 1995, Mosby.)

A pneumothorax greater than 20% requires intervention to evacuate the air from the pleural space and facilitate reexpansion of the collapsed lung. Interventions include aspiration of the air with a needle, placement of a percutaneous catheter attached to a Heimlich valve, insertion of a thoracic vent, and insertion of a chest tube with underwater-seal suction drainage. The Heimlich valve, a small, one-way valve device that is easily secured to a catheter placed in the chest, allows air to exit from but not enter the pleural space. A thoracic vent is similar to a Heimlich valve in that it is a one-way valve, but it comes attached to the catheter.[52] Chest tubes are usually inserted in the 4th or 5th intercostal space on the midaxillary line. Once the tubes are inserted and connected to an underwater chest drainage system with at least 20 cm of suction, a chest x-ray examination is performed to confirm reexpansion of the lung.[55]

Two conditions that require emergency intervention for immediate relief are a tension pneumothorax and a tension pneumopericardium.

Tension pneumothorax. A tension pneumothorax develops when air enters the pleural space on inhalation and cannot exit on exhalation. As pressure inside the pleural space increases, it results in collapse of the lung and shifting of the mediastinum and trachea to the unaffected side. The resultant effect is decreased venous return and compression of the unaffected lung. Treatment is comprised of the administration of supplemental oxygen and the insertion of a large-bore needle or catheter into the 2nd intercostal space at the midclavicular line of the affected side. This action relieves the pressure within the chest. The needle must remain in place until the patient is stabilized and a chest tube is inserted.[53,55]

Tension pneumopericardium. A tension pneumopericardium develops when air enters the pericardial space and has no outlet for exiting. As pressure inside the pericardium increases, it results in compression of the heart and the development of cardiac tamponade. A pericardiocentesis must be immediately performed to relieve the pressure within the pericardial sac.[53]

Nursing Management

Nursing management of the patient with air leak disorders incorporates a variety of nursing diagnoses (Box 22-14). Nursing interventions focus on optimizing oxygenation and ventilation, maintaining the chest tube system, providing comfort and emotional support, and maintaining surveillance for complications.

Optimizing oxygenation and ventilation. Nursing interventions to optimize oxygenation and ventilation include positioning, preventing desaturation, and promoting secretion clearance. For further discussion on these interventions, see Nursing Management of Acute Respiratory Failure earlier in this chapter.

Maintaining the chest tube system. Maintaining the chest tube system (Figure 22-4) involves careful attention to the suction applied and to maintenance of unobstructed drainage tubes. Kinks and large loops of tubing must be prevented, because they impede drainage and air evacuation, which in turn may prevent timely lung reexpansion or may result in a tension pneumothorax. Retained drainage also becomes an excellent medium for bacterial growth.[56]

The water-seal chamber must routinely be observed for unexpected bubbling caused by an air leak in the system. When unexpected bubbling is present, the source must be identified. To determine whether the source is within the system or within the patient, systematic brief clamping of the drainage tube is performed. The nurse places a padded clamp on the drainage tubing as close to the occlusive dressing as possible. If the bubbling stops, the air leak is located between the patient and the clamp. The leak can be within the patient or at the insertion site. Therefore the clamp is removed and the chest tube site exposed. The tube is inspected at the site where it enters the chest to ensure that all the eyelets are within the patient. If an eyelet port is outside the chest, it can be a source of an air leak and must be occluded, which may require the attention of the physician. When the insertion site has been eliminated as a leakage source, the chest dressing is reapplied, completely and securely covering the site.[56] If the air bubbling does not stop when a clamp is placed on the chest tube, the leak is located between the clamp and the drainage collector. By releasing the clamp and moving it down the tubing a few inches at a time to a point where the bubbling stops, the leak will be found. Once located, the area of the leak can be taped to reestablish a seal or the system can be replaced.[56]

Sterile petroleum gauze and a bottle of sterile water must be available at all times. If the chest tube system is inadvertently interrupted, the tube must be placed a few centimeters into the bottle of water while the drainage system is reestablished. Sterile petroleum gauze is applied to the chest wall if the chest tube is accidentally removed. Implementing both of these techniques immediately minimizes or prevents the formation of a pneumothorax and other complications.

Throughout the duration of chest tube placement, the patient is assessed periodically for reexpansion of the lung and for complications of chest tube drainage. The nurse assesses the thorax and lungs, paying particular attention to any tracheal deviation; asymmetry of chest movement; presence of subcutaneous emphysema; characteristics of breathing; quality of lung sounds; and presence of tympany or percussion sounds, which are indicative of pneumothorax.

BOX 22-14 NURSING DIAGNOSIS AND MANAGEMENT

AIR LEAK DISORDERS

- Impaired Gas Exchange related to ventilation/perfusion mismatching or intrapulmonary shunting, p. 725
- Ineffective Breathing Pattern related to decreased lung expansion, p. 723
- Acute Pain related to transmission and perception of cutaneous, visceral, muscular, or ischemic impulses, p. 197
- Anxiety related to threat to biologic, psychologic, and/or social integrity, p. 99
- Ineffective Family Coping related to critically ill family member, p. 97

Chest Tube Review

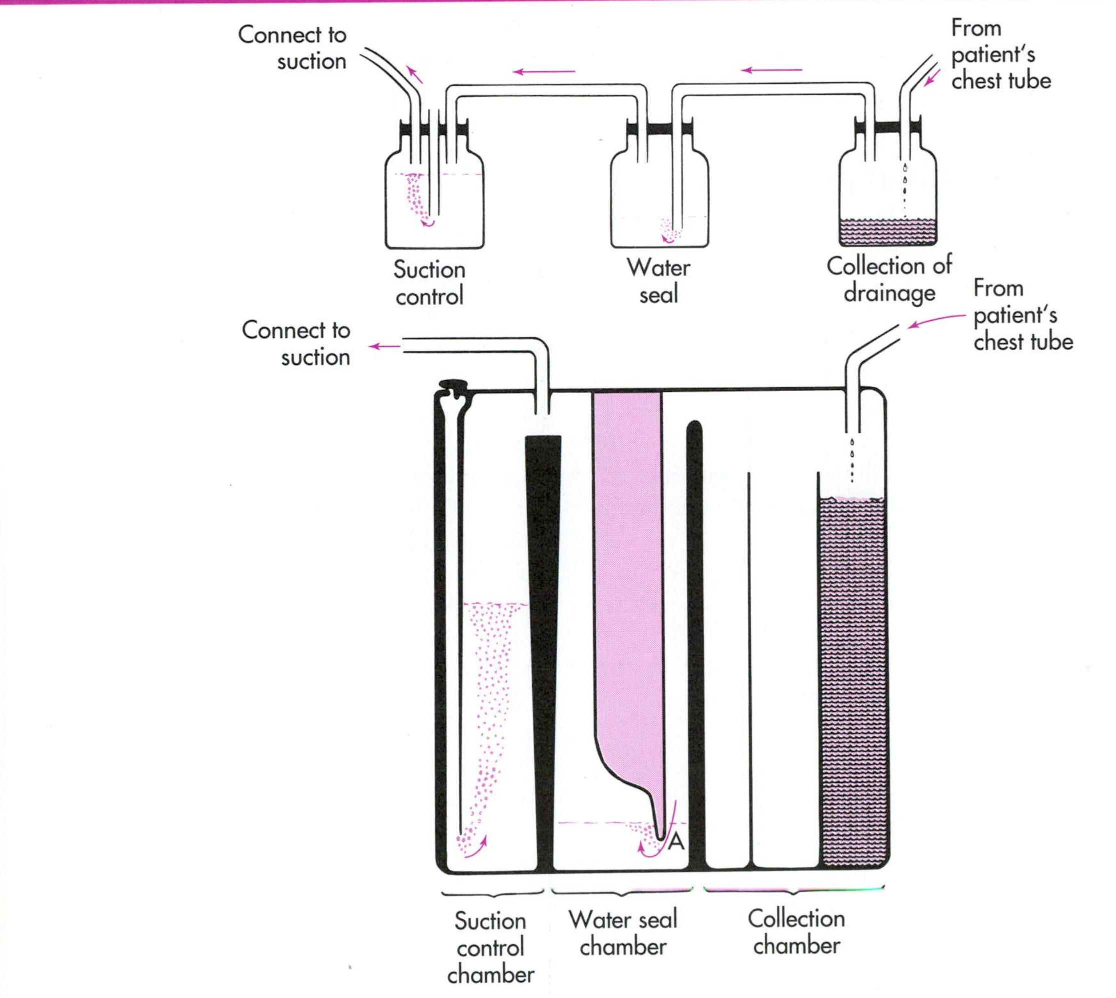

FIGURE 22-4. Chest tube review. (From Daitch JS: Post anesthesia care after thoracic surgery. In Frost EAM, editor: *Post anesthesia care unit: current practices,* ed 2, St Louis, 1990, Mosby.)

Chest tubes are inserted into the pleural space to remove fluid or air and thus reinstate the negative intrapleural pressure and reexpand a collapsed lung. Once a chest tube is inserted, it is connected to a water-seal drainage system. Water-seal drainage systems have evolved from separate glass bottles of one, two, or three containers into a self-contained disposable plastic unit. The drainage system is aseptically prepared for use, with sterile water placed in the water seal and suction control chambers. Usually the water-seal chamber is filled to the 2 cm level and the suction-control chamber is filled to the desired level of suction. The water-seal chamber acts as a one-way valve, allowing air to escape from the chest but not enter it. Once the chest tubes are placed, the suction control chamber is attached to an external suction regulator, which is adjusted until gentle bubbling occurs in the chamber. Any fluid draining from the chest will be evident in the collection chamber. Connection points of the drainage tubing are sealed with tape, and an occlusive dressing is applied over the chest tube insertion site. Nursing measures are aimed at maintaining the patency and sterility of the system.

THORACIC SURGERY

Types of Surgery

Thoracic surgery refers to a number of surgical procedures that involve opening the thoracic cavity (thoracotomy) and/or the organs of respiration. Indications for thoracic surgery range from tumors and abscesses to repair of the esophagus and thoracic vessels.[57] Table 22-5 describes thoracic surgical procedures and their indications.[58-60] This discussion focuses only on the surgical procedures that involve the removal of lung tissue.

TABLE 22-5 Thoracic Surgeries

Procedure	Definition	Indications
Segmental resection (also called segmentectomy)	Resection of bronchovascular segment of lung lobe	Small peripheral lesions Patients with borderline lung function who would not tolerate a more extensive procedure
Wedge resection	Removal of small section of lung tissue	Small peripheral lesions (without lymph node involvement) Peripheral granulomas Pulmonary blebs
Lobectomy	Resection of one or more lobes of lung	Lesions confined to a single lobe Pulmonary tuberculosis Bronchiectasis Lung abscesses or cysts Trauma
Pneumonectomy	Removal of entire lung with or without resection of the mediastinal lymph nodes	Malignant lesions Unilateral tuberculosis Extensive unilateral bronchiectasis Multiple lung abscesses Massive hemoptysis Bronchopleural fistula
Bronchoplastic reconstruction (also called sleeve resection)	Resection of lung tissue and bronchus with end-to-end reanastomosis of bronchus	Small lesions involving the carina or major bronchus without evidence of metastasis May be combined with lobectomy
Decortication	Removal of fibrous membrane from pleural surface of lung	Fibrothorax resulting from hemothorax or empyema
Bullectomy	Resection of large bullae	Severe emphysema with large bullae compressing surrounding tissue
Lung reduction volume surgery (also called reduction pneumoplasty or pneumectomy)	Resection of the most damaged portions of lung tissue, allowing more normal chest-wall configuration	Emphysema
Tracheal resection	Resection of portion of trachea with end-to-end reanastomosis of trachea	Tracheal stenosis Tumors Trauma
Thoracoscopy	Endoscopic procedure performed through small incisions in the chest	Evaluation of pulmonary, pleural, mediastinal, or pericardial conditions Biopsy of lung, pleural, or mediastinal lesions Recurrent spontaneous pneumothorax Evacuation of emphysema, hemothorax, pleural effusion, or pericardial effusion Thymectomy Blebectomy/bullectomy Pleurodesis Sympathectomy Closure of bronchopleural fistula Lysis of adhesions

Thoracic surgery falls under three DRGs, depending on the type of surgery and whether the patient develops complications or comorbid conditions (CC). DRG 75 (Major chest procedures), DRG 76 (Other respiratory system OR procedures with CC), and DRG 77 (Other respiratory system OR procedures without CC) have average lengths of stay of 11.2 days, 12.5 days, and 5.5 days, respectively.[4]

Preoperative Care

Before surgery, a complete evaluation of the patient is needed to determine the appropriateness of surgery as a treatment and to determine whether removal of lung tissue can be done without jeopardizing respiratory function. This is especially important when a lobectomy or pneumonectomy is being considered. When resection is being undertaken for tumor treatment, preoperative care includes evaluation of the type and extent of tumor and the physical condition of the patient.[58]

The evaluation of the patient's physical status focuses on the adequacy of cardiopulmonary function. The preoperative evaluation includes pulmonary function tests to determine the patient's ability to lose lung tissue. Cardiac function also is evaluated. Uncontrolled dysrhythmias, acute myocardial infarction, severe congestive heart failure, and unstable angina are all contraindications to surgery.[58]

Surgical Considerations

The type and location of surgery will dictate the type of surgical approach used. The most common approach is the posterolateral thoracotomy, which allows for exposure of both the lung and mediastinum. Other approaches that are used include anterolateral thoracotomy, axillary incision, and median sternotomy.[59]

Special care is taken to avoid drainage of blood or secretions into the unaffected lung during surgery, because such an occurrence could cause hypoxemia and cardiac dysfunction. A double-lumen endotracheal tube is used during the surgery to protect the unaffected lung from secretions and necrotic tumor fragments. In addition, the deflated lung is suctioned and ventilated every 20 to 30 minutes during the procedure.[60]

After a pneumonectomy the mediastinal position requires evaluation. This is done on closure of the operative site and involves manometric measurement and a chest x-ray examination. With the patient lying in the supine position, pressure in the empty chest cavity should be −4 to −6 cm of H_2O pressure. When the pressure is abnormal, air or fluid can be added or withdrawn. If the abnormality is not corrected, a mediastinal shift can occur, resulting in hemodynamic compromise and cardiac dysfunction. A chest x-ray examination will show the location of the mediastinum.[59]

Complications and Medical Management

A number of complications are associated with a lung resection. These include acute respiratory failure, bronchopleural fistula, hemorrhage, cardiovascular disturbances, and mediastinal shift.

Acute respiratory failure. In the postoperative period, acute respiratory failure may result from atelectasis or pneumonia. Atelectasis can occur as a result of anesthesia, the surgical procedure, immobilization, and pain. Treatment is aimed at correcting the underlying problems and supporting gas exchange. Supplemental oxygen and mechanical ventilation with PEEP may be necessary.[60]

Bronchopleural fistula. Development of a postoperative bronchopleural fistula is a major cause of mortality after a lung resection. A bronchopleural fistula develops when the suture line fails to secure occlusion of the bronchial stump and an opening develops. This can result from an imperfect stump closure; perforation of the stump (e.g., with a suction catheter); high pressure within the airways (e.g., caused by mechanical ventilation)[61]; or infection.[62] During surgery, careful attention is given to isolating and closing the bronchus in an attempt to secure a lasting seal with subsequent stump healing.[59] In addition, early extubation is encouraged to eliminate the possibility of perforation of the stump and high airway pressures.[61] Clinical manifestations of a bronchopleural fistula include shortness of breath and coughing up serosanguineous sputum. Immediate surgery is usually necessary to close the stump to prevent flooding of the remaining lung with fluid from the residual space resulting in aspiration.[62] If this occurs, the patient is placed with the operative side down (remaining lung up), and a chest tube is inserted to drain the residual space.

Hemorrhage. Hemorrhage is an early, life-threatening complication that can occur after a lung resection. It can result from bronchial or intercostal artery bleeding or disruption of a suture or clip around a pulmonary vessel.[61] Excessive chest tube drainage can signal excessive bleeding. During the immediate postoperative period, chest tube drainage is measured every 15 minutes, and this frequency is decreased as the patient's condition stabilizes. If chest tube loss is greater than 100 ml/hour, fresh blood is noted, or a sudden increase in drainage occurs, hemorrhage must be suspected.

Cardiovascular disturbances. Cardiovascular complications after thoracic surgery include dysrhythmias and pulmonary edema. Resections of a large lung area or a pneumonectomy may be followed by a rise in central venous pressure. With the loss of one lung, the right ventricle must empty its stroke volume into a vascular bed that has been reduced by 50%. This means a higher pressure system is created, which increases right ventricular workload, precipitating right ventricular failure. Depending on previous heart function, acute decompensation of both ventricles can result. Measures are aimed at supporting cardiac function and avoiding intravascular volume excess. These measures include optimizing preload, afterload, and contractility with vasoactive agents.[60,61] (∞Heart Failure, p. 502; Cardiovascular Drugs, p. 574.)

Mediastinal shift. The pneumonectomy patient also is monitored for a shift in the mediastinum. The mediastinal position can be determined by palpating for tracheal deviation, palpating and auscultating the position of the apex of the heart, and performing a chest x-ray examination. If a mediastinal shift occurs, it must be corrected by injecting or withdrawing air or fluid.[62]

BOX 22-15 NURSING DIAGNOSIS AND MANAGEMENT

THORACIC SURGERY

- Ineffective Breathing Pattern related to decreased lung expansion, p. 723
- Impaired Gas Exchange related to ventilation/perfusion mismatching or intrapulmonary shunting, p. 725
- Impaired Gas Exchange related to alveolar hypoventilation, p. 726
- Acute Pain related to transmission and perception of cutaneous, visceral, muscular, or ischemic impulses, p. 197
- Anxiety related to threat to biologic, psychologic, and/or social integrity, p. 99
- Body Image Disturbance related to actual change in body structure, function, or appearance, p. 87
- Ineffective Family Coping related to critically ill family member, p. 97

Postoperative Nursing Management

Nursing care of the patient after thoracic surgery incorporates a number of nursing diagnoses (Box 22-15). Nursing management involves interventions aimed at optimizing oxygenation and ventilation, preventing atelectasis, monitoring chest tubes, assisting the patient to return to an adequate activity level, and maintaining surveillance for complications.

Optimizing oxygenation and ventilation. Nursing interventions to optimize oxygenation and ventilation include positioning, preventing desaturation during procedures, and promoting secretion clearance. For further discussion on these interventions, see Nursing Management of Acute Respiratory Failure earlier in this chapter.

Preventing atelectasis. Nursing interventions to prevent atelectasis include proper patient positioning and early ambulation, deep breathing exercises, incentive spirometry (IS), and pain management. The goal is to promote maximal lung ventilation and prevent hypoventilation.

Patient positioning and early ambulation. The nurse needs to consider the surgical incision site and the type of surgery when positioning the patient.

Lobectomy. After a lobectomy the patient is turned onto the nonoperative side to promote V/Q matching. When the good lung is dependent, blood flow is greater to the area with better ventilation and V/Q matching is better. V/Q mismatching results when the affected lung is positioned down, because of the increase in blood flow to an area with less ventilation. The patient is turned frequently to promote secretion removal but must have the affected lung dependent as little as possible.[61]

Pneumonectomy. The patient who has had a pneumonectomy is positioned supine or on the operative side during the initial period. Turning the patient onto the operative side promotes splinting of the incision and facilitates deep breathing exercises. Positioning the patient on the unaffected side can result in the drainage of secretions from the operative side and a shift in the mediastinum, adversely affecting the remaining lung. Tilting the patient slightly toward the unaffected side is possible, but the surgeon must indicate when free side-to-side positioning is safe.[62]

When sitting at the bedside or ambulating, patients must be encouraged to keep the thorax in straight alignment while they breathe deeply. This position best accommodates diaphragmatic descent and intercostal muscle action. The sitting or standing position provides enhanced ventilation to areas of the lung that are dependent in the supine position, thus accommodating maximal inflation and promoting gas exchange. Ambulation is essential in restoring lung function and is initiated as soon as possible.[63]

Deep breathing and incentive spirometry. Deep breathing and incentive spirometry are performed regularly by patients who have undergone a thoracotomy. Deep breathing involves having the patient take a deep breath and hold it for approximately 3 seconds or longer. Incentive spirometry involves having the patient take at least 10 deep, effective breaths per hour using an incentive spirometer. These activities help reexpand collapsed lung tissue, thus promoting early resolution of the pneumothorax in patients with partial lung resections. The chest is auscultated during inflation to ensure that all dependent parts of the lung are well-ventilated and to help the patient understand the depth of breath necessary for optimal effect. Coughing, which is encouraged only when secretions are present, assists in mobilizing secretions for removal.[63]

Pain management. Pain can be a major problem after thoracic surgery. Pain can increase the workload of the heart, precipitate hypoventilation, and inhibit mobilization of secretions. Clinical manifestations of pain include tachypnea, tachycardia, elevated blood pressure, facial grimacing, splinting of the incision, hypoventilation, moaning, and restlessness. There are several alternatives for pain management after thoracic surgery. The two most common methods are systemic narcotic administration and epidural narcotic administration. Systemic narcotics can be administered intravenously, intramuscularly, or via patient-controlled analgesia (PCA). In addition, the patient is assisted with splinting the incision with a pillow or blanket when deep breathing and coughing. Splinting stabilizes the area and reduces pain when moving, deep breathing, or coughing.[60,62,64] (∞Pain Management, p. 180.)

Maintaining the chest tube system. Chest tubes are placed after all thoracic surgery procedures (except a pneumonectomy) to remove air and fluid. The drainage will initially appear bloody, becoming serosanguineous and then serous over the first 2 to 3 days postoperatively. There will be approximately 100 to 300 ml of drainage during the first 2 hours postoperatively, which will decrease to less than 50 ml/hour over the next several hours. Routine "milking," or stripping, of chest tubes is not recommended, because excessive negative pressure can be generated in the chest. If blood clots are present in the drainage tubing or an obstruction is present, the chest tubes may be carefully "milked."[64]

During auscultation of the lungs, air leaks are evaluated. In the early phase, an air leak is commonly heard over the affected area, because the pleura has not yet tightly sealed. As healing occurs, this leak should disappear. An increase in an air leak or appearance of a new air leak must prompt investigation of the chest drainage system to discover whether the air is originating from outside the system or from within the patient. Increased air leaks not related to the chest drainage system may indicate disruption of sutures.[64]

Assisting patient to return to adequate activity level. Within a few days after surgery, range of motion to the shoulder on the operative side is initiated. The patient frequently splints the operative side and avoids shoulder movement because of pain. If immobility is allowed, stiffening of the shoulder joint can result. This is referred to as *frozen shoulder* and may require physical therapy and rehabilitation to regain satisfactory range of motion of the shoulder joint.[59,62]

Usually, on the day after surgery, the patient is able to sit in a chair. Activity is systematically increased, with attention to the patient's activity tolerance. With adequate pulmonary function before surgery and a surgical approach designed to preserve respiratory function, full return to previous activity levels is possible. This may take as long as 6 months to 1 year, depending on the tissue resected and the patient's general condition.[58]

LONG-TERM MECHANICAL VENTILATION

Description

Long-term mechanical ventilation (LTMV) is a secondary disorder that occurs when a patient requires assisted ventilation for more than 3 days. It is the result of complex medical problems that do not allow the normal weaning process to take place in a timely manner and results in ventilator dependence. Ventilator dependence can be described as a state in which the patient is mechanically ventilated longer than expected, given the patient's underlying condition,[65] and has usually failed at least one weaning attempt.[66]

Long-term mechanical ventilation falls under DRG 475 (Respiratory system diagnosis with ventilator support), if the patient does not have a tracheostomy, and DRG 483 (Tracheostomy except for face, mouth, and neck diagnoses), if the patient does have a tracheostomy, with anticipated lengths of stay of 12.3 days and 46.4 days, respectively.[4]

Etiology and Pathophysiology

There are a variety of physiologic and psychologic factors that contribute to the development of LTMV. Physiologic factors include conditions that result in decreased gas exchange, increased ventilatory workload, increased ventilatory demand, decreased ventilatory drive, and increased respiratory muscle fatigue (Box 22-16).[66-70] Psychologic factors include conditions that result in loss of breathing pattern control, lack of motivation and confidence, and delirium (Box 22-17).[67,71] The development of LTMV is also affected by the severity and duration of the patient's current illness and any underlying chronic health problems.[71]

Medical and Nursing Management

The goal of medical and nursing management of the patient requiring LTMV is successful weaning.

BOX 22-16 Physiologic Factors Contributing to the Development of LTMV

Decreased Gas Exchange
- Ventilation/perfusion mismatching
- Intrapulmonary shunting
- Alveolar hypoventilation
- Anemia
- Acute heart failure

Increased Ventilatory Workload
- Decreased lung compliance
- Increased airway resistance
- Small endotracheal tube
- Decreased ventilator sensitivity
- Improper positioning
- Abdominal distention
- Dyspnea

Increased Ventilatory Demand
- Increased pulmonary dead space
- Increased metabolic demands
- Improper ventilator mode/settings
- Metabolic acidosis
- Overfeeding

Decreased Ventilatory Drive
- Respiratory alkalosis
- Metabolic alkalosis
- Hypothyroidism
- Sedatives
- Malnutrition

Increased Respiratory Muscle Fatigue
- Increased ventilatory workload
- Increased ventilatory demand
- Malnutrition
- Hypokalemia
- Hypomagnesemia
- Hypophosphatemia
- Hypothyroidism
- Critical illness polyneuropathy
- Inadequate muscle rest

BOX 22-17 Psychologic Factors Contributing to the Development of LTMV

Loss of Breathing Pattern Control
- Anxiety
- Fear
- Dyspnea
- Pain
- Ventilator asynchrony
- Lack of confidence in ability to breathe

Lack of Motivation and Confidence
- Inadequate trust in staff
- Depersonalization
- Hopelessness
- Powerlessness
- Depression
- Inadequate communication

Delirium
- Sensory overload
- Sensory deprivation
- Sleep deprivation
- Pain
- Medications

The Third National Study Group on Weaning from Mechanical Ventilation, sponsored by the American Association of Critical Care Nurses, proposed a conceptual model that divides weaning into three phases: preweaning, weaning process, and weaning outcome (Figure 22-5).[65] It is within this framework that the management of the long-term ventilator dependent patient is described. In addition, the common nursing diagnoses for this patient population are listed in Box 22-18.

Preweaning phase. For the long-term ventilator dependent patient, the preweaning phase consists of resolving the precipitating event that necessitated ventilatory assistance and preventing the physiologic and psychologic factors that can interfere with weaning. Before any attempts at weaning, the patient must be assessed for weaning readiness, an approach must be determined, and a method must be selected.[65]

Weaning preparedness. The patient must be physiologically and psychologically prepared to initiate the weaning process by addressing those factors that can interfere with weaning. Aggressive medical management to prevent and treat ventilation/perfusion mismatching, intrapulmonary shunting, anemia, cardiac failure, decreased lung compliance, increased airway resistance, acid-base disturbances, hypothyroidism, abdominal distention, and electrolyte imbalances must be initiated. In addition, interventions to decrease the work of breathing are implemented, such as replacing a small endotracheal tube with a larger tube or a tracheostomy; suctioning airway secretions; administering bronchodilators; optimizing the ventilator settings and trigger sensitivity; and positioning the patient in straight alignment, with the head of the bed elevated at least 30 degrees. Enteral or parenteral nutrition should be started and the patient's nutritional state optimized. Physical therapy is initiated for the patient with critical illness polyneuropathy, because increased

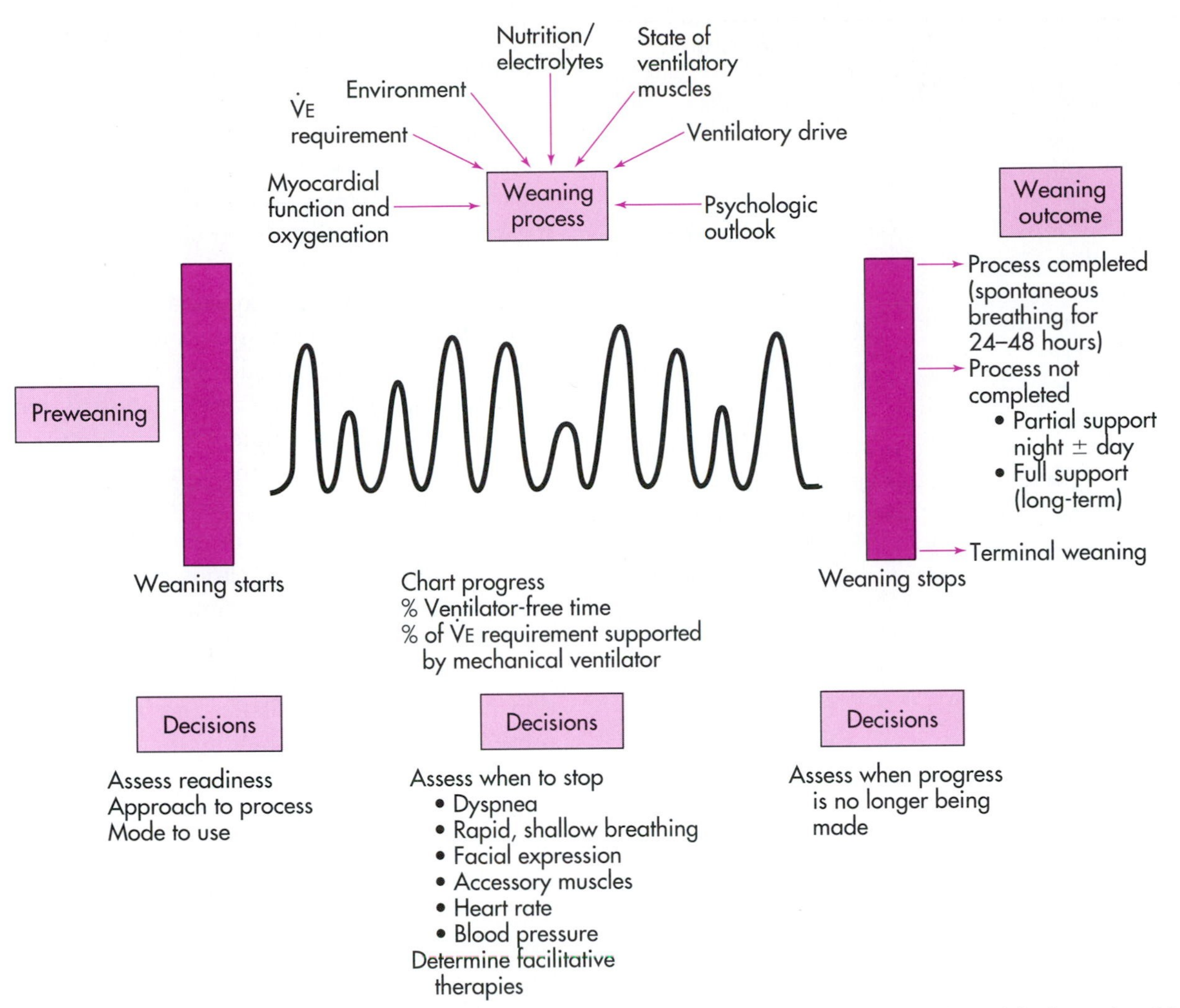

FIGURE 22-5. The Third National Study Group on Weaning from Mechanical Ventilation conceptual model of weaning. Note the three phases of weaning: preweaning, weaning process, and weaning outcome. (From Knebel AR and others: Weaning from mechanical ventilation: concept development, *Am J Crit Care* 3:416, 1994.)

mobility facilitates weaning. A means of communication is established with the patient. Sedatives can be administered to provide anxiety control, but the avoidance of respiratory depression is critical.[72,73]

Weaning readiness. Though a variety of different methods for assessing weaning readiness have been developed, none of them have proved to be very accurate in predicting weaning success in the patient requiring LTMV.[73] One study did indicate that the presence of left ventricular dysfunction, fluid imbalance, and nutritional deficiency increased the duration of mechanical ventilation.[74] Another study suggested that the upward trending of the albumin level may be predictive of weaning success.[75] Because so many variables can affect the patient's ability to wean, any assessment of weaning readiness must incorporate these variables.[76] Cardiac function, gas exchange, pulmonary mechanics, nutritional status, electrolyte and fluid balance, and motivation must all be considered when making the decision to wean. This assessment must be ongoing to reflect the dynamic nature of the process.

Weaning approach. Though weaning the patient requiring short-term mechanical ventilation is a relatively simple process that can usually be accomplished with a nurse and respiratory therapist, weaning the patient requiring LTMV is a much more complex process that usually requires a multidisciplinary team approach.[65,73] Multidisciplinary weaning teams who use a coordinated and collaborative approach to weaning have demonstrated improved patient outcomes and decreased weaning times.[73] The team consists of a physician; nurse; respiratory therapist; dietitian; physical therapist; and a case manager,

BOX 22-18 NURSING DIAGNOSIS AND MANAGEMENT

LONG-TERM MECHANICAL VENTILATION

- Inability to Sustain Spontaneous Ventilation related to respiratory muscle fatigue or neuromuscular impairment, p. 724
- Dysfunctional Ventilatory Weaning Response related to physical, psychosocial, or situational factors, p. 728
- Risk for Aspiration, p. 727
- Altered Nutrition: Less than Body Requirements related to lack of exogenous nutrients and increased metabolic demand, p. 165
- Risk for Infection, p. 1119
- Acute Confusion related to sensory overload, sensory deprivation, and sleep pattern disturbance, p. 99
- Body Image Disturbance related to functional dependence on life-sustaining technology, p. 86
- Anxiety related to threat to biologic, psychologic, and/or social integrity, p. 99
- Powerlessness related to lack of control over current situation or disease progression, p. 89
- Ineffective Family Coping related to critically ill family member, p. 97

clinical outcomes manager, or clinical nurse specialist. Additional members, if possible, include an occupational therapist, speech therapist, discharge planner, and social worker. Working together, team members develop a comprehensive plan of care for the patient that is efficient, consistent, progressive, and cost-effective.[73]

Weaning method. There are a variety of weaning methods available, but no one method has consistently proved to be superior to the others.[73] These methods include T-tube (T-piece), constant positive airway pressure (CPAP), pressure support ventilation (PSV), and synchronized intermittent mandatory ventilation (SIMV).[65] One recent multicenter study lends evidence to support the use of PSV weaning over T-tube or SIMV weaning.[77] Often these weaning methods are used in combination with each other, such as SIMV with PSV, CPAP with PSV, or SIMV with CPAP.[65]

Weaning process phase. For the long-term ventilator dependent patient, the weaning process phase consists of initiating the weaning method selected and minimizing the physiologic and psychologic factors that can interfere with weaning.[65] It is imperative that the patient not become exhausted during this phase, because this can result in a setback in the weaning process.[78] During this phase the patient is assessed for weaning progress and signs of weaning intolerance.[65]

Weaning initiation. Weaning is initiated in the morning while the patient is rested. Before starting the weaning process, the patient is provided with an explanation of how the process works, a description of the sensations he or she can expect, and reassurances that he or she will be closely monitored and returned to the original ventilator mode and settings if he or she is having difficulty.[67] This information is reinforced with each weaning attempt.

T-tube and CPAP weaning are accomplished by removing the patient from the ventilator and placing him or her on a T-tube or on CPAP mode for a specified duration of time (known as a *weaning trial*) for a specified number of times per day. When the weaning trial is finished, the patient is placed on the assist/control mode (continuous mandatory ventilation mode) of the ventilator and allowed to rest to prevent respiratory muscle fatigue. Gradually the frequency and duration of time spent weaning is increased until the patient is able to breathe spontaneously for 24 hours. If PSV is used in conjunction with CPAP, the PSV is initially set to provide the patient with an assisted tidal volume of 10 to 12 ml/kg, and the patient is gradually weaned of this until a level of 6 to 8 cm H_2O of pressure support is achieved. SIMV and PSV weaning are accomplished by gradually decreasing the number of breaths or the amount of pressure support the patient receives by a specified amount until the patient is able to breathe spontaneously for 24 hours.[78]

Weaning progress. Weaning progress can be evaluated using various methods. Evaluation of progress when using a weaning method that gradually withdraws ventilatory support, such as SIMV or PSV, can be accomplished by measuring the percentage of the minute ventilation requirement provided by the ventilator. If the percentage steadily decreases, weaning is progressing. Evaluation of progress when using a weaning method that removes ventilatory support, such as T-tube or CPAP, can be accomplished by measuring the amount of time the patient remains free from support. If the time steadily increases, weaning is progressing.[65]

Weaning intolerance. Once the weaning process has begun the patient is continuously assessed for signs of intolerance. When present, these signs indicate when to place the patient back on the ventilator or to return

TABLE 22-6 Indicators of and Interventions to Control or Prevent Weaning Intolerance

Indicator	Etiology	Intervention
PULMONARY SIGNS (EMOTIONAL)		
Altered breathing pattern Dyspnea intensity Change in facial expression	Inadequate understanding of weaning process Inability to control breathing pattern Environmental factors	Build trust in staff/consistent care providers Encouragement/concrete goals for extubation Involve patient in process/planning daily activities Efficient communication established Organizing care/avoid interruptions during weaning Adequate sleep Calm, caring presence of nurse/nonsedating anxiolytics Measure dyspnea Fan/music Biofeedback/relaxation/breathing control Family involvement/normalizing daily activities
PULMONARY SIGNS (PHYSIOLOGIC)		
Accessory muscle use Prolonged expiration	Airway obstruction Secretions/atelectasis Bronchospasm Patient position/kinked ET tube	Suction/air-mask bag unit ventilation Bronchodilators Sitting upright in bed or chair or patient preference
Asynchronous movements of chest and abdomen Retractions Facial expression changes Dyspnea	Increased workload or muscle fatigue Caloric intake Electrolyte imbalances Inadequate rest on ventilator Patient/ventilator interactions	Dietary assessment Assess electrolytes/replacements as necessary Rest between weaning trials (i.e., IMV frequency rate >5) Assess ventilator settings (i.e., flow rate, trigger sensitivity) Muscle training if appropriate
Shortened inspiratory time Increased breathing frequency, decreased V_T	Increased V_E requirement Infection Overfeeding Respiratory alkalosis Anxiety Pain	Check for infection (treat if indicated) Appropriate caloric intake Baseline ABGs achieved (ventilate according to pH) Coaching to regularize breathing pattern/nonsedating anxiolytics Judicious use of analgesics
CNS CHANGES		
Restless/irritable Decreased responsiveness	Hypoxemia/hypercarbia	Increase FIO_2 Return to mechanical ventilation Discern etiology and treat
CV DETERIORATION		
Excessive change in BP or HR Dysrhythmias Angina Dyspnea	Heart failure Increased venous return Ischemia	Diuretics as ordered Beta-blockers Increase FIO_2 Return to mechanical ventilation Discern etiology and treat

Modified from Knebel AR: *Am J Crit Care* 1(3):19, 1992.

the patient to his or her previous ventilator settings. Commonly used indicators include dyspnea; accessory muscle use; restlessness; anxiety; change in facial expression; changes in heart rate and blood pressure; rapid, shallow breathing; and discomfort.[65,67,73] Table 22-6 lists weaning intolerance indicators and actions that can be taken to control or prevent them. These signs and symptoms, however, have not been validated by research.[73] Thus a patient may exhibit some of these indicators and still tolerate the weaning process.

Facilitative therapies. Additional therapies may be needed to facilitate weaning in the patient who is having difficulty making weaning progress. These therapies include ventilatory muscle training and biofeedback.[65,67,73] Inspiratory muscle training is used to enhance the strength and endurance of the respiratory muscles.[73,78] Biofeedback can be used to promote relaxation and assist in the management of dyspnea and anxiety.[72,73]

Weaning outcome phase. There are three possible outcomes for a patient requiring LTMV: successful weaning, incomplete weaning, or terminal weaning.[65,66]

Successful weaning. Weaning is deemed successful when a patient is able to breathe spontaneously for 24 hours without ventilatory support. Once this occurs the patient may be extubated or decannulated at anytime, though this is not necessary for weaning to be considered successful.[65]

Incomplete weaning. Weaning is deemed incomplete when a patient has reached a plateau (5 days at the same ventilatory support without any changes) in his or her weaning process despite managing the physiologic and psychologic factors that impede weaning. Thus the patient is unable to breathe spontaneously for 24 hours without full or partial ventilatory support. Once this occurs the patient is placed in a subacute ventilator facility or discharged home on a ventilator with home care nursing follow-up.[65]

Terminal weaning. The withdrawal of ventilatory support, knowing it will result in the patient's death, at the request of the patient/family or because of the futility of continuing therapy is known as *terminal weaning.*[65,79] Terminal weaning can be accomplished either by removing the patient from the ventilator and placing the patient on a T-tube or by rapidly decreasing the rate, tidal volume, and/or fraction of inspired oxygen on the ventilator. If the patient shows signs of shortness of breath, pain, or anxiety, a continuous morphine or sedative infusion is started and adjusted to relieve the patient's symptoms of respiratory distress.[79] Once the terminal weaning process is completed and the patient is withdrawn from ventilatory support, death may occur within a several minutes, hours, or days.

REFERENCES

1. Op't Holt TB, Scanlan CL: Respiratory failure and the need for ventilatory support. In Scanlan CL, Spearman CB, Sheldon RL, editors: *Egan's fundamentals of respiratory care,* ed 6, St Louis, 1995, Mosby.
2. Bone RC: Acute respiratory failure. In Burton GG, Hodgkin JE, Ward JJ, editors: *Respiratory care: a guide to clinical practice,* ed 3, Philadelphia, 1991, JB Lippincott.
3. Balk R, Bone RC: Classification of acute respiratory failure, *Med Clin North Am* 67:551, 1983.
4. *St Anthony's DRG guidebook 1997,* Reston, Va, 1996, St Anthony.
5. Curtis JR, Hudson LD: Emergent assessment and management of acute respiratory failure in COPD, *Clin Chest Med* 15:481, 1994.
6. Pratter MR, Irwin RS: Extrapulmonary causes of respiratory failure, *J Intens Care Med* 1:197, 1986.
7. Green KE, Peters JI: Pathophysiology of acute respiratory failure, *Clin Chest Med* 15:1, 1994.
8. Misasi RS, Keyes JL: The pathophysiology of hypoxia, *Crit Care Nurse* 14(4):55, 1994.
9. Higgins TL, Yared JP: Clinical effects of hypoxemia and tissue hypoxia, *Respir Care* 38:603, 1993.
10. Vaughan P: Acute respiratory failure in the patient with chronic obstructive lung disease, *Crit Care Nurse* 1(6):46, 1981.
11. Misasi RS, Keyes JL: Matching and mismatching ventilation and perfusion in the lung, *Crit Care Nurse* 16(3):23, 1996.
12. Meduri GU and others: Noninvasive positive pressure ventilation via face mask, *Chest* 109:179, 1996.
13. Slutsky AS and others: American College of Chest Physicians' consensus conference: mechanical ventilation, *Chest* 104:1833, 1993.
14. American Thoracic Society: Standards for the diagnosis and care of patients with chronic obstructive pulmonary disease, *Am J Respir Crit Care Med* 152:S77, 1995.
15. Sapirstein A, Hurford WE: Neuromuscular blocking agents in the management of respiratory failure: indications and treatment guidelines, *Crit Care Clin* 10:831, 1994.
16. Doering LV: The effect of positioning on hemodynamics and gas exchange in the critically ill: a review, *Am J Crit Care* 2:208, 1993.
17. Lasater-Erhand M: The effect of patient position on arterial saturation, *Crit Care Nurse* 15(5):31, 1995.
18. Norton LC, Conforti C: The effect of body position on oxygenation, *Heart Lung* 14(1):45, 1985.
19. Cosenza JJ, Norton LC: Secretion clearance: state-of-the-art from a nursing perspective, *Crit Care Nurse* 6(4):23, 1986.
20. Bernard GR and others: The American-European consensus conference on ARDS: definitions, mechanisms, relevant outcomes, and clinical trial coordination, *Am J Respir Crit Care Med* 149:818, 1994.

21. Hammer J: Challenging diagnosis: adult respiratory distress syndrome, *Crit Care Nurse* 15(5):46, 1995.
22. Hanley ME, Repine JC: Pathogenetic aspects of the adult respiratory distress syndrome, *Semin Respir Crit Care Med* 15:260, 1994.
23. Milberg JA and others: Improved survival of patients with acute respiratory distress syndrome (ARDS): 1983-1993, *JAMA* 273:306, 1995.
24. Garber BG and others: Adult respiratory distress syndrome: a systematic overview of incidence and risk factors, *Crit Care Med* 24:687, 1996.
25. Marinelli WA, Ingbar DH: Diagnosis and management of acute lung injury, *Clin Chest Med* 15:517, 1994.
26. Vollman KM: Adult respiratory distress syndrome, *Crit Care Nurs Clin North Am* 6:341, 1994.
27. Kollef MH, Schuster DP: The acute respiratory distress syndrome, *New Engl J Med* 332:27, 1995.
28. Gleeson K, Reynolds HY: Life-threatening pneumonia, *Clin Chest Med* 3:581, 1994.
29. Kollef MH, Silver P: Ventilator-associated pneumonia, *Respir Care* 40:1130, 1995.
30. Cunha B: The antibiotic treatment of community-acquired, atypical, and nosocomial pneumonia, *Med Clin North Am* 79:581, 1995.
31. Huang L, Stansell JD: AIDS and the lung, *Med Clin North Am* 80:775, 1996.
32. Leeper KV, Torres A: Community-acquired pneumonia in the intensive care unit, *Clin Chest Med* 16:155, 1995.
33. Nelson S and others: Pathophysiology of pneumonia, *Clin Chest Med* 16:1, 1995.
34. Tablan OC and others: Guideline for prevention of nosocomial pneumonia. I. Issues on prevention of nosocomial pneumonia-1994, *Am J Infect Control* 22:247, 1994.
35. American Thoracic Society: Hospital-acquired pneumonia in adults: diagnosis, assessment of severity, initial antimicrobial therapy, and preventable strategies—a consensus statement, *Am J Respir Crit Care Med* 153:1711, 1995.
36. Dal Nogare AR: Nosocomial pneumonia in the medical surgical patient, *Med Clin North Am* 78:1081, 1994.
37. DePaso WJ: Aspiration pneumonia, *Clin Chest Med* 12:269, 1991.
38. Tietjen PA, Kaner RJ, Quinn CE: Aspiration emergencies, *Clin Chest Med* 15:117, 1994.
39. Chokshi S, Asper R, Khandheria B: Aspiration pneumonia: a review, *Am Fam Physician* 33:195, 1986.
40. Goodwin RS: Prevention of aspiration pneumonia: a research-based protocol, *DCCN* 15(2):58, 1996.
41. Wagenvoort CA: Pathology of pulmonary thromboembolism, *Chest* 107:11S, 1995.
42. King MB, Harmon KR: Unusual forms of pulmonary embolism, *Clin Chest Med* 15:561, 1994.
43. Cowen JC, Kelley MA: An organized approach to detecting pulmonary embolism in the critically ill, *J Crit Illn* 9:551, 1994.
44. Kelley MA, Abbuhl S: Massive pulmonary embolism, *Clin Chest Med* 15:547, 1994.
45. Manganelli D and others: Clinical features of pulmonary embolism: doubts and certainties, *Chest* 107:25S, 1995.
46. Davis LA, O'Rouke NC: Pulmonary embolism: early recognition and management in the postanesthesia care unit, *J Post Anesth Nurs* 8:338, 1993.
47. Agnelli G: Anticoagulation in the prevention and treatment of pulmonary embolism, *Chest* 107:39S, 1995.
48. Goldhaber SZ: Contemporary pulmonary embolism thrombolysis, *Chest* 107:45S, 1995.
49. Borkgren MW, Grankeiwicz CA: Update your asthma care from hospital to home, *Am J Nurs* 95(1):25, 1995.
50. Abou-Shala N, MacIntyre N: Emergency management of acute asthma, *Med Clin North Am* 80:677, 1996.
51. Leatherman J: Life-threatening asthma, *Clin Chest Med* 15:453, 1994.
52. Corbridge TC, Hall JB: The assessment and management of adults with status asthmaticus, *Am J Respir Crit Care Med* 151:1296, 1995.
53. Jantz M, Pierson DJ: Pneumothorax and barotrauma, *Clin Chest Med* 15:75, 1994.
54. Des Jardins T, Burton GC: *Clinical manifestations and assessment of respiratory disease,* ed 3, St Louis, 1995, Mosby.
55. Kirby TJ, Ginsberg RJ: Management of the pneumothorax and barotrauma, *Clin Chest Med* 13:97, 1992.
56. Gordon PA, Norton JM, Merrell R: Refining chest tube management: analysis of the state of practice, *DCCN* 14(11):6, 1995.
57. Litwack K: Practical points in the care of the thoracic surgery patient, *Post Anesth Nurs* 5:276, 1990.
58. Cottrell JJ, Ferson PF: Preoperative assessment of the thoracic surgery patient, *Chest* 14:47, 1992.
59. Langston W: Surgical resection of lung cancer, *Nurs Clin North Am* 27:665, 1992.
60. Boysen PG: Perioperative management of the thoracotomy patient, *Clin Chest Med* 14:321, 1993.
61. Daitch JS: Post anesthesia care after thoracic surgery. In Frost EAM, editor: *Post anesthesia care unit: current practices,* ed 2, St Louis, 1990, Mosby.
62. Brenner Z, Addona C: Caring for the pneumonectomy patient: challenges and changes, *Crit Care Nurse* 15(5):65, 1995.
63. Brooks-Braun JA: Postoperative atelectasis and pneumonia, *Heart Lung* 24:94, 1995.
64. Whitman GR, Weber MM: Postoperative care after thoracic surgery, *Curr Rev PACU* 14:137, 1992.
65. Knebel AR and others: Weaning from mechanical ventilation: concept development, *Am J Crit Care N* 3:416, 1994.
66. Pierson DJ: Long-term mechanical ventilation and weaning, *Respir Care* 40:289, 1995.
67. Knebel AR: When weaning from mechanical ventilation fails, *Am J Crit Care* 1(3):19, 1992.
68. MacIntyre NR: Respiratory factors in weaning from mechanical ventilatory support, *Respir Care* 40:244, 1995.
69. Pierson DJ: Nonrespiratory aspects of weaning from mechanical ventilation, *Respir Care* 40:263, 1995.

70. Hund EF and others: Critical illness polyneuropathy: clinical findings and outcomes of a frequent cause of neuromuscular weaning, *Crit Care Med* 24:1328, 1996.
71. MacIntyre NR: Psychological factors in weaning from mechanical ventilatory support, *Respir Care* 40:277, 1995.
72. Criner GJ, Tzouanakis A, Kreimer DT: Overview of improving tolerance of long-term mechanical ventilation, *Crit Care Clin* 10:845, 1994.
73. Burns SM and others: Weaning from long-term mechanical ventilation, *Am J Crit Care* 4:4, 1995.
74. Clochesy JM: Weaning chronically critically ill adults from mechanical ventilatory support: a descriptive study, *Am J Crit Care* 4:93, 1995.
75. Sapijaszko MJA and others: Nonrespiratory predictor of mechanical ventilation dependency in intensive care unit patients, *Crit Care Med* 24:601, 1996.
76. Ingersoll GL and others: Measurement issues in mechanical ventilation weaning research, *Online J Knowledge Synthesis Nurs* 2(12):24, 1995.
77. Brochard L and others: Comparison of three methods of gradual withdrawal from ventilatory support during weaning from mechanical ventilation, *Am J Respir Crit Care Med* 150:898, 1994.
78. Brochard LJ, Lessard MR: Weaning from ventilatory support, *Clin Chest Med* 17:475, 1996.
79. Daly BJ and others: Withdrawal of mechanical ventilation: ethical principles and guidelines for terminal weaning, *Am J Crit Care* 2:217, 1993.

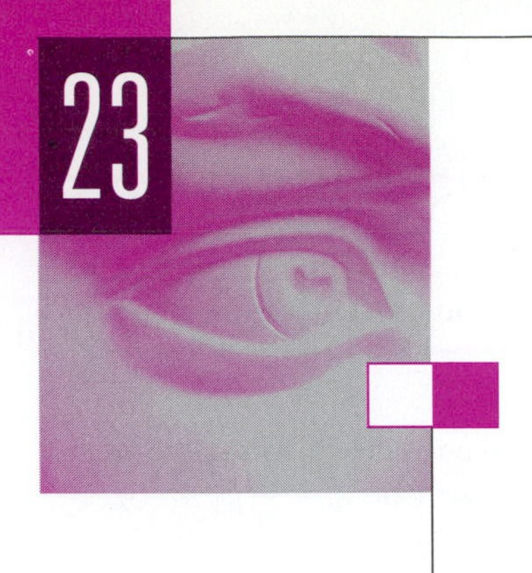

Pulmonary Therapeutic Management

OXYGEN THERAPY

Goals of Therapy

NORMAL CELLULAR FUNCTION depends on an adequate supply of oxygen to meet metabolic needs. The primary indications for oxygen administration are hypoxemia and tissue hypoxia. The goal of oxygen administration is to provide a sufficient concentration of inspired oxygen to permit full use of the oxygen-carrying capacity of the arterial blood, thus ensuring adequate tissue oxygenation if the cardiac output (CO) is adequate and if the hemoglobin (Hgb) concentration and structure are normal.[1,2]

Principles of Therapy

Oxygen is an atmospheric gas that must also be considered a drug, because—like most other drugs—oxygen has both detrimental and beneficial effects. Oxygen is one of the most commonly used and misused drugs. As a drug, it must be administered for good reason and in a proper, safe manner. Oxygen is generally ordered in liters per minute (L/min); as a concentration of oxygen expressed as a percent, such as 40%; or as a fraction of inspired oxygen (FIO_2), such as 0.4.[3]

The amount of oxygen administered depends on the pathophysiologic mechanisms affecting the patient's oxygenation status. In most cases the amount required should provide an arterial partial pressure of oxygen (PaO_2) of 60 to 90 mm Hg, so that a Hgb saturation (SaO_2) of greater than 90% is achieved.[3] The concentration of oxygen given to an individual patient is a clinical judgment based on the many factors that influence oxygen transport, such as Hgb concentration, CO, and the arterial oxygen tension.[1,2]

Once oxygen therapy has begun, the patient is continuously assessed for level of oxygenation and the factors affecting it. The patient's oxygenation status is evaluated several times daily until the desired oxygen level is reached and has stabilized. If the desired response to the amount of oxygen delivered is not achieved, the oxygen supplementation is adjusted and the patient's condition reevaluated. It is important to use this dose-response method, so that the lowest possible level of oxygen is administered that will still achieve a satisfactory PaO_2 or SaO_2.[3] (Oxygenation: Clinical Assessment and Evaluation; Pulmonary Care IVD.)

Methods of Delivery

Oxygen therapy can be delivered by many different devices (Table 23-1). These devices are classified as either low-flow or high-flow delivery systems. A low-flow system supplies an amount of oxygen that is insufficient to meet all inspiratory volume requirements and depends on the existence of a reservoir of oxygen, dilution with room air, and the patient's ventilatory pattern. The anatomic reservoir in this case is composed of the nasopharynx and the oropharynx. As the patient's ventilatory pattern changes, the inspired oxygen concentration varies because of differing amounts of air mixing with the reservoir gas and the constant flow of oxygen. With a high-flow system, the oxygen flows out of the device into the patient's airways in amounts sufficient to meet all inspiratory volume requirements. This type of system is not affected by the patient's ventilatory pattern. Examples of low-flow systems are nasal cannulas, simple oxygen masks, partial rebreathing masks, and nonrebreathing masks. An air-entrainment (Venturi) mask is an example of a high-flow oxygen delivery system.[1,3,4]

TABLE 23-1 Oxygen Administration Devices

Equipment	Objective	L/min	FIO_2 (%)	Advantages/Disadvantages
LOW FLOW-SYSTEMS				
Nasal cannula	Provides oxygen through a low-flow oxygen delivery system	1 2 3 4 5 6	24 28 32 36 40 44	Can be used with mouth breathers Convenient Comfortable Good low flow Allows for talking and eating FIO_2 not really accurate because it depends on patient's respiratory pattern May cause sinus pain >2 L/min requires added humidity Easily displaced Nasal passages must be patent
Simple face mask*	Provides oxygen through a mask and low-flow oxygen delivery system	5 6 8	40 50 60	Simple set-up; good for emergency situations Can get uncomfortable Poor patient tolerance FIO_2 not really accurate because it depends on patient's respiratory pattern Cannot provide enough humidity for prolonged use Must be removed at meals Tight fitting mask can cause pressure sores Aspiration of vomitus is a potential problem
Partial rebreathing mask	Provides a high oxygen concentration through a low-flow delivery system	6 8 10-15	35 45-50 In excess of 60 depending on patient's ventilatory pattern	Simple set-up; good in emergency situations Can be uncomfortable Does not provide adequate humidity for long-term use
Nonrebreathing mask	Provides high oxygen concentration	6 8 10-15	55-60 60-80 80-90	Delivers the highest possible oxygen concentration (55%-90%) possible from a low-flow system Good for short-term therapy and transport Has three one-way valves Requires a tight seal May irritate skin

Complications of Oxygen Therapy

Oxygen, like most drugs, has adverse effects and complications resulting from its use. The old adage "if a little is good, a lot is better" does not apply to oxygen. The lung is designed to handle a concentration of 21% oxygen, with some adaptability to higher concentrations, but adverse effects and oxygen toxicity can result if a high concentration is administered for too long.[2]

Oxygen toxicity. The most detrimental effect of breathing a high concentration of oxygen is the development of oxygen toxicity. It can occur in any pa-

TABLE 23-1 **Oxygen Administration Devices—cont'd**

Equipment	Objective	L/min	FIO_2 (%)	Advantages/Disadvantages
HUMIDIFYING SYSTEMS				
Aerosol mask (high humidity face mask)	Delivers a specific FIO_2 through an aerosol device		28-100 (variable)	High humidity Accurate FIO_2 Does not dry mucous membranes Can be uncomfortable May need extra equipment for higher FIO_2 Moisture build-up in tube
Face tent	Delivers high humidity		21-55	Used for patients with facial trauma Does not dry mucous membranes Can function as high-flow system when attached to Venturi system Interferes with eating and talking Impractical for long-term use Possible to rebreathe CO_2
Trach mask T-tube	Delivers a specific FIO_2 through an aerosol system		28-100 (variable)	High humidity Accurate FIO_2 Can control oxygen Does not need vent May need extra equipment for higher FIO_2
HIGH-FLOW SYSTEMS				
Air-entrainment (Venturi) mask†	Provides high-flow oxygen with a precise FIO_2 in a selected range	Blue-4 Yellow-4 White-6 Green-8 Pink-8	24 28 31 35 40	Can provide humidity Accurate oxygen levels Simple set-up; good for emergency situations Well-tolerated Can only have FIO_2 in selected range Hot and confining Must fit snugly
CONSTANT POSITIVE AIRWAY PRESSURE (CPAP)				
CPAP mask	Provides continual positive airway pressure through a mask without the use of a ventilator		30-100	Do not need ventilator Do not need to be intubated Can get gastric distention Mask is uncomfortable Not useful if patient becomes apneic

From Flynn JBM, Bruce NP: *Introduction to critical care nursing skills,* St Louis, 1993, Mosby.
*A minimum flow rate of 5 L/min to flush expired carbon dioxide from the mask is needed.
†Jet adapters on Venturi masks are color coded.

tient breathing oxygen concentrations of greater than 50% for more than 24 hours. Patients most likely to develop oxygen toxicity are those who require intubation, mechanical ventilation, and high oxygen concentrations for extended periods.[1,3,5]

Hyperoxia, or the administration of higher-than-normal oxygen concentrations, produces an overabundance of oxygen-free radicals. These radicals, toxic metabolites of oxygen metabolism, are responsible for the initial damage to the alveolar-capillary membrane. Normally, enzymes neutralize the radicals, which prevents any damage from occurring. However, during the administration of high levels of oxygen, the large number of oxygen-free radicals produced exhausts the supply of neutralizing enzymes. Thus damage to the lung parenchyma and vasculature occurs.[1,5]

The pathologic features of oxygen toxicity can be divided into an early exudative stage and a late proliferative stage. Within 24 to 48 hours of oxygen exposure, exudative changes appear. Initially, the capillary endothelial cells become damaged, and they leak serum protein and fluid into the interstitial space of the alveolar wall. This fluid is collected by the lymphatic system, which empties it into the general circulation. As the capillary damage progresses, the flow of fluid out of the capillaries increases and exceeds the lymphatic system's ability to drain it. With continued exposure to hyperoxia, the Type I alveolar cells become damaged, allowing the escaped alveolar-capillary fluid to pass directly into the alveolar spaces and causing "flooding" of the alveoli and severe gas exchange impairment.[5]

The lung will respond with cellular proliferation if it survives the aforementioned process and the disease process originally responsible for the hypoxemia. Cellular proliferation occurs in an attempt to repair the alveolar damage, and the alveolar walls become filled with fibroblasts. Alveolar Type II cells, which are relatively tolerant to hyperoxia, replicate and reestablish the damaged alveolar wall. Endothelial cell repair and replacement occurs, and the pulmonary edema is reabsorbed. The final result is irregular scarring that can lead to pulmonary fibrosis.[5]

A number of clinical manifestations are associated with oxygen toxicity. The first symptom is substernal chest pain that is exacerbated by deep breathing. A dry cough and tracheal irritation follow. Eventually, definite pleuritic pain occurs on inhalation, followed by dyspnea. Upper airway changes may include a sensation of nasal stuffiness, sore throat, and eye and ear discomfort. Chest radiographs and pulmonary function tests show no abnormalities until symptoms are severe. Complete, rapid reversal of these symptoms occurs as soon as normal oxygen concentrations return.[5]

As oxygen toxicity progresses, objective pulmonary damage becomes evident. A chest radiograph reveals atelectatic streaks and patches of bronchopneumonia, and bronchoscopy reveals tracheobronchitis but no infection. As atelectasis develops, there is evidence of decreased vital capacity, decreased compliance, reduced functional residual capacity, and increased intrapulmonary shunting. These abnormalities are reversible several days after normal oxygen concentrations return. If high oxygen concentrations are still needed, permanent damage may occur.[5]

Carbon dioxide retention. In patients with severe chronic obstructive pulmonary disease (COPD), carbon dioxide (CO_2) retention may occur as a result of administering oxygen in higher concentrations. There are a number of possible theories for this phenomenon. One theory states that in patients with COPD the normal stimulus to breathe (increasing CO_2 levels) is muted and decreasing oxygen levels become the stimulus to breathe. When oxygen is administered and hypoxemia corrected, the stimulus to breathe is abolished and hypoventilation develops, resulting in a further increase in the arterial partial pressure of carbon dioxide ($Pa{CO_2}$).[2,3] Another theory is that the administration of oxygen abolishes the compensatory response of hypoxic pulmonary vasoconstriction. This results in an increase in perfusion of underventilated alveoli and the development of dead space producing ventilation/perfusion mismatching. As alveolar dead space increases so does the retention of CO_2.[3,6] One other theory states the rise in CO_2 is related to the proportion of deoxygenated hemoglobin to oxygenated hemoglobin (Haldane effect). Since deoxygenated hemoglobin carries more CO_2 than oxygenated hemoglobin, when oxygen is administered it increases the amount of oxygenated hemoglobin, which results in an increase in the release of CO_2 at the lung level.[6] Because of the risk of carbon dioxide accumulation, chronically hypercapnic patients require careful, controlled low-flow oxygen administration.[2]

Absorption atelectasis. Another adverse effect of high concentrations of oxygen is absorption atelectasis. Breathing high concentrations of oxygen washes out the nitrogen that normally fills the alveoli and helps hold them open (residual volume). As oxygen replaces the nitrogen in the alveoli, the alveoli start to shrink and collapse because oxygen is absorbed into the blood stream faster than it can be replaced in the alveoli, particularly in areas of the lungs that are minimally ventilated.[1]

Nursing Management

Nursing interventions for the management of the patient receiving oxygen therapy are outlined in Box 23-1.

ARTIFICIAL AIRWAYS

Oropharyngeal and Nasopharyngeal Airways

Pharyngeal airways are made of rubber or plastic and are used to maintain airway patency by keeping the tongue from obstructing the upper airway. An oral

NURSING INTERVENTION CLASSIFICATIONS

BOX 23-1 Oxygen Therapy

DEFINITION: Administration of oxygen and monitoring of its effectiveness

ACTIVITIES:

Clear oral, nasal, and tracheal secretions, as appropriate
Restrict smoking
Maintain airway patency
Set up oxygen equipment and administer through a heated, humidified system
Administer supplemental oxygen, as ordered
Monitor the oxygen liter flow
Monitor position of oxygen delivery device
Instruct patient about importance of leaving oxygen delivery device on
Periodically check oxygen delivery device to ensure that the prescribed concentration is being delivered
Ensure replacement of oxygen mask/cannula whenever the device is removed
Monitor patient's ability to tolerate removal of oxygen while eating
Change oxygen delivery device from mask to nasal prongs during meals, as tolerated
Observe for signs of oxygen-induced hypoventilation
Monitor for signs of oxygen toxicity and absorption atelectasis
Monitor oxygen equipment to ensure that it is not interfering with the patient's attempts to breathe
Monitor patient's anxiety related to need for oxygen therapy
Monitor for skin breakdown from friction of oxygen device
Provide for oxygen when patient is transported
Instruct patient to obtain a supplementary oxygen prescription before air travel or trips to high altitude, as appropriate
Consult with other health care personnel about use of supplemental oxygen during activity and/or sleep
Instruct patient and family about use of oxygen at home
Arrange for use of oxygen devices that facilitate mobility and teach patient accordingly
Convert to alternate oxygen delivery device to promote comfort, as appropriate

From McCloskey JC, Bulechek GM: *Nursing interventions classification,* ed 2, St Louis, 1996, Mosby.

airway is placed by inserting it upside down and rotating it 180 degrees as it is passed into the mouth. It is used only in an unconscious patient who has an absent or diminished gag reflex. A nasal airway is placed by lubricating the tube and inserting it midline along the floor of the naris into the posterior pharynx. Respirations are assessed after placement of either airway to ensure proper position. Complications of these airways include trauma to the oral or nasal cavity, obstruction of the airway, laryngospasm, and gagging and vomiting.[7-9]

Endotracheal Tubes

An endotracheal tube (ETT) is the most commonly used artificial airway for providing short-term airway management. Indications for endotracheal intubation include airway maintenance and protection, secretion control, oxygenation, and ventilation.[10] An endotracheal tube may be placed through the orotracheal or nasotracheal route. In most situations involving emergency placement, the orotracheal route is used, because the approach is simpler and affords the use of a larger diameter endotracheal tube. Nasotracheal intubation provides greater patient comfort over time and is preferred in situations in which the patient has a jaw fracture.[9-11] The advantages of orotracheal intubation and nasotracheal intubation are presented in Table 23-2.[9-11]

ETTs are available in a variety of sizes, according to the inner diameter of the tube, and have a radiopaque marker that runs the length of the tube. On one end of the tube is a cuff that is inflated using the pilot balloon. Because of the high incidence of cuff-related problems, low-pressure, high-volume cuffs are preferred. On the other end of the tube is a 15 mm adaptor that facilitates the connection of the tube to a manual resuscitation bag (MRB), T-tube, or ventilator (Figure 23-1).[12]

Intubation. Before intubation, equipment must be organized to facilitate the procedure. Equipment that must be readily available includes a suction system with catheters and tonsil suction, an MRB with a mask connected to 100% oxygen, a laryngoscope handle with

TABLE 23-2 Advantages of Orotracheal, Nasotracheal, and Tracheostomy Tubes

Orotracheal Tubes	Nasotracheal Tubes	Tracheostomy Tubes
Easier access	Easily secured and stabilized	Easily secured and stabilized
Avoid nasal and sinus complications	Reduced risk of unintentional extubation	Reduced risk of unintentional decannulation
Allow for larger diameter tube, which facilitates:	Well-tolerated by patient	Well-tolerated by patient
Work of breathing	Enable swallowing and oral hygiene	Enable swallowing, speech, and oral hygiene
Suctioning	Facilitate communication	Avoid upper airway complications
Fiberoptic bronchoscopy	Avoid need for bite block	Allow for larger diameter tube, which facilitates:
		Work of breathing
		Suctioning
		Fiberoptic bronchoscopy

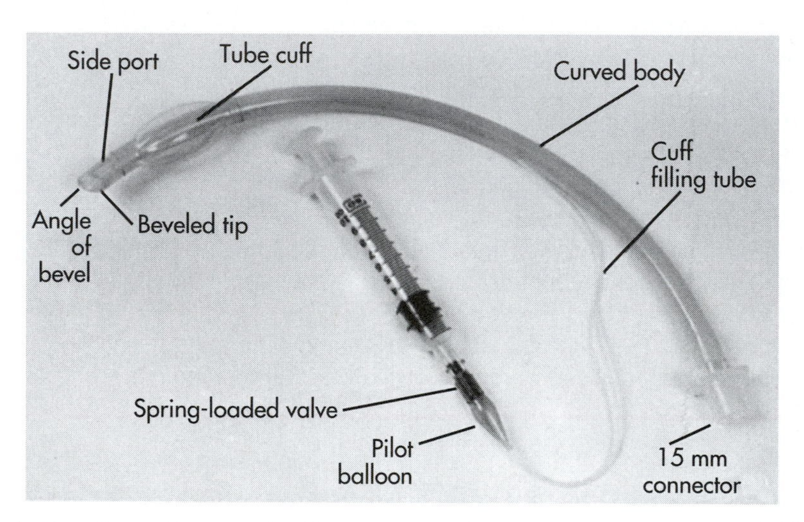

FIGURE 23-1. Endotracheal tube. (From Simmons K: Airway care. In Scanlan CL, Spearman CB, Sheldon RL, editors: *Egan's fundamentals of respiratory care,* ed 6, St Louis, 1995, Mosby.)

assorted blades, a variety of sizes of ETTs, and a stylet. Before the procedure is initiated, all equipment must be inspected to ensure it is in working order. The patient must be prepared for the procedure, if possible, with an intravenous catheter in place and be monitored with a pulse oximeter. The patient is sedated before the procedure, and a topical anesthetic is applied to facilitate placement of the tube. In some cases a paralytic agent may be necessary if the patient is extremely agitated.[7-9]

The procedure is initiated by positioning the patient with the neck flexed and head slightly extended in the "sniff" position. The oral cavity and pharynx are suctioned, and any dental devices are removed. The patient is preoxygenated and ventilated using the MRB and mask with 100% oxygen. Each intubation attempt is limited to 30 seconds. Once the ETT is inserted, the patient is assessed for bilateral breath sounds and chest movement. A disposable end-tidal CO_2 detector can be used to initially verify correct airway placement,[10] after which the cuff of the tube is inflated, the tube secured, and a chest radiograph obtained to confirm placement.[7,9,10] The tip of the endotracheal tube must be approximately 5 to 7 cm above the carina when the patient's head is in the neutral position.[13] Once final adjustment of the position is complete, the level of insertion (marked in centimeters on side of tube) is noted.[10]

Complications. There are a number of complications with intubation. These include gastric intubation; right mainstem bronchus intubation; vomiting with aspiration; trauma to the mouth, nose, pharynx, trachea, esophagus, eyes, or facial tissue; laryngospasm; hypoxemia; and hypercapnia. Hypoxemia and hypercapnia can cause bradycardia, tachycardia, dysrhythmias, hypertension, and hypotension.[7,10,14]

A number of factors predispose a patient to the development of complications while he or she is intubated—particularly prolonged intubation. Complications that can occur include tube obstruction and displacement, sinusitis, nasal injury, and tracheoesophageal fistulas. A number of complications can occur days to weeks after the ETT is removed; these include mucosal lesions, laryngeal and/or tracheal stenosis, and cricoid abscess (Table 23-3).[9,11,14] Delayed complications usually require some form of surgical intervention to correct.[14]

Tracheostomy Tubes

A tracheostomy tube is the preferred method of airway maintenance in the patient requiring intubation for more than 21 days. It is also indicated in several other situations, including upper airway obstruction or malformation, failed intubation, repeated intubations, presence of complications of endotracheal intubation, glottic incompetence, sleep apnea, and chronic inability to clear secretions.[9,11,15]

A tracheostomy tube provides the best route for long-term airway maintenance and avoids the oral, nasal, pharyngeal, and laryngeal complications of endotracheal intubation. The tube is shorter, of wider diameter, and less curved than is the endotracheal tube; thus the resistance to airflow is less, and breathing is easier. The tracheostomy has other advantages over endotracheal intubation, including easier secretion removal; increased patient acceptance and comfort; the possibility of the patient being able to eat and talk; and the facilitation of ventilator weaning, because a tracheostomy tube is easier to breathe through, decreasing the work of breathing.[9,15] Table 23-2 presents the advantages of tracheostomy tubes.

Tracheostomy tubes are made of plastic or metal and may be single-lumen or double-lumen tubes. Single-lumen tubes consist of the tube and a built-in cuff, which is connected to a pilot balloon for inflation purposes, and an obturator, which is used during tube insertion. The double-lumen tubes consist of the tube with the attached cuff; the obturator; and an inner cannula that can be removed for cleaning and reinserted or, if disposable, replaced by a new sterile inner cannula. The inner cannula can quickly be removed if it becomes obstructed, making the system safer for patients with significant secretion problems. Single-lumen tubes provide a larger inside diameter for airflow than do double-lumen tubes, thus reducing airflow resistance and allowing the patient to ventilate through the tube with greater ease. Plastic tracheostomy tubes also have a 15 mm adaptor on the end (Figure 23-2).[16]

Tracheostomy tubes are inserted either surgically or percutaneously. Placement complications include hemorrhage, pneumothorax, pneumomediastinum, tracheoesophageal fistula, laryngeal nerve injury, and cardiopulmonary arrest. Immediate postprocedural complications include hemorrhage, wound infection, subcutaneous emphysema, tube obstruction, and tube displacement. Later complications of a tracheostomy tube include tracheal stenosis, tracheoesophageal fistula, tracheoinnominate artery fistula, and tracheocutaneous fistula (Table 23-4).[10,17,18]

Airway Management

The patient with an endotracheal or tracheostomy tube requires some additional measures that address the effects associated with tube placement on the respiratory and other body systems (Box 23-2). The tube bypasses the upper airway system; therefore warming and humidifying of air must be performed by external means. Because the cuff of the tube can cause damage to the walls of the trachea, proper cuff inflation and management is imperative. In addition, the normal defense mechanisms are impaired and secretions may accumulate; thus suctioning may be needed to promote secretion clearance. Because the tube does not allow airflow over the vocal cords, developing a method of communication is also very important.

Unintentional extubation. Observing the patient to ensure proper placement of the tube and patency of the airway is essential. In the event of unintentional extubation or decannulation, the patient's airway is opened with the head tilt–chin lift maneuver and maintained with an oropharyngeal or nasopharyngeal airway. If the patient is not breathing, he or she is manually ventilated with an MRB and face mask with 100% oxygen. In the case of a tracheostomy, the stoma is covered to prevent air from escaping through it.

Humidification. Humidification of air normally is performed by the mucosal layer of the upper respiratory tract. When this area is bypassed, such as occurs in endotracheal intubation and tracheostomy or when supplemental oxygen is used, humidification by external means is necessary. Various humidification devices add water to inhaled gas to prevent drying and irritation of the respiratory tract, to prevent undue loss of body water, and to facilitate secretion removal.[19]

(Text continues on page 699.)

TABLE 23-3 Endotracheal Tubes: Complications, Causes, and Treatment

Complication	Causes	Prevention/Treatment
Tube obstruction	Patient biting tube Tube kinking during repositioning Cuff herniation Dried secretions, blood, or lubricant Tissue from tumor Trauma Foreign body	***Prevention:*** Place bite block. Sedate patient PRN. Suction PRN. Humidify inspired gases. ***Treatment:*** Replace tube.
Tube displacement	Movement of patient's head Movement of tube by patient's tongue Traction on tube from ventilator tubing Self-extubation	***Prevention:*** Secure tube to upper lip. Restrain patient's hands. Sedate patient PRN. Ensure that only 2 inches of tube extend beyond lip. Support ventilator tubing. ***Treatment:*** Replace tube.
Sinusitis and nasal injury	Obstruction of the paranasal sinus drainage Pressure necrosis of nares	***Prevention:*** Avoid nasal intubations. Cushion nares from tube and tape/ties. ***Treatment:*** Remove all tubes from nasal passages. Administer antibiotics.
Tracheoesophageal fistula	Pressure necrosis of posterior tracheal wall resulting from overinflated cuff and rigid nasogastric tube	***Prevention:*** Inflate cuff with minimal amount of air necessary. Monitor cuff pressures every 8 hours. ***Treatment:*** Position cuff of tube distal to fistula. Place gastrostomy tube for enteral feedings. Place esophageal tube for secretion clearance proximal to fistula.
Mucosal lesions	Pressure at tube and mucosal interface	***Prevention:*** Inflate cuff with minimal amount of air necessary. Monitor cuff pressures every 8 hours. Use appropriate size tube. ***Treatment:*** May resolve spontaneously. Perform surgical intervention.

TABLE 23-3 Endotracheal Tubes: Complications, Causes, and Treatment—cont'd

Complication	Causes	Prevention/Treatment
Laryngeal or tracheal stenosis	Injury to area from end of tube or cuff, resulting in scar tissue formation and narrowing of airway	***Prevention:*** Inflate cuff with minimal amount of air necessary. Monitor cuff pressures every 8 hours. Suction area above cuff frequently. ***Treatment:*** Perform tracheostomy. Place laryngeal stint. Perform surgical repair.
Cricoid abscess	Mucosal injury with bacterial invasion	***Prevention:*** Inflate cuff with minimal amount of air necessary. Monitor cuff pressures every 8 hours. Suction area above cuff frequently. ***Treatment:*** Perform incision and drainage of area. Administer antibiotics.

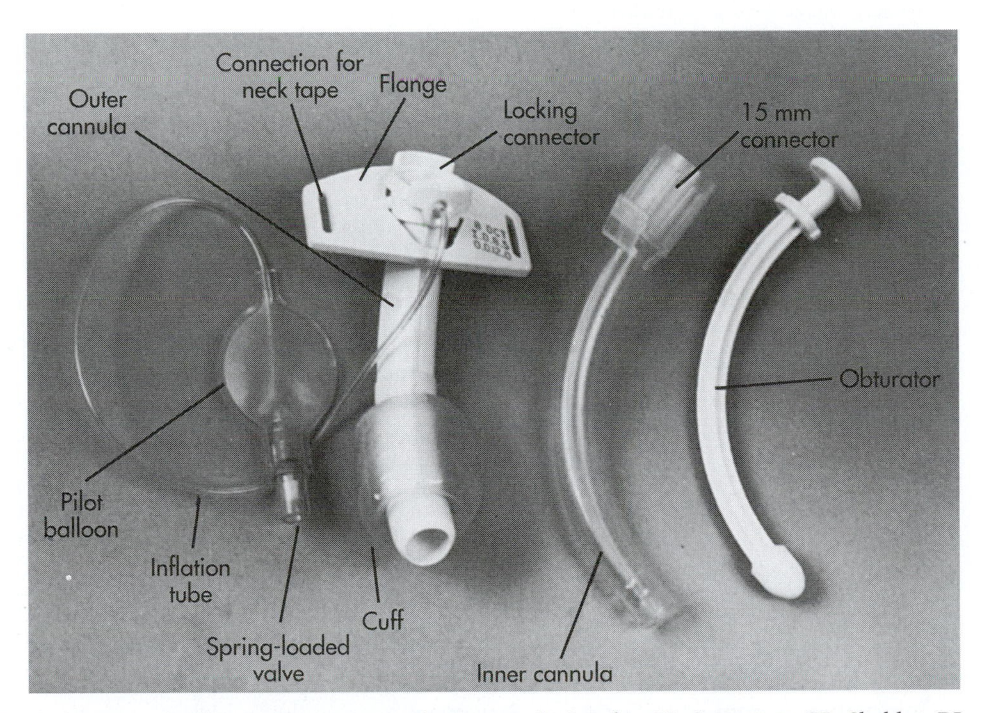

FIGURE 23-2. Tracheostomy tube. (From Simmons K: Airway care. In Scanlan CL, Spearman CB, Sheldon RL, editors: *Egan's fundamentals of respiratory care,* ed 6, St Louis, 1995, Mosby.)

TABLE 23-4 Tracheostomy Tubes: Complications, Causes, and Treatment

Complication	Causes	Prevention/Treatment
Hemorrhage	Vessels' opening after surgery Vessel erosion caused by tube	***Prevention:*** Use appropriate size tube. Treat local infection. Suction gently. Humidify inspired gases. Position tracheal window not lower than third tracheal ring. ***Treatment:*** Pack lightly. Perform surgical intervention.
Wound infection	Colonization of stoma with hospital flora	***Prevention:*** Perform routine stoma care. ***Treatment:*** Remove tube, if necessary. Perform aggressive wound care and debridement. Administer antibiotics.
Subcutaneous emphysema	Positive pressure ventilation Coughing against a tight, occlusive dressing or sutured or packed wound	***Prevention:*** Avoid suturing or packing wound closed around tube. ***Treatment:*** Remove any sutures or packing if present.
Tube obstruction	Dried blood or secretions False passage into soft tissues Opening of cannula positioned against tracheal wall Foreign body Tissue from tumor	***Prevention:*** Suction PRN. Humidify inspired gases. Use double-lumen tube. Position tube so that opening does not press against tracheal wall. ***Treatment:*** Remove/replace inner cannula. Replace tube.
Tube displacement	Patient movement Coughing Traction on ventilatory tubing	***Prevention:*** Tie tapes to allow only one finger width between the tape and neck. Suture tube in place. Use tubes with adjustable neck plates for patients with short necks. Support ventilator tubing. Sedate patient PRN. Restrain patient PRN. ***Treatment:*** Cover stoma and manually ventilate patient via mouth. Replace tube.
Tracheal stenosis	Injury to area from end of tube or cuff, resulting in scar tissue formation and narrowing of airway	***Prevention:*** Inflate cuff with minimal amount of air necessary. Monitor cuff pressures every 8 hours. ***Treatment:*** Perform surgical repair.

TABLE 23-4 Tracheostomy Tubes: Complications, Causes, and Treatment—cont'd

Complication	Causes	Prevention/Treatment
Tracheoesophageal fistula	Pressure necrosis of posterior tracheal wall resulting from overinflated cuff and rigid nasogastric tube	***Prevention:*** Inflate cuff with minimal amount of air necessary. Monitor cuff pressures every 8 hours. ***Treatment:*** Perform surgical repair.
Tracheoinnominate artery fistula	Direct pressure from the elbow of the cannula against the innominate artery Placement of tracheal stoma below fourth tracheal ring Downward migration of the tracheal stoma resulting from traction on tube High-lying innominate artery	***Prevention:*** Position tracheal window no lower than third tracheal ring. ***Treatment:*** Hyperinflate cuff to control bleeding. Remove tube and replace with endotracheal tube and apply digital pressure through stoma against the sternum. Perform surgical repair.
Tracheocutaneous fistula	Failure of stoma to close after removal of tube	***Treatment:*** Perform surgical repair.

Bubble humidifiers commonly are used to provide moisture to inhaled gas. They may be warm or cold humidifiers. With a cold humidifier, the gas diffuses out of a stem submerged in water, breaks into small bubbles, and vaporizes. At room temperature, the gas provides only approximately 50% of the humidification needed by the body. Therefore this method of humidification can lead to drying and irritation of mucous membranes when used for a significant length of time. Bubble humidifiers cannot humidify gas adequately at higher rates of flow, making them more suitable for low-flow oxygen delivery over short time spans. Cold humidifiers are relatively simple and reliable devices and are available as disposable units, thus decreasing maintenance time and eliminating the potential for infection associated with reusable equipment. Warm humidifiers provide better humidification than do cold humidifiers, because warm humidification supplies both heat and moisture and breaks gas into smaller particles at higher flow rates. Heated cascade humidifiers are preferred for use with intubated patients, because 100% humidification of inhaled gas can be ensured.[19]

Aerosol therapy. An aerosol is a liquid particle suspended in a gas. Distilled water or saline solutions often are used as liquid aerosol, but other solutions such as medications may be used. The inhalation of aerosols increases secretion clearance and liquefies mucus, but continuous administration of water aerosol can lead to water retention and fluid overload. Aerosol therapy must be used cautiously in patients with heart failure, respiratory distress, or decreased ability to clear secretions.[19]

The effects of aerosols on the respiratory tract depend on the level to which the aerosol penetrates the lungs. Penetration is related to particle size: particles of greater than 5 μm in diameter are deposited in the upper airway, whereas particles of less than 5 μm can reach the smaller airways. The patient's breathing pattern can affect penetration. Slower breathing results in more fallout deposition in the upper airways, whereas larger tidal volumes and mouth breathing can encourage deeper aerosol penetration. Aerosol deposition increases with momentary breath holding at peak inhalation.[19]

Aerosols are cleared from the lungs by the mucociliary blanket or by phagocytosis. Nebulizers often are used to deliver aerosols to patients with a respiratory disease involving mucus production. Nebulizers are classified by power source, aerosol production, and water production. The two most commonly used nebulizers are the jet nebulizer and the ultrasonic nebulizer. These devices may become a source of bacterial contamination of the respiratory tract and therefore require disinfection between patient uses.[19]

Cuff management. Because the cuff of the endotracheal or tracheostomy tube is a major source of the complications associated with artificial airways, proper

NURSING INTERVENTION CLASSIFICATIONS

BOX 23-2 Artificial Airway Management

DEFINITION: Maintenance of endotracheal and tracheostomy tubes and preventing complications associated with their use

ACTIVITIES:

Provide an oropharyngeal airway or bite block to prevent biting on the endotracheal tube, as appropriate
Provide 100% humidification of inspired gas/air
Provide adequate systemic hydration via oral or intravenous fluid administration
Inflate endotracheal/tracheostoma cuff using minimal occlusive volume technique or minimal leak technique
Maintain inflation of the endotracheal/tracheostoma cuff at 15 to 20 mm Hg during mechanical ventilation and during and after feeding
Suction the oropharynx and secretions from the top of the tube cuff before deflating cuff
Monitor cuff pressures every 4 to 8 hr during expiration using a three-way stopcock, calibrated syringe, and mercury manometer
Check cuff pressure immediately after delivery of any general anesthesia
Change endotracheal tapes/ties every 24 hr, inspect the skin and oral mucosa, and move ET tube to the other side of the mouth
Loosen commercial endotracheal tube holders at least once a day, and provide skin care
Auscultate for presence of lung sounds bilaterally after insertion and after changing endotracheal/tracheostomy ties
Note the centimeter reference marking on endotracheal tube to monitor for possible displacement
Assist with chest x-ray examination, as needed, to monitor position of tube
Minimize leverage and traction on the artificial airway by suspending ventilator tubing from overhead supports, using flexible catheter mounts and swivels, and supporting tubes during turning, suctioning, and ventilator disconnection and reconnection
Monitor for presence of crackles and rhonchi over large airways
Monitor for decrease in exhale volume and increase in inspiratory pressure in patients receiving mechanical ventilation
Institute endotracheal suctioning, as appropriate
Institute measures to prevent spontaneous decannulation: secure artificial airway with tape/ties; administer sedation and muscle paralyzing agent, as appropriate; and use arm restraints, as appropriate
Provide additional intubation equipment and ambu bag in a readily available location
Provide trach care every 4 to 8 hr as appropriate: clean the inner cannula, clean and dry the area around the stoma, and change tracheostomy ties
Inspect skin around tracheal stoma for drainage, redness, and irritation
Maintain sterile technique when suctioning and providing tracheostomy care
Shield the tracheostomy from water
Provide mouth care and suction oropharynx, as appropriate
Tape the tracheostomy obturator to head of bed
Tape a second tracheostomy (same type and size) and forceps to head of bed
Institute chest physiotherapy, as appropriate
Ensure that endotracheal/tracheostomy cuff is inflated during feedings, as appropriate
Elevate head of the bed or assist patient to a sitting position in a chair during feedings, as appropriate
Add food coloring to enteral feedings, as appropriate

From McCloskey JC, Bulechek GM: *Nursing interventions classification,* ed 2, St Louis, 1996, Mosby.

cuff management is essential. To prevent the complications associated with cuff design, only low-pressure, high-volume cuffed tubes are used in clinical practice.[9,20] Even with these tubes, cuff pressures can be generated that are high enough to lead to tracheal ischemia and injury. Both cuff-inflation techniques and cuff-pressure monitoring are critical components to the care of the patient with an artificial airway.[20]

Cuff-inflation techniques. Two different cuff-inflation techniques currently are being used—the minimal leak (ML) technique and the minimal occlusion volume (MOV) technique. The ML technique consists of injecting air into the cuff until no leak is heard and then withdrawing the air until a small leak is heard on inspiration.[21] Problems with this technique include difficulty maintaining positive end-expiratory pressure (PEEP),[9] aspiration around the cuff,[9,21] and increased movement of the tube in the trachea.[21] The MOV technique consists of injecting air into the cuff until no leak is heard, then withdrawing the air until a small leak is heard on inspiration, and then adding more air until no leak is heard on inspiration.[21] The problem with this technique is that it generates higher cuff pressures than does the ML technique.[22] The selection of one technique over the other must be determined for the individual patient. If the patient needs a seal to provide adequate ventilation and/or is at risk for aspiration, the MOV technique is used. If these are not concerns, the ML technique is used.[22]

Cuff-pressure monitoring. Cuff pressures are monitored at least every 8 hours with a mercury or aneroid manometer.[9,21,22] Cuff pressures are maintained at 18 to 22 mm Hg (25 to 30 cm H_2O), because greater pressures decrease blood flow to the capillaries in the tracheal wall and lesser pressures increase the risk of aspiration. Pressures in excess of 22 mm Hg (30 cm H_2O) must be reported to the physician. In addition, cuffs must not be routinely deflated, because this increases the risk of aspiration.[22]

Foam cuff tracheostomy tubes. One type of tracheostomy tube on the market has a cuff made of foam that is self-inflating. It is deflated during insertion, after which the pilot port is opened to atmospheric pressure (room air) and the cuff self-inflates. Once inflated the foam cuff conforms to the size and shape of the patient's trachea, thereby reducing the pressure against the tracheal wall. The pilot port is either left open to atmospheric pressure or attached to the mechanical ventilator tubing, thus allowing the cuff to inflate and deflate with the cycling of the ventilator. Routine maintenance of a foam cuff tracheostomy tube includes aspirating the pilot port every 8 hours to measure cuff volume, removing any condensation from the cuff area, and assessing the integrity of the cuff. Removal is accomplished by deflating the cuff and can be complicated if the plastic sheath covering the foam is perforated. When perforation occurs, the foam may not be deflatable because the air cannot be totally aspirated.[23]

Suctioning. Suctioning is often required to maintain a patent airway in the patient with an endotracheal or tracheostomy tube. Suctioning is a sterile procedure that is performed only when the patient needs it and not on a routine schedule. Indications for suctioning include coughing, respiratory distress, presence of rhonchi on auscultation, increased peak airway pressures on the ventilator, and decreasing Sao_2 or Pao_2 levels.[24] A number of complications are associated with suctioning, including hypoxemia, atelectasis, bronchospasms, cardiac dysrhythmias, hemodynamic alterations, increased intracranial pressure,[25] and airway trauma.[9]

Complications. Hypoxemia can result from disconnecting the oxygen source from the patient and/or removing the oxygen from the patient's airways when the suction is applied.[25] Atelectasis is thought to occur when the suction catheter is larger than one half of the diameter of the ETT. Excessive negative pressure occurs when suction is applied, promoting collapse of the distal airways.[25] Bronchospasms are the result of the stimulation of the airways with the suction catheter.[25] Cardiac dysrhythmias, particularly bradycardias, are attributed to vagal stimulation.[26] Some hemodynamic alterations—such as increases in mean arterial pressure, cardiac output, and pulmonary artery pressure—are the result of lung hyperinflation during the procedure.[27] Airway trauma occurs with impaction of the catheter in the airways and excessive negative pressure applied to the catheter.[25]

Suctioning protocol. A number of protocols regarding suctioning have been developed. Several different practices have been found helpful in limiting the complications of suctioning. Hypoxemia can be minimized by giving the patient three hyperoxygenated breaths (breaths at 100% Fio_2) with the ventilator before the procedure and after each pass of the suction catheter.[28] If the patient exhibits signs of desaturation, hyperinflation (breaths at 150% tidal volume) is added to the procedure.[29] Atelectasis can be avoided by using a suction catheter with an external diameter less than one half of the internal diameter of the ETT.[24,25] Using 100 mm Hg of suction or a flow rate of 15 to 20 L/minute will decrease the chances of hypoxemia and airway trauma.[25] Limiting the duration of each suction pass to 10 seconds and the number of passes to three or less also will help minimize hypoxemia, airway trauma, cardiac dysrhythmias, and hemodynamic alterations.[25,30] The process of applying intermittent, instead of continuous, suction has been shown to be of no benefit.[31] In addition, the instillation of normal saline to help remove secretions has not proved to be of any benefit[32] and may actually contribute to lower airway colonization with bacteria and development of nosocomial pneumonia.[33]

Closed tracheal suction system. One of the newer devices to facilitate suctioning the airway of a patient on the ventilator is the closed tracheal suction system (CTSS) (Figure 23-3). This device consists of

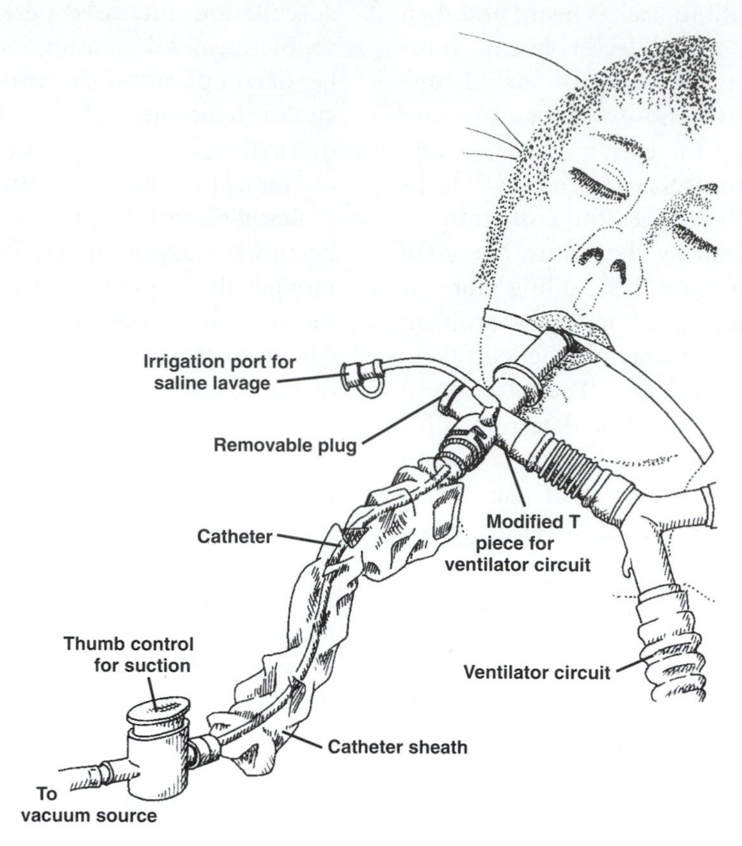

FIGURE 23-3. Closed tracheal suction system. (Sills JR: *Respiratory care certification guide,* St Louis, 1991, Mosby.)

a suction catheter in a plastic sleeve that attaches directly to the ventilator tubing. It allows the patient's airways to be suctioned while the patient remains on the ventilator. Advantages of the CTSS include the maintenance of oxygenation and PEEP during suctioning, the reduction of hypoxemia-related complications, and the protection of staff members from the patient's secretions. The CTSS is convenient to use, requiring only one person to perform the procedure. Concerns related to the CTSS include autocontamination, inadequate removal of secretions, and increased risk of unintentional extubation resulting from the extra weight of the system on the ventilator tubing. Autocontamination has been shown not to be an issue if the catheter is cleaned properly after every use and is changed every 24 hours. Inadequate removal of secretions may or may not be a problem, and further investigation is required to settle this issue.[34]

Communication. One of the major stressors for the patient with an artificial airway is impaired communication. This is related to the inability to speak, insufficient explanations from staff members, inadequate understanding, fear of being unable to communicate, and difficulty with communication methods.[35] A number of interventions can facilitate communication in the patient with an endotracheal or tracheostomy tube. These include performing a complete assessment of the patient's ability to communicate, teaching the patient how to communicate, using a variety of methods to communicate, and facilitating the patient's ability to communicate by providing the patient with his or her eyeglasses or hearing aid.[36]

A number of methods are available to facilitate communication in this patient population. These include the use of verbal and nonverbal language and a variety of devices to assist the short-term and long-term ventilator-assisted patient. Nonverbal communication may include the use of sign language, gestures, lip reading, pointing, facial expressions, or eye blinking. Simple devices available include pencil and paper; magic slates; magnetic boards with plastic letters; picture, alphabet, or symbol boards; and flash cards. More sophisticated devices include typewriters, computers, talking tracheostomy and endotracheal tubes, and external hand-held vibrators. Regardless of the method selected, the patient must be taught how to use the device.[36] Patients with ETTs are encour-

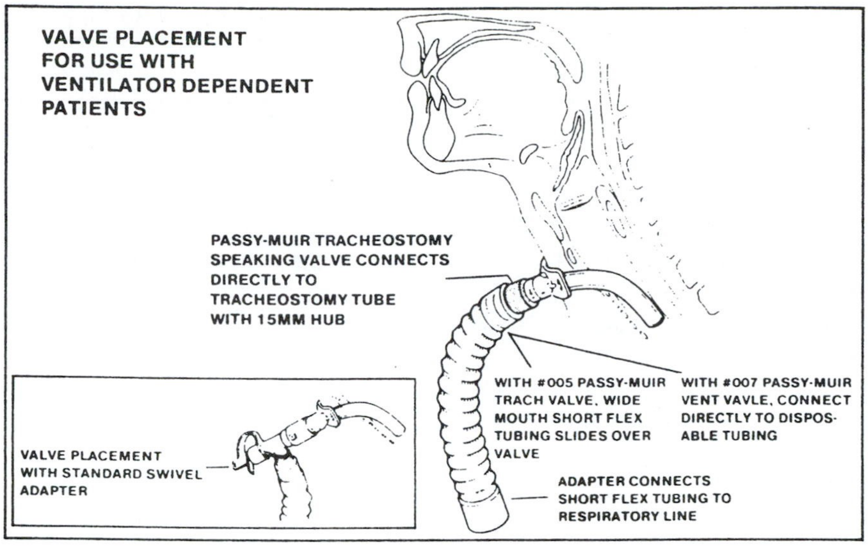

VALVE PLACEMENT FOR USE WITH VENTILATOR DEPENDENT PATIENTS

PASSY-MUIR TRACHEOSTOMY SPEAKING VALVE CONNECTS DIRECTLY TO TRACHEOSTOMY TUBE WITH 15MM HUB

WITH #005 PASSY-MUIR TRACH VALVE, WIDE MOUTH SHORT FLEX TUBING SLIDES OVER VALVE

WITH #007 PASSY-MUIR VENT VAVLE, CONNECT DIRECTLY TO DISPOSABLE TUBING

VALVE PLACEMENT WITH STANDARD SWIVEL ADAPTER

ADAPTER CONNECTS SHORT FLEX TUBING TO RESPIRATORY LINE

FIGURE 23-4. Passy-Muir valve. (Courtesy Passy-Muir, Inc., Irvine, Calif)

aged to communicate in writing, because attempts at speech cause tube movement and increase tracheal injury.[9]

Passy-Muir valve. One of the newer devices designed to assist the mechanically ventilated patient with a tracheostomy to speak is the Passy-Muir valve (Figure 23-4). This one-way valve opens on inhalation, allowing air to enter the lungs through the tracheostomy tube, and closes on exhalation, forcing air over the vocal cords and out the mouth, thus permitting the patient to speak. Before placing the valve on a tracheostomy tube, the cuff must be deflated to allow air to pass around the tube, and the tidal volume of the ventilator must be increased to compensate for the air leak. In addition to assisting the patient to communicate, the Passy-Muir valve can assist the ventilator-dependent patient with relearning normal breathing patterns. The valve is contraindicated in patients with laryngeal and pharyngeal dysfunction, excessive secretions, and poor lung compliance.[37]

Extubation. Once the airway is no longer needed, it is removed. Extubation is the process of removing an endotracheal tube. It is a simple procedure that can be accomplished at the bedside (Box 23-3).[9] Complications of extubation include glottic edema, laryngeal dysfunction, sore throat and hoarseness, and vocal cord paralysis. Decannulation is the process of removing a tracheostomy tube. It is also a simple process that can be performed at the bedside. After the removal of a tracheostomy tube, the stoma is usually covered with a dry dressing, with the expectation that it will close within several days.[38]

INVASIVE MECHANICAL VENTILATION

Indications

Mechanical ventilation is indicated for a variety of physiologic and clinical reasons. Physiologic objectives include supporting cardiopulmonary gas exchange (alveolar ventilation and arterial oxygenation), increasing lung volume (end-expiratory lung inflation and functional residual capacity), and reducing the work of breathing. Clinical objectives include reversing hypoxemia and acute respiratory acidosis, relieving respiratory distress, preventing or reversing atelectasis, reversing ventilatory muscle fatigue, permitting sedation and/or neuromuscular blockade, decreasing systemic or myocardial oxygen consumption, reducing intracranial pressure, and stabilizing the chest wall.[39] (Mechanical Ventilation Concepts; Mechanical Ventilation: Nursing Management.)

Types of Ventilators

The two main types of ventilators currently available are positive-pressure ventilators and negative-pressure ventilators. Negative-pressure ventilators are applied externally to the patient and decrease the atmospheric pressure surrounding the thorax to initiate inspiration. They are not commonly used in the critical care environment. Positive-pressure ventilators use a mechanical drive mechanism to force oxygen into the patient's lungs through an endotracheal or tracheostomy tube to initiate respiration.[40]

Phase variables. There are four phases of ventilation that the ventilator must complete to properly ventilate a patient: (1) change from expiration to

NURSING INTERVENTION CLASSIFICATIONS

BOX 23-3 Endotracheal Extubation

DEFINITION: Purposeful removal of the endotracheal tube from the nasopharyngeal or oropharyngeal airway

ACTIVITIES:

Position the patient for best use of ventilatory muscles, usually with the head of the bed elevated 75 degrees
Instruct patient about the procedure
Hyperoxygenate the patient and suction the endotracheal airway
Suction the oral airway
Deflate the endotracheal cuff and remove the endotracheal tube
Encourage the patient to cough and expectorate sputum
Administer oxygen as ordered
Encourage coughing and deep breathing
Suction the airway, as needed
Monitor for respiratory distress
Observe for signs of airway occlusion
Monitor vital signs
Encourage voice rest for 4 to 8 hr, as appropriate
Monitor ability to swallow and talk

From McCloskey JC, Bulechek GM: *Nursing interventions classification,* ed 2, St Louis, 1996, Mosby.

inspiration; (2) inspiration; (3) change from inspiration to expiration; and (4) expiration. The ventilator uses four different variables to begin, sustain, and terminate each of these phases. These phase variables are known as *volume, pressure, flow,* and *time.*

The variable that causes inspiration is called the *trigger.* Breaths may be pressure-triggered or flow-triggered, based on the sensitivity setting of the ventilator and the patient's inspiratory effort (patient-triggered), or breaths may be time-triggered, based on the rate setting of the ventilator (machine-triggered). The variable that changes inspiration to expiration is called the *cycle.*[41] There are four classifications of positive-pressure ventilators based on the cycle variable: volume-cycled, pressure-cycled, flow-cycled, and time-cycled.[40,41] Volume-cycled ventilators are designed to deliver a breath until a preset volume is delivered. Pressure-cycled ventilators deliver a breath until a preset pressure is reached within the patient's airway. Flow-cycled ventilators deliver a breath until a preset inspiratory flow rate is achieved. Time-cycled ventilators deliver a breath over a preset time interval. Most of the newer ventilators are capable of using a variety of cycling mechanisms.[40] Figure 23-5 depicts three commonly used ventilators in critical care.

Modes of Ventilation

The term *ventilator mode* refers to how the machine ventilates the patient. In other words, selection of a particular mode of ventilation determines how much the patient will participate in his or her own ventilatory pattern. The choice depends on the patient's situation and the goals of treatment. A large variety of modes are available (Table 23-5).[39,40,43-45] Many of these modes may be used in conjunction with each other. Because brands of ventilators vary in their ability to perform certain functions, not all modes are available on all ventilators.[42]

Ventilator Settings

A variety of settings on the ventilator allows the ventilator parameters to be individualized to the patient and the mode of ventilation selected (see Table 23-6).[39,46] In addition, each ventilator has a patient-monitoring system that allows all aspects of the patient's ventilatory pattern to be assessed, monitored, and displayed. These monitoring capabilities include exhaled minute volume, exhaled tidal volume, total respiratory rate, peak pressure, plateau pressure, PEEP, mean airway pressure, spontaneous minute volume, spontaneous respiratory rate, circuit temperature, FIO_2, inspired tidal volume, pressure waveform, flow waveform, auto-PEEP, and respiratory mechanics. Monitoring capabilities vary slightly from one brand of ventilator to another.[43]

Complications

Mechanical ventilation is often lifesaving, but similar to other interventions, it is not without complications. Some complications are preventable, whereas

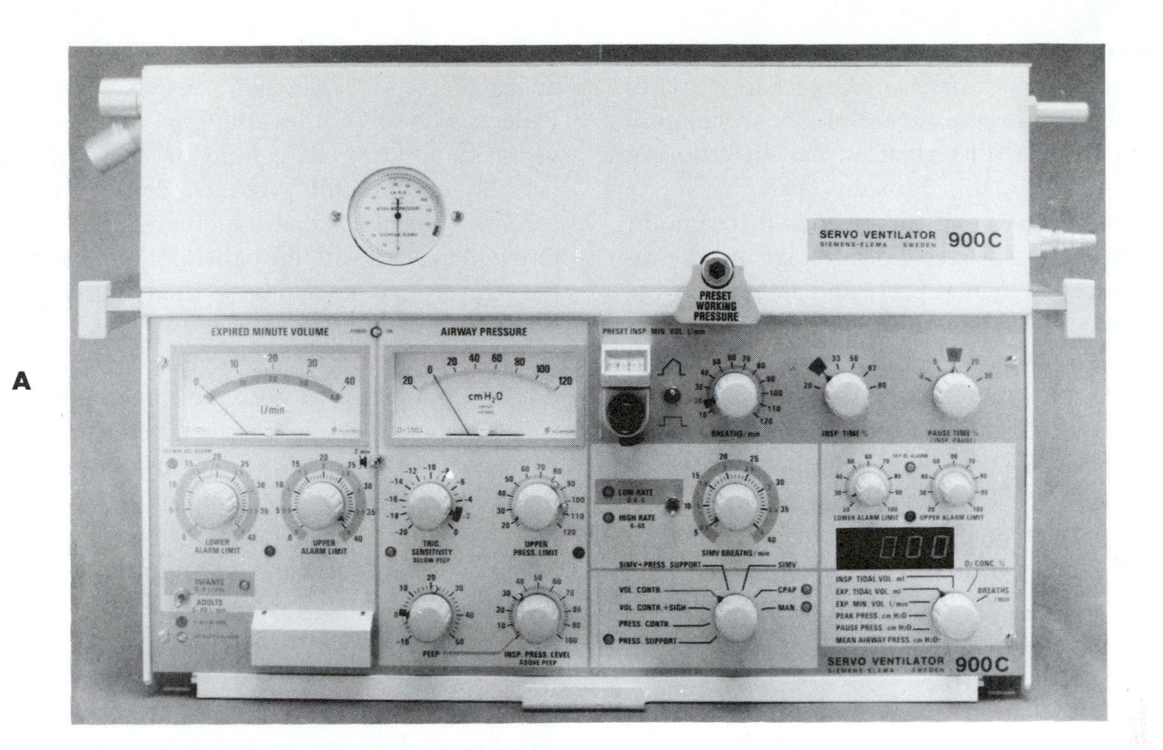

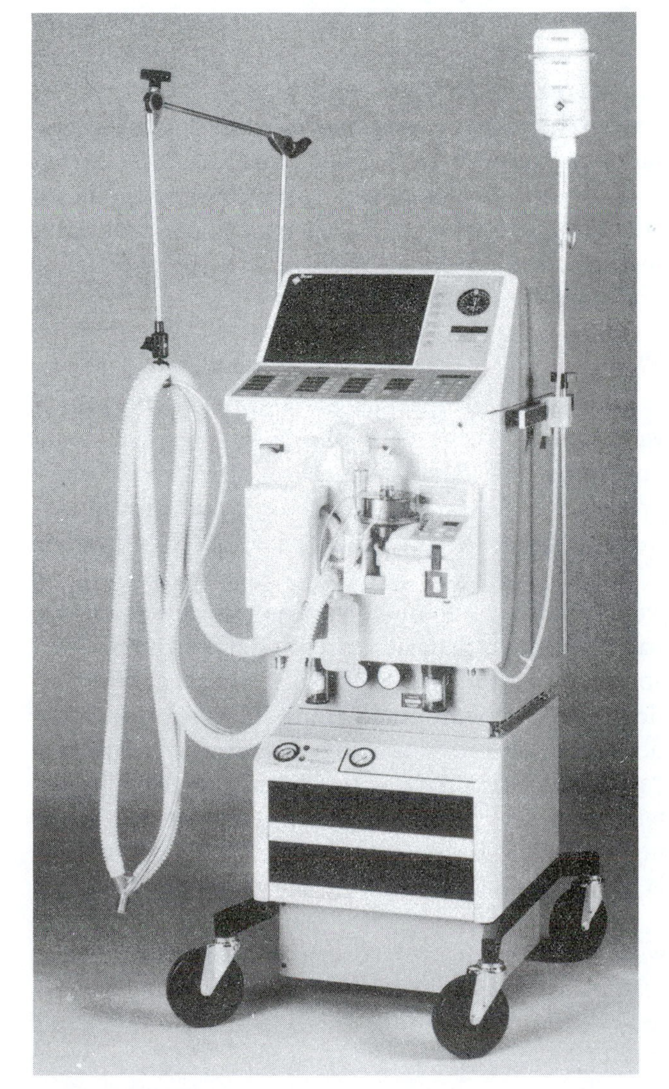

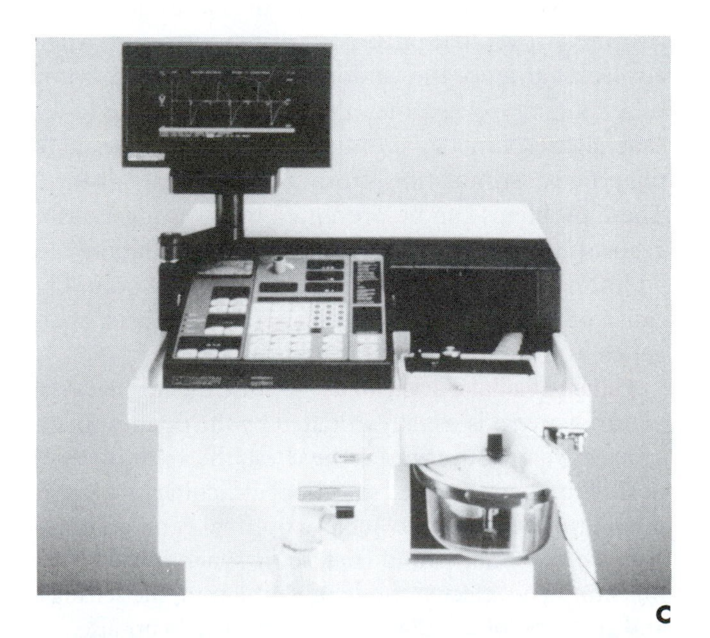

FIGURE 23-5. Three types of volume-cycled ventilators. **A,** Servo 900C ventilator. **B,** BEAR 5 ventilator. **C,** Puritan-Bennett 7200 microprocessor ventilator. (From Dupuis YG: *Ventilators: theory and clinical application,* ed 2, St Louis, 1992, Mosby.)

others can be minimized but not eradicated. Physiologic complications associated with mechanical ventilation include barotrauma, cardiovascular compromise, gastrointestinal disturbances, patient-ventilator asynchrony, and nosocomial pneumonia.

Barotrauma. Barotrauma occurs in mechanically ventilated patients as a result of alveolar overdistention. This causes alveolar rupture and air leakage into the pulmonary interstitial space. Once in the space, the air travels out through the hilum and into the mediastinum (pneumomediastinum), pleural space (pneumothorax), subcutaneous tissues (subcutaneous emphysema), pericardium (pneumopericardium), peritoneum (pneumoperitoneum), and retroperitoneum (pneumoretroperitoneum). The resultant disorders vary from the fairly benign to the potentially lethal. The two most lethal of which are a pneumothorax and a pneumopericardium resulting in cardiac tamponade.[39,47,48] (∞Air Leak Syndromes, p. 673.)

Cardiovascular compromise. Positive-pressure ventilation increases intrathoracic pressure, which decreases venous return to the right side of the heart. Impaired venous return decreases preload, which results in a decrease in CO. As a secondary consequence, hepatic and renal dysfunction may occur. In addition, positive-pressure ventilation impairs cerebral venous return. In patients with impaired autoregulation, positive-pressure ventilation can result in increased intracranial pressure.[39,47,48]

Gastrointestinal disturbances. A number of gastrointestinal disturbances can also occur as a result of positive pressure ventilation. Gastric distention occurs when air leaks around the endotracheal or tracheostomy tube cuff and overcomes the resistance of the lower esophageal sphincter.[48] Vomiting can occur as a result of pharyngeal stimulation from the artificial airway.[39] These problems can be prevented by inserting a nasogastric tube and ensuring appropriate cuff inflation.[48] In addition hypomotility and constipation may occur because of the administration of paralytic agents, analgesics, and sedatives and immobility.[39]

Patient-ventilator asynchrony. Because the normal ventilatory pattern is usually initiated by the establishment of negative pressure within the chest, the application of positive pressure can lead to patient difficulties in breathing on the ventilator. To achieve optimal ventilatory assistance, the patient should breathe in synchrony with the machine. The selected mode of ventilation, the settings, and the type of ventilatory circuitry used can also increase the work of breathing and lead to the patient breathing out of synchrony with the ventilator. Patient-ventilator asynchrony can result in a decrease in effectiveness of mechanical ventilation, the development of auto-PEEP, and psychologic distress for the patient. Patients who are not breathing in synchrony with the ventilator appear to be fighting or "bucking" the ventilator. To minimize this problem, adjust the ventilator to accommodate the patient's spontaneous breathing pattern and to work with the patient. If this is not possible, the patient may need to be sedated and/or pharmacologically paralyzed.[39]

Nosocomial pneumonia. There is great potential for the development of nosocomial pneumonia after the placement of an artificial airway, because the tube bypasses or impairs many of the lungs' normal defense mechanisms. Once an artificial airway is placed, contamination of the lower airways follows within 24 hours. This results from a number of factors that directly and indirectly promote airway colonization. The use of respiratory therapy devices (e.g., ventilators, nebulizers, and intermittent positive-pressure breathing machines) can also increase the risk of pneumonia. The severity of the patient's illness, presence of acute lung injury, or malnutrition significantly increases the likelihood that an infection will ensue. In addition, therapeutic measures such as nasogastric tubes, antacids, and histamine inhibitors facilitate the development of pneumonia. Nasogastric tubes promote aspiration by acting as a wick for stomach contents, whereas antacids and histamine inhibitors increase the pH level of the stomach, thus promoting the growth of bacteria that can then be aspirated.[20] (∞Pneumonia, p. 663.)

Weaning

Weaning is the gradual withdrawal of mechanical ventilation and the reestablishment of spontaneous breathing.[39] Weaning begins only after the original process that necessitated ventilator support for the patient has been corrected and patient stability has been achieved.[49] Other factors to consider when weaning are length of time on ventilator, sleep deprivation, and nutritional status. Major factors that affect the patient's ability to wean include the ability of the lungs to participate in ventilation and respiration, cardiovascular performance, and psychologic readiness.[39] This discussion focuses on weaning the patient from short-term (3 or fewer days) mechanical ventilation. Weaning the patient from long-term mechanical ventilation is discussed in Chapter 22.

Readiness to wean. Once the decision is made to wean the patient, an assessment of the patient's readiness to wean is performed. Two strong predictors for weaning readiness are vital capacity (VC)/kg

TABLE 23-5 Modes of Mechanical Ventilation

Mode of Ventilation	Clinical Application	Nursing Implications
Control (volume or pressure) ventilation (CV)—delivers gas at preset rate and tidal volume or pressure (depending on selected cycling variable), regardless of patient's inspiratory efforts	CV is used as the primary ventilatory mode in patients who are apneic	Used in patients unable to initiate a breath Spontaneously breathing patients must be sedated and/or paralyzed
Assist-control (volume or pressure) ventilation (A/C) or continuous mandatory ventilation (CMV)—delivers gas at preset tidal volume or pressure (depending on selected cycling variable) in response to patient's inspiratory efforts and will initiate breath if patient fails to do so within preset time	A/C or CMV is used as the primary mode of ventilation in spontaneously breathing patients with weak respiratory muscles	Hyperventilation can occur in patients with increased respiratory rates Sedation may be necessary to limit the number of spontaneous breaths
Synchronous intermittent mandatory (volume or pressure) ventilation (SIMV)—delivers gas at preset tidal volume or pressure (depending on selected cycling variable) and rate while allowing patient to breathe spontaneously; ventilator breaths are synchronized to patient's respiratory effort	SIMV is used both as a primary mode of ventilation in a wide variety of clinical situations and as a weaning mode	May increase the work of breathing and promote respiratory muscle fatigue
Positive end-expiratory pressure (PEEP)—positive pressure applied at the end of expiration of ventilator breaths (used with CV, A/C, and SIMV) Constant positive airway pressure (CPAP)—positive pressure applied during spontaneous breaths	PEEP and CPAP are used in patients with hypoxemia refractory to oxygen therapy; they increase functional residual capacity and improve oxygenation by opening collapsed alveoli at end expiration	Side effects include decreased cardiac output, barotrauma, and increased intracranial pressure No ventilator breaths are delivered in PEEP and CPAP mode unless it is used with CV, A/C, or SIMV
Pressure support ventilation (PSV)—preset positive pressure used to augment patient's inspiratory efforts; patient controls rate, inspiratory flow, and tidal volume Volume-assured pressure support ventilation (VAPSV)—tidal volume is set to ensure patient receives minimum tidal volume with each pressure support breath	PSV is used as the primary mode of ventilation in patients with stable respiratory drive, is used with SIMV to support spontaneous breaths, and is used as a weaning mode in patients who are difficult to wean	Advantages include increased patient comfort, decreased work of breathing and respiratory muscle fatigue, and promotion of respiratory muscle conditioning
Independent lung ventilation (ILV)—each lung is ventilated separately	ILV is used in patients with unilateral lung disease, bronchopleural fistulas, and bilateral asymmetric lung disease	Requires a double-lumen endotracheal tube, two ventilators, sedation, and/or pharmacologic paralysis

Continued

TABLE 23-5 Modes of Mechanical Ventilation—cont'd

Mode of Ventilation	Clinical Application	Nursing Implications
High frequency ventilation (HFV)—delivers a small volume of gas at a rapid rate High-frequency positive-pressure ventilation (HFPPV)—delivers 60-100 breaths/min High-frequency jet ventilation (HFJV)—delivers 100-600 cycles/min High-frequency oscillation (HFO)—delivers 900-3000 cycles/min	HFV is used in situations in which conventional mechanical ventilation compromises hemodynamic stability, with bronchopleural fistulas, during short-term procedures, and with diseases that create a risk of barotrauma	Patients require sedation and/or pharmacologic paralysis Inadequate humidification can compromise airway patency Assessment of breath sounds is difficult
Inverse ratio ventilation (IRV)—proportion of inspiratory to expiratory time is greater than 1:1; can be initiated using pressure-controlled breaths (PC-IRV) or volume controlled breaths (VC-IRV)	IRV is used in patients with hypoxemia refractory to PEEP; the longer inspiratory time increases functional residual capacity and improves oxygenation by opening collapsed alveoli, and the shorter expiratory time induces auto-PEEP that prevents alveoli from recollapsing	Requires sedation and/or pharmacologic paralysis because of discomfort Increased intrathoracic pressure can result in excessive air trapping and decreased cardiac output

TABLE 23-6 Ventilator Settings

Parameter	Description
Respiratory rate (f)	Number of breaths the ventilator delivers per minute; usual setting is 4-20 breaths/min
Tidal volume (V_T)	Volume of gas delivered to patient during each ventilator breath; usual volume is 5-15 ml/kg
Oxygen concentration (FIO_2)	Fraction of inspired oxygen delivered to patient; may be set between 21% and 100%; usually adjusted to maintain PaO_2 level greater than 60 mm Hg or SaO_2 level greater than 90%
I:E ratio	Duration of inspiration to duration of expiration; usual setting is 1:2 to 1:1.5 unless IRV is desired
Flow rate	Speed with which the tidal volume is delivered; usual setting is 40-100 L/min
Sensitivity/trigger	Determines the amount of effort the patient must generate to initiate a ventilator breath; it may be set for pressure-triggering or flow-triggering; usual setting for a pressure-trigger is 0.5-1.5 cm H_2O below baseline pressure and for a flow-trigger is 1-3 L/min below baseline flow
Pressure limit	Regulates the maximal pressure the ventilator can generate to deliver the tidal volume; when the pressure limit is reached, the ventilator terminates the breath and spills the undelivered volume into the atmosphere; usual setting is 10-20 cm H_2O above peak inspiratory pressure

IRV, Inverse ratio ventilation.

greater than or equal to 15 ml and a negative inspiratory pressure (NIP) of −30 cm H_2O or less. Other weaker predictors of weaning readiness include a spontaneous minute volume greater than or equal to 10 L/minute, maximum voluntary ventilation (MVV) equal to at least twice the minute ventilation (V_E), a PaO_2 level of 50 mm Hg or greater, a low mean arterial pressure, an arterial pH level greater than 7.35, a respiratory rate (f) of less than 25 breaths/minute, a tidal volume (V_T) greater than 300 ml (rapid, swallow breathing index), inspiratory work per minute (W_I/minute) less than or equal to 1.6 kg-m, and inspiratory work per liter of minute ventilation (W_I/L) less than or equal to 0.14 kg-m (work of breathing indices).[50]

Once readiness to wean has been established, the patient is prepared for the weaning trial. The patient is positioned upright to facilitate breathing and the airway suctioned to ensure airway patency. In addition, the process is explained to the patient and the patient is offered reassurance and diversional activities. The patient is assessed immediately before the start of the trial and frequently during the weaning period for signs of weaning intolerance (Box 23-4).[49]

Weaning methods. A number of methods can be used to wean a patient from the ventilator. The method selected depends on the patient, his or her pulmonary status, and the length of time on the ventilator. The three main methods for weaning are T-tube (T-piece) trials, synchronous intermittent mandatory ventilation (SIMV), and pressure support ventilation (PSV).[39]

T-tube. T-tube trials consist of alternating periods of ventilatory support (usually on assist/control [A/C] or continuous mandatory ventilation [CMV]) with periods of spontaneous breathing. The trial is initiated by removing the patient from the ventilator and having him or her breathe spontaneously on a T-tube. After a duration of time, the patient is placed back on the ventilator. The goal is to progressively increase the duration of time spent off the ventilator. During the weaning process the patient is observed closely for respiratory muscle fatigue.[39,49] Constant positive airway pressure (CPAP) may be added to prevent atelectasis and to improve oxygenation.[49]

SIMV. The goal of SIMV weaning is the gradual transition from ventilatory support to spontaneous breathing. It is initiated by placing the ventilator in the SIMV mode and slowly decreasing the rate until zero (or close) is reached. The rate is usually decreased one to three breaths at a time, and an arterial blood gas (ABG) analysis is usually obtained 30 minutes afterward. This method of weaning can increase the work of breathing, and thus the patient is closely monitored for signs of respiratory muscle fatigue.[39,49]

PSV. PSV weaning consists of placing the patient on the pressure support mode and setting the pressure support at a level that facilitates the patient achieving a spontaneous tidal volume of 10 to 12 ml/kg. PSV augments the patient's spontaneous breaths with a positive-pressure "boost" during inspiration. During the weaning process the level of pressure support is gradually decreased in increments of 3 to 5 cm H_2O while maintaining a tidal volume or 10 to 15 ml/kg until a level of 5 cm H_2O is achieved. If the patient is able to maintain adequate spontaneous respirations at this level, extubation is considered. PSV can also be used with SIMV weaning to help overcome the resistance in the ventilator system.[49]

BOX 23-4 Weaning Intolerance Indicators

Decrease in level of consciousness
Diastolic blood pressure >100 mm Hg
Fall in systolic blood pressure
Heart rate > 110 beats/min or > 20 beats/min increase over baseline
f > 30/min or > 10/min increase over baseline
VT < 250-300 ml
pH level < 7.35
Pa_{CO_2} level increased by 8 mm Hg
Premature ventricular contractions > 6 per minute or salvos
Changes in ST segment (usually elevation)
Ventricular conduction changes

From Weilitz PB: *Crit Care Nurs* 13(4):33, 1993.

Nursing Management

Nursing management of the patient on a ventilator is outlined in Box 23-5. Routine assessment of a patient on a ventilator includes monitoring the patient for both patient-related and ventilator-related complications. It includes a routine total assessment, with particular emphasis on the pulmonary system, placement of the endotracheal tube, and observation for subcutaneous emphysema and synchrony with the ventilator. Assessment of the ventilator includes a review of all the ventilator settings and alarms.

Bedside evaluation of vital capacity, minute ventilation, ABG values, and other pulmonary function tests may be warranted, according to the patient's condition. The use of pulse oximetry can facilitate continuous, noninvasive assessment of oxygenation. Static and dynamic compliance is also monitored to assess for changes in lung compliance (see Appendix D).

Some additional measures are required to maintain a trouble-free ventilator system. These include maintaining a functional MRB connected to oxygen at the bedside, ensuring that the ventilator tubing is free of water, positioning the ventilator tubing to avoid kinking, maintaining the patency of ventilator tubing and connections, changing ventilator tubing per hospital

NURSING INTERVENTION CLASSIFICATIONS

BOX 23-5 Mechanical Ventilation

DEFINITION: Use of an artificial device to assist a patient to breathe

ACTIVITIES:

Monitor for respiratory muscle fatigue
Monitor for impending respiratory failure
Consult with other health care personnel in selection of a ventilator mode
Initiate setup and application of the ventilator
Instruct the patient and family about the rationale and expected sensations associated with use of mechanical ventilators
Routinely monitor ventilator settings
Monitor for decrease in exhale volume and increase in inspiratory pressure
Ensure that ventilator alarms are on
Administer muscle-paralyzing agents, sedatives, and narcotic analgesics, as appropriate
Monitor the effectiveness of mechanical ventilation on patient's physiological and psychological status
Initiate calming techniques, as appropriate
Provide patient with a means for communication (e.g., paper and pencil or alphabet board)
Check all ventilator connections regularly
Empty condensed water from water traps, as appropriate
Ensure change of ventilator circuits every 24 hr, as appropriate
Use aseptic technique, as appropriate
Monitor ventilator pressure readings and breath sounds
Stop NG feedings during suctioning and 30 to 60 min before chest physiotherapy
Silence ventilator alarms during suctioning to decrease frequency of false alarms
Monitor patient's progress on current ventilator settings and make appropriate changes as ordered
Monitor for adverse effects of mechanical ventilation: infection, barotrauma, and reduced cardiac output
Position to facilitate ventilation/perfusion matching ("good lung down"), as appropriate
Collaborate with physician to use CPAP or PEEP to minimize alveolar hypoventilation, as appropriate
Perform chest physical therapy, as appropriate
Perform suctioning, based on presence of adventitious sounds and/or increased ventilatory pressures
Promote adequate fluid and nutritional intake
Provide routine oral care
Monitor effects of ventilator changes on oxygenation: ABG, Sa_{O_2}, Sv_{O_2}, end-tidal CO_2, Q_{sp}/Q_t, and $A\text{-}a_{DO_2}$ levels and patient's subjective response
Monitor degree of shunt, vital capacity, V_D/V_T, MVV, inspiratory force, and FEV_1 for readiness to wean from mechanical ventilation, based on agency protocol

From McCloskey JC, Bulechek GM: *Nursing interventions classification,* ed 2, St Louis, 1996, Mosby.

policy, and monitoring the temperature of the inspired air. In addition, a clear understanding of the alarms and their related problems is important (Table 23-7). In the event that the ventilator malfunctions, the patient is removed from the ventilator and ventilated manually with an MRB.

NONINVASIVE MECHANICAL VENTILATION

Noninvasive mechanical ventilation is a relatively new method of ventilation that uses a mask, instead of an endotracheal tube, to administer positive pressure. Advantages of this type of ventilation include decreased frequency of nosocomial pneumonia; increased comfort; and its noninvasive nature, which allows easy application and removal. It is indicated in a variety of situations, including acute hypercapnia respiratory failure, acute hypoxemic respiratory failure, and when intubation is not an option. Contraindications to noninvasive mechanical ventilation include hemodynamic instability; dysrhythmias; apnea; uncooperativeness; intolerance of the mask; and the inability to maintain a patent airway, clear secretions, and properly fit the mask.[51]

RESEARCH ABSTRACT

Interactions between nurses and patients on ventilators.

Hall D: *Am J Crit Care,* 5(4):293, 1996.

PURPOSE

The purpose of this study was to examine the interactions between nurses and patients on ventilators and the relationship between characteristics of these nurses and their communication with patients.

DESIGN

Cross-sectional, experimental.

SAMPLE

The sample consisted of 30 registered nurses who were not in orientation, did not have any communication handicaps, and were assigned to a patient on a ventilator in a medical or surgical intensive care unit of a university-affiliated hospital. Only 10% of the nurses were the primary nurse for the patient; 50% were prepared at the baccalaureate or graduate level.

PROCEDURE

Nurse communication was measured by the Categories of Nurse-Patient Interaction Content scale, and patient responsiveness was assessed using the Glasgow Coma Scale (GCS). One data collector gathered information for a 30-minute interval during mornings or evenings. The data collector was positioned to easily observe the nurse-patient interaction, but the data collection was not obvious to the study subjects. After being observed, subjects were asked to complete a demographic questionnaire and to evaluate the patient's responsiveness using the GCS.

RESULTS

Significant correlations were found between the nurse's perceptions of the patient's degree of responsiveness and the number of positive and negative interactions with the patient ($p < .05$) and between the length of time the nurse had cared for the patient and the number of positive reactions from nurse to patient ($p < .05$). There was no significant difference between the length of time the nurse was assigned to the patient and the number of positive and negative actions by the nurse. Higher GCS scores were associated with more positive reactions from the nurse to the patient ($p < .05$). Higher GCS scores were also related to fewer negative actions from nurse to patient ($p < .05$). Positive actions were the most common pattern of communication (63%); negative actions were less common (25%); positive reactions occurred 11% of the time, and negative reactions occurred only 0.2% of the time.

DISCUSSION/IMPLICATIONS

Findings from this study indicate that nurses' positive interactions with ventilated patients are related to the degree of perceived responsiveness from those patients. Patterns of communication illustrate that nurses spend more time giving information to patients that nurses feel is important, rather than assessing and responding to patients' needs. Nurses displayed few positive actions and reactions, even with those patients who had higher GCS scores. It is important to identify and address patient needs to provide patient-centered care. Facilitating communication between nurse and patient is an essential element of care and needs to be supported through the identification of factors that may hinder communication. By identifying barriers to communication and enhancing communication, quality of care and services will be maintained or increased.

Noninvasive mechanical ventilation can be applied using a nasal or facial mask and ventilator or a BiPAP (trademark of Respironics) machine. This mode of therapy uses a combination of PSV (ventilator) or inspiratory positive airway pressure (IPAP) (BiPAP machine) and PEEP (ventilator) or expiratory positive airway pressure (EPAP) (BiPAP machine) to assist the spontaneously breathing patient with ventilation. On inspiration the patient receives PSV or IPAP to increase tidal volume and minute ventilation, which results in increased alveolar ventilation, a decreased $Paco_2$ level, relief of dyspnea, and reduced accessory muscle use. On expiration the patient receives PEEP or EPAP to increase functional residual capacity, which results in an increased Pao_2 level. Humidified supplemental oxygen is administered to maintain a clinically acceptable Pao_2 level, and timed breaths may be added if necessary.[51]

Nursing Management

As with invasive mechanical ventilation, the patient must be closely monitored while receiving noninvasive mechanical ventilation. Respiratory rate, accessory muscle use, and oxygenation status are continually assessed to ensure that the patient is tolerating this method of ventilation. Continued pulse oximetry with a set alarm parameter is initiated.[51]

The key to ensuring adequate ventilatory support is a properly fitted mask. Either a nasal mask or a full face mask may be used, depending on the patient. A

TABLE 23-7 Troubleshooting Ventilator Alarms

Problem	Causes	Interventions
Low exhaled VT	Altered settings; any condition that triggers high or low pressure alarm; patient stops spontaneous respirations; leak in system preventing VT from being delivered; cuff insufficiently inflated; leak through chest tube; airway secretions; decreased lung compliance; spirometer disconnected or malfunctioning	Check settings; evaluate patient, check respiratory rate; check all connections for leaks; suction patient's airway; check cuff pressure; calibrate spirometer
Low inspiratory pressure	Altered settings; unattached tubing or leak around ET tube; ET tube displaced into pharynx or esophagus; poor cuff inflation or leak; tracheal-esophageal fistula; peak flows that are too low; low VTs; decreased airway resistance resulting from decreased secretions or relief of bronchospasm; increased lung compliance resulting from decreased atelectasis; reduction in pulmonary edema; resolution of ARDS; change in position	Reset alarm; reconnect tubing; modify cuff pressures; tighten humidifier; check chest tube; adjust peak flow to meet or exceed patient demand and correct for the patient's VT; reposition or change ET tube
Low exhaled minute volume	Altered settings; leak in system; airway secretions; decreased lung compliance; malfunctioning spirometer; decreased patient-triggered respiratory rate resulting from drugs; sleep; hypocapnia; alkalosis; fatigue; change in neurological status	Check settings; assess patient's respiratory rate, mental status, and work of breathing; evaluate system for leaks; suction airway; assess patient for changes in disease state; calibrate spirometer
Low PEEP/CPAP pressure	Altered settings; increased patient inspiratory flows; leak; decreased expiratory flows from ventilator	Check settings and correct; observe for leaks in system; if unable to correct problem, increase PEEP setting
High respiratory rate	Increased metabolic demand; drug administration; hypoxia; hypercapnia; acidosis; shock; pain; fear; anxiety	Evaluate ABGs; assess patient; calm and reassure patient
High pressure limit	Improper alarm setting; airway obstruction resulting from patient fighting ventilator (holding breath as ventilator delivers VT); patient circuit collapse; tubing kinked; ET tube in right mainstem bronchus or against carina; cuff herniation; increased airway resistance resulting from bronchospasm, airway secretions, plugs, and coughing; water from humidifier in ventilator tubing; decreased lung compliance resulting from tension pneumothorax; change in patient position; ARDS; pulmonary edema; atelectasis; pneumonia; or abdominal distention.	Reset alarms; clear obstruction from tubing; unkink and reposition patient off of tubing; empty water from tubing; check breath sounds; reassure patient and sedate if necessary; check ABGs for hypoxemia; observe for abdominal distention that would put pressure on the diaphragm; check cuff pressures; obtain chest x-ray and evaluate for ET tube position, pneumothorax, and pneumonia; reposition ET tube; give bronchodilator therapy
Low pressure oxygen inlet	Improper oxygen alarm setting; oxygen not connected to ventilator; dirty oxygen intake filter	Correct alarm setting; reconnect or connect oxygen line to a 50 psi source; clean or replace oxygen filter
I:E ratio	Inspiratory time longer than expiratory time; use of an inspiratory phase that is too long with a fast rate; peak flow setting too low while rate too high; machine too sensitive	Change inspiratory time or adjust peak flow; check inspiratory phase, or hold; check machine sensitivity
Temperature	Sensor malfunction; overheating resulting from too low or no gas flow; sensor picking up outside airflow (from heaters, open doors or windows, air conditioners); improper water levels	Test or replace sensor; check gas flow; protect sensor from outside source that would interfere with readings; check water levels

Modified from Flynn JBM, Bruce NP: *Introduction to critical care nursing skills,* St Louis, 1993, Mosby.

properly fitted mask minimizes discomfort for the patient and air leakage. Transparent dressings placed over the pressure points of the face help minimize air leakage and prevent facial skin necrosis from the mask. The BiPAP machine is able to compensate for air leaks.[51]

The patient is positioned with the head of the bed elevated at 45 degrees to minimize the risk of aspiration and facilitate breathing. Insufflation of the stomach is a complication of this mode of therapy and places the patient at risk for aspiration. In addition, the patient is closely monitored for gastric distention. Often, patients are very anxious with high levels of dyspnea before the initiation of noninvasive mechanical ventilation. Once adequate ventilation has been established, anxiety and dyspnea are usually sufficiently relieved. Heavy sedation is avoided, but if needed constitutes the need for intubation and invasive mechanical ventilation. Spending 30 minutes with the patient after the initiation of noninvasive ventilation is important, because the patient needs reassurance and must learn how to breathe on the machine.[15]

PHARMACOLOGY

There are a number of pharmacologic agents used in the care of the critically ill patient with pulmonary dysfunction. Table 23-8 reviews the various agents and special considerations necessary for administering them.[52-57]

Bronchodilators and Adjuncts

Medications to facilitate removal of secretions and dilate airways are of major benefit in the treatment of various pulmonary disorders. Mucolytics are administered to help liquefy secretions, which facilitates their removal.[52] Bronchodilators, such as xanthines, $beta_2$ agonists, and anticholinergic agents, aid in smooth muscle relaxation and are of particular benefit to patients with airflow limitations.[53-55] Steroids are also often used in conjunction with $beta_2$ agonists to decrease airway inflammation and to enhance the effects of $beta_2$ agonists.[56]

Neuromuscular Blocking Agents

Sedation is necessary in many patients to assist with maintaining adequate ventilation. It can be used to comfort the patient and decrease the work of breathing, particularly if the patient is fighting the ventilator. In some patients, sedation does not decrease spontaneous respiratory efforts enough to allow for adequate ventilation, and patient-ventilator asynchrony may develop. Neuromuscular paralysis may be necessary to facilitate optimal ventilation. Paralysis also may be necessary to decrease oxygen consumption in the severely compromised patient.[57]

Nursing Management

Nursing management of the patient receiving a neuromuscular blocking agent incorporates a number of additional interventions. Because paralytic agents only halt skeletal muscle movement and do not inhibit pain or awareness, they are administered with a sedative or anxiolytic agent. Pain medication is administered if the patient has a pain-producing illness or surgery. Reorientation and explanations for all procedures are critical because the patient can still hear but not move or see. The patient is also at risk for developing the complications of immobility. Interventions related to the prevention of skin breakdown, atelectasis, and deep vein thrombosis are implemented. Patient safety is another concern, because the patient cannot react to the environment. Special precautions are taken to protect the patient at all times.[58]

Peripheral nerve stimulator. Long-term use of neuromuscular blocking agents can result in prolonged neuromuscular blockade and skeletal muscle weakness. To avoid these complications the patient's level of paralysis is carefully monitored using a peripheral nerve stimulator (PNS). The PNS delivers an electrical stimulus (single, tetanic, or train-of-four) to a preselected nerve (ulnar, facial, posterior tibial, or peroneal) via electrodes (needle, ball, or pre-gelled), and the response is monitored to gauge the level of paralysis.[58]

Usually the ulnar nerve is used, with pre-gelled electrodes placed 2 to 3 inches proximal to the crease of the wrist (Figure 23-6). The train-of-four (TOF) stimulation test, which delivers four electrical stimuli in a row, is the most commonly used test. When the ulnar nerve is stimulated with TOF the expected response is four twitches (adduction) of the thumb medially across the palm of the hand. The number of twitches correlates to the level of paralysis; four twitches indicate 75% blockade; three twitches, 80%; two twitches, 85%; one twitch, 90%; and zero twitches, 100%. Usually, the neuromuscular blocking agent is titrated to maintain a 90% blockade, or one out of four twitches. The goal is to administer the smallest dose possible of the paralytic agent to avoid prolonged weakness after therapy is discontinued.[58]

Use of the PNS for estimating the degree of paralysis is not without problems. Poor skin contact, improper electrode placement, edema in the extremity being monitored, and malfunction of the device can

TABLE 23-8 Pharmacologic Agents Used in the Management of Pulmonary Disorders

Drug	Dosage	Actions	Special Considerations
NEUROMUSCULAR BLOCKING AGENTS (NMBAs)			
Vecuronium (Norcuron)	Loading dose 0.08-0.10 mg/kg IV IV infusion: 0.8-1.2 μg/kg/min	Used to paralyze patient to decrease oxygen demand and avoid ventilator asynchrony	Administer sedative and analgesic agents concurrently, because NMBAs have no sedative or analgesic properties Evaluate the level of paralysis q 4 hr using a peripheral nerve stimulator Monitor patients for immobility complications Protect patients from the environment because they are unable to respond Prolonged muscle paralysis may occur after discontinuation of the paralytic agent
Pancuronium (Pavulon)	Loading dose: 0.06-0.08 mg/kg IV IV infusion: 0.02-0.03 mg/kg/hr		
MUCOLYTICS			
N-acetylcysteine (Mucomyst)	Aerosol: 20% solution mixed in equal parts normal saline	Used to decrease the viscosity and elasticity of mucus by breaking down disulfide bonds within the mucus	May be administered with a bronchodilator, because drug can cause bronchospasms and inhibit ciliary function Treatment is considered effective when bronchorrhea develops and coughing occurs Antidote for acetaminophen overdose
BETA-AGONISTS			
Albuterol (Proventil, Ventolin)	Aerosol: 2.5-5 mg q 4-6 hr Metered-dose inhaler (MDI): 1-2 puffs q 4-6 hr	Used to relax bronchial smooth muscle and dilate airways and prevent bronchospasms	May cause skeletal muscle temors Higher doses may cause tachycardia, palpitations, increased blood pressure, dysrhythmias, and angina May increase serum glucose and decrease serum potassium levels Treatment is considered effective when breath sounds improve and dyspnea is lessened Only approximately 10% of the administered dose reaches the site of action within the lungs
Bitolterol (Tornalate, Produral)	MDI: 1-3 puffs q 4-6 hr		
Isoetharine (1%) (Bronkosol)	Aerosol: 3-5 mg q 2-4 hr MDI: 1-2 puffs q 2 - 4hr		
Metaproterenol (5%) (Alupent, Metaprel)	Aerosol: 15 mg q 2-4 hr diluted in 2.5 ml normal saline MDI: 2-3 puffs q 3-4 hr		
Terbutaline (Brethaire, Brethine)	Aerosol: 2-5 mg q 2-6 hr MDI: 2 puffs q 4-6 hr		

TABLE 23-8 Pharmacologic Agents Used in the Management of Pulmonary Disorders—cont'd

Drug	Dosage	Actions	Special Considerations
ANTICHOLINERGIC AGENTS			
Ipratropium (Atrovent)	Aerosol: 0.25-0.5 mg q 4-6 hr MDI: 2-4 puffs q 4-6 hr	Used to block the constriction of bronchial smooth muscle and reduce mucus production	Relatively few adverse effects because systemic absorption is poor
XANTHINES			
Theophylline	Loading dose: 5 mg/kg IV IV infusion: 0.5-0.7 mg/kg/hr	Used to dilate bronchial smooth muscle and reverse diaphragmatic muscle fatigue	Administer loading dose over 30 min Monitor serum blood levels; therapeutic level is 10-20 μg/dL Administer with caution in patients with cardiac, renal, or hepatic disease Signs of toxicity include central nervous system excitation, seizures, confusion, irritability, hyperglycemia, headache, nausea, hypotension, and dysrhythmias
Aminophylline	Loading dose: 6 mg/kg IV IV infusion: 0.5-0.7 mg/kg/hr		
STEROIDS			
Beclomethasone (Vanceril, Beclovent)	MDI: 2 puffs q 4-6 hr	Used to decrease airway inflammation and enhance effectiveness of beta-agonists	Suppresses inflammatory response and interfers with ability to fight infection Oral candidiasis is a side effect that can be minimized by having patients rinse their mouths after treatment
Flunisolide (AeroBid)	MDI: 2 puffs q 8-12 hr		
Triamcinolone (Azmacort)	MDI: 2 puffs q 6-8 hr		

lead to overestimation of the degree of blockade. For instance, the patient may appear to have a zero-out-of-four twitch response, but evidence of muscle movement is present. More problematic is underestimation of the degree of blockade. Direct stimulation of the muscle or mistaking finger responses (instead of the thumb) can result in a false positive twitch response. This can lead to the unnecessary administration of additional doses of the paralytic agent. It is imperative that the patient's twitch response be correlated with clinical observations of patient movement.[58]

NEW FRONTIERS IN TREATMENT

Extracorporeal/Intracorporeal Gas Exchange

Extracorporeal and intracorporeal gas exchange are last-resort techniques currently being used in the treatment of severe acute respiratory distress syndrome (ARDS) when conventional therapy has failed. These methods allow the lungs to rest by facilitating the removal of carbon dioxide and the provision of oxygen external to the lungs via an "artificial lung" or membrane/fiber oxygenator. Extracorporeal membrane oxygenation (ECMO), extracorporeal carbon dioxide removal ($ECCO_2R$), and intravascular oxygenation (IVOX) are three techniques that currently use this type of technology.[59] ECMO is similar to cardiopulmonary bypass in that blood is removed from the body, pumped through a membrane oxygenator where CO_2 is removed and O_2 is added, and then returned to the body.[60] $ECCO_2R$ is a variation of ECMO with the primary focus of removing CO_2.[61] IVOX facilitates oxygenation and ventilation using a fiber oxygenator that is implanted in the inferior vena cava.[59] All of

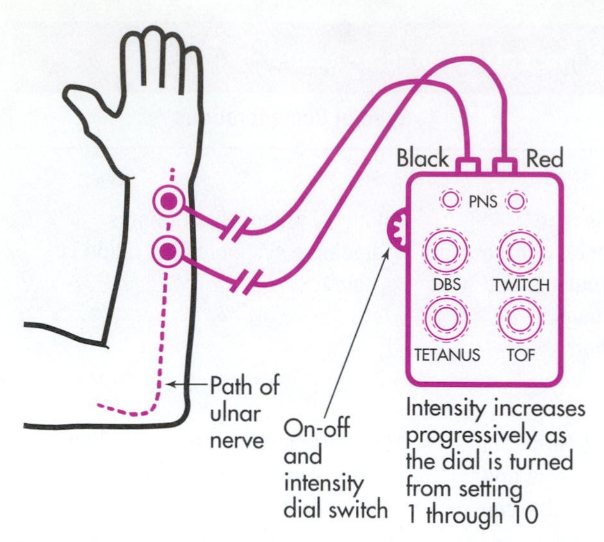

FIGURE 23-6. Peripheral nerve stimulator. Note placement of electrodes along ulnar nerve.

these techniques pose serious bleeding problems to the patient, and none of them has been shown to improve patient outcome.[59]

Surfactant Therapy

One of the newer drugs currently being tested in adults with severe ARDS is exogenous surfactant. The two main types of exogenous surfactant available are natural, either from amniotic fluid or animals (Alveofact, a calf-lung surfactant extract, and surfactant-TA), and synthetic (colfosceril palmitate, an artificial lung-expanding compound). Currently, doses of 2 to 16 ml/kg are being administered, either via direct instillation or nebulization. Though proven to be extremely beneficial in neonates, exogenous surfactant has not yet been proven to be of any benefit to adults.[62]

Inhaled Nitric Oxide

Nitric oxide is a potent bronchodilator and selective pulmonary vasodilator that has been used in the treatment of ARDS and other disorders resulting in pulmonary hypertension. When inhaled, nitric oxide is distributed to the well-ventilated regions of the lungs, resulting in vasodilation and increased blood flow to these areas. This leads to improved matching of ventilation to perfusion and enhanced oxygenation. Dosing guidelines for nitric oxide have not yet been established nor has a standard delivery system. Toxic effects include the production of nitric dioxide, which can cause pulmonary parenchymal damage, and methemoglobinemia, which can interfere with the delivery of oxygen to the cells. Adverse effects include platelet inhibition, increased left ventricular filling pressure because of increased right ventricular stroke volume, and rebound hypoxemia and pulmonary hypertension upon discontinuing the gas.[63]

Partial Liquid Ventilation

Partial liquid ventilation involves the instillation of perfluorocarbon into the lungs via an endotracheal tube. Perfluorocarbon is a liquid that has a low surface tension and a high solubility for oxygen and carbon dioxide. Once instilled the liquid flows down into the dependent regions of the lungs where it facilitates the patency of functioning alveoli and helps open collapsed alveoli. The low surface tension of perfluorocarbon decreases alveolar surface tension, which increases alveolar compliance and in turn decreases airway pressures. The high solubility of the liquid enhances gas exchange through the liquid. Partial liquid ventilation is accomplished by instilling a volume of perfluorocarbon equal to the patient's functional residual capacity (approximately 30 ml/kg) into the patient's lungs and then instituting conventional gas ventilation.[64,65]

REFERENCES

1. O'Connor BS, Vender JS: Oxygen therapy, *Crit Care Clin* 11:67, 1995.
2. Carlton TJ, Anthonisen NR: A guide for judicious use of oxygen in critical illness, *J Crit Ill* 7:1744, 1992.
3. Scanlan CL, Thalken FR: Medical gas therapy. In Scanlan CL, Spearman CB, Sheldon RL, editors: *Egan's fundamentals of respiratory care,* ed 6, St Louis, 1995, Mosby.
4. Branson RD: The nuts and bolts of increasing arterial oxygenation: devices and techniques, *Respir Care* 38:672, 1993.
5. Durbin CG, Wallace KK: Oxygen toxicity in the critically ill patient, *Respir Care* 38:739, 1993.
6. Hanson CW and others: Causes of hypercarbia with oxygen therapy in patients with chronic obstructive pulmonary disease, *Crit Care Med* 24:23, 1996.
7. Kharasch M, Graff J: Emergency management of the airway, *Crit Care Clin* 11:53, 1995.
8. Somerson SJ, Sicilia MR: Emergency oxygen administration and airway management, *Crit Care Nurse* 12(4):23, 1992.
9. Stauffer JL: Medical management of the airway, *Clin Chest Med* 12:449, 1991.
10. Einarsson O, Rochester CL, Rosenbaum S: Airway management in respiratory emergencies, *Clin Chest Med* 15:13, 1994.
11. Stone DJ, Bogdonoff DL: Airway considerations in the management of patients requiring long-term endotracheal intubation, *Anesth Anal* 74:276, 1992.

12. Colice GL: Technical standards for tracheal tubes, *Clin Chest Med* 12:433, 1991.
13. Zarshenas Z, Sparschu RA: Catheter placement and misplacement, *Crit Care Clin* 10:417, 1994.
14. McCulloch TM, Bishop MJ: Complications of translaryngeal intubation, *Clin Chest Med* 12:507, 1991.
15. Wenig BL, Applebaum EL: Indications for and techniques of tracheotomy, *Clin Chest Med* 12:545, 1991.
16. Weilitz PB, Dettenmeier PA: Back to basics: test your knowledge of tracheostomy tubes, *Am J Nurs* 94(2):46, 1994.
17. Myers EN, Carrau RL: Early complications of tracheotomy: incidence and management, *Clin Chest Med* 12:589, 1991.
18. Wood DE, Mathisen DJ: Late complications of tracheotomy, *Clin Chest Med* 12:597, 1991.
19. Fink J: Humidity and aerosol therapy. In Scanlan CL, Spearman CB, Sheldon RL, editors: *Egan's fundamentals of respiratory care,* ed 6, St Louis, 1995, Mosby.
20. Chang VM: Protocol for prevention of complications of endotracheal intubation, *Crit Care Nurse* 15(5):19, 1995.
21. Goodnough SKC: Reducing tracheal injury and aspiration, *DCCN* 7:324, 1988.
22. Tyler DO, Clark AP, Ogburn-Russell L: Developing a standard for endotracheal tube cuff care, *DCCN* 10:54, 1991.
23. Bivona: *Fome-Cuf users manual,* Gary, Indiana, 1991, Bivona.
24. Glass CA, Grap MJ: Ten tips for safer suctioning, *Am J Nurs* 95(5):51, 1995.
25. Stone KS: Endotracheal suctioning in the critically ill, *Crit Care Nurs Curr* 7:5, 1989.
26. Gunderson LP, Stone KS, Hamlin RL: Endotracheal suctioning-induced heart rate alterations, *Nurs Res* 40:139, 1991.
27. Stone KS and others: The effect of lung hyperinflation and endotracheal suctioning on cardiopulmonary hemodynamics, *Nurs Res* 40:76, 1991.
28. Grap MJ and others: Endotracheal suctioning: ventilator vs manual delivery of hyperoxygenation breaths, *Am J Crit Care* 1(3):62, 1992.
29. Mancinelli-Van Atta J, Beck SL: Preventing hypoxemia and hemodynamic compromise related to endotracheal suctioning, *Am J Crit Care* 1(3):62, 1992.
30. Stone KS: Ventilator versus manual resuscitation bag as the method of delivering hyperoxygenation before endotracheal suctioning, *AACN Clin Issues Crit Care Nurs* 1:289, 1990.
31. Czarnik RE and others: Deferential effects of continuous versus intermittent suction on tracheal tissue, *Heart Lung* 20:144, 1991.
32. Raymond SJ: Normal saline instillation before suctioning: helpful or harmful? A review of the literature, *Am J Crit Care* 4:267, 1995.
33. Hagler DA, Traver GA: Endotracheal saline and suction catheters: sources of lower airway contamination, *Am J Crit Care* 3:444, 1994.
34. Johnson KL and others: Closed versus open endotracheal suctioning: costs and physiologic consequences, *Crit Care Med* 22:658, 1994.
35. Jablonski RS: The experience of being mechanically ventilated, *Qual Health Res* 4:186, 1994.
36. Williams ML: An algorithm for selecting a communication technique with intubated patients, *DCCN* 11:222, 1992.
37. Bell SD: Use of Passy-Muir tracheostomy speaking valve in mechanically ventilated neurological patients, *Crit Care Nurse* 16(1):63, 1996.
38. Godwin JE, Heffner JE: Special critical care considerations in tracheostomy management, *Clin Chest Med* 12:573, 1991.
39. American College of Chest Physicians: ACCP consensus conference: mechanical ventilation, *Chest* 194:1833, 1993.
40. Scanlan CL, Blazer C: Physics and physiology of ventilatory support. In Scanlan CL, Spearman CB, Sheldon RL, editors: *Egan's fundamentals of respiratory care,* ed 6, St Louis, 1995, Mosby.
41. Kacmarek RM, Meklaus GJ: The new generation of mechanical ventilators, *Crit Care Clin* 6:551, 1990.
42. Dupuis YG: *Ventilators: theory and clinical application,* ed 2, St Louis, 1992, Mosby.
43. Bone RC, Eubanks DH: Second- and third-generation ventilators: sorting through available options, *J Crit Ill* 7:399, 1992.
44. Herridge MS, Slutsky AS: High frequency ventilation: a ventilatory technique that merits revisiting, *Respir Care* 41:385, 1996.
45. Brochard L: Pressure-limited ventilation, *Respir Care* 41:447, 1996.
46. Scanlan CL: Initiating and adjusting ventilatory support. In Scanlan CL, Spearman CB, Sheldon RL, editors: *Egan's fundamentals of respiratory care,* ed 6, St Louis, 1995, Mosby.
47. Parker JC, Hernandez LA, Peevy KJ: Mechanisms of ventilatory-induced lung injury, *Crit Care Med* 21:131, 1993.
48. Pierson DJ: Complications associated with mechanical ventilation, *Crit Care Clin* 6:711, 1990.
49. Weilitz PB: Weaning a patient from mechanical ventilation, *Crit Care Nurse* 13(4):33, 1993.
50. Hanneman SKG and others: Weaning from short-term mechanical ventilation: a review, *Am J Crit Care* 3:421, 1994.
51. Abou-Shola N, Meduri GU: Noninvasive mechanical ventilation in patients with acute respiratory failure, *Crit Care Med* 24:705, 1996.
52. Connolly MA: Mucolytics and the critically ill patient: help or hindrance? *AACN Clin Issues Crit Care Nurs* 6:307, 1995.
53. Sterling LP: Beta adrenergic agonists, *AACN Clin Issues Crit Care Nurs* 6:271, 1995.
54. Geiger-Bronsky MJ: Anticholinergic therapy in the critically ill patient with bronchospasm, *AACN Clin Issues Crit Care Nurs* 6:287, 1995.

55. Perry AG: Aminophylline use in the critically ill: an old ally or new foe, *AACN Clin Issues Crit Care Nurs* 6:297, 1995.
56. Peters JA, Peters BA: Pharmacology for respiratory care. In Scanlan CL, Spearman CB, Sheldon RL, editors: *Egan's fundamentals of respiratory care,* ed 6, St Louis, 1995, Mosby.
57. Shapiro BA and others: Practice parameters for sustained neuromuscular blockade in the adult critically ill patient: an executive summary, *Crit Care Med* 23:1601, 1995.
58. Ford EV: Monitoring neuromuscular blockade in the adult ICU, *Am J Crit Care* 4:122, 1995.
59. Wilson BG: Extracorporeal and intracorporeal techniques for the treatment of severe respiratory failure, *Respir Care* 41:306, 1996.
60. Dirkes S, Dickinson S, Valentine J: Acute respiratory failure and ECMO, *Crit Care Nurse* 12(5):39, 1992.
61. Chillcott S, Sheridan PS: $ECCO_2R$: an experimental approach to treating ARDS, *Crit Care Nurse* 15(2):50, 1995.
62. Haas CF, Weg JG: Exogenous surfactant therapy: an update, *Respir Care* 41:397, 1996.
63. Hess D and others: Use of inhaled nitric oxide in patients with acute respiratory distress syndrome, *Respir Care* 41:424, 1996.
64. Hurst JM, Branson RD: Liquid breathing—partial liquid ventilation, *Respir Care* 41:416, 1996.
65. Dirkes S: Liquid ventilation: new frontiers in the treatment of ARDS, *Crit Care Nurse* 16(30):53, 1996.

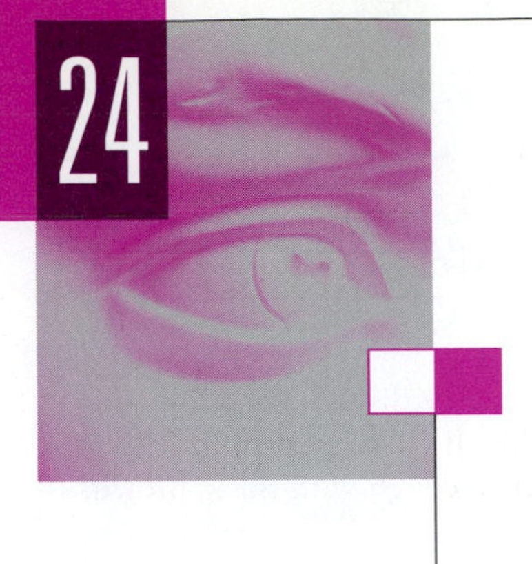

Pulmonary Nursing Diagnosis and Management

THIS CHAPTER IS designed to supplement the preceding chapters in the *Pulmonary Alterations* unit by integrating theoretic content into clinically applicable case studies and nursing management plans.

The case study is designed to illustrate clinical problem solving and patient care management occurring in actual patients. The case, reviewed retrospectively, demonstrates how medical and nursing diagnoses may be effectively used in critical care. The case study also demonstrates revisions to the plan of care and the nursing and medical management outcomes that are apt to occur during the course of a complicated hospitalization as the patient responds physiologically to treatment. Often in a short case anecdote, such as that which is presented in this chapter, the clinical answer may appear to be obvious from the day of admission. In practice, however, critical care patient management is sometimes investigative and the "correct" diagnosis for an individual patient may not become apparent until midway into the hospitalization. Or a patient with an apparently straightforward diagnosis may develop an unexpected complication, and the plan of care and potential outcomes will then require revision. Many of the case studies demonstrate this principle.

The nursing management plans, which—unlike the case study—are not patient-specific, provide a basis nurses can use to individualize care for their patients. In the previous *Pulmonary Alterations* chapters, each medical diagnosis is assigned a Nursing Diagnosis and Management Box. Using this box as a page guide, the reader can access relevant nursing management plans for each medical diagnosis. For example, nursing management of *acute respiratory failure,* described on p. 655, may involve several nursing diagnoses and management plans outlined in this chapter and in other Nursing Diagnosis and Management chapters. Specific examples are (1) *Impaired Gas Exchange related to ventilation/perfusion mismatching or intrapulmonary shunting,* on p. 725; (2) *Impaired Gas Exchange related to alveolar hypoventilation,* on p. 726; (3) *Altered Nutrition: Less than Body Requirements related to lack of exogenous nutrients or increased metabolic demand,* on p. 165; and (4) *Risk for Infection,* on p. 1119. These examples highlight the interrelationship of the various physiologic systems in the body and the fact that pathology often has a multisystem impact in the critically ill.

Use of the case study and management plans can enhance the understanding and application of the *Pulmonary* content in clinical practice.

CASE STUDY

PULMONARY

CLINICAL HISTORY

Mr. B is a 63-year-old obese man. He has a long history of chronic obstructive pulmonary disease (COPD) associated with smoking two packs of cigarettes a day for 40 years. During the past week Mr. B has experienced a "flulike" illness with fever, chills, malaise, anorexia, diarrhea, nausea, vomiting, and a productive cough with thick, brown, purulent sputum.

CURRENT PROBLEMS

Mr. B was admitted to the critical care unit from the emergency department with acute respiratory insufficiency. He sat up in bed, leaning forward, with his elbows resting on the overbed table. Mr. B breathed through his mouth, taking rapid, shallow breaths, using his accessory muscles to ventilate. On inhalation, his nostrils flared and his intercostal muscles retracted. During exhalation, Mr. B used pursed-lip breathing, and his intercostal muscles bulged. He appeared anxious and irritable and could speak only one or two barely audible words between each breath. Auscultation revealed crackles anteriorly and posteriorly in both right and left lower lung fields. Rhonchi were heard in the right upper lung field. His admission chest x-ray film revealed infiltrates in the right upper lobe, right middle lobe, right lower lobe, and left lower lobe. Gram stain of Mr. B's sputum contained numerous gram-positive diplococci. His baseline vital signs were: blood pressure (BP), 110/60; heart rate (HR), 114 (sinus tachycardia); respiratory rate (RR), 30; temperature (T), 101.3° F. His baseline arterial blood gas (ABG) values on a 50% nonrebreather mask were $Pa{O_2}$, 50 mm Hg; $Pa{CO_2}$, 33 mm Hg; pH, 7.42; HCO_3, 28 mEq/L; O_2 saturation, 88%.

MEDICAL DIAGNOSIS

Pneumococcal pneumonia

NURSING DIAGNOSES

Ineffective Airway Clearance related to excessive secretions or abnormal viscosity of mucus

Ineffective Breathing Pattern related to musculoskeletal fatigue or neuromuscular impairment

Anxiety related to threat to biologic, psychologic, and/or social integrity

PLAN OF CARE

1. Promote secretion clearance by humidifying supplemental oxygen, encouraging deep breathing, facilitating frequent position changes, providing chest physical therapy (postural drainage, chest percussion and vibration, and coughing techniques), ensuring adequate systemic hydration, and performing nasotracheal suctioning if necessary.
2. Promote an effective ventilatory pattern by encouraging pursed-lip and diaphragmatic breathing, positioning with the head of the bed up, and reducing energy demands.
3. Decrease anxiety by providing orientation and education to environment and illness, supporting existing coping mechanisms, speaking slowly and calmly, removing excess stimulation, and promoting presence of and comforting significant other.

MEDICAL AND NURSING MANAGEMENT AND PATIENT OUTCOME

Mr. B was started on antibiotic therapy and systemic and nebulized bronchodilators, his oxygen concentration was increased to 100%, and he was systemically hydrated with intravenous fluids. Six hours after admission Mr. B's condition continued to deteriorate. He was very confused and combative. Crackles and rhonchi were heard throughout both lung fields, respirations were shallow, and he no longer could produce an effective cough. Mr. B was diaphoretic and had marked cyanosis around his lips. His vital signs were: BP, 90/60; HR, 130 (sinus tachycardia with occasional premature ventricular contractions); RR, 30; T, 103.1° F. His ABG values on a 100% nonrebreather mask were: $Pa{O_2}$, 40 mm Hg; $Pa{CO_2}$, 70 mm Hg; pH, 7.22; HCO_3, 28 mEq/L; O_2 saturation, 78%.

CASE STUDY—CONT'D

PULMONARY

MEDICAL DIAGNOSIS

Acute respiratory failure

NURSING DIAGNOSES

Impaired Gas Exchange related to ventilation/perfusion mismatching or intrapulmonary shunting

Inability to Sustain Spontaneous Ventilation related to respiratory muscle fatigue and metabolic factors

REVISED PLAN OF CARE

1. Support oxygenation by ensuring supplemental oxygen administration, preventing desaturation during procedures, encouraging deep breathing, facilitating frequent position changes, providing chest physical therapy, and suctioning nasotracheally if necessary.
2. Support adequate breathing by maintaining upper airway patency (positioning and use of an oropharyngeal or nasopharyngeal airway) and assisting with ventilation (using a manual resuscitation bag) if necessary.

MEDICAL AND NURSING MANAGEMENT AND PATIENT OUTCOME

Mr. B was intubated and placed on a ventilator with the following settings: mode, synchronized intermittent mandatory ventilation (SIMV); rate, 10; tidal volume (V_T), 1100 ml; fraction of inspired oxygen (FIO_2), 100%; positive end-expiratory pressure (PEEP), 5 cm H_2O; pressure support (PS), 10 cm H_2O. ABG values on current ventilator settings were: PaO_2, 80 mm Hg; $PaCO_2$, 43 mm Hg; pH, 7.37; HCO_3, 28 mEq/L; O_2 saturation, 95%.

During the next 4 days Mr. B was maintained on the ventilator. The FIO_2 was weaned down to 40% to maintain an O_2 saturation $> 90\%$. On the fifth day he was awake and alert and following commands appropriately. Lung sounds were clear and with minimal secretions, and temperature was normal. Tube feedings were started at 50 ml/hr. The decision was made to wean Mr. B from mechanical ventilation. His weaning parameters were: minute ventilation (V_E), 9 L/min; static compliance, 35 cm H_2O; maximum inspiratory pressure, -18 cm H_2O; vital capacity, 11 ml/kg; spontaneous tidal volume, > 3.5 ml/kg.

Weaning was initiated by decreasing the rate on the ventilator from 10 to 6 breaths per minute. Mr. B's baseline vital signs were: BP, 135/65; HR, 90 (sinus rhythm); spontaneous RR, 22; T, 98.4° F. Within 1 hour his vital signs were: BP, 165/75; HR, 115 (sinus tachycardia with premature ventricular contractions); spontaneous RR, 35. Mr. B was diaphoretic and restless and complained of dyspnea. His ABG values were: PaO_2, 75 mm Hg; $PaCO_2$, 60 mm Hg, pH, 7.33; HCO_3, 24 mEq/L; O_2 saturation, 93%. The weaning attempt was terminated, and his rate on the ventilator was increased back to 10. Over the next 5 days, three more unsuccessful attempts were made to wean Mr. B from the ventilator.

MEDICAL DIAGNOSIS

Chronic ventilatory failure

NURSING DIAGNOSES

Dysfunctional Ventilatory Weaning Response related to physical, psychologic, or situational factors

Risk for Aspiration risk factor: impaired laryngeal closure or elevation

REVISED PLAN OF CARE

1. Facilitate weaning by ensuring availability of energy substrates (oxygen and nutrition); promoting rest; using appropriate training techniques; teaching, modifying, and normalizing the environment; coaching and supporting all efforts; establishing trust; controlling and enhancing social support; and ensuring that staff and others respond appropriately to the patient's needs or wishes.
2. Prevent aspiration by maintaining the head of the bed elevated, frequently checking placement of nasogastric tube, checking amount of residual, and assessing bowel function.

Continued

CASE STUDY—CONT'D

PULMONARY

MEDICAL AND NURSING MANAGEMENT AND PATIENT OUTCOME

On the tenth day Mr. B was taken to the operating room and a tracheostomy was performed. He was moved to the intermediate care unit for long-term ventilator management. During the next 3 days constant positive airway pressure (CPAP) weaning trials were successfully carried out. On the fourteenth day Mr. B was placed on a 40% humidified T-piece, with no signs of respiratory distress. On the fifteenth day Mr. B's tracheostomy tube was buttoned, and the following day the tracheostomy tube was removed. Mr. B was transferred to the pulmonary floor and entered into a pulmonary rehabilitation program.

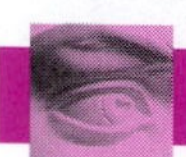

NURSING MANAGEMENT PLAN

INEFFECTIVE AIRWAY CLEARANCE

DEFINITION:

The state in which an individual is unable to clear obstructions or secretions from the respiratory tract to maintain airway patency.

Ineffective Airway Clearance Related to Excessive Secretions or Abnormal Viscosity of Mucus

DEFINING CHARACTERISTICS

- Abnormal breath sounds (displaced normal sounds, adventitious sounds, diminished or absent sounds)
- Ineffective cough with or without sputum
- Tachypnea, dyspnea
- Verbal reports of inability to clear airway

OUTCOME CRITERIA

- Cough produces thin mucus.
- Lungs are clear to auscultation.
- Respiratory rate, depth, and rhythm return to baseline

NURSING INTERVENTIONS AND *RATIONALE*

1. Assess sputum for color, consistency, and amount.
2. Assess for clinical manifestations of pneumonia.
3. Provide for maximal thoracic expansion by repositioning, deep breathing, splinting, and pain management ***to avoid hypoventilation and atelectasis.*** If hypoventilation is present, implement "Ineffective Breathing Pattern Related to Decreased Lung Expansion" Management Plan, p. 723.
4. Maintain adequate hydration by administering oral and intravenous fluids (as ordered) ***to thin secretions and facilitate airway clearance.***
5. Provide humidification to airways via oxygen delivery device or artificial airway ***to thin secretions and facilitate airway clearance.***
6. Administer bland aerosol every 4 hours ***to facilitate expectoration of sputum.***
7. Collaborate with the physician regarding the administration of the following:
   - Bronchodilators ***to treat or prevent bronchospams and facilitate expectoration of mucus***
   - Mucolytics and expectorants ***to enhance mobilization and removal of secretions***
   - Antibiotics ***to treat infection***
8. Assist with directed coughing exercises ***to facilitate expectoration of secretions.*** If patients are unable to perform cascade cough, consider using huff cough (patients with hyperactive airways), end-expiratory cough (patients with secretions in distal airways), or augmented cough (patients with weakened abdominal muscles).
   - Cascade cough—Instruct patients to do the following:
     a. Take a deep breath and hold it for 1 to 3 seconds
     b. Cough out forcefully several times until all air is exhaled
     c. Inhale slowly through the nose
     d. Repeat once
     e. Rest and then repeat as necessary
   - Huff cough—Instruct patients to do the following:
     a. Take a deep breath and hold it for 1 to 3 seconds
     b. Say the word "huff" while coughing out several times until air is exhaled
     c. Inhale slowly through the nose
     d. Repeat as necessary
   - End-expiratory cough—Instruct patients to do the following:
     a. Take a deep breath and hold it for 1 to 3 seconds
     b. Exhale slowly
     c. At the end of exhalation, cough once

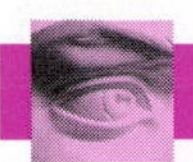
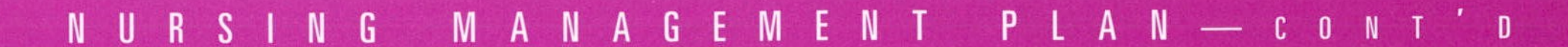

Ineffective Airway Clearance Related to Excessive Secretions or Abnormal Viscosity of Mucus

NURSING INTERVENTIONS AND *RATIONALE*—cont'd

d. Inhale slowly through the nose
e. Repeat as necessary or follow with cascade cough

- Augmented cough—Instruct patients to do the following:
  a. Take a deep breath and hold it for 1 to 3 seconds
  b. Perform one or more of the following maneuvers to increase intraabdominal pressure:
     1) Tighten knees and buttocks
     2) Bend forward at the waist
     3) Place a hand flat on the upper abdomen just under the xiphoid process and press in and up abruptly during coughing
     4) Keep hands on the chest wall and press inward with each cough
  c. Inhale slowly through the nose
  d. Rest and repeat as necessary

9. Suction nasotracheally or endotracheally as necessary ***to assist with secretion removal.***
10. Reposition patients at least every 2 hours or use continuous lateral rotation therapy ***to mobilize and prevent stasis of secretions.***
11. Consider chest physiotherapy (postural drainage and/or chest percussion) three to four times per day in patients with large amounts of sputum ***to assist with the expulsion of retained secretions.***
12. Allow rest periods between coughing sessions, chest physiotherapy, suctioning, or any other demanding activities ***to promote energy conservation.***

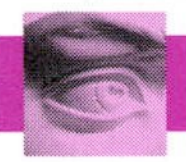

NURSING MANAGEMENT PLAN

INEFFECTIVE BREATHING PATTERN

DEFINITION:

The state in which an individual's inhalation and/or exhalation pattern does not enable adequate pulmonary inflation or emptying.

Ineffective Breathing Pattern Related to Decreased Lung Expansion

DEFINING CHARACTERISTICS

Abnormal respiratory patterns (hypoventilation, hyperventilation, tachypnea, bradypnea, obstructive breathing)

- Abnormal ABG values (increased $Pa{CO_2}$, decreased pH)
- Unequal chest movement
- Shortness of breath, dyspnea

OUTCOME CRITERIA

- Respiratory rate, rhythm, and depth return to baseline.
- Minimal or absent use of accessory muscles.
- Chest expands symmetrically.
- ABG values return to baseline.

NURSING INTERVENTIONS AND *RATIONALE*

1. Treat pain, if present, ***to prevent hypoventilation and atelectasis.*** Implement "Acute Pain Related to Transmission and Perception of Cutaneous, Visceral, Muscular, or Ischemic Impulses" Management Plan, p. 197.
2. Position patients in high-Fowler's or semi-Fowler's position ***to promote diaphragmatic descent and maximal inhalation.***
3. Assist with deep breathing exercises and incentive spirometry with sustained maximal inspiration 5 to 10 times/hr ***to help reinflate collapsed portions of the lung.***
   - Deep breathing—Instruct patients to do the following:
     a. Sit up straight or lean forward slightly while sitting on edge of bed or chair (if possible)
     b. Take a slow, deep breath in
     c. Pause slightly or hold breath for at least 3 seconds
     d. Exhale slowly
     e. Rest and repeat
   - Incentive spirometry—Instruct patients to do the following:
     a. Exhale normally
     b. Place lips around the mouthpiece and close mouth tightly around it
     c. Inhale slowly and as deeply as possible, noting the maximum volume of air inspired
     d. Hold maximum inhalation for 3 seconds
     e. Take the mouthpiece out of mouth and slowly exhale
     f. Rest and repeat
4. Assist physician with intubation and initiation of mechanical ventilation as indicated.

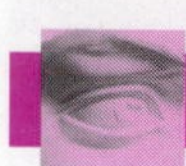

NURSING MANAGEMENT PLAN

Ineffective Breathing Pattern Related to Musculoskeletal Fatigue or Neuromuscular Impairment

DEFINING CHARACTERISTICS

- Unequal chest movement
- Shortness of breath, dyspnea
- Use of accessory muscles
- Tachypnea
- Thoracoabdominal asynchrony
- Abnormal ABG values (increased $PaCO_2$, decreased pH)
- Nasal flaring
- Assumption of 3-point position

OUTCOME CRITERIA

- Respiratory rate, rhythm, and depth return to baseline.
- Minimal or absent use of accessory muscles.
- Chest expands symmetrically.
- ABG values return to baseline.

NURSING INTERVENTIONS AND *RATIONALE*

1. Prevent unnecessary exertion ***to limit drain on patients' ventilatory reserve.***
2. Instruct patients in energy-saving techniques ***to conserve patients' ventilatory reserve.***
3. Assist with pursed-lip and diaphragmatic breathing techniques ***to facilitate diaphragmatic descent and improved ventilation.***
   - Diaphragmatic breathing—Instruct patients to do the following:
     a. Sit in the upright position
     b. Place one hand on the abdomen just above the waist and the other on the upper chest
     c. Breathe in through the nose and feel the lower hand push out; the upper hand should not move
     d. Breathe out through pursed lips and feel the lower hand move in
4. Position patients in high-Fowler's or semi-Fowler's position ***to promote diaphragmatic descent and maximal inhalation.***
5. Assist physician with intubation and initiation of mechanical ventilation as indicated.

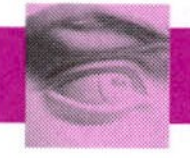

NURSING MANAGEMENT PLAN

INABILITY TO SUSTAIN SPONTANEOUS VENTILATION

DEFINITION:

A state in which the response pattern of decreased energy reserves results in an individual's inability to maintain breathing adequate to support life.

Inability to Sustain Spontaneous Ventilation Related to Respiratory Muscle Fatigue or Metabolic Factors

DEFINING CHARACTERISTICS

- Dyspnea and apprehension
- Increased metabolic rate
- Increased restlessness
- Increased use of accessory muscles
- Decreased tidal volume
- Increased heart rate
- Abnormal arterial blood gas (ABG) values (decreased PaO_2, increased $PaCO_2$, decreased pH, decreased SaO_2)
- Decreased cooperation

OUTCOME CRITERIA

- Metabolic rate and heart rate are within patients' baseline.
- Eupnea.
- ABG values are within patients' baseline.

NURSING INTERVENTIONS AND *RATIONALE*

1. Collaborate with the physician regarding the application of pressure support to the ventilator ***to assist patients in overcoming the work of breathing imposed by the ventilator and endotracheal tube.***
2. Carefully snip excess length from the proximal end of the endotracheal tube ***to decrease dead space and thereby decrease the work of breathing.***
3. Collaborate with the physician and dietitian to ensure that at least 50% of the diet's nonprotein caloric source is in the form of fat versus carbohydrates ***to prevent excess carbon dioxide production.***
4. Collaborate with the physician and respiratory therapist regarding the best method of weaning for individual patients ***because each situation is different, and a variety of weaning options are available.***

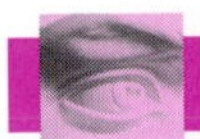

NURSING MANAGEMENT PLAN—CONT'D

Inability to Sustain Spontaneous Ventilation Related to Respiratory Muscle Fatigue or Metabolic Factors

NURSING INTERVENTIONS AND *RATIONALE*—cont'd

5. Collaborate with the physician and physical therapist regarding a progressive ambulation and conditioning plan ***to promote overall muscle conditioning and respiratory muscle functioning.***
6. Determine the most effective means of communication for patients ***to promote their independence and reduce their anxiety.***
7. Develop a daily schedule and post it in patients' rooms ***to coordinate care and facilitate patients' involvement in the plan.***
8. Treat pain, if present, ***to prevent respiratory splinting and hypoventilation.*** Implement "Acute Pain Related to Transmission and Perception of Cutaneous, Visceral, Muscular, or Ischemic Impulses" Management Plan, p. 197.
9. Ensure that patients receive at least 2- to 4-hour intervals of uninterrupted sleep in a quiet, dark room. Collaborate with the physician and respiratory therapist regarding the use of full ventilatory support at night ***to provide respiratory muscle rest.***
10. Place patients in semi-Fowler's position or in a chair at the bedside ***for best use of ventilatory muscles and to facilitate diaphragmatic descent.***
11. Explain the weaning procedure to patients before the initial trial ***so that patients will understand what to expect and how to participate.***
12. Monitor patients during the weaning trial for evidence of respiratory muscle fatigue ***to avoid overtiring patients.***
13. Provide diversional activity during the weaning trial ***to reduce patients' anxiety.***
14. Collaborate with physician and respiratory therapist regarding the removal of the ventilator and artificial airway when patients have been successfully weaned.

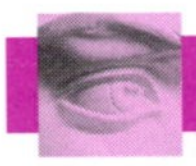

NURSING MANAGEMENT PLAN

IMPAIRED GAS EXCHANGE

DEFINITION:

A state in which an individual experiences an imbalance between oxygen uptake and carbon dioxide elimination at the alveolar-capillary membrane gas exchange area.

Impaired Gas Exchange Related to Ventilation/Perfusion Mismatching or Intrapulmonary Shunting

DEFINING CHARACTERISTICS

- Abnormal ABG values (decreased PaO_2, decreased SaO_2)
- Somnolence
- Neurobehavioral changes (restlessness, irritability, confusion)
- Central cyanosis

OUTCOME CRITERIA

- ABG values are within patients' baseline.
- Absence of central cyanosis.

NURSING INTERVENTIONS AND *RATIONALE*

1. Initiate continuous pulse oximetry or monitor SpO_2 every hour.
2. Collaborate with physician on the administration of oxygen to maintain an $SpO_2 > 90\%$
   a. Administer supplemental oxygen via appropriate oxygen delivery device ***to increase driving pressure of oxygen in the alveoli.***
   b. If supplemental oxygen alone is not effective, administer constant positive airway pressure or mechanical ventilation with positive end-expiratory pressure ***to open collapsed alveoli and increase the surface area for gas exchange.***
3. Position patients to optimize ventilation/perfusion matching
   a. For patients with unilateral lung disease, position with the good lung down ***because gravity will improve perfusion to this area, and this will best match ventilation with perfusion.***

Continued

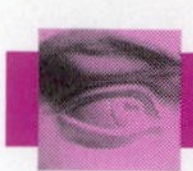

NURSING MANAGEMENT PLAN—CONT'D

Impaired Gas Exchange Related to Ventilation/Perfusion Mismatching or Intrapulmonary Shunting

NURSING INTERVENTIONS AND *RATIONALE*—cont'd

b. For patients with bilateral lung disease, position with the right lung down ***because this lung is larger than the left and affords a greater area for ventilation and perfusion,*** or change position every 2 hours, favoring positions that improve oxygenation.
c. Avoid any position that seriously compromises oxygenation status.

4. Perform procedures only as needed and provide adequate rest and recovery time in between ***to prevent desaturation.***
5. Collaborate with the physician regarding the administration of the following:
   - Sedatives ***to decrease ventilator asynchrony and facilitate patients' sense of control***
   - Neuromuscular blocking agents ***to prevent ventilator asynchrony and decrease oxygen demand***
   - Analgesics ***to treat pain if present;*** implement "Acute Pain Related to Transmission and Perception of Cutaneous, Visceral, Muscular, or Ischemic Impulses" Management Plan, p. 197.
6. If secretions are present, implement "Ineffective Airway Clearance Related to Excessive Secretions or Abnormal Viscosity of Mucus" Management Plan, p. 722.

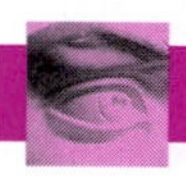

NURSING MANAGEMENT PLAN

Impaired Gas Exchange Related to Alveolar Hypoventilation

DEFINING CHARACTERISTICS

- Abnormal ABG values (decreased PaO_2, increased $PaCO_2$, decreased pH, decreased SaO_2)
- Somnolence
- Neurobehavioral changes (restlessness, irritability, confusion)
- Tachycardia or dysrhythmias
- Central cyanosis

OUTCOME CRITERIA

- ABG values within patients' baseline.
- Absence of central cyanosis.

NURSING INTERVENTIONS AND *RATIONALE*

1. Initiate continuous pulse oximetry or monitor SpO_2 every hour.
2. Collaborate with physician on the administration of oxygen to maintain an $SpO_2 > 90\%$
   a. Administer supplemental oxygen via appropriate oxygen delivery device ***to increase driving pressure of oxygen in the alveoli.***
   b. If supplemental oxygen alone is not effective, administer constant positive airway pressure or mechanical ventilation with positive end-expiratory pressure ***to open collapsed alveoli and increase the surface area for gas exchange.***
3. Prevent hypoventilation
   a. Position patients in high-Fowler's position or semi-Fowler's position ***to promote diaphragmatic descent and maximal inhalation.***
   b. Assist with deep breathing exercises and/or incentive spirometry with sustained maximal inspiration 5 to 10 times/hr ***to help reinflate collapsed portions of the lung.*** See "Ineffective Breathing Pattern Related to Decreased Lung Expansion" Management Plan, p. 723, for further instructions.
   c. Treat pain, if present, ***to prevent hypoventilation and atelectasis.*** Implement "Acute Pain Related to Transmission and Perception of Cutaneous, Visceral, Muscular, or Ischemic Impulses" Management Plan, p. 197.
4. Assist physician with intubation and initiation of mechanical ventilation as indicated.

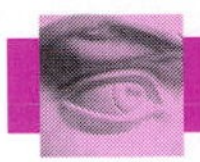

NURSING MANAGEMENT PLAN

RISK FOR ASPIRATION

DEFINITION:

A state in which an individual is at risk for entry of gastric secretions, oropharyngeal secretions, or exogenous food or fluids into tracheobronchial passages because of dysfunction of normal protective mechanisms.

RISK FACTORS

- Impaired laryngeal sensation or reflex
  - Reduced level of consciousness
  - Immediately after extubation
- Impaired pharyngeal peristalsis or tongue function
  - Neuromuscular dysfunction
  - Central nervous system dysfunction
  - Head or neck surgery
- Impaired laryngeal closure or elevation
  - Laryngeal nerve dysfunction
  - Artificial airways
  - Gastrointestinal tubes
- Increased gastric volume
  - Delayed gastric emptying
  - Enteral feedings
  - Medication administration
- Increased intragastric pressure
  - Upper abdominal surgery
  - Obesity
  - Pregnancy
  - Ascites
- Decreased lower esophageal sphincter pressure
  - Increased gastric acidity
  - Gastrointestinal tubes
- Decreased antegrade esophageal propulsion
  - Trendelenburg or supine position
  - Esophageal dysmotility
  - Esophageal structural defects or lesions

OUTCOME CRITERIA

- Normal breath sounds or no change in patients' baseline breath sounds.
- ABG values remain within patients' baseline.
- No evidence of gastric contents in lung secretions.

NURSING INTERVENTIONS AND *RATIONALE*

1. Assess gastrointestinal function ***to rule out hypoactive peristalsis and abdominal distention.***
2. Position patients with head of bed elevated 30 degrees ***to prevent gastric reflux through gravity.*** If head elevation is contraindicated, position patients in right lateral decubitus position ***to facilitate passage of gastric contents across the pylorus.***
3. Maintain patency and functioning of nasogastric suction apparatus ***to prevent accumulation of gastric contents.***
4. Provide frequent and scrupulous mouth care ***to prevent colonization of the oropharynx with bacteria and inoculation of the lower airways.***
5. Ensure that endotracheal/tracheostomy cuff is properly inflated ***to limit aspiration of oropharyngeal secretions.***
6. Treat nausea promptly; collaborate with physician on an order for antiemetic ***to prevent vomiting and resultant aspiration.***

Additional interventions for patients receiving continuous or intermittent enteral tube feedings

1. Position patients with head of bed elevated 45 degrees ***to prevent gastric reflux.*** If a head-down position becomes necessary at any time, interrupt the feeding 30 minutes before the position change.
2. Check placement of feeding tube either by auscultation or radiographically at regular intervals (e.g., before administering intermittent feedings and after position changes, suctioning, coughing episodes, or vomiting) ***to ensure proper placement of the tube.***
3. Instill blue food coloring to feeding solutions ***to assist with identification of gastric contents in pulmonary secretions.***
4. Monitor patients for signs of delayed gastric emptying ***to decrease potential for vomiting and aspiration***
   a. For large-bore tubes, check residuals of tube feedings before intermittent feedings and every 4 hours during continuous feedings. Consider withholding feedings for residuals greater than 150% of the hourly rate (continuous feeding) or greater than 50% of the previous feeding (intermittent feeding).
   b. For small-bore tubes, observe abdomen for distention, palpate abdomen for hardness or tautness, and auscultate abdomen for bowel sounds.

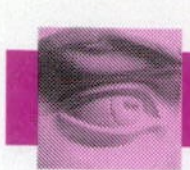

NURSING MANAGEMENT PLAN

DYSFUNCTIONAL VENTILATORY WEANING RESPONSE

DEFINITION:

A state in which a patient cannot adjust to lowered levels of mechanical ventilator support, which interrupts and prolongs the weaning process.

Dysfunctional Ventilatory Weaning Response (DVWR) Related to Physical, Psychologic, or Situational Factors

DEFINING CHARACTERISTICS

Mild DVWR

Responds to lowered levels of mechanical ventilator support with:

- Restlessness
- Slight increased respiratory rate from baseline
- Expressed feelings of increased need for oxygen; breathing discomfort; fatigue; warmth
- Queries about possible machine malfunction
- Increased concentration on breathing

Moderate DVWR

Responds to lowered levels of mechanical ventilator support with:

- Slight baseline increase in blood pressure < 20 mm Hg
- Slight baseline increase in heart rate < 20 beats/min
- Baseline increase in respiratory rate < 5 breaths/min
- Hypervigilence to activities
- Inability to respond to coaching
- Inability to cooperate
- Apprehension
- Diaphoresis
- Eye widening "wide-eyed look"
- Decreased air entry on auscultation
- Color changes; pale, slight cyanosis
- Slight respiratory accessory muscle use

Severe DVWR

Responds to lowered levels of mechanical ventilator support with:

- Agitation
- Deterioration in arterial blood gases from current baseline
- Baseline increase in blood pressure > 20 mm Hg
- Baseline increase in heart rate > 20 beats/min
- Respiratory rate increases significantly from baseline
- Profuse diaphoresis
- Full respiratory accessory muscle use
- Shallow, gasping breaths
- Paradoxical abdominal breathing
- Discoordinated breathing with the ventilator
- Decreased level of consciousness
- Adventitious breath sounds, audible airway secretions
- Cyanosis

OUTCOME CRITERIA

- Airway is clear.
- Underlying disorder is resolving.
- Patients are rested, and pain is controlled.
- Nutritional status is adequate.
- Patients have feelings of perceived control, situational security, and trust in the nurses.
- Patients are able to adapt to selected level of ventilator support without undue fatigue.

NURSING INTERVENTIONS AND *RATIONALE*

1. Communicate interest and concern for the patients' well-being and demonstrate confidence in ability to manage weaning process ***to instill trust in the patient.***
2. Use normalizing strategies (e.g., grooming, dressing, mobilizing, social conversation) ***to reinforce patients' self-esteem and feelings of identity.***
3. Identify parameters of the patients' usual functioning before the weaning process begins ***to facilitate early identification of problems.***
4. Identify patients' strengths and resources that can be mobilized ***to enhance the patients' coping and maximize their weaning effort.***
5. Note concerns that adversely affect the patients' comfort and confidence, and manage them discretely ***to facilitate the patients' ease.***
6. Praise successful activities, encourage a positive outlook, and review the patients' positive progress to date ***to increase patients' perceived self-efficacy.***
7. Inform patients of their situation and weaning progress ***to permit the patients as much control as possible.***
8. Teach patients about the weaning process and how they can participate in the process.
9. Negotiate daily weaning goals with patients ***to gain cooperation.***
10. Position patients with the head of the bed elevated ***to optimize their respiratory efforts.***
11. Coach patients in breath control by regular demonstrations of slow, deep, rhythmic patterns of breathing ***to assist with dyspnea.***
12. Remain visible in the room and reassure patients that help is immediately available if needed ***to reduce the patients' anxiety and fearfulness.***

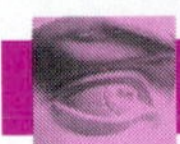

NURSING MANAGEMENT PLAN—CONT'D

Dysfunctional Ventilatory Weaning Response (DVWR) Related to Physical, Psychologic, or Situational Factors

13. Encourage patients to view weaning trials as a form of training, regardless of whether the weaning goal is achieved ***to avoid discouragement.***
14. Encourage patients to maintain emotional calmness by reassuring, being present, comforting, talking down if emotionally aroused, and reinforcing the idea that they can and will succeed.
15. Monitor the patients' status frequently ***to avoid undue fatigue and anxiety.***
16. Provide regular periods of rest by reducing activities, maintaining or increasing ventilator support, and providing oxygen as needed before fatigue advances.
17. Provide distraction (e.g., visitors, radio, television, conversation) when the patients' concentration starts to create tension and increases their anxiety.
18. Ensure adequate nutritional support, sufficient rest and sleep time, and sedation or pain control ***to promote the patients' optimal physical and emotional comfort.***
19. Start weaning early in the day ***when patients are most rested.***
20. Restrict unnecessary activities and visitors who do not cooperate with weaning strategies ***to minimize energy demands on patients during the weaning process.***
21. Coordinate necessary activities ***to promote adequate time for rest or relaxation.***
22. Monitor the patients' underlying disease process ***to ensure it is stabilized and under control.***
23. Advocate for additional resources (e.g., sedation, analgesia, rest) needed by patients ***to maximize their comfort status.***
24. Develop and adhere to an individualized plan of care ***to promote the patients' feelings of control.***

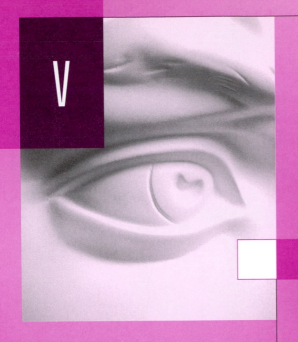

NEUROLOGIC ALTERATIONS

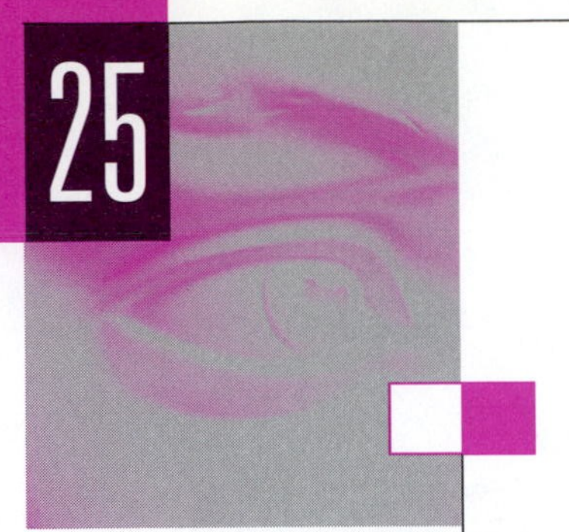

Neurologic Anatomy and Physiology

The nervous system is a unique, complex, and still somewhat mysterious network of fibers running throughout the body. It has the task of directing body systems and functions. Receiving thousands of bits of information each second from different sensory organs, this system transmits, analyzes, interprets, and integrates responses throughout the billions of nervous system cells. A basic understanding of the anatomy and physiology of the nervous system is essential to the delivery of quality critical care nursing. Although the roles and functions of the nervous system are diverse, a few principles and concepts apply to all. This chapter reviews the divisions of the nervous system and its microstructure, or cellular level, and functions. Mechanisms that provide protection to the nervous system also are presented. Finally, the anatomy and physiology of all the components of the central nervous system are outlined.

DIVISIONS OF THE NERVOUS SYSTEM

The nervous system is the most highly organized system of the body, with all of its parts functioning as an inseparable unit. For review, this system may be classified in terms of location or according to function.

Anatomic Divisions

The central nervous system (CNS) comprises all the portions of the brain and spinal cord. The peripheral nervous system (PNS) comprises the 12 pairs of cranial nerves plus the 32 pairs of spinal nerves and the peripheral nerves that connect the CNS with the body wall and the viscera.

Physiologic Divisions

The somatic, or voluntary, nervous system is composed of fibers that connect the CNS with structures of the skeletal muscles and the skin. The autonomic, or involuntary, nervous system is composed of fibers that connect the CNS with smooth muscle, cardiac muscle, internal organs, and glands. It includes both sympathetic and parasympathetic branches.

Most activities of the nervous system originate from sensory receptors, such as visual, auditory, or tactile receptors. This sensory information is transmitted to the CNS by afferent fibers (sensory fibers). Efferent fibers (motor fibers) transmit the CNS response to the periphery to produce a motor response, such as contraction of skeletal muscles, contraction of the smooth muscles of organs, or secretion by endocrine glands. Transmission of both afferent (sensory) and efferent (motor) information in the CNS is performed by internuncial fibers. To better understand the macrostructure and functions of the nervous system, it is essential to look first at the microstructure, or cellular level.[1]

MICROSTRUCTURE OF THE NERVOUS SYSTEM

The cellular units of the nervous system are the neurons and the neuroglia.[2-4] The neurons are the functional units of the nervous system and are responsible for conduction of nerve impulses. The neuroglial cells provide support, repair, and protection for the delicate neurons.

Neurons

More than 10 billion neurons are in the CNS alone. The cellular appearance of a neuron varies, depending

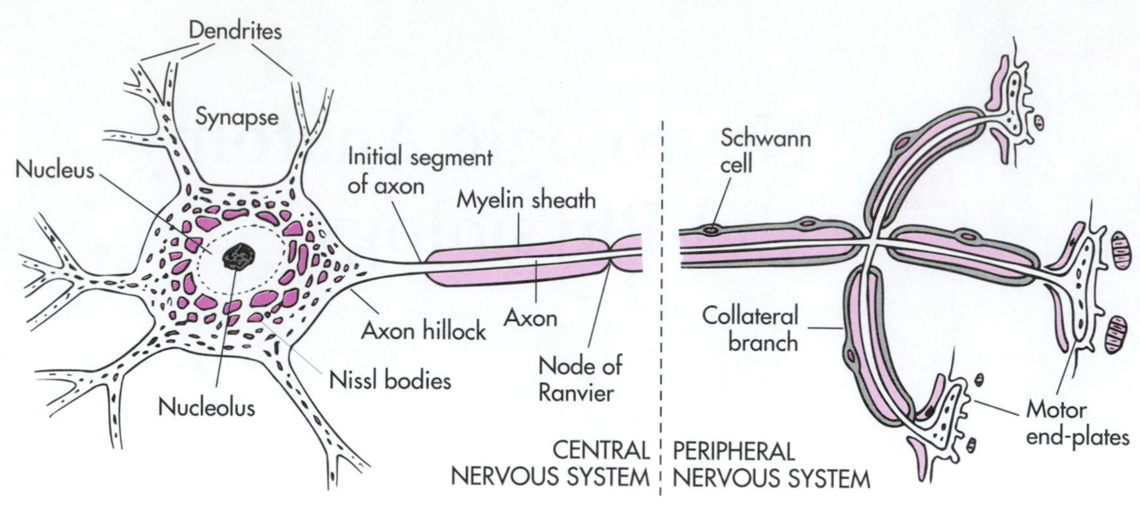

FIGURE 25-1. Diagram of the neuron with composite parts.

on its specific function, but each cell contains three basic components (Figure 25-1). The first component is the cell body (soma), which controls the metabolic activity of the cell. Inside the cell body is the nucleus, which stores ribonucleic acid (RNA) and deoxyribonucleic acid (DNA) and also contains the nucleolus for synthesis of RNA. The cell body also contains Nissl bodies for storage of RNA and synthesis of protein; Golgi apparati for storage of protein and synthesis of cell membranes; neurofibrils for support; and lysosomes, which function as intracellular scavengers. An intact, well-nourished cell body is essential to the life of the neuron as a whole. If the cell body dies, the rest of the neuron also dies and cannot be replaced. These specialized cells cannot reproduce themselves; therefore cell bodies are grouped together in relatively protected areas. Cell bodies form the gray matter in the brain, the brainstem, and the spinal cord. Ganglia, small nodules of nervous tissue lying close to the CNS, are cell bodies in the peripheral nervous system.

Dendrites, the second component of a neuron, are branched fibers extending only a short distance from the cell body. Each neuron may have several dendrites, which carry impulses to the cell body. The third component of a neuron is the axon. Each neuron contains only one axon, which carries information away from the cell. Axons can be microscopic in length or extend up to 4 feet. Many axons are protected by a myelin sheath, which is a white protein-lipid complex laid down by Schwann cells in the PNS and by oligodendroglia in the CNS. Myelin sheath acts as insulation for the conduction of nerve impulses. Fibers enclosed in the sheath are called *myelinated fibers;* those not enclosed are called *unmyelinated fibers.* The white matter of the CNS is composed of myelinated fiber tracts.

Myelin is not a continuous layer but has gaps called *nodes of Ranvier.* Nerve impulses are conducted from node to node; therefore conduction is more rapid. Loss of myelin sheath integrity disrupts nerve impulse transmission. Multiple sclerosis, for example, is a disease that causes degeneration of myelin.

Neurons are structurally classified as unipolar, a cell body with one process that divides into a central branch (the axon) and a peripheral branch (the dendrite); as bipolar, a cell body with two processes (one axon and one dendrite); and as multipolar, a cell body with one axon and several dendrites.

Neuroglia

Neuroglial cells are the support cells to the neuron. There are four types of neuroglial cells: astroglia, oligodendroglia, ependyma, and microglia (Figure 25-2). These cells provide structural support, nourishment, and protection for the neurons (Table 25-1).[4] In the nervous system there are 6 to 10 times more neuroglial cells than neurons. It is of clinical significance that neuroglia retain their mitotic abilities. Therefore neuroglia can become the source of nonmetabolic CNS primary neoplasms.[4]

Physiology of Nervous Tissue

The nervous system consists of chains of neurons with no actual anatomic continuity. Each neuron is a separate unit in contact with another neuron or target cell through synapses (Figure 25-3).

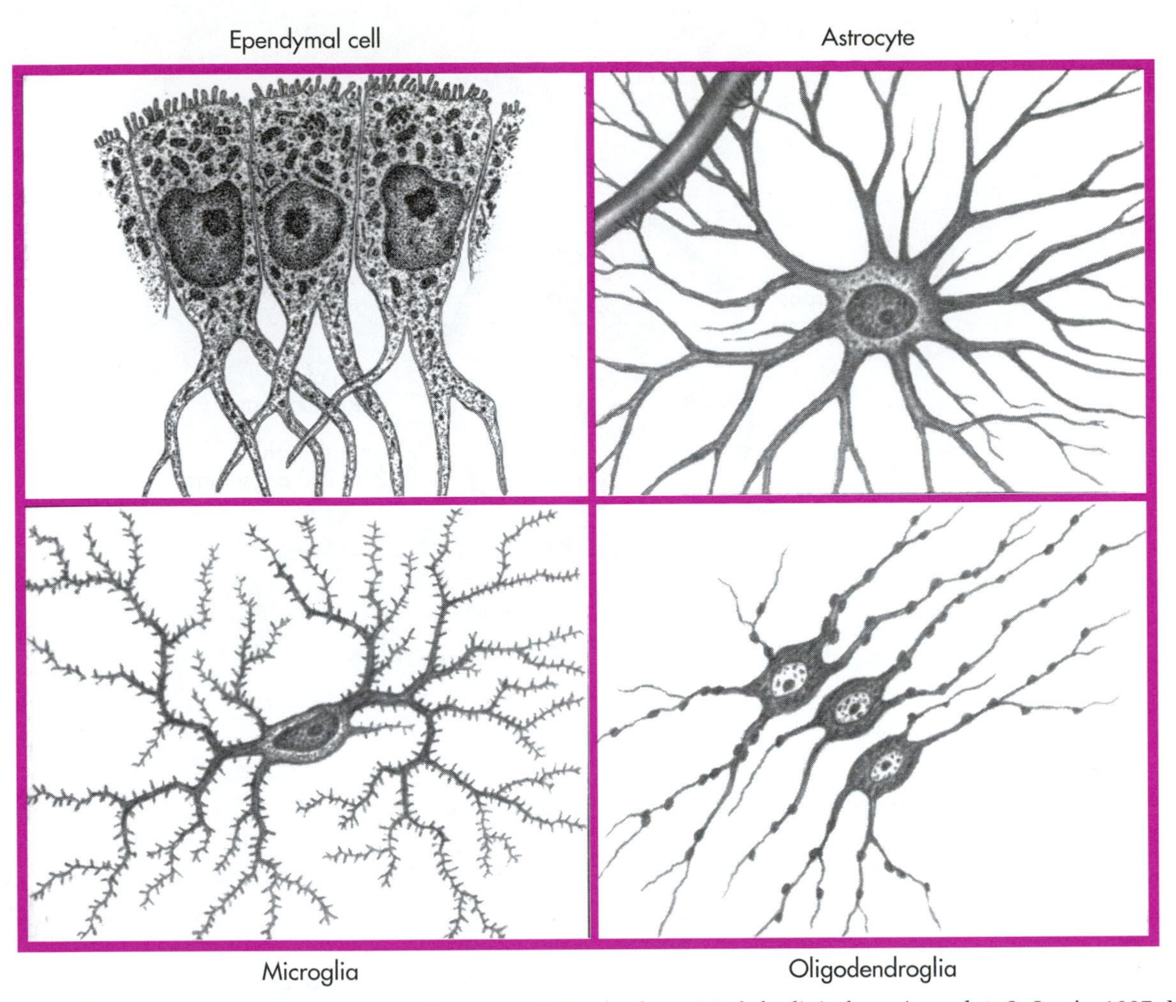

FIGURE 25-2. Types of neuroglial cells. (From Thompson JM and others: *Mosby's clinical nursing,* ed 4, St Louis, 1997, Mosby.)

TABLE 25-1 Types of Neuroglial Cells

Cell Type	Function
Astroglia (astrocyte)	Supplies nutrients to neuron structure and to support framework for neurons and capillaries; forms part of the blood-brain barrier
Oligodendroglia	Forms the myelin sheath in the CNS
Ependyma	Lines the ventricular system; forms the choroid plexus, which produces cerebrospinal fluid (CSF)
Microglia	Occurs mainly in the white matter; phagocytizes waste products from injured neurons

The generation of a nerve impulse, as with other cells of the body, begins with the depolarization of the cell membrane. The speed of the impulse conduction depends on whether the nerve is myelinated or unmyelinated. In an unmyelinated nerve, depolarization must travel the entire length of the fiber. In myelinated nerves, impulses "jump" from one node of Ranvier to another. This node-to-node conduction, called *saltatory transmission,* increases the velocity of impulse transmission and decreases energy demands. Impulses are transmitted away from cell bodies by axons and pass from the axon of one cell body to the dendrite or cell body of another neuron through the synapse.

Actual synaptic transmission is a chemical process involving the release of neurotransmitters. Anatomically, a synapse travels from the presynaptic terminal, or knob, at the end of an axon, across the synaptic cleft, to the postsynaptic membrane.

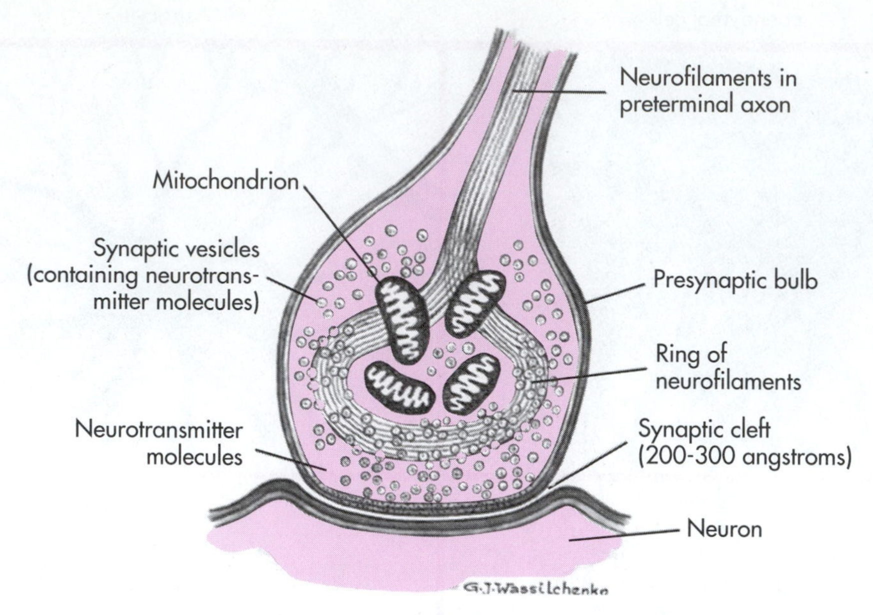

FIGURE 25-3. Schematic diagram of a synapse.

Neurotransmitters. Neurotransmitters, chemical substances secreted by the presynaptic terminal, provide the connection from axon to dendrite or target cell for transmission of the nerve impulse.[4] As a nerve impulse reaches the presynaptic terminal, neurotransmitters are secreted into the microscopic synaptic cleft, causing a change in the permeability of the postsynaptic membrane and therefore passage of the impulse across the synaptic cleft.

More than 30 different chemical substances have been identified as neurotransmitters and can be divided into two types—excitatory and inhibitory. Excitatory neurotransmitters promote the conduction of the impulse from one cell to the next. When inhibitor neurotransmitters are released, the neuron's internal charge becomes more negative and the resistance to depolarization is increased. The most commonly known neurotransmitters are acetylcholine, dopamine, norepinephrine, serotonin, γ-aminobutyric acid, glycine, and glutamic acid.

After synaptic transmission, binding of the neurotransmitters to the postsynaptic membrane continues until the neurotransmitter is inactivated by an enzyme (acetylcholine is inactivated by acetylcholinesterase), reabsorbed by the presynaptic terminal, or diffused away from the postsynaptic membrane.

Dysfunction of synaptic pathways results in poor or absent transmission of the nerve impulse. Parkinson's disease, resulting from the lack of dopamine in the basal ganglia, allows excitatory neurotransmitters to go unchecked. Symptoms of Parkinson's disease include tremors, rigidity of limbs, and difficulty initiating movement. Myasthenia gravis, a disease characterized by generalized weakness and fatigability of voluntary muscles, is caused by a reduction of acetylcholine receptors on the postsynaptic membrane.

Intentional pharmacologic blockade of synaptic transmission at the neuromuscular junction is often used in critical care units to produce temporary motor paralysis in patients who require mechanical ventilation, control of metabolic demands, or restriction of movement.[5,6]

CENTRAL NERVOUS SYSTEM

The CNS, composed of the spinal cord, brainstem, and brain, is the control unit for all physiologic functions. Review of the anatomy and physiology of the CNS begins with the most basic functions of the brainstem and progresses through the diencephalon to the highly developed cerebrum. The spinal cord is reviewed at the end of this section. Maintaining a healthy CNS is challenged by the delicateness of the nerves and tissues involved. Therefore several mechanisms are in place to provide protection and support to these fragile structures. The brain and spinal cord have similar protective mechanisms,[4,7] but because of the distinct anatomic differences of these two portions of the CNS, protective mechanisms specific to the spinal cord are discussed separately (see the Spinal Cord section in this chapter).

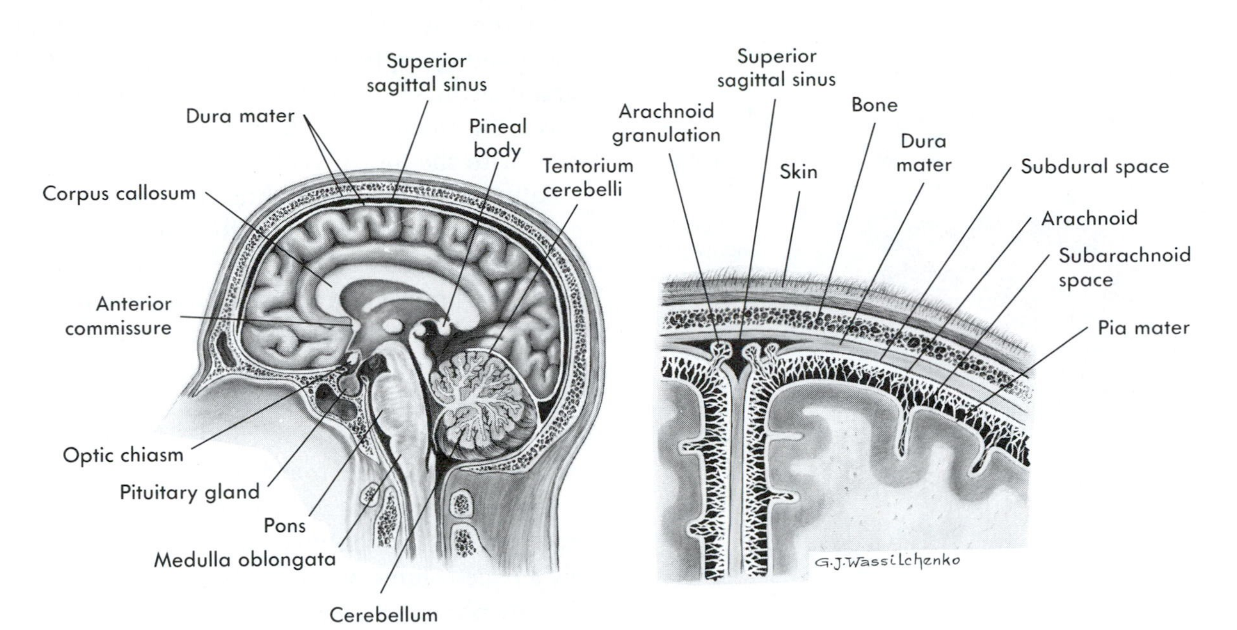

FIGURE 25-4. Meningeal layers of the brain.

Cranial Protective Mechanisms

Bony structures. The outermost protective measures underneath the integument are the bony structures that encase the CNS. The skull, or cranium, forms the bony container that surrounds the brain. Composed of eight flat, irregular bones fused through suture lines, the skull protects the brain from direct force or superficial trauma. Excessive force causing fracture of the skull can destroy this protective mechanism and push bony fragments into the fragile brain tissue.

Viewing the skull from the inside, the superior surfaces form a smooth inner wall, whereas the basilar skull contains ridges and folds with sharp edges that provide structure for the support of different portions of the brain. Sharp blows to the head that cause shifting of intracranial contents can lead to brain tissue laceration and contusion across these sharp edges.

The cranium is an enclosed vault except for one large opening at the base called the *foramen magnum,* through which the brainstem projects and connects to the spinal cord. Several other very small openings in the base of the skull allow entrance and exit of blood vessels and cranial nerves.

Meninges. Beneath the skull lies the second layer of intracranial protection, the meninges. The three layers of meninges are the dura mater, the arachnoid, and the pia mater (Figure 25-4).

Dura mater. The first of the meninges beneath the skull is the dura mater. Consisting of two layers, this tough, fibrous membrane provides several functions. The outermost layer comprises the periosteum for the cranial bones and therefore adheres to the skull. The inner, meningeal layer of the dura extends into the cranial space. The four extensions of the dural layer are the falx cerebri, tentorium cerebelli, falx cerebelli, and diaphragma sellae.

The falx cerebri divides the right and left hemispheres of the brain vertically through the longitudinal fissures extending from the frontal lobe to the occipital lobe. The tentorium cerebelli forms a tent between the occipital lobes and the cerebellum and separates the cerebral hemispheres from the brainstem and cerebellum. Intracranial terminology labels all structures above the tentorium as *supratentorial* and all structures below as *infratentorial.* Structures below the tentorium are also located in the area referred to as the *posterior fossa.*

The falx cerebelli forms the division between the two lateral lobes of the cerebellum. The final extension of the dura mater is the diaphragma sellae, which forms a roof over the sella turcica. Inside the sella turcica is the pituitary gland.

Further dural separations form the venous sinuses located throughout the intracranial space. These venous sinuses, which collect blood from intracerebral and meningeal veins, drain into the internal jugular vein to return venous blood to the heart.

The main blood supply for the dura, the middle meningeal artery, courses above the dura in the epidural space. Traumatic interruption of this vessel is a

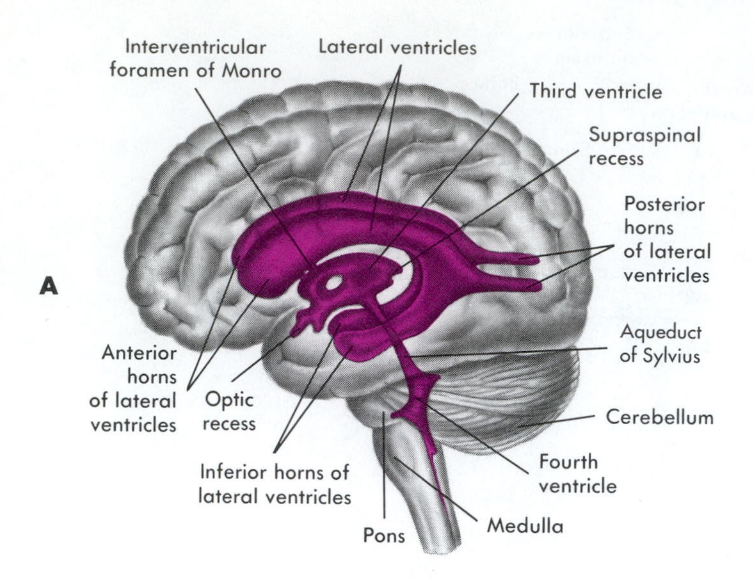

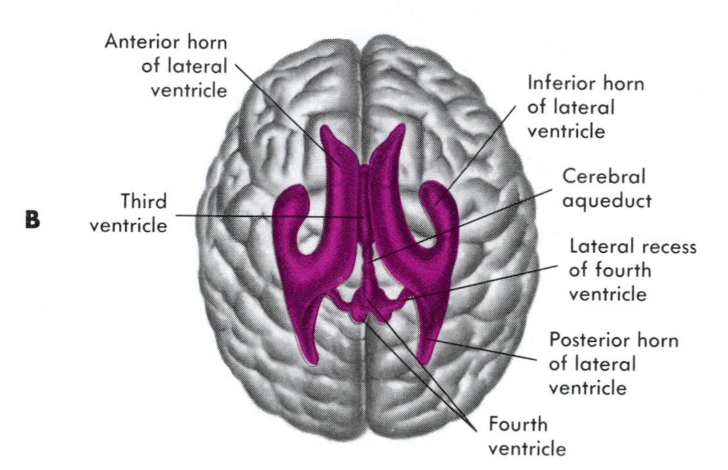

FIGURE 25-5. Cerebral ventricles. **A,** Lateral view. **B,** Superior view. (From Thompson JM and others: *Mosby's clinical nursing,* ed 4, St Louis, 1997, Mosby.)

common cause of epidural hematoma. Between the dura mater and the arachnoid lies the subdural space. This narrow space has a large number of unsupported small veins connecting the arachnoid and dura, so this area is highly susceptible to injury. When the small vessels are stretched and torn, a subdural hematoma is formed.

Arachnoid membrane. The arachnoid membrane is a delicate, fragile membrane that loosely surrounds the brain. Fine threads of elastic tissue called *trabeculae* connect the arachnoid to the pia mater, creating a spongy, weblike structure called the *subarachnoid space.* Located in the subarachnoid space are cerebrospinal fluid (CSF) and a variety of cerebral arteries and veins. Subarachnoid hemorrhage occurs when one of these vessels is disrupted.

At the base of the brain, widened areas of subarachnoid space form cisterns, or pools, of CSF. The largest of these cisterns, the cisterna magna, lies between the medulla and the cerebellum and communicates with the fourth ventricle.

Tufts of arachnoid membrane, called *arachnoid villi,* or granulations, project into the superior sagittal and transverse venous sinuses. This communication between arachnoid villi and sinuses allows reabsorption of CSF from the subarachnoid space into the venous space. Several conditions, such as meningitis or subarachnoid hemorrhage, can obstruct these arachnoid villi and decrease the rate of CSF reabsorption. This arachnoid villi obstruction is termed *communicating hydrocephalus.*

Pia mater. The innermost of the meninges is the delicate pia mater. Rich in small blood vessels that supply a large volume of arterial blood to cerebral tissues, this membrane closely follows all folds and convolutions of the brain's surface. Tufts or folds of the pia mater in the lateral, third, and fourth ventricles form a portion of the choroid plexus that is responsible for the production of CSF.

Ventricular system. A central CSF-filled core of the brain is called the *ventricular system* (Figure 25-5). Made of four connected chambers lined with ependymal cells, the ventricles provide the anatomic structure around which the brain and brainstem are formed.

The two largest ventricles, one within each of the cerebral hemispheres, are called the lateral ventricles. Extending from the frontal lobe to the occipital lobe, the lateral ventricles consist of a body and a frontal, temporal, and occipital horn. When cannulation of the ventricular system is required for intracranial pressure monitoring, CSF drainage, or placement of a CSF shunt, the frontal horn of the lateral ventricle is most often selected.

The foramen of Monro connects the two lateral ventricles with a central cavity, the third ventricle. Located directly above the midbrain, the third ventricle lies between the structures of the thalamus in the diencephalon.

The cerebral aqueduct (aqueduct of Sylvius) provides communication with the fourth ventricle, which lies between the brainstem and the cerebellum. At the base of the fourth ventricle, two openings, the foramen of Luschka and the foramen of Magendie, open the ventricular system into the subarachnoid space. Any blockage of CSF flow in the ventricular system, such as a blood clot in the cerebral aqueduct or a mass pressing against the cerebral aqueduct, causes dilation of the ventricles, termed *noncommunicating hydrocephalus.*

Cerebrospinal fluid. CSF fills the ventricular system and surrounds the brain and spinal cord in the sub-

TABLE 25-2 Normal CSF Profile Values

Property	Values
pH	7.35-7.45
Specific gravity	1.007
Appearance	Clear and colorless
Cells	0 white blood cells (WBCs) 0 red blood cells (RBCs) 0-10 lymphocytes
Glucose	50-75 mg/dL (two thirds of blood sugar value)
Protein	5-25 mg/dL
Volume	135-150 ml
Pressure	70-200 mm H_2O (lumbar puncture) 3-15 mm Hg (ventricular)

arachnoid space. Protection of the CNS is thereby accomplished because the CSF system acts as a "shock absorber" and participates in the removal of waste products from cerebral tissue.

CSF is normally a clear, colorless, odorless solution secreted by the choroid plexuses (95%) located in all four ventricles and also in small amounts by ependymal cells and capillaries of the pia mater. Believed to be a filtrate of blood, CSF contains some unique properties that make the actual secretion process still a mystery (Table 25-2).

The production of CSF occurs at a rate of approximately 20 ml/hour, or 500 ml/day. With a circulating volume of 135 to 150 ml, CSF must be reabsorbed daily to prevent development of hydrocephalus. The CSF system does not have any feedback mechanism for volume regulation; CSF is continually produced at the rate of 20 ml/hour, regardless of the total circulating volume and the rate of reabsorption. Because CSF is essentially a filtrate of blood and occurs by diffusion, blood pressure is an important component in the overall CSF-production process. Cerebral metabolism and serum osmolality also affect CSF production. Flow of CSF occurs through a closed system between the ventricles and the subarachnoid space (Figure 25-6). CSF formed in the lateral ventricles flows through the foramen of Monro into the third ventricle. This fluid, plus the additional CSF formed by the choroid plexus of the third ventricle, flows through the cerebral aqueduct and joins the CSF produced by the fourth ventricle. CSF exit from the ventricular system occurs medially through the foramen of Magendie and laterally through the two foramina of Luschka. Once out of the ventricles, CSF flows in

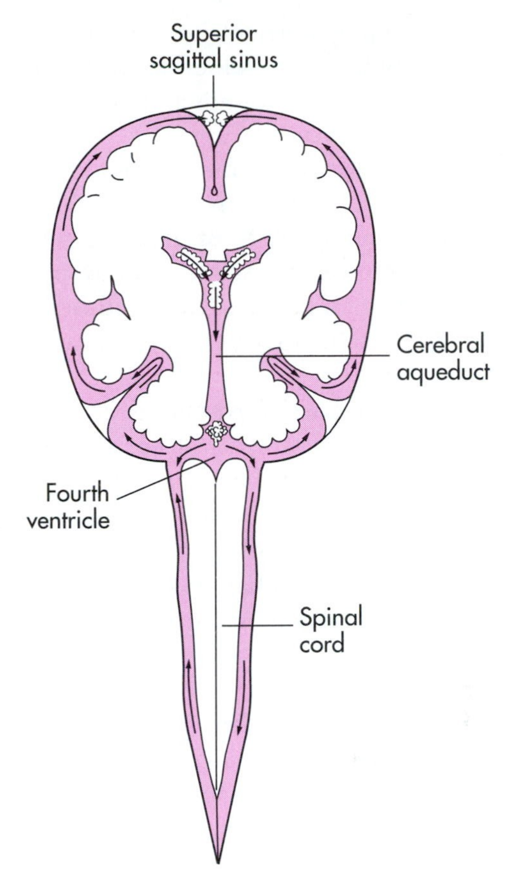

FIGURE 25-6. Path of circulation of cerebrospinal fluid from its formation in the ventricles to its absorption into the superior sagittal sinus. (From Waxman SG, deGroot J: *Correlative neuroanatomy*, ed 23, Norwalk, Conn, 1996, Appleton & Lange.)

the subarachnoid space, down around the spinal cord, and up over the surface of the brain, where it is reabsorbed into the venous circulation through the arachnoid villi.

Blood-brain barrier. The final protective mechanism is a physiologic mechanism that helps maintain a delicate balance in the brain's internal environment. The blood-brain barrier regulates the transport of nutrients, ions, water, and waste products through selective permeability.[1]

Stabilization of the physical and chemical environment surrounding the neurons of the CNS is the goal of the blood-brain barrier. Many substances, such as metabolites or toxic compounds, cannot cross the blood-brain barrier. Other substances, such as antibiotics, cross slowly, thus have a lesser concentration in the brain than in other areas of the body.

The blood-brain barrier operates on the concept of "tight junctions" between adjacent capillary endothelial cells and astrocytes of the CNS. In contrast to other capillaries in the body, cerebral capillaries are surrounded by astrocyte end feet. One function of the astrocyte is to supply nutrients to the neuron. The selective permeability of the blood-brain barrier keeps out toxic or harmful compounds and protects the fragile, irreplaceable neuron.

Passage of substances across the blood-brain barrier is a function of particle size, lipid solubility, and protein-binding potential. Most drugs or compounds that are lipid-soluble and stable at body pH rapidly cross the blood-brain barrier. The blood-brain barrier is also very permeable to water, oxygen, carbon dioxide, and glucose.

The blood-brain barrier exists only in certain areas of the CNS. The areas in which it does not exist—the pineal region, the hypothalamus, and the floor of the fourth ventricle—require contact with plasma to sense changes in concentration of glucose, carbon dioxide, and serum osmolality. Initiation of feedback mechanisms by the hypothalamus in response to these changes regulates the internal environment of the rest of the body.

Of clinical significance, disruption or alteration of blood-brain barrier permeability occurs with injury to cerebral tissue. This injury could be mechanical from trauma, chemical from toxins or drugs, or functional from intracranial tumors. Brain irradiation also may alter the permeability of the blood-brain barrier. Systemic chemotherapeutic agents can be administered because they do not cross the blood-brain barrier, thus preventing destruction of the neuronal tissue by these harsh agents. The obvious disadvantage is that use of chemotherapy in CNS neoplasms is often ineffective.

Two other weaker barrier systems also exist. The blood-CSF barrier existing in the capillary endothelium, pial membranes, and ependymal cells of the choroid plexus permits selective transport of substances into the CSF. Finally, the brain-CSF barrier is a weak barrier between CSF and interstitial fluid. Because this barrier is weaker, drugs placed directly into CSF (intrathecal injection) will pass into interstitial CNS fluid.

Brainstem

Medulla oblongata. As the spinal cord extends through the foramen magnum of the skull, it becomes the lowermost portion of the brainstem, the medulla oblongata. In the caudal portion of the medulla, decussation (crossing) of the motor fibers occurs. Below the point of decussation, stimuli from the right side of the brain control movement in the left side of the body and vice versa.[1]

The medulla also contains groups of neurons, or "centers," that control involuntary functions such as swallowing, vomiting, hiccoughing, coughing, vasoconstriction, and respirations. The medullary respiratory center works in conjunction with the apneustic and pneumotaxic centers of the pons to control respirations. It is responsible for the basic involuntary rhythm of respirations but cannot maintain a smooth, life-sustaining respiratory pattern without stimuli from other higher centers of the brain (Figure 25-7).

Also located in the medulla are the origins of cranial nerves IX (glossopharyngeal), X (vagus), XI (spinal accessory), and XII (hypoglossal) (Table 25-3). The reticular formation begins in the medulla.

Pons. Located above the medulla, the pons continues to relay information to and from the brain and spinal cord along fiber tracts. The ventral surface of the pons contains fibers that connect to the cerebellum. These pathways allow the transmission of influences from the cerebellum to the cerebral cortex, ensuring efficiency and smoothness of movement. Located in the pons are two respiratory control centers—the apneustic and pneumotaxic—which communicate with the medullary respiratory center. The apneustic center controls the length of inspiration and expiration, and the pneumotaxic center controls the rate of respirations. Behind the pons lies the fourth ventricle.[1,2]

The origins of cranial nerves V (trigeminal), VI (abducens), VII (facial), and VIII (acoustic) are in the pons.[2,4] The medial longitudinal fasciculus is an important fiber tract in the pons. In a normally functioning brainstem, the medial longitudinal fasciculus connects cranial nerves III, IV, and VI with the vestibular and pontine paramedian reticular formation, allowing coordinated and appropriate movements of the eyes in response to noise, motion, position, and arousal. Portions of the reticular formation are also in the pons.

Midbrain. The midbrain forms the junction between the pons and diencephalon. Cranial nerves III and IV originate in this region. The aqueduct of Sylvius, which connects the third and fourth ventricles, is in the midbrain. Again, fibers of the reticular formation are present.

The major function of the midbrain is to relay stimuli involved in voluntary motor movement of the body. Also arising in the midbrain are the tectospinal and rubrospinal tracts of the extrapyramidal (involuntary) motor functions.[4] The tectospinal tract controls reflex motor movements in response to visual and auditory stimuli, and the rubrospinal tract controls tone of flexor muscles.[1]

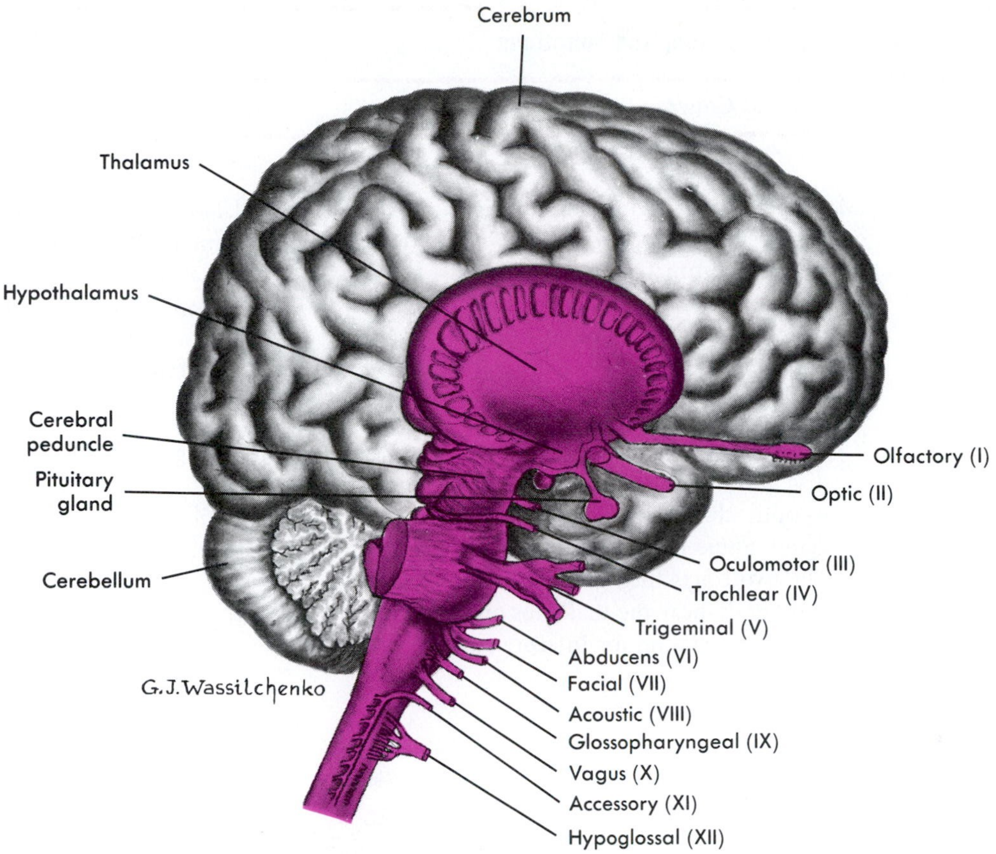

FIGURE 25-7. Lateral view of the brain, showing brainstem, diencephalon, and cranial nerves.

Reticular Formation

The reticular formation is a diffuse set of neurons, both gray matter nuclei and white matter fiber tracts, that extends from the upper level of the spinal cord, through the medulla, pons, and midbrain into the thalamus and cerebral cortex.[4,7] Composed of both motor and sensory tracts, the reticular formation is closely tied to functions of the basal ganglia, thalamus, cerebellum, and cerebral cortex. This formation of neural fibers has many excitatory and some inhibitory capabilities, achieving the capacity to regulate the activity from the sources mentioned and to enhance, suppress, or modify impulse transmission. The main role of the reticular formation is to provide a balance between the excitatory and inhibitory stimuli to maintain normal muscle tone, which supports the body against gravity. Damage to the inhibitory areas above the reticular formation (cerebellum and basal ganglia) leads to an excitatory response of the body. Decorticate (abnormal flexion) or decerebrate (abnormal extension) posturing is a result of such an injury. Also located in the reticular formation are centers for blood pressure, respiration, and heart rate function.

Reticular activating system. Located within the same region as the reticular formation is the reticular activating system (RAS). Also a diffuse network of fibers extending from the lower brainstem to the cerebral cortex, the RAS has two main levels. The lower portion of the RAS in the brainstem assists with the control of wake-sleep cycles and consciousness. The upper portion in the thalamus region allows the ability to focus attention on a specific task. When the upper RAS is damaged, the patient exhibits a vegetative state, exhibiting sleep-wake cycles and other brainstem functions but no upper levels of cerebration. Although the RAS is not the "center" of consciousness, communication between the cerebral cortex and the RAS is apparently necessary for consciousness to occur.[4,7]

Cerebellum

The cerebellum, separated from the cerebrum by the tentlike structure of the tentorium cerebelli, has also been called the "little brain" or the "hind brain." Approximately one fifth the size of the brain, the cerebellum is composed of two lateral hemispheres and a central portion called the *vermis.* As is the cerebrum,

TABLE 25-3 Cranial Nerves, Origins, Course, and Functions

Cranial Nerve	Origin and Course	Function
I OLFACTORY		
Sensory	Mucosa of nasal cavity; only cranial nerve with cell body located in peripheral structure (nasal mucosa). Passes through cribriform plate of ethmoid bone and goes on to olfactory bulbs at floor of frontal lobe. Final interpretation is in temporal lobe.	Smell. However, system is more than receptor/interpreter for odors; perception of smell also sensitizes other body systems and responses, such as salivation, peristalsis, and even sexual stimulus. Loss of sense of smell is termed *anosmia*.
II OPTIC		
Sensory	Ganglion cells of retina converge to the optic disc and form optic nerve. Nerve fibers pass to optic chiasm, which is above pituitary gland. Some fibers decussate; others do not. The two tracts then go to the lateral geniculate body near the thalamus and then on to the end station for interpretation in the occipital lobe.	Vision (Figure 25-8).

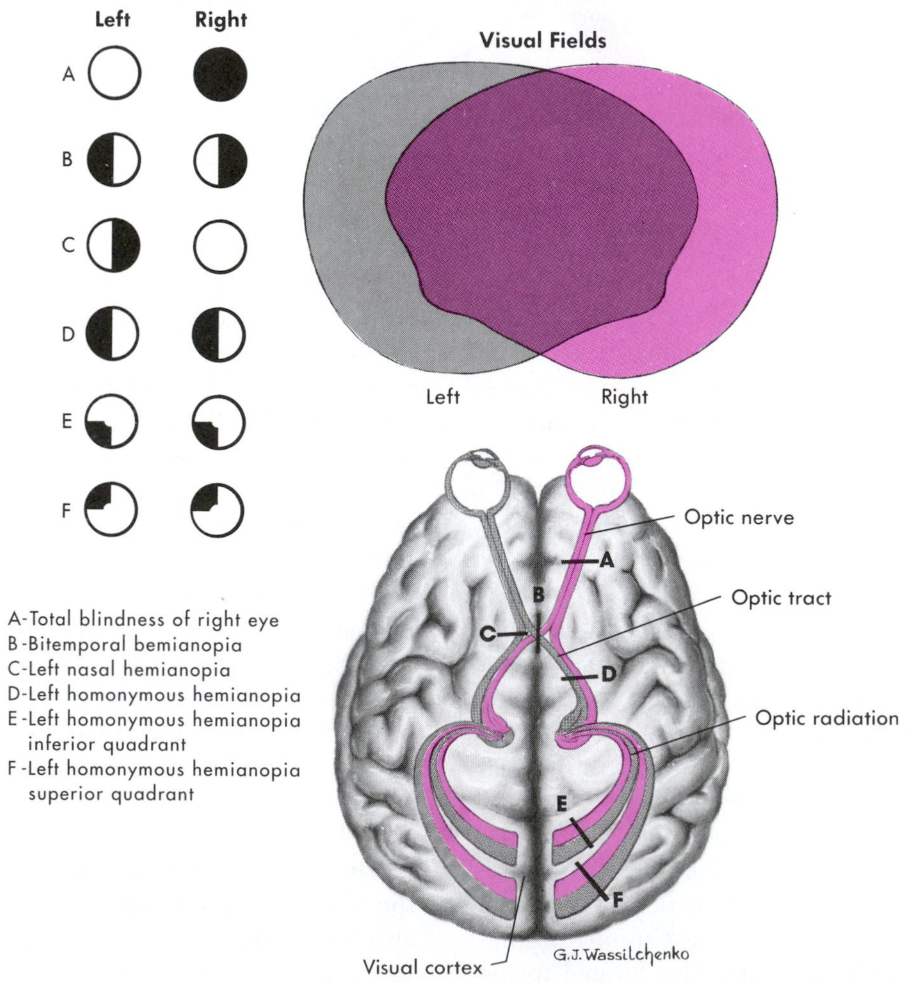

A-Total blindness of right eye
B-Bitemporal hemianopia
C-Left nasal hemianopia
D-Left homonymous hemianopia
E-Left homonymous hemianopia inferior quadrant
F-Left homonymous hemianopia superior quadrant

FIGURE 25-8. Visual fields showing optic nerve, optic chiasm, optic tracts, and optic radiations. Examples of various visual field defects. (From Rudy E: *Advanced neurological and neurosurgical nursing,* St Louis, 1984, Mosby.)

TABLE 25-3 Cranial Nerves, Origins, Course, and Functions—cont'd

Cranial Nerve	Origin and Course	Function
III OCULOMOTOR		
Motor	Originates in midbrain and emerges from brainstem at the upper pons. Motor fibers to superior, medial, inferior recti, and inferior oblique for eye movement; levator muscle of the eyelid.	Extraocular movement of eyes (Figure 25-9). Raises eyelid.
Parasympathetic	Parasympathetic fibers to ciliary muscles and iris of eye.	Constricts pupil; changes shape of lens.

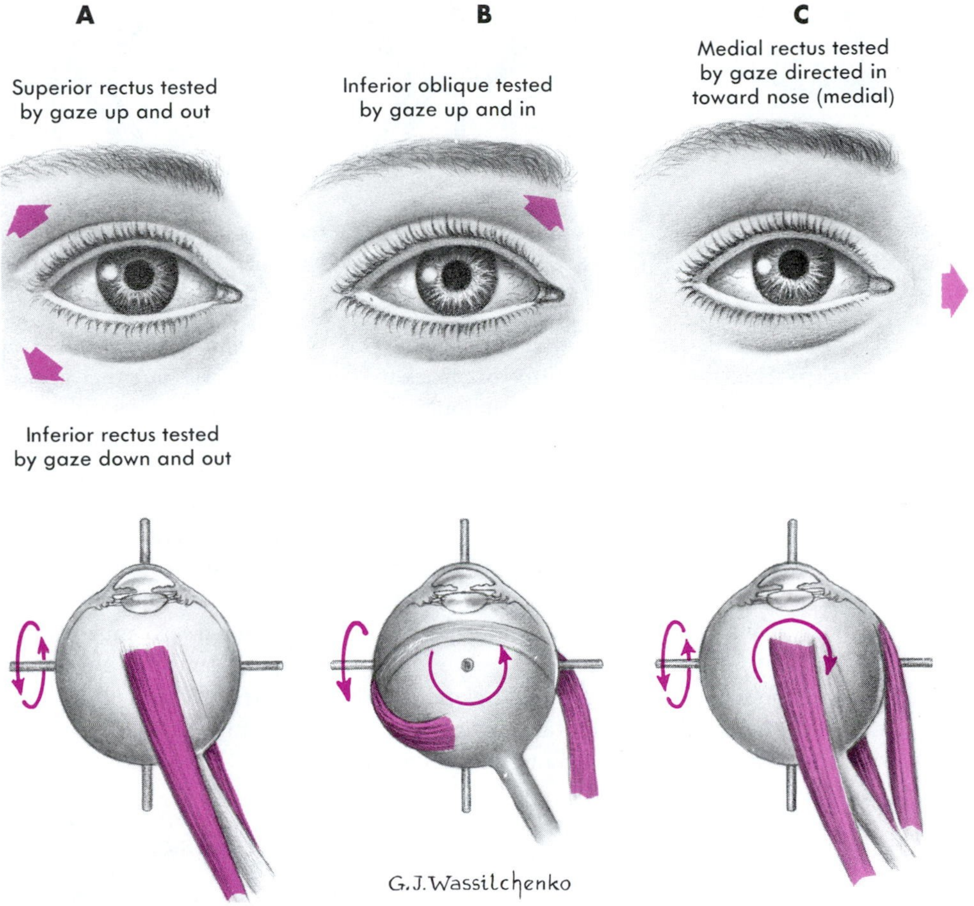

FIGURE 25-9. A, Superior and inferior rectus muscles. Superior rectus moves eye upward; inferior rectus moves eye down and in. **B,** Inferior oblique muscle elevates and abducts the eye. **C,** Medial rectus muscle adducts eye toward the nose.

Continued

the cerebellum is composed of a thin outer layer of gray matter, or cortex, and a core of white matter, or fiber tracts. Four pairs of nuclei are located deep in the white matter.

The cerebellum influences muscle tone associated with equilibrium, orientation in space, locomotion, and posture to ensure synchronization of muscle action. Input is received from sensory pathways of the spinal cord, the brainstem, and the cerebrum. Output is communicated through descending motor pathways, such as the corticospinal, vestibulospinal, and reticulospinal tracts.

Cerebellar influences work through continual excitatory and inhibiting stimuli from deep nuclei of the white matter. The balancing of these two opposing

(Text continues on p. 746)

TABLE 25-3 Cranial Nerves, Origins, Course, and Functions—cont'd

Cranial Nerve	Origin and Course	Function
IV TROCHLEAR		
Motor	Midbrain origin near oculomotor, emerges at the upper pons near cerebral peduncle. Motor fibers to superior oblique muscle of eyeball.	Extraocular movement of eyes (Figure 25-10).

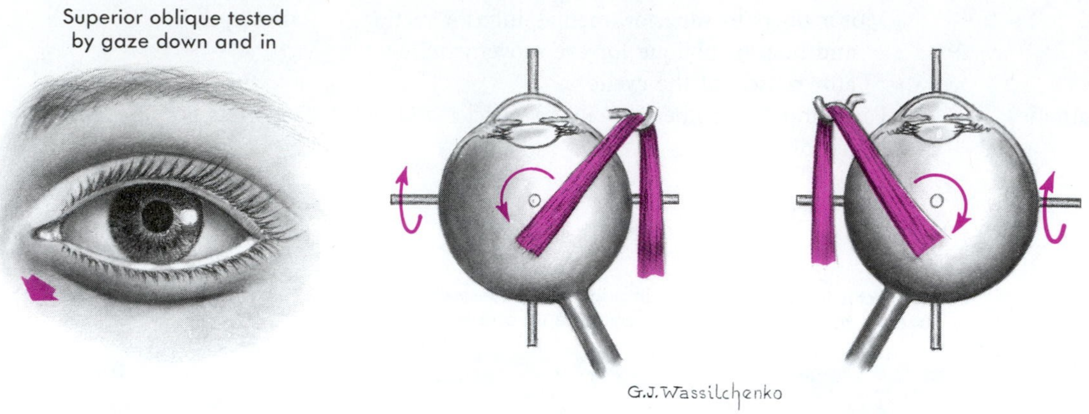

FIGURE 25-10. Superior oblique muscle, which rotates the eye down and out at the same time it causes intorsion, or inward rotation, of the eyeball. The strongest primary action of this muscle is adduction; thus the gaze for testing this muscle is in and down.

Cranial Nerve	Origin and Course	Function
V TRIGEMINAL		
Sensory	Originates in fourth ventricle and emerges at the lateral parts of the pons. Has three branches to face: ophthalmic, maxillary, and mandibular.	*Ophthalmic branch:* Sensation to cornea, ciliary body, iris, lacrimal gland, conjunctiva, nasal mucosal membranes, eyelids, eyebrows, forehead, and nose. *Maxillary branch:* Sensation to skin of cheek, lower lid, side of nose and upper jaw, teeth, mucosa of mouth, sphenopolative-pterygoid region, and maxillary sinus. *Mandibular branch:* Sensation to skin of lower lip, chin, ear, mucous membrane, teeth of lower jaw, and tongue.
Motor	Goes to temporalis, masseter, pterygoid gland, anterior part of digastric muscles (all for mastication), and the tensor tympani and tensor veli palatini muscles (clench jaws).	Muscles of chewing and mastication and opening jaw (Figure 25-11).

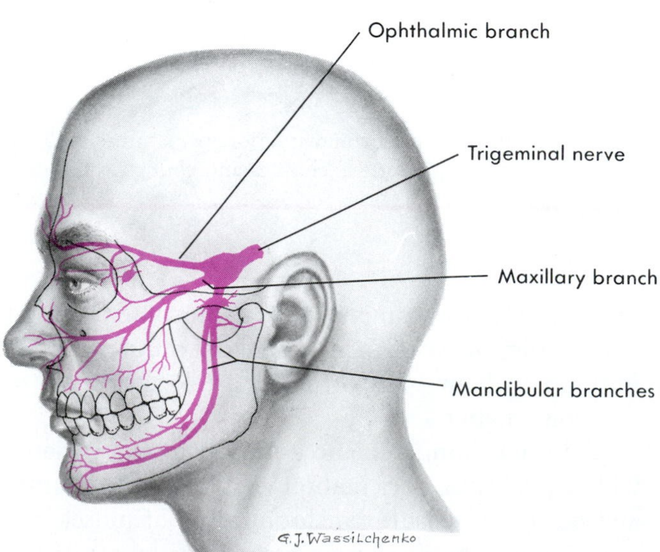

FIGURE 25-11. Trigeminal nerve with innervation to face by ophthalmic, maxillary, and mandibular branches.

TABLE 25-3 Cranial Nerves, Origins, Course, and Functions—cont'd

Cranial Nerve	Origin and Course	Function
VI ABDUCENS		
Motor	Posterior part of the pons goes to lateral rectus muscle for eye movement.	Extraocular eye movement; rotates eyeball outward (Figure 25-12).
VII FACIAL		
Sensory	Lower portion of the pons goes to anterior two thirds of tongue and soft palate.	Taste in anterior two thirds of tongue. Sensation to soft palate.
Motor	Pons to muscles of forehead, eyelids, cheeks, lips, ears, nose, and neck.	Movement of facial muscles to produce facial expressions, close eyes.
Parasympathetic	Pons to salivary gland and lacrimal glands.	Secretory for salivation and tears.
VIII ACOUSTIC	Two divisions:	
Sensory	*Cochlear division:* Originates in spinal ganglia of the cochlea, with peripheral fibers to the organ of Corti in the internal ear. Goes to the pons, and impulses transmitted to the temporal lobe.	Hearing.
	Vestibular division: Originates in otolith organs of the semicircular canals in the inner ear and in the vestibular ganglion. Terminates in the pons, with some fibers continuing to cerebellum. The only cranial nerve that originates wholly within a bone, the petrous portion of the temporal bone.	Equilibrium.
IX GLOSSOPHARYNGEAL		
Sensory	Posterior one third of tongue for taste sensation and sensations from soft palate, tonsils, and opening to mouth in back of oral pharynx (fauces). Fibers go to medulla and then to the temporal lobe for taste and sensory cortex for other sensations.	Taste in posterior one third of tongue. Sensation in back of throat; stimulation elicits a gag reflex.
Motor	Medulla to constrictor muscles of pharynx and stylopharyngeal muscles.	Voluntary muscles for swallowing and phonation.
Parasympathetic	Medulla to parotid salivary gland via otic ganglia.	Secretory, salivary glands. Carotid reflex.

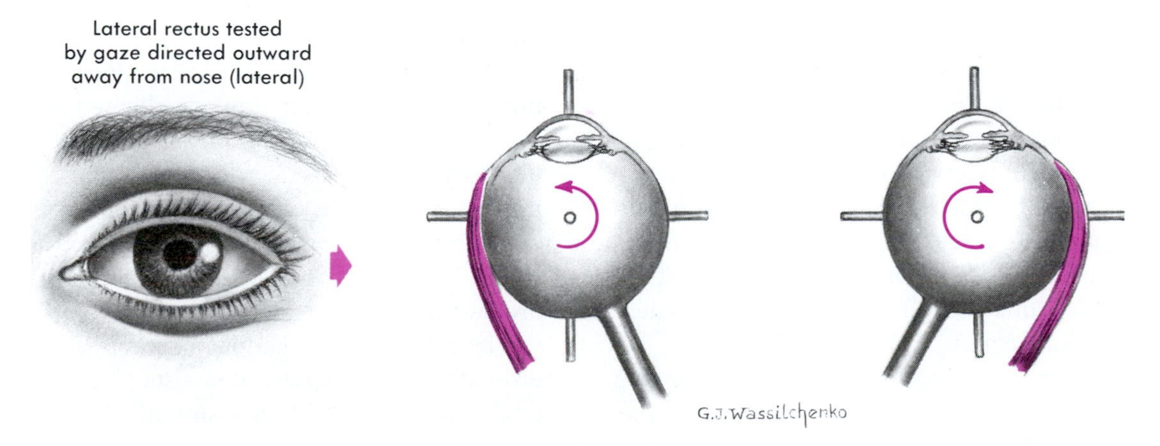

FIGURE 25-12. Lateral rectus muscle, which abducts the eye away from the nose to the temporal side of the head.

Continued

TABLE 25-3 Cranial Nerves, Origins, Course, and Functions—cont'd

Cranial Nerve	Origin and Course	Function
X VAGUS		
Sensory	Sensory fibers in back of ear and posterior wall of external ear go to medulla oblongata and on to sensory cortex.	Sensation behind ear and part of external ear meatus.
Motor	Fibers go from medulla oblongata through jugular foramen with glossopharyngeal nerve and on to pharynx, larynx, esophagus, bronchi, lungs, heart, stomach, small intestines, liver, pancreas, kidneys.	Voluntary muscles for phonation and swallowing. Involuntary activity of visceral muscles of heart, lungs, and digestive tract.
Parasympathetic	Medulla oblongata to larynx, trachea, lungs, aorta, esophagus, stomach, small intestines, and gallbladder.	Carotid reflex. Autonomic activity of respiratory tract, digestive tract including peristalsis and secretion from organs.
XI SPINAL ACCESSORY		
Motor	This nerve has two roots, cranial and spinal. Cranial portion arises at several rootlets at side of medulla, runs below vagus, and is joined by spinal portion from motor cells in cervical cord. Some fibers go along with vagus nerve to supply motor impulse to pharynx, larynx, uvula, and palate. Major portion to sternomastoid and trapezius muscles, branches to cervical spinal nerves C2-C4.	Some fibers for swallowing and phonation. Turns head and shrugs shoulders.
XII HYPOGLOSSAL		
Motor	Arises in medulla oblongata and goes to muscles of tongue.	Movement of tongue necessary for swallowing and phonation.

forces results in smooth motor movements instead of rapid, jerky, erratic movements. This complex system in the cerebellum monitors and adjusts motor activity simultaneously with the performance of the activity.

Diencephalon

The diencephalon, the lowest structure of the cerebrum, lies at the top of the brainstem surrounding the third ventricle.[1,2] It is divided into four regions: the thalamus, hypothalamus, epithalamus, and subthalamus (see Figure 25-7). Also located in this area are the pituitary gland and the internal capsule. The first two cranial nerves, I (olfactory) and II (optic), originate in the diencephalon region.

Thalamus. The largest region of the diencephalon, the thalamus, consists of two connected ovoid masses of gray matter forming the lateral walls of the third ventricle deep in the cerebral hemispheres. The thalamus is a relay station for both motor and sensory activity, basic neuronal activity such as processing of brain activity (measured by electroencephalogram) and memory, thought, emotion, and complex behavior (Figure 25-13).

The thalamus's role as a relay station for sensory input is a complex function coordinated with the parietal lobe of the cerebrum. All sensory pathways except olfactory communicate with some area of the thalamus. With the assistance of stimuli from the cerebral cortex, the thalamus sorts and sends sensory impulses to the appropriate area of the cerebral cortex for final processing.

The role of the thalamus in motor activity is to coordinate and integrate. It assists the cerebrum and cerebellum in providing a smooth, integrated motor response.

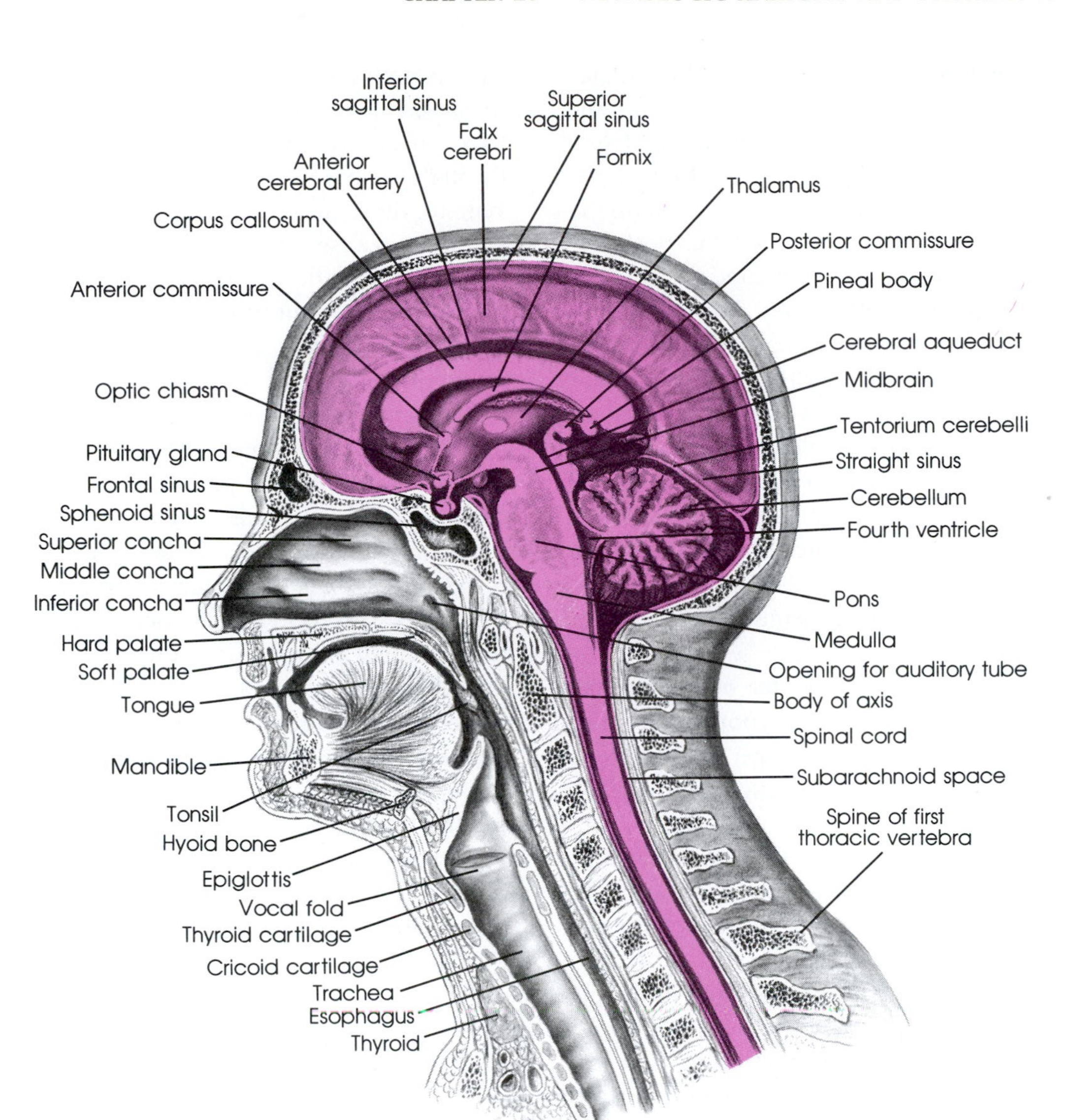

FIGURE 25-13. Schematic drawing of sagittal section of head.

Hypothalamus. The hypothalamus, located below the thalamus, forms the floor and anterior lateral walls of the third ventricle. Other landmarks around the hypothalamus are the optic chiasm, which is located behind the hypothalamus, and the pituitary gland, which sits below the hypothalamus in the sella turcica. The pituitary stalk connects the hypothalamus to the pituitary gland.

Functions of the hypothalamus include regulating and maintaining internal body environment and interacting with the limbic system to generate actual physical responses to emotions, such as blushing when embarrassed. Areas of the internal environment regulated and maintained by the hypothalamus include (1) temperature regulation, (2) autonomic nervous system responses, (3) regulation of food and water intake, (4) control of hormonal secretions of the pituitary, and (5) behavioral responses.

Temperature regulation. Temperature regulation is achieved by the anterior and posterior parts of the hypothalamus. As blood with increased temperature flows through the anterior region of the hypothalamus, stimuli travel to sweat glands to produce perspiration; to peripheral vessels to cause vasodilation, which allows heat loss through the skin; and to respiratory centers to increase respiratory rate. Low blood temperature stimulates the posterior region of the hypothalamus and causes vasoconstriction; piloerection, or "goose bumps;" and shivering, which increases cell metabolism and produces heat.

Autonomic nervous system responses. The hypothalamus serves as the "brain" for the autonomic, or involuntary, nervous system. The parasympathetic (resting) system response is elicited by stimulation of the anterior region of the hypothalamus. The sympathetic (fight or flight) system responds when the posterior region of the hypothalamus is stimulated.

Regulation of food and water intake. Food intake is regulated by two centers: the hunger center, which causes the sensation of hunger when stimulated, and the satiety center, which decreases the desire for food when the stomach is full or the blood glucose is high. Water intake is regulated through the secretion of antidiuretic hormone (ADH). A change in serum osmotic pressure is the stimulus for ADH response. An increase in serum osmotic pressure stimulates the release of ADH, and a decrease in serum osmotic pressure depresses the release of ADH.

Control of hormonal secretions by the pituitary gland. The interrelationships between the hypothalamus and the pituitary in the production, storage, and secretion of hormones are discussed in the section on the pituitary gland later in this chapter.

Behavioral responses. Behavioral responses influenced by the hypothalamus and interacting with the limbic system include behaviors associated with aggression, pleasure, punishment, and sexual activities.

Epithalamus. Located in the dorsal portion of the diencephalon, the epithalamus contains the pineal gland, which is believed to play a role in physical growth and sexual development. This gland often calcifies in early adulthood and can be identified on a computed tomographic scan or radiographic films.

Subthalamus. The subthalamus is located below the thalamus. It is integrated with extrapyramidal tracts of the autonomic nervous system and the basal ganglia.

Pituitary gland. The pituitary gland, also known as the *hypophysis,* has been called the "master gland" because of its role in the regulation of hormone production of all other endocrine organs. Lying in the sella turcica, the pituitary gland is connected to the hypothalamus by the pituitary or hypophyseal stalk. The pituitary gland itself is divided into two lobes, the anterior (adenohypophysis) and the posterior (neurohypophysis). The anterior and posterior lobes of the pituitary are different and are described individually.

Anterior lobe. The anterior lobe constitutes 75% of the pituitary gland and is responsible for regulation of the majority of endocrine function. Hormone and electrolyte levels in the blood are sensed by the hypothalamus. The hypothalamus then sends neurosecretory substances (releasing or inhibiting factors) through the blood supply of the pituitary stalk portal vein to the anterior pituitary. These neurosecretory substances cause the anterior pituitary gland to release or inhibit specific hormones. The seven major hormones of the anterior pituitary are adrenocorticotropic hormone (ACTH), thyroid-stimulating hormone (TSH), growth hormone (GH), prolactin (PRL), follicle-stimulating hormone (FSH), luteinizing hormone (LH), and melanocyte-stimulating hormone (MSH). Hormones are produced, stored, and then secreted from the pituitary when stimulated by the hypothalamus. Once the anterior pituitary hormone is released, it travels to the target endocrine gland and stimulates secretion of endocrine hormone, which then circulates through the blood supply back to the hypothalamus where an increased hormonal level is sensed. The hypothalamus stops the release of neurosecretory substances, and the stimulating cycle is broken. See Box 25-1 for an example of this cycle, using the thyroid gland and thyroxin.

Posterior lobe. The posterior lobe constitutes the other 25% of the pituitary gland and is directly connected to the hypothalamus by the pituitary stalk. The posterior lobe does not produce any hormones.

BOX 25-1 Hormone-Stimulating Cycle

Thyroxin level is low in blood
↓
Hypothalamus senses low level
↓
Hypothalamus releases thyrotropin-releasing factor (TRF)
↓
TRF travels through portal venous system to anterior pituitary
↓
Anterior pituitary secretes thyroid-stimulating hormone (TSH) into blood
↓
TSH travels to thyroid gland and stimulates production of thyroxin
↓
Hypothalamus senses circulating amount of thyroxin
↓
TRF is not released

However, the posterior lobe does secrete two hormones, ADH and oxytocin, which are produced by cells in the hypothalamus and trickle down fiber tracts through the pituitary stalk for storage in the posterior pituitary. When ADH or oxytocin release is required, the hypothalamus stimulates the pituitary to release these hormones rapidly in response to a variety of stimuli.

Internal capsule. Fiber tracts from many portions of each half of the cerebrum converge in the area of the diencephalon on their way to the brainstem and spinal cord to form the internal capsule. The internal capsule contains both afferent and efferent fibers but is mainly considered a motor, or efferent, pathway (Figure 25-14). All afferent (sensory) fibers traveling to the cortex travel through the internal capsule in the following succession: brainstem to thalamus to internal capsule to cerebral cortex. All efferent (motor) fibers leaving the cortex also pass through the internal capsule. Because of the collection of all major motor and sensory fibers through this small area, a tiny area of damage to the internal capsule causes major loss of motor and some sensory function on the opposite side of the body.

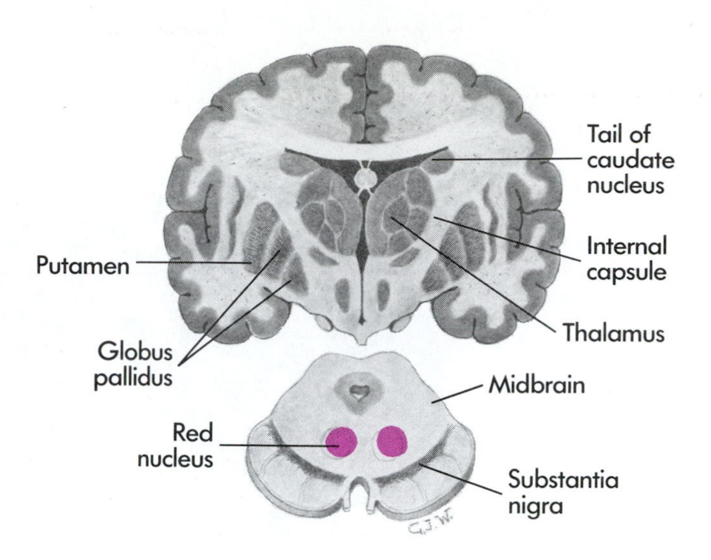

FIGURE 25-14. Coronal section of brain.

Basal Ganglia

The main role of the basal ganglia is associated with motor function.[2,4,7] They provide a pathway and assist in processing information from the cerebral motor cortex and the thalamus. The basal ganglia are composed of several subcortical nuclei located deep within the white matter of the cerebral hemispheres. These paired sets of nuclei include the corpus striatum (composed of the caudate nuclei, the putamen, and the globus pallidus); the amygdala; the claustrum; the subthalamic nuclei; and the substantia nigra (see Figure 25-14).

Much of the basal ganglia's function is through the extrapyramidal (involuntary) motor pathways. It influences motor activity to integrate voluntary movement with associated movements and postural adjustments and suppresses skeletal muscle tone and postural reflexes. The basal ganglia also process input from visual, labyrinthine, and proprioceptive sources, resulting in smooth, coordinated movements of the body without loss of balance.

Cerebrum

The cerebrum is the largest portion of the brain, comprising 80% of its weight. It is composed of two cerebral hemispheres (right and left) incompletely divided by the longitudinal fissure. The cerebral hemispheres are connected at the base of the longitudinal fissure by the corpus callosum. The corpus callosum is a large tract of transverse, or commissural, fibers that provides a communication link between the two hemispheres.

The outside of the cerebrum is covered with a thin layer of gray matter (multiple layers of unmyelinated cell nuclei) called the *cerebral cortex.* Underneath the cerebral cortex are the white matter (myelinated) tracts, which communicate impulses from the cerebral cortex to other areas of the brain. Three types of fibers—commissural (transverse), projection, and association—are in the white matter and are named for the role they play in communication of information. Commissural fibers are tracts that communicate between corresponding parts of the two hemispheres. The corpus callosum is the largest of these fiber tracts. Projection fibers communicate between the cerebral cortex and lower regions of the brain and spinal cord. Association fibers communicate between various regions of the same hemisphere.

The cerebral hemispheres are divided into four surface lobes, based on anatomic divisions or fissures. The four paired lobes are the frontal lobes, the parietal lobes, the temporal lobes, and the occipital lobes (Figure 25-15). Another area deeper inside the cerebrum can also be classified as a lobe and is called the *limbic lobe.*

Classification of different areas of the cerebral cytoarchitecture, based on minute histologic differences of

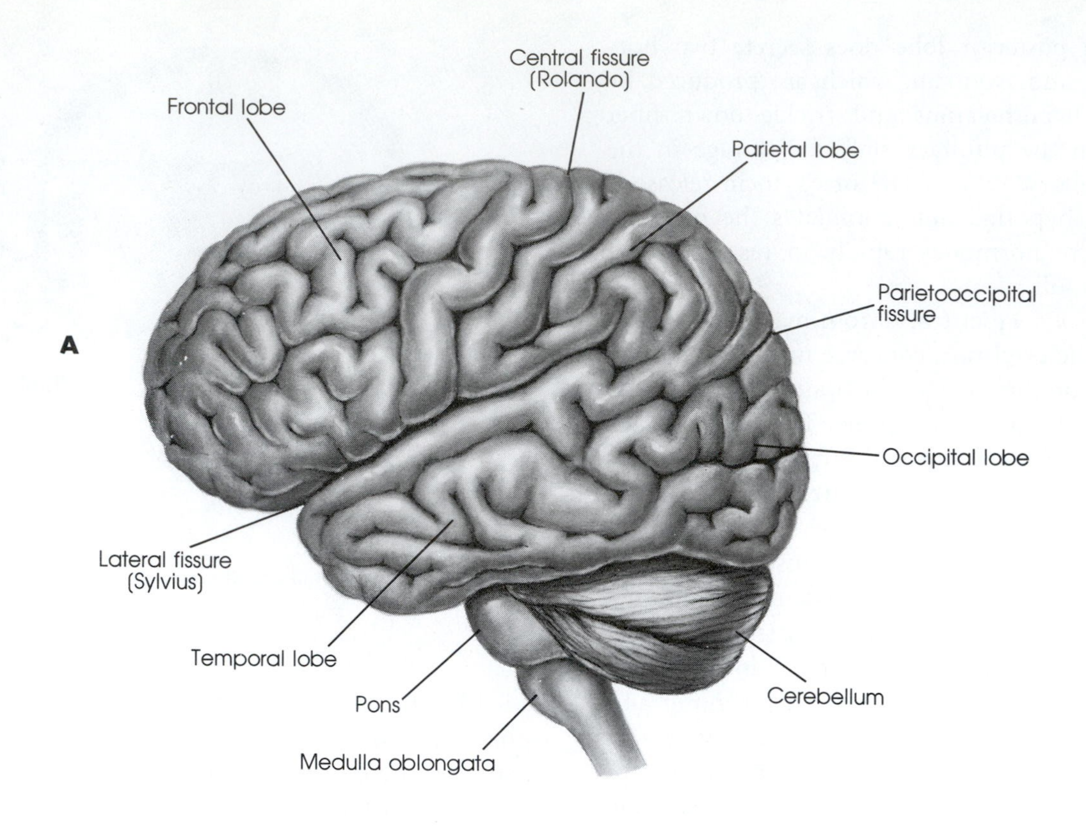

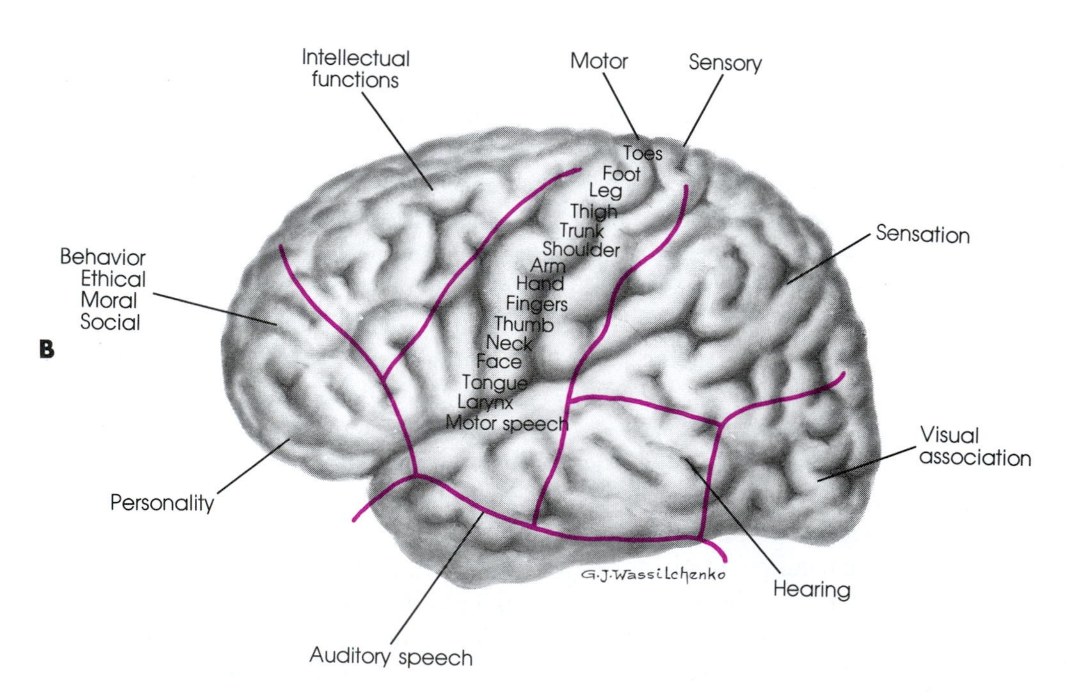

FIGURE 25-15. A, Lateral view of cerebral hemisphere (showing lobes and principal fissures), cerebellum, pons, and medulla oblongata. **B,** Principal functional subdivisions of cerebral hemisphere.

the cell, is credited to Brodmann. More than 100 of these numbered areas have been identified (Figure 25-16). See Table 25-4 for a summary of the cerebral lobes and their major functions.

Frontal lobe. The largest of the four lobes of the cerebral hemispheres is the frontal lobe. The frontal lobe lies underneath the frontal bone of the skull and is separated posteriorly from the parietal lobe by the cen-

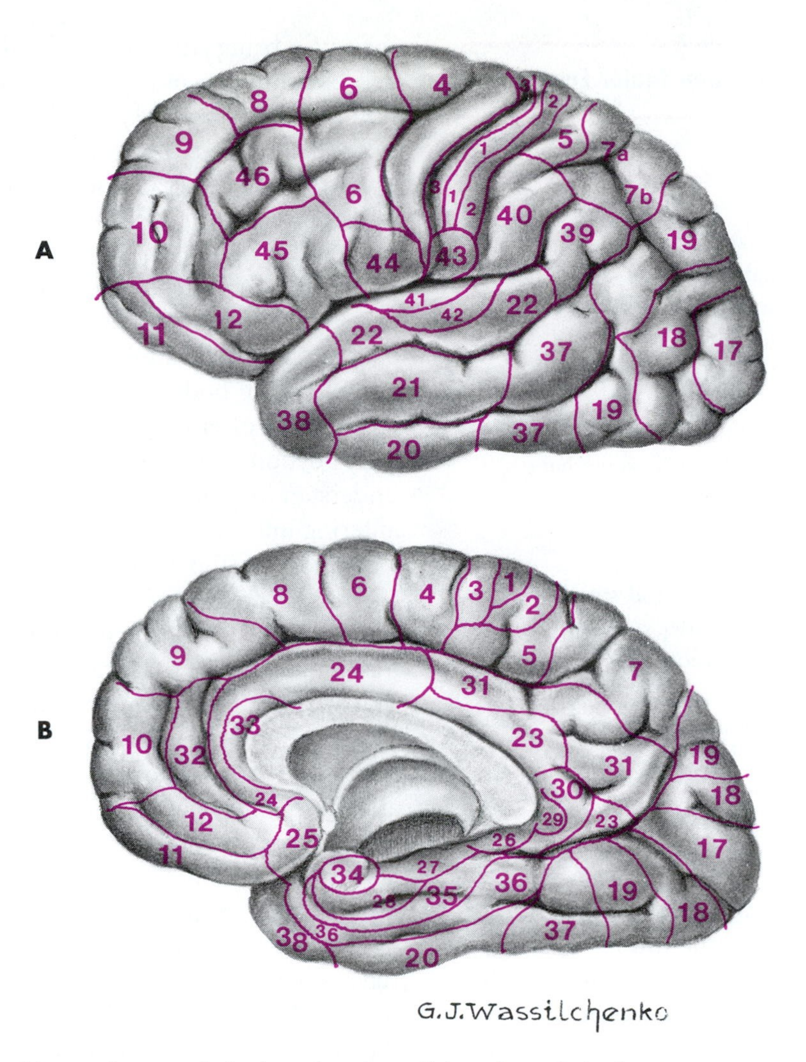

FIGURE 25-16. Cytoarchitectural map of the lateral and medial surface of the human cortex according to Brodmann's map. **A,** Lateral surface. **B,** Medial surface.

tral fissure (fissure of Rolando) and inferiorly from the temporal lobe by the lateral fissure (Sylvian fissure). The major functions of the frontal lobe are voluntary motor function, higher mental functions, cognition, memory, personality, and language. Some of the higher control centers for autonomic nervous system function also lie in the frontal lobe.

The prefrontal area of the frontal lobe (areas 9 to 12) is concerned with the process of cerebration (or thought), affect, feeling, and emotion, as well as autonomic nervous system response in relation to emotional changes. The rationale behind the use of biofeedback techniques and relaxation techniques correlates with the prefrontal area's influence on the autonomic nervous system.

The premotor area (areas 6 and 8) is an association area for the motor area lying adjacent to it. When stimulated, the premotor area provides general body movements, such as turning the eyes and head and turning the trunk with the head. A connection exists between the premotor area and cranial nerves III, IV, VI, IX, X, and XII to allow coordination of the movements described.

The motor area, or motor strip (area 4), contains the cells for voluntary (pyramidal) motor functions of the opposite side of the body. The motor-strip functions are drawn spatially by the homunculus (Figure 25-17, *A*). The appearance is of an upside-down man with a foot on the medial aspect of the frontal lobe. The knees, hips, trunk, and shoulders extend over the outer surface of the cortex and the hands, thumb, head, face, and tongue down the side to the lateral fissure, which is the border of the frontal lobe. The size of the area for each body part along this strip is proportional to the amount of dexterity associated with the body part's function. Therefore the large surface area of the

TABLE 25-4 Cerebral Lobes and Their Major Functions

Cerebral Lobe	Major Functions
Frontal	Personality Moral, ethical, and social values Abstract thought Long-term memory Motor strip for opposite side of body
Parietal	Sensory strip for opposite side of body Two-point discrimination Recognition of object by size, shape, weight, or texture Body part awareness
Temporal	Hearing Special senses of taste and smell Interpretive area—integrates sounds, thoughts, and emotions
Occipital	Vision Visual recognition of objects Reading comprehension

trunk occupies a relatively small part of the motor strip. The smaller areas, such as the thumb or tongue, that involve a great deal of dexterity and fine motor movement occupy a larger area of this strip.

Broca's area (areas 44 and 45) is located at the inferior frontal gyrus. Part of the speech center, this area is responsible for the motor aspects of speech and is involved in coordination of activities for the formulation of verbal speech. Damage to this area results in expressive or nonfluent aphasia.

Parietal lobe. The parietal lobe is directly posterior to the frontal lobe on the other side of the central fissure. The posterior border of the parietal lobe is the parietooccipital fissure, which separates it from the occipital lobe. The inferior border is incompletely defined by the posterior portion of the lateral fissure. The main function of the parietal lobe is sensory, including integration of sensory information; awareness of body parts; interpretation of touch, pressure, and pain; and recognition of object size, shape, and texture.

The parietal lobe contains a sensory strip (areas 1, 2, and 3) that lies adjacent to the motor strip of the frontal lobe. Similar to the homunculus of the motor strip, the sensory homunculus re-creates a caricature of an upside-down man (Figure 25-17, *B*). Sensory areas of body parts lie close to motor areas of the same parts. Also, areas of the body with greater tactile response occupy larger areas on the sensory strip. Fibers going to the sensory strip bring stimuli associated with cutaneous and deep sensibility sensations, as well as cutaneous sensation of touch, pressure, position, and vibration. Input from the thalamus also reaches the sensory strip.

Associative areas of the parietal lobe (areas 5 and 7) interpret sensory input in terms of size, shape, texture, and weight. The parietal lobe provides the ability to localize a sensation and define it in terms of pressure, temperature, or vibration. Interpretive aspects of the parietal lobe's response to stimuli include awareness of body parts, orientation in space, and recognition of environmental spatial relationships.

A portion of the sensory aspect of speech and the understanding of the written word is located in the anterior-inferior area of the parietal lobe. Along with a portion of the temporal lobe, this area is called Wernicke's area (area 22).

Temporal lobe. The temporal lobe lies beneath the temporal bone in the lateral portion of the cranium. The anterior, lower border of the temporal lobe is encased in the sphenoid wing. With a strong blow to the head the temporal lobe is easily contused and lacerated as it moves against this hard, irregular surface. Separated from the frontal and parietal lobes by the lateral fissure, this lobe has the primary functions of hearing, speech, behavior, and memory.

The primary auditory areas (areas 41 and 42) receive sound impulses and assist in determining the source of the sound and interpreting the meaning of the sound. These areas are closely linked with Wernicke's area, which is located in both the parietal and temporal lobes. Responsible for the comprehension of both spoken and written language, Wernicke's area, in the dominant hemisphere, is called an *associative area.* Disruption of this area leads to receptive (fluent) aphasia—the individual can hear but is unable to interpret the message.

In the superior portion of the temporal lobe where the frontal, parietal, and temporal lobes meet is an essential interpretive area in which auditory, visual, and somatic association areas are integrated into complex thought and memory. Seizures in this region of the temporal lobe cause auditory, visual, and sensory hallucinations.

Occipital lobe. The occipital lobe of the cerebrum forms the most posterior portion. It is separated from the cerebellum by the tentorium. Primary responsibility of the occipital lobe is vision and the interpretation of visual stimuli.

The primary visual cortex (area 17) receives impulses from projections of the optic tract. These impulses are then referred to the visual associative areas (areas 18 and 19) for interpretation and integration.

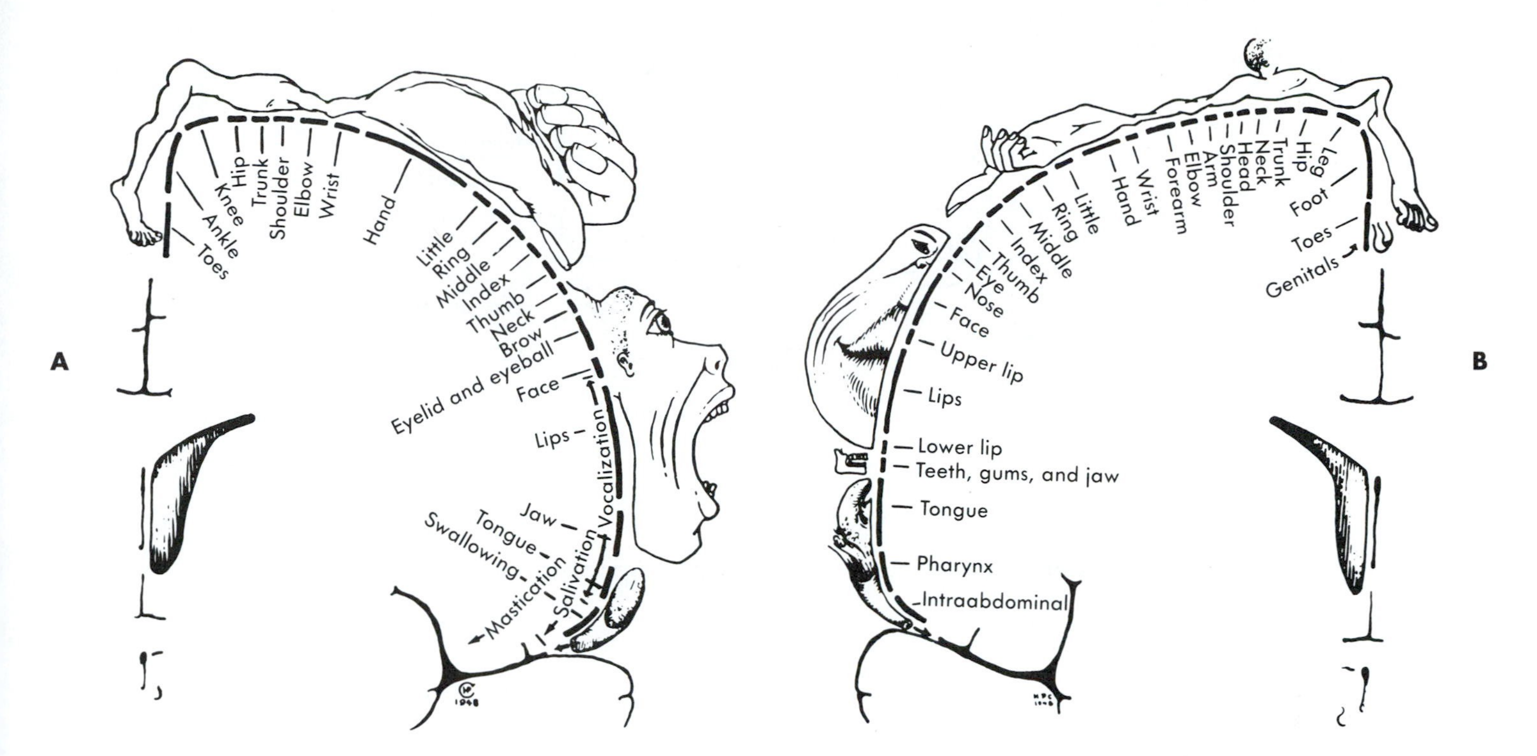

FIGURE 25-17. Classic drawing of **A,** motor homunculus and **B,** sensory homunculus. (From Penfield W, Rasmussen T: *The cerebral cortex of man,* New York, 1950, Macmillan; renewed 1978 by Theodore Rasmussen.)

Limbic lobe. One other cerebral section, which is anatomically part of the temporal lobe, is often separated from the temporal lobe for discussion of function and is called (although sometimes controversially) the limbic lobe. Also called the rhinencephalon, this lobe forms the border of the lateral ventricles and contains the hippocampus, the uncus, primary olfactory cortex, and the amygdaloid nucleus. The functions of the limbic lobe are self-preservation, primitive behavior, moods, the visceral processes associated with emotion, short-term memory, and the interpretation of smell.

Cerebral Circulation

The brain constitutes 2% of the body's weight but uses 20% of the body's cardiac output. It requires approximately 750 ml of cerebral blood flow per minute. The role of cerebral circulation is to provide enough blood to supply oxygen, glucose, and nutrients to the cerebral tissues. There is no reserve of either oxygen or glucose in the cerebral tissues, and a lack or inadequate amount of either one rapidly disrupts cerebral function and produces irreversible damage. Two pairs of arteries, the internal carotids and the vertebral arteries, are responsible for supplying blood to the brain. Anatomically they can be separated into the arteries of the anterior circulation and the posterior circulation (Figure 25-18).[7] These two circulations are connected at the base of the brain by the circle of Willis.

Anterior circulation. The anterior circulation begins with the common carotid arteries (Figure 25-19). The left common carotid originates from the arch of the aorta, and the right common carotid originates from the innominate artery. At the level of the crycothyroid junction, the common carotid splits to form the external and internal carotid arteries. The external carotid feeds the face, the scalp, and the skull and includes the branch called the *middle meningeal artery,* which lies between the skull and the dura. When the middle meningeal artery is torn or lacerated, the blood can develop into an epidural hematoma.

The internal carotid artery continues upward through the carotid siphon and enters the base of the skull through an opening in the petrous bone. At the base of the brain the internal carotid connects with the circle of Willis and then branches into the anterior and middle cerebral arteries, which are primarily responsible for anterior circulation. One major branch of the internal carotid, the ophthalmic artery, exits before the circle of Willis and supplies blood to the optic nerve and eye.

Posterior circulation. Posterior circulation begins with the two vertebral arteries, which originate from the subclavian arteries and travel posteriorly through

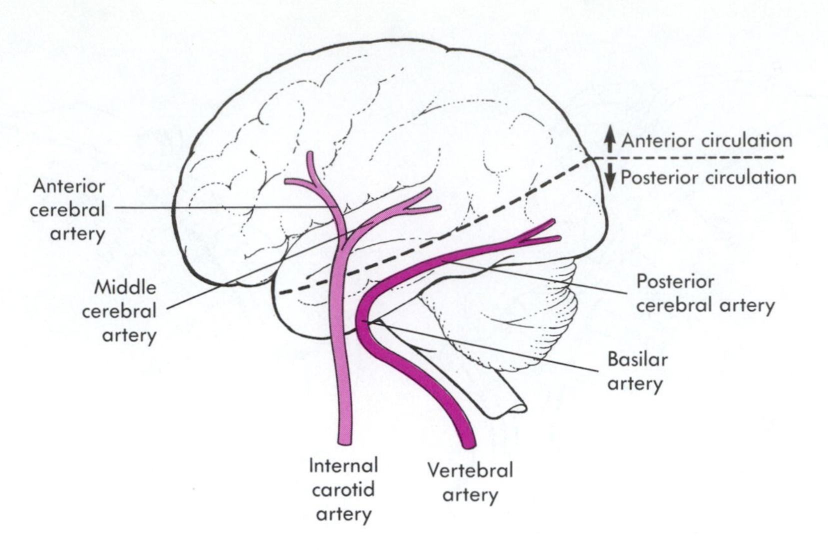

FIGURE 25-18. Arteries of anterior and posterior cerebral circulation.

small openings in the lateral spinous processes of the cervical spine. They enter the skull through the foramen magnum, and at the level of the pons the two vertebral arteries join to form the basilar artery.

Branches of the basilar artery feed the brainstem and the cerebellum. The basilar artery continues upward into the posterior portion of the circle of Willis and into the two posterior cerebral arteries.

Circle of Willis. The circle of Willis is a vascular supply system unique to cerebral circulation (Figure 25-20). Located in a small area above the optic chiasm in the subarachnoid space, the circle is fed by the internal carotid and basilar arteries. The three cerebral arteries (anterior, middle, and posterior) supplying each hemisphere are connected by communicating arteries to form a complete circle. The anterior communicating artery connects the right and left anterior cerebral arteries, and the two posterior communicating arteries connect the middle cerebral and posterior cerebral artery in each of the hemispheres.

In a normal situation the left internal carotid artery supplies blood to the left anterior and middle cerebral arteries, and the right internal carotid artery supplies blood to the right anterior and middle cerebral arteries, thus constituting anterior circulation. In the posterior circulation the basilar artery feeds both posterior cerebral arteries.

When an artery such as the right internal carotid is blocked with atherosclerotic material so that an inadequate amount of blood is flowing to the right anterior and middle cerebral arteries, blood from the left internal carotid will flow across the anterior communicating artery and assist with the vascular supply to the right hemisphere. Also, blood flow from the right posterior cerebral artery will flow through the right posterior communicating artery to supply blood to the right middle cerebral artery. Thus supply of oxygen and nutrients to the brain is not disrupted.

It is not unusual to have an anatomically incomplete circle of Willis.[4] Autopsy and angiographic studies have supplied evidence that up to 50% of individuals have absent or hypoplastic communicating vessels.[7]

Anterior cerebral artery. The anterior cerebral artery runs anteriorly along the base of the brain and supplies the longitudinal fissure and therefore the medial surfaces of the frontal and parietal lobes. It also feeds the basal ganglia, portions of the internal capsule, and the corpus callosum (Figure 25-21).

Middle cerebral artery. The middle cerebral artery is the largest of the cerebral arteries. As a direct branch from the internal carotid, it travels laterally and feeds the surface of the frontal, parietal, and temporal lobes and the internal capsule.

Posterior cerebral artery. The posterior cerebral artery, a branch of the basilar artery, runs along the tentorium and feeds the occipital lobes and the medial and lateral aspects of the temporal lobe (see Figure 25-21).

Venous circulation. Venous drainage is accomplished by the venous sinuses of the dura. Capillary flow moves to venules and then to cerebral veins, which empty into the sinuses located throughout the cranium. Blood from these sinuses empties into the internal jugular vein, which empties into the superior vena cava and then back into the right atrium.

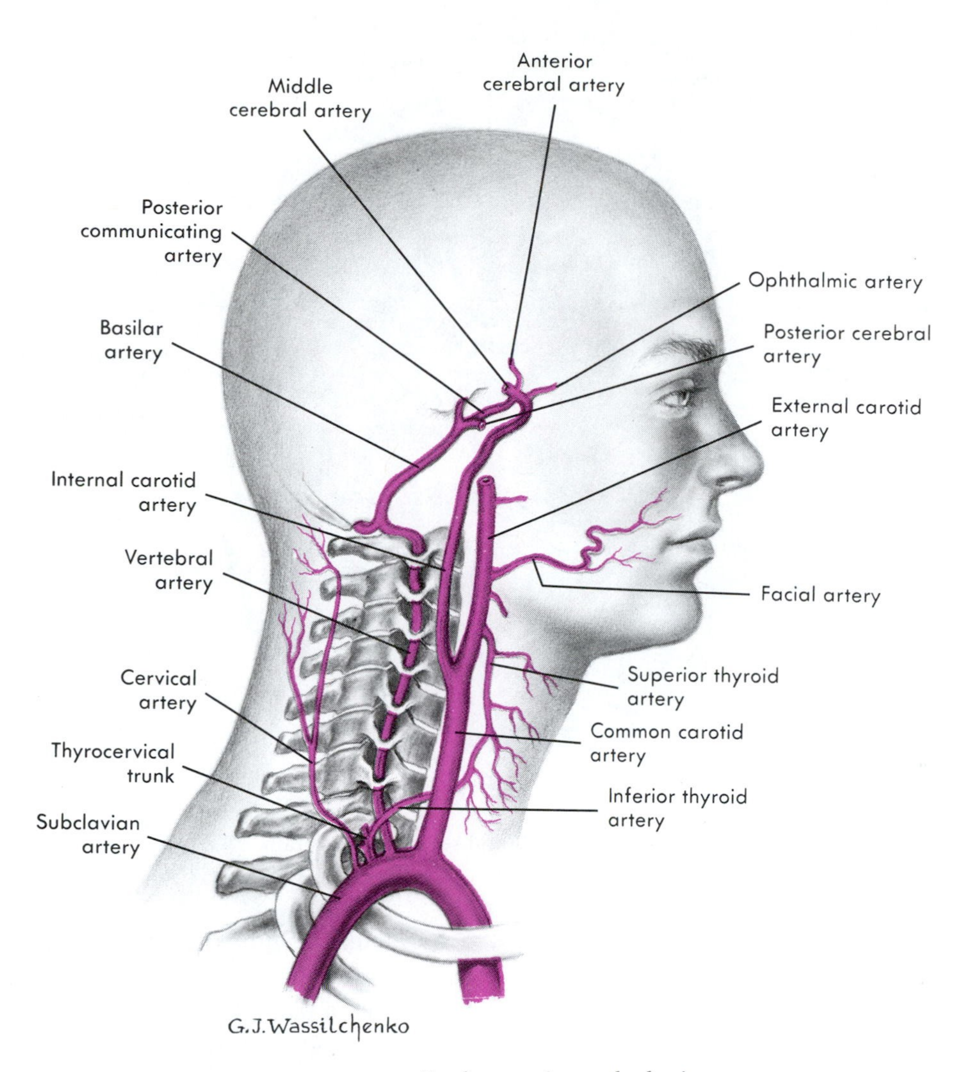

FIGURE 25-19. Feeder arteries to the brain.

Spinal Cord

The spinal cord is the extension of the medulla after its exit from the foramen magnum.[3] It is a long, ropelike structure composed of white and gray matter. The spinal cord itself tapers down to an end or conus medullaris at the level of the first or second lumbar vertebra. Exiting from the spinal cord are 31 pairs of spinal nerve roots, which travel through the intervertebral foramina. Because the spinal cord ends at L1 and the final nerve roots do not exit until the coccyx, long lengths of nerve roots, called the *cauda equina,* extend through the space in the lumbar and sacral regions. Most of the protective mechanisms for the cranium also exist, with slight modification, for the spinal cord.

Protective mechanisms

Bony structures. The bony structure that encases the spinal cord is the vertebral column. Comprising 33 vertebrae and 24 intervertebral disks, this column, held together by ligaments and tendons, provides support and protection for the spinal cord plus structure and flexibility for body movement. The vertebrae are divided into sections in relation to their appearance. There are 7 cervical vertebrae, 12 thoracic vertebrae, 5 lumbar vertebrae, 5 sacral vertebrae (fused as 1), and 4 coccygeal vertebrae (fused as 1).

Although differences in vertebral appearance exist, the basic structure includes a vertebral body connected by two pedicles to the transverse processes (Figure 25-22). Two laminae connect the transverse processes to the posterior segment of the vertebrae, the spinous process, forming a ring. In the center of the spinal foramen is the canal, which houses the spinal cord.

Intervertebral disk. The bodies of the vertebrae are separated by an intervertebral disk. These fibrocartilaginous structures are between each vertebral body from the first cervical vertebra to the beginning of

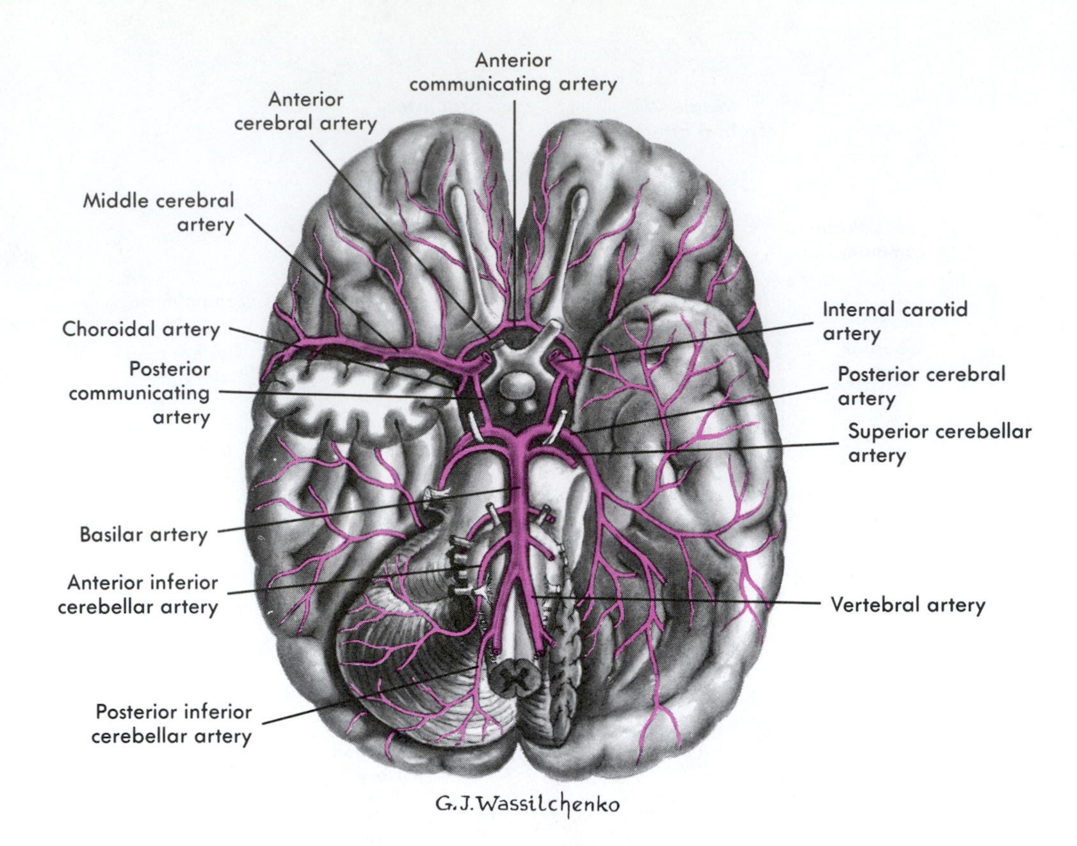

FIGURE 25-20. Blood supply of the brain.

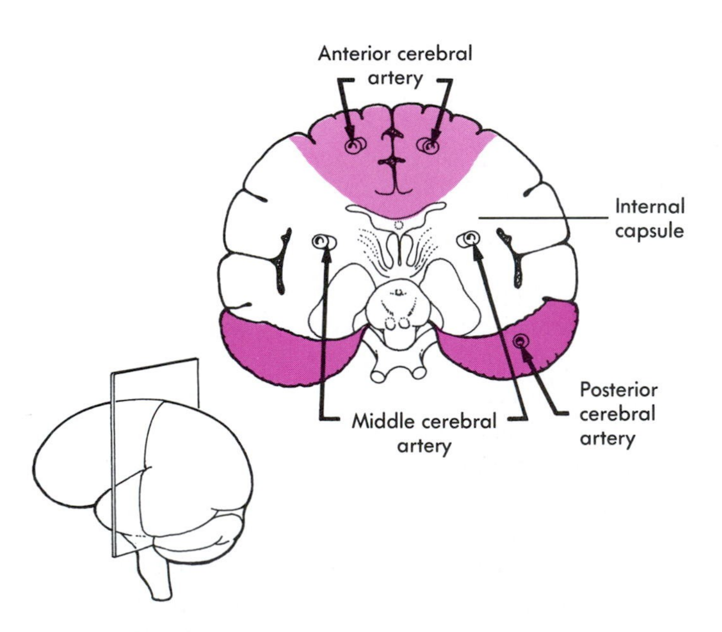

FIGURE 25-21. Distribution of arterial blood supply.

the sacrum. The intervertebral disk is composed of two layers. The inner core, the nucleus pulposus, is a soft, gelatinous material, which assists in shock absorbency along the spinal column. Surrounding the nucleus pulposus is the annulus fibrosus. This thick, tough outer layer provides firmer structure to assist the spinal column in supporting the weight of the body when upright.

When a patient suffering from severe back and leg pain is diagnosed as having a herniated disk, the annulus fibrosus has usually torn and a portion of the nucleus pulposus has herniated into the spinal foramen, pressing against the spinal nerve root as it exits the spinal cord across the pedicle. If surgery is required, a laminectomy or diskectomy is performed. It involves removal of one lamina to gain entrance to the spinal foramen. The herniated portion of the disk is then removed and pressure relieved.

Meninges. The meninges of the spinal cord are similar to those in the cranium (Figure 25-23). The dura is a continuation of the inner layer of the intracranial dura. The dura of the spinal cord encases the cord, the nerve roots, and the spinal nerves until they exit from the vertebral column. The dura extends to the level of the second sacral vertebra, even though the spinal cord itself ends at the L1 or L2 level.

The arachnoid membrane is the same weblike, delicate tissue that is in the cranium. Cerebrospinal fluid (CSF) flows in the subarachnoid space of the spinal cord also. Because the spinal cord terminates at L2 and the meninges continue to S2, a volume of CSF is contained in this space and can be tapped

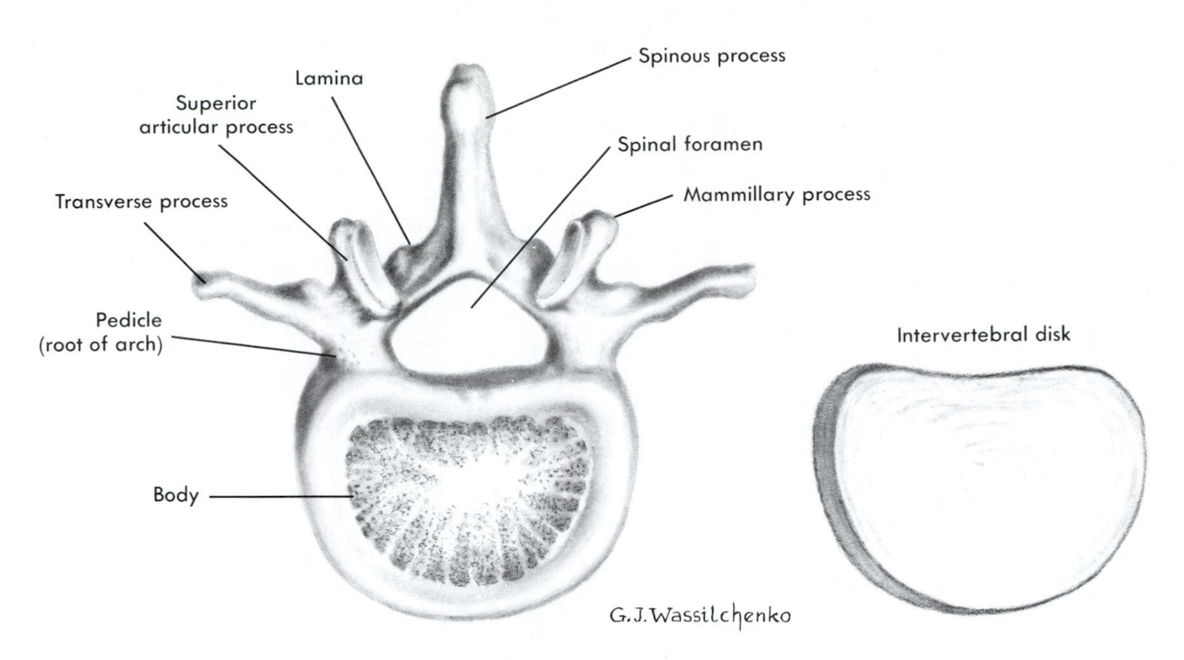

FIGURE 25-22. Vertebra and intervertebral disk.

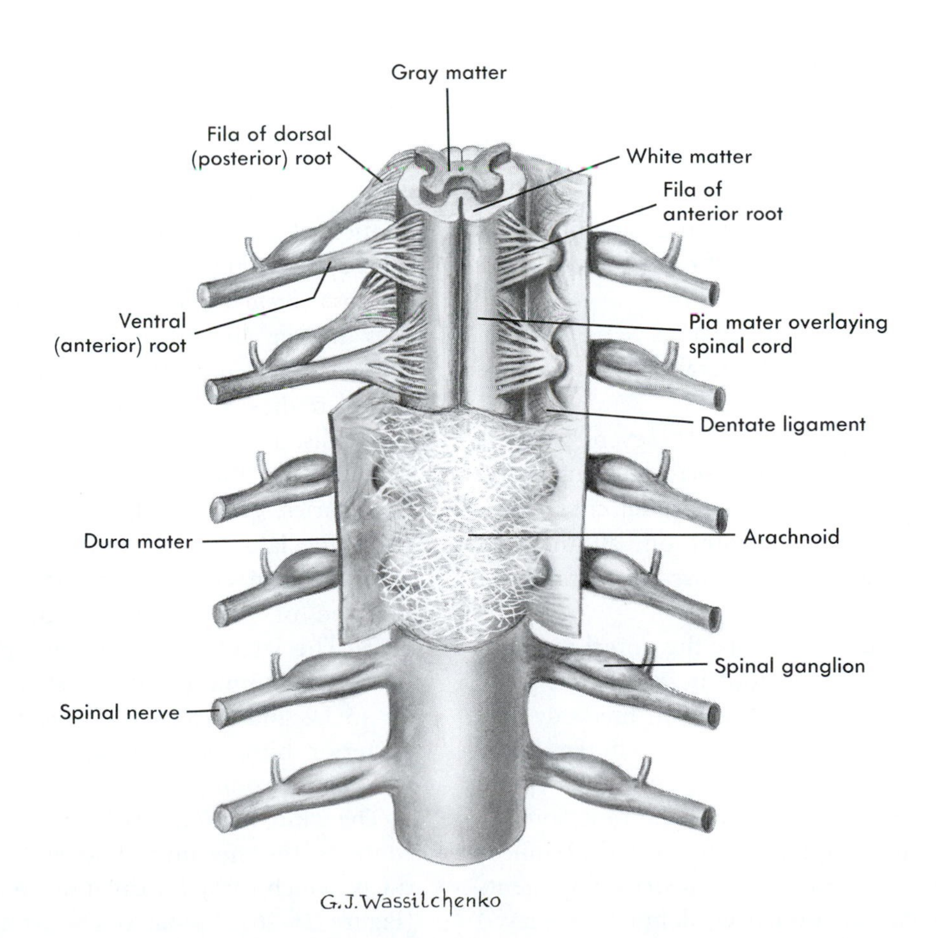

FIGURE 25-23. Meningeal layers of the spinal cord. Segment of spinal cord is viewed from behind with portions of dura mater and arachnoid removed.

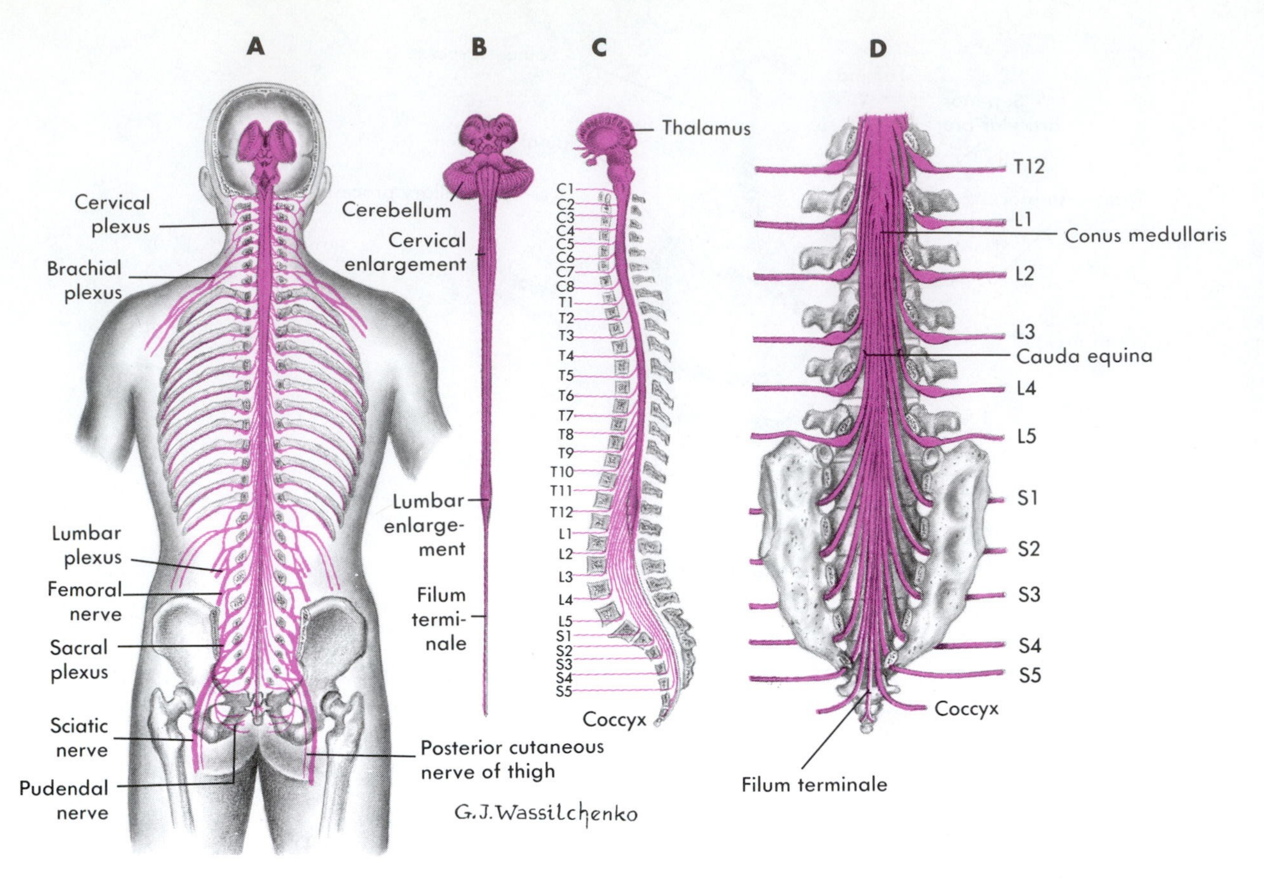

FIGURE 25-24. Spinal cord within vertebral canal and exiting spinal nerves. **A,** Posterior view in situ. **B,** Anterior view. **C,** Lateral view. **D,** Cauda equina.

through a lumbar puncture procedure. The pia mater of the spinal cord is a thicker, firmer, less vascular membrane than that in the cranium.

Spinal nerves. There are 31 spinal nerve pairs: 8 cervical, 12 thoracic, 5 lumbar, 5 sacral, and 1 coccygeal (Figure 25-24).

In the cervical region the first seven pairs of nerves exit the cord above the corresponding vertebrae. The C8 nerve pair exits the spinal cord below the C7 vertebra. From this point on, all thoracic, lumbar, and sacral nerves exit below the corresponding vertebrae.

The spinal nerve has two roots: the dorsal root and the ventral root. The dorsal root is an afferent pathway and carries sensory impulses from the body into the spinal cord. The ventral root is an efferent pathway and carries motor information from the spinal cord to the body. The dorsal and ventral roots join together as they exit the spinal foramen and become a spinal nerve. Distribution of the sensory components of the spinal nerve has been well-defined. Displayed as sensory dermatomes, these diagrams allow identification of sensory innervation in the peripheral nervous system (Figure 25-25).

Cross section. The spinal cord is composed of both gray matter and white matter.[2,4,7] The central gray matter, which appears in the shape of an H, consists of cell bodies, small projection fibers, and glial support cells. The gray matter has been divided into areas based on the cell body type located within their boundaries. The three basic divisions are the anterior horn, the lateral horn, and the posterior horn. The anterior horn contains motor cells and is the final junction of motor information before it exits the CNS. The lateral horn contains preganglionic fibers of the autonomic nervous system: sympathetic fibers T1 to L2 and parasympathetic fibers S2 to S4. The posterior horn contains axons from the peripheral sensory neurons.

The white matter, which surrounds the gray matter, contains the myelinated ascending and descending tracts, which carry information to and from the brain (Figure 25-26). Spinal tracts are named so that the prefix denotes the origin of the tract and the suffix

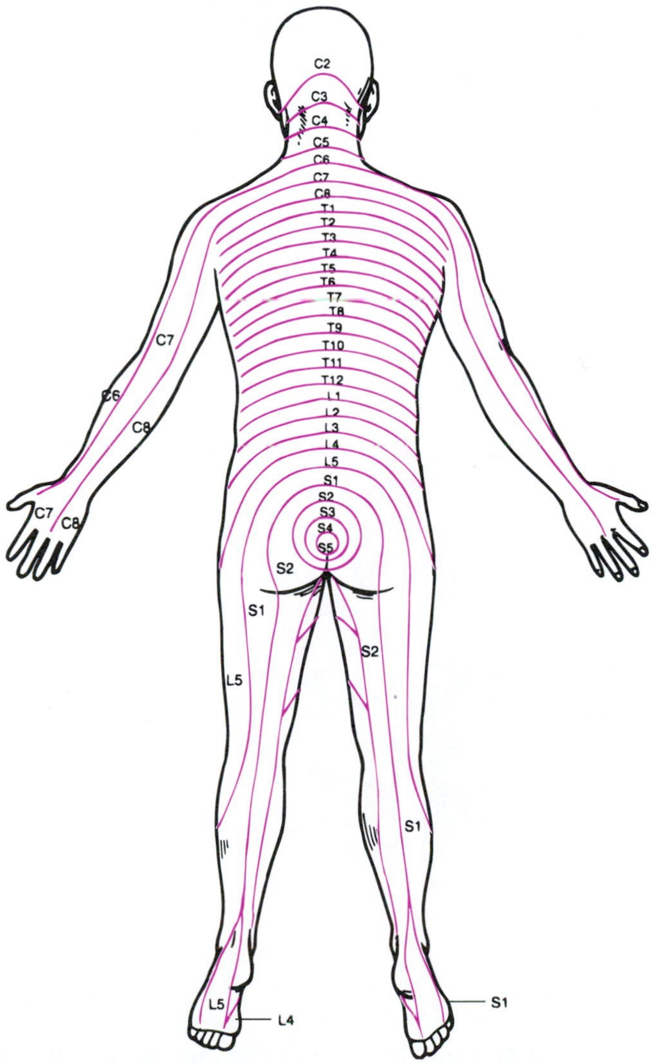

FIGURE 25-25. Dermatomes. **A,** Anterior view, **B,** Posterior view.

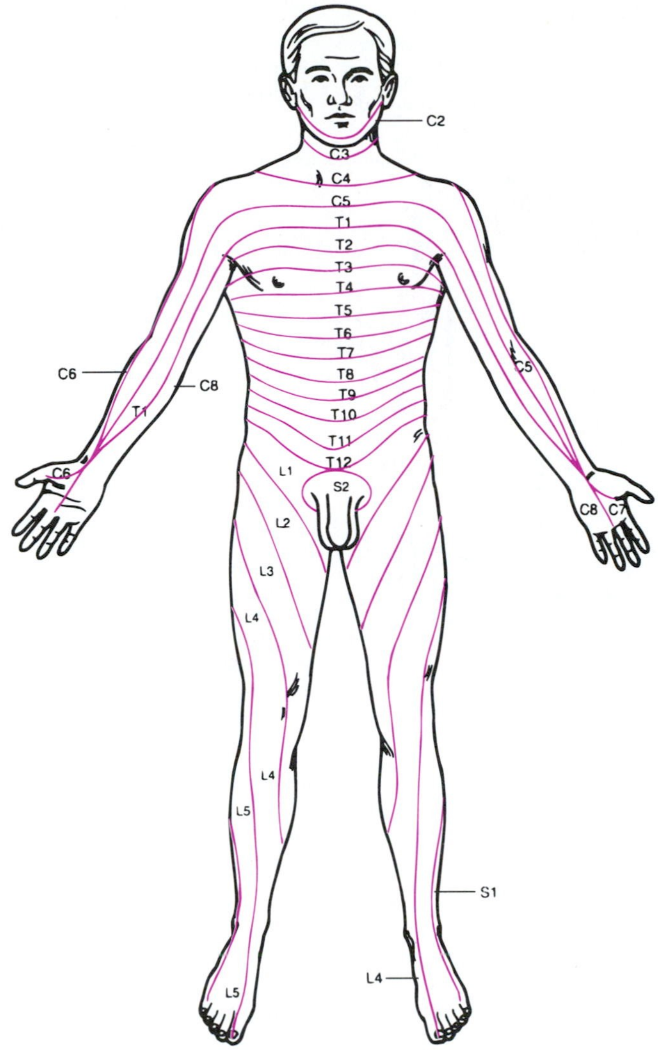

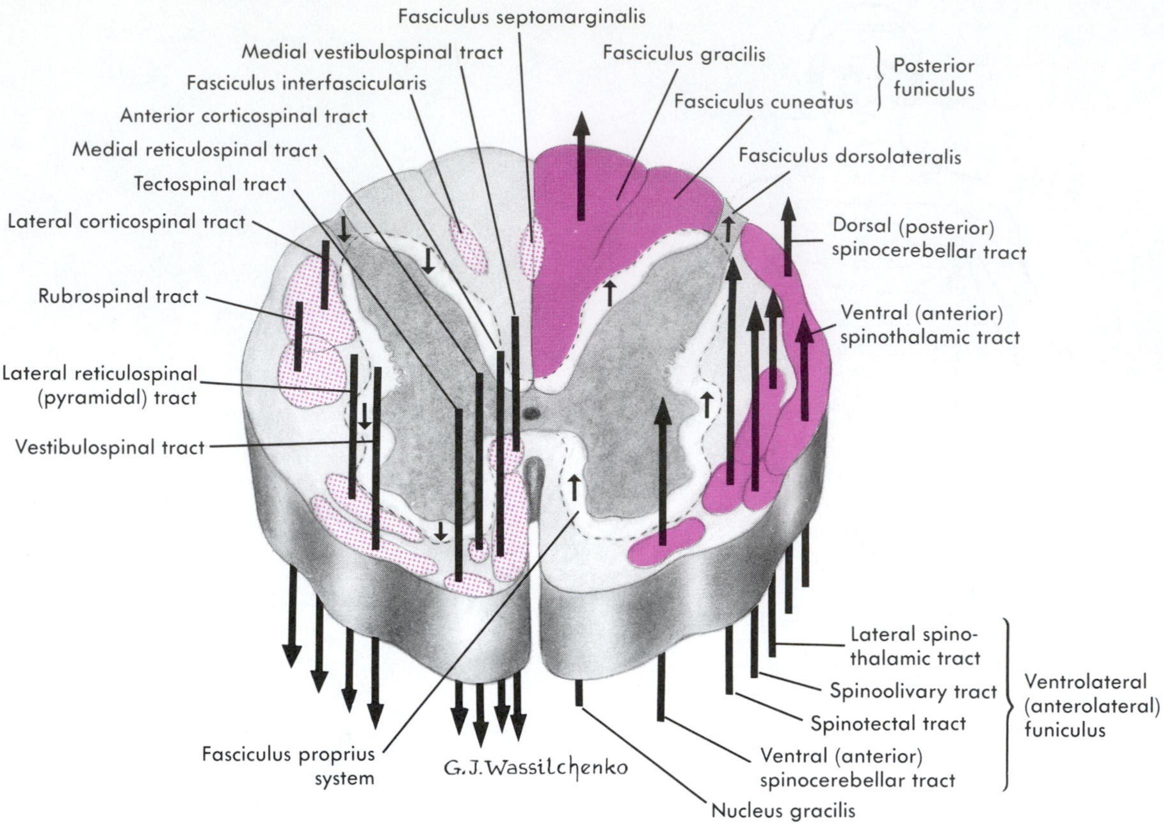

Fasciculus septomarginalis
Medial vestibulospinal tract
Fasciculus gracilis
Posterior funiculus
Fasciculus interfascicularis
Fasciculus cuneatus
Anterior corticospinal tract
Medial reticulospinal tract
Fasciculus dorsolateralis
Tectospinal tract
Lateral corticospinal tract
Dorsal (posterior) spinocerebellar tract
Rubrospinal tract
Ventral (anterior) spinothalamic tract
Lateral reticulospinal (pyramidal) tract
Vestibulospinal tract
Lateral spino-thalamic tract
Spinoolivary tract
Ventrolateral (anterolateral) funiculus
Spinotectal tract
Fasciculus proprius system
G.J.Wassilchenko
Ventral (anterior) spinocerebellar tract
Nucleus gracilis

FIGURE 25-26. Spinal cord tracts of the white matter.

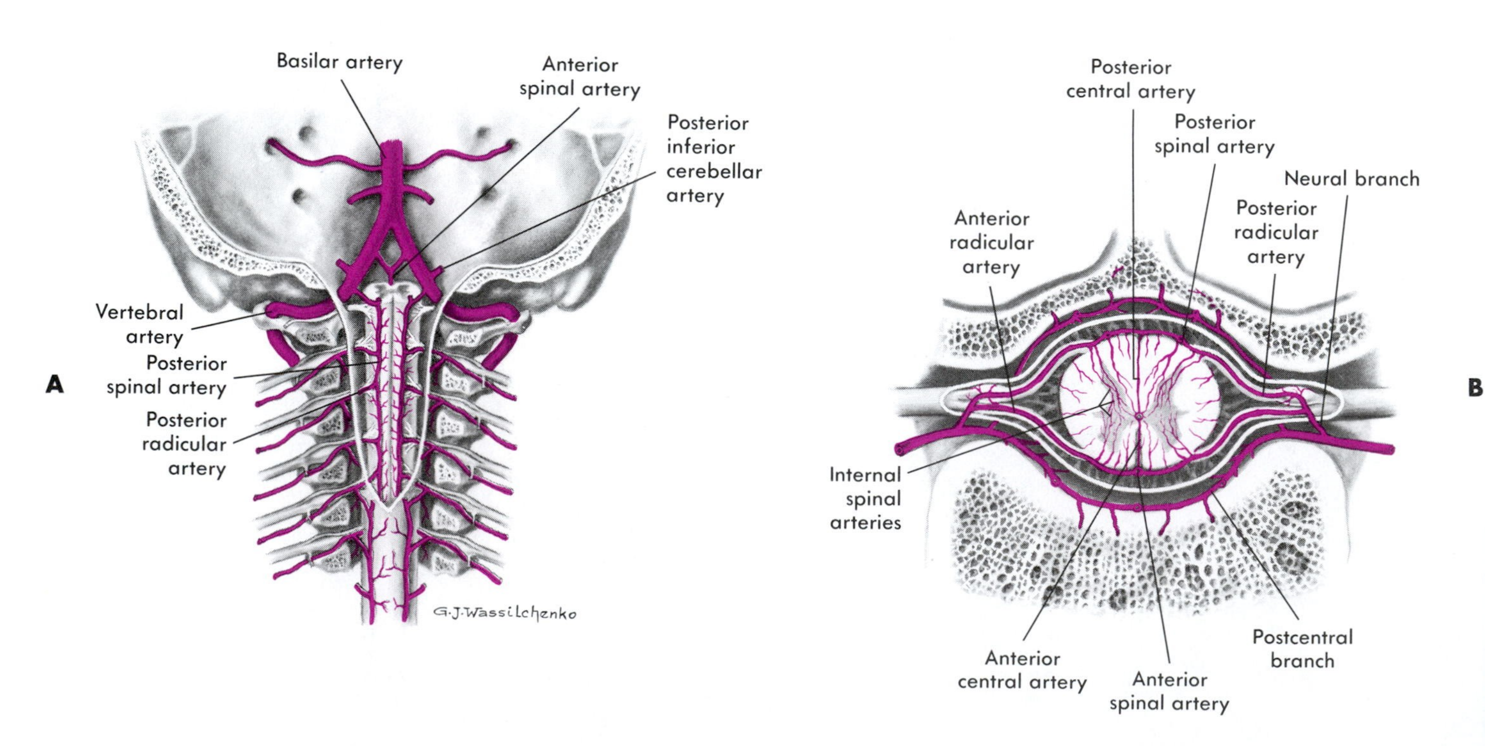

FIGURE 25-27. Arteries of spinal cord. **A,** Cervical cord arteries. **B,** Vascular distribution in spinal cord.

BOX 25-2 Sensory and Motor Tracts

ASCENDING, OR SENSORY, TRACTS

Lateral spinothalamic tract: ascension of pain and thermal sensations

Anterior spinothalamic tract: ascension of light touch and pressure sensation

Posterior white columns: ascension of discriminatory touch

DESCENDING, OR MOTOR, TRACTS

Ventral and lateral corticospinal tracts: descending voluntary motor tracts

Rubrospinal tract: originates in the nucleus of the midbrain; receives fibers from cerebellum and descends in the lateral and anterior funiculi; conveys impulses to control muscle synergy and tone

is the destination, thus allowing easy identification of sensory or motor tracts. Sensory tracts begin with the prefix spino and motor tracts end with the suffix spinal (Box 25-2).

Many other motor and sensory tracts are within the spinal cord, but only those presented here can be clinically tested.

Vascular supply. Supply of arterial blood to the spinal cord comes from branches of the vertebral arteries plus small radicular arteries that enter at the intervertebral foramina. They combine to form the anterior spinal and two posterior spinal arteries. These three arteries, along with some additional radicular arterial flow from cervical, intercostal, lumbar, and sacral arteries, feed the entire length of the spinal cord (Figure 25-27).

Arterial supply to the spinal cord is segmented at best; therefore certain portions of the spinal cord that receive their blood supply from two separate sources are vulnerable areas. These vulnerable areas are C2 to C3, T1 to T4, and L1 to L2. Evidence of this tenuous blood supply can occasionally be noted in a patient after open heart surgery or abdominal aortic aneurysm repair who becomes paraplegic because of loss of the small arterial feeders from the aorta responsible for spinal cord circulation.

REFERENCES

1. Guyton A: *Textbook of medical physiology,* ed 9, Philadelphia, 1996, WB Saunders.
2. Waxman SG, deGroot J: *Correlative neuroanatomy,* ed 23, Norwalk, 1996, Appleton & Lange.
3. Snell R: *Clinical neuroanatomy for medical students,* ed 3, Boston, 1992, Little, Brown.
4. Hickey JV: *The clinical practice of neurological and neurosurgical nursing,* ed 3, Philadelphia, 1992, JB Lippincott.
5. Dickens MD: Pharmacology of neuromuscular blockade: interactions and implications for concurrent drug therapies, *Crit Care Nurs Q* 18(2):1, 1995.
6. Miller JN: Comprehensive review: neuromuscular blocking agents in critical care, *Crit Care Nurs Q* 18(2):60, 1995.
7. Gilman S, Winans S: *Manter and Gatz's essentials of clinical neuroanatomy and neurophysiology,* ed 8, Philadelphia, 1992, FA Davis.

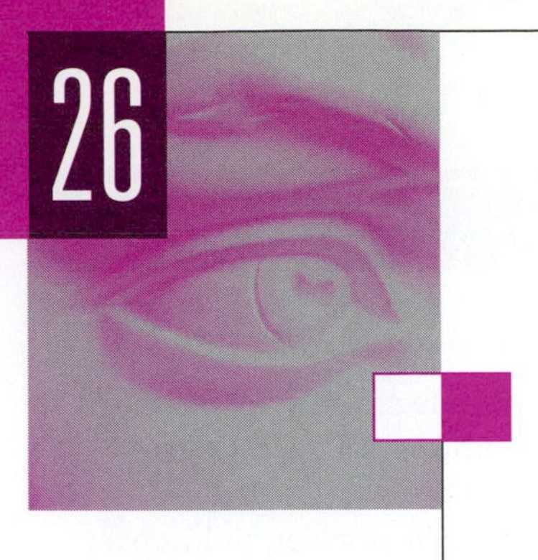

26 Neurologic Clinical Assessment

ASSESSMENT OF THE patient with actual or potential neurologic dysfunction is the essential beginning point in the nursing process and forms the basis for nursing diagnosis. Only when the nurse is aware of all components of a patient's physiologic dysfunction can appropriate diagnosing, planning, intervention, and evaluation take place. This chapter presents a basic introduction to a neurologic examination in the critical care environment.

HISTORY

Neurologic assessment encompasses a wide variety of applications and a multitude of techniques. This chapter focuses on the type of assessment performed in a critical care environment. The one factor common to all neurologic assessments is the need to obtain a comprehensive history of events preceding hospitalization. An adequate neurologic history includes information about clinical manifestations, associated complaints, precipitating factors, progression, and familial occurrences (Box 26-1). If the patient is incapable of providing this information, family members or significant others must be contacted as soon as possible. When someone other than the patient is the source of the history, it must be an individual who was in contact with the patient on a daily basis. Frequently, valuable information is gained, which directs the caregiver to focus on certain aspects of the patient's clinical assessment.

PHYSICAL EXAMINATION

Five major components make up the neurologic examination of the critically ill patient. They are evaluation of (1) level of consciousness, (2) motor function, (3) pupillary function and eye movement, (4) respiratory patterns, and (5) vital signs. Until all five components have been assessed, a complete neurologic examination has not been performed. At any time primary responsibility for patient care is passed from one nurse to another, joint completion of this examination by both nurses will greatly enhance the accuracy and consistency of both the assessment and the evaluation of findings.

Level of Consciousness

Assessment of the level of consciousness is the most important aspect of the neurologic examination. In most situations a patient's level of consciousness deteriorates before any other neurologic changes are noted. This deterioration often is subtle and must be monitored carefully.

Level-of-consciousness assessment is a component of the mental status, or cognition, assessment. Other components of the cognitive assessment include speech and language, memory, general information, calculation, and abstraction and judgment. In the critical care environment assessment of these additional components may occur initially but usually is not a part of an ongoing evaluation.

Components of consciousness. There are two major components of consciousness: arousal, or alertness, and content of consciousness, or awareness.[1]

Arousal. Assessment of the arousal component of consciousness is an evaluation of the reticular activating system and its connection with the thalamus and the cerebral cortex. Arousal is the lowest level of consciousness, and observation centers on the patient's ability to respond to verbal or noxious stimuli in an appropriate manner.

Awareness. Content of consciousness is a higher-level function and is concerned with assessment of the

BOX 26-1 DATA COLLECTION FOR NEUROLOGIC HISTORY

COMMON NEUROLOGIC SYMPTOMS
- Fainting
- Dizziness
- Blackouts
- Seizures
- Headache
- Memory loss
- Weakness
- Paralysis
- Tremors or other involuntary movements
- Pain
- Numbness
- Tingling
- Speech disturbances
- Vision disturbances

EVENTS PRECEDING ONSET OF SYMPTOMS
- Travel
- Animal contact
- Falls
- Infection
- Dental problems or procedures
- Sinus or middle ear infections
- Prodromal symptoms
- Food or drugs ingested

PROGRESSION OF SYMPTOMS
- Initial onset
- Evolution
- Frequency
- Severity
- Duration
- Associated activities/aggravating factors

FAMILY HISTORY
- Stroke (AV malformation, aneurysm)
- Diabetes mellitus
- Hypertension
- Seizures
- Tumors
- Headaches
- Emotional problems or depression

MEDICAL HISTORY
- Childhood
  - Birth injuries, congenital defects, encephalitis, meningitis, bed wetting, fainting, seizures, trauma
- Adult
  - Diabetes; hypertension; cardiovascular, pulmonary, kidney, liver, or endocrine disease; tuberculosis; tropical infection; sinusitis; visual problems; tumors; psychiatric disorders
- Surgical history
  - Neurologic, ear-nose-throat, dental, eye
- Traumatic history
  - Motor vehicle accidents; falls; blows to the head, neck or back; being knocked out
- Allergies
  - Drug, food, environmental

PATIENT PROFILE
- Personal habits
  - Use of alcohol, recreational drugs, over-the-counter drug use, smoking, dietary habits, sleeping patterns, elimination patterns, exercise habits
- Recent life changes
- Living conditions
- Working conditions
  - Exposure to toxins, chemicals, fumes; occupational duties
- General temperment

CURRENT MEDICATION USAGE
- Sedatives, tranquilizers
- Antiepileptics
- Psychotropics
- Anticoagulants
- Antibiotics
- Calcium channel blockers
- Beta-blockers
- Nitrates
- Oral contraceptives

AV, Arteriovenous.

patient's orientation to person, place, and time. Assessment of content of consciousness requires the patient to give appropriate answers to a variety of questions. Changes in the patient's answers that indicate increasing degrees of confusion and disorientation may be the first sign of neurologic deterioration.

Categories of consciousness. It is necessary to view consciousness as a continuum ranging from full alertness to deep coma. Universally accepted definitions for various levels of consciousness do not exist. The categories outlined in Box 26-2, although vague, are often used to describe the patient's level of consciousness.[1-3]

Frequently it is difficult to categorize patients under these descriptions, and communication of patient condition often is misinterpreted. Because of the dif-

BOX 26-2 Categories of Consciousness

Alert—responds immediately to minimal external stimuli.
Lethargic—state of drowsiness or inaction in which the patient needs an increased stimulus to be awakened, but is still easily arousable. Verbal, mental, and motor responses are slow and sluggish.
Obtunded—very drowsy when not stimulated. Follows simple commands when stimulated. A duller indifference to external stimuli exists, and response is minimally maintained.
Stuporous—minimal spontaneous movement. Arousable only by vigorous and continuous external stimuli. Motor responses to tactile stimuli are appropriate. Verbal responses are minimal and incomprehensible.
Comatose—vigorous stimulation fails to produce any voluntary neural response. Both arousal and awareness are absent. No verbal responses. Motor responses may be purposeful withdrawal to pain (light coma), nonpurposeful, or absent (deep coma).

ficulty in communicating level of consciousness, a variety of assessment tools have been devised to assist in this evaluation. Even when these tools are used, optimal care can be facilitated by assessment and documentation of complete descriptions of the patient's state of arousal and awareness before, during, and after stimulation; the type and degree of stimulation used to obtain response; and verbal, motor, and physiologic responses to stimuli.

Tools for assessment of consciousness. The general rule for evaluation of an altered level of consciousness is to determine systematically the type and degree of noxious stimuli required to produce a response. This concept is incorporated into a variety of clinical assessment tools.

The most widely recognized level-of-consciousness assessment tool is the Glasgow Coma Scale (GCS).[4] This scored scale is based on evaluation of three categories: eye opening, verbal response, and best motor response (Table 26-1). The best possible score on the GCS is 15, and the lowest score is 3. Generally a score of 7 or less on the GCS indicates coma.

Originally the scoring system was developed to assist general communication concerning the severity of neurologic injury. Adapted and modified, this scale has become the basis of many neurologic assessment flow sheets. Recent testing of the GCS revealed a moderate to high agreement rating among both physicians and nurses.[5] Several points must be kept in mind when the GCS is used for serial assessment. It provides data about level of consciousness only and never must be considered a complete neurologic examination. It is not a sensitive tool for evaluation of an altered sensorium. The GCS does not account for possible aphasia, nor is it a good indicator of lateralization of neurologic deterioration. Lateralization involves decreasing motor response on one side or unilateral changes in pupillary reaction.

Whatever assessment tool is chosen to measure level of consciousness, the goal is to identify subtle changes in consciousness responses. Communication of small signs of deteriorating consciousness may allow early intervention and thus prevent neurologic disaster.

Motor Function

Motor assessment techniques. Correct technique and accurate description of findings are imperative for appropriate interpretation and evaluation of motor assessment. Evaluation of motor function must first include observation for spontaneous movement. The second step is to elicit movement in response to a stimulus. The type and degree of stimuli applied to produce a motor response is a key element in the assessment of motor function.

Verbal stimuli. Next to the assessment of orientation and awareness, the assessment of the patient's ability to follow commands is one of the highest levels of functioning evaluated. Several points must be recognized in assessing ability to follow commands. Commands given to a patient with an altered level of consciousness must be phrased in simple and direct statements, such as: "Show me your thumb." A common error made by clinicians in assessing the patient's ability to respond to commands is to include the simple command along with other verbal communication. To prevent sensory overload and therefore the patient's inability to respond to command, the command must not be included as part of any other conversation. An example of the *inappropriate* use of a simple command is: "Robert, your mother is here. Let's show her how much better you are doing. Robert, show her your thumb. Come on Robert, you did it for me an hour ago. Robert, show your mother your thumb. She will be very excited if she could see you do this. Robert, I know you can do it." As a patient is emerging from an unconscious state, the brain is less capable of simultaneous processing and sorting of multiple stimuli. The key to assessment of the patient's ability to follow

TABLE 26-1 Glasgow Coma Scale

Category	Score	Response
Eye opening	4	Spontaneous—eyes open spontaneously without stimulation
	3	To speech—eyes open with verbal stimulation but not necessarily to command
	2	To pain—eyes open with noxious stimuli
	1	None—no eye opening regardless of stimulation
Verbal response	5	Oriented—accurate information about person, place, time, reason for hospitalization, and personal data
	4	Confused—answers not appropriate to question, but use of language is correct
	3	Inappropriate words—disorganized, random speech, no sustained conversation
	2	Incomprehensible sounds—moans, groans, and incomprehensible mumbles
	1	None—no verbalization despite stimulation
Best motor response	6	Obeys commands—performs simple tasks on command; able to repeat performance
	5	Localizes to pain—organized attempt to localize and remove painful stimuli
	4	Withdraws from pain—withdraws extremity from source of painful stimuli
	3	Abnormal flexion—decorticate posturing spontaneously or in response to noxious stimuli
	2	Extension—decerebrate posturing spontaneously or in response to noxious stimuli
	1	None—no response to noxious stimuli; flaccid

commands is to reduce surrounding stimuli or distractors and to keep the command simple and direct.

Another error commonly made in the assessment of the patient's ability to follow commands involves the type of command given. Appropriate commands are those that do not elicit random or reflex responses. "Squeeze my hand" is a common command used by caregivers and family alike. In low levels of consciousness, the reflex of hand grasp, if present, is initiated when the assessor's hand is placed within the patient's hand. If this is the case, it often is difficult to assess accurately whether the patient is responding to command or exhibiting a reflex response. Asking the patient to "Let go of my hand" after hand grasp also is difficult to assess accurately. Relaxation of the reflex can mimic the command: "Let go." Use of hand grasp in assessment of the patient's motor strength is discussed separately.

Acceptable commands include: "Show me your thumb" or "Stick out your tongue." When these commands are used, care must be taken that the command is not followed by visual or tactile stimuli. It is not uncommon to observe an assessment in which the nurse asks the patient to "show me your thumb" while tapping the patient's thumb. With this scenario it is impossible to determine whether the patient is following a verbal command or withdrawing from tactile stimuli.

Noxious stimuli. Once it has been determined that the patient is incapable of comprehending and following a simple command, the use of noxious stimuli is required to determine motor responses. A variety of acceptable and unacceptable ways of administering painful stimuli are presented in Box 26-3.

Levels of motor movements. A simple way of organizing the assessment of motor movements is to use the categories defined in the Glasgow Coma Scale[4] as a guide. The difference in this part of the assessment is that now each extremity is evaluated and recorded individually. It is also necessary to include the presence or absence of spontaneous movement and seizure activity, because these components of motor movement evaluation are not included in the GCS. The following are categories of motor movement:

Obeys commands—performs simple tasks on command and is able to repeat performance

Localizes to pain—organized attempt to localize and remove painful stimuli

Withdraws from pain—withdraws extremity from source of painful stimuli

Abnormal flexion—decorticate posturing spontaneously or in response to noxious stimuli

Extension—decerebrate posturing spontaneously or in response to noxious stimuli

Flaccid—no response to noxious stimuli

In addition, a comparison of function is made with that of the opposite extremity. In the evaluation of a patient with spinal cord injury or dysfunction, a sep-

BOX 26-3 Methods of Noxious Stimuli

1. **Nailbed pressure**—requires use of an object such as a pen to apply firm pressure to the nailbed. Pressure applied to each extremity allows evaluation of individual extremity function. The patient's movement must not be interrupted while the nurse is applying the nailbed pressure. If no response is elicited from nailbed pressure, other noxious stimuli measures are employed.
2. **Trapezius pinch**—performed by squeezing the trapezius muscle, this method allows for observation of total body response to stimuli. Trapezius pinch often is difficult to perform on large or obese adults.
3. **Sternal rub**—firm pressure is applied to the sternum in a rubbing motion, usually with the assessor's knuckles. If used repeatedly, the sternum could become excoriated, open, and infected. Open-handed firm patting of the sternal area to arouse the patient is acceptable.
4. **Supraorbital pressure**—must be avoided in patients with head injuries, frontal craniotomies, or facial surgery because of the possibility of underlying fractured or unstable cranium.
5. **Nipple pinching and testicle pinching**—for obvious reasons this type of noxious stimuli is inappropriate and unnecessary.

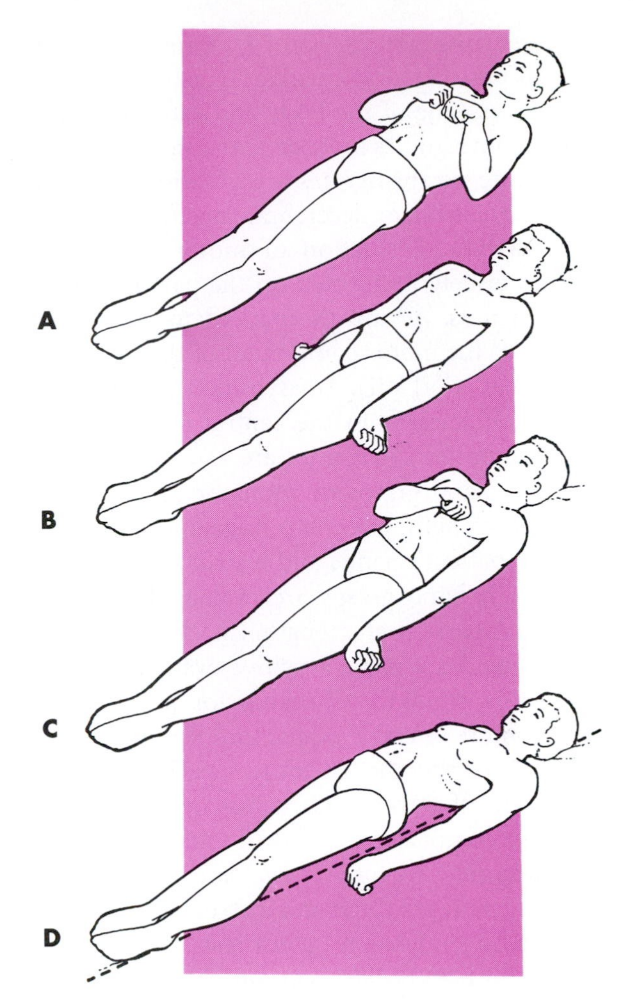

FIGURE 26-1. Abnormal motor responses. **A,** Decorticate posturing. **B,** Decerebrate posturing. **C,** Decorticate posturing on right side, and decerebrate posturing on left side of body. **D,** Opisthotonic posturing.

arate scale is used with more detail about motor strength of particular muscle groups.

Seizure activity may occur spontaneously or in response to stimuli in the patient with neurologic impairment. *Tonus* refers to a steady state of muscular contraction. *Clonus* refers to an ongoing rhythmic pattern of muscle spasm followed by relaxation. Grand mal seizures are composed of a tonic phase followed by a clonic phase.[2] It is important to identify and describe any seizure activity. It is also important to identify possible stimuli precipitating seizure activity.

Abnormal motor responses. In the unconscious patient noxious stimuli may elicit an abnormal motor response (Figure 26-1). These responses are identified as abnormal flexion (decorticate posturing) or extension (decerebrate posturing). The assessment of abnormal flexion and extension is an integral part of the motor component of the GCS. The exact anatomic location of these abnormal responses remains a mystery. Generally the severity of damage to the brain precludes localization of the lesion that causes these abnormal movements.[1]

Abnormal flexion. Abnormal flexion also is known as *decorticate posturing.* In response to painful stimuli, the upper extremities exhibit flexion of the arm, wrist, and fingers with adduction of the limb. The lower extremity exhibits extension, internal rotation, and plantar flexion.

Abnormal extension. Abnormal extension also is known as *decerebrate rigidity,* or *posturing.* When the patient is stimulated, the teeth clench and the arms are stiffly extended, adducted, and hyperpronated. The legs are stiffly extended with plantar flexion of the feet.

Because abnormal flexion and extension appear similar in the lower extremities, the upper extremities are used to determine the presence of these abnormal movements. It is possible for the patient to exhibit abnormal flexion on one side of the body and extension on the other. Outcome studies indicate that abnormal flexion, or decorticate posturing, has a less serious prognosis than does extension, or decerebrate posturing.[1]

Motor strength. Evaluation of motor strength can only be accurately performed on the patient who follows commands. Asking the patient to smile allows evaluation of the motor component of the facial nerve (cranial nerve [CN] VII). An asymmetrical smile is associated with a lesion in the central nervous system (CNS). The upper extremities are assessed by checking bilateral hand grasps or pronator drift. To assess hand grasp strength, place two fingers in the palm of each of the patient's hands and instruct the patient to squeeze. Both hand grasps are evaluated simultaneously for comparison of strength. Checking for pronator drift provides a more sensitive evaluation of upper extremity strength. Checking for pronator drift provides a more sensitive evaluation of upper extremity strength. Instruct the patient to close his or her eyes and to extend the arms with palms upturned. Check for evidence of unilateral arm drift within 30 seconds. Lower extremity strength is evaluated by placing a hand on the patient's thigh and instructing him or her to raise the leg straight up against resistance. Next, ask the patient to planter flex (step on gas) and dorsiflex (pull toes toward nose) against resistance. A key element in evaluation of motor strength is comparison with the same muscle group on the opposite side of the body. Subtle changes in motor strength between the right and left sides of the body, lateralizing, may indicate an impending neurologic emergency.

Lateralizing signs. Lateralizing signs are neurologic findings that occur only on one side of the body, such as unilateral deterioration in motor movements or changes in pupillary response. Lateralizing signs help to localize the lesion to one side of the brain. For example, a patient who was withdrawing to painful stimuli with both arms at the last examination is now withdrawing on the right but exhibiting abnormal flexion on the left. This change in response on the left side points to an expanding intracranial lesion on the right side of the brain.

The occurrence of lateralizing signs indicates an emergency situation. Unilateral deterioration of motor movements and pupillary response may herald herniation. Notification of the physician and immediate intervention are imperative.

Reflexes

Muscle-stretch reflexes (deep tendon reflexes). Deep tendon reflexes (DTRs) are usually evaluated by a physician when a complete neurologic evaluation is performed. DTRs are tested by tapping the appropriate tendon using a reflex or percussion hammer. The muscle needs to be relaxed and the joint at midposition for reflex testing to be accurate. The four reflexes tested are the achilles (ankle jerk), the quadriceps (knee jerk), the biceps, and the triceps. DTRs are graded on a scale from 0 (absent) to 4 (hyperactive). A DTR grade of 2 is normal.[2] Hyperreflexia is associated with upper motor neuron interruption, and areflexia is associated with lesions of the lower motor neurons.

Superficial reflexes. Superficial reflexes are normal if present and abnormal if absent. Superficial reflexes are tested by stimulating cutaneous receptors of the skin, cornea, or mucous membrane. Stroking, scratching, or touching can be used as the stimulus. The corneal reflex is present if the eyelids quickly close when the cornea is lightly stroked with a wisp of cotton. The pathway for the corneal reflex is formed by the trigeminal (CN V) and facial (CN VII) nerves and the pons. The gag reflex is present if retching or gagging occurs with stimulation of the back of the pharynx. The swallowing reflex is present if the uvula elevates when touched. Observation of visible swallowing is also indicative of the swallowing reflex. The gag and swallow reflexes are a function of the glossopharyngeal (CN IX) and vagus (CN X) nerves. The swallowing reflex and the gag reflex are often stimulated during routine oral and pulmonary hygiene in the critical care environment. The presence of these reflexes must be noted and documented during completion of these activities.

Pathologic reflexes. The presence of pathologic reflexes is an abnormal neurologic finding. The grasp reflex is present when tactile stimulation of the palm of the hand produces a grasp response that is not a conscious voluntary act. The grasp reflex is a primitive reflex that normally disappears with maturational development. Presence of the grasp reflex indicates cortical damage. The Babinski reflex is a pathologic sign in any individual older than 2 years. The presence of this reflex is tested by slow, deliberate stroking of the lateral half of the sole of the foot. Sustained extensor response of the big toe is indicative of a positive Babinski reflex. This response is sometimes accompanied by fanning out of the other four toes. Flexor response of all the toes in response to the same stimuli is a normal finding and indicates absence of the Babinski reflex. The Babinski reflex is an extremely important neurologic finding, significantly indicative of CNS disease in either the brain, brainstem, or spinal cord. The disease may be degenerative, neoplastic, inflammatory, vascular, or posttraumatic.[6,7]

BOX 26-4 Pathways of Pupillary Response

SYMPATHETIC

Brainstem
 Dilates

PARASYMPATHETIC

CN III
 Constricts

The Babinski reflex may also become positive during transtentorial herniation.[2]

Pupillary Function and Eye Movement

The assessment of pupillary function and eye movement is an important component of the neurologic examination. Pupillary response may be one of the few neurologic signs that can be assessed, especially in the unconscious patient or the patient receiving neuromuscular blocking agents and sedation. Serial evaluation, appropriate technique, recognition of abnormalities, and good documentation are all important.

Anatomy of pupillary response. Pupil size and reaction to light are a function of the autonomic nervous system. Parasympathetic control of the pupil occurs through innervation of the oculomotor nerve (CN III), which exits from the brainstem in the midbrain area. When the parasympathetic fibers are stimulated, the pupil constricts. Sympathetic control originates in the hypothalamus and travels down the entire length of the brainstem. When the sympathetic fibers are stimulated, the pupil dilates (Box 26-4). The pupillary light reflex is mediated by the retina and optic nerve (CN II) as the sensory pathway and the oculomotor nerve (CN III) as the motor pathway.

Pupillary changes provide a valuable tool to assessment because of pathway location (Figure 26-2). The oculomotor nerve lies at the junction of the midbrain and the tentorial notch. Any increase of pressure that exerts force down through the tentorial notch compresses the oculomotor nerve. Oculomotor nerve compression results in a dilated, nonreactive pupil. Sympathetic pathway disruption occurs with involvement in the brainstem. Loss of sympathetic control leads to pinpoint, nonreactive pupils. Pupillary reactivity also is affected by medications, particularly sympathetic and parasympathetic agents; direct trauma; and eye surgery. Pupillary reactivity is relatively resistant to metabolic dysfunction and can be used to differentiate between metabolic and structural causes of decreased levels of consciousness.

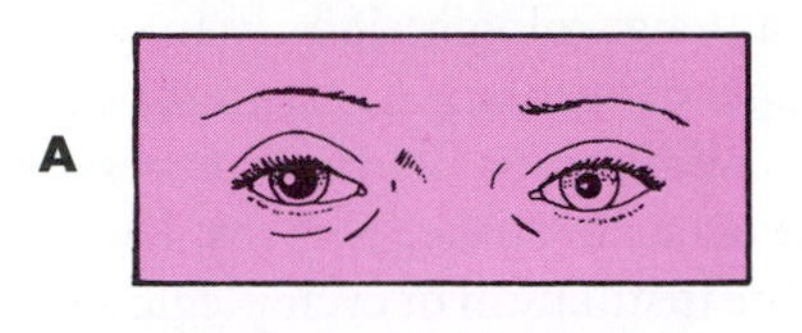

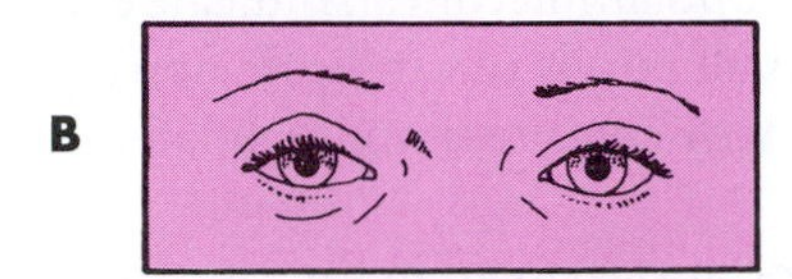

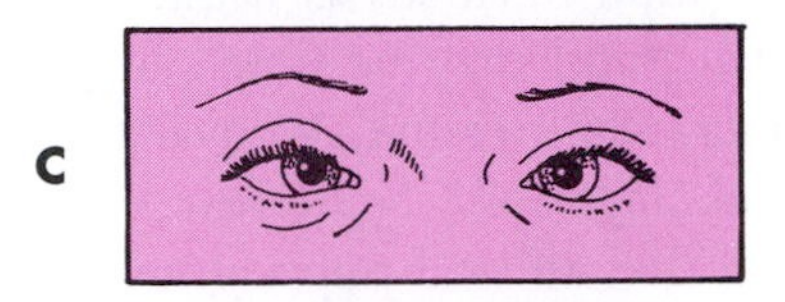

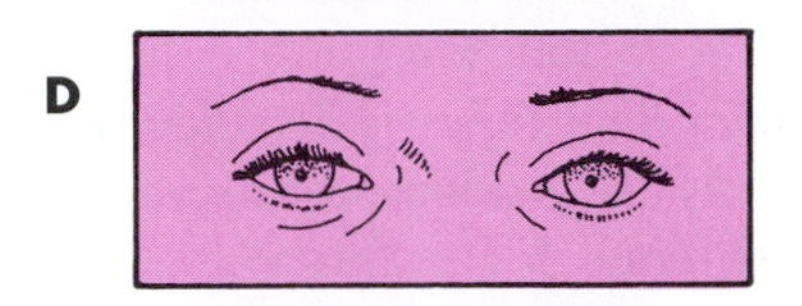

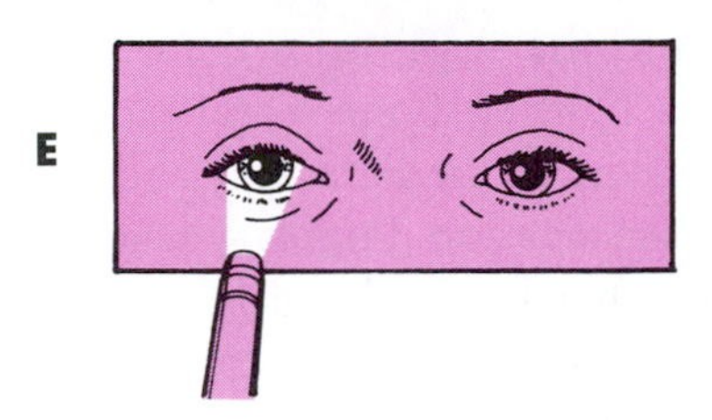

FIGURE 26-2. Abnormal pupillary responses. **A,** Oculomotor nerve compression. **B,** Bilateral diencephalon damage. **C,** Midbrain damage. **D,** Pontine damage. **E,** Dilated, nonreactive pupils.

Assessment of pupillary response. Evaluation of pupillary response includes assessment of size; shape (round, irregular, or oval); and degree of reactivity to light. The two pupils are compared for equality. Since any of these components of the pupil assessment could change in response to increasing pressure on the oculomotor nerve at the tentorium, pupillary assessment plays a key role in the physical assessment of intracranial pressure changes and herniation syndromes.

Pupil size is documented in millimeters with the use of a pupil gauge to reduce the subjectivity of describing the pupil as small, medium, large, dilated, and so on. Although the pupils of most persons are of equal size, a discrepancy of up to 1 mm between the two pupils is normal. Inequality of pupils is known as *anisocoria* and occurs in 15% to 17% of the human population.

Change or inequality in pupil size, especially in patients who previously have not shown this discrepancy, is a significant neurologic sign. It may indicate impending danger of herniation and must be reported immediately. In addition to CN III compression, changes in pupil size occur for other reasons. Large pupils can result from the instillation of cycloplegic agents, such as atropine or scopolamine, or can indicate extreme stress. Extremely small pupils can indicate narcotic overdose, lower brainstem compression, or bilateral damage to the pons.

Pupil shape also is noted in the assessment of pupils. Although the pupil normally is round, an irregularly shaped or oval pupil may be noted in patients with elevated intracranial pressure. An oval pupil can indicate the initial stages of CN III compression.[2] It has been observed that an oval pupil almost always is associated with an elevated intracranial pressure (ICP) between 18 and 35 mm Hg.[8]

The pupillary light reflex is dependent on both optic nerve (CN II) and oculomotor nerve (CN III) function. The technique for evaluation of the pupillary light response involves use of a narrow-beamed bright light shone into the pupil from the outer canthus of the eye. If the light is shone directly onto the pupil, glare or reflection of the light may prevent the assessor's proper visualization. Pupillary reaction to light is identified as either brisk, sluggish, or nonreactive or fixed. Each pupil is evaluated both for direct light response and for consensual response. The consensual pupillary response is constriction in response to a light shone into the opposite eye. This reflex occurs as a result of crossing of nerve fibers at the optic chiasm. Evaluation of consensual response is necessary to rule out optic nerve dysfunction as a cause for lack of a direct light reflex. Since the optic nerve is the afferent pathway for the light reflex, shining a light into a blind eye will produce neither a direct light response in that eye nor a consensual response in the opposite eye. A consensual response in the blind eye produced by shining a light into the opposite eye demonstrates an intact oculomotor nerve. Oculomotor compression associated with transtentorial herniation affects both the direct light response and the consensual response in the affected pupil.[2,6,9]

Anatomy of eye movement. Control of eye movements occurs with interaction of three cranial nerves: oculomotor (CN III), trochlear (CN IV), and abducens (CN VI) (Figure 26-3). The pathways for these cranial nerves provide integrated function through the internuclear pathway of the medial longitudinal fasciculus (MLF) located in the brainstem. The MLF provides coordination of eye movements with the vestibular (CN VIII) nerve and reticular formation.

Assessment of eye movements

Extraocular movements. In the conscious patient the function of the three cranial nerves of the eye and their MLF innervation can be assessed by asking the patient to follow a finger through the full range of eye motions (see Figure 26-3). If the eyes move together into all six fields, extraocular movements (EOM) are intact.[6]

Oculocephalic reflex (doll's eyes). In the unconscious patient, assessment of ocular function and innervation of the MLF is performed by eliciting the doll's eyes reflex. If the patient is unconscious as a result of trauma, the nurse must ascertain the absence of cervical injury before performing this examination.

To assess the oculocephalic reflex, the nurse holds the patient's eyelids open and briskly turns the head to one side while observing the eye movements, then briskly turns the head to the other side and observes. If the eyes deviate to the opposite direction in which the head is turned, doll's eyes are present and the oculocephalic reflex arc is intact. If the oculocephalic reflex arc is not intact, the reflex is absent. This lack of response, in which the eyes remain midline and move with the head, indicates significant brainstem injury. The reflex may also be absent in severe metabolic coma.[3] An abnormal oculocephalic reflex is present when the eyes rove or move in opposite directions. Abnormal oculocephalic reflex indicates some degree of brainstem injury (Figure 26-4).

Oculovestibular reflex (cold caloric test). The oculovestibular reflex is performed by a physician, often as one of the final clinical assessments of brainstem function. After confirmation that the tympanic membrane is intact, the head is raised to a 30 degree angle. Then, 20 to 100 ml of ice water is injected into the external auditory canal. The normal eye movement response is a conjugate, slow, tonic, nystagmus deviating toward the irrigated ear and lasts 30 to 120 seconds. This response indicates brainstem integrity. Rapid nystagmus returns the eyes back to the midline only in the conscious patient with cortical functioning (Figure 26-5).[2,3] An abnormal response is dysconjugate eye movement, which indicates a brainstem lesion, or no response, which indicates little to no brainstem function. The oculovestibular reflex may also be temporarily absent in reversible metabolic encephalopathy.[3] This test is an extremely noxious stimulation and may produce a decorticate or decerebrate posturing response in the comatose patient. In the conscious patient, this procedure may produce nausea, vomiting, or dizziness.[2]

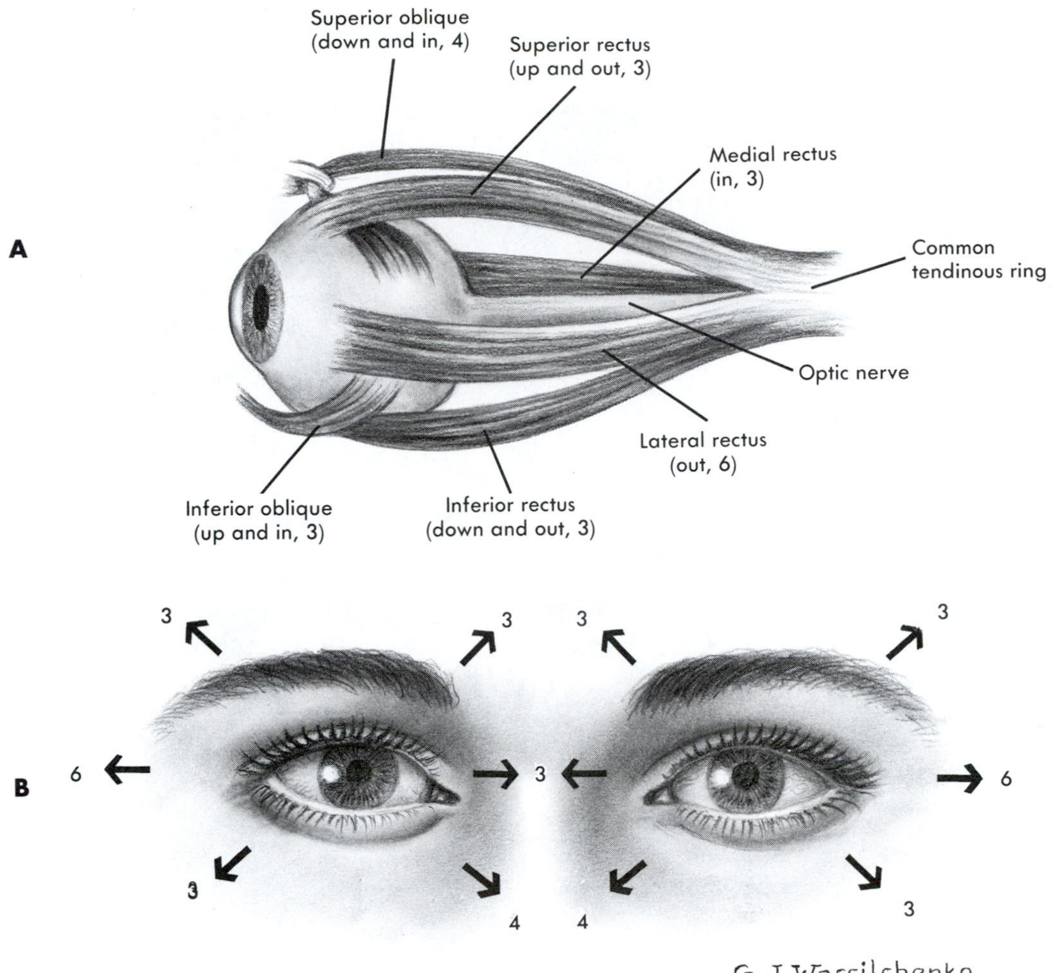

FIGURE 26-3. Extraocular eye movements. **A,** Extraocular muscles. **B,** The six cardinal directions of gaze with each associated cranial nerve supply.

Respiratory Patterns

Control of respirations. The activity of respiration is a highly integrated function that receives input from the cerebrum, brainstem, and metabolic mechanisms. A close correlation exists in clinical assessment among altered levels of consciousness, the level of brain or brainstem injury, and the respiratory pattern noted (Figure 26-6).

Under the influence of the cerebral cortex and the diencephalon, three brainstem centers control respirations. The lowest center, the medullary respiratory center, sends impulses through the vagus nerve to innervate muscles of inspiration and expiration. The apneustic and pneumotaxic centers of the pons are responsible for the length of inspiration and expiration and the underlying respiratory rate.

Respiratory patterns. Changes in respiratory patterns assist in identifying the level of brainstem dysfunction or injury. The respiratory patterns are defined in Table 26-2.

Several respiratory patterns have been noted to occur with metabolic disorders, such as Kussmaul's respirations. These respiratory patterns are initiated in the cerebral cortex in response to metabolic alterations and are a compensatory mechanism. Respiratory patterns of metabolic disorders are not identified in the same terms as the level of dysfunction of a structural injury.

Evaluation of respiratory pattern also must include evaluation of the effectiveness of gas exchange in maintaining adequate oxygen and carbon dioxide levels. Hypoventilation is not uncommon in the patient with an altered level of consciousness. Alterations in oxygenation or carbon dioxide levels can result in further neurologic dysfunction. ICP increases with hypoxemia or hypercapnia.

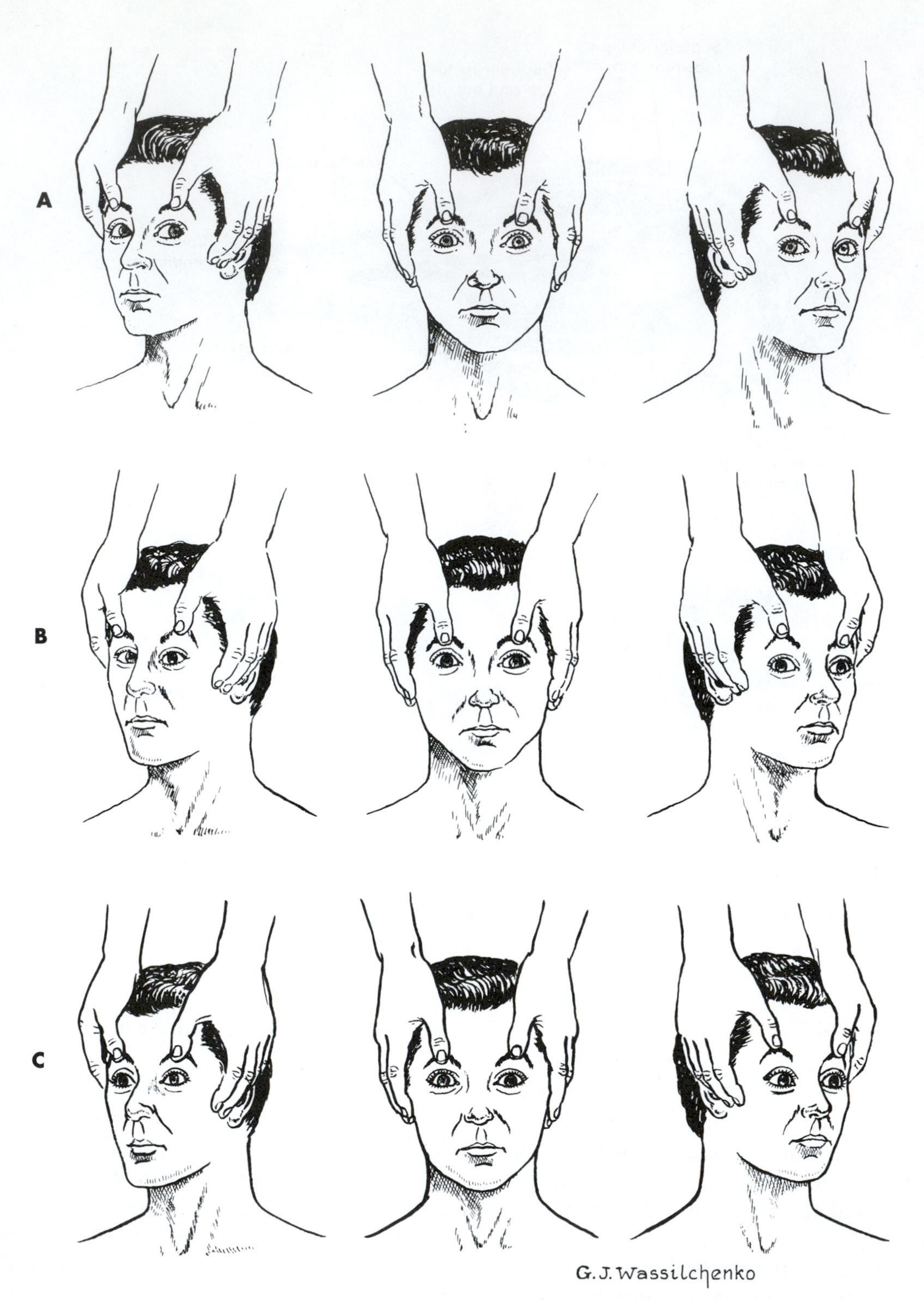

FIGURE 26-4. Oculocephalic reflex (doll's eyes). **A,** Normal. **B,** Abnormal. **C,** Absent.

Finally, assessment of respiratory function in a patient with neurologic deficit must include assessment of airway maintenance and secretion control. Cough, gag, and swallow reflexes responsible for protection of the airway may be absent or diminished.

Vital Signs

The final portion of the neurologic examination is the evaluation of vital signs. As a result of the brain and brainstem influences on cardiac, respiratory, and body temperature functions, changes in vital signs can

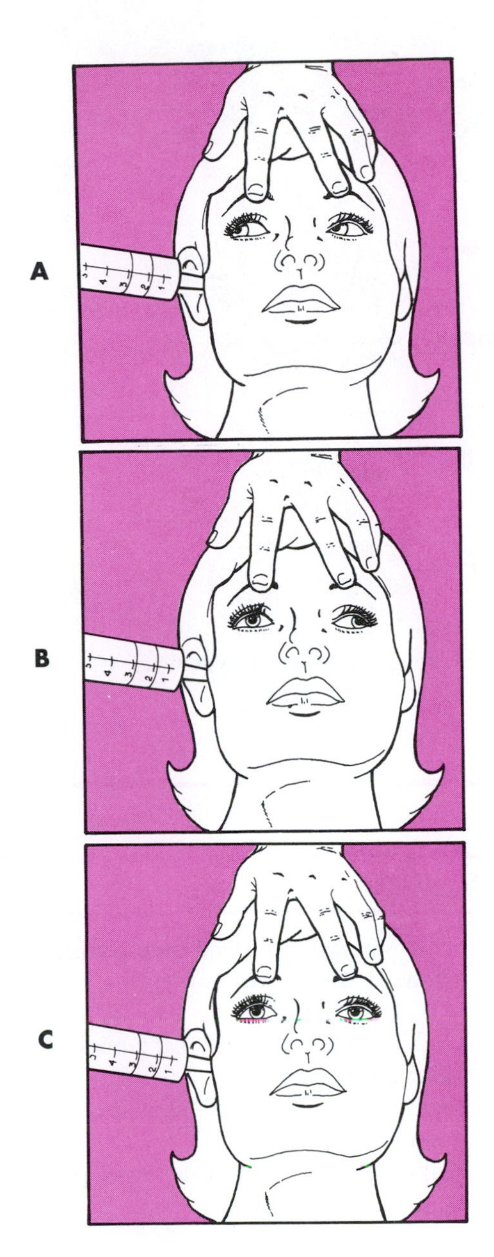

FIGURE 26-5. Oculovestibular reflex (cold caloric test). **A,** Normal. **B,** Abnormal. **C,** Absent.

indicate deterioration in neurologic status. Alterations in cardiopulmonary and thermal status caused by non-neurologic problems can also induce neurologic deterioration. Although a vital sign in the neurologic patient, ICP measurement is not included in this discussion.

Cardiac. The brain's tremendous metabolic demand requires an adequate supply of blood for continual perfusion. Evaluation of the cardiovascular system identifies inappropriate supply for the known cerebral demand and activation of compensatory mechanisms to protect threatened cerebral perfusion.

Hypotension. Cerebral injury rarely produces hypotension except as a terminal event. Regardless of cause (vasodilation, bradycardia, tachycardia, hypovolemia, or inadequate pump), inadequate systemic arterial pressure leads to decreased perfusion of cerebral tissue, hypoxia, and neurologic injury. In the presence of increased ICP, hypotension is even more detrimental because low blood pressure must overcome the additional resistance of ICP to provide blood to the brain.

Hypertension. A common manifestation of intracranial injury is systemic hypertension. Cerebral autoregulation, responsible for the control of cerebral blood flow, frequently is lost with any type of intracranial injury. After cerebral injury the body often is in a hyperdynamic state (increased heart rate, blood pressure, and cardiac output) as part of a compensatory response. With the loss of autoregulation, as blood pressure increases, cerebral blood flow and cerebral blood volume increase, and therefore ICP increases. Control of systemic hypertension is necessary to stop this cycle. However, caution must be exercised. The mean arterial pressure must be maintained at a level sufficient to produce adequate cerebral blood flow in the presence of elevated ICP. Attention must also be paid to the pulse pressure because widening of this value may occur in the late stages of intracranial hypertension.

Dysrhythmias. The medulla and the vagus nerve provide parasympathetic control to the heart. When stimulated, this lower brainstem system produces bradycardia. Sympathetic stimulation increases the rate and contractility. Various intracranial pathologies and abrupt ICP changes can produce cardiac dysrhythmias, such as bradycardia, premature ventricular contractions (PVCs), atrioventricular (AV) block, or ventricular fibrillation and myocardial damage.[10]

Cushing's triad. Cushing's triad is a set of three clinical manifestations (bradycardia, systolic hypertension, and widening pulse pressure) related to pressure on the medullary area of the brainstem. These signs often occur in response to intracranial hypertension or a herniation syndrome. The appearance of Cushing's triad is a late finding that may be absent in neurologic deterioration. Attention must be paid to alteration in each component of the triad and intervention initiated accordingly.

Respiratory. Respiratory function sufficient to maintain adequate cerebral oxygenation and carbon dioxide elimination is essential for neurologic viability. The respiratory rate usually becomes rapid and noisy as intracranial pressure increases. Changes in respiratory pattern also occur with intracranial hypertension.

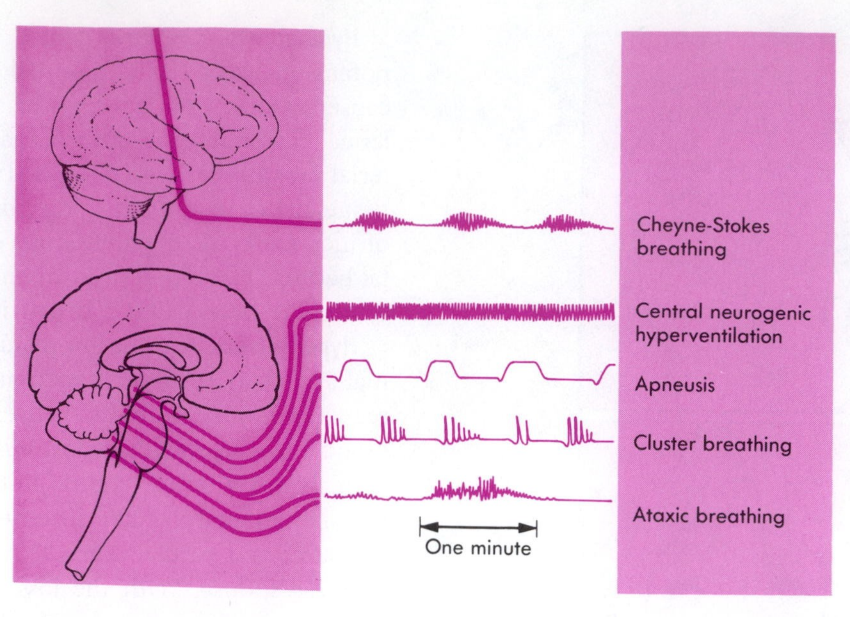

FIGURE 26-6. Abnormal respiratory patterns with corresponding level of central nervous system activity.

TABLE 26-2 Respiratory Patterns

Pattern of Respiration	Description of Pattern	Significance
Cheyne-Stokes	Rhythmic crescendo and decrescendo of rate and depth of respiration; includes brief periods of apnea	Usually seen with bilateral deep cerebral lesions or some cerebellar lesions
Central neurogenic hyperventilation	Very deep, very rapid respirations with no apneic periods	Usually seen with lesions of the midbrain and upper pons
Apneustic	Prolonged inspiratory and/or expiratory pause of 2-3 sec	Usually seen in lesions of the mid to lower pons
Cluster breathing	Clusters of irregular, gasping respirations separated by long periods of apnea	Usually seen in lesions of the lower pons or upper medulla
Ataxic respirations	Irregular, random pattern of deep and shallow respirations with irregular apneic periods	Usually seen in lesions of the medulla

Temperature. Various CNS conditions can produce an elevation in body temperature. Hyperthermia must be controlled to prevent increased production of metabolic by-products such as carbon dioxide and lactic acid. Nonneurologic causes must always be investigated to prevent delay in medical intervention. Hypothermia may occur with metabolic or toxic coma, spinal shock, and brainstem or hypothalamic lesions.

RAPID NEUROLOGIC EXAMINATION

An adequate neurologic examination focuses on covering all major areas of neurologic control. Any abnormalities identified can then be further evaluated and investigated. Findings must always be evaluated in light of those of previous examinations. A neurologic examination must be organized, thorough, and simple so that it can be performed accurately and easily at each assessment point.

BOX 26-5 Rapid Neurologic Assessment of the Conscious Patient

1. **Level of consciousness**—address the patient and ask a variety of orientation questions. Avoid the obvious, overused questions about name, date, and place, and focus on questions about recent and past events from the patient's experiences, such as spouse's name, home address, what was eaten at the previous meal. Be sure that, as examiner, you are aware of the correct answers to all questions asked.
2. **Facial movements**—during assessment of level of consciousness, observe the patient's facial movements for symmetry. Listen to speech patterns for evidence of slurred speech.
3. **Pupillary function and eye movements**—perform pupil check and assess extraocular eye movements.
4. **Motor assessment**—assess upper and lower extremity movement and strength.
5. **Sensory**—with a finger, stroke the patient bilaterally on the face, upper aspect of the arm, hand, leg, and foot. Ask the patient to identify what is touched and whether there is any difference in sensation between the two sides.
6. **Vital signs**—note any alterations in blood pressure, heart rate or rhythm, respiratory pattern, or temperature.
7. **Change in status**—ask the patient whether he or she feels any differences between this and the previous examination.

BOX 26-6 Rapid Neurologic Assessment of the Unconscious Patient

1. **Level of consciousness**—perform the Glasgow Coma Scale assessment.
2. **Pupillary assessment**—perform pupillary assessment with special attention to size, reactivity, and shape of pupil in comparison with the opposite eye.
3. **Motor examination**—assess each extremity individually by means of a predetermined coding score of motor movement.
4. **Respiratory pattern**—if the patient is not receiving mechanical ventilation, observe respiratory patterns for evidence of deteriorating level of function.
5. **Vital signs**—include comparison of preassessment vital signs with postassessment vital signs, paying special attention to arterial blood pressure and ICP if these parameters are being monitored.

The Conscious Patient

An example of a rapid neurologic examination that can be performed in the critical care unit on a conscious patient with known or potential neurologic deficit is outlined in Box 26-5. This examination, which usually takes less than 4 minutes, is meant to provide a starting point. If any neurologic deficit is identified that is new or different from that of the last assessment, attention must be focused in more detail on that abnormality.

The Unconscious Patient

In the assessment of the unconscious patient (Box 26-6), initial efforts are directed at achieving maximal arousal of the patient. Calling the patient's name, patting him or her on the chest, or shaking his or her shoulder accomplishes this task. Once the patient has been stimulated, the examiner can proceed with the neurologic examination. As in the assessment of the conscious patient, if any abnormalities or changes from previous assessment are noted, further investigation must occur. This assessment takes 3 to 4 minutes.

Neurologic Changes Associated With Intracranial Hypertension

Assessment of the patient for signs of increasing intracranial pressure is an important responsibility of the critical care nurse. Increasing ICP can be identified by changes in level of consciousness, pupillary reaction, motor response, vital signs, and respiratory patterns.

Level of consciousness. As ICP increases, the level of consciousness deteriorates. Increased restlessness and confusion, agitation, or decreased responsiveness can all indicate deterioration in neurologic status. For the most part, level of consciousness is the first sign of deterioration in a conscious patient. Subtle changes that are identified and acted on may prevent the serious consequences associated with neurologic decline.

Pupillary reaction. Any changes in pupillary size, shape, or reactivity are ominous signs. In the unconscious patient, pupils are the most sensitive indication that deterioration is in progress.

LEGAL REVIEW

Coma, Persistent Vegetative State, and Brain Death

To maintain full consciousness, both the reticular activating system (RAS)—a brainstem regulatory system—and the cerebral hemispheres need to be reciprocally sustaining. Consciousness has two features: arousal and awareness.

Arousal is simply wakefulness and reflects activation of the RAS. It manifests by eye opening, either spontaneously or in response to stimuli. It may occur in the presence of complete destruction of the hemispheres.

Awareness implies functioning cerebral hemispheres and manifests by cognition of self and the environment. The patient demonstrates goal-directed or purposeful motor behavior and language.

Coma is a pathologic state in which neither arousal nor awareness is present. The patient maintains a sleep-like unresponsiveness from which he or she cannot be aroused. Nonpurposive, reflex movements, such as flexor (decorticate) or extensor (decerebrate) posturing, may be present.

In some cases after head trauma or ischemic-anoxic injury as a result of cardiac arrest, both hemispheres are severely damaged but the RAS is preserved. After a period of hours to days of coma, wakefulness returns without evidence of purposive behavior or cognition. This functionally decorticate state is distinct from coma and is known as the *vegetative state,* which may be persistent. Ventilation may remain spontaneous, and circulation is maintained. In the case of *In Re Quinlan,* Plum described a person in a chronic persistent vegetative state as one who retains the capacity to maintain the vegetative parts of neurologic function but no longer has any cognitive function.

However, Karen Ann Quinlan was not brain dead as defined by the ad hoc committee of the Harvard Medical School. The committee's definition included absence of response to pain or other stimuli; absence of pupillary, corneal, pharyngeal, and other reflexes; and absence of blood pressure and spontaneous respiration, as well as isoelectric or flat electroencephalograms, with testing repeated at least 24 hours later with no change.

Patients who are brain dead have irreversible loss of brain function and compose a small percentage of those who are comatose. In *brain death,* coma of established cause exists, with no evidence of cerebral function (absence of appropriate response to noxious stimulation and absence of decerebrate and decorticate reflex responses) or brainstem reflexes (pupils fixed in response to light stimulation, corneal blink reflex absent, doll's eyes reflex and ice-water caloric responses absent, and apnea without spontaneous ventilation) for 24 or more hours, with absent cerebral circulation and/or electrical activity confirmed by sequential angiography and/or electroencephalography.

A larger percentage of comatose patients are those with severe brain damage in whom prognosis is uncertain. For some of these persons the provision of comprehensive critical care ultimately promotes survival in a vegetative state, which may become persistent and chronic even as care is reduced to maintenance levels.

Most states have adopted statutes that define death and brain death. Similarly, most major medical institutions have hospital ethics committees (HECs) or institutional ethics committees (IECs) that (1) educate about medical-ethical issues; (2) develop the criteria, policies, and procedures that are used to define, diagnose, and manage these various clinical conditions; and (3) resolve particular issues and cases. It is imperative for the critical care nurse to be intimately conversant with state law and the institution's established standards.

Ad Hoc Committee of the Harvard Medical School to Examine the Definition of Brain Death: *JAMA* 205:337, 1968; Bates D and others: *Ann Neurol* 2:211, 1977; Beresford HR: *Ann Neurol* 15(5):409, 1984; Caronna JJ: Approach to the patient with impairment of consciousness. In Kelley WN, editor: *Textbook of internal medicine,* Philadelphia, 1989, JB Lippincott; Cranford R: *Hastings Cent Rep* 18:27, 1988; Davis KM and others: *J Neurosci Nurs* 19(1):36, 1987; Fischer CM: *Acta Neurol Scand* 45(suppl 36):4, 1969; Fost N, Cranford R: *JAMA* 253:2687, 1985; *Idem.* APACHE II: *Crit Care Med* 13:818, 1985; *In Re Quinlan,* 70 NJ 10, 355 A2d 647, 654; *cert denied,* 429 US 922 (1976); Jennett B, Bond M: *Lancet* 1:480, 1975; Jennett B, Plum F: *Lancet* 7:734, 1972; Knaus WA and others: *Ann Surg* 202:685, 1985; Levy DE and others: *Ann Intern Med* 94:293, 1981; Longstreth WT Jr, Diehr P, Inui TS: *N Engl J Med* 308:1378, 1983; Medical consultants on the diagnosis of death to the President's Commission for the Study of Ethical Problems in Medicine and Biomedical and Behavioral Research: *JAMA* 246:2184, 1981; Murphy CA: *Specialty L Dig: Health Care* 158:7, Apr 1992; Narayan RK and others: *J Neurosurg* 54:751, 1981; Plum F, Posner JB: *The diagnosis of stupor and coma,* ed 3, Philadelphia, 1980, FA Davis; Teasdale G, Jennett B: *Lancet* 2:81, 1974; Ventura MG, Masser PG: Defining death: developments in recent law. In Rogers MC, Traystman RJ, editors: *Critical care clinics: symposium on neurologic intensive care,* vol 1, Philadelphia, 1985, WB Saunders; National Conference of Commissioners on Uniform State Laws: *Uniform brain death act,* 1978; National Conference of Commissioners on Uniform State Laws: 1978; Uniform determination of death act, 1980.

Motor response. Deterioration in motor strength or the appearance of lateralizing signs may indicate increasing ICP. Even subtle changes in motor response can be highly predictive of neurologic deterioration.

Vital signs. As described, vital signs play a variable role in the evaluation of deteriorating neurologic status. A change in respiratory rate, respiratory pattern, increasing systolic blood pressure, or development of dysrhythmia is a signal for the evaluator to further assess for potential deterioration in function.

Respiratory patterns. Change in respiratory patterns can be a sensitive indicator of decreasing levels of function. The assessment of this parameter usually is lost, because most patients with critical neurologic injury are intubated and ventilated to prevent the serious neurologic damage caused by hypoxia and hypercapnia.

REFERENCES

1. Plum F, Posner JB: *The diagnosis of stupor and coma,* ed 3, Philadelphia, 1980, FA Davis.
2. Hickey JV: *The clinical practice of neurological and neurosurgical nursing,* ed 3, Philadelphia, 1992, JB Lippincott.
3. Topel JL, Lewis SL: Examination of the comatose patient. In Weiner WJ, Goetz CG, editors: *Neurology for the non-neurologist,* ed 3, Philadelphia, 1994, JB Lippincott.
4. Teasdale G, Jennett W: Assessment of coma and impaired consciousness: a practical scale, *Lancet* 2:81, 1974.
5. Juarez VJ, Lyons M: Interrater reliability of the Glascow Coma Scale, *J Neurosci Nurs* 27:283, 1995.
6. Haerer AF: *DeJong's The neurologic examination,* ed 5, Philadelphia, 1992, JB Lippincott.
7. Singer C, Weiner WJ: The neurologic examination. In Weiner WJ, Goetz CG, editors: *Neurology for the non-neurologist,* ed 3, Philadelphia, 1994, JB Lippincott.
8. Marshall LF and others: The oval pupil: clinical significance and relationship to intracranial hypertension, *J Neurosurg* 58:566, 1983.
9. Goodwin JA: Eye signs in neurologic diagnosis. In Weiner WJ, Goetz CG, editors: *Neurology for the non-neurologist,* ed 3, Philadelphia, 1994, JB Lippincott.
10. Keller C, Williams A: Cardiac dysrhythmias associated with central nervous system dysfunction, *J Neurosci Nurs* 25:349, 1993.

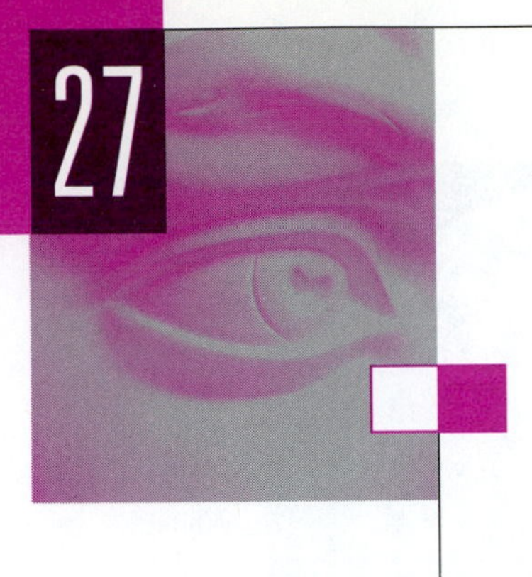

Neurologic Diagnostic Procedures

A WIDE ARRAY OF diagnostic tests is available to assist the nurse in identifying the cause of neurologic dysfunction. Improved technology has increased the sophistication of assessment, especially in the area of radiographic procedures and electrophysiology studies. Neurodiagnostic testing is performed as an adjunct to a thorough neurologic examination. When clinical findings are identified on examination, the nurse begins the process of diagnosing the problem. Results of diagnostic testing should provide the examiner with data to further refine and locate the cause of the abnormality identified during the neurologic assessment of the patient. Management is based on clinical manifestations, pathologic conditions, and the results of the diagnostic tests.

The role of the nurse in neurologic diagnostic testing is varied, but four functions are always present: (1) patient/family education, (2) physical preparation, (3) continued observation of neurologic status, and (4) observation for complications.

It is essential that the patient be aware of the reason for a procedure, the procedural process, any preprocedure preparation, and postprocedural monitoring. Emphasis is placed on the sensations that the patient will experience, including the level of discomfort involved. Once the physician has discussed the risks of the procedure with the patient, the nurse is available to listen to the patient's fears or concerns and to attempt to lessen anxiety.

The nurse assists in the physical preparation by providing medications, scrubs, or dye solutions. During the procedure the nurse also might assist in maintaining patient position or compliance with the procedure. (∞Conscious Sedation, p. 193.)

In addition to discussing concerns about risk factors, the nurse assesses the patient for potential development of any complications associated with the procedure. Proper observation and intervention, if necessary, are nursing responsibilities.

The goal of this chapter is to focus on the tests frequently performed on the critically ill patient, rather than review all available diagnostic studies. Discussion of each test includes a definition and purpose of the test, a review of the procedure, and the patient care needs both before and after the procedure.

RADIOLOGIC PROCEDURES

Skull and Spine Films

The purpose of radiographs of the skull or spine is to identify fractures, anomalies, or possibly tumors. The role of skull radiographs in trauma has diminished with the advent of computerized axial tomography (CT). If the patient is to undergo a CT scan during the initial assessment process, a skull radiograph may not be necessary.

The procedure for obtaining skull and spine radiographs is relatively painless. Proper patient positioning is essential, especially for spine radiographs. When searching for spine fractures it frequently is difficult to obtain a clear view of C1-2 and C6-7. A C1-2 view is obtained by taking the x-ray through the open mouth of the patient (Water's view). Intubation, however, usually prevents this approach. For C6-7 views, adequate visualization often requires the nurse or technician to pull down firmly on the patient's arms while the film is being taken. Spinal precautions (i.e., cervical collar and strict maintenance of head alignment) must be maintained until lateral films confirm integrity of the cervical structures.

Nursing care involves positioning of the patient to obtain adequate films. In any situation in which traumatic injury, especially head injury, is the cause of the patient's admission to the critical care unit, the cervical spine must be treated as unstable until proved otherwise.

Computerized Tomography

CT scanning provides the nurse with a mathematically reconstructed view of multiple sections of the head and body. This is accomplished by passage of intersecting x-ray beams through the examined area and measurement of the density of substances through which the x-ray beams pass. The denser the substance through which an x-ray beam passes, the whiter it appears on the finished film. The less dense a substance, the blacker it appears. Therefore with normal findings in a CT scan of the head, bone appears white, blood appears off-white, brain tissue appears shaded gray, cerebral spinal fluid (CSF) appears off-black, and air appears black (Figure 27-1).

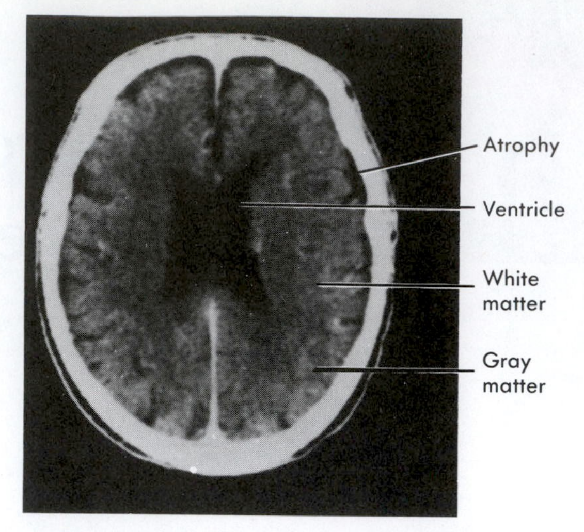

FIGURE 27-1. CT scan image. (From Ballinger PW: *Merrill's atlas of radiographic positions and radiologic procedures,* ed 7, St Louis, 1991, Mosby.)

The purpose of the CT scan is to obtain rapid, noninvasive visualization of structures. CT scanning is indicated in the diagnostic work up of severe headache, head trauma with associated loss of consciousness; seizures; hydrocephalus; suspicion of space-occupying lesions, hemorrhage, or vascular lesions; and edema. There are two types of CT scans—contrast and noncontrast scans. The noncontrast scan is noninvasive, requires no premedication of the patient, and is good for analysis and location of normal brain structures. Noncontrast CT scans of the head are appropriate in trauma patients in whom the goal is to view the intracranial area for evidence of intracranial hemorrhage, cerebral edema, or shift of structures. Noncontrast CT scan is also appropriate in the diagnosis of hydrocephalus.

The contrast CT scan involves the use of an intravenously injected contrast medium. The use of contrast enhances the vascular areas and allows for detection of vascular lesions or the further definition of lesions noted on a noncontrast scan.

Nursing management of the patient receiving a CT scan can be divided into two areas of focus: observation of patient tolerance of the procedure and observation of patient reaction to the dye in contrast scanning. Because of the associated activity and positioning, transporting and scanning of a critically ill patient with known or suspected intracranial hypertension can cause a deterioration in the patient's condition. The nurse must always remain with the patient during the CT scan and closely observe the neurologic status, vital signs, and, if monitored, intracranial pressure (ICP).

If the patient is to receive a contrast CT scan, questions about possible sensitivity to iodine-based dye must be asked beforehand if at all possible. During the infusion of the dye and for 10 to 30 minutes after, the patient is observed closely for anaphylactic reaction. Of all patients receiving contrast CT scans, fewer than 1% per year have severe anaphylactic reactions, shock, or cardiac arrest.

Magnetic Resonance Imaging

Magnetic resonance imaging (MRI) is a relatively new procedure. The patient is placed in a large magnetic field that stimulates the nuclei of the atoms of the body. Introduction of radio frequency waves causes resonance of the nuclei, which is emitted as the nuclei relax. A computer then constructs an image of the tissue[1] (Figure 27-2).

In MRI, small tumors, whose tissue densities differ from those of the surrounding cells, can be identified before they would be visible on any other radiographic test. MRI also can identify small hemorrhages deep in the brain that are invisible on CT scan. Finally, MRI can detect areas of cerebral infarct within a few hours of the incident, as well as small areas of plaque in patients with multiple sclerosis.

Nursing management involves patient teaching and preparation. The procedure is lengthy and requires the patient to lie motionless in a tight, enclosed space. Many patients experience anxiety, panic, and an acute sense of claustrophobia. Mild sedation or a blindfold, or both, may be necessary. The neurologically impaired

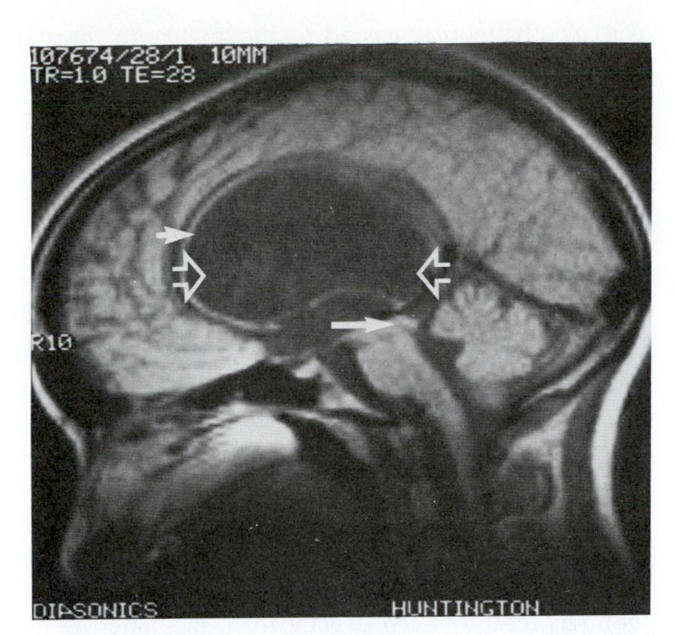

FIGURE 27-2. Magnetic resonance image of the brain. Sagittal section demonstrating marked enlargement of the lateral ventricle *(open arrows)* with stretching of the corpus callosum *(arrowhead)* as a result of aqueductal stenosis *(arrow)* (SE 1000/28). (From Stark DD, Bradley WG: *Magnetic resonance imaging,* ed 2, St Louis, 1992, Mosby.)

patient may not be able to comprehend the instructions, and sedation, possibly combined with neuromuscular blockade, will be required. Removal of all metal from the patient's body and clothing is essential because the basis of MRI is a magnetic field. In the past it was believed that any metal material, such as dental filling, prostheses, or internal clips or staples, would prevent scanning. Further study and changes in the type of metals used for many procedures have made the test safer. Any questions about specific devices or metals must be directed to the neuroradiologist before testing. The test is considered relatively safe and noninvasive, but all risks have not yet been identified in this procedure.

Cerebral Angiography

Cerebral angiography involves the injection of radiopaque contrast medium into the intracranial or extracranial vasculature.[1,2] With the use of serial radiologic filming, an angiogram traces the flow of blood from the arterial circulation through the capillary bed to the venous circulation. Cerebral angiography allows visualization of the lumen of vessels to provide information about patency, size (narrowing or dilation), any irregularities, or occlusion. The use of angiography is necessary in the diagnosis of cerebral aneurysm, arteriovenous malformation, carotid artery disease, and some vascular tumors. Information obtained from the angiogram guides the surgeon in choosing the operative approach or provides information on which to make medical management decisions other than surgery.

The procedure involves placement of a catheter in the femoral artery and threading it up the aorta and into the origin of the cerebral circulation. Other injection sites include a direct carotid or vertebral artery puncture or placement of a catheter in the brachial, axillary, or subclavian artery. Several views of vessels can be studied by means of angiogram. A four-vessel angiogram involves injections into the right and left internal carotid arteries and the right and left vertebral arteries. If the area of suspected disease already has been identified, a single-vessel study may be all that is required. This is particularly true when angiography is used as a follow-up in the evaluation of intracranial vascular surgery. Also, if carotid artery disease is a working diagnosis, the angiogram may include views of the arch of the aorta, plus the external and internal carotid arteries.

Once the catheter is appropriately placed, the contrast medium is injected. Then a rapid succession of radiographs is taken as the contrast medium progresses through the cerebral circulation. Separate contrast medium injections are administered for each vessel being studied.

Nursing management associated with this invasive procedure is comprehensive. Patient instruction and education are essential to patient preparation. The patient's complete understanding of the role this procedure plays in diagnosis, as well as the process itself, relieves anxiety about the unknown and also ensures cooperation in what commonly is an uncomfortable procedure. Discomforts include the need to lie still on a cold, hard table and the possibility of pain during preparation and insertion of the groin catheter. The patient often experiences a hot, burning sensation when the contrast medium is injected, especially if it is injected into the external carotid system. Preparation of patients for this burning sensation assures them that it is not an abnormal occurrence. Finally, the patient must be aware of the postprocedure assessment. Before and after the procedure, adequate hydration is necessary to assist the kidneys in clearing the heavy dye load. Inadequate hydration may lead to an acute tubular necrosis (ATN) and renal shutdown. If the patient is unable to tolerate oral fluids, an intravenous line is placed before the procedure is begun.

Postprocedure assessment involves vital sign measurement, neurologic evaluation, observation of the injection site, and assessment of neurovascular integrity distal to the injection site every 15 minutes for the first 1 to 2 hours. Any abnormalities noted must be immediately reported.

Complications associated with cerebral angiography include (1) cerebral embolus caused by the catheter dislodging a segment of atherosclerotic plaque in the vessel, (2) hemorrhage or hematoma formation at the insertion site, (3) vasospasm of a vessel caused by the irritation of catheter placement, (4) thrombosis of the extremity distal to the injection site, and (5) allergic or adverse reaction to the contrast medium.

Digital Subtraction Angiography

Digital subtraction angiography is a newer method of visualizing the arteriovenous circulation of the intracranial space.[1,2] Radiographic dye is injected into either the venous or the arterial circulation, but significantly less dye is necessary for this procedure than for arterial angiography. Films taken before and after dye injection are superimposed on each other and all matching images are subtracted. Thus only the dye-enhanced cerebral vessels are left for study and evaluation. Digital subtraction angiography eliminates the shadows and distortions of bone or other material that sometimes block the viewing of the cerebral vessels.

The major disadvantage of digital subtraction angiography involves the patient's ability to remain motionless during the entire procedure. Even swallowing interferes significantly with the imaging process. Complications and nursing management are similar to those described for cerebral angiography. The risk of embolism is decreased with the intravenous route.

Interventional Angiography

Angiography recently has advanced from a purely diagnostic tool to an interventional tool. Interventional angiography changes cerebral blood flow by two different methods, occlusion and dilation. Interventional angiography is used to alter the blood supply of a tumor or arteriovenous malformation by embolizing feeding vessels to reduce the size of the abnormal structure. This procedure involves the use of small beads of glue, resin, or silicone that are directed by the angiography catheter to the feeding vessels where they occlude blood flow. Two recently developed embolic agents have been designed for use in intracranial aneurysms.[3] Surgically inaccessible aneurysms can be occluded by either a specially designed, detachable, inflatable balloon or a platinum coil. The balloon is passed to the aneurysm through uniquely designed microcatheters that can enter vessels well less than 1 mm in diameter. When the catheter enters the aneurysm, the balloon is inflated with material that will solidify and is detached. The platinum coil is placed in a similar fashion. The same technique can be used to preoperatively reduce blood flow in arteriovenous malformations.[3]

Dilation of cerebral vessels is accomplished in much the same manner as for cardiac vessels. Angioplasty and stent techniques, which are well-established for the cardiac vasculature, are still under investigation for cerebral circulation. These techniques are limited to the carotid, internal carotid, and vertebral vessels; the greatest risk with the use of either angioplasty or stenting is the dislodging of debris that then could lodge distally in critical areas of the brain. A new microballoon has recently been developed to facilitate the use of cerebral angioplasty in the treatment of cerebral vasospasm after subarachnoid hemorrhage. This technique is still being investigated.[3]

Nursing management after the patient has undergone interventional angiography is similar to that for diagnostic cerebral angiography. Because the risk of complications, especially stroke, is greater with interventional angiography, the nurse must be especially meticulous and thorough in the postprocedure assessments.

Myelography

Myelography is radiographic examination of the spinal cord and vertebral column after injection of a contrast material into the subarachnoid space by lumbar or cisternal puncture.[1] Myelography allows visualization of the spinal canal, the subarachnoid space around the spinal cord, and the spinal nerve roots. Indications for myelography include identification of spinal canal blockage caused by herniated intervertebral disks, spinal cord tumors, bony fragments or growths, and congenital anomalies (Figure 27-3).

The procedure involves a lumbar or cisternal puncture followed by an injection of contrast medium. It is performed fluoroscopically; the infusion of the dye is observed, and radiographic films are taken. Oil-based preparations such as Pantopaque have been replaced by water-based preparations. Use of the water-based preparations, which are lighter than CSF, allows for better visualization of nerve roots and projections off the spinal cord. These agents are absorbed by the arachnoid system and therefore do not require removal after the procedure. Disadvantages of a water-based preparation include rapid dissolution of the dye into

A

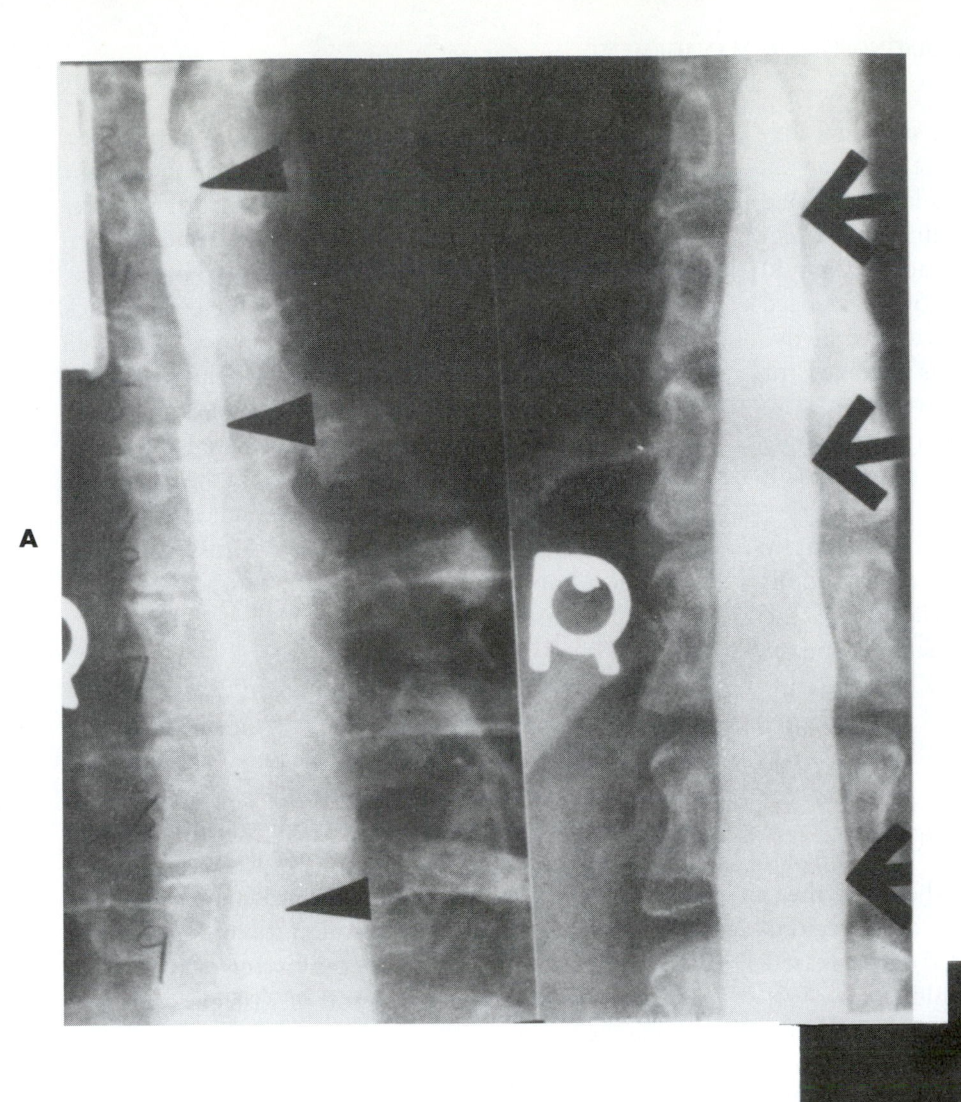

B

FIGURE 27-3. **A,** Normal myelogram finding, with dorsal thoracic view on left and lumbar view on right. Pointers and arrows indicate normal flow of radiographic dye (Pantopaque). **B,** Abnormal myelogram finding, with obstruction of dye column caused by metastatic tumor compressing the canal. (From Pagana KD, Pagana TJ: *Diagnostic testing and nursing implications: a case study approach,* ed 3, St Louis, 1990, Mosby.)

the subarachnoid space. Because of the potential toxicity of water-based preparations to the cerebral tissue, care must be taken to ensure that a large dye load does not reach the surface of the brain. This is accomplished by keeping the patient's head elevated 30 to 45 degrees after the procedure. Toxicity is evidenced by grand mal seizures. To assist the clearance of dye through the urine, adequate hydration is necessary for patients who undergo a metrizamide myelogram. Use of phenothiazines is to be avoided after a metrizamide myelogram because of the increase in symptoms of toxicity.

Possible risks involved with the use of myelography include injection of the dye outside the subarachnoid space, arachnoiditis as a result of irritation of the arachnoid membranes from a foreign material, and allergic reaction. Other adverse reactions include confusion, hallucinations, headache, grand mal seizure, chest pain, and dysrhythmias.[1]

CEREBRAL BLOOD FLOW STUDIES

The goal of cerebral blood flow studies is to measure the amount of blood flow overall or in regions of the brain to detect areas of increased or decreased cerebral circulation. Normal cerebral blood flow values average 50 to 55 ml of flow per 100 g of cerebral tissue per minute. Studies to determine the actual amount of cerebral blood flow in the injured brain would be a valuable addition to the planning of interventions. Some techniques are available, but as yet none of the procedures has achieved wide acceptance in clinical practice.

Uses of cerebral blood flow (CBF) studies include evaluation of cerebral vasospasm after subarachnoid hemorrhage; evaluation of cerebral blood flow during operative procedures that require extreme hypotension, such as aneurysm clipping; and evaluation of the changes in cerebral blood flow after cerebral vascular surgery, such as carotid endarterectomy, cerebral revascularization (superficial temporal artery-middle cerebral artery bypass), or arteriovenous malformation excision. Blood flow studies are also used to evaluate changes in cerebral flow associated with transient ischemic attacks (TIAs), strokes, increased intracranial pressure, and brain death.[4]

Xenon

The gold standard for clinical bedside evaluation of cerebral blood flow is the xenon washout technique.[5,6] Xenon-133 is administered by inhalation or injection into a peripheral vein. Scintillation detectors, or probes, placed on the outside of the skull monitor the uptake and clearance, or washout, of the xenon from the cerebral circulation. Information from the probes is then passed to a computer that calculates global or regional cerebral blood. A CT scanner also may be used to track the xenon. One difficulty with this method is that all body tissues take up xenon and then clear it, including the skin and muscles of the scalp under the detectors. Although mathematic calculations are factored in, cerebral blood flow results are an estimated value at best. Another limitation of xenon washout is that small regional variations in blood flow are missed, a phenomenon known as "look through."[6]

Doppler Ultrasound

Ultrasound technology, although not an absolute measure of cerebral blood flow, provides information about the flow velocity of blood through cerebral vessels using a noninvasive technique. A Doppler probe is placed externally over the vessel where ultrasonic waves are generated and blood flow velocities are calculated. As the diameter of the vessel changes, the velocity of the flow of blood through the vessel changes. The higher the flow velocity, the narrower the vessel. This narrowing can be the result of vasospasm or vessel plaque.

Extracranial Doppler Studies

Extracranial Doppler studies are used as a routine screening procedure for intraluminal narrowing of the common and internal carotid arteries as a result of arteriosclerotic plaques or atheromata.[1] Extracranial Doppler studies are noninvasive, relatively inexpensive, and painless. When changes in flow velocities are noted that may indicate significant occlusion of the vessel, a cerebral angiogram often is indicated to verify the degree of severity of the narrowed vessel.

Transcranial Doppler Studies

Transcranial Doppler (TCD) studies monitor cerebral blood flow velocity through cranial "windows" or thinned areas of the skull. Three areas commonly used are the temporal bone (transtemporal), the eye (transorbital), and the foramen magnum (transoccipital). Depending on the angle of the Doppler probe, flow velocities can be measured in the anterior, middle, or posterior cerebral arteries and the vertebral and basilar arteries. TCD studies are frequently used in critical care for postintracranial aneurysm rupture, in which concern about vasospasm development is a factor. The

RESEARCH ABSTRACT

Letting go: family willingness to forgo life support.

Swigart V and others: *Heart Lung* 25(6):483, 1996.

PURPOSE

The purpose of this study was to describe the process of family decision making about life support for critically ill family members.

DESIGN

Descriptive, explorative, using grounded theory methods.

SAMPLE

Thirty family members of 16 critically ill medical intensive care unit (MICU) patients participated in the study. Sixteen of the family members were women; the average age was 50 years; and 28 were high school and college graduates. Six families dealt primarily with decisions regarding cardiopulmonary resuscitation; physicians recommended removal of life support in 10 cases. The average age of the patients was 60 years; average length of stay in the MICU was 9.6 days. Nine of the patients had multiple organ dysfunction syndrome; 5 had primary neurologic conditions; and 2 had primary pulmonary failure.

PROCEDURE

Family members were interviewed individually by two trained interviewers, who used open-ended questions. Questions focused on family members' perceptions of the reason for admission, the diagnosis, treatment and prognosis; family relationships before the admission; family experiences and interactions during the hospital experience; previous knowledge of patient's preferences regarding end-of-life treatment; and religious beliefs of the patient and family. Data collection took place over 7 months with concurrent data analysis.

RESULTS

Three interrelated processes for letting go were identified. Family members sought out, obtained, and tried to understand information about the critical condition. They also reviewed the life of the patient, searching for meaning in the patient's life and current illness. And finally, they struggled to maintain family roles and relationships. During the process, there was a reframing of issues related to the critical illness in three areas: (1) they believed that all they could do had been done and that they could then concentrate on a peaceful death; (2) upon review of the patient's life and wishes, they determined that the patient would not want anything else done; and (3) they were able to bring about a "sense of doing the right thing" with family members. Family members who were unable to move through these stages experienced conflict and prolongation of the end-of-life period and decision-making time.

DISCUSSION/IMPLICATIONS

It is important to be cognizant of issues facing family members as they react to the critical illness of their loved ones and the possibility or reality of needing to make end-of-life decisions. This study provided information on the cognitive, emotional, and moral experiences of family members. Although families and individual family members react differently, health care professionals can support families during these stressful periods and facilitate the process of end-of-life decision making. The small number of subjects, sampling procedure, and setting do not allow for generalization to other settings. Additional research is needed to more deeply explore decision-making issues and interventions that will support and facilitate families.

noninvasive technique and portability of the equipment allow for frequent bedside monitoring of flow velocity and therefore vascular diameter. Use of serial transcranial Doppler studies for the detection of cerebral vasospasm greatly reduces the need for cerebral angiograms to verify and follow postsubarachnoid hemorrhage vasospasm. In response to the increasing use of TCD, many advanced critical care nurses and clinical nurse specialists are finding it useful to learn to perform the procedure as a component of their nursing responsibilities.[4]

Limitations of the TCD study must be understood. Accuracy of the TCD study is operator-dependent. Correct location and angle of the probe are essential. A small percentage of patients have temporal bones too thick for ultrasound penetration. Finally, a normal TCD study does not completely rule out the presence of vasospasm, because vasospasm may not be evident in the particular vessel examined.[7] TCD results are always evaluated in conjunction with clinical assessment findings.

During the TCD study, the patient will experience only mild pressure at the transducer site. No pain is involved. The patient must remain still during the study, which lasts 15 to 90 minutes. Activity restrictions must be considered if the transoccipital approach is desired, because neck flexion is required. Sterile gel is available if an incisional area is to be used as the acoustic window.[4]

Emission Tomography

Positron emission tomography (PET) and single photon emission computed tomography (SPECT) use injection and tracking of radioactive radionuclides to calculate global and regional cerebral blood flow.[5] PET uses paired radiation sensitive detectors, and SPECT uses unpaired detectors. The ability of the SPECT and PET scanners to measure cerebral metabolic use of oxygen and glucose permits them to distinguish between brain tumor recurrence and brain or tumor necrosis. Emission tomography offers a qualitative, rather than an absolute, measure of cerebral blood flow. It is useful to compare the sides of the brain. Clinical use of emission tomography is extremely limited because of the significant cost, lack of portability, and unavailability of the technology at many hospitals.[5] Nursing management of the patient undergoing PET or SPECT involves transportation of the patient to the scanning area and observation during the procedure.

Continuous Bedside Cerebral Blood Flow Monitoring

CBF monitoring by thermal diffusion is an innovative technology currently under evaluation.[5] An invasive Silastic catheter is placed directly on a gyrus of the cerebral cortex during a craniotomy procedure. The pathophysiologic reason for monitoring dictates the exact placement of the tip of the catheter. Two gold discs are embedded in the catheter. One disc monitors the cortical temperature, and the other serves as a heat source. The proximal end of the catheter is connected to a monitor or computer. Cerebral blood flow is calculated by comparing the difference in temperature between the two discs and measuring the rate of heat dissipation. Continuous CBF monitoring by thermal diffusion measures regional cortical blood flow in the area where the catheter is placed. The major limitations and complications of this procedure include need for intracranial placement, risk of intracranial infection, and erroneous readings related to catheter displacement or loss of catheter contact with the cortex. Nursing management of continuous CBF monitoring is similar to that of other invasive modalities such as intracranial pressure monitoring.[5] A similar technique using laser energy is being developed and refined.[6]

ELECTROPHYSIOLOGY STUDIES

Two basic electrophysiologic studies are used in the critical care setting. Both studies can be performed intermittently to evaluate symptoms or review progress or can be used continuously to assist in ongoing assessment of neurologic function.

Electroencephalography

Electroencephalography (EEG) is the recording of electrical impulses, commonly called *brain waves,* generated by the brain. This test has been in existence for many years and is well-known to the general public. It is important for the nurse caring for a patient with a neurologic dysfunction to be aware of the appropriate indications for use of this testing procedure. The purpose of the EEG is to detect and localize abnormal electrical activity. This abnormal activity can be defined as slowing, which occurs in areas of injury or infarct, or as the spikes and waves seen in irritated tissue. Indications for the use of EEG include seizure focus identification, infarct, metabolic disorders, confirmation of brain death (electrocerebral silence), and some head injuries.

Noninvasive electrodes are placed on the head, and the electrical impulses detected are transferred to a central recording device that records the information in waveform. Six types of waves or rhythms may be present (Table 27-1).[8]

Continuous generalized slowing in the delta or theta range is associated with anoxic damage. Intermittent slowing is associated with metabolic encephalopathy. The combination of alpha waves that do not change with stimulation and a coma state is associated with a poor prognosis.[9]

In preparing the patient for an EEG, the nurse must stress the noninvasive aspects of this procedure. The awake patient may be asked to perform certain simple tasks during the procedure, such as blinking, closing the eye, or swallowing. Occasionally, testing needs to be performed during sleep or after a period of sleep deprivation.

Continuous monitoring of the EEG is becoming more common in the critical care environment. The neuroscience critical care nurse monitors the computerized continuous EEG signals to detect neurologic changes and to assess responses to treatment.[8] The goal of computerized continuous EEG monitoring is to

TABLE 27-1 Types of Electrical Brain Waves

Wave	Duration	Description
Delta	1-4 cycles/second	Normal, seen in stages 3 and 4 of sleep
Alpha	8-13 cycles/second	Normal, relaxed state with eyes closed; seen often in occipital leads
Theta	4-7 cycles/second	Less common in adults than in children, characteristic of coma in brain injury
Beta	12-40 cycles/second	Fast waves, indicating mental or physical activity
Sleep spindles	12-14 cycles/second	Seen in stage 2 sleep, not REM
Spike and slow waves	Variable	Seen in irritable brain tissue (such as seizure)

identify changes in electrical activity that could indicate cerebral ischemia or provide evidence of subclinical seizures. Computerized EEG reflects insufficient cerebral blood flow related to hemorrhage, trauma, increased ICP, or seizure activity within seconds, providing the opportunity for intervention before irreversible cell death occurs.[8] Subclinical seizures are evidenced by sharp spike and wave electrical activity that is not evident by visual observation of the patient. Subclinical seizures increase cerebral metabolic rate in response to the greatly increased cellular activity. This increased metabolic rate requires increasing supply of oxygen and nutrients to an already compromised vascular supply system. Detection and treatment of subclinical seizures may prevent secondary brain injury. Computerized EEG can also be used in brain death determination.

Evoked Potentials

Evoked potentials involve the recording of electrical impulses generated by a sensory stimulus as it travels through the brainstem and into the cerebral cortex.[9] Measuring evoked potentials is a sophisticated way of observing the status of sensory pathways as they enter the central nervous system, travel through the brainstem, and reach the cerebral cortex. Evoked potentials also can be used during therapeutically induced comas, such as barbiturate coma, inasmuch as these sensory pathways are unaffected by the depressive activity of such drugs. Another use of evoked potentials is in the determination of the existence of brainstem or spinal cord injury in the traumatically injured patient.

The three types of evoked potential tests are (1) visual evoked responses (VERs), (2) brainstem auditory evoked responses (BAERs), and (3) somatosensory evoked responses (SSERs). VER involves monitoring of the visual pathways through the brainstem and cortex in response to the patient's viewing a shifting geometric pattern on a screen or by placing a mask, which sends a flashing light stimulus, over the eye. BAER involves monitoring the auditory pathway through the brainstem and cortex in response to a rhythmic clicking sound sent through earphones placed over the patient's ears. BAERs are useful in assessing brainstem integrity in the critical care unit when cranial nerve testing cannot be performed or is inconclusive.[9] SSER involves monitoring of sensory pathways from the extremities ascending the spinal cord through the brainstem and into the cortex. This is performed by administering a small electrical shock to a nerve root in the periphery, such as the ulnar or radial nerve. SSER can be used to evaluate cortical functioning after cardiac arrest or head trauma.[9]

Preparation of awake patients involves appropriate teaching so that they cooperate with the instructions for the procedure. No pain or discomfort is involved in the administration of these tests, except for the irritation of the small electrical shock used for SSER.

LUMBAR PUNCTURE

The main purpose of lumbar puncture (LP) is to enter the subarachnoid space to obtain diagnostic information or to provide therapeutic intervention. Diagnostic information comes from samples of CSF evaluated for the presence of subarachnoid blood or infection, or for laboratory analysis. Pressure readings also are obtained for diagnostic use. Therapeutic modalities of an LP include removal of bloody or purulent CSF that the arachnoid villi are unable to clear,

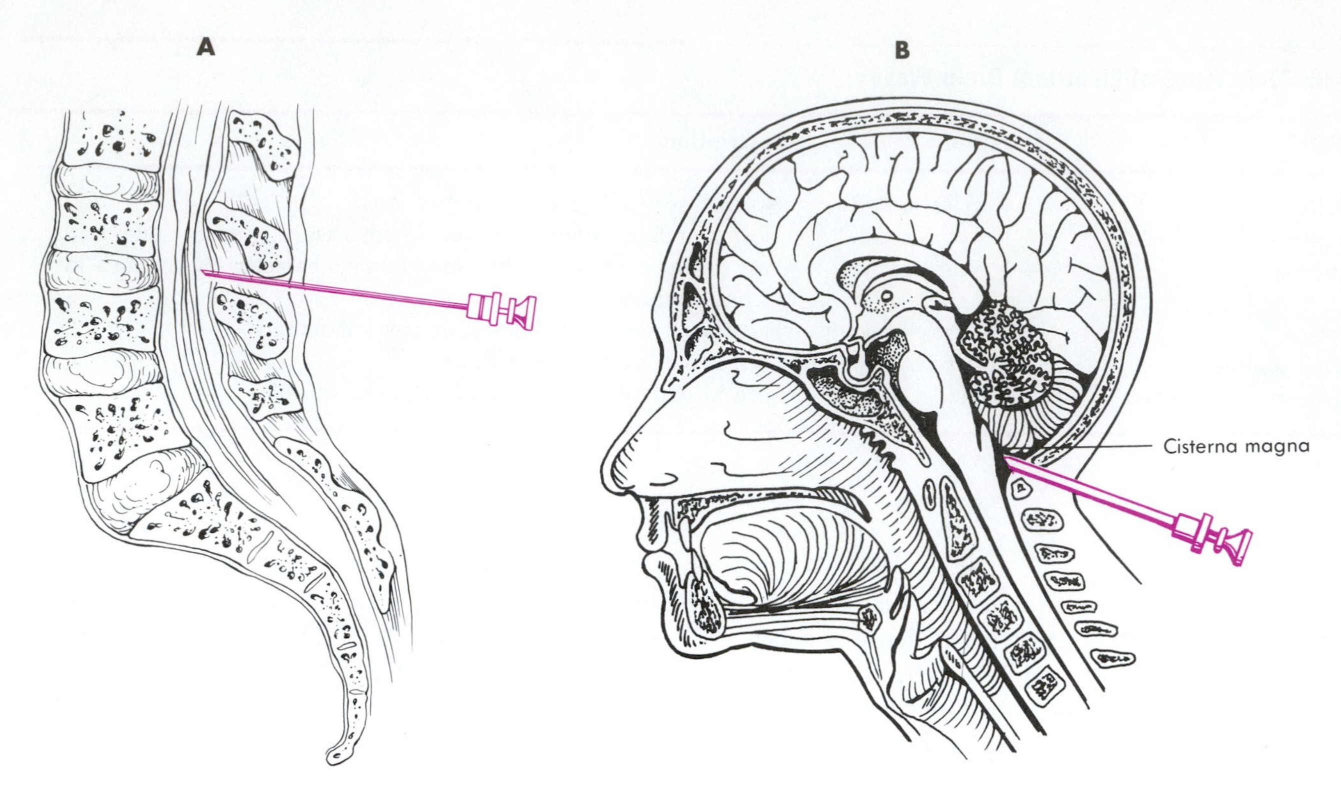

FIGURE 27-4. A, Lumbar puncture. **B,** Cisternal puncture. (From Long BC, Phipps WJ, Cassmeyer VL: *Medical-surgical nursing: a nursing process approach,* ed 3, St Louis, 1993, Mosby.)

injection of medications into the subarachnoid space to bypass the blood-brain barrier (antibiotics or analgesics), or the introduction of spinal anesthesia.

An LP involves the introduction of an 18- to 22-gauge hollow needle into the subarachnoid space at L4-5 below the end of the spinal cord, which usually is at L1-2. The patient can be placed either in the lateral recumbent position with the knees and head tightly tucked or in the sitting position leaning over a bedside table or some other support (Figure 27-4).

Two life-threatening risks associated with LP include possible brainstem herniation if intracranial pressure is elevated or respiratory arrest associated with neurologic deterioration. During the procedure the nurse must monitor the patient's neurologic and respiratory status. Also, if the patient is not fully alert and cooperative, the nurse may need to assist the patient in maintaining the position necessary for performance of the LP.[1,2] The longstanding routine of keeping the patient flat in bed for several hours after diagnostic LP has been recently refuted by scientific study.[10] The usual incidence of post LP headache, approximately 32%, is unaffected by activity. It is important to note that mentioning the possibility of post LP headache during preprocedure patient teaching has been related to an increased incidence in this complication. (∞Assessment of Intracranial Pressure: Signs and Symptoms, p. 823.)

Cisternal puncture, which is the introduction of a needle into the cisterna magna at the C1-2 level, is another method for obtaining access to the subarachnoid space. Risks of cisternal puncture are slightly higher than those associated with an LP, but cisternal puncture is necessary if there is inability to enter the lumbar space because of scar tissue or some other physical barrier or if there is a total blockage of the CSF pathway somewhere along the spinal column.

REFERENCES

1. Hickey JV: *The clinical practice of neurologic and neurosurgical nursing,* ed 3, Philadelphia, 1992, JB Lippincott.
2. Mason PJB: Neurodiagnostic testing in critically injured adults, *Crit Care Nurse* 12(4):64, 1992.
3. Barnwell SL: Interventional neuroradiology, *West J Med* 158:162, 1993.
4. Fearon M, Rusy KL: Transcranial Doppler: advanced technology for assessing cerebral hemodynamics, *DCCN* 13:241, 1994.

5. Lucke KT, Kerr ME, Chovanes GI: Continuous bedside cerebral blood flow monitoring, *J Neurosci Nurs* 27:164, 1995.
6. Martin NA, Doberstein C: Cerebral blood flow measurement in neurosurgical intensive care, *Neurosurg Clin N Am* 5:607, 1994.
7. Maurer PK, Malkoff MD: Cerebral protective measures and brain injury, *Controver Crit Care* 2(2):1, 1995.
8. Buzea CE: Understanding computerized EEG monitoring in the intensive care unit, *J Neurosci Nurs* 27:292, 1995.
9. Nuwer MR: Electroencephalograms and evoked potentials: monitoring cerebral function in the neurosurgical intensive care unit, *Neurosurg Inten Care* 5:647, 1994.
10. Spriggs DA and others: Is bedrest useful after diagnostic lumbar puncture? *Postgrad Med J* 68:581, 1992.

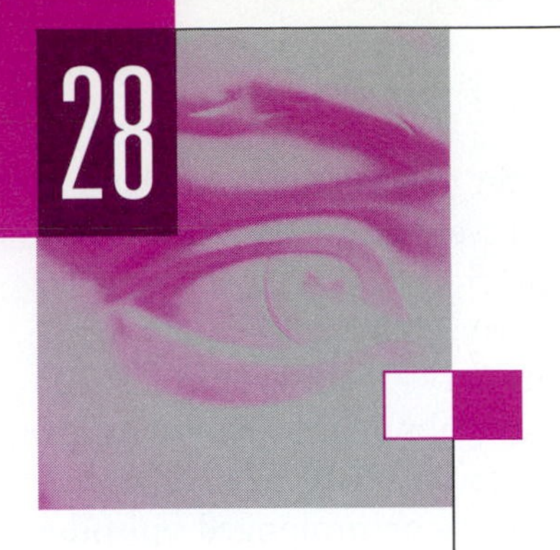

28

Neurologic Disorders

An understanding of the pathology of a disease or condition, the areas of assessment on which to focus, and the usual medical management allows the critical care nurse to more accurately anticipate and plan nursing interventions. Although a wide array of neurologic disorders exists, only a few routinely require care in the critical care environment. This chapter presents a review of coma, persistent vegetative state, cerebral vascular accidents, Guillain-Barré syndrome, and craniotomy.

COMA

Description

Coma is a state of unconsciousness in which both wakefulness and awareness are lacking.[1] The patient cannot be aroused and demonstrates no voluntary movement.[2] Like consciousness, the state of coma comprises a continuum of many levels. The patient in a light coma demonstrates purposeful withdrawal in response to noxious stimuli. The patient in deep coma lacks any response, even to noxious stimuli. Between these two extremes, levels of coma are difficult to clearly differentiate.

The state of coma is actually a symptom, rather than a disease. It occurs as a result of some underlying process. And yet like any other life-threatening condition, coma requires identification and therapeutic management even when the cause cannot be determined or treated.

The incidence of coma is difficult to ascertain. Since a wide variety of both neurologic and nonneurologic conditions can produce coma, this state of unconsciousness is unfortunately very common in critical care. Of the survivors of severe head injury, 59% experience a period of coma.[3] Ten percent of patients with head injury remain in coma.[4]

Though any number of diagnosis-related groups (DRGs) may apply to the patient in a coma, depending on the underlying cause and subsequent treatment, usually DRG 27 (Traumatic stupor and coma, coma greater than 1 hour) or DRG 23 (Nontraumatic stupor and coma) is used, with anticipated lengths of stay of 6.3 days and 5.1 days, respectively.[5]

Etiology

The causes of coma can be divided into three general categories: structural neurologic lesions, metabolic and toxic conditions, and psychiatric disorders. Psychiatric disorders are not discussed in this chapter. Box 28-1 provides a brief list of the possible causes of coma.

Structural lesions. Structural lesions that can result in coma include vascular lesions, trauma, brain tumors, and brain abscesses.

Vascular lesions. Ischemic and hemorrhagic strokes are common structural lesions that can produce coma. (∞Cerebrovascular Accident, p. 798.)

Trauma. Trauma is a common cause of coma. The loss of consciousness may occur immediately, or it may develop several days to weeks after injury, as often seen with subdural hematoma. Epidural hematoma often presents with an immediate loss of consciousness, followed by a period of lucidity, and then gradual onset of coma. (∞Head Injuries, p. 1057.)

Brain tumors and brain abscesses. Brain tumors and abscesses are mass lesions that produce changes in level of consciousness by compressing neurologic structures. The coma associated with a focal brain tumor or brain abscess is often accompanied by motor paralysis. The typical history reveals a gradual onset of headache, vomiting, focal signs, convulsions, apathy, stupor, failing vision, and personality changes. Sudden onset of coma can occur with sudden hemorrhage into

BOX 28-1 Causes of Coma

STRUCTURAL LESIONS

Subarachnoid hemorrhage
Intracerebral hemorrhage
Subdural hematoma
Epidural hematoma
Thrombotic or embolic brain infarction
Brain tumor
Brain abscess
Trauma

METABOLIC OR TOXIC CONDITIONS

Meningitis
Encephalitis
Alcohol
Hepatic failure
Renal failure (uremia)
Cardiac failure
Ischemia, hypoxemia, anoxia
Hypercapnia
Hypoglycemia or hyperglycemia
Electrolyte imbalance (sodium, calcium, magnesium, phosphorus)
Water imbalance
Acidosis or alkalosis
Hypothyroidism (myxedema)
Addisonian crisis
Thiamine deficiency (Wernicke's encephalopathy)
Sepsis
Poisoning (lead, mushroom, cyanide, methanol, carbon monoxide)
Drug overdose
Lactic acidosis
Hypertensive encephalopathy
Hypothermia or hyperthermia
Postictal state

a tumor or sudden obstruction of cerebrospinal fluid (CSF) flow. Coma may also result from a secondary increase in intracranial pressure (ICP).[2]

Metabolic and toxic conditions. Metabolic and diffuse brain dysfunction accounts for more than half of all cases of coma.[6] Metabolic and toxic conditions that can result in coma include cardiopulmonary decompensation, poisoning, alcohol, hypertensive encephalopathy, meningitis, encephalitis, postconvulsive states, and other metabolic conditions.

Cardiopulmonary decompensation. Cardiopulmonary decompensation and arrest are the primary causes of anoxic and ischemic encephalopathies and coma in the critical care environment. Progress in cardiopulmonary resuscitation is far more advanced than in cerebral resuscitation. Essentially any cardiopulmonary condition can precipitate a state of coma by threatening the state of oxygenation of cerebral tissue. Dysrhythmias, coronary insufficiency, aortic stenosis or insufficiency, pulmonary hypertension, and chronic pulmonary insufficiency related to emphysema may cause transient or prolonged episodes of loss of consciousness.

Poisoning and alcohol. Coma from poisoning may occur as a result of self-administration, accidental ingestion, industrial exposure, or homicidal administration of an endogenous substance. The symptoms that accompany the altered level of consciousness depend on the substance ingested. Alcohol is a direct central nervous system (CNS) depressant. The patient in coma from alcohol ingestion can usually be aroused slightly, has dilated but reactive pupils, and has diminished or absent reflexes. Convulsions may also occur. It must be remembered that alcohol ingestion may not be the cause of coma in the inebriated patient. Trauma, cerebral hemorrhage, and subdural hematoma are all associated with intoxication. Thiamine deficiency is a common complication in the undernourished alcoholic patient and may also produce coma. Thiamine is a harmless drug that is administered to anyone in coma of uncertain cause.[2]

Hypertensive encephalopathy or acute hypertensive crisis. The coma associated with hypertensive encephalopathy or acute hypertensive crisis has a sudden onset, usually following a history of kidney disease, severe hypertension (HTN), or both. Preceding symptoms include severe headache, irritability, fatigue, drowsiness, vomiting, and failing vision. The presence of severe hypertensive retinopathy with papilledema supports the diagnosis. The possibility of disruption of the cerebral vasculature (intracerebral hemorrhage) or a structural lesion must also be investigated in any patient in coma with a history of hypertension. (∞Intracerebral Hemorrhage, p. 807.)

Meningitis. Meningitis is a relatively common cause of coma.[2] Meningococcal meningitis produces an abrupt onset of symptoms including a severe headache followed by a loss of consciousness. A history of an infectious process affecting the middle ear or paranasal sinuses should raise suspicion of streptococcal, pneumococcal, or staphylococcal meningitis. Two other signs and symptoms are evidence of infection and the presence of a skin rash. The rash, especially common in meningococcal meningitis, appears as petechial hemorrhages in the skin and mucous membranes. The rash often blends into purpuric patches that occasionally become necrotic. Signs of meningeal irritation such as nuchal rigidity, Kernig's sign, and Brudzinski's sign are the most important diagnostic indicators of meningitis. Lumbar puncture (LP) is used to confirm meningitis as the cause of coma. Common LP findings are increased pressure, pleocytosis, increased protein, marked decrease in glucose, and presence of infectious organisms.[2]

Encephalitis. Encephalitis may produce either coma or hypersomnia. The patient in a coma related to encephalitis is frequently arousable for short periods. In addition to coma, viral encephalitis may produce dissociated eye movements, cranial nerve abnormalities, and hyperkinetic phenomena. Other types of encephalitis that cause coma are toxic and hemorrhagic encephalitis after exposure to toxins; demyelinating encephalitis associated with vaccinia, smallpox, or measles; and Reye's syndrome.

Postconvulsion. The postictal stage after a grand mal seizure is characterized by a brief period of stupor or coma. Evidence that the patient may have experienced a recent convulsion includes incontinence, frothing at the mouth, bloody sputum, and lacerations or other injuries to the body. Sleep, confusion, or irrational behavior may follow arousal from the postconvulsive coma.[2]

Other metabolic disturbances. Numerous metabolic disturbances can cause coma, including hyperglycemia and hypoglycemia. Uremic coma occurs as a result of complex metabolic disturbances associated with renal dysfunction. Hepatic coma results from acute or chronic liver failure and portal or hepatic circulatory disorders. Pneumonia and other infections may produce coma as a result of the infectious process itself or as a result of endogenous toxic substances, such as mediators or cellular by-products, released as part of the inflammatory-immune response. Other metabolic disturbances that may produce coma are eclampsia; various endocrine disorders; hyperthermia; and electrolyte, acid-base, or water imbalance.

Pathophysiology

Consciousness involves both arousal, or wakefulness, and awareness. Neither of these functions is present in the patient in coma. Ascending fibers of the reticular activating system in the pons, hypothalamus, and thalamus maintain arousal as an autonomic function. Neurons in the cerebral cortex are responsible for awareness. Diffuse dysfunction of both cerebral hemispheres and/or diffuse or focal dysfunction of the reticular activating system is necessary to produce coma.[7] Small focal lesions in the posterior hypothalamic and midbrain regions can also produce coma, whereas unilateral cerebral lesions usually do not, unless they increase ICP. Alterations in cerebral function that can also produce coma include ischemia, hypoxia, infection, metabolic imbalance, toxic exposure, and structural disruption.

The pathophysiologic continuum of coma is comparable with the stages of anesthesia. Slight or moderate cortical depression produces clouding of consciousness, impairment of contact with the environment, loss of discrimination, and euphoria. In complete cortical suppression, motor and reflex functions are controlled solely by subcortical structures. Midbrain depression produces a loss of reflex response and a loss of several visceral functions. Finally, brainstem depression results in gradual abolition of respiratory and circulatory control.[2]

Assessment and Diagnosis

Diagnosis of the coma state is a clinical one, readily established by assessment of the level of consciousness. Determining the full nature and cause of coma, however, requires a thorough history and physical examination. A past medical history is essential, because events immediately preceding the change in level of consciousness can often provide valuable clues as to the origin of the coma. When limited information is available and the coma is profound, the response of the patient to emergency treatment may provide clues to the underlying diagnosis, such as the patient who becomes responsive with the administration of naloxone can be presumed to have ingested some type of opiate.

Detailed serial neurologic examinations are essential for all patients in coma. Assessment of motor function, pupil responses, and respiratory pattern provides valuable diagnostic information.[6,8] Pupillary light responses are often the key to differentiating between structural and metabolic causes of coma, because they are usually intact in metabolic-induced coma, with the exceptions of anoxic encephalopathy, barbiturate intoxication, and hypothermia. Focal or asymmetrical motor deficits usually indicate structural lesions. (∞Neurologic Physical Examination, p. 763.)

Structural causes of coma are usually readily apparent with computerized tomography (CT) scanning or magnetic resonance imaging (MRI). Lumbar puncture, unless contraindicated by signs of increased ICP, facilitates the analysis of CSF pressure and content. Lumbar puncture must always be preceded by CT scanning to identify patients at high risk for brain herniation. The risk of herniation with lumbar puncture in the patient with increased ICP is estimated at 1% to 12%.[6] Laboratory studies are also used to identify metabolic or endocrine abnormalities. Occasionally, the cause of coma is never clearly determined.

Medical Management

The goal of medical management of the patient in a coma is identification and treatment of the underlying cause of the condition. Initial medical management includes emergency measures to support vital functions and prevent further neurologic deterioration. Protection of the airway and ventilatory assistance are frequently needed. Administration of thiamine (100 mg), glucose, and a narcotic antagonist is suggested whenever the cause of coma is not immediately known.[2,6,8] Thiamine is administered before glucose since the coma produced by thiamine deficiency, Wernicke's encephalopathy, can be precipitated by a glucose load.[2] The cervical neck is stabilized until traumatic injury is ruled out.

The patient who remains in coma after emergency treatment requires supportive measures to maintain physiologic body functions and prevent complications. Continued airway protection and nutritional support are essential. Fluid and electrolyte management is often complex because of alterations in the neurohormonal system. Anticonvulsant therapy may be necessary to prevent further ischemic damage to the brain.

Decision making regarding the level of medical management to be provided is made jointly by the health care team and the patient's family. Family members require informational support in terms of probable cause of the coma and prognosis for recovery of both consciousness and function. Prognosis is dependent on the cause of the coma and the length of time unconsciousness persists. As a general rule, metabolic coma has a better prognosis than coma caused by a structural lesion.

Much research has been directed toward identifying prognostic indicators for the patient in a coma after a cardiopulmonary arrest. As with all types of coma, the best prognosis is associated with early arousal. There is a 20% to 30% chance of survival with a good outcome in the comatose patient who responds to pain with reflex posturing (decorticate or decerebrate) within 1 to 3 hours after an arrest. Survival is unlikely in the coma patient who has absent pupillary light reflexes for more than 6 hours after cardiopulmonary resuscitation.[9]

Nursing Management

Nursing management of the patient in a coma incorporates a variety of nursing diagnoses (Box 28-2). Nursing management is directed by the specific etiology of the coma, although some common interventions are used. One of the most important things to remember is that the patient in a coma is totally dependent on the health care team.

BOX 28-2 NURSING DIAGNOSIS AND MANAGEMENT

COMA

- Decreased Adaptive Capacity: Intracranial related to failure of normal intracranial compensatory mechanisms, p. 843
- Ineffective Airway Clearance related to excessive secretions or abnormal viscosity of mucus, p. 722
- Ineffective Breathing Pattern related to decreased lung expansion, p. 723
- Altered Nutrition: Less than Body Requirements related to lack of exogenous nutrients or increased metabolic demand, p. 165
- Risk for Aspiration, p. 727
- Risk for Infection, p. 1119
- Ineffective Family Coping related to critically ill family member, p. 97

Nursing management includes frequent assessment for changes in neurologic status and clues to the origin of the coma, supportive care of all body functions, prophylactic measures to prevent complications, psychosocial and informational support of the family, and initial rehabilitation measures such as coma stimulation therapy. Because a complete description of the nursing management of the comatose patient is beyond the scope of this text, only two key nursing measures are addressed: eye care and coma stimulation therapy.

Eye care. The blink reflex is often diminished or absent in the comatose patient. The eyelids may be flaccid and dependent on body positioning to remain in a closed position, and edema may prevent complete closure. Loss of these protective mechanisms results in drying and ulceration of the cornea, which can lead to permanent scarring and blindness.

Two interventions that are commonly used to protect the eyes are instilling saline or methyl cellulose lubricating drops and taping the eyelids in the shut position. Recent evidence suggests that an alternative technique may be more effective in preventing corneal epithelial breakdown. In addition to instilling saline drops every 2 hours, a polyethylene film is taped over the eyes, extending beyond the orbits and eyebrows. The film creates a moisture chamber around the cornea and assists in keeping the eyes moist and in the closed position.[10] This technique also prevents damage to the eyes that results from tape or gauze being placed directly on the delicate skin of the eyelids.

BOX 28-3 Sensory Stimulation Used in Coma Stimulation Therapy

AUDITORY	VISUAL	OLFACTORY	GUSTATORY	TACTILE	KINESTHETIC
Verbal orientation	Photographs	Vinegar	Mouthwash swabs	Hand holding	Turning
Music	Penlight	Spices	Lemon juice	Rubbing lotion	Range of motion
Bells	Familiar objects	Perfume	Sweet or salty solutions	Heat/cold	Chair
Clapping	Faces	Potpourri		Cotton balls	Tilt table
Tuning fork	Flashcards	Orange/lemon peel		Rough surfaces	
				Familiar objects	

From Sosnowski C, Ustik M: *J Neurosci Nurs* 26:336, 1994.

Coma stimulation therapy. Coma stimulation has been used in rehabilitation settings for many years.[3,4,11] This therapy is based on the belief that structured brain stimulation fosters brain recovery. The purpose of coma stimulation is to stimulate the reticular activating system and increase the patient's level of alertness.

Preliminary research suggests that coma stimulation therapy may reduce the duration of coma and enhance functional recovery. Based on the belief that maximal reorganization of the brain takes place in the early weeks after an insult, coma stimulation therapy must begin in the critical care unit to increase the possibility for maximal recovery.

The methods of stimuli used in coma stimulation therapy and the anticipated neurologic responses are listed in Boxes 28-3 and 28-4, respectively. Simple auditory and tactile stimulation are most often used in the critical care environment. Stimuli must be meaningful, rather than random. Taped voices of family and friends talking to the patient have been found to be particularly effective.[11]

The family must be included in all aspects of planning and implementing the coma stimulation program. Some experts advocate bombarding the patient with stimuli up to 16 hours a day, whereas others support providing stimulation every hour. In the critical care unit, a program consisting of a single stimulation activity lasting no more than 10 to 30 minutes per session two to four times a day allows time for necessary patient care activities and rest periods.[4] Family visits and nursing activities will naturally augment this program with additional auditory and tactile stimulation. Medical stability, including normal ICP and hemodynamic values, is required before initiation of coma stimulation, and the therapy is usually not started until the second week after neurologic insult. Any increase in ICP; sustained increase in blood pressure, heart rate, or respiratory rate; or development of seizure activity is considered unfavorable and reason to terminate or revise the stimulation program.[3]

PERSISTENT VEGETATIVE STATE

Description

Persistent vegetative state (PVS) is a state of unconsciousness in which wakefulness is present but awareness is lacking. The term vegetative state is used to describe the state of unconsciousness in which sleep-wake cycles and complete or partial hypothalamic and brainstem autonomic functions are present, but there is complete unawareness of self and the surrounding environment because of the absence of any ascertainable cerebral cortical function. A patient may transiently progress through a vegetative state during recovery from coma.

A vegetative state is considered persistent when present for 1 month or more after acute traumatic or nontraumatic brain injury, metabolic or degenerative disorders, and developmental malformations.[1] The incidence of PVS is uncertain because, until recently, there were no accepted diagnostic criteria for identifying this disorder. It is estimated that there are 10,000 to 25,000 adults and 4,000 to 10,000 children in the United States in a PVS.[1]

Etiology

Persistent vegetative state is caused by acute traumatic and nontraumatic brain injuries, degenerative or metabolic brain disorders, and severe congenital malformations of the nervous system.[1]

Pathophysiology

The two components of consciousness are arousal and awareness. Arousal, or wakefulness, is a function of the diencephalon and brainstem. Awareness is dependent on cerebral cortical neurons. PVS is a combination of absent cortical function and the presence

BOX 28-4 Responses to Stimulation

AUDITORY	VISUAL	OLFACTORY	GUSTATORY	TACTILE	KINESTHETIC
Startle reaction	Eye blink	Grimacing	Grimacing	Localization	Spasticity of joints
Visual tracking toward sound	Visual tracking	Tearing	Spitting	Withdrawal	Assisted ROM
Follows commands		Head turning	Swallowing	Posturing	Follows commands

From Sosnowski C, Ustik M: *J Neurosci Nurs* 26:336, 1994.

of at least some hypothalamic or brainstem function. The lack of cortical function produces the lack of awareness. The presence of hypothalamic or brainstem function produces the state of wakefulness.[1]

Research regarding the pathology associated with PVS is extremely limited. Two major patterns of neuropathology have been identified in patients in PVS associated with acute traumatic and nontraumatic brain injury. The first pattern is diffuse laminar cortical necrosis after acute, global hypoxia and ischemia, and the second is diffuse axonal injury resulting from shearing after acute trauma. The cortex is isolated from the rest of the brain because of extensive subcortical axonal injury.[1]

Assessment and Diagnosis

The diagnosis of PVS is a clinical one based on a detailed and thorough neurologic examination. The diagnostic criteria for PVS is listed in Box 28-5. Many of the assessment findings in the patient in PVS are misleading. The patients may move their limbs or trunk in meaningless ways and may smile, shed tears, utter grunts, or even moan or scream.[1] The nurse must focus the evaluation of these activities on their purposefulness. The lack of purposefulness of these motor activities confirms the diagnosis.

Pupillary reflexes and eye movement are usually normal. The eyes of the PVS patient open and close appropriately during the wake-sleep cycles. It is necessary to assess fixation and tracking. Most patients in PVS do not fixate on a visual target, do not track moving objects with their eyes, and have no response to threatening gestures. When a patient does regain awareness after being in a vegetative state, sustained visual pursuit is one of the first signs to appear.

The differentiating feature between PVS and coma is the wakefulness of the PVS patient. The most difficult differential diagnosis is between PVS and a locked-in state. The patient in a locked-in state is conscious but unable to communicate because of severe paralysis. The inability to communicate must not be confused with lack of awareness. Table 28-1 lists the differentiating characteristics of PVS and other related conditions.

BOX 28-5 Criteria for Diagnosis of Vegetative State

- No evidence of awareness of self or environment
- Inability to interact with others
- No evidence of sustained, reproducible, purposeful, or voluntary behavioral response to visual, auditory, tactile, or noxious stimuli
- No evidence of language comprehension or expression
- Intermittent wakefulness manifested by presence of sleep-wake cycles
- Sufficiently preserved hypothalamic and brainstem autonomic functions to permit survival with medical and nursing management
- Bowel and bladder incontinence
- Variably preserved cranial nerve reflexes (pupillary, oculocephalic, corneal, vestibuloocular, and gag) and spinal reflexes

The diagnosis of PVS must be made by a specialist with expertise in differentiating these conditions. Positron-emission tomography and electroencephalography are used to provide laboratory support for the appropriate diagnosis.

Medical Management

There is no known treatment to reverse PVS.[12] Coma sensory stimulation has not been found to be effective in this condition. The primary role of medical management is to provide an accurate diagnosis and appropriate prognostic evaluation. Recovery from PVS encompasses two dimensions: recovery of consciousness and recovery of function. Functional recovery is characterized by the ability to communicate,

TABLE 28-1 Characteristics of the Persistent Vegetative State and Related Conditions*

Condition	Self-Awareness	Sleep-wake Cycles	Motor Function	Experience of Suffering	Respiratory Function	EEG Activity	Cerebral Metabolism†	Prognosis for Neurologic Recovery
Persistent vegetative state	Absent	Intact	No purposeful movement	No	Normal	Polymorphic delta or theta, sometimes slow alpha	Reduced by 50% or more	Depends on cause (acute traumatic or nontraumatic injury, degenerative or metabolic condition, or developmental malformation)
Coma	Absent	Absent	No purposeful movement	No	Depressed, variable	Polymorphic delta or theta	Reduced by 50% or more (depends on cause)	Usually recovery, persistent vegetative state, or death in 2 to 4 weeks
Brain death	Absent	Absent	None or only reflex spinal movements	No	Absent	Electrocerebral silence	Absent	No recovery
Locked-in syndrome	Present	Intact	Quadriplegia and pseudobulbar palsy; eye movement preserved	Yes	Normal	Normal or minimally abnormal	Minimally or moderately reduced	Recovery unlikely; persistent quadriplegia with prolonged survival possible
Akinetic mutism	Present	Intact	Paucity of movement	Yes	Normal	Nonspecific slowing	Unknown	Recovery very unlikely (depends on cause)
Dementia	Present but lost in late stages	Intact	Variable; limited with progression	Yes but lost in late stages	Normal	Nonspecific slowing	Variably reduced	Irreversible (ultimate outcome depends on cause)

From Multi-Society Task Force on PVS: *N Engl J Med* 330:1499, 1994.

*This table provides a general overview of the persistent vegetative state and related neurologic conditions. Because of the overlap between clinical and laboratory findings, these characteristics will not apply to every patient. Neuroimaging studies (magnetic resonance imaging or computed tomography) may be useful in the clinical evaluation of patients but may not always be helpful in differentiating among these conditions.

†Determined by positron-emission or single-photon-emission computed tomography.

learn, and perform adaptive tasks and self-care. Prognosis for both levels of recovery is dependent on the cause of the underlying brain disease. Patients who remain in a PVS for 12 months after traumatic injury or 3 months after nontraumatic injury are unlikely to regain consciousness.[12] There is no chance for recovery for the patient in a PVS that resulted from degenerative or metabolic brain disease. When the prognosis is that the state is irreversible, the term *permanent vegetative state* is used.

The average life expectancy for the patient in PVS is 2 to 5 years.[12] Collaboration between the physicians and the family is necessary to determine the appropriate level of medical management. Decisions must be made regarding resuscitation status, medications (including antibiotics and oxygen), hydration, nutrition, and long-term placement either in a skilled nursing facility or at home. Aggressive therapy usually includes placing a feeding tube; monitoring and treating infections; and performing a tracheostomy, if necessary, to maintain airway patency. Guidelines for the termination of treatment in the adult patient in a PVS are available in the literature.[13-15]

Nursing Management

Nursing management of the patient in a PVS incorporates a variety of nursing diagnoses (Box 28-6). Nursing management is primarily comprised of performing a detailed neurologic assessment, providing supportive and hygienic measures, and preventing the complications of immobility.

Psychosocial and informational support of the family is essential because of the devastating nature of this diagnosis. Flexible visitation provides for proximal needs. It is important to communicate to the family that the patient in a PVS lacks the cortical capacity to feel pain. This belief is based on neurodiagnostic studies and neuropathologic examination and is supported by the Multi-Society Task Force on PVS, composed of leading neurologic experts throughout the United States.[12]

BOX 28-6 NURSING DIAGNOSIS AND MANAGEMENT

PERSISTENT VEGETATIVE STATE

- Altered Nutrition: Less than Body Requirements related to lack of exogenous nutrients or increased metabolic demand, p. 165
- Ineffective Airway Clearance related to excessive secretions or abnormal viscosity of mucus, p. 722
- Ineffective Breathing Pattern related to decreased lung expansion, p. 723
- Risk for Aspiration, p. 727
- Risk for Infection, p. 1119
- Ineffective Family Coping related to critically ill family member, p. 97

BRAIN DEATH

Brain death is the term used to describe complete, irreversible cessation of function of the cerebrum, cerebellum, and brainstem.[1,2,16] At the point this occurs, the patient is dead, regardless of the presence of a heartbeat, maintenance of respiration via mechanical means, or functioning of other vital organs.[2,8] The diagnosis of brain death is made by physical examination of the patient, usually by a neurologist. National guidelines describing the clinical criteria for brain death have been available for many years. Absence of hypothermia and any CNS depressant drugs in the blood are necessary to make the diagnosis of brain death. Several diagnostic procedures may be used to confirm the clinical diagnosis. Cessation of cerebral blood flow can be confirmed by transcranial Doppler or angiography. Cessation of electrophysiologic function can be confirmed by electroencephalography or evoked potential testing.[2]

CEREBROVASCULAR ACCIDENT

Cerebrovascular accident, commonly known as *stroke,* is a descriptive term for the onset of neurologic symptoms caused by the interruption of blood flow to the brain. Stroke is the third leading cause of death in the United States, preceded by heart disease and cancer. The number of survivors of stroke in the United States is estimated at 3 million people. The morbidity associated with stroke is the leading cause of adult disability.[17] The annual cost for care and loss of productivity is nearly $20 billion.[18]

The national concern for the incidence and effects of stroke are illustrated by the inclusion of emergent stroke care in the American Heart Association guidelines for basic and advanced life support. Major public education programs, stroke appraisal screening programs, development of stroke centers, and algorithms for stroke management are based on the success these same approaches have had with coronary artery disease.

CULTURAL INSIGHTS 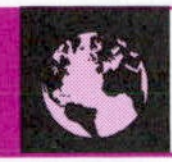 Death-Related Behaviors in Seven Cultural Groups

CULTURAL GROUP	RELIGIOUS ATTITUDES	GRIEF EXPRESSIONS	DEATH RITUALS
Japanese-Americans	May be Buddhist, Shinto, and/or Christian; parents may be of different religious affiliation than children; DNR is a difficult choice decided by the entire family	Not publicly expressive	Use of prayer and offerings prevalent in Shinto and Buddhist religions, cremation common; issei (first generation) less likely to agree to organ donation or autopsy because of strong feelings that when person dies, the body should be kept intact
Chinese-Americans	May be fatalistic when faced with terminal illness and death; family may prefer that patient is not told about terminal illness	Not publicly expressive	Some families prefer to bathe their family member after death; believe that body should be kept intact: hence, organ donation and autopsies are not common
Vietnamese-Americans	May be Buddhist or Catholic or other Christian religion; DNR is a sensitive decision made by entire family	May weep/wail aloud	For Catholic patient, a spiritual object such as a rosary or figure of a saint may be kept close to patient For Buddhist families, incense is lit in room; important to allow extra time for families to be with deceased patient while monk performs religious rite in the deceased person's room Body is given great respect; organ donation and autopsy not allowed by older generations
African-Americans	Commonly recognized Western concept of heaven and hell	Open and public expression is expected but varies	Funeral rite is an informal gathering, including prayers, scripture reading, songs, screaming/crying; donating organs or blood except for immediate family needs is taboo; when the need for an autopsy is explained, families usually concur
Mexican-Americans	Illness and death are God's will	Very expressive; wailing is common and socially acceptable as a sign of respect	Extended family obligated to pay respects to dying—except pregnant women, who are usually prohibited from caring for sick or attending funerals Roman Catholic priest performs "Anointing of the Sick"; praying is commonly practiced at bedside of dying; family member may help clean the body after death Majority of Catholics do not permit organ donation or autopsy, and if so, it is a full family decision

Modified from Lipson JG, Dibble SL, Minarik PA: *Culture and nursing care: a pocket guide,* 1996 San Francisco, UCSF Nursing Press; York C, Stickler J: *DCCN* 4(2):122, 1985.

Continued

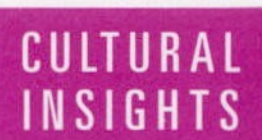
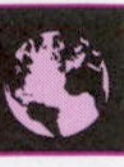

CULTURAL INSIGHTS Death-Related Behaviors in Seven Cultural Groups—cont'd

CULTURAL GROUP	RELIGIOUS ATTITUDES	GRIEF EXPRESSIONS	DEATH RITUALS
American-Indians	Some families may wish the body to rest at place of death for up to 36 hours, when soul is believed to depart	May or may not be publicly expressive	Traditional practices include turning and/or flexing body, use of sweet-grass smoke or other purification; family may choose to stay in room with the deceased person; some tribes avoid contact with the deceased person and his or her possessions; some families take the body home the night before burial to be cleansed and dressed; nurses should ask families if it is appropriate to cleanse and prepare the body before individual visits; some may prefer to have an open window or orient patient's body toward a cardinal direction before death; organ donation and autopsy generally are not desired
Arab-Americans	Some are Moslem, some are Christian; anticipatory grief work not acceptable; Moslems do not need an imam to be present before or during the dying process; imam reads from the Koran after death	Express grief openly; much touching of deceased person's body	Inform head of family of impending death and allow him to inform rest of family; in some families, young women are prohibited from being with dying or dead members of the family DNR decision very difficult; family may lose trust in health team if option is offered Special rituals are followed after death, such as washing the body and all its orifices May not allow organ donation or autopsy because of respect for burying the body whole and meeting the creator with integrity

There are two basic types of stroke: ischemic and hemorrhagic. Hemorrhagic strokes are divided into subarachnoid hemorrhage and intracerebral hemorrhage. Cerebrovascular accident falls under DRG 14 (Specific cerebrovascular disorders, except transient ischemic attack), with an average length of stay of 7.5 days. If the patient has surgery to correct the underlying cause of the hemorrhage, then DRG 1 (Craniotomy, age greater than 17 years except for trauma) or DRG 2 (Craniotomy, age 0-17 years) is used, with average lengths of stay of 11.1 and 11.6 days, respectively.[5]

Ischemic Stroke

Description. Ischemic stroke is a stroke that results from low cerebral flow, usually because of occlusion of a blood vessel. The occlusion can be either thrombotic or embolic in nature. Eighty percent of the 500,000 Americans that suffered a stroke in 1991 suffered an ischemic stroke.[18] The 30-day survival rate after ischemic stroke is approximately 67% to 85%.

Etiology. Strokes are preventable. Most thrombotic strokes are the result of the accumulation of atherosclerotic plaque in the vessel lumen, especially at bifurcations, or curves, of the vessel. The pathogenesis of cerebrovascular disease is identical to that of coronary vasculature. The greatest risk factor for ischemic stroke is hypertension. Other risk factors are diabetes, elevated blood lipids, obesity, smoking, stress, and family history. Common sites of atherosclerotic plaque are the bifurcation of the common carotid artery, the origins of the middle and anterior cerebral arteries, and the origins of the vertebral arteries.[19] Elderly women are at greater risk for cardioembolic stroke.[20]

An embolic stroke occurs when a small embolus from the heart or lower cerebral circulation travels distally and lodges in a small vessel, resulting in loss of blood supply. Up to one third of ischemic strokes are attributed to a cardioembolic phenomenon.[20,21] Risk factors include atrial fibrillation, coronary artery disease, and an enlarged heart. Aspirin and warfarin therapy are currently under investigation as preventive measures to guard against this complication in patients with chronic atrial fibrillation.

Pathophysiology. Ischemic stroke is a cerebral hemodynamic insult. When cerebral blood flow is reduced to a level insufficient to maintain neuronal viability, ischemic injury occurs. In focal stroke, an area of marginally perfused tissue surrounds a core of ischemic cells. Five minutes of anoxic insult initiates a chain of events producing brain infarction. Irreversible neuronal injury soon follows.[19] If infarction occurs, the affected brain tissue eventually softens and liquefies.

The phenomenon of a focal ischemic stroke is identical to that associated with myocardial infarction. Cerebral blood flow is diminished by either atherosclerotic vascular disease or embolus. Often a history of transient ischemic attacks (TIAs), brief episodes of neurologic symptoms, offers clues to the progressive severity of cerebrovascular disease. Sudden onset indicates embolism as the final insult to flow.[19] The size of the stroke is dependent on the size and location of the occluded vessel and the availability of collateral blood flow. Global ischemia results when severe hypotension or cardiopulmonary arrest produces a transient drop in blood flow to all areas of the brain.

Cerebral edema sufficient to produce clinical deterioration develops in 10% to 20% of patients with ischemic stroke and can result in intracranial hypertension. The edema results from a loss of normal metabolic function of the cells and peaks at 3 to 5 days. This process is commonly the cause of death during the first week after a stroke.[19] Secondary hemorrhage at the site of the stroke lesion, known as *hemorrhagic conversion,* and seizures are the two other major acute neurologic complications of ischemic stroke. Mortality rates in the first 20 days after ischemic stroke range from 8% to 30%.[19]

Assessment and diagnosis. The characteristic sign of an ischemic stroke is the sudden onset of focal neurologic signs.[18] These signs usually occur in combination. Box 28-7 lists common patterns of neurologic symptoms associated with an ischemic stroke. Hemiparesis, aphasia, and hemianopia are common. Changes in level of consciousness usually only occur with brainstem or cerebellar involvement, seizure, hypoxia, hemorrhage, or elevated ICP. These changes may be exhibited as stupor, coma, confusion, and agitation. The reported frequency of seizures in patients with ischemic stroke is variable, ranging from 4% to 43%. If seizures occur, they are usually seen within 24 hours of insult.[18]

Confirmation of the diagnosis of ischemic stroke is the first step in the emergent evaluation of these patients. Differentiation from intracranial hemorrhage is vital. Noncontrast CT scanning is the method of choice for this purpose and is considered the most important initial diagnostic study. In addition to excluding intracranial hemorrhage, CT can also assist in identifying early neurologic complications and the etiology of the insult. An MRI will demonstrate actual infarction of cerebral tissue earlier than a CT, but is less useful in the emergent differential diagnosis. Because of the strong correlation between acute ischemic stroke and heart disease, electrocardiography, chest x-ray, and cardiac monitoring are suggested to detect a cardiac etiology or co-existing condition. Echocardiography is also valuable in identifying a cardioembolic phenomenon when a sufficient index of suspicion warrants.[20] Laboratory evaluation of hematologic function, electrolyte and glucose levels, and renal and hepatic function is also recommended. Arterial blood gas analysis is performed if hypoxia is suspected, and an electroencephalogram is obtained if seizures are suspected. Lumbar puncture is only performed if subarachnoid hemorrhage is suspected and the CT is negative.[18]

Medical management. After confirming the diagnosis of ischemic stroke, the next step is to determine the possibility for reversal of the pathology. Emergent care must include airway protection and ventilatory assistance to maintain adequate tissue oxygenation. Hypertension is often present in the early period as a compensatory response and in most cases must not be lowered. Antihypertensive therapy is considered only if the mean blood pressure (BP) is greater than 130 mm Hg or the systolic BP is greater than 220 mm Hg.[18] Oral agents or easily titratable intravenous agents are recommended in this instance. Body temperature and glucose levels must also be normalized.

BOX 28-7 Common Patterns of Neurologic Abnormalities in Patients with Acute Ischemic Strokes

LEFT (DOMINANT) HEMISPHERE

Aphasia; right hemiparesis; right-sided sensory loss; right visual field defect; poor right conjugate gaze; dysarthria; difficulty in reading, writing, or calculating

RIGHT (NONDOMINANT) HEMISPHERE

Neglect of the left visual space, left visual field defect, left hemiparesis, left-sided sensory loss, poor left conjugate gaze, extinction of left-sided stimuli, dysarthria, spatial disorientation

BRAINSTEM/CEREBELLUM/POSTERIOR HEMISPHERE

Motor or sensory loss in all four limbs, crossed signs, limb or gait ataxia, dysarthria, dysconjugate gaze, nystagmus, amnesia, bilateral visual field defects

SMALL SUBCORTICAL HEMISPHERE OR BRAINSTEM (PURE MOTOR STROKE)

Weakness of face and limbs on one side of the body without abnormalities of higher brain function, sensation, or vision

SMALL SUBCORTICAL HEMISPHERE OR BRAINSTEM (PURE SENSORY STROKE)

Decreases sensation of face and limbs on one side of the body without abnormalities of higher brain function, motor function, or vision

From Adams HP and others: *Circ* 90(3):1588, 1994.

Medical management must also include the identification and treatment of acute complications, such as cerebral edema or seizure activity. Prophylaxis for these complications is not recommended. Surgical decompression is recommended if a large cerebellar infarction compresses the brainstem.

There is much conflicting evidence regarding a variety of interventions for the patient with acute ischemic stroke.[18] Heparin therapy has been used for years to prevent recurrent embolism, however, recent scientific studies have demonstrated conflicting results. The Stroke Council of the American Heart Association (AHA) has determined that evidence regarding the role of heparin in the patient with ischemic stroke is insufficient to make any recommendation regarding its use.[18]

Clot lysis by thrombolytic therapy is currently under intense study. Conflicting evidence and the danger of intracranial hemorrhage have prevented generalized use of this therapy. It is expected that, as in myocardial infarction, thrombolytic therapy will become standard once specific indications are refined. The following is a list of additional therapies that are currently under investigation but are not recommended at this time for routine use because of insufficient evidence: emergent carotid endarterectomy; embolectomy or angioplasty; hemodilution of the blood; and the administration of steroids, barbiturates, calcium channel blockers, nimodipine, naloxone, glutamate antagonists, or amphetamines.[18,21] The immediacy of treatment after insult is probably a major factor in the documented effectiveness of several of these therapies.

Subarachnoid Hemorrhage

Description. Subarachnoid hemorrhage (SAH) is bleeding into the subarachnoid space, usually caused by rupture of a cerebral aneurysm or arteriovenous malformation (AVM). Subarachnoid hemorrhage accounts for 6% to 7% of all strokes—with nontraumatic SAH affecting more than 30,000 Americans each year. The incidence of SAH is greater in women and increases with age. The overall mortality rate is 25%, with most patients dying on the first day after insult. The rate of significant morbidity approximates 50% of all survivors.[22] Unfortunately, no appreciable decrease in the incidence of SAH has occurred over time. Approximately 2 million people in the United States are believed to have an unruptured cerebral aneurysm, the congenital anomaly responsible for most cases of SAH. The risk for rupture is 1% to 2% annually. The known risk factors for SAH include hypertension, smoking, alcohol use, and stimulant use.[22] As in ischemic stroke, the single most important risk factor is hypertension.

Etiology. Causes of SAH include cerebral aneurysms, AVMs, hypertensive intracerebral hemorrhages, and bleeding from a cerebral tumor.

Cerebral aneurysm rupture accounts for more than 50% of all cases of spontaneous SAH.[23] An aneurysm is an outpouching of the wall of a blood vessel that results from weakening of the wall of the vessel. Ninety percent of aneurysms are congenital—the cause of which is unknown. The other 10% can be a result of traumatic injury (that stretches and tears the muscular middle layer of the arterial vessel), infectious material (most often from infectious vegetation on valves of the left side of the heart after bacterial endocardi-

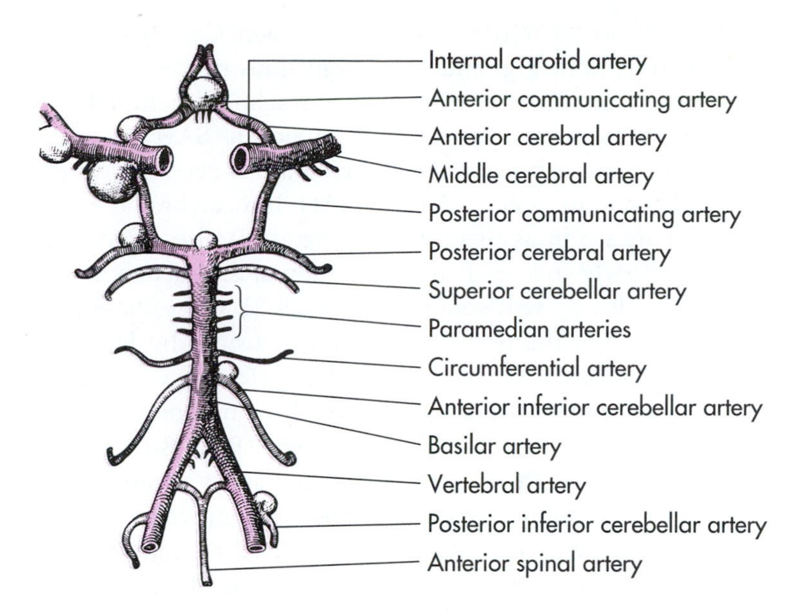

FIGURE 28-1. The common sites of berry aneurysms. The size of the aneurysm in the drawing is proportional to the frequency of occurrence at the various sites. (From Wyngaarden JB, Smith LH, editors: *Cecil's textbook of medicine,* ed 16, Philadelphia, 1982, WB Saunders.)

tis) that lodges against a vessel wall and erodes the muscular layer, or of undetermined cause. Multiple aneurysms occur in 20% to 25% of the cases and often are bilateral, occurring in the same location on both sides of the cerebral vascular system. It is possible for an individual to live a full life span with an unruptured cerebral aneurysm. Aneurysm rupture usually occurs between 30 and 60 years of age, with peak incidence during the fifth decade of life.[23]

Arteriovenous malformation rupture is responsible for less than 10% of all SAHs.[8] An AVM is a tangled mass of arterial and venous blood vessels that shunt blood directly from the arterial side into the venous side, bypassing the capillary system. They may be small, focal lesions or large diffuse lesions that occupy almost an entire hemisphere. AVMs are always congenital, though the exact embryonic cause for these malformations is unknown. They also occur in the spinal cord and renal, gastrointestinal, and integumentary systems. Small superficial AVMs are seen as port-wine stains of the skin. In contrast to the middle-aged population with SAH from aneurysm, SAH from an AVM usually occurs before the third decade of life.[8]

Pathophysiology. The pathophysiology of the two most common causes of SAH are distinctly different.

Cerebral aneurysm. As the individual with a congenital cerebral aneurysm matures, blood pressure rises and more stress is placed on the poorly developed and thin vessel wall. Ballooning out of the vessel occurs, giving the aneurysm a berry-like appearance. Most cerebral aneurysms are saccular or berry-like with a stem or neck. Aneurysms are usually small, 2 to 7 mm in diameter, and frequently occur at the base of the brain on the circle of Willis. Figure 28-1 illustrates the usual distribution between the vessels. Most cerebral aneurysms occur at the bifurcation of blood vessels.

The aneurysm becomes clinically significant when the vessel wall becomes so thin that it ruptures, sending arterial blood at a high pressure into the subarachnoid space. For a brief moment after the aneurysm ruptures, intracranial pressure is believed to approach mean arterial pressure and cerebral perfusion falls. In other situations, the unruptured aneurysm expands and places pressure on surrounding structures. This is particularly true with posterior communicating artery aneurysms, as they put pressure on the oculomotor nerve (CN III) causing ipsilateral pupil dilation and ptosis.

Arteriovenous malformation. The pathophysiologic features of an AVM are related to the size and location of the malformation. An AVM is fed by one or more cerebral arteries, also known as *feeders.* These feeder arteries tend to enlarge over time and increase the volume of blood shunted through the malformation, as well as increase the overall mass effect. Large, dilated, tortuous draining veins also develop as a result of increasing arterial blood flow being delivered at a higher than normal pressure. Normal vascular flow has a mean arterial pressure of 70 to 80 mm Hg, a mean arteriole pressure of 35 to 45 mm Hg, and a mean capillary pressure that drops from 35 to 10 mm Hg as it connects with the venous side. Lack of this capillary bridge allows blood with a mean pressure of 35 to 45 mm Hg to flow into the venous system. Because there is no muscular layer in a vein as there is in an artery, the veins become extremely engorged and rupture easily. Cerebral atrophy is also present sometimes in the patient with an AVM. It is the result of chronic ischemia because of the shunting of blood through the AVM and away from normal cerebral circulation.

Assessment and diagnosis. The patient with an SAH characteristically has an abrupt onset of pain, described as the "worst headache of my life." A brief loss of consciousness, nausea, vomiting, focal neurologic deficits, and a stiff neck may accompany the headache. The SAH may result in coma or death.

Patient history may reveal one or more incidences of sudden onset of headache with vomiting in the weeks preceding a major SAH. These are "warning leaks" of an aneurysm in which small amounts of blood ooze from the aneurysm into the subarachnoid space. The presence of blood is an irritant to the meninges, particularly the arachnoid membrane. This irritation causes headache, stiff neck, and photophobia. These small "warning leaks" seldom are detected because the condition is not severe enough for the patient to seek medical attention. If a neurologic deficit, such as third cranial nerve palsy, develops before aneurysm rupture, medical intervention is sought and the aneurysm may be surgically secured before the devastation of a rupture can occur. Symptoms of unruptured AVM—headaches with dizziness or syncope or fleeting neurologic deficits—may also be found in the history.

Diagnosis of SAH is based on clinical presentation, CT scan, and lumbar puncture. Noncontrast CT is the cornerstone of definitive SAH diagnosis.[22] In 92% of the cases, CT scan can demonstrate a clot in the subarachnoid space, if performed within 24 hours of the onset of the hemorrhage. On the basis of the appearance and the location of the SAH, diagnosis of cause—aneurysm or AVM—may be made from the CT scan. MRI is relatively insensitive for detecting blood in the subarachnoid space.

If the initial CT scan is negative, an LP is performed to obtain CSF for analysis. CSF after SAH is bloody in appearance with a red blood cell count greater than $1000/mm^3$. If the lumbar puncture is performed more than 5 days after the SAH, CSF fluid is xanthochromic (dark amber), because the blood products have broken down. Cloudy CSF usually indicates some type of infectious process, such as bacterial meningitis, not a subarachnoid hemorrhage.

Once the SAH has been documented, a cerebral angiogram is necessary to identify the exact cause of the SAH. If a cerebral aneurysm rupture is the cause, angiogram is also essential for identifying the exact location of the aneurysm in preparation for surgery (Figure 28-2). Once the aneurysm has been located, it is graded using the Hunt and Hess classification scale. This scale categorizes the patient based on the severity of the neurologic deficits associated with the hemorrhage (Box 28-8).[24] If AVM rupture is the cause, an angiogram is necessary to identify the feeding arteries and draining veins of the malformation.

Medical management. SAH is a medical emergency, and time is of the essence. Preservation of neurologic function is the goal. Initial treatment must always support vital functions. Airway management and ventilatory assistance may be necessary. Early diagnosis is also essential. A ventriculostomy is performed to control ICP if the patient's level of consciousness is depressed.[22]

Evidence suggests that only 19% of the deaths attributable to aneurysmal SAH are related to the direct effects of the initial hemorrhage.[25] In a recent major multicenter study, rebleeding accounted for 22% of deaths from aneurysmal SAH, cerebral vasospasm accounted for 23%, and nonneurologic medical complications accounted for 23%.[25] Therefore, once initial intervention has provided necessary support for vital physiologic functions, medical management of acute SAH is primarily aimed toward the prevention and treatment of the complications of SAH that can produce further neurologic damage and death.

Rebleeding. Rebleeding is the occurrence of a second SAH in an unsecured aneurysm or, less commonly, an AVM.[6] The incidence of rebleeding with conservative therapy is 20% to 30% in the first month, with the highest occurrence on the first day after initial hemorrhage.[22] Mortality with aneurysmal rebleeding is 48% to 78%.[23]

Historically, conservative measures to prevent rebleeding have included BP control and SAH precautions (see section on nursing management of cerebrovascular accident). An elevation in BP is a normal compensatory response to maintain adequate cerebral perfusion after a neurologic insult. In the belief that hypertension contributes to rebleeding, nitroprusside, propranolol, or hydralazine have been commonly used to maintain a systolic BP no greater than 150 mm Hg.[26] Recent evidence suggests that rebleeding has more to do with variations in BP rather than absolute values and that BP control does not lower the incidence of

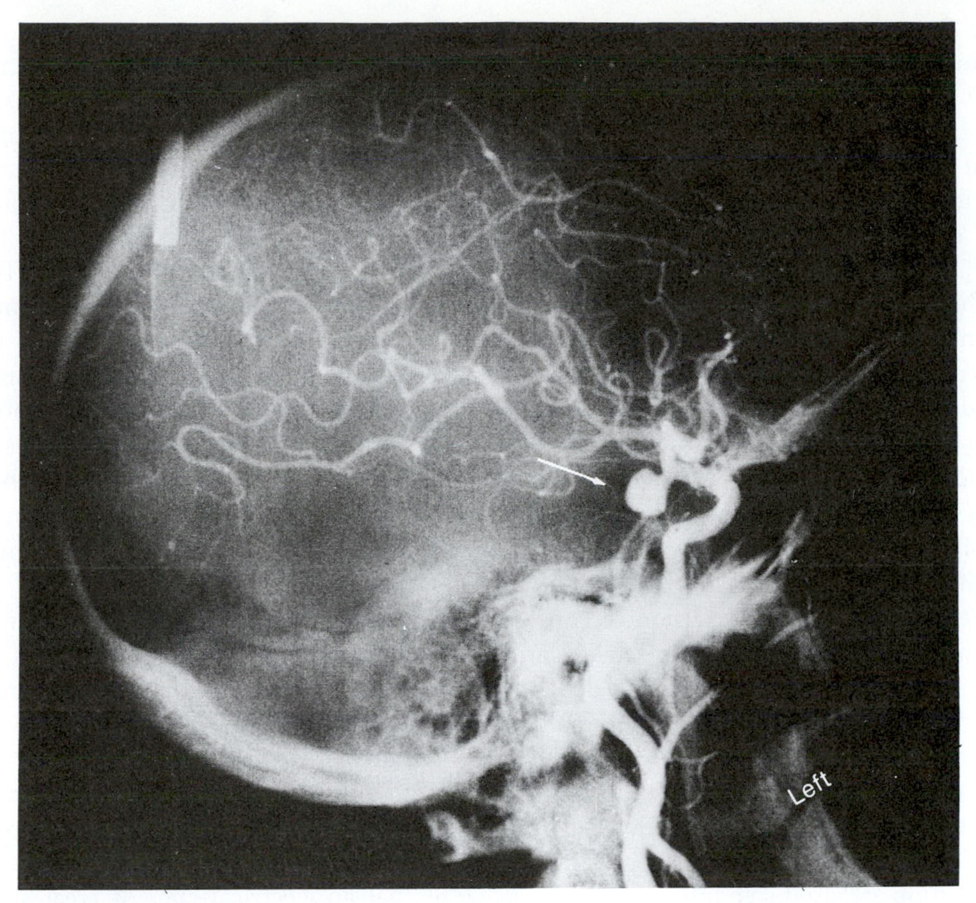

FIGURE 28-2. Cerebral angiography showing location of aneurysm at posterior communicating artery. (From Tortorici M: *Fundamentals of angiography,* St Louis, 1982, Mosby.)

BOX 28-8 Hunt and Hess Classification of Subarachnoid Hemorrhage

Grade I	Asymptomatic or minimal headache and slight nuchal rigidity
Grade II	Moderate to severe headache, nuchal rigidity, no neurologic deficit other than cranial nerve palsy
Grade III	Drowsiness, confusion, or mild focal deficit
Grade IV	Stupor, moderate to severe hemiparesis, possible early decerebrate rigidity, and vegetative disturbances
Grade V	Deep coma, decerebrate rigidity, moribund appearance

rebleeding.[22] Prophylactic anticonvulsant therapy is recommended to prevent seizures.[22]

Surgical aneurysm clipping. Definitive treatment for the prevention of rebleeding is surgical clipping with complete obliteration of the aneurysm. Timing of the surgery is a key medical management issue. Since the introduction of microsurgery and improved surgical techniques, patients commonly are taken to the operating room within the first 48 hours after rupture. This early surgical intervention to secure the aneurysm eliminates the risk of rebleeding and allows more aggressive therapy to be used in the postoperative period for the treatment of vasospasm. Early surgery also allows the neurosurgeon to flush out the excess blood and clots from the basal cisterns (reservoir of CSF around the base of the brain and circle of Willis) to reduce the risk of vasospasm. Early surgery is recommended for patients with a Grade I or Grade II SAH and some patients with Grade III. In patients with a Grade III SAH, the initial hemorrhage did not produce significant neurologic deficit, but the risk of rebleeding with a tragically high incidence of mortality is present until the aneurysm is secured. Because of the patient's clinical condition and the technical difficulty of the surgery, early surgical repair of the aneurysm is not always possible. Early surgery continues to be controversial for patients with Grade IV or V SAH and those demonstrating vasospasm. However, recent studies have not supported the fear of worse ischemic sequelae with early surgery in these patients.[23] Careful consideration of the patient's clinical situation is necessary in determining the optimal time for surgery.

The surgical procedure involves a craniotomy to expose and isolate the area of aneurysm. A clip is placed over the neck of the aneurysm to eliminate the area of weakness. This is a technically difficult procedure that requires the skill of an experienced neurosurgeon. It is not uncommon, particularly in early surgery, for the clot to break away from the aneurysm as it is surgically exposed. Extensive hemorrhage into the craniotomy site results, and cessation of the hemorrhage often causes increased neurologic deficits. Deficits may also occur as a result of surgical manipulation to gain access to the site of the aneurysm.

Surgical AVM excision. Medical management of AVM traditionally has involved surgical excision or conservative management of such symptoms as seizures and headache. The decision for surgical excision depends on the location and size of the AVM. Some malformations are located so deep in the cerebral structures (the thalamus or midbrain) that attempts to remove the AVM would cause severe neurologic deficits. History of a previous hemorrhage and the patient's age and overall condition are also taken into account when making the decision regarding surgical intervention.

Surgical excision of large AVMs includes the risk of reperfusion bleeding. As feeding arteries of the AVM are clamped off, the arterial blood that usually flowed into the AVM is now diverted into the surrounding circulation. In many cases the surrounding tissue has been in a state of chronic ischemia and the arterial vessels feeding these areas are maximally dilated. As arterial blood begins to flow at a higher volume and pressure into these dilated arteries, seeping of blood from the vessels may occur. Evidence of reperfusion bleeding in the operating room is an indication that no more arterial blood can be diverted from the AVM without risk of serious intracerebral hemorrhage. In the postoperative phase, a low blood pressure is maintained to prevent further reperfusion bleeding. In large AVMs, two to four stages of surgery may be required over 6 to 12 months.

Embolization. Embolization is used to secure a cerebral aneurysm or AVM that is surgically inaccessible because of size, location, or medical instability of the patient. Embolization involves several new interventional neuroradiology techniques. All of the techniques use a percutaneous transfemoral approach in a manner similar to an angiogram. Under fluoroscopy, the catheter is threaded up to the internal carotid artery. Specially developed microcatheters are then manipulated into the area of the vascular anomaly and embolic materials are placed endovascularly. Three different embolization techniques are used, depending on the underlying pathological derangement.

The first type of embolization is used to embolize an AVM. Small silastic beads or glue are slowly introduced into the vessels feeding the AVM. Blood flow then carries the material to the site and embolization is achieved. This procedure may be used in combination with surgery. One to three sessions of embolization of the feeding vessels are performed to reduce the size of the lesion before a craniotomy is performed for total excision. The primary risk of this procedure is lodging of the embolic substance in a vessel that feeds normal tissue. This occurrence creates an embolic stroke with the immediate onset of neurologic symptoms.

The second type of embolization involves placement of one or more detachable balloons into an aneurysmal sac or AVM. A liquid polymerizing agent is used to inflate the balloon. The material then solidifies within approximately 45 minutes.[26] The third techniques involves placement of one or more detachable platinum coils into an aneurysm to produce an endovascular thrombus. The advantage of this technique is that an electrical current creates positive charging of the coil, which induces electrothrombosis.[27,28] The most common complication of these two techniques is the development of distal ischemia resulting from emboli. Again, the onset of neurologic symptoms is immediate. Other risks include subtotal occlusion and intraprocedural rupture of the vasculature and death.

Pharmacologic therapy. For years the use of antifibrinolytic agents (aminocaproic acid) has been suggested in situations in which early surgery is not an option. Antifibrinolytic agents prevent the production of fibrin, which is responsible for the eventual dissolution of the clot at the tip of the aneurysm. Controversy continues to surround the use of these agents. Results of studies reporting a reduced incidence of rebleeding have been minimally positive. The main issue with the use of antifibrinolytic agents is the tendency of these drugs to increase the incidence and severity of the other common SAH complication—vasospasm. Clinical trials continue to evaluate the efficacy of this treatment.[22]

Cerebral vasospasm. The presence or absence of cerebral vasospasm significantly affects the outcome of aneurysmal SAH. This complication does not occur with SAH resulting from AVM rupture. Cerebral vasospasm is a narrowing of the lumen of the cerebral arteries. It is believed to be a response to subarachnoid blood clots coating the outer surface of the blood vessels.[29] Inasmuch as aneurysms occur at the circle of Willis, the major vessels responsible for feeding the cerebral circulation are affected by vasospasm. Depending on the arterial vessels involved in the vasospasm reaction, decreased arterial flow occurs in large areas of the cerebral hemispheres.

It is estimated that 50% of all SAH patients develop vasospasm, which is demonstrable by angiography. Thirty-two percent of these patients develop symptomatic vasospasm, resulting in ischemic stroke and/or death for 15% to 20% of them despite the use of maximal therapy.[22] The onset of vasospasm is usually 3 to 5 days after the initial hemorrhage, with maximal narrowing occurring at 5 to 14 days.[22] Vasospasm can last for 3 to 4 weeks.

A variety of therapies have been evaluated in an attempt to reverse or overcome cerebral vasospasm. To date, three treatments seem to have potential benefit: induced hypertensive, hypervolemic, hemodilution therapy; oral nimodipine; and transluminal cerebral angioplasty.

Hypertensive, hypervolemic, hemodilution therapy. Hypertensive, hypervolemic, hemodilution (HHH) therapy involves increasing the patient's blood pressure and cardiac output with vasoactive medications and diluting the patient's blood with fluid and volume expanders. Systolic BP is maintained between 150 and 160 mm Hg. The increase in volume and pressure forces blood through the vasospastic area at higher pressures. Hemodilution facilitates flow through the area by reducing blood viscosity. Many anecdotal reports exist of patients' neurologic deficits improving as systolic pressure increases from 130 mm Hg to between 150 and 160 mm Hg. The Stroke Council of the AHA has recommended this therapy for prevention and treatment of vasospasm.[22]

The obvious deterrent to use of induced hypertension is the risk of rebleeding in an unsecured aneurysm. Surgical clipping of the aneurysm before HHH therapy is preferred. Cerebral edema, elevated intracranial pressure, cardiac failure, and electrolyte imbalance are also risks of HHH therapy. Careful monitoring of the patient's neurologic status, hemodynamic parameters, ICP, and serum electrolytes is necessary.[22]

Oral nimodipine. Oral nimodipine is strongly recommended to reduce the poor outcomes associated with vasospasm. The exact nature of the effect of nimodipine is not clear, but use of the drug has demonstrated consistently positive effects on outcome without any demonstrable effect on the incidence or severity of vasospasm. Nimodipine is administered by mouth or nasogastric tube prophylactically in all patients with SAH. Nimodipine may produce hypotension, especially when administered concurrently with other antihypertensive agents. The drug is not effective if administered sublingually.[30] To administer nimodipine via a nasogastric tube (NGT), the soft capsule is punctured at both ends and the contents are withdrawn and then squirted down the NGT, followed by flushing. Intravenous administration of other calcium channel blockers is under investigation.[22] (∞Neurologic Pharmacologic Agents, p. 834.)

Transluminal cerebral angioplasty. Transluminal cerebral angioplasty is used when pharmacologic management of cerebral vasospasm has failed.[31] It is only performed when CT or MRI provides evidence that infarction has not yet occurred. The procedure is performed by an interventional neuroradiologist, and the patient is under either local, general, or neuroleptic analgesia. The technique of cerebral angioplasty is very similar to that used in the coronary vasculature. Risks include intimal perforation or rupture, cerebral artery thrombosis or embolism, recurrence of stenosis, and severe diffuse vasospasm unresponsive to therapy. Hemorrhage at the femoral site may also occur. Early evidence is promising, and this procedure is recommended when conventional therapy is unsuccessful.[22]

Hyponatremia. Hyponatremia develops in 10% to 43% of patients with SAH. It usually occurs around the same timeframe as vasospasm, several days after initial hemorrhage. There is strong evidence that the use of fluid restriction to treat hyponatremia is associated with poor outcome in the SAH patient. The AHA Stroke Council has strongly recommended that fluid restriction not be used in this instance and instead recommends sodium replenishment with isotonic fluids.[22]

Hydrocephalus. The development of hydrocephalus is a late complication that commonly occurs after SAH. Blood that has circulated in the subarachnoid space and has been absorbed by the arachnoid villi may obstruct the villi and reduce the rate of CSF absorption. Over time, increasing volumes of CSF in the intracranial space produce communicating hydrocephalus.

Treatment consists of placing a drain to remove CSF. This can be accomplished temporarily by inserting a ventriculostomy or permanently by placing a ventriculoperitoneal shunt.

Intracerebral Hemorrhage

Description. Intracerebral hemorrhage (ICH) is bleeding directly into cerebral tissue, usually from a small artery. Causes of intracerebral hemorrhage are aneurysm or AVM rupture, trauma, or hypertensive hemorrhage. This section concentrates on hypertensive hemorrhage. Intracerebral hemorrhage destroys cerebral tissue, causes cerebral edema, and increases ICP.

The incidence of hypertensive hemorrhage accounts for 2% of all deaths in the United States and is responsible for about 10% to 15% of all strokes annually .[20] ICH usually occurs in patients between 55 and 75 years old.

Etiology. Intracerebral hemorrhage is most often caused by hypertensive rupture of a cerebral vessel. The cause of a hypertensive stroke is largely a longstanding history of hypertension. Blood dyscrasia (leukemia, hemophilia, sickle cell disease); anticoagulation therapy; and hemorrhage into brain tumors are other possible causes of intracerebral hemorrhage. Many patients develop headache and neurologic symptoms after straining to have a bowel movement. Often on questioning, the patient with a hypertensive hemorrhage admits to having discontinued antihypertensive medication 2 to 3 weeks before the hemorrhage.

Pathophysiology. The pathophysiology of intracerebral hemorrhage is caused by continued elevated blood pressure exerting force against smaller arterial vessels that have become damaged from arteriosclerotic changes. Eventually, these arteries break, and blood bursts from the vessels into the surrounding cerebral tissue, creating a hematoma. ICP rises precipitously in response to the increase in overall intracranial volume.

Assessment and diagnosis. Initial assessment usually reveals a critically ill patient who often is unconscious and requires ventilatory support. History from a relative or significant other describes a sudden onset of severe headache with rapid neurologic deterioration. Diagnosis is established easily with CT.

Vital signs usually reveal a severely elevated blood pressure (200/100 to 250/150 mm Hg); slow pulse; and deep, labored respirations. The patient arrives in the emergency room with many of the signs of increased ICP. Airway, breathing, and circulation must be addressed first to make sure that the airway is adequate, breathing patterns are acceptable, and circulation is present.

An antihypertensive medication usually is administered immediately to reduce the blood pressure to a relatively normal reading. If the hemorrhage is significant enough to cause increased ICP, the blood pressure must not be allowed to drop too rapidly or too low. If the blood pressure drops below 140 mm Hg systolic and ICP remains high, cerebral perfusion may be compromised.

Medical management. Medical management of a hypertensive hemorrhage is similar to that for a traumatic hemorrhage. Surgical removal of the clot depends on the size and location of the hematoma, the patient's ICP, and other neurologic symptoms. If the hematoma is large and causes a shift in cerebral structures or if ICP is elevated despite routine methods to lower it, a craniotomy for removal of the hematoma is performed.

Nonsurgical management includes measures to maintain the ICP within normal limits and to support all other vital functions until the patient regains consciousness. The case fatality rate for intracerebral hemorrhagic strokes is approximately 50%.[20]

Nursing Management of Cerebrovascular Accident

Nursing management of the patient with a cerebrovascular accident incorporates a variety of nursing diagnoses (Box 28-9). Nursing measures include performing frequent neurologic and hemodynamic assessments and monitoring and preventing complications.

Assessments. The goal of frequent assessments is early recognition of neurologic and/or hemodynamic deterioration. Close monitoring of the patient's neurologic signs and vital signs is essential and requires almost continuous observation. Automatic noninvasive devices, such as a blood pressure cuff and a pulse oximeter, are helpful. Seizure activity must be identified and treated immediately. It is essential that all personnel working with the patient be aware of the desired hemodynamic and neurologic parameters set by the physician and that the physician be notified at the first sign of any changes.

Complications. The patient with a cerebrovascular accident should be monitored closely for signs of bleeding, vasospasm, and increased intracranial pressure. Other complications of stroke include aspiration, malnutrition, pneumonia, deep vein thrombosis, pulmonary embolism, decubitus ulcers, contractures, and joint abnormalities.[18] Nursing measures to prevent these complications are well-known.

Additional complications that may be seen in the patient with a cerebrovascular accident are related to the area of the brain that has been damaged. Damage to the temporoparietal area can create a variety of disturbances that affect the patient's ability to interpret sensory information.[32] Damage to the dominant hemisphere (usually left) produces problems with speech and language and abstract and analytical skills. Damage to the nondominant hemisphere (usually right) produces problems with spatial relationships. The resulting deficits include agnosia, apraxia, and visual field defects. Perceptual deficits are not as readily noticeable as are motor deficits, but they may be more

BOX 28-9 NURSING DIAGNOSIS AND MANAGEMENT

CEREBROVASCULAR ACCIDENT

- Decreased Adaptive Capacity: Intracranial related to failure of normal intracranial compensatory mechanisms, p. 843
- Altered Cerebral Tissue Perfusion related to vasospasm or hemorrhage, p. 842
- Acute Pain related to transmission and perception of cutaneous, visceral, muscular, or ischemic impulses, p. 197
- Unilateral Neglect related to perceptual disruption, p. 844
- Impaired Verbal Communication related to cerebral speech center injury, p. 845
- Impaired Swallowing related to neuromuscular impairment, fatigue, and limited awareness, p. 976
- Activity Intolerance related to prolonged immobility or deconditioning, p. 597
- Risk for Aspiration, p. 727
- Risk for Infection, p. 1119
- Anxiety related to threat of biologic, psychologic, and/or social integrity, p. 99
- Body Image Disturbance related to actual change in body structure, function, or appearance, p. 87
- Ineffective Family Coping related to critically ill family member, p. 97
- Knowledge Deficit: Discharge Regimen related to lack of previous exposure to information, p. 61 (see Patient Education Box 28-10.)

BOX 28-10 PATIENT EDUCATION

CEREBROVASCULAR ACCIDENT

- Pathophysiology of disease
- Specific etiology
- Risk factor modification
- Importance of taking medications
- Activities of daily living
- Measures to prevent injuries of impaired limbs
- Measures to compensate for residual deficits
- Basic rehabilitation techniques
- Importance of participating in neurologic rehabilitation program and/or support group

debilitating and can lead to the inability to perform skilled or purposeful tasks.[33] In addition, the patient may develop impaired swallowing.[34]

Bleeding and vasospasm. In the patient with a cerebral aneurysm, sudden onset of or an increase in headache, nausea and vomiting, increased BP, and changes in respiration herald the onset of rebleeding. The first indication of vasospasm is usually the appearance of new focal or global neurologic deficits. SAH precautions must be implemented to prevent any stress or straining that could potentially precipitate rebleeding. Precautions include bedrest; a dark, quiet environment, and stool softeners. Short-acting analgesics and sedatives are used to relieve pain and anxiety. The patient must be kept calm. Limb restraints cause straining and must be avoided. If restraint is necessary, only a vest or jacket type of restraint is used. The head of the bed should be elevated to 35 to 45 degrees at all times. The patient is taught to avoid any activities that create the Valsalva maneuver, such as pushing with the legs to move up in bed, straining for a bowel movement, or holding his or her breath during procedures or discomfort. Deep vein thrombosis precautions are routinely implemented. Historically, family visitation has been limited, but with the vast research available documenting the benefit of family visitation, the nurse must develop an individualized visitation plan to meet the needs of each patient. Often, family members at the bedside can assist the patient to remain calm.

Increased intracranial pressure. There are numerous signs and symptoms of increased ICP. These include decreased level of consciousness; Cushing's triad (bradycardia, systolic hypertension, and bradypnea); diminished brainstem reflexes; papilledema; decerebrate posturing (abnormal extension); decorticate posturing (abnormal flexion); unequal pupil size; projectile vomiting; decreased pupillary response to light; altered breathing patterns; and headache.[35] (∞Management of Intracranial Hypertension, p. 808.)

Damage to nondominant hemisphere. Patients with nondominant hemispheric pathologic conditions may exhibit emotional lability, with periods of euphoria, impulsiveness, and inattention. A short attention span, lack of insight, and poor judgment may lead to injuries as the patient attempts to perform activities beyond his or her capabilities. In addition, these patients may suffer from agnosia, visual field defects, and apraxia.

Agnosia. Agnosia is a disturbance in the perception of familiar sensory (verbal, tactile, visual) information. Unilateral neglect is a form of agnosia characterized by an unawareness or denial of the affected half of the body. This denial may range from inattention to refusing to acknowledge a paralysis by neglecting the involved side of the body or by denying ownership of the side, attributing the paralyzed arm or leg to someone else. This neglect also may extend to extrapersonal space. This defect most often results from right hemispheric brain damage that causes left hemiplegia.[33,36]

A variety of other types of agnosia exist in addition to unilateral neglect. Some patients are unable to recognize objects visually (visual object agnosia), whereas others cannot recognize faces (prosopagnosia) and may have to rely on the voice or characteristic mannerisms of a familiar person to identify that person. Tactile agnosia is a perceptual disorder in which a patient is unable to recognize by touch alone an object that has been placed in his or her hand. This may occur even in the presence of an intact sense of touch. If allowed to see or hear the object, the patient usually recognizes it.[32,33]

Spatial orientation is also affected, resulting in interference with the patient's ability to judge position, distance, movement, form, and the relationship of his or her body parts to surrounding objects. Patients may confuse concepts such as up and down and forward and backward. They may have difficulty following a route from one place to another and may even get lost in areas that were once familiar. Stroke patients may also experience reading and writing problems related to visual perception and visuospatial deficits. One type of spatial dyslexia is related to unilateral spatial neglect. The patient may not look at the beginning of a line of written material that appears on the left. Instead the patient fixes attention on a point to the right of the beginning of the line and reads to the end of the line. If asked to draw a design, the person completes only half a design or drawing.[36]

Visual field defects. Visual field defects may accompany agnosia, although they do not cause it. A hemispheric lesion can interrupt the visual pathways, with the resulting visual defect dependent on the location and extent of the lesion. At the optic chiasm, nerve fibers coming from the nasal half of each retina cross to the opposite side, whereas fibers coming from the temporal half of each retina do not cross. This partial crossing allows binocular vision. In the optic chiasm, fibers from the nasal half of each retina join the uncrossed fibers from the temporal half of the retina to form the optic tract. Impulses conducted to the right hemisphere by the right optic tract represent the left field of vision, and those conducted to the left hemisphere by the left optic tract represent the right field of vision. Optic radiations extend back to the occipital lobes. Visual defects restricted to a single field, right or left, are termed *homonymous hemianopsia.*[34]

The nurse may be the first person to detect that the patient has this defect. The patient with hemianopsia may neglect all sensory input from the affected side and initially may appear unresponsive if approached from the affected side. If the nurse approaches the patient from the healthy side, the patient actually may be quite alert. Another clue to hemianopsia is observing that the patient eats food only from one half of the tray.[33] Hemianopsia may recede gradually with time. Many patients can learn to scan their environment visually to compensate for the defect, although in the acute stage of stroke the patient may be too lethargic to follow instructions in methods of visual scanning. This visual defect can lead to fear and confusion and present a risk to the patient's safety.[34]

Apraxia. Lesions in the parietal lobe, as well as in other cortical structures, can result in apraxia, an inability to perform a learned movement voluntarily. Even though the patient may understand the task to be performed and may have intact motor ability, he or she is unable to perform the task and often fumbles and makes mistakes. The patient suffering from dressing apraxia, for example, may not be able to orient clothing in space, becoming tangled in his or her clothes when attempting to dress.[32,33]

Damage to dominant hemisphere. Damage to the dominant hemisphere produces problems with speech and language. Impaired communication is a condition that results from a patient's difficulty in expressing and exchanging thoughts, ideas, or desires. The posterior temporoparietal area contains the receptive speech center known as *Wernicke's area.* The center for the perception of written language lies anterior to the visuoreceptive areas. Located at the base of the frontal lobe's motor strip and slightly anterior to it is Broca's area, also known as the *motor speech center.* These sensory and motor areas are connected by a large bundle of nerve fibers. Rather than receptive and motor language functions being entirely within discrete areas, it is believed that language is an integrated sensorimotor process, roughly located in these areas in the dominant cerebral hemisphere. It also is recognized that the elaborately complex functions of speech and language depend on other associative areas of the cerebrum and their thalamic connections. Consequently there is much inconsistency in the degree of communication impairment among patients with lesions located in the same area of the brain.[37]

Aphasia is a loss of language abilities caused by brain injury, usually to the dominant hemisphere. It involves more than just understanding speech or expressing oneself through verbal means. Language is a much broader term, referring to what the individual is attempting to interpret or convey through listening, speaking, reading, writing, and gesturing. Most cases of aphasia are partial, rather than complete. The severity of the disorder depends on the area and the extent of the cerebral damage.[37]

Receptive aphasia. Receptive aphasia, also referred to as *sensory, Wernicke's,* or *fluent aphasia,* occurs when the connection between the primary auditory cortex in the temporal lobe and the angular gyrus in the parietal lobe is destroyed. The patient's comprehension of speech is impaired, but he or she can still talk if the motor area for speech, Broca's area, is intact. The patient may in fact talk excessively, with many errors in the use of words. The patient is able to hear the examiner but cannot comprehend what is being said and cannot repeat the examiner's words. Such patients may talk nonsense, with rambling speech that gives little information. Patients with receptive aphasia also cannot read words, although they can see them.[37]

Expressive aphasia. Expressive aphasia, also known as *motor, Broca's,* or *nonfluent aphasia,* is primarily a deficit in language output or speech production. Depending on the lesion's size and exact location, a wide variation in the motor deficit can result. Expressive aphasia can range from a mild dysarthria (imperfect articulation as a result of weakness or lack of coordination of speech musculature) to incorrect tonation and phrasing, and, in its most severe form, to complete loss of ability to communicate through verbal and written means. In this severe form of aphasia, there also is a loss of ability to communicate through conventional gestures, such as nodding or shaking the head for "yes" or "no." In most cases of expressive aphasia, the muscles of articulation are intact. If speech is possible at all, occasionally the words "yes" or "no" are uttered, sometimes appropriately. In some cases the words of well-known songs may be sung. Other patients, when excited or angered, may utter expletives. Some patients with expressive aphasia struggle or hesitate in trying to express words. They struggle to form words while using motor musculature (verbal apraxia), an articulatory disorder that is a feature of some expressive types of aphasia. All these difficulties lead to exasperation and despair for the patient. Most patients with expressive aphasia also have severely impaired writing ability. Even though penmanship may be intact, they are unable to express themselves through writing—a deficit termed *agraphia.* If the right hand is paralyzed, as is often the case, the patient still cannot write or print with the left hand.[37] In the recovery phase of severe expressive aphasia, patients become able to speak aloud to some degree, although words are uttered slowly and laboriously. Many patients, however, are able to learn to communicate ideas to some extent.

Global aphasia. Global aphasia results when a massive lesion affects both the motor and sensory speech areas. The patient is unable to transform sounds into words and is unable to comprehend spoken words. All language modalities are affected, and impairment may be so severe that the patient may be unable to communicate on any level. These patients generally have severe hemiplegia and also homonymous hemianopsia. In these patients, language function rarely recovers to a significant degree unless the lesion is caused by some transient disorder, such as cerebral edema or a metabolic derangement.[37]

Impaired swallowing. Normal swallowing occurs in four phases that are controlled by the cranial nerves. Damage to the brain, brainstem, or cranial nerves can result in a variety of swallowing deficits that can place the patient at risk for aspiration. The stroke patient is observed for signs of dysphagia including drooling; difficulty handling oral secretions; absence of gag, cough, or swallowing reflexes; moist, gurgly voice quality; decreased mouth and tongue movements; and the presence of dysarthria. A speech therapy consult is initiated if any of these signs are present and the patient must not be orally fed. In the absence of these warning signs, the patient may be fed, as ordered by the physician, though he or she must be continually monitored for signs of aspiration.[38]

Patient Education

Rehabilitation starts in the critical care area, with a multidisciplinary team designing and implementing an individualized plan for maximizing the patient's potential for neurologic rehabilitation. Early in the patient's hospital stay, the patient and family must be taught about cerebrovascular accident, its etiologies, and its treatment. As the patient moves toward discharge, teaching focuses on the interventions necessary for preventing the reoccurrence of the event and on maximizing the patient's rehabilitation potential. The patient's family must be encouraged to participate in the patient's care; learn how to feed, dress, and bathe the patient; and learn some basic rehabilitation techniques. In addition, the importance of participating in a neurologic rehabilitation program and/or a support group must be stressed (see Box 28-10).

GUILLAIN-BARRÉ SYNDROME

Description

Guillain-Barré syndrome (GBS), also known as *Landry-Guillain-Barré syndrome,* is an inflammatory peripheral polyneuritis characterized by a rapidly progressive, ascending peripheral nerve dysfunction leading to paralysis. It is 90% to 100% reversible and is one of the most common peripheral nervous system diseases. Because of the need for ventilatory support, GBS is one of the few peripheral neurologic diseases that necessitates a critical care environment.

The annual incidence of GBS is 1.6 to 1.9 per 100,000 persons. It occurs equally in males and females and is the most commonly acquired demyelinating neuropathy.[39] The incidence of GBS increased slightly for a period after the 1977 swine flu vaccinations.[40]

GBS falls under a variety of different DRGs, depending on whether the patient develops comorbid conditions (CC) or the need for continuous ventilatory support. DRG 18 (Cranial and peripheral nerve disorders with CC) or DRG 19 (Cranial and peripheral nerve disorders without CC) are usually used and have average lengths of stay of 6.4 days and 4.5 days, respectively. If the patient requires mechanical ventilation or a tracheostomy, DRG 475 (Respiratory system diagnosis with ventilator support) or DRG 483 (Tracheostomy except for face, mouth, and neck diagnoses) are used, with anticipated lengths of stay of 12.3 days and 46.4 days, respectively.[5]

Etiology

The cause of GBS is unknown, but more than 60% of patients report a viral infection 2 to 4 weeks before the onset of clinical manifestations. The result is a possible autoimmune response of the peripheral nervous system.[41]

Pathophysiology

This disease affects the motor and sensory pathways of the peripheral nervous system, as well as the autonomic nervous system functions of the cranial nerves. The major finding in GBS is a segmental demyelination process of the peripheral nerves. GBS is believed to be an autoimmune response to antibodies formed against a recent viral illness, usually upper respiratory or gastrointestinal. T-cells migrate to the peripheral nerves, resulting in edema and inflammation. Macrophages then invade the area and break down the myelin.[42] Inflammation around this demyelinated area causes further dysfunction.[41]

The myelin sheath of the peripheral nerves is generated by Schwann's cells and acts as an insulator for the peripheral nerve. Myelin promotes rapid conduction of nerve impulses by allowing the impulses to jump along the nerve via nodes of Ranvier. Disruption of the myelin fiber slows and may eventually stop the conduction of impulses along the peripheral nerves. In GBS, the more thickly myelinated fibers of motor pathways and the cranial nerves are more severely affected than are the thinly myelinated sensory fibers of cutaneous pain, touch, and temperature.[42]

Once the temporary inflammatory reaction stops, myelin-producing cells begin the process of reinsulating the demyelinated portions of the peripheral nervous system. When remyelination occurs, normal neurologic function should return. In some instances the axon may be damaged during the inflammatory process. The degree of axonal damage is responsible for the degree of neurologic dysfunction that persists after recovery.[41]

Assessment and Diagnosis

Symptoms of GBS include motor weakness; paresthesias and other sensory changes; cranial nerve dysfunction (especially oculomotor, facial, glossopharyngeal, vagal, spinal accessory, and hypoglossal); and some autonomic dysfunction. The usual course of GBS begins with an abrupt onset of lower extremity weakness that progresses to flaccidity and ascends over a period of hours to days. Motor loss usually is symmetric, bilateral, and ascending. In the most severe cases, complete flaccidity of all peripheral nerves, including spinal and cranial nerves, occurs.[42]

Admission to the hospital occurs when lower extremity weakness prevents mobility. Admission to the critical care unit occurs when progression of the weakness threatens respiratory muscles. As the patient's weakness progresses, close observation is essential. Frequent assessment of the respiratory system, including ventilatory parameters such as inspiratory force and tidal volume, is necessary. The most common cause of death in patients with GBS is from respiratory arrest. As the disease progresses and respiratory effort weakens, intubation and mechanical ventilation are necessary. Continued, frequent assessment of neurologic deterioration is required until the patient reaches the peak of the disease and plateau occurs.[41]

The diagnosis of GBS is based on clinical findings plus CSF analysis and nerve conduction studies. CSF analysis demonstrates a normal protein initially, which elevates in the fourth to sixth week. No other changes in CSF occur. Nerve conduction studies that test the velocity at which nerve impulses are conducted show significant reduction, as the demyelinating process of the disease suggests.[41]

Medical Management

With no curative treatment available, the medical management of GBS is limited. The disease simply must run its course, which is characterized by ascending paralysis that advances over 1 to 3 weeks and then remains at a plateau for several weeks. The plateau stage is followed by descending paralysis and return to normal or near-normal function. The main focus of medical management is the support of bodily functions and the prevention of complications.[41]

Plasmapheresis is often used in an attempt to limit the severity and duration of the syndrome. Plasmapheresis involves plasma exchanges or washes that remove the antibodies that cause GBS. Exchanges are given over 10 to 15 days.[43] Controversy exists over the benefit of plasmapheresis. It is contraindicated in patients with hemodynamic instability. In a recently published study of 220 patients in a multicenter clinical trial, the long-term benefit of plasmapheresis demonstrated that 71% of the treatment group versus 52% of the control group had full muscular strength recovery at 1 year.[44] Research suggests that intravenous immunoglobulin may have beneficial effects in treating GBS. A recent large multicenter randomized trial has demonstrated promising results.[45] Immunoglobulin is a blood product; close monitoring during its administration and during plasmapheresis is necessary. Some physicians support the use of steroids for their antiinflammatory effect, though their effectiveness remains unclear.

Nursing management. The nursing management of the patient with GBS incorporates a variety of nursing diagnoses and interventions (Box 28-11). The goal of nursing management is to support all normal body functions until the patient can do so on his or her own. Although the condition is reversible, the patient with GBS requires extensive long-term care, because recovery can be a long process. Nursing management focuses on immobility, nutritional support, pain management, and psychological support.

In patients with GBS, immobility may last for months. The usual course of GBS involves an average of 10 days of symptom progression and 10 days of maximum level of dysfunction, followed by 2 to 48 weeks of recovery. Although GBS is usually completely reversible, the patient will require physical and occupational rehabilitation because of the problems of long-term immobility. Rehabilitation starts in the critical care area, with a multidisciplinary team designing and implementing an individualized plan for maximizing the patient's potential for rehabilitation.

Nutritional support is implemented early in the course of the disease. Because GBS recovery is a long process, adequate nutritional support will be a problem for an extended period. Nutritional support usually is accomplished through the use of enteral feeding, which is preferable to the use of total parenteral nutrition because it is less invasive and

BOX 28-11 NURSING DIAGNOSIS AND MANAGEMENT

GUILLAIN-BARRÉ SYNDROME

- Ineffective Breathing Pattern related to musculoskeletal fatigue or neuromuscular impairment, p. 724
- Acute Pain related to transmission and perception of cutaneous, visceral, muscular, or ischemic impulses, p. 197
- Activity Intolerance related to prolonged immobility or deconditioning, p. 597
- Risk for Aspiration, p. 727
- Altered Nutrition: Less than Body Requirements related to lack of exogenous nutrients or increased metabolic demand, p. 165
- Risk for Infection, p. 1119
- Anxiety related to threat to biologic, psychologic, and/or social integrity, p. 99
- Powerlessness related to lack of control over current situation or disease progression, p. 89
- Ineffective Individual Coping related to situational crisis and personal vulnerability, p. 95
- Ineffective Family Coping related to critically ill family member, p. 97
- Knowledge Deficit: Discharge Regimen related to lack of previous exposure to information, p. 61 (see Patient Education Box 28-12.)

BOX 28-12 PATIENT EDUCATION

GUILLAIN-BARRÉ SYNDROME

- Pathophysiology of disease
- Importance of taking medications
- Measures to compensate for residual deficits
- Basic rehabilitation techniques
- Importance of participating in neurologic rehabilitation program (if necessary)

reduces the risk of infection in a patient who is highly vulnerable.

Pain control is another important component in the care of the patient with GBS. Although patients may have minimal to no motor function, most sensory functions remain, causing patients considerable muscle ache and pain. Because of the length of this illness, a safe, effective, long-term solution to pain management must be identified (∞Pain Management, p. 180.)

These patients also require extensive psychological support. Although the illness is almost 100% reversible, lack of control over the situation, constant pain or discomfort, and the long-term nature of the disorder create coping difficulties for the patient. GBS does not affect the level of consciousness or cerebral function. Patient interaction and communication are essential elements of the nursing management plan.

Patient Education

Early in the patient's hospital stay, the patient and family must be taught about GBS and its different treatments. As the patient moves toward discharge, teaching focuses on the interventions to maximize the patient's rehabilitation potential. The patient's family must be encouraged to participate in the patient's care and to learn some basic rehabilitation techniques. In addition, the importance of participating in a neurologic rehabilitation program (if necessary) must be stressed (see Box 28-12).

CRANIOTOMY

Types of Surgery

A craniotomy is performed to gain access to portions of the CNS inside the cranium, usually to allow removal of a space-occupying lesion. Common procedures include tumor resection or removal, cerebral decompression, evacuation of hematoma or abscess, and clipping or removal of an aneurysm or arteriovenous malformation. Box 28-13 provides definitions of common neurosurgical terms. This section provides a generalized discussion of craniotomy care.

Most patients who undergo craniotomy for tumor resection or removal do not require care in a critical care unit. Those who do usually need intensive monitoring or are at greater risk of complications because of underlying cardiopulmonary dysfunction or the surgical approach used. One common procedure requiring routine postoperative care in the critical care unit is hypophysectomy or pituitary adenomectomy using either a transcranial or transsphenoidal approach (Figure 28-3).

BOX 28-13 Operative Terms

Term	Definition
Burr hole	Hole made into the cranium using a special drill
Craniotomy	Surgical opening of the skull
Craniectomy	Removal of a portion of the skull without replacing it
Cranioplasty	Plastic repair of the skull
Supratentorial	Above the tentorium, separating the cerebrum from the cerebellum
Infratentorial	Below the tentorium; includes the brainstem and the cerebellum; an infratentorial surgical approach may be used for temporal or occipital lesions

Preoperative Care

Protection of the integrity of the CNS is a major priority of care for the patient awaiting a craniotomy. Optimal arterial oxygenation, hemodynamic stability, and cerebral perfusion are essential to maintaining adequate cerebral oxygenation. Management of seizure activity is essential to controlling metabolic needs.

Detailed assessment and documentation of the patient's preoperative neurologic status are imperative for accurate postoperative evaluation. Specific attention is placed on identifying and describing the nature and extent of any preoperative neurologic deficits. (∞Neurologic Clinical Assessment, p. 763.)

Current trends in health care demand judicious use of routine preoperative studies. Depending on the type of surgery to be performed and the general health of the patient, preoperative screening may include a complete blood count (CBC), blood urea nitrogen (BUN), creatinine, fasting blood sugar (FBS), chest x-ray, and electrocardiogram. A type and crossmatch for blood may also be ordered.

Preoperative teaching is necessary to prepare both the patient and family for what to expect in the postoperative period. A description of the intravascular lines and intracranial catheters used during the postoperative period allows the family to focus on the patient, rather than be overwhelmed by masses of tubing. Some or all of the patient's hair is shaved off in the operating room and a large, bulky, turban-like craniotomy dressing is applied. Most patients experience some degree of postoperative eye or facial swelling and perior-

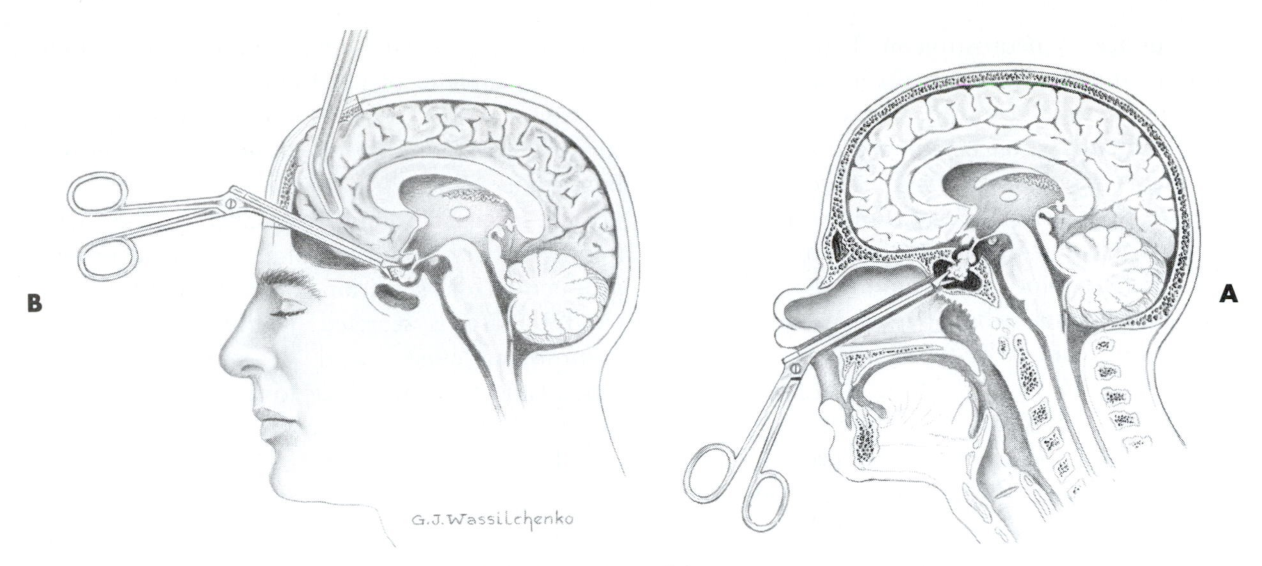

FIGURE 28-3. Hypophysectomy. **A,** Transcranial. **B,** Transsphenoidal.

bital ecchymosis. An explanation of these temporary changes in appearance helps alleviate the shock and fear many patients and families experience in the immediate postoperative period.

All craniotomy patients require instruction to avoid activities known to produce sudden changes in intracranial pressure. These activities include bending, lifting, straining, and avoiding the Valsalva maneuver. Patients commonly elicit the Valsalva maneuver during repositioning in bed by holding their breath and straining with a closed epiglottis. Teaching the patient to continue to breathe deeply through the mouth during all position changes is an effective deterrent.

The patient undergoing transsphenoidal surgery requires preparation for the sensations associated with nasal packing. The patient often awakens with alarm because of the inability to breathe through the nose. Preoperative instruction in mouth breathing and avoidance of coughing, sneezing, or blowing of the nose facilitates postoperative cooperation.[45]

The psychosocial issues associated with the prospect of neurosurgery cannot be overemphasized. Few procedures are as threatening as those involving the brain or spinal cord. For some patients the fear of permanent neurologic impairment may be as or more ominous than the fear of death. Steps to meet the needs of the patient, as well as the family, include collaboration with clergy and social services personnel, patient controlled visitation, and provision of as much privacy as the patient's condition permits. Both the patient and the family must be provided with the opportunity to express their fears and concerns apart from each other as well as jointly.

Surgical Considerations

While the emphasis in surgical approach for most other types of surgery is to gain adequate exposure of the surgical site, the neurosurgeon must select a route that also produces the least amount of disruption to the intracranial contents. Neural tissue is unforgiving. A significant portion of neurologic trauma and postoperative deficits is related to the surgical pathway through the brain tissue, rather than to the procedure performed at the site of pathology. Depending on the location of the lesion and the surgical route decided upon, either a transcranial or a transsphenoidal approach is used to open the skull.

Transcranial. In the transcranial approach a scalp incision is made and a series of burr holes are drilled into the skull to form an outline of the area to be opened. A special saw is then used to cut between the holes. In most cases the bone flap is left attached to the muscle to create a hinge effect. In some cases the bone flap is removed completely and either placed in the abdomen for later retrieval and implantation or discarded and replaced with synthetic material. Next the dura is opened and retracted. After the intracranial procedure, the dura and the bone flap are closed, the muscles and scalp are sutured, and a turban-like dressing is applied.[26]

Transsphenoidal. The transsphenoidal approach is the technique of choice for removal of a pituitary tumor without extension into the intracranial vault.[46] This approach involves making a microsurgical entrance into the cranial vault via the nasal cavity. An otorhinolaryngologist performs the necessary steps to enter the sphenoid sinus and reach the anterior wall of the sella turcica. A neurosurgeon then opens the sphenoid bone and the dura to gain intracranial access. After removal of the tumor, the surgical bed is packed with a small section of adipose tissue grafted from the patient's abdomen or thigh. After closure of the intranasal structures, the otorhinolaryngologist places nasal splints and soft packing or nasal tampons impregnated with antibiotic ointment in the nasal cavities. Occasionally, epistaxis balloons are used instead. A nasal drip pad or mustache-type dressing is placed at the base of the nose to catch surgical drainage.[46]

The patient may be placed in a supine, prone, or even sitting position for a craniotomy procedure. A skull clamp connected to skull pins is used to position and secure the patient's head throughout the surgery. During a transsphenoidal approach or a transcranial approach into the infratentorial area, the patient's head is elevated during the surgery. This position places the patient at risk for an air embolism. Air can enter the vascular system either through the edges of the dura or a venous opening. Continuous monitoring of the patient's heart sounds by Doppler signal allows immediate recognition of this complication. If it occurs, an attempt may be made to withdraw the embolus from the right atrium through a central line. An immediate barrier to any further air entrance is created by flooding the surgical field with irrigation fluid and placing a moistened sterile surgical sponge over the surgical site.[26,46]

Several other procedures are used intraoperatively during a craniotomy to either facilitate the surgery or to prevent surgical complications. Hypothermia is used to decrease the metabolic needs of the brain. Controlled hypotension lessens blood loss during resection of an AVM or cerebral aneurysm. Hyperventilation is used to reduce the size or bulk of the brain through reduction in cerebral blood flow.[26]

Complications and Medical Management

Complications associated with a craniotomy include intracranial hypertension, surgical hemorrhage, fluid imbalance, CSF leak, deep vein thrombosis, gastric stress ulceration, and pulmonary infection.

Intracranial hypertension. Postcraniotomy management of intracranial hypertension is usually accomplished through CSF drainage, hyperventilation, patient positioning, and steroid administration. (∞Management of Intracranial Hypertension, p. 826.)

Surgical hemorrhage. Surgical hemorrhage after a transcranial procedure can occur in the intracranial vault and is manifested by signs and symptoms of increasing ICP. Hemorrhage after a transsphenoidal craniotomy may be evident from external drainage, patient complaint of persistent postnasal drip, or excessive swallowing. Postoperative hemorrhage requires surgical reexploration. (∞Assessment of Intracranial Pressure, p. 821.)

Fluid imbalance. Fluid imbalance in the postcraniotomy patient usually results from a disturbance in production or secretion of antidiuretic hormone (ADH). ADH is secreted by the posterior pituitary (neurohypophysis) gland. It stimulates the renal tubules and collecting ducts to retain water in response to low circulating blood volume or increased serum osmolality. Inoperative trauma or postoperative edema of the pituitary gland or hypothalamus can result in insufficient ADH secretion. The outcome is unabated renal water loss even when blood volume is low and serum osmolality is high. This condition is known as *diabetes insipidus (DI)*. The polyuria associated with DI is often greater than 200 ml/hour. Urine specific gravity of 1.005 or less and elevated serum osmolality provide evidence of insufficient ADH. The loss of volume may produce hypotension and inadequate cerebral perfusion. DI is usually self-limiting, with fluid replacement being the only necessary therapy. In some cases, however, it may be necessary to administer vasopressin intravenously once or twice a day to control the loss of fluid.[47] (∞Diabetes Insipidus, p. 1021.)

The syndrome of inappropriate antidiuretic hormone (SIADH) commonly occurs with neurologic insult and results from excessive ADH secretion.[47] SIADH is manifested by inappropriate water retention with hyponatremia in the presence of normal renal function. Urine specific gravity is elevated and urine osmolality is greater than serum osmolality. The dangers associated with SIADH include circulating volume overload and electrolyte imbalance, both of which may impair neurologic functioning. SIADH is usually self-limiting, with the mainstay of treatment being fluid restriction.[47] (∞Syndrome of Inappropriate Antidiuretic Hormone, p. 1027.)

CSF leak. Leakage of CSF fluid results from an opening in the subarachnoid space, as evidenced by clear fluid draining from the surgical site. When this complication occurs after transsphenoidal surgery, it is evidenced by excessive, clear drainage from the nose or persistent postnasal drip. To differentiate CSF drainage from postoperative serous drainage, a specimen is tested for glucose content. A CSF leak is confirmed by glucose values of 30 mg/dL or greater. Management of the patient with a CSF leak includes bedrest and head elevation. Lumbar puncture or placement of a lumbar subarachnoid catheter may be used to reduce CSF pressure until the dura heals. Rarely, surgical reexploration is necessary.

Deep vein thrombosis. Deep vein thrombosis (DVT) has been reported to occur in 29% to 46% of all neurosurgical patients, as compared with a 25% incidence in general surgical patients. The risk is greater after removal of a supratentorial tumor and is increased twofold for patients whose surgery lasts for more than 4 hours.[48] Clinical manifestations of DVT include leg or calf pain, edema, localized tenderness, and pain with dorsiflexion or plantar flexion (Homan's sign). Unfortunately the patient with a DVT is often asymptomatic and the diagnosis is not made until the patient experiences a pulmonary embolus. (∞Pulmonary Embolus, p. 668.)

The primary treatment for DVT is prophylaxis. Graduated elastic stockings and sequential pneumatic compression boots or stockings have been demonstrated to be effective in reducing the incidence of DVT. These devices are commonly used in the care of the neurosurgical patient, either alone or in combination. Effectiveness is enhanced when these devices are initiated in the preoperative period.[48,49] Low-dose heparin may also be used prophylactically in high risk patients. Recent evidence suggests that a combination of pneumatic compression therapy applied in the operating room and postoperative low-dose heparin is both safe and effective in preventing DVT in the neurosurgical patient.[50]

If a DVT develops in the postcraniotomy patient, the physician must weigh the risk of therapeutic heparinization versus the risk of pulmonary embolus (PE). There is evidence that a DVT in the distal circulation below the knee carries a much lower risk of PE than a DVT in the proximal circulation.[47] Even when a PE occurs, the use of therapeutic heparin doses in the neurosurgical patient is controversial.[49]

Stress ulcers. Historically, stress ulcers have been a common complication in neurosurgical patients, especially in those requiring long-term mechanical ventilation. Effective prophylactic measures for this complication include intravenous histamine$_2$ antagonists and early enteral feeding. (∞Stress Ulcers, p. 945.)

Pneumonia. The risk of pneumonia in the postoperative craniotomy patient is significantly increased if the patient remains in the critical care unit for more than 5 days because of prolonged intubation.[47] Adequate pulmonary hygiene and strict infection control measures are helpful to prevent this complication. Treatment consists of antibiotics and appropriate pulmonary management. Acute respiratory distress syndrome and neurogenic pulmonary edema may also occur in the postcraniotomy patient, possibly related to intracranial hypertension. (∞Pneumonia, p. 663.)

Numerous other complications may also occur after a craniotomy. Focal or grand mal seizure activity is common and is managed prophylactically with anticonvulsant therapy. Postoperative meningitis may result from surgical infection or CSF leak and is treated with antibiotics.[47] Cranial nerve dysfunction may occur either transiently or permanently as a result of surgical manipulation, edema, or anatomic disruption.[51] Compression of the optic chiasm with complete or partial visual loss may result from migration of the adipose tissue packing placed in a pituitary tumor bed and requires surgical reexploration.[46]

Postoperative Nursing Management

Types of agents used in routine postoperative drug therapy are listed in Box 28-14. As in preoperative care, the primary goal of postcraniotomy nursing management is protection of the integrity of the CNS. Maintenance of cerebral oxygenation is accomplished through preservation of adequate cerebral perfusion, arterial oxygenation, and hemodynamic stability. Frequent neurologic assessment is necessary to evaluate accomplishment of this objective and to identify and quickly intervene if complications do arise. Often a ventriculostomy is placed to facilitate ICP monitoring and/or CSF drainage.

Postoperative cerebral edema may be expected to peak 48 to 72 hours after surgery. If the bone flap is not replaced at the time of surgery, intracranial hypertension will produce bulging at the surgical site. Close monitoring of the surgical site is important so that integrity of the incision can be maintained.

Patient positioning is an important component of care for the craniotomy patient. The head of the bed should be elevated 30 to 45 degrees at all times to reduce the incidence of hemorrhage, facilitate venous drainage, and control ICP. Other positioning measures to control ICP include maintaining the patient's head in a neutral position at all times and avoiding neck or hip flexion. It is vital to adhere to these rules of positioning throughout all nursing activities, including linen changes and transporting the patient for diagnostic evaluation.

Most craniotomy patients can still be turned from side to side within these restrictions, using pillows for support, except in some cases of extensive tumor removal, cranioplasty, and when the bone flap is not replaced. Specific orders from the surgeon must be obtained in these instances. The patient with an infratentorial incision may be restricted to only a very

BOX 28-14 Postoperative Drug Therapy

- Anticonvulsants
- Antibiotics
- Histamine$_2$ antagonists
- Analgesics
- Corticosteroids
- Antiemetics
- Antipyretics
- Neuromuscular blocking agents and sedatives (rare)

small pillow under the head to prevent strain on the incision. Avoidance of anterior or lateral neck flexion also protects the integrity of this type of incision.

Routine pulmonary care is used to maintain airway clearance and prevent pulmonary complications. To prevent dangerous elevations in ICP, this care must be performed using proper technique and at time intervals that are adequately spaced from other patient care activities. If pulmonary complications do arise, consideration must be given to maintaining adequate oxygenation during repositioning. It may be necessary to restrict turning to only the side that places the good lung down.

Care of the incision and surgical dressings is institution- and physician-specific. The rule of thumb for a craniotomy dressing is to reinforce it as needed and change it only with a physician's order. Often times a drain is left in place to facilitate decompression of the surgical site. If a ventriculostomy is present, it is treated as a component of the surgical site. All drainage devices must be secured to the dressing to prevent unintentional displacement with patient movement. Sterile technique is required to prevent infection and resultant meningitis.

Fluid management is another important component of postcraniotomy care. Hourly monitoring of fluid intake and output facilitates early identification of fluid imbalance. Urine specific gravity must be measured if DI is suspected. Fluid restriction may be ordered as a routine measure to lessen the severity of cerebral edema or as treatment for the fluid and electrolyte imbalances associated with SIADH.

Pain management in the postcraniotomy patient primarily involves control of headache. Small doses of intravenous morphine may be used in the intensive care setting. As soon as oral analgesics can be tolerated, acetaminophen with codeine is used. Both of these analgesics cause constipation. Administration of stool softeners and initiation of a bowel program are important components of postcraniotomy care. Constipation is hazardous, because straining to have a bowel movement can create significant elevations in blood pressure and ICP. (∞Pain Management, p. 180.)

Postoperative vomiting must be avoided to prevent sharp spikes in ICP and possibly surgical hemorrhage. Antiemetics are administered as soon as nausea is apparent. The patient is usually given nothing by mouth for at least 24 hours; then the diet is progressed as tolerated.

Postoperative fever may also adversely affect ICP and increase the metabolic needs of the brain. Acetaminophen is administered either orally, rectally, or via a feeding tube. External cooling measures, such as a hypothermia blanket, may also be necessary.

Routine eye care may be necessary to prevent corneal drying and ulceration. Periorbital edema interferes with normal blinking and eyelid closure, which are essential to adequate corneal lubrication. Saline drops are instilled every 2 hours. If the patient remains in a coma state, the eyes must also be covered with a polyethylene film extending over the orbits and eyebrows.[10]

The postcraniotomy patient may also experience periods of altered mentation. Protection from injury may require use of restraint devices. The side rails of the bed must also be padded to protect the patient from injury. Having a family member stay at the bedside and/or use of music therapy is often helpful to keep the patient calm during periods of restlessness. In rare circumstances, neuromuscular blockade and sedation may be necessary to control patient activity and metabolic needs on a short-term basis.

Increased patient activity, including ambulation, is begun as soon as tolerated in the postoperative period. Rehabilitation measures and discharge planning may begin in the critical care unit, but are beyond the scope of this text. Transfer to a general care or rehabilitation unit is usually accomplished as soon as the patient is considered to be stable and without complication.

REFERENCES

1. Multi-Society Task Force on PVS: Medical aspects of the persistent vegetative state (first of two parts), *N Engl J Med* 330:1499, 1994.
2. Haerer AF: *DeJong's the neurologic examination,* ed 5, Philadelphia, 1992, JB Lippincott.
3. Sosnowski C, Ustik M: Early intervention: coma stimulation in the intensive care unit, *J Neurosci Nurs* 26:336, 1994.

4. Helwick LD: Stimulation programs for coma patients, *Crit Care Nurse* 14(4):47, 1994.
5. *St Anthony's DRG guidebook 1997,* Reston, Va, 1996, St Anthony Publishing.
6. Berger JR: Clinical approach to stupor and coma. In Bradley WG and others, editors: *Neurology in clinical practice: principles of diagnosis and management,* vol 1, ed 2, Boston, 1996, Butterworth-Heinemann.
7. Topel JL, Lewis SL: Examination of the comatose patient. In Weiner WE, Goetz CG, editors: *Neurology for the non-neurologist,* ed 3, Philadelphia, 1994, JB Lippincott.
8. Brust JCM: Coma. In Rowland LP, editor: *Merritt's textbook of neurology,* ed 9, Baltimore, 1995, Williams & Wilkins.
9. Snyder BD, Tulloch JW: Anoxic and ischemic encephalopathies. In Bradley WG and others, editors: *Neurology in clinical practice: principles of diagnosis and management,* vol 2, ed 2, Boston, 1996, Butterworth-Heinemann.
10. Cortese D, Capp L, McKinley S: Moisture chamber versus lubrication for the prevention of corneal epithelial breakdown, *Am J Crit Care* 4:425, 1995.
11. Jones R and others: Auditory stimulation effect on a comatose survivor of traumatic brain injury, *Arch Phys Med Rehabil* 75:164, 1994.
12. Multi-Society Task Force on PVS: Medical aspects of the persistent vegetative state (second of two parts), *N Engl J Med* 330:1572, 1994.
13. ANA Committee on Ethical Affairs: Persistent vegetative state: report of the American Neurological Association Committee on Ethical Affairs, *Ann Neurol* 33:386, 1993.
14. Bernat JL: Ethical issues in neurology. In Joynt RJ, editor: *Clinical neurology,* vol 1, Philadelphia, 1991, JB Lippincott.
15. Position of the American Academy of Neurology on certain aspects of the care and management of the persistent vegetative state patient: adopted by the Executive Board, American Academy of Neurology, April 1, 1988, Cincinnati, Ohio, *Neurology* 39:125, 1989.
16. Day L: Practical limits to the uniform determination of death act, *J Neurosci Nurs* 27:319, 1995.
17. Gwynn M: tPA in acute stroke—risk or reprieve? *J Neurosci Nurs* 25:180, 1993.
18. Adams HP and others: Guidelines for the management of patients with acute ischemic stroke: a statement for healthcare professionals from a special writing group of the Stroke Council, American Heart Association, *Circulation* 90:1588, 1994.
19. Sacco RL: Pathogenesis, classification, and epidemiology of cerebrovascular disease. In Rowland LP, editor: *Merritt's textbook of neurology,* ed 9, Baltimore, 1995, Williams & Wilkins.
20. Hart RG: Cardiogenic embolism to the brain, *Lancet* 339:589, 1992.
21. Camarata PJ, Heros RC, Latchaw RE: "Brain attack": the rationale for treating stroke as a medical emergency, *Neurosur* 34:144, 1994.
22. Mayberg MR and others: Guidelines for the management of aneurysmal subarachnoid hemorrhage: a statement for healthcare professionals from a special writing group of the Stroke Council, American Heart Association, *Circulation* 25:2315, 1994.
23. Rusy KL: Rebleeding and vasospasm after subarachnoid hemorrhage: a critical care challenge, *Crit Care Nurse* 16(1):41, 1996.
24. Hunt WE, Hess RM: Surgical risks as related to time of intervention in the repair of intracranial aneurysms, *J Neurosurg* 28:14, 1968.
25. Solenski NJ and others: Medical complications of aneurysmal subarachnoid hemorrhage: a report of the multicenter, cooperative aneurysm study, *Crit Care Med* 23:1007, 1995.
26. Hickey JV: *The clinical practice of neurological and neurosurgical nursing,* ed 3, Philadelphia, 1992, JB Lippincott.
27. Coleman R, Sifri-Steele P: Treatment of posterior circulation aneurysms using platinum coils, *J Neurosci Nurs* 26:367, 1994.
28. Guglielmi G and others: Carotid-cavernous fistula caused by a ruptured intracavernous aneurysm: endovascular treatment by electrothrombosis with detachable coils, *Neurosurgery* 31:591, 1992.
29. Findlay JM, Macdonald RL, Weir BK: Current concepts of pathophysiology and management of cerebral vasospasm following aneurysmal subarachnoid hemorrhage, *Cerebrovasc Brain Metab Rev* 3:336, 1991.
30. Counsell C, Gilbert M, Snively C: Nimodipine: a drug therapy for treatment of vasospasm, *J Neurosci Nurs* 27:54, 1995.
31. Grimes CM: Cerebral balloon angioplasty for treatment of vasospasm after subarachnoid hemorrhage, *Heart Lung* 20:431, 1991.
32. Olson E: Perceptual deficits affecting the stroke patient, *Rehabil Nurs* 16:213, 1991.
33. Baggerly J: Sensory perceptual problems following stroke: the "invisible" deficits, *Nurs Clin North Am* 26:997, 1991.
34. Phipps MA: Assessment of neurologic deficits in stroke: acute and rehabilitation implications, *Nurs Clin North Am* 26:957, 1991.
35. Wall BM, Philips JP, Howard JC: Validation of increased intracranial pressure and high risk of increased intracranial pressure, *Nurs Diagnosis* 5:74, 1994.
36. Kalbach LR: Unilateral neglect: mechanisms and nursing care, *J Neurosci Nurs* 23:125, 1991.
37. Boss BJ: Managing communication disorders in stroke, *Nurs Clin North Am* 26:985, 1991.
38. Baker DM: Assessment and management of impairments in swallowing, *Nurs Clin North Am* 28:793, 1993.
39. Lange DJ, Latov N, Trojaborg C: Acquired neuropathies. In Rowland LP, editor: *Merritt's textbook of neurology,* ed 9, Baltimore, 1995, Williams & Wilkins.
40. Keenlyside R, Brezman D: Fatal Guillain-Barré syndrome after the national influenza immunization program, *Neurology* 30:929, 1980.
41. Hund EF and others: Intensive management and treatment of severe Guillain-Barré syndrome, *Crit Care Med* 21:433, 1993.

42. Ross AP: Nursing interventions for persons receiving immunosuppressive therapies for demyelinating pathology, *Nurs Clin North Am* 28:829, 1993.
43. Murray DP: Impaired mobility: Guillain-Barré syndrome, *J Neurosci Nurs* 25:100, 1993.
44. French Cooperative Group on Plasma Exchange: Plasma exchange in Guillain-Barré syndrome: one year follow-up, *Ann Neurol* 32:94, 1992.
45. Chipps E, Skinner C: Intravenous immunoglobulin: implications for use in the neurological patient, *J Neurosci Nurs* 26:8, 1994.
46. McEwen DR: Transsphenoidal adenomectomy, *AORN J* 61:321, 1995.
47. Levin AB: Intensive care. In Wilkins RH, Rengachary SS, editors: *Neurosurgery,* ed 2, vol 1, New York, 1996, McGraw-Hill.
48. Powers SK, Maliner LI: Prevention and treatment of thromboembolic complications in neurosurgical patients. In Wilkins RH, Rengachary SS, editors: *Neurosurgery,* ed 2, vol 1, New York, 1996, McGraw-Hill.
49. Fowler SB: Deep vein thrombosis and pulmonary emboli in neuroscience patients, *J Neurosci Nurs* 27:224, 1995.
50. Frim DM and others: Postoperative low-dose heparin decreases thromboembolic complications in neurosurgical patients, *Neurosurgery* 30:830, 1992.
51. Geary SM: Nursing management of cranial nerve dysfunction, *J Neurosci Nurs* 27:102, 1995.

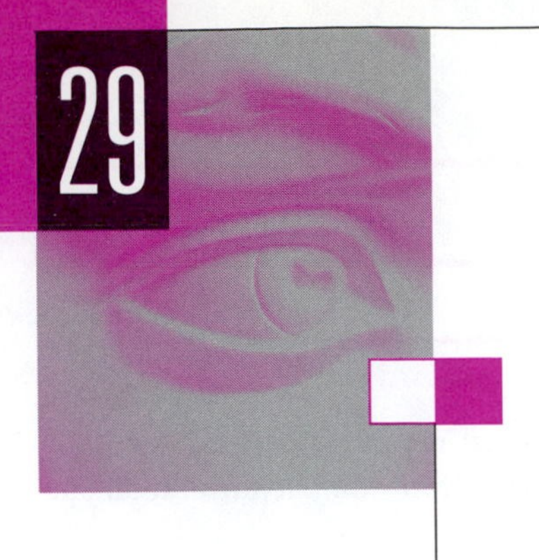

29 Neurologic Therapeutic Management

DESPITE THE DIVERSITY of neurologic abnormalities, there is one aspect of the critical care management of patients with neurologic disorders that is common to a wide variety of these pathologic conditions. This chapter focuses on the concepts of intracranial pressure (ICP) and the types of ICP monitoring. Also discussed are the therapies for management of intracranial hypertension. (ICP: Concepts and Nursing Management; Neurologic Care IVD.)

ASSESSMENT OF INTRACRANIAL PRESSURE

Monro-Kellie Hypothesis

The intracranial space comprises three components: brain substance (80%), cerebrospinal fluid (CSF) (10%), and blood (10%).[1] Under normal physiologic conditions, the ICP is maintained below 15 mm Hg mean pressure.[2] Essential to understanding the pathophysiology of ICP, the Monro-Kellie hypothesis proposes that an increase in volume of one intracranial component must be compensated by a decrease in one or more of the other components, so that total volume remains fixed. This compensation, although limited, includes displacing CSF from the intracranial vault to the lumbar cistern, increasing CSF absorption, and compressing the low-pressure venous system. Pathophysiologic alterations that can elevate ICP are outlined in Table 29-1.

Volume-Pressure Curve

When capable of compliance, the brain can tolerate significant increases in intracranial volume without much increase in ICP. The amount of intracranial compliance, however, is limited. Once this limit has been reached, a state of decompensation with increased ICP results. As the ICP rises, the relationship between volume and pressure changes, and small increases in volume may cause major elevations in ICP (Figure 29-1). The exact configuration of the volume-pressure curve and the point at which the steep rise in pressure occurs vary among patients. The configuration of this curve also is influenced by the cause and the rate of volume increases within the intracranial vault; for example, neurologic deterioration occurs more rapidly in a patient with an acute epidural hematoma than in a patient with a meningioma of the same size.[3] Monitoring these changes in intracranial dynamics and continuous clinical assessment of the patient's neurologic status have proved beneficial in diagnosing and treating sustained rises in ICP. Such elevations of ICP often precede evidence of neurologic deterioration obtained through the clinical assessment.

Cerebral Blood Flow and Autoregulation

Cerebral blood flow (CBF) corresponds to the metabolic demands of the brain and is normally 50 ml/100 g of brain tissue/minute. Although the brain makes up only 2% of body weight, it requires 15% to 20% of the resting cardiac output and 15% of the body's oxygen demands. The normal brain has a complex capacity to maintain constant CBF, despite wide ranges in arterial pressure—an effect known as *autoregulation.* Mean arterial pressure (MAP) of 50 to 150 mm Hg does not alter CBF when autoregulation is present. Outside the limits of this autoregulation, CBF becomes passively dependent on the perfusion pressure.[3]

Factors other than arterial blood pressure that affect CBF are conditions that result in acidosis, alkalosis, and changes in metabolic rate. Conditions that cause acidosis (e.g., hypoxia, hypercapnia, and ischemia) result in cerebral vascular dilation. Conditions causing alkalosis (e.g., hypocapnia) result in cerebral

TABLE 29-1 Mechanisms of ICP Elevation

Pathophysiology	Example	Treatment
DISORDERS OF CSF SPACE		
Overproduction of CSF	Choroid plexus papilloma	Diuretics, surgical removal
Communicating hydrocephalus from obstructed arachnoid	Old subarachnoid hemorrhage	Surgical drainage from lumbar intrathecal site
Noncommunicative hydrocephalus	Posterior fossa tumor obstructing aqueduct	Surgical drainage by ventricular drainage
Interstitial edema	Any of above	Surgical drainage of CSF
DISORDERS OF INTRACRANIAL BLOOD		
Intracranial hemorrhage causing increased ICP	Epidural hematoma	Surgical drainage
Vasospasm	Subarachnoid hemorrhage	Hypervolemia and hypertensive therapy Calcium channel antagonists
Vasodilation Increasing cerebral blood volume and ICP	Elevated $Paco_2$ Hypoxia	Hyperventilation and adequate oxygenation
DISORDERS OF BRAIN SUBSTANCE		
Expanding mass lesion with local vasogenic edema causing increased ICP	Brain tumor	Steroids Surgical removal
Ischemic brain injury with cytotoxic edema increasing ICP	Anoxic brain injury from cardiac or respiratory arrest	Resistant to therapy
Increased cerebral metabolic rate increasing cerebral blood flow and ICP	Seizures, hyperthermia	Anticonvulsant medications, especially barbiturates; control fever

From: Helfaer MA, Kirsch JR: *Crit Care Rep* 1:12, 1989.

vascular constriction. Normally, a reduction in metabolic rate (e.g., from hypothermia or barbiturates) decreases CBF, and increases in metabolic rate (e.g., from hyperthermia) increase CBF.[4]

Arterial blood gases exert a profound effect on CBF. Carbon dioxide, which affects the pH of the blood, is a potent vasoactive substance. Carbon dioxide retention (hypercapnia) leads to cerebral vasodilation, with increased cerebral blood volume, whereas hypocapnia leads to cerebral vasoconstriction and a reduction in cerebral blood volume.[3] Prolonged hypocapnia, however, especially at an arterial partial pressure of carbon dioxide ($Paco_2$) level less than 20 mm Hg, can produce cerebral ischemia.[5] Low arterial partial pressure of oxygen (Pao_2) levels, especially below 40 mm Hg, lead to cerebral vasodilation, which increases the intracranial blood volume and can contribute to increased ICP. High Pao_2 levels have not been shown to affect CBF in either direction.

Metabolic activity in the brain significantly influences CBF. Normally, when cerebral metabolic activity increases, CBF also increases to meet the demand. Any pathologic process that decreases CBF could lead to a mismatch between metabolic demand and blood supply, resulting in cerebral ischemia.[5]

Cerebral Perfusion Pressure

Measuring CBF in the clinical setting is difficult. Cerebral perfusion pressure (CPP), an estimated pressure, is the blood pressure gradient across the brain and is calculated as the difference between the incoming MAP and the opposing ICP on the arteries:

$$(CPP = MAP - ICP)$$

The CPP in the average adult is approximately 80 to 100 mm Hg, with a range of 60 to 150 mm Hg. The CPP must be maintained near 80 mm Hg to provide adequate blood supply to the brain. If the CPP drops below this point, ischemia may develop. A sustained CPP of 30 mm Hg or less usually results in neuronal hypoxia and cell death. When the mean systemic arterial pressure equals the ICP, CBF may cease.[6]

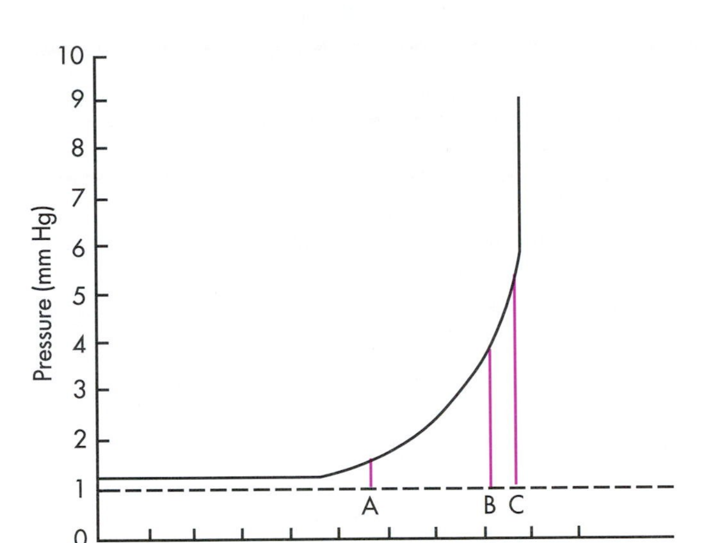

FIGURE 29-1. Intracranial volume-pressure curve. **A,** Pressure is normal, and increases in intracranial volume are tolerated without increases in intracranial pressure. **B,** Increases in volume may cause increases in pressure. **C,** Small increases in volume may cause larger increases in pressure.

Cerebral Metabolism

The measurements of CBF and CPP do not address the brain's metabolic need for oxygen. The determination that flow CBF matches the brain's metabolic needs is expressed as *cerebral metabolic rate* ($CMRo_2$), the normal value of which is 3.4 ml/100 g brain tissue/minute. This value is not easily attained for technical reasons, though it can be calculated. It is the product of the measured CBF and calculated arteriojugular oxygen difference ($AJDo_2$):

$$(CMRo_2 = CBF \times AJDo_2)^7$$

CBF can be measured using a variety of complex techniques (e.g., clearance of xenon after inhalation or intraarterial injection using multiple detectors, resolving ∝ camera, computed tomography, or positron emission tomography). Most recently, continuous bedside monitoring of regional cerebrocortical blood flow has become available but is not widely used, because it is cost-prohibitive.[7] Arteriojugular oxygen difference is the amount of oxygen extracted by the brain and is reflected in the difference between the arterial oxygen content and the jugular bulb (venous) oxygen content (Appendix D). The normal value is 5.0 to 7.5 vol%.[7]

Jugular bulb monitor. One method that has been developed allows on-line measurement of oxygenation within the jugular system through the use of the jugular bulb monitor. A catheter placed into one of the jugular veins measures jugular bulb oxygen saturation (S_jO_2). The normal value is 55% to 70%. Patients with values below 50% to 55% are considered oligemic (CBF inadequate for metabolic need). Patients with values above 75% to 80% are often considered hyperemic (CBF high in comparison to metabolic need). Both oligemic cerebral hypoxia and hyperemia place the patient at risk for ischemia and/or infarction.[7] Cerebral $AJDo_2$ and S_jO_2 can be used to reflect cerebral oxygen supply and demand balance (Table 29-2).

Assessment Techniques

Signs and symptoms. The numerous signs and symptoms of increased ICP include decreased level of consciousness; Cushing's triad (bradycardia, systolic hypertension, and bradypnea); diminished brainstem reflexes; papilledema; decerebrate posturing (abnormal extension); decorticate posturing (abnormal flexion); unequal pupil size; projectile vomiting; decreased pupillary reaction to light; altered breathing patterns; and headache.[8] Patients may exhibit one or all of these symptoms, depending on the underlying cause of the elevation in ICP. One of the earliest and most important signs of increased ICP is a decrease in level of consciousness. This change must be reported immediately to the physician.

Monitoring techniques. The common sites for monitoring ICP are the intraventricular space, the subarachnoid space, the epidural space, and the parenchyma. Each system has advantages and disadvantages for monitoring ICP (Table 29-3). The type of monitor chosen depends on both the suspected pathologic condition and physician's preferences.

Ventriculostomy. The type of monitor placed in the ventricular system usually is a small catheter known as a *ventriculostomy catheter.* It is inserted through a burr hole with the patient under local anesthesia and usually is placed in the anterior horn of the lateral ventricle. If at all possible, the side chosen for placement of the ventriculostomy is the nondominant hemisphere (Figure 29-2, *A*).

Subarachnoid bolt. The second type of monitor commonly used is the subarachnoid bolt or screw. This small, hollow device is placed in a patient under local anesthesia through a burr hole, with the distal end lying in the subarachnoid or subdural space. Inserting this device (Figure 29-2, *B*) is easier than the ventriculostomy catheter.[1,9]

Epidural monitor. Another type of device commonly used is the epidural monitor, which is also placed through a burr hole while the patient is under local anesthesia. The physician strips the dura away from the inner table of the skull before inserting the epidural

TABLE 29-2 Cerebral Oxygen Balance

Cerebral Oxygen Balance	$AJDO_2$	S_jO_2	Significance
Supply = demand	5.0%-7.5%	55%-70%	No global cerebral ischemia
Supply > demand	< 5.0%	> 70%	Cerebral hyperemia or compensated hypoperfusion
Demand > supply	> 7.5%	< 55%	Cerebral oligemia

Modified from Sikes PJ, Segal J: *Crit Care Nurs Q 17(1):9,* 1994.

TABLE 29-3 Comparison of ICP Monitoring Systems

System	Advantages	Disadvantages
Ventricular catheter	Access for CSF drainage and sampling Access for determination of volume-pressure curve Direct measurement of pressure Access for medication instillation	Difficulty locating lateral ventricle Risk of intracerebral bleeding or edema at cannula track Risk of infection Need for transducer repositioning with head movement
Subarachnoid bolt/screw	Useful if ventricles are small No penetration of brain Decreased risk of infection Access for CSF sampling Direct measurement of pressure	Unable to drain CSF Unreliable pressure when high ICP herniates brain into bolt Requires intact skull Need for transducer repositioning with head movement
Epidural sensor	Ease of insertion No dural penetration Lower risk of infection No adjustment of transducer needed with head movement	Unable to drain CSF Unable to recalibrate or rezero after placement Questionable accuracy of sensing ICP through dura Separate large monitoring system required
Fiberoptic transducer-tipped catheter	Versatile system, which can be placed in ventricle, subarachnoid space, or brain tissue Able to monitor intraparenchymal pressure No adjustment of transducer needed with head movement	Catheter relatively fragile Unable to recalibrate or rezero after placement Separate monitoring system required

monitor. The most common type of epidural monitor is the fiberoptic, or pneumatic, sensor, although other implantable epidural transducers often are used for long-term monitoring (Figure 29-2, *C*).[1,9]

Fiberoptic catheter. The fourth type of ICP monitoring system is the fiberoptic transducer-tipped catheter (Figure 29-2, *D*). This small (4F) catheter can be placed intraventricularly, intraparenchymally, in the subarachnoid space, or in the subdural space.[1,9]

Intracranial pressure waves. The ICP pulse waveform is observed on a continuous, real time pressure display and corresponds to each heartbeat. The waveform arises primarily from pulsations of the major intracranial arteries, receiving retrograde venous pulsations as well.[10]

Normal ICP waveform. The normal ICP wave has three or more defined peaks (Figure 29-3). The first peak, or P_1, is called the percussion wave. Originating from the pulsations of the choroid plexus, it has a sharp peak and is fairly consistent in its amplitude. The second peak, or P_2, is called the tidal wave. The tidal wave is more variable in shape and amplitude, ending on the dicrotic

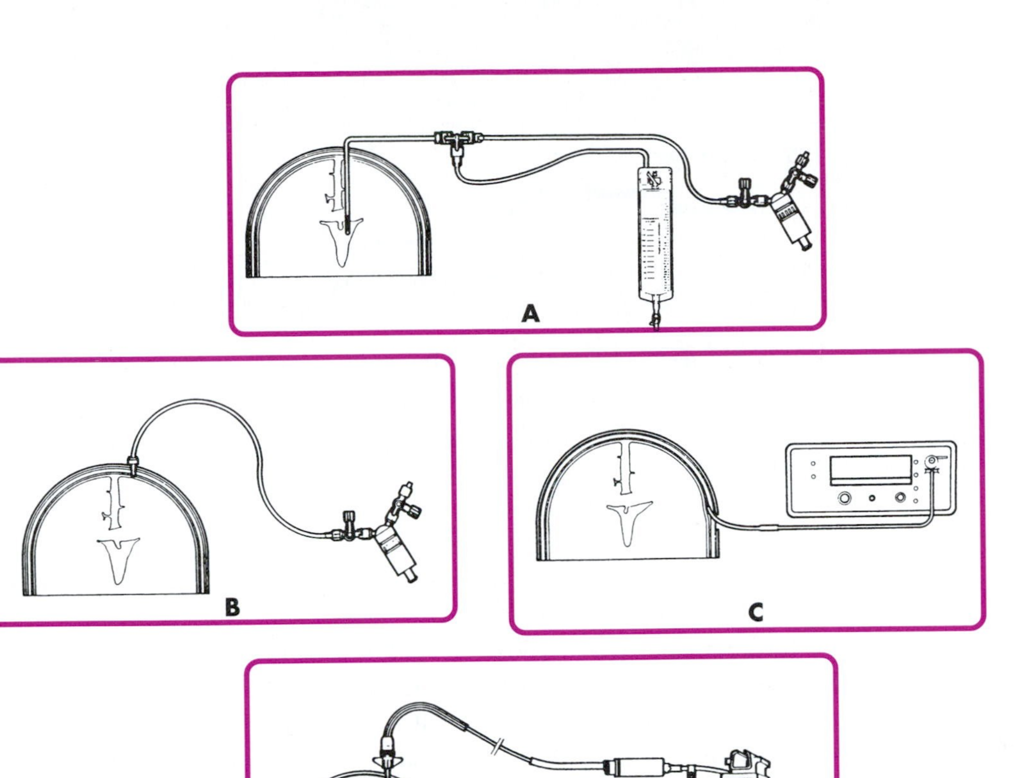

FIGURE 29-2. **A,** Ventricular pressure monitoring system. **B,** Subarachnoid pressure monitoring system. **C,** Epidural pressure monitoring system. **D,** Intraparenchymal pressure monitoring system. (Courtesy Camino NeuroCare, San Diego, Calif.)

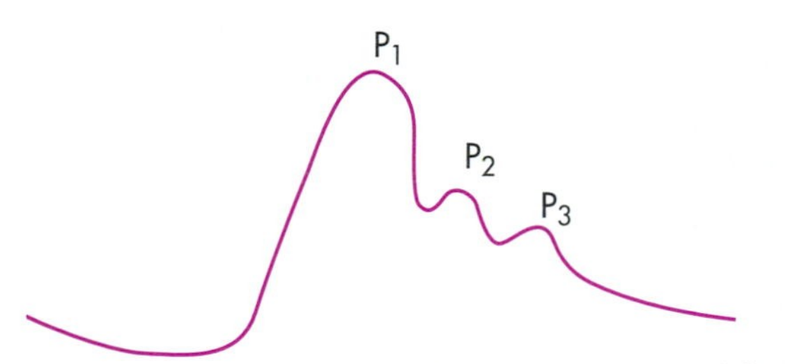

FIGURE 29-3. Components of a normal intracranial pressure waveform. (From Barker E: Intracranial pressure and monitoring. In Barker E, editor: *Neuroscience nursing,* St Louis, 1994, Mosby.)

notch. The P_2 portion of the pulse waveform has been most directly linked to the state of decreased compliance. When the P_2 component is equal to or higher than P_1, decreased compliance occurs. Immediately after the dicrotic notch is the third wave, P_3, which is called the *dicrotic wave.* After the dicrotic wave, the pressure usually tapers down to the diastolic position, unless retrograde venous pulsations add a few more peaks.

A, B, and C pressure waves are not true waveforms (Figure 29-4). Rather they are the graphically displayed trend data of ICPS over time. These waves reflect spontaneous alterations in ICP associated with respiration, systemic blood pressure, and deteriorating neurologic status.

A waves. Also called *plateau waves* because of their distinctive shape, A waves are the most clinically significant of the three types. They usually occur in an already elevated baseline ICP (greater than 20 mm Hg) and are characterized by sharp increases in ICP of 30 to 69 mm Hg, which plateau for 2 to 20 minutes and then return to baseline. The actual cause of A waves is unknown, but they may result from vasodilation and increased CBF, decreased venous outflow (and therefore increased cerebral blood volume), fluctuations in Pa_{CO_2} (and therefore changes in cerebral blood volume), or decreased CSF absorption. B waves frequently precede A waves. Plateau waves are considered significant because of the reduced cerebral perfusion pressure associated with ICP in the 50 to 100 mm Hg

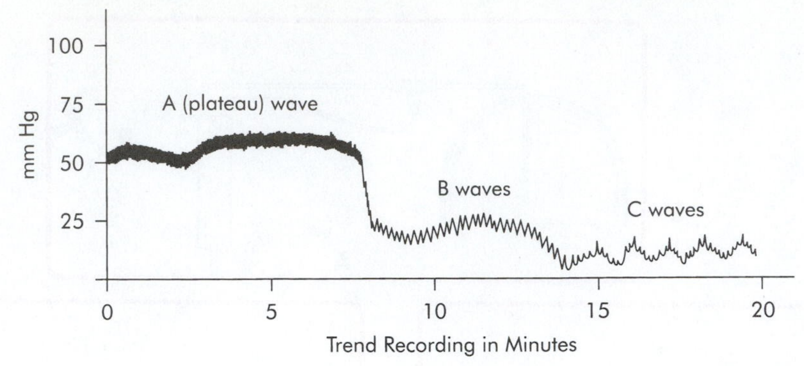

FIGURE 29-4. Abnormal intracranial pressure waveforms. (From Barker E: Intracranial pressure and monitoring. In Barker E: *Neuroscience nursing,* St Louis, 1994, Mosby.)

range. Transient signs of intracranial hypertension such as a decreased level of consciousness, bradycardia, pupillary changes, or respiratory changes may accompany these waves. Some research suggests that prolonged increases in ICP associated with plateau waves could result in transient as well as permanent cell damage from ischemia.[1,9]

There are some clear clinical correlations for A waves, such as sudden spontaneous posturing; diaphoresis; and elevated heart rate, blood pressure, and respiratory rate. In the event that clinical presentation cannot be monitored for increased intracranial pressure, such as in the chemically paralyzed patient, it helps to remember that A waves are often preceded by B waves.[6] Management of A waves is directed at the reduction of the high pressure and prevention of other plateau waves.[1,9]

B waves. B waves are sharp, rhythmic oscillations with a sawtooth appearance that occur every 30 seconds to 2 minutes and can raise the ICP from 5 to 70 mm Hg. They are a normal physiologic phenomenon that can occur in any patient, but they are amplified in states of low intracranial compliance. B waves appear to reflect fluctuations in cerebral blood volume. Decompensation of normal intracranial volume compensatory capacity is indicated by B waves with a high amplitude (greater than 15 mm Hg pressure change from peak to trough of wave).[1,9]

In the clinical setting B waves often precede A waves, so their occurrence cannot be lightly dismissed. If B waves occur during a procedure, the procedure is stopped and the patient's response evaluated. Sedation and/or pain medication may be necessary to avert intracranial hypertension.[6]

C waves. C waves are smaller, rhythmic waves that occur every 4 to 8 minutes and at normal levels of ICP. They are related to normal fluctuations in respiration and systemic arterial pressure. C waves are considered clinically insignificant.

MANAGEMENT OF INTRACRANIAL HYPERTENSION

Once intracranial hypertension is documented, therapy must be prompt to prevent secondary insults. Although the exact pressure level denoting intracranial hypertension remains uncertain, most current evidence suggests that ICP generally must be treated when it exceeds 20 mm Hg.[4] All therapies are directed toward reducing the volume of one or more of the components (blood, brain, CSF) that lie within the intracranial vault. A major goal of therapy is to determine the cause of the elevated pressure and, if possible, to remove the cause.[11] In the absence of a surgically treatable mass lesion, intracranial hypertension is treated medically. Nurses play an important role in rapid assessment and implementation of appropriate therapies for reducing ICP (Boxes 29-1 and 29-2).

Nursing interventions for the management of intracranial hypertension include keeping the patient's head elevated 30 to 45 degrees and in the neutral plane; maintaining normothermia and controlled ventilation to ensure a $PaCO_2$ level of 25 to 30 mm Hg and a PaO_2 level greater than 70 mm Hg; administering diuretic agents, anticonvulsants, and medications to ensure systolic blood pressure between 140 to 160 mm Hg; and performing ventricular drainage (if a ventriculostomy catheter is present).

NURSING INTERVENTION CLASSIFICATIONS

BOX 29-1 Intracranial Pressure (ICP) Monitoring

DEFINITION: Measurement and interpretation of patient data to regulate intracranial pressure

ACTIVITIES:

Assist with ICP monitoring device insertion
Provide information to family/significant others
Calibrate and level the transducer
Irrigate flush system
Set alarms
Obtain cerebrospinal fluid (CSF) drainage samples, as appropriate
Record ICP pressure readings and analyze waveforms
Monitor cerebral perfusion pressure
Note patient's change in response to stimuli
Monitor patient's ICP and neurological response to care activities
Monitor amount/rate of cerebrospinal fluid drainage
Monitor intake and output
Restrain patient, as needed
Monitor pressure tubing for bubbles
Change transducer/flush system
Change and/or reinforce insertion site dressing, as necessary
Monitor insertion site for infection
Monitor temperature and WBC count
Check patient for nuchal rigidity
Administer antibiotics
Position the patient with head elevated 30 to 45 degrees and with neck in a neutral position
Minimize environmental stimuli
Space nursing care to minimize ICP elevation
Alter suctioning procedure to minimize increase in ICP with catheter introduction (e.g., give lidocaine and limit number of suction passes)
Maintain controlled hyperventilation, as ordered
Maintain systemic arterial pressure within specified range
Administer pharmacological agents to maintain ICP within specified range
Notify physician for elevated ICP that does not respond to treatment protocols

From McCloskey JC, Bulechek GM: *Nursing interventions classification,* ed 2, St Louis, 1996, Mosby.

Patient Positioning

Positioning of the patient is a significant factor in the prevention and treatment of elevated ICP. Positions that keep the head and neck elevated 30 to 45 degrees and in a neutral position at all times allow proper venous drainage. In these positions, gravity enhances venous drainage from the brain and head.[12,13] Positions that impede venous return from the brain cause elevations in ICP. Obstruction of jugular veins or an increase in intrathoracic or intraabdominal pressure is communicated as increased pressure throughout the open venous system, thereby impeding drainage from the brain and increasing ICP. Positions that decrease venous return from the head (e.g., Trendelenburg, prone, extreme flexion of the hips, angulation of the neck) must be avoided if possible. If changes to positions such as Trendelenburg are necessary to provide adequate pulmonary care, critical care nurses must closely monitor ICP and vital signs. Mechanisms to reduce intracranial pressure (e.g., sedation, ventricular drainage) also may be used while the patient is in Trendelenburg's position.[14] Other impediments to cerebral venous drainage are

NURSING INTERVENTION CLASSIFICATIONS

BOX 29-2 Cerebral Edema Management

DEFINITION: Limitation of secondary cerebral injury resulting from swelling of brain tissue

ACTIVITIES:

Assess for confusion, changes in mentation, complaints of dizziness, and syncope
Establish means of communication: ask yes or no questions; provide magic slate, paper and pencil, picture board, flashcards, and vocaid device
Monitor neurological status closely and compare to baseline
Monitor CSF drainage characteristics: color, clarity, and consistency
Record CSF drainage
Decrease stimuli in patient's environment
Give sedation, as needed
Note patient's change in response to stimuli
Monitor respiratory status: rate, rhythm, and depth of respirations; Pao_2, $Paco_2$, pH, and bicarbonate levels
Allow ICP to return to baseline between nursing activities
Screen conversation within patient's hearing
Administer anticonvulsants, as appropriate
Avoid neck flexion or extreme hip/knee flexion
Avoid Valsalva maneuvers
Administer stool softeners
Hyperventilate patient
Position with head of bed up 30 degrees or greater
Avoid use of PEEP
Analyze ICP waveform
Plan nursing care to provide rest periods
Monitor patient's ICP and neurological response to care activities
Administer paralyzing agent
Encourage family/significant other to talk to patient
Restrict fluids
Avoid hypotonic IV fluids
Adjust ventilator settings to keep $Paco_2$ at prescribed level
Limit suction passes to less than 15 seconds
Monitor for CSF rhinorrhea/otorrhea
Monitor lab values: serum and urine osmolality, sodium, and potassium levels
Monitor volume pressure indices
Perform passive range of motion
Monitor CVP
Monitor ICP and CPP
Monitor PAWP and PAP
Monitor P and BP
Monitor intake and output
Drain CSF, according to standing orders
Hyperventilate before suctioning
Maintain normothermia
Administer loop active or osmotic diuretics
Implement seizure precautions
Titrate barbiturate to achieve suppression or burst suppression of EEG, as ordered

From McCloskey JC, Bulechek GM: *Nursing interventions classification*, ed 2, St Louis, 1996, Mosby.

positive end-expiratory pressure (PEEP) greater than 5 to 10 cm H_2O pressure, coughing, suctioning, tight tracheostomy tube ties, and the Valsalva maneuver.[3]

Hyperventilation

Controlled hyperventilation has been an important adjunct of therapy for the patient with increased ICP. If the $Paco_2$ can be reduced from its normal level of 35 to 40 mm Hg to a range of 25 to 30 mm Hg in the patient with intracranial hypertension, vasoconstriction of cerebral arteries, reduction of cerebral blood flow, and increased venous return will result. Reducing the intracranial blood volume results in a general reduction in ICP.[4] The use of controlled hyperventilation is currently under investigation. Research indicates that in certain situations of increased ICP, vasoconstriction of the cerebral vessels already has occurred. In these cases further application of controlled hyperventilation could cause vasoconstriction to such an extent that cerebral ischemia occurs.[15] Documentation shows that high levels of $Paco_2$ cause cerebral vasodilation and contribute to elevated ICP. For this reason $Paco_2$ levels greater than 40 mm Hg are considered dangerous.[2]

Although hypoxemia must obviously be avoided, excessively high levels of oxygen offer no benefits.[3] In fact, increasing inspired oxygen concentrations (FIO_2) above 60% may lead to toxic changes in lung tissue. The increasing use of devices that monitor oxygen saturation (e.g., pulse oximeter) has led to greater awareness of the circumstances, such as suctioning and restlessness, that can cause oxygen desaturation and therefore elevate ICP.

Sedation and Neuromuscular Blocking Agents

Any treatment modality that increases the incidence of noxious stimulation to the patient carries with it the potential for increasing ICP. Such noxious stimuli include pain as a result of injuries sustained with the initial trauma, the presence of an endotracheal tube, coughing, suctioning, repositioning, bathing, and many routine nursing management procedures. To ensure adequate ventilation ($Paco_2$ level of 25 to 30 mm Hg and Pao_2 level greater than 70 mm Hg) and in anticipation of the deleterious effects of noxious stimuli on ICP, nurses may use sedatives alone or in combination with neuromuscular blocking agents. Use of these medications is recommended only in patients who have an ICP monitor in place, because sedation and neuromuscular blocking agents affect the reliability of neurologic assessment. Although sedation of the unconscious patient can obscure portions of the neurologic examination, its benefits may outweigh the risks.[16] Neuromuscular blocking agents without sedation is not recommended. These agents, such as pancuronium (Pavulon), have no analgesic effect and do not adequately protect patients from pain and the physiologic responses that can occur from pain-producing procedures.

Temperature Control

Directly proportional to body temperature, cerebral metabolic rate increases 5% to 7% per degree centigrade of increase in body temperature.[5] This fact is significant because as the cerebral metabolic rate increases, blood flow to the brain must increase to meet the tissue demands. To avoid the increase in blood volume associated with an increased cerebral metabolic rate, nurses must prevent hyperthermia in the patient with a brain injury. Antipyretics and cooling devices must be used when appropriate while the source of the fever is being determined.[16]

Conversely, hypothermia reduces cerebral metabolic rate. Research done in severely injured head injury patients who were unresponsive to barbiturate therapy for control of intractable intracranial hypertension demonstrated a significant decrease in ICP when subjected to mild hypothermia between 33.5° C and 34.5° C.[17]

Persistent fluctuation and/or hypothermia or hyperthermia in conjunction with head injury is a grave prognostic sign and usually has been associated with death or a persistent vegetative state. These patients may represent a group with severe hypothalamic injury.

Blood Pressure Control

Maintenance of arterial blood pressure in the high normal range is essential in the brain-injured patient. Inadequate perfusion pressure decreases the supply of nutrients and oxygen requirements for cerebral metabolic needs. On the other hand, a blood pressure too high increases cerebral blood volume and may increase ICP.

Sustained systolic arterial hypertension (greater than 160 mm Hg) in conjunction with elevated ICP must be vigorously treated. Control of systemic arterial hypertension may require nothing more than the administration of a sedative agent. Small, frequent doses may be sufficient to blunt noxious stimuli and prevent them from triggering rises in blood pressure. When sedation proves inadequate in controlling systemic arterial hypertension, primary antihypertensive agents are used. Care must be taken in choosing these agents because many of the peripheral vasodilators also

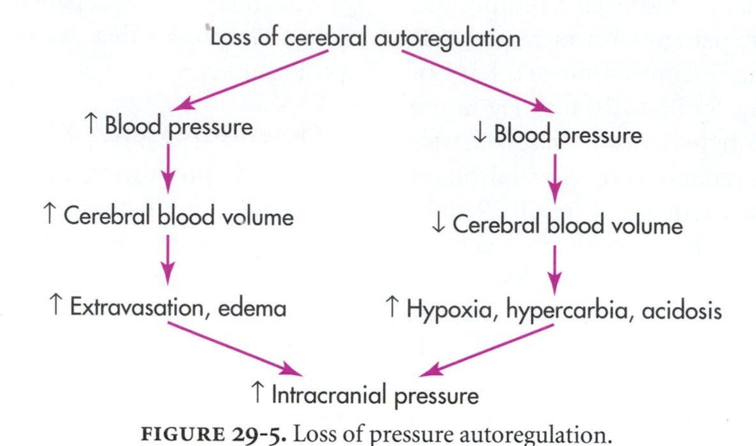

FIGURE 29-5. Loss of pressure autoregulation.

are cerebral vasodilators (e.g., nitroprusside and nitroglycerin). However, all antihypertensives are believed to cause some degree of cerebral vasodilation. To reduce this vasodilating effect, co-treatment with beta-blockers (e.g., propranolol and labetalol) may be beneficial.[16] Figure 29-5 shows the relationship between blood pressure and ICP.

Seizure Control

The incidence of posttraumatic seizures in the head-injured population has been estimated at 5%. Because of the risk of a secondary ischemic insult associated with seizures, many physicians prescribe anticonvulsant medications prophylactically. Seizures cause metabolic requirements to increase, which results in elevation of cerebral blood flow, cerebral blood volume, and ICP, even in paralyzed patients. If blood flow cannot match demand, ischemia develops, cerebral energy stores are depleted, and irreversible neuronal destruction occurs. The usual anticonvulsant regimen for seizure control includes phenytoin or phenobarbital, or both, in therapeutic doses.[16]

Lidocaine

Various forms of sensory stimulation (e.g., tracheal intubation, laryngoscopy, and endotracheal suctioning) may provoke marked increases in ICP and MAP. One therapy used to prevent cerebral ischemia and acute intracranial hypertension has been the administration of lidocaine through an endotracheal tube or through intravenous infusion before nasotracheal suctioning.[4] Lidocaine is believed to be effective in blunting ICP spikes secondary to tracheal stimulation. Studies have found that peak lidocaine concentrations are linearly related to the administered dose and that the rate of absorption depends on the vascularity of the site of administration.[4] It also has been documented that lidocaine is initially distributed to the lungs, then to the heart and kidneys, and then to muscle and adipose tissue.[18]

Prophylactic administration of lidocaine before endotracheal suctioning is widely practiced. Lidocaine protects the patient from the associated increases in ICP that occur with suctioning. A number of studies investigating the usefulness of lidocaine in this area are in progress.[18]

Cerebrospinal Fluid Drainage

Cerebrospinal fluid drainage for intracranial hypertension may be used with other treatment modalities. CSF drainage is accomplished by the insertion of a pliable catheter into the anterior horn of the lateral ventricle (ventriculostomy), preferably on the nondominant side. Such drainage can help support the patient through periods of cerebral edema by controlling spikes in ICP. One of the major advantages of the

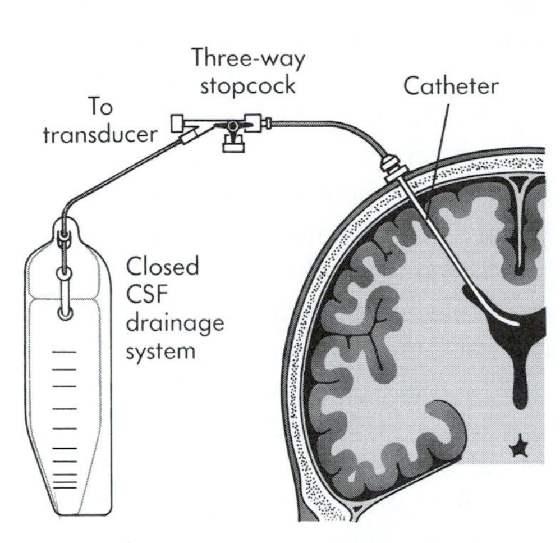

FIGURE 29-6. Intermittent drainage system. Intermittent drainage involves draining CSF via a ventriculostomy when ICP exceeds the upper pressure parameter set by the physician. Intermittent drainage involves opening the three-way stopcock to allow CSF to flow into the drainage bag for brief periods (30 to 120 seconds) until the pressure is below the upper pressure parameter. (From Barker E: Intracranial pressure and monitoring. In Barker E: *Neuroscience nursing,* St Louis, 1994, Mosby.)

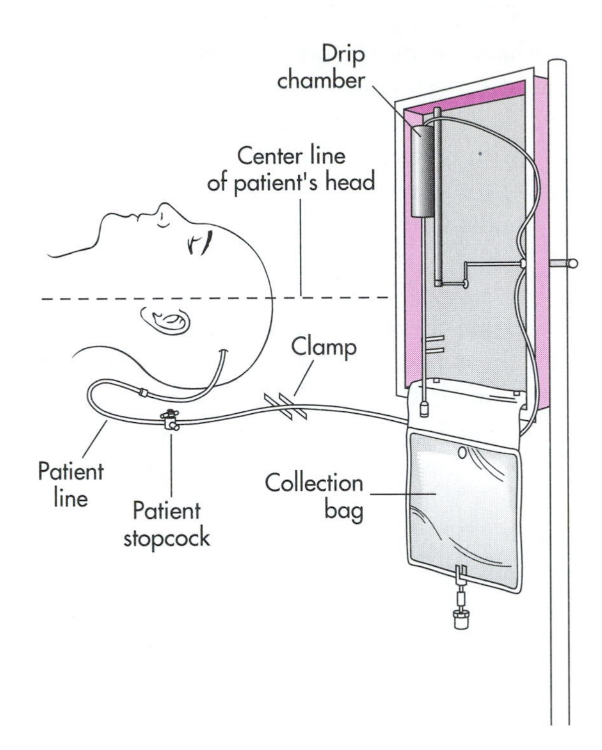

FIGURE 29-7. Continuous drainage system. Continuous drainage involves placing the drip chamber of the drainage system at a specified level above the foramen of Monro (usually 15 cm). The system is left open to allow continuous drainage of CSF into the chamber (which drains into a collection bag) against a pressure gradient that prevents excessive drainage and ventricular collapse. (Courtesy Codman/Johnson & Johnson Professional Inc., Raynham, Mass.)

ventriculostomy is its dual role as both a monitoring device and a treatment modality. Because CSF provides a favorable medium for the development of infection, flawless aseptic technique must be followed during insertion and maintenance of the system. The ventricular system is connected to a drainage bag and is then maintained as a closed system for the period the ventriculostomy remains in place—usually 3 to 5 days (Figures 29-6 and 29-7).[9]

Diuretics

Osmotic agents. Clinicians have known for decades that osmotic agents effectively reduce ICP. The mechanism by which these diuretics reduce ICP continues to be a subject of investigational interest. One theory is that these agents act by remaining relatively impermeable to the blood-brain barrier, thereby drawing water from normal brain tissue to plasma. The direction of flow is from the hypoconcentrated tissue to the hyperconcentrated cerebral vasculature. If the situation becomes reversed and the tissue becomes hyperconcentrated in relation to the cerebral vasculature, a rebound phenomenon could occur. These agents have little direct effect on edematous cerebral tissue situated in an area of defective blood-brain barrier; instead, they require an intact blood-brain barrier for osmosis to occur.[16]

The most widely used osmotic diuretic is mannitol, a large molecule that is retained almost entirely in the extracellular compartment and has little to no rebound effect noted with other osmotic diuretics. Mannitol may improve perfusion to ischemic areas of the brain, producing cerebral vasoconstriction and resulting in a reduction of ICP.[16]

Perhaps the most common difficulty associated with the use of osmotic agents is the production of electrolyte disturbances. Careful attention must be paid to body weight and fluid and electrolyte stability. Serum osmolality must be kept between 300 and 320 mOsm/L. Hypernatremia and hypokalemia are frequently associated with repeated administration of osmotic agents. Central venous pressure readings must be monitored to prevent hypovolemia.[16] Smaller doses of mannitol simplify fluid and electrolyte management, and their use is encouraged whenever possible.[4]

Nonosmotic agents. Loop diuretics have also been used to decrease ICP. Furosemide, one such nonosmotic diuretic, may act differently from osmotic agents by pulling sodium and water from edematous areas and, perhaps, by decreasing CSF production. One advantage of furosemide administration over the use of osmotic diuretics is that its effect is not generally associated with increases in serum osmolality. Therefore electrolyte imbalances may not be as severe with the use of nonosmotic diuretics.[16]

High-Dose Barbiturate Therapy

Barbiturate therapy is a treatment protocol developed for the management of uncontrolled intracranial hypertension that has not responded to the conventional treatments previously described. Uncontrolled ICP is defined as ICP greater than 20 mm Hg for 30 minutes or ICP greater than 40 mm Hg for 15 minutes or more or CPP lower than 50 mm Hg that does not respond to aggressive use of conventional therapies.[5]

Although the specific action of barbiturates in the reduction of ICP is unclear, several theories explain their effect on the central nervous system (CNS) and the subsequent cerebral protection they provide. Barbiturates increase the cerebral vascular resistance in the undamaged portions of the brain, resulting in a decreased cerebral blood flow and shunting of blood to the damaged portions of the brain. Systemic blood pressure also is lowered, reducing hydrostatic pressure in the damaged cerebral tissue and helping arrest edema formation. Barbiturates also slow cerebral metabolism by reducing the functional electrical generation of the neurons. This decreased cerebral metabolism thus lessens the glucose and oxygen demands of the brain. Barbiturates are also effective anticonvulsants and may suppress subclinical seizure activities. Finally, some researchers postulate that barbiturates are scavengers of free radicals and thereby prevent cell membrane damage and destruction.[16]

The two most commonly used drugs in high-dose barbiturate therapy are pentobarbital and thiopental. The goal with either of these drugs is a reduction of ICP to 15 to 20 mm Hg while a MAP of 70 to 80 mm Hg is maintained. Patients are maintained on high-dose barbiturate therapy until ICP has been controlled within the normal range for 24 hours. Barbiturates must never be stopped abruptly but are tapered slowly over approximately 4 days.[5]

Complications of high-dose barbiturate therapy can be disastrous without a specific and organized approach. The most frequent complications are hypotension, hypothermia, and myocardial depression. If any complications occur and are allowed to persist unchecked, they may cause secondary insults to an already damaged brain. Hypotension, the most common complication, results from peripheral vasodilation and can be compounded in an already dehydrated patient who has received large doses of an osmotic diuretic in an attempt to control ICP. Careful monitoring of fluid status by central venous pressure or a pulmonary artery catheter can help in preventing this complication. Myocardial depression results from cardiac muscle suppression and can be avoided by frequent monitoring of fluid status, cardiac output, and serum drug levels. If an adequate cardiac output cannot be maintained in the presence of normothermia, barbiturates must be reduced, regardless of serum levels.[16]

The major unresolved issue in the use of high-dose barbiturates is their effect on outcome after head injury. Several laboratory and clinical trials have been undertaken to address this issue. Results of a multicenter randomized trial of barbiturates found that most elevations of ICP could be controlled with aggressive use of standard therapies of ICP management. For the small subset of patients in whom standard therapy fails to achieve ICP control, judicious, carefully monitored and administered high-dose barbiturate therapy is beneficial.[19]

HERNIATION SYNDROMES

The goal of neurologic evaluation, ICP monitoring, and treatment of increased ICP is to prevent herniation. Herniation of intracerebral contents results in the shifting of tissue from one compartment of the brain to another and places pressure on cerebral vessels and vital function centers of the brain. If unchecked, herniation rapidly causes death as a result of the cessation of cerebral blood flow and respirations.

Supratentorial Herniation

There are four types of supratentorial herniation syndrome: central, or transtentorial; uncal; cingulate; or transcalvarial (Figure 29-8).

Uncal herniation. Uncal herniation is the most frequently noted herniation syndrome. In uncal herniation, a unilateral, expanding mass lesion, usually of the temporal lobe, increases ICP, causing lateral displacement of the tip of the temporal lobe (uncus). Lateral displacement pushes the uncus over the edge of the tentorium, puts pressure on the oculomotor nerve (cranial nerve III) and posterior cerebral artery ipsilateral to the lesion, and flattens the midbrain against the opposite side.[3,20]

Clinical manifestations of uncal herniation include ipsilateral pupil dilation, decreased level of conscious-

RESEARCH ABSTRACT

Therapeutic intervention scoring system used in the care of patients in pentobarbital-induced coma to determine nurse-patient ratios.

Myles G and others: *Am J Crit Care* 5(1):74, 1996.

PURPOSE

The purpose of this study was to use the Therapeutic Intervention Scoring System (TISS) to analyze and quantify how interventions affect nurse-patient ratios in the management of patients in pentobarbital coma for refractory increased intracranial pressure.

DESIGN

Descriptive, medical record review.

SAMPLE

The medical records of all patients (n = 62) with the diagnosis of subarachnoid hemorrhage from aneurysmal rupture with subsequent increased intracranial pressure (ICP) who were admitted over a 3-year period to a Midwest trauma center were reviewed. The average age was 46.7 years; patients were in a pentobarbital coma an average of 10.7 days with an average ICP of 19.4 mm Hg and an average TISS score of 41.7, necessitating a 1:1 nurse-patient ratio during the therapy.

PROCEDURE

The TISS was modified for use in the neurologic critical care setting. Interventions specific to the patient population were selected and rearranged on the tool for congruency with the critical care flow sheets. The modified tool was then subjected to content validity assessment, and the tool was pilot-tested for internal consistency reliability (test-retest = .94). The retrospective medical record review was then conducted using the modified TISS.

RESULTS

The intensity of interventions correlated with the level of coma, length of time in coma, and associated complications ($p < .001$). As serum pentobarbital levels increased, TISS scores increased. The greatest significance ($p < .05$) occurred between the precoma and coma group, and between the precoma and postcoma group.

DISCUSSION/IMPLICATIONS

Findings from this study indicate that the TISS modified for use in the neurologic critical care setting appropriately captured the intensity of nursing interventions for this patient population. Nursing care and complications involved in this therapy were quantified, and nurse-patient ratios were established. It is important to measure nursing resources quantitatively so that an accurate assessment of nursing management can be documented. This study demonstrated that there is a marked increase in nursing workload related to a medical management decision. By validating reliable instruments that measure patient acuity, staffing needs can be projected and appropriate resources allocated that respond to the specific care required.

ness, respiratory pattern changes leading to respiratory arrest, and contralateral hemiplegia leading to decorticate or decerebrate posturing. If no intervention occurs, uncal herniation results in fixed and dilated pupils, flaccidity, and respiratory arrest.[3,20]

Central, or transtentorial, herniation. In central herniation an expanding mass lesion of the midline, frontal, parietal, or occipital lobes results in downward displacement of the hemispheres, basal ganglia, and diencephalon through the tentorial notch. Central herniation often is preceded by uncal and cingulate herniation.[3,20]

Clinical manifestations of central, or transtentorial, herniation include loss of consciousness; small, reactive pupils progressing to fixed, dilated pupils; respiratory changes leading to respiratory arrest; and decorticate posturing progressing to flaccidity. In the late

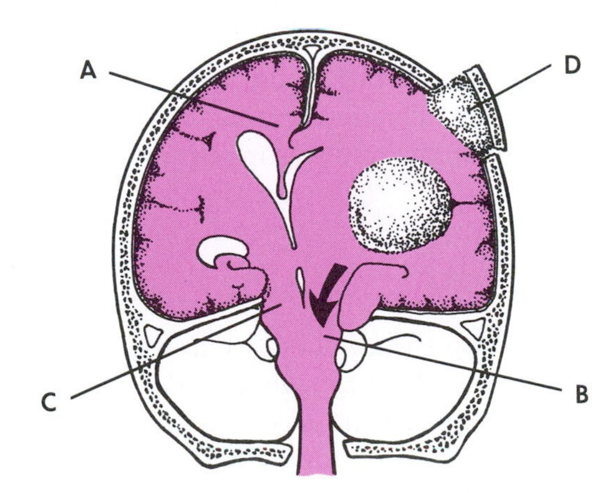

FIGURE 29-8. Supratentorial herniation. **A,** Cingulate. **B,** Uncal. **C,** Central. **D,** Transcalvarial.

stages, uncal and central herniation syndromes affect the brainstem similarly.[3,20]

Cingulate herniation. Cingulate herniation occurs when an expanding lesion of one hemisphere shifts laterally and forces the cingulate gyrus under the falx cerebri. Cingulate herniation occurs frequently. Whenever a lateral shift is noted on computed tomography (CT) scan, cingulate herniation has occurred. Little is known about the effects of cingulate herniation, and there are no clinical manifestations that assist in its diagnosis. Cingulate herniation is not in itself life threatening, but if the expanding mass lesion that caused cingulate herniation is not controlled, uncal or central herniation will follow.[3,20]

Transcalvarial herniation. Transcalvarial herniation is the extrusion of cerebral tissue through the cranium. In the presence of severe cerebral edema, transcalvarial herniation occurs through an opening from a skull fracture or craniotomy site.[3]

Infratentorial Herniation

There are two infratentorial herniation syndromes: upward transtentorial herniation and downward cerebellar herniation.

Upward transtentorial herniation. Upward transtentorial herniation occurs when an expanding mass lesion of the cerebellum causes protrusion of the vermis (central area) of the cerebellum and the midbrain upward through the tentorial notch. Compression of the third cranial nerve and diencephalon occur. Blockage of the central aqueduct and distortion of the third ventricle obstruct CSF flow. Deterioration progresses rapidly.[3,20]

Downward cerebellar herniation. Downward cerebellar herniation occurs when an expanding lesion of the cerebellum exerts pressure downward, sending the cerebellar tonsils through the foramen magnum. Compression and displacement of the medulla oblongata occur, rapidly resulting in respiratory and cardiac arrest.[3,20]

PHARMACOLOGIC AGENTS

A number of pharmacologic agents are used in the care of patients with neurologic disorders. Table 29-4 reviews the various agents used and any special considerations necessary for administering them.[21]

NEW FRONTIERS IN TREATMENT

Cerebral Resuscitation

Cerebral resuscitation refers to brain-oriented resuscitation therapies that are centered around neuronal compromise after circulatory arrest. Factors that influence neuronal survival include time of ischemia, hyperglycemia, CPP, and brain temperature.[22] The goals of cerebral resuscitation are to ameliorate CNS damage that has occurred, reverse ongoing mechanisms of injury, and protect uninjured but endangered neurons. Therapy designed to improve cerebral resuscitation after cardiac arrest includes maintaining adequate CNS perfusion, improving cerebral metabolism, and reducing cerebral metabolic demands (Table 29-5).

A great deal of research has focused on metabolic derangements secondary to injury or ischemia and the brain's sensitivity to the ischemic damage.

Free radicals. A free radical can be defined as a molecule that has an unpaired electron in its structure, thus making it highly reactive and unstable. Oxygen free radicals occur as a by-product of cellular metabolism.[23] Various enzymes and endogenous free radical scavengers control the presence and circulation of these metabolic by-products. Trauma, hypoxia, or an ischemic event can overwhelm the intrinsic ability of the body to deal with free radicals. Unchecked free radicals will destroy the cell's lipid membrane and impair the cell's ability to function.

Experimental therapies are aimed at halting the destruction caused by free radicals. Synthetic steroids, once commonly known as *lazaroids* and now referred to as *tirilazads,* act as scavengers of free radicals.[24] On the forefront of pharmacology is superoxide dismutase, which directly scavenges free radicals but has an extremely short half-life.[25]

Glutamide. Glutamide is a neurotransmitter widely distributed in the brain that is released through damaged ionic channels in the neurons in the presence of trauma and ischemia. This release results in an unstable membrane. Consequently, calcium ions flood into the cell, and potassium leaks out. The by-product of lactic acid quickly builds. The result is cellular edema and neuronal death.[24] Investigators are focusing on investigational drugs such as CGS 19755 that minimize the effects of glutamate release in the acute stroke population.[26]

Lactate. Lactate occurs as a normal by-product of intracellular metabolism, and jugular bulb monitoring has made the measurement of cerebral lactate levels possible. In a head injured patient with hypoxia and ensuing ischemia, oxygen demand rises. To meet the demand, the body shifts from aerobic to anaerobic metabolism. The resultant cellular acidosis can potentiate further cellular injury and impair the return of ionic homeostasis, ultimately leading to the formation of free radicals.[24] An option that may be available in

TABLE 29-4 Pharmacologic Agents Used in the Management of Neurologic Disorders

Drug	Dosage	Actions	Special Considerations
ANTICONVULSANTS			
Phenytoin (Dilantin)	Loading dose: 18 mg/kg IV Maintenance dose: 3-5 mg/kg q 12 h IV	Used to prevent the influx of sodium at the cell membrane and inhibit cell depolarization; blocks the spread of a seizure, rather than preventing initial neuronal discharge.	Infuse no faster than 50 mg/min. Administer with normal saline only as it precipitates with other solutions. Monitor serum levels closely; therapeutic level is 10-20 μg/ml.
BARBITURATES			
Phenobarbital	Loading dose: 6-8 mg/kg IV Maintenance dose: 3-4 mg/kg q 12-24 h IV	Used to produce CNS depression and reduce the spread of an epileptic focus.	Administer at a rate of 60 mg/min. Monitor serum levels closely; therapeutic level is 15-40 μg/ml. May depress cardiac and respiratory function.
OSMOTIC DIURETICS			
Mannitol	0.5-2.0 g/kg IV	Used to treat cerebral edema by pulling fluid from the extravascular space into the intravascular space; requires intact blood-brain barrier.	Side effects include hypovolemia and increased serum osmolality. Monitor serum osmolality, and notify the physician if > 310 mOsm/L. Warm and shake before administering to ensure crystals are dissolved.
LOOP DIURETICS			
Furosemide (Lasix)	0.1-2.0 mg/kg IV	Used to decrease sodium transport within the brain and thereby reduce cerebral edema; may inhibit CSF production.	Side effects include hypovolemia and hypokalemia.
CALCIUM CHANNEL BLOCKERS			
Nimodipine (Nimotop)	60 mg q 4 h NG or PO	Used to decrease cerebral vasospasm.	Side effects include hypotension, palpitations, headache, and dizziness. Monitor blood pressure frequently when implementing therapy.
LOCAL ANESTHETIC			
Lidocaine	50-100 mg IV or 2 ml of 4% solution	Effective in blunting ICP spikes secondary to tracheal stimulation.	Must be administered not longer than 5 minutes before suctioning.
PLATELET INHIBITORS			
Acetylsalicylic acid (aspirin)	1.3 g daily in 2-4 divided doses	Used in the prevention of stroke.	Side effects include tinnitus, hearing loss, dyspepsia, hemorrhage, and hepatotoxicity. Prolongs bleeding time for 5-7 days; may prolong prothrombin time and interfere with urine glucose test. Administer after meals or with food.

TABLE 29-5 **Goals of Cerebral Resuscitation**

Maintain CNS Perfusion and Oxygenation	Decrease Cerebral Metabolism	Prevent Chemical Damage to the Brain
BP at normal or higher levels	Prevent seizures	Scavenger free radicals
CVP and ICP as low as possible	Barbiturates	Mannitol
PaO_2 > 80-100 mm Hg	Prevent hyperthermia	
CPP > 70-90 mm Hg		

the future is the administration of an alkalinizing agent such as tromethamine (THAM) in head injured patients. This buffering agent can raise the brain's cellular pH level and thus promote cellular homeostasis and a significant difference in the control of ICP.[27]

Treatment of Ischemic Stroke

Some patients with ischemic stroke deteriorate because of the development of increased ICP. Cytotoxic edema is common after a stroke and usually reaches a peak 3 to 5 days after the initial insult. As the brain swells the ICP can increase and cause further neurologic deficits.

Antiplatelet therapy in the form of aspirin (ASA) has become increasingly recommended for reduction of stroke risk and completed ischemic strokes.[28] In the patient with a stroke in evolution (a progressive worsening of neurologic symptoms), heparin has been of benefit. A CT scan is mandatory to rule out intracerebral hemorrhage or hemorrhagic stroke before starting heparin therapy. If the CT is negative, current therapeutic standards advise using intravenous (IV) heparin within 48 hours. Close monitoring of prothrombin (PT) is important to maintain a range of 1.3 to 1.5 times the control. Long-term oral anticoagulant therapy is usually begun in the acute setting by tapering the heparin and adding a warfarin (Coumadin) compound on an increasing schedule related to the method of dosing (3 to 10 days). Warfarin (Coumadin) is commonly used with hypoprothrombinemia occurring 36 to 72 hours after the initial dose. The dosing is individually adjusted with a partial thromboplastin time (PTT) of 1.5 to 2.0 times normal as an indicator of appropriate therapy. Treatment is usually continued for 3 to 6 months.[29]

Investigation into the use of thrombolytic therapy within 3 hours of an ischemic stroke is also under way. Multicenter trials with tissue plasminogen activator (t-PA)[30] and ancrod[29] have demonstrated clinical improvement in the ischemic stroke patient.

REFERENCES

1. Richmond TS: Intracranial pressure monitoring, *AACN Clin Issues Crit Care Nurs* 4:148, 1993.
2. Boss BJ: Concepts of neurologic dysfunction. In McCance K, Huether S, editors: *Pathophysiology: the biologic basis for disease in adults and children,* ed 2, St Louis, 1994, Mosby.
3. Barker E: Intracranial pressure and monitoring. In Barker E, editor: *Neuroscience nursing,* St Louis, 1994, Mosby.
4. Chestnut RM, Marshall LF: Management of head injury: treatment of abnormal intracranial pressure, *Neurosurg Clin N Am* 2:267, 1991.
5. Hickey JV: *The clinical practice of neurological and neurosurgical nursing,* ed 3, Philadelphia, 1991, JB Lippincott.
6. Vos HR: Making headway with intracranial hypertension, *Am J Nurs* 93(2):28, 1993.
7. Sikes PJ, Segal J: Jugular bulb oxygen saturation monitoring for evaluating cerebral ischemia, *Crit Care Nurs Q* 17(1):9, 1994.
8. Wall BM, Philips JP, Howard JC: Validation of increased intracranial pressure and high risk for increased intracranial pressure, *Nurs Diag* 5:74, 1994.
9. Cummings R: Understanding ventricular drainage, *J Neurosci Nurs* 24:84, 1992.
10. McQuillan KA: Intracranial pressure monitoring: technical imperatives, *AACN Clin Issues Crit Care Nurs* 2:623, 1991.
11. Wrobel CJ, Marshall LF: Closed head injury management dilemmas. In Long DM, editor: *Current therapy in neurological surgery,* ed 3, St Louis, 1992, Mosby.
12. Andrus C: Intracranial pressure: dynamics and nursing management, *J Neurosci Nurs* 23:85, 1991.
13. Feldman Z and others: Effect of head elevation on intracranial pressure, cerebral perfusion, and cerebral blood flow in head-injured patients, *J Neurosurg* 76:207, 1992.

14. Fontaine DK, McQuillan K: Positioning as a nursing therapy in trauma care, *Crit Care Nurs Clin North Am* 1:105, 1990.
15. Muizelaar JP and others: Adverse effects of prolonged hyperventilation in patients with severe head injury: a randomized clinical trial, *J Neurosurg* 75:731, 1991.
16. Frank JI: Management of intracranial hypertension, *Med Clin North Am* 77:61, 1993.
17. Nikas DL: Commentary on the effect of mild hypothermia on uncontrolled hypertension after severe head injury and the use of moderate therapeutic hypothermia for patients with severe head injuries: a preliminary report, *AACN-Nurs Scan Crit Care* 4(1):14, 1994.
18. Brucia JJ, Owen DC, Rudy EB: The effects of lidocaine on intracranial hypertension, *J Neurosci Nurs* 24:205, 1992.
19. Lee M and others: The efficacy of barbiturate coma in the management of uncontrolled intracranial hypertension following neurosurgical trauma, *J Neurotrauma* 11(3):325, 1994.
20. Morrison CAM: Brain herniation syndromes, *Crit Care Nurs* 7(5):34, 1987.
21. Rose BA: Neurologic therapies in critical care, *Crit Care Nurs Clin North Am* 5:237, 1993.
22. Emergency brain resuscitation: a group working on emergency brain resuscitation, *Ann Intern Med* 122:622, 1995.
23. Grade G and others: Pathology and pathophysiology of head injury. In Youmans J, editor: *Neurological surgery,* ed 3, Philadelphia, 1990, WB Saunders.
24. Prendergast V: Current trends in research and treatment on intracranial hypertension, *Crit Care Nurs Q* 17:1, 1994
25. Allison M: Metabolic effects of brain injury: searching for moving targets, *Headlines* 4(1):2, 1993.
26. Grotta J for the CGS 19755 study group: Safety and tolerability of the glutamate agonist CGS 19755 in acute stroke patients, *Stroke* 25:12, 1994.
27. Wolf A and others: Effects of THAM upon outcome in severe head injury: a randomized prospective clinical trial, *J Neurosurg* 78:54, 1993.
28. Barnett HJM and others: Aspirin dose in stroke prevention: beautiful hypothesis slain by ugly facts, *Stroke* 27:588, 1996.
29. Whitney F: Stroke. In Barker E, editor, *Neuroscience nursing,* St Louis, 1994, Mosby.
30. The National Institute of Neurological Disorders and Stroke rt-PA Study Group: Tissue plasminogen activator for acute ischemic stroke, *New Engl J Med* 333:1581, 1995.

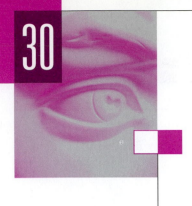

30 Neurologic Nursing Diagnosis and Management

THIS CHAPTER IS designed to supplement the preceding chapters in the Neurologic Alterations unit by integrating theoretic content into clinically applicable case studies and nursing management plans.

The case study is designed to illustrate clinical problem solving and patient care management occurring in actual patients. The case study, reviewed retrospectively, demonstrates how medical and nursing diagnoses may be effectively used in critical care. The case study also demonstrates revisions to the plan of care and the nursing and medical management outcomes that are apt to occur during the course of a complicated hospitalization as the patient responds physiologically to treatment. Often in a short case anecdote, such as presented in this chapter, the clinical answer may appear to be obvious from the day of admission. In practice, however, critical care patient management is sometimes investigative and the "correct" diagnosis for an individual patient may not become apparent until midway in the hospitalization, or a patient with an apparently straightforward diagnosis may develop an unexpected complication, and the plan of care and potential outcomes will then require revision. Many of the case studies demonstrate this principle.

The nursing management plans, which—unlike the case study—are not patient-specific, provide a basis nurses can use to individualize care for their patients. In the previous *Neurologic Alterations* chapters, each medical diagnosis is assigned a Nursing Diagnosis and Management box. Using this box as a page guide, the reader can access relevant nursing management plans for each medical diagnosis. For example, nursing management of *subarachnoid hemorrhage,* described on p. 802, may involve several nursing diagnoses and management plans outlined in this chapter and in other Nursing Diagnosis and Management chapters. Specific examples are (1) *Ineffective Breathing Pattern related to decreased lung expansion,* on p. 723; (2) *Altered Nutrition: Less than Body Requirements related to lack of exogenous nutrients or increased metabolic demand,* on p. 165; (3) *Risk for Infection risk factor: invasive monitoring devices,* on p. 598; and (4) *Anxiety related to threat of biologic, psychologic, and/or social intergrity,* on p. 99. These examples highlight the interrelationship of the various physiologic systems in the body and the fact that pathology often has a multisystem impact in the critically ill.

Use of the case study and management plans can enhance the understanding and application of the *Neurologic* content in clinical practice.

CASE STUDY

NEUROLOGIC

CLINICAL HISTORY

Mrs. T is a 66-year-old white woman with a medical history of hypertension controlled by diet and medication. Her health otherwise has been good. Premorbid vital signs are not available.

CURRENT PROBLEMS

While leaving a grocery store with her husband, Mrs. T suddenly complained of severe headache and almost immediately collapsed to the floor. An ambulance transported her to the hospital. On arrival to the emergency department she was conscious, disoriented, and complaining of severe, diffuse headache. Her Glasgow Coma Scale (GCS) score was as follows: eye opening, 4; best verbal, 4; best motor, 6. The pupils were round and equal and reacted briskly to light. No nuchal rigidity was evident, and the motor examination was symmetric. Her blood pressure (BP) was 210/124; heart rate, 98 (normal sinus rhythm [NSR] with occasional premature ventricular contractions [PVCs]); and respiratory rate, 24 and regular.

MEDICAL DIAGNOSIS

Probable subarachnoid hemorrhage (SAH), grade II

NURSING DIAGNOSIS

Acute Pain related to transmission and perception of cutaneous, visceral, muscular, or ischemic impulses

PLAN OF CARE

1. Perform a computed tomography (CT) scan to definitively determine the nature of cerebral vascular accident (CVA).
2. Reduce blood pressure.

MEDICAL AND NURSING MANAGEMENT AND PATIENT OUTCOME

Nifedipine (Procardia) 10 mg was administered sublingually as Mrs. T was prepared for an emergency CT scan of the head. Her neurologic status rapidly deteriorated, she became stuporous and difficult to arouse, and her respirations became irregular. Her pupils were midposition and sluggish in reaction to light. Intubation, oxygenation, and manual hyperventilation were carried out, and she was transported to the CT scanner. Based on the results of the CT scan, the following diagnoses were made.

MEDICAL DIAGNOSIS

SAH extending into the ventricles with acute, obstructive hydrocephalus, grade IV

NURSING DIAGNOSES

Decreased Adaptive Capacity: Intracranial related to failure of normal intracranial compensatory mechanisms

Ineffective Breathing Pattern related to decreased lung expansion

REVISED PLAN OF CARE

Mrs. T was taken directly to the operating room (OR) for placement of a ventriculostomy for drainage of cerebrospinal fluid (CSF) to relieve the intracranial hypertension and to monitor the intracranial pressure (ICP).

MEDICAL AND NURSING MANAGEMENT AND PATIENT OUTCOME

Mrs. T was stable at the end of the procedure and was extubated in the OR. She was transferred to the critical care unit and was soon alert, but disoriented to time, and was experiencing short-term memory difficulty. Her GCS was 14. Pupils were equal and reactive to light, and the motor examination findings were symmetric. Her ICP was 10 cm H_2O; BP, 155/88; pulse, 85 (NSR); and respirations, 18 (regular). She was placed on nimodipine to lessen the potential for cerebral vasospasm, and precautions were taken to prevent subarachnoid rebleeding (bedrest; analgesics; stool softener; quiet, darkened room). An IV of $D_5{}^1/_2NS$ was maintained.

CASE STUDY—CONT'D

NEUROLOGIC

REVISED PLAN OF CARE

The following day Mrs. T underwent cerebral angiography followed by a right frontal craniotomy for clipping of an anterior communicating artery aneurysm.

MEDICAL AND NURSING MANAGEMENT AND PATIENT OUTCOME

Mrs. T was continued on nimodipine postoperatively. Her BP averaged 150 to 160 mm Hg systolic, and her ICP averaged 10 to 12 cm H_2O with bloody CSF drained in small amounts. Hydration was maintained with $D_5$1/2NS. Her serum Na1 was 133 mEq/L, and other electrolytes, blood urea nitrogen (BUN), and creatinine were within normal limits. After 3 uneventful days the ventriculostomy was removed. Later that night Mrs. T became obtunded and developed a slight right lower facial droop and weakness of the left arm and leg. Because recurrent obstructive hydrocephalus was suspected, mannitol was administered. An emergency CT scan was done and revealed no recurrent hydrocephalus and no new bleeding. Her serum Na1 at this time was 114 mEq/L.

MEDICAL DIAGNOSES

Cerebral vasospasm affecting both cerebral hemispheres
Severe hyponatremia

NURSING DIAGNOSIS

Altered Cerebral Tissue Perfusion related to vasospasm or hemorrhage

REVISED PLAN OF CARE

Hypertensive-hypervolemic therapy was warranted to combat the severe cerebral vasospasm, improve cerebral perfusion, and prevent cerebral infarction.

MEDICAL AND NURSING MANAGEMENT AND PATIENT OUTCOME

Nimodipine was continued. Mrs. T was placed with the head of bed elevated no higher than 10 degrees to improve cerebral perfusion. Her BP was maintained at 200 to 210 mm Hg systolic with IV crystalloids and colloids and a dopamine infusion. A pulmonary artery catheter was inserted to monitor and maintain the pulmonary capillary wedge pressure between 14 and 16 mm Hg. Hypertonic NaCl was administered IV to correct the severe hyponatremia, since fluid restriction is contraindicated in the presence of cerebral vasospasm. Mrs. T's Na^+ slowly rose to 132 mEq/L, and after several days of hypertensive-hypervolemic therapy she became more alert and was able to follow simple commands. The right facial droop persisted, and her left extremities were now flaccid, indicating that cerebral infarctions had occurred in both hemispheres. After 12 days this therapy was slowly withdrawn, and she was transferred from the critical care unit.

Two weeks later, while sitting in a chair, she became obtunded and aspirated. Right facial focal seizures were noted. Her serum Na^+ was again found to be 116 mEq/L. Her electrolyte imbalance was corrected, but she never fully regained consciousness. Mrs. T was later transferred to a skilled nursing facility. Her disease progression is unknown.

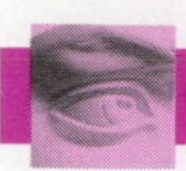

NURSING MANAGEMENT PLAN

ALTERED TISSUE PERFUSION

DEFINITION

The state in which an individual experiences a decrease in nutrition and oxygenation at the cellular level due to a deficit in arterial capillary blood supply.

Altered Cerebral Tissue Perfusion Related to Vasospasm or Hemorrhage

DEFINING CHARACTERISTICS

Hemorrhage

- Aneurysm grading system according to Hunt and Hess
  - Grade I: minimal bleed
    - Asymptomatic or minimal headache
    - Slight nuchal rigidity
  - Grade II: mild bleed
    - Moderate-to-severe headache
    - Nuchal rigidity
    - Minimal neurologic deficit (for example, possible cranial nerve palsies—oculomotor [cranial nerve III] most common; unilateral pupillary dilation, ptosis, and dysconjugate gaze)
  - Grade III: moderate bleed
    - Drowsiness
    - Confusion
    - Nuchal rigidity
    - Possible mild focal neurologic deficits
  - Grade IV: moderate-to-severe bleed
    - Extremely decreased level of consciousness, stupor
    - Possible moderate-to-severe hemiparesis
    - Possible early posturing (decorticate or decerebrate)
  - Grade V: severe bleed
    - Profound coma
    - Posturing
    - Moribund appearance
- Pathological reflexes resulting from meningeal irritation
  - Kernig's sign: resistance to full extension of the leg at the knee when the hip is flexed
  - Brudzinski's sign: flexion of the hip and knee during passive neck flexion
  - Photophobia
  - Nausea and vomiting

Vasospasm

Worsening headache
Confusion and decreasing level of consciousness
Focal motor deficits such as unilateral weakness of extremities
Speech deficits such as slurring, receptive, or expressive aphasia
Increasing BP

OUTCOME CRITERIA

- Patient is oriented to time, place, person, and situation.
- Pupils are equal and normoreactive.
- BP is within patient's norm.
- Motor function is bilaterally equal.
- Headache, nausea, and vomiting are absent.
- Patient verbalizes importance of and displays compliance with reduced activity.

NURSING INTERVENTIONS AND *RATIONALE*

1. Assess for indicators of increased intracranial pressure (ICP) and brain herniation (see Decreased Adaptive Capacity: Intracranial related to failure of normal intracranial compensatory mechanism, p. 843). ***ICP will increase during vasospasm only when caused by the edema resulting from brain infarction.***
2. If hypertensive-hypervolemic therapy is prescribed, administer crystalloid and colloid IV fluids and monitor pulmonary artery wedge pressure (PAWP), pulmonary artery diastolic (PAD) pressure, systemic vascular resistance (SVR), and BP to achieve and maintain prescribed parameters. Systolic blood pressure is usually maintained at 150-160 mm Hg.
3. Monitor lung sounds and chest x-ray reports because of ***the risk of pulmonary edema associated with fluid overload.***
4. Anticipate administration of calcium channel blockers such as nifedipine ***to decrease peripheral vascular resistance and cause vasodilation.***
5. Rebleeding is a potential complication of aneurysm rupture; to prevent rebleeding, the following interventions constitute subarachnoid precautions:
   - Ensure bedrest in a quiet environment ***to lessen external stimuli.***
   - Maintain a darkened room ***to lessen symptoms of photophobia.***
   - Restrict visitors and instruct them to keep conversation as nonstressful as possible.
   - Administer prescribed sedatives as needed ***to reduce anxiety and promote rest.***
   - Administer analgesics as prescribed ***to relieve or lessen headache.***
   - Provide a soft, high-fiber diet and stool softeners ***to prevent constipation, which can lead to straining and increased risk of rebleeding.***
   - Assist with activities of daily living (feeding, bathing, dressing, toileting).
   - Avoid any activity that could lead to increased ICP; ensure that patient does not flex hips beyond 90 degrees and avoids neck hyperflexion, hyperextension, or lateral hyperrotation ***that could impede jugular venous return.***

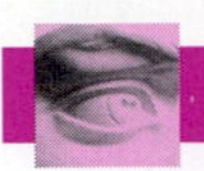

DECREASED ADAPTIVE CAPACITY: INTRACRANIAL

DEFINITION

A clinical state in which intracranial fluid dynamic mechanisms that normally compensate for increases in intracranial volumes are compromised, resulting in repeated disproportional increases in intracranial pressure (ICP) over baseline in response to a variety of noxious and nonnoxious stimuli.

Decreased Adaptive Capacity: Intracranial Related to Failure of Normal Intracranial Compensatory Mechanisms

DEFINING CHARACTERISTICS

- ICP >15 mm Hg, sustained for 15-30 minutes
- Headache
- Vomiting, with or without nausea
- Seizures
- Decrease in Glasgow Coma Scale score of two or more points from baseline
- Alteration in level of consciousness, ranging from restlessness to coma
- Change in orientation: disoriented to time and/or place and/or person
- Difficulty or inability to follow simple commands
- Increasing systolic blood pressure of more than 20 mm Hg with widening pulse pressure
- Bradycardia
- Irregular respiratory pattern (e.g., Cheyne-Stokes, central neurogenic hyperventilation, ataxic, apneustic)
- Change in response to painful stimuli (e.g., purposeful to inappropriate or absent response)
- Signs of impending brain herniation:
  - Hemiparesis or hemiplegia
  - Hemisensory changes
  - Unequal pupil size (1 mm or more difference)
  - Failure of pupil to react to light
  - Dysconjugate gaze and inability to move one eye beyond midline if third, fourth, or sixth cranial nerves involved
  - Loss of oculocephalic or oculovestibular reflexes
  - Possible decorticate or decerebrate posturing

OUTCOME CRITERIA

- ICP is ≤15 mm Hg.
- Cerebral perfusion pressure (CPP) is >60 mm Hg.
- Absence of clinical signs of increased ICP as previously described.

NURSING INTERVENTIONS AND *RATIONALE*

1. Maintain adequate CPP.
   a. With physician's collaboration, maintain BP within patient's norm by administering volume expanders, vasopressors, or antihypertensives.
   b. Reduce ICP.
      - Elevate head of bed 30 to 45 degrees ***to facilitate venous return.***
      - Maintain head and neck in neutral plane (avoid flexion, extension, or lateral rotation) ***to enhance venous drainage from the head.***
      - Avoid extreme hip flexion.
      - With physician's collaboration, administer steroids, osmotic agents, and diuretics.
      - Drain cerebrospinal fluid (CSF) according to protocol if ventriculostomy is in place.
      - Assist patient to turn and move self in bed (instruct patient to exhale while turning or pushing up in bed) ***to avoid isometric contractions and Valsalva maneuver.***
2. Maintain patent airway and adequate ventilation and supply oxygen ***to prevent hypoxemia and hypercarbia.***
3. Monitor arterial blood gas (ABG) values and maintain PaO_2 >80 mm Hg, $PaCO_2$ at 25-35 mm Hg, and pH at 7.35-7.45. ***to prevent cerbral vasodilation.***
4. Avoid suctioning beyond 10 seconds at a time; hyperoxygenate and hyperventilate before and after suctioning.
5. Plan patient care activities and nursing interventions around patient's ICP response. Avoid unnecessary additional disturbances and allow patient up to 1 hour of rest between activities as frequently as possible. ***Studies have shown the direct correlation between nursing care activities and increases in ICP.***
6. Maintain normothermia with external cooling or heating measures as necessary. Wrap hands, feet, and male genitalia in soft towels before cooling measures ***to prevent shivering and frostbite.***
7. With physician's collaboration, control seizures with prophylactic and as necessary (PRN) anticonvulsants. ***Seizures can greatly increase the cerebral metabolic rate.***
8. With physician's collaboration, administer sedatives, barbiturates, or paralyzing agents ***to reduce cerebral metabolic rate.***
9. Counsel family members to maintain calm atmosphere and avoid disturbing topics of conversation (e.g., patient condition, pain, prognosis, family crisis, financial difficulties).
10. If signs of impending brain herniation are present, do the following:
    - Notify physician at once.

Continued

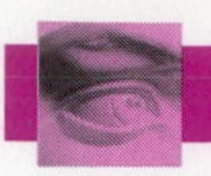

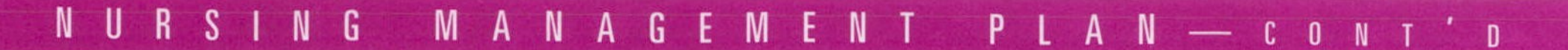

Decreased Adaptive Capacity: Intracranial Related to Failure of Normal Intracranial Compensatory Mechanisms

NURSING INTERVENTIONS AND *RATIONALE*—cont'd

- Be sure head of bed is elevated 45 degrees and patient's head is in neutral plane.
- Slow mainline intravenous (IV) infusion to keep open rate.
- If ventriculostomy catheter is in place, drain CSF as ordered.
- Prepare to administer osmotic agents and/or diuretics.
- Prepare patient for emergency computed tomographic (CT) head scan and/or emergency surgery.

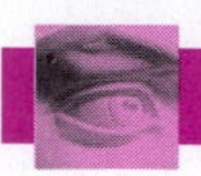

NURSING MANAGEMENT PLAN

UNILATERAL NEGLECT

DEFINITION

The state in which an individual is perceptually unaware of and inattentive to one side of the body.

Unilateral Neglect Related to Perceptual Disruption

DEFINING CHARACTERISTICS

- Neglect of involved body parts and/or extrapersonal space
- Denial of the existence of the affected limb or side of body
- Denial of hemiplegia or other motor and sensory deficits
- Left homonymous hemianopia
- Difficulty with spatial-perceptual tasks
- Left hemiplegia

OUTCOME CRITERIA

- Patient is safe and free from injury.
- Patient is able to identify safety hazards in the environment.
- Patient recognizes disability and describes physical deficits present (e.g., paralysis, weakness, numbness).
- Patient demonstrates ability to scan the visual field to compensate for loss of function or sensation in affected limb(s).

NURSING INTERVENTIONS AND *RATIONALE*

1. Adapt environment to patient's deficits ***to maintain patient safety.***
   - Position the patient's bed with the unaffected side facing the door.
   - Approach and speak to the patient from the unaffected side. If the patient must be approached from the affected side, announce your presence as soon as entering the room ***to avoid startling the patient.***
   - Position the call light, bedside stand, and personal items on the patient's unaffected side.
   - If the patient will be assisted out of bed, simplify the environment ***to eliminate hazards*** by removing unnecessary furniture and equipment.
   - Provide frequent reorientation of the patient to the environment.
   - Observe the patient closely and anticipate his or her needs. In spite of repeated explanations, the patient may have difficulty retaining information about the deficits.
   - When patient is in bed, elevate his or her affected arm on a pillow ***to prevent dependent edema and support the hand in a position of function.***
2. Assist the patient to recognize the perceptual defect.
   - Encourage the patient to wear any prescription corrective glasses or hearing aids ***to facilitate communication.***
   - Instruct the patient to turn the head past midline to view the environment on the affected side.
   - Encourage the patient to look at the affected side and to stroke the limbs with the unaffected hand. Encourage handling of the affected limbs ***to reinforce awareness of the affected side.***
   - Instruct the patient to always look for the affected extremity or extremities when performing simple tasks ***to know where it is at all times.***
   - After pointing to them, have the patient name the affected parts.
   - Encourage the patient to use self-exercises (e.g., lifting the affected arm with the good hand).
   - If the patient is unable to discriminate between the concepts of "right" and "left," use descriptive adjectives such as "the weak arm," "the affected leg," or "the good arm" to refer to the body. Use gestures not just words to indicate right and left.
3. Collaborate with the patient, physician, and rehabilitation team ***to design and implement a beginning rehabilitation program for use during critical care unit stay.***
   - Use adaptive equipment (braces, splints, slings) as appropriate.

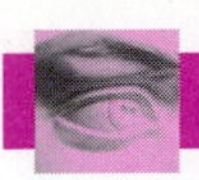

Unilateral Neglect Related to Perceptual Disruption

NURSING INTERVENTIONS AND *RATIONALE*—cont'd

- Teach the patient the individual components of any activity separately, then proceed to integrate the component parts into a completed activity.
- Instruct the patient to attend to the affected side, if able, and to assist with the bath or other tasks.
- Use tactile stimulation ***to reintroduce the arm or leg to the patient.*** Rub the affected parts with different textured materials ***to stimulate sensations (warm, cold, rough, soft).***
- Encourage activities that require the patient to turn the head toward the affected side and retrain the patient to scan the affected side and environment visually.
- If patient is allowed out of bed, cue him or her with reminders to scan visually when ambulating. Assist and remain in constant attendance because ***the patient may have difficulty maintaining correct posture, balance, and locomotion.*** There may be vertical-horizontal perceptual problems, with the patient leaning to the affected side to align with the perceived vertical. Provide sitting, standing, and balancing exercises before getting the patient out of bed.
- Assist patient with oral feedings.
  a. Avoid giving patient any very hot food items that could cause injury.
  b. Place the patient in an upright sitting position if possible.
  c. Encourage the patient to feed himself or herself; if necessary, guide the patient's hand to the mouth.
  d. If the patient is able to feed himself or herself, place one dish at a time in front of the patient. When the patient is finished with the first, add another dish. Tell the patient what he or she is eating.
  e. Initially place food in the patient's visual field; then gradually move the food out of the field of vision and teach the patient to scan the entire visual field.
  f. When the patient has learned to visually scan the environment, offer a tray of food with various dishes.
  g. Instruct the patient to take small bites of food and to place the food in the unaffected side of the mouth.
  h. Teach the patient to sweep out pockets of food with the tongue after every bite ***to eliminate retained food in the affected side of the mouth.***
  i. After meals or oral medications, check the patient's oral cavity for pockets of retained material.

4. Initiate patient and family health teaching.
   - Assess to ensure that both the patient and the family understand the nature of the neurologic deficits and the purpose of the rehabilitation plan.
   - Teach the proper application and use of any adaptive equipment.
   - Teach the importance of maintaining a safe environment and point out potential environmental hazards.
   - Instruct family members how to facilitate relearning techniques (e.g., cueing, scanning visual fields).

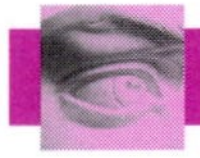

NURSING MANAGEMENT PLAN

IMPAIRED VERBAL COMMUNICATION

DEFINITION

The state in which an individual experiences a decreased or absent ability to use or understand language in human interaction.

Aphasia Related to Cerebral Speech Center Injury

DEFINING CHARACTERISTICS

- Inappropriate or absent speech or responses to questions
- Inability to speak spontaneously
- Inability to understand spoken words
- Inability to follow commands appropriately through gestures
- Difficulty or inability to understand written language
- Difficulty or inability to express ideas in writing
- Difficulty or inability to name objects

OUTCOME CRITERION

- Patient is able to make basic needs known.

Continued

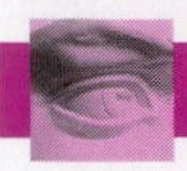

NURSING MANAGEMENT PLAN—CONT'D

Aphasia Related to Cerebral Speech Center Injury

NURSING INTERVENTIONS AND *RATIONALE*

1. Consult with physician and speech pathologist ***to determine the extent of the patient's communication deficit (e.g., if fluent, nonfluent, or global aphasia is involved).***
2. Have the speech therapist post a list of appropriate ways to communicate with the patient in the patient's room ***so that all nursing personnel can be consistent in their efforts.***
3. Assess the patient's ability to comprehend, speak, read, and write.
   - Ask questions that can be answered with a "yes" or a "no." If a patient answers "yes" to a question, ask the opposite (e.g., "Are you hot?" "Yes." "Are you cold?" "Yes."). ***This may help determine if in fact the patient understands what is being said.***
   - Ask simple, short questions, and use gestures, pantomime, and facial expressions to give the patient additional clues.
   - Stand in the patient's line of vision, giving a good view of your face and hands.
   - Have the patient try to write with a pad and pencil. Offer pictures and alphabet letters at which to point.
   - Make flash cards with pictures or words depicting frequently used phrases (e.g., glass of water, bedpan).
4. Maintain an uncluttered environment, and decrease external distractions ***that could hinder communication.***
5. Maintain a relaxed and calm manner, and explain all diagnostic, therapeutic, and comfort measures before initiating them.
6. Do not shout or speak in a loud voice. ***Hearing loss is not a factor in aphasia, and shouting will not help.***
7. Have only one person talk at a time. ***It is more difficult for the patient to follow a multisided conversation.***
8. Use direct eye contact, and speak directly to the patient in unhurried, short phrases.
9. Give one-step commands and directions, and provide cues through pictures or gestures.
10. Try to ask questions that can be answered with a "yes" or a "no," and avoid topics that are controversial, emotional, abstract, or lengthy.
11. Listen to the patient in an unhurried manner, and wait for his or her attempt to communicate.
    - Expect a time lag from when you ask the patient something until the patient responds.
    - Accept the patient's statement of essential words without expecting complete sentences.
    - Avoid finishing the sentence for the patient if possible.
    - Wait approximately 30 seconds before providing the word the patient may be attempting to find (except when the patient is very frustrated and needs something quickly, such as a bedpan).
    - Rephrase the patient's message aloud ***to validate it.***
    - Do not pretend to understand the patient's message if you do not.
12. Encourage the patient to speak slowly in short phrases and to say each word clearly.
13. Ask the patient to write the message, if able, or draw pictures if only verbal communication is affected.
14. Observe the patient's nonverbal clues for validation (e.g., answers "yes" but shakes head "no").
15. When handing an object to the patient, state what it is, ***since hearing language spoken is necessary to stimulate language development.***
16. Explain what has happened to the patient, and offer reassurance about the plan of care.
17. Verbally address the problem of frustration over inability to communicate, and explain that patience is needed for both the nurse and the patient.
18. Maintain a calm, positive manner, and offer reassurance (e.g., "I know this is very hard for you, but it will get better if we work on it together").
19. Talk to the patient as an adult. Be respectful, and avoid talking down to the patient.
20. Do not discuss the patient's condition or hold conversations in the patient's presence without including him or her in the discussion. ***This may be the reason some aphasic patients develop paranoid thoughts.***
21. Do not exhibit disapproval of emotional utterances or spontaneous use of profanity; instead, offer calm, quiet reassurance.
22. If the patient makes an error in speech, do not reprimand or scold but try to compliment the patient by saying, "That was a good try."
23. Delay conversation if the patient is tired. ***The symptoms of aphasia worsen if the patient is fatigued, anxious, or upset.***
24. Be prepared for emotional outbursts and tears in patients who have more difficulty in expressing themselves than with understanding. The patient may become depressed, refuse treatment and food, ignore relatives, and push objects away. Comfort the patient with statements such as, "I know it's frustrating and you feel sad, but you are not alone. Other people who have had strokes have felt the way you do. We will be here to help you get through this."

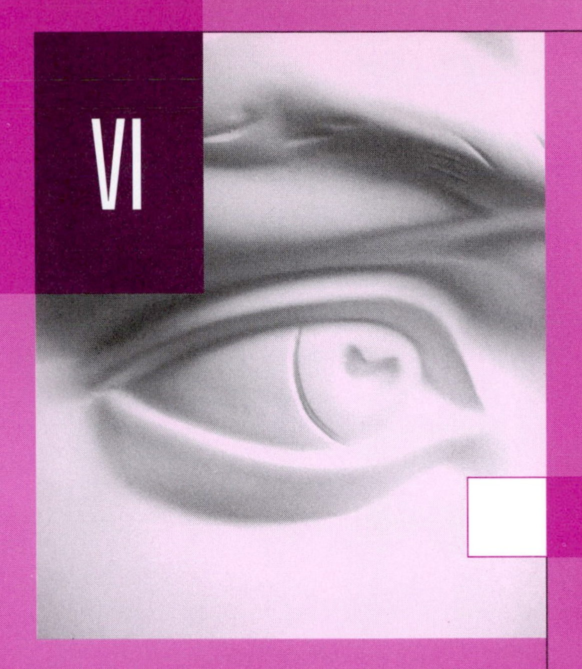

RENAL ALTERATIONS

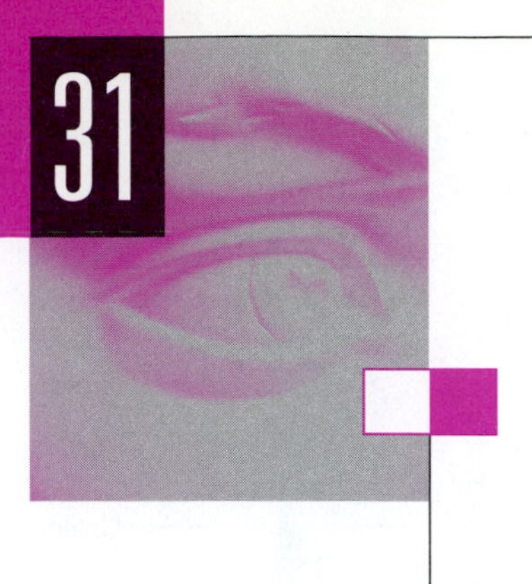

Renal Anatomy and Physiology

THE KIDNEYS ARE complex organs responsible for several functions necessary to maintain homeostasis. Although the primary role of the kidneys is to maintain fluid and electrolyte balance, the kidneys are also important for metabolic waste removal, blood pressure control, red blood cell synthesis, bone metabolism, and acid-base balance. Without adequate kidney function, homeostasis in all of these functions is affected.

The purpose of this chapter is to provide an overview of the anatomy and physiologic processes of the kidneys. An understanding of normal renal function is an important background for understanding pathophysiology, symptoms, and therapeutic management of renal system dysfunction.

MACROSCOPIC ANATOMY

The kidneys are paired organs located retroperitoneally with one on each side of the vertebral column between T12 and L3. The right kidney is positioned slightly lower than the left because of the presence of the liver. The bean-shaped organs weigh about 120 to 170 g each and in the adult measure approximately 12 cm long, 6 cm wide, and 2.5 cm thick.[1] The kidneys are protected anteriorly and posteriorly by the rib cage and by a tough fibrous capsule that encloses each kidney. Additional protection is provided by a cushion of perirenal fat and the support of the renal fascia.[1]

Internally the kidneys are made up of two distinct layers: the cortex and the medulla. The cortex is the outer layer and contains the glomeruli, the proximal tubules, the cortical portions of the loops of Henle, the distal tubules, and the cortical collecting ducts.[2,3] The inner layer, the medulla, is made up of the renal pyramids, which contain the medullary portions of the loops of Henle, and the medullary portions of the collecting ducts. After urine leaves the renal pyramids, it travels through increasingly larger structures that carry the urine to the bladder. Numerous pyramids taper and join to form a minor calyx. Several minor calyces combine to form a major calyx. The major calyces then join and enter the funnel-shaped renal pelvis, which directs the urine into the ureter (Figure 31-1). The capacity of the renal pelvis measures only about 5 to 10 ml, so this structure functions as a conduit, not a storage area for urine.

The renal system is also made up of the ureters, bladder, and urethra (Figure 31-2). The ureters are fibromuscular tubes that exit the renal pelvis and enter the bladder at an oblique angle. As urine is formed by the kidneys, the urine flows through the ureters by peristalsis. The peristaltic action of the ureters and the angle at which the ureters enter the bladder posteriorly under the epithelium help prevent reflux of urine from the bladder back up into the kidneys.[4] The urinary bladder is a muscular sac in the pelvic region with a fluid capacity of approximately 300 to 500 ml. Urine leaves the bladder through the urethral orifice and is excreted from the body via the urethra. In the male the urethra is about 20 cm long; in the female the urethra is 3 to 5 cm long.[3]

VASCULAR ANATOMY

The kidneys receive 20% to 25% of the cardiac output, about 1200 ml/minute. Blood enters the kidneys through the renal arteries, which branch bilaterally from the abdominal aorta. The renal artery divides into arterial branches that split into interlobular arteries,[3] which are located between the pyramid structures and

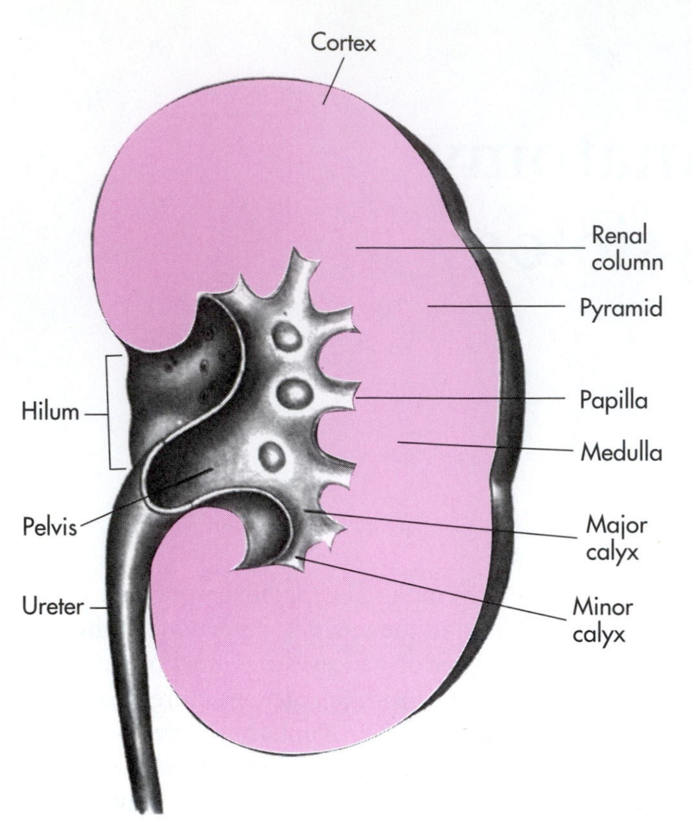

FIGURE 31-1. Cross-section of the kidney. (From Thompson JM and others: *Mosby's clinical nursing,* ed 4, St Louis, 1997, Mosby.)

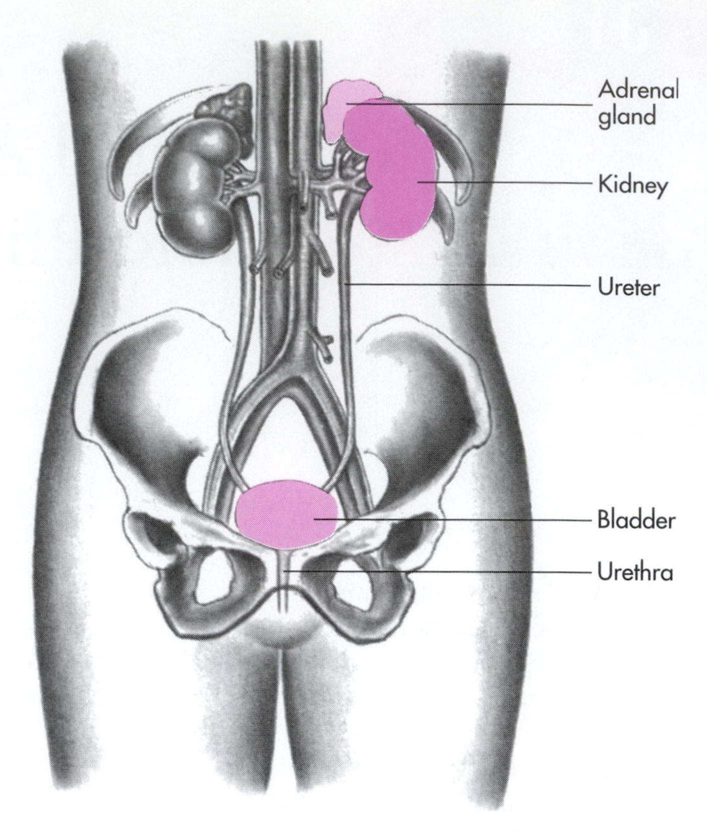

FIGURE 31-2. Structures of the urinary system. (From Thompson JM and others: *Mosby's clinical nursing,* ed 4, St Louis, 1997, Mosby.)

branch into the afferent arterioles. A single afferent arteriole supplies blood to each glomerulus, a tuft of capillaries that is the first structure of the nephron, the functional unit of the kidneys. Blood exits the glomerulus by the efferent arteriole, which divides into the vasa recta and the peritubular capillaries. The vasa recta extends into the medulla to supply the long medullary loops of Henle; the peritubular capillaries provide blood to the cortical portions of the nephron tubules. This intricate capillary network surrounds the tubules and allows water and solutes to move between the tubules and the capillaries for urine formation. The capillaries then rejoin the gradually enlarging venous vessels until the blood finally leaves each kidney through the renal vein and enters the general circulation by the inferior vena cava.

MICROSCOPIC STRUCTURE AND FUNCTION

Each kidney is made up of about one million nephrons, the functional units of the kidney. Not all of the nephrons function at the same level. As a result, the kidneys can continue to function even when several thousand nephrons are destroyed or damaged by disease or injury. Each nephron consists of the glomerulus, Bowman's capsule, the proximal convoluted tubule, the loop of Henle, the distal convoluted tubule, and the collecting duct (Figure 31-3).

There are two types of nephrons: the cortical nephrons and the juxtamedullary nephrons.[3] Approximately 85% of the nephrons are cortical nephrons, with the glomeruli located in the outer renal cortex. Cortical nephrons have short loops of Henle and perform only excretory and regulatory functions. The remaining 15% of the nephrons are juxtamedullary nephrons with glomeruli located deep in the cortex and extending into the medullary layer of the kidney. The juxtamedullary nephrons have long loops of Henle that are responsible for the concentration and dilution of urine.

Glomerulus. The first structure of each nephron is the glomerulus, a knot of capillaries that branches off from the afferent arteriole. The glomerulus is a high-pressure

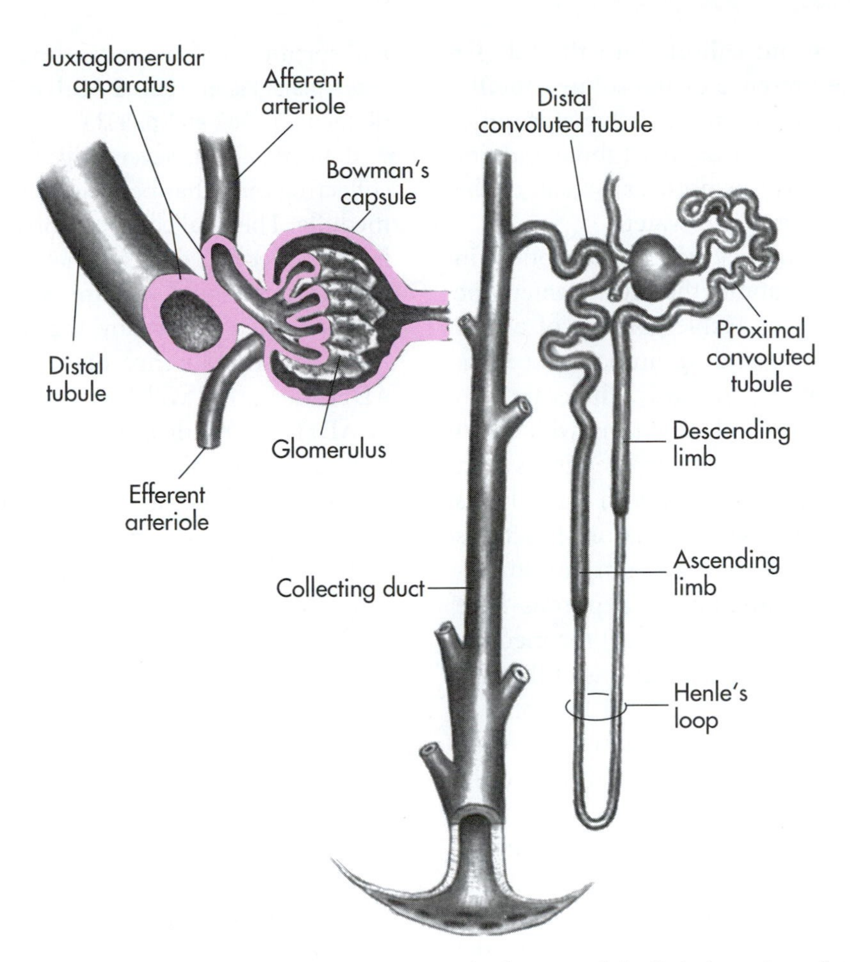

FIGURE 31-3. Components of the nephron. (From Thompson JM and others: *Mosby's clinical nursing,* ed 4, St Louis, 1997, Mosby.)

capillary bed and serves as the filtering point for the blood. Blood enters the glomerulus via the afferent arteriole and exits via the efferent arteriole. Positive filtration pressure in the glomerulus is achieved as a result of the high arterial pressure as the blood enters the afferent arteriole and the resistance created by the smaller efferent arteriole as the blood exits the glomerulus. As a result of the positive pressure gradient, excess fluid and solutes are filtered through the glomerular capillary walls. The basement membrane lining the glomerulus allows fluid and small molecules to be filtered from the blood and form a filtrate that eventually becomes urine. Large molecules such as albumin and red blood cells are prevented from entering the filtrate. The presence of large molecules in the urine is a signal that the glomerular membrane is damaged or affected by disease. In addition to the size of the molecules, the electrical charge, protein binding, and shape of molecules determine which molecules are filtered.[1,5]

Bowman's capsule. The filtrate (also known as ultrafiltrate) enters Bowman's capsule, a tough membranous layer of epithelial cells that completely surrounds the glomerular capillary bed. Bowman's space is located between the capillary walls of the glomerulus and the inner layer of Bowman's capsule and is a small holding area for the initial filtrate from the blood. Fluid, solutes, and other substances filtered by the glomerulus collect in the space. The space connects with the first portion of the nephron's tubular system, the proximal convoluted tubule.

Proximal convoluted tubule. The proximal convoluted tubule is located in the cortex of the kidney and reabsorbs most of the solutes the body does not routinely excrete in the urine. Solutes that are usually completely reabsorbed include glucose, amino acids, and bicarbonate. In addition, a large percentage of the water and solutes such as potassium, sodium, and calcium filtered by the glomerulus are also reabsorbed. Solutes such as urea, nitrogen, and creatinine are not reabsorbed and are thus excreted in the urine. In addition to a major role in reabsorbing water and solutes from the filtrate, the proximal convoluted tubule also secretes organic anions and cations into the tubular lumen. Because of the presence of the solutes, the filtrate that enters the proximal tubule is hyperosmotic. When the filtrate leaves the proximal tubule and enters the loop of Henle, it is isosmotic as a result of the reabsorption of both solutes and water.

Loop of Henle. Following selective reabsorption in the proximal convoluted tubule, the filtrate enters the loop of Henle. The loop of Henle consists of a thin descending limb, a thin ascending limb, and a thick ascending limb.[3] As noted previously, there are two types of nephrons: the cortical nephrons with short loops of Henle and the juxtamedullary nephrons with long loops of Henle. The nephrons with short loops of Henle perform excretory and regulatory functions but participate minimally in the concentration or dilution of urine. The juxtamedullary nephrons have glomeruli that are next to (juxtaposed to) the medulla near where the cortex and medulla sections of the kidney join, and these nephrons are critical for concentrating and diluting the urine. Major control of urine concentration and dilution occurs through the countercurrent mechanism. The thin descending limb is very permeable to water but fairly impermeable to urea, sodium, and other solutes. As a result, water is reabsorbed and the filtrate changes from isosmotic to more hyperosmotic or concentrated as it enters the thin ascending and thick ascending limbs. As the filtrate moves up the ascending limb into the collecting duct, it becomes more dilute. The thick ascending limb is impermeable to water but allows reabsorption of potassium, sodium, calcium, and bicarbonate. As solutes are reabsorbed without water, the filtrate becomes hypoosmotic.

Distal convoluted tubule. The hypoosmotic filtrate leaves the ascending portion of the loop of Henle and enters the distal convoluted tubule in the cortex of the kidney. The first portion of the distal tubule contains the cells of the macula densa, specialized cells that are a component of the juxtaglomerular apparatus important in blood pressure control. The first section of the distal tubule is impermeable to water, reabsorbs solutes such as sodium, bicarbonate, and calcium, and excretes potassium.[2,3] The later section of the distal tubule regulates sodium, bicarbonate, potassium, and calcium, depending on hormonal, acid-base, and electrolyte balance influences. For example, in the presence of antidiuretic hormone (ADH), the late distal tubule reabsorbs water and some solutes and the filtrate changes from hypoosmotic to isosmotic. In the absence of ADH the filtrate remains hypoosmotic because the distal tubule is impermeable to water and reabsorption of solutes without water occurs. (∞Diabetes Insipidus, p. 1021; SIADH, p. 1027; Serum Antidiuretic Hormone, p. 983 and p. 993.)

Collecting duct. Several distal tubules join to form a collecting duct that begins in the cortex and enters the medulla. The final composition of the urine is achieved in the collecting duct, primarily because of the transport of potassium, sodium, and water. Water permeability is determined by the absence or presence of ADH.[3] In the absence of or with small amounts of ADH, the urine will be dilute, while larger amounts of ADH will result in a very concentrated urine. The filtrate is generally more concentrated when it leaves the collecting duct than when it entered. Acidification of the urine is accomplished by the transport of bicarbonate and hydrogen in the collecting duct. Several collecting ducts then combine to form the pyramids. After the urine leaves the collecting ducts, no change in the composition of the filtrate occurs. Box 31-1 summarizes tubular reabsorption and secretion in the various portions of the nephron.[2,3]

NEURAL INNERVATION

The autonomic nervous system provides the primary innervation to the kidneys and urinary system. The kidneys receive messages from the lowest splanchnic and inferior splanchnic nerves, which form the renal plexus. The inferior mesenteric plexus, the hypogastric plexus, and the pudic nerve from the sacral region serve the bladder, ureters, and urethra.[4]

Nervous system control in the urinary tract is reflected in the process of micturition, or the release of urine. Bladder fullness stimulates stretch receptors in the bladder wall and a portion of the urethra. Signals are sent through nerves in the sacral area and return as parasympathetic messages to contract the detrusor muscle of the bladder. With a full bladder, contractions usually are powerful enough to relax the external sphincter. Sympathetic stimulation returns the external sphincter to contraction after the urine is released. Nervous system control is also present from the central nervous system in the cerebral cortex and brainstem. The central nervous system regulates the micturition reflex, frequency, and external sphincter tone and allows conscious control over urinary release.

PROCESSES OF URINE FORMATION

The nephrons are responsible for clearing the blood of unwanted metabolic substances and wastes and re-

BOX 31-1 Tubular Reabsorption and Secretion

GLOMERULUS	PROXIMAL CONVOLUTED TUBULE	LOOP OF HENLE	DISTAL TUBULE	COLLECTING DUCT
• Filters fluid and solutes from blood	• Reabsorbs Na^+, K^+, Cl^-, HCO_3^-, urea, glucose, amino acids • Filtrate leaves isosmotic	• Reabsorbs Na^+, K^+, Cl^- • Blocks reabsorption of H_2O from ascending limb • Countercurrent mechanism dilutes/concentrates urine • Filtrate leaves hypoosmotic	• Na^+, K^+, Ca^{++}, PO_4 selectively reabsorbed • H_2O reabsorbed in presence of ADH • Na^+ reabsorbed in presence of aldosterone • Filtrate leaves hypoosmotic	• Reabsorption similar to that in distal tubule • H_2O reabsorbed in presence of ADH • HCO_3^- and H^+ reabsorbed/secreted to acidify urine • Filtrate leaves hyperosmotic or hypoosmotic, depending on body needs

taining essential electrolytes and water as needed by the body. The entire blood volume of an individual is filtered by the kidneys 60 to 70 times each day. As a result, about 180 L of fluid is filtered from the plasma and enters Bowman's space.[1] The glomerular filtration rate (GFR), or the amount of filtrate formed in the nephrons, is therefore about 125 ml/minute. The kidneys must reduce the 180 L of filtrate to an average of 1 to 2 L of urine per day. Thus, although 180 L of filtrate is formed, 99% is reabsorbed and only 1% is excreted as urine. There are three processes necessary for the formation of urine: glomerular filtration, tubular reabsorption, and tubular secretion.[1,3]

Glomerular filtration. The first process in urine formation, glomerular filtration, depends on glomerular blood flow, the pressure in Bowman's space, and plasma oncotic pressure.[2,3] Glomerular blood flow is the most important of these three factors. The afferent and efferent arterioles of the glomeruli have the ability to increase or decrease the glomerular blood flow rate through selective dilation and/or constriction. To function effectively, a constant arterial blood pressure is needed in the glomerulus. For example, when the mean arterial blood pressure is decreased, the afferent arteriole dilates and the efferent arteriole constricts to maintain a higher pressure in the glomerular capillary bed and therefore maintain the GFR at 125 ml/minute. The ability of the kidneys to autoregulate blood flow fails when the mean arterial blood pressure is less than 80 mm Hg or greater than 180 mm Hg.[5]

The second factor that influences the GFR is the pressure in Bowman's space. An increase in pressure in the space will decrease filtration because the increased pressure resists the movement of solutes and water from the capillaries into the space. For example, if the tubules of the nephrons are blocked by cellular debris, backward pressure is exerted on Bowman's space, the GFR drops below 125 ml/minute, and a decreased urine output results.

The final factor that influences GFR is plasma oncotic pressure. When the oncotic pressure in the blood is decreased, as in disease states that result in low plasma protein levels, pressure in the capillary bed is decreased. Therefore, although the mean arterial pressure in the bed favors filtration, decreased amounts of fluid and solutes will leave the capillaries and enter Bowman's space because the oncotic pressure gradient in the plasma is less favorable. Filtration will still occur, but it is decreased from the normal 125 ml/minute, leading to a decrease in filtrate formation and therefore urine output.

The status of the glomerular filtration system is assessed by measuring the GFR. To measure this, the clearance of a substance from the plasma into the filtrate is assessed. The term *clearance of a substance* refers to the volume of plasma from which the substance is completely cleared by the kidneys and is expressed in milliliters per minute.[3,6] To measure clearance, three factors must be known: the concentration of the substance in the urine (U), the volume of urine produced over a specific time period (V), and the concentration of the substance in the plasma (P). The relationship between these factors is expressed as the following formula:

$$\text{Clearance} = U \times V/P$$

Every substance in the blood has a distinct clearance, the most useful of which is creatinine. Creatinine is used as a measure of the GFR because it is a waste product produced at a fairly constant rate by the muscles, is freely filtered by the glomerulus, and is not reabsorbed or secreted by the tubules. Therefore most of the creatinine produced by the body is excreted by the kidneys, making the creatinine clearance a good screening and follow-up test for estimating the GFR. In general, the creatinine clearance mirrors the GFR, so that a normal creatinine clearance is 125 ml/minute. A creatinine clearance less than 100 ml/minute indicates a GFR of less than 100 ml/minute and is a signal of insufficient renal function. A creatinine clearance (and GFR) less than 20 ml/minute results in symptoms of renal failure.[6]

Tubular reabsorption. The second process in the formation of urine is tubular reabsorption, the movement of a substance from the tubular lumen (filtrate) into the peritubular capillaries (blood). Tubular reabsorption allows the 180 L of solutes and water that were filtered by the glomerulus to be taken back into the circulation and decreases the 180 L of filtrate to 1 to 2 L of urine per day. Tubular reabsorption occurs by both passive and active transport processes.[3]

Passive transport. Passive transport of substances in the tubule depends on changes in concentration gradients and does not require energy. Diffusion and osmosis are the primary passive transport processes in the nephrons. Diffusion is the spontaneous movement of molecules from an area of higher concentration to an area of lower concentration across a semipermeable membrane ("semi" permeable because not all substances will cross, primarily because of the large size of a molecule). For example, when water is reabsorbed by the tubules, the concentration of urea in the tubules is increased. Urea then diffuses across the semipermeable membrane of the tubule and reenters the plasma to achieve balance in the concentration gradient.

Osmosis is the movement of water from an area of lower solute concentration to an area of higher solute concentration. Osmosis occurs any time the concentration of solutes on one side of a semipermeable membrane is greater than the concentration of solutes on the other side of the membrane. For example, when the concentration of sodium is greater in the peritubular capillaries than in the tubules, water passively moves from the tubules into the capillaries to balance the concentration gradient.

Active transport. Active transport of substances into or out of the tubules requires energy in the form of adenosine triphosphate (ATP).[3] In active transport a substance must combine with a carrier and then diffuse across the semipermeable tubular membrane. Substances that are actively reabsorbed include glucose, amino acids, calcium, potassium, and sodium. The rate at which substances can be actively reabsorbed depends on availability of the carriers, saturation of the carriers, and availability of energy. The transport maximum refers to the maximum rate at which substances can be reabsorbed and varies according to each individual substance.[3]

The threshold concentration of a substance is also important in active transport. The threshold of a substance is the plasma level of a substance at which none of the substance appears in the urine.[3] When the threshold of a substance in the plasma is exceeded, progressively larger amounts of the substance appear in the urine because the large amounts cannot be reabsorbed. For example, the threshold concentration for glucose is about 200 mg/dL. At or below a plasma glucose concentration of 200 mg/dL, all glucose is actively reabsorbed from the tubules back into the circulation and none is excreted in the urine. When the plasma glucose concentration is above 200 mg/dL, the threshold concentration is exceeded, and some of the glucose cannot be reabsorbed from the tubules and is excreted in the urine.

Tubular secretion. The third process in urine formation is tubular secretion, the transport of substances into the tubules from the peritubular capillaries. Tubular secretion occurs by both diffusion and active transport and is dependent on the needs of the body. For example, potassium, hydrogen, and drugs are secreted into the tubules to decrease their concentration in the body. Tubular secretion plays a lesser role than tubular reabsorption in changing the filtrate into urine.

FUNCTIONS OF THE KIDNEYS

The formation of urine through the processes described above is one of the major functions of the kidneys. The kidneys are also responsible for a number of other functions that are essential to maintaining homeostasis. These additional functions include the elimination of metabolic wastes, blood pressure regulation, the regulation of erythrocyte production, the activation of vitamin D, prostaglandin synthesis, acid-base balance, and fluid-electrolyte balance.[2,3]

Elimination of metabolic wastes. Metabolic processes in the body produce waste products that are selectively filtered out of the circulation by the kidneys. Urea, uric acid, and creatinine are by-products of protein metabolism that the kidneys filter out of the circulation and excrete in the urine. In addition, metabolic acids (ammonium chloride, for example), bilirubin, and drug metabolism by-products are also eliminated as waste products.[2]

Urea. Urea and creatinine are the primary waste products that are measured in determining renal function. Urea is measured as blood urea nitrogen (BUN) and is the end product of protein metabolism resulting from the breakdown of ammonia in the liver. The level of urea in the blood is influenced by protein metabolism, the amount of protein in the diet, and renal excretion. The body forms at least 25 to 30 g of urea per day.[2] More urea is formed if protein intake is high or if the individual is in a catabolic state and is breaking down body protein stores. Urea is primarily excreted in the urine and will therefore accumulate in the blood if the glomerulus is unable to filter it.

Creatinine. Creatinine is an end product of protein metabolism by the muscles. Normally, creatinine is completely filtered by the kidneys and excreted in the urine. As a result, the level of creatinine in the blood provides an index of renal function.

Blood pressure regulation. The kidneys regulate arterial blood pressure by maintaining the circulating blood volume through fluid balance and by altering peripheral vascular resistance via the renin-agiotensin-aldosterone system. Regulation by the renin-angiotensin-aldosterone system occurs in the juxtaglomerular apparatus (JGA), a group of specialized cells located around the afferent arteriole where the distal convoluted tubule makes contact (see Figure 31-3). This group of specialized cells is called the macula densa and provides a feedback message system from the distal tubule to control blood flow through the afferent arteriole.[3] An increase in tubular filtrate in the macula densa causes the afferent arteriole to constrict and therefore decrease the GFR and the amount of filtrate. Conversely, a decrease in the amount of tubular filtrate results in afferent arteriole dilation, an increased GFR, and an increased amount of filtrate.

The JGA synthesizes, stores, and releases renin.[2,3] Renin is released in response to reduced pressure in the glomerulus, sympathetic stimulation of the kidneys, and a decrease in the amount of sodium in the distal convoluted tubule. Renin enters the lumen of the afferent arteriole and is released into the general circulation. Renin is then converted to angiotensin I, which is further converted to angiotensin II as the blood circulates through the lungs. Angiotensin II is a powerful vasoconstrictor that causes increased systemic vascular resistance and therefore increased arterial blood pressure.

Angiotensin II also stimulates the release of aldosterone by the adrenal cortex. Aldosterone acts on the distal tubule to cause sodium and water reabsorption, resulting in an expanded circulating blood volume and therefore increased blood pressure. When the arterial blood pressure increases, the JGA stops releasing renin and the renin-angiotensin-aldosterone system is no longer in effect. Figure 31-4 summarizes the major aspects of the renin-angiotensin-aldosterone mechanism.

Erythrocyte production. The kidneys secrete erythropoietin, the hormone that controls erythrocyte (red blood cell) production in the bone marrow. Erythropoietin is released in response to a decrease in the amount of oxygen delivered to the kidneys, such as in anemia or hypoxia.[7] The hormone is active for about 24 hours after release and stimulates the bone marrow to increase the production of erythrocytes. The absence of erythropoietin, which occurs in individuals with renal failure, results in a profound anemia that must be treated by administering synthetic erythropoietin or by blood transfusion therapy.

Vitamin D activation. The kidneys convert vitamin D from food sources into an active form for use by the body. Active vitamin D is essentially a hormone that stimulates the absorption of calcium by the intestine and reabsorption of calcium by the renal tubules so that calcium is available for bone and tooth metabolism.[7] When the kidneys fail, the body is unable to convert dietary vitamin D to its active form, calcium is poorly absorbed, and bone disease results.

Prostaglandin synthesis. Prostaglandins are vasoactive substances that dilate or constrict the arteries. The prostaglandins produced by the kidneys produce only local renal blood flow effects and have minimal if any systemic effects.[8] The primary prostaglandins produced by the kidneys are vasodilators, PGE_1 and PGI_2, which act on the afferent arteriole to maintain blood flow and glomerular perfusion and filtration. The vasodilating effects of the prostaglandins also counteract the effects of angiotensin II and the sympathetic nervous system on the kidneys. As a result, renal perfusion is protected. See Box 31-2 for the effects of prostaglandins.

Acid-base balance. The nephron is involved in acid-base regulation by reabsorbing or excreting acids and bases.[2,3] The renal mechanism is not as rapid in altering acid-base concentrations as the lungs; therefore the

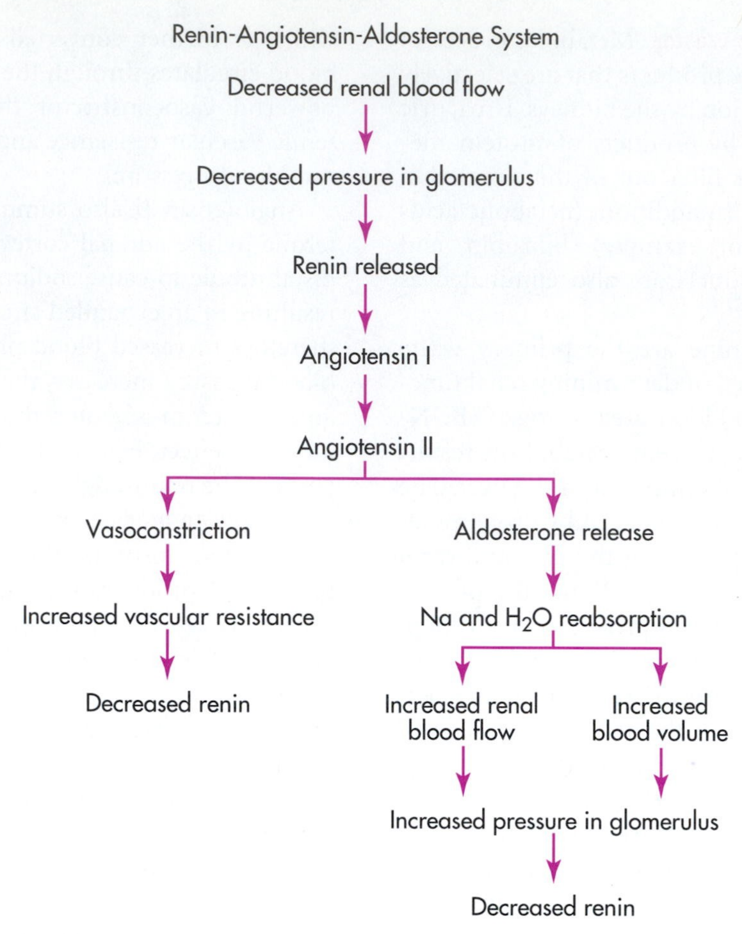

FIGURE 31-4. Renin-angiotensin-aldosterone system.

BOX 31-2 Effects of Prostaglandins

- Vasodilation
- Increased sodium and water excretion
- Stimulation of renin release
- Bronchoconstriction
- Vasoconstriction (PGF_2 in volume depletion)

kidneys regulate the day-to-day balance rather than coping with emergencies requiring quick response. (∞Arterial Blood Gases, p. 641.)

Bicarbonate, the principal blood buffer, is reabsorbed from the tubules, and hydrogen, a potent organic acid, is secreted into the tubules. Carbonic acid (H_2CO_3) in the renal tubular cells splits and sends hydrogen ions (H^+) to the tubular lumen and bicarbonate (HCO_3^-) to the blood. Recombination and then further splitting of carbonic acid in the tubules produces carbon dioxide for perpetuation of the bicarbonate/ hydrogen cycle and water for excretion. Hydrogen ions combine with either phosphates or ammonia and are transported into the tubular filtrate and excreted in the urine.

FLUID BALANCE

Regulation of the total amount of water in the body is vital for homeostasis and is one of the most important functions of the kidneys. In the absence of renal function, fluid volume overload occurs and threatens homeostasis. Similarly, if the renal system is unable to preserve adequate amounts of fluid, a severe volume deficit occurs that also disrupts homeostasis.

Fluid compartments. The fluid of the body is captured in distinct internal spaces or compartments. The compartments are separated from each other by membranes or thin sheets of tissue. The membranes are semipermeable, with openings (pores) that allow molecules of specific size and molecular weight to pass through while preventing larger, heavier molecules from doing so. As a result of the semipermeable membrane that separates

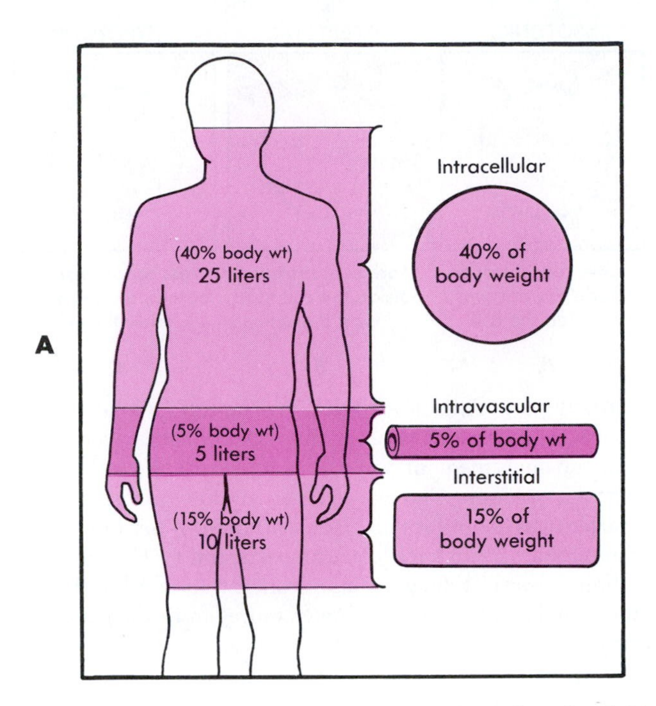

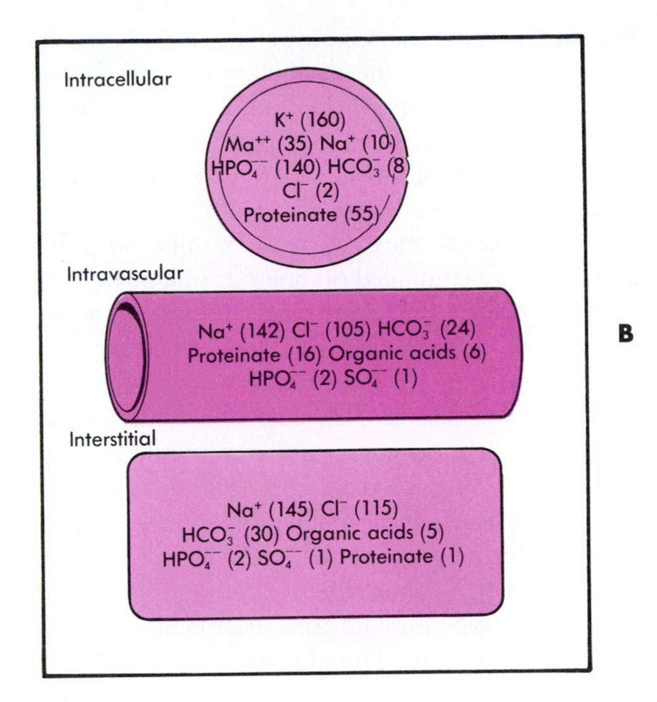

FIGURE 31-5. A, Fluid compartments. **B,** Electrolytes by fluid compartment.

the compartments, fluid movement between the compartments is dynamic and constant.

The body has two basic fluid compartments: intracellular and extracellular.[7] The intracellular compartment refers to the fluids inside each of the body's cells and accounts for 40% of a person's weight. The remaining fluid is outside the cells in the spaces referred to as the extracellular compartment. This compartment comprises two distinct subcompartments: intravascular and interstitial. The intravascular compartment, or the fluid within the blood supply, accounts for 5% of the body's weight. The fluid in the tissue spaces, or interstitial compartment, is outside both the body cells and the blood vessels and accounts for the remaining 15% of the body weight that is fluid. Approximate amounts of fluid contained in each compartment are listed in Figure 31-5, *A*.

The percentage of total body water varies slightly from individual to individual in relationship to gender, age, and body fat content. For instance, an adult male usually has a 60% body water content, whereas an adult female has closer to 50%. Infants have a body fluid content estimated at 77%, while body fluids may represent only 46% to 52% of body weight in elderly persons.[9] Also, with any increase in body fat, the body fluid percentage decreases because fat does not contain a significant amount of water.

Composition. Any information about body fluids by necessity must involve a description of the substances contained within the fluids. Movement of fluids within the body does not occur without simultaneous movement of these substances.

Electrolytes are elements or compounds that, when dissolved in water, dissociate into parts known as ions and give the fluid the ability to conduct an electrical current. The ions carry either a positive or a negative charge. Positive ions are known as cations, and negative ions are known as anions. Electrolytes exist in differing amounts in each of the fluid compartments. The primary electrolytes and other substances of importance in fluid and electrolyte balance are listed by fluid compartment in Figure 31-5, *B*.

A balance exists between cations, anions, and other substances in the fluid compartments. Maintaining this balance is important to the normal function of all body systems. For example, one of the differences between the intravascular and interstitial compartments is the amount of protein in the vascular compartment.[9] This difference helps maintain a balance between these two compartments. Finally, there are obvious differences in electrolyte composition between the fluids of the intracellular and extracellular compartments.

Fluid physiology. An overall understanding is needed of both the structures containing or balancing fluids and electrolytes and the physiologic forces that govern movement and balance. In addition, factors that inhibit or enhance the transfer of fluids and electrolytes are discussed.

Tonicity. The terms *isotonic, hypotonic,* and *hypertonic* all refer to tonicity, or the osmolality of body fluids.[3] Osmolality is a measure of the number of particles in a solution and is stated in milliosmoles. The normal osmolality of body fluids is 275 to 295 mOsm/kg of body weight.[10] (∞Serum Osmolality, p. 992.)

The term *isotonic* means that the number of particles in a solution contained on one side of a membrane approximates the number of particles in solution on the other side of the membrane. In the body an isotonic solution is one that has roughly the same tonicity as the blood plasma. Therefore cells bathed in an isotonic solution maintain consistency and do not lose or gain fluid to their surroundings (Figure 31-6, *A*).

The term *hypertonic* means that the number of particles in a solution is greater on one side of the membrane than on the other side of the membrane. Hypertonic fluid contains a concentration of particles greater than that inside the cell (Figure 31-6, *B*). When a hypertonic fluid is infused into the body for a prolonged time, fluid may be drawn out of the cells, causing a withering of the cell called crenation. If used appropriately, hypertonic solutions (such as the osmotic diuretic mannitol) can draw excess fluid from the cells and interstitial spaces into the intravascular space.

The term *hypotonic* means that the number of particles in a solution is less on one side of the membrane than on the other side of the membrane. A hypotonic solution contains fewer particles than does the solution inside the cell (Figure 31-6, *C*). As a result, cells suspended in a hypotonic fluid take on water, swell, and can eventually burst, a condition known as hemolysis. In dehydration states, hypotonic solutions such as 0.45% saline solution replenish the fluids and some of the lost electrolytes because fluids (and electrolytes) move from the intravascular space into the interstitial and intracellular spaces to rehydrate the cells.

Hydrostatic pressure. The force of left ventricular contraction of the heart pushes the blood through the circulatory system, causing pressure to be exerted by the blood against the vessel walls. This force is hydrostatic pressure. Hydrostatic pressure creates the tendency for fluids and dissolved substances to move into the interstitial spaces via filtration (movement of fluid and substances from an area of high pressure to one of low pressure).[2] Without other forces counteracting the hydrostatic pressure, fluid would leave the intravascular space until that space was depleted. However, while hydrostatic pressure favors fluid and electrolyte movement out of the intravascular compartment, the colloid osmotic pressure of the plasma tends to hold the fluid and substances in the intravascular space.[11]

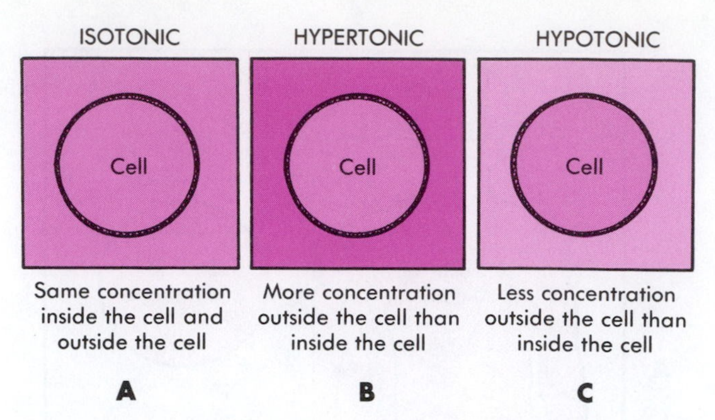

FIGURE 31-6. **A,** Isotonic solution. The extracellular solution concentration is the same as the intracellular concentration, with no movement of water into or out of the cell. **B,** Hypertonic solution. The extracellular solution concentration is greater than the intracellular concentration. Water moves from the cell into the extracellular compartment. **C,** Hypotonic solution. The extracellular solution concentration is less than the intracellular concentration. Water moves from the extracellular compartment into the cell.

Colloid osmotic pressure is created primarily by the presence of plasma proteins in the intravascular space.

Diffusion, osmosis, and active transport. Fluid balance within the compartments is also achieved through the processes of diffusion, osmosis, and active transport. Just as in the renal tubular cells, these three processes are constantly at work in other parts of the body to facilitate the movement of water and solutes to maintain homeostasis between the intracellular and extracellular compartments.

Movement of water. The forces generated by cardiac contraction, the plasma protein content in the intravascular space, and the solute content of both the extracellular fluid (ECF) and the intracellular fluid (ICF) result in a constant movement and balance of fluid throughout the fluid compartments. Movement of fluid between the intracellular space and the extracellular space is also a function of the osmotic pressure of the two spaces.

Fluid movement at the capillary level between the intravascular and interstitial spaces is a function of protein content in the plasma (capillary colloid osmotic pressure) and the pressure generated through cardiac contraction (capillary hydrostatic pressure). Similarly, the solute and protein content of the tissue space (interstitium) results in the generation of interstitial colloid osmotic pressure. An increase in plasma volume results in increased capillary hydrostatic pressure, forcing fluid into the interstitial space and creating edema. Conversely, a decrease in plasma volume causes the movement of fluid from the interstitium into the vascular space because the interstitial hydrostatic pressure is greater than the capillary hydrostatic pressure.

While the primary function of protein is to maintain basic cell structure and enzyme formation, an important secondary function is the maintenance of fluid balance. Protein is especially needed to control the movement of fluid between the intravascular and interstitial compartments. The plasma proteins (albumin, globulin, fibrinogen) are contained within the intravascular compartment. These plasma proteins exert a pull on water molecules and therefore produce a force called oncotic or osmotic pressure, which retains fluid within the intravascular compartment. This force is maintained because proteins are large and cannot travel across the membrane unless the permeability of the membrane is changed by disease (for example, burns or infections). A decrease in serum protein lessens the osmotic pressure in the intravascular space so that the tissue oncotic pressure is greater and pulls fluid from the vascular space into the interstitial space, causing edema.

The normal total protein content is 6.0 to 8.0 g/dL, of which 68% is albumin.[12] With normal kidney function, intact proteins are not filtered through the glomerulus because of their large size. In some disease states of the kidney, however, glomerular membrane permeability is altered, and protein molecules pass into the glomerular filtrate and appear in the urine.[6] (∞Nutrition and Renal Disorders, p. 137.)

FACTORS CONTROLLING FLUID BALANCE

Antidiuretic hormone. ADH is secreted by the posterior pituitary gland and functions as the primary controller of ECF volume. ADH acts on the distal convoluted tubule and the collecting ducts to reabsorb water. In the presence of ADH, water is reabsorbed and the ECF volume remains high; in the absence of ADH, water reabsorption does not occur and the ECF volume is diminished.[3] Several mechanisms stimulate or inhibit the release of ADH (Box 31-3). In addition to the usual stimuli, the presence of severe stress, either emotional or physical, can initiate ADH release through the limbic system that surrounds the hypothalamus.[10]

The strongest messages for release of ADH are sent by the osmoreceptors located in the hypothalamus.[10] As serum osmolality rises above 285 mOsm/kg (normal, 275 to 295 mOsm/kg), ADH is released and carried through the circulation to the nephrons. There, ADH attaches to receptor sites in the distal convoluted tubule and the collecting ducts and increases the permeability of the tubular structures to water. Water therefore can be reabsorbed into the circulatory system at a greater rate, leading to normalization of the serum osmolality and a steep rise in the urinary osmolality as less water in comparison to solutes is excreted.[10] ADH can sustain the effect on the renal tubules to a urinary osmolality of 1200 to 1400 mOsm/kg (normal, 500 to 800 mOsm/kg).[9] (∞Serum Antidiuretic Hormone, p. 993; Diabetes Insipidus, p. 1021; SIADH, p. 1027.)

BOX 31-3 Factors Stimulating Release of ADH

- Hyperosmolality of ECF
- Hypovolemia
- Increased body temperature
- Medications
  - Narcotics
  - Antineoplastics
  - Oral hypoglycemics
  - Beta-adrenergics

Renin-angiotensin-aldosterone system. The relationship between sodium and water plays an important role in the influence of the renin-angiotensin-aldosterone system on body water regulation. As noted in Figure 31-4, a reduction in vascular volume stimulates the release of renin. Renin converts to angiotensin I, which converts to the powerful vasoconstrictor angiotensin II. In turn, angiotensin II stimulates the adrenal glands to secrete aldosterone, a mineralocorticoid. Aldosterone acts on the distal tubules to reabsorb sodium from the tubular lumen into the circulation. In addition to hypernatremia, aldosterone is secreted in response to hypovolemia and hyperkalemia (Box 31-4). When sodium is retained, so is water. Angiotensin II also constricts the renal vasculature, reducing renal blood flow and available glomerular filtrate, thus sending a signal to the posterior pituitary to release ADH. In this way the two systems intertwine, not only to maintain fluid balance, but also to maintain electrolyte balance.[5]

Atrial natriuretic peptide. An additional influence on fluid and electrolyte regulation comes from the synthesis of atrial natriuretic peptide (ANP).[2,3] This hormone is secreted from atrial cells through the coronary sinus in response to hypernatremia, hypervolemia, and increased pressure in the heart (Box 31-5). ANP exerts many effects on sodium and water balance, among which are blocking aldosterone and ADH production, initiating vasodilation, and stimulating increased sodium and water excretion by the kidneys. Sites for

BOX 31-4 Factors Stimulating Release of Aldosterone

- Hypovolemia
- Hyponatremia
- Hyperkalemia
- Stress—emotional, physical

BOX 31-5 Factors Stimulating Release of ANP

- Hypernatremia
- Hypervolemia
- Vasoconstriction
- Decreased cardiac output
- Increased cardiac preload and afterload
- Increased systemic vascular resistance

stimulation of ANP production exist in the atrial walls, kidneys, lungs, vessel walls, eyes, brain, and adrenal glands. Production and release of ANP occur in response to the stimulation of stretch receptors as a result of increased volume.[13]

The beneficial effects of ANP production include a reduction in fluid overload through diuresis, decreased cardiac workload, and reduction in cardiac preload and afterload. The primary effects of ANP are circulatory volume control and blood pressure regulation. (∞Atrial Natriuretic Factor [ANF], p. 352.)

ELECTROLYTE BALANCE

Potassium. Potassium is the primary intracellular electrolyte. For this reason, it is difficult to accurately measure true body stores. Changes in the intracellular potassium concentration, however, are quickly reflected by the measurement of the extracellular amount. For example, during tissue breakdown, potassium leaves the cells, resulting in an elevated serum potassium level. The normal serum levels of potassium are 3.5 to 5.0 mEq/L.[9]

Diffusion and active transport across the cell membrane maintain potassium balance. Potassium leaves the cell by diffusion, moving toward the area of lesser concentration outside the cell, but it must be actively transported back into the cell to maintain cellular stability. With this movement the cell membrane is made ready to accept neural messages, leading to one of the most important potassium functions in the body—that of aiding nervous impulse conduction and muscle contraction.[9]

Potassium is also responsible for enzyme activity that helps in protein and carbohydrate metabolism for energy production. Additionally, because it is so abundant in the ICF, potassium controls the maintenance of intracellular osmolality (Box 31-6).

The gastrointestinal (GI) tract and skin excrete small amounts of potassium, but the major controllers of the body's potassium stores are the kidneys. Potassium is reabsorbed by the proximal tubules and secreted into the distal tubules as needed to maintain balance. Of the estimated 50 to 100 mEq/day ingested by an individual, 90% of the potassium is reabsorbed before arriving at the distal convoluted tubule, where the remainder is usually excreted. Reabsorption and secretion of potassium are influenced by many factors, which are presented in Box 31-7.

Potassium and sodium are in a constant state of competition within the body despite the need for both electrolytes and despite their differing functions. Because both electrolytes are cations, one intracellular and one extracellular, potassium and sodium must remain in balance to preserve electrical neutrality at the cell membrane. As a result, when sodium level is elevated, potassium level will decrease, and vice versa. For example, in the presence of aldosterone, potassium is excreted by the tubules while sodium is retained. Therefore potassium wasting may occur despite the body's need for potassium. (∞Potassium, p. 377.)

Sodium. Sodium is the most abundant extracellular electrolyte and is primarily responsible for shifts in body water and the amount of water retained or excreted by the kidneys. In addition to water regulation, sodium plays a role in the transmission of nerve impulses through the "sodium pump," or active transport mechanism at the cellular level. Sodium also combines with either chloride or bicarbonate to maintain acid-base balance. The normal serum value for sodium is 135 to 145 mEq/L[9] (Box 31-8).

The body contains a complex system of safeguards and feedback mechanisms to protect the level of sodium in the ECF. The three organs responsible for regulating sodium balance are the kidneys, the adrenal glands (aldosterone secretion), and the posterior pituitary gland (ADH secretion). Most sodium reabsorption occurs in the proximal tubule under the influence of aldosterone. Because of the extremely sensitive mechanism for retaining sodium, ingestion of large amounts of sodium is not necessary.

BOX 31-6 Potassium

NORMAL SERUM VALUE

3.5-5.0 mEq/L

FUNCTIONS

Transmission of nerve impulses
Intracellular osmolality
Enzymatic reactions
Acid-base balance
Myocardial, skeletal, and smooth muscle contractility

BOX 31-7 Factors Affecting Reabsorption and Secretion of Potassium

- Sodium balance—sodium deficit results in potassium loss
- Acid-base balance—acidosis moves hydrogen into the cell and potassium out, with potassium excreted in the urine
- Diuretics—increase loss of potassium in distal tubule
- GI losses—vomiting and GI suction remove potassium
- Insulin—promotes movement of potassium into the cell
- Epinephrine—enhances potassium reabsorption from distal tubule

BOX 31-8 Sodium

NORMAL SERUM VALUE

135-145 mEq/L

FUNCTIONS

Body fluid movement and retention
Extracellular osmolality
Active transport mechanism (with potassium)
Neuromuscular activity
Enzyme activities
Acid-base balance

Calcium. Calcium is the electrolyte of greatest quantity in the body, with stores estimated at 1200g.[4] Of the total body calcium, 99% is contained in the bones.[14] The remaining 1% is contained primarily in the ECF in the vascular space. The calcium contained within bone is in an inactive form that maintains bone strength and is a ready storehouse for mobilization of calcium to the serum in cases of depletion. The mobilization of calcium is accomplished through the influence of parathyroid hormone (PTH). The calcium in the intravascular space is either bound to protein or circulates freely in an ionized form.[15] Ionized calcium is the active form and functions in cell membrane stability and blood clotting. Protein-bound calcium awaits use during immediate crisis and ionizes more quickly than the calcium in the bone.

In the ionized (active) form, calcium plays an important role in maintaining the internal integrity of the cell. The amount of ionized calcium in the serum depends on changes in serum pH and on the availability of plasma protein, primarily albumin. Because changes in pH and albumin levels occur with relative frequency, the measurement of serum calcium can be deceptive. For instance, a change in the serum albumin level affects the calcium level. As serum albumin levels rise, ionized calcium becomes bound to the available protein, thus lowering the ionized calcium level. However, because total calcium is measured rather than only the ionized fraction, the actual decrease in the ionized and therefore immediately active calcium may not be accurately reflected.[14] Conversely, when albumin levels fall, calcium is split free of the protein and creates an actual rise in the ionized calcium level. Under the influence of the hormone calcitonin, however, the ionized calcium may be returned to the bone, and the actual availability of the calcium again may not be accurately reflected.

The normal serum calcium level ranges from 8.5 to 10.5 mg/dL.[9] For every increase or decrease in serum albumin of 1 g/dL, a change of 0.8 mg/dL occurs in the total serum calcium level. Therefore any serum calcium level measurement should be accompanied by a measurement of serum albumin level.

In addition to bone metabolism, calcium is responsible for other important functions. Myocardial contractility is influenced primarily by calcium. Neuromuscular activity, cell permeability, thickness of cell membranes, coagulation of blood, and hardness of bones and teeth all depend on calcium levels (Box 31-9).

Calcium levels are highly dependent on individual dietary intake and on a variety of physiologic mechanisms related to absorption.[14] The uptake of calcium is influenced by the amount of phosphorus, magnesium, vitamin D and its breakdown products, PTH, and calcitonin. Other factors, such as changes in acid-base

BOX 31-9 Calcium

NORMAL SERUM VALUE

8.5-10.5 mg/dL

FUNCTIONS

Hardness of bone and teeth
Skeletal muscle contraction
Blood coagulation
Cellular permeability
Heart muscle contraction

BOX 31-10 Phosphorus

NORMAL SERUM VALUE

2.5-4.5 mg/dL

FUNCTIONS

Intracellular energy production (ATP)
Bone hardness
Structure of cellular membrane
Oxygen delivery to tissues
Enzyme regulation (ATPase)

balance, affect calcium levels in the ECF. For example, acidosis ionizes or splits calcium free from albumin, resulting in "ionized" hypercalcemia, whereas alkalosis enhances the binding of calcium to proteins, thereby creating a deficit of ionized calcium.[15]

Phosphorus. The normal serum phosphorus level is 2.5 to 4.5 mg/dL. As with calcium and magnesium, the serum values of phosphorus represent a minute portion of the actual body stores.[9] Approximately 75% of the phosphorus is found in the bones, and part of the remaining amount is intracellular, making it difficult to measure. Serum phosphorus levels change frequently and dramatically, particularly in response to the ingestion of phosphate-rich foods such as milk, red meats, poultry, and fish.

The primary function of phosphorus is in the formation of ATP, which provides intracellular energy. The active transport mechanism across the cell membrane cannot function without the energy provided by ATP. Additional functions of phosphorus include cell membrane structure, acid-base balance, oxygen delivery to the tissues, cellular immunity, and bone strength (Box 31-10).

Absorption of phosphorus takes place in the GI tract, and excretion, for the most part, occurs in the kidney. Phosphorus is reabsorbed from the distal convoluted tubules of the kidney when body stores are low.[3] Acid-base balance is also influenced by the availability of phosphorus. Phosphates in the renal tubular filtrate combine with sodium and excess hydrogen ions to form sodium diphosphate ($NaHPO_4$). This complex then dissociates into its component parts. Sodium combines with the available bicarbonate and is reabsorbed into the peritubular capillary network. The remaining hydrogen and phosphates are excreted into the urine.

An important reciprocal relationship exists between phosphorus and calcium.[14] High levels of phosphorus result in low levels of calcium, and, conversely, high levels of calcium result in low levels of phosphorus. PTH secretion, vitamin D functions, and the processes of reabsorption and secretion in the renal tubules are all involved in this complex relationship.

Magnesium. Magnesium is primarily an intracellular electrolyte with about 60% located in the bone.[12] The ECF contains only about 1%, and the remaining body magnesium resides in the ICF. The normal serum value for magnesium is 1.3 to 2.1 mEq/L.[9] The levels of other intracellular electrolytes, such as calcium and potassium, are affected by the level of magnesium. For example, calcium and magnesium compete for absorption in the GI tract. If the dietary intake is higher in calcium than magnesium, calcium will be preferentially reabsorbed, and vice versa. The most important function of magnesium is ensuring the transport of sodium and potassium across the cell membrane. Magnesium in the ICF helps maintain potassium stores on both sides of the cell membrane inasmuch as magnesium is required for appropriate function of the intracellular "carrier substances" that transport sodium and potassium across the cell membrane. A depletion of magnesium liberates potassium to the ECF, which causes an increase in the renal excretion of potassium and hypokalemia.[16] In addition, magnesium plays a role in transmitting central nervous system messages, maintaining neuromuscular activity, and activating enzymes for the metabolism of carbohydrates and proteins (Box 31-11).

Chloride. Chloride is rarely found in the body without being in combination with one of the major cations. Therefore changes in serum chloride levels

BOX 31-11 Magnesium

NORMAL SERUM VALUE

1.3-2.1 mEq/L

FUNCTIONS

Neuromuscular transmission
Contraction of heart muscle
Activation of enzymes for cellular metabolism
Active transport at cellular level
Transmission of hereditary information

BOX 31-12 Chloride

NORMAL SERUM VALUE

97-110 mEq/L

FUNCTIONS

Body fluid osmolality (with sodium)
Body water balance (with sodium)
Acid-base balance
Acidity of body fluids

usually indicate changes in the other electrolytes or in acid-base balance.

Chloride combines most frequently with sodium; therefore it plays a major role in maintaining serum osmolality and water balance. Also, because it competes with bicarbonate for combination with sodium, it affects acid-base balance. In addition, chloride combines with hydrogen ions to form the hydrochloric acid present in gastric secretions (Box 31-12).

Red blood cell oxygenation and the transport of carbon dioxide also depend on adequate chloride levels. The dissociation of carbonic acid inside red blood cells creates hydrogen and bicarbonate ions. The hydrogen usually combines with hemoglobin, and the bicarbonate leaves the cell in exchange for the chloride ions that move into the cell (chloride shift).[4] Therefore carbon dioxide in the form of bicarbonate is liberated to travel to the lungs for excretion.

The normal serum chloride level is 97 to 110 mEq/L.[9] Most often chloride is ingested with sodium in the form of salt and is reabsorbed or excreted in the proximal tubules of the kidney. Chloride is actively transported out of the tubule into the interstitium, again with sodium, to help maintain the high tubular interstitial osmolality and the mechanism for concentrating the urine.[3]

Bicarbonate. Bicarbonate (HCO_3^-), an anion in the ECF, performs the single function of maintaining acid-base balance. Although bicarbonate is not solely responsible for acid-base balance, it is the major ECF buffer. Bicarbonate levels in the body are in balance with carbonic acid (H_2CO_3) levels. The ratio between the two must remain proportional at 1 mEq of carbonic acid to 20 mEq of bicarbonate or acid-base disturbances will result. When the carbonic acid level is elevated, acidosis results. When the bicarbonate level is high, alkalosis results. The normal serum level of bicarbonate is 24 to 28 mEq/L, and the normal value for carbonic acid is 1.2 to 1.4 mEq/L.[11]

The amount of bicarbonate available in the ECF is regulated by the kidneys.[3] Reabsorption of bicarbonate occurs primarily from the proximal tubule into the peritubular capillaries. Bicarbonate is also reconstructed in the distal tubule and reabsorbed into the blood in response to acid-base balance and body requirements. In addition, the kidneys either reabsorb or excrete bicarbonate in response to the number of hydrogen ions present as part of the body buffer system. More bicarbonate will be reabsorbed when there is a large number of hydrogen ions and excreted when few hydrogen ions are present.

As described in this chapter, the kidneys provide many functions that assist in the maintenance of homeostasis. While fluid balance is one of the most important functions that the kidney provides, an understanding of the numerous other roles the kidneys play provides clues to total body function.

REFERENCES

1. Chmielewski C: Renal anatomy and overview of nephron function, *ANNA J* 19(1):34, 1992.
2. Brundage D: *Renal disorders,* St Louis, 1992, Mosby.
3. Lancaster L: Renal anatomy and physiology. In Lancaster L, editor: *Core curriculum for nephrology nursing,* ed 3, Pitman, NJ, 1995, American Nephrology Nurses Association.
4. Guyton A, Hall, J: *Textbook of medical physiology,* ed 9, Philadelphia, 1996, WB Saunders.
5. Holechek M: Glomerular filtration and renal hemodynamics, *ANNA J* 19(3):237, 1992.

6. Richard D: Assessment of renal structure and function. In Lancaster L, editor: *Core curriculum for nephrology nursing,* ed 3, Pitman, NJ, 1995, American Nephrology Nurses Association.
7. Lancaster L: Systemic manifestations of renal failure. In Lancaster L, editor: *Core curriculum for nephrology nursing,* ed 3, Pitman, NJ, 1995, American Nephrology Nurses Association.
8. Spilman P, Whelton A: Nonsteroidal antiinflammatory drugs: effects on kidney function and implications for nursing care, *ANNA J* 19(1):19, 1992.
9. Metheny N: *Fluid and electrolyte balance—nursing considerations,* ed 2, Philadelphia, 1992, JB Lippincott.
10. Porth C, Erickson M: Physiology of thirst and drinking: implication for nursing practice, *Heart Lung* 21(3):274, 1992.
11. Soltis B, Cassmeyer V: Fluid and electrolyte imbalance. In Phipps WJ and others, editors: *Medical-surgical nursing: concepts and clinical practice,* ed 4, St Louis, 1991, Mosby.
12. Kavanagh JM: Assessment of the cardiovascular system. In Phipps WJ and others, editors: *Medical-surgical nursing: concepts and clinical practice,* ed 4, St Louis, 1991, Mosby.
13. Birney M, Penney D: Atrial natriuretic peptide: a hormone with implications for clinical practice, *Heart Lung* 19(2):174, 1990.
14. Brunier G: Calcium/phosphate imbalances, aluminum toxicity, and renal osteodystrophy, *ANNA J* 21(4):171, 1994.
15. Zaloga G: Hypocalcemia in critically ill patients, *Crit Care Med* 20(2):251, 1992.
16. Workman M: Magnesium and phosphorus: the neglected electrolytes, *AACN Clin Issues Crit Care Nurs* 3(3):655, 1992.

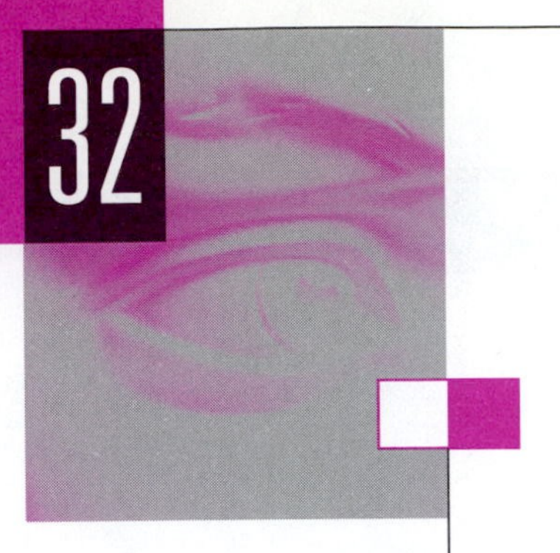

Renal Clinical Assessment and Diagnostic Procedures

Understanding the anatomic location and physiologic workings of the renal system provides a good basis for understanding the clinical manifestations that signal renal system dysfunction. The body presents a variety of clinical manifestations that demonstrate renal disorders. A methodic history and careful physical examination furnish data that help pinpoint the actual problem and often the cause of the problem.

HISTORY

A renal history begins with a description of the chief symptom, stated in the patient's own words. A description of the chief complaint includes the onset, location, duration, and factors that lessen or aggravate the problem.[1] Descriptions of any treatment sought by the individual, medications taken to alleviate symptoms (both prescription and nonprescription), or procedures performed to improve the problem often are helpful in determining the extent of the current complaint.

Predisposing factors for acute renal dysfunction are elicited during the history, including the use of over-the-counter medicines, recent infections requiring antibiotic therapy, and any diagnostic procedures performed using radiopaque contrast media.[2] Nonsteroidal antiinflammatory drugs (such as ibuprofen), antibiotics (especially aminoglycosides), and iodine-based dyes are potentially nephrotoxic, and it is important to assess for them when an individual has renal-related symptoms. In addition, the individual is questioned about any recent strenuous physical exercise. Exercise-induced rhabdomyolysis and resulting acute renal failure symptoms are much more likely in an individual who is unconditioned or poorly conditioned for strenuous physical activity.[3] A history of recent onset of nausea and vomiting or appetite loss caused by taste changes (uremia causes a metallic taste) may also provide clues to the rapid onset of renal problems.[2] Finally, symptoms that indicate rapid fluid volume gains are also sought. For example, rapid weight gains of more than 2 pounds per day or sleeping on additional pillows or sitting in a chair to sleep are signals of volume overload and potential kidney dysfunction.

In addition to outlining the current reason for admission to the critical care unit, a complete medical history is important. Similar symptoms, problems, or treatment for complaints in the past may help establish the cause of the problem or provide clues for treatment. The patient and/or family or significant other must provide as much detail as possible during the history.

The family history may also provide important information to aid in identifying and treating the patient's disorder. For example, the patient may reveal that one or two close family members have always had swelling of the extremities or high blood pressure. These symptoms should lead to questions about any history of kidney problems in the family. Box 32-1 summarizes the information gained when obtaining a renal history.

PHYSICAL EXAMINATION

In the critical care area, nursing assessment does not routinely include a full physical examination of the renal system. However, many of the assessment parameters for the renal system provide information related to the volume status of the individual and can be used in a large number of patients regardless of renal function or status. While not often performed in

BOX 32-1 DATA COLLECTION FOR RENAL HISTORY

COMMON RENAL SYMPTOMS
Dyspnea
Peripheral dependent edema
Nocturia
Nausea
Metallic taste in mouth
Loss of appetite
Headache
Rapid weight gain
Itching
Dry, scaly skin
Weakness, fatigue

PATIENT PROFILE
Personal habits
 Use of over-the-counter drugs
 Change in employment caused by illness
Financial problems resulting from illness—cost, time off work, etc.
Sex—decreased libido, amenorrhea
Recent strenuous exercise

RISK FACTORS
Family history
Hypertension
Diabetes mellitus

FAMILY HISTORY
Hypertension
Diabetes mellitus
Polycystic kidney disease
Kidney disease
Headaches
Chronically swollen extremities

RENAL STUDIES IN PAST
KUB x-ray
Intravenous pyelogram
Renal ultrasound
Renal arteriography
Kidney biopsy

MEDICAL HISTORY
Childhood
 Nephrotic syndrome, streptococcal infection
Adult
 Frequent urinary tract infections
 Use of iodine-based radiographic contrast media
 Use of nonsteroidal antiinflammatory drugs

CURRENT MEDICATION USAGE
Nonsteroidal antiinflammatory drugs
Antibiotics
Antihypertensives
Diuretics

the depth described in the following sections, the critical care nurse must be aware of how to perform a renal assessment in stable patients and as needed in patients with renal dysfunction.

Inspection

Bleeding. Visual inspection related to the kidneys generally focuses on the flank and abdomen. Renal trauma is suspected if a purplish discoloration is present on the flank (Grey-Turner's sign) or near the posterior eleventh or twelfth ribs.[4] Bruising, abdominal distention, and abdominal guarding may also signal renal trauma or a hematoma around a kidney.

Volume. Inspection is especially helpful in looking for signs of volume depletion or overload that might signal kidney problems. Fluid volume assessment begins with an inspection of the patient's neck veins. The supine position facilitates normal venous distention. An absence of distention (or flat neck veins) indicates hypovolemia. Assessment continues with the head of the bed elevated 45 to 90 degrees.[1] If the neck veins remain distended more than 2 cm above the sternal notch when the bed is at 45 degrees, fluid overload may be present.[5] (∞External Jugular Vein, p. 358.)

Hand vein inspection is also helpful in assessing volume status and is performed by observing for venous distention when the hand is held in the dependent position. Venous filling that takes longer than 5 seconds suggests hypovolemia. When the hand is elevated, the distention should disappear within 5 seconds. If distention does not disappear within 5 seconds after the hand is elevated, fluid overload is suspected.

Assessment of skin turgor provides additional data for identifying fluid-related problems. As the skin over the forearm is picked up and released, the rapidity of its return to its normal position is observed. Normal elasticity and fluid status allow an almost immediate return to shape once the skin is released. In fluid volume deficit, however, the skin remains raised and does not return to its normal position for several seconds. Because of the loss of skin elasticity in elderly persons, skin turgor assessment in the forearm is not accurate for fluid assessment of this age group. Rather, skin turgor can be assessed in the shoulder area, which retains elasticity.[5]

Finally, inspection of the oral cavity also provides clues to fluid volume status. When a fluid volume deficit exists, the mucous membranes of the mouth become dry. However, mouth breathing can also dry the mucous membranes temporarily. Therefore a more accurate way to assess the oral cavity is to inspect the mouth with the use of a tongue blade. Dryness of the oral cavity is more indicative of fluid volume deficit than are complaints of a dry mouth.[5]

Edema. Edema is the presence of excess fluid in the interstitial space and can be a symptom of volume overload. In the presence of volume excess, edema may be present in dependent areas of the body such as the feet and legs. The presence of edema, however, does not always indicate fluid volume overload. A loss of albumin from the vascular space can cause peripheral edema in the presence of hypovolemia or normal fluid states. For example, a critically ill patient may have a low serum albumin level because of inadequate nutrition following surgery, a burn, or a head injury. In addition, edema may signal circulatory difficulties. For example, an individual in fluid balance but with poor venous return may experience pedal edema after prolonged sitting in a chair with the feet dependent. Similarly, an individual with heart failure may experience edema because the left ventricle is unable to pump blood effectively through the vessels.

Edema can be assessed by applying fingertip pressure on the skin over a bony prominence, such as the ankles, pretibial areas (shins), and sacrum. If the indentation made by the fingertip does not disappear within 30 seconds, "pitting" edema is present. Pitting edema indicates increased interstitial volume and is not evident until a weight gain of approximately 10% has occurred.[6] Edema may also appear in the hands and feet, around the eyes, and in the cheeks. Dependent areas, such as the feet and sacrum, are the most likely to demonstrate edema in patients confined to a wheelchair or bed. One way of measuring the extent of edema is by a subjective scale of 1 to 4, with +1 indicating only minimal pitting and +4 indicating severe pitting (Table 32-1). Other scales for assessing and measuring edema are also used. (∞Edema, p. 363, Box 14-7.)

TABLE 32-1 Pitting Edema Scale

Rating	Approximate Equivalent
+1	5 mm depth
+2	8-10 mm depth
+3	>10 mm (lasting up to 30 sec)
+4	>20 mm (lasting longer than 30 sec)

Auscultation

Auscultation of the kidneys yields virtually no useful information. However, the renal arteries are auscultated for a bruit, a blowing or swishing sound that resembles a cardiac murmur (Figure 32-1). The examiner listens for bruits above and to the left and right of the umbilicus.[4] A renal artery bruit generally indicates stenosis, which may lead to acute or chronic renal dysfunction resulting from compromised blood flow to the kidney(s).

Auscultation is especially helpful in providing information about extracellular fluid (ECF) volume status. Listening for specific sounds in the heart and lungs provides information about the presence or absence of increased fluid in the interstitium or vascular space.

Heart. Auscultation of the heart requires not only assessing rate and rhythm but also listening for extra sounds. Fluid overload is often accompanied by a third or fourth heart sound, which may be heard with the bell of the stethoscope. Increased heart rate alone offers few data about fluid volume, but combined with a low blood pressure, it may indicate hypovolemia. (∞Third and Fourth Heart Sounds, p. 367.)

The heart is also auscultated for the presence of a pericardial friction rub. A rub can best be heard at the third intercostal space to the left of the sternal border, with the individual leaning slightly forward. The presence of a pericardial friction rub indicates pericarditis and may result from uremia in a patient with renal failure. (∞Pericardial Friction Rub, p. 371.)

Blood pressure. Blood pressure and heart rate changes are very useful in assessing fluid volume deficit. In stable critically ill patients or in patients on a telemetry unit, orthostatic vital sign measurements provide clues to blood loss, dehydration, unexplained syncope, and the effects of some antihypertensive medications.[7] A drop in blood pressure of more than 20 mm Hg or a rise in pulse rate of more than 20 beats per minute from lying to sitting or from sitting to standing represents

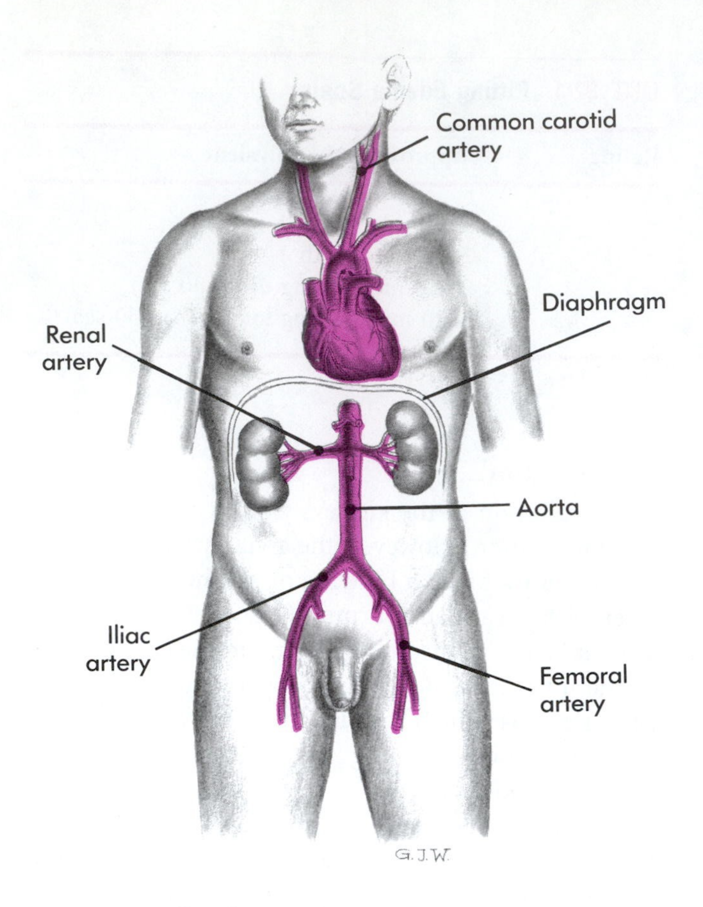

FIGURE 32-1. Sites for auscultation of bruits.

orthostatic hypotension. The drop in blood pressure occurs because the venous circulation is so volume depleted that a sufficient preload is not immediately available after the position change. The heart rate increases in an attempt to maintain cardiac output and circulation. Orthostatic hypotension produces subjective feelings of weakness, dizziness, or faintness. Although orthostatic hypertension is often a sign of hypovolemia, peripheral vascular disease may also be responsible. Peripheral vascular disease often damages the venous circulation of the lower extremities and therefore decreases blood return to the heart, leading to a blood pressure drop in a normovolemic individual.

Lungs. Lung assessment is also extremely important in gauging fluid status. Crackles indicate fluid overload. Dyspnea with mild exertion or dyspnea at night that prevents sleeping in a supine position may also indicate pooling of fluid in the lungs. Shallow, gasping breaths with periods of apnea reflect severe acid-base imbalances. (∞Abnormal Breath Sounds, p. 632.)

Palpation

Although rarely performed in critically ill patients, palpation of the kidneys in stable patients provides information about the kidneys' size and shape. Palpation of the kidneys is achieved through the bimanual capturing approach. Capturing is accomplished by placing one hand posteriorly under the flank of the supine patient with fingers pointing to the midline, while placing the opposite hand just below the rib cage anteriorly. The patient is asked to inhale deeply while pressure is exerted to bring the hands together (Figure 32-2). As the patient exhales, the examiner should feel the kidney between the hands. After each kidney is palpated in this manner, the two should be compared for size and shape. Each kidney should be firm and smooth, and they should be of equal size.[8] The examiner is usually unable to palpate a normal left kidney. The right kidney is more easily palpated because of its lower position, being displaced downward by the liver. Problems should be suspected if a mass (trauma or cancer) or an irregular surface (polycystic kidneys) is palpated, a size difference is detected, or the kidney extends significantly lower than the rib cage on either side.

Percussion

Percussion is performed to detect pain in the area of a kidney or to determine excess accumulation of air, fluid, or solids around the kidneys. Percussion of the kidneys also provides information about kidney location, size, and possible problems. Like palpation, percussion of the kidneys is not a routine part of a nursing assessment in critical care. However, the information gained through percussion can provide important patient care data.

Kidneys. Percussion of a kidney is performed with the patient in a side-lying or sitting position, with the examiner's hand placed over the costovertebral angle (lower border of the rib cage on the flank).[1] Striking the back of the hand with the opposite fist produces a dull thud, which is normal. Pain may indicate infection (such as a urinary tract infection that has extended into the kidneys) or injury resulting from trauma. Traumatic injury to the kidneys should be suspected in the presence of a penetrating abdominal wound, with blunt abdominal trauma, or with a fractured pelvis or ribs.[4,9] (∞Posttraumatic Renal Failure, p. 1090.)

Abdomen. Observation and percussion of the abdomen are of value in assessing fluid status. Percussing the abdomen (using the same procedure as for the kidneys but placing the patient supine) can result in a dull sound (solid bowel contents or fluid) or a hollow sound (gaseous bowel).[1,10]

Ascites, severe fluid distention of the abdominal cavity, is an important observation in determining fluid imbalances. Differentiating ascites from distortion caused by solid bowel contents is accomplished

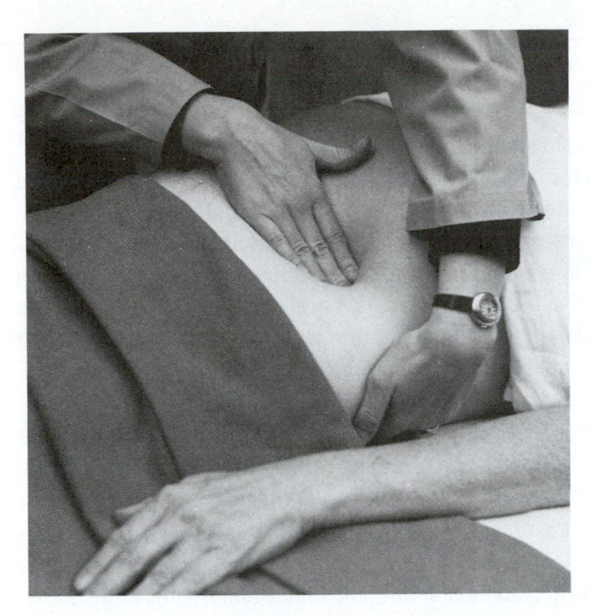

FIGURE 32-2. Palpation of the kidney. (From Malasanos L, Barkauskas V, Stoltenberg-Allen K: *Health assessment,* ed 4, St Louis, 1990, Mosby.)

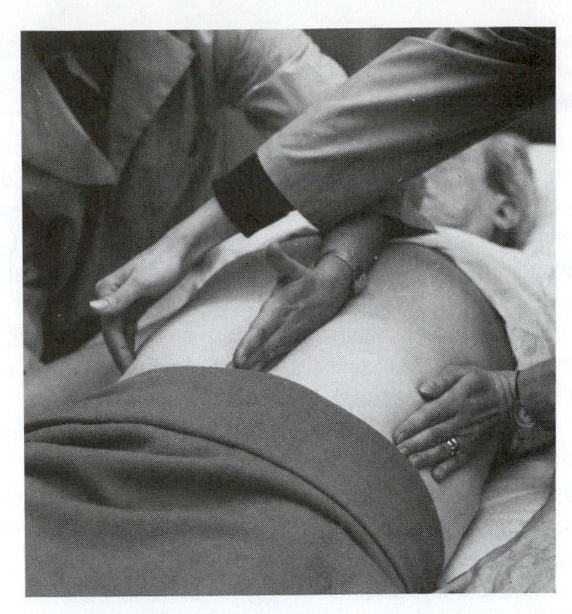

FIGURE 32-3. Test for the presence of a fluid wave. (From Malasanos L, Barkauskas V, Stoltenberg-Allen K: *Health assessment,* ed 4, St Louis, 1990, Mosby.)

by producing a fluid wave. A fluid wave is elicited by exerting pressure to the abdominal midline while one hand is placed on the right or left flank. Tapping the opposite flank produces a wave in the accumulated fluid that can be felt under the hands (Figure 32-3). Other signs of ascites include a protuberant, rounded abdomen and abdominal striae.[10]

Individuals with renal failure may have ascites caused by volume overload, which forces fluid into the abdomen because of increased capillary hydrostatic pressures. However, ascites may or may not represent fluid volume excess. Severe ascites in persons with compromised hepatic function may result from hypovolemia. The ascites occurs because the increased vascular pressure associated with hepatic dysfunction forces fluid and plasma proteins from the vascular space into the interstitial space and abdominal cavity.

ADDITIONAL ASSESSMENT PARAMETERS

Weight. One of the most important assessments of renal and fluid status is the patient's weight. In the critical care unit, weight is monitored on every patient and is an important vital sign measurement. Significant fluctuations in body weight over a 1 to 2-day period indicate fluid gains and losses. Rapid weight gains or losses of greater than 2 pounds per day generally indicate fluid rather than nutritional factors. One liter of fluid equals 1 kg, or approximately 2.2 pounds.

Whenever possible, the patient is weighed during admission to the critical care unit. It is important to note whether the current weight differs significantly from the weight 1 to 2 weeks before admission. When stable, the patient is weighed daily for comparison with the previous day's weight. The weight is obtained at the same time each day, with the patient wearing the same amount of clothing.

The individual's weight is of critical importance to the dialysis nurse caring for a patient with acute or chronic renal failure. The differences in weight from day to day are used to calculate the amount of fluid to remove during a dialysis treatment.

Intake and output. Like patient weight, intake and output are monitored on all patients in the critical care unit. Intake and output can be compared with the patient's weight to evaluate accurately the gain or loss of fluid. Urinary output plus insensible fluid losses (perspiration, stool, and water vapor from the lungs) can range widely from 750 to 2400 ml/day. When intake exceeds output (excessive intravenous fluid, decreased renal output), a positive fluid balance exists. In impaired renal function the positive fluid balance results in fluid volume overload. Conversely, if output exceeds intake (fever, increased respiration, profuse sweating, vomiting, diarrhea, gastric suction, diuretic therapy), a negative fluid balance exists and volume deficit results. During a 24-hour period, fever can increase skin and respiratory losses by as much as 75 ml/degree of Fahrenheit temperature rise.

CULTURAL INSIGHTS 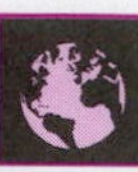 **Family Involvement in Care**

A Chinese-American female patient in the intensive care unit after a liver transplant appeared to have a sudden drop in urinary output. Intravenous fluids and albumin were administered, but instead of improving her urinary output, the woman developed pulmonary edema and had to be reintubated. Later, the staff was surprised to learn that the patient's Chinese-American friend, in an attempt to fulfill her role as helpful caretaker, had been emptying the patient's Foley catheter bag and discarding the urine.

In this case there was a serious transcultural misunderstanding. The staff was upset, the patient's friend was upset, and the patient incurred harm. The nurses' understanding of the role the family plays when a member is ill would have been useful in this case.

Traditionally, particularly among Chinese men, the sick family member *expects* to be cared for by other family members, close family friends, and the health care staff. It is the family's responsibility and *duty* to care for their relative. Shirking this responsibility is a violation of filial piety, one of the highest ranking of Confucian tenets.

Conversely, the duty of the "good patient" is to not resist the ministrations of the caregivers. This can be reflected in a seemingly passive behavior of the patient and can cause frustration among the nursing staff when they are attempting to encourage the Chinese-American patient to perform more self-care activities. Whereas the American nurses are working toward making the patient more independent, the patient may be striving to be more dependent, a highly valued characteristic in the Chinese culture.

In cases such as this, the nurses might try to involve the family and friends in permissible activities such as bathing the patient, combing his or her hair, massaging his or her arms or back, reading to the patient, and pushing the IV pole during ambulation to the commode. Of equal importance, the nursing staff must inform the family and friends of the activities that only the nurses can carry out and give reassurance that the staff will perform these for the patient. These explanations will help assure the family that the patient's needs are being addressed and satisfied and that their responsibility for overseeing the care of their relative is being met.

See Lepler M: *Nurseweek* 9(16):1, 1996; Lipson JG, Dibble SL, Minarik PA: *Culture and nursing care,* San Francisco, 1996, UCSF Nursing Press.

In many cases, individuals with acute renal failure (ARF) will exhibit a decrease in urine output, or oliguria (less than 400 ml/day). However, in most patients with ARF, as in those with early intrarenal ARF, there may be a fairly normal or only slightly decreased urine output that reflects water removal without solute removal. Therefore renal function cannot be accurately determined by urine output alone.[11]

Abnormal output of body fluids creates not only fluid imbalances but also electrolyte and acid-base disturbances. For example, gastrointestinal suction or loss by diarrhea can result in fluid deficit, sodium and potassium deficits, and metabolic acidosis from excessive loss of bicarbonate.

In maintaining daily records of intake and output, all gains or losses must be recorded. A standard list of the fluid volume held in various containers (e.g., milk cartons and juice containers) expedites this process. Discussions about the importance of accurate intake and output with the patient and family or friends are necessary and can improve the accuracy of record keeping.

Hemodynamic monitoring. Body fluid status is accurately reflected in measurements of cardiovascular hemodynamics. Measurements such as central venous pressure (CVP), pulmonary artery wedge pressure (PAWP), cardiac index (CI), and mean arterial pressure (MAP) provide a clear picture of the increases or decreases in vascular volume returning to and being ejected from the heart. Indeed, both volume depletion and overload are easily detected by use of central venous or arterial catheters from which pressure measurements can be obtained (Table 32-2).

A central venous catheter is often inserted to evaluate fluid volume status, and measure the CVP. The CVP represents the filling pressure of the right atrium and is a measurement of right ventricular preload. The CVP will change with fluctuations in volume status. A normal CVP is 2 to 6 mm Hg.[12] In volume depletion the CVP is less than 2 mm Hg, whereas volume overload is reflected by readings of more than 6 mm Hg. (∞Central Venous Pressure Monitoring, p. 451.)

If the patient has co-existing cardiopulmonary disease, or if more information about hemodynamic function is required, a pulmonary artery catheter may be inserted. This catheter provides information about left ventricular filling pressures and cardiac output. The PAWP represents the left atrial pressure required

TABLE 32-2 Hemodynamic Assessment of Fluid Status

Measurement	Volume Depletion	Volume Overload
CVP	<2 mm Hg	> 6 mm Hg
PAWP	<8 mm Hg	>12 mm Hg
CI	<2.2 L/min/m^2	>4.4 L/min/m^2
MAP	Decreased	Increased

BOX 32-2 Important Aspects of Fluid and Electrolyte Assessment

FLUID STATUS

- Skin turgor
- Mucous membranes
- Intake and output
- Presence of edema/ascites
- Diaphoresis
- Low-grade fever
- Neck and hand vein engorgement
- Lung sounds—crackles
- Dyspnea
- CVP <2 mm Hg, >6 mm Hg
- PAWP < 8 mm Hg, >12 mm Hg
- Tachycardia
- Hypertension, hypotension
- CI <2.2 L/min/m^2
- S_3, S_4 heart sounds
- Headache
- Blurred vision
- Vertigo on rising
- Papilledema
- Mental changes

ELECTROLYTE STATUS

- Serum osmolality
- Complete blood count (CBC)
- Serum electrolyte level
- Electrocardiogram tracings (potassium, calcium, magnesium levels)
- Behavioral and/or mental changes
- Chvostek's, Trousseau's signs (calcium levels)
- Changes in peripheral sensation (numbness, tremor)
- Muscle strength
- Gastrointestinal changes (nausea and vomiting)
- Therapies that can alter electrolyte status (gastrointestinal suction, diuretics, antihypertensives, calcium channel blockers)

to fill the left ventricle. When the left ventricle is full at the end of diastole, this represents the volume of blood available for ejection. It is also known as left ventricular preload and is measured by the PAWP. The normal PAWP is 8 to 12 mm Hg.[12] In fluid volume excess, PAWP rises. In fluid volume deficit, PAWP is low. (∞Pulmonary Artery Pressure Monitoring, p. 459.)

The CI demonstrates the cardiac output, or ejection volume of the left ventricle over 1 minute standardized for body size.[12] The normal CI is 2.2 to 4.4 L/minute/m^2. Compensatory mechanisms in early hypovolemic shock maintain the CI at or near normal. With prolonged loss, however, the CI falls. Fluid volume overload increases heart rate, which in turn increases cardiac output, but only to a point. Pump failure may result from massive volume overload, such as with acute heart failure secondary to renal failure, in which case the CI falls.[12] (∞Cardiac Output, p. 467; Cardiac Index, p. 446 and p. 473.)

MAP is the product of systemic vascular resistance (SVR) times the cardiac output and represents an average of blood pressure within the cardiac system. Changes in SVR or cardiac output inevitably result in corresponding MAP changes. For example, an increase in SVR during the early stages of hypovolemic shock leads to elevation of the MAP. Ongoing losses eventually lead to a decreased cardiac output, which leads to a reduction in MAP.[12] The net effect of a decreased MAP to the kidneys is a reduction in blood flow, leading to prerenal ARF. (∞Intraarterial Blood Pressure Monitoring, p. 444; Prerenal Failure, p. 878.)

Other observations. Renal system dysfunction often leads to fluid and electrolyte imbalances. Some of the disturbances in fluid and electrolyte levels are accompanied by clinical manifestations less measurable than those previously mentioned but that, nonetheless, indicate a change from normal function. Box 32-2 summarizes the important aspects to consider during fluid and electrolyte assessment.

Sudden or slowly developing changes in mental status must be investigated. For example, acidosis often results in disorientation. Lethargy, coma, and confusion may result from sodium, calcium, or magnesium excess or deficit. Apprehension or anxiety may be secondary to sodium deficit, a shift of fluid from the plasma to the interstitium, or respiratory changes caused by fluid volume overload.[10]

Finally, apathy and withdrawal often accompany hypovolemic states.[10] Patients with renal failure with systemic increases in electrolytes, fluids, and nitrogenous waste products can also exhibit apathy, restlessness, confusion, and withdrawal.[2] The speed of onset will vary according to how rapidly (or slowly) the renal failure progresses and alters homeostasis. In some patients, it may be difficult to separate the emotional component of critical illness from the physiologic mechanism; therefore both mechanisms are considered by the critical care nurse.

LABORATORY ASSESSMENT

Serum

Blood urea nitrogen. In addition to history and physical examination, laboratory data are extremely helpful in the diagnosis and therapeutic management of renal system dysfunction. Blood urea nitrogen (BUN) is a by-product of protein metabolism. The normal value for BUN is 9 to 20 mg/dL and is increased when renal function deteriorates.[13] With renal dysfunction the BUN is elevated because of a decrease in the glomerular filtration rate (GFR) and therefore a fall in urea excretion. Elevations in the BUN can be correlated with the clinical manifestations of uremia; as the BUN rises, symptoms of uremia become more pronounced.[2] However, a drop in the GFR and therefore an increase in the BUN may also be caused by hypovolemia, nephrotoxic drugs, or a sudden hypotensive episode. In these cases the rise in BUN is caused by a decreased GFR in the presence of normal kidney function. BUN is also increased by changes in the rate of protein metabolism such as excessive protein intake and catabolism.[14] A catabolic state may occur with starvation (or chronic poor nutrition in a critically ill patient), severe infection, surgery, or trauma. The BUN may also be elevated as the result of hematoma resorption, GI bleeding, or steroid or tetracycline therapy.[14]

Creatinine. Creatinine is also a by-product of protein and normal cell metabolism and appears in serum in amounts proportional to the body muscle mass. Although slightly higher in males than females, the normal serum creatinine level is about 0.7 to 1.5 mg/dL.[13] Creatinine is easily excreted by the renal tubules and is not reabsorbed or secreted in the tubules. Measuring the amount of creatinine in the excreted urine and the amount of creatinine in the blood over 24 hours provides accurate information about kidney function (creatinine clearance).[2,9]

Creatinine levels are fairly constant and are affected by fewer factors than BUN. As a result, the serum creatinine level is a better indicator of renal function than BUN. Creatinine excess occurs most often in persons with renal failure resulting from impaired excretion. Non-renal failure elevations in creatinine may occur in muscle growth disorders such as acromegaly or with skeletal muscle injury (such as in a trauma patient).[11] Also, malnutrition can result in transient increases in creatinine levels as the rapid muscle catabolism associated with malnutrition causes "dumping" of increased amounts of creatinine into the circulation. Decreased levels of creatinine are rare and usually are associated with muscular dystrophy.[13]

In general, there is a 10:1 ratio of BUN to creatinine. A change in the ratio can indicate renal dysfunction and help identify the etiology of the renal dysfunction.[15] For example, if both BUN and creatinine are elevated and maintain an approximate 10:1 ratio, the disorder is intrarenal, or affecting the tubules of the kidneys. If the ratio of BUN to creatinine is greater than 10:1, the etiology is most likely prerenal (such as hypovolemia). In prerenal kidney failure the creatinine is excreted by functioning tubules, but the urea nitrogen is retained because of the poor GFR and hemoconcentration, leading to the increased ratio.

Osmolality. The serum osmolality reflects the concentration or dilution of vascular fluid. The normal serum osmolality is 275 to 295 mOsm/L.[13] When the serum osmolality level increases (e.g., with insufficient fluid intake or excessive losses), antidiuretic hormone (ADH) is released from the pituitary gland and stimulates increased water reabsorption. This expands the vascular space, brings the serum osmolality back to normal, and results in a more concentrated urine (and thus an elevated urine osmolality). The opposite occurs with a decreased serum osmolality level, which inhibits the production of ADH. The decreased ADH results in increased excretion of water through the kidneys, producing dilute urine with a low osmolality, and brings the serum osmolality back to normal. Measurement of serum osmolality is a useful parameter in determining fluid balance and fluid replacement therapy in critically ill patients. (∞Serum Osmolality, p. 992.)

Anion gap. The anion gap is a calculation of the difference between the measurable cations (sodium and potassium) and the measurable anions (chloride and bicarbonate).[5] The value represents the remaining unmeasurable anions present in the ECF (phosphates, sulfates, ketones, lactate). The formula generally used in the calculation of the anion gap is as follows:

$$Na^{+} - (Cl^{-} + HCO_3^{-}).$$

A normal anion gap is 1 to 12 mEq/L and should not exceed 14 mEq/L. An increased anion gap level reflects overproduction or decreased excretion of acid products and correlates with serum pH measurement.

Acute and chronic renal failure can increase the anion gap because of retention of acids and altered bicarbonate reabsorption. The anion gap is also increased in diabetic ketoacidosis caused by ketone production. The measurement of the anion gap is a rapid method for identifying acid-base imbalance but cannot be used to pinpoint the source of the acid-base disturbance specifically.

Hemoglobin and hematocrit. The hemoglobin (Hgb) and hematocrit (Hct) levels can indicate increases or decreases in intravascular fluid volume. Both Hgb and Hct vary between genders, with the Hgb in males normally 13.5 to 17.5 g/dL and in females 12 to 16 g/dL. The Hct ranges from 40% to 54% in males and 37% to 47% in females. Hgb transports oxygen and carbon dioxide and is important in maintaining cellular metabolism and acid-base balance.[13]

The Hct is the percentage of red blood cells (RBCs) in a volume of whole blood. An increase in the Hct often indicates a fluid volume deficit, which results in hemoconcentration. Although rare, true disorders of RBC production, such as polycythemia, can result in an increased Hct.

Conversely, a decreased Hct can indicate fluid volume excess because of the dilutional effect of the extra fluid load. Decreases, however, can also result from anemias, blood loss, liver damage, or hemolytic reactions.[13] In individuals with acute renal failure, anemia may occur early in the disease, so that a decreased Hct may either indicate the anemia of renal failure or reflect fluid volume overload. If the Hct is dropping but the Hgb remains constant, then the cause is fluid volume overload. If both the Hct and the Hgb are decreased, this indicates a true loss of RBCs. The history and bedside assessment, including hemodynamic monitoring data, aid in determining whether fluid imbalances, disease states, or both are responsible for changes in Hct in the critically ill patient.

Albumin. Slightly more than 50% of the total plasma protein is serum albumin. It is manufactured in the liver, with a normal blood level of 3.5 to 5.5 g/dL.[13] Albumin is primarily responsible for the maintenance of colloid osmotic pressure, which functions to hold fluid in the vascular space. The blood vessel walls, because of their impermeability to plasma proteins, prevent albumin from leaving the vascular space. However, in some disease states such as third-degree burns (cell membrane destruction) or ARF resulting from the nephrotic syndrome (increased glomerular capillary permeability to protein), albumin escapes from the vascular space and enters the interstitial space.

Decreased albumin levels result in a plasma-to-interstitium fluid shift, which creates peripheral edema. A decreased albumin level can occur as a result of protein-calorie malnutrition, which occurs in many critically ill patients in whom available stores of albumin are depleted. A decrease in the plasma oncotic pressure results, and fluid shifts from the vascular space to the interstitial space. Liver disease or severe injury to the liver also causes a fall in albumin levels as the diseased liver fails to synthesize sufficient albumin. Furthermore, severe portal hypertension can force albumin and other plasma proteins into the abdominal cavity, resulting in ascites.

Increased albumin levels are rare. The body uses a fixed amount of protein for energy and body cell replacement and converts excess protein into stored fat. If all plasma protein levels are elevated, fluid volume deficit (hemoconcentration) is suspected.

Urine Analysis

Analysis of the urine provides excellent information about the patient's renal function and condition relative to fluids and electrolytes. Specific tests and abnormal indications are presented in Table 32-3.[4,8,9,11,15] In many cases, urinalysis in the critically ill patient aids in locating the site of renal damage or disease and therefore guides therapeutic management.

pH. Urine pH indicates the acidity or alkalinity of the urine. The normal urinary pH level is 6.0, which is acidic, but may range from 4.5 to 8.0. The kidney regulates acid-base balance; therefore more hydrogen ions are excreted than bicarbonate ions, creating the acidity of the urine. Changes in renal function produce changes in urinary pH.

An increase in urinary acidity (decreased pH) indicates retention of sodium and acids by the body, which would be present in intrarenal ARF. Conversely, a decrease in urinary acidity (increased pH or more alkaline) means the body is retaining bicarbonate. However, in the presence of normal renal function, urinary pH levels are greatly affected by diet and medications. Certain food groups, such as citrus fruits and vegetables, lead to an alkaline urine, whereas a diet high in protein can produce an acid urine. In the critical care unit, patients receiving total parenteral nutrition or a high-protein tube-feeding formula may have an acidic urine caused by high protein intake. (∞TPN, p. 159.)

Specific gravity. Specific gravity measures the density or weight of urine compared with that of distilled water. The normal urinary specific gravity is 1.003 to 1.030 as compared to the normal specific gravity of distilled water at 1.000. Because urine is composed of many solutes and substances suspended in water, the specific gravity should always be higher than that of water.

The specific gravity indicates the ability of the kidneys to dilute or concentrate the urine. Decreases in

TABLE 32-3 Urinalysis Results

Test	Normal	Increased	Decreased
pH	4.5-8.0	Alkalosis	Acidosis
Specific gravity	1.003-1.030	Volume deficit Glycosuria Proteinuria Prerenal ARF (>1.020)	Intrarenal ARF Volume overload
Osmolality	300-1200 mOsm/kg	Volume deficit Prerenal ARF (urine osmolality >serum osmolality)	Volume excess Intrarenal ARF (urine osmolality <serum osmolality)
Protein	30-150 mg/24 hr	Trauma Infection Intrarenal ARF Transient with exercise Glomerulonephritis	
Sodium	27-287 mEq/24 hr	High sodium diet Intrarenal ARF	Prerenal ARF
Creatinine	1-2 g/24 hr		Intrarenal ARF Chronic renal failure
Urea	6-17 g/24 hr		Intrarenal ARF Chronic renal failure
Myoglobin	Absent	Crush injury Rhabdomyolysis	
RBCs	0-5	Trauma Intrarenal ARF Infection Strenuous exercise Renal artery thrombus	
WBCs	0-5	Infection	
Bacteria	None-few	Infection	
Casts	None-few	RBC: Glomerular disease WBC: Pyelonephritis Glomerular disease Nephrotic syndrome Epithelial: Glomerular disease	

specific gravity reflect the inability of the kidneys to excrete the usual solute load into the urine (less dense with fewer solutes). Increases in specific gravity (a more concentrated urine) occur with fluid volume deficit as the result of fever, vomiting, or diarrhea. An increased specific gravity can also occur with diabetes or glomerular membrane disease, both of which allow glucose and protein to pass into the urine, thereby increasing urine density.

Osmolality. The urinary osmolality more accurately pinpoints fluid balance than does the serum osmolality value. The serum osmolality reflects serum sodium concentration and therefore is subject to more influences than the urinary osmolality. The simultaneous measurement of both the serum and urinary osmolality levels provides an accurate assessment of fluid status. Normal urinary osmolality is 300 to 1200 mOsm/kg and depends on reabsorption or excretion of water in the kidney tubules. The urinary osmolality level increases (and urine output decreases) during fluid volume deficit because of the retention of fluid by the body. Conversely, the urinary osmolality level decreases (and urine output increases) during volume excess because fluid is excreted by the kidneys.

In intrarenal ARF, however, the urinary osmolality value and urine output are both decreased because solutes and fluids are being retained.[2]

Glucose. Glucose normally is completely reabsorbed by the renal tubules; therefore the urine should be free of glucose. The appearance of glucose in the urine, however, may be transient, brought on by ingestion of a heavy carbohydrate load (as in patients on total parenteral nutrition), caused by stress (trauma, surgery), or resulting from the renal changes that accompany pregnancy.

Consistent appearance of glycosuria occurs during hyperglycemic episodes of diabetes when the renal threshold for glucose is exceeded and the excess glucose spills into the urine. In the presence of ARF or chronic renal failure, glycosuria is not a reliable indicator of the level of hyperglycemia because of the erratic excretion of glucose by the damaged nephrons.

Protein. Protein, like glucose, normally is absent from urine because the large protein molecule cannot pass across the normal glomerular capillary membrane. Thus consistent appearance of protein in urine suggests compromise of the glomerular membrane and possible intrarenal acute renal failure. The amount of protein in the urine is often directly correlated with the severity of the damage and may exceed 4.0 g/day.

Transient appearance of protein in the urine can occur as the result of efferent arteriole constriction caused by extreme exercise but should decrease within 24 hours.[3] Also, proteinuria can occur after ingestion of a high protein meal or can accompany the renal changes associated with pregnancy.

Electrolytes. Levels of electrolytes in the urine are not as frequently measured as are levels in serum but can also yield information about kidney function. To measure urinary electrolyte levels, a 24-hour urine sample is often required. Urine electrolyte levels are highly variable, and the electrolytes depend on the kidneys for adequate excretion. Consequently, changes in urinary electrolyte levels are highly suggestive of renal failure and generally indicate intrarenal ARF.

Sediment. The presence of sediment such as epithelial cells and casts aids in identifying problems related to the kidneys. In addition, the presence or absence of urine sediment can be helpful in identifying the etiology of ARF.[9,15] In prerenal ARF the kidneys are not damaged and urinary sediment is normal. However, in intrarenal ARF the kidney tubules are damaged and urine sediment is abnormal, with the presence of casts and epithelial cells. Casts are shells or clumps of cellular breakdown or protein materials that form in the renal tubular system and are washed out in the urinary flow. Casts differ in composition and size, and both characteristics correlate with the severity and type of renal damage. White blood cell (WBC) casts indicate pyelonephritis or may occur during acute glomerulonephritis. RBC casts indicate glomerulonephritis, whereas hyaline casts are associated with renal parenchymal disease and glomerular capillary membrane inflammation. Consistent appearance of epithelial cells shed by the lining of the nephron may indicate nephritis. Although small numbers of epithelial cells normally appear in the urine and an occasional cast may be found, their consistent appearance is abnormal.

Hematuria. Both obvious and microscopic hematuria may signal renal damage. Although a few RBCs in the urine are normal, apparently bloody urine indicates bleeding within the urinary tract or renal trauma.[4,9] Microscopic hematuria may occur normally after strenuous exercise or the insertion of a retention catheter but should disappear within 48 hours.

The presence of myoglobin can also make the urine appear red. However, microscopic examination of the urine fails to reveal RBCs, with myoglobin present instead.[3] Myoglobin in the urine may be present as a result of skeletal muscle damage (traumatic crush injury) or rhabdomyolysis. Rhabdomyolysis may develop in patients admitted to a critical care unit for heat prostration or collapse during intense physical exercise (such as running a marathon race on a hot day). Myoglobin is released by the muscle cells and blocks the tubules, resulting in intrarenal ARF. (∞Posttraumatic Renal Failure, p. 1090; Renal Trauma, p. 1083.)

RADIOLOGIC ASSESSMENT

Although laboratory assessment is used most often in diagnosing renal problems in the critically ill patient, radiologic assessment can confirm or clarify causes of particular disorders. Radiologic assessment ranges from basic to more complex (Table 32-4) and provides information about abnormal masses, abnormal fluid collection, obstructions, vascular supply alterations, and other disorders of the kidneys and urinary tract.[2]

Some of the radiologic studies require the use of contrast medium or injection of a radiopaque dye. Many of the dyes used in radiology are potentially nephrotoxic and must therefore be used carefully in patients with ARF or chronic renal failure. For example, an individual with ARF undergoing a test using contrast medium may experience an even further worsening of renal function caused by the dye. In general,

TABLE 32-4 Renal Imaging Tests

Test	Comments
KUB (kidney-ureter-bladder)	Flat plate x-ray of abdomen; determines position, size, and structure of kidneys and urinary tract. Usually followed by additional tests.
Intravenous pyelogram (IVP)	Intravenous injection of contrast medium with x-ray; allows visualization of internal kidney tissues.
Renal angiography	Injection of contrast medium into arterial blood perfusing the kidneys; allows visualization of renal blood flow. May also visualize stenosis, cysts, clots, trauma, infarctions.
Renal computed tomography (CT)	Radioisotope administered IV and absorbed by kidneys; scintillation photography is then performed in several planes. Density of the image helps determine renal perfusion, tumors, cysts, hemorrhage, necrosis.
Renal ultrasound	High-frequency sound waves are transmitted to the kidneys and urinary tract and image is viewed on an oscilloscope. Identifies fluid accumulation or obstruction.
Magnetic resonance imaging (MRI)	A scanner produces three-dimensional images in response to the application of high-energy radiofrequency waves to the tissues. Produces clear images; the density of the image may indicate trauma, lesions, malformation of the vessels or tubules, and necrosis.

adequate hydration before and after the test and careful monitoring of renal status are indicated any time a contrast medium is used.

Renal biopsy. Renal biopsy is the definitive tool for diagnosing disease processes of the kidney. Two methods are used: closed biopsy and open biopsy. Percutaneous needle biopsy (closed method) involves inserting a needle via the flank to obtain a specimen of cortical and medullary kidney tissue. An open biopsy is a surgical procedure and is rarely done in critically ill patients. In either case, biopsy is often the last choice for diagnostic assessment in the critically ill patient because of the postprocedural risks of bleeding, hematoma formation, and infection.

REFERENCES

1. Bates B: *A guide to physical examination and history taking,* ed 6, Philadelphia, 1995, JB Lippincott.
2. Richard C: Assessment of renal structure and function. In Lancaster L, editor: *Core curriculum for nephrology nursing,* ed 3, Pitman, NJ, 1995, American Nephrology Nurses Association.
3. Fishbane S: Exercise-induced renal and electrolyte changes, *Phys Sportsmed* 23(8):39, 1996.
4. Talbot L, Meyers-Marquardt M: *Critical care assessment,* ed 2, St Louis, 1993, Mosby.
5. Metheny NM: *Fluid and electrolyte balance—nursing considerations,* Philadelphia, 1987, JB Lippincott.
6. Grimes J, Burns E: *Health assessment in nursing practice,* ed 3, Boston, 1992, Jones & Bartlett.
7. Roper M: Back to basics. Assessing orthostatic vital signs, *Am J Nurs* 96(8):43, 1996.
8. Brundage D: *Renal disorders,* St Louis, 1992, Mosby.
9. Weems J: *Quick reference to renal critical care nursing,* Gaithersburg, Md, 1991, Aspen.
10. Malasanos L, Barkauskas V, Stoltenberg-Allen K: *Health assessment,* ed 4, St Louis, 1990, Mosby.
11. Anderson R: Prevention and management of acute renal failure, *Hosp Pract* 27(8):61, 1993.
12. Chulay M, Guzzetta C, Dossey B: *AACN handbook of critical care nursing,* 1997, Appleton & Lange.
13. Fischbach F: *A manual of laboratory diagnostic tests,* ed 5, Philadelphia, 1996, JB Lippincott.
14. Stark J: Interpreting BUN/creatinine levels. It's not as simple as you think, *Nurs 94* 24(9):58, 1994.
15. Waite L, Krumberger J: *Noncardiac critical care nursing,* Albany, NY, 1994, Delmar.

Renal Disorders and Therapeutic Management

ACUTE RENAL FAILURE

Description

ACUTE RENAL FAILURE (ARF) is a clinical syndrome that is characterized by an abrupt decline in glomerular filtration rate (GFR) with subsequent retention of metabolic waste products from protein catabolism (azotemia) and an inability to maintain electrolyte and acid-base homeostasis.[1,2] This change in renal function also disturbs the regulation of fluid volume. Oliguria, or a urine output less than 400 ml/day, is a classic finding in ARF[3] (Box 33-1) and occurs in about half of the patients admitted to critical care units.[1,4] ARF is usually reversible if the appropriate treatment is initiated promptly.

However, if the condition goes untreated or if the patient does not respond to treatment, the acute condition may lead to chronic renal failure, with significant morbidity and mortality. ARF is a serious complication in the critically ill patient, and mortality remains high, ranging from 35% to 86%, even with advanced critical care and dialysis techniques.[5] Insults from gastrointestinal (GI) bleeding, sepsis, burns, trauma injuries (rhabdomyolysis), multisystem organ dysfunction syndrome (MODS), and central nervous system (CNS) changes often are implicated in deaths related to ARF.[2,4] ARF is covered under DRG 316, with an anticipated length of stay of 8.1 days.[6]

Etiology

To establish a differential diagnosis and management plan, ARF is classified into three major categories according to the location of the cause: prerenal, intrarenal, or postrenal (Box 33-2).

Prerenal azotemia is a physiologic response to an insult that occurs before blood reaches the kidney. This results in renal hypoperfusion, yet initially the integrity of the kidney's structure and function is preserved.[4,7] The hypoperfusion decreases the GFR, leading to oliguria. The nephrons remain normal, and a return to normal renal function is possible with prompt treatment of the underlying cause of the prerenal condition.[1,7] About 70% of critical care patients suffer from a sequela of events that can precipitate prerenal azotemia.[7] The term *azotemia* is used to describe an acute rise in blood urea nitrogen (BUN). For example, in trauma injuries, damage to the skeletal muscle tissue and loss of cell membrane integrity results in hypovolemia. The body sequesters large amounts of fluid as edema in damaged muscle, decreasing the circulating blood volume, which is a prerenal factor in the development of ARF.[8] In sepsis a systemic inflammatory response or infection triggers the cascade of sequelae that results in sepsis with hypoperfusion leading to oliguria.[8] (∞Renal Trauma, p. 1083; MODS, p. 1124.)

BOX 33-1 Urine Volumes in ARF

Anuria: urine volume < 100 ml/24 hr
Oliguria: urine volume 100-400 ml/24 hr
Polyuria: urine volume excessive/24 hr

Intrarenal azotemia, also known as *intrinsic*, *primary*, or *parenchymal damage*, is the physiologic response to an insult that occurs at the site of the nephrons. It may involve both the glomeruli and the tubular epithelium. This is more commonly known as acute tubular necrosis (ATN). About 25% of patients admitted to critical care units suffer from this ischemic/toxic condition. ATN accounts for approximately 90% of intrarenal azotemia.[1,7] Examples of intrarenal processes include glomerulonephritis, hypertension,

BOX 33-2 Etiology of Acute Renal Failure

PRERENAL

Hemorrhage
Severe gastrointestinal losses
Burns
Shock
Cirrhosis
Renal trauma
Volume depletion (actual loss or "third-spacing")
Heart failure
Renal losses (diuretics, diabetes insipidus, osmotic diuresis)

INTRARENAL

Thrombus
Stenosis
Hypertensive sclerosis
Glomerulonephritis
Pyelonephritis
Acute tubular necrosis
Diabetic sclerosis
Toxic damage

POSTRENAL

Obstructions (stenosis, calculi)
Prostatic disease
Tumors

diabetes mellitus, crush injuries, rhabdomyolysis, and nephrotoxic drugs and poisons.[1,7,8] Acute intrarenal problems involve primarily the glomerulus or the tubules.[1,7] However, renal injury can sometimes be limited by prompt restoration of blood flow.

Postrenal azotemia is the physiologic response caused by the disruption of the normal flow of urine from the urinary tract. Fewer than 5% of patients suffer from this.[7] Causes usually are obstructive disorders occurring beyond the kidney in the remainder of the urinary tract. Anuria or urine output less than 400 ml over 24 hours[3] occurs more commonly in postrenal obstruction[6] (see Box 33-2). As with prerenal conditions, prompt treatment aimed at alleviating the obstruction will restore normal kidney function and prevent permanent kidney damage.[4,7]

ACUTE TUBULAR NECROSIS

Description

ATN results from either nephrotoxic or ischemic injury that damages the renal tubular epithelium and, in severe cases, extends to the basement membrane.[1,3,7] Injury that is limited to the epithelial layer recovers sooner than injury that also involves the basement membrane. ATN is the most common form of intrarenal failure, making up approximately 75% of cases, and accounts for the vast majority of cases of hospital-acquired ARF.[1,7] Damage to the cellular structures in this area prevents normal concentration of urine, filtration of wastes, and regulation of acid-base, electrolyte, and water balance. A number of disorders can result in ATN, and several contributing factors may work together to bring about tubular damage.[1] (∞Glomerular Filtration, p. 853; Tubular Reabsorbtion, p. 854.)

Etiology

Common causes of ATN are shown in Box 33-3. Causes are usually divided into two categories: ischemic and toxic.

Ischemic acute tubular necrosis. Ischemic damage occurs irregularly along the tubular membranes, causing areas of tubular cell damage and cast formation. Perfusion to the kidneys is obliterated or severely reduced, which causes the autoregulation properties of the afferent and efferent arterioles, which regulate GFR, to be lost.[8] Ischemia results if the ischemic episode is prolonged.

Toxic acute tubular necrosis. Toxic damage results from nephrotoxins, usually drugs, chemical agents, or bacterial endotoxins, which cause uniform, widespread damage. The renal tubular cells are constantly at risk for damage because of their normally high blood flows, high oxygen requirements, and the constant reabsorption and secretion of metabolites. Because the basement membrane is not injured as severely as with ischemic ATN, the healing is more rapid and there is a better chance for full recovery from ATN.[8]

Pathophysiology

The mechanisms responsible for tubular dysfunction in ischemic ATN are multifactorial and explain the pathophysiology behind ATN. Accumulation of "cellular debris" in the tubular lumen (tubular obstruction) from interstitial edema or from an accumulation of casts and sloughing tissue can create an obstruction. Filtration ceases when tubular hydrostatic pressure reaches that of glomerular filtration pressure. This decreases the formation of urine because of the nonavailability of filtrate to process.[9,10] The result of tubular cell swelling causes an obstruction that decreases capillary blood flow, leading to further ischemia and cell injury.[9] Adenosine triphosphate (ATP) decreases, causing cellular dysfunction. This results in

BOX 33-3 Etiology of Acute Tubular Necrosis

ISCHEMIC

Hemorrhage
Excessive diuretic use
Burns
Peritonitis
Sepsis
Heart failure
Myocardial ischemia
Pulmonary emboli
Transfusion reactions
Obstetric complications (severe toxemia, abruptio placentae, placenta previa, uterine rupture)

TOXIC

Rhabdomyolysis
Hypercalcemia
Gram-negative sepsis
Nephrotoxic medications (aminoglycosides, cephalosporins, antimicrobials, antineoplastic agents, analgesics containing phenacetin)
Heavy metals
Radiocontrast media
Insecticides
Carbon tetrachloride
Methanol
Street drugs such as phencyclidine (PCP)

an accumulation of intracellular calcium and the production of oxygen free radicals that can cause tubular cell injury.[9]

Phases of Acute Tubular Necrosis

The clinical course of ATN can be divided into four phases: the initiation phase, the maintenance phase, the diuretic phase, and the recovery phase.[7,10]

Onset phase. The onset (initiating) phase is the period of time from which an insult occurred until cell injury. Ischemic injury is evolving during this time. The GFR is decreased because of impaired renal blood flow and decreased glomerular ultrafiltration pressure. This disrupts the integrity of the tubular epithelium, which backleaks the glomerular filtrate.[7] The phase lasts from hours to days, depending on the cause, with toxic factors lasting longer. If treatment is initiated during this time, irreversible damage can be alleviated. Only 50% of patients are oliguric, and the remainder are nonoliguric with a urine output greater than 600 ml/8 hours.[10]

Oliguric/anuric phase. The oliguric/anuric phase, the second phase of ATN, lasts 5 to 8 days in the nonoliguric patient and 10 to 16 days in the oliguric patient.[10] This phase is also referred to as the maintenance phase because total support of renal function is often required during this period. ATN is often reversible and may last from a few hours to several weeks, depending on the cause and severity of renal tubular cell injury.[10] Oliguria is encountered more commonly in ischemic damage, whereas nonoliguria is seen most often when toxins have damaged the kidney.[4,11] The mortality in patients with nonoliguric ATN is 25%, whereas it is 66% if oliguria is present.[1,2] During the oliguric/anuric phase the GFR is greatly reduced, which leads to increased levels of BUN, elevated creatinine levels, electrolyte abnormalities (hyperkalemia, hyperphosphatemia, hypocalcemia), and metabolic acidosis.[1,4,11]

Diuretic phase. The third phase, the diuretic phase, lasts 7 to 14 days and is characterized by an increase in GFR and sometimes polyuria with a urine output as high as 2 to 4 L/day.[1,4] If the patient is receiving hemodialysis during this phase, the polyuria will not be evident because excess volume will be removed by dialysis. During the diuretic phase, tubular function returns slowly and tubular reabsorption may not increase as quickly as GFR. The kidneys can clear volume but not solutes, which, with a large diuresis, can lead to volume depletion.[1]

Recovery phase. The last phase of ATN is the recovery or convalescent phase. Both oliguric and nonoliguric patients will increase their urine output.[10] During this stage, renal function slowly returns to normal or near normal, with GFR 70% to 80% of normal within 1 to 2 years.[4] If significant renal parenchymal damage has occurred, BUN and creatinine levels may never return to normal.[1,4] For patients surviving ATN, approximately 62% will recover normal renal function, 33% will be left with residual renal insufficiency, and at least 5% will require long-term hemodialysis.[12]

ASSESSMENT AND DIAGNOSIS

Acute Renal Failure

In the critically ill patient with ARF, the first step in the diagnostic process is to determine whether the ARF is the result of a prerenal, intrinsic, or postrenal event.[2] Assessment of ARF can be divided into evaluation of laboratory, radiologic, and fluid balance.

Laboratory assessment. Laboratory assessment usually includes both serum and urinary values. Normal serum electrolyte values are listed in Table 33-1. Electrolyte

TABLE 33-1 Normal Serum Electrolyte Values

Serum Electrolyte	Normal Serum Value
Sodium	135-145 mEq/L
Potassium	3.5-5.0 mEq/L
Chloride	98-108 mEq/L
Calcium	8.5-10.5 mg/dL or 4.5-5.8 mEq/L
Phosphorus	2.7-4.5 mg/dL
Magnesium	1.5-2.5 mEq/L
Bicarbonate	24-28 mEq/L

disturbances in ARF are discussed in Table 33-2. Normal and abnormal urinalysis findings and significance are summarized in Table 32-3 in the previous chapter. (∞Laboratory Assessment: Serum, p. 872; Laboratory Assessment: Urine, p. 873.)

Blood urea nitrogen and creatinine levels. Laboratory assessments always include a test of BUN and serum creatinine levels. BUN is neither the sole indicator of ARF nor the most reliable indicator of renal damage because, although it reflects cellular damage, the BUN level is easily changed by protein intake, blood in the GI tract, or cell catabolism.[2,9]

Creatinine, on the other hand, is an accurate reflection of renal damage because it is almost totally excreted by the renal tubules. Elevated levels of serum creatinine can reflect damage to 50% of the nephrons or more.[9] If the patient is making sufficient urine, the creatinine clearance can be measured from the urine. A normal urine creatinine clearance is 120 ml/minute. It decreases in renal failure. However, many critical care patients in ARF do not make urine; therefore the health care team must depend on the serum creatinine level instead.

Urinalysis. The urine sodium level, urine osmolality, and specific gravity reflect the concentrating and diluting ability of the kidney and help to distinguish between prerenal and intrarenal failure. In the early stages of ATN the kidneys lose the ability to concentrate urine.[9] The renal tubules cannot effectively control urine concentration and the urine is dilute; urine osmolality is less than 300 mOsm/kg and specific gravity is less than 1.010. In ATN the urine sodium level is greater than 20 mEq/L; in prerenal failure it is generally less than 20 mEq/L. However, its usefulness is limited because there is an overlap in the 20 to 40 mEq/L range that may represent either prerenal failure or ATN.[9]

Electrolyte levels. Most of the electrolytes in the blood stream will become increasingly elevated in ARF.[13] As oliguria develops, the patient with renal failure becomes hyperkalemic. Moreover, the rise in extracellular potassium levels results from the loss of the tubule's ability to concentrate the urine with potassium. Trauma also elevates extracellular potassium levels because of the related tissue destruction that damages the cells, releasing potassium from the intracellular space into the extracellular space.[8,9] Other affected electrolytes include calcium and phosphorus. The serum calcium level may be reduced during ATN, whereas the serum phosphorus level is elevated.[15] In fact, serum phosphorus level can be more dramatically elevated in the presence of the traumatized, catabolic patient as well as in the setting of rhabdomyolysis. Conversely, as the serum phosphorus level rises, the serum calcium level declines.[8,9]

Radiologic findings. Radiographic information provides another perspective in assessment. Radiologic tests used in diagnosing renal disorders have become increasingly sophisticated and valuable tools. Sonography, tomography, and angiography can help pinpoint the causal mechanism and even help differentiate between acute diseases and chronic renal failure. Radiologic contrast media have been implicated in the development and worsening of renal disorders. For example, patients with a history of coronary artery disease, diabetes, or renal disease can suffer from acute renal problems when contrast medium is not adequately cleared because of an already compromised circulatory or renal system.[14] (∞Radiologic Assessment, p. 384.)

Hemodynamic monitoring and fluid balance. Hemodynamic monitoring is important for the analysis of fluid volume status in ARF. Hemodynamic monitoring includes surveillance of central venous pressure (CVP), pulmonary artery wedge pressure (PAWP), cardiac output (CO), and cardiac index (CI). Hemodynamic monitoring is valuable in tracking fluid balance and the need for fluid removal (dialysis), or replacement (intravenous [IV] fluids). (∞Bedside Hemodynamic Monitoring, p. 442.)

Hemodynamic pressure monitoring guides tolerance of IV volume replacement when infused to prevent prerenal failure. Assessment of ATN usually involves tracking losses, compartmental fluid shifts, and cardiovascular function and monitoring the patient's general physical condition.[9] Because hypovolemia is the usual precursor of ischemic tubular damage, careful assessment of fluid losses from all potential sources is important. Frequent blood pressure measurements and monitoring hemodynamic values are other means of evaluating fluid status. Changes in CO and PAWP

TABLE 33-2 Serum Electrolyte Disturbances in Acute Renal Failure

Electrolyte Disturbance	Serum Value	Findings
POTASSIUM		
Hypokalemia	Less than 3.5 mEq/L (rare)	Muscular weakness Cardiac irregularities on ECG Abdominal distention and flatulence Paresthesia Decreased reflexes Anorexia Dizziness Confusion Increased sensitivity to digitalis
Hyperkalemia	Greater than 5.0 mEq/L	Irritability and restlessness Anxiety Nausea and vomiting Abdominal cramps Weakness Numbness and tingling (fingertips and circumoral) Cardiac irregularities on ECG
SODIUM		
Hyponatremia	Less than 135 mEq/L	Disorientation Muscle twitching Nausea and vomiting Abdominal cramps Headaches Seizures Dizziness Postural hypotension Cold, clammy skin Decreased skin turgor Tachycardia Oliguria
Hypernatremia	Greater than 145 mEq/L	Extreme thirst Dry, sticky mucous membranes Altered mentation Seizures (later stages)
CALCIUM		
Hypocalcemia	Less than 8.5 mg/dL or 4.5 mEq/L	Irritability Muscular tetany Muscle cramps Decreased cardiac output (decreased contractions) Bleeding (decreased ability to coagulate) ECG changes Positive Chvostek's sign Positive Trousseau's sign
Hypercalcemia	Greater than 10.5 mg/dL or 5.8 mEq/L	Deep bone pain Excessive thirst Anorexia Lethargy Weakened muscles

Continued

TABLE 33-2 **Serum Electrolyte Disturbances in Acute Renal Failure—cont'd**

Electrolyte Disturbance	Serum Value	Findings
MAGNESIUM		
Hypomagnesemia	Less than 1.4 mEq/L	Choroid and athetoid muscle activity Facial tics Spasticity Cardiac dysrhythmias
Hypermagnesemia	Greater than 2.5 mEq/L	CNS depression Respiratory depression Lethargy Coma Bradycardia ECG changes
PHOSPHATE		
Hypophosphatemia	Less than 3.0 mg/dL	Hemolytic anemias Depressed white cell function Bleeding (decreased platelet aggregation) Nausea, vomiting, and anorexia
Hyperphosphatemia	Greater than 4.5 mg/dL	Tachycardia Nausea Diarrhea Abdominal cramps Muscle weakness Flaccid paralysis Increased reflexes
CHLORIDE		
Hypochloremia	Less than 98 mEq/L	Hyperirritability Tetany or muscular excitability Slow respirations
Hyperchloremia	Greater than 108 mEq/L	Weakness Lethargy Deep, rapid breathing Possible unconsciousness (later stages)
ALBUMIN		
Hypoalbuminemia	Less than 3.8 g/dL	Muscle wasting Peripheral edema (fluid shift) Decreased resistance to infection Poorly healing wounds

values will indicate decreases or increases in intravascular volume.

The patient's weight is indicative of fluid gains or losses over a 1- to 2-day period. Additional signs and symptoms, such as thirst, decreased skin turgor, and apathy, suggest extracellular fluid (ECF) depletion.[5,11] Measurement of abdominal girth for ascites and testing for pitting edema over body prominences and in dependent body areas is performed frequently. (∞Palpation: Abdomen, p. 868; Inspection: Edema, p 867.)

Cardiopulmonary system. The pulmonary system responds to the metabolic acidosis of ARF by deep, rapid breathing (Kussmaul's respirations). Fluid overload caused by excess fluid shifts into the lungs leads the nurse to assess for bilateral crackles, or even pulmonary edema. Pulse oximetry is used to frequently assess the oxygen saturation, especially if there is pulmonary congestion from fluid overload. The cardiovascular system responds to renal failure by sinus tachycardia. Dysrhythmias can occur secondary to electrolyte imbalance. The blood pressure can be normal or elevated. A friction rub from uremic pericarditis is often heard on auscultation.[14] (∞Pericardial Friction Rub, p. 371.)

Other systems. The neurologic system is adversely affected by ARF. The critically ill patient may experience confusion, lethargy, decreased level of consciousness, and stupor secondary to increases in the BUN and creatinine.[15]

In the integumentary system the renal failure causes dry skin, pruritus, edema, bruising, and pallor. In terminal renal failure, uremic frost may occur.[14]

The patient with ARF experiences many GI symptoms, including nausea, vomiting, anorexia, abdominal distention, constipation, or diarrhea.[14]

Medical management. Treatment goals for patients experiencing ARF focus on compensating for the deterioration of renal function. Medical interventions for ARF are directed toward three basic goals: (1) prevention, (2) correcting the causative mechanism, and (3) promoting regeneration of the remaining functional capacity. Medical management is based on the three categories or causes of ARF.[2]

Acute renal failure prevention. The only truly effective remedy for ARF is prevention. For effective prevention the patient's risk for ARF must be known. Principles of prevention include avoiding the use of nephrotoxic drugs in the elderly and in those with chronic renal failure as well as avoiding the use of nonsteroidal antiinflammatory drugs for pain relief in patients taking antibiotics or recovering from major surgery. Delaying the use of intravascular x-ray contrast medium until the patient is rehydrated and antibiotics have been discontinued can help preserve kidney function in the high-risk patient. If this is not possible, low-dose dopamine can be infused to improve diuresis or dobutamine given to help increase creatinine clearance.[2] (∞Cardiac Drugs: Dopamine, p. 577; Cardiac Drugs: Dobutamine, p. 577.)

Fluid balance. Prerenal failure is caused by decreased perfusion and is often associated with trauma, hemorrhage, or other fluid losses. Prerenal failure requires two specific methods of management: fluid and electrolyte restoration and stimulation of urinary output with diuretics.[2]

The objectives of fluid replacement are to replace losses of fluids and electrolytes and to prevent fluid imbalance in the face of ongoing loss.[14] Maintenance fluid therapy is initiated only when oral fluid intake is clinically inadvisable.[1] Maintenance fluids are calculated with consideration for individual body surface area. Adults require approximately 1500 ml/m^2/24 hours.[14] Requirements may be altered by fever, burns, environmental temperature, humidity changes, and other injuries.[14] The rate of replacement depends on cardiopulmonary reserve, adequacy of renal mechanisms, ongoing loss, and type of fluid required.

Crystalloids and colloids. Crystalloids and colloids refer to two different types of intravenous fluids that are frequently used for volume management in the critically ill. Crystalloid solutions, which are balanced salt solutions, are in widespread use for both maintenance infusions and replacement therapy. Crystalloid fluids include dextrose in water (D_5W, $D_{10}W$); normal saline solution (0.9 NaCl); half-strength saline solution (0.45 NaCl), and lactated Ringer's (LR) solution, as described in Table 33-3. LR solution is used frequently in the intraoperative environment, but should be avoided in patients with renal failure.[15]

Colloids are solutions containing oncotically active particles that are employed to expand intravascular volume to achieve and maintain hemodynamic stability. Albumin (5% and 25%) and Hetastarch are examples of colloids (see Table 33-3). The effect from colloid volume expansion can last as long as 24 hours. The goal is to increase PAWP, mean arterial pressure (MAP) and CI to a therapeutic level.

Adequacy of IV fluid replacement depends on strict ongoing evaluation and frequent adjustment. Frequent monitoring of serum electrolyte levels is required, and strictly regulated intake and output are correlated with daily weight records. Finally, hemodynamic readings are frequent and ongoing. If, following a fluid challenge, the increase in CVP is only minimal, this indicates the need for fluid replacement. Continued decreases in CVP, PAWP, and CI indicate ongoing volume losses. Significant rises in CVP and PAWP, with a fall in CI, may indicate hypervolemia with underlying cardiac failure. (∞Bedside Hemodynamic Monitoring, p. 442.)

Fluid restriction. Fluid restriction constitutes a large part of the medical treatment for renal failure. Fluid restriction is used to prevent circulatory overload and interstitial edema when excess volume cannot be removed by the kidneys. The fluid requirements are calculated on the basis of daily urinary volumes and insensible losses. Obtaining daily weights and keeping accurate intake and output records are essential. Renal failure patients are usually restricted to 1 L of fluid if urinary output is 500 ml or less and insensible losses range from 500 to 750 ml/day.

Fluid removal. Intrarenal failure involves the introduction of increased amounts of water, solutes, and potential toxins into the circulation; thus prompt measures are needed to decrease their levels. Diuretics are used to stimulate the urinary output. However, hemodialysis or hemofiltration are the treatments of choice,

TABLE 33-3 Frequently Used Intravenous Solutions

Name	Electrolytes		Indications
CRYSTALLOIDS*			
Dextrose in water (D_5W)—isotonic	None		To maintain volume
			To replace mild loss
			To provide minimal calories
Normal saline solution (0.9% NaCl)	Sodium	154 mEq/L	To maintain volume
	Chloride	154 mEq/L	To replace mild loss
	Osmolality	308 mEq/L	To correct mild hyponatremia
Half-strength saline solution (0.45% NaCl)	Sodium	77 mEq/L	For free water replacement
	Chloride	77 mEq/L	To correct mild hyponatremia
			For free water and electrolyte replacement (used in fluid- and electrolyte-restricted conditions)
Lactated Ringer's solution	Sodium	130 mEq/L	For fluid and electrolyte replacement (contraindicated for patients with renal or liver disease or in lactic acidosis)
	Potassium	4 mEq/L	
	Calcium	2.7 mEq/L	
	Chloride	107 mEq/L	
	Lactate	27 mEq/L	
	pH	6.5	
COLLOIDS			
5% Albumin (Albumisol)	Albumin	50 g/L	For volume expansion
	Sodium	130 to 160 mEq/L	For moderate protein replacement
	Potassium	300 mOsm/L	For achievement of hemodynamic stability in shock states
	Osmolality		
	Osmotic pressure	20 mm Hg	
	pH	6.4 to 7.4	
25% Albumin (salt-poor)	Albumin	240 g/L	Concentrated form of albumin sometimes used with diuretics to move fluid from tissues into the vascular space for diuresis
	Globulins	10 g/L	
	Sodium	130 to 160 mEq/L	
	Osmolality	1500 mOsm/L	
	pH	6.4 to 7.4	
Hetastarch	Sodium	154 mEq/L	Synthetic polymer (6% solution) used for volume expansion
	Chloride	154 mEq/L	
	Osmolality	310 mOsm/L	For hemodynamic volume replacement after cardiac surgery, burns, sepsis
	Colloid osmotic pressure	30-35 mm Hg	
Low molecular weight dextran (LMWD)	Glucose polysaccharide molecules with an average molecular weight of 40,000, no electrolytes		For volume expansion and support (contraindicated for patients with bleeding disorders)
High molecular weight dextran (HMWD)	Glucose polysaccharide molecules with an average molecular weight of 70,000, no electrolytes		Used prophylactically in some cases to prevent platelet aggregation, available in either saline or glucose solutions

*For the crystalloid solutions that contain electrolytes, specific concentrations of electrolytes and pH will vary according to manufacturers.

particularly if volume overload creates pulmonary and cardiac compromise. Severe hyperkalemia almost always necessitates hemodialysis because of the life-threatening cardiac dysrhythmias resulting from hyperkalemia.[16] Hemodialysis may also be initiated for severe azotemia when other treatments are contraindicated.

Electrolyte balance

Potassium. Electrolyte levels require frequent observation, especially in the critical phases of renal failure. Potassium may quickly reach levels of 6.0 mEq/L and above. Specific ECG changes are associated with hyperkalemia, specifically peaked T waves, a widening of the QRS interval, and ultimately ventricular tachycardia or fibrillation.[16] If hyperkalemia is present, all potassium supplements are stopped.[13] If the patient is producing urine, IV diuretics can be administered. Acute hyperkalemia can be treated temporarily by an IV infusion of insulin and glucose. An infusion of 100 ml of 50% dextrose accompanied by 20 units of regular insulin forces potassium out of the serum and into the cells. Sodium bicarbonate (40 to 160 mEq) may be infused to promote higher excretion of potassium in the urine, particularly if the serum pH is below 7.10. Finally, sodium polystyrene sulfonate (Kayexalate), a cation-exchange resin, is mixed in water and sorbitol and given orally, rectally, or through a nasogastric (NG) tube. The resin binds potassium in the bowel, which eliminates it in the feces. Kayexalate and dialysis are the only permanent methods of potassium removal.[13,16] (∞Laboratory Assessment: Potassium p. 377 and p. 860.)

Sodium. Dilutional hyponatremia, associated with renal failure, can be corrected with fluid restriction.[17] If, however, sodium stores actually are depleted, hypertonic 3% saline solution is sometimes administered intravenously as a replacement. In addition, sodium levels may be raised during dialysis by changing the amount of sodium in the dialysate bath.[3]

Calcium and phosphorus. Calcium levels are reduced in renal failure. This reduction results from multiple factors, among which is hyperphosphatemia. At the renal level, calcium and phosphorus are regulated in part by parathyroid hormone (PTH). Normally, PTH helps calcium be reabsorbed into the proximal tubule and distal nephron and promotes excretion of phosphate by the kidney to maintain homeostasis. Aluminum hydroxide preparations are administered orally or via an NG tube to bind phosphorus in the bowel and thus eliminate it from the body. This lowers the serum phosphorus level and increases the calcium blood level. Calcium may also be increased by use of calcium supplements, vitamin D preparations, and synthetic calcitrol.[18]

Nutrition. The nutritional aspects of renal failure involve replacement as well as restriction. If the patient is anorexic and malnourished, total parenteral nutrition (TPN) can be provided and the excess TPN fluid volume removed during hemodialysis or hemofiltration. The renal diet restricts protein, potassium, sodium, and phosphorus. Protein restriction may vary to limit azotemia (increased BUN). Carbohydrates are encouraged, primarily to provide needed energy for healing.[9] (∞Nutrition and Renal Alterations, p. 137.)

Medications. Care must be taken in the use of diuretics to avoid creating secondary electrolyte abnormalities. Diuretic therapy is thought to increase renal blood flow, GFR, and intratubular pressure while decreasing the possibility of tubular obstruction and dysfunction. Both osmotic and loop diuretics may be effective in decreasing the initial insult to the renal system if given promptly at the onset of oliguria.[2]

A number of clinicians have advocated the use of vasodilators to increase renal blood flow. Also, a combination of dopamine and furosemide (Lasix) is used to convert the oliguric to nonoliguric ARF.[2] Other studies suggest that calcium channel blockers can prevent the intracellular calcium overload observed in ischemic ARF, possibly offering some protection against renal ischemia.[2]

Nursing management. Nursing management of ARF patients involves several nursing diagnoses related to fluid volume management (Box 33-4). Some individuals have an increased risk of acquiring ARF as a complication during their hospitalization, and the alert critical care nurse recognizes potential risk factors. The critical care nurse caring for the elderly client recognizes that the GFR in this age-group may be decreased and that dehydration can result in hypoperfusion of the kidneys, with subsequent development of ATN. Other patients at risk are those with increased creatinine levels before their hospitalization. Hemodynamic parameters (PAWP and CI), urine output, and serum creatinine and BUN values provide information about fluid balance and kidney function.

Infection control. The critical care patient with ARF is at risk for infectious complications. Signs of infection, such as increased WBC count, redness at a wound or IV site, or increased temperature, are a cause for concern. Pulmonary hygiene is maintained by asking the patient to cough and deep breathe frequently, by suction if the person is intubated and ventilated, and by frequent position changes. Should the patient be immobile, frequent turning and observation of potential sites for skin breakdown enhance the chances of avoiding infection. If significant anasarca (severe generalized edema) has developed, the use of a circulating or air-fluid mattress may help prevent skin breakdown.

Fluid balance. Frequent assessment of intake and output, particularly in response to diuretics, is a necessary part of nursing management for the patient in renal failure. Hemodynamic values and daily weights are correlated with the intake and output to confirm fluid overload. Urinary output is measured throughout all phases of ARF. During the diuretic phase as urinary function returns, it may be necessary to replace the fluids and electrolytes that are lost during this phase.

BOX 33-4 NURSING DIAGNOSIS AND MANAGEMENT

ACUTE RENAL FAILURE

- Fluid Volume Excess related to renal dysfunction, p. 915
- Altered Renal Tissue Perfusion related to decreased renal blood flow, p. 916
- Anxiety related to threat to biologic, psychologic, and/or social integrity, p. 99
- Decreased Cardiac Output related to alterations in preload, p. 590
- Risk for Infection risk factors: protein-calorie malnourishment, invasive monitoring devices, p. 598
- Body Image Disturbance related to functional dependence on life-sustaining technology, p. 86
- Ineffective Individual Coping related to situational crisis and personal vulnerability, p. 95
- Sleep Pattern Disturbance related to fragmented sleep, p. 118
- Knowledge Deficit: Fluid Restriction, Reportable Symptoms, and Medications related to lack of previous exposure to information, p. 61 (see Patient Education Box 33-5)

Electrolyte balance. Hyperkalemia, hypocalcemia, hyponatremia, hyperphosphatemia, and acid-base imbalances all occur during ARF.[2] Clinical manifestations of these electrolyte imbalances must be prevented and their associated side effects controlled. The imbalances with the most potential hazard are hyperkalemia and hypocalcemia, which can result in life-threatening cardiac dysrhythmias. Dilutional hyponatremia may develop as fluid overload worsens in the patient with oliguria. Monitoring the serum sodium level is important to prevent this complication. Hyperphosphatemia results in severe pruritus. Nursing care is directed at soothing the itching by performing frequent skin care with emollients, discouraging scratching, and administering phosphate-binding medications. The acid-base imbalances that occur with renal failure are monitored by arterial blood gas analysis. The goal of treatment is to maintain the pH within the normal range. (∞Laboratory Assessment: Arterial Blood Gases, p. 641.)

Anemia. Anemia is an expected side effect of renal failure that occurs because the kidney no longer produces the hormone erythropoietin. Thus the bone marrow is not stimulated to produce red blood cells. Care is taken to prevent blood loss in the patient with ARF, and blood withdrawal is minimized as much as possible. Irritation of the GI tract from metabolic waste accumulation is expected, and GI bleeding is a possibility. Stool, NG drainage, and emesis are routinely tested for occult blood. Anemia is treated by red blood cell replacement, or pharmacologically by the administration of Epogen to stimulate erythrocyte production by the bone marrow.

Patient education. The nurse gives accurate and uncomplicated information to the patient and family about ARF, including its prognosis, treatment, and possible complications. Education can be challenging because elevations of BUN and creatinine can negatively impact level of consciousness. Also, sleep-rest disorders and emotional upset often occur as complications of ARF and can disrupt short-term memory. Encouraging the patient and family to voice concerns, frustrations, or fears and allowing the patient to control some aspects of the acute care environment and treatment also are essential (see Patient Education Box 33-5).

DIALYSIS

A wide range of options is available for the treatment of ARF, including the following: hemodialysis, peritoneal dialysis, and continuous renal replacement therapy.[3,11] It is essential for the nurse to become familiar with each type of dialysis, the potential problems that each can develop, and the nursing interventions each requires. The dialysis patient is taught that the dialysis access is a "lifeline" and that care on the part of the patient and nurse can prevent complications.

Vascular Access

Acute access

Subclavian and femoral vein catheters. A dual-lumen venous catheter is the most commonly used form of vascular access for acute hemodialysis. It has a central partition running the length of the catheter. The outflow catheter pulls the blood flow through openings that are proximal to the inflow openings on the opposite side. This design avoids dialyzing the same blood just returned to the area (recirculation), which can severely reduce the procedure's efficiency.[19,20] A silicone rubber, dual-lumen catheter with a Dacron cuff that is designed to decrease the incidence of catheter-related infections is also available.[20]

Subclavian and femoral veins are usually catheterized in cases of ARF when short-term access is required or when vascular access is nonfunctional in a patient requiring immediate hemodialysis. Both subclavian and femoral catheters can be inserted at the bedside. When the subclavian vein is not available, a shorter dialysis catheter is used for placement into the femoral vein.

Chronic access. Hemodialysis can be performed only by obtaining access to the blood stream. Over many

BOX 33-5 PATIENT EDUCATION

ACUTE RENAL FAILURE

- Explain pathophysiology:
  "ARF is a sudden, severe impairment of renal function, causing an acute build-up of toxins in the blood"
- Explain etiology:
  Prerenal (before the kidneys)
  Hemorrhage
  Severe GI losses
  Burns
  Volume depletion
  Acute heart failure
  Hypoxia
  Intrarenal (within the kidneys)
  Thrombus
  Stenosis
  Rhabdomylosis
  Toxic damage
  Glomerulonephritis
  Pyelonephritis
  Toxic damage
  Postrenal (past the kidneys)
  Obstructions (stones)
  Prostatic disease
  Tumors
- Identify predisposing factors:
  Hypotensive episodes
  Hypovolemia
  Sepsis, burns, jaundice
  Advanced age
  Recent surgery
  Preexisting renal disease or diabetes
  Drug therapy
- Explain the level of renal function after the acute phase is over.
- Explain diet and fluid restrictions.
- Demonstrate how to check blood pressure, pulse, respirations, and weight.
- Discuss good hygiene and how to avoid infections.
- Emphasize need for exercise and rest.
- Describe medications and adverse effects.
- Explain need for ongoing follow-up with health care professional.
- Explain purpose of dialysis and importance of regular treatments.

years, various types of accesses, such as arteriovenous fistulas, shunts, and grafts and femoral and subclavian catheters, have been created. The common denominator in most chronic access devices is access to the arterial circulation and return to the venous circulation. This type of access is most frequently used for patients with chronic renal failure who require long-term access.[3,11,20]

Arteriovenous fistula. The arteriovenous (A-V) fistula is created by surgically visualizing a peripheral artery and vein, creating an opening in the artery and the vein, and anastomosing the two open areas. Anastomoses may be side-to-side, end-to-side, or end-to-end.[3,11,19] The high arterial flow creates swelling of the vein, or a *pseudoaneurysm,* at which point—when healed—a large-bore needle can be inserted to obtain outflow. Inflow is accomplished through a second large-bore needle inserted into a peripheral vein distal to the fistula (Figure 33-1, *A*). If the patient's vessels are adequate, fistulas are the preferred mode of access because of the durability of blood vessels and the relatively few complications in comparison to the other accesses. Development of sufficient flow to the fistula, however, may require weeks to months. Attempting to obtain flow from the underdeveloped fistulas often causes painful vascular spasm and reduced flow.

Arteriovenous fistulas have the potential for creating arterial insufficiency because of the high arterial blood flow diverted for dialysis purposes. The arterial insufficiency produces a set of symptoms known as *vascular steal syndrome,* wherein the extremity becomes pale, cold, and painful.[3,11,20] Additional complications that can occur are thrombosis, infection, or venous hypertension.[13]

The critical care nurse frequently assesses the quality of blood flow through the fistula. A patent fistula has a thrill when palpated gently with the fingers and a bruit if auscultated with a stethoscope. The extremity should be pink and warm to the touch.

Arteriovenous grafts. Arteriovenous (A-V) grafts are the most frequently used access for treating chronic renal failure. The graft is a tube formed of Gortex, which is surgically implanted in the limb. The area is surgically opened, and an artery and a vein are located. A tunnel is created, either straight or U-shaped, in the tissue where the graft is placed. Anastomoses are made with the graft ends connected to the artery and vein. The blood is allowed to flow through the graft, and the surgical area is closed. The graft creates a raised area that looks like a large peripheral vein just under the skin and peripheral tissue layers (Figure 33-1, *B*). Two large-bore needles are used for outflow and inflow to the graft. For both grafts and fistulas, after needle removal at the end of the hemodialysis treatment, firm pressure must be applied to stem bleeding.

Arteriovenous shunt. Because of the advent of subclavian and femoral catheters, arteriovenous (A-V) shunts are used infrequently today in critical care. If,

CULTURAL INSIGHTS 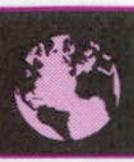

Self-Care and Decision Making

Some of the greatest challenges ethnic and cultural diversity presents to the critical care nurse arise out of differing attitudes toward health care and toward the health care professional. These variations in attitude include differing views on the position and responsibility of the health care professional and differing beliefs about the patient's ability to control health and destiny.

It is impossible to generalize about patient attitudes toward health care professionals. However, two perspectives vary so dramatically from those found among mainstream, native-born Americans that they must be mentioned. They are the patient's perception of the health professional as (1) an authority figure and (2) the individual who is ultimately responsible for the success or failure of treatment.

One manifestation of this perception is the tendency for some patients—and their families—to resist, when given the opportunity, to make choices about their treatment, such as whether to initiate chemotherapy or how radical of a mastectomy should be performed. During recent years in the United States, there has been a growing trend toward patient involvement and patient responsibility in the treatment process. Indeed, the provision of choice, whenever possible, has become one of the basic tenets of sound, effective nursing care.

In many nations of the world the movement toward patient involvement and decision making has yet to manifest itself. The patient, instead, looks to the health professional to make decisions and accept full responsibility for these decisions. In short, it cannot be assumed that the patient and family are uncooperative, lazy, or unintelligent when its members do not wish to participate in the decision-making process. This behavior quite simply reflects a different health care hierarchy.

Fatalism—the view that the course of life is dictated by a higher power—is a positive version of powerlessness. The difference between the two is that feelings of powerlessness arise out of discrimination, poverty, and historical adversity, and fatalism is generated out of faith in a higher power and in the preordained perfection of the universe. Although the impact of fatalism on health care can sometimes be adverse (e.g., resistance to invoking heroic measures during critical illness), the effect is a positive one, because it leaves the patient and family in a more peaceful, accepting state of mind.

The impact of fatalism is seen most dramatically in those who are critically ill. The notion of calling on the individual's "will to live" is an important feature of American health care attitudes. The fatalistic attitudes found among Hispanic and Middle Eastern immigrants, on the other hand, hold that the will of God dictates the fate of the critically ill. The Arabic phrase *in shallah* (if God wills it) sums up this perspective and illustrates the importance of critical care nurses' recognizing and honoring this distinction.

To speak, for example, to the Hispanic patient of his or her "will to live" will, in all probability, be fruitless and misunderstood. To speak, on the other hand, of the importance of relying on and having faith in God's will may prove both comforting and productive. However, this reliance on God's will among the terminally ill can create problems for the nursing staff. Because in many cultures it is considered God's will whether a person lives or dies, many family members will not want the patient told that he or she is terminally ill because this, in their eyes, would be second-guessing God and therefore defying His will. There is little that the critical care nurse can or should do about this preference. However, awareness is necessary so that misunderstandings that could result in family alienation can be avoided.

however, long-term hemodialysis is required, a permanent vascular access is necessary to permit rapid blood access to be obtained through an external arteriovenous shunt (Figure 33-1, *C*). The arteriovenous shunt requires a peripheral artery, usually radial or ulnar, and a peripheral vein, such as the cephalic or basilic. A cutdown is performed on each vessel. The vessel tips are sutured in place. When not being used for dialysis, a straight connector or a heparin T device connects the peripheral artery and vein. Blood flows in a U-shaped fashion from the higher arterial pressure to the lower venous system. Shunts may also be inserted in the thigh or ankle areas. Complications common to arteriovenous shunts are thrombosis, infection, and skin erosion, as listed in Table 33-4.

Medical management. Medical management involves the decision to place a vascular access device and the most appropriate type and location for each patient. Patients in the critical care setting require vascular access if they suffer from ARF or chronic renal failure and require hemodialysis.[14]

Some patients with chronic renal failure are admitted to the hospital to receive lytic therapy (streptokinase, or urokinase) to lyse a thrombus in the vascular access. In some cases this may require invasive procedures such as angiography or surgery to remove clots. (∞Thrombolytic Therapy, p. 561.)

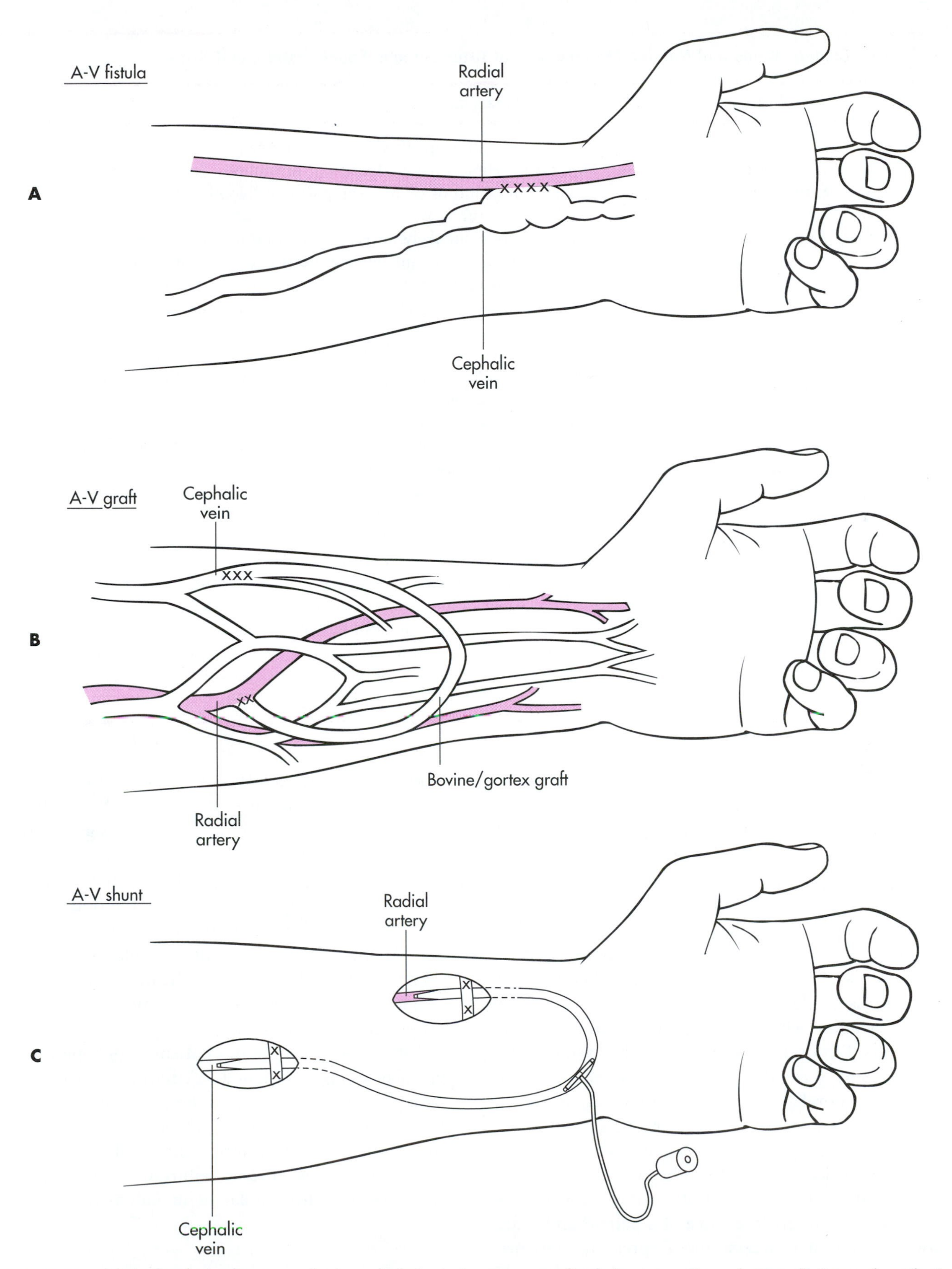

FIGURE 33-1. Methods of vascular access for hemodialysis. **A,** Arteriovenous fistula between vein and artery. **B,** Internal synthetic graft corrects artery and vein. **C,** External synthetic cannula, or shunt, with T-connector.

TABLE 33-4 Complications and Nursing Management of Arteriovenous Shunt, Fistula, and Graft

Type	Complications	Nursing Management
Shunt	Clotting Dislodgment Skin erosion Infection Bleeding	Monitor for clinical manifestations of infection. Monitor for clinical manifestations of thrombosis (darkening of blood, separation of serum or cellular compartment blood in tubing, decreased temperature of tubing). Assess insertion site daily for erosion around insertion sites. Use strict aseptic technique during dressing changes at insertion sites. Teach patients to avoid sleeping on or prolonged bending of accessed limbs. Keep two shunt clamps attached to patients' clothing or access dressing at all times.
Fistula	Thrombosis Infection Pseudoaneurysm Vascular steal syndrome Venous hypertension Carpal tunnel syndrome Inadequate blood flow	Teach patients to avoid wearing constrictive clothing on limbs containing access. Teach patients to avoid sleeping on or prolonged bending of accessed limb. Use aseptic technique when cannulating access. Avoid repetitious cannulation of one segment of access. Offer comfort measures, such as warm compresses and ordered analgesics, to lessen pain of vascular steal. Teach patients to develop blood flow in the fistulas through exercises (squeezing a rubber ball) while applying mild impedance to flow just distal to the access (at least once per day for 10 to 15 minutes).
Graft	Bleeding Thrombosis False aneurysm formation Infection Arterial or venous stenosis Vascular steal syndrome	Avoid too early cannulation of new access. Teach patients to avoid wearing constrictive clothing on accessed limbs. Avoid repeated cannulation of one segment of access. Use aseptic technique when cannulating access. Monitor for changes in arterial or venous pressure while patients are on dialysis. Provide comfort measures to reduce pain of vascular steal (e.g., warm compresses, analgesics as ordered).

Nursing management. Nursing management of the patient with a subclavian or femoral central line relates to central line placement and hemodialysis. The location of a subclavian access is always confirmed by chest x-ray film to evaluate the possibility of pneumothorax or hemothorax resulting from catheter insertion. Following insertion, the patient is closely monitored for signs and symptoms of respiratory distress caused by a pneumothorax or hemothorax, elevations in heart rate or blood pressure, decrease in oxygen saturation, and tracheal deviation, which could indicate a tension pneumothorax. Femoral catheter sites are observed carefully for any signs of rapidly developing hematomas resulting from femoral artery puncture. Ongoing care of the acute access site involves monitoring for signs of infection, such as redness, swelling, increased white blood cell count, or erosion around the catheter site.

The nursing management of chronic access devices is focused on the maintenance of a patient and infection-free vascular access. Blood pressure measurements or venipunctures are never performed on the arm that has the chronic access site. For those patients who require anticoagulants to remove clots from the chronic devices, the nurse assists with the titration of these medications, monitoring of vital signs, and assessing for the return of a bruit or thrill.

Patient education. Patient teaching in the acute phase describes the changes that occur in the body as a result of ARF and explains the need for hemodialysis and the purpose of the acute vascular access. Fluid limits, nutritional restrictions, the importance of daily weight measurements, and how to measure intake and output are also explained.

Patient teaching for the patient with a permanent vascular access is designed to educate the patient and family about care of the peripheral vascular access and to decrease the incidence of thrombosis, infection, or pseudoaneurysm. The importance of fluid and nutritional restrictions in renal failure is reemphasized, as is the necessity for regular hemodialysis treatments.

Hemodialysis

Hemodialysis roughly translates as "separating from the blood."[20] Indications and contraindications for hemodialysis are listed in Box 33-6. As a treatment, hemodialysis literally separates and removes from the blood the excess electrolytes, fluids, and toxins by use of a dialyzer (Figure 33-2). Although efficient in removing chemicals, it does not remove all metabolites. Furthermore, electrolytes, toxins, and fluids increase between treatments, requiring hemodialysis on a regular basis. Each dialysis treatment takes 3 to 4 hours. In the acute phases of renal failure, dialysis is performed daily. The dialysis frequency gradually decreases to three times per week as the patient moves into a more chronic phase of renal failure. Indications for hemodialysis include BUN greater than 90 mg/dL, serum creatinine greater than 9 mg/dL, hyperkalemia, drug toxicity, intravascular fluid overload, and metabolic acidosis.[2] The level of BUN should decrease at least 60% with each dialysis or to 30 mg/dL.[2] Other uremia-related symptoms that may improve after hemodialysis include uremic pericarditis, GI bleeding, and encephalopathy with decreased level of consciousness. Contraindications for hemodialysis include hemodynamic instability, inability to anticoagulate, and lack of access to the circulation.[7,8,10]

Hemodialyzer. Hemodialysis works by circulating blood outside the body through synthetic tubing to a *dialyzer,* which consists of hollow-fiber tubes as shown in Figure 33-2. The components of a hemodialysis system appear in Figure 33-3. While the blood flows through the membranes, which are semipermeable, a fluid known as the *dialysate* bath bathes the membranes and, through osmosis and diffusion, performs exchanges of fluid, electrolytes, and toxins from the blood to the bath.[19] The blood and bath are shunted in opposite directions (countercurrent flow) through the dialyzer to maintain the osmotic and chemical gradients at their highest.

Ultrafiltration. To remove fluid, a positive hydrostatic pressure is applied to the blood and a negative hydrostatic pressure is applied to the dialysate bath. The two forces together, called *transmembrane pressure,* pull and squeeze the excess fluid from the blood. The difference between the two values (expressed in millimeters of mercury) represents the transmembrane pressure and results in fluid extraction, known as *ultrafiltration,* from the vascular space.[19]

Anticoagulation. Heparin is added to the system just before the blood enters the dialyzer. Without the heparin the blood would clot because its presence outside the body and its passage through foreign substances initiate the clotting mechanism. Heparin can be administered by bolus injection or intermittent infusion. Administration is determined on the basis of patient weight. The dosage is calculated in units per kilogram of weight, followed by monitoring of the response to the particular dose by measuring clotting times.[19] Heparin has a very short half-life; thus its effects subside within 2 to 4 hours. Also, the effects of heparin are easily reversed through the injection of protamine.

Dialysis process. The dialysis process moves the blood from the body through synthetic tubing to the dialyzer, where dialysis and ultrafiltration occur. The blood returns via artificial tubing to the body. Because the systemic blood pressure is not sufficient to propel the blood through this extracorporeal (outside the vessels) circuit, a pump is used to provide a consistent flow of blood (200 to 400 ml/minute) through the system. Various monitoring devices prevent blood loss, air embolus, vascular access collapse, or high-pressure destruction of the dialyzer or access site. The dialyzer, or artificial kidney, mimics the action of the renal tubules. Active transport and other physiologic mechanisms are not possible with synthetic membranes. Thus the artificial kidney provides for only partial normalization of the blood abnormalities.

The dialysis process moves blood through either microscopic hollow tubes or thin membranous pockets (see Figure 33-2). The membranes have fixed-sized pores, which allow passage of small molecules such as water, glucose, and electrolytes while preventing passage

BOX 33-6 Indications and Contraindications for Hemodialysis

INDICATIONS

BUN >90 mg/dL
Serum creatinine >9 mg/dL
Hyperkalemia
Drug toxicity
Intravascular and extravascular fluid overload
Metabolic acidosis
Symptoms of uremia:
- Pericarditis
- GI bleeding
- Mental changes

Contraindications to other forms of dialysis

CONTRAINDICATIONS

Hemodynamic instability
Inability to anticoagulate
Lack of access to circulation

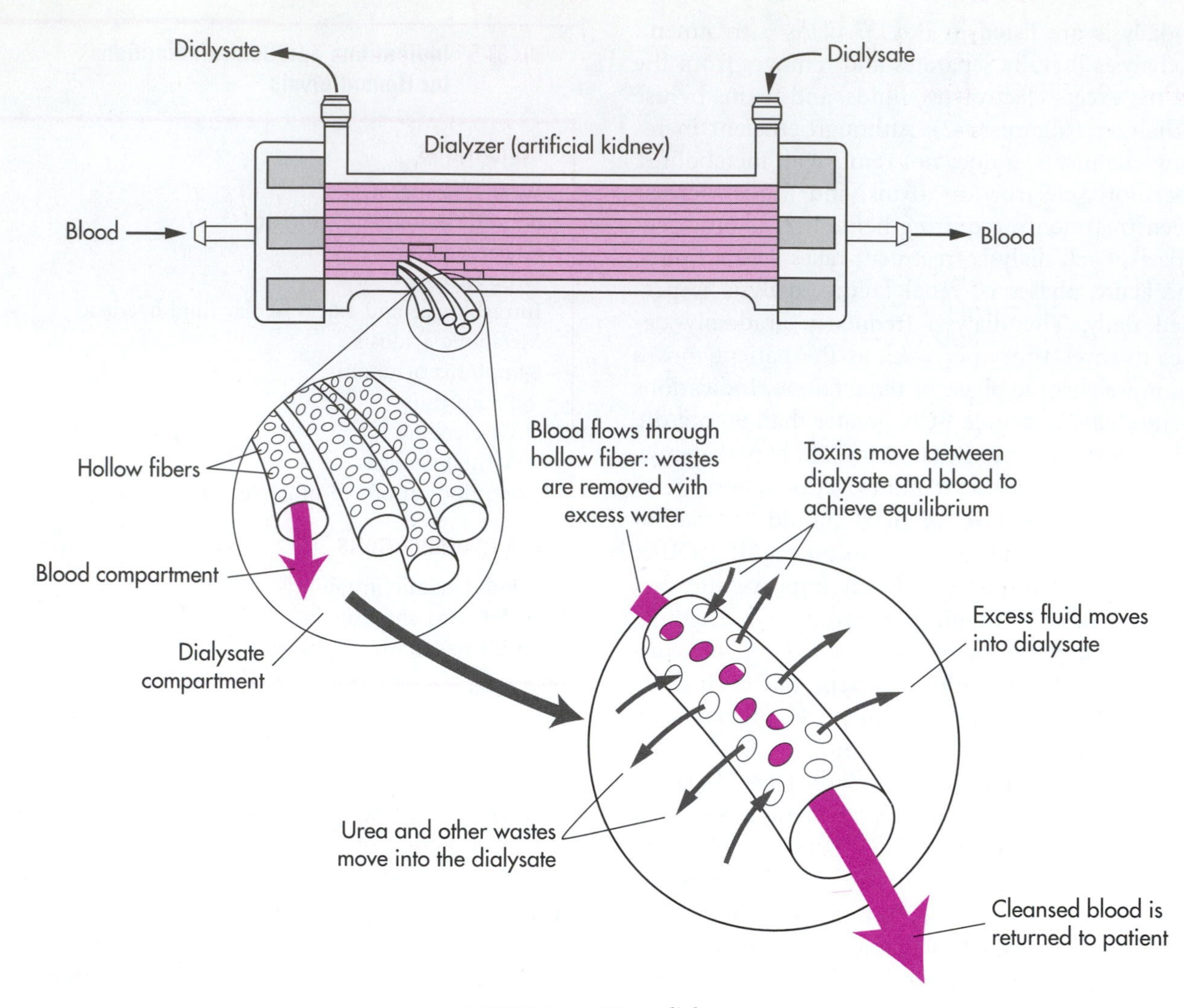

FIGURE 33-2. Hemodialyzer.

of large molecules, including bacteria. The dialysate bath is composed of electrolytes, blood buffers, and water in quantities that create a diffusion gradient across the membranes. For instance, the potassium content may be 2.0 mEq/L in the dialysate to enhance diffusion from the hyperkalemic blood of the renal patient to the dialysate. Calcium absorption is also enhanced by this process. Higher amounts of ionized calcium are placed in the dialysate than are present in the patient's serum. The calcium travels from the dialysate to the patient's vascular space, thereby improving calcium stores.

Several factors affect the efficiency of the dialysis treatment. Blood flow rate must be constant and sufficiently fast to provide the solute and fluid load that maintain the chemical and osmotic gradient on either side of the membrane. The dialysate flow rate should be 2 to $2^1/_2$ times that of the blood flow rate.[11] The dialysate temperature is the same as the blood temperature to maintain the ability of solutes to diffuse. The dialysate composition maintains a concentration gradient between the dialysate and the blood fluid laden with solute. In addition, the direction of flow of the dialysate should be countercurrent, with dialysate flowing in one direction and the blood in the opposite direction. Finally, differences in the pore size, membrane thickness, available membrane surface area, and composition of the membrane can affect the relative efficiency of the dialysis treatment. Nursing management of extracorporeal passage of the patient's blood through the dialyzer is described in Box 33-7.

Tap water is not safe for use in dialysis; the prevalence of calcium, magnesium, organic and inorganic matter, bacteria, and chloramines in tap water can jeopardize effective dialysis. Therefore purification methods must be undertaken to remove these mate-

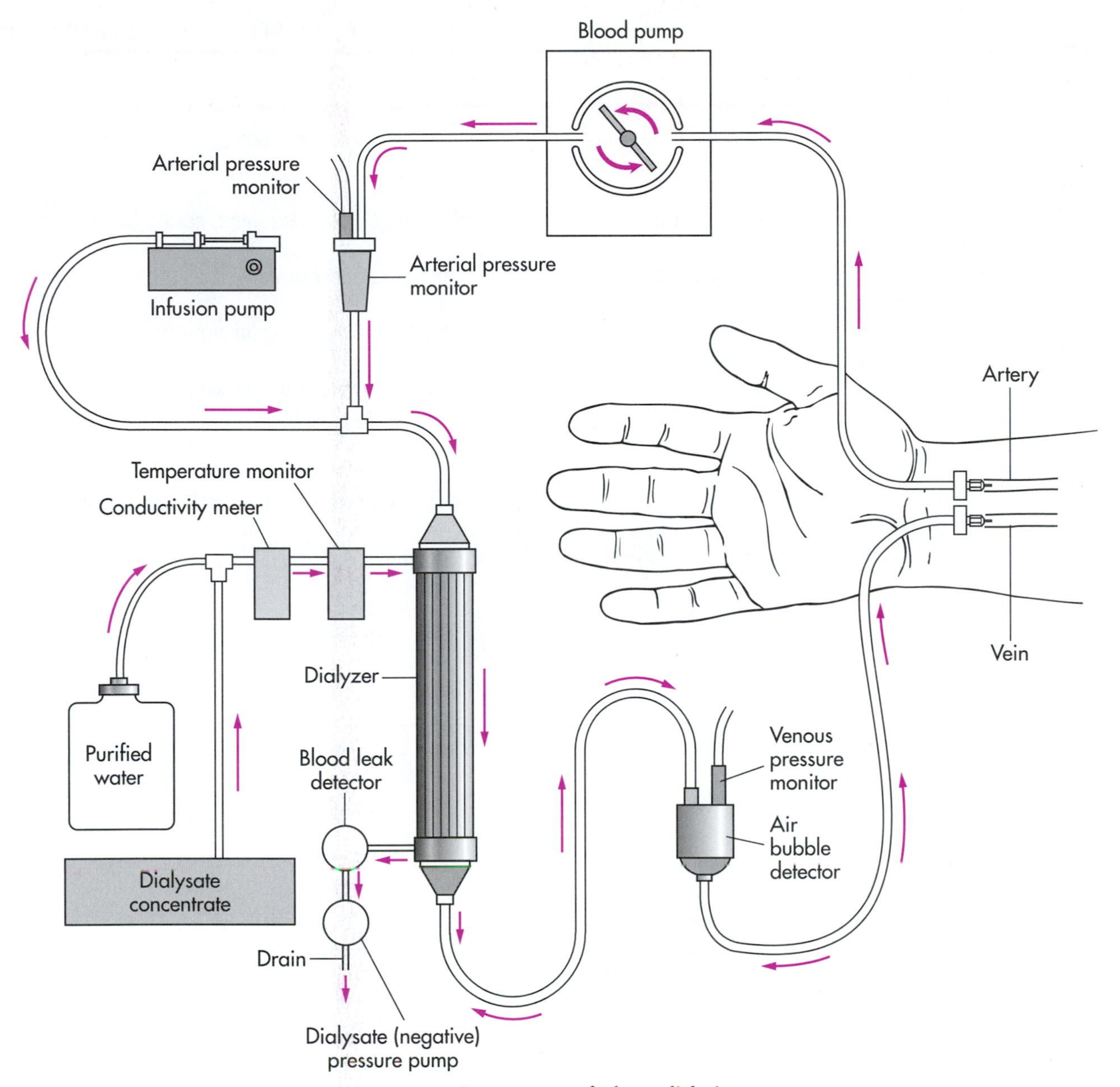

FIGURE 33-3. Components of a hemodialysis system.

rials, as well as salts contained in the tap water. Distillation, reverse osmosis purification, and carbon filtering are the currently used methods for obtaining safe water for use in the dialysis treatment.

Continuous Renal Replacement Therapy

Continuous renal replacement therapy (CRRT) is a newer mode of dialysis that is the treatment of choice in many institutions.[18] CRRT is a continuous therapy lasting 12 hours or longer in which blood is circulated from an artery to a vein—or from vein to vein—through a highly porous hemofilter.[11,18,21] The system allows for continuous fluid removal from the plasma, the amount ranging from 5 to 45 ml/minute, depending on the particular CRRT system used, plus removal of urea, creatinine, and electrolytes.[18,22] If large amounts of fluid are removed, replacement solutions are infused. If fluid removal is low, this is not required.

In an ideal situation, the hydrostatic pressure exerted by the patient's MAP forms the basis for the continuous flow of blood through the hemofilter. To maintain this flow a MAP greater than 70 mm Hg is desirable. The removed ultrafiltrate can be drained by gravity flow or by a suction-assisted collection system.[18] However, because many critically ill patients do

NURSING INTERVENTION CLASSIFICATIONS

BOX 33-7 Hemodialysis Therapy

DEFINITION: Management of extracorporeal passage of the patient's blood through a dialyzer

ACTIVITIES:

Draw blood sample and review blood chemistries (e.g., blood urea nitrogen, serum creatinine, serum Na, K, and PO_4 levels) pretreatment
Record baseline vital signs: weight, temperature, pulse, respirations, and blood pressure
Explain hemodialysis procedure and its purpose
Monitor for AV fistula patency at frequent intervals (e.g., palpate for thrill and auscultate for a bruit)
Check equipment and solutions, according to protocol
Use sterile technique to initiate hemodialysis and for needle insertions and catheter connections
Use gloves, eyeshield, and clothing to prevent direct contact with blood
Initiate hemodialysis, according to protocol
Anchor connections and tubing securely
Check system monitors (e.g., flow rate, pressure, temperature, pH level, conductivity, clots, air detector, negative pressure for ultrafiltration, and blood sensor) to ensure patient safety
Monitor blood pressure, pulse, respirations, temperature, and patient response during dialysis
Administer heparin, according to protocol
Monitor clotting times and adjust heparin administration appropriately
Adjust filtration pressures to remove an appropriate amount of fluid
Institute appropriate protocol, if patient becomes hypotensive
Discontinue hemodialysis according to protocol
Compare postdialysis vitals and blood chemistries to predialysis values
Avoid taking blood pressure or doing intravenous punctures in arm with fistula
Provide catheter or fistula care, according to protocol
Work collaboratively with patient to adjust diet regulations, fluid limitations, and medications to regulate fluid and electrolyte shifts between treatments
Teach patient to self-monitor signs and symptoms that indicate need for medical treatment (e.g., fever, bleeding, clotted fistula, thrombophlebitis, and irregular pulse)
Work collaboratively with patient to relieve discomfort from side effects of the disease and treatment (e.g., cramping, fatigue, headaches, itching, anemia, bone demineralization, body image changes, and role disruption)
Work collaboratively with patient to adjust length of dialysis, diet regulations, and pain and diversion needs to achieve optimal benefit of the treatment

From McCloskey JC, Bulechek GM: *Nursing interventions classification*, ed 2, St Louis, 1996, Mosby.

not have a MAP greater than 70 mm Hg—sufficient to provide adequate flow through the system—in many critical care units a roller pump is added to the system to augment flow. The various CRRT systems are shown in Figure 33-4.

Indications. Indications for the use of CRRT include the need for large fluid volume removal in hemodynamically unstable patients, hypervolemic or edematous patients unresponsive to diuretic therapy, patients with MODS, or fluid removal in patients requiring large daily fluid volumes from TPN. CRRT may also be used in some patients who are too hemodynamically unstable for hemodialysis. A hematocrit greater than 45% is a contraindication for the use of CRRT[3,11,18,21] (Box 33-8).

Because controlled removal and replacement of fluid are possible with CRRT, hemodynamic stability is maintained. This makes CRRT highly advantageous for use in the patient with MODS.[3,21] The four most frequently seen forms of CRRT are as follows:

1. Slow continuous ultrafiltration (SCUF)
2. Continuous arteriovenous hemofiltration (CAVH)
3. Continuous arteriovenous hemodialysis (CAVHD)
4. Continuous venovenous hemodialysis (CVVHD)

The first three types of CRRT require an arterial access (SCUF, CAVH, CAVHD)[21]; the fourth requires only venous access (CVVHD).[23] The decision as to which type of therapy to initiate is based on myriad

BOX 33-8 Indications and Contraindications for Continuous Renal Replacement Therapy

INDICATIONS

- Need for large fluid volume removal in the hemodynamically unstable patient
- Hypervolemic or edematous patients unresponsive to diuretic therapy
- Patients with MODS
- Ease of fluid management in patients requiring large daily fluid volume, such as replacement for oliguria, TPN administration
- Contraindications to hemodialysis and peritoneal dialysis
- Inability to anticoagulate

CONTRAINDICATIONS

- Hematocrit >45%
- Lack of arterial access (for SCUF, CAVH, CAVHD only)

factors, including clinical assessment, metabolic status, severity of uremia, and whether a particular treatment modality is available at that institution. A comparison of CRRT approaches is found in Table 33-5, and a discussion of each of these methods follows.

Slow continuous ultrafiltration. SCUF, as the name implies, slowly removes fluid, 100 to 300 ml/hour, through a process of ultrafiltration.[12,21,22] This process consists of an exchange of fluid, solutes, and solvents across a semipermeable membrane.[21] Because small amounts of fluid are removed via this process, it is a treatment of choice for patients with acute heart failure and diminished renal perfusion who are unresponsive to diuretics.

SCUF system setup. The SCUF system setup is illustrated in Figure 33-4, *A*. This system provides the basic setup on which the other systems build. The blood leaves the patient's body from a cannulated artery such as the femoral artery. The hemofilter and tubing are anticoagulated with a continuous infusion of heparin. The blood is propelled toward the hemofilter by the arterial pressure if the patient's MAP is adequate; otherwise a roller pump can be added to the system to ensure sufficient flow. Outflow ultrafiltrate is collected in a large urometer bag.[21] The ultrafiltrate volume is regulated either by gravity—raising or lowering the height of the bag—or by a negative pressure outflow pump or wall suction added to the system as shown in Figure 33-4, *A*. After passing through the hemofilter, the blood is returned to a cannulated vein such as the femoral vein. An air filter and a pressure monitoring device are added to the venous return line to increase patient safety.

Ultrafiltration. Ultrafiltration is defined as filtration through a semipermeable membrane or any filter that separates colloid solutions from crystalloids or separates particles of different size in a colloid mixture. It occurs through the combination of the hydrostatic pressure of the blood (blood pressure) and the negative hydrostatic pressure of the outflowing ultrafiltrate. The two pressures are opposed by the oncotic pressure created by the plasma proteins. The volume that is removed from the blood is called *ultrafiltrate*. The ultrafiltrate is collected in a closed urometer system that exits from the hemofilter.

With SCUF, fluid removal can be accomplished, if the patient has an adequate MAP, by simply allowing the blood pressure to push the blood continuously through the circuit. If the blood pressure is not sufficient, a roller pump is added to ensure adequate flow and fluid removal. Because large amounts of fluid are not removed, volume replacement is not required.

Anticoagulation. Anticoagulation is important because blood is traveling through an extracorporeal circuit. Commonly, a 2000 unit bolus of heparin is given before the initiation of CRRT. Thereafter continuous infusion at a rate of 5 to 10 units/kg/hour via an IV infusion pump or syringe pump is used throughout the treatment. Clotting times are frequently assessed to monitor anticoagulation. The blood sample is taken from the in-line venous return port. The goal is to anticoagulate the hemofilter but not the patient.

Solute removal. Hemofilters are designed to clear solutes and unbound molecules of up to 50,000 daltons. Typical hemodialysis can clear only particles of up to 10,000 daltons. Therefore the hemofilter clears many drugs that dialysis cannot remove, along with large amounts of fluids that cannot be removed in as great a quantity through hemodialysis.

Continuous arteriovenous hemofiltration. CAVH is indicated when the patient's clinical condition warrants removal of significant volumes of fluid and solutes. Fluid is removed by ultrafiltration in volumes of 5 to 20 ml/minute or 7 to 30 L in 24 hours.[24] Increased removal of solutes such as urea, creatinine, or other nonprotein-bound toxins is accomplished by increasing flow through the hemofilter via the addition of a prehemofilter replacement fluid, as shown in Figure 33-4, *B*.

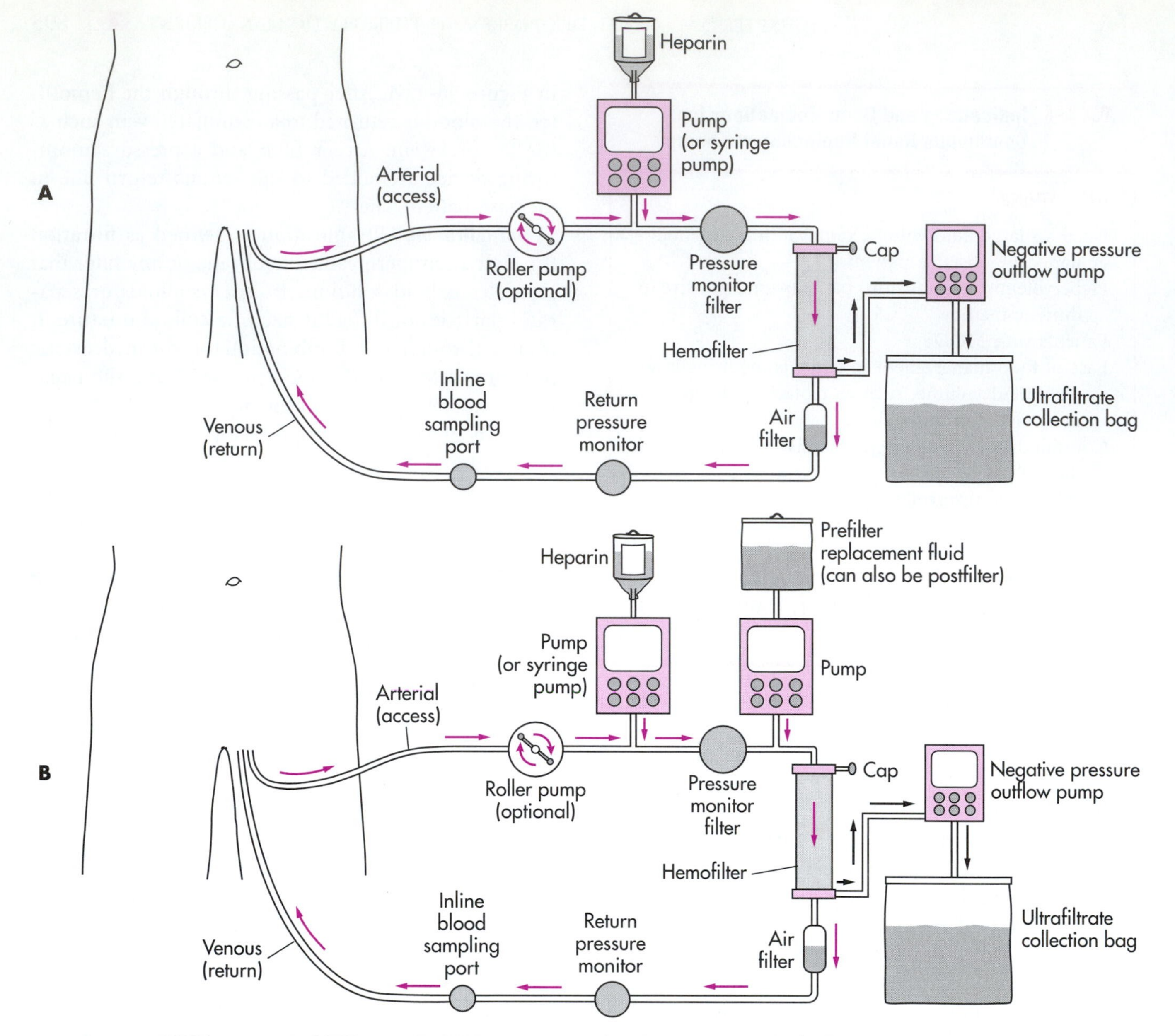

FIGURE 33-4. CRRT systems. **A,** SCUF setup. **B,** CAVH setup. Note that the systems are similar but vary in complexity, depending on what function is to be performed. For example, the CVAH setup differs from the SCUF setup in that it contains prefilter replacement fluid and a pump so that significant blood volume can be removed. (The purple arrows indicate blood flow, and the black arrows indicate ultrafiltrate flow.)

CAVH set-up. The CAVH system requires arterial access. The setup is similar to that for SCUF, with the addition of a prehemofilter fluid replacement on an IV pump to the system before the blood reaches the hemofilter. The additional volume increases flow and pressure through the hemofilter and thus increases removal of both fluid and solutes.[21] As with other systems, the blood is anticoagulated and the ultrafiltrate collected in a large urometer bag, either by gravity or by the addition of negative pressure suction. After passage through the hemofilter, the blood is returned into the venous circulation. CAVH also provides ultrafiltration, requires therapeutic anticoagulation, and has an air filter, a return pressure monitor, and an in-line sampling port. The CAVH system setup is illustrated in Figure 33-4, *B*.

Replacement solution. Because large volumes of fluid may be removed in CAVH, some of the ultrafiltrate volume is replaced hourly with a continuous infusion. In addition to maintaining appropriate fluid balance, fluid replacement lowers the plasma concentration of solutes by dilution.

The amount of fluid replacement is based on fluid losses and electrolyte values, with consideration given to achieving a therapeutic reduction in the ECF volume. Replacement fluids may consist of standard solutions of bicarbonate, potassium-free LR solution, acetate, or dextrose. Electrolytes such as potassium, sodium,

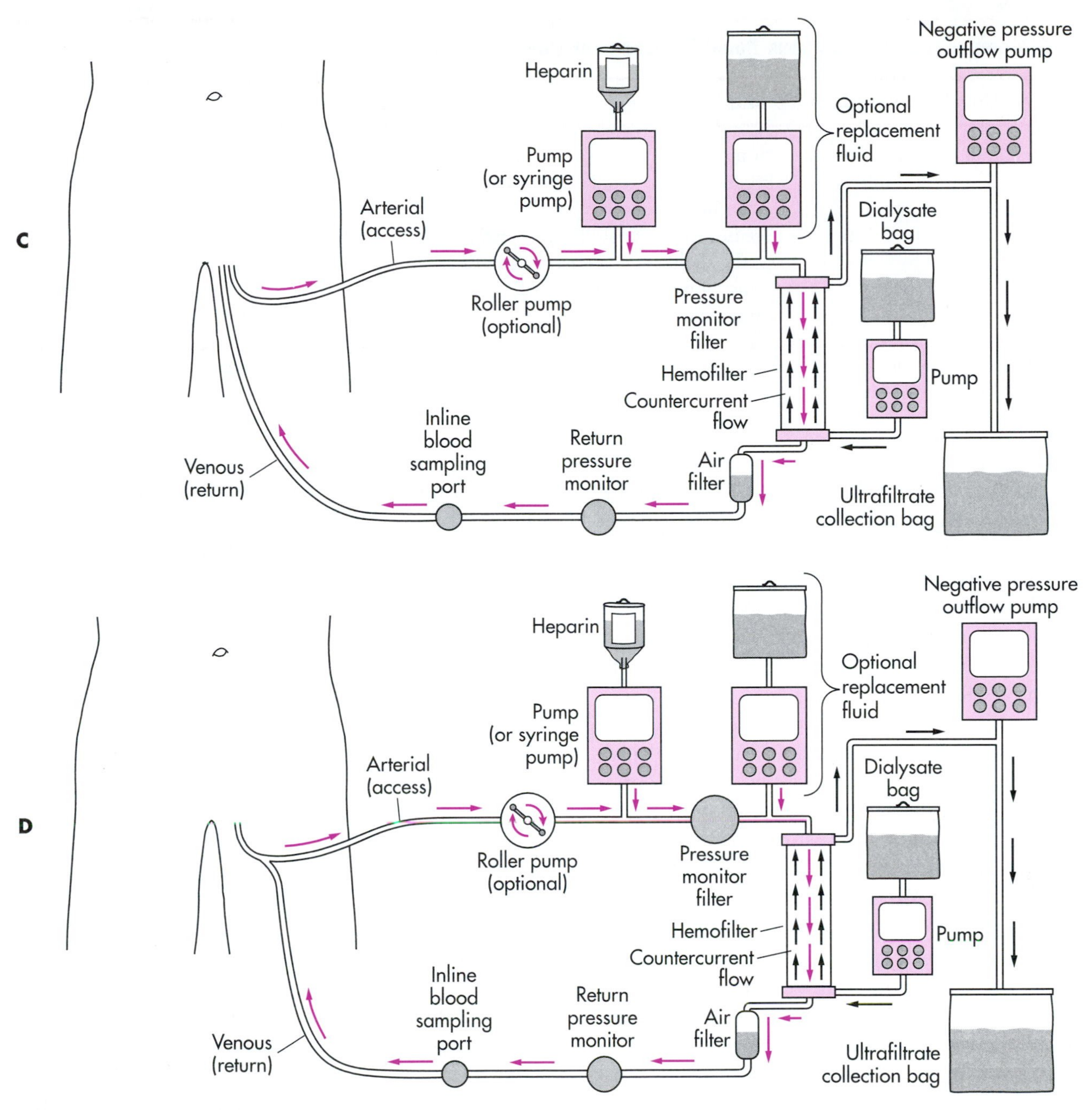

FIGURE 33-4—Cont'd. **C,** CAVHD setup. **D,** CVVHD setup.The CAVHD setup and CVVHD setup differ from the SCUF setup and CAVH setup in that they have additional countercurrent flow. (The purple arrows indicate blood flow, and the black arrows indicate ultrafiltrate flow.)

calcium chloride, magnesium sulfate, or sodium bicarbonate may also be added.[18,21] The replacement solution can be infused as a posthemofilter or a prehemofilter infusion,[18] as shown in Figure 33-4, *B.* The difference between the total ultrafiltrate volume removed and the replacement fluid (plus any other IV fluid and oral intake) determines the fluid that has actually been taken from the patient. An example of a formula that can be used to calculate the volume removed follows:

Formula:

Outflow − replacement = output/hour
(Ultrafiltrate in bag) − (CAVH replacement + IV and oral intake) = output/hour

Example:

1000 ml − 800 ml = 200 ml output/hour

Continuous arteriovenous hemodialysis. CAVHD requires arterial access but is technically different from the two previously described methods because it contains a slow (15 to 30 ml/minute) countercurrent

TABLE 33-5 Comparison of Continuous Renal Replacement Therapy Methods

Type	Ultrafiltration Rate	Fluid Replacement	Indication
SCUF	100 to 300 ml/hr	None	Fluid removal
CAVH	500 to 800 ml/hr	Predilution or postdilution, calculating an hourly net loss	Fluid removal, moderate solute removal
CAVHD	500 to 800 ml/hr	Predilution or postdilution, subtracting the dialysate and then calculating an hourly net loss	Fluid removal, maximum solute removal
CVVHD		Same as CAVHD	Fluid removal and solute removal

SCUF, Slow continuous ultrafiltration; *CAVH,* continuous arteriovenous hemofiltration; *CAVHD,* continuous arteriovenous hemodialysis, *CVVHD,* continuous venovenous hemodialysis.

drainage flow on the membrane side of the hemofilter, as shown in Figure 33-4, *C.*[24] The countercurrent flow is through the hemodialyzer. Countercurrent means the blood flows in one direction and the dialysate flows in the opposite direction. This increases its clearance of uremic toxins and makes it more like traditional hemodialysis.[21] CAVHD is the most efficient form of CRRT.[18]

CAVHD is indicated in patients who require large-volume removal for severe uremia or critical acid-base imbalances or who are diuretic resistant. A MAP of at least 70 mm Hg is desirable for effective volume removal and dialysis, and it is most effective when used over days, not hours.

CAVHD set-up. In CAVHD, arterial access is required. If the blood pressure is adequate, the arterial hydrostatic pressure can push the blood through the system. Usually, however, the anticoagulated blood is moved by a roller pump to provide more consistent flow through the hemofilter. What makes this system technically different from CVAH is that a dialysate solution is infused via countercurrent flow into the hemofilter to accomplish removal of fluids and solutes. Also, as illustrated in Figure 33-4, *C,* the ultrafiltrate collection tubing position is changed to the top of the hemofilter. Dialysate enters the hemofilter at the bottom to allow for countercurrent flow. In other words, as blood moves down the hemofilter, it encounters dialysate moving upward in the opposite direction. The dialysate is pulled through the hemofilter by the negative outflow pump. The dialysate solution is then removed with the ultrafiltrate and collected in the ultrafiltrate collection bag.[21] After the blood has passed through the hemofilter, it is returned to the patient via the venous catheter. In the CAVHD system there is always an air filter, a return pressure monitor, and an in-line sampling port. The CAVHD setup is shown in Figure 33-4, *C.*

Fluid replacement. The CAVHD system can be set up with or without additional replacement fluid similar to CAVH. A replacement fluid setup may be added to the system to give the critical care team more control over fluid balance. The use of replacement fluid is optional. If the amount of ultrafiltrate removed is large, some of the ultrafiltrate is replaced. If the volume removed is low, replacement is not required. As with CAVHD, the nurse is responsible for calculating the hourly intake and output, noting fluid trends, and replacing excessive losses.

Continuous venovenous hemodialysis. CVVHD is a newer method of renal replacement therapy. The advantage of CVVHD is that arterial access is not required. The CVVHD system is set up in the same way as CAVHD and also includes a slow countercurrent drainage flow on the membrane side of the hemofilter. The indications for CVVHD are the same as for CAVHD.

CVVHD setup. The CVVHD setup is identical to that for CAVHD except that a dual lumen venous access catheter is used and therefore arterial access is not required.[23,25] A roller pump is mandatory because the low-pressure venous circulation does not have the force to push the blood through the system. The blood enters the hemofilter at the top, and the dialysate is infused at the bottom. The blood moves downward, and the dialysate moves upward toward the collection tubing. Once the blood has passed through the hemofilter, it is returned to the venous circulation. As with other systems, the blood is anticoagulated, ultrafiltration is effective, and there is an air filter, a return pressure monitor, and an in-line sampling port. The CVVHD setup is shown in Figure 33-4, *D.*

Dialysate. A dialysate solution is infused into the hemofilter to increase fluid and solute removal. Prehemofilter or posthemofilter fluid replacement may also be infused. This is in addition to the dialysate. In both CAVHD and CVVHD a countercurrent mechanism is employed. The blood enters the hemofilter at the top. The dialysate enters at the bottom of the hemofilter and exits at the top via the ultrafiltration collection tubing. The ultrafiltrate is then collected in a collection bag. The dialysate is pulled through the system by either wall suction or a negative pressure outflow pump.

Fluid replacement. In CVVHD, volume is replaced only if the amount of ultrafiltrate is large; otherwise it is not required. When volume replacement is needed, it is added either as a prehemofilter or as a posthemofilter solution, as shown in Figure 33-4, *C* and *D*. As discussed earlier, the nurse is responsible for calculating the amount of fluid removed each hour. The formula described in the section on CAVH can also be used with CVVHD to determine hourly fluid balance. Table 33-5 compares all four CCRT methods.

Complications of CRRT. Although CRRT is a successful treatment for ARF, potential complications are numerous: dehydration, hypotension, electrolyte imbalance, acid-base abnormalities, hypothermia, hyperglycemia, decreased ultrafiltrate, inadequate blood flow through the hemofilter, clotted hemofilter, blood leak with blood in the ultrafiltrate, and disconnection at the catheter or hemofilter causing hemorrhage. The patient with ARF undergoing CRRT presents unique challenges to the critical care nurse. The nurse's role is crucial to early detection and treatment of any complications that result from CRRT therapy.[18,22,24] Table 33-6 describes problems, etiologies, clinical manifestations, and nursing management related to CRRT.

Medical management. The choice of blood purification to use in ARF is a medical decision. Age, sex, and preexisting chronic conditions are of little help in determining the need for hemofiltration or hemodialysis, and often it is the acute clinical diagnosis that is the deciding factor.[2] In trauma the location of injury is important. For example, patients with head and abdominal injury have a poorer prognosis than those with chest and limb damage. Multisystem organ failure often involves the kidneys; however, the number of organ systems involved and the severity of their involvement have been shown to be of very limited prognostic importance, at least at the onset of ARF.[2] Infectious complications are associated with a grave prognosis. Dialysis is prescribed for almost anyone who develops severe ARF unless the patient is clearly dying.[2]

Intermittent hemodialysis or CCRT is usually begun before the BUN level exceeds 90 mg/dL or the creatinine exceeds 9 mg/dL. It is controversial whether daily treatment is more effective than treatment every other day.[2] The patient's serum creatinine, BUN, and fluid volume status are the deciding factors. CCRT is often prescribed when the BUN level is approximately 60 mg/dL. CRRT is more effective in the early stages of ARF. If severe electrolyte imbalance or fluid overload is present, even earlier intervention may be required.[2]

Nursing management. Critical care nurses play a vital role in monitoring the patient receiving hemodialysis and hemofiltration. Side effects include hypotension, hypertension, nausea, vomiting, muscle cramps, headaches, dyspnea, and chest and back pain. Accurate fluid balance, including the measurement of intake and output as well as daily weights, is imperative. Also, daily laboratory values are recorded, noting the trends in electrolytes, blood count, bleeding times, and chemistry panels to comprehensively assess the patient's status.

Assessment for catheter patency is ongoing. Signs of clotting include a cool hemofilter, separation of blood in the blood lines, and a decrease in the ultrafiltration rate.[24] If the IV access is in the femoral artery, circulation to the affected extremity is assessed and documented hourly, including warmth, color, and presence of pedal pulses. If large-bore arterial catheters are used, hemorrhage can occur if the system becomes disconnected. For this reason the filtering lines are positioned to be secure and visible at all times. If patients are restless, their activity may need to be restricted to prevent accidental disconnection or displacement of catheters.[24] A sterile dressing is maintained over the insertion site, which is assessed daily for signs or symptoms of infection such as localized redness or swelling. Other indications of infection include increased white blood cell count or fever.

Patient education. The purpose of the CRRT system is described to the patient and family in uncomplicated terms. It is helpful to explain anticipated outcomes and the laboratory and fluid volume indicators that are being monitored.

Peritoneal Dialysis

Peritoneal dialysis (PD) involves the introduction of sterile dialyzing fluid through an implanted catheter into the abdominal cavity. The dialysate bathes the peritoneal membrane, which covers the abdominal organs and overlies the capillary beds that support the organs. By the processes of osmosis, diffusion, and active transport, excess fluid and solutes travel from the peritoneal capillary fluid through the capillary

TABLE 33-6 Problems, Etiologies, Clinical Manifestations, and Nursing Interventions Related to CRRT

Problem	Etiology	Clinical Manifestations	Nursing Management
Decreased ultrafiltration rate	Hypotension Dehydration Kinked lines Bending of catheters Clotting of filter	Ultrafiltration rate decreased Minimal flow through blood lines	Observe filter and arteriovenous system. Control blood flow. Control coagulation time. Position patients on back. Lower height of collection container.
Filter clotting	Obstruction Insufficient heparinization	Ultrafiltration rate decreased, despite height of collection container being lower	Control heparinization. Maintain continuous heparinization. Call physicians. Remove system. Prime catheters with heparin. Prime a new system and connect it. Start predilution with 1000 ml saline 0.9% solution per hour. Do not use three-way stopcocks.
Hypotension	Increased ultrafiltration rate Blood leak Disconnection of one of lines	Bleeding	Control amount of ultrafiltration. Control access sites. Clamp lines. Call physician.
Fluid and electrolyte changes	Too much/little removal of fluid Inappropriate replacement of electrolytes Inappropriate dialysate	Changes in mentation ↑ or ↓ CVP, PAWP ECG change ↑ or ↓ BP and heart rate Abnormal electrolyte levels	Observe for changes in central venous pressure or pulmonary capillary wedge pressure. Observe for changes in vital signs. Observe electrocardiogram for changes in result of electrolyte abnormalities. Monitor output values every hour. Control ultrafiltration.
Bleeding	System disconnection ↑ Heparin dose	Oozing from catheter insertion site or connection	Monitor ACT no less than once every hour. Adjust heparin dose within specifications to maintain ACT. Observe dressing on vascular access for blood loss. Observe for blood in filtrate (filter leak).
Access dislodgment or infection	Catheter/connections not secured Break in sterile technique Excessive patient movement	Bleeding from catheter site or connections Inappropriate flow/infusion Fever Drainage at catheter site	Observe access site at least once every 2 hr. Ensure that clamps are available within easy reach at all times. Observe strict sterile technique when dressing vascular access.

walls, through the peritoneal membrane, and into the dialyzing fluid. After a selected time period, the fluid is drained out of the abdomen by gravity (Figure 33-5). The process is then repeated at regular prescribed intervals.

Indications for PD include uremia, volume overload, electrolyte imbalances, hemodynamic instability, lack of access to circulation, and removal of high molecular weight toxins. In the critical care unit, patients who have PD at home may be admitted with a non-

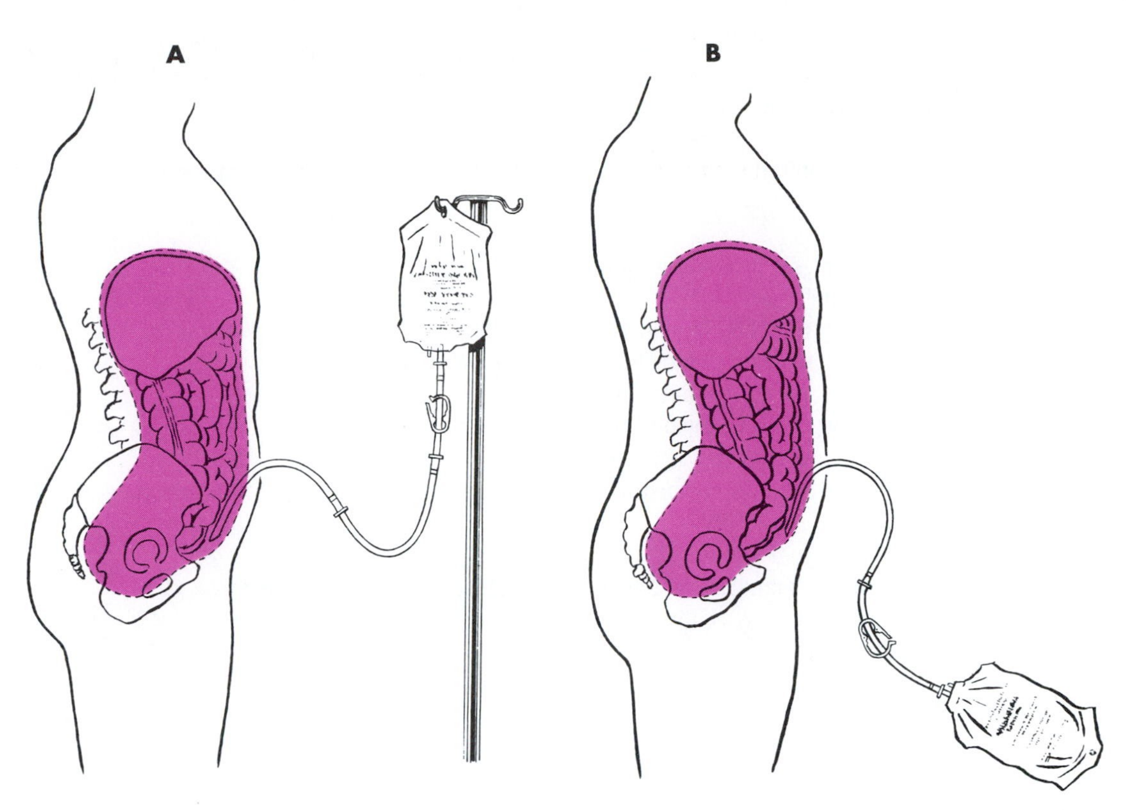

FIGURE 33-5. Peritoneal dialysis. **A,** Inflow. **B,** Outflow (drains by gravity). (From Thompson JM and others: *Mosby's clinical nursing,* ed 4, St Louis, 1997, Mosby.)

renal critical illness, but will continue to receive PD for chronic renal failure in the critical care unit (Box 33-9). Contraindications for PD include recent abdominal surgery, history of abdominal surgeries with adhesions and scarring, significant pulmonary disease, need for rapid fluid removal, and peritonitis.[3,12,26]

The peritoneal membrane's structure and capillary blood flow to the peritoneum account for the relatively slow nature of PD. The small capillary pores, the capillary membrane, the interstitium, the mesothelium of the peritoneum, and the fluid film layers in the capillary and the peritoneal cavity provide formidable barriers to fluid and solute passage.[26]

Much about the nature of the peritoneal membrane is still a mystery, but several factors are implicated in changing the performance of the membrane. For instance, any change in the capillary blood flow changes solute removal but not to a great degree. This is probably a result of the relatively poor vasculature of the area, in which not all capillaries are perfused at the same time and in which there exists resistance of the capillary membrane to solute transfer. The volume of dialysate instilled into the abdomen affects the clearance. During acute PD, 3.5 L/hour provides a urea clearance of 26 ml/minute. During chronic,

BOX 33-9 Indications and Contraindications for Peritoneal Dialysis

INDICATIONS

Uremia
Volume overload
Electrolyte imbalances
Hemodynamic instability
Lack of access to circulation
Removal of high molecular weight toxins
Patients with nonrenal critical illness who are receiving PD for chronic renal failure
Severe cardiovascular disease
Inability to anticoagulate
Contraindication to hemodialysis

CONTRAINDICATIONS

Recent abdominal surgery
History of abdominal surgeries with adhesions and scarring
Significant pulmonary disease
Need for rapid fluid removal
Peritonitis

NURSING INTERVENTION CLASSIFICATIONS

BOX 33-10 Peritoneal Dialysis Therapy

DEFINITION: Administration and monitoring of dialysis solution into and out of the peritoneal cavity

ACTIVITIES:
Explain the selected peritoneal dialysis procedure and purpose
Warm the dialysis fluid before instillation
Assess patency of catheter, noting difficulty in inflow/outflow
Maintain record of inflow/outflow volumes and individual/cumulative fluid balance
Have patient empty bladder before peritoneal catheter insertion
Monitor blood pressure, pulse, respirations, temperature, and patient response during dialysis
Ensure aseptic handling of peritoneal catheter and connections
Draw laboratory samples and review blood chemistries (e.g., blood urea nitrogen, serum creatinine, and serum Na, K, and PO_4 levels)
Obtain cell count cultures of peritoneal effluent, if indicated
Record baseline vital signs: weight, temperature, pulse, respirations, and blood pressure
Measure and record abdominal girth
Measure and record daily weight
Anchor connections and tubing securely
Check equipment and solutions, according to protocol
Administer dialysis exchanges (inflow, dwell, and outflow), according to protocol
Monitor for signs of infection (e.g., peritonitis and exit site inflammation/drainage)
Monitor for signs of respiratory distress
Monitor for bowel perforation or fluid leaks
Work collaboratively with patient to adjust length of dialysis, diet regulations, and pain and diversion needs to achieve optimal benefit of the treatment
Teach patient to monitor self for signs and symptoms that indicate need for medical treatment (e.g., fever, bleeding, respiratory distress, irregular pulse, cloudy outflow, and abdominal pain)
Teach procedure to patient requiring home dialysis

From McCloskey JC, Bulechek GM: *Nursing interventions classification,* ed 2, St Louis, 1996, Mosby.

continuous PD, 2 L exchanges every 4 hours provide a clearance of 7 ml/minute. The dialysate should be instilled at body temperature to be comfortable, provide some vasodilation, and provide increased solute transport in the peritoneum. The length of time the solution remains in the peritoneal cavity (dwell time) and the solution composition affect the outcome. The dwell time affects the amount of fluid removed from the peritoneal capillaries, although a longer dwell time will not remove proportionately more fluid because of osmotic equilibration across the membranes. The various glucose concentrations of the dialysate provide for different rates of fluid removal. See Box 33-10 for information about administration and monitoring of dialysis solutions into and out of the peritoneal cavity.

Peritoneal dialysis catheter placement. Two types of catheters are used for PD: the rigid stylet and the silicone catheter. The single-use *rigid stylet catheter* can be inserted at the bedside for immediate initiation of dialysis. Patient mobility is limited when the rigid stylet is in place because of the possibility of perforation.[26] The *silicone catheter* usually is inserted surgically, although it can be inserted at the bedside. This catheter is designed for multiple treatments over extended periods. Because the catheter is extremely flexible, the patient is able to move freely with minimal discomfort.[26]

Most catheters have an external segment, a tunnel segment that passes through subcutaneous tissue and muscle, a cuff for stabilization at the peritoneal membrane, and an external segment with numerous holes for fast delivery and drainage of dialysate (Figure 33-6).

Peritoneal dialysis complications. Complications of PD can be numerous. The complications, which range from annoying to severe, require careful observation and intervention to control or even prevent further problems.[27] With the exception of peritonitis, however,

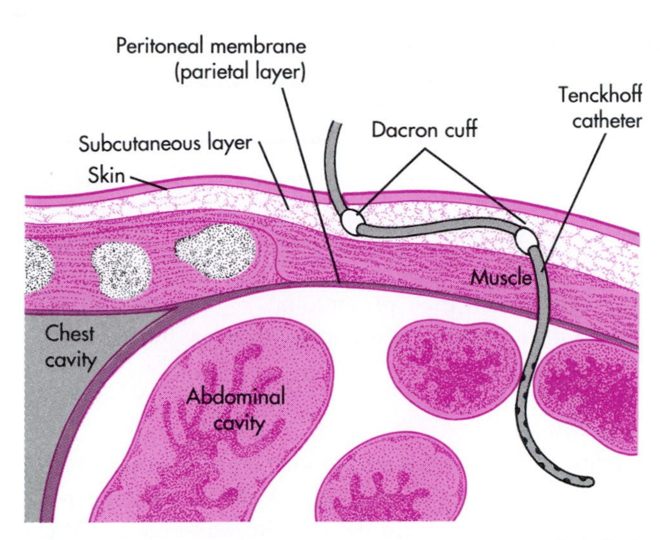

FIGURE 33-6. Tenckhoff catheter used in peritoneal dialysis. (From Lewis SM, Collier IC: *Medical-surgical nursing assessment and management of clinical problems,* ed 3, St Louis, 1992, Mosby.)

the complications from PD are less severe than those associated with hemodialysis.

Medical management. PD is generally used for long-term chronic renal failure. One acute clinical situation that may have application for PD is patients with a head injury. In this case, PD is advised because no anticoagulation is needed, the osmolality changes are not pronounced, and pressure changes in the CNS are avoided.[27]

Nursing management. The patient undergoing PD is at risk of contracting peritonitis. For this reason the infusion and removal of the dialysate fluid are sterile procedures. If the effluent looks cloudy, or if the patient complains of abdominal pain or tenderness, samples of effluent are sent for bacterial culture.

If sufficient effluent does not come out following the dwell time, the patient should be asked to change position. If no fluid exits the abdomen, the catheter may need to be irrigated. This is a sterile procedure, and the utmost care must be taken not to contaminate the catheter. If fibrin clots have blocked the peritoneal catheter, heparin may be prescribed by the physician. Complications and nursing management related to PD are listed in Table 33-7.

Patient education. Patients and their families are taught about chronic renal failure and the purpose of the PD. Symptoms to report to a health care professional and signs and symptoms of infection are explained. Care of the catheter and how to perform PD are demonstrated before discharge or sometimes at an outpatient setting soon after discharge from the acute care hospital. Education that allows the patient to perform these activities under supervision will decrease the risks of catheter contamination and peritonitis at a later time.

PHARMACOLOGY

Diuretics

Diuretics are frequently prescribed in the critical care setting, as they are used to increase water excretion via the kidneys. Several classes of diuretics are available as listed in Table 33-8. These medications are usually administered by IV bolus, although they are also effective by continuous direct infusion.[28,29]

Interactions of Medications with Renal Failure

Medications are eliminated from the body by renal excretion or metabolized by the liver. In determining whether renal failure will affect drug clearance from the body, the amount of unchanged drug that is excreted by the kidney is a major factor. If medications are secreted primarily by the liver, they will not be significantly affected by changes in renal function, unless there is a pharmacologic reaction that causes the drug to be excreted by the kidney. If the kidney is the normal place in which the drug is excreted, the health care team must look at the dose, interval between doses, or combination of drug actions to avoid accumulation of the drug in the serum (Table 33-9).

The critical care nurse is cognizant of those drugs which are eliminated by the kidney and which are dialyzed during hemodialysis. Some of the drugs more frequently encountered in critical care and that are affected by renal failure or hemodialysis are listed in Table 33-9. The molecular weight of medications, the higher water solubility of some medications that make them easily removed by dialysis, or the ability of the medications to bind with proteins and therefore not be removed by dialysis are factors that affect the blood level of the medication.

TABLE 33-7 Complications and Nursing Management of Peritoneal Dialysis

Complications	Nursing Management
Peritonitis	Assess for signs and symptoms: cloudy effluent, abdominal pain, rebound tenderness, nausea and vomiting, and fever. Obtain effluent sample for culture. Administer antibiotics as ordered. Teach patients and families signs and symptoms and their prevention.
Exit site infection	Monitor site daily for signs and symptoms of infection: enduration, erythema, purulence, and hyperthermia. Increase daily cleaning of site. Apply topical antibiotics as ordered (controversial). Teach patients and families to avoid agents such as creams and lotions around exit site.
Catheter-tunnel infection	Assess for signs and symptoms of infection: pain along tunnel, enduration for several centimeters away from catheter, erythema leading away from the exit site, and drainage at exit site or as tunnel is "milked" toward exit site. Teach patients and families signs and symptoms of infection. Teach patients and families to avoid pulls or tugs on the catheter or trauma to the exit site. Emphasize the need to maintain cleansing regimen at exit site.
Fluid obstruction	Change position of patients (i.e., standing, lying, side-lying, knee chest). Relieve patients' constipation. Irrigate the catheter. Ensure that sufficient fluid is in abdomen (sometimes requires a residual reservoir of approximately 50 ml).
Rectal pain	Ensure a sufficient reservoir of fluid. Use slow infusion rate.
Shoulder pain	Ensure that all air is primed from infusion tubing. Attempt draining the effluent with patients in knee-chest position. Administer mild analgesics as ordered.
Hernias	Monitor for increase in size of or pain in area of hernia. Decrease volume of exchanges as ordered. Dialyze with patients in the supine position. Use abdominal binder or support for patients (as long as not binding on catheter exit site). Avoid initiation of PD until exit site healing has taken place (approximately 1 to 2 weeks) if possible.
Fluid overload	Increase use of hypertonic solutions. Decrease by-mouth (PO) fluid intake. Shorten dwell times. Weigh patients frequently. Monitor lung sounds and peripheral edema.
Dehydration	Assess patients for decreased skin turgor, muscle cramps, hypotension, tachycardia, and dizziness. Discontinue hypertonic solutions. Increase PO fluid intake. Lengthen dwell times.
Blood-tinged effluent	Monitor for change in effluent color (clear yellow to pink or rusty). Administer heparin, as ordered, to avoid fibrin formation. Obtain patient history about catheter trauma and patient activity before appearance of complication.

TABLE 33-8 Renal Drugs

Drug	Dosage	Actions	Special Considerations
DIURETICS			
Loop diuretics			
Lasix, Bumex	20-80 mg/day (Lasix) 0.5-2 mg/day (Bumex)	Acts on loop of Henle to Inhibit sodium and chloride	Ototoxicity if administered too rapidly or with other otoxic drugs Monitor intake/output, hydration, watch for hypotension
Thiazide diuretics			
Diuril	500 mg-2 g/day	Inhibit sodium, chloride reabsorption in distal tubule	Enhanced with low-sodium diet Absorption of thiazides decreased by lipid-lowering drugs cholestyramine and colestipol Synergistic effect with loop diuretics
Potassium-sparing diuretics			
Aldactone	100 mg/day for 5 days	Exert effects on collecting tubule; reduce potassium, hydrogen and increase sodium	Weak diuretic effect, so given with other diuretics Potassium supplements not required; monitor for hyperkalemia
Osmotic diuretics			
Mannitol (Osmitrol, Resectial)	0.25-2.0 g/kg IV infusion as a 15%-20% solution over 30-90 min	Increases urine output because of increased plasma osmolality, increasing flow of water from tissues Increases sodium, potassium	Often used in head injury to decrease cerebral edema Can be used to promote urinary secretion of toxic substances Use in-line 5 micron IV filter with $>$ 20% solutions
METHYLXANTHINES			
Aminophylline (Phylocontin; Truphylline)	300 mg/day PO/IV Maximum infusion rate 20 mg/ml	Acts similarly to the thiazide diuretics but on proximal tubule Decreases sodium, potassium, chloride	Increase heart rate (monitor ECG) Increase blood pressure (monitor BP) Target serum aminophylline level 10-15 mg/ml
Phosphate binding			
Amphojel, AlternaGel	30-40 ml/meals	Reduces phosphate absorption in the gut	Causes constipation Stop if hypercalcemia present
Erythrocyte-stimulating hormone			
Epogen	50-100 U/kg 3 times/week	Promotes the production of RBCs	May increase blood pressure Not used to correct anemia

TABLE 33-9 Impact of Renal Failure and Hemodialysis on Selected Drugs Used in Critical Care

Drug	Normal Drug Metabolism and Excretion	% of Normal Dose Adjustment in Renal Failure Caused by Decreased Creatinine Clearance (ml/minute)*	Effect of Hemodialysis
ANTIINFECTIVES			
Antibiotics			
Amikacin†	94%-99% renal excretion	—	Dialyzed
Ampicillin	73%-92% renal excretion 12%-24% hepatic metabolism	Creatinine clearance 10-50: 100% of normal dose every 6-12 hours Creatinine clearance <10: 50%-100% of normal dose every 12 hours	Moderately dialyzed
Clindamycin	10% renal excretion 85% hepatic metabolism (some active metabolites)	No change	Not dialyzed
Cefazolin	>95% renal excretion	Creatinine clearance 10-50: 50%-100% of normal dose every 12 hours Creatinine clearance <10: 50% of normal dose every 24 hours	Moderately dialyzed
Cefotaxime	40%-65% renal excretion 40%-60% hepatic metabolism (active metabolite has 25% activity of parent)	Creatinine clearance 10-50: 50%-100% of normal dose every 8-12 hours Creatinine clearance <10: 50% of normal dose every 8-12 hours	Moderately dialyzed
Ceftriaxone	40%-67% renal excretion 40% hepatic metabolism	Creatinine clearance 10-50: no change Creatinine clearance <10: decrease dose only with hepatic failure	Questionably dialyzed
Cefoxitin	78%-99% renal excretion	Creatinine clearance 10-50: 50%-100% of normal dose every 12-24 hours Creatinine clearance <10: 25% of normal dose every 24 hours	Moderately dialyzed
Ceftazidime	>85% renal excretion	Creatinine clearance 10-50: 50% of normal dose every 6-8 hours Creatinine clearance <10: 25% of normal dose every 12-24 hours	Dialyzed
Ciprofloxacin	62% renal excretion 38% hepatic metabolism	Creatinine clearance 10-50: 75% of normal dose every 12 hours Creatinine clearance < 10: 50%-75% of normal dose every 24 hours	Slightly dialyzed

Modified from Bubp JL, Rodondi LC, Gamberloglio JG: Renal dialysis. In Koda-Kimble MA, Young LY, editors: *Applied therapeutics: the clinical use of drugs,* ed 5, Vancouver, Wash, 1992, Applied Therapeutics; and Aweeka FT: Drug dosing in renal failure. In Koda-Kimble MA, Young LY: *Applied therapeutics: the clinical use of drugs,* ed 5, Vancouver, Wash, 1992, Applied Therapeutics.

*The degree of renal failure is assessed by the creatinine clearance. Normal creatinine clearance is 120 ml/minute; it decreases in renal failure. In renal failure, drug dosages are reduced either by decreasing the amount of drug administered each dose, lengthening the time between doses, or both.

†Aminoglycosides (amikacin, gentamycin, and tobramycin): these drugs have a narrow therapeutic window, which means that the range between the therapeutic level and the toxic level is small, and they require close monitoring. In addition, drug clearance is affected by multiple factors. Refer to a pharmacist or pharmacokinetic text for recommendations.

TABLE 33-9 Impact of Renal Failure and Hemodialysis on Selected Drugs Used in Critical Care—cont'd

Drug	Normal Drug Metabolism and Excretion	% of Normal Dose Adjustment in Renal Failure Caused by Decreased Creatinine Clearance (ml/minute)*	Effect of Hemodialysis
ANTIINFECTIVES—cont'd			
Antibiotics			
Cefotetan	50%-89% renal excretion 12% hepatic metabolism	Creatinine clearance 10-50: 50%-100% of normal dose every 12-24 hours Creatinine clearance <10: 25%-50% of normal dose every 24 hours	Moderately dialyzed
Erythromycin	5%-15% renal excretion 85%-95% hepatic metabolism	No change	Slightly dialyzed
Gentamycin†	90%-97% renal excretion		Dialyzed
Imipenem	60%-75% renal excretion 22% hepatic metabolism	Creatinine clearance 10-50: 50%-75% of normal dose every 8-12 hours Creatinine clearance <10: 25%-50% of normal dose every 12 hours	Moderately dialyzed
Mezlocillin	45%-65% renal excretion 35%-55% hepatic metabolism	Creatinine clearance 10-50: 100% of normal dose every 6-8 hours Creatinine clearance <10: 50% of normal dose every 8 hours	Slightly dialyzed
Nafcillin	25%-30% renal excretion Up to 70% hepatic metabolism	No change	Not dialyzed
Penicillin‡	50% renal excretion 19% hepatic metabolism		Moderately dialyzed
Piperacillin	50%-60% renal excretion Up to 30%-40% hepatic metabolism	Creatinine clearance 10-50: 100% of normal dose every 6-8 hours Creatinine clearance <10: 50%-75% of normal dose every 8 hours	Moderately dialyzed
Sulfamethoxazole	10% renal excretion 65%-80% hepatic metabolism	Creatinine clearance 10-50: 100% of normal dose every 12-24 hours Creatinine clearance < 10: 100% of normal dose every 24 hours	Slightly dialyzed
Tobramycin†	90%-97% renal excretion		Dialyzed
Trimethoprim	20%-35% renal excretion 53%-80% hepatic metabolism	Creatinine clearance 10-50: 100% of normal dose every 12-24 hours Creatinine clearance < 10: 100% of normal dose every 24 hours	Slightly dialyzed
Vancomycin	80%-90% renal excretion 10%-20% hepatic metabolism	Requires individualized dosing regimens	Not dialyzed

‡Penicillin G: methods have been developed to calculate dosage based on changes in creatinine clearance. However, none of these methods have been subjected to careful clinical trials. Other factors can also affect patients' responses to therapy. Refer to a pharmacist or pharmacokinetic text for recommendations.

Continued

TABLE 33-9 Impact of Renal Failure and Hemodialysis on Selected Drugs Used in Critical Care—cont'd

Drug	Normal Drug Metabolism and Excretion	% of Normal Dose Adjustment in Renal Failure Caused by Decreased Creatinine Clearance (ml/minute)*	Effect of Hemodialysis
ANTIINFECTIVES—cont'd			
Antifungal			
Amphotericin B	3%-5% renal excretion 95%-97% hepatic metabolism	Creatinine clearance 10-50: 100% of normal dose every 24 hours Creatinine clearance <10: 100% of normal dose every 24-48 hours	Not dialyzed
Fluconazole	70% renal excretion Some hepatic metabolism	Creatinine clearance 10-50: 50% of normal dose every 24 hours Creatinine clearance <10: 25% of normal dose every 24 hours	Moderately dialyzed
Ketoconazole	3% renal excretion 51% hepatic metabolism	No change	Not dialyzed
Antiviral			
Acyclovir	70-80% renal excretion 14% hepatic metabolism	Creatinine clearance 10-50: 100% of normal dose every 12-24 hours Creatinine clearance <10: 50% of normal dose every 24 hours	Dialyzed
Gancyclovir	>90% renal excretion	Creatinine clearance 10-50: 1.25-2.5 mg/kg every 24 hours Creatinine clearance <10: 1.25 mg/kg every 24 hours	Dialyzed
CARDIOVASCULAR DRUGS			
Beta blockers			
Atenolol	75% renal excretion 10% hepatic metabolism	Creatinine clearance <50: 50% dose reduction and titrate as needed	Moderately dialyzed
Labetalol	5% renal excretion 95% hepatic excretion	No change	Not dialyzed
Metoprolol	10% renal excretion 90% hepatic metabolism	No change	Metabolites dialyzed
Nadolol	75% renal excretion 25% hepatic metabolism	Creatinine clearance <50: 50% dose reduction and titrate as needed	Moderately dialyzed
Propranolol	<1% renal excretion Primarily hepatic metabolism	No change	Not dialyzed
ACE inhibitors			
Captopril	36%-42% renal excretion 50% hepatic metabolism	Creatinine clearance 10-50: No change Creatinine clearance < 10: 25% dose reduction and titrate as needed	Moderately dialyzed
Enalapril	61% renal excretion 33% hepatic metabolism	Creatinine clearance < 50: 50% dose reduction and titrate as needed	Moderately dialyzed
Calcium channel blockers			
Nifedipine	100% hepatic metabolism	No change	Not known
Verapamil	100% hepatic metabolism	No change	Not dialyzed

TABLE 33-9 Impact of Renal Failure and Hemodialysis on Selected Drugs Used in Critical Care—cont'd

Drug	Normal Drug Metabolism and Excretion	% of Normal Dose Adjustment in Renal Failure Caused by Decreased Creatinine Clearance (ml/minute)*	Effect of Hemodialysis
CARDIOVASCULAR DRUGS—cont'd			
Antidysrhythmics			
Digoxin	70% renal excretion	Creatinine clearance 10-50: 50% dose reduction and titrate as needed Creatinine clearance <10: 75% dose reduction and titrate as needed	Moderately dialyzed
Lidocaine	100% hepatic metabolism	No change	Not dialyzed
Procainamide	50%-60% renal excretion Hepatic metabolism to active NAPA metabolite	Creatinine clearance 10-50: 100% of normal dose every 6-12 hours Creatinine clearance <10: 100% of normal dose every 12-24 hours	Moderately dialyzed
ANALGESICS			
Codeine	Hepatic metabolism	Creatinine clearance 10-50: 25% of normal dose and titrate as needed Creatinine clearance <10: 50% of normal dose and titrate as needed	Not known
Ibuprofen	45%-60% excreted unchanged and as metabolites	No change	Not dialyzed
Meperidine	10% renal excretion Hepatic metabolism	Creatinine clearance 10-50: 75%-100% of normal dose every 6 hours Creatinine clearance <10: 50% of normal dose every 6-8 hours and use with caution	Not known
ANTICONVULSANTS/SEDATIVES			
Anticonvulsants			
Phenobarbital	10%-40% renal excretion Hepatic metabolism	Creatinine clearance 10-50: No change Creatinine clearance <10: Slight dosage decrease	Moderately dialyzed
Phenytoin	Hepatic metabolism	No change	Not dialyzed
Sedatives			
Diazepam	Renal excretion of active metabolites	Reduction of dose and titration as needed	Not dialyzed
	Hepatic metabolism	Not known	Not dialyzed
Midazolam	Not known		
H_2 BLOCKERS			
Cimetidine	40%-80% renal excretion	Creatinine clearance 10-50: 25% dose reduction Creatinine clearance <10: 50% dose reduction	Slightly dialyzed
Famotidine	Significant renal excretion Small hepatic metabolism	Creatinine clearance <10: 100% of normal dose every 24-48 hours	
Ranitidine	70% renal excretion	Creatinine clearance 10-50: 25% dose reduction	Slightly dialyzed

NAPA, N-acetylprocainamide.

REFERENCES

1. Douglas S: Acute tubular necrosis: diagnosis, treatment and nursing implications, *AACN Clin Issues Crit Care Nurs* 3(3): 688, 1992.
2. Kjellstrand C, Barsoum R: Management of acute renal failure. In Jacobson H, Sinker G, Klohr S, (editors: *The principles and practice of nephrology,* ed 2, St Louis, 1995, Mosby.
3. Baer C, Lancaster LE: Acute renal failure, *Crit Care Nurs Q* 14(4):1, 1992.
4. Lancaster LE: Renal response to shock, *Crit Care Nurs Clin North Am* 2(2):221, 1990.
5. Jochimsen F and others: Impairment of renal function in medical intensive care: predictability of acute renal failure, *Crit Care Med* 18(5):480, 1990.
6. *St. Anthony's DRG guidebook 1996,* Reston, Va, 1996, St Anthony.
7. Brady H, Singer G: Acute renal failure, *Lancet* 346:1533, 1995.
8. Cheney P: Early management and physiologic changes in crush syndrome, *Crit Care Nurs Q* 17(2):62, 1994.
9. Toto K: Acute renal failure: a question of location, *Am J Nurs* 92(11):44, 1992.
10. Tisher C, Wilcox C, editors: *Nephrology for the house officer,* ed 2, Baltimore, 1993, Williams & Wilkins.
11. Stark JL: Acute tubular necrosis: differences between oliguria and nonoliguria, *Crit Care Nurs Q* 14(4):22, 1992.
12. Bonaventure J: Mechanisms of ischemic acute renal failure, *Kidney Int* 43:1160, 1993.
13. Innerarity SA: Electrolyte emergency in critically ill renal patient, *Crit Care Nurs Clin North Am* 2(1):89, 1990.
14. Brundage D, editor: Renal disorders, St Louis, 1995, Mosby.
15. Innerarity SA: Hyperkalemic emergency, *Crit Care Nurs Q* 14(4):32, 1992.
16. Braxmeyer DL, Keyes JL: The pathophysiology of potassium balance, *Crit Care Nurs* 16(5):59, 1995.
17. Cluitman FH: Management of severe hypernatremia: rapid or slow corrections, *Am J Med* 88:161, 1990.
18. Price CA: Continuous renal replacement therapy: the treatment of choice for acute renal failure, *ANNA J* 18(3):239, 1992.
19. Pechman P: Acute hemodialysis: issues in critical illness, *AACN Clin Issues Crit Care Nurs* 3(3):545, 1992.
20. Gutch C, Stoner M, Corea A: *Review of hemodialysis for nurses and dialysis personnel,* ed 5, St Louis, 1993, Mosby.
21. Bosworth C: SCUF/CAVH/CAVHD. Critical differences, *Crit Care Nurs Q* 14(4):45-55, 1992.
22. Price CA: An update on continuous renal replacement therapies, *AACN Clin Issues Crit Care Nurs* 3(3):597, 1992.
23. Forni LG, Hilton PJ: Continuous hemofiltration in the treatment of acute renal failure, *N Engl J Med* 336(18): 1303-1309, 1997.
24. Higley RR: Continuous arteriovenous hemofiltration; a case study, *Crit Care Nurs* 16(5):37, 1996.
25. Bressolle F, Kinowski J: Clinical pharmacokinetics during continuous hemofiltration, *Clin Pharmacokinet* 26(6):457, 1994.
26. Smith LJ: Peritoneal dialysis in the critically ill, *AACN Clin Issues Crit Care Nurs* 3(3):558, 1992.
27. Graham-Macaluso M: Complications of peritoneal dialysis: nursing care plans to document teaching, *ANNA J* 18(5):479, 1991.
28. Yelton SL, Gaylor MA, Murray KM: The role of continuous infusion loop diuretics, *Ann Pharmocother* 29(10):1010-1014, 1995.
29. Martin S, Danzinger L: Continuous infusion of loop diuretics in the critically ill: a review of the literature, *Crit Care Med* 22(8):1323, 1994.

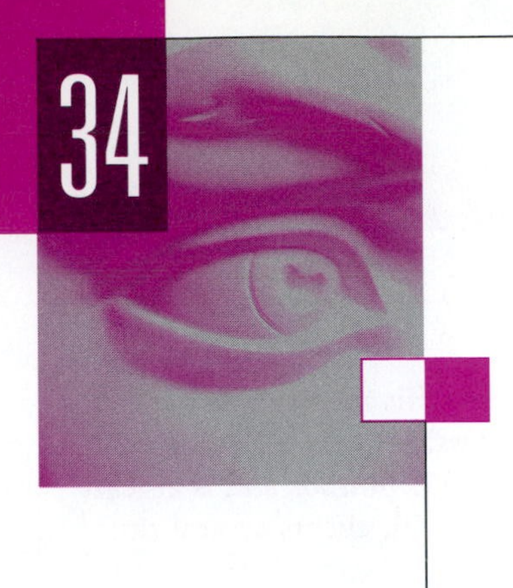

Renal Nursing Diagnosis and Management

THIS CHAPTER IS designed to supplement the preceding chapters in the *Renal Alterations* unit by integrating theoretic content into clinically applicable case studies and nursing management plans.

The case study is designed to illustrate clinical problem solving and patient care management occurring in actual patients. The case, reviewed retrospectively, demonstrates how medical and nursing diagnoses may be effectively used in critical care. The case study also demonstrates revisions to the plan of care and the nursing and medical management outcomes that are apt to occur during the course of a complicated hospitalization as the patient responds physiologically to treatment. Often in a short case anecdote, such as that presented in this chapter, the clinical answer may appear to be obvious from the day of admission. In practice, however, critical care patient management is sometimes investigative and the "correct" diagnosis for an individual patient may not become apparent until midway in the hospitalization. Or a patient with an apparently straightforward diagnosis may develop an unexpected complication, and the plan of care and potential outcomes will then require revision. Many of the case studies demonstrate this principle.

The nursing management plans, which—unlike the case study—are not patient-specific, provide a basis nurses can use to individualize care for their patients. In the previous *Renal Alterations* chapters, each medical diagnosis is assigned a Nursing Diagnosis and Management box. Using this box as a page guide, the reader can access relevant nursing management plans for each medical diagnosis. For example, nursing management of *acute renal failure,* described on pp. 877, may involve several nursing diagnoses and management plans outlined in this chapter and in other Nursing Diagnosis and Management chapters. Specific examples are (1) *Risk for Fluid Volume Excess risk factors: renal dysfunction,* on p. 915; (2) *Anxiety related to threat to biologic, physiologic, and/or social integrity,* on p. 99; (3) *Risk for Infection risk factors: invasive monitoring devices,* on p. 598; and (4) *Ineffective Individual Coping related to situational crisis and personal vulnerability,* on p. 95. These examples highlight the interrelationship of the various physiologic systems in the body and the fact that pathology often has a multisystem impact in the critically ill.

Use of the case study and management plans can enhance the understanding and application of the *Renal* content in clinical practice.

CASE STUDY

RENAL

CLINICAL HISTORY

JT is a 55-year-old white man who was diagnosed with severe hypertension 3½ years ago. His medication regimen includes at least two potent antihypertensive drugs, as well as furosemide (Lasix) and a potassium supplement. He admits to frequent omissions of his medications because of a hectic work schedule. He weighs 235 pounds and is at least 40 pounds overweight. JT smokes at least one pack of cigarettes per day and drinks socially with clients several times each week.

CURRENT PROBLEMS

After a stressful day at work and several hundred miles of travel, JT arrived at his hotel room for the night. While sitting on the bed to remove his shoes, he experienced a sudden, intense midabdominal to lower abdominal pain. He began to feel faint and nauseated but was able to summon help. Paramedics arrived to find JT alert, ashen, and dyspneic. He complained of accelerating midabdominal pain radiating to his thoracic spine. Paramedics noted the following: blood pressure (BP), 88/40 mm Hg; pulse (P), 126; respiratory rate (RR), 32 (despite receiving 6 L O_2); and tense, distended abdomen without bowel sounds.

EMERGENCY MEDICAL MANAGEMENT

En route to the hospital, JT's systolic BP fell to 74 mm Hg despite rapid IV infusion of lactated Ringer's solution. When the patient arrived at the hospital, an arterial line was placed, oxygen was continued, and a dopamine drip was initiated for blood pressure support at 90/50 mm Hg. Before dopamine initiation, JT's blood pressure was unstable for 45 minutes. A diagnosis of ruptured abdominal aortic aneurysm was made and immediate surgery was scheduled. Before surgery, JT received 1200 ml of intravenous (IV) fluids.

MEDICAL DIAGNOSES

Ruptured abdominal aortic aneurysm
Class III hemorrhagic shock

NURSING DIAGNOSES

Fluid Volume Deficit related to absolute loss: blood
Acute Pain related to transmission and perception of visceral and ischemic impulses
Anxiety related to threat to biologic, psychologic, and/or social integrity
Knowledge Deficit: Impending Surgery and Risks related to lack of previous exposure to information

PLAN OF CARE

Surgery was scheduled to repair abdominal aortic aneurysm with synthetic graft.

MEDICAL AND NURSING MANAGEMENT AND PATIENT OUTCOME

During surgery, JT experienced active blood loss of approximately 9 L, which was replaced with lactated Ringer's (LR), Plasmanate, and whole blood. He returned to the critical care unit (CCU) in stable condition with the following assessment:

Neuro: Lethargic but responsive. Moves all extremities. Hand grasps equal but weak bilaterally, as are pedal pushes. Pupils equal and react to light and accommodation (PEARLA).

Resp: Rhythmic respirations at 26/min. Decreased excursion and diminished breath sounds throughout lung bases. O_2 continues per mask at 4 L/min. PaO_2, 90 mm Hg; $PaCO_2$, 40 mm Hg; pH, 7.40; O_2 saturation, 96%.

CV: BP, 118/60 mm Hg; P, 98; mean arterial pressure (MAP), 80 mm Hg; right atrial pressure (RAP), 4 mm Hg; cardiac output (CO), 6 L/min; pulmonary artery wedge pressure (PAWP), 8 mm Hg; systemic vascular resistance (SVR), 1014 dynes/sec/cm^{-5}. Regular heart rate with no extra sounds. Peripheral pulses are 1+.

GI Integument/Temperature: Skin cool and mottled over extremities, but upper body warm and dry. Nasogastric (NG) tube in right naris draining pink-tinged fluid. Abdomen soft and nondistended. Bowel sounds absent. Bulky dressing at midabdomen is clean, dry, intact.

GU: Urinary catheter in place draining clear, dark amber urine. Approximately 500 ml urine in bag.

Laboratory: Hct, 28%; Hgb, 8.4 g/dL; Na^+, 136 mEq/L; K^+, 3.8 mEq/L; Cl^-, 108 mEq/L.

CASE STUDY—CONT'D

RENAL

MEDICAL DIAGNOSES

Status post abdominal aortic aneurysm repair
Anemia

NURSING DIAGNOSES

Hypothermia related to cold environment (operating room [OR], trauma [ruptured aortic aneurysm])
Fluid Volume Deficit related to absolute loss: blood
Acute Pain related to transmission and perception of cutaneous, visceral, or muscular impulses
Anxiety related to threat to biologic, psychologic, and/or social integrity

REVISED PLAN OF CARE

1. Increase body temperature through the use of blankets.
2. Replace fluid through infusion of IV fluids as ordered.
3. Reposition patient frequently, and instruct and encourage use of the incentive spirometer. Have patient perform passive and semiactive range of motion (ROM).
4. Accurately measure and record intake and output (I&O). Weigh patient daily. Monitor hemodynamic parameters hourly.
5. Explain surgery, CCU routine, and other care procedures. Encourage patient and family to ask questions.
6. Administer analgesics per physician order. Assess pain level every 2 to 3 hours. Assess response to all analgesics.

MEDICAL AND NURSING MANAGEMENT AND PATIENT OUTCOME

On the third postoperative day JT was transferred to the medical/surgical unit. On day 4 he began to experience decreased renal output to 50 ml/hr. Output continued to drop to 30 ml/hr. By day 5 his weight had increased 5½ pounds. 3+ edema was present in both lower extremities. JT complained of mild dyspnea and nausea. Despite furosemide (Lasix) administration, his renal output had not increased.

Laboratory values were as follows: K^+, 5.4 mEq/L; Na^+, 138 mEq/L; Cl^-, 110 mEq/L; creatinine, 7.0 mg/dL; blood urea nitrogen (BUN), 73 mg/dL. Cardiac ECG shows peaked T waves. Sodium polystyrene sulfonate (Kayexalate) was administered, and a subclavian catheter was placed to initiate hemodialysis.

MEDICAL DIAGNOSES

Status post abdominal aortic aneurysm repair
Acute renal failure
Electrolyte imbalances
Anemia
Fluid overload

NURSING DIAGNOSES

Altered Renal Tissue Perfusion related to decreased renal blood flow
Fluid Volume Excess related to renal dysfunction
Acute Pain related to transmission and perception of cutaneous, visceral, and muscular impulses
Altered Nutrition: Less than Body Requirements related to lack of exogenous nutrients
Knowledge Deficit: Dialysis Initiation, Prognosis for Recovery, and Return to Previous Life-style related to lack of previous exposure to information

REVISED PLAN OF CARE

1. Limit oral fluids to 1500 ml/24 hrs. Accurately measure and record I&O. Weigh patient before and after dialysis.
2. Assess for edema and changes in abdominal girth and circumferences of lower extremities.
3. Observe strict asepsis and monitor for clinical manifestations of infection.
4. Refer patient and family to nutritionist for instruction in fluid restriction and renal diet.
5. Structure treatment regimen to provide increased rest periods for patient.
6. Administer analgesics for pain relief, and instruct patient in use of adjunctive relief techniques (distraction, guided imagery, deep breathing, massage).
7. Educate patient regarding basic principles of dialysis treatment and self-care.

Continued

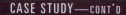

CASE STUDY—CONT'D

RENAL

MEDICAL AND NURSING MANAGEMENT AND PATIENT OUTCOME

During the following 12 days, JT received 7 hemodialysis treatments. On the thirteenth postoperative day, he experienced a sudden, dramatic return of urinary output to 125 ml/hr by day's end. On day 18, JT was discharged to home with the following laboratory values: creatinine, 2.2 mg/dL; BUN, 36 mg/dL; Na^+, 140 mEq/L; K^+, 4.0 mEq/L. JT and his family received discharge teaching regarding nutritional intake, infection prevention, exercise, and relationship of life-style and adherence to medical regimen to subsequent health events.

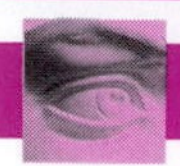

NURSING MANAGEMENT PLAN

FLUID VOLUME DEFICIT

DEFINITION

The state in which an individual experiences vascular, cellular, or intracellular dehydration.

Fluid Volume Deficit Related to Absolute Loss

DEFINING CHARACTERISTICS

- Cardiac output (CO) <4 L/min
- Cardiac index (CI) <2.2 L/min
- Pulmonary artery wedge pressure (PAWP), pulmonary artery diastolic pressure (PAD) less than normal or less than baseline, central venous pressure (CVP) less than normal or less than baseline (PAWP <6 mm Hg)
- Tachycardia
- Narrowed pulse pressure
- Systolic blood pressure (BP) <100 mm Hg
- Urinary output <30 ml/hour
- Pale, cool, moist skin
- Apprehensiveness

OUTCOME CRITERIA

- Patient's CO is >4 L/min and CI is >2.2 L/min.
- Patient's PAWP, PAD, and CVP are normal or back to baseline level.
- Patient's pulse is normal or back to baseline.
- Patient's systolic blood pressure is >90.
- Patient's urinary output is >30 ml/hour.

NURSING INTERVENTIONS AND *RATIONALE*

1. Continue to monitor the assessment parameters listed under "Defining Characteristics." In addition, a serum lactate level > 2 mOsm/L is believed to represent cellular perfusion failure at its earliest stage.
2. Secure airway and administer high-flow oxygen.
3. Place patient in supine position with legs elevated ***to increase preload.*** Consider using low-Fowler's position with legs elevated for patient with head injury.
4. For fluid repletion use the 3:1 rule, replacing three parts of fluid for every unit of blood lost.
5. Administer crystalloid solutions using the fluid challenge technique: infuse precise aliquots of fluid (usually 5 to 20 ml/min) over 10-minute periods; monitor cardiac loading pressures serially ***to determine successful challenging.*** If the PAWP or PAD elevates more than 7 mm Hg above beginning level, the infusion should be stopped. If the PAWP or PAD rises only to 3 mm Hg above baseline or falls, another fluid challenge should be administered.
6. Replete fluids first before considering use of vasopressors, ***since vasopressors increase myocardial oxygen consumption out of proportion to the reestablishment of coronary perfusion in the early phases of treatment.***
7. When blood is available or its need is indicated, replace it with fresh packed red cells and fresh frozen plasma ***to keep clotting factors intact.***
8. Move or reposition patient minimally ***to decrease or limit tissue oxygen demands.***
9. Evaluate patient's anxiety level and intervene through patient education or sedation ***to decrease tissue oxygen demands.***
10. Be alert for the possibility of acute respiratory distress syndrome (ARDS) development in the ensuing 72 hours.

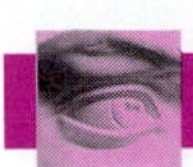

NURSING MANAGEMENT PLAN

Fluid Volume Deficit Related to Relative Loss

DEFINING CHARACTERISTICS

- Pulmonary artery wedge pressure (PAWP), pulmonary artery diastolic pressure (PAD), central venous pressure (CVP) less than normal or less than baseline
- Tachycardia
- Narrowed pulse pressure
- Systolic blood pressure (BP) <100 mm Hg
- Urinary output <30 ml/hour
- Increased hematocrit level

OUTCOME CRITERIA

- The patient's PAWP, PAD, and CVP are normal or back to baseline.
- Systolic BP is >90 mm Hg.
- Urinary output is >30 ml/hour.
- The patient's hematocrit level is normal.

NURSING INTERVENTIONS AND *RATIONALE*

1. Continue to monitor the assessment parameters listed under "Defining Characteristics." In addition, inspect soft tissues ***to determine the presence of edema.***
2. With physician's collaboration, administer intravenous (IV) fluid replacements (usually normal saline solution or lactated Ringer's solution) at a rate sufficient ***to maintain urinary output >30 ml/hour.*** Colloid solutions are avoided in the initial phases (but can be used later) because of the possibility of increased edema formation ***as a result of the increased capillary permeability.***

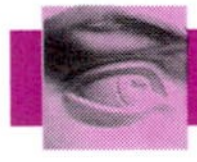

NURSING MANAGEMENT PLAN

FLUID VOLUME EXCESS

DEFINITION

The state in which an individual experiences increased fluid retention and edema.

Fluid Volume Excess Related to Renal Dysfunction

DEFINING CHARACTERISTICS

- Weight gain that occurs during a 24- to 48-hour period
- Dependent pitting edema
- Ascites in severe cases
- Fluid crackles on lung auscultation
- Exertional dyspnea
- Oliguria or anuria
- Hypertension
- Engorged neck veins
- Decrease in urinary osmolality as renal failure progresses
- Central venous pressure (CVP) >15 cm of H_2O
- Pulmonary artery wedge pressure (PAWP) 20-25 mm Hg

OUTCOME CRITERIA

- Weight returns to baseline.
- Edema or ascites is absent or reduced to baseline.
- Lungs are clear to auscultation.
- Exertional dyspnea is absent.
- Blood pressure returns to baseline.
- Heart rate returns to baseline.
- Neck veins are flat.
- Mucous membranes are moist.

NURSING INTERVENTIONS AND *RATIONALE*

1. Continue to monitor the assessment parameters listed under "Defining Characteristics."
2. Promote skin integrity of edematous areas by frequent repositioning and elevation of areas where possible. Avoid massaging pressure points or reddened areas of skin ***because this results in further tissue trauma.***
3. Plan patient care to provide rest periods ***to not heighten exertional dyspnea.***
4. Weigh patient daily at same time in same clothing, preferably with the same scale.
5. Instruct the patient about the correlation between fluid intake and weight gain, using commonly understood fluid measurements such as ingesting 4 cups (1000 ml) of fluid results in an approximate 2-pound weight gain in the anuric patient.

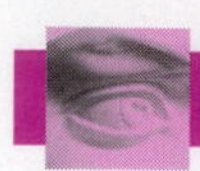

NURSING MANAGEMENT PLAN

ALTERED RENAL TISSUE PERFUSION

DEFINITION

The state in which an individual experiences altered renal blood flow.

Altered Renal Tissue Perfusion Related to Decreased Renal Blood Flow

DEFINING CHARACTERISTICS

Initial Stages

- Decreased mean arterial pressure (MAP) <60 mm Hg
- Low cardiac output (CO) 4.0 L/min
- Low cardiac index (CI) 2.2 L/min/m^2
- Decreased urinary output

Later Stages

- Anuria or oliguria
- Decreased urinary creatinine clearance
- Increased serum creatinine
- Increased blood urea nitrogen (BUN)
- Electrolyte abnormalities: ↑ K^+, ↓ Na^+
- Increased MAP, pulmonary artery wedge pressure (PAWP), pulmonary artery diastolic (PAD) pressure, central venous pressure (CVP) secondary to fluid overload
- Sinus tachycardia
- Metabolic acidosis
- Crackles on lung auscultation
- Engorged neck veins
- Fluid weight gain
- Pitting edema
- Mental status changes
- Anemia

OUTCOME CRITERIA

- CO is >4.0 L/min.
- CI is >2.2 L/min/m^2.
- MAP, PAWP, PAD, CVP are within normal limits for patient.
- Electrolytes are within normal range.
- Serum creatinine and BUN are within normal range.
- Normal acid-base imbalance.
- Normal level of consciousness.
- Lungs are clear on auscultation.
- Urinary output to normal limits or patient stable on dialysis.
- Hemoglobin and hematocrit values are stable.

NURSING INTERVENTIONS AND RATIONALE

Initial Stages

1. Increase MAP 70 mm Hg to restore renal perfusion pressure.
2. Increase CO > 4.0 L/min to increase renal blood flow.
3. Increase CI > 2.5 L/min to increase renal blood flow.

Later Stages

1. Monitor hourly urinary output.
2. Administer prescribed diuretics.
3. Measure daily weight.
4. Restrict fluids as appropriate for urine output or dialysis/CRRT filtrate removal.
5. Assist with hemodialysis (if required by patient) to remove excess fluid.
6. Assist with hemodialysis (if required by patient) to maintain electrolyte balance.
7. Maintain oxygenation by keeping lungs clear of fluid.
8. Maintain skin integrity by frequent repositioning or air mattress bed.
9. Minimize risk of infection by sterile dialysis catheter care.
10. Orient patient to time and place.
11. Minimize blood withdrawals.
12. Monitor blood levels of drugs cleared by kidneys or dialysis.
13. Educate patient and family about renal failure, medications, and dialysis.

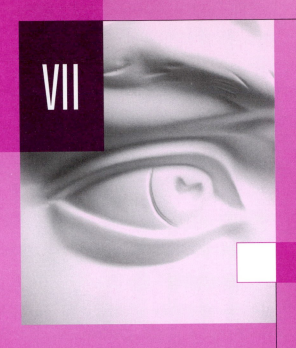

GASTROINTESTINAL ALTERATIONS

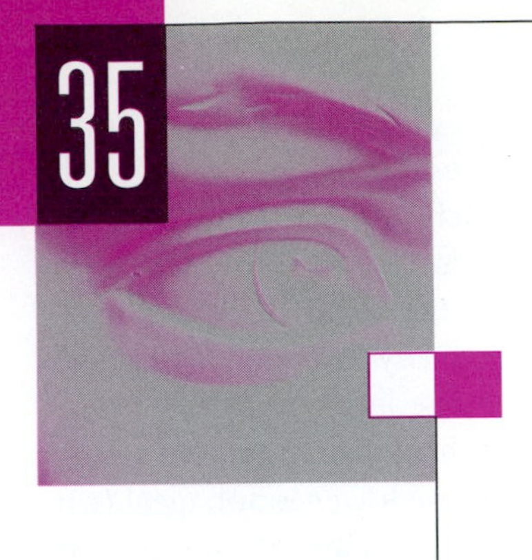

Gastrointestinal Anatomy and Physiology

THE MAJOR FUNCTION of the gastrointestinal (GI) tract is digestion—that is, to convert ingested nutrients into simpler forms that can be transported from the tract's lumen to the portal circulation and used in metabolic processes. The GI system also plays a vital role in detoxification and elimination of bacteria, viruses, chemical toxins, and drugs. Disturbances of the GI system itself or of the complex hormonal and neural controls that regulate it can severely upset homeostasis and compromise the overall nutritional status of the patient. Furthermore, any circumvention of the normal feeding mechanism can alter digestive processes or contribute to malabsorption. Thus it is vital for the critical care nurse to have an active knowledge of the normal function of the GI tract to facilitate assessment, diagnosis, and intervention in patients with GI dysfunction.

ROLE OF THE BRAIN

Feeding actually begins with the sensation of hunger—the intrinsic desire for food—which is under the control of the feeding center in the lateral nuclei of the hypothalamus. Activation of the feeding center initiates a search for food. The satiety center, which provides the sensation of satisfaction and fulfillment after a meal and inhibits the feeding center, is located in the ventromedial nuclei of the hypothalamus. The nutritional status of the body is a primary concern of the hypothalamus, which also excites the lower centers and the brainstem, in which the mechanics of feeding, such as chewing and mastication, are controlled.

GASTROINTESTINAL TRACT

The GI tract consists of the mouth, esophagus, stomach, small intestine, and large intestine (Figure 35-1).

Mouth

The mouth and accessory organs, which include the lips, cheeks, gums, tongue, palate, and salivary glands, perform the initial phases of digestion, which are ingestion, mastication, and salivation.

Ingestion and mastication. The mouth is the beginning of the alimentary canal (see Figure 35-1) and is the means for ingestion and entry of nutrients. The teeth cut, grind, and mix food, transforming it into a form suitable for swallowing and increasing the surface area of food available to salivary secretions. Healthy dentition is vital for this process. Mucous glands located behind the tip of the tongue and serous glands located at the back of the tongue aid in the lubrication of food and in its distribution over the taste buds.

Salivation. Salivation has an important role in the first stage of digestion because saliva lubricates the mouth, facilitates the movement of the lips and the tongue during swallowing, and washes away bacteria. Saliva consists of approximately 99% water and 1% mucin and amylase. It also contains a large amount of ions, such as potassium and bicarbonate, as well as protein antibodies and thiocyanate ions, which are vital in destroying oral bacteria. Approximately 1000 to 1500 ml of saliva is produced each day by three pairs of salivary glands: the submaxillary glands, the sublingual glands, and the parotid glands. Parotid gland secretions are enzymatic, containing amylase, which begins the chemical

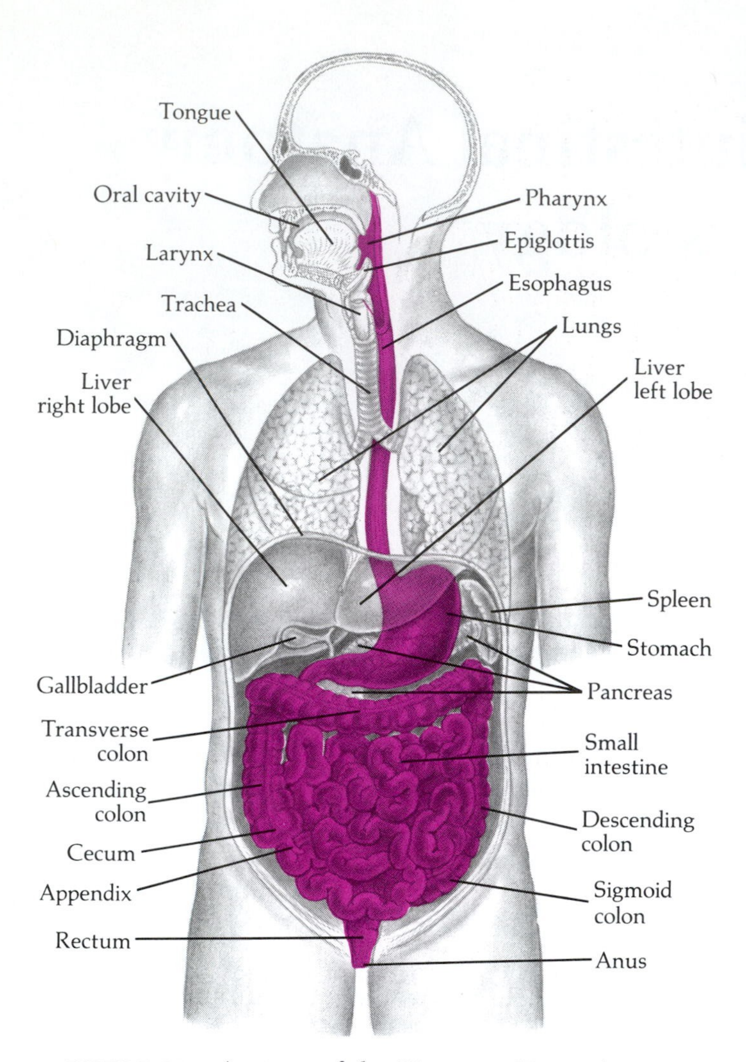

FIGURE 35-1. Anatomy of the GI system. (From Thompson JM and others: *Mosby's clinical nursing,* ed 4, St Louis, 1997, Mosby.)

breakdown of large polysaccharides into dextrins and sugars.

The mouth and pharynx are also lined with small salivary glands that provide additional lubrication. Parasympathetic stimulation results in profuse secretions of watery saliva. Sympathetic stimulation causes release of small amounts of saliva with organic constituents from the submaxillary glands. Anticholinergic drugs reduce salivary secretion and a number of GI hormones, such as secretin, cholecystokinin, vasoactive intestinal peptide, and gastric inhibitory peptide.

Esophagus

The esophagus is a collapsible tube that lacks cartilage. In adults it measures 23 to 25 cm (9 to 10 inches) long and 1 to 2 cm (to 1 inch) wide. It is the narrowest part of the digestive tube and lies posterior to the trachea and heart, with attachments at the hypopharynx and at the cardiac portion of the stomach below the diaphragm. It begins at the level of the C6 to T1 vertebrae and extends vertically through the mediastinum and diaphragm to the level of T11.

The esophagus has two sphincters: the upper esophageal (hypopharyngeal) and the lower esophageal (cardiac). The upper esophageal sphincter inhibits air from entering the esophagus during breathing. In the lower esophageal sphincter, which is located in the distal 3 to 5 cm of the esophagus, a pressure of approximately +25 mm Hg is maintained, although it may reach 15 to 20 mm Hg higher than the pressure in the fundus of the stomach. This pressure difference prevents reflux of gastric contents and erosion of the esophageal mucosa from gastric secretions.

Swallowing. The functions of the esophagus are to accept a bolus of food from the oropharynx, to transport the bolus through the esophageal body by gravity and peristalsis, and to release the bolus into the stomach through the cardiac sphincter. The esophagus also serves as an antireflex barrier and as a vent for increased gastric pressure. The esophageal phase of swallowing is a visceral response and is reflexive in nature. Peristalsis consists of waves of circular contractions and relaxations in which a bolus of food is propelled. A peristaltic wave takes 5 to 10 seconds to reach the stomach from the pharynx. Secondary peristalsis begins in the upper thoracic esophagus and is caused by distention from foods remaining in the esophagus. Body position, the acidity of the food bolus, pain, anxiety, anger, and age can affect transit time.

Stomach

The stomach is an elongated pouch approximately 25 to 30 cm (10 to 12 inches) long and 10 to 13 cm (4 to 5 inches) wide at the maximal transverse diameter. It lies obliquely beneath the cardiac sphincter at the esophagogastric junction and above the pyloric sphincter, next to the small intestine. The anatomic divisions of the stomach are the cardia (proximal end), the fundus (portion above and to the left of the cardiac sphincter), the body (middle portion), the antrum (elongated constricted portion), and the pylorus (distal end connecting the antrum to the duodenum) (Figure 35-2). The greater curvature, which begins at the cardiac orifice and arches backward and upward around the fundus, is in contact with the transverse colon and the pancreas at the posterior edge. The lesser curvature extends from the cardia to the pylorus. Two sphincters control the rate of food passage: the car-

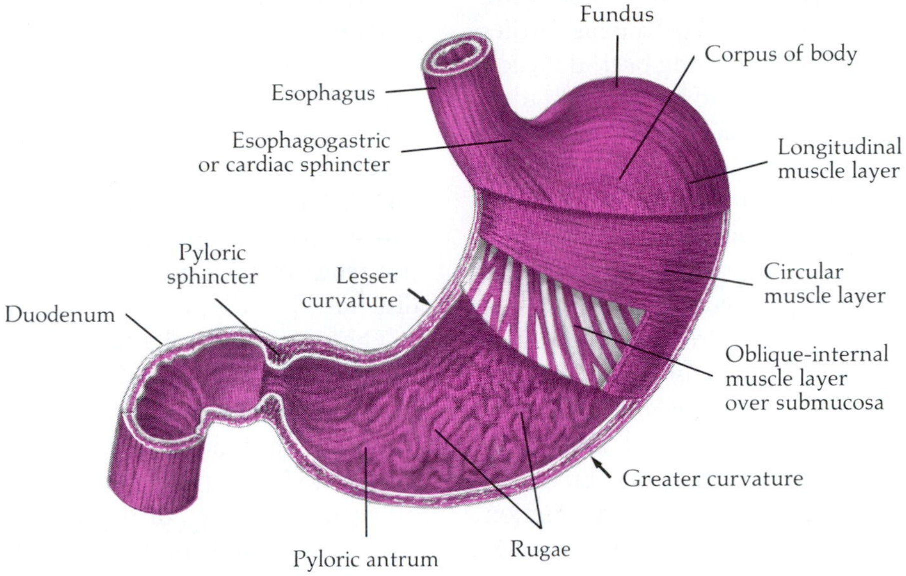

FIGURE 35-2. Gross anatomy of the stomach. (From Thompson JM and others: *Mosby's clinical nursing,* ed 4, St Louis, 1997, Mosby.)

diac at the esophagogastric junction and the pyloric at the gastroduodenal junction.

The shape and size of the stomach vary with body build, body position, contents, digestive stage, development of gastric muscles, gender, and condition of adjacent intestine. Its capacity is approximately 1 quart (1 L) of food or liquid. When distended, it may impede the descent of the diaphragm during inhalation.

The stomach wall has four layers (Figure 35-3). The outermost layer, the serous coat (tunica serosa), consists of squamous epithelial tissue and continues as a double fold from the lower edge of the stomach to cover the intestine. The second layer, the muscular coat (tunica muscularis), extends from the fundus to the antrum and consists of three smooth muscle layers, specifically, the longitudinal layer, the circular layer, and the oblique layer. The third layer, the submucous coat (tunica submucosa), consists of connective tissue that contains blood vessels, lymphatics, and nerve plexuses. The innermost layer, the mucous coat (tunica mucosa), consists of a muscular layer that is arranged in longitudinal folds, or rugae, that can expand as the stomach fills. This layer also contains 35 million glands that secrete up to 3000 ml of gastric juice per day.[1,2]

The celiac artery provides the blood supply required for the motor and secretory activity of the stomach. The splenic vein provides venous drainage for the right side of the stomach, while the gastric vein provides it for the left. Numerous lymphatic channels arise in the submucosa and terminate in the thoracic duct. The stomach is innervated by the autonomic nervous system. Sympathetic fibers arises from the celiac plexus, whereas parasympathetic fibers arise from the gastric branch of the vagus nerve.

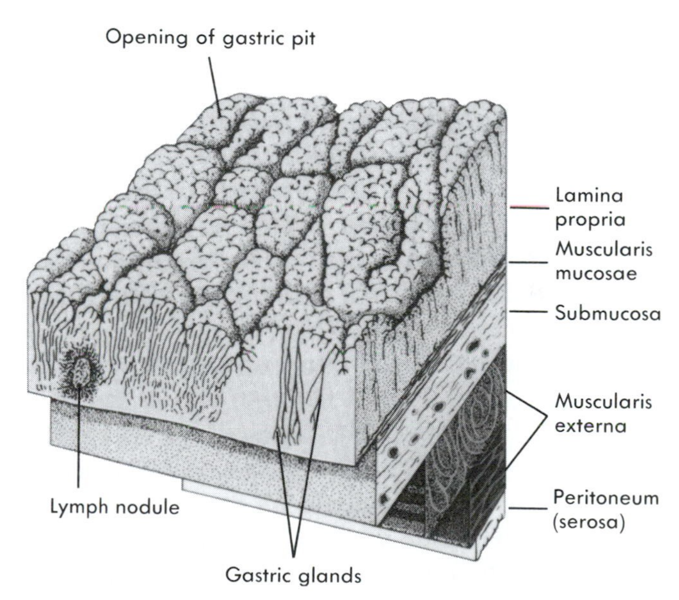

FIGURE 35-3. Structure of the gastric mucosa. (From Berne RM, Levy MN, editors: *Principles of physiology,* ed 3, St Louis, 1993, Mosby.)

The epithelial cells of the gastric mucosa are packed very close together and serve as a protective barrier, preventing diffusion of hydrogen ions into the mucosa.

The surface epithelial cells produce alkaline mucus and secrete a bicarbonate-laden fluid. The mucus further protects the gastric mucosa by delaying back-diffusion of hydrogen ions and trapping them for neutralization by the secreted bicarbonate. In addition, gastric mucosal cells can compensate for cell destruction. Epithelial cells are in a constant state of growth, migration, and desquamation and are shed at a rate of one-half million cells per minute. The gastric mucosa also has the ability to increase blood flow, providing an additional buffer for acid neutralization and aiding in the removal of toxic metabolites and chloride ions from injured mucosa. Finally, the gastric mucosal cells synthesize a family of unsaturated fatty acids known as prostaglandins. Prostaglandins facilitate mucosal bicarbonate secretion and inhibit acid secretion by preventing the activation of parietal cells by histamine (a local biochemical mediator).[3-6] Certain lipid-soluble substances can break the mucosal barrier and penetrate the cells, causing their destruction, edema, and eventual bleeding. These substances include alcohol, regurgitated bile acids, and other aliphatic acids, such as acetic, butyric, propionic, salicylic, and acetylsalicylic acids.

Gastric secretion. The stomach has approximately 35 million glands of various types that secrete 1500 to 3000 ml of gastric juice into the lumen per day, depending on the diet and other stimuli. Gastric juice is composed of hydrochloric acid (HCl), pepsinogen, which converts to pepsin (an enzyme that breaks down protein) in the presence of acid, mucus, intrinsic factor (necessary for vitamin B_{12} absorption), sodium, and potassium. Digestive hormones, which are released into the blood stream instead of into the gastric juice, are also produced by these glands (Table 35-1). The gastric glands contain parietal cells, which secrete HCl and intrinsic factor, and chief cells, which secrete pepsinogen. Gastric glands are stimulated by the parasympathetic impulses and gastrin and are inhibited by gastric-inhibitory peptide and enterogastrone. In addition, histamine and entero-oxyntin also stimulate the parietal cells to produce acid, while secretin also stimulates the chief cells to produce pepsinogen.

The pH of gastric juice is 1.0, but when mixed with food, it rises to 2.0 to 3.0. Gastric juice dissolves soluble foods and has bacteriostatic action against swallowed microorganisms. The composition of gastric secretions varies depending on several factors, including flow rate, volume, and time of day. In addition, pain, fear, or rage inhibit gastric secretion, while aggression or hostility stimulate it.[5]

Gastric motility. The functions of the stomach include relaxation for food storage, digestion, and emptying. Gastric motility is regulated by the autonomic nervous system, digestive hormones, and neural reflexes. Gastrin, motilin, and parasympathetic stimulation increase gastric motility, while secretin, cholecystokinin, enterogastrone, gastric-inhibitory peptide, and sympathetic stimulation decrease it. The ileogastric reflex inhibits gastric motility when the ileum is distended.[5]

The stomach receives food from the cardiac sphincter, stores it for a period of time, and mixes it with gastric secretions. The food is then ground into a substance of semifluid consistency called *chyme,* which is delivered via the pylorus to the duodenum. The rate of gastric emptying, or the movement of gastric contents in the duodenum, is influenced by the volume, chemical composition, acidity, osmolality, caloric density, and temperature of the chyme. Larger volumes of food increase gastric emptying, while highly acidic chyme inhibits emptying. Liquids empty before solids, and this emptying occurs faster in the sitting or right side-lying position. Hyperosmolar and hypoosmolar solutions slow gastric emptying; temperature extremes retard emptying. Greater amounts of fatty acids in the chyme also retard emptying, with unsaturated fatty acids affecting the rate more than saturated fatty acids.

Small Intestine

The small intestine, a coiled, folded tube approximately 7 m (22 to 23 feet) long, extends from the pyloric sphincter to the cecum and fills most of the abdominal cavity. It has three anatomic divisions: duodenum, jejunum, and ileum. The duodenum, shaped like the letter C, begins at the pyloric sphincter of the stomach. It is 25 cm (10 inches) long and 4 cm (1 to 1.5 inches) wide. The jejunum, which is 250 cm (8 to 9 feet) long and 4 cm (1 to 1 inches) wide, lies in the left iliac and umbilical regions. The ileum, which is 375 cm (12 feet) long and 2.5 cm (1 inch) wide, lies in the hypogastric, right iliac, and pelvic regions. Although the demarcating line between the jejunum and the ileum is somewhat arbitrary, the ileum is narrower than the jejunum. The ileocecal valve, located at the terminal end of the ileum at the junction of the cecum and colon, controls the flow of small bowel contents into the large intestine and prevents reflux (Figure 35-4).

The small intestine has four layers (Figure 35-5). The outermost layer, the serous coat (tunica serosa), is a continuation of the serous coat surrounding the

TABLE 35-1 Digestive Hormones

Source	Hormone	Stimulus for Secretion	Action
Mucosa of the stomach	Gastrin	Presence of partially digested proteins in the stomach	Stimulates gastric glands to secrete HCl and pepsinogen
Mucosa of the small intestine	Motilin	Presence of acid and fat in the duodenum	Increases GI motility
	Secretin	Presence of chyme (acid, partially digested proteins, and fats) in the duodenum	Stimulates pancreas to secrete alkaline pancreatic juice and liver to secrete bile; decreases GI motility
	Cholecystokinin	Same as for secretin	Stimulates gallbladder to eject bile and pancreas to secrete alkaline fluid; decreases gastric motility
	Enterogastrone	Presence of fat in the duodenum	Inhibits gastric secretion and motility
	Entero-oxyntin	Presence of chyme in the small intestine	Stimulates gastric glands to secrete HCl
	Gastric-inhibitory peptide	Stretching of the duodenum and fatty acids	Decreases gastric motility and secretion of pepsin and HCl

From Huether SE: Structure and function of the digestive system. In McCance KL, Huether SE, editors: *Pathophysiology: the biologic basis for disease in adults and children,* ed 2, St Louis, 1994, Mosby.

stomach. The second layer, the muscular coat (tunica muscularis), consists of two smooth muscle layers, which are the longitudinal and circular layers. The third layer, the submucous coat (tunica submucosa), consists of connective tissue and contains blood vessels, lymphatics, glands, and nerve plexuses. The innermost layer, the mucous coat (tunica mucosa), is arranged in visible circular folds, which are largest and most numerous in the distal duodenum and proximal jejunum and disappear in the lower ileum. These folds are covered by a second series of projectile-like folds called villi that are in constant motion—constricting, lengthening, and shortening (villous movement). The four to five million villi (see Figure 35-4) give the intestine a velvety appearance and are more numerous and larger in the jejunum than in the ileum. Villi contain a network of capillaries and blind lymphatic vessels called *lacteals.* The outer layer of the villus is composed of microvilli. The circular folds of the small intestine, along with the villi and microvilli, increase the digestive-absorptive surface of the small intestine 600 times.

The gastroduodenal artery provides the blood supply for the duodenum, while branches of the superior mesenteric artery provide for the jejunum and ileum. The superior mesenteric vein provides for venous drainage of the small intestine. Numerous lymphatic channels arise in the submucosa and terminate in the thoracic duct. The small intestine is extrinsically innervated by the autonomic nervous system. Sympathetic fibers arise from the celiac plexus, while parasympathetic fibers arise from the gastric branch of the vagus nerve. Intrinsic innervation, which initiates motor functions, is provided by two plexuses (Auerbach's and Meissner's) located in the intestinal wall.

Intestinal secretion. The small intestine has two major types of glands: Brunner's glands and intestinal glands. Brunner's glands lie in the mucosa of the duodenum and secrete mucus, an alkaline fluid (pH of 9) that neutralizes chyme and protects the mucosa. Intestinal glands are found in pits of the submucosa and are called the *crypts of Lieberkühn.* These crypts secrete 2 to 3 L/day of yellow fluid containing enzymes that assist in nutrient digestion.

Intestinal motility. Intestinal motility consists of two separate motions: peristalsis and haustral segmentation. Peristalsis is sequential contraction and relaxation of short segments of the small intestine that facilitate digestion and absorption. Haustral segmentation consists of rhythmic contractions that facilitate the mixing and forward movement of chyme. It is controlled

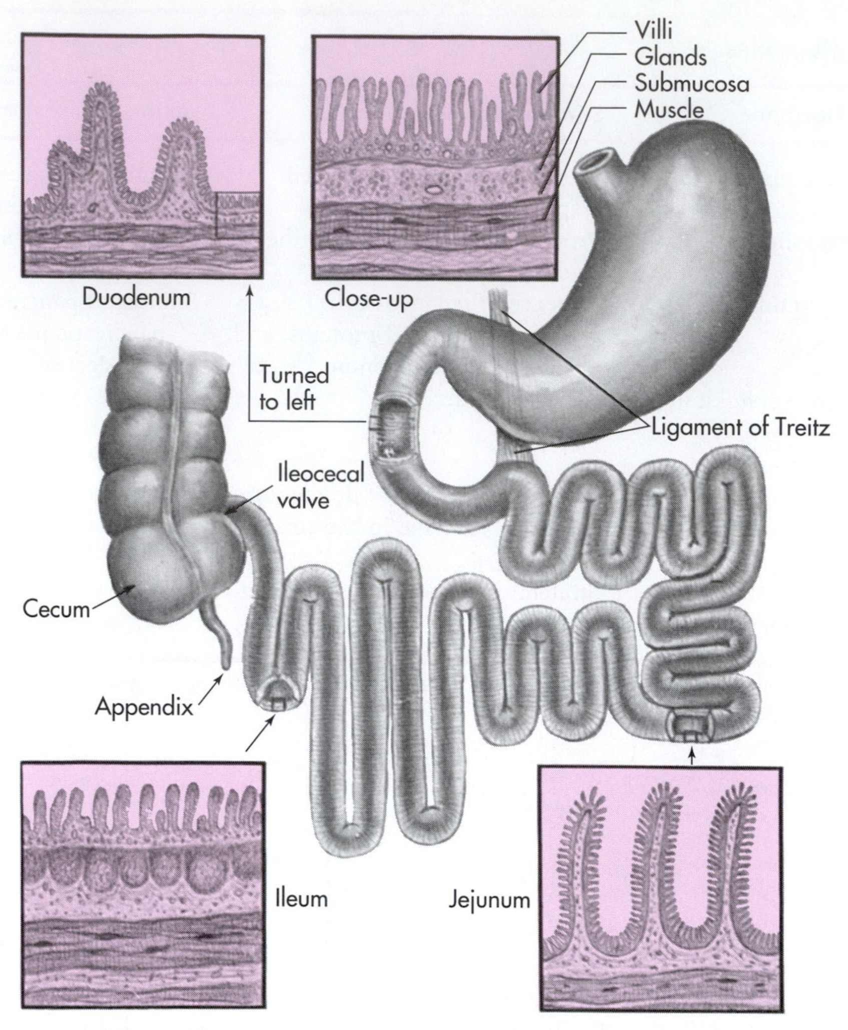

FIGURE 35-4. Clinical anatomy of the small intestine. (From Thompson JM and others: *Mosby's clinical nursing,* ed 4, St Louis, 1997, Mosby.)

by Auerbach's plexus. Intestinal motility is also affected by neural reflexes located along the length of the small intestine. Motility is inhibited by the intestinointestinal reflex, which is activated by distention of the small intestine, and stimulated by the gastroileal reflex, which is initiated by an increase in gastric motility.

Digestion and absorption. The functions of the small intestine include digestion and absorption. Digestion, which involves breaking down large molecules into smaller ones, is essential for nutrient absorption from the small intestine. Maintenance of pH and osmolality is crucial for digestion in the small intestine. The entry of chyme into the duodenum stimulates the production of secretin, which in turn stimulates the pancreas to secrete a highly alkaline fluid into the duodenum. Once in the small intestine, the chyme mixes with pancreatic enzymes, intestinal enzymes, and bile from the liver and gallbladder, where it is reduced to absorbable elements of proteins, fats, and carbohydrates. The nutrients are absorbed through the villi and transported to the liver via the portal system for further processing (Table 35-2). The small intestine absorbs up to 8 L of fluid each day, passing only a small part of this fluid into the large intestine. In addition to the nutrients, electrolytes, water, components of saliva, gastric juice, bile, and intestinal and pancreatic secretions are also absorbed.

Large Intestine

The large intestine, or colon, is approximately 150 cm (5 feet) long and extends from the ileocecal valve to the anus. The divisions of the colon are the ascending colon, hepatic flexure, transverse colon, splenic flexure, descending colon, sigmoid colon, rec-

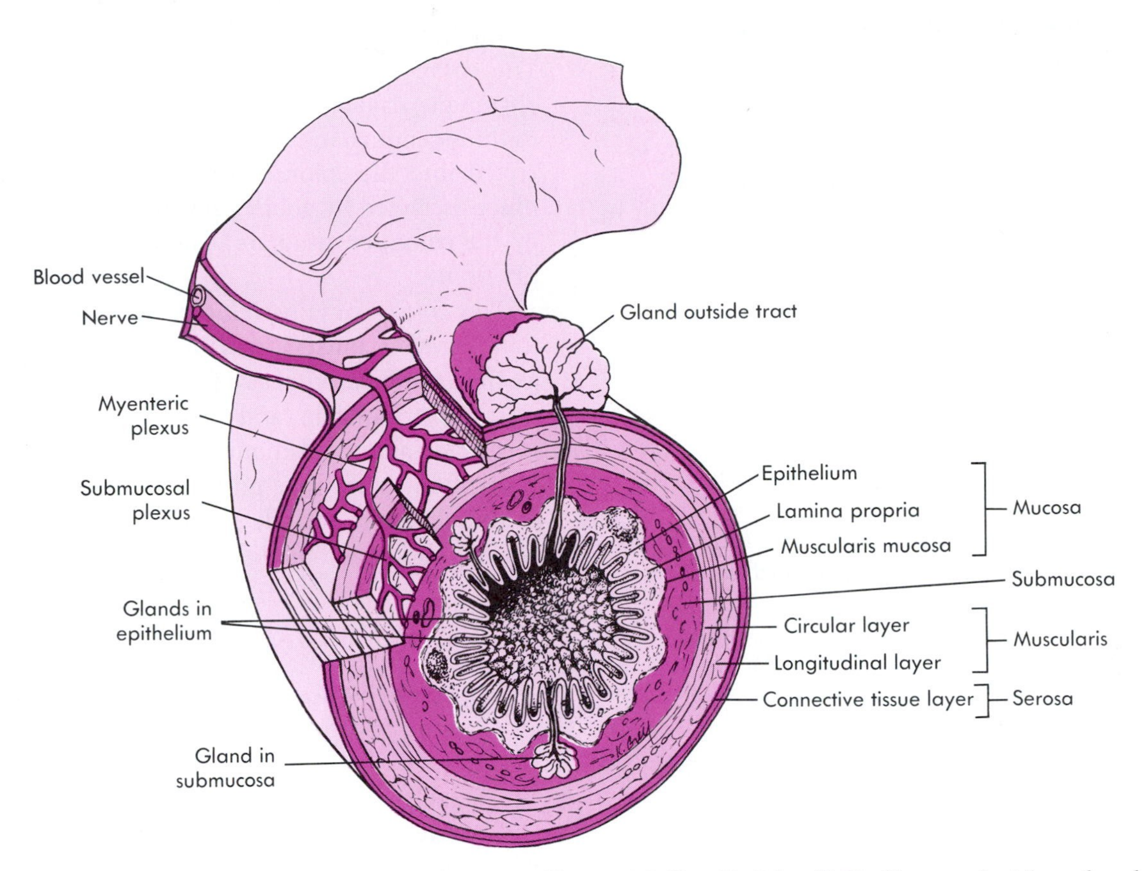

FIGURE 35-5. Cross section of the small intestine. (From Moffett DF, Moffett SB, Schauff CL: *Human physiology: foundations and frontiers,* ed 2, St Louis, 1993, Mosby.)

tum, and anal canal. The diameter of the colon decreases as it proceeds distally and averages 2.5 to 5 cm (1 to 2 inches) in width.

The colon has four layers. The outermost layer, the serous coat (tunica serosa), is formed from the visceral peritoneum and covers most of the large intestine, with the exclusion of the sigmoid colon. The second layer, the muscular coat (tunica muscularis), consists of two smooth muscle layers; the longitudinal and the circular. These muscles work together to propel fecal matter through the colon and to "knead" the stool into a compact bolus. The longitudinal muscle consists of three muscular bands that stretch from the cecum to the distal sigmoid colon. These muscular bands create sacculations of haustra, important clinical features that normally are apparent on a barium enema radiograph. Haustra aid segmentation so that absorption of fluid from the fecal bolus is achieved. The third layer, the submucous coat (tunica submucosa), consists of connective tissue, which contains blood vessels, lymphatics, glands, and nerve plexuses. The innermost layer, the mucous coat (tunica mucosa), is lined with simple columnar epithelial cells and contains deep crypts of Lieberkühn that are lined with mucus-producing goblet cells. Mucus is produced to ease the passage of the fecal material and to protect the mucosal surface from trauma.

The rectum begins midsacrum, is 12 to 15 cm (5 inches) long, and is quite angulated. These angles, also known as *Houston's valves,* are important in the defecation process because they tend to slow the passage of fecal material in the rectal vault, thus assisting the continence mechanism.

Arterial blood is supplied to the colon from branches of the superior and inferior mesenteric arteries. Venous drainage occurs via the branches of the superior and inferior mesenteric veins into the portal system. The colon is intrinsically innervated by the Auerbach's plexus, which controls secretion and motility, and extrinsically innervated by the autonomic nervous system. Both the sympathetic and parasympathetic branches of the autonomic system innervate the colon, which regulates motility. Sympathetic stimulation inhibits colonic activity and relaxes

TABLE 35-2 Nutrient Digestion and Absorption

	Digestive Enzymes	Site of Action/Absorption
Carbohydrates	Amylase	Produced in mouth/(salivary glands) Absorbed in stomach (limited) Produced in small intestine (pancreas) Absorbed in small intestine
	Disaccharidases (sucrase, maltase, isomaltase, lactase)	Produced in small intestine (brush border) Absorbed in small intestine
Proteins	Pepsin	Produced in stomach (chief cells) Absorbed in small intestine
	Trypsin, chymotrypsin	Produced in small intestine (pancreas) Absorbed in small intestine
	Carboxypeptidase Peptidases	Produced in small intestine (brush border) Absorbed in small intestine
Lipids	Bile (not enzyme)	Produced in liver and delivered to duodenum Absorbed in small intestine
	Lipase	Produced in small intestine (pancreas, brush border) Absorbed in small intestine
	Esterase	Produced in small intestine (pancreas) Absorbed in small intestine

From Doughty DB, Jackson DB: *Gastrointestinal disorders,* St Louis, 1993, Mosby.

the anal sphincters, while parasympathetic stimulation increases colonic activity and secretion but relaxes the anal sphincter.

Colonic motility. Colonic motility consists of both haustral shuttling and peristalsis. Haustral shuttling, a variation of haustral segmentation, consists of the contraction and relaxation of the circular muscle. It moves the contents of the colon back and forth to facilitates the grinding of food masses and fluid absorption. Peristalsis is produced primarily by the longitudinal muscles and propels the fecal bolus forward. Mass peristalsis is a strong, slow contraction in which the distal left colon contracts en masse to move the fecal bolus into the rectum.

Reabsorption. The major functions of the colon are reabsorption of water, sodium, chloride, glucose, and urea; dehydration of undigested residue; putrefaction of contents by bacteria; movement of the fecal bolus through the colon; and elimination of the fecal mass. The colon receives approximately 500 to 700 ml of chyme per day; all but 100 to 150 ml of it is absorbed in the ascending and transverse colon. Potassium is secreted into the colonic lumen in the potassium-rich mucus secreted by goblet cells. Bicarbonate is secreted by the colon, creating an alkaline fecal matter with a pH of 7.8.

The colon contains billions of anaerobic bacteria that serve to putrefy remaining proteins and indigestible residue; synthesize folic acid, vitamin K, nicotinic acid, riboflavin, and some B vitamins; and convert urea salts to ammonium salts and ammonia for absorption into the portal circulation. Common colonic bacteria include *Escherichia coli, Clostridium welchii,* and anaerobic lactobacilli.[5]

ACCESSORY ORGANS OF DIGESTION

The accessory organs of digestion are the liver, biliary system, and pancreas (Figure 35-6).

Liver

The liver is the largest internal organ in the body. Weighing 1200 to 1600 g (3 to 4 pounds), it is friable, dark red, and of a soft-solid consistency. Located in the right upper abdominal quadrant, it fits snugly against the right inferior diaphragm. The liver is surrounded by connective tissue known as *Glisson's capsule,* which is covered by serosa and contains blood vessels and lymphatics. The peritoneum covering the liver forms the falciform ligament, which attaches the liver to the anterior portion of the abdomen between the diaphragm and umbilicus and divides the liver into two main lobes: right and left (Figure 35-6). The right lobe, which is six times larger than the left, has three sections: the right lobe proper, the caudate lobe, and the quadrate lobe. The left lobe is divided into two sections. Each lobe is divided into numerous lobules.

The liver receives one third of the total cardiac output from two major sources: the hepatic artery, which provides oxygenated blood, and the portal vein, which is supplied with nutrient-rich blood from the gut, pancreas, spleen, and stomach (Figure 35-7). The portal vein, which accounts for 75% of the total liver blood flow, branches into sinusoids to transport blood to each lobule. Unlike capillaries, sinusoids lack a definite cell wall but contain a lining of phagocytic (Kupffer's) cells and some nonphagocytic cells of modified epithelium. Sinusoids empty blood into an intralobular vein in the

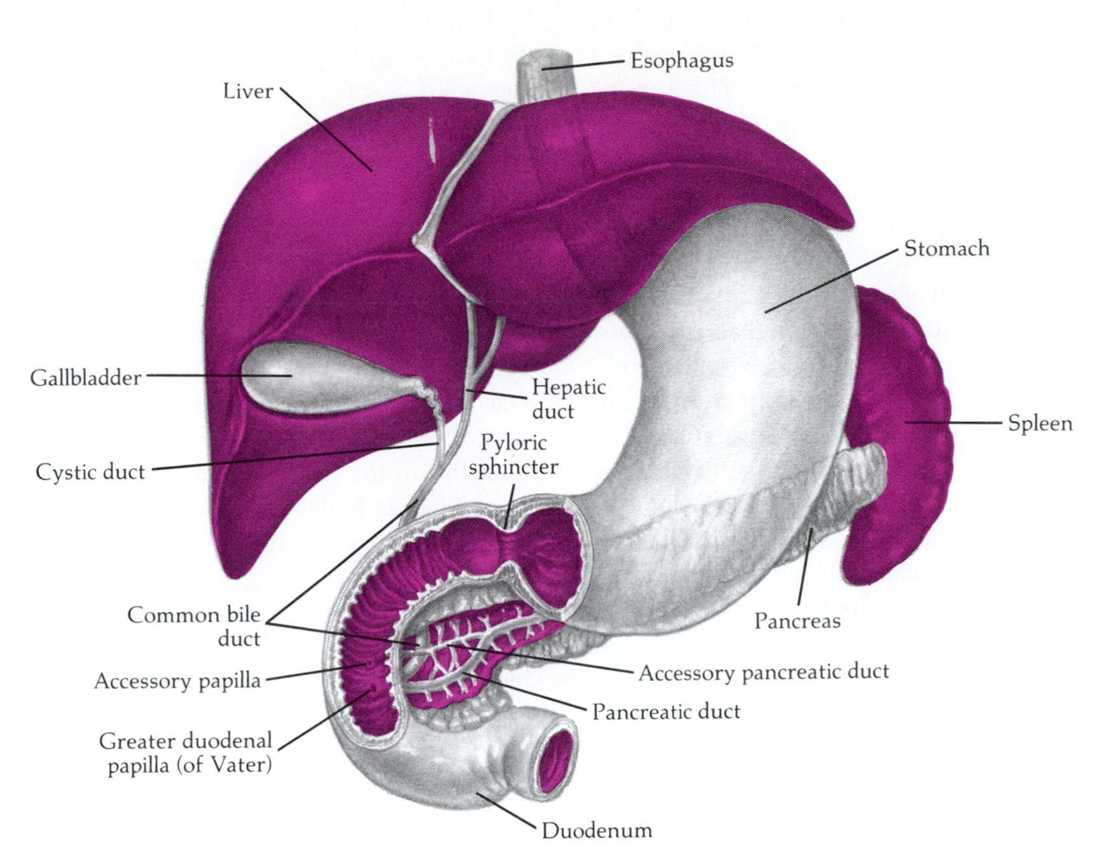

FIGURE 35-6. Liver, gallbladder, and pancreas. (From Thompson JM and others: *Mosby's clinical nursing,* ed 4, St Louis, 1997, Mosby.)

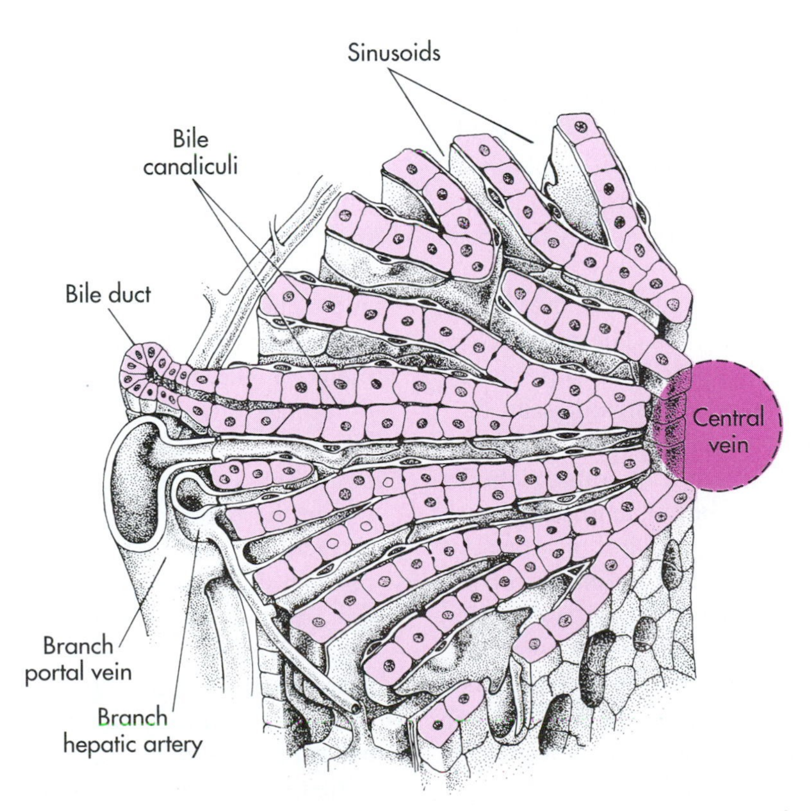

FIGURE 35-7. Cross section of a liver lobule. (From Berne RM, Levy MN: *Principles of physiology,* ed 3, St Louis, 1993, Mosby.)

center of the lobule. Intralobular veins empty into larger veins and finally into the hepatic vein, which empties eventually into the vena cava. The hepatic artery also divides and subdivides between the lobules, supplying sinusoids with oxygenated blood before emptying into the hepatic vein. Lymphatic spaces are between liver cells. Lymph drains into lymphatic vessels that surround the hepatic veins and bile ducts.

Nutrient metabolism. The liver plays a key role in metabolizing and storing carbohydrates, fats, proteins, and vitamins. Glycogen, the stored form of glucose, can be synthesized from glucose or from protein, fat, or lactic acid. Glycogen is broken down to glucose by the liver to maintain normal blood glucose levels. The liver also has a vital role in amino acid metabolism and can synthesize amino acids from metabolites of carbohydrates and fats or can deaminate amino acids to produce ketoacids and ammonia, from which urea is formed. In fat metabolism the liver hydrolyzes triglycerides to glycerol and fatty acids in the process of ketogenesis and synthesizes phospholipids, cholesterol, and lipoproteins.

Hematologic function. The liver synthesizes plasma proteins, such as globulins and albumin, which are important in maintaining the normal osmotic balance of blood. It also synthesizes a number of clotting factors, including fibrinogen and prothrombin. Kupffer's cells destroy worn red blood cells, and hepatocytes conjugate bilirubin (by-product of red cell destruction) for excretion.

Detoxification and storage. Steroid hormones are conjugated, and polypeptide hormones are inactivated by the liver. In addition, the liver stores fat-soluble vitamins, vitamin B_{12}, and the minerals iron and copper. Finally, detoxification of drugs and toxins occurs in the Kupffer's cells.

Bile. The production of bile makes the liver a vital organ in digestion and absorption. The major components of bile are bile pigments, bile salts, cholesterol, neutral fats, phospholipids, inorganic salts, fatty acids, mucin, conjugated bilirubin, lecithin, and water. There are also traces of albumin, gamma globulin, urea, nitrogen, and glucose in bile. The principal electrolytes of bile are sodium chloride and bicarbonate.

Bile functions to emulsify fat globules and absorb fat-soluble vitamins. Bile salts also serve as an excretion route for bilirubin, cholesterol, and various hormones. Approximately 80% of bile salts are actively reabsorbed in the distal ileum and are recycled to the liver through the enterohepatic circulation; only 20% are lost in the feces.

Bilirubin, the primary bile pigment, is formed from the heme portion of hemoglobin during the degradation of red blood cells by Kupffer's cells. When released into the blood stream, bilirubin binds to albumin as fat-soluble, unconjugated bilirubin. Taken up by liver hepatocytes, unconjugated bilirubin is conjugated with glucuronic acid to form water-soluble, conjugated bilirubin, which is then excreted through hepatic ducts into the large intestine. If the amount of bilirubin sent to the liver is in excess, the ability of the liver to conjugate the bilirubin may be taxed; thus free, unconjugated indirect bilirubin will appear in the blood. High levels of unconjugated bilirubin in the blood suggest hepatocellular dysfunction, whereas high levels of conjugated bilirubin suggest biliary tract obstruction.

Biliary System

The biliary system (Figure 35-8) consists of the gallbladder and its related ductal system, including the hepatic, cystic, and common bile ducts. The hepatic duct, from the liver, joins the cystic duct, from the gallbladder, to form the common bile duct, which empties into the duodenum. The common bile duct is surrounded by Oddi's sphincter, which pierces the wall of the duodenum and controls the flow of bile into the duodenum. The gallbladder is a pear-shaped organ that is 7 to 10 cm (3 to 4 inches) long and 2.5 to 3.5 cm (1 to 1.5 inches) wide, lying on the underside of the liver (see Figure 35-6). It is attached to the liver by connective tissue, peritoneum, and blood vessels.

Bile. The main functions of the gallbladder are to collect, concentrate, acidify, and store bile. Bile is continuously formed in the liver and excreted into the hepatic duct for transport to the gallbladder via the cystic duct. The gallbladder can store up to 90 ml of bile and concentrate it about 15 to 29 times by removing approximately 90% of the water. Cholesterol and pigment are likewise concentrated. Bile, which is golden or orange-yellow in the liver, becomes dark brown when concentrated in the gallbladder. By altering its shape and volume, the gallbladder regulates pressure within the biliary system. Relaxation of the sphincter of Oddi is coordinated with gallbladder contraction through the regulatory action of cholecystokinin. Factors such as sight, smell, and taste can stimulate gallbladder contraction, whereas fear or excitement can decrease contraction. After a meal the amount of bile entering the duodenum increases as a result of enhanced liver secretion and gallbladder contraction. Intestinal secretion of cholecystokinin and secretin, high

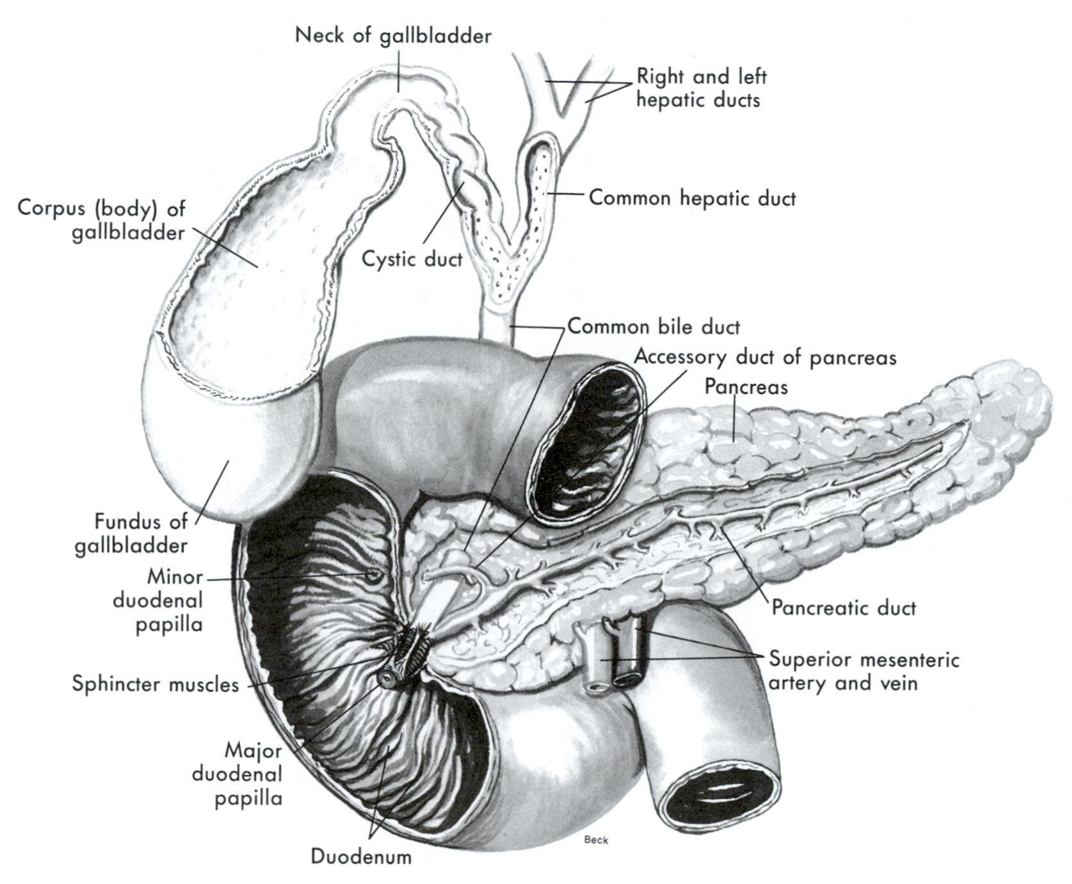

FIGURE 35-8. Gallbladder and pancreas. (From Huether SE: Structure and function of the digestive system. In McCance KL, Huether SE, editors: *Pathophysiology: the biologic basis for disease in adults and children,* ed 2, St Louis, 1994, Mosby.)

levels of bile salts in the blood, and vagal stimulation increase biliary secretion.

Pancreas

The pancreas is a soft, lobulated, fish-shaped gland (see Figure 35-8) lying beneath the duodenum and spleen (see Figure 35-6). It is a pink-yellow color, 10 to 22 cm (5 to 10 inches) long, and 5 cm (2 inches) wide. Its anatomic divisions include the head, which lies in the C-shaped curve of the duodenum to which it is attached; the body, the main part of the gland, which extends horizontally across the abdomen and is largely hidden behind the stomach; and the tail, a thin, narrow portion in contact with the spleen. The main pancreatic duct, called the *duct of Wirsung,* traverses the entire length of the organ. Wirsung's duct empties exocrine secretions into the ampulla of Vater, which is the same lumen draining the common bile duct, at the entrance to the duodenum.

The internal structural unit of the pancreas is the lobule, consisting of numerous small ducts with secretory cells called *tubuloacinar cells.* Each acinus has a small duct that empties into lobular ducts. Lobules are joined by connective tissue into lobes, which unite to form the gland. The ducts from each lobule empty into the duct of Wirsung.

Arterial blood supply to the pancreas is provided by branches of the superior mesenteric artery and celiac arteries. Venous drainage of the head of the pancreas is via the portal vein, and drainage of the body and tail is via the splenic vein. The pancreas is innervated by the autonomic nervous system. Sympathetic stimulation decreases pancreatic secretion, and parasympathetic stimulation increases it.

Exocrine functions. Exocrine functions of the pancreas are limited to digestion. Acinar cells secrete pancreatic juice, which consists of water, sodium bicarbonate, and electrolytes at a highly alkaline pH. Enzymes produced in the pancreas include trypsin, chymotrypsin, carboxypeptidase, amylase, and lipase. The pancreas also produces a trypsin inhibitor that prevents the activation of trypsinogen (inactive form of trypsin), which inhibits autodigestion, the underlying cause of acute pancreatitis. Pancreatic exocrine function is regulated by digestive hormones. Signals provided primarily by the intestinal hormones secretin and cholecystokinin stimulate the pancreas to secrete pancreatic juice. The two hormones potentiate each other's effects on the pancreas.

Endocrine functions. Endocrine tissue in the pancreas consists of spherical islets called *islets of Langerhans,* which are embedded within the lobules of acinar tissue throughout the pancreas, especially in the distal body and tail. Endocrine products include insulin, which is produced in beta cells; glucagon, which is produced in alpha cells; and gastrin. All of these hormones are secreted directly into the blood stream. (∞The Pancreas, p. 979.)

REFERENCES

1. Guyton AC: *Textbook of medical physiology,* ed 9, Philadelphia, 1996, WB Saunders.
2. Powell LW, Piper DW: *Fundamentals of gastroenterology,* ed 6, New York, 1995, McGraw-Hill.
3. Moran JR, Greene HL: Digestion and absorption. In Rombeau JL, Caldwell MD, editors: *Enteral and tube feeding: clinical nutrition,* vol 2, ed 2, Philadelphia, 1990, WB Saunders.
4. Porth CM: *Pathophysiology: concepts of altered health states,* ed 4, Philadelphia, 1994, JB Lippincott.
5. Huether SE: Structure and function of the digestive system. In McCance KL, Huether SE, editors: *Pathophysiology: the biologic basis for disease in adults and children,* ed 2, St Louis, 1994, Mosby.
6. Rowlands BJ, Miller TA: The physiology of eating. With particular reference to the role of gastrointestinal hormones in the regulation of digestion. In Rombeau JL, Caldwell JD, editors: *Enteral and tube feeding: clinical nutrition,* vol 1, ed 2, Philadelphia, 1990, WB Saunders.

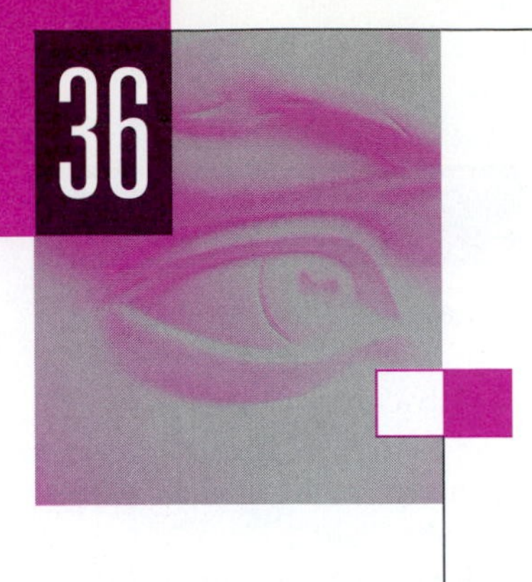

Gastrointestinal Clinical Assessment and Diagnostic Procedures

ASSESSMENT OF THE critically ill patient with gastrointestinal (GI) dysfunction includes a review of the patient's history, a thorough physical examination, and analysis of the patient's laboratory data. Numerous invasive and noninvasive diagnostic procedures may also be performed to help identify the disorder.

CLINICAL ASSESSMENT

A thorough clinical assessment of the patient with GI dysfunction is imperative for the early identification and treatment of GI disorders. Once completed, the assessment serves as the foundation for developing the management plan for the patient. The assessment process can be brief or can involve a detailed history and examination, depending on the nature and immediacy of the patient's situation.[1]

HISTORY

Taking a thorough and accurate history is extremely important to the assessment process. The patient's history provides the foundation and direction for the rest of the assessment. The overall goal of the patient interview is to expose key clinical manifestations that will facilitate the identification of the underlying cause of the illness. This information will then assist in the development of an appropriate management plan.[2]

The initial presentation of the patient determines the rapidity and direction of the interview. For a patient in acute distress the history should be curtailed to just a few questions about the patient's chief complaint and precipitating events. For a patient in no obvious distress the history should focus on current symptoms, patient medical history, and family history. Specific items regarding each of these areas are outlined in Box 36-1.[3,4]

PHYSICAL EXAMINATION

The physical examination helps establish baseline data about the physical dimensions of the patient's situation.[3] The abdomen is divided into four quadrants (left upper, right upper, left lower, and right lower), with the umbilicus as the middle point, to facilitate the identification of the location of examination findings (Figure 36-1 and Box 36-2). The assessment should proceed when the patient is as comfortable as possible and in the supine position; however, the position may need readjustment if it elicits pain. To prevent stimulation of GI activity, the order for the assessment should be changed to inspection, auscultation, percussion, and palpation.[4]

Inspection

Inspection should be performed in a warm, well-lighted environment with the patient in a comfortable position with the abdomen exposed. Although assessment of the GI system classically begins with inspection of the abdomen, the patient's oral cavity also must be inspected to determine any unusual findings. Abnormal findings of the mouth include joint tenderness, inflammation of the gums, missing teeth, dental caries, ill-fitting dentures, and mouth odor.[5]

The skin is observed for pigmentation, lesions, striae, scars, petechiae, signs of dehydration, and venous pattern. Pigmentation may vary considerably within normal because of race and ethnic background, although the abdomen is generally lighter in color than other exposed areas of the skin. Abnormal findings include jaundice, skin lesions, and a tense

BOX 36-1 DATA COLLECTION FOR GASTROINTESTINAL HISTORY

DEMOGRAPHIC DATA

(Name, address, phone number, birth date, sex, race, marital status, occupation, education, religious preference)

CHIEF COMPLAINT/REASON FOR VISIT

(In patient's own words)

PRESENT PROBLEM/CURRENT HEALTH STATUS

Description to include onset, duration, severity, associated factors, associated symptoms, exacerbating or relieving factors, patient's concerns

MEDICAL HISTORY

Chronic illnesses
Previous weight gain or loss
Tooth extractions or orthodontic work
Gastrointestinal (GI) disorders (e.g., peptic ulcer, inflammatory bowel disease, polyps, cholelithiasis, diverticular disease, pancreatitis, intestinal obstruction)
Hepatitis or cirrhosis
Abdominal surgery
Abdominal trauma
Cancer affecting GI system
Spinal cord injury
Women: episiotomy or fourth-degree laceration during delivery

FAMILY HISTORY

(Investigate for history of following disorders, and document [+ or −] responses)
Hirschsprung's disease
Obesity
Metabolic disorders
Inflammatory disorders
Malabsorption syndromes
Familial Mediterranean fever
Rectal polyps
Polyposis syndromes
Cancer of the GI tract

PERSONAL AND SOCIAL HISTORY

Dietary habits
- Usual number of meals or snacks per day
- Usual fluid intake per day

Exercise patterns
Oral care patterns
- Frequency of toothbrushing/denture care
- Frequency of flossing

Alcohol intake (frequency and usual amounts)

REVIEW OF GI SYSTEM

General data

Usual height and weight
Nutrient intake
- Types of food usually eaten at each meal or snack
- Food likes and dislikes
- Religious or medical food restrictions
- Food intolerances
- Patient's perceptions and concerns about adequacy of diet and appropriateness of weight
- Effects of life-style on food intake, weight gain or loss
- Vitamins or nutritional supplements (type, amount, frequency)

Oral hygiene
- Last visit to dentist
- Presence of braces, dentures, bridges, or crowns

Bowel elimination
- Usual frequency of bowel movements
- Usual consistency and color of stool
- Ability to control elimination of gas and stool
- Any changes in bowel elimination patterns
- Use of enemas or laxatives (reason for use, frequency, type, response)

Medications (e.g., laxatives, stool softeners, antiemetics, antidiarrheals, antacids, frequent or high doses of aspirin, acetaminophen, corticosteroids)

Specific data

Oral lesions
Appetite
Digestion or indigestion (heartburn)
Dysphagia
Nausea
Vomiting
Hematemesis
Change in stool color or contents (clay colored, tarry, fresh blood, mucus, undigested food)
Constipation
Diarrhea
Flatulence
Hemorrhoids
Abdominal pain
Hepatitis
Jaundice
Ulcers
Gallstones
Polyps
Tumors
Anal discomfort
Fecal incontinence
Exposure to infectious agents (e.g., foreign travel, water source, other exposure)

From Doughty DB, Jackson DB: *Gastrointestinal disorders,* St Louis, 1993, Mosby.

A

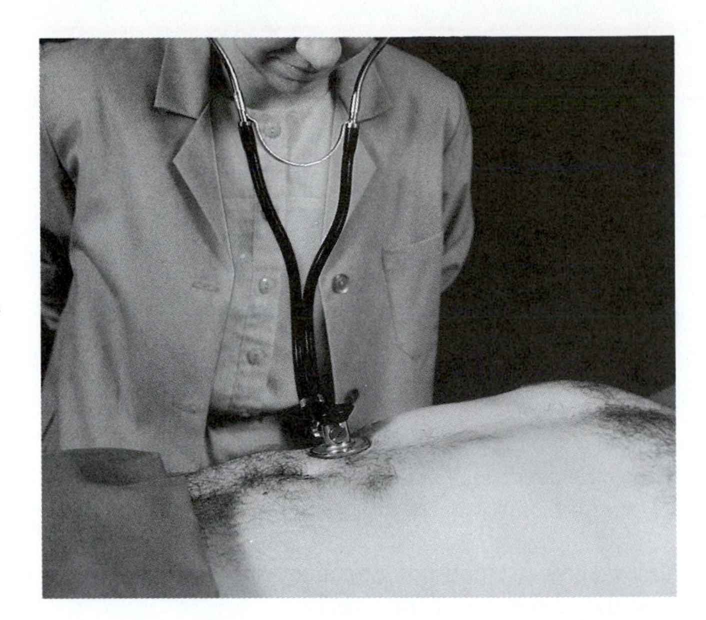

B

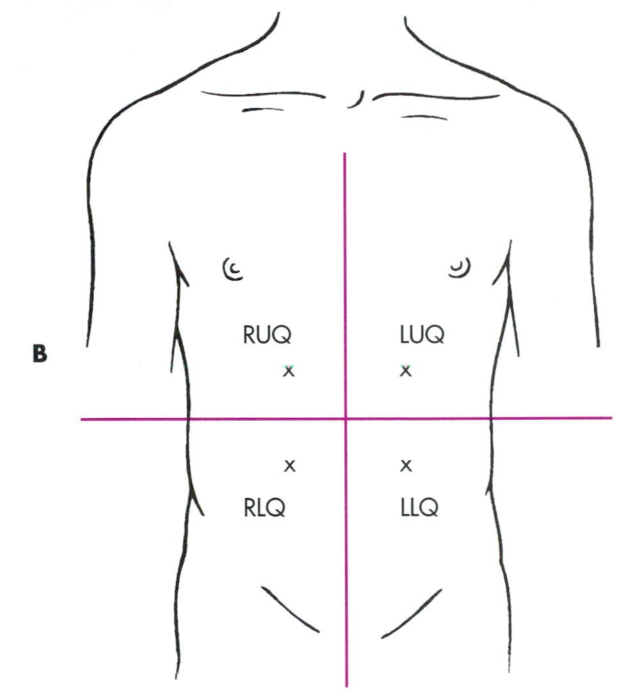

FIGURE 36-1. A, Auscultation for bowel sounds. **B** shows correct placement of the stethoscope in each quadrant. (**A** from Barkauskas V and others: *Health and physical assessment,* 1994, St Louis, Mosby.)

BOX 36-2 Anatomic Correlates of the Four Quadrants of the Abdomen

RIGHT UPPER QUADRANT	LEFT UPPER QUADRANT
Liver and gallbladder	Left lobe of liver
Pylorus	Spleen
Duodenum	Stomach
Head of pancreas	Body of pancreas
Right adrenal gland	Left adrenal gland
Portion of right kidney	Portion of left kidney
Hepatic flexure of colon	Splenic flexure of colon
Portions of ascending and transverse colon	Portions of transverse and descending colon

RIGHT LOWER QUADRANT	LEFT LOWER QUADRANT
Lower pole of right kidney	Lower pole of left kidney
Cecum and appendix	Sigmoid colon
Portion of ascending colon	Portion of descending colon
Bladder (if distended)	Bladder (if distended)
Ovary and salpinx	Ovary and salpinx
Uterus (if enlarged)	Uterus (if enlarged)
Right spermatic cord	Left spermatic cord
Right ureter	Left ureter

From Malasanos L, Barkauskas V, Stoltenberg-Allen K: *Health assessment,* ed 4, St Louis, 1990, Mosby.

and glistening appearance of the skin. Old striae (stretch marks) are generally silver in color, while pink purple striae may be indicative of Cushing's syndrome.[4] A bluish discoloration of the umbilicus (Cullen's sign) or of the flank (Grey Turner's sign) is indicative of intraperitoneal bleeding.[1]

The abdomen is observed for contour, noting if it is flat, slightly concave, or slightly round, for symmetry, and for movement. Marked distention is an abnormal finding. In particular, ascites may cause generalized distention and bulging flanks. Asymmetric distention may be indicative of organ enlargement or a mass. Peristaltic waves should not be visible except in very thin patients. In the case of intestinal obstruction, hyperactive peristaltic waves may be noted. Pulsation in the epigastric area is frequently a normal finding, but increased pulsation may be indicative of an aortic aneurysm. Symmetric movement of the abdomen with respirations is usually seen in men.[4,5]

Auscultation

Auscultation of the abdomen provides clinical data regarding the status of the motility of the bowel. Initially, the examiner must listen with the diaphragm of the stethoscope below and to the right of the umbilicus. Proceeding methodically through all four quadrants, the examiner lifts and places the diaphragm of the stethoscope lightly against the abdomen (see Figure 36-1). Normal bowel sounds include high-pitched, gurgling sounds that occur approximately every 5 to 15 seconds or at a rate of 5 to 34 times each minute. Colonic sounds are low pitched and have a rumbling quality. A venous hum may also be audible

TABLE 36-1 Abnormal Abdominal Sounds

Sound	Cause
Hyperactive bowel sounds (borborygmi) Loud and prolonged	Hunger, gastroenteritis, or early intestinal obstruction
High-pitched, tinkling sounds	Intestinal air and fluid under pressure; characteristic of early intestinal obstruction
Decreased (hypoactive) bowel sounds Infrequent and abnormally faint	Possible peritonitis or ileus
Absence of bowel sounds (confirmed only after auscultation of all four quadrants and continuous auscultation for 5 min)	Temporary loss of intestinal motility, as occurs with complete ileus
Friction rubs High-pitched sounds heard over liver and spleen (RUQ and LUQ), synchronous with respiration	Pathologic conditions such as tumors or infection that cause inflammation of organ's peritoneal covering
Bruits Audible swishing sounds that may be heard over aortic, iliac, renal, and femoral arteries	Abnormality of blood flow (requires additional evaluation to determine specific disorder)
Venous hum Low-pitched, continuous sound	Increased collateral circulation between portal and systemic venous systems

From Doughty DB, Jackson DB: *Gastrointestinal disorders,* St Louis, 1993, Mosby.
RUQ, Right upper quadrant; *LUQ,* left upper quadrant.

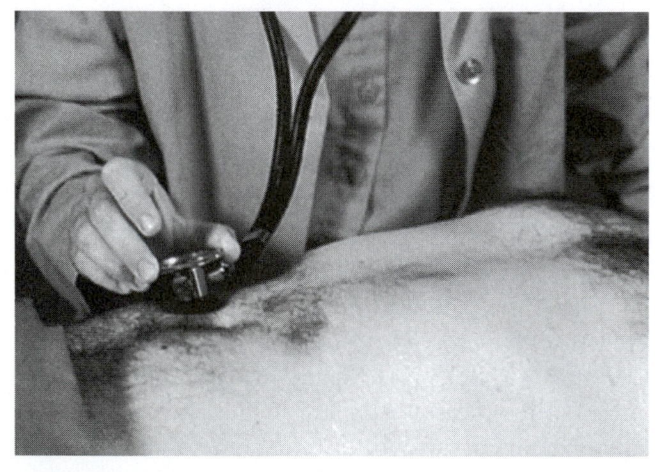

FIGURE 36-2. Auscultation for bruits. (From Barkauskas V and others: *Health and physical assessment,* St Louis, 1994, Mosby.)

at times.[6] See Table 36-1 for list of abnormal abdominal sounds.

Abnormal findings include the absence of bowel sounds throughout a 5-minute period, extremely soft and widely separated sounds, and increased sounds with a high-pitched, loud rushing sound (peristaltic rush). Absent bowel sounds may occur as a result of inflammation, ileus, electrolyte disturbances, and ischemia. Bowels sounds may be increased with diarrhea and early intestinal obstruction.[6]

The abdomen should also be auscultated for the presence of bruits using the bell of the stethoscope (Figure 36-2). Bruits are created by turbulent flow over a partially obstructed artery and are always considered an abnormal finding. The aorta, right and left renal arteries, and iliac arteries should be auscultated.[5,6]

Percussion

Percussion is used to elicit information about deep organs, such as the liver, spleen, and pancreas (Figure 36-3). As the abdomen is a sensitive area, muscle tension may interfere with this part of the assessment. Because percussion often helps relax tense muscles, it is performed before palpation. Percussion, in the absence of disease, is most helpful in delineating the position and size of the liver and spleen, and it also assists in the detection of fluid, gaseous distention, and masses in the abdomen.[5]

Percussion should proceed systemically and lightly in all four quadrants. Normal findings include tympany over the stomach when empty, tympany or hyperresonance over the intestine, and dullness over the liver and spleen. Abnormal areas of dullness may indicate an underlying mass. Solid masses, enlarged organs, and

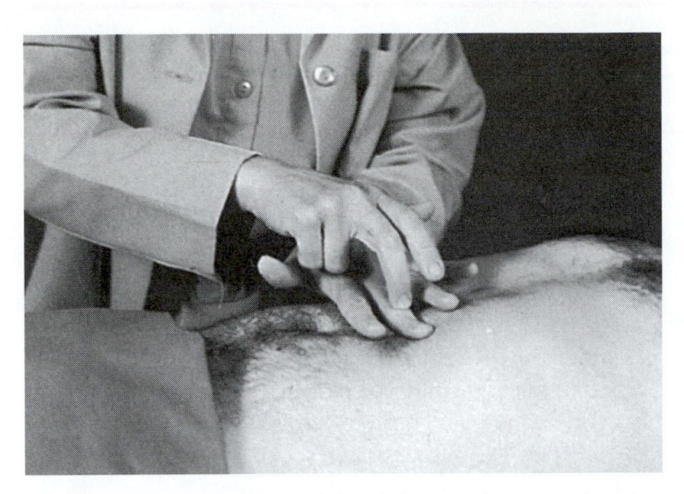

FIGURE 36-3. Percussion of the abdomen. (From Barkauskas V, and others: *Health and physical assessment,* St Louis, 1994, Mosby.)

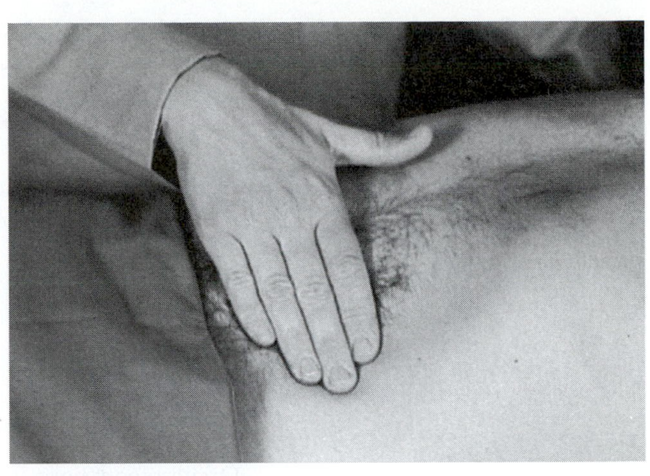

FIGURE 36-4. Light palpation of the abdomen. (From Barkauskas V, and others: *Health and physical assessment,* St Louis, 1994, Mosby.)

a distended bladder also produce areas of dullness. Dullness over both flanks may be indicative of ascites and requires further assessment.[6]

Palpation

Palpation is the assessment technique most useful in detecting abdominal pathologic conditions. Both light and deep palpation of each organ and quadrant should be completed. Light palpation assesses the depth of skin and fascia, which has a depth of palpation of approximately 1 cm (Figure 36-4). Deep palpation assesses the rectus abdominis muscle and is performed bimanually to a depth of 4 to 5 cm (Figure 36-5). Deep palpation is most helpful in detecting abdominal masses. Areas in which the patient complains of tenderness should be palpated last.[6]

Normal findings include no areas of tenderness or pain, no masses, and no hardened areas. Persistent involuntary guarding may indicate peritoneal inflammation, particularly if it continues even after relaxation techniques are used. Rebound tenderness, in which pain increases with quick release of palpated area, is indicative of an inflamed peritoneum.[4]

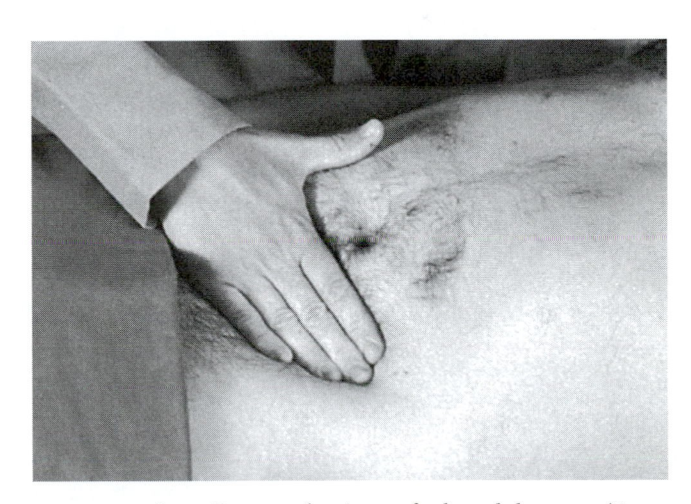

FIGURE 36-5. Deep palpation of the abdomen. (From Barkauskas V, and others: *Health and physical assessment,* St Louis, 1994, Mosby.)

LABORATORY STUDIES

The value of various laboratory studies used to diagnose and treat diseases of the GI system has often been emphasized. No single study, however, provides an overall picture of the various organs' functional state. Also, no single value is predictive by itself. More than 100 laboratory studies have been proposed for the study of the GI system.[7] Laboratory studies used in the assessment of GI function, liver function, and pancreatic function are found in Tables 36-2, 36-3, and 36-4, respectively.

TABLE 36-2 Selected Laboratory Studies of GI Function

Test	Normal Findings	Clinical Significance of Abnormal Findings
Stool studies	Resident microorganisms: clostridia, enterococci, *Pseudomonas*, a few yeasts	Detection of *Salmonella typhi* (typhoid fever), *Shigella* (dysentery), *Vibrio cholerae* (cholera), *Yersinia* (enterocolitis), *Escherichia coli* (gastroenteritis), *Staphylococcus aureus* (food poisoning), *Clostridium botulinum* (food poisoning), *Clostridium perfringens* (food poisoning), *Aeromonas* (gastroenteritis)
	Fat: 2-6 g/24 hr	Steatorrhea (increased values) can result from intestinal malabsorption or pancreatic insufficiency
	Pus: none	Large amounts of pus are associated with chronic ulcerative colitis, abscesses, and anal-rectal fistula
	Occult blood: none (Ortho-Tolidin or guaiac test)	Positive tests associated with bleeding
	Ova and parasites: none	Detection of *Entamoeba histolytica* (amebiasis), *Giardia lamblia* (giardiasis), and worms
D-Xylose absorption	5-hr urinary excretion: r4.5 g/L Peak blood level: >30 mg/dL	Differentiation of pancreatic steatorrhea (normal D-xylose absorption) from intestinal steatorrhea (impaired D-xylose absorption)
Gastric acid stimulation	11-20 mEq/hr after stimulation	Detection of duodenal ulcers, Zollinger-Ellison syndrome (increased values), gastric atrophy, gastric carcinoma (decreased values)
Manometry (use of water-filled catheters connected to pressure transducers passed into the esophagus, stomach, colon, or rectum to evaluate contractility)	Values vary at different levels of the intestine	Inadequate swallowing, motility, sphincter function
Culture and sensitivity of duodenal contents	No pathogens	Detection of *Salmonella typhi* (typhoid fever)

From Huether SE: Structure and function of the digestive system. In McCance KL, Huether SE, editors: *Pathophysiology: the biologic basis for disease in adults and children,* ed 2, St Louis 1994, Mosby.

DIAGNOSTIC PROCEDURES

Fiberoptic Endoscopy

Available in several forms, fiberoptic endoscopy is a diagnostic and therapeutic procedure for the direct visualization and evaluation of the GI tract. The main difference between the various diagnostic forms is the length of the anatomic area that can be examined. Fiberoptic endoscopy is the procedure of choice for the diagnosis of upper GI (UGI) bleeding, having replaced barium contrast studies, and is also used to evaluate the status of surgical anastomoses. An esophagogastroduodenoscopy (EGD) allows viewing of the esophagus, stomach, and upper duodenum and is used to survey esophageal and gastric bleeding sites and lesions. A proctosigmoidoscopy is used to examine the sigmoid colon, rectum, and anus and is used to evaluate rectosigmoidal bleeding. A colonoscopy permits viewing of the colon and rectum and is used to evaluate lower GI (LGI) bleeding, inflammatory bowel disease, and polyps.[8] In addition, endoscopy provides therapeutic benefits for a variety of conditions, including the sclerotherapy to control UGI bleeding (see Therapeutic Management section of Chapter 38).[9]

Fiberoptic endoscopy may present risks for the patient. Although rare, potential complications include bowel perforation, hemorrhage, vasovagal stimulation, and oversedation. Signs of perforation include abdominal pain and distention, rectal bleeding, and fever.[9]

Angiography

Angiography is used as both a diagnostic and a therapeutic procedure (Figure 36-6). Diagnostically, it is used to evaluate the status of the GI circulation. Therapeutically, it is used to achieve transcatheter control

TABLE 36-3 **Common Laboratory Studies of Liver Function**

Test	Normal Value	Interpretation
SERUM ENZYMES		
Alkaline phosphatase	13-39 U/ml	Increases with biliary obstruction and cholestatic hepatitis
Aspartate amino transferase (AST; previously SGOT)	5-40 U/ml	Increases with hepatocellular injury
Alanine amino transferase (ALT; previously SGPT)	5-35 U/ml	Increases with hepatocellular injury
Lactate dehydrogenase (LDH)	200-500 U/ml	Isoenzyme LD_5 is elevated with hypoxic and primary liver injury
5'-Nucleotidase	2-11 U/ml	Increases with increase in alkaline phosphatase and cholestatic disorders
BILIRUBIN METABOLISM		
Serum bilirubin		
Indirect (unconjugated)	<0.8 mg/dL	Increases with hemolysis (lysis of red blood cells)
Direct (conjugated)	0.2-0.4 mg/dL	Increases with hepatocellular injury or obstruction
Total	<1.0 mg/dL	Increases with biliary obstruction
Urine bilirubin	0	Decreases with biliary obstruction
Urine urobilinogen	0-4 mg/24 hr	Increases with hemolysis or shunting of portal blood flow
SERUM PROTEINS		
Albumin	3.5-5.5 g/dL	Reduced with hepatocellular injury
Globulin	2.5-3.5 g/dL	Increases with hepatitis
Total	6-7 g/dL	
A/G ratio	1.5:1-2.5:1	Ratio reverses with chronic hepatitis or other chronic liver disease
Transferrin	250-300 μg/dL	Liver damage with decreased values, iron deficiency with increased values
Alpha-fetoprotein	6-20 ng/ml	Elevated values in primary hepatocellular carcinoma
BLOOD CLOTTING FUNCTIONS		
Prothrombin time	11.5-14 sec or 90%-100% of control	Increases with chronic liver disease (cirrhosis) or vitamin K deficiency
Partial thromboplastin time	25-40 sec	Increases with severe liver disease or heparin therapy
Bromsulphalein (BSP) excretion	<6% retention in 45 min	Increased retention with hepatocellular injury

From Huether SE: Structure and function of the digestive system. In McCance KL, Huether SE, editors: *Pathophysiology: the biologic basis for disease in adults and children,* ed 2, St Louis 1994, Mosby.

TABLE 36-4 **Common Laboratory Studies of Pancreatic Function**

Test	Normal Value	Clinical Significance
Serum amylase	60-180 Somogyi units/ml	Elevated levels with pancreatic inflammation
Serum lipase	1.5 Somogyi units/ml	Elevated levels with pancreatic inflammation (may be elevated with other conditions; differentiates with amylase, isoenzyme study)
Urine amylase	35-260 Somogyi units/hr	Elevated levels with pancreatic inflammation
Secretin test	Volume r1.8 ml/kg/hr Bicarbonate concentration: >80 mEq/L Bicarbonate output: >10 mEq/L/30 sec	Decreased volume with pancreatic disease as secretin stimulates pancreatic secretion
Stool fat	2-5 g/25 hr	Measures fatty acids; decreased pancreatic lipase increases stool fat

From Huether SE: Structure and function of the digestive system. In McCance KL, Huether SE, editors: *Pathophysiology: the biologic basis for disease in adults and children,* ed 2, St Louis, 1994, Mosby.

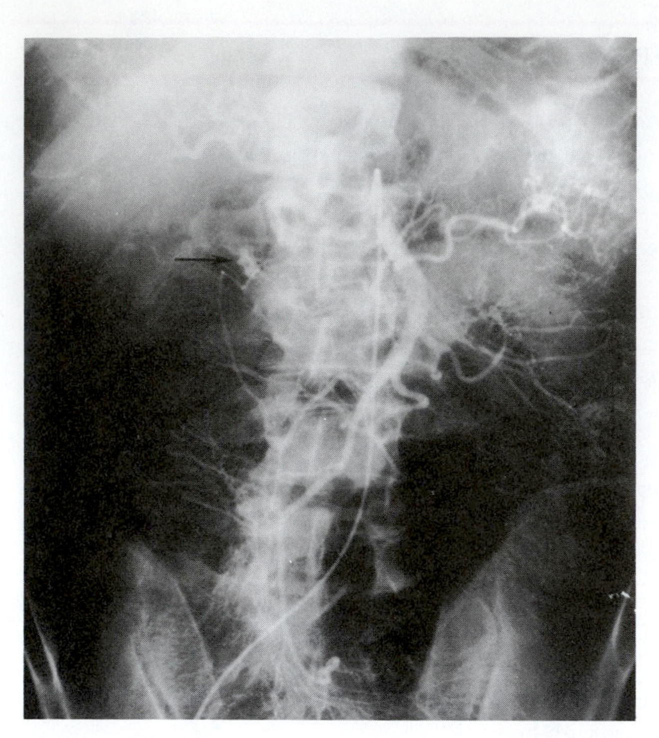

FIGURE 36-6. Arteriogram of superior mesenteric artery showing diverticular bleeding. Note area of contrast extravasation. (From Doughty DB, Jackson DB: *Gastrointestinal disorders,* St Louis, 1993, Mosby.)

of GI bleeding.[10,11] Angiography is used in the diagnosis of UGI bleeding only when endoscopy fails,[10] and it is used to treat those patients (approximately 15%) whose GI bleeding is not stopped with medical measures or endoscopic treatment.[11] In addition, angiography is also used to evaluate cirrhosis, portal hypertension, intestinal ischemia, and other vascular abnormalities.[8]

The radiologist cannulates the femoral artery with a needle and passes a guide wire through it into the aorta. The needle is removed, and an angiographic catheter is inserted over the guide wire. The catheter is advanced into the vessel supplying the portion of the GI tract that is being studied. Once in place, contrast medium is injected and serial x-rays are taken.[11] If the procedure is undertaken to control bleeding, vasopressin (Pitressin) or embolic material (Gelfoam) is injected once the site of the bleeding is located.[10,11]

Complications include overt and covert bleeding at the femoral puncture site, neurovascular compromise of the affected leg, and sensitivity to the contrast medium. Before the procedure the patient should be asked about any sensitivities to contrast. Postprocedural assessment involves monitoring vital signs, observing the injection site for bleeding, and assessing neurovascular integrity distal to the injection site every 15 minutes for the first 1 to 2 hours. The patient should remain flat for at least 12 hours. Any evidence of bleeding or neurovascular impairment must be immediately reported to the physician.[8]

Abdominal Plain Film Radiologic Studies

Numerous radiologic studies are available to investigate large bowel disease further. The most noninvasive studies are the plain films, such as abdominal x-rays (Figure 36-7). Air in the bowel serves as a contrast medium to aid in the visualization of the bowel. Gas patterns (the presence of gas inside or outside the bowel lumen and the distribution of gas in dilated and nondilated bowel) are best revealed by plain films. An abdominal film is useful in the diagnosis and evaluation of a bowel obstruction, perforated bowel, ruptured esophagus, and an ileus. In addition, the abdominal films are used to verify nasogastric or feeding tube placement.[12]

Plain films can be obtained at the patient's bedside using a portable x-ray machine. An anteroposterior film of the abdomen is usually obtained. A left lateral decubitus view may also be obtained to evaluate for free air or fluid. No special preparation is required for plain films.[12]

Ultrasound

Ultrasound is useful in evaluating the status of the gallbladder and biliary system, liver, spleen, and pancreas. It plays a key role in the diagnosis of many acute abdominal conditions, such as acute cholecystitis and biliary obstructions, because it is sensitive in detecting obstructive lesions, as well as ascites. Ultrasound is used to identify gallstones and hepatic abscesses, candidiasis, and hematomas. Intestinal gas, ascites, and extreme obesity can interfere with transmission of the sound waves and thus limit the usefulness of the procedure.[13]

Ultrasound is easily performed, noninvasive, and well-tolerated by critically ill patients. The procedure uses sound waves to produce echoes that are converted into electrical energy and transferred to a screen for visual viewing. A transducer that emits and receives sound waves is moved slowly over the area of the abdomen to be studied. Tissues of varying densities produce different echoes that translate into different structures.[13]

Computed Tomography

Computed tomography (CT) scan is a radiographic examination that provides cross-sectional images of internal anatomy.[14] It may be used to evaluate abdominal vasculature and identify focal points found

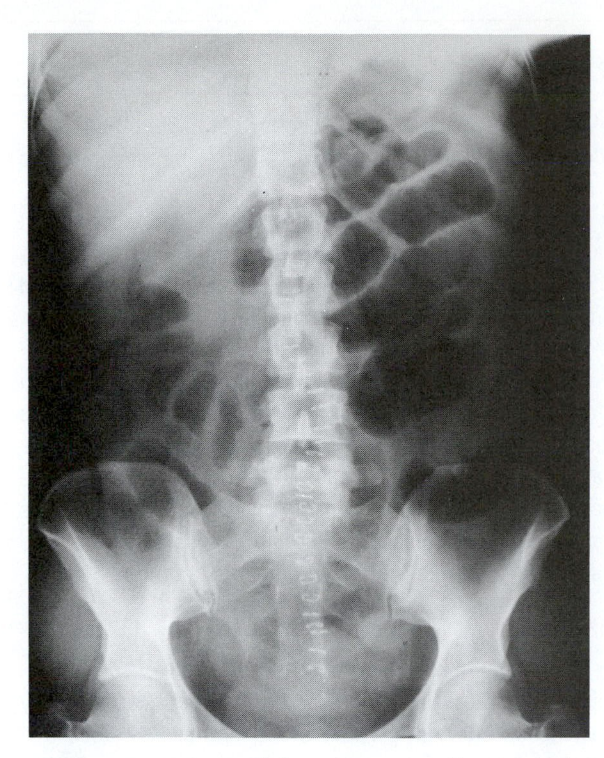

FIGURE 36-7. Abdominal flat plate x-ray film. Note the dilated loops of small bowel consistent with a postoperative ileus. (From Doughty DB, Jackson DB: *Gastrointestinal disorders,* St Louis, 1993, Mosby.)

on nuclear scans as solid, cystic, inflammatory, or vascular.[8] CT detects mass lesions more than 2 cm in diameter and allows visualization and evaluation of many different aspects of GI disease.[14] It is particularly useful in identifying pancreatic pseudocysts, abdominal abscesses, biliary obstructions, and a variety of GI neoplastic lesions.[15,16]

The procedure involves taking the patient to the CT scanner, placing him or her on the table, and inserting the area to be studied into the opening of the scanner. Multiple x-rays are then taken at a variety of angles. A computer then synthesizes images of the structures being studied.[15] Intravenous or GI contrast may also be used to facilitate the imaging of the blood vessels or GI tract, respectively.[8]

Liver Scans

A liver scan is used to assess the patient's hepatic status and is useful in detecting various abnormalities of the liver and spleen. A liver scan yields information about the size, vascularity, and blood flow of the organs. Little or no uptake occurs in patients with cirrhosis or splenomegaly secondary to portal hypertension. Uptake results can indicate cirrhosis, hepatitis, tumors, abscesses, and cysts while nonvisualization indicates obstruction.[17]

The scan involves injecting intravenous radioisotopes, the uptake of which is primarily in the liver. The liver cells take up 80% to 90% of the isotope, which is then secreted into the bile and transported throughout the system, allowing visualization of the biliary system, gallbladder, and duodenum. The patient is usually not sedated but must be able to lie flat for 60 minutes during the scanning.[17]

Percutaneous Liver Biopsy

Liver biopsy is a diagnostic procedure that is used to evaluate liver disease. Morphologic, biochemical, bacteriologic, and immunologic studies are performed on the tissue sample to diagnose a variety of liver disorders such as cirrhosis, hepatitis, infections, or cancer. The biopsy also can yield information about the progression of the patient's disease and response to therapy.[18]

Percutaneous liver biopsy can be performed at the bedside or in the imaging department using an imaging-guided needle approach. Prior to the test the patient should be allowed nothing orally (NPO) for 8 hours and have coagulation studies drawn. The procedure is performed by anesthetizing the pericapsular tissue, inserting either a coring or suction needle between the eighth and ninth intercostal space into the liver while the patient holds his or her breath on exhalation, withdrawing the needle with the sample, and applying pressure to stop any bleeding. During the procedure the patient may experience a deep pressure sensation or dull pain that radiates to the right shoulder. Afterward, the patient is positioned on the right side for 2 hours and kept on complete bedrest for 6 hours.[18]

Hemorrhage is the major complication associated with a liver biopsy, although it occurs in less than 1% of the patients. Other complications include damage to neighboring organs (kidney, lung, colon, gallbladder) and infection at the needle site. Puncturing the gallbladder can result in leakage of the bile in the abdominal cavity, resulting in peritonitis.[18]

Nursing Management

The nursing management of a patient undergoing a diagnostic procedure involves a variety of interventions. Nursing actions include preparing the patient psychologically and physically for the procedure, monitoring the patient's responses to the procedure, and assessing the patient after the procedure. Preparing the patient includes teaching the patient about the procedure, answering any questions, and transporting and/or positioning the patient for the procedure. Monitoring the patient's responses to the procedure

CULTURAL INSIGHTS 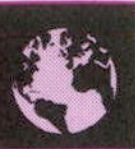 Cultural Diversity in Ethical Decision Making

Ethical problems in the United States have been framed in terms of the Western philosophical principles of autonomy, beneficence, nonmaleficence, and distributive justice. These principles represent the values of the American society and are used to guide treatment decisions, particularly in end-of-life situations.

From the anthropologic perspective, ethical problems are culturally constructed. An ethical dilemma and its resolution are seen as bound to a culture's world view, which defines health and illness as concepts of life's phenomena. Therefore if a patient ascribes to a cultural group other than that of the dominant American society, there is the possibility that a conflict can occur when an ethical dilemma is identified in a US intensive care unit. The following case study illustrates an example of this conflict.

Rev. E is a 72-year-old Japanese Buddhist priest suffering from postpolio syndrome quadriplegia. At the time his case was brought to the Ethics Committee, Rev. E had been a patient in the intensive care unit (ICU) for more than 3 months, having sustained two myocardial infarctions, respiratory arrest, intubation, cardiac arrest, resuscitation, massive gastrointestinal bleeding, and a splenectomy. He remained totally ventilator dependent, with no possibility of weaning because of his quadriplegia. The patient had appointed his wife, also a Buddhist who was born and raised in Japan, as his agent for health care decision making if he were unable to provide informed consent.

Although Rev. E was intubated and remained totally ventilator dependent, he was able to make his wishes known to the staff. He had instructed the medical staff that if he should suffer a cardiac arrest again, he should not receive cardiopulmonary resuscitation. In other words, he consented to a "No Code" order. However, this was vetoed by his wife. When the medical team again approached her about code status, she responded with a lawyer's letter telling the ICU team to desist from further discussions of this nature, since these would be construed as harassment. The lawyer stated that continued requests of Rev. E to clarify his wishes regarding his code status would be viewed as assaultive behavior by the ICU staff, under the logic that if continued requests caused Rev. E anxiety and agitation, harm would be done. The patient's wife stated her intent on "everything possible" being done for her husband and considered "any shortening of his suffering to be an avoidance of his karma."

When the ICU team attempted to develop a treatment plan based on the patient's wishes, his wife claimed he was incompetent to make that decision. Psychiatry was called to consult and declared him incompetent. This left the wife as the legally recognized surrogate.

A Buddhist, Japanese-speaking chaplain was called in to attempt to break the deadlock between the medical team's frustration over "futile" treatment and Mrs. E's insistence that everything be done to allow her husband's karma to be realized. Ultimately, the patient survived the ICU, but remains completely ventilator dependent and hospitalized on a general medical-surgical unit now 8 months later.

DISCUSSION

Ironically, the treating of a condition such as cardiac arrest with cardiopulmonary resuscitation was not viewed by the wife as interfering with natural processes, since this action is helping the patient survive the incident. On the other hand, stopping of treatment that is life sustaining, such as discontinuation of mechanical ventilation, was viewed as actively and directly interfering in the process of life and his "karma" (fate) and resulting in the direct causation of death.

The principle of autonomy, which ranks very high on the hierarchy of American values, is not viewed with the same importance by many Eastern cultural groups. "The peg that stands up gets hammered down," is a common lesson Japanese parents teach their children. Individuality is looked on with disfavor, whereas subjugating one's own personal wishes in lieu of the goals of the society as a whole is the preferred behavior. Hence, with such contrasting value systems between the patient's family and the health care providers, it is understandable that staff members wrestled with the feelings that they were possibly not acting according to the wishes of the patient with regard to the extent to which treatment was delivered. From the patient's wife's perspective, though, the patient's value to his community as a priest superseded his own personal desires.

includes observing the patient for signs of pain, anxiety, or hemorrhage and monitoring vital signs. Assessing the patient after the procedure includes observing for complications of the procedure and medicating the patient for any postprocedure discomfort. Any evidence of GI bleeding should be immediately reported to the physician, and emergency measures to maintain circulation must be initiated. (∞Conscious Sedation, p. 193; Acute Gastrointestinal Hemorrhage, p. 945.)

ASSESSMENT FINDINGS OF COMMON DISORDERS

Table 36-5 presents a variety of common GI disorders and their associated assessment findings.

TABLE 36-5 Assessment Findings of Common GI Disorders

Condition	History	Symptoms	Signs
RIGHT LOWER QUADRANT OF THE ABDOMEN			
Appendicitis	Children (except infants) and young adults	Anorexia Nausea Pain: early vague epigastric, periumbilical, or generalized pain after 12-24 hours; RLQ at McBurney's point	Signs may be absent early Vomiting Localized RLQ guarding and tenderness after 12-24 hours Rovsing's sign: pain in RLQ with pressure RLQ, iliopsoas sign Obturator sign White blood cell count 10,000 mm^3 or shift to left Low-grade fever Cutaneous hyperesthesia in RLQ Signs highly variable
Perforated duodenal ulcer	Prior history	Abrupt onset pain in epigastric area or RLQ	Tenderness in epigastric area or RLQ Signs of peritoneal irritation Heme-positive stool Increased white blood cell count
Cecal volvulus	Seen most frequently in the elderly	Abrupt severe abdominal pain	Distention Localized tenderness Tympany
Strangulated hernia	Any age Women: femoral Men: inguinal	Severe localized pain If bowel obstructed, generalized pain	If bowel obstructed, distention
RIGHT UPPER QUADRANT OF THE ABDOMEN			
Liver hepatitis	Any age, often young blood product user Drug addict	Fatigue Malaise Anorexia Pain in RUQ Low-grade fever May have severe fulminating disease with liver failure	Hepatic tenderness Hepatomegaly Bilirubin elevated Jaundice Lymphocytosis in one third of cases Liver enzymes elevated Hepatitis A or B or antibodies to the viruses may be found
Acute hepatic congestion	Usually elderly with congestive heart failure Pericardial disease Pulmonary embolism	Symptoms of congestive heart failure	Hepatomegaly Congestive heart failure
Biliary stones, colic	"Fair, fat, forty" (90%) but can be 30 to 80 years of age	Anorexia Nausea Pain severe in RUQ or epigastric area Episodes lasting 15 minutes to hours	Tenderness in RUQ Jaundice

Modified from Malasanos L, Barkauskas V, Stoltenberg-Allen K: *Health assessment*, ed 4, St Louis, 1990, Mosby.

Continued

TABLE 36-5 Assessment Findings of Common GI Disorders—cont'd

Condition	History	Symptoms	Signs
RIGHT UPPER QUADRANT OF THE ABDOMEN—cont'd			
Acute cholecystitis	"Fair, fat, forty" (90%) but may be 30 to 80 years of age	Severe RUQ or epigastric pain Episodes prolonged up to 6 hours	Vomiting Tenderness in RUQ Peritoneal irritation signs Increased white blood cell count
Perforated peptic ulcer	Any age	Abrupt RUQ pain	Tenderness in epigastrium and/or right quadrant Peritoneal irritation signs Free air in abdomen
LEFT UPPER QUADRANT OF THE ABDOMEN			
Splenic trauma	Blunt trauma to LUQ of abdomen	Pain: LUQ pain of the abdomen often referred to the left shoulder (Kehr's sign)	Hypotension Syncope Increased dyspnea X-ray studies show enlarged spleen
Pancreatitis	Alcohol abuse Pancreatic duct Obstruction Infection Cholecystitis	Pain in LUQ or epigastric region radiating to the back or chest	Fever Rigidity Rebound tenderness Nausea Vomiting Jaundice Cullen's sign Turner's sign Abdominal distention Diminished bowel sounds
Pyloric obstruction	Duodenal ulcer	Weight loss Gastric upset Vomiting	Increasing dullness in LUQ Visible peristaltic waves in epigastric region
LEFT LOWER QUADRANT OF THE ABDOMEN			
Ulcerative colitis	Family history Jewish ancestry	Chronic, watery diarrhea with bloody mucus Anorexia Weight loss Fatigue	Fever Cachexia Anemia Leukocytosis
Colonic diverticulitis	Over age 39 years Low-residue diet	Pain that recurs in LUQ	Fever Vomiting Chills Diarrhea Tenderness over descending colon

REFERENCES

1. O'Toole MT: Advanced assessment of the abdomen and gastrointestinal problems, *Nurs Clin North Am* 24:771, 1990.
2. Gehring PE: Physical assessment begins with a history, *RN* 54(11):26, 1991.
3. Bates B: *A guide to physical examination,* ed 6, Philadelphia, 1995, JB Lippincott.
4. Malasanos L, Barkauskas V, Stoltenberg-Allen K: *Health assessment,* ed 4, St Louis, 1990, Mosby.
5. Thompson JM and others: *Mosby's clinical nursing,* ed 3, St Louis, 1993, Mosby.
6. Holmgren C: Perfecting the art: abdominal assessment, *RN* 55(3):28, 1992.
7. Normal reference values, *N Engl J Med* 327(10):718, 1992.
8. Doughty DB, Jackson DB: *Gastrointestinal disorders,* St Louis, 1993, Mosby.
9. Kovacs TOG, Jensen DM: Therapeutic endoscopy for upper gastrointestinal bleeding. In Taylor MB, editor: *Gastrointestinal emergencies,* Baltimore, 1992, Williams & Wilkins.
10. Porter DH, Kim D: Angiographic intervention in upper gastrointestinal bleeding. In Taylor MB, editor: *Gastrointestinal emergencies,* Baltimore, 1992, Williams & Wilkins.
11. Elta GH: Approach to the patient with gross gastrointestinal bleeding. In Yamada T, editor: *Textbook of gastroenterology,* vol 1, Philadelphia, 1991, JB Lippincott.
12. Roszler MH: Plain film radiologic examination of the abdomen, *Crit Care Clin* 10:277, 1994.
13. Ramano WM, Platt JF: Ultrasound of the abdomen, *Crit Care Clin* 10:297, 1994.
14. Dobranowski J and others: *Procedures in gastrointestinal radiology,* New York, 1990, Springer-Verlag.
15. Eisenberg RL: *Gastrointestinal radiology,* ed 2, Philadelphia, 1990, JB Lippincott.
16. Zingas AP: Computed tomography of the abdomen in the critically ill, *Crit Care Clin* 10:321, 1994.
17. Davis LR, Fink-Bennet D: Nuclear medicine in the acutely ill patient. I. *Crit Care Clin* 10:265, 1994.
18. Niedzwick L, Stringer C: Liver biopsy and nursing intervention, *Gastroenterol Nurs* 17(1):17, 1994.

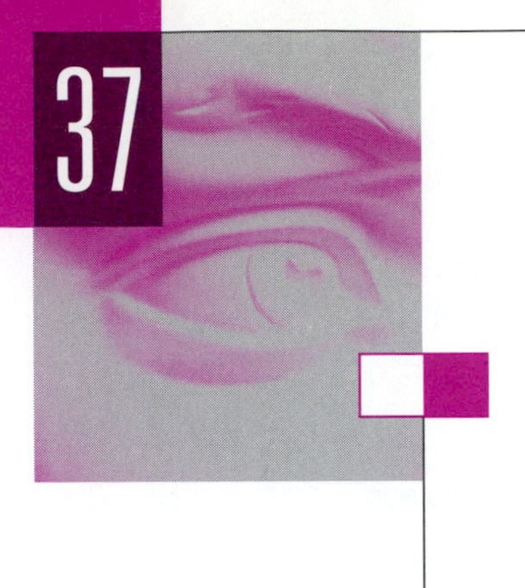

Gastrointestinal Disorders and Therapeutic Management

UNDERSTANDING THE PATHOLOGY of a disease, the areas of assessment on which to focus, and the usual medical management allows the critical care nurse to more accurately anticipate and plan nursing interventions. This chapter focuses on gastrointestinal (GI) disorders commonly seen in the critical care environment.

ACUTE GASTROINTESTINAL HEMORRHAGE

Description

GI hemorrhage is a medical emergency that remains a very common complication of critical illness[1] and results in almost 300,000 hospital admissions yearly.[2] Despite advances in medical knowledge and nursing care, the mortality for acute GI bleeding has not changed in more than 50 years[2]; it remains approximately 10%.[3]

GI hemorrhage falls under two different diagnosis-related groups (DRGs), depending on whether the patient develops complications or comorbid conditions (CC). DRG 174 (GI hemorrhage with CC) and DRG 175 (GI hemorrhage without CC) have average lengths of the stay of 5.6 days and 3.5 days, respectively.[4]

Etiology

GI hemorrhage can occur from bleeding in the lower or upper GI tract. Causes for acute lower GI hemorrhage include ulcerative colitis, diverticulosis, angiodysplasis, and trauma.[5] Most cases of GI hemorrhage, though, result from bleeding in the upper GI tract as a result of a variety of disorders, including peptic ulcers, stress ulcers, and esophagogastric varices.[3,6]

Peptic ulcer. Peptic ulcers (gastric and duodenal ulcers), resulting from the breakdown of the gastromuscosal lining, are the leading cause of upper GI hemorrhage, accounting for approximately 50% of cases.[2,7] Normally, protection of the gastric mucosa from the digestive effects of gastric secretions is accomplished in several ways. First, the gastroduodenal mucosa is coated by a glycoprotein mucus. The mucus forms a gel that prevents the back diffusion of acid and pepsin and helps to maintain a mucosal-luminal pH gradient. Second, gastroduodenal epithelial cells secrete bicarbonate, which augments the actions of the glycoprotein mucus in maintaining this pH gradient. Finally, gastroduodenal epithelial cells are protected structurally against damage from acid and pepsin inasmuch as they are connected by tight junctions that help prevent acid penetration. Through these mechanisms, gastroduodenal mucosal pH is maintained above 6, even when the luminal pH is as low as 1.5.[7]

Peptic ulceration occurs when these protective mechanisms cease to function, thus allowing gastroduodenal mucosal breakdown. Once the mucosal lining is penetrated, gastric secretions autodigest the layers of the stomach, resulting in damage to the mucosal and submucosal layers of the stomach or duodenum. This results in damage to blood vessels and subsequent hemorrhage. A number of factors can disrupt gastroduodenal mucosal resistance, including the use of nonsteroidal antiinflammatory drugs, the bacterial action of *Helicobacter pylori,* decreased mucosal bicarbonate secretion, and cigarette smoking.[8]

Stress ulcers. Stress ulcers, also known as *hemorrhagic erosive gastritis,* is a term used to describe the gastric mucosal abnormalities often found in the critically ill patient. These abnormalities develop rapidly, within hours of admission; range from superficial mucosal erosions to deep ulcers; and are usually limited to the stomach.[1,9] GI hemorrhage is estimated

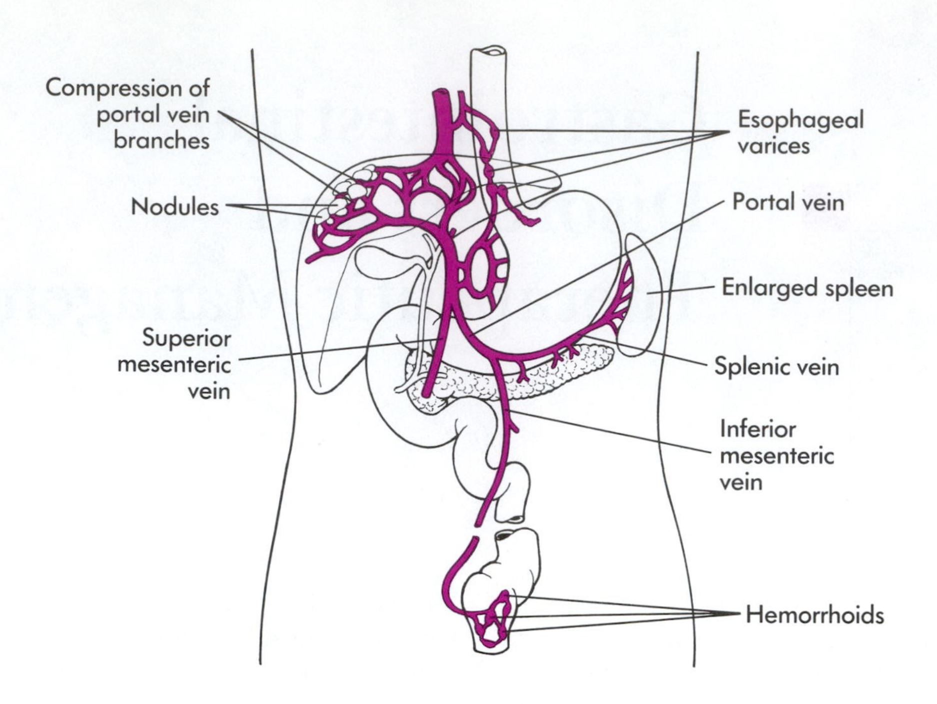

FIGURE 37-1. Esophageal varices caused by cirrhosis. (Modified from Powell LW, Piper DW: *Fundamentals of gastroenterology,* NY, 1991, McGraw-Hill.)

to occur in 2% to 6% of patients who develop stress ulcers, with an associated mortality of 50% to 80%. Stress ulcers are the second leading cause of upper GI hemorrhage, accounting for approximately 20% of cases.[9]

Stress ulcers occur from the same mechanisms as peptic ulcers, but the contributing factor is thought to be decreased mucosal blood flow, which results in ischemia and degeneration of the mucosal lining.[9,10] Patients at risk include those in high physiologic stress situations, such as those which occur with thermal injury, head trauma, extensive surgery, shock, or acute neurologic disease.[1] In the burn patient, stress ulcers are often referred to as Curling's ulcers; in the brain-injured patient, they are often called Cushing's ulcers. In addition to decreased mucosal blood flow, excessive acid secretion resulting from overstimulation of the parasympathetic nervous system contributes to the development of Cushing's ulcers.[1,10]

Esophagogastric varices. Esophagogastric varices develop as a result of portal hypertension secondary to hepatic cirrhosis. Rupture and hemorrhage occur in 19% to 40% of the patients with varices and have an associated mortality of 40% to 70%.[11] Variceal bleeding is the third leading cause of GI hemorrhage, accounting for approximately 15% of cases.[3]

Engorged and distended blood vessels of the esophagus and proximal stomach are referred to as *esophagogastric* varices (Figure 37-1). Varices are the result of hepatic cirrhosis, a chronic disease of the liver that results in damage to the liver sinusoids. Without adequate sinusoid function, resistance to portal blood flow is increased and pressures within the liver are elevated. This leads to a rise in portal venous pressure (portal hypertension), causing collateral circulation to divert portal blood from areas of high pressure within the liver to adjacent areas of low pressure outside the liver, such as into the veins of the esophagus, spleen, intestines, and stomach. The tiny thin-walled vessels of the esophagus and proximal stomach that receive this diverted blood lack sturdy mucosal protection. The vessels become engorged and dilated, forming gastroesophageal varices that are vulnerable to damage from gastric secretions, resulting in subsequent rupture and hemorrhage.[11,12]

Pathophysiology

GI hemorrhage is a life-threatening disorder characterized by acute, massive GI bleeding. Regardless of the etiology, acute GI hemorrhage results in hypovolemic shock, initiation of the shock response, and the development of multiple organ dysfunction syndrome if left untreated (Figure 37-2).[10] The most common cause of death in GI hemorrhage is exacerbation of the underlying disease, not intractable hypovolemic shock.[2] (∞Hypovolemic Shock, p. 1100.)

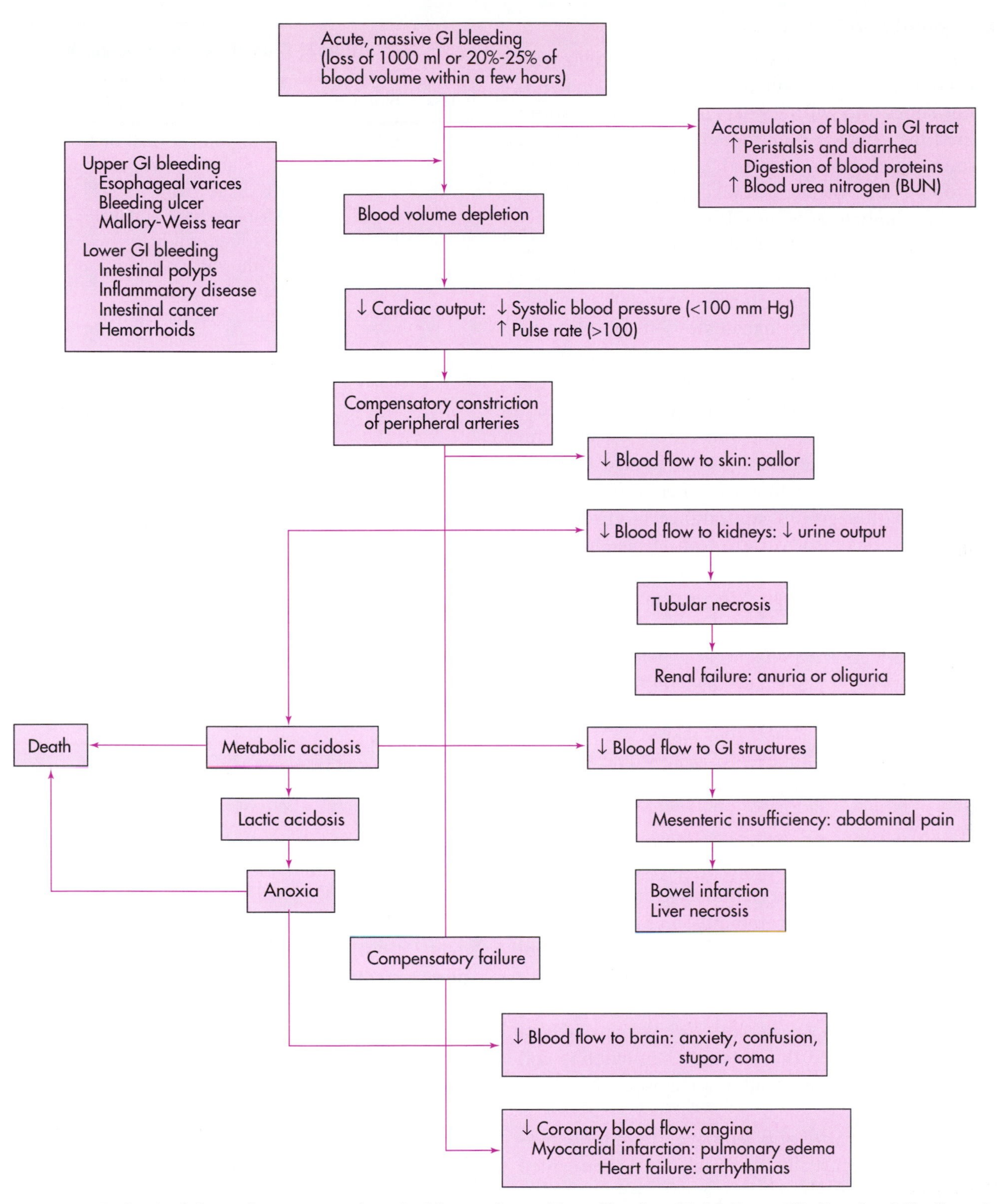

FIGURE 37-2. Pathophysiology of acute gastrointestinal hemorrhage. (From Huether SE, McCance KL, Tarmina MS: Alterations of digestive function. In McCance KL, Huether SE, editors: *Pathophysiology: the biologic basis for disease in adults and children,* ed 2, St Louis, 1994, Mosby.)

Assessment and Diagnosis

The initial clinical presentation of the patient with acute GI hemorrhage will be as a patient in hypovolemic shock and will vary depending on the amount of blood lost (Table 37-1).[13] Hematemesis (bright red or brown coffee-ground emesis), hematochezia (bright red stools), and melena (black, tarry, or dark red stools) are the hallmarks of GI hemorrhage.[10]

Hematemesis. The patient who is vomiting blood is usually bleeding from a source above the duodenojejunal junction, since reverse peristalsis is seldom sufficient to cause hematemesis if the bleeding point is below this area. The emesis may be bright red or coffee-ground in appearance, depending on the amount of gastric contents at the time of the bleeding and the length of time the blood has been in contact with gastric secretions. Gastric acid converts bright red hemoglobin to brown hematin, accounting for the coffee-ground appearance of the emesis. Bright red emesis results from profuse bleeding with little contact with gastric secretions.[2]

Hematochezia and melena. The presence of blood in the GI tract results in increased peristalsis and diarrhea. Hematochezia occurs from massive lower GI hemorrhage and, if rapid enough, upper GI hemorrhage. Melena occurs from digestion of blood from an upper GI hemorrhage, and it may take several days after the bleeding has stopped to clear.[10] The effect of gastric blood loss on stool characteristics is shown in Table 37-2.

Laboratory tests can help determine the extent of bleeding, although it is important to realize that the patient's hemoglobin and hematocrit are poor indicators of the severity or rapidity of blood loss. As whole blood is lost, plasma and red blood cells are lost in the same proportion; thus if the patient's hematocrit is 45% before a bleeding episode, it will still be 45% several hours later.[1,6,10] It may take as long as 48 hours for the patient's hemoglobin and hematocrit to equilibrate after an episode of blood loss.[10]

To isolate the source of bleeding, an urgent fiberoptic endoscopy is usually undertaken. If performed within 12 hours of the bleeding event, endoscopy has a 90% accuracy rate. Before initiating the endoscopy the patient must be hemodynamically stabilized and the area to be visualized cleared of blood. Angiography is done when the endoscopy fails to identify the source of bleeding or it is impossible to clearly view the GI tract because of continued active bleeding.[13] (∞Fiberoptic Endoscopy, p. 936.)

TABLE 37-1 Clinical Classification of Hemorrhage

Class	Blood Loss	Clinical Signs/Symptoms
1	≤15%	Pulse rate: normal or <100 beats/min (supine) Capillary refill: <3 sec Urine output: adequate (30-35 ml/hr) Orthostatic hypotension Apprehensive
2	15%-30%	Pulse rate: increased (>100 beats/minute) Capillary refill: sluggish Pulse pressure: decreased Blood pressure: normal (supine) Tachypnea Urine output: low (25-30 ml/hr)
3	30%-40%	Pulse/rate: 120+ beats/min (supine) Hypotension Skin: cool, pale Confused Hyperventilating Urine output: low (5-15 ml/hr)
4	≥40%	Profoundly hypotensive Pulse rate: 140+ beats/min Confused, lethargic Urine output minimal

From Klein DG: *AACN Clin Issues Crit Care Nurs* 1:508, 1990.

Medical Management

To reduce mortality related to GI hemorrhage, patients at risk should be identified early and interventions to reduce gastric acidity and support the gastric mucosal defense mechanisms should be implemented. Management of the patient at risk for GI hemorrhage should include prophylactic administration of pharmacologic agents for gastric acid neutralization. These agents include antacids, histamine$_2$ (H_2) antagonists, cytoprotective agents, and gastric proton pump inhibitors.[1,9] (∞Gastrointestinal Pharmacologic Agents, p. 970.)

The goals of medical management of the patient with GI hemorrhage are fluid resuscitation to achieve hemodynamic stability, therapeutic procedures to control and/or stop bleeding, and diagnostic procedures to determine the exact etiology of the bleeding.

The initial treatment priority is the restoration of adequate circulating blood volume to treat or prevent shock. This is accomplished with the administration

TABLE 37-2 Effect of Gastric Blood Loss on Stool Characteristics

Volume Lost	Stool Characteristics
20 ml	Normal appearance, occult positive
100-200 ml	Melena
1000 ml (<4-hr transit)	Bloody
1000 ml (>4-hr transit)	Melena

From Gogel HK, Tandberg D: *Am J Emerg Med* 4:153, 1986.

of intravenous infusions of crystalloids, blood, and blood products. A pulmonary artery catheter should be placed to provide a more decisive guide to fluid replacement therapy. A large nasogastric (NG) tube should be inserted and lavaged till clear with water or normal saline solution. Lavaging is used to confirm the diagnosis of active bleeding, slow the bleeding, and prepare the esophagus, stomach, and proximal duodenum for endoscopic evaluation.[13]

Interventions to control bleeding are the next priority. In the patient with GI hemorrhage related to peptic ulcer disease, bleeding hemostasis may be accomplished via endoscopic thermal therapy or endoscopic injection therapy. Endoscopic thermal therapy uses heat to cauterize the bleeding vessel while endoscopic injection therapy uses a variety of agents, such as hypertonic saline solution, epinephrine, and dehydrated alcohol, to induced localized vasoconstriction of the bleeding vessel.[14] Intraarterial infusion of vasopressin into the gastric artery or intraarterial injection of an embolizing agent (Gelfoam pledgets, stainless steel coils, platinum microcoils, and polyvinyl alcohol particles) can also be performed during arteriography to control bleeding once the site has been identified.[15] Intraarterial administration of vasopressin is less effective for duodenal lesions because of the dual blood supply of the duodenum. GI hemorrhage caused by stress ulcers is managed in a similar fashion.[1] (∞Gastrointestinal Pharmacologic Agents, p. 970.)

In acute variceal hemorrhage, control of bleeding may be initially accomplished by endoscopic sclerotherapy, endoscopic variceal band ligation, and/or intravenous vasopressin administration. If these therapies fail, esophagogastric balloon tamponade and/or transjugular intrahepatic portosystemic shunting (TIPS) may become necessary. Endoscopic sclerotherapy controls bleeding via the injection of a sclerosing agent in or around the varices. This creates an inflammatory reaction that induces vasoconstriction and results in the formation of a venous thrombosis. During endoscopic variceal band ligation, latex bands are placed around the varices to create an obstruction to stop the bleeding. Intravenous administration of vasopressin reduces portal venous pressure and slows blood flow by constricting the splanchnic arteriolar bed. Balloon tamponade tubes (Sengstaken-Blakemore, Linton, and Minnesota tubes) halt hemorrhaging by applying direct pressure against bleeding vessels while decompressing the stomach. During a TIPS procedure a channel between the systemic and portal venous systems is created to redirect portal blood, thereby reducing portal hypertension and decompressing the varices to control bleeding.[12,16] (∞Endoscopic Sclerotherapy, p. 968; Esophagogastric Balloon Tamponade Tubes, p. 966; Transjugular Intrahepatic Portosystemic Shunt, p. 968; Endoscopic Variceal Band Ligation, p. 968.)

The patient who remains hemodynamically unstable despite volume replacement needs urgent surgery. Indications for surgery include poor prognosis, loss of 30% of estimated blood volume within 24 hours, administration of blood transfusions greater than 1500 ml within 24 hours, massive hemorrhage to the point of shock, and rebleeding despite medical and endoscopic interventions.[13] Operative procedures to control bleeding from gastric or duodenal ulcers include vagotomy, pyloroplasty, partial gastrectomy, subtotal gastrectomy, and Billroth I and II procedures.[10] Operative procedures to control bleeding gastroesophageal varices include portacaval shunt, mesocaval shunt, spenorenal shunt, and liver transplantation.[12] Operative procedures to control bleeding from stress ulcers include total gastrectomy (bleeding generalized) and oversewing of the ulcers (bleeding localized).[13]

Nursing Management

All critically ill patients should be considered at risk for stress ulcers and thus GI hemorrhage. Routine assessments should include gastric fluid pH monitoring every 2 to 4 hours, with a goal of keeping the pH greater than 5. Gastric pH measurements, via either litmus paper or direct nasogastric tube probes, may be used to assess gastric fluid pH and the need for or effectiveness of prophylactic agents. In addition, patients at risk should be assessed for the presence of bright red or coffee-ground emesis, bloody nasogastric aspirate, and bright red, black, or dark red stools. Any signs

BOX 37-1 NURSING DIAGNOSIS AND MANAGEMENT

ACUTE GASTROINTESTINAL HEMORRHAGE

- Fluid Volume Deficit related to absolute loss, p. 914
- Decreased Cardiac Output related to alterations in preload, p. 590
- Risk for Aspiration, p. 727
- Altered Nutrition: Less Than Body Requirements related to lack of exogenous nutrients and increased metabolic demand, p. 165
- Risk for Infection, p. 1119
- Powerlessness related to health care environment or illness-related regimen, p. 89
- Ineffective Family Coping related to critically ill family member, p. 97
- Knowledge Deficit: Discharge Regimen related to lack of previous exposure to information, p. 61 (see Patient Education Box 37-2)

BOX 37-2 PATIENT EDUCATION

ACUTE GASTROINTESTINAL HEMORRHAGE

- GI hemorrhage
- Specific etiology
- Precipitating factor modification
- Interventions to reduce further bleeding episodes
- Importance of taking medications
- Life-style changes
- Stress management
- Diet modifications
- Alcohol cessation
- Smoking cessation

of bleeding should be promptly reported to the physician.[1] (∞Intramucosal pH Monitoring, p. 968.)

Nursing management of a patient experiencing acute GI hemorrhage incorporates a variety of nursing diagnoses (Box 37-1). Nursing interventions are directed toward administering volume replacement and controlling the bleeding. Measures to facilitate volume replacement include obtaining intravenous access and administering prescribed fluids and blood products. Two large-diameter peripheral intravenous catheters should be started to facilitate the rapid administration of prescribed fluids.

One measure to control active bleeding is gastric lavage. It is used to decrease gastric mucosal blood flow and evacuate blood from the stomach. Gastric lavage is performed by inserting a large-bore nasogastric tube into the stomach and irrigating it with normal saline solution or water until the returned solution is clear. It is important to keep accurate records of the amount of fluid instilled and aspirated as to ascertain the true amount of bleeding. Historically, iced saline solution was favored as a lavage irrigant.[13] Research has shown, however, that low-temperature fluids shift the oxyhemoglobin dissociation curve to the left, decrease oxygen delivery to vital organs, and prolong bleeding time and prothrombin time. Iced saline solution may also further aggravate bleeding; therefore room-temperature water or saline solution is the currently preferred irrigant for use in gastric lavage.[2]

In addition to monitoring the patient's response to care, the patient should also be continuously observed for signs of gastric perforation. Although a rare complication, gastric perforation constitutes a surgical emergency. Signs and symptoms include sudden, severe, generalized abdominal pain, with significant rebound tenderness and rigidity. Perforation should be suspected when fever, leukocytosis, and tachycardia persist despite adequate volume replacement.[2]

Early in the patient's hospital stay, the patient and family should be taught about acute GI hemorrhage, its etiologies, and its treatments. As the patient moves toward discharge, teaching should focus on the interventions necessary for preventing the recurrence of the precipitating disorder. If the patient is an alcohol abuser, he or she should be encouraged to stop drinking and referred to an alcohol cessation program (Box 37-2).

ACUTE PANCREATITIS

Description

Pancreatitis is an inflammation of the pancreas that produces exocrine and endocrine dysfunction, and it can be classified as acute or chronic. Acute pancreatitis is best described as an acute onset of mild or severe abdominal pain, accompanied by a rise in pancreatic enzymes indicating inflammation. No permanent damage to the pancreas occurs, and once the primary cause is eliminated, complete resolution should occur. Chronic pancreatitis results in progressive destruction of the pancreatic cells and is characterized by recurrent or persistent abdominal pain and evidence of functional insufficiency. Chronic pancreatitis persists despite elimination of the cause.[17]

BOX 37-3 Ranson's Criteria for Estimating the Severity of Acute Pancreatitis

AT ADMISSION

Age >55 years
Hypotension
Abnormal pulmonary findings
Abdominal mass
Hemorrhagic or discolored peritoneal fluid
Increased serum LDH levels (>350 U/L)
AST >250 U/L
Leukocytosis (>16,000/mm^3)
Hyperglycemia (>200 mg/dL; no diabetic history)
Neurologic deficit (confusion, localizing signs)

DURING INITIAL 48 HOURS OF HOSPITALIZATION

Fall in hematocrit >10% with hydration or hematocrit <30%
Necessity for massive fluid and colloid replacement
Hypocalcemia (<8 mg/dL)
Arterial Po_2 <60 mm Hg with or without acute respiratory distress syndrome
Hypoalbuminemia (<3.2 mg/dL)
Base deficit >4 mEq/L
Azotemia

From Latifi R, McIntosh JK, Dudrick SJ: *Surg Clin North Am* 71:583, 1991.

BOX 37-4 Drugs Associated With Acute Pancreatitis

DEFINITE

Azathioprine	Sulfonamides
Thiazide diuretics	Tetracycline
Furosemide	Estrogens
Ethacrynic acid	Valproic acid

PROBABLE

Chlorthalidone	Iatrogenic hypercalcemia
Procainamide	L-Asparaginase
Methyldopa	

EQUIVOCAL

Acetaminophen	Corticosteroids
Isoniazid	Propoxyphene
Rifampin	

From Steer ML: Acute pancreatitis. In Taylor MB, editor: *Gastrointestinal emergencies,* Baltimore, 1992, Williams & Wilkins.

The severity of the acute pancreatitis can be estimated with Ranson's criteria (Box 37-3). If the patient has no to two factors present, there is a 2% predicted mortality; three to four factors present, a 15% predicted mortality; five to six factors, a 40% predicted mortality; and with seven to eight factors present, there is a 100% predicted mortality.[18] Acute pancreatitis falls under DRG 204 (Disorders of pancreas except malignancy), with an average length of stay of 6.8 days.[4]

Etiology

The two most common causes of acute pancreatitis are biliary disease (gallstones) and alcoholism.[19,20] Other much less common causes include peptic ulcer disease, surgical trauma, hyperparathyroidism,[21] vascular disease, and the use of certain drugs (Box 37-4).[22] In 10% to 25% of patients with acute pancreatitis, no etiologic factor can be determined.[23]

Pathophysiology

In acute pancreatitis the normally inactive digestive enzymes become prematurely activated within the pancreas itself, creating the central pathophysiologic mechanism of acute pancreatitis, namely, autodigestion.[21] The enzymes become activated through a variety of mechanisms, including obstruction or damage to the pancreatic duct system, alterations in the secretory processes of the acinar cells, infection, ischemia, and other idiopathic factors.[24]

Trypsin is the enzyme that becomes activated first and initiates the autodigestion process by triggering the secretion of proteolytic enzymes phospholipase A, elastase, and kallikrein. Phospholipase A, in the presence of bile, digests the phospholipids of cell membranes. This causes severe pancreatic parenchymal and adipose tissue necrosis, with subsequent release of free fatty acids. Elastase activation causes dissolution of the elastic fibers of blood vessels and ducts, leading to hemorrhage. Kallikrein activation causes the release of bradykinin and kallidin, resulting in decreased peripheral vascular resistance, vasodilation, and increased vascular permeability.[21,24]

Together these proteases and phosopholipases cause pancreatic inflammation and swelling. Extravasation of plasma and red blood cells in the area surrounding the pancreas causes fluid to be redistributed from the intravascular space to the retroperitoneum and bowel. With large amounts of plasma volume sequestration, hypovolemia and hypotension occur and the patient goes into shock.[18,21] (∞Hypovolemic Shock, p. 1100.)

Assessment and Diagnosis

The clinical manifestations of acute pancreatitis range from mild to severe and often mimic other disorders (see Box 37-5). Epigastric to midabdominal pain may vary from mild and tolerable to severe and incapacitating. Many patients report a twisting or knifelike sensation that radiates to the low dorsal region of the back. Nausea, vomiting, or both may accompany the pain.[24] The patient may obtain some comfort by leaning forward or by lying down with the knees drawn up. Other clinical findings include abdominal guarding, distention, hypertension, abdominal mass, jaundice, hematemesis, and melena.[24]

The results of GI auscultation vary according to the presence or absence of bowel sounds; abdominal palpitation reveals tenderness and guarding. Uncommon inspection findings that could indicate pancreatic hemorrhage include Grey Turner's sign (gray-blue discoloration of the flank) and Cullen's sign (discoloration of the umbilical region).[24] Neuromuscular irritability may result from electrolyte deficiencies, but although muscle weakness or tremors may appear, tetany rarely develops.[21]

Assessment of laboratory data usually demonstrates elevated levels of serum amylase and lipase. Serum lipase level is more pancreas specific than amylase level and a more accurate marker for acute pancreatitis. Amylase is present in other body tissues, and other disorders, such as cerebral trauma, mumps, renal insufficiency, burns, and shock, may contribute to an elevated level. However, amylase is excreted in urine, unlike other serum enzymes, and this clearance increases with acute pancreatitis. Measurement of urinary versus serum amylase level should be considered in light of the patient's creatinine clearance. In addition, serum amylase level may be elevated for only 2 days in mild cases. If the patient delays seeking treatment and the amylase level is not measured within 2 to 7 days after the onset of the symptoms, a normal level (false negative) may be noted. Leukocytosis, hypocalcemia, hyperglycemia, hyperbilirubinemia, and hypoalbuminemia may also be present (Table 37-3).[23]

Medical Management

The major goals in treating the patient with acute pancreatitis include ensuring adequate circulating volume, minimizing pancreatic function, and correcting metabolic alterations.[24] In addition, the management of systemic and local complications is critical.

Intravenous crystalloids, typically Ringer's lactate, and colloids are administered immediately to prevent

(Text continues on p. 957)

BOX 37-5 Presenting Clinical Manifestations of Acute Pancreatitis

- Pain
- Vomiting
- Nausea
- Fever
- Abdominal distention
- Abdominal guarding
- Abdominal tympany
- Hypoactive/absent bowel sounds
- Severe disease
  - Peritoneal signs
  - Ascites
  - Jaundice
  - Palpable abdominal mass
  - Grey Turner's sign
  - Cullen's sign
  - Signs of hypovolemic shock

From Krumberger JM: *Crit Care Nurs Clin North Am* 5:185, 1993.

TABLE 37-3 Laboratory Tests and Diagnostic Procedures in Acute Pancreatitis

Study	Finding in Pancreatitis
Laboratory	
Serum amylase	Elevated
Serum isoamylase	Elevated
Urine amylase	Elevated
Serum lipase (if available)	Elevated
Serum triglycerides	Elevated
Glucose	Elevated
Calcium	Decreased
Magnesium	Decreased
Potassium	Decreased or increased
Albumin	Decreased
White blood cell count	Elevated
Bilirubin	May be elevated
Liver enzymes	May be elevated
Prothrombin time	Prolonged
Arterial blood gases	Hypoxemia, metabolic acidosis
Radiographic	
Abdominal computed tomography	
Ultrasonography	
Magnetic resonance imaging	
ERCP	
Abdominal films (flat plate and upright or decubitus)	
Chest films (posteroanterior and lateral)	

From Krumberger JM: *Crit Care Nurs Clin North Am* 5:185, 1993.
ERCP, Endoscopic retrograde cholangiorpancreatograph

CULTURAL INSIGHTS 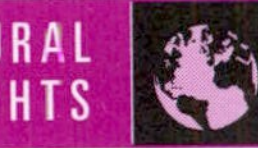 Symptom Management in Eight Cultures

CULTURE	PAIN	DYSPNEA	NAUSEA/ VOMITING	CONSTIPATION/ DIARRHEA	FATIGUE	DEPRESSION	SELF-CARE FOR SYMPTOM MANAGEMENT
American-Indian	Pain generally undertreated in this group; may complain of pain in terms like "I don't feel so good" or "something doesn't feel right"	May complain of dyspnea in subtle expression, such as "the air is heavy" or "the air is not right"	Vomiting may be source of embarrassment	When describing symptoms or accepting treatment, patient is matter-of-fact but modest	May reflect psychosocial issues as well as physical problems; in general, a high level of activity is maintained despite a high level of poor health	Often presented as vague physical complaints; may report as "being out of harmony" or having problems with social or physical universe	Traditional medicine possibly used first or in combination with Western medicine; self-care and self-healing integral to wellness-oriented health concepts
Arab-American	Very expressive about pain, especially in presence of family members; express pain metaphorically, such as fire, iron, knives; pain feared and causes panic when it occurs; better able to cope with pain if source and prognosis known; some can respond to 1-10 scale, others cannot	Panic attached to being unable to breathe; tend to hyperventilate; need careful coaching about meaning of oxygenation	Many embarrassed when they vomit; most do not differentiate between nausea and vomiting: they will say "I will vomit" but not "I am nauseated;" Vomiting is serious for them because of loss of nutrition; need to be assured that vomiting not as devastating as it seems	Expect routine bowel movement and become very distressed if it does not occur at specific time; may not volunteer information because of modesty, but will be uncomfortable and distressed; constipation prevalent as a result of low fluid intake, lack of mobility, and low roughage in American diet; some use laxatives—ask about their use	Expressions of fatigue are "tired, dizzy, fatigued, can't open my eyes, my blood pressure is low"; encourage afternoon nap; ask family to allow patient to rest; give family permission to be away from patient so everyone can rest	Fatigue, sadness, restlessness, oversleeping, and flat affect are all expressions of depression; will not acknowledge because emotional well-being is believed to be a family matter; encourage patient to discuss; give permission to feel depressed	Prefer Western medicine for treatment of symptoms; may use home remedies simultaneously

Adapted from Lipson JG, Dibble SL, Minarik PA: *Culture and nursing care: a pocket guide,* San Francisco, 1996, UCSF Nursing Press.

Continued

CULTURAL INSIGHTS 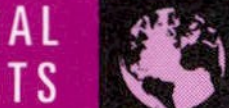 Symptom Management in Eight Cultures—cont'd

CULTURE	PAIN	DYSPNEA	NAUSEA/ VOMITING	CONSTIPATION/ DIARRHEA	FATIGUE	DEPRESSION	SELF-CARE FOR SYMPTOM MANAGEMENT
African-American	Expression of pain generally open and public but can vary; avoid pain medication for fear of addiction; pain scales helpful to rate discomfort levels	"Difficulty catching breath"; will accept oxygen and/or opiates to control dyspnea if explained (fear of addiction is strong)	Prefer nonpharmacologic methods, such as ginger ale and soda crackers, teas; with severe symptoms, intravenous medications welcomed	Open attitude about reporting constipation; state, "bowels blocked up"; accept nutritional controls such as fruits, roughage, especially prunes; will welcome enema for control of symptoms; elderly become upset if lack of daily bowel movement	Report feeling fatigued or tired; will take sleeping medication to aid in sleep	Seldom acknowledge depression; may view as a "tired" state; accepting of medications to assist with symptoms	Home remedies used first; usually role of mother or wife is to provide or obtain remedy from a "knowing person"
Chinese-American	Patient may not complain of pain; be aware of nonverbal cues to assess pain; offer pain medications instead of waiting for patient to ask for them; some patients may use acupressure or acupuncture to treat pain or illness	Caused by too much yin; some patients will treat with hot soups or broths and will wear warm clothing	Caused by too much yin; some patients will treat with hot soups or broths	Caused by too much yang; some patients will treat with fruits, vegetables, and other yin foods	Caused by too much yin; some patients will treat with hot soups or broths; ginseng a common remedy	Mental health problems and depression viewed as shameful and not readily discussed	Most Chinese treat minor illness with corresponding yin and yang food remedies; however, many major illnesses (i.e., heart disease and cancer) are ignored until advanced; some patients will seek Western medicine for treatment

CULTURAL INSIGHTS

Symptom Management in Eight Cultures—cont'd

CULTURE	PAIN	DYSPNEA	NAUSEA/ VOMITING	CONSTIPATION/ DIARRHEA	FATIGUE	DEPRESSION	SELF-CARE FOR SYMPTOM MANAGEMENT
Filipino-American	Can be stoic; some have high pain threshold; understand numerical pain rating scale; fearful of becoming addicted to narcotics; hate intramuscular administration of medications, prefer to take medications by mouth or intravenously; offer warm compress when necessary; some moan as a way of expressing pain	State, "can't breathe"; get frantic when dyspneic; will hyperventilate, but use oxygen after some explanation; some more anxious about using oxygen, associating it with gravity of disease	Because of modesty and shame, will alert nurse after vomiting; some will clean up or throw away vomitus; some will ask nurse for nausea medication	Become uncomfortable if bowel routine disrupted; will only disclose this to nurse if asked (because of modesty); will accept measures to correct alteration in bowel functions; enema only as last resort	State, "tired," naps in early afternoon; hesitant to use sleeping medication for fear of addiction	State, "Sad"; because of shame, will not acknowledge to nurse unless asked	Does not respond to illness until advanced, is taken to bed, or is in severe pain
Japanese-American	Can be stoic in expression of pain or discomfort; offer pain medication, as ordered; some have high pain threshold but others may refrain from asking for medication; elderly especially concerned about becoming addicted and may refuse; prefer medications by mouth to injections; may refuse rectal medications	State, "can't breathe"; will accept oxygen	Loss of control of bodily functions embarrassing; some individuals or family members may clean up after event	Uncomfortable when routine is disrupted; may disclose if asked; may prefer to take own remedies before taking medication; enema last resort	Generally will tolerate fatigue; if needed, may resort to foods thought to relieve fatigue	Psychologic state or mood may not be expressed by patient because of fear of social stigma or shame	Older generation may not respond to illness until advanced; younger generations more open to self-care for symptom management and more likely to listen to health care professional than to family member in pursuing self-care

Continued.

CULTURAL INSIGHTS

Symptom Management in Eight Cultures—cont'd

CULTURE	PAIN	DYSPNEA	NAUSEA/ VOMITING	CONSTIPATION/ DIARRHEA	FATIGUE	DEPRESSION	SELF-CARE FOR SYMPTOM MANAGEMENT
Mexican-American	Patients tend not to complain of pain; assess pain by nonverbal cues; Mexican-Americans prize inner control and self-endurance; for some men, expressing pain shows weakness and possible loss of respect; expression of pain socially more acceptable in women; however, stoicism common	Tendency to feel that something is very wrong if oxygen is required	Symptom disclosed if asked	Symptom disclosed if asked; some believe diarrhea beneficial purging of cause of illness and may not agree to use of medications to stop it; information about dehydration required; herbal teas well-accepted as healing agents and may be effective means of correcting dehydration	Accustomed to siesta rest period after midday meal; many Mexican-American women report exhaustion because of multiple roles without the traditional grandmother in the home in the United States to help with child care and domestic work	Not easily disclosed; see mental illness as a sign of weakness and embarrassment to family; depression the most common response to stress in Mexican-Americans	Informal health care system in Mexico and many Latin American countries is self-medication; in theory, prescriptions required for all medications such as antibiotics and steroids, but in practice, sale of drugs is uncontrolled; pharmacist is, in effect, the physician-surrogate
Vietnamese-American	May be stoic; will not voluntarily request pain medication for fear of addiction and side effects; some may understand numerical pain scale; if not, use facial expression of pain and inquire about its intensity; facial expression is good way to assess patient's pain; prefer medications by mouth or intravenously	State, "difficulty in breathing"; patient's family will report more than patient; will get anxious and begin to hyperventilate; offer oxygen and reassurance	Because of modesty, will alert nurse after vomiting; some will clean up or dispose of vomitus; some might accept medication only after many episodes of vomiting; will use home remedy first, such as the external analgesic "tiger balm" placed under the nose	Patient will not report any disruption until problematic or if nurse asks; will accept measures to correct alteration in bowel function; home remedies include consumption of fluids or green leafy vegetables; use enema for constipation only as last resort	Will not report or take any pills; however, will resist aggressive activities when fatigued; sleep part of healing process	Because of social stigma of mental illness, will not acknowledge unless the nurse asks; will seek help from mental health professional only when problems become very severe or obvious; family will try to cheer up by telling funny stories or something to distract patient's mind from sadness	First will try home remedies, spiritual consultations, or take Chinese herbs; will not acknowledge problem until advanced or in severe pain; will take bed rest for a few days

hypovolemic shock and to maintain hemodynamic stability. Assessment of fluid replacement therapy should include blood pressure, heart rate, capillary refill, and strict intake and output records. In severe forms of the disease the use of a pulmonary artery catheter guides such fluid management.[18]

To minimize pancreatic function the pancreas should be placed "at rest." Interventions to suppress pancreatic stimulation include insertion of a nasogastric tube and initiation of gastric suction, restricting all oral food and fluids, and bed rest.[24] In addition, antacids or H_2 antagonists should be administered to elevate the pH of gastric secretions.[17] Electrolytes are monitored closely, and abnormalities, such as hypocalcemia, hypokalemia, and hypomagnesemia, should be treated. If hyperglycemia develops, exogenous insulin is given. Total parenteral nutrition should be started as soon as possible for patients with severe pancreatitis who show two or more of Ranson's factors (see Box 37-3). Supplemental oxygen is also needed.[24] (∞Gastrointestinal Pharmacologic Agents, p. 970; Electrolyte Disturbances, p. 881.)

Acute pancreatitis can affect every organ system (Box 37-6), with recognition and treatment of complications being of vital importance in the management of the patient. The most serious complications are hypovolemic shock, acute respiratory distress syndrome (ARDS), acute renal failure, and GI hemorrhage. Hypovolemic shock is the result of relative hypovolemia caused by third spacing of intravascular volume and vasodilation resulting from the release of inflammatory-immune mediators. These mediators also contribute to the development of ARDS and acute renal failure. Additional pulmonary complications that may be seen include pleural effusions, atelectasis, pneumonia, and diaphragmatic elevation. Stress ulcers and bleeding gastroesophageal varices (in the alcoholic patient) can precipitate GI hemorrhage.[24] (∞Systemic Inflammatory Response, p. 1121; Acute Respiratory Distress Syndrome, p. 660; Acute Renal Failure, p. 877; Acute Gastrointestinal Hemorrhage, p. 945.)

Pancreatic complications include phlegmon, necrosis and abscess, and pseudocyst. A phlegmon is a space-occupying mass that is best described as an inflamed hardened area of the pancreas. Although it can spontaneously resolve, a phlegmon can cause damage to the surrounding organs, resulting in necrosis. The necrotic areas of the pancreas can lead to the development of a widespread pancreatic infection (infected pancreatic necrosis) or a localized infection (pancreatic abscess). An abscess is a collection of purulent inflammatory exudate either within or around the pancreas. It can perforate, resulting in hemorrhage or peritonitis.[18] Ranson states that virtually all patients with fever and/or leukocytosis, after 21 days of continuous treatment, have a pancreatic infection.[23] A pseudocyst is a collection of pancreatic fluid enclosed in a fibrous capsule, resulting from an obstruction in the main pancreatic duct. A pancreatic pseudocyst can resolve spontaneously, rupture resulting in peritonitis, erode a major blood vessel resulting in hemorrhage, become infected resulting in sepsis, or evade surrounding structures resulting in obstruction. If the patient develops an infected necrotic pancreas, infected pseudocyst, or abscess, surgery is usually indicated. A variety of surgical procedures may be performed, including wide sump drainage and debridement and open packing and drainage.[25]

Nursing Management

Nursing management of the patient with pancreatitis incorporates a variety of nursing diagnoses (see Box 37-7). Nursing interventions include correcting fluid and electrolyte imbalances, facilitating pain management, promoting gas exchange and tissue oxygenation, and monitoring the patient's response to care.

Assisting with insertion of a pulmonary artery catheter and/or central venous catheter to guide fluid replacement therapy is an important nursing function, as is the continuous assessment of the patient's hemodynamic status once the catheter is in place. Monitoring for signs of hypovolemia, electrolyte imbalances (hypocalcemia, hypokalemia, and hypomagnesemia), hyperglycemia, and sepsis, as well as implementing aggressive measures, as ordered, to correct these problems are also key nursing measures. Signs of a pancreatic infection are listed in Box 37-8.

Pain management is a major priority for the patient with acute pancreatitis because the patient may be in severe pain. The administration of analgesics to achieve pain relief is of critical importance. For years, meperidine (Demerol) has been thought to be the preferred agent in the patient with acute pancreatitis because morphine may produce spasms at the sphincter of Oddi. This belief is now being seriously questioned, as morphine is the more effective analgesic, has been found to have minimal effects on the sphincter of Oddi,[24] and as long as pancreatic stimulation is controlled, the issue is no longer important.[17] Positioning the patient in the knee-to-chest position and implementing measures to rest the pancreas (nothing by mouth and nasogastric suction) also assist in pain control. Relaxation techniques may augment analgesia.

BOX 37-6 Complications of Acute Pancreatitis

RESPIRATORY

Early hypoxemia
Pleural effusion
Atelectasis
Pulmonary infiltration
ARDS
Mediastinal abscess

CARDIOVASCULAR

Hypotension
Pericardial effusion
ST-T changes

RENAL

Acute tubular necrosis
Oliguria
Renal artery or vein thrombosis

HEMATOLOGIC

DIC
Thrombocytosis
Hyperfibrinogenemia

ENDOCRINE

Hypocalcemia
Hypertriglyceridemia
Hyperglycemia

NEUROLOGIC

Fat emboli
Psychosis
Encephalopathy

OPHTHALMIC

Purtscher's retinopathy—sudden blindness

DERMATOLOGIC

Subcutaneous fat necrosis

GI/HEPATIC

Hepatic dysfunction
Obstructive jaundice
Erosive gastritis
Paralytic ileus
Duodenal obstruction
Pancreatic
- Pseudocyst
- Phlegmon
- Abscess
- Ascites

Bowel infarction
Massive intraperitoneal bleed
Perforation
- Stomach
- Duodenum
- Small bowel
- Colon

From Ranson JHC: Complications of pancreatitis. In Taylor MB, editor: *Gastrointestinal emergencies,* Baltimore, 1992, Williams & Wilkins.

Accurate pulmonary assessment is vital because abdominal pain often results in shallow, rapid breathing, which can precipitate respiratory insufficiency. Pulmonary crackles, shortness of breath, and hypoxemia indicate the development of atelectasis, pneumonia, and/or acute respiratory failure. Mediators released as part of the inflammatory-immune response can facilitate the development of ARDS. Measures to improve oxygenation and ventilation are of critical importance. (∞Acute Respiratory Failure, p. 655.)

Early in the patient's hospital stay, the patient and family should be taught about acute pancreatitis, its etiologies, and its treatment. As the patient moves toward discharge, teaching should focus on the interventions necessary for preventing the reccurrence of the precipitating disorder. If the patient has sustained permanent damage to the pancreas, the patient will require teaching specific to diet modification and supplemental pancreatic enzymes. Diabetes education may also be necessary. If the patient is an alcohol abuser, he or she should be encouraged to stop drinking and referred to an alcohol cessation program (Box 37-9).

ACUTE INTESTINAL OBSTRUCTION

Description

Acute intestinal obstruction occurs when bowel contents fail to move forward and can be classified as either functional (nonmechanical) or mechanical. Functional obstruction, also known as a *neurogenic obstruction* or a *paralytic ileus,* results from the absence of peristalsis resulting from either ischemia or neuromuscular dysfunction.[26] A functional obstruction pre-

BOX 37-7 NURSING DIAGNOSIS AND MANAGEMENT

ACUTE PANCREATITIS

- Acute Pain related to transmission and perception of cutaneous, visceral, muscular, ischemic impulses, p. 197
- Fluid Volume Deficit related to relative fluid loss, p. 915
- Decreased Cardiac Output related to alterations in preload, p. 590
- Ineffective Breathing Pattern related to decreased lung expansion, p. 723
- Altered Nutrition: Less than Body Requirements related to lack of exogenous nutrients or increased metabolic demand, p. 165
- Anxiety related to threat to biologic, psychologic, and/or social integrity, p. 99
- Ineffective Family Coping related to critically ill family member, p. 97
- Knowledge Deficit: Discharge Regimen related to lack of previous exposure to information, p. 61 (see Patient Education Box 37-9)

sents as a mechanical obstruction except for the bowel sounds, which are decreased or absent.[27] Mechanical obstruction results from occlusion of the small or large bowel lumen[28] and can be further classified as strangulated or simple, depending on the presence or absence of blood flow to surrounding bowel wall.[26] Mechanical obstructions can also be classified as high small intestinal, low small intestinal, and colonic, depending on their location.

Acute intestinal obstruction falls under two different DRGs, depending on whether the patient develops complications or CC. DRG 180 (GI obstruction with CC) and DRG 181 (GI obstruction without CC) have average lengths of stay of 6.1 days and 4.0 days, respectively.[4]

Etiology

Functional obstructions can be the result of an intraabdominal problem or an extraabdominal problem. Specific causes include the postoperative state, sepsis, electrolyte imbalances, trauma, and the use of opiates, chemotherapeutic agents, or cardiac drugs.[26] Mechanical obstructions can be the result of extrinsic lesions, intrinsic lesions, and objects blocking the intestinal lumen.[26] Most mechanical obstructions occur in the small intestine, with abdominal adhesions generally the causative factor.[27] Obstructions of the large intestine result generally from malignant tumors.[28] Box 37-10 lists the etiologies of functional and mechanical obstructions.[26-28]

BOX 37-8 Signs of Pancreatic Infection

Symptoms
- Persistent abdominal pain
- Abdominal tenderness

Signs
- Prolonged fever
- Abdominal distention
- Palpable abdominal mass
- Vomiting

Diagnostics
- Laboratory
  - Increased white blood cell count
  - Persistent elevation of serum amylase
  - Hyperbilirubinemia
  - Elevated alkaline phosphatase
  - Positive culture and Gram stain
- Radiography/CT
  - Pancreatic inflammation or enlargement
  - Necrosis
  - Cystic or mass lesions
  - Fluid accumulations
  - Pseudocyst abscess

From Krumberger JM: *Crit Care Nurs Clin North Am* 5:185, 1993.

BOX 37-9 PATIENT EDUCATION

ACUTE PANCREATITIS

- Pancreatitis
- Specific etiology
- Precipitating factor modification
- Interventions to reduce further episodes
- Importance of taking medications
- Life-style changes
- Diet modification
- Stress management
- Alcohol cessation
- Diabetes management (if present)

Pathophysiology

Regardless of the etiology once an obstruction develops, fluid and gas accumulate in the bowel lumen proximal to the point of obstruction (Figure 37-3). Trapped fluids cause bowel distention and bowel wall edema, triggering the secretion of more fluid and electrolytes into the lumen and resulting in progressive distention. Typically, the fluid and electrolyte shifts are much more pronounced in mechanical obstructions,

BOX 37-10 Etiologies of Intestinal Obstructions

FUNCTIONAL OBSTRUCTIONS

Intraabdominal

Peritonitis
Pancreatitis
Bowel ischemia
Abdominal surgery or trauma

Extraabdominal

Rib, spine, or pelvic trauma
Retroperitoneal surgery or trauma
Myocardial infarction
Pneumonia
Electrolyte abnormalities (hypokalemia, hypomagnesemia)
Metabolic disturbances
Sepsis
Drugs

MECHANICAL OBSTRUCTION

Extrinsic lesions

Adhesions
Hernias
Volvulus
Tumors

Intrinsic lesions

Tumors
Intussusception
Congenital atresia or stenosis
Bowel ischemia
Bowel inflammation (radiation enteritis, Crohn's disease)
Diverticulitis

Blockage of intestinal lumen

Gallstones
Impaction (fecal, barium, bezoars, worms)
Tumors

as opposed to functional obstructions. Large losses of sodium, potassium, and chloride occur, as well as a loss of hydrogen ions from the stomach. As the obstruction continues, the vascular space becomes rapidly depleted, which results in dehydration, hypotension, and hypovolemic shock. If intestinal distention progresses, bowel wall edema will ultimately impede venous and arterial supply, causing ischemia (strangulation), bowel necrosis, and perforation. Once the bowel perforates, peritonitis and sepsis ensue.[29] (∞Hypovolemic Shock, p. 1100.)

Assessment and Diagnosis

Patients with acute intestinal obstruction may initially present with vague warning symptoms such as abdominal distention, nausea, vomiting, obstipation, constipation, cramping abdominal pain, and abnormal bowel sounds. In the patient with a mechanical obstruction, bowel sounds are high-pitched, tinkling, and hyperactive proximal to the obstruction site and hypoactive or absent distal to the obstruction, as opposed to the patient with a functional obstruction where the bowel sounds are low-pitched and hypoactive or absent.[26-28] The patient may also exhibit signs of dehydration such as dry mucous membranes, poor skin turgor, tachycardia, and hypotension.[29]

Small bowel obstructions, which comprise about two thirds of mechanical obstructions, usually present with rapid onset of cramplike abdominal pain, nausea, vomiting (may be projectile), and abdominal distention. The patient may continue to pass small amounts of stool or flatus. Abdominal pain is severe and frequent, with short quiet periods between peristaltic rushes. The higher the obstruction's location in the intestine, the more intense is the pain.[27]

Large bowel obstructions, about one third of mechanical obstructions, generally have an insidious onset of low-grade, crampy pain, marked abdominal distention, and obstipation. Nausea and vomiting are rare, and the patient's history frequently includes a change in bowel habits and report of weight loss. Vomiting may occur late and contain fecal material, requiring immediate attention.[28]

Diagnosis of intestinal obstruction is aided by radiologic examination. A chest x-ray and serial abdominal flat-plate films taken with the patient standing or sitting and supine reveal dilated loops of gas-filled bowel. Barium or meglumine diatrizoate (Gastrografin) enemas are used to locate the exact site and degree of obstruction. Laboratory data may reveal an elevated serum amylase level, an elevated white blood cell count (marked elevation with complete or necrotic obstructions), hyponatremia, and hypokalemia.[29]

Medical Management

Medical interventions for both functional and mechanical obstructions include decompression of the intestine with nasogastric suctioning, correction and maintenance of fluid and electrolyte balance, and relief or removal of the obstruction. Antibiotic prophy-

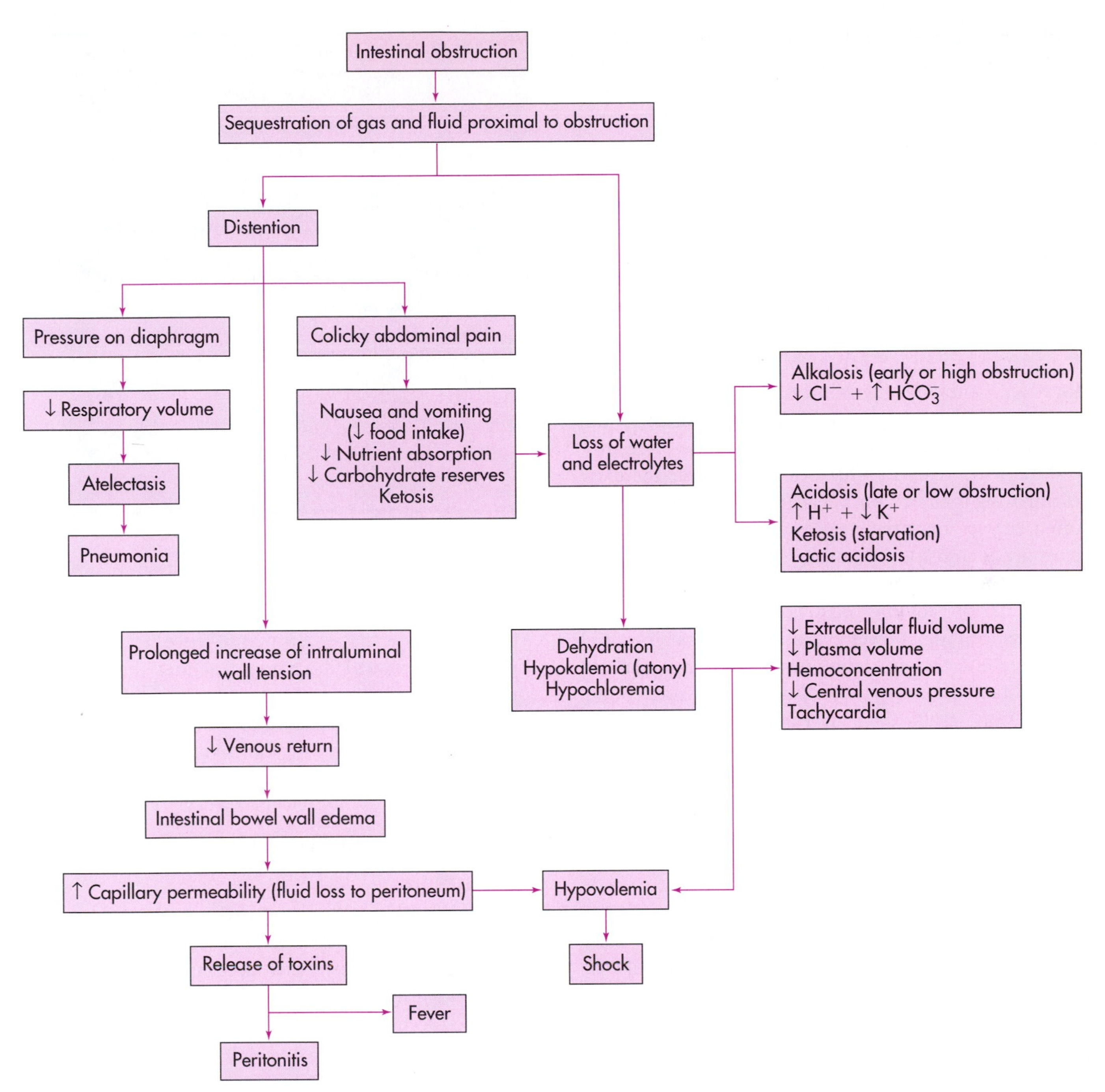

FIGURE 37-3. Pathophysiology of intestinal obstruction. (From Huether SE, McCance KL, Tarmina MS: Alterations of digestive function. In McCance KL, Huether SE, editors: *Pathophysiology: the biologic basis for disease in adults and children,* ed 2, St Louis, 1994, Mosby.)

laxis should also be initiated for patients with large bowel obstructions.[29]

Much controversy exists over whether a nasogastric tube or a nasointestinal tube should be placed for decompressing small bowel mechanical obstructions.[29] Nasointestinal tubes are contraindicated for large bowel mechanical obstructions.[26] Decompression of the upper GI tract of gas and fluids relieves abdominal distention and controls nausea and vomiting. In addition, the patient should receive nothing by mouth.

Fluid and electrolyte balance is most often achieved with normal saline solution and potassium supplement administration.[26,29]

Functional obstructions generally resolve within 24 to 72 hours with conservative therapy that includes giving the patient nothing by mouth, decompressing the upper GI tract with nasogastric suction, stimulating motility pharmacologically, and eliminating underlying aggravating factors. Partial small bowel obstructions may also resolve with this conservative therapy.[27]

Surgical intervention is required when the obstruction fails to resolve within a reasonable time or if there is evidence of a strangulation, bowel necrosis, and perforation. Complete mechanical obstructions also require surgical intervention.[26] When the patient is not acutely ill, surgical resection can be a one-stage procedure with reanastomosis of the bowel, therefore eliminating the need for a temporary colostomy. More often, a two- or three-stage procedure is used and a temporary colostomy created.[29]

Bowel necrosis and perforation are potential complications of colonic obstruction, and both can progress to sepsis. Bowel necrosis occurs as a result of impaired circulation to the bowel wall (strangulation) and sustained excessive intraluminal pressure. Bowel perforation results from overdistention of the bowel lumen and is a sequela to bowel necrosis. These complications carry a high mortality and can be avoided by astute clinical observations, followed by prompt surgical intervention.[26]

Nursing Management

Nursing management of the patient with an acute intestinal obstruction incorporates a variety of nursing diagnoses (Box 37-11). The patient should be closely monitored for signs of bowel necrosis and perforation, such as leukocytosis, fever, tachycardia, localized tenderness, and absence of bowel sounds.[29]

Once a nasogastric tube is inserted, it should be checked regularly for placement and patency to ensure adequate decompression. Outputs greater than 1000 ml/8 hours can occur; therefore the patient should be monitored closely for electrolyte imbalances (hyponatremia and hypokalemia) and fluid volume deficit. Accurate intake and output must be maintained. Intravenous fluid and electrolyte solutions should be administered to prevent dehydration and replace lost electrolytes. Administration of antipyretics is necessary for the treatment of fever.

Early in the patient's hospital stay, the patient and family should be taught about acute intestinal obstruction, its etiologies, and its treatments. As the patient moves toward discharge, teaching should focus on the interventions necessary for preventing the recurrence of the precipitating etiology. If the patient has either a temporary or a permanent colostomy, he or she will also require ostomy teaching (Box 37-12).

BOX 37-11 NURSING DIAGNOSIS AND MANAGEMENT

ACUTE INTESTINAL OBSTRUCTION

- Acute Pain related to transmission and perception of cutaneous, visceral, muscular, ischemic impulses, p. 197
- Ineffective Breathing Pattern related to decreased lung expansion, p. 723
- Fluid Volume Deficit related to relative fluid loss, p. 915
- Altered Nutrition: Less Than Body Requirements related to lack of exogenous nutrients or increased metabolic demand, p. 165
- Anxiety related to threat to biologic, psychologic, and/or social integrity, p. 99
- Ineffective Family Coping related to critically ill family member, p. 97
- Knowledge Deficit: Discharge Regimen related to lack of previous exposure to information, p. 61 (see Patient Education Box 37-12)

FULMINANT HEPATIC FAILURE

Description

Fulminant hepatic failure (FHF) is a medical emergency that is best described as severe acute liver failure (hepatocellular necrosis) accompanied by hepatic encephalopathy. It has a mortality as high as 90% and generally occurs in patients without preexisting liver disease, although it is occasionally seen in patients with compensated chronic liver disease. As liver transplantation is one of the few definitive treatments for FHF, the patient with FHF should be transferred to a critical care unit and strongly considered for referral to a major medical center where transplant services are available.[30,31]

Fulminant hepatic failure falls under two different DRGs, depending on whether the patient develops complications or CC. DRG 205 (Disorders of liver except malignancy, cirrhosis, and alcoholic hepatitis with CC) and DRG 206 (Disorders of liver except malignancy, cirrhosis, and alcoholic hepatitis without CC) have average lengths of stay of 7.3 days and 4.7 days, respectively.[4]

BOX 37-12 PATIENT EDUCATION

ACUTE INTESTINAL OBSTRUCTION

- Acute intestinal obstruction
- Specific etiology
- Precipitating factor modification
- Interventions to reduce further episodes
- Importance of taking medications
- Life-style changes
- Diet modification

Etiology

The etiologies of FHF include infections, drugs, toxins, hypoperfusion, metabolic disorders, and surgery (Box 37-13). Patients presenting with FHF are usually healthy before the onset of symptoms, as it tends to occur in patients with no known liver history. Therefore it is imperative that a thorough medication and health history be explored to determine a possible etiology. The patient should be questioned about exposure to environmental toxins, hepatitis, intravenous drug use, and sexual history. Viral hepatitis, drug toxicity, poisoning, and metabolic disorders, such as Reye's syndrome and Wilson's disease, should be considered.[30-32]

Pathophysiology

FHF is a syndrome characterized by the development of acute liver failure over 1 to 3 weeks, followed by the development of hepatic encephalopathy within 8 weeks, in a patient with a previously healthy liver. Generally the interval between the actual failure of the liver and the onset of hepatic encephalopathy is less than 2 weeks. The underlying cause is massive necrosis of the hepatocytes.[30-32]

Acute liver failure results in a number of derangements, including impaired bilirubin conjugation, decreased production of clotting factors, depressed glucose synthesis, and decreased lactate clearance. This results in jaundice, coagulopathies, hypoglycemia, and metabolic acidosis.[31] Other effects of acute liver failure include increased risk of infection and altered carbohydrate, protein, and glucose metabolism. Hypoalbuminemia, fluid and electrolyte imbalances, and acute portal hypertension contribute to the development of ascites.[31,33] Hepatic encephalopathy is thought to result from failure of the liver to detoxify various substances in the blood stream and may be worsened by metabolic and electrolyte imbalances.[31]

BOX 37-13 Etiologies of Fulminant Hepatic Failure

INFECTIONS

Hepatitis A, B, C, D, E, non-A, non-B, non-C
Herpes simplex virus (types 1 and 2)
Epstein-Barr virus
Varicella zoster
Dengue fever virus
Rift Valley fever virus

DRUGS/TOXINS

Industrial substances (chlorinated hydrocarbons, phosphorus)
Amanita phalloides (mushrooms)
Aflatoxin (herb)
Medications (isoniazid, rifampin, halothane, methyldopa, tetracycline, valproic acid, monoamine oxidase inhibitors, phenytoin, nicotinic acid, tricyclic antidepressants, isoflurane, ketoconazole, co-trimethoprim, sulfasalazine, pyrimethamine, octreotide)
Acetaminophen toxicity
Cocaine

HYPOPERFUSION

Venous obstructions
Budd-Chiari syndrome
Veno-occlusive disease
Ischemia

METABOLIC DISORDERS

Wilson's disease
Tyrosinemia
Heat stroke
Galactosemia

SURGERY

Jejunoileal bypass
Partial hepatectomy
Liver transplant failure

OTHER

Reye's syndrome
Acute fatty liver of pregnancy
Massive malignant infiltration
Autoimmune hepatitis

The patient may also experience a variety of other complications, including cerebral edema, cardiac dysrhythmias, acute respiratory failure, and acute renal failure. Cerebral edema develops as a result of breakdown of the blood-brain barrier and astrocyte

BOX 37-14 Staging of Hepatic Encephalopathy

I Euphoria or depression, mild confusion, slurred speech, disordered sleep rhythm; slight asterixis and normal electroencephalogram (EEG)
II Lethargy, moderate confusion; marked asterixis and abnormal EEG
III Marked confusion, incoherent speech, sleeping but arousable; asterixis present and abnormal EEG
IV Coma; initially responsive to noxious stimuli, later unresponsive; asterixis absent and abnormal EEG

swelling. Hypoxemia, acidosis, electrolyte imbalances, and/or cerebral edema can precipitate the development of cardiac dysrhythmias. Acute respiratory failure, progressing to ARDS, can result from pulmonary edema, aspiration pneumonia, and atelectasis. Acute renal failure caused by acute tubular necrosis, hypotension, or hemorrhage may also develop.[31] (∞Acute Respiratory Failure, p. 655; Acute Renal Failure, p. 877.)

Assessment and Diagnosis

Early recognition of FHF is extremely important. The diagnosis should include potentially reversible conditions, such as autoimmune hepatitis, as well as differentiate from decompensating chronic liver disease. Prognostic indicators such as coma grade, serum bilirubin, prothrombin time, coagulation factors, pH, and investigation of potential etiologies should be noted.

Signs and symptoms of FHF include headache, hyperventilation, jaundice, personality changes, palmar erythema, spider nevi, bruises, and edema. The patient should be evaluated for the presence of asterixis or "liver flaps," best described as the inability to voluntarily sustain a fixed position of the extremities. Asterixis is best demonstrated by having the patient extend the arms and dorsiflex the wrists, resulting in downward flapping of the hands. Hepatic encephalopathy is assessed using a grading system that stages the encephalopathy according to the patient's clinical manifestations (Box 37-14).[32] Diagnostic findings include elevated serum bilirubin, AST, alkaline phosphatase, serum ammonia, and decreased serum albumin. Arterial blood gases reveal respiratory alkalosis and/or metabolic acidosis. Hypoglycemia, hypokalemia, and hyponatremia may also be present.[31]

Factors I (fibrinogen), II (prothrombin), V, VII, IX, and X are produced by the liver exclusively. Of these, the prothrombin time may be the most useful test in the evaluation of acute FHF, as levels may be 40 to 80 seconds above control values. Decreased levels of plasmin and plasminogen and increased levels of fibrin and fibrin split products are also noted. Platelet counts are often decreased, sometimes to less than 80,000/mm^3.[34]

Medical Management

Medical interventions are directed toward management of the multiple system impact of FHF. Neomycin or lactulose is administered to remove or decrease production of nitrogenous wastes in the large intestine. Neomycin, which is given orally or rectally, reduces the bacterial flora of the colon. This aids in decreasing ammonia formation by reducing bacterial action on protein in the feces. Side effects include renal toxicity and hearing impairment. Lactulose is a synthetic ketoanalog of lactose and is split into lactic acid and acetic acid in the intestine. It is given orally, via nasogastric tube, or as a retention enema. The result is the creation of an acidic environment that decreases bacterial growth. Lactulose also traps ammonia and has a laxative effect that promotes expulsion.[33]

Bleeding is best controlled through prevention. As these patients are at risk for acute GI hemorrhage, stress ulcer prophylaxis is essential. If the patient develops active bleeding, vitamin K, fresh frozen plasma (to maintain reasonable prothrombin time), and platelet transfusions are necessary. Metabolic disturbances such as hypoglycemia, metabolic acidosis, hypokalemia, and hyponatremia should be monitored and treated appropriately. Prophylactic antibiotic administration may be initiated because the patient is at high risk for an infection. The development of cerebral edema necessitates intracranial pressure monitoring. Mannitol (although not suggested for patients experiencing associated renal failure), albumin, and hyperventilation may be used to decrease intracranial pressure. If renal failure develops, continuous renal replacement therapy should be initiated. Intubation and mechanical ventilation are necessary as hypoxemia develops. Hemodynamic instability is a common complication requiring fluid administration and vasoactive medications to avoid prolonged episodes of hypotension.[30-33] (∞Management of Intracranial Hypertension, p. 826; Continuous Renal Replacement Therapy, p. 893.)

If FHF continues and the patient shows no immediate signs of improvement or reversal, the patient should be considered for a liver transplant. Prompt referral to a transplant center should be a high priority for patients experiencing fulminant hepatic failure.[31] (∞Liver Transplantation, p. 1191.)

BOX 37-15 NURSING DIAGNOSIS AND MANAGEMENT

FULMINANT HEPATIC FAILURE

- Ineffective Breathing Pattern related to decreased lung expansion, p. 723
- Impaired Gas Exchange related to ventilation/perfusion mismatching or intrapulmonary shunting, p. 725
- Decreased Cardiac Output related to alterations in preload, p. 590
- Decreased Cardiac Output related to alterations in heart rate, p. 593
- Decreased Adaptive Capacity: Intracranial related to failure of normal compensatory mechanisms, p. 843
- Altered Renal Tissue Perfusion related to decreased renal blood flow, p. 916
- Risk for Infection, p. 1119
- Altered Nutrition: Less Than Body Requirements related to lack of exogenous nutrients or increased metabolic demand, p. 165
- Body Image Disturbance related to actual change in body structure, function, or appearance, p. 87
- Ineffective Family Coping related to critically ill family member, p. 97
- Knowledge Deficit: Discharge Regimen related to lack of previous exposure to information, p. 61 (see Patient Education Box 37-16)

Nursing Management

Nursing management of the patient with FHF incorporates a variety of nursing diagnoses (Box 37-15). Nursing management is directed toward maintenance of airway and ventilatory status, neurologic assessment and management, and maintenance of fluids and electrolytes. Continuous oxygen saturation monitoring and arterial blood gas analysis are helpful in assessing the adequacy of respiratory efforts. Strict monitoring of intake and output and electrolyte balance is essential.

As neurologic condition worsens, the nurse should be aware that respiratory depression and arrest can occur quickly. Use of benzodiazepines and other sedatives is discouraged in the FHF patient because of the "masking" of pertinent neurologic changes and further potentiating of hepatic encephalopathy. This is often difficult for the nurse to understand, since these patients may be extremely agitated and combative and require restraints for patient protection. A thorough neurologic assessment should be performed at least every hour. (∞Neurologic Physical Examination, p. 763.)

Early in the patient's hospital stay, the patient and family should be taught about fulminant hepatic failure, its etiologies, and its treatment. As the patient moves toward discharge, teaching should focus on the interventions necessary for preventing the recurrence of the precipitating etiology. If the patient is considered a liver transplant candidate, the patient and family will need significant information regarding the procedure and care. Liver transplant evaluation may include screening for medical contraindications, human immunodeficiency virus (HIV) serology, anticipated compliance, and assessment of the social support system. Psychiatric and other specialty team consultations are necessary for a thorough evaluation of the patient's suitability for a transplant (Box 37-16). (∞Liver Transplantation, p. 1191.)

BOX 37-16 PATIENT EDUCATION

FULMINANT HEPATIC FAILURE

- Fulminant hepatic failure
- Specific etiology
- Precipitating factor modification
- Interventions to reduce further episodes
- Importance of taking medications
- Life-style changes
- Diet modification
- Alcohol cessation

THERAPEUTIC MANAGEMENT

Gastrointestinal Intubation

Because GI intubation is so commonly used in critical care units, it is important for nurses to know the clinical indications and responsibilities inherent in its use. The four categories of GI tubes are based on function: nasogastric suction tubes, long intestinal tubes, esophagogastric balloon tamponade tubes, and feeding tubes. (∞Enteral Nutritional Support, p. 155.)

Nasogastric suction tubes. Nasogastric suction tubes (Levin, Salem sump) remove fluid regurgitated into the stomach, prevent accumulation of swallowed air, may partially decompress the bowel, and reduce the patient's risk for aspiration. These tubes can also be used for collecting specimens and administering tube feedings. The tube is passed through the nose into the nasopharynx and then down through the pharynx into the esophagus and stomach. The length of time the nasogastric tube remains in place depends on its use. The tube is then placed to gravity, low-intermittent suction, or low continuous suction, or, in rare instances, it is clamped.

NURSING INTERVENTION CLASSIFICATIONS

BOX 37-17 Tube Care: Gastrointestinal

DEFINITION: Management of a patient with a gastrointestinal tube

ACTIVITIES:

Monitor for correct placement of the tube by inspecting oral cavity, checking pH level of aspirate, and noting placement per x-ray, as appropriate
Connect tube to suction, as appropriate
Secure tube to appropriate body part with consideration for patient comfort and skin integrity
Irrigate tube, as appropriate
Monitor for sensations of fullness, nausea, and vomiting
Monitor bowel sounds
Monitor for diarrhea
Monitor fluid and electrolyte status
Monitor amount, color, and consistency of nasogastric output
Replace the amount of gastrointestinal output with the appropriate IV solution, as ordered
Provide nose and mouth care 3 to 4 times daily or as needed
Provide hard candy or chewing gum to moisten mouth, as appropriate
Initiate and monitor delivery of enteral tube feedings, as appropriate
Teach patient and family how to care for tube, as appropriate
Provide skin care around tube insertion site
Remove tube, as indicated

From McCloskey JC, Bulechek GM: *Nursing interventions classification,* ed 2, St Louis, 1996, Mosby.

Nursing management is focused on preventing complications common to this therapy, such as ulceration and necrosis of the nares, esophageal reflux, esophagitis, esophageal erosion and stricture, gastric erosion, and dry mouth and parotitis from mouth breathing. In addition, interference with ventilation and coughing, aspiration, and loss of fluid and electrolytes can also be critical problems. Interventions include irrigating the tube every 4 hours with normal saline solution, ensuring the blue air vent of the Salem sump is patent and maintained above the level of the patient's stomach, and providing frequent mouth and nare care. Box 37-17 outlines the nursing activities for managing a patient with a GI tube.

Long intestinal tubes. Miller-Abbott, Cantor, Johnston, and Baker tubes are examples of long intestinal tubes that are placed either preoperatively or intraoperatively. The long length allows the removal of contents from the intestine that cannot be accomplished by a nasogastric tube. These tubes can decompress the small bowel and splint it intraoperatively or postoperatively. Because progression of the tubes depends on bowel peristalsis, their use is contraindicated in patients with paralytic ileus and severe mechanical bowel obstructions.

Interventions used in the care of the patient with a long intestinal tube are similar to those with a nasogastric tube. The patient should be observed for gaseous distention of the balloon section, which makes removal difficult; rupture of the balloon or spillage of mercury into the intestine; overinflation of the balloon, which can lead to intestinal rupture; and reverse intussusception if the tube is removed rapidly. Intestinal tubes should be removed slowly; usually 6 inches of the tube is withdrawn every hour (Box 37-17).

Esophagogastric balloon tamponade tubes. Currently there are three different types of balloon tamponade tubes available: the Sengstaken-Blakemore tube, Linton tube, and Minnesota tube. The Sengstaken-Blakemore tube has three lumens: one for the gastric balloon, one for the esophageal balloon, and one for gastric suction (Figure 37-4, *A*). The Linton tube also has three lumens: one for the gastric balloon, one for gastric suction, and one for esophageal suction (Figure 37-4, *B*). The Minnesota tube has four lumens: one for the gastric balloon, one for the esophageal balloon, one for gastric suction, and one for esophageal suction (Figure 37-4, *C*). The Minnesota tube is preferable to the other tubes because it offers both a gastric and an esophageal balloon and allows suction to be applied both above and below the balloons (in the stomach and in the esophagus).[35]

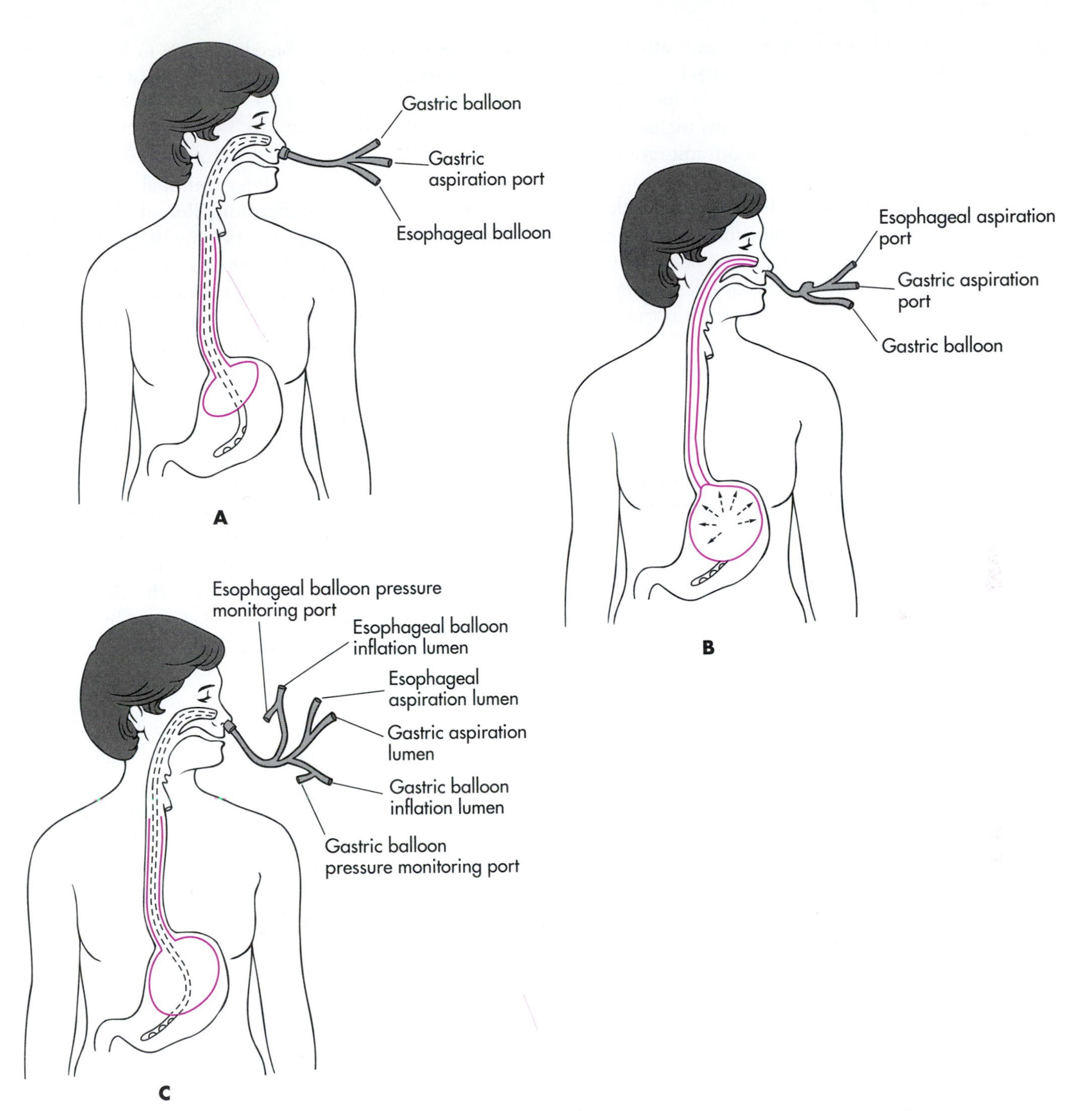

FIGURE 37-4. Esophageal tamponade tubes. **A,** Sengstaken-Blakemore tube. **B,** Linton tube. **C,** Minnesota tube.

Balloon tamponade tubes are inserted by the physician. Once the tube is passed into the stomach and placement assessed, the gastric balloon is inflated with 250 to 300 ml of air (or as specified by the tube manufacturer). The tube is then placed under tension so that the gastric balloon places pressure on the gastroesophageal junction. Two to three pounds of tension is usually applied using a helmet with a constant traction spring device. Once secured in place, the esophageal balloon is inflated to a pressure of 25 to 45 mm Hg. Low intermittent suction is applied to both the gastric and esophageal ports. Once the patient's bleeding has stopped for 24 hours, the esophageal balloon is deflated; if rebleeding does not occur over the next 24 hours, the gastric balloon is deflated. If there is no further bleeding, the tube is discontinued 24 hours later.[35]

Nursing management of the patient with a balloon tamponade tube includes monitoring for rebleeding and observing for complications of the tube. The most common complication is pulmonary aspiration, which can be limited by emptying the stomach and placing an endotracheal tube before passing the balloon tamponade tube. Additional complications include esophageal erosion and rupture, balloon migration, and nasal necrosis. Balloon migration can be a potentially life-threatening complication. If the gastric balloon is allowed to slowly deflate or ruptures, the esophageal balloon migrates upward where it can occlude the patient's airway. If the patient develops respiratory distress, the gastric and esophageal balloon ports should be cut immediately.[35]

Endoscopic Sclerotherapy

Endoscopic sclerotherapy is used to control the bleeding of acute or chronic varices. It may be performed emergently, electively, or prophylactically. An endoscope is introduced through the patient's mouth, and panendoscopy is performed of the esophagus and stomach to identify the bleeding varices. An injector with a retractable needle is introduced through the biopsy channel of the endoscope. Once in place, the needle is inserted into a varix and/or into an area around the varix and the sclerosing agent is injected. The sclerosing agent causes an inflammatory reaction in the vessel that results in thrombosis and eventually a fibrous band. Repeated sclerotherapy results in the development of supportive scar tissue around the varices.[12]

Sclerotherapy controls acute variceal bleeding in 71% to 96% of patients, with bleeding recurring in approximately 20% to 30% of these cases and a complication rate of approximately 22%. Complications can vary from mild to severe and include fever, tachycardia, temporary dysphagia, chest pain, esophageal perforation, and anaphylaxis.[3]

Endoscopic Variceal Band Ligation

Endoscopic variceal band ligation involves applying latex bands or clips (endoscopic clipping) around the circumference of the bleeding varices to induce venous obstruction and control bleeding. In 1 to 2 days after the procedure, necrosis and scar formation promote band and tissue sloughing. Fibrinous deposits within the healing ulcer potentiate vessel obliteration. Band ligation is accomplished via endoscopy, with five to 10 bands being placed initially. The procedure may be repeated on an inpatient or outpatient basis over 1 to 4 weeks, until all the varices are obliterated.[12]

Endoscopic variceal band ligation controls bleeding approximately 86% of the time. This procedure has a lower complication rate (2%) than sclerotherapy but a higher incidence of rebleeding (40% to 50%).[3] Complications include transient dysphagia and chest pain.[12]

Transjugular Intrahepatic Portosystemic Shunt

A transjugular intrahepatic portosystemic shunt (TIPS) is an angiographic interventional procedure for decreasing portal hypertension. Recent data suggest that TIPS is advocated in patients with portal hypertension who are also experiencing active bleeding or poor liver reserve, in transplant patients, or in patients with other operative risks.[34] The TIPS procedure is usually performed by a gastroenterologist, vascular surgeon, or interventional radiologist.

Portal hypertension is first confirmed via direct measurement of the pressure in the portal vein (gradient greater than 10 mm Hg). Cannulation is achieved via the internal jugular vein, and an angiographic catheter is advanced into the middle or right hepatic vein. The midhepatic vein is then catheterized, and a new route is created connecting the portal and hepatic veins, using a needle and guidewire with a dilating balloon. A expandable stainless steel stent is then placed in the liver parenchyma to maintain that connection (Figure 37-5). The increased resistance in the liver is therefore bypassed.[36]

TIPS may be performed on patients with bleeding varices or refractory bleeding varices, or it may be used as a "bridge" to liver transplant if the candidate becomes hemodynamically unstable. Postprocedure care should include observation for overt (cannulation site) or covert (intrahepatic site) bleeding, hepatic or portal vein laceration (resulting in rapid loss of blood volume), and inadvertent puncture of surrounding organs. Other complications include bile duct trauma, stent migration, and stent thrombosis. Loss of shunt patency occurs 5% to 75% of the time as a result of shunt thrombosis or stenosis. The 30-day mortality for this procedure is approximately 24% to 45%.[36]

Intramucosal pH Monitoring

Intramucosal pH (pHi) refers to the indirect tonometric measurement of the pH of the gastric mucosa. This relatively noninvasive measurement is obtained via a standard vented nasogastric sump tube that has been combined with a silicone balloon system. It is important to note that pHi is not the same measurement as gastric fluid pH. pHi provides the clinician with an indirect measurement of gastric mucosal pH, which yields helpful cellular and metabolic data.

The nasogastric tonometer (NGT) is primed to clear all air, then inserted as a normal nasogastric tube (Figure 37-6). Once inserted, the balloon lies close to the

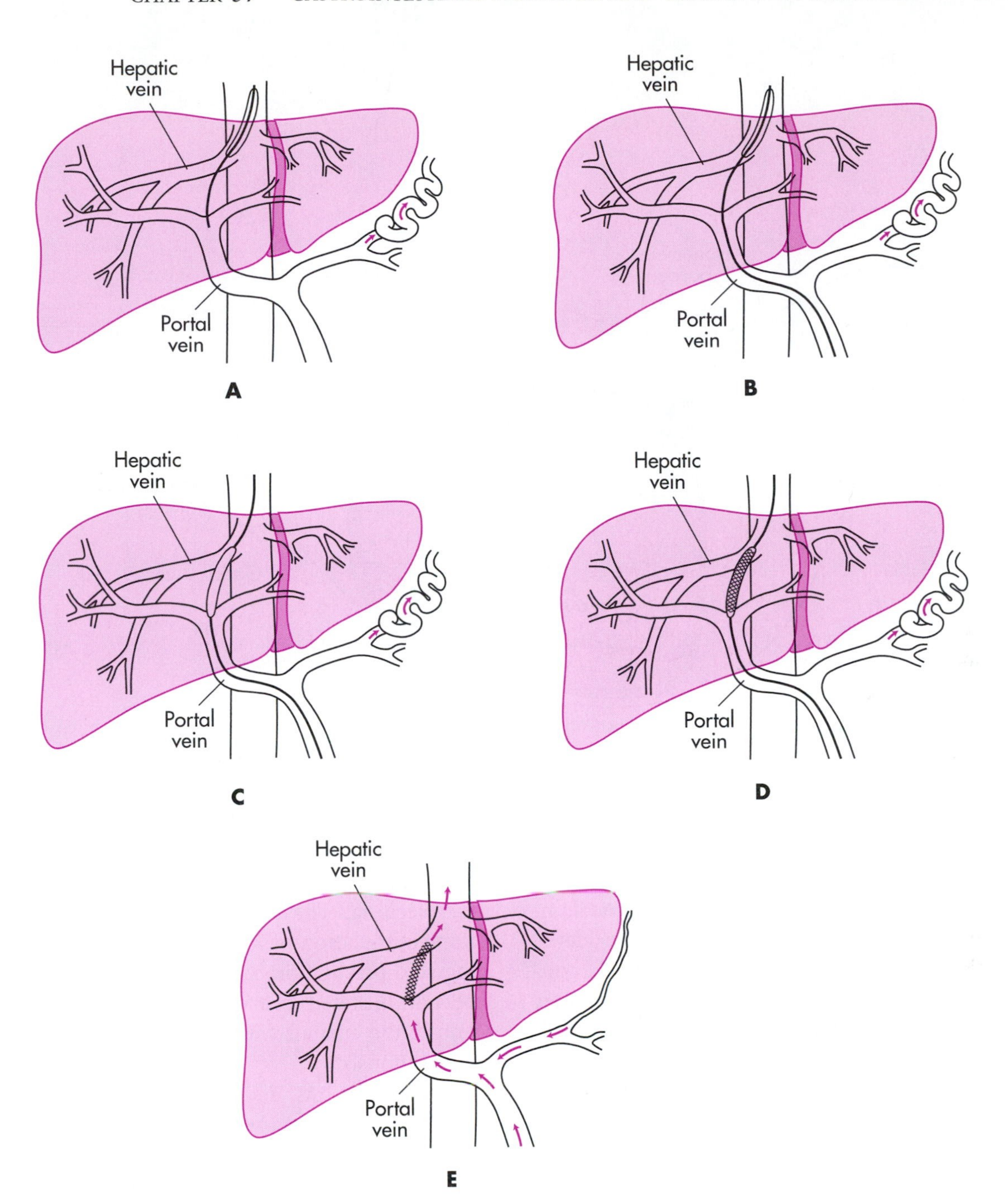

FIGURE 37-5. Transjugular intrahepatic portosystemic shunt (TIPS). **A,** Needle directed through liver parenchyma to portal vein. **B,** Needle and guidewire passed down to midportal vein. **C,** Balloon dilation. **D,** Deployment of stent. **E,** Intrahepatic shunt from portal to hepatic vein. (From Zemel G and others: Percutaneous transjugular portosystemic shunt, *JAMA* 266:391, 1991.)

gastric mucosa. The balloon is then infused with 2.5 ml of anaerobic saline solution. The balloon is semipermeable to carbon dioxide (CO_2), which is produced by cells during the normal metabolic process. The level of CO_2 in the saline solution in the balloon equilibrates with the level of CO_2 in the gastric mucosal cells after 30 to 90 minutes. The saline solution is then withdrawn anaerobically and sent along with an arterial blood gas sample to the blood gas laboratory. The CO_2 from the saline solution and the HCO_3^- from the arterial blood gas sample are then correlated in the Henderson-Hasselbalch equation to determine pHi.[37]

A normal pHi is 7.35 to 7.45, the same as a normal arterial blood gas value. This value may decrease (indicating acidosis) in the presence of decreased gastric/splanchnic perfusion, as in vascular shunting

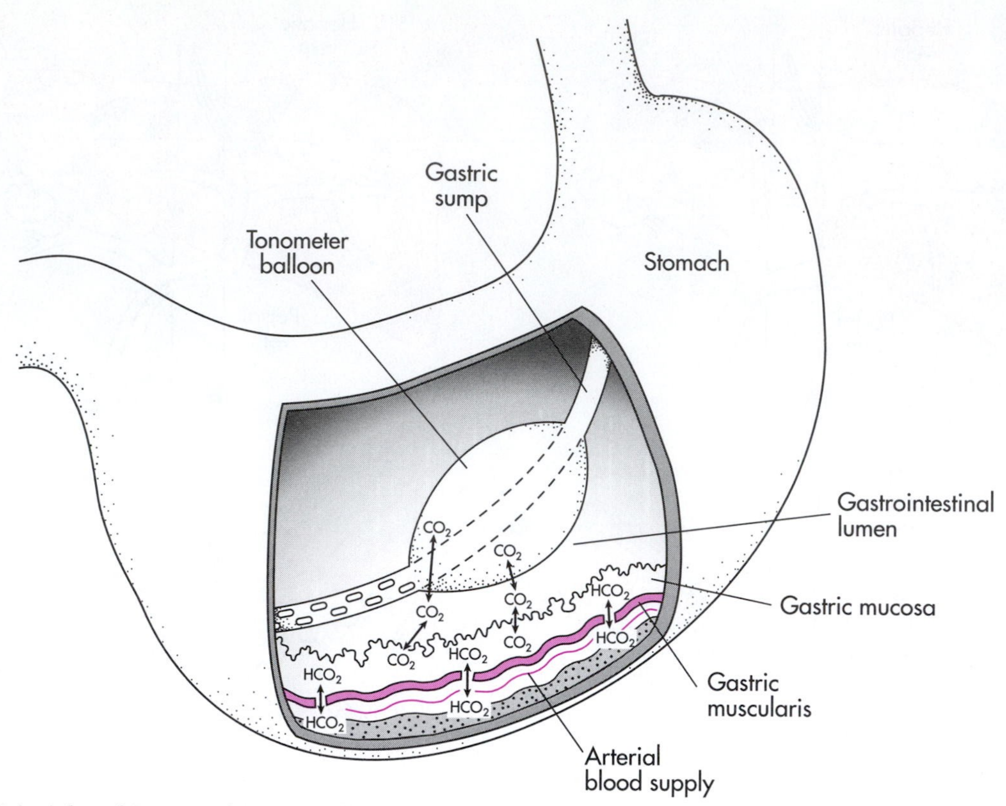

FIGURE 37-6. Principles of $Paco_2$ and HCO_3^- diffusion in gastric tonometry. (From Clark CH, Gutierrez G: Gastric intramucosal pH: a noninvasive method for the indirect measurement of tissue oxygenation, *Am J Crit Care* 1:53, 1992.)

associated with shock. pHi is considered a "window" to the gut, providing the clinician with regional instead of global monitoring. Since the gut is considered a sensitive indicator of early shunting in shock, continued development and use of this technology may result in an enhanced clinical picture in the recognition and early treatment of shock.[37]

Nursing considerations with the use of pHi monitoring include strict user sampling procedures, particularly emphasizing the need for strict anaerobic technique during sampling, and waiting at least 90 minutes between samples. The reproducibility of the value is enhanced by ensuring the patient is taking H_2 antagonists.[38] In addition, all antacids and gastric feedings should be discontinued at least 2 hours before sampling.

Pharmacologic Agents

Various pharmacologic agents are used in the care of patients with GI disorders. Table 37-4 reviews the various agents and any special considerations necessary for administering them.[39]

H_2 antagonists. H_2 antagonists are commonly used in the critical care setting to decrease volume and concentration of gastric secretions and control gastric pH, thus decreasing the incidence of stress-related upper GI bleeding. These agents work by blocking histamine stimulation of acid-secreting cells, thus decreasing acid production. Although all of these drugs may be administered orally, intramuscularly, or intravenously the current trend is to administer these drugs intravenously.[1]

Vasopressin. As discussed earlier, vasopressin is a treatment modality used to control gastric ulcer and variceal bleeding. It is administered intraarterially, through a catheter inserted into the right or left gastric artery (via the femoral artery, aorta, and celiac trunk), or intravenously.[15] It reduces mesenteric blood flow and subsequently portal pressure.[12]

A major side effect of the drug is systemic vasoconstriction, which can result in cardiac ischemia and chest pain, hypertension, congestive heart failure, dysrhythmias, phlebitis, bowel ischemia, and cerebral vascular accident. These side effects can be offset with the concurrent administration of nitroglycerin.[3] Other complications include bradycardia and fluid retention.[12] Nursing responsibilities with the use of this therapy include maintenance of a patent infusion system and continuous monitoring for vasoconstrictive complications of therapy.

TABLE 37-4 Pharmacologic Agents Used in the Management of GI Disorders

Drug	Dosage	Actions	Special Considerations
Antacids	30-90 ml q 1-2 hr PO or NG; possibly titrated to NG pH	Used to buffer stomach acid and raise gastric pH	Can cause diarrhea or constipation and electrolyte disturbances Irrigate NG tube with water after administration because antacids can clog tube
Histamine$_2$ antagonist		Used to reduce volume and concentration of gastric secretions	Side effects include CNS toxicity (confusion or delirium) and thrombocytopenia Separate administration of antacids and histamine$_2$ antagonists by 1 hr
Cimetidine (Tagamet)	300 mg q 6 hr IV or PO		
Ranitidine (Zantac)	150 mg q 12 hr PO or 50 mg q 8 hr IV		
Famotidine (Pepcid)	40 mg qd PO or 20 mg q 12 hr IV		
Cytoprotective agents		Form an ulcer-adherent complex with proteinaceous exudate; cover the ulcer and protect against acid, pepsin, and bile salts	Requires an acid medium for activation; do not give with histamine$_2$ antagonists May cause severe constipation May cause decreased absorption of certain drugs (e.g., phenytoin)
Sucralfate (Carafate)	1 g q 6 hr NG or PO		
Gastric proton pump inhibitors		Inactivate hydrogen pump, thus blocking secretion of hydrochloric acid by gastric parietal cells	Capsules should be swallowed intact May increase levels of phenytoin, diazepam, or warfarin May administer concomitantly with antacids
Omeprazole (Prilosec)	20-40 mg q 12 hr PO		
Vasopressin (Pitressin)	Loading dose of 20 units over 20 minutes IV followed by 0.2 to 0.8 units/min IV infusion	Vasoconstrictor used to lower portal pressure by decreasing blood flow to the splanchnic bed	Side effects include coronary, mesenteric, and peripheral vasoconstriction May be administered concurrently with nitroglycerin to minimize side effects

REFERENCES

1. Prevost SS, Oberle A: Stress ulceration in the critically ill patient, *Crit Care Nurs Clin North Am* 5:163, 1993.
2. Lichtenstein DR, Berman MD, Wolfe MM: Approach to the patient with acute upper gastrointestinal hemorrhage. In Taylor MB, editor: *Gastrointestinal emergencies,* Baltimore, 1992, Williams & Wilkins.
3. Brewer TG: Treatment of acute gastroesophageal variceal hemorrhage, *Med Clin North Am* 77:993, 1993.
4. *St Anthony's DRG guidebook 1997,* Reston, Va, 1996, St Anthony Publishing.
5. DeMarkles MP, Murphy JR: Acute lower gastrointestinal bleeding, *Med Clin North Am* 77:1085, 1993.
6. Gupta PK, Fleischer DE: Nonvariceal upper gastrointestinal bleeding, *Med Clin North Am* 77:973, 1993.
7. Mertz HR, Walsh JH: Peptic ulcer pathophysiology, *Med Clin North Am* 75:799, 1991.
8. McQuaid KR, Isenberg JI: Medical therapy of peptic ulcer disease, *Surg Clin North Am* 72:885, 1992.
9. Fisher RL, Pipkin GA, Wood JR: Stress-related mucosal disease: pathophysiology, prevention, and treatment, *Crit Care Clin* 11:323, 1995.

10. Huether SE, McCance KL, Tarmina MS: Alterations of digestive function. In McCance KL, Huether SE, editors: *Pathophysiology: the biologic basis for disease in adults and children,* ed 2, St Louis, 1994, Mosby.
11. Joff DL, Chung RT, Friedman LS: Management of portal hypertension and its complications, *Med Clin North Am* 80:1021, 1996.
12. McEwen DR: Management of alcoholic cirrhosis of the liver, *AORN J* 64:214, 1996.
13. Geier DL, Cooke AR: Upper GI bleeding: a five step approach to diagnosis and treatment, *J Crit Illness,* 7:1676, 1992.
14. Sugawa C, Joseph AL: Endoscopic interventional management of bleeding duodenal and gastric ulcers, *Surg Clin North Am* 72:317, 1992.
15. Rosen RJ, Sanchez G: Angiographic diagnosis and management of gastrointestinal hemorrhage: current concepts, *Radiol Clin North Am* 32:951, 1994.
16. Jutabha R, Jensen DM: Management of upper gastrointestinal bleeding in the patient with chronic liver disease, *Med Clin North Am* 80:1035, 1996.
17. Smith SL, Butler RW: *Acute pancreatitis. Part I. An overview,* Aliso Viejo, Ca, 1993, American Association of Critical Care Nurses.
18. Forsmark CC, Toskes PP: Acute pancreatitis: medical management, *Crit Care Clin* 11:295, 1995.
19. Steer ML: Acute pancreatitis. In Taylor MB, editor: *Gastrointestinal emergencies,* Baltimore, 1992, Williams & Wilkins.
20. Singh M, Simsek H: Ethanol and the pancreas, *Gastroenterology* 98:1051, 1990.
21. Brown A: Acute pancreatitis: pathophysiology, nursing diagnoses, and collaborative problems, *Focus Crit Care* 18(2):121, 1991.
22. Ranson JHC: Complications of pancreatitis. In Taylor MB, editor: *Gastrointestinal emergencies,* Baltimore, 1992, Williams & Wilkins.
23. Ranson J: The current management of acute pancreatitis, *Adv Surg* 28:93, 1995.
24. Krumberger JM: Acute pancreatitis, *Crit Care Nurs Clin North Am* 5:185, 1993.
25. Butler RW, Smith: *Acute pancreatitis. Part II. Complications and surgical management,* Aliso Viejo, Ca, 1993, American Association of Critical Care Nurses.
26. McConnell EA: Loosening the grip of intestinal obstructions, *Nursing* 24(3):34, 1994.
27. Scovill WA: Small bowel obstruction. In Cameron JL, editor: *Current surgical therapy,* ed 5, St Louis, 1995, Mosby.
28. Choti MA: Obstruction of the large bowel. In Cameron JL, editor: *Current surgical therapy,* ed 5, St Louis, 1995, Mosby.
29. Steinhagen RM, Aufses AH: Acute abdominal obstruction: when to consider nonoperative therapy, *J Crit Illness* 8:209, 1993.
30. Ganger D and others: Hepatic failure. In Parrillo JE, Bone RC, editors: *Critical care medicine: principles of diagnosis and management,* St Louis, 1995, Mosby.
31. Lidofsky SD: Fulminant hepatic failure, *Crit Care Clin* 11:415, 1995.
32. Kucharski SA: Fulminant hepatic failure, *Crit Care Nurs Clin North Am* 5:141, 1993.
33. Elrod R: Problems of the liver, biliary tract, and pancreas. In Lewis SM, Collier IC, Heitkemper MM, editors: *Medical-surgical nursing: assessment and management of clinical problems,* ed 4, St Louis, 1996, Mosby.
34. Becker YT and others: The role of elective operation in the treatment of portal hypertension, *Ann Surg* 62:171, 1996.
35. Amato EJ: A nursing reference: gastrointestinal tubes and drains. II. Esophageal tubes, *Crit Care Nurs* 3(1):46, 1983.
36. Bouley G and others: Transjugular intrahepatic portosystemic shunt: an alternative, *Crit Care Nurs* 16(1):26, 1996.
37. Clark CH, Gutierrez G: Gastric intramucosal pH: a noninvasive method for the indirect measurement of tissue oxygenation, *Am J Crit Care* 1:53, 1992.
38. Taylor DE, Gutierrez G: Tonometry: a review of clinical studies, *Crit Care Clin* 12:1007, 1996.
39. McEvoy GK, editor: *American hospital formulary service drug information,* Bethesda, Md, 1996, American Society of Health-System Pharmacists.

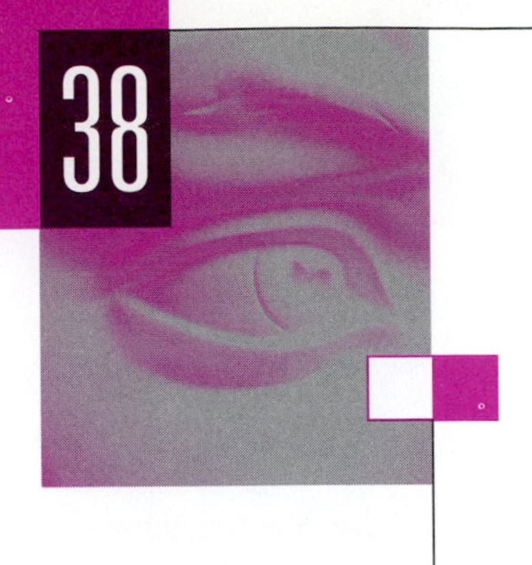

Gastrointestinal Nursing Diagnosis and Management

THIS CHAPTER IS designed to supplement the preceding chapters in the *Gastrointestinal Alterations* unit by integrating theoretic content into clinically applicable case studies and nursing management plans.

The case study is designed to illustrate clinical problem solving and patient care management occurring in actual patients. The case, reviewed retrospectively, demonstrates how medical and nursing diagnoses may be effectively used in critical care. The case study also demonstrates revisions to the plan of care and the nursing and medical management outcomes that are apt to occur during the course of a complicated hospitalization as the patient responds physiologically to treatment. Often in a short case anecdote, such as that presented in this chapter, the clinical answer may appear to be obvious from the day of admission. In practice, however, critical care patient management is sometimes investigative and the "correct" diagnosis for an individual patient may not become apparent until midway in the hospitalization. Alternatively, a patient with an apparently straightforward diagnosis may develop an unexpected complication, and the plan of care and potential outcomes will then require revision. Many of the case studies demonstrate this principle.

The nursing management plans, which—unlike the case study—are not patient specific, provide a basis nurses can use to individualize care for their patients. In the previous *Gastrointestinal Alterations* chapters, each medical diagnosis is assigned a Nursing Diagnosis and Management box. Using this box as a page guide, the reader can access relevant nursing management plans for each medical diagnosis. For example, nursing management of *acute gastrointestinal hemorrhage,* described on p. 945, may involve several nursing diagnoses and management plans outlined in this chapter and in other Nursing Diagnosis and Management chapters. Specific examples are (1) *Fluid Volume Deficit related to absolute loss,* on p. 914; (2) *Powerlessness related to lack of control over current situation or disease progression,* on p. 89; (3) *Risk for Aspiration,* on p. 727; and (4) *Knowledge Deficit: Discharge Regimen related to lack of previous exposure to information,* on p. 61. These examples highlight the interrelationship of the various physiologic systems in the body and the fact that pathology often has a multisystem impact in the critically ill.

Use of the case study and management plans can enhance the understanding and application of the *Gastrointestinal* content in clinical practice.

CASE STUDY

GASTROINTESTINAL

CLINICAL HISTORY

Mrs. M is a 47-year-old Native American woman about whom little is known.

CURRENT PROBLEMS

Mrs. M was brought by automobile to the hospital because she vomited blood earlier in the day. She was intoxicated on arrival at the hospital. Her friends, who were also intoxicated, left immediately. The patient promptly vomited more blood in the emergency room and became hypotensive. During the brief period when the patient could give a history, she said she had been in the hospital earlier and someone had put a tube in her stomach. No other direct medical history was available.

MEDICAL DIAGNOSES

Acute upper gastrointestinal (GI) bleed
Hypovolemic shock

NURSING DIAGNOSES

Fluid Volume Deficit related to absolute loss: blood
Acute Confusion related to sensory overload, sensory deprivation, and sleep pattern disturbance
Risk for Aspiration risk factor: increased intragastric pressure

PLAN OF CARE

1. Admit patient to the critical care unit (CCU) for medical and nursing management of acute upper GI bleeding.
2. Achieve hemostasis.
3. Replace lost blood volume.
4. Correct hypovolemic shock.
5. Maintain adequacy of oxygenation status.

MEDICAL AND NURSING MANAGEMENT AND PATIENT OUTCOME

To deal with a presumed variceal bleed, Mrs. M was started on intravenous vasopressin at 0.4 units/minute. A Sengstaken-Blakemore tube was inserted, and after an x-ray film was obtained, both gastric and esophageal balloons were inflated with 40 mm Hg pressure. Because Mrs. M's systolic blood pressure (BP) decreased to 50 mm Hg, fluid resuscitation was begun. She received a total of 8 units of packed red blood cells, 4 units of fresh frozen plasma, and 7 L of crystalloid solution (lactated Ringer's and normal saline solution). Dopamine infusion at 2-5 μg/kg/min was initiated to help raise her blood pressure. Because of massive vomiting of blood and hypotension, Mrs. M was intubated to protect her airway. After initiation of these treatments, the nursing assessment revealed the following:

Neuro: Mrs. M was very agitated while being ventilated and was given a sedative and paralytic agent. She was able to move all extremities before a paralytic state was induced.

Resp: She was intubated and ventilated. Lungs remarkable for crackles at both bases. Ventilator settings: FIO_2, 40%; tidal volume, 900 ml; intermittent mandatory ventilation (IMV) mode, respiratory rate, 8; no positive end-expiratory pressure (PEEP) or pressure support ventilation (PSV).

CV: Sinus tachycardia with rate of 140. Blood pressure up to 136/80 mm Hg after fluid resuscitation. Extremities without edema. Heart without murmur, gallop, rub, or click. Large-bore IV in the right femoral venous position.

Integument/Temp: Skin cool and dry with palpable peripheral pulses. No jaundice. Rectal temperature 100° F.

Medications: Because Mrs. M's blood pressure rose so quickly after fluid resuscitation, dopamine was weaned off. After insertion of the Sengstaken-Blakemore tube, bleeding seemed stopped; therefore vasopressin infusion was also weaned off. Because of mild pulmonary congestion after fluid administration, Mrs. M was given 20 mg of intravenous furosemide to promote diuresis.

GI: Sengstaken-Blakemore tube in place. Abdomen soft, bowel sounds present. No stigmata of chronic liver disease.

GU: Foley catheter intact, draining 20 to 30 ml/hour of clear, amber-colored urine.

Lab: Blood alcohol level, 130 mg/dL; prothrombin time, 15.1 seconds with an international normalized ratio (INR) of 1.9; potassium, 3.1 mEq/L (replaced); O_2 saturation, 96%; hematocrit, 46% (hematocrit takes up to 72 hours to equilibrate after an acute bleeding episode.)

CASE STUDY—CONT'D

GASTROINTESTINAL

MEDICAL DIAGNOSES

Acute upper GI bleed (resolving)
Volume overload

NURSING DIAGNOSIS

Fluid Volume Deficit related to absolute loss: blood

REVISED PLAN OF CARE

1. Discontinue the Sengstaken-Blakemore tube.
2. Continue to monitor for fluid volume and electrolyte imbalances, and replace fluids and electrolytes as needed.
3. Localize the site of bleeding by endoscopy, and provide endoscopic sclerotherapy if necessary.
4. Monitor for delirium tremens (DTs) related to alcohol withdrawal.
5. Ensure adequacy of oxygenation via monitoring of respiratory status and ventilator settings.

MEDICAL AND NURSING MANAGEMENT AND PATIENT OUTCOME

Sixteen hours after CCU admission, Mrs. M's Sengstaken-Blakemore tube was removed without difficulty. No further bleeding ensued. Endoscopy verified esophageal varices. No other bleeding sites were found. She received sclerotherapy (9.5 ml of 5% sodium morrhuate) to prevent further bleeding. Fluid volume balance was maintained effectively, with urine output 50 to 100 ml/hour and electrolytes within normal limits. Blood urea nitrogen (BUN) and creatinine also were within normal limits. Mrs. M still required quite a bit of sedation while she was on the ventilator; she demonstrated agitation and thrashing about in bed as the sedation wore off. Although vital signs were stable (BP, 102/47; respiratory rate [RR], 14; pulse [P], 114), Mrs. M's rectal temperature rose to 100.4° F and rhonchi were audible in both lung fields. White blood cell count was 11,000, and arterial blood gases measured as follows: pH, 7.52; $Paco_2$, 36 mm Hg; Pao_2, 69 mm Hg; O_2 saturation, 96%.

MEDICAL DIAGNOSES

Acute GI bleed (resolving)
Pneumonia
Delirium tremens/alcohol withdrawal syndrome

NURSING DIAGNOSES

Impaired Gas Exchange related to ventilation/perfusion mismatching
Sensory/Perceptual Alterations related to alcohol withdrawal

REVISED PLAN OF CARE

1. Culture sputum, urine, and blood.
2. Remove right femoral IV and start new IV.
3. Begin empiric antibiotic therapy.
4. Continue to provide sedation as needed until delirium tremens lessens.
5. Continue ventilatory support until respiratory status more stable.

MEDICAL AND NURSING MANAGEMENT AND PATIENT OUTCOME

The remainder of Mrs. M's stay in CCU was uneventful. Her urine culture was positive for *Escherichia coli,* blood culture was positive for *Staphylococcus aureus,* and sputum culture was positive for *S. aureus,* as well as *Haemophilus influenzae.* She was started on antibiotics and was given aggressive pulmonary toilet by her nurses. A new triple-lumen central venous catheter was placed without difficulty. Sedation was decreased, and ventilatory support was lessened. On day 4, agitation was decreasing, allowing less sedation. Mrs. M was effectively coughing up copious pulmonary secretions, temperature had decreased to 100° F, and she was placed on a T-tube with 40% oxygen. On day 5, Mrs. M continued to need less sedation and was demonstrating less agitation. Temperature was down to 99.8° F, and she was extubated without difficulty. With no further evidence of GI bleeding, she was transferred to the stepdown unit.

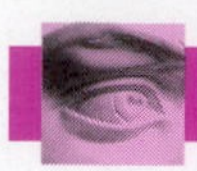

NURSING MANAGEMENT PLAN

IMPAIRED SWALLOWING

DEFINITION:

The state in which an individual has decreased ability to voluntarily pass fluids and/or solids from the mouth to the stomach.

Impaired Swallowing Related to Neuromuscular Impairment, Fatigue, and Limited Awareness

DEFINING CHARACTERISTICS

- Evidence of difficulty swallowing
  - Drooling
  - Difficulty handling oral secretions
  - Absence of gag, cough, and/or swallow reflex
  - Moist, wet, gurgling voice quality
  - Decreased tongue and mouth movements
  - Presence of dysarthria
  - Difficulty handling solid foods:
    - Uncoordinated chewing or swallowing
    - Stasis of food in the oral cavity
    - Wet-sounding voice or change in voice quality
    - Sneezing, coughing, or choking with eating
    - Delay in swallowing for more than 5 seconds
    - Change in respiratory pattern
  - Difficulty handling liquids:
    - Momentary loss of voice or change in voice quality
    - Nasal regurgitation of liquids
    - Coughing with drinking
- Evidence of aspiration
  - Hypoxemia
  - Productive cough
  - Frothy sputum
  - Wheezing, crackles, or rhonchi
  - Temperature elevation

OUTCOME CRITERIA

- Absence of evidence of swallowing difficulties.
- Absence of evidence of aspiration.

NURSING INTERVENTIONS AND *RATIONALE*

1. Collaborate with physician and speech therapist regarding a swallowing evaluation and rehabilitation program ***to decrease the incidence of aspiration.***
2. Collaborate with physician and dietitian regarding a nutritional assessment and nutritional plan ***to ensure that the patient is receiving enough nutrition.***
3. Place the patient in an upright position with the head midline and the chin slightly down ***to keep food in the anterior portion of the mouth and to prevent it from falling over the base of the tongue into the open airway.***
4. Provide patient with single-textured soft foods (e.g., cream cereals) that maintain their shape ***because these foods require minimal oral manipulation.***
5. Avoid particulate foods (e.g., hamburger) and foods containing more than one texture (e.g., stew) ***because these foods require more chewing and oral manipulation.***
6. Avoid dry foods (e.g., popcorn, rice, crackers) and sticky foods (e.g., peanut butter, bananas) ***because these foods are difficult to manipulate orally.***
7. Provide patients with thick liquids (e.g., fruit nectar, yogurt) ***because thick liquids are more easily controlled in the mouth.***
8. Thicken thin liquids (e.g., water, juice) with a thickening preparation or avoid them ***because thin liquids are easily aspirated.***
9. Place foods in the uninvolved side of the mouth ***because oral sensitivity and function are greatest in this area.***
10. Avoid the use of straws ***because they can deposit the liquid too far back in the mouth for the patient to handle.***
11. Serve foods and liquids at room temperature ***because the patient may be overly sensitive to heat or cold.***
12. Offer solids and liquids at different times ***to avoid swallowing solids before being properly chewed.***
13. Provide oral hygiene after meals ***to clear food particles from the mouth that could be aspirated.***
14. Collaborate with physician and pharmacist regarding oral medication administration ***to adjust medication regimen to prevent aspiration and choking and to ensure all prescribed medications are swallowed.***
15. Crush tablets (if appropriate) and mix with food that is easily formed into a bolus, use thickened liquid medications (if available), and/or embed small capsules into food ***to facilitate oral medication administration.***
16. Inspect mouth for residue following all medication administration ***to ensure medication has been swallowed.***
17. Educate patient and family on the swallowing problem, rehabilitation program, and emergency measures for choking ***H***

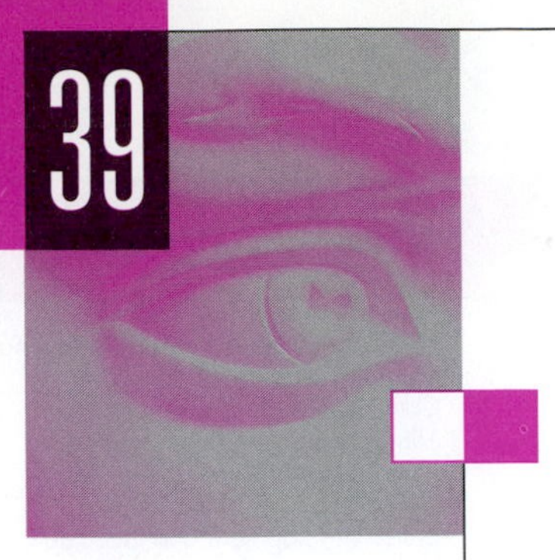

39 Endocrine Anatomy and Physiology

MAINTAINING DYNAMIC EQUILIBRIUM among the various cells, tissues, organs, and systems of the human body is a highly complex and specialized process. Two systems regulate these critical relationships: the nervous system and the endocrine system. The nervous system communicates by nerve impulses that control skeletal muscle, smooth muscle tissue, and cardiac muscle tissue. The endocrine system controls and communicates by distributing potent hormones throughout the body (Figure 39-1 lists the endocrine glands and their hormones, target tissues, and actions). When stimulated, the endocrine glands secrete hormones into surrounding body fluids. Once in circulation, these hormones travel to specific target tissues where they exert a pronounced effect. Receptors found on or within these specialized target tissue cells are equipped with molecules that recognize the hormone and bind it to the cell, producing a specific response.

Specific hormones either stimulate or inhibit a physiologic response. Hormone actions are either organ specific or generalized. The hormone prolactin is targeted to one organ only. Prolactin maintains milk production for breast-feeding. An example of a hormone with a generalized effect is thyroxine, which maintains the rate of metabolism throughout the body.

The endocrine alterations unit will discuss nursing management of endocrine disorders in a critical care setting. The typical patient in the critical care unit has undergone massive disruption to his or her homeostasis as a result of the admitting diagnosis. The degree to which this imbalance can be rectified will depend, in part, on the proper functioning of the patient's endocrine system. If the endocrine hormones cannot restore oxygen to the cells, compensate for fluid and electrolyte imbalance, and restore metabolic demands, the patient may be faced with an additional life-threatening complication.

Not all endocrine problems will require critical care interventions. Most clients with common endocrine abnormalities are diagnosed by their primary care provider, followed up with periodic laboratory tests to determine subtle endocrine changes and perhaps given a replacement hormone or other medication to compensate for any persistent imbalance.

The critical care nurse may not be aware of endocrine dysfunction in the patient newly admitted to the intensive care unit. Clinical manifestations of the underlying pathologic endocrine conditions may initially be overshadowed by the presenting systems' failures. The critical care nurse will need to focus on admitting the patient or collecting data relating to the primary diagnosis. The patient's history may not be inclusive; perhaps an endocrine imbalance was diagnosed in the past but because the imbalance was thought to be well controlled with daily replacement therapy, the patient and/or family may feel that the disorder is not worthy of mention. The endocrine disorder may be a chronic, undiagnosed problem whereby the patient has coped with abnormal signs and symptoms by attributing them to the "aging process." It is also possible that the endocrine system may have been functioning adequately, but now it may be unable to tolerate the illness that caused admission to the critical care environment.

Clinical and laboratory data reflecting endocrine responses to nonendocrine life-threatening diseases must be acknowledged and adequately treated. Without prompt interventions, death may occur as a result of endocrine dysfunction rather than the primary disease.

Selected endocrine disorders of the pancreas, pituitary, and thyroid are presented in this chapter.

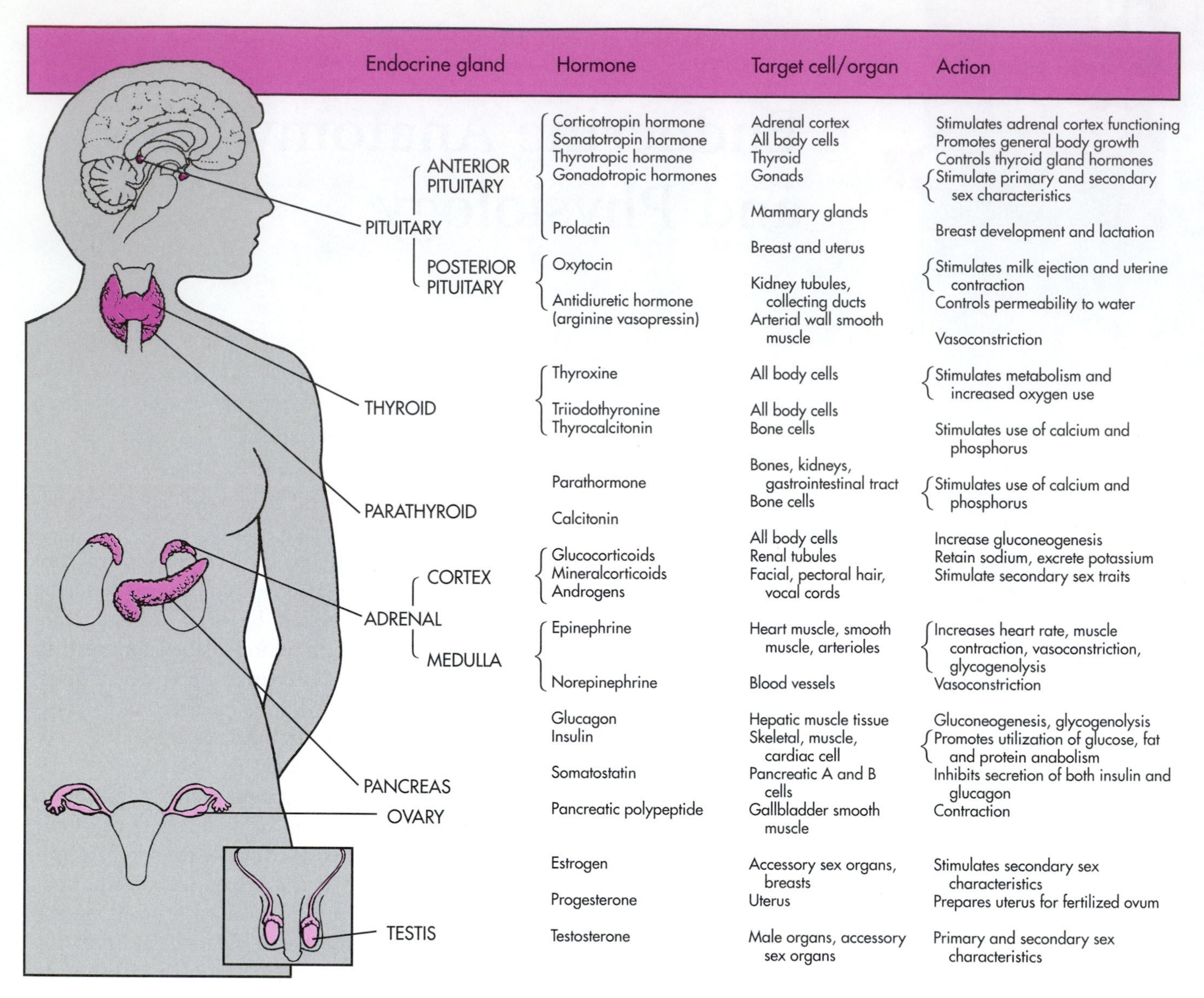

Endocrine gland
Hormone
Target cell/organ
Action
ANTERIOR PITUITARY
PITUITARY
POSTERIOR PITUITARY
Corticotropin hormone
Somatotropin hormone
Thyrotropic hormone
Gonadotropic hormones
Prolactin
Oxytocin
Antidiuretic hormone (arginine vasopressin)
Adrenal cortex
All body cells
Thyroid
Gonads
Mammary glands
Breast and uterus
Kidney tubules, collecting ducts
Arterial wall smooth muscle
Stimulates adrenal cortex functioning
Promotes general body growth
Controls thyroid gland hormones
Stimulate primary and secondary sex characteristics
Breast development and lactation
Stimulates milk ejection and uterine contraction
Controls permeability to water
Vasoconstriction
THYROID
Thyroxine
Triiodothyronine
Thyrocalcitonin
All body cells
All body cells
Bone cells
Stimulates metabolism and increased oxygen use
Stimulates use of calcium and phosphorus
PARATHYROID
Parathormone
Calcitonin
Bones, kidneys, gastrointestinal tract
Bone cells
Stimulates use of calcium and phosphorus
CORTEX
ADRENAL
MEDULLA
Glucocorticoids
Mineralcorticoids
Androgens
All body cells
Renal tubules
Facial, pectoral hair, vocal cords
Increase gluconeogenesis
Retain sodium, excrete potassium
Stimulate secondary sex traits
Epinephrine
Norepinephrine
Heart muscle, smooth muscle, arterioles
Blood vessels
Increases heart rate, muscle contraction, vasoconstriction, glycogenolysis
Vasoconstriction
PANCREAS
Glucagon
Insulin
Somatostatin
Pancreatic polypeptide
Hepatic muscle tissue
Skeletal, muscle, cardiac cell
Pancreatic A and B cells
Gallbladder smooth muscle
Gluconeogenesis, glycogenolysis
Promotes utilization of glucose, fat and protein anabolism
Inhibits secretion of both insulin and glucagon
Contraction
OVARY
Estrogen
Progesterone
Accessory sex organs, breasts
Uterus
Stimulates secondary sex characteristics
Prepares uterus for fertilized ovum
TESTIS
Testosterone
Male organs, accessory sex organs
Primary and secondary sex characteristics

FIGURE 39-1. Location of endocrine glands with hormones, target cell/organ, and hormone action.

Diabetic ketoacidosis (DKA) is a complication of Type I diabetes, or insulin-dependent diabetes mellitus, and is an endocrine emergency. DKA occurs when cells, starved for glucose, rely on protein and fat for their energy needs. A dangerous shift in the acid-base balance occurs when the noncarbohydrate substances are catabolized and, unless corrected, coma and death follow. DKA is one of the most common endocrine disorders seen in the critical care unit. (∞DKA, p. 1003.)

Hyperglycemic hyperosmolar nonketotic syndrome (HHNS), previously referred to as hyperglycemic hyperosmolar nonketotic coma[1] is a potentially lethal metabolic disorder, with a mortality between 10% and 50%.[2] It involves undetected high levels of blood glucose, the absence of acidosis, increased osmolality of the blood, and profound dehydration. Unless the events are interrupted, coma and death quickly ensue. When HHNS is seen in critical care, it is typically seen as a complication of the primary diagnosis. (∞HHNS, p. 1015.)

Diabetes insipidus (DI) and syndrome of inappropriate antidiuretic hormone (SIADH) are two pituitary disorders that disrupt the body's regulation of plasma osmotic pressure and circulating blood volume. These diseases are rarely seen as sole admitting diagnoses to critical care. These dysfunctions either precipitate or develop along with the patient's life-threatening illnesses. (∞Diabetes Insipidus, p. 1021; SIADH, p. 1027.)

Thyroid crisis, also called thyrotoxic crisis or thyrotoxic storm, is an uncommon emergency caused by an excess of thyroid hormones that carries a high mortality. Crisis occurs when a sudden rise in the body's metabolic processes leads to tachydysrhythmias and hyperthermia. This extreme form of hyperthyroidism jeopardizes vital homeostasis. (∞ Thyroid Crisis, p. 1031.)

Myxedema coma is a serious but rare abnormality that occurs as a result of an extreme deficiency in thyroid hormones. Severe hypothyroidism prevents the body's metabolism from adjusting to the increasing demands of the precipitating critical nonthyroid disease. The resulting extreme metabolic slowing usually results in coma and death if untreated. (∞Myxedema Coma, p. 1038.)

Disorders of the adrenal glands will not be presented in this unit. Adrenal insufficiency (Addison's disease) and adrenal cortical excess (Cushing's syndrome) are not discussed because of their extreme rarity in the critical care unit.

THE PANCREAS

Description

The pancreas is generally triangular in shape. The base end of the organ lies in the C-shaped curvature of the duodenum, and the apex extends behind and below the stomach toward the spleen. It is approximately 15 cm (6 inches) long and 4 cm (1 to 2 inches) wide. Specialized exocrine cells within the pancreas secrete digestive enzymes into a 3 mm duct that transverses the pancreas and empties into the duodenum. Figure 39-2 shows the pancreatic duct, known also as the *duct of Wirsung,* which forms the passageway for pancreatic juice during intestinal digestion.

Function

The endocrine functions of the pancreas are accomplished by many clusters of cells that appear to form tiny islands among the exocrine cells. These islets of Langerhans are composed of four distinct cell types. The cells are known as *A, B, D,* and *F cells* (see Figure 39-2). *A cells* secrete glucagon, *B cells* secrete insulin, *D cells* secrete somatostatin, and *F cells* secrete pancreatic polypeptide hormone.

Glucagon, insulin, somatostatin, and polypeptide hormones are released into the surrounding capillaries to empty into the portal vein, where they are distributed to target cells in the liver. They then go into general circulation to reach other target cells.

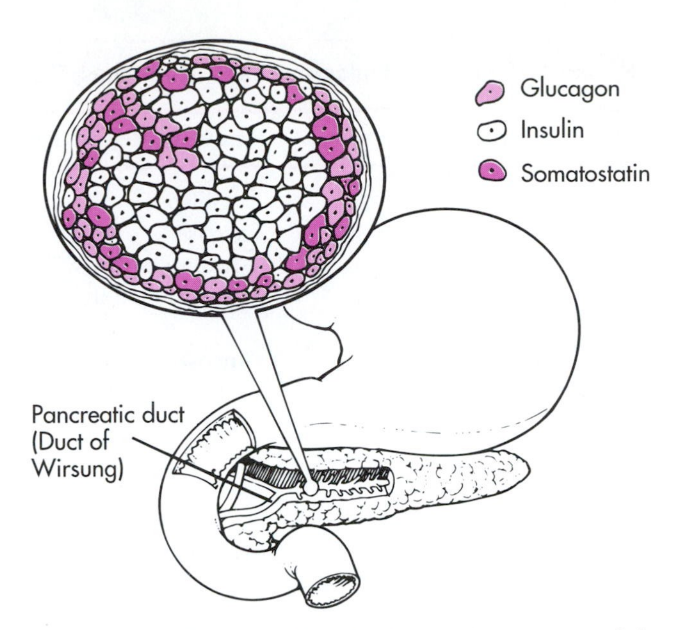

FIGURE 39-2. Macroscopic and microscopic structure of the pancreas.

Pancreatic Hormones

Insulin. Insulin is responsible for the storage of carbohydrate, protein, and fat nutrients. It is a potent anabolic hormone that is stimulated by the presence of glucose. It is the only hormone produced in the body that directly lowers glucose levels in the blood stream. Insulin also augments the transport of potassium into the cells, decreases the mobilization of fats, and stimulates protein synthesis (Table 39-1). (See Box 39-1 for terms and definitions frequently used when discussing glucose/insulin balance.)

The major stimulant for insulin secretion is glucose (Box 39-2). When serum glucose levels are within 80 to 90 mg/dL, the serum insulin levels are approximately 25 ng/minute/kg of body weight. When glucose levels rapidly rise to 200 mg, as would occur during a meal, insulin secretion rises to 11 times the baseline.[3]

Functions of insulin

Anabolism. Glucose is admitted to the skeletal, cardiac, and adipose cells for use as energy in the presence of effective insulin. Excess glucose, in the form of glycogen, is stored in the hepatic and muscle cells for use as fuel at a later time. The movement of glucose from the circulation into the intracellular compartment reduces the presence of glucose in the blood stream and helps preserve the blood's osmolality. Simultaneously, glucose is available to the cell as its main energy source.

TABLE 39-1 Pancreatic Endocrine Cells, Hormones, Stimulant Release Factor, Target Tissue, and Response/Action

Cell	Hormone	Stimulant Release Factor	Target Tissue	Response/Action
A	Glucagon	↓ Glucose Exercise ↑ Amino acids SNS stimulation	Hepatocyte Myocyte	↑ Glucose in blood stream ↑ Gluconeogenesis ↑ Glycogenolysis Fat mobilization Protein mobilization
B	Insulin	Glucose	Skeletal cells Muscle cells Cardiac cells	↓ Blood glucose ↓ Fat mobilization ↑ Fat storage ↓ Protein mobilization ↑ Protein synthesis ↑ Glucogenesis
D	Somatostatin	Hyperglycemia	A cells B cells	↓ Blood glucose ↓ Glycogen secretion ↓ Insulin secretion
F	Pancreatic polypeptide	Acute hypoglycemia	Gallbladder Smooth muscle	↑ Gallbladder contraction ↓ Pancreatic enzyme

SNS, Sympathetic nervous system.

BOX 39-1 Frequently Used Terms When Discussing Insulin/Glucose Imbalance

Anabolism—constructive phase of metabolism where the body converts simple substances into more complex compounds in the presence of energy.
Catabolism—destructive phase of metabolism where the body breaks down complex substances to form simpler substances in the presence of energy.
Gluconeogenesis—formation of glucose from noncarbohydrate nutrients (i.e., fats, protein). It occurs in the liver.
Glycogenolysis—conversion of stored glucose (called glycogen and typically stored in the liver and muscles) into usable, free state.
Ketonemia—production of ketone bodies more rapid than the body can process through the liver. Acetone, beta-hydroxybutyric acid, and acetoacetic acid buildup in the blood stream.
Ketonuria—excess of ketone bodies filtered from the blood stream and excreted in the urine.
Osmolality—measurement of number of particles in a solution or the concentration of a solution.

BOX 39-2 Agents That Release or Inhibit Insulin

INSULIN RELEASE* (MAJOR STIMULANT: ELEVATED BLOOD GLUCOSE LEVEL)	INSULIN INHIBITION (MAJOR INHIBITOR: LOW BLOOD GLUCOSE LEVEL)
HORMONES	
Glucagon	Somatostatin
Corticotropic hormone	Norepinephrine
Thyrotropin	Epinephrine
Somatotropin	
Glucocorticoids	
Secretin	
Gastrin	
DRUGS	
Beta-adrenergic stimulators	Beta-adrenergic blocking agents
Sulfonylurea	Diazoxide
Theophylline	Phenytoin
Acetylcholine	Thiazide/sulfonamide diurectics

*NOTE: Vagal stimulation can affect insulin release also.

Central nervous system glucose uptake. The central nervous system is freely permeable to glucose. It does not rely on insulin for the transport of glucose across the cell membrane. Brain cells store only a minimum of glycogen for energy release. These cells are unable to use the end product of gluconeogenesis for energy. Decreased insulin levels alone (hyperglycemia) do not damage brain cells; however, these cells cannot survive the glucose deficiency (hypoglycemia) that occurs from hypersecretion of insulin.[4]

BOX 39-3 Insulin/Glucagon Ratio and its Effect on Carbohydrate, Fat, and Protein Metabolism

BALANCED INSULIN/ GLUCAGON	DECREASED INSULIN/ INCREASED GLUCAGON
↑ Use of glucose by cells	↓ Use of glucose by cells
↑ Movement of potassium intracellularly	↓ Movement of potassium intracellularly
↑ Carbohydrate metabolism	↑ Blood glucose
↓ Gluconeogenesis	↑ Gluconcogenesis
↑ Glycogen storage	↓ Glycogen storage
↓ Glycogenolysis	↑ Glycogenolysis
↓ Lipolysis	↑ Lipolysis
↓ Fat mobilization	↑ Fat mobilization
↑ Fat storage	↓ Fat stores
↓ Protein mobilization	↑ Hepatic metabolism fats
↑ Protein synthesis	↑ Ketogenesis
	↑ Mobilization of protein
	↑ Proteolysis
	↑ Lipoprotein

Lipid anabolism. Fat metabolism is also affected by adequate, effective insulin levels. In the presence of insulin, fat is stored in connective tissues, thereby reducing fat mobilization and fat catabolism. Protein metabolism also benefits from adequate insulin supply.

Protein sparing. Insulin admits the transfer of glucose across the cell wall to the cell receptor site. By having glucose (carbohydrate) available as the body's fuel source, protein is spared from use as energy. Protein is then available for critical protein synthesis for amino acid active transport into the cells, for construction of blood proteins, and for the conversion of ribonucleic acid (RNA) into new protein.

Abnormal insulin levels. Insufficient or ineffective insulin levels lead to hyperglycemia, which deprives cells of their energy source. This forces the body to shift from using glucose as fuel to using fat and protein as fuel. Fats and protein are catabolized in an attempt to provide a reserve source of glucose through a process called *gluconeogenesis.* Fats are broken down to fatty acids and glycerol. The glycerol is oxidized as carbohydrate, whereas the fatty acids are converted to ketone bodies. Ketosis occurs when the ketone bodies accumulate faster than they are metabolized.

Protein is catabolized when the body's stores of carbohydrate and fat are depleted. As part of this process, amino acids are broken down to form ammonia and ketoacids. Nitrogen is removed from the amino groups, and the resulting ammonia is detoxified by the liver and removed by the kidneys in the form of urea. Through gluconeogenesis, the ketoacids are converted to glucose.

In a catabolic state the body is unable to maintain the protein synthesis needed for healthy functioning and blood proteins are used for energy. Without necessary insulin to act on the cell receptor site, blood glucose levels increase. In addition, the end products of fat and protein catabolism collect in the blood stream.

Glucagon. Glucagon, synthesized by the A cells, has the opposite effect of insulin. Glucagon counterregulates insulin levels and raises blood sugar levels. It is a potent gluconeogenic hormone. By means of gluconeogenesis, it forms glucose from noncarbohydrate sources, such as fat and protein. Glucagon release is stimulated by such factors as a decrease in circulating insulin, an increase in blood amino acids, a fall in blood sugar level, starvation, exercise, or stimulation of the sympathetic nervous system (see Box 39-2). Glucagon is released to protect the body from the hypoglycemia that may result from these conditions.

Initially, glucagon stimulates the release of glycogen stored in the liver and muscle cells to meet short-term energy needs. Through a process called *glycogenolysis,* the glycogen stored in the liver and muscles is converted back into a glucose form to be used by the cells. If the energy needs are long-term, the glucagon stimulates glucose release through the more complex process of gluconeogenesis. In gluconeogenesis, fat and protein nutrients are rapidly broken down into end products that are then changed into glucose.

A normal blood glucose level is maintained in the healthy body by the insulin/glucagon ratio. When the blood glucose level is high, insulin is released and glucagon is inhibited. When blood glucose levels are low, glucagon rather than insulin is released (Box 39-3). The insulin/glucagon ratio is considered more important in the overall metabolism of fuel sources than is the absolute level of either hormone.

Somatostatin. Somatostatin is a protein hormone that inhibits the release of both insulin and glucagon. Somatostatin is synthesized by the pancreatic D cells, the hypothalamus, gastric mucosa, and elsewhere. The hormone decreases glucagon secretion, and in high quantities it decreases insulin release (see Table 39-1).

Hyperglycemia stimulates the activity of the D cells. It is theorized that the release of insulin causes somatostatin to keep the B cells under control. It also is believed that somatostatin allows the gradual influx of glucose into the cell after ingestion of a meal, thus preventing postprandial hyperglycemia.

Pancreatic polypeptide. Pancreatic polypeptide synthesized by the F cells within the islets of Langerhans is not yet completely understood. While levels of pancreatic polypeptide are stimulated by acute hypoglycemia and by ingestion of a balanced, nutrient-dense meal, the effect of hypersecretion or hyposecretion of this hormone is not yet identified.[5] The hormone represses pancreatic enzyme secretion, and, less importantly, it also relaxes the smooth muscle tissue of the gallbladder. Pancreatic polypeptide release can be stimulated by acute hypoglycemia or by an intake that is high in protein and low in carbohydrate.[6]

PITUITARY GLAND AND HYPOTHALAMUS

The hypothalamus is linked to the pituitary gland in two distinct ways: a vascular network connects the anterior portion of the pituitary with the hypothalamus, while a separate pathway of nerve fibers connects the posterior pituitary with the hypothalamus. Understanding the proximity of the hypothalamus and the pituitary gland is necessary to appreciate the correlation that exists between these organs.

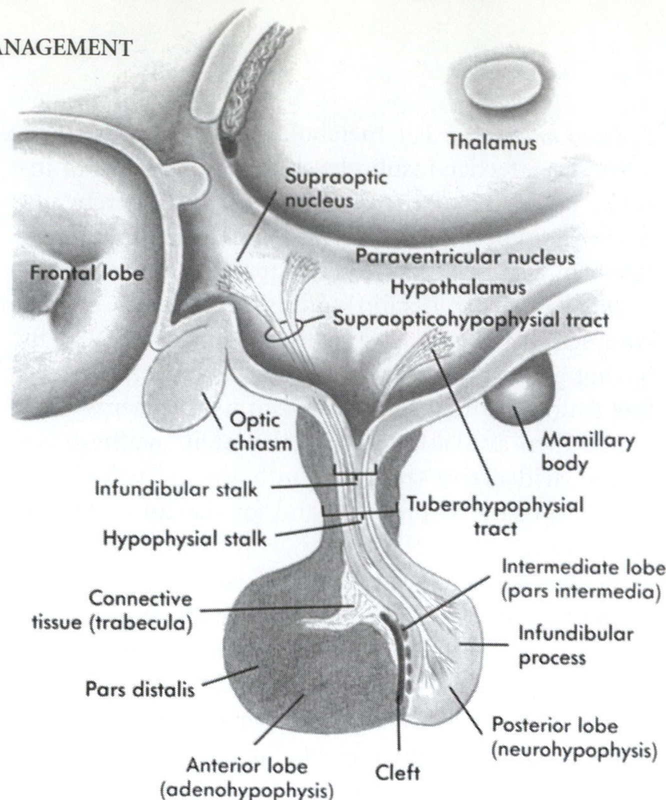

FIGURE 39-3. Anatomy of the hypothalamus and the pituitary gland and their location in the skull. (Modified from Thompson JM and others: *Mosby's clinical nursing,* ed 4, St Louis, 1997, Mosby.

Hypothalamus

The hypothalamus lies in the base of the brain, superior to the pituitary gland. It is composed of specialized nervous tissue responsible for the integrated functioning of the nervous system and endocrine system, which is termed *neuroendocrine control.* The hypothalamus weighs approximately 4 g and forms the walls and lower portion of the third ventricle of the brain. The area composing the floor of the ventricle thickens in the center and elongates. It is from this funnel-shaped portion, called the *infundibular stalk* (or stem), that the pituitary gland is suspended (Figure 39-3). The infundibular stalk contains a rich vascular supply and a network of communicating neurons that travels from the hypothalamus to the pituitary. The vascular network and neural pathways transport chemical and neural signals and maintain constant communication between the nervous system and the endocrine system.

Pituitary gland

Description. The pituitary gland, also called the *hypophysis* because it is attached below the hypothalamus, is found recessed in the base of the cranial cavity in a hollow depression of the sphenoid bone known as the *sella turcica.* Secured in such a protected environment, the pituitary is one of the most inaccessible endocrine glands in humans. Yet it is because of this very location that the pituitary gland is susceptible to injury from surgical and accidental trauma of the face and head.

Function. The pituitary gland has been known as the *master gland* because of the major influence it has over all areas of body functioning. It is now known, however, that the pituitary does not act independently. Rather, the release and inhibition of its hormones are actually controlled by the hypothalamus. The hypothalamus controls pituitary response by secreting substances termed *release-inhibiting factors.* These factors then control the release or inhibition of hormones. Thyrotropin-releasing hormone (TRH) is an example of a release-inhibiting factor. Virtually every function necessary to maintaining the human body in a state of dynamic equilibrium is regulated in this manner. The pituitary is composed of three parts (see Figure 39-3): the anterior lobe, the intermediate lobe, and the posterior lobe. Each component within the pituitary has its own origin, morphology, and function.

Anterior pituitary. The anterior lobe of the pituitary, also called the *adenohypophysis,* is the largest portion of the gland. It communicates with the hypothalamus by means of a vascular network. Several hormones are produced by the glandular tissue of the anterior pituitary.

Although the exact number of hormones produced here is uncertain, it is known that adrenocorticotropic hormone (ACTH), thyroid-stimulating hormone (TSH), follicle-stimulating hormone (FSH), luteinizing hormone (LH), growth hormone, and prolactin are manufactured here. Information about all the hormones, their target tissue, and their action is found in Figure 39-1.

Intermediate pituitary. The intermediate lobe of the pituitary, the *pars intermedia,* is located in the central portion of the pituitary between the anterior and posterior lobes. Although the pars intermedia is present in the fetus, it gradually merges with and becomes indistinct from the posterior lobe in the adult. The functions of the pars intermedia in humans are poorly understood.

Posterior pituitary. The posterior lobe of the pituitary is called the *neurohypophysis.* It retains its continuity with the hypothalamus by means of neural fibers running through the infundibular stalk. The neurohypophysis has no glandular properties but functions as an extension of the hypothalamus. It collects, stores, and later releases hormones that are produced in the hypothalamus.

After hormones are synthesized in the hypothalamus, they are transported to the posterior pituitary until the hypothalamus signals their release. Oxytocin (Pitocin) and arginine vasopressin (antidiuretic hormone) are both manufactured in the hypothalamus and stored in the posterior pituitary.

Pituitary hormones

Oxytocin. Oxytocin stimulates smooth muscle contraction of the uterus and causes the myoepithelial cells of the breast to contract and force milk from the alveoli into the secretory ducts. Pathologic conditions caused by hypersecretion or hyposecretion of oxytocin have not been identified.[7] Insufficient amounts of oxytocin are known to result in delayed labor and delivery. Exogenous oxytocin is used clinically to induce labor, to augment contractions during the first and second stages of labor, and to manage postpartum hemorrhage.

Antidiuretic hormone. Antidiuretic hormone (ADH), known also as *arginine vasopressin (AVP),* has been identified as the single most important hormone responsible for regulating fluid balance within the body. ADH has two functions: it constricts smooth muscles within the arterial wall (pharmacologic doses may elevate blood pressure), and, more importantly, it maintains the osmolality of the blood in a very narrow range. ADH regulates fluid balance by altering the permeability of the kidney tubule.

ADH also contributes to control of the sodium level in the extracellular fluid by control of plasma osmolality. Plasma osmolality is determined largely by the sodium ion concentration process in the plasma. Osmoreceptors, believed to be sodium receptors,[3] are located in the hypothalamus and are sensitive to changes in the circulating plasma osmolality. When sodium levels rise, plasma osmolality increases. ADH is released to stimulate fluid reabsorption at the nephron to retain water and maintain sodium balance. Permeability of the kidney tubules is increased, and water is reabsorbed from the renal filtrate in the presence of ADH. This process decreases water loss from the body and subsequently concentrates and reduces urine volume. Fluid conserved in this manner is returned to the circulating plasma, where it dilutes the concentration (osmolality) of plasma (Figure 39-4).

The release of ADH increases with hypovolemia. The release of ADH is regulated primarily by the plasma osmotic pressure and the volume of circulating blood. Stretch receptors located in the left atrium are sensitive to volume changes in the plasma, as may be caused by vomiting, diarrhea, or blood loss. Hemorrhage, sufficient to lower the blood pressure, and emesis, sufficient to reduce fluid volume, will stimulate the release of ADH. Other factors capable of influencing ADH secretion are pain, stress, malignant disease, surgical intervention, alcohol, and drugs (see Box 39-4 for additional factors that affect ADH levels).

THE THYROID GLAND

Description

The thyroid gland, considered the largest endocrine gland, weighs from 15 to 30 g. (The size of the adult gland varies according to the availability of dietary iodine in different parts of the world.[8]) The gland partially encases the trachea, is wrapped around the second to fourth tracheal rings anteriorly and laterally, and is located at the level of the sixth and seventh cervical vertebrae posteriorly. The thyroid gland lies below the thyroid cartilage and the articulating surface of the cricoid cartilage.

This bow tie–shaped gland has two lateral lobes that are partially covered by the sternohyoid and sternothyroid muscles. The thyroid isthmus, the band of narrow thyroid tissue that connects the lateral lobes, lies directly below the cricoid cartilage (Figure 39-5). The richly vascularized thyroid tissue receives about 5 ml of blood/gram/minute. (This perfusion exceeds the normal 3 ml/gram/minute perfusion to the nephron.[9]) The basic functional units of the thyroid gland are spherical-shaped cells called *follicles.* Follicles are filled with a protein thyroglobulin.

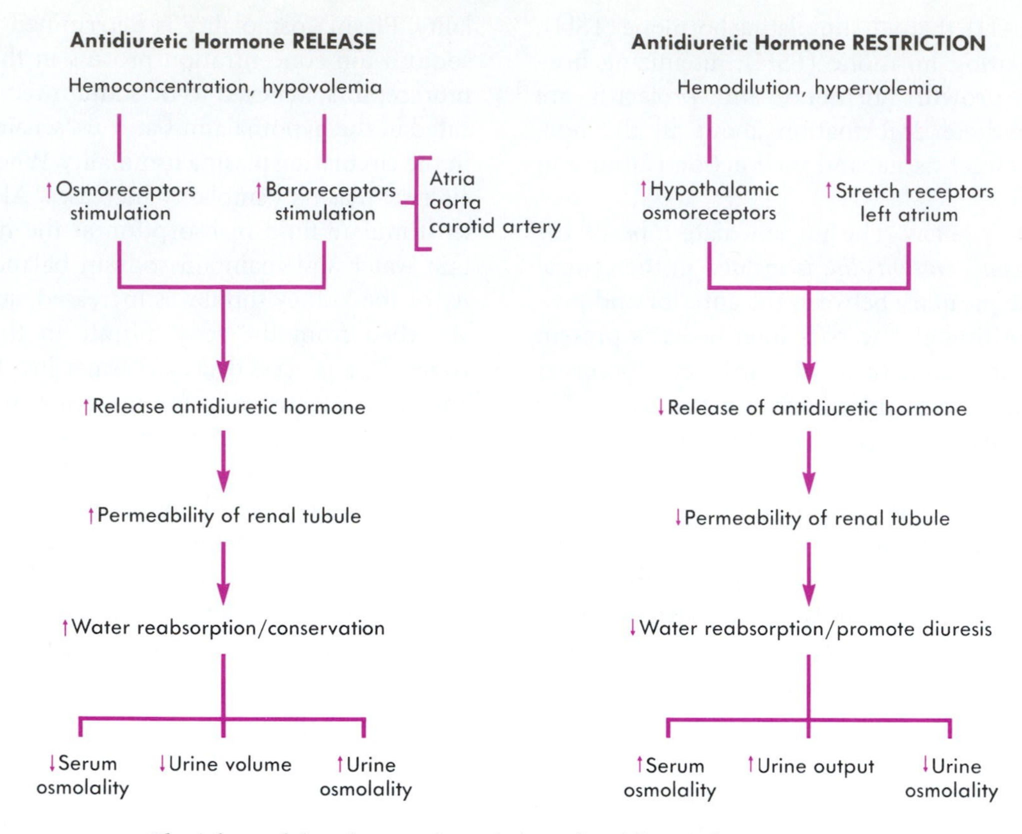

FIGURE 39-4. Physiology of the release and restriction of antidiuretic hormone.

Function

The functioning of the thyroid gland depends in part on the hypothalamus, anterior pituitary, dietary intake of iodine, and circulating protein bodies in the blood. The anterior lobe of the pituitary gland secretes thyrotropin (TSH), which prompts the thyroid cells to produce thyroid hormones. Through a complex process, dietary iodine is absorbed and concentrated in the thyroid follicles. The iodine is oxidized to iodide, and, through active transport, the amino acid tyrosine binds the iodide to the thyroglobulin and eventually yields triiodothyronine (T_3) and thyroxine (T_4). More than 99% of T_3 and T_4 circulates through the blood supply bound to the serum transporting proteins, thyroxin-binding globulin, prealbumin, and albumin.[10] The minute amount of free thyroid hormone that is not protein bound is responsible for activating thyroid responses throughout the body.

Whereas both T_4 and T_3 are produced by the thyroid gland, T_3 is primarily the result of the conversion of T_4 to T_3 in the peripheral tissues of the liver, kidneys, heart, and other tissues. (This conversion can be slowed by certain drugs, such as beta-adrenergic blocking agents.) T_3 acts more rapidly on target tissues in the body than does T_4 and is more actively potent than T_4. Both thyroid hormones affect the rate at which oxygen is used in the body and therefore affect all metabolic processes in the body.

The thyroid gland also produces a third hormone, thyrocalcitonin, also called *calcitonin.* This hormone is produced by the parafollicular cells or C cells found scattered among the follicular cells. Calcitonin reduces levels of calcium in the blood stream by augmenting calcium absorption in the bone. Throughout this unit, discussion of thyroid hormone refers collectively to T_3 and T_4, not calcitonin.

The hypothalamus-pituitary-thyroid axis describes the mechanism for the synthesis and secretion of thyroid hormone (Figure 39-6). The entire production and secretion of thyroid hormone is regulated by a feedback mechanism that limits the amount of hormone circulating to the cellular need at that time. This regulatory cycle prevents the unwanted increase in metabolism caused by a rise in circulating hormones and, conversely, a lethargy or slowness in reaction caused by a decreased secretion of hormones.[10]

BOX 39-4 Factors Affecting Antidiuretic Hormone

ANTIDIURETIC HORMONE STIMULATION	ANTIDIURETIC HORMONE RESTRICTION
Increased serum osmolality	Decreased serum osmolality
Emesis	Hypervolemia
Hypovolemia	Water intoxication
Hemorrhage	
Pain	Cold
	Congenital defect
	CO_2 inhalation
Trauma to hypothalamic-hypophyseal system	Trauma to hypothalamic-hypophyseal system
Accidental	Accidental
Surgical	Surgical
Pathologic	Pathologic
Stress	
Physical	
Emotional	
Acute infections	
Malignancies	
Nonmalignant pulmonary disorders	
Stimulated pulmonary baroreceptors	
Nocturnal sleep	
Drugs	Drugs
Nicotine	Phenytoin
Barbiturates	Chlorpromazine
Oxytocin	Reserpine
Glucocorticoids	Norepinephrine
Anesthetics	Ethanol
Acetaminophen	Narcotics
Amitriptyline	Lithium
Carbamazepine	Demeclocycline
Cyclophosphamide	Tolazamide
Chlorpropamide	
K^+-depleting diuretics	
Vincristine	
Isoproterenol	

Thyroid functioning presents a clear example of the hypothalamus, pituitary, and thyroid axis and a negative feedback loop (Figure 39-6). The negative feedback loop includes the hypothalamus, which, when stimulated by neural mechanisms in response to decreased circulating T_3 and T_4, secretes TRH. The TRH activates thyrotropin, TSH, in the anterior pituitary. TSH then stimulates the thyroid gland to manufacture and release the thyroid hormones T_3 and T_4. When serum blood levels of T_3 and T_4 become high, the pituitary inhibits the production of additional TSH. When levels of T_3 and T_4 become too low, the pituitary is stimulated to secrete additional TSH.

Hormones

Thyroid hormone stimulates oxygen consumption, increases the metabolic processes in almost all cells, and activates heat production. Thyroxine prompts the activation of beta-adrenergic receptors in widespread areas of the body.[11] These receptors trigger a sympathetic nervous system response and release epinephrine at various nerve endings. The effect is stimulation of the cardiac tissue, nervous tissue, and smooth muscle tissue, as well as an increase in metabolism and thermogenesis, or increased body heat. Box 39-5, Major Functions of Thyroid Hormones, offers additional detail.

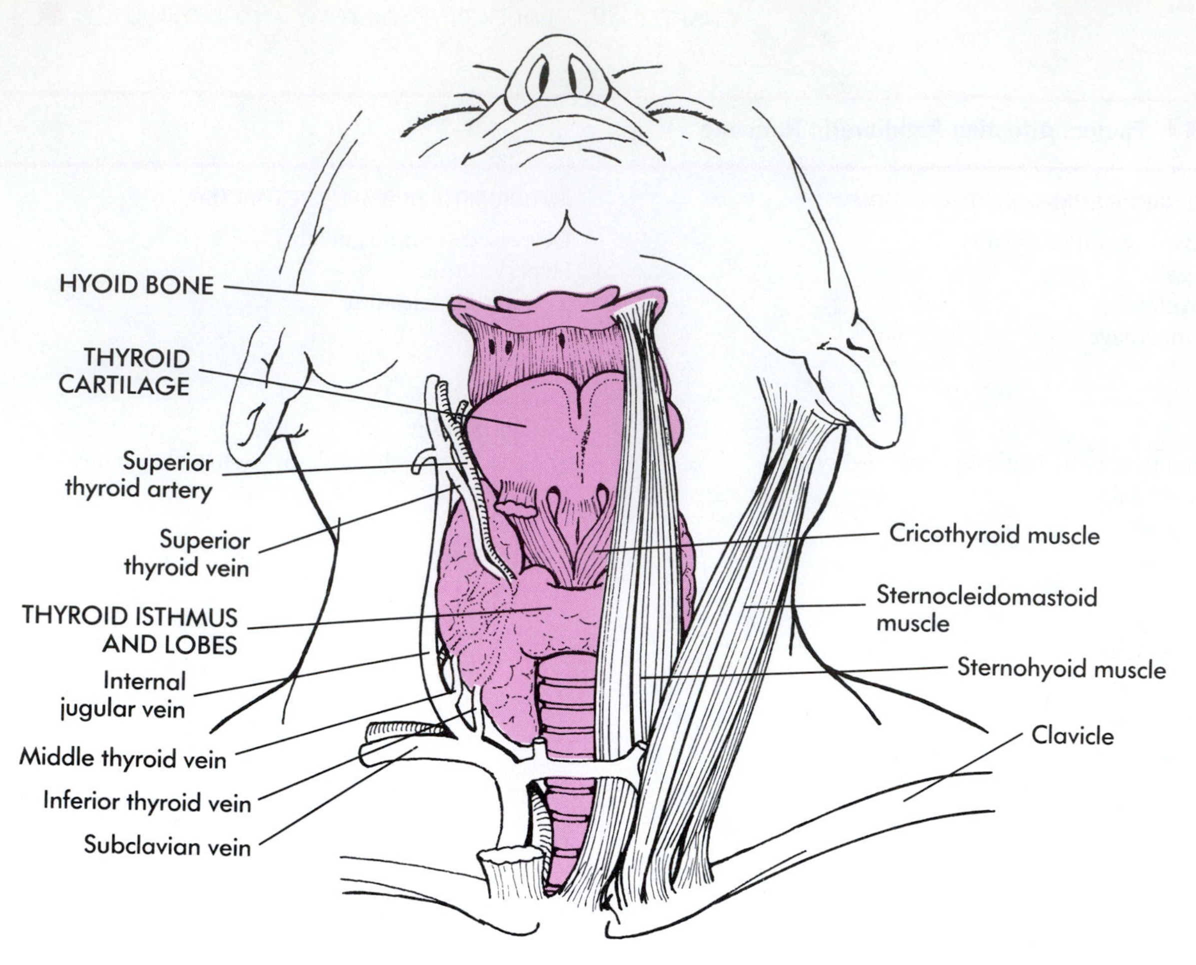

FIGURE 39-5. Gross anatomy of the human thyroid.

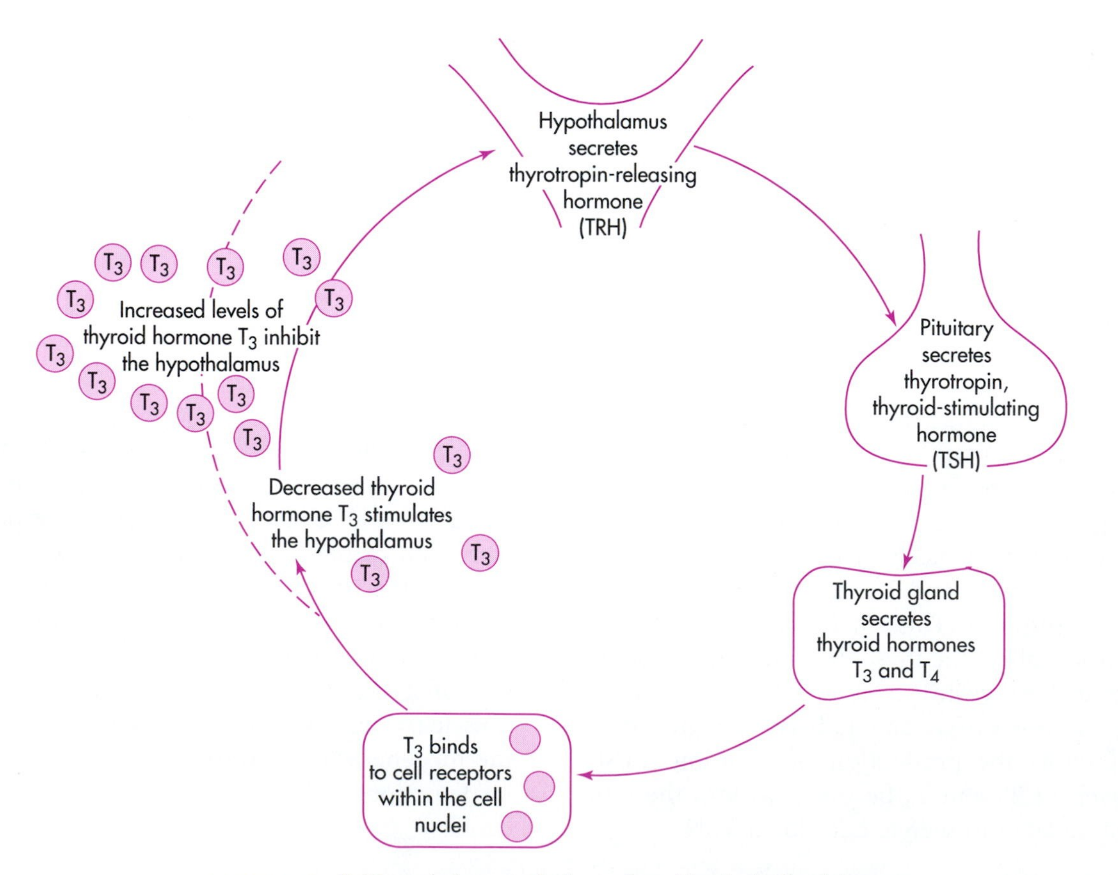

FIGURE 39-6. Hypothalamus-pituitary-thyroid axis feedback loop.

BOX 39-5 Major Functions of Thyroid Hormones

- Interact with growth hormone
  - Maturation of skeletal system
  - Development of central nervous system
- Stimulate carbohydrate metabolism
  - Increase the rate of glucose absorption from the gastrointestinal tract
  - Increase the rate of glucose use by the cells
- Accelerate the rate of fat metabolism
  - Increase cholesterol degradation in the liver
  - Decrease serum cholesterol levels
- Increase protein anabolism and catabolism
  - Mobilize protein and release amino acids into circulation
  - Increase energy from protein nutrients through gluconeogenesis
- Increase body's demand for vitamins
- Increase oxygen consumption and utilization
- Increase basal metabolic rate
- Have marked chronotropic and inotropic effects on heart
- Increase cardiac output
- Stimulate contractility and excitability of myocardium
- Increase blood volume
- Expand respiratory rate and depth necessary for normal hypoxic and hypercapnic drive
- Promote sympathetic overactivity
- Boost crythropoiesis
- Increase metabolism and clearance of various hormones and pharmacologic agents
- Stimulate bone resorption

REFERENCES

1. American Diabetes Association: Clinical practice recommendations 1995, *Diabetes Care,* 18 (suppl 1), 1995.
2. Harris MI and others, editors: *Diabetes in America, National Diabetes Data Group,* ed 2, NIH Publication, No. 95-1468, 1995, National Institutes of Health, National Institutes of Diabetes & Digestive & Kidney Diseases.
3. Guyton AC, Hall JE: *Textbook of medical physiology,* ed 9, Philadelphia, 1996, WB Saunders.
4. Recker B, Copstead LE: Alterations in endocrine control of growth. In Copstead LE, editor: *Perspectives on pathophysiology,* Philadelphia, 1995, WB Saunders.
5. Ganong WF: *Review of medical physiology,* ed 16, Philadelphia, 1996, WB Saunders.
6. Mulvihill S, Debas H: Regulatory peptides of the gut. In Greenspan F, Baxter J, editors: *Basic & clinical endocrinology,* Norwalk, CT, 1994, Appleton & Lange.
7. Hadley M: *Endocrinology,* ed 4, Englewood Cliffs, NJ, 1995, Prentice-Hall.
8. Carcangiu ML, Dellis RA: Thyroid gland. In Damjanov I, Linder J, editors: *Anderson's pathophysiology,* vol 2, ed 10, St Louis, 1996, Mosby.
9. Larsen P, Ingbar S: The thyroid gland. In Wilson J, Foster D, editors: *William's textbook of endocrinology,* Philadelphia, 1992, WB Saunders.
10. Dillman W: The thyroid. In Bennett J, Plum F, editors: *Cecil textbook of medicine,* vol 2, ed 20, Philadelphia, 1996, WB Saunders.
11. Genuth S: The endocrine system. In Berne RM, Levy MN, editors: *Physiology,* ed 3, St Louis, 1993, Mosby.

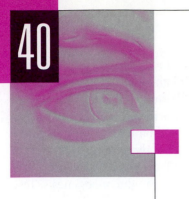

40

Endocrine Clinical Assessment and Diagnostic Procedures

Most of the endocrine glands are deeply encased in the human body. This protected position safeguards the glands against injury and trauma. Although the placement of the glands provides security for the glandular functions, their resulting inaccessibility prevents the glands from being physically appraised by palpation, percussion, or auscultation. The thyroid gland and male gonads are unusual in that the anatomic position of these endocrine glands permits palpation. An enlarged thyroid can also be auscultated for a systolic bruit or continuous venous hum.

Nevertheless, the endocrine glands whose anatomic placement precludes physical inspection can be assessed in an indirect manner. The nurse who understands the metabolic actions of the hormones produced by those glands assesses the physiology of the gland by monitoring that gland's target tissue.

Frequently the initial manifestation of a hormonal disturbance is not on the gland itself, but rather on the specific cell receptor or target of the hormonal action. For example, a nurse may suspect posterior pituitary dysfunction when a patient has decreased urine output, clinical manifestations of hypervolemia (bounding pulse, increased blood pressure, elevated pulmonary artery or central venous pressure reading, engorged neck veins), and serum hyponatremia with hypertonic urine. A nurse's understanding that the target cell for antidiuretic hormone (ADH) is the kidney tubule and reabsorption of urine filtrate is the action of ADH leads him or her to suspect a compromise in ADH or posterior pituitary functioning.

Similarly, pancreatic disorders often are first recognized by noting imbalances in the B cell hormone, insulin, and its systemic effects. The cell receptor site of insulin is found on the adipose and muscle cells. The major action of insulin is to increase the uptake and use of glucose by the muscle and fat cells and to decrease blood glucose levels. When glucose is used for cellular energy, insulin prevents fat and protein from being broken down for fuel. The nurse who understands the metabolic effects of insulin may suspect a dysfunctioning pancreas in a patient who is lethargic, has a long-standing infected wound, has hot dry skin, exhibits oliguria, and has a sweet-smelling breath.

The nurse can also assess the hormonal effect of the thyroid glandular secretions, thyroxine (T_4) and triiodothyronine (T_3), indirectly. Each hormone affects the metabolism of almost every cell in the body. Increasing levels of the hormone may induce spiking fever and tachycardia, especially tachydysrhythmia with escalating restlessness and anxiety. These changes alert the knowledgeable caregiver to look deeper for alterations in the body's metabolic processes controlled by the thyroid gland. Conversely, the patient with a laboratory report of decreased T_4, hypoventilation, severe hypothermia, and bradycardia is at serious risk for developing coma related to hypothyroidism.

Collecting clues that may signal a dysfunctioning gland poses a challange to the nurse because target tissues of insulin (adipose and muscle cells), ADH (kidney tubule), and T_4 (almost all body cells) are influenced by numerous other factors. Therefore the nurse starts with a pertinent data base, including history, when available, and precipitating factors. The patient in the critical care unit may not be able to provide an adequate history for the nurse's assessment data base. Changes in level of consciousness and urgent medical/nursing procedures may delay communication of the patient's personal perspective of the current problem. This initial phase of the nursing process should not be ignored, however, and sources other than the patient (family, friends, previous medical records) can be used to supply vital information.

CLINICAL ASSESSMENT

Pancreas

Insulin, which is produced by the pancreas, is responsible for glucose metabolism. The clinical assessment provides information about pancreatic functioning. Clinical manifestations of abnormal insulin levels identify the patient's response to altered glucose metabolism.

History. A complete health history includes the patient's chief complaint and current health history. Chronic and episodic diseases are discussed. Also included in the data collection is the patient's history. Family history is assessed with respect to present illness, as carbohydrate metabolic imbalance is commonly influenced by hereditary factors. For further detail on history collection for diabetic complications, see Box 40-1.

Physical examination. Since the glucose level is a key factor in determining extracellular and intracellular fluid balance, observation of hydration status and skin assessment can provide additional information about pancreatic functioning. Satisfactory fluid balance is easily identified by the presence of moist, shiny buccal membranes. Skin turgor that is resilient and returns to its original position in less than 3 seconds after being pinched or lifted indicates adequate skin elasticity. (Skin over the forehead, clavicle, and sternum is the most reliable for testing tissue turgor because it is less affected by aging and thus more easily assessed for changes related to fluid balance.) A well-hydrated patient has skin in the groin and axilla that is slightly moist to touch. A balanced intake and output, absence of thirst, absence of edema, stable weight, and urine specific gravity that falls within the normal range (1.005 to 1.030) all serve as indicators that the patient's hydration status is adequate for metabolic demands.

PANCREATIC LABORATORY ASSESSMENT

Pancreas

Pertinent laboratory tests for the pancreas measure the amount of insulin produced by the pancreatic B cells and the effectiveness of insulin in transporting glucose from the blood stream into the cell. The test results reveal whether insulin can maintain a constant serum glucose level, as well as contribute to the metabolism of fats and protein. When adequate insulin is unavailable to permit glucose to be used for fuel, the body is forced to break down noncarbohydrate sources, such as fat and protein, as alternate energy sources. The liver, which normally contributes to protein and fat metabolism, is unable to complete gluconeogenesis as rapidly as the body requires fuel sources. The end result is accumulation of "waste products" from incomplete protein and fat gluconeogenesis. Tests to determine the osmolality, glucose level, and ketone level identify the residual effects of incomplete glucose uptake and use by the cells.

Insulin. The normal value of serum insulin is 5 to 20 μU/ml. This measurement of insulin levels, obtained by a sensitive radioimmunoassay test, indicates the amount of insulin circulating in the blood stream during a period of fasting. The release of insulin depends on the concentration of blood glucose; in the healthy person, when glucose levels rise, insulin levels also rise. Conversely, when serum glucose levels are low, insulin secretion is inhibited. A fasting blood sample is preferred for evaluation of serum insulin levels, although insulin levels are not typically measured to determine diabetes mellitus. (∞Insulin, p. 979.)

Glucose. The normal fasting serum or plasma value of glucose, when measured by a blood test, is 70 to 110 mg/dL. The fasting whole blood value is 60 to 100 mg/dL. The nonfasting value is 85 to 125 mg/dL. A fasting blood sample is read as a simple, numeric value, but it actually measures many complex, interrelated processes. The circulating blood glucose level is derived from three sources: exogenous intake of glucose, release of glycogen stores (glycogenolysis), and breakdown of noncarbohydrate sources (gluconeogenesis). The glucose reading measures the ability of the pancreatic A cells to balance the release of glucagon with the B-cell release of insulin. The circulating glucose level also depends on the peripheral uptake of glucose and the functioning of the liver and its role in gluconeogenesis. Consistently elevated glucose levels signal both an increase in glucagon production and an insufficient amount of effective insulin.

Fingerstick glucose test. Fingerstick glucose tests are used at the bedside for immediate readings that serve as a basis for insulin coverage. The test involves a technique that makes frequent glucose testing rapid, economical, and convenient. The test involves a reagent strip and a monitor or reflectance meter. Numerous devices are available, each with its own specific instructions and guarantee of accuracy. Some strips can be read by comparing the color left by a drop of blood with a color chart. Strips may also be placed into a meter or monitor for an exact reading. Obtaining fre-

BOX 40-1 DATA COLLECTION FOR DIABETIC COMPLICATIONS

Current health status

The body may not be able to adjust to increased insulin needs from sudden physiologic changes such as infection, injury, or surgery, among others. The nurse would assess whether the patient had a severe infection, surgical wound, or traumatic injury.

Recent/current signs and symptoms
- Unexplained changes in weight, thirst, hunger
- Headache, blurred vision
- Long-standing, unhealed infection
- Vaginitis, pruritus
- Leg pain, numbness

Unexplained change in urinary patterns, (i.e., daytime and night time, frequency, and volume)
- Energy/stamina changes
- Endurance level
- Weakness
- Unexplained, excessive fatigue

Behavior/mental changes (also ask family member or significant other for input)
- Memory loss
- Disorientation

History of present illness—onset, characteristics, course

Chronic illness—physiologic or psychologic stress could increase endogenous glucose

Recent treatments that could be a source of exogenous glucose
- Hyperalimentation
- Peritoneal dialysis
- Hemodialysis

Medications—prescription and over-the-counter preparations (Pharmacologic agents can alter pancreatic function by either increasing or decreasing release of the endocrine hormones. Drugs may also interfere with hormonal action at the receptor site on the target cell.)

Past history—previous pancreatic surgery?

Ever been told you
- Had too much sugar in the urine?
- Had too much sugar in the blood?
- Would probably develop too much sugar later in life?

If "yes" answer to any of the above, what treatment if any was prescribed?

Are you currently following such a treatment?

Family history—has a family member ever been diagnosed with diabetes/sugar in the blood?

If so, how did he or she treat the condition?

quent bedside glucose levels allows early identification of situations that cause hyperglycemia or hypoglycemia, permit tighter control over glucose levels, and keep the glucose level as close to normal as possible with intensive insulin therapy.

Fingerstick glucose testing is not appropriate for every patient. A recent critical care and emergency room nursing study questioned the accuracy of results obtained from a capillary blood sample obtained by a fingerstick versus results obtained from a venous blood sample. The study postulated that clients with inadequate peripheral perfusion were poor candidates for fingerstick samples for glucose monitoring. The authors demonstrated that hypoperfusion alters the validity of a fingerstick test. The authors showed that clients in shock and those with cardiovascular collapse, hypotension, or hypovolemia who required close glucose tracking for insulin coverage required blood samples from traditional sources (blood vessel or venous or arterial line) and glucose testing by the laboratory for accuracy.[1]

Glycosylated hemoglobin. A normal glycosylated hemoglobin level is 4% to 7%, with acceptable values within 1% of the upper limit of normal,[2] that is, 4% to 7% of the person's hemoglobin contains a glucose group. This laboratory test provides information about the average amount of glucose that has been present in the patient's blood stream over the previous 3 to 4 months. During the 120-day life span of erythrocytes the hemoglobin within each cell binds to the available blood glucose through a process known as *glycosylation.* The result is Hgb_{1A} and Hgb_{1C}. Through this irreversible process, increased levels of circulating glucose cause an increase in glycosylation. This test is not routinely performed as a pancreatic screening tool but rather used for patients previously diagnosed with diabetes mellitus. It provides information about the degree of hyperglycemia, including the actual increased values over a specific period of time. This test eliminates many variables that normally could affect the accurate interpretation of a glucose test result. Fasting state, exercise, stress, and medications do not interfere with this test result, nor will the test outcome be influenced by patient compliance or changes in a patient's usual habits initiated only to have a fasting blood glucose value read closer to normal than usual.

Serum ketones. In a serum blood test the normal ketone levels are 2 to 4 mg/dL of blood and acetone is 0.3 to 3 mg/dL of blood. Ketones are by-products of fat metabolism. In most cases, when the body uses carbohydrate as its main sorce of energy, fat metabolism is completed by the liver and only a trace of ketones is found in the blood. Ketone bodies in the blood (ketonemia) is observed by a fruity, sweet-smelling odor on the exhaled breath. This odor is the result of the body's attempt to keep the pH within the normal range. A sweet-smelling breath occurs when the lungs release carbon dioxide in an attempt to decrease the accumulated acids.

Urine ketones. Normally ketones are not present in the urine; thus the results of urine tests would be negative. As mentioned previously, in the absence of glucose, fats are burned for energy. Lipolysis (fat breakdown) occurs so rapidly that fat metabolism is incomplete, and ketone bodies (acetone, beta-hydroxybutyric acid, and acetoacetic acid) collect in the blood (ketonemia) and are excreted in the urine (ketonuria).

Both blood and urine specimens can be tested in the laboratory or with reagent strips. Urine samples can also be tested with specially prepared tablets. Both reagent strips and tablets are compared with a color chart. These bedside urine tests are easily performed and provide immediate information regarding ketoacidosis in a person with hyperglycemia.

Serum osmolality. Osmolality is a measurement of the number of particles in a solution or the concentration of the solution (this differs from the size or weight of particles in a solution). A search of laboratory data identifies an all-inclusive range for serum osmolality to be 270 to 300 mOsm/kg of water. The literature shows that while the different laboratories report various extremes for their ranges, the range itself remained narrow. See Box 40-2 (Serum Osmolality Ranges) for examples of acceptable ranges.[3-10] Serum osmolality is not a routine screening tool for pancreatic dysfunction. It is used commonly to identify the effects of an imbalance in carbohydrate metabolism and to assess fluid volume status.

An accumulation of ketone bodies and ketoacids results from the rapid, incomplete breakdown of fat and protein. The ketone bodies and ketoacids collect in the plasma as metabolic "debris" and, along with the increasing levels of glucose that cannot enter the cell, drastically increase the number of particles that normally circulate in the plasma. This increase in circulating particles, coupled with the fluid loss from osmotic diuresis, significantly raises the plasma osmolality.

BOX 40-2 Acceptable Serum Osmolality Ranges

270-290 mOsm/kg H_2O (see reference No. 3)
275-295 mOsm/kg H_2O (see reference No. 4)
278-295 mOsm/kg H_2O (see reference No. 5)
280-296 mOsm/kg H_2O (see reference No. 6)
280-300 mOsm/kg H_2O (see reference No. 7)
285-293 mOsm/kg H_2O (see reference No. 8)
285-295 mOsm/kg H_2O (see reference No. 9)
285-295 mOsm/kg H_2O (see reference No. 10)

Pituitary Gland

The pituitary gland, recessed in the base of the cranium, is not accessible to physical assessment. Therefore the clinician must be aware of the systemic effects of a normally functioning pituitary to identify dysfunction. (∞Pituitary Gland, p. 982.)

History. When possible, the patient and/or significant other is asked about the patient's chief complaint and current health history. (See Box 40-3 for additional questions.)

Physical examination. ADH controls the amount of fluid lost and retained within the body. The nurse determines the effectiveness of ADH function by conducting a hydration assessment.

Hydration assessment. A hydration assessment includes observations of skin integrity, skin turgor, and buccal membrane moisture. Blood pressure and pulse are monitored frequently. Decreased blood pressure with an increased pulse is characteristic of hypovolemia, whereas elevated blood pressure and rapid, bounding pulse may indicate hypervolemia. Orthostatic hypotension, which occurs when extracellular fluid volume decreases, is identified by a drop in systolic blood pressure of 20 mm Hg and a drop in diastolic blood pressure of 10 mm Hg when the patient changes position from lying to standing.

Weight. Daily weight changes coincide with fluid retention and fluid loss. Sudden changes in weight could result from a change in fluid balance; 1 L of fluid lost or retained is equal to approximately 2.2 pounds (2 pounds, 2 ounces or 1 kg) of weight gained or lost. To use weight as a true determinant of the body's weight changes, all extraneous variables are eliminated

BOX 40-3 DATA COLLECTION FOR DIABETIC INSIPIDUS AND SYNDROME OF INAPPROPRIATE ANTIDIURETIC HORMONE

CHIEF COMPLAINT

Recent/current signs and symptoms

Physical: Unexplained weight loss
Excessive urination interfering with sleep or activities of daily living
Increase in thirst? Easily satiated?
Headache
Fatigue
Active blood loss (decreased or increased fluid levels affected by circulating antidiuretic hormone [ADH] also affect sodium levels; changes in cerebral hydration and serum sodium levels will lead to further neurologic damage if not corrected)

Behavioral: (may also ask family member or significant other for information)Obsessional neurosis, especially those involving water drinking?

History of present illness—onset, characteristics, course

Has patient been treated for another endocrine dysfunction that could potentially interfere with ADH? (Hypothyroidism and adrenal insufficiency stimulate release of ADH regardless of serum osmolality or volume deficit.10)

Is a head injury or neurologic disorder present that could interfere with synthesis of ADH in the hypothalamus or its passage down to the posterior pituitary before its release?

Does the patient have a concurrent cancer or a pulmonary disease that would be capable of autonomous production of ADH (tuberculosis, pneumonia, duodenal carcinoma, oat cell carcinoma)?

What medications are in use—several medications affect ADH imbalance (see Box 39-4, p. 985 for a more complete listing)

Decreased ADH release	Increased ADH release
Phenytoin	Barbiturates
Chlorpromazine	Anesthetics
Reserpine	Glucocorticoids

Past history

Congenital anomaly involving infundibular stalk?

and the same scale is used at the same time each day. The patient must also wear similar clothing so as not to affect the reading.

Intake and output. Measuring and recording intake and output is a simple task that, when performed accurately and conscientiously on all routes of fluid intake and loss, provides information about the body's fluid balance. Precise intake and output records are used as criteria for fluid replacement therapy. Physical characteristics of urine, such as concentration, color, and specific gravity, are significant factors in assessing the patient's fluid balance.

Neurologic assessment. The patient's neurologic system frequently is evaluated in an assessment of the pituitary gland. Alterations in serum sodium levels adversely affect brain tissue and disrupt the patient's behavioral patterns. Muscle coordination, deep tendon reflexes, and muscle strength are included in the neurologic assessment.

LABORATORY ASSESSMENT

Pituitary

No single diagnostic test identifies dysfunctioning of the posterior pituitary gland. Diagnosis usually is made through an array of laboratory tests combined with the clinical profile of the patient.

The tests include both a measurement of the serum antidiuretic hormone that is produced by the hypothalamus and tests that gauge the subsequent release of ADH by the posterior pituitary. Serum and urine osmolality tests measure the effectiveness of ADH in maintaining the correct solute concentration for the particular sample of fluid.

Serum antidiuretic hormone. The result of a blood test for normal levels of serum ADH is 1 to 13.3 pg/ml (picogram = trillionth of a gram). The serum ADH test measures the amount of ADH present in a frozen sample of blood. The direct measurement of ADH is possible by means of a laboratory radioimmunoassay. This diagnostic procedure can help distinguish between central diabetes insipidus (DI) and the syndrome of inappropriate antidiuretic hormone. This test provides accurate results and is used in preference to two other tests, water load and water deprivation tests, both discussed later in this chapter.

To prepare a patient for the antidiuretic hormone radioimmunoassay testing, all drugs that may alter the release of ADH are withheld for a minimum of 8 hours. Medications that affect ADH levels are morphine sulfate, lithium carbonate, chlorothiazide, carbamazepine, oxytocin, and certain neoplastic and anesthetic agents (see Box 39-4 for additional drugs). Nicotine, alcohol, both positive- and negative-pressure ventilation, and emotional stress can also influence the ADH levels and must be considered in the interpretation of values.

The test, read by comparing serum ADH levels with the blood and urine osmolality, is helpful in differentiating the syndrome of antidiuretic hormone (SIADH) from central DI. The presence of increased ADH in the blood stream compared with a low serum osmolality and elevated urine osmolality confirms the diagnosis of SIADH. Reduced levels of serum ADH in a patient with high serum osmolality, hypernatremia, and reduced urine concentration signal central diabetes insipidus.

Urine and blood osmolality. As previously presented, the literature values for serum osmolality range from 270 to 300 mOsm/kg H_2O, with an normal variance from 285 to 300 mOsm/kg H_2O (see Box 40-2, Serum Osmolality Range). Osmolality measurements determine the concentration of dissolved particles in a solution. In a healthy person a change in the concentration of solutes triggers a chain of events to maintain proper dilution. The average value for urine osmolality is within 300 to 800 mOsm/kg H_2O, with the outermost range of 50 to 1200 mOsm/kg H_2O.

Increased serum osmolality stimulates the release of ADH, which in turn reduces the amount of water lost at the nephron tubules. Body fluid thereby is retained to dilute the particle concentration in the blood stream. Decreased serum osmolality inhibits the release of ADH, the kidney tubules increase their permeability, and fluid is eliminated from the body in an attempt to regain normal concentration of particles in the blood stream. The most accurate results of the body's ability to maintain a fluid balance are obtained when urine and blood samples are collected simultaneously.

Water deprivation test. Normal values for the water deprivation test are urine osmolality, 800 mOsm/kg H_2O and serum osmolality, 285 to 300 mOsm/kg H_2O. This test is based on the premise that ADH is released to conserve urinary water when a patient is at risk of becoming dehydrated. The results of this test are useful in diagnosing central diabetes insipidus and SIADH. The procedure for this test purposely withholds all fluid for 24 hours while serum and urine laboratory tests determine the body's response to the pending dehydration. The water deprivation test is rarely done in the intensive care unit because of the time involved and the risks of dehydration to an already severely compromised patient. (The sensitive radioimmunoassay serum ADH test, discussed earlier, is a preferred test.)

Synthetic ADH test. Another test done in place of water deprivation is the administration of a subcutaneous injection of aqueous vasopressin (Pitressin) (synthetic ADH). This test provides information to differentiate the type of diabetes insipidus. The test is performed by measuring urine volume and osmolality on serial urine collections over a 2-hour period. The patient with normal posterior pituitary functioning responds to the exogenous ADH by reabsorbing water at the tubule and raising the urine osmolality slightly. In cases of severe central diabetes insipidus, the urine osmolality has a significant rise. (Values are established by the associated laboratory.) A significant rise indicates that the cell receptor sites on the renal tubules are responsive to Pitressin. Test results in which urine osmolality remains unchanged are suggestive of nephrogenic diabetes insipidus, indicating that the target tissue or cell receptor sites are no longer receptive to ADH.

Water load test. The water load test is based on the premise that changes in the concentration of particles in the blood stream will affect the release of ADH as the body strives to maintain a homeostatic balance. The water load test is helpful in evaluating the function of ADH in both diabetes insipidus and syndrome of inappropriate antidiuretic hormone. In this test the patient is overhydrated and then a series of blood and urine samples are taken to monitor the sequence of physiologic events leading to a fluid balance. Because of the serious risks of overhydrating the critically ill patient and the potentially lethal effect on patients with cardiac or renal dysfunction, this test is rarely seen in the critical care environment. The ADH radioimmunoassay test, discussed previously, is preferred.

DIAGNOSTIC PROCEDURES

Pituitary

In addition to laboratory tests, radiographic examination, computerized tomography (CT), and magnetic resonance imaging (MRI) are helpful in diagnosing hypothalamic-pituitary disease. Although these tests may not definitively diagnose diabetes insipidus or syndrome of inappropriate antidiuretic hormone, they are useful in diagnosing the primary causes of these diseases. Cranial bone fractures that injure the hypophyseal stalk and space-occupying masses, such as tumors or blood clots that interfere with pituitary circulation, are examples of abnormalities identified and studied in diagnostic tests.

Radiologic examination. A basic x-ray examination of the inferior skull views the sella turcica and surrounding bone formation. Bone fractures or tissue swelling at the base of the brain, which are apparent on a radiograph, suggest interference with the vascular supply and nerve impulses to the hypothalamic-pituitary system. Dysfunction may occur if the hypothalamus, the infundibular stalk, or the pituitary is impaired.

Computerized axial tomography. Computed tomography (CT) of the base of the skull (sella turcica) identifies pituitary tumors, blood clots, cysts, nodules, or other tissue masses. A skull CT scan provides more definitive results than does an x-ray test and, whenever possible, is obtained in preference to a skull x-ray film. The 40-minute procedure causes no discomfort except that it requires the patient to be perfectly still. A radiopaque sodium iodine solution may be given intravenously to highlight the hypothalamus, infundibular stalk, and pituitary gland. This dye may cause allergic reactions in iodine-sensitive persons, and the patient must be carefully questioned before the start of the test. Multiple x-ray beams pass through the head from specific angles while detectors record the attenuation (absorption or scattering) of the x-ray beam. The x-rays pass through the head on a predetermined axis, producing images of minute slices or layers of brain tissue. As the x-rays pass through bone, soft tissue, and body fluid, a portion of the beam is absorbed or scattered, depending on the density of the tissue. A computer then calculates the degree of attenuated x-rays over very small areas and identifies tissue density changes. Size and shape of the sella turcica and position of the hypothalamus, infundibualr stalk, and pituitary gland are identified. The resulting data are then projected on a viewing screen as an image of the head.

Magnetic resonance imaging. Magnetic resonance imaging (MRI) enables the radiologist to visualize internal organs, as well as examine the cellular characteristics of specific tissue. MRI uses a magnetic field rather than radiation to produce images of internal structures of the body. The body part under examination is presented in cross-sectional slices as a high-resolution image.

The soft fluid tissue in and immediately surrounding the brain makes the brain especially responsive to MRI scanning. Although MRI is not a definitive diagnostic test for posterior pituitary hormonal imbalance, its use identifies anatomic disruption of the gland and the surrounding area suggestive of primary causes of diabetes insipidus and syndrome of inappropriate antidiuretic hormone.

Thyroid

Increased circulating thyroid hormone results in hyperthyroidism, also known as *thyrotoxicosis.* The hyperthyroid condition increases the breakdown of nutrients and the synthesis of organic compounds within the cells. This increased metabolism requires energy to yield energy. They body responds with an effort to replenish the oxygen and energy used in a hypermetabolic state and exhibits an increased appetite, tachycardia, and tachypnea. The increased nutrient intake, however, is insufficient to meet accelerated needs of the cells, and weight loss occurs. Most characteristic of thyrotoxicosis is the hyperpyrexia and heightened state of nervousness. (∞The Thyroid Gland, p. 983.)

Thyroid crisis. Thyroid crisis is a rare and potentially lethal medical condition. It is the most extreme, severe response to an overactive thyroid hormone. Manifestations include **extremes** of hypermetabolism, hyperpyrexia, tachycardia, and a heightened sense of nervousness. The thyroid hormone produces an intensified sympathetic nervous system response in the body. T_3 and T_4 increase beta-adrenergic receptor activity in the body, and the cardiovascular system becomes especially sensitive to catecholamines.[3] Additional clinical manifestations of thyroid abnormalities are listed in Box 40-4. It is important to recognize that there are no distinct signs or symptoms in thyroid crisis that distinguish it from hyperthyroidism (thyrotoxicosis) except for the severity of the signs and symptoms. No separate laboratory values identify thyroid crisis or differentiate it from hyperthyroidism. Therefore the responsibility rests on the clinician who is assessing the body's presentation of a covertly worsening condition.

Hypothyroidism. Hypothyroidism (myxedema) occurs when there is an insufficient amount of circulating thyroid hormone. Decreased thyroid hormone results in sluggish or decreased metabolism throughout the body systems. Fatigue, weight gain, intolerance to cold, and impaired decision making are characteristic of this disorder. Additional clinical manifestations of hypothyroidism are listed in Box 40-4. The depressed functioning of each body system caused by hypothyroidism is usually amenable to replacement therapy.

Severe hypothyroidism. Untreated hypothyroidism, however, once combined with a life-threatening nonthyroid disease, could progress to myxedema coma.

BOX 40-4 Clinical Manifestations of Thyroid Abnormalities

HYPOTHYROIDISM

Decreased basal metabolic rate
Lethargy
Myxedema
Severe muscle cramps
Chronic anemia
Decreased bowel activity, constipation
Menstrual irregularities
Bradycardia
Bradypnea
Paresthesia
Muscle weakness
Decreased glomerular filtration
Decreased cardiac output

THYROTOXICOSIS

Increased basal metabolic rate
Fatigue, exhaustion
Diaphoresis
Intolerance to heat
Goiter
Diarrhea
Ophthalmopathy
Hyperkinesis
Increased cardiac output
Tachydysrhythmias
Frequent urination
Emotion lability
Fine tremors

Myxedema coma is a condition of severely decreased thyroid hormone level that, as the name implies, leads to a comatose state (myxedema coma) and death if not treated. (∞Box 41-23, p. 1038.)

History. The history of a patient in the critical care area should be as detailed as possible. Information regarding the clinical manifestations of either hypothyroidism or hyperthyroidism must be obtained from the patient, family, or others with knowledge about the patient. Sample questions considered pertinent to thyroid disease are presented in Box 40-5.

Physical examination. The normal-size thyroid gland is not visible or apparent in the anterior neck. Palpation of the neck to reveal a goiter or enlargement of the thyroid gland would be done before the initial diagnosis of hyperthyroidism and is not necessary in the assessment of thyrotoxic storm. Auscultation of the thyroid is accomplished by use of the bell portion of the stethescope to identify a bruit or blowing noise from the circulation through the thyroid gland. Although the presence of a bruit indicates increased blood flow through the glandular tissue, it is not a proven method to differentiate the presence of thyrotoxic crisis from thyrotoxicosis.

Hyperthyroidism clinical assessment. Critical assessments for hyperthyroidism include observations of patient responses to increased metabolism, heightened sensitivity to adrenergic receptors, and loss of thermoregulation. Cardiac functioning, including stroke volume and cardiac output, is monitored. Appetite, nausea, vomiting, and diarrhea are assessed as the body attempts to increase food intake and replenish fuel for energy expenditure. Hyperglycemia may result from the change in mobilization of nutrients and imbalance of insulin release. In addition, motility of the gastrointestinal tract is affected by increased thyroid hormones. Observation of the client's tolerance of heat is also important. The patient who complains of profuse sweating from being too hot often follows this report with turning off room heat, opening all windows, and taking off all but minimal clothing and bed linens, even on the coldest days. (∞Box 41-23, p. 1038.)

Hypothyroidism clinical assessment. Clinical monitoring of the patient with hypothyroidism includes an assessment similar to that for the patient with hyperthyroidism but with different expected outcomes. Critical assessments for hypothyroidism include observations of patient responses to a slowed body metabolism because of decreased oxygen consumption by the tissues. Mental impairment influences judgment, comprehension, and awareness. Bradycardia and reduced cardiac contractility result in diminished cardiac output. The patient is carefully evaluated for heart failure. Hypoventilation and decreased respiratory capacity occur. A distended abdomen, decreased intestinal peristalsis, and constipation are common. The patient with hypothermia has sensations of being cold, wearing layers of clothing and blankets even on the warmest/hottest days. (∞Box 41-23, p. 1039.)

Thyroid laboratory assessment. Tests most commonly performed on a thyroid panel are listed Table 40-1. The tests measure the hormonal negative feedback response within the hypothalamic-pituitary axis. Laboratory diagnosis of hyperthyroidism and hypothyroidism is usually based on the ultrasensitive thyroid-stimulating hormone (TSH) (also known as *serum thy-*

BOX 40-5 DATA COLLECTION FOR THYROTOXICOSIS (HYPERTHYROIDISM) AND MYXEDEMA (HYPOTHYROIDISM)

NOTE: **The patient would be the best source from whom to obtain the following information. However, if the patient is unable to respond, the following questions are directed to family, friends, significant other, and/or those involved in admission of the patient to the intensive care unit.**

1. Have you every been diagnosed with overactive thyroid, increased metabolism, or hyperthyroidism? What about underactive thyroid, slowed metabolism, or hypothyroidism?
2. Have you ever been treated for hyperthyroidism or hypothyroidism?
3. Have you ever had an operation for thyroid disease?
4. Have you ever received radioactive iodine for thyroid disease?
5. Were you taking any medicine for thyroid disease? If so, what is the name of the medicine, dose, frequency?
6. When did you first notice the constant restlessness and/or extreme fatigue?
7. Has your weight been the same or changed over the last year?
   Has your appetite changed over the last 6 months?
   Have you lost weight even though your appetite has increased? (May indicate hyperthyroidism.)
   Have you gained weight or stayed at the same weight even though you haven't felt like eating over the last 6 months? (May indicate hypothyroidism.)
8. Are you always feeling warm? (May indicate hyperthyroidism.)
   Do you open windows in house, even in winter months?
   Do you wear lightweight clothing, even when everyone around is wearing layers of heavier clothing?
9. Are you always feeling cold? (May indicate hypothyroidism.)
   Do you wear multiple layers of clothing despite warm weather or the use of a heater/furnace?
   Do you use several blankets with closed windows, even in warm weather?
   Does patient complain of never being able to "warm-up"?
10. Over the last six months to 1 year ago have you developed any of the following?

Indicators for Hypothyroidism	Indicators for Hyperthyroidism
Hair thinning	Tremors
Facial puffiness	Insomnia
Decreased appetite	Increased appetite
Severe constipation	Diarrhea
Pain when moving hands, wrist, feet	Muscle weakness/wasting
Change in menstruation	Change in menstruation

rotropin assay, which has the same initials), and free T_4[5]. (∞Thyroid Function, p. 984.)

The outcome of TSH and free T_4 may be inconclusive in the critically ill patient, however, because hormonal adaptation to the stress of the illness and common problems of protein malnutrition in critical care situations influence the thyroid hormone production[11] and distribution throughout the body. Additional disadvantages inherent in the thyroid laboratory tests are the adjustments that need to be made for the individual variables in serum protein levels—for example, the elderly patient,[11] the pregnant woman, and persons with hepatitis and acute intermittent porphyria.[12] Concomitant use of certain drugs also must be considered. Heparin, corticosteroids, and dopamine interfere with thyroid test results. Additional interfering drugs are found in Box 40-6.[7,11,13]

Thyrotoxicosis, the precursor of thyrotoxic crisis, is diagnosed in part by elevated T_4 and T_3 serum levels. Laboratory levels of TSH and TRH are measured to confirm thyrotoxicosis, as well as to identify the cause as thyroid or extrathyroid. Extrathyroid conditions implicate a source other than the thyroid gland as the cause of the increased hormones. Interference with the feedback system, pituitary dysfunction, and thyroid malignancy that produces hormones despite the body's needs are examples of these conditions.

Thyroid diagnostic procedure

Thyroid scanning. Thyroid scanning involves the use of oral radioactive iodine. ^{123}I is the preferred isotope because of its low-energy, 13-hour output. This short half-life minimizes the patient's exposure to radioactive material. The thyroid-scanning procedure is useful in detecting the presence of ectopic thyroid tissue and thyroid carcinomas. Thyroid scans also identify the presence and amount of viable thyroid glandular tissue after irradiation treatment.

TABLE 40-1 Tests Most Commonly Performed on a Thyroid Panel

Test	Normal Adult Value	Conditions with Abnormal Values		Special Consideration
		Decreased	Increased	
Serum thyroxine (T_4)	T_4, 4.5-11.5 μg/dL T_4RIA, 5-12 μg/dL	Hypothyroidism Protein malnutrition Anterior pituitary hypofunction	Hyperthyroidism Viral hepatitis Acute/chronic illness	Simple peripheral blood withdrawal Identifies amount of hormone in circulation Bound by serum protein, therefore affected by TBG Affected by pregnancy
Free thyroid index (FT_4I)	Free T_4, 0.8-2.3 ng/dL	Hypothyroidism	Hyperthyroidism	Same as above, except this measures amount of free T_4, the unbound portion of which enters the cells T_3 uptake multiplied by T_4 equals FTI
Serum triiodothyronine (T_3) (T_3RIA)	110-230 ng/dL	Hypothyroidism Malnutrition Trauma Critical illness	Thyrotoxicosis Toxic adenoma Thyroiditis	Simple peripheral blood withdrawal Measured directly by RIA Direct measurement of both bound and free T_3 Values increase in pregnancy
T_3 uptake ratio (T_3 UR) T_3 resin uptake	25%-35% uptake 0.8-1.30 ratio of laboratory result to standard control	Hypothyroidism Active hepatitis Thyroiditis	Hyperthyroidism Nephrosis Malignancy Protein malnutrition	Does not measure T_3 as name implies Indirectly measure TBG available to bind T_3 and T_4; increase in thyrotoxicosis related to increase in thyroid hormone binding Affected by pregnancy Affected by diseases that alter these proteins
Serum thyroid-stimulating hormone (TSH) test	2-5.4 mU/L <3 ng/ml	Secondary hypothyroidism Anterior pituitary disorder, very low levels, 0.005 mU/L, indicate hyperthyroidism	Primary hypothyroidism Cirrhosis	Identifies thyroid versus pituitary hypothalamus disorder
Serum thyrotropin-releasing hormone (TRH), stimulation test, or thyrotropin-releasing factor (TRF) test	Serum TSH rises approximately twice its normal level 30 min after IV TRH			Test confirms presence of thyrotoxicosis by measuring response of the pituitary gland's production of TSH 3-4 wk before test, thyroid medication should be discontinued 500 μg of TRH is given IV to mimic the hypothalamus Venous blood samples are taken at intervals as stated by processing laboratory; peak response occurs in 20 min and returns to normal within 2 hr

FTI, Free thyroid index; *RIA,* radioimmunoassay; *TBG,* thyroxine-binding globulin.

BOX 40-6 Drugs That Influence Diagnostic Thyroid Levels

TRIIODOTHYRONINE (T_3)

Increase	Decrease
Methadone	Anabolic steroid
Estrogens	Androgens
Progestins	Salicylates
Amiodarone	Phenytoin
	Lithium
	Reserpine
	Propranolol
	Sulfonamides
	Propylthiouracil
	Methylthiouracil

THYROXINE (T_4)

Increase	Decrease
Oral contraceptives	Phenytoin
Heparin	Steroids
Aspirin	Diphenylhydantoin
Furosemide	Chlorpromazine
Clofibrate	Lithium
Phenylbutazone	Sulfonylurea
Some nonsteroidal antiinflammatory drugs (NSAIDs)	Sulfonamides
Propranolol	Reserpine
Corticosteroids	Chlordiazepoxide
Amiodarone	

THYROID-STIMULATING HORMONE (TSH)

Increase TSH	Decrease TSH and TSH Response to TRH
Metoclopramide	Glucocorticoids
Iodides	Dopamine
Lithium	Heparin
Potassium iodide	Aspirin
Morphine sulfate	Carbamazepine

THYROXINE-BINDING GLOBULIN (TBG)

Increase	Decrease
Opiates	Androgen therapy
Oral contraceptives	L-Asparaginase
Estrogens	
Clofibrate	
5-Fluorouracil (5-FU)	
Perphenazine	

REFERENCES

1. Sylvain HF: Accuracy of fingerstick glucose values in shock patients, *Am J Crit Care* 4(1):44, 1995.
2. Peterson KA, Smith CK: The DCCT (Diabetes Control and Complications Trial), *Am Fam Physician* 52(4):1092-1098, 1995.
3. Ewald MA, McKenzie CR, editors: *Manual of medical therapeutics,* ed 28, Boston, 1995, Little, Brown.
4. Fischbach F: *A manual of laboratory and diagnostic tests,* ed 5, Philadelphia, 1996, JB Lippincott.
5. Ravel R: *Clinical laboratory medicine: clinical application of laboratory data,* ed 6, St Louis, 1995, Mosby.
6. *Massachusetts General Hospital normal reference laboratory values, N Engl J Med* 327:718-724 (Sept 3), 1992.
7. LeFever Kee J: *Laboratory and diagnostic tests with nursing implications,* ed 4, Norwalk, Conn, 1995, Appleton & Lange.
8. Tierney LM, McPhee SJ, Papadakis MA, editors: *Current medical diagnosis and treatment,* ed 35, Stamford, Conn, 1996, Appleton & Lange.
9. Noe DA, Rock RC, editors: *Laboratory medicine: the selection and interpretation of clinical laboratory studies,* Baltimore, 1994, Williams & Wilkins.
10. Isselbacher KJ and others, editors: *Harrison's principles of internal medicine,* ed 13, New York, 1994, McGraw-Hill.
11. Shoemaker W and others, editors: *Textbook of critical care,* ed 3, Philadelphia, 1995, WB Saunders.
12. Pagana KD, Pagana TJ: *Mosby's diagnostic and laboratory test reference,* ed 2, St Louis, 1995, Mosby.
13. Tietz N and others, editors: *Clinical guide to laboratory tests,* ed 3, Philadelphia, 1995, WB Saunders.

Endocrine Disorders and Therapeutic Management

STRESS AND CRITICAL ILLNESS

PHYSIOLOGIC CHANGES OCCUR when the individual is confronted with the threat of illness, trauma, or psychologic sress. These changes are initiated when, in an attempt to protect itself from the harm of the stressor, the body mobilizes energy to the cardiopulmonary, endocrine, and nervous systems; the liver; and the muscles. Other systems, such as the reproductive, integumentary, and genitourinary system, are slowed in an attempt to conserve energy. The body's response to stress has a profound effect on both the endocrine and nervous systems. The combined systems' characteristic response pattern to stressors is described as the neuroendocrine stress response. The physiologic responses to the stress of critical illness frequently observed by the practitioner are listed in Table 41-1.[1-4]

DIABETES MELLITUS

Diabetes mellitus (DM) involves several chain reactions. The problem begins when absent or ineffective insulin limits the entry of glucose into the muscle and adipose cells. Without glucose the body loses access to its optimal source of energy. Consequently, the body uses noncarbohydrate products, such as protein and fats, for energy. This breakdown of noncarbohydrate sources of energy depletes the body of nutrients needed for other functions and further compromises the individual.

The two types of diabetes mellitus discussed in this unit are Type I, insulin-dependent diabetes (IDDM), and Type II, non–insulin-dependent diabetes (NIDDM). (It has been suggested that the Roman numerals used in Type I and Type II be changed to Arabic numerals [i.e., Type 1, Type 2] to prevent confusion with the abbreviation for insulin in IDDM and NIDDM.) The two diseases are different in nature, etiology, treatment, and prognosis and deserve to be discussed as two entirely separate diseases. DM is covered by two diagnostic related groups (DRGs): DRG 295 if the age is between 0 and 35 years, with an anticipated length of stay of 5.1 days, or DRG 294 if the person is 35 years or older, with an anticipated length of stay of 6.2 days.[5] Many factors impact length of stay in the hospital; increased acuity prolongs the hospital stay, as does the presence of diabetic ketoacidosis (DKA) and associated underlying conditions such as renal insufficiency or cardiopulmonary compromise.

Type I

Type I, IDDM, is most likely, although not proven to be, an autoimmune disease, resulting in progressive destruction of the B cells of the islets of Langerhans. The disease occurs at any age but especially during youth. Type I DM is believed to be genetically coded.[6] The B cells can no longer secrete insulin, resulting in impaired carbohydrate, protein, and fat metabolism. Ultimately, the insulin deficiency results in blood hyperosmolality, severe dehydration, and a lack of glucose to the brain tissue. Treatment requires exogenous replacement of parenteral insulin to restore normal serum osmolality and entry of glucose into the cells. Without insulin as a treatment the rapid breakdown of noncarbohydrate substances leads to ketonemia and ketonuria. DKA is a severe life-threatening complication associated with IDDM.

Type II

The widespread differences in the number of people with NIDDM among various cultures suggests a critically important environmental component to the epidemiology of NIDDM.[6] This form of diabetes is characterized by B cells, which function actively but produce ineffective or insufficient insulin to move glucose out of circulation and into selected cells. NIDDM

TABLE 41-1 Endocrine Response During Stress

	Hormone	Response
Adrenal cortex	Cortisol	↑ Insulin resistance→ ↑ glycogenolysis→ ↑ glucose circulation
		↑ Hepatic gluconeogenesis→ ↑ glucose available
		↑ Lipolysis
		↑ Protein catabolism
		↑ Sodium,→ ↑ water retention to maintain blood plasma osmolality by movement of extravascular fluid to intravascular space
		Connective tissue fibroblasts→ collagen for poor wound healing
	Glucocorticoid	↓ Histamine release→ suppresses immune system
		↓ Lymphocytes, monocytes, eosinophils, basophils
		↑ Polymorphonuclear leukocytes→ ↑ risk infection
		↑ Glucose
		↓ Gastric acid secretion
	Mineralocorticoids	↑ Aldosterone→ ↓ sodium excretion→ ↓ water excretion↓ ↑ intravascular volume↓ ↑ vasoconstriction↓ ↑ blood pressure
		↑ Potassium excretion→ hypokalemia→
		↑ Hydrogen ion excretion→metabolic alkalosis
Adrenal medulla	Epineprhine	↑ Endorphins→ ↓ pain
	Norepineprhine, Epinephrine	↑ Metabolic rate to accommodate stress response
		↑ Liver glycogenolysis→ ↑ glucose
		↑ Insulin (cells are insulin resistant)
		↑ Cardiac contractility
		↑ Cardiac output
		↑ Dilation coronary arteries
		↑ Blood pressure
		↑ Heart rate
		↑ Bronchodilation→ ↑ respirations
		↑ Perfusion to heart, brain, lungs, liver, muscle
		↓ Perfusion to periphery of body
		↓ Peristalsis
	Norepinephrine	↑ Peripheral vasoconstriction
		↑ Blood pressure
		↑ Sodium retention
		↑ Potassium excretion
Pituitary	All hormones	↑ Endogenous opioids→ ↓ pain
Anterior pituitary	Adrenocorticotropic hormone	↑ Aldosterone→ ↓ sodium excretion→ ↓ water excretion ↑ intravascular volume→ ↑ blood pressure
		↑ Cortisol to ↑ blood volume
	Growth hormones	↑ Protein anabolism of amino acids to protein
		↑ Lipolysis→ ↑ gluconeogenesis
Posterior pituitary	Antidiuretic hormone	↑ Vasoconstriction
		↑ Water retention→restoration circulating blood volume
		↓ Urinary output
		↑ Hypoosmolality
Pancreas	Insulin	Insulin resistance→hyperglycemia
	Glucagon	Directly opposes action of insulin→↑ glycolysis
		↑ Glucose for fuel
		↑ Glycogenolysis
		↑ Gluconeogenesis
		↑ Lipolysis
Thyroid	Thyroxine	↓ Routine metabolic demands during stress
Gonads	Sex hormones	Energy and oxygen supply diverted to brain, heart, muscles, liver

↑, Increased; →, causes; ↓, decreased.

is initially treated with diet management and physical exercise to promote weight loss.

The majority of patients with Type II diabetes are adults and have a body mass index that exceeds 30%.[7] If the patient's glucose level remains unaffected by a change in diet and exercise regimen, oral hypoglycemic medications and antihyperglycemic drugs may be used. Hypoglycemic and antihyperglycemic drugs are not oral forms of insulin, as insulin is destroyed by gastric juices. Table 41-2 lists oral medications and nursing considerations for the person with Type II diabetes.[8-10] It is not uncommon that after a period of time the hypoglycemic agents fail to increase sensitivity at the cell receptor site and the patient requires insulin to control blood sugar levels.

The patient with NIDDM secretes some insulin; therefore a certain amount of glucose is available to the cells for energy. This passage of glucose into brain, muscle, and adipose tissue prevents the continuous breakdown of noncarbohydrate substances for use as energy. It is believed that the ability of glucose to enter the cells for energy and the decreased degree of catabolism in the body prevents or limits DKA. DKA is not an expected sequela for the patient with Type II diabetes. However, another serious complication of Type II diabetes is hyperglycemic hyperosmolar nonketotic syndrome[9] (previously known as *hyperglycemic hyperosmolar nonketotic coma*). The case study in Box 41-1 presents a patient with NIDDM and a primary diagnosis that resulted in the patient being admitted to the critical care unit.

DIABETIC KETOACIDOSIS

Description

DKA is a significant community health problem with a major financial impact. Approximately 45,000 to 130,000 hospitalizations for DKA occur annually, based on a population of 10 million persons with diabetes. Of DKA episodes, 20% occur in persons with newly diagnosed diabetes, whereas the other 80% occur after the diagnosis has been made. Individuals 40 years of age and older are most commonly affected by this complication.[11,12] Of all deaths attributed to diabetes, 9% to 14% result from DKA.[7] It is estimated, however, that these deaths occur not from the ketoacidotic state alone, but rather from late complications (pneumonia, myocardial infarction, infection) resulting from DKA.[13] Available statistics show that the mortality for patients hospitalized for DKA is 9%, with DKA and mortality for females higher than that for males. The death rate from DKA is three times higher

BOX 41-1 Non–Insulin Dependent Diabetes Mellitus Case Study

Mrs. S is a 70-year-old female with non–insulin dependent diabetes mellitus (NIDDM) and acute heart failure with underlying ischemic cardiomyopathy. She is moderately obese. Mrs. S was placed on a ventilator the first day of admission and given diuretics: Bumex 1 mg/hr to help eliminate fluid and ease the cardiac workload. She developed decreased gastrointestinal (GI) motility along with increased nasogastric tube feeding residuals. She had decreased urinary output with the urine specific gravity and hemodynamic central venous pressure readings within the normal range. She began receiving total parenteral nutrition (TPN) via central venous catheter with a sliding scale of subcutaneous (SQ) regular human insulin. Mrs. S then developed pneumonia with increasing temperatures. Blood glucose levels also increased.

Hyperglycemia: Mrs S was switched from her sliding scale SQ insulin doses to an insulin drip of 5 units intravenous (IV) bolus and 3 to 4 units/hr titrated to q 1-2 hr blood glucose results. The plan was to lower the blood sugar level without causing a sudden hypoglycemia. Following a typical course of management, later Mrs. S's IV insulin was stopped when her glucose reached 250 mg/dL blood.

Dehydration: Several days later Mrs. S had decreased urine output and was unresponsive to furosemide or to a Bumex drip. A nephrology consultation was called. Slow fluid replacement was given, and the Bumex was changed to smaller doses (2 mg). This resulted in increased urine output and lowered blood urea nitrogen (BUN) and creatinine values over the next few days.

Infection: The pneumonia was treated with antibiotics and aggressive pulmonary care. Gradually, Mrs. S's chest x-rays and temperatures improved to normal and she was weaned off the ventilator.

Two weeks after her admission into acute care Mrs. S was transferred to a skilled nursing facility (SNF). Her laboratory tests had greatly improved, and she was tolerating her American Dietetic Association (ADA) diet. Mrs. S was taking NPH human insulin 45 units SQ every morning and 30 units SQ every evening. Highlights of the laboratory tests follow:

		Day 5	Day 14
	Normal (mg/dL)	Critical Care Unit (mg/dL)	SNF (mg/dL)
Blood glucose	70-110	315	150
BUN	7-18	84	46
Creatinine	0.6-1.2	3.9	1.5

TABLE 41-2 Oral Medications and Nursing Implications for NIDDM

Drug	Dosage	Action	Onset, Peak, and Duration	Special Considerations
FIRST-GENERATION HYPOGLYCEMICS				
Tolbutamide (Orinbase)	0.5-2.0 g bid-tid	Hypoglycemic Stimulates release of insulin from functioning pancreatic beta cells	Onset: rapid absorption: 30 min to 1 hr Peak concentration: 3-5 hr Duration: 6-12 hr	Not to be used during pregnancy (parenteral insulin is used to maintain serum glucose level within normal limits.) Drug is metabolized in liver and eliminated in kidneys. Patients with renal insufficiency are started with lower dose and observed for signs of hypoglycemia. Numerous drug interactions exist. Only a few are related.
Acetohexamide (Dymelor)	0.25-1.5 g single dose or bid	Hypoglycemic	Onset: 1 hr Peak concentration: 3 hr Duration: 10-24 hr	
Tolazamide (Tolinase)	0.1-1.0 g single dose or bid	Hypoglycemic	Onset: 4 hr Peak concentration: 4 hr Duration: 10 hr	
Chlorpropamide (Diabinese)	0.1-0.5 g single dose	Hypoglycemic Antidiuretic	Onset: 1 hr Peak concentration: 2-4 hr Duration: 48 hr	Precautions—Disulfiram-like reaction with alcohol. Frequent monitoring for patients with fluid retention or cardiac dysfunction.
SECOND-GENERATION HYPOGLYCEMICS*				
Glipizide (Glucotrol) (Glucotrol XL)	0.1 mg bid qd	Hypoglycemic	Onset: 1 hr Peak concentration: 1-3 hr Duration: 12-24 hr	
Glyburide (Micronase, DiaBeta)	5 mg single dose or bid	Hypoglycemic	Onset: 1 hr Peak concentration: 4 hr Duration: 24 hr	
Glimepiride (Amaryl)	1-4 mg qd	Hypoglycemic		
BIGUANIDE				
Metformin (Glucophage)	Maximum dose: 2500 mg divided dose	Antihyper-glycemic	Plasma concentration: 24-48 hr Duration: 24 hr	Temporarily withhold in patients receiving parenteral iodinated contrast materials for x-rays. Adverse effects—lactic acidosis, gastrointestinal upset; not to be used in pregnancy. Nonsulfonylurea drug. Directly lowers serum glucose level by reduction of hepatic glucose output. Promotes weight loss. Contraindicated in patients with renal insufficiency; acute or chronic acidosis, including diabetic ketoacidosis; hepatic dysfunction, including excessive alcohol intake.

TABLE 41-2 Oral Medications and Nursing Implications for NIDDM—cont'd

Drug	Dosage	Action	Onset, Peak, and Duration	Special Considerations
THIAZOLIDINEDIONES				
Troglitazone (Rezulin)	400 mg single dose	Enhances insulin action by increasing cell receptors to exogenous and endogenous insulin	Peak concentration: 2-3 hr	Used for patients with Type II DM currently on therapy whose hyperglycemia is inadequately controlled ($HgA_{1c} > 85\%$) despite > 30 U insulin qd. Take with meals to increase absorption. Reduces BP, triglycerides. Administration with oral contraceptives reduces efficacy of both troglitazone and contraception by 30%.
ALPHA GLUCOSIDASE INHIBITORS				
Acarbose (Precose)	100 mg tid, with meals	Inhibits activity of several intestinal enzymes that metabolize carbohydrates	Peak concentration: 2-3 hr	Suggested administration with "first bite" each main meal. First drug to effectively reduce peak past prandial glucose. Delays CHO digestion by blocking absorption of complex carbohydrates in small intestines. Does not promote weight loss as CHO is absorbed in distal small intestines, and perhaps colon. Does not seem to affect lactose absorption; therefore lactose-containing substances should be used to treat hypoglycemia rather than sucrose. Major side effects: flatulence, abdominal pain, diarrhea. Side effects minimized with slow titration. Not recommended with severe renal impairment. Safety in pregnancy not established.
Miglitol (Glyset)	50-100 mg tid, with meals	Alpha glucosidase inhibitor Inhibits activity of several intestinal enzymes that metabolize carbohydrates	Peak concentration: 2-3 hr	Same considerations as with acarbose, plus: Administration with digoxin reduces average plasma concentration of digoxin. Administration with propranolol or ranitidine greatly reduces bioavailability of propranolol and ranitidine. Do not take concomitantly with digestive enzymes (e.g., amylase, pancreatin).

** The second-generation hypoglycemics in this table are considered second-generation oral hypoglycemics. These medications are considered more potent. The dosage is lower than that for the first-generation drugs, yet there are fewer side effects associated with the second-generation oral hypoglycemics.*

in the nonwhite population than in the white population.[7]

DKA may develop over several hours in a person who has had diabetes for a period of time. In an undiagnosed diabetic patient, it may take days to develop and signal an abrupt onset of the disease.

Etiology

Ketoacidosis is a result of hyperglycemia, ketosis, and acidemia without treatment. Counterregulatory hormones, such as glucagon, growth hormone, cortisol, and catecholamines, respond in an attempt to reverse the imbalance, yet only add to the continuing cycle. Box 41-2 lists the etiology of DKA in terms of decreased insulin availability and the presence of increased glucose in the blood stream. Changes in self-management of diabetes can influence this ratio, such as a decrease in insulin intake, an increase in dietary intake, or a decrease in routine exercise without adequate adjustment in insulin or diet. Life-style changes, such as growth spurts in the adolescent, require an increase in insulin intake, as do surgery, infection, and trauma. Emotional stress can increase glucose levels by releasing epinephrine or norepinephrine, or both, which triggers increased glucagon secretion. The person may be continuing a routine insulin dose that is then inadequate for the rate of glucose entry into the blood stream from gluconeogenesis and glycogenolysis triggered by the stress hormones. (∞Box 39-1, p. 980.)

DKA is seen in patients who use the subcutaneous insulin pump. This device can provide tighter glucose control than subcutaneous injections. Improper functioning resulting in insulin leakage or pump failure[6,13] initially causes subtle changes in glucose levels. The patient, believing that his or her glucose is adequately controlled by the pump, attributes the physical symptoms to extraneous health problems. Tending to trust the functioning of the pump, the patient delays testing serum glucose and urine ketone levels while DKA is progressively developing.

BOX 41-2 Etiology of Diabetic Ketoacidosis

DECREASED EXOGENOUS INSULIN INTAKE

- Lack of knowledge, poor compliance
  - Omitting dose
  - Insufficient dose to meet glucose requirement (e.g., hyperalimentation)
- Malfunctioning insulin pump
- Pharmacologic drugs
  - Phenytoin
  - Thiazide/sulfonamide diuretics

INCREASED ENDOGENOUS GLUCOSE

- Diabetes management changes
  - Decreased exercise without decreasing food or increasing insulin
  - Increased dietary intake
- Sympathetic nervous system responses
  - Stressful events
    - Injury
    - Surgery
    - Infections
      - Respiratory tract
      - Urinary tract
      - Pancreatitis
    - Emotional trauma
- Increased glucagon
- Increased growth hormone
- Pharmacologic drugs
  - Steroid therapy
  - Epinephrine/norepinephrine

Pathophysiology

Insulin deficiency. Insulin is the metabolic key to the transfer of glucose from the blood stream into the cell where it can be used immediately for energy or stored to be used at a later time. Without insulin, glucose remains in the blood stream and cells are deprived of their energy source. A complex pathophysiologic chain of events follows (Figure 41-1). The release of glucagon is stimulated when insulin is ineffective in providing the cells with glucose for energy. Glucagon increases the amount of glucose in the blood stream by breaking down stored glucose (glycogenolysis) and converting noncarbohydrate molecules into glucose (gluconeogenesis). Blood glucose levels for the patient in DKA typically range from 300 to 800 mg/dL of blood. (Blood glucose levels alone do not indicate DKA; ketoacidosis, which is discussed later, is a major determining factor).

Hyperglycemia. Hyperglycemia increases the plasma osmolality, and blood becomes hyperosmolar. Cellular dehydration occurs as the hyperosmolar extracellular fluid draws the more dilute intracellular and interstitial fluid into the vascular space in an attempt to return the plasma osmolality to normal. Dehydration stimulates catecholamine production for further glycogenolysis, lipolysis, gluconeogenesis, and ketogenesis.

Fluid volume deficit. Excessive urination (polyuria) and glycosuria occur as a result of the osmotic diuresis. The excess glucose, filtered at the glomeruli, cannot be reabsorbed at the renal tubule and "spills" into the urine. The unreabsorbed solute exerts its own

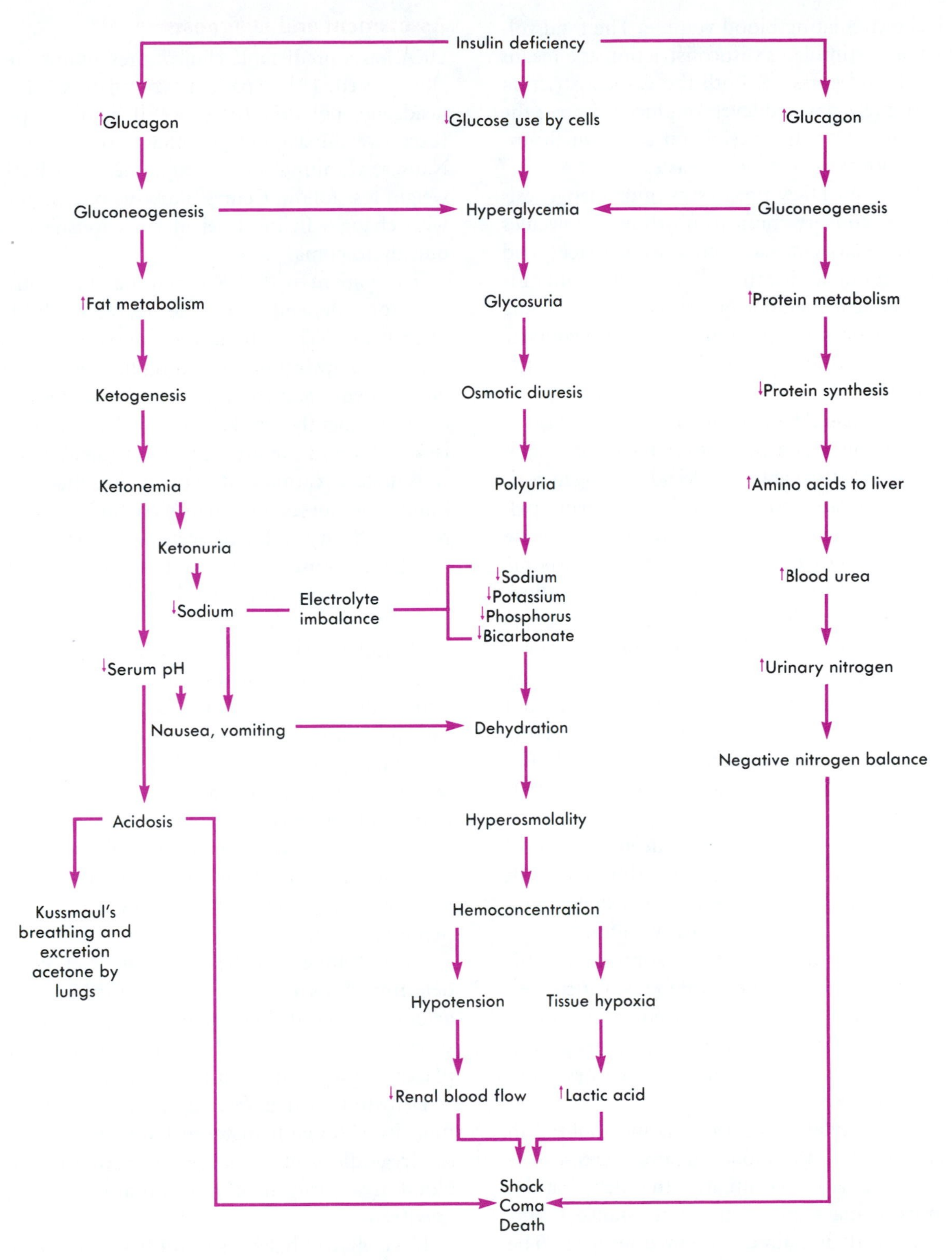

FIGURE 41-1. Pathophysiology of diabetic ketoacidosis (DKA). A carbohydrate derangement affects the metabolism of both protein and fat.

osmotic pull in the renal tubules, and less water is returned to circulation via the collecting ducts. As a result, large volumes of water, along with sodium, potassium, and phosphorus, are excreted in the urine, causing fluid volume deficit and electrolyte imbalance.

Thirst. Excessive thirst (polydipsia) occurs as the decrease in circulating blood volume stimulates the osmoreceptors in the hypothalamus and promotes the release of angiotensin II. The strong thirst sensation is intended to compensate for the loss of fluids and replenish the circulating blood volume. The fluid volume deficit also stimulates vasoconstriction as a means to preserve blood pressure. Both the vasoconstriction and the extremely elevated levels of glucose impair the delivery of oxygen to the peripheral cells, which impedes the removal of metabolic wastes.

Ketoacidosis. As DKA progresses, gluconeogenesis continues to convert noncarbohydrate molecules into glucose. Ketoacidosis occurs as ketoacid end products accumulate in the blood and rapid, incomplete fatty acid metabolism releases highly acidic substances (acetoacetic acid and beta-hydroxybutyric acid) into the blood stream (ketonemia) and the urine (ketonuria).

Acid base balance. The patient with moderate to severe DKA typically has a pH between 7.2 and 7.36.[14] The acid ketones dissociate and yield hydrogen ions (H^+) that accumulate and cause a drop in serum pH. Normally the hydrogen ions react with bicarbonate (HCO_3^-) to produce carbonic acid (H_2CO_3). Carbonic acid dissociates to form water (H_2O) and carbon dioxide (CO_2), which are eliminated through the kidneys and the lungs, respectively. In gluconeogenesis, however, ketones accumulate in the blood stream faster than they can be metabolized. The bicarbonate and sodium loss through osmotic diuresis prevents the formation of sodium bicarbonate needed to buffer the increasing carbonic acid. The respiratory rate is altered in an attempt to compensate for the carbonic acid build-up. Breathing becomes deep and rapid (Kussmaul's respirations) to release carbonic acid in the form of carbon dioxide. Acetone is exhaled, giving the breath its characteristic "fruity" odor.

Gluconeogenesis. Gluconeogenesis stimulates mobilization of protein, and protein catabolism increases. Protein is broken down and converted to glucose in the liver. Continuous, uninterrupted gluconeogenesis leaves no reserve protein available for synthesis and repair of vital body tissues.

Nitrogen accumulates as protein is metabolized to urea. Urea, added to the blood stream, increases the osmotic diuresis and accentuates the dehydration. Loss of muscle mass and reduced resistance to infection occur with impaired protein utilization. The combined states of acidosis and osmotic diuresis lead to a significant loss of phosphorus (yet laboratory serum phosphorus level may not change), further compromising peripheral tissue perfusion. Hypophosphatemia impairs the oxygen function of the hemoglobin by increasing hemoglobin's affinity for oxygen and thereby reducing delivery of oxygen to the cells.[15]

Assessment and Diagnosis

DKA has a predictable clinical presentation. It is usually preceded by patient complaints of malaise, headache, polyuria (excessive urination), polydipsia (excessive thirst), and polyphagia (excessive hunger). Nausea, vomiting, extreme fatigue, dehydration, and weight loss follow. Central nervous system depression, with changes in the level of consciousness, can lead quickly to coma.

The patient with DKA may be stuporous or unconscious, depending on the degree of fluid-balance disturbance. The physical examination reveals evidence of dehydration, including flushed, dry skin, dry buccal membranes, and skin turgor greater than 3 seconds. Frequently, "sunken eyeballs," resulting from the lack of fluid in the interstitium of the eyeball, are observed. Tachycardia and hypotension may signal profound fluid losses. Kussmaul's air hunger continues to reveal a "fruity" odor of acetone. Normal or subnormal temperatures exist despite volume depletion. An increased temperature at this point may indicate the presence of infection.[12]

Considering the complexity and potential seriousness of DKA, the diagnosis is straighforward. With a known diabetic patient, a diagnosis of DKA is determined by heavy ketonuria and glycosuria in the presence of hyperglycemia and ketonemia. If the patient is not known to have diabetes, other causes of metabolic acidosis must be differentiated before a course of therapy is begun. Starvation, alcoholism, certain toxic chemicals, lactic acid, and uremia may result in a ketoacidotic state.[13] The treatment plan varies, depending on the cause.

Urine ketones and bedside fingerstick blood sugar determinations provide rapid confirmation of ketoacidosis in the diabetic patient. Laboratory evidence supporting the ketoacidosis includes low arterial blood pH and low plasma bicarbonate levels.[16]

Dehydration manifests by an increased serum osmolality, elevated hematocrit level, marked leukocytosis (regardless of presence of infection), increased blood urea nitrogen (BUN), and a high urine specific gravity.

Electrolyte imbalances result from osmotic diuresis, fluid depletion, and the acidosis driving potassium out of the cells. Vomiting and polyuria cause a decrease in serum sodium and potassium levels. Hyponatremia also occurs from the shift of extracellular sodium to intracellular as the potassium is depleted.

Serum potassium levels vary, depending on the phase of ketoacidosis. Potassium levels may be elevated as potassium moves from the intercellular compartment to the extracellular compartment in an exchange for hydrogen ions. Hyperkalemia is reduced quickly as potassium is lost from the body by the vomiting, diarrhea, and osmotic diuresis. Potassium is also decreased with the replacement of insulin. Phosphorus levels also may be low, normal, or elevated despite actual serum depletion. Assessment of electrolyte levels must continue throughout the treatment phase inasmuch as both potassium and phosphorus rapidly reenter the cell when fluid and insulin therapy are provided.

Medical Management

Diagnosis of DKA is based on the combination of presenting symptoms, patient history, medical history (Type I diabetes mellitus), precipitating factors if known, and results of serum glucose and urine ketone testing. Additional information is obtained from laboratory serum electrolyte values, arterial blood gases, urinalysis, and a baseline electrocardiogram. Emergency medical treatment is aimed at reversing the ketoacidosis. Once diagnosed, DKA requires aggressive medical and nursing management to prevent progressive decompensation. Treatment is needed to accomplish the following:

- Reverse dehydration
- Restore the insulin-glucagon ratio to achieve the following:
  - Promote cellular use of glucose
  - Reduce the counterregulatory hormone glucagon
  - Break the ketotic cycle
- Treat and prevent circulatory collapse
- Replenish electrolytes

In addition to vigorous medical treatment, the practitioner investigates the precipitating causes of ketoacidosis. Unless the precipitating factors are known and resolved, DKA probably will recur. After 10 to 12 hours of effective treatment, the patient's hydration and neurologic and metabolic status should improve drastically.

Hydration. The patient with DKA is significantly dehyrated, may have lost 5% to 10% of body weight in fluids, and may have a fluid deficit of 3 to 5 L.[8] There is no consensus among medical practitioners on the use of isotonic or hypotonic solution as a replacement for lost fluid. Initially, normal physiologic saline solution may be given to reverse the vascular deficit, hypotension, and extracellular fluid losses. During the first hour of severe dehydration, 1 L is infused. The rate varies, however, depending on urinary output, secondary illnesses, and precipitating factors. To dilute the serum osmolality, infusions of half-strength sodium chloride may follow the initial saline replacement. Because the water deficit exceeds the sodium loss, half-strength sodium chloride can be given at a rate of 300 to 500 ml/hour until the serum osmolality returns to normal and the blood glucose levels decrease.

Intravenous glucose. Once the serum glucose level is 250 to 300 mg/dL of blood, a 5% dextrose solution is infused.[8] Intravenously administered glucose is necessary to replenish glucose stores because muscle and liver glycogen reserves may have been depleted during gluconeogenesis. Perhaps more importantly, it is necessary to prevent hypoglycemia, which may result from a relative drop in circulating glucose from the infusion of exogenous insulin. In addition, glucose is given to prevent cerebral edema, which may result when free water is drawn across the blood-brain barrier into brain tissue (although several theories exist, the exact mechanism involved in this alteration in the blood-brain barrier is not known).[17] Intravenous glucose level is maintained until the patient no longer requires intravenous fluids and is taking liquids by mouth.

Insulin administration. Insulin is given simultaneously with intravenous fluids. Refer to Table 41-3 for types of insulin medication and nursing considerations in their administration.[8,10,12,15] A reversal of the ketoacidotic metabolic abnormalities gradually occurs as the patient becomes hydrated and receives insulin. The serum glucose level falls as large quantities of glucose are perfused through the kidneys and removed in the urine. The exogenous insulin complements the fluid therapy and promotes the entry of glucose into the cell (insulin also permits potassium and phosphorus to reenter the cell). Insulin inhibits the release of glucagon, and glucose no longer is poured into the circulation as a result of gluconeogenesis and glycogenolysis. The ketoacidotic cycle gradually is broken because ketoacids no longer are produced as a by-product of incomplete fat metabolism. The serum osmolality is reduced with vigorous fluid replacement, coupled with the reduction of glucose, urea, and ketones circulating in the blood stream. Osmotic diuresis is reversed as the continuous fluids replace fluid losses, and serum glucose levels return to normal.

Insulin resistance. The patient who does not respond to insulin may have a problem with insulin resistance at the cell receptor site. These patients require a more aggressive approach. A one-time bolus of 0.3 U/kg may be given to saturate the insulin cell receptor sites and compete with the insulin resistance. Replacement of low-dose insulin, 0.1 U/kg/hour (approximately 5 U/hour), is given intravenously (or

TABLE 41-3 Parenteral* Insulins and Nursing Implications for Use in Diabetes Mellitus

Type of Insulin	Dosage†	Action	Onset, Peak, and Duration	Special Considerations
Regular insulin (crystalline zinc)	Intravenously (IV) or subcutaneously (SQ)	Insulin replacement therapy; regulates storage and metabolism of protein, carbohydrate, and fats; potent hypoglycemic agent	Onset: within 1 hr Peak: 2-4 hr Duration: 5-8 hr	Only type of insulin suitable for IV use. Also available as regular insulin, human insulin. Do not use if cloudy, colored, or unusually viscous. Insulins prepared from bovine, pork, and human sources. Source determined by patient sensitivity. Human source has least intolerance. Several drugs interact or have potentially related problems with insulin. The reader is referred to a drug information text for further information. Side effect—hypoglycemia
Insulin Lispro	SQ	Insulin replacement	Onset: 10-15 min Peak: 45-60 min Duration: 1.5-3.5 hrs	First available synthetic insulin almost *immediately* absorbed. Shorter duration of action than human regular insulin, therefore should be used with longer-acting insulins. Reliable treatment of postprandial hyperglycemia with decreased risk of hypoglycemia.
Insulin zinc suspension (Lente Insulin, Semilente Insulin)	SQ; not for IV use	Insulin replacement hormone	Onset: 1-3 hr Peak: 8-12 hr Duration: 18-28 hr	Also available as insulin zinc, human suspension
Isophane insulin suspension (NPH Insulin)	SQ; not for IV use	Insulin replacement hormone	Onset: 3-4 hr Peak: 6-12 hr Duration: 18-28 hr	Also available as isophane insulin, human
Insulin zinc supsension (Ultralente Insulin)	SQ; not for IV use	Extended action; insulin replacement hormone	Onset: 4-6 hr Peak: 18-24 hr Duration: 36 hr	Also available as extended insulin zinc, human
Isophane insulin, human suspension and insulin human injection	SQ; not for IV use	Rapid and intermediate acting	Varies	Combination of insulins: 50% isophane insulin human with 50% insulin human Humulin 50/50 (biosynthetic) 70% isophane insulin, human with 30% insulin human injection (Humulin 70/30 biosynthetic) and Novolin

*Parenteral refers to a route other than by mouth (PO).
†Doses are individualized according to patient's age and size.

intramuscularly depending on circulatory perfusion) until acidosis is reversed. Low-dose insulin results in a few serious cases of hypoglycemia.[17]

Potassium and phosphorus administration. Hypokalemia may occur as insulin promotes the return of potassium into the cell and acidosis is reduced. Replacement of potassium begins as soon as the potassium shift has stabilized. Insulin treatment also precipitates hypophosphatemia as serum phosphate returns to the cell. Although the need to administer phosphate currently is debated, its use does seem to improve tissue oxygenation and promote the renal excretion of hydrogen ions.[13]

Bicarbonate administration. Replacement of lost bicarbonate is closely monitored. It is given to replace depleted bicarbonate stores in association with a severely acidotic pH. It generally is agreed that bicarbonate is started for clinically severe acidotic states (pH <7.0)[18] and stopped when the pH level reaches 72.0.[19] An indwelling arterial line provides access for hourly sampling of blood gases to evaluate pH and bicarbonate.

Prevention of abdominal distention. Intubated or comatose patients may require a nasogastric tube to decompress stomach contents and to prevent vomiting and subsequent aspiration. The use of nasogastric tube also reduces impaired ventilation that results from an elevated diaphragm caused by abdominal distention.

Nursing Management

The management of the patient with DKA demands astute assessments, critical thinking, and quick decision making. Use of the nursing process helps to organize activities and to promote reversal of symptoms. (See Box 41-3 for a summary of Nursing Diagnoses.) An accurately maintained flow sheet is a necessity because the nurse simultaneously monitors several system functions, collects multiple laboratory values, and provides various interventions.

Hydration status. The patient's hydration status is severely compromised in ketoacidosis. Osmotic diuresis and increased insensible loss of fluid from Kussmaul's breathing can result in loss of 10% of total body water.[13] Nausea, vomiting, and changes in level of consciousness interfere with the person's ability to ingest or retain fluids (see Box 41-4 for more detail on hydration assessment).

Fluid replacement. Rapid intravenous fluid replacement requires the use of a volumetric pump. Accurate intake and output measurements must be maintained to record the body's use of fluid. Hourly urine output measures renal functioning and also provides information that helps prevent overhydration or underhydration. Vital signs, especially pulse rate, hemodynamic findings, and blood pressure, are constantly monitored to assess cardiac response to the fluid replacement. Evidence that fluid replacement is effective includes normal central venous pressure (CVP), decreased heart rate, and normal pulmonary artery pressure (PAP). Further evidence of hydration includes a change from the previously weak, thready pulse to a pulse that is strong and full and a change from a previously low blood pressure to a gradual elevation of systolic blood

BOX 41-3 NURSING DIAGNOSIS AND MANAGEMENT

DIABETIC KETOACIDOSIS

- Decreased Cardiac Output related to alterations in preload, p. 590
- Fluid Volume Deficit related to absolute loss, p. 914
- Anxiety rleated to threat to biologic, psychologic, and/or social integrity, p. 99
- Body Image Disturbance related to functional dependence on life-sustaining technology, p. 87
- Ineffective Individual Coping related to situational crisis and personal vulnerability, p. 95
- Powerlessness related to lack of control over current situation and/or disease progression, p. 89
- Knowledge Deficit: Discharge Regimen related to lack of previous exposure to information, p. 61 (see Patient Education Box 41-8)

BOX 41-4 Hydration Assessment for the Patient in Diabetic Ketoacidosis and Hyperglycemic Hyperosmolar Nonketotic Syndrome

Hydration status assessment includes the following:
Hourly intake
Blood pressure changes
  Orthostatic hypotension
  Pulse pressure
  Pulse rate, character, rhythm
Neck vein filling
Skin turgor
Skin moisture
Body weight
Central venous pressure
Pulmonary arterial wedge pressure
Hourly output
Complaints of thirst

pressure. Reduced respirations also signal a return to adequate fluid balance.

Overhydration. Circulatory overload from the rapid fluid volume infusion is a serious complication that can occur in the patient with a compromised cardiovascular or renal system, or both. Neck vein engorgement, dyspnea without exertion, and elevated CVP and PAP, as well as moist lung sounds, signal circulatory overload. Reduction in the rate and volume of infusion, elevation of the head, and administration of oxygen may be required to manage the increased intravascular volume. Measuring hourly urine is mandatory to assess renal output and adequacy of fluid replacement. Catheterizing the alert patient remains controversial because of the risk of secondary infection.

Laboratory analysis. Tests for blood glucose are performed every 30 to 60 minutes at the bedside. Urine specific gravity determination is performed every 2 hours. Once ketonuria is established and treatment is monitored, and BUN and creatinine levels are assessed for possible renal impairment related to decreased renal perfusion.

Insulin/glucose balance. Insulin is given intravenously to the severely dehydrated patient to ensure absorption when inadequate tissue perfusion is present. The insulin dose must be calculated to accommodate the binding that causes insulin to be absorbed by the glass or plastic container and tubing. Inert materials are used in collapsible intravenous containers that minimize this binding. The institution's pharmacy department protocol should be followed so that the prepared solution provides maximum absorption relative to the container and tubing. As glucose levels, dehydration, and hypotension diminish, insulin is given subcutaneously.

Throughout the insulin therapy, both patient response and laboratory data are assessed for changes relating to glucose levels. Reduction in glucose levels is fairly consistent with low-dose therapy, as previously discussed. In most patients, serum glucose levels decline approximately 100 mg/dL/hour.[15] Respirations frequently are assessed for changes in rate, depth, and fruity "acetone" odor. When the blood glucose level falls to 250 to 300 mg/dL of blood, a 5% dextrose solution is infused to prevent hypoglycemia. At this time, insulin dosage may be decreased. Administration of regular insulin drip is not discontinued until ketoacidosis subsides, as identified by the arterial blood gases.[15] Signs of hypoglycemia, such as unexpected behavioral changes, diaphoresis, and tremors (see Box 41-5), may occur from a relative drop in glucose level. Should hypoglycemia occur, insulin is stopped and the physician notified (see Box 41-6 for management of hypoglycemia).

BOX 41-5 Clinical Manifestations of Hypoglycemia and Hyperglycemia

HYPOGLYCEMIA	HYPERGLYCEMIA
Restlessness	Excessive thirst
Apprehension	Excessive urination
Irritability	Hunger
Trembling	Weakness
Weakness	Listlessness
Diaphoresis	Mental fatigue
Pallor	Flushed, dry skin
Paresthesia	Itching
Headache	Headache
Hunger	Nausea
Difficulty thinking	Vomiting
Loss of coordination	Abdominal cramps
Difficulty walking	Dehydration
Difficulty talking	Weak, rapid pulse
Visual disturbances	Postural hypotension
Blurred vision	Hypotension
Double vision	Acetone breath odor
Tachycardia	Kussmaul's respirations
Shallow respirations	Rapid breathing
Hypertension	Changes in level of consciousness
Changes in level of consciousness	Stupor
Seizures	Coma
Coma	

Signs of hyperglycemia (see Box 41-5), such as Kussmaul's respirations; dry skin; and fruity, acetone breath odor, also may be related to both physical and emotional stressors that the patient experiences before or during the stay in the critical care unit. Reducing these stressors and their hyperglycemic effects is a worthy challenge for the nurse (see Box 41-7 for management of hyperglycemia).

Electrolytes. Electrolytes fluctuate throughout the rehydration phase. Standard critical care protocols for administering electrolytes on the basis of laboratory criteria are usually followed. The nurse must be aware of both the obvious and the obscure signs that indicate changing electrolyte levels.

Potassium. Hypokalemia can occur within the first 4 hours of the rehydration-insulin treatment. Continuous cardiac monitoring is required because potassium affects the heart's electrical condition, and hyperkalemia or hypokalemia may lead to lethal cardiac

NURSING INTERVENTION CLASSIFICATIONS

BOX 41-6 Hypoglycemia Management

DEFINITION: Preventing and treating below normal blood glucose levels

ACTIVITIES:

Identify patient at risk for hypoglycemia
Monitor blood glucose levels, as indicated
Monitor for signs and symptoms of hypoglycemia: pallor, diaphoresis, tachycardia, palpitations, hunger, paresthesia, shakiness, inability to concentrate, confusion, slurred speech, irrational or uncontrolled behavior, blurred vision, somnolence, inability to arouse from sleep, or seizures
Provide simple carbohydrate, as indicated
Provide complex carbohydrate and protein, as indicated
Maintain IV access, as appropriate
Administer intravenous dextrose, as appropriate
Administer glucagon, as appropriate
Consult physician if signs and symptoms of hypoglycemia persist or worsen
Maintain patient airway, as necessary
Protect from injury, as necessary
Identify possible cause of hypoglycemia
Recommend changes in regimen to prevent hypoglycemia (e.g., reduction in insulin when NPO)
Instruct patient and significant others on prevention, recognition, and treatment of hypoglycemia
Instruct significant others on use and administration of glucagon, as appropriate
Instruct patient to obtain and carry appropriate emergency medical identification
Encourage patient to have simple carbohydrate available at all times
Encourage self-monitoring of blood glucose levels
Provide assistance to patient in making self-care decisions to prevent hypoglycemia (e.g., eating additional food or reducing insulin when exercising)

From McCloskey JC, Bulechek GM: *Nursing interventions classification*, ed 2, St Louis, 1996, Mosby.

dysrhythmias. Hypokalemia is depicted on the cardiac monitor by ventricular dysrythmias, a prolonged QT interval, a flattened or depressed T wave, and depressed ST segments. Physical signs of hypokalemia include muscle weakness, decreased gastrointestinal motility (evidenced by abdominal distention or paralytic ileus), hypotension, and a weak pulse. Respiratory arrest can occur as a result of severe hypokalemia. (∞ Potassium, p. 377 and p. 860.)

Hyperkalemia occurs with acidosis or when potassium deficit is treated too aggressively in patients with renal insufficiency. Hyperkalemia is noted on a cardiac monitor by a large, peaked T wave, flattened P wave, and a broad, slurred QRS complex. Ventricular fibrillation can follow. Additional changes related to increased potassium levels include bradycardia, increased gastrointestinal motility (with nausea and diarrhea), and oliguria. Neuromuscular signs of hyperkalemia include weakness, impaired muscle activity, flaccid paralysis, respiratory arrest, and ventricular asystole.

Sodium. Serum sodium levels fall as the sodium replaces the potassium that moves out of the cells. Sodium is eliminated from the body as a result of the osmotic diuresis. In addition, the hyponatremia is compounded by the vomiting and diarrhea that occur during ketoacidosis. Clinical manifestations of hyponatremia include abdominal cramping, apprehension, postural hypotension, and unexpected behavioral changes. Sodium chloride is infused as the initial intravenous solution. Maintenance of the saline infusion depends on clinical manifestations of sodium imbalance plus serum laboratory values.

Basic assessments. Skin care takes on new dimensions for the patient with DKA. Dehydration, hypovolemia, and hypophosphatemia interfere with oxygen delivery at the cell site and contribute to inadequate perfusion and tissue breakdown. Patients must be repositioned every hour to relieve capillary pressure and promote adequate perfusion to body tissues. The typical patient with Type I diabetes is either of normal weight or underweight. Bony

NURSING INTERVENTION CLASSIFICATIONS

BOX 41-7 Hyperglycemia Management

DEFINITION: Preventing and treating above normal blood glucose levels

ACTIVITIES:

Monitor blood glucose levels, as indicated
Monitor for signs and symptoms of hyperglycemia: polyuria, polydipsia, polyphagia, weakness, lethargy, malaise, blurring of vision, or headache
Monitor urine ketones, as indicated
Monitor ABG, electrolyte, and betahydroxybutyrate levels, as available
Monitor orthostatic blood pressure and pulse, as indicated
Administer insulin, as prescribed
Encourage oral fluid intake
Monitor fluid status (including I&O), as appropriate
Maintain IV access, as appropriate
Administer IV fluids, as needed
Administer potassium, as prescribed
Consult physician if signs and symptoms of hyperglycemia persist or worsen
Assist with ambulation if orthostatic hypotension is present
Provide oral hygiene, if necessary
Identify possible causes of hyperglycemia
Anticipate situations in which insulin requirements will increase (e.g., intercurrent illness)
Restrict exercise when blood glucose levels are > 250 mg/dL, especially if urine ketones are present
Instruct patient and significant others on prevention, recognition, and management of hyperglycemia
Encourage self-monitoring of blood glucose levels
Instruct on urine ketone testing, as appropriate
Instruct on indications for, and significance of, urine ketone testing, if appropriate
Instruct patient to report moderate or large urine ketone levels to the health professional
Instruct patient and significant others on diabetes management during illness, including use of insulin and/or oral agents, monitoring, fluid intake, carbohydrate replacement, and when to seek health professional assistance, as appropriate
Provide assistance in adjusting regimen to prevent and treat hyperglycemia (e.g., increasing insulin or oral agent), as indicated
Facilitate adherence to diet and exercise regimen

From McCloskey JC, Bulechek GM: *Nursing interventions classification,* ed 2, St Louis, 1996, Mosby.

prominences must be assessed for tissue breakdown and body weight repositioned every hour. Irritation of skin from adhesive tape, shearing force, and detergents is to be avoided. Maintenance of skin integrity prevents unwanted portals of entry for microorganisms.

Skin assessment for hydration. Skin assessment for degree of moisture indicates the body's distribution and use of fluid within body tissues. The patient with ketoacidosis has flushed, dry skin, dry buccal membranes, parched lips, and ropy saliva. The lips and tongue may adhere to the teeth because of decreased fluids. The conscious patient complains of intense thirst, but consumption of large quantities of water may be unwise if there is a concurrent problem with abdominal distention. Quickly drinking a large volume of fluid may add to the distended abdomen and stimulate vomiting. Ice chips may be used as an alternative to quench the patient's thirst, along with reassurance that the intravenous fluids will soon satisfy the thirst.

Mouth care. Oral care, including lip balm, helps keep lips supple and prevents cracking. Prepared sponge sticks or moist gauze pads can be used to moisten oral membranes of the unconscious patient. Swabbing the mouth moistens the tissue and displaces the bacteria that collect when saliva, which has a bacteriostatic action, is curtailed by dehydration. The conscious patient removes bacteria and provides oral comfort with frequent tooth brushing and oral rinsing.

Pulmonary care. Lung sounds are assessed every 8 hours or as needed. Encouraging the conscious patient to breathe deeply every hour promotes full ventilation of the lungs and helps prevent pulmonary complications.

Sterile technique. Strict sterile technique is used to maintain all intravenous systems. All venipuncture sites are checked every 4 hours for signs of inflammation, phlebitis, or infiltration. Strict surgical asepsis is used for all invasive procedures. Careful sterile technique is used if urinary catheterization is necessary to obtain urine samples for testing. Catheter care is given every 8 hours.

Neurologic status. Changes in the patient's neurologic status may be insidious. Alterations in level of consciousness, pupil reaction, and motor function may be the result of fluctuating glucose levels and cerebral fluid shifts. Confusion and sudden complaints of headache are ominous signs that may signal cerebral edema. These observations require immediate action to prevent neurologic damage. Neurologic assessments performed every 4 hours or as needed, coupled with serum osmolality values, serve as an index of the patient's response to the rehydration therapy.

Patient education. For patients with previously diagnosed diabetes the knowledge level and compliance history are important in formulating a teaching plan. Learning objectives include a definition of hyperglycemia and its causes, harmful effects, and symptoms. Additional objectives include a definition of ketoacidosis and its causes, symptoms, and harmful consequences. The patient and family are expected to learn the principles of diabetes management during illness. They also are expected to know the warning signs that must be brought to the attention of a health care practitioner. Education of the patient and family or other persons involved in the patient's supportive care is the goal of the teaching process.

The patient whose diabetes is newly diagnosed requires teaching about the disease process and self-care management. This instruction is provided once the acute illness is controlled. Comprehensive instruction for patients and families involves various health care personnel, including the nurse, nutritionist, and physician. It is helpful if family members or a specific friend/caregiver attend diabetic sessions as a backup for the client when needed. During this instruction, emphasis is placed on daily maintenance of a chronic disease as well as factors that led to DKA and required admission to a critical care unit. See Patient Education Box 41-8 for a summary of patient education needs after diabetic ketoacidosis. The long-term patient education needs will focus on management of diabetes mellitus. (∞Nutrition and Endocrine Alterations, p. 149.)

BOX 41-8 PATIENT EDUCATION

DIABETIC KETOACIDOSIS (DKA)

- Acute Phase
  - Explain rationale for critical care unit admission
  - Reduce anxiety associated with critical care unit
- Predischarge
  - Assess knowledge level
  - Assess compliance history
  - Diabetes disease process
  - Definition of hyperglycemia
  - Causes of DKA
  - Pathophysiology of DKA
  - Self-care of diabetics
  - Signs and symptoms to report to health care practitioner

HYPERGLYCEMIC HYPEROSMOLAR NONKETOTIC SYNDROME

Description

Hyperglycemic hyperosmolar nonketotic syndrome[16] (HHNS) is a frequently lethal complication of DM. The hallmarks of HHNS are extremely high levels of plasma glucose with resulting elevations in hyperosmolality and osmotic diuresis. Ketosis is mild or absent. Inability to replace fluids lost through diuresis or severe diarrhea leads to profound dehydration and changes in level of consciousness. HHNS has a 10% to 50% mortality,[7] which is heightened by other existing disease processes. The severity of symptoms, plus minimal or absent ketosis, distinguishes HHNS from DKA (Table 41-4).

Etiology

HHNS occurs when the pancreas produces a relatively insufficient amount of insulin for the high levels of glucose that flood the blood stream (see Box 41-9, Etiology of HHNS). The disorder occurs mainly, although not exclusively, in elderly obese persons with underlying conditions that require medical treatment. The patient may have Type II non–insulin-dependent diabetes that is treated with diet and oral hypoglycemic agents. HHNS also can occur in persons with previously undiagnosed and therefore untreated diabetes.

TABLE 41-4 General Comparison of DKA and HHNS

	Diabetic Ketoacidosis	Hyperglycemic Hyperosmolar Nonketotic Syndrome
Cause	Insufficient exogenous insulin for glucose needs	Insufficient exogenous/endogenous insulin for glucose needs
Onset	Sudden (hours)	Slow, insidious (days, weeks)
Predisposing factors	Noncompliance to Type I DM, illness, surgery, decreased activity	Elderly with recent acute illness; therapeutic procedures
Mortality	9% to 14%	10% to 50%
Population affected	Type I DM	Type II DM, age > 65 yr
Clinical manifestations	Similarities: dry mouth, polydipsia, polyuria, polyphagia, dehydration, dry skin, hypotension, weakness, mental confusion, tachycardia, changes in level of consciousness	
	Differences: ketoacidosis: air hunger, acetone breath odor, respirations rapid and deep, nausea, vomiting	No ketosis, no breath odor, respirations rapid and shallow, usually mild nausea and vomiting
Laboratory tests		
Serum glucose	300-800 mg/dL	600-2000 mg/dL
Serum ketones	Strongly positive	Normal or mildly elevated
Serum pH	<7.3	Normal
Serum osmolality	<350 mOsm/L	>350 mOsm/L
Serum sodium	Normal or low	Normal or elevated
Serum potassium	Low, normal, or elevated (total body K^+ is depleted)	Low, normal, or elevated
Serum bicarbonate	<15 mEq/L	Normal
Serum phosphorus	Low, normal, or elevated (may decrease after insulin therapy)	Low, normal, or elevated (may decrease after insulin therapy)
Urine acetone	Strong	Absent or mild

DM, Diabetes mellitus.

In either situations, it is possible that some of the manufactured insulin is effective in admitting glucose into the cells for energy. This is a major difference between DKA and HHNS. In HHNS, protein and fats are not used to the same degree as in DKA and the ketotic cycle is either never started or is very mild. HHNS is covered by the same DRGs as diabetes mellitus: DRG 295 if the age is between 0 and 35 years, with an anticipated length of stay of 5.1 days, and DRG 294 if the person is 35 years older, with an anticipated length of stay of 6.2 days.[5]

The extreme hyperglycemia of HHNS can be precipitated by the stress of extensive burns, infection, or other major illness, such as myocardial infarction. The syndrome also may be precipitated by iatrogenic treatments that may increase the serum glucose levels and cause an imbalance in the insulin/glucagon ratio. Such treatments include hyperalimentation, high-calorie enteral feedings, hemodialysis, and peritoneal dialysis. Prescription medications that interfere with pancreatic insulin production may precipitate HHNS, including phenytoin, thiazide diuretics, and diazoxide. Other medications, such as sympathomimetic agents, stimulate gluconeogenesis by increasing glucose levels through the metabolism of protein and fats.

Pathophysiology

HHNS represents a deficit of insulin and an excess of glucagon. Figure 41-2 schematically presents the pathophysiology. Reduced insulin levels prevent the movement of glucose into the cells, thus allowing glucose to accumulate in the plasma. Glucagon release is triggered by the decreased insulin, and hepatic glucose from glycogenolysis is poured into the circulation. Glucagon also stimulates the metabolism of fat and protein through gluconeogenesis in an attempt to provide cells with an energy source. Excessive glucose, along with the end products of incomplete fat and protein metabolism, collects as debris in the blood stream. As the number of particles increases in the blood, hyperosmolality increases. In an effort to decrease the serum osmolality, fluid is drawn from the intracel-

BOX 41-9 Etiology of Hyperglycemic Hyperosmolar Nonketotic Syndrome

INSUFFICIENT INSULIN

Diabetes mellitus
Pancreatic disease
Pancreatectomy
Pharmacologic
- Phenytoin
- Thiazide/sulfonamide diuretics

INCREASED ENDOGENOUS GLUCOSE

Acute stress
- Extensive burns
- Myocardial infarction
- Infection

Pharmacologic
- Glucocorticoids
- Steroids
- Sympathomimetics
- Thyroid preparations

INCREASED EXOGENOUS GLUCOSE

Hyperalimentation (total parenteral nutrition)
High-calorie enteral feedings
Hemodialysis
Peritoneal dialysis

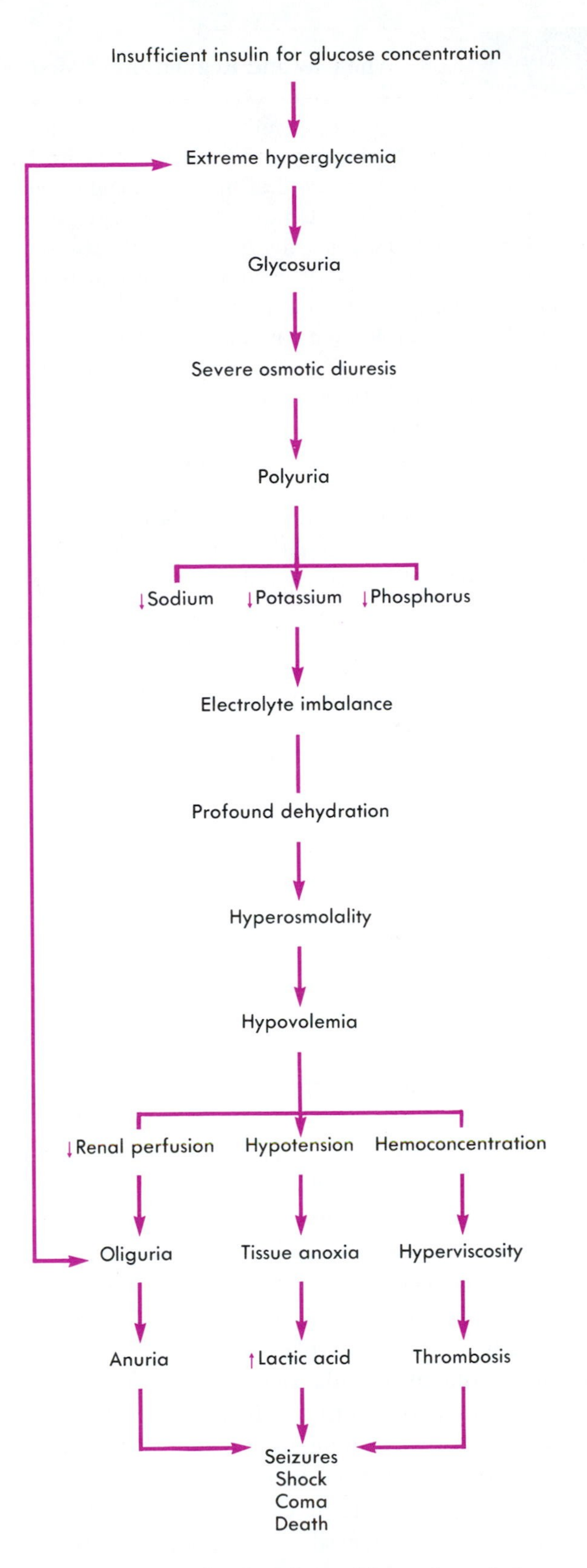

FIGURE 41-2. Pathophysiology of hyperglycemic hyperosmolar nonketotic syndrome (HHNS).

lular compartment into the vascular bed. Profound intracellular volume depletion occurs if the patient's thirst sensation is absent or decreased, if the patient is unable to respond to thirst, or if the fluids are inaccessible.

Hemoconcentration persists despite removal of large amounts of glucose in the urine (glycosuria). The glomerular filtration and elimination of glucose by the kidney tubules are ineffective in reducing the serum glucose level sufficiently to maintain normal glucose levels. The hyperosmolality and reduced blood volume stimulate the release of ADH to increase the tubular reabsorption of water. ADH, however, is powerless in overcoming the osmotic pull exerted by the glucose load. Excessive fluid volume is lost at the kidney tubule with simultaneous loss of potassium, sodium, and phosphate in the urine.

Hypovolemia reduces renal circulation, and oliguria develops. Although this process conserves water and preserves the blood volume, it prevents further glucose loss, and hyperosmolality increases. Ketoacidosis is absent or very mild in HHNS despite the level of

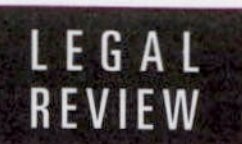

The Law and Regulation of Medical Records

Documentation in the patient's medical record must be (1) complete, (2) accurate, and (3) timely. The medical record provides legal proof of the nature and extent of care delivered to the patient. The critical care nurse has a legal duty to maintain the record in sufficient detail; insufficient or improper documentation may result in nursing liability or nonreimbursement by a third-party payer. The general rule, "What isn't in the medical record didn't occur," continues to prevail. The courts have held fairly consistently that failure to document care infers failure to provide care.

Federal regulations (including Medicare and Medicaid provisions under the Social Security Act), state laws and regulations (including hospital, medical, and nursing licensure statutes), accrediting organization (such as the Joint Commission on Accreditation of Healthcare Organizations) standards, professional organization standards, institutional policies and procedures, and custom all contribute to define documentation standards and to determine the form and content of the medical record.

As a general rule of law, the medical record is presumed to be accurate, absent evidence of tampering or fraud. Correcting an entry is lawful if the corrected portion remains legible; obliterating an entry may expose one to liability. Loss of the medical record raises a rebuttable presumption of negligence. Other documentation errors include factual omissions, unreasonably late entries, unauthorized entries, vague or ambiguous recordings, abbreviations not in common usage, personal opinions and subjectivity, failure to sign or time the record, and illegibility.

See *Battochi v Wash. Hosp. Center,* 581 A 2d 759 (DC App 1990); *Brookover v Mary Hitchcock Memorial Hosp.,* 893 F. 2d 411 (1st Cir 1990); *Collins V Westlake Community Hosp.,* 312 NE 2d 614 (Ill 1974); *Joseph Brant Memorial Hosp. v Koziol,* 2 CCLT 170 (SC 1978); Morrissey-Ross M: *Documentation: if you haven't written it, you haven't done it, Nurs Clin North Am* 23(2):363, 1988: Roach WH Jr: *Legal review: incentive for completing medical records–the legal risks, Top Health Rec Manage* 10(3):78, 1990; *Rogers v Kasdan,* 612 SW 2d 133 (Ky 1981); *Stack v Wapner,* 368 A 2d 292 (Pa Super 1976); Staggers N: *Comput Nurs,* 6(4):164, 1988; *St. Paul Fire and Marine Ins. Co. v Prothro,* 590 SW 2d 35 (Ark App 1979); Tomes JP: *Healthcare records: a practical legal guide,* Westchester, Ill, 1990, Healthcare Financial Management Association; *Villetto v Weilbaecher,* 377 So 2d 132 (La App 1979); *Whalen v Roe,* 429 US 589, 97 S Ct 869 (1977).

free fatty acids resulting from gluconeogenesis. It is surmised that the patient may have sufficient insulin present to prevent ketosis.[20]

Failure of the body to regain homeostatic balance further accelerates the life-threatening cycle brought about by hyperglycemia, hyperosmolality, osmotic diuresis, and profound dehydration. To restore homeostasis the sympathetic nervous system reacts to the body's stress response. Epinephrine, a potent stimulus for gluconeogenesis, is released, and additional glucose is added to the blood stream. Unless the glycemic diuresis cycle is broken with aggressive fluid replacement, the intracellular dehydration affects fluid and oxygen transport to the brain cells. Central nervous system dysfunctioning may result and lead to coma. Hemoconcentration increases the blood viscosity, which may result in clot formation, thromboemboli, and cerebral, cardiac, and pleural infarcts.[13]

Assessment and Diagnosis

HHNS has a slow, subtle onset. Initially, the symptoms may be nonspecific and may be ignored or attributed to the patient's concurrent disease processes. History reveals polyuria, polydipsia (depending on patient's thirst sensation), and advancing weakness. Medical attention may not be obtained for these nonspecific, nonacute symptoms until the patient is unable to take sufficient fluids to offset the fluid losses. Progressive dehydration follows and leads to mental confusion, convulsions, and coma.

The physical examination may reveal obtundation, with a profound fluid deficit. Signs of severe dehydration include longitudinal wrinkles in the tongue, decreased salivation, and decreased central venous pressure, with increases in pulse and respirations (Kussmaul's air hunger is not present).

Serum glucose levels are strikingly elevated, often to double the levels seen in ketoacidosis (reaching 2000 mg/dL). Serum osmolality may reach 340 mOsm/kg, averaging 320 mOsm/kg.[20] Elevated hematocrit and depleted potassium and phosphorus levels result from the osmotic diuresis. Studies have identified an increased hematocrit as a risk factor for both increased insulin resistance and NIDDM.[21] Serum electrolyte levels vary, depending on the activity and position of the electrolyte when the laboratory test is performed.

Serial laboratory tests keep the clinician apprised of the fluctuating serum electrolyte levels and provide the basis for electrolyte replacement. Intracellular potassium usually is depleted as dehydration progresses. Increased potassium in the extracellular fluid quickly reenters the cells, however, when insulin is administered. Phosphate levels also are carefully monitored and replaced according to insulin activity.

Kidney impairment as a result of the severe reduction in renal circulation is suggested by elevated BUN and creatinine levels. Metabolic acidosis usually is absent. When acidosis is present, it tends to be mild and attributed to other factors. The mild acidosis may be a result of starvation ketosis, a relative increase in lactic acid circulating in the reduced blood volume, or azotemia caused by impaired renal function.[13]

BOX 41-10 NURSING DIAGNOSIS AND MANAGEMENT

HYPERGLYCEMIC HYPEROSMOTIC NONKETOTIC SYNDROME

- Decreased Cardiac Output related to alterations in preload, p. 590
- Fluid Volume Deficit related to absolute loss, p. 914
- Anxiety related to threat to biologic, psychologic, and/or social integrity, p. 99
- Knowledge Deficit: Discharge Regimen related to previous lack of exposure to information, p. 61 (see Patient Education Box 41-11)

Medical Management

Medical management is necessary to interrupt the glycemic diuresis and to prevent vascular collapse. The underlying cause of HHNS must then be sought. The same basic principles used to treat DKA are used for the patient with hyperglycemic hyperosmolar coma: rehydration, electrolyte replacement, restoration of insulin/glucagon ratio, and prevention/treatment of circulatory collapse.

Rapid rehydration is the primary intervention. The fluid deficit may be as much as 150 ml/kg of body weight. The average 150-pound adult may lose more than 7 to 10 L of fluid a day.[12,22] Debate continues regarding whether isotonic or hypotonic solutions are more appropriate for treating the severe fluid deficit. Although an isotonic solution would expand the extracellular fluid and treat hypotension, it could compound the serum osmolality and exceed the body's requirement for sodium. A hypotonic solution would reduce the serum osmolality and provide free water for excretion; however, it could result in hypotonic expansion of the cells. The consensus is to use physiologic normal saline solution (0.9%) for the first 2 L during the first hour of treatment,[22] especially for the patient undergoing circulatory collapse.[13] Once blood pressures are within normal range for the patient, a hypotonic solution may follow. Half-strength hypotonic saline solution (0.45%) subsequently can be used to reduce the serum osmolality. The patient may need replacement of 6 to 10 L of fluid in the first 10 hours.[8] Another parameter for changing from 0.9% to 0.45% is the serum sodium level. Patients with sodium levels equal to or less than 140 mEq/L receive 0.9% normal saline solution;[22] those with levels greater than 140 mEq/L receive 0.45% normal saline solution.[22] Sodium input should not exceed that required to replace the losses. Careful monitoring for sodium and water balance is required to prevent hemolysis as hemoconcentration is reduced.

To prevent relative hypoglycemia, the hydrating solution is changed to 5% dextrose in water, in 0.9% saline solution, or in 0.45% saline solution when the serum glucose levels fall to 250 to 300 mg/dL.

Vigorous fluid therapy can reverse hyperglycemia; however, it may not reverse ketoacidosis. Intravenously administered insulin usually is given to facilitate the cellular use of glucose and to decrease the serum osmolality more rapidly.[13] Muscle, liver, and adipose cells tend to be receptive to exogenous insulin levels in the patient with HHNS, and the insulin needs are minimal; 10 to 15 U of regular insulin is given intravenously as a bolus. Maintenance doses of insulin to control hyperglycemia vary according to the practitioner. A common practice is to give insulin intravenously at the rate of 0.1 U/kg/hour (this dose mimics the normal physiologic secretion of 30 U/day, which includes upsurges at mealtime)[23] until the glucose falls between 250 and 300 mg. Once glucose levels are at 250 mg/dL, insulin treatment usually is discontinued. Aggressive treatment of the underlying causees of HHNS (severe infection, therapeutic procedures, medications) is included in the medical treatment to prevent HHNS recurrence.

Diagnostic procedures to identify and plan the treatment of HHNS are the same as those for DKA (see Table 41-4), with differences only in the frequency performed. Although arterial blood gas testing is not repeated as often in HHNS as in DKA, the serum osmolality determination is performed more frequently in HHNS than in ketoacidosis.

Nursing Management

Nursing management of patients with HHNS incorporates a variety of nursing diagnoses, which are listed in Box 41-10.

Fluid balance. Hyperglycemic hyperosmolar coma occurs most frequently in the patient with a precipitating stressor or illness; thus it is not unlikely for the nurse to be the first person to recognize its development. Nursing management of the patient at risk for HHNS involves prompt recognition of changes in the patient's osmolar state. A hydration assessment is outlined in Box 41-4. The assessment provides beginning signs and symptoms of fluid imbalance that signal dehydration from the increased number of glucose molecules in the blood stream. Blood values for hematocrit, osmolality, glucose, sodium, and potassium are monitored. Urine values for osmolality and ketones also are followed.

A convenient formula used at the bedside to identify the osmolality of blood on the basis of known laboratory values is the following:

$$\text{Serum osmolality} = 2\,(Na^{+} + K^{+}) + \frac{\text{Glucose mg/dL}}{18} + \frac{\text{BUN mg/dL}}{2.8}$$

Changes in the patient's personality provide neurologic clues to the impact of fluid imbalance on the central nervous system. When unexplained behavior changes are coupled with changing laboratory values and other signs of dehydration, hyperosmolality is to be suspected.

Once HHNS is identified, the nurse manages the alterations brought about by the fluid deficit, the increase in glucose, and the electrolyte imbalances. Because HHNS occurs most often in elderly persons, special care of this age-group is emphasized. Throughout the critical care period the nurse collects information necessary to identify the precipitating cause of HHNS and educates the patient and family in prevention of its recurrence. Hemodynamic monitoring, including CVP, pulmonary arterial wedge pressure, and PAP, evaluates the degree of dehydration, the effectiveness of the hydration therapy, and the patient's fluid tolerance. Symptoms of circulatory overload include elevated CVP and PAP levels, tachycardia, bounding pulse, dyspnea, tachypnea, lung crackles, and engorged neck veins. Decreasing cardiac output is signaled by hypotension and urine output less than 0.5 ml/kg/hr. Because a preexisting cardiopulmonary or renal problem may exist in the elderly patient, the hemodynamic criteria must be based on the values normal for that patient's age and current medical condition. The nurse is alerted for the clinical manifestations of fluid overload while rehydrating the older patient. (∞Age-Associated Changes in Hemodynamics and Electrocardiogram, p. 274)

Intravenous replacement considerations. Rigorous fluid replacement and low-dose insulin administration are best controlled with electronic volumetric pump devices.

Electrolytes. Electrolyte replacement orders are based on the patient's response to the treatment plan. Rapid fluctuations of serum potassium and phosphorus levels further compromise the patient with cardiac or renal problems. Increasing the circulating levels of insulin with therapeutic doses of intravenous insulin will promote the rapid return of potassium and phosphorus into the cell. Potassium imbalances disturb the electrocardiographic tracings (Table 41-5). Continuous cardiac monitoring provides information necessary to maintain or modify electrolyte dosages. Physical changes, such as alterations in gastrointestinal motility and neuromuscular control, also signal the effectiveness of electrolyte replacement.

Laboratory assessments. Bedside reflectometer glucose monitoring is performed every 30 to 60 minutes to determine effectiveness of treatment. Serum laboratory glucose measurements are usually done every 2 hours along with serum electrolyte determinations. Arterial blood gases are measured at the bedside to rule out the presence of ketoacidosis.

Neurologic assessment. Alteration in the level of consciousness is directly related to osmotic diuresis and resulting intracellular dehydration. Neurologic assessments, including level of consciousness, pupillary response, motor function, and reflexes, are performed frequently to monitor the patient's response to treatment. Seizure activity may occur as a result of the hyperosmolar state, which interferes with oxygen delivery to the brain cells. Seizure precautions include nursing actions to protect the patient from injury (padded side rails, bed in low position) and to provide an open airway (oral airway, head turned to side without forcibly restraining the patient, suction equipment available). Oxygen is administered, if required, to maintain oxygen saturation (Spo_2) above 90%.

Anticonvulsants, with the exception of phenytoin (which interferes with endogenous insulin [see Table 41-3]), may be ordered. Documentation of seizures includes onset, duration, and description of seizure activity.

Skin integrity. Interference with tissue perfusion by hypovolemia and hypophosphatemia is a serious problem for the severely compromised, dehydrated patient. Fluid replacement, range of motion, frequent positioning, and assessing skin turgor, color, temperature, and peripheral pulses are used to maintain and monitor skin integrity. Elastic support hose, elastic wraps, or antimetabolism stockings may be used in an effort to prevent lower extremity venous stasis.

TABLE 41-5 Clinical Manifestations of Hypokalemia and Hyperkalemia

Hypokalemia	Hyperkalemia
Generalized muscle weakness	Impaired muscle activity
Fatigue	Weakness
Diminished to absent reflexes	Muscle pain/cramps
Decreased GI motility	Increased GI motility
Anorexia	Nausea
Abdominal distention	Diarrhea
Paralytic ileus	Intestinal colic
Vomiting	Oliguria
Hypotension	Dizziness
Decreased stroke volume	Bradycardia
Dysrhythmias	Ventricular fibrillation
Weak pulse	Irritability
Respiratory muscle weakness	ECG changes
Shallow respirations	Flattened P wave
Shortness of breath	Large, peaked T wave
Apathy	Broad, slurred QRS complex
Drowsiness	
Depression	
Irritability	
Tetany	
Coma	
ECG changes	
Prolonged QT interval	
Flattened, depressed T wave	
Depressed ST segments	

Patient education. As the patient's condition improves and the patient and family have received assistance regarding coping strategies, the patient and family become more ready to learn.[24] Patient education needs are listed in Box 41-11. Prevention of recurrence is the major goal. Patients admitted to the critical care area with HHNS and undiagnosed diabetes and those with HHNS with previously diagnosed diabetes will require a teaching plan to include a description of diabetes and how it relates to HHNS. Dietary restrictions, exercise requirements, and medication protocols are all necessary for the patient and/or family member to learn. Additionally, the patient needs to know how a change in daily activities or an illness, such as the flu with nausea or vomiting will alter the daily diabetes management. Home testing of blood for glucose and signs and symptoms of hyperglycemia and hypoglycemia are part of the learning defense against the complication of diabetes. Patients who use the insulin pump are to have the instructions reviewed. A malfunctioning pump will need to be repaired and recalibrated for accuracy. Effective teaching can be accomplished in momentary, informal opportunities or through structured, formal class presentations. New skills, such as insulin administration, may take longer to master than the length of a patient's stay in the intensive care unit. The nurse who recognizes the need for frequent, short teaching/practice sessions and the time constraints on the critical care unit staff would do well to collaborate with a diabetic nurse educator or patient educator in the hospital. Continued alertness to the signs and symptoms of diabetes so that necessary interventions can take place is needed to help prevent complications. (∞Nutrition and Endocrine Alterations, p. 149.)

BOX 41-11 PATIENT EDUCATION

HYPERGLYCEMIC HYPEROSMOTIC NONKETOTIC SYNDROME

- Acute phase
  - Explain rationale for critical care unit admission
- Predischarge
  - Assess knowledge level
  - Assess compliance history
  - Diabetes disease process
  - Definitions of HHNS
  - Causes of HHNS
  - Self-care of diabetes
  - Signs and symptoms to report to health care practitioner

DIABETES INSIPIDUS/HYPOSECRETION OF ANTIDIURETIC HORMONE

Description

Diabetes insipidus (DI) occurs when there is an insufficiency or a hypofunctioning of antidiuretic hormone (ADH). ADH normally stimulates the kidney tubules to reabsorb filtered water when the body needs to increase fluid stores. ADH stimulates the tubules to increase permeability to water when particles in the blood stream increase in number (rising osmolality) or when blood pressure falls (see Table 39-4 for additional events that affect ADH). Persons with inadequately functioning ADH develop unrestricted serum hyperosmolality. An intense thirst and the passage of excessively large quantities of very dilute urine add to the characteristics of the disease.

DI is covered under two DRGs: DRG 300, endocrine disorders with co-morbid conditions, which has an anticipated length of stay of 7.9 days, and DRG 301, endocrine disorders without co-morbid conditions, with an anticipated length of stay of 4.8 days.[5]

Etiology

Diabetes insipidus is categorized into three types according to cause: central DI, nephrogenic DI, and psychogenic DI. Box 41-12 lists each category of DI and the related etiology.

Central DI occurs when there is an interruption in the synthesis and release of ADH. Central DI is further divided into primary and secondary categories. Primary DI occurs when structural abnormalities within the hypothalamus, infundibular stalk, and posterior pituitary prevent the release of ADH according to the body's inherent signals. Primary DI may result from an inherited familial disorder or from a posterior pituitary system that fails to develop at birth. Primary DI also may be idiopathic or sporadic and occur without apparent cause.[18]

Secondary DI occurs as a result of trauma to or a pathologic condition of the posterior pituitary functioning unit. Surgery or irradiation to the pituitary gland, traumatic head injury, tumors (malignant and benign), and infections, such as encephalitis, tuberculosis, and meningitis, can potentially interfere with the structure and physiology of the unit and compromise the release of ADH. This is a condition frequently seen in critical care units in patients with head injury or certain types of neurosurgery.

Nephrogenic DI results from the inability of the kidney nephrons to respond to circulating ADH. This may result from diseased kidneys and insensitive or inadequate numbers of receptors on the nephron. Drugs can promote nephrogenic DI by decreasing the responsiveness of the kidney tubules to ADH. Long-term lithium carbonate use is a common cause of nephrogenic NDI.[25]

Psychogenic DI is a rare form of the disease that occurs with compulsively drinking more than 5 L of water a day.[25] The infundibular stalk is functioning adequately in psychogenic DI, as are the receptor sites on the kidney nephrons. Long-standing psychogenic DI may closely mimic nephrogenic DI because the kidney tubules develop decreased responsiveness to ADH as a result of prolonged conditioning to hypotonic urine.

BOX 41-12 Etiology of Diabetes Insipidus

CENTRAL DI

Primary

ADH deficiency from hypothalamic-hypophyseal malformation
- Congenital defect
- Idiopathic

Secondary

ADH deficiency from destruction to the hypothalamic-hypophyseal system
- Trauma
- Infection
- Surgery
- Primary neoplasms
- Metastatic malignancies
- Autoimmune response

NEPHROGENIC DI

Inability of kidney tubles to respond to circulating ADH
- Decrease or absence of ADH receptors
- Cellular damage to nephron, especially loop of Henle
- Kidney damage (e.g., hydronephrosis, pyelonephritis, polycystic kidney)
- Untoward response to drug therapy (e.g., lithium carbonate, demeclocycline)

PSYCHOGENIC DI

Rare form of water intoxication
- Compulsive water drinking

Pathophysiology

ADH is released in an effort to maintain blood tonicity and circulating blood volume. (∞Antidiuretic Hormone, p 983.)

Injury to the hypothalamus, infundibular stalk, or posterior pituitary can lead to a disruption in the normal neuroendocrine communication system and resultant secretion of ADH. When ADH is absent, inefficient, or secreted in insufficient amounts, the kidney tubules prevent the reabsorption of urinary substrate and an excessive amount of water is lost to the body, a pathologic condition known as *diabetes insipidus.* (Figure 41-3 is a diagram of the events postulated to occur with primary DI.)

In DI, as free water is excreted in urine, the serum osmolality rises and excessive sodium concentration (hypernatremia) in the vascular space stimulates the thirst receptors. Polyuria develops as the kidneys fail to reabsorb tubular fluid and to concentrate the urine. Extremely dilute urine is excreted, and the body is de-

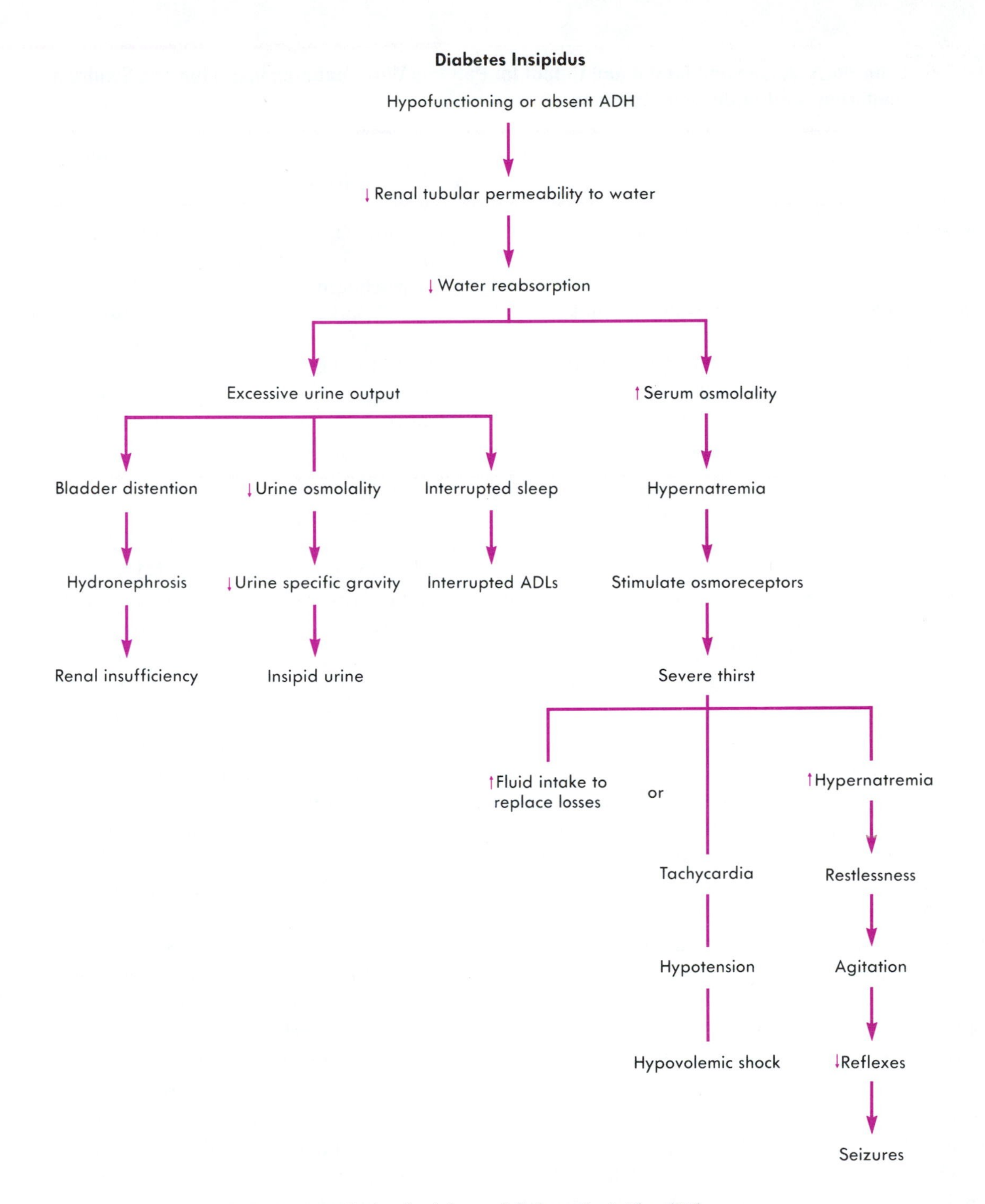

FIGURE 41-3. Pathophysiology of diabetes insipidus (DI).

pleted of the fluid necessary for hydration. Urine osmolality and specific gravity decrease. Rising serum osmolality triggers the synthesis and release of ADH. However, the ADH that is released is ineffective or insufficient. Without ADH the kidney tubules are incapable of conserving enough water to reduce serum sodium.

As the extracellular dehydration ensues, hypotension and hypovolemic shock can occur. Extreme polydipsia develops as the individual attempts to replace lost fluids. The excessive intake of water reduces the serum osmolality to a more normal level and prevents dehydration. The dramatic cycle of polydipsia and polyuria interferes with the person's ability to work, eat, or sleep. Unless the lost fluids are replaced, severe hypernatremia, decreased cerebral perfusion, and severe dehydration lead to seizures, loss of consciousness and death.

TABLE 41-6 Laboratory Values and Intake and Output for Patients With Diabetes Insipidus and Syndrome of Inappropriate Antidiuretic Hormone

Value	Normal	Diabetes Insipidus	Syndrome of Inappropriate Antidiuretic Hormone
Serum ADH	1-5 pg/ml	↓ in central DI, may be normal with nephrogenic or psychogenic DI	Elevated
Serum osmolality	285-300 mOsm/kg	>300 mOsm/kg	<250 mOsm/kg
Serum sodium	135-145 mEq/L	>145 mEq/L	<120 mEq/L
Urine osmolality	300-1400 mOsm/kg	<300 mOsm/kg	Increased
Urine specific gravity	1.005-1.030	<1.005	>1.030
Urine output	1-1.5 L/24 hr	30-40 L/24 hr	Below normal
Fluid intake	1-1.5 L/24 hr	≥50 L 24 hr	Unchanged

Assessment and Diagnosis

Clinical manifestations of DI may develop gradually or may occur suddenly after head injury or other precipitating diseases. Initially, urine production may exceed 300 ml/hr, accompanied by an abnormally low urine osmolality.[26] The diluted urine in DI is "insipid" or tasteless, as opposed to the sweet, honey "mellitus" taste of urine associated with DM.

Diagnostic tests used to establish the presence of DI evaluate the body's innate ability to balance fluid and electrolytes. Although these tests are early markers for the disease, most are routinely performed and not specific to the endocrine system (Table 41-6). The tests performed most frequently include a comparison of serum osmolality, urine osmolality, and serum sodium values.

Serum and urine osmolality. The serum osmolality has a narrow range, between 285 and 300 mOsm/kg. Urine osmolality can fluctuate between 300 and 800 mOsm/kg, with extremes ranging from 50 to 1200 mOsm/kg.[26] Severe DI could raise serum osmolality to 330 mOsm/kg, while urine osmolality falls well below normal.[27,28] (∞Serum Osmolality, p. 992; Urine and Blood Osmolality, p. 994.)

The bedside measurement of urine output identifies polyuria. Urine specific gravity can be measured more conveniently than can urine osmolality because the procedure can take place at bedside and does not require patient preparation. Osmolality tests, however, are preferred because they give a more accurate measurement of the renal tubules' reabsorption of water and resulting concentration or dilution of urine.[29]

In the patient with ineffective, absent, or decreased ADH, the urine osmolality is expected to be decreased while the serum osmolality is increased. The degree of serum osmolality is directly related to the degree of urine osmolality. Its measurement can provide data to support the diagnosis of DI. For a more accurate relfection of the ADH influence on water balance, the urine sample should be collected and tested simultaneously with the blood sample.

Sodium. Serum sodium levels mirror the high solute concentration within the blood stream. Unconscious patients or patients unable to respond to the thirst mechanism that accompanies polyuria are at risk of rapid dehydration and hypovolemia if DI is not diagnosed and treated. For these patients a gradual rise in serum sodium level signals the fluid imbalance. Suspect DI in the unconscious patient with hypoosmotic polyuria when the serum sodium level reaches 143 mEq/L before more serious problems with hemoconcentration develop.[28]

Laboratory tests are useful in differentiating DI according to cause. In a water deprivation or dehydration test, the patient is deprived of fluids for a 24-hour period. During this time, urine and plasma osmolality measurements are taken. In patients with ADH deficiency the urine is minimally concentrated after dehydration, whereas plasma osmolality rises above 300 mOsm/kg and serum sodium is greater than 145 mEq/L. This test is seldom done in critical care settings because of the potentially serious consequence to the patient who is already volume depleted with an elevated plasma osmolality. Exogenous ADH can be used in urine concentration testing without depriving the patient of fluids. The ADH is given parenterally, after which urine and blood osmolality tests are recorded. While the exogenous ADH test is preferred over the water deprivation test, there are still inherent fluid and sodium risks with this test, and patients with cardiac dysfunction are to be observed cautiously.[30] (∞Water Deprivation Test, p. 994; Synthetic ADH Test, p. 994; Water Load Test, p. 994.)

Alternate tests (see Table 41-6) may include quantitative analysis of serum ADH. Absent or decreased levels of serum ADH in the presence of hyperosmolar serum and hypoosmolar urine indicate primary and secondary ADH deficiency. Normal serum ADH levels (1.0 to 13.3 pg/ml)[31] accompanying clinical manifestations of DI may indicate nephrogenic DI, in which the kidney tubule is insensitive to ADH.

Normal ADH levels with elevated blood osmolality and increased urine output also may suggest pharmacologically induced DI or excessive or compulsive water drinking. The vasopressin (ADH) concentration level may be measured to differentiate the type of DI present.

Medical Management

Treatment involves management of the primary condition that is creating the interference in ADH circulation. Fluid replacement is provided in the initial phase of the treatment to prevent circulatory collapse. Patients who are able to drink are given voluminous amounts of fluid orally to balance output. For those unable to take sufficient fluids orally, hypotonic intravenous solutions are rapidly infused and carefully monitored to restore the hemodynamic balance.

Medications have been used successfully to treat DI[10,14,16,18] (see Table 41-7). Patients with primary and secondary DI who are unable to synthesize ADH require exogenous ADH (vasopressin) replacement therapy. One form of the hormone available for short-term substitution is aqueous, synthetic Pitressin. It is administered intramuscularly or subcutaneously or applied topically to the nasal mucosa. Onset of antidiuresis is rapid and lasts up to 8 hours. This drug constricts smooth muscle and can elevate systemic blood pressure. Water intoxication also can occur if the dose is higher than the therapeutic level.

Another drug for patients with mild forms of DI is a synthetic analogue of vasopressin, desmopressin acetete (DDAVP). It is administered parenterally or topically, via the nasal mucosa (not inhaled). The drug has fewer side effects than do other vasopressin preparations. It has minimal effects on the smooth muscle tissue and rarely causes hypertension. It is, however, expensive, costing the patient up to $2500/year.[8] Minute doses of pituitary extract provide greater control of the patient's fluid balance with minimal side effects. Recent trial studies have found that ultra-low doses of bovine posterior pituitary extract of combined oxytocin and vasopressin (Pituitrin) have satisfactorily regulated urine output and promoted cardiovascular stability. The dose is scrupulously measured with a syringe pump to ensure the exact amount of the hormone for the patient's hydration status.[26]

Nursing Management

The basic nursing management of DI involves a continual, conscientious assessment of the patient's hydration status; DI, however, may be complicated by the primary reason for which the patient was admitted to the critical care unit. Nursing care includes management of several dysfunctioning systems and incorporates a variety of nursing diagnoses and interventions (Boxes 41-13 and 41-14).

Rehydration. Critical assessment and management of the fluid status are the most important concerns for the patient with DI. Intake and output measurement, condition of buccal membranes, skin turgor, daily weights, presence of thirst, and temperature provide a basic assessment list that is vital for the patient unable to regulate fluid needs and fluid lost.

A formula that assists the caregiver to estimate the amount of fluid lost to the body, based on normal fluid stores and usual body weight, is given here.

$$\text{Liters body water deficit} = \frac{0.6\ (\text{kg wt}) \times ([\text{measured serum sodium}] - 140)}{140}$$

The formula assumes that 60% of an individual's weight is fluid, although this is not always exact.[32] Also, the patient or family member may not be able to provide the patient's usual body weight. Nevertheless, the formula provides an approximation of the fluid weight and the fluid loss. The resulting liters of body water deficit can then be used for planning replacement fluids. A hypotonic intravenous solution is used to replace fluids lost and reduce the serum hyperosmolality.

Laboratory tests. Urine and blood specimens are simultaneously collected for osmolality studies. Bedside specific gravity analysis gives immediate information regarding variations in the kidney tubules' reabsorption of water. Serum sodium and potassium levels are monitored and relayed to the physician as necessary (Box 41-15).

Daily nursing care. Meticulous skin care is necessary to preserve skin integrity and to prevent breakdown caused by dehydration. If the patient has an indwelling urinary catheter, scrupulous asepsis is required to prevent a nosocomial infection.

Constipation and diarrhea are common problems in the patient with DI. Constipation results from fluid

TABLE 41-7 Medications and Nursing Implications for DI

Drug	Dosage	Actions	Special Considerations
Desmopressin acetate (DDAVP, nasal spray, Rhinal tube, Rhinyle drops, Stimate)	Nasally, 10-40 μg hs or in divided doses 10 mg/0.1 ml; 100 mg/ml Parenteral, 2-4 mg bid	Treatment of central diabetes insipidus (DI) Antidiuretic—increases water reabsorption in nephron Prevents and controls polydipsia, polyuria Preferred treatment for chronic, long-term DI	Few side effects Observe for nasal congestion, URI, allergic rhinitis Monior intake and output, urine osmolality, serum sodium level
Vasopressin (Pitressin, Pressyn)	Parenteral, IM, IV, SQ, intrarterial Topical nasal mucosa	Treatment of central DI Antidiuretic Promotes reabsorption of water at kidney tubule Decreases urine output Increases urine osmolality Diagnostic aid Increases gastrointestinal peristalsis	Monitor fluid volume status frequently, especially of elderly Assess cardiac status May precipitate angina, hypertension, myocardial infarction if increased dose given to patient with cardiac history Parenteral extravasation may cause skin necrosis
Lypressin (Diapid)	Intranasal, 1-2 sprays (7-14 μg) each nostril qid	Treatment of central DI Synthetic antidiuretic hormone Increases reabsorption of sodium and water in nephron	Proper instillation important for absorption and action of drug Patient to sit upright while holding bottle upright for administration Repeated sprays (>2-3) are ineffective and wastful; if dose is increased to 2-3 sprays, the time interval between dosing is to be shortened Cough, tightness in chest, shortness of breath
Thiazide diuretics	Varies according to diuretic chosen and size and age of patient	Treatment of nephrogenic DI Leads to mild fluid depletion; incresaed water and sodium is reabsorbed in the proximal nephron and less fluid travels on to the distal nephron, thereby excreting less water	Varies according to diuretic chosen
Anticompulsive disorder medications, anxietolytics, psychopharmacologic medications	Varies	Treatment of psychogenic DI	Varies according to medication chosen

loss and, depending on the patient's status, is treated with dietary fiber, stool softeners, or both. Diarrhea may accompany the abdominal cramping and intestinal hyperactivity associated with vasporessin drug therapy. Untoward effects are brought to the attention of the physician for dose modification. The nurse must recognize the patient's reluctance to engage in any activity because of the polyuria. Having a bedpan or commode constantly available will reduce anxiety for the alert patient who does not have an indwelling urinary catheter.

ADH replacement. ADH replacement is accomplished with extreme caution in the patient with a history of cardiac disease because vasopressin may cause hyper-

BOX 41-13 NURSING DIAGNOSIS AND MANAGEMENT

DIABETES INSIPIDUS

- Fluid Volume Deficit related to decreased secretion of ADH, p. 1049
- Decreased Cardiac Output related to alterations in preload, p. 590
- Anxiety related to threat to biologic, psychologic, and/or social integrity, p. 99
- Knowledge Deficit: Discharge Regimen related to lack of previous exposure to information, p. 61 (see Patient Education Box 41-14)

BOX 41-14 PATIENT EDUCATION

DIABETES INSIPIDUS

- Acute phase
    - Explain the reasons for critical care unit admission
- Predischarge
    - Assess knowledge base
    - Measurement of fluid intake and output
    - Urine specific gravity
    - Causes of DI
    - Disease process of DI
    - Nutritional information to prevent constipation and diarrhea
    - Signs and symptoms to report to a health care professional
    - Medications
        - Explain purpose, side effects, dosage, and how often to use

tension and overhydration. At the first signs of cardiovascular impairment the drug is discontinued and fluid intake is restricted until urine specific gravity is less than 1.015 and polyuria resumes.

Emotional support. The patient who is unable to satisfy sensations of thirst or to complete any task or self-care activity without the need to urinate is confused and frightened. For patients who are able to verbalize their fears, having someone who is interested and nonjudgmental may help reduce the emotional turmoil.

Patient education. Educating the patient and the family about the disease process and how it affects thirst, urination, and fluid balance will encourage patients to participate in their care and reduce the feelings of hopelessness. Patients who are discharged with the disease are taught, along with their families, the signs and symptoms of dehydration and overhydration. They are taught the procedures for correct daily weight and urine specific gravity measurements. Printed information pertaining to drug actions, side effects, dosages, and timetable is given to the patient, as well as an outline of factors that need to be reported to the physician.

BOX 41-15 Diabetes Insipidus Case Study

Mrs. LM, a 54-year-old woman, was admitted for a bowel resection. She had a history of DI after a motor vehicle accident 20 years ago. She was taking Desmopressin (DDAVP) 0.1% per Rhinatube bid. She missed her usual doses postoperatively and was admitted to the critical care unit with altered level of consciousness, acute confusion, severe electrolyte imbalance, and dehydration. Her intake and output were negative 5000 ml over 2 days. The patient was given intravenous fluid replacement with potasium protocols, restarted on DDAVP, and transferred to a medical/surgical unit the following day. She was coherent and reoriented easily, but did not remember her transfer to the critical care unit or the preceding 3 days. Her laboratory results before and after the DDAVP, as follow, are of interest:

	Normal Value	Before DDAVP	After DDAVP
Na^+	135-145 mEq/L	169 mEq/L	145 mEq/L
K^+	3.5-5.0 mEq/L	2.5 mEq/L	3.6 mEq/L
Cl^-	98-106 mEq/L	127 mEq/L	103 mEq/L
BUN	7-18 mg/dL	5 mg/dL	9 mg/dL
Creatinine	0.6-1.2 mg/dL	0.5 mg/dL	0.5 mg/dL

SYNDROME OF INAPPROPRIATE ANTIDIURETIC HORMONE/ HYPERSECRETION OF ANTIDIURETIC HORMONE

Description

The opposite of DI is the syndrome of inappropriate/increased antidiuretic hormone (SIADH). The patient with SIADH has ADH secreted into the blood stream exceeding the amount needed to maintain blood volume and serum osmolality. Excessive water is reabsorbed at the kidney tubule, leading to dilutional hyponatremia. The patient becomes water intoxicated. SIADH is covered under two DRGs: DRG 300, endocrine disorders with comorbid conditions, which has an anticipated length of stay of 7.9 days, and DRG 301, endocrine disorders without co-morbid conditions, with the anticipated length of stay of 4.8 days.[5]

BOX 41-16 Etiology of Syndrome of Inappropriate Antidiuretic Hormone (ADH)

Malignant disease associated with autonomous production of ADH
- Bronchogenic oat cell carcinoma
- Pancreatic adenocarcinoma
- Duodenal, bladder, ureter, prostatic carcinomas
- Lymphosarcoma, Ewing's sarcoma
- Acute leukemia, Hodgkin's disease
- Cerebral neoplasm, thymoma

Central nervous system diseases that interfere with the hypothalamic-hypophyseal system and increase the production and/or release of ADH
- Head injury
- Brain abscess
- Hydrocephalus
- Pituitary adenoma
- Subdural hematoma
- Subarachnoid hemorrhage
- Cerebral atrophy
- Guillain-Barré syndrome
- Tuberculosis meningitis
- Purulent meningitis
- Herpes simplex encephalitis
- Acute intermittent porphyria

Neurogenic stimuli capable of increasing ADH
- Decreased glomerular filtration rate
- Physical and/or emotional stressors
  - Pain
  - Fear
  - Trauma
  - Surgery
  - Myocardial infarction
  - Acute infection
  - Hypotension
  - Hemorrhage
  - Hypovolemia

Pulmonary diseases believed to stimulate the baroreceptors and increase ADH
- Pulmonary tuberculosis
- Viral and bacterial pneumonia
- Empyema
- Lung abscess
- Chronic obstructive lung disease
- Status asthmaticus
- Cystic fibrosis

Endocrine disturbances that hormonally influence ADH
- Myxedema
- Hypothyroidism
- Hypopituitarism
- Adrenal insufficiency—Addison's disease

Medications that mimic, increase the release of, or potentiate ADH
- Hypoglycemics
  - Insulin
  - Tolbutamide
  - Chlorpropamide
- Potassium-depicting thiazide diuretics
- Tricyclic antidepressants
  - Imipramine
  - Amitriptyline
- Phenothiazine
  - Fluphenazine
  - Thioridazine
- Thioxanthenes
  - Thiothixene
  - Chlorprothixene
- Chemotherapeutic agents
  - Vincristine
  - Cyclophosphamide
- Narcotics
- Carbamazepine
- Clofibrate
- Acetaminophen
- Nicotine
- Oxytocin
- Vasopressin
- Anesthetics

Etiology

Of the numerous causes of SIDAH, many are seen in patients who are critically ill (Box 41-16). Central nervous system injury or disease interfering with the normal functioning of the hypothalamic-pituitary system may cause SIADH. The most common cause, however, is malignant bronchogenic oat cell carcinoma. This type of malignant cell is capable of synthesizing and releasing ADH. Other carcinomas capable of this autonomous production of ADH involve the pancreas, prostate, duodenum, and thymus. ADH levels also have been elevated in Hodgkin's disease and leukemia. In addition, ectopic endocrine production of ADH is identified in certain nonmalignant pulmonary conditions, such as tuberculosis and pneumonia. Levels of ADH are also increased by positive pressure ventilators that decrease venous return to the thorax, thus stimulating pulmonary baroreceptors to release ADH.[18]

Other causes of SIADH are neurologic disorders, such as tetanus, meningitis, and Guillain-Barré syndrome. Anesthesia, stress, pain, and such drugs as cyclophosphamide and chlorpropamide also have been implicated.

Pathophysiology

ADH (vasopressin) is a powerful, complex polypeptide compound. When released into the circulation by the posterior pituitary gland, ADH regulates water and electrolyte balance. (∞Antidiuretic Hormone, p. 983.)

Fluid balance. In SIADH, profound fluid and electrolyte disturbances result from the unsolicited, continuous release of the hormone into the blood stream (Figure 41-4). Rather than providing a water balance within the body, excessive ADH stimulates the kidney tubules to retain fluid, regardless of need. This results in severe overhydration.

Sodium balance. Excessive ADH also alters the extracellular fluid's sodium balance. The overhydration causes a dilutional hyponatremia and reduces the sodium concentration to critically low levels.[33] In the healthy adult, hyponatremia inhibits the release of ADH; however, in SIADH the increased levels of circulating ADH are unrelated to the serum sodium.

Aldosterone. The hyponatremia continues as aldosterone, which is normally released by the adrenal glands to retain sodium at the tubules, is suppressed. Serum hypoosmolality leads to a shift of fluid from the extracellular fluid space into the intracellular fluid compartment in an attempt to equalize osmotic pressure. Because minimal sodium is present in this fluid, edema usually does not result. Without ADH and aldosterone, water is retained, urine output is diminished, and further sodium is excreted in the urine.

Urine. The urine has an increased osmolality from the decreased water excretion. Urinary concentration is also elevated by excess sodium in the urine.[18] It is believed that despite the serum hyponatremia, the increased release of ADH promotes sodium loss through the kidneys into the urine.

Assessment and Diagnosis

The clinical manifestations of SIADH relate to the excess fluids in the extracellular compartment and the proportionate dilution of the circulating sodium. Although edema usually is not present, slight weight gain may occur from the expanded extracellular fluid volume.

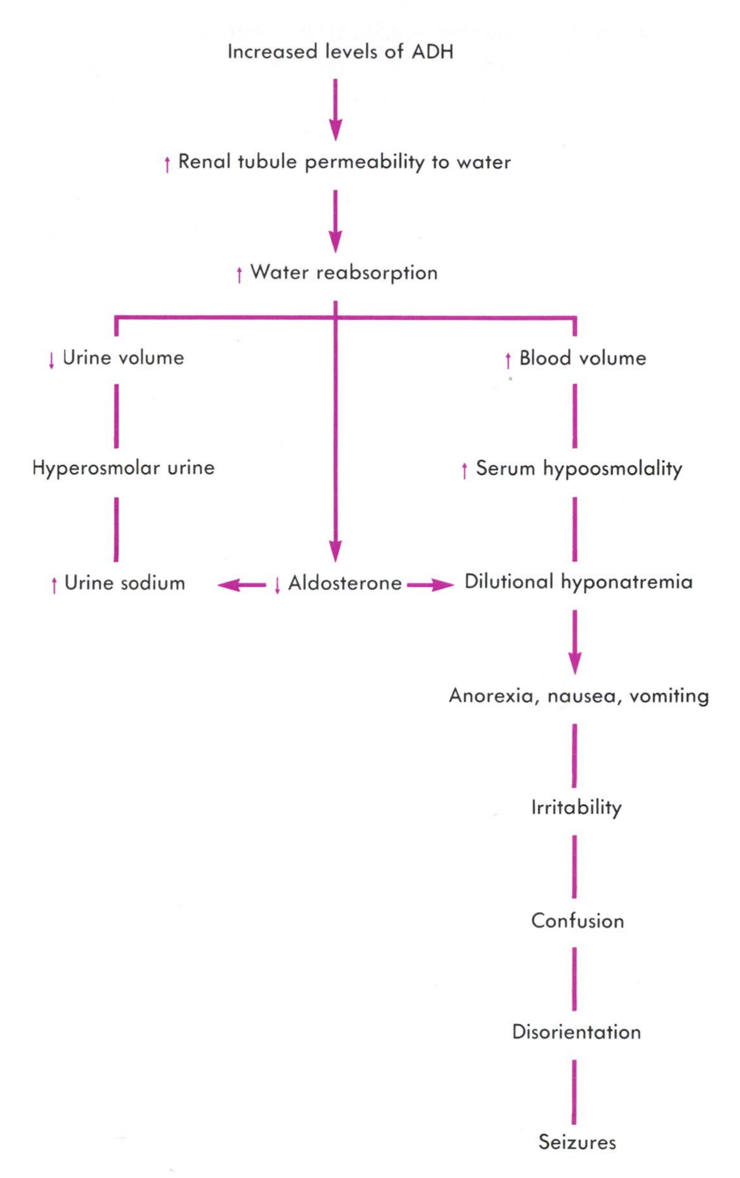

FIGURE 41-4. Pathophysiology of syndrome of inappropriate antidiuretic hormone (SIADH).

Hyponatremia. Hyponatremia initially may be asymptomatic. Early clinical manifestations of dilutional hyponatremia include lethargy, anorexia, nausea, and vomiting. The water and sodium imbalance progresses, with the sodium levels dropping below 120 mEq/L.[17] Progressively deteriorating neurologic signs of hyponatremia then predominate, and the patient is admitted to the critical care unit. Symptoms of severe hyponatremia include the inability to concentrate, mental confusion, apprehension, seizures, loss of consciousness, coma, and death.

The medical diagnosis is based on various factors. Primary disorders (oat cell carcinoma, central nervous system disturbance), clinical manifestations, and laboratory tests provide data to verify the presence of SIADH.

Laboratory values. Laboratory values provide the clinical hallmarks of SIADH: serum hypoosmolality with hyponatremia and a urine osmolality greater than would be expected of the hypotonic blood (see Table 43-6 for typical laboratory results for patient with SIADH). The patient with SIADH characteristically displays a serum hypoosmolality less than 275 mOsm/kg, with urine osmolality that is les than maximally dilute or less than 100 mOsm/kg water.[18] Urine osmolality that is equal to or that exceeds serum osmolality, with urinary sodium greater than 20 mEq/L, demonstrates the SIADH paradox of a very dilute serum with a concentrated urine output.

To confirm the diagnosis, a water-load test may be performed. After a period of fasting, a dehydrated patient is overhydrated with water. The urine output and serum osmolality are carefully monitord to discover a decline in serum osmolality resulting from peak moments of overhydration. Patients with SIADH show a decrease in serum osmolality regardless of the fasting state and an inability to secrete dilute urine despite the hydration resulting from the water load.[18] This test is identified as very useful in identifying changes in free water excretion. The test, however, requires that the patient withstand the physical insult of overhydration and for that reason is almost never done in a critical care unit. (∞Water Load Test, p. 994.)

Medical Management

In the critical care unit, SIADH often occurs as a secondary disease. Ideally, recognition and treatment of the primary disease will reduce the production of ADH. If the patient is receiving any of the chemical agents suspected of causing the disease, discontinuing the drug may return ADH levels to normal.

Fluid restriction and diuresis. The medical therapy that is the most successful (along with treatment of the primary disease) is simple reduction of fluid intake. This is done most successfully for the patient with a moderate increase in the body fluid volume, with hyponatremia. Although fluid restrictions are to be calculated on the basis of individual needs and losses, a general criterion is to restrict fluids to 500 ml less than average daily output.[18]

Sodium replacement. Patients with severe hyponatremia (less than 115 mEq/L) or those with seizures are cautiously infused with 3% to 5% hypertonic saline solution[32] for rapid but temporary correction of the hemodilution caused by the retention of fluid at the tubules and severe sodium loss. It is considered safe to raise serum sodium levels up to 12 mEq/day for the first 24 to 48 hours while avoiding fatal consequences from neurologic complications. Furosemide may be added to further increase the diuresis of free water and to prevent the risk of pulmonary edema related to the hypertonic saline solution. Hypertonic saline solution is administered very slowly and with extreme caution (1 to 2 ml/kg/hour) until the patient's serum sodium level is increased no greater than 1 to 2 mEq/L/hour.[34] Treatment with a hypertonic saline solution is temporary inasmuch as the sodium is continuously removed from the body through the urine.

Medications. Certain drugs reduce the effectiveness of ADH on the kidney tubule. Narcotic agonists, such as oxilorphan and butorphanol, are used to reduce the secretion of ADH in many patients with SIADH. The drugs, however, do not seem to be effective in patients with SIADH caused by lung malignancies. Patients with lung malignancies are treated with demeclocycline hydrochloride, an antibacterial tetracycline, and lithium carbonate, an alkali metal salt primarily used to alter psychogenic behavior. These drugs inhibit the tubule response to ADH and decrease the water reabsorption at the tubules.[8]

Nursing Management

Assessment. Thorough, astute nursing assessments are required for care of the patient with SIADH while an attempt is made to correct the fluid and sodium imbalance; the systemic effects of hyponatremia occur rapidly and can be lethal. Evaluation of the patient's neurologic status, especially level of consciousness, occurs every 1 to 2 hours. Frequent assessment of the patient's hydration status is accomplished with serial measurements of urine output, blood and urine sodium levels, urine specific gravity, and urine and blood osmolality. Elimination patterns are assessed because constipation may occur when fluids are restricted. Several nursing diagnoses are associated with nursing management of SIADH and are listed in Box 41-17.

Neurologic assessment. Seizure precautions for the patient with SIADH are provided regardless of the degree of hyponatremia. Serum sodium levels may fluctuate rapidly, and neurologic impairment may occur with no apparent warning. The patient's altered neurologic response may also be influenced by the acuity of the primary disease (i.e., central nervous system disease) and not soley by the result of low sodium levels. Seizure precautions include nursing actions to protect the patient from injury (padded side rails, bed in low position when patient is unattended) and to provide an open airway (oral airway, head turned to side without forcibly restraining the patient, suction apparatus). Oxygen is administered as needed.

BOX 41-17 NURSING DIAGNOSIS AND MANAGEMENT

SYNDROME OF INAPPROPRIATE ANTIDIURETIC HORMONE (SIADH)

- Fluid Volume Excess related to increased secretion of ADH, p. 1049
- Anxiety related to lack of control over current situation or disease progression, p. 99
- Knowledge Deficit: Discharge Regimen related to lack of previous exposure to information, p. 61 (see Patient Education Box 41-18)

BOX 41-18 PATIENT EDUCATION

SYNDROME OF INAPPROPRIATE ANTIDIURETIC HORMONE (SIADH)

- Acute phase
  - Explain reasons for admission to the critical care unit
  - Explain reasons for neurologic changes
- Predischarge
  - Assess knowledge level
  - Causes of SIADH
  - Disease process of SIADH
  - Measuring intake and output
  - Measuring urine specific gravity
  - Signs and symptoms to report to a health care professional

Hydration. Accurate intake and output measurement is required to calculate fluid replacement for the patient with excessive ADH. All fluids are restricted as ordered. Intake that equals urine output may be given until serum sodium level returns to normal. Frequent mouth care through moistening the buccal membrane may give comfort during the perid of fluid restriction. Weights may be taken every 12 hours to gauge fluid retention or loss. Weight gain could signify continual fluid retention, whereas weight loss could indicate loss of body fluid.

Parenteral therapy. Hypertonic saline solution is infused very cautiously. A volumetric pump is used to deliver 1 ml/kg/hour or it is set to deliver a flow rate determined by the serum sodium levels. Hypertonic expansion of the vascular space is a complication of the rapid infusion of hypertonic saline solution that must be avoided. Hypertonic expansion occurs when the hypertonic solution is infused so rapidly that it creates an immediate hyperosmolality of the blood stream. Fluid is drawn from the more diluted intracellular spaces to the blood stream in an effort to equalize the concentration of particles. The hypertonic solution is discontinued if any signs or symptoms of fluid overload occur, such as pulmonary edema, increased CVP and increased PAP, and increased cardiac output and cardiac index. Other symptoms of fluid overload such as hypertension, lung crackles, and bounding pulse are reasons to discontinue the hypertonic saline infusion.

Fluid volume overload. Blood pressure, CVP, and pulmonary arterial wedge pressure are all expected to be within the normal range of the patient. Clinical manifestations of acute heart failure and pulmonary edema, such as elevated blood pressure, pulmonary artery wedge pressure, and CVP are causes to discontinue the hypertonic saline infusion. Apprehension, abrupt position changes to an upright position to breathe, dyspnea, moist cough, and increased respiratory and pulse rates also indicate the inability of the cardiopulmonary system to accommodate the increased fluid load. (∞Bedside Hemodynamic Monitoring, p. 440.)

Elimination. An alteration in bowel elimination resulting in constipation may occur from decreased fluid intake and inactivity. Cathartics or low-volume hypertonic enemas may be given to stimulate peristalsis. Tap water or hypotonic enemas should not be given because the water in the enema solution may be absorbed through the bowel and potentiate water intoxication.

Patient education. Rapidly occurring changes in the patient's neurologic status may frighten visiting family members. Sensitivity to the family's unspoken fears can be shown by words that express empathy and by providing time for the patient and family to communicate their feelings. The nurse may discuss the course of the disease, its effect on water balance, the reasons for fluid restrictions, and the family's role in treating SIADH. Teaching the patient and the family to be alert to severe thirst and measure intake and output along with parameters to notify the physician will encourage independence and involve the family in the patient's care. (See Patient Education Box 41-18 for further details.)

THYROTOXIC CRISIS

Description

To describe thyrotoxic crisis, it is necessary to include comments about hyperthyroidism. Hyperthyroidism, also called thyrotoxicosis, occurs when the thyroid gland produces thyroid hormone in excess of the body's need. Hyperthyroid conditions may also result from ingestion of excessive thyroid replacement

BOX 41-19 Conditions Associated with Thyrotoxicosis

GLANDULAR DYSFUNCTION

Grave's disease (Basdeow's disease, diffuse toxic goiter)
Toxic nodular goiter
Plummer's disease (toxic multinodular adenoma)
Giant cell thyroiditis (subacute thyroiditis)
Radiation-induced thyroiditis

DRUG THERAPY

Hormonal therapy
- Iatrogenic thyroid replacement
- Thyrotoxicosis factitia (purposeful ingestion of unphysiologic doses to produce weight loss)
- Accidental ingestion of thyroid (foods or medications)

Antidysrhythmic drug
- Amiodarone (may cause thyroid dysfunction)
- Propranolol

TUMORS

The following cause hyperthyroidism only rarely:
- Metastatic thyroid carcinoma
- Hypophyseal tumors (increasing TSH)
- Hypothalamus tumors (increasing TRH)
- Trophoblastic tumors (malignancies with circulating thyroid stimulants), such as hyadtidiform mole, testicular tumors, and choriocarcinoma

drugs. Although rare, excess thyroid hormone may be produced by a neoplasm of ectopic thyroid tissue. Conditions associated with thyrotoxicosis are presented in Box 41-19.

Thyrotoxic crisis, also called thyroid storm, is a critical stage of hyperthyroidism. It is an uncommon, life-threatening condition which occurs when the overactive thyroid has not been diagnosed or adequately treated. It is known that thyrotoxic crisis does not occur because of a sudden increase in the amount of circulating thyroid hormone during hyperthyroidism. Rather, it is believed that there is an increase in the number of receptor sites responding to catecholamine that heightens the response of all body systems and results in thyroid crisis. Thyrotoxic crisis often is precipitated by a major stressor, such as an acute infection or a severe trauma. See Box 41-20 for additional conditions known to precipitate thyrotoxic crisis. The signs and symptoms of hyperthyroidism are exaggerated in the crisis stage, and, unless emergency treatment is provided, death occurs from heart failure.

BOX 41-20 Conditions Precipitating Thyrotoxic Crisis

- Systemic infections
- Diabetes out of control
- Trauma
- Myocardial infarction
- Thyroid medication overdose
- Thyroid ablations (surgical or radioiodine)
- Surgery
- Parturition in patient with poorly controlled hyperthyroidism

Etiology

In hyperthyroidism, excessive uptake of thyroid hormone causes cellular dysfunction in the body regardless of etiologic factors in the hypersecretion. Increased thyroid hormone causes increased metabolic activity and stimulates the beta-adrenergic receptors, which results in a heightened sympathetic nervous system response. In addition to the effects of the hypermetabolism, the increased number of epinephrine-binding sites hyperactivates cardiac tissue, nervous tissue, smooth muscle tissue metabolism, and heat production.

Pathophysiology

Thyroid hormone increases cellular oxgyen consumption in almost all metabolically active cells. It is generally believed that thyroid hormones increase the rate of sodium and potassium movement through permeable membranes by stimulation of the sodium pump. It is likely, therefore, that increased thyroid hormone levels increase the sodium-potassium-linked pumping and accelerate metabolism and heat production even more.[35] Much energy in the form of heat is lost rather than used by the cell. Cellular oxygen demands are incrased in the patient with a hyperthyroid condition, and the cardiac response is to increase the cardiac output and pump more blood more rapidly to deliver oxygen and to expel carbon dioxide. Hypertension and tachycardia follow. The oxygen demands in the hypermetabolic state are so great that the cardiac system cannot compensate adequately. Fatigue and tachydysrhythmias ensure, along with a critically high fever. Increased metabolic rate requires increased oxygen and sufficient energy sources. In hyperthyroidism the patient's appetite increases to meet metabolic demands. Generally the patient is unable to take in enough food to meet the demands and prevent mobilization of carbohydrates, fats, and protein for energy sources. As a result of rapidly broken-down nutrients, negative nitrogen balance occurs and uric acid excretion increases.[7] Metabolic acidosis is a potential problem. Intestinal peristalsis increases, often resulting in diarrhea, nausea, and vomiting. These all lead to dehydration and compound the problem of malnutrition and weight loss. Excess metabolism generates heat, and the body temperature may rise as high as 41° C (106° F). Inefficient use of oxygen also affects the muscular system. Muscular contraction and relaxation increase more rapidly and is referred to as the hyperreflexia of hyperthyroidism. Muscular weakness occurs and is compounded by the excessive protein breakdown.

Hypersensitivity to the increased adrenergic-binding sites potentiates the cardiovascular and nervous system response to the hypermetabolic state. Tachydysrhythmias often progress to pulmonary edema and acute heart failure. Increased beta-adrenergic activity manifests in emotional lability, fine muscular tremors, and delirium.

Assessment and Diagnosis

Thyrotoxic crisis is a potentially lethal complication of thyrotoxicosis. It is insidious in nature, with an almost paradoxically abrupt presentation of symptoms. Thyrotoxic crisis lacks a "textbook" profile that signals its presence. The presenting symptoms and severity of the disease differ from one patient to another and change during the course of the disease, posing a profound threat to the patient's survival. Metabolic pathways are accelerated, thermoregulation is impaired, and hyperactivity of the nervous and cardiovascular system can lead to cardiac collapse and death.

Of the patients diagnosed with thyrotoxicosis, 15% are older than 65 years, yet diagnosis of a thyroid disorder in elderly persons may present more difficulties than in any other age-group. The aging process and decrease in the serum albumin level reduces the circulating thyroid levels. These levels can be further reduced during hospitalization, when the patient is adapting to a major illness and to the effects of medications. In addition, symptoms associated with thyrotoxicosis, such as hyperkinesia, often are absent in elderly persons.[36] When these symptoms are present, they frequently are attributed to senescence.

Clinical manifestations of thyrotoxicosis are exaggerated in thyrotoxic crisis. An important exception, however, is that the laboratory values of patients with thyrotoxic crisis will not show any sudden changes as a result of thyrotoxicosis. Serum triiodothyronine (T_3) and thyroxine (T_4) remain at their elevated thyrotoxic levels. No diagnostic test is available to differentiate thyrotoxic crisis from its predecessor, thyrotoxicosis.[18]

Clinical manifestations of thyroid are exaggerated signs and symptoms of thyrotoxicosis. The clinical manifestations are listed in Box 41-21.

Medical Management

The medical management of thyrotoxicosis is of an acute, emergency nature. Various abnormal processes are occurring in the body that, if left untreated, could quickly lead to coma and death from cardiac failure. Production of thyroid hormone and conversion of T_4 to more active, potent T_3 needs to be reduced.

The body's heightened sensitivity to the increased adrenergic and catecholamine receptors must be suppressed. Cardiac irregularities need to be controlled and progression of heart failure halted. Pyrexia must be treated with hypothermia measures such as cooling blanket and acetaminophen (aspirin is to be avoided because it is believed to free the thyroid hormone from its protein state, thus rendering it more active).[15] Vigorous fluid replacement needs to be instituted to treat or prevent dehydration. Antibiotic therapy may be warranted in the presence of systemic infection. Other existing pathologic conditions need to be treated appropriately. Table 41-8 lists the most commonly used medications and their nursing implication of the patient in thyrotoxic crisis. Pharmacologic treatment consists of blocking the synthesis and release of thyroid hormone into circulation, inhibiting the conversion of T_4 to T_3 and decreasing the body's sensitivity to the sympathetic adrenergic receptors.

Blocking the synthesis of thyroid hormone is accomplished by the administration of antithyroid thioamide drugs. These drugs include propylthiouracil (PTU) and methimazole (Tapazole). Neither drug is available in parenteral form and must be given by mouth or via a nasogastric tube. PTU is especially therapeutic because it also blocks the conversion of T_4 to T_3. Methimazole has a slower action rate, but it is more potent than PTU. The antithyroid drugs do not block the release of previously synthesized thyroid hormone; therefore in a crisis state they are given with iodide preparations.

Drugs that reduce thyroid hormone release into circulation are the iodides and a similarly acting glucocorticoid, dexamethasone. The iodide preparations are rapid acting, with a short duration. They are given 1 hour after the administration of the antithyroid drugs to prevent the iodide from being used for thyroid hormone and possibly worsening the clinical state. The iodides

BOX 41-21 Clinical Manifestations of Thyrotoxic Crisis

CARDIOVASCULAR SYSTEM

Prompted by increased number and affinity of beta-adrenergic receptors in the heart:
Tachycardia
Systolic murmur
Increased stroke volume
Increased cardiac output
Increased systolic blood pressure
Decreased diastolic blood pressure
Extra systoles
Paroxysmal atrial tachycardia
Premature ventricular contraction
Palpitations
Chest pain
Increased cardiac contractility
Congestive heart failure
Pulmonary edema
Cardiogenic shock

CENTRAL NERVOUS SYSTEM

Resulting from an increased catecholamine response:
Hyperkinesis
Nervousness
Muscle weakness
Confusion
Convulsions
Heat intolerance
Fine tremor
Emotional lability
Frank psychosis
Apathy
Stupor
Diaphoresis

GASTROINTESTINAL SYSTEM

Nausea
Vomiting
Diarrhea
Liver enlargement
Abdominal pain
Weight loss
Increased appetite

INTEGUMENTARY SYSTEM

Pruritus
Hyperpigmentation of skin
Fine, straight hair
Alopecia

THERMOREGULATORY SYSTEM

Hyperthermia
Heat dissipation
Diaphoresis

SERUM/URINE

Hypercalcemia
Hyperglycemia
Hypoalbuminemia
Hypoprothrombinemia
Hypocholesterolemia
Creatinuria

maintain and increase the levels of protein-bound thyroid hormone, thereby decreasing the levels of free active thyroid. The iodide most frequently used for thyrotoxic crisis is sodium iodide. Potassium iodide, saturated solution of potassium iodide, or strong iodide solution also may be used. Patients who cannot take iodides because of allergies may be given lithium carbonate, which inhibits release of the thyroid hormone.[20]

A powerful glucocorticoid, dexamethasone suppresses the release of thyroid hormone.[15] Beta-adrenergic blocking agents are used to decrease the catecholamine effects of excessive thyroid hormone. Propranolol, used in thyrotoxic crisis, has no effect on the thyroid hormone but effectively reduces the exaggerated myocardial stimulation, reduces myocardial contraction force, and slows the atrioventricular (AV) conduction rate. Doses vary from patient to patient, but typically higher doses are required to affect the number of receptor sites active in the crisis. Esmolol, a short-acting beta-blocker specifically used for short-term-rapid control of atrial fibrillation, also can be used. Currently clinicians disagree on the use of beta-blockers for patients with overt heart failure. Drugs that can be used when beta-adrenergic blocking agents are contraindicated[20] include reserpine and guanethidine. These drugs, used infrequently because of their numerous side effects, deplete or inhibit norepinephrine release at the adrenergic nerve endings.

Calcium channel blockers such as verapamil also are effective in controlling heart rate in patients for whom beta-blockers are contraindicated.

Medical management is concurrently directed at reducing critical multiple organ dysfunction syndrome that results from the hypermetabolic effects of thyrotoxic crisis. Reduction in body temperature is managed by use of a cooling blanket and antipyretic agent,

TABLE 41-8 Medications and Nursing Implications for Thyrotoxic Crisis[8,10,18,20]

Drug	Dosage	Actions	Special Considerations
BLOCKS SYNTHESIS OF THYROID HORMONE			
Propylthiouracil	Loading dose: 800-1200 mg maintenance dose: 100-400 mg q 4-6 hr PO or gavage	Blocks synthesis of thyroid hormone Blocks conversion of T_3 to T_4	Monitor thyrotoxic response (i.e., heart rate, nervousness, fever, diarrhea, diaphoresis). Observe for sudden conversion to hypothyroidism: headache, sluggish responses. Assess for skin rash. Administer with meals to reduce gastrointestinal (GI) effects. May cause rash, nausea, vomiting, agranulocytosis, skin hyperpigmentation, prothrombin deficiency.
Methimazole	10-20 mg q 6-8 hr PO or gavage	Blocks synthesis of thyroid hormone	More toxic than propylthiouracil. Presence of rash may be reason to discontinue drug. Monitor signs listed for propylthiouracil. May cause rash, agranulocytosis.
SUPPRESSES RELEASE OF THYROID HORMONE			
Sodium iodide	1 g/L q 12 hr IV	Suppresses release of thyroid hormone	Give iodide 1 hr after propylthiouracil or methimazole. Toxic iodinism poisoning: edema, mucosal stomatitis, hemorrhage, metallic taste, skin lesions, severe GI upset.
Potassium iodide	2-5 gtt q 8 hr PO	Suppresses release of thyroid hormone	Discontinue if rash appears. Signs of toxic iodinism as above.
Saturated solution of potassium iodide (SSKI)	10 gtt q 8 hr PO	Suppresses release of thyroid hormone	Give through a straw to prevent teeth discoloration. Mix with juice or milk to lessen GI upset. Signs of toxic iodinism as above.
Dexamethasone	2 mg q 6 hr, variable, IV	Suppresses thyroid hormone release Blocks conversion of T_4 to T_3	Monitor intake and ouput; monitor serum glucose levels. May cause hypertension, nausea, vomiting, anorexia, increased susceptibility to infection.
BETA-BLOCKERS			
Propranolol	1-3 mg q 1-4 hr IV 40-80 mg q 4-6 hr PO	Beta-adrenergic blocking agent to counter sympathetic activity Decreases conversion of T_4 to T_3	Monitor cardiac activity, CVP, PAWP, bradycardia, hypotension, pending CHF. Hold if heart rate < 50 beats/min Have atropine available, may cause GI upset, weakness, fatigue.
Esmolol	500 μg/kg/min for first minute, then 50 μg/kg/min for 4 minutes IV	Beta-adrenergic blocker	Monitor for bradycardia, orthostatic hypotension, dysrhythmia. Measure intake and output. May cause edema, diarrhea, diaphoresis, vertigo.
ALPHA BLOCKERS			
Reserpine	1.0-2.5 mg q 24 hr PO	Depletes stores of catecholamine in sympathetic nerve endings	Monitor BP, heart rate changes in hyperthyroid conditions. May cause bradycardia, drowsiness, GI bleeding, diarrhea.
Guanethidine sulfate	50-150 mg q 24 hr PO	Antiadrenergic Inhibits norepinephrine release in response to sympathetic nerve stimulation	Monitor orthostatic hypotension. Measure and record intake and output. Monitor diarrhea. May cause GI upset, edema, fatigue, drowsiness.

acetaminophen. Intravenous infusion of dantrolene, used to prevent or treat malignant hyperthermia, has been used successfully in the management of pyrexia from thyrotoxic crisis. Dantrolene appears to block the calcium release in select myocytes and inhibit the intense catabolism in these muscle cells. Preventing rapid breakdown of metabolites within the cells prevents the production of heat, which is believed to stimulate the critical rise in body temperature.[9] Digitalis and diuretics may be required to treat symptoms of acute heart failure, with doses possibly increased to achieve the desired effect.

When dehydration and metabolic acidosis are present, they are treated with large volumes of glucose and sodium solutions to replace circulating fluid and sodium and to provide calories used by the hypermetabolism. Sodium bicarbonate replacement may be ordered to reverse the metabolic acidosis. Its use is controversial, however, because it can cause further tissue hypoxia.

Oxygen is given to reduce the patient's work of breathing. Oxygen titration is based on pulse oximeter readings or on arterial blood gas values obtained to determine the metabolic acidosis.

BOX 41-22 NURSING DIAGNOSIS AND MANAGEMENT

THYROTOXIC CRISIS

- Hyperthermia related to increased thyroid hormone, p. 1049
- Altered Nutrition: Less Than Body Requirements related to lack of exogenous nutrients or increased metabolic demand, p. 165
- Decreased Cardiac Output related to alterations in heart rate, p. 593
- Anxiety related to threat to biologic, psychologic, and/or social integrity, p. 99
- Sleep Pattern Disturbance related to fragmented sleep, p. 118
- Knowledge Deficit: Self-care of Thyrotoxicosis related to lack of previous exposure to information, p. 61 (see Patient Education Box 41-23)

Nursing Management

It is the patient who is hospitalized for a major illness—the person with either undiagnosed or previously controlled thyrotoxicosis—who is at greatest risk of experiencing the complication of thyrotoxic crisis. Thyrotoxic crisis may be precipitated by increased physical stress on the body in the form of a major illness and hospitalization. Currently no diagnostic tests specific for thyrotoxic crisis are available. Standard laboratory tests are inconclusive. The results of thyroid function tests, such as those that measure T_4 and T_3, show understandably elevated levels caused by thyrotoxicosis, but they do not reflect the increased sensitivity of the catecholamine receptors. The condition, therefore, is identified by a combination of past medical history and current clinical manifestations. The nursing history is of great importance for this patient.

Nursing management includes constant vigilance over hypermetabolic effects on the body's temperature, cardiac functioning, and nervous system responses. Hydration must be preserved, hyperglycemia treated if present, metabolic acidosis prevented and/or treated, and weight loss curtailed. A variety of nursing diagnoses are associated with thyrotoxic crisis and are listed in Box 41-22.

Hyperthermia. In thyrotoxic crisis the patient has hyperthermia related to a hypermetabolic state as evidenced by critically high body temperature; diaphoresis; hot, flushed skin; intolerance to heat; tachycardia; and tachypnea. Temperature is to be assessed every 15 minutes and frequency gradually tapered after the temperature reaches safe levels and stabilizes. Core temperature is identified most accurately with an invasive pulmonary arterial line (The arterial line also is least disruptive to the patient, who is in an agitated, restless state). The second choice is to use a temperature-sensitive catheter for patients requiring indwelling urinary catheters. Research has shown that the urinary catheter thermistor reading is identical to pulmonary arterial readings.[37] Safety hazards and the invasive nature of rectal thermometers disqualify the rectal method as a option for use with the agitated, restless patient with thryoid storm. The next choice would be the ear-based infrared thermometer for ear canal temperature. Although ear readings do not provide accuracy as compared with the standard urinary catheter thermistor, it is considered sensitive to variations in temperature above 37.8°C.[37,38] To maximize the sensitivity of the ear probe, many variables are to be considered: ear canal anatomy, absence of cerumen between the probe and the tympanic membrane, and holding the probe securely against the tympanic membrane. The accuracy of the ear probe is determined by the fact that the eardrum (against which the sensor is held) shares the blood supply and is in proximity to the hypothalamus, the body's "thermostat."

Nursing measures to provide comfort while the patient is intolerant to heat include a room with a cool environment and a fan to circulate air, lightweight bed coverings, and comfortable, nonrestrictive bed clothes. A tepid sponge bath helps to reduce heat by evaporation, and ice application to the groin and axilla increases heat loss at major blood vessels through conduction.

Changes in cardiac functioning relate to the high metabolic activity and adrenergic response. The resulting tachydysrhythmia and heart failure, coupled with the hyperthermia, eventually causes death.

Cardiovascular management. Cardiovascular assessment includes rate, rhythm, irregularities, blood pressure changes, pulse pressure variances, decrease in quality of peripheral pulses, and patient reports of chest pain and palpitations. Hemodynamic monitoring includes atrial blood pressure, CVP, pulmonary artery wedge pressure (PAWP) and cardiac output readings. High-output cardiac failure may occur with the demands of the hypermetabolic activity within the body, far exceeding the ability of the myocardium to pump oxygenated blood to meet those demands. Heart failure ensues as the catecholamine-driven receptors produce abnormal conduction patterns and weakening rapid contractions. The rapid heart rate allows little time for the coronary arteries to fill and supply oxygen to the cardiac tissue. In this hyperdynamic state, atrial fibrillation with rapid ventricular response, premature ventricular contractions, and other ventricular dysrhythmias can occur.

Nursing management includes the administration of the prescribed beta-adrenergic blocking agents to decrease the catecholamine effects of the thyroid hormone. Reduction in heart rate, decreased cardiac irritability, and decreased contractile force of the myocardium should result. An increase in the refractory period prolongs AV conduction, allowing the heart a longer diastole for rest and an increased time to fill coronary arteries to supply oxygen to the myocardium. Bradycardia and hypotension are to be closely monitored as potential untoward effects of the beta-blocking agents.

Fluid and electrolyte considerations. Hyperthermia, tachypnea, diaphoresis, vomiting, and diarrhea predispose the patient to a fluid volume deficit. Fluids and electrolytes are as vigorously replaced as the decompensated cardiovascular system can manage. Glucose solutions are given to replace glycogen stores. Insulin may be administered to treat the hyperglycemia that results from mobilization of nutrients and high doses of glucocorticoids. Serum glucose tests may be performed to identify the level of glucose in the blood stream and to use as a reference point for insulin dose. Hyponatremia from active loss, such as vomiting, is monitored by means of laboratory serum values. Hyponatremia is prevented and/or treated with appropriate sodium concentrations of intravenous fluids. Additional nursing measures focus on hourly hydration assessments. Intake and output measurements include estimating diaphoretic fluid loss through the number of gown and linen changes, checking buccal membranes for moisture, and recording daily weights. (See Box 41-4 for additional hydration assessments.)

Nursing assessments include CVP, PAP, breath sounds, neck vein engorgement, and hourly urine output. A serious complication is circulatory overload. It is signaled by increased CVP, increased PAP, moist lung sounds, neck vein engorgement, and dyspnea without exertion. Reduction in fluid volume infusion, elevation of the head of the bed, and administration of diuretics and oxygen may be needed to support the patient's breathing and to alleviate the increased fluid load.

Neurologic assessment. The patient in thyrotoxic crisis is agitated, anxious, and unable to rest and thus requires intensive care that is quiet, restful, and calm. Phenobarbital, previously given to minimize tremors and promote sedation, has been found to displace thyroxine from plasma proteins and can actually exacerbate hyperthyroid symptoms.[39] Gradually the antithyroid medications and beta-adrenergic blocking drugs will decrease the neurologic symptoms related to the catecholamine sensitivity. The patient needs to be told that his or her extreme agitation is the result of the disease process and that the medications will help to control the nonstop fidgeting and tremors. Frequent reassurance and clear, simple explanations regarding the patient's condition help decrease the fear brought on by the strange surroundings.

Rest and sleep. Sleep deprivation as a result of the intense neuroexcitation is another challenge for the critical care nurse. The patient needs uninterrupted blocks of time to rest even if he or she is unable to sleep during that time. The primary nurse is responsible for encouraging all members of the medical, nursing, and paramedical staff to respect these rest periods. Family and other visitors are to adhere to the treatment plan as well. (∞Sleep Deprivation, p. 109.)

The goal of intense medical and nursing management of thyrotoxic crisis is to reduce thyroid hormone levels within 24 to 48 hours. During this time the life-threatening symptoms of hyperpyrexia, cardiac excitation, and nervous system dsyfunction are brought under control.

Patient education. During the critical events surrounding the thyroid crisis the patient and family are given information according to their emotional state and cognitive level of understanding. In terms that are understandable, the cause of the high fever, anxiety, and cardiac dysrhythmias is presented. Often the patient and family are relieved to know that the agitation and nervousness result from circulating chemicals that may be decreased by taking daily medications. Side effects of drug therapy are taught before discharge. Patients treated with beta-blockers or antiadrenergic medications are taught to report signs of bradycardia, unexplained fatigue, and orthostatic hypotension, among other untoward effects. Patients discharged with antithyriod drugs are alerted to the main side effect: agranulocytosis. Symptoms of agranulocytosis include sudden cough, fever, rash, and inflammation. These symptoms must be brought to the attention of the primary care provider. Patients are instructed to use acetaminophen rather than salicylates, as the salicylate increases the free thyroid hormone in circulation. Table 41-8 describes other medications and special considerations. Also refer to Box 41-23 for Thyrotoxic Crisis patient education.

BOX 41-23 PATIENT EDUCATION

THYROTOXIC CRISIS

- Acute phase
  - Explain reasons for critial care unit admission
  - Explain reasons for extreme hypermetabolism
- Predischarge
  - Assess knowledge level
  - Disease process of thyrotoxicosis
  - Causes of thyrotoxic crisis
  - Signs and symptoms to report to a health care professional
  - Medications
    - Explain purpose, side effects, dosage, and how often to use

MYXEDEMA COMA

Description

Manifestation of hypothyroidism depends, in part, on the severity of the nonfunctioning thyroid and the age of the individual at the onset of the disease. A severe deficiency or absence of thyroid hormone during the embryonic development results in a newborn infant with mental and physical retardation. This hypothyroidism is referred to as cretinism. Deficiency in thyroid functioning in an older child is referred to as juvenile hypothyroidism. A severe deficiency or absence of thyroid hormone later in life is called hypothyroidism or myxedema.[14,40] Unrecognized, untreated, or inadequately treated myxedema (hypothyroidism) in an adult will result in a comatose state, called myxedema coma, and lead to death. Discussion of myxedema coma necessitates frequent reference to its precursor state, hypothyroidism. Additionally, for the sake of clarity, the following presentation will use the term hypothyroidism in mentioning the state of inadequate or absent thyroid hormone. The term myxedema will be used only as myxedema coma, in referring to the progressive worsening or terminal stage of hypothyroidism.

Hypothyroidism is caused by a deficiency of circulating thyroid hormons. The lack of hormone, or the insufficient amount of hormone, affects all body cells, organs, and systems. Since thyroid hormone is responsible for increased protein synthesis in all cells and increased oxgyen consumption in every organ, a deficiency of thyroid hormone leads to a decrease in the energy metabolic rate or a slowing of response time in every system.

Myxedema coma is found in 5% of the geriatric population and has a mortality above 50%.[8,14,25] Ten time more women are affected than men.[18] Myxedema coma is rarely seen as a single disease entity in the intensive care unit. Its underlying presence is frequently revealed by an acute primary disease, which may result in increased metabolic demands. Cardiorespiratory disease, systemic infection, and exposure to extreme cold are a few of the physiologic stressors that require an increase in the body's metabolic activity. Hypothyroidism and myxedema coma are covered under the same two DRGs as many of the other endocrine conditions: DRG 300, endocrine disorders with co-morbid conditions, which has an anticipated length of stay of 7.9 days, and DRG 301, endocrine disorders without co-morbid conditions, with an anticipated length of stay of 4.8 days.[5]

Metabolism. The effects of hypothyroidism are widespread and varied. When the basic metabolic rate of oxygen consumption is reduced, the cell is unable to maintain the processes necessary to sustain life. Without thyroid hormone, protein synthesis is severely curtailed and amino acid production, manufacture of blood proteins, and repair of tissues are halted. Metabolism of carbohydrate and fat is incomplete, and gluconeogensis is not able to supply the counterregulatory source of glucose. Lipolysis is ineffective, and cholesterol collects in the blood stream. A more complete list of the effects of decreased thyroid hormones on the body is provided in Box 41-24.

Skin. The composition of the skin changes as hyaluronic acid deposits (gel-like substance capable of hold-

BOX 41-24 Conditions Associated With Myxedema

Chronic autoimmune thyroiditis (i.e., Hashimoto's thyroiditis)
Iodine deficiency
- Nontoxic goiter
- Surgical removal of gland
- Surgical removal of pituitary
- Intrathyroid chemical defect with impaired capacity to secrete thyroxine
- Ingestion antithyroid agents
  - Drugs: nitroprusside, sulfonamides, sulfonylureas, iodides, lithium, paraminosalicylic acid
  - Foods: turnips, cabbage, rutabagas, kale

Iodine excess
Pituitary thyroid stimulating hormone secretion deficiency
Hereditary defects in thyroid hormone biosynthesis

ing large amounts of fluid) accumulate in the interstitial spaces giving rise to a full, puffy appearance of face, hands, and feet. The face is dull and masklike. The skin is pale, with an overall yellowish appearance resulting from the increase of carotene deposits. The nails and hair are thin and brittle. Absence of thyroid hormone also leads to decreased or absent sweat production. The hyaluronic acid deposits are evident in cardiac muscle tissue, skeletal muscles, and muscles of the tongue, pharynx, and proximal esophagus. These striated muscular changes of the tongue, pharynx, and esophagus most probably contribute to the hoarse, husky voice and dull facial expression of hypothyroid patients.

Cardiopulmonary system. Interstitial edema impairs cardiac myocytes, resulting in bradycardia and diminished cardiac output (Box 41-25). The heart appears to be enlarged, but its size may be exaggerated by serous fluid accumulation in the pericardial sac. There is a decreased sensitivity to catecholamines. The resting heart rate and stroke volume are reduced. The force of myocardial contraction is weakened with a decrease in the systolic blood pressure and an increase in diastolic pressure, causing a narrowed pulse pressure. Electrocardiogram typically reveals shallow, weak QRS complex and PT waves.

Pulmonary system. Pleural effusions and muscular changes affect gas exchange. The basal rate of oxygen consumption decreases with a resulting insensitivity to CO_2. The hypoventilation increases the CO_2 serum content, which increases cerebral hypoxia. Pleural effusion, reduced vital capacity, and shallow respirations occur as the patient manifests dyspnea with exertion and decreased exercise tolerance. Airway obstruction

BOX 41-25 Clinical Manifestations of Hyperthyroidism, Thyroid Crisis, as Compared With Hypothyroidism, Myxedma Coma

HYPERTHYROIDISM (THYROTOXICOSIS)	HYPOTHYROIDISM (MYXEDEMA)
Thyroid crises	Myxdema Coma
Thyrotoxic storm	
Elevated T_4, T_3	Decreased T_4, T_3
Decreased TSH	Elevated TSH
Hypercalcemia	Hyponatremia
Hyperglycemia	Hypoglycemia
Metabolic acidisis	Respiratory acidosis
	Metabolic acidosis
	Hypercholesterolemia
	Anemia
Tachycardia	Bradycardia
Angina	Enlarged heart
Palpitations	Decreased stroke volume
Atrial fibrillation	Decreased cardiac output
ST wave changes	Flattened, inverted T waves
Shortened QT	Prolonged QT and PR intervals
Hypertension	Increased total body fluid with decreased effective aterial blood volume
AV block	
Hypovolemia	Peripheral vasoconstriction
Angina	Pericardial effusion
Acute heart failure	
Tachypnea	Hypoventilation
SOB	Possible CO_2 retention
Hypermetabolism	Depressed metabolism
Polyphagia	Decreased lipolysis
Weight loss	Increased cholesterol
Nausea, vomiting	Weight gain
Increased peristalsis	Constipation
Tremor	Depression
Extreme restlessness	Seizures
Insomina	Slowness
Anxiety	Hypothermia
Uneasiness	Impaired short-term memory
Emotional instability	Slow, deliberate speech
Despondency	Thickened tongue
Diaphoresis	Coarse, dry, scaly, edematous skin
Heat intolerance	Frank delirium (myxedema madness)
	Lethargy→stupor→coma (myxedema coma)
Increased deep tendon reflexes (DTRs)	Diminished DTRs
Muscle weakness/muscle wasting	Paresthesia of hands
Oligoamenorrhea	Menorrhagia

→, Leading to.

or choking may occur from the interstitial edema causing the thickened tongue and the slowed activation time of the tongue muscles.

Elimination. Abdominal distention, decreased intestinal peristalsis, and eventual paralytic ileus lead to extreme constipation, called obstipation. Understandably, a lack of appetite and inability to eat co-exist.

Nutrients. Food utilization and nutrient mobilization decrease with insufficient thyroid hormone. When carbohydrate, protein, and fat are ingested, they are incompletely metabolized, and therefore, unavailable for cellular needs of growth and repair. Intestinal hypomotility and abdominal distention prevent absorption of food nutrients in the small intestine. Lipolysis decreases while serum cholesterol increases.

Thermoregulation. Heat production decreases as a result of insufficient energy for the base metabolic rate within the cells. The inability to maintain body heat is further restricted by the hypoglycemia. Sweating and insensible water loss diminish.

Kidney. Renal blood flow is reduced with decreased glomerular filtration rate (GFR), decreased urine specific garvity, and decreased urine osmolality. Without sufficient thyroid hormone, urea production is diminished.

Erythropoiesis. Anemia is a common problem associated with hypothyroidism, as is the fatigue and depression associated with the iron deficiency. Decreased thyroid hormones prevent normal iron absorption, storage, and use. Insufficient amount of the hormone also interferes with hemoglobin synthesis and leads to an impaired folic acid absorption in the interstitial mucosa. The resulting erythropoiesis is impaired and inadequate against the excessive blood loss through yet another common hypothyroidism symptom in females, menorrhagia.

Assessment and Diagnosis

The diagnosis of myxedema coma is based on the clinical manifestations of end-stage hypothyroidism. There are no specific laboratory tests to differentiate between hypothyroidism and myxedema coma. Thyroid function laboratory values support hypothyroidism and report a decreased T_4[41] and an elevated or a normal thyroid-stimulating hormone level.[42]

The diagnosis of end-stage hypothyroidism is based on the clinical presentation of the patient. Increasing signs of somnolence, depression, and diminished mental acuity signal diminished cellular functioning. Interstitial edema collects in most all tissues. Organs become infiltrated with the mucoidal rich substrate, mucopolysaccharides. Collection of this fluid further compromises organ functioning. Patients manifest cardiovascular collapse, hypothermia, decreased renal functioning, fluid excess, hypoventilation, and severe metabolic disorders.

Weight gain is attributed to the collection of mucopolysaccharides in the interstitium, increase in fluid retention, and decrease in metabolism. Hand and feet paresthesia is caused by the hyaluronic acid accumulation in the synovial sacs, which leads to the compression of nerves and carpal tunnel syndrome. The compression of nerves interferes with the simplest hand grasp and the ability to raise one's hands. Reflexes contract briskly but take extended seconds to relax.

Hypothermia is a very distressing symptom. The patient is seemingly unable to keep the body warm. Temperatures are reported to be as low as 24° C (80° F) to 35° C (95° F).[34]

The myxedematous patient has hypotension, reduced total blood volume, decreased cardiac output, and bradycardia—all related to a decrease in the beta-adrenergic stimulation.[23]

Neuropsychiatric symptoms of depression, confusion, and decreased mental acuity may degenerate to a psychosis aptly termed "myxedema madness."

Medical Management

The patient's primary admitting diagnosis may mask an underlying hyothyroidism. However, clinical manifestations can trigger the alert clinician to suspect a hypofunctioning thyroid. Both the primary disease condition and the myxedema coma must be treated immediately to improve the patient's chances for recovery. A complete blood count and differential are done to establish the presence of infection. Hypothyroidism produces a characteristically low white blood count. A normal white blood count and a differential with elevated and immature neutrophils indicates an ongoing acute infection. Severe systemic infection, often a precipitating factor for the myxedema coma, must be treated to decrease the stress on the thyroid-pituitary axis. Empiric antibiotic therapy may be required.

Once the nonthyroid diseases that warranted the initial admission to an intensive care unit are diagnosed, the patient is treated for the myxedema coma. The goal for the treatment of end-stage or decompensating hypothyroid condition is to restore the patient to an euthyroid condition. This is accomplished with thyroid hormone replacement and support measures for the multisystem involvement.

Immediaely after the diagnosis of myxedema coma is made, the patient is intubated in preparation for mechanical ventilation. Respiratory failure is a common occurrence in myxedema coma. Initiating mechanical ventilation depends on arterial blood gas reports of hypercapnea and cerebral hypoxia. (∞Invasive Mechanical Ventilation, p. 703; Arterial Blood Gases, p. 641.)

Medications. Methods of treating end-stage hypothyroidism with medications vary among practitioners. A common method is the use of levothyroxine 300 to 500 mg intravenously to saturate the previously empty T_4 binding sites[8,14,15,18,19,28] and to correct hyponatremia. The thyroid binding globulin must be saturated before any free thyroxine can circulate. The loading dose is followed by daily administration of 50 to 200 mg of levrothyroxine.[8,14,15,18,19,28] The elderly patient with concurrent heart disease necessitating treatment with replacement hormones would start slow so as not to precipitate heart failure or angina.

Medications such as vasopressors may be given to improve cardiac circulation. However, this is done with great caution because of the possibility of stimulating ventricular tachycardia in a patient with compromised cardiac contractions. Dopamine may be the preferred vasopressor agent, yet even this must be given with great vigilance and caution.[42] Glucocorticoids may be necessary to assist the patient to respond to the stress state of hypothyroidism until a co-existing adrenal insufficiency is ruled out.[18]

Nursing Management

Nursing care of the patient with myxedema coma focuses on management of the precipitating disease as well as the severe hypothyroid condition. Many nursing diagnoses are associated with management of myxedema coma and are listed in Box 41-26.

Pulmonary care. Patients are usually intubated and, depending on the degree of ventilatory insufficiency, attached to mechanical assistance. Individuals who are not intubated are closely observed for changes in respiratory rate, depth, and muscle use. Frequent arterial blood gas measurements are done to determine possible CO_2 retention and respiratory acidosis.

Cardiac concerns. Dysrhythmias, common in the myxedematous patient with impaired myocardial - contraction, can quickly be identified by continous electrocardiogram monitoring. Expected signs of myxedema such as flattened or inverted T waves or prolonged QT and PR intervals resolve in a positive response to replacement therapy. Hypotension management requires cautious fluid replacement of 5% to 10% glucose in 0.45% sodium chloride or 0.9% sodium chloride, depending on serum sodium levels.

Thermoregulation. Hypothermia will show gradual improvement as the patient is treated with thyroid hormone. Several warm blankets comfortably wrapped around the patient (with mild hypothermia) may be sufficient to help raise the body temperature to normal. Passive warming blankets are used to minimize heat loss and avoid rapid rewarming. Rewarming too abruptly could cause further vasodilation, leading to hypotension and shock. Patients with more severe hypothermia may require active rewarming devices along with continuous assessments to avoid rapid vasodilation. Temperatures are to be measured with electronic devices because these devices can measure temperatures at the extreme lower range of body temperatures.

Fluid needs. Parenteral intravenous solutions are given slowly and with caution, avoiding free water, which would compound the circulatory status.

Replacement therapy. Elderly patients or those with a cardiac history are to receive intravenous thyroxine with due precautions. Increased doses of thyroxine could precipitate angina and dysrhythmias. Hemodynamic monitoring includes heart rate, arterial blood pressure, electrocardiogram reading, CVP, and PAWP. (∞Bedside Hemodynamic Monitoring, p. 442.)

Medication concerns. Patients with overall decreased metabolism have a slowed drug inactivation time. This decreased biotransformation requires that drug dosages be reduced. Also, the frequency of administration of a drug is prolonged to avoid an increase in the circulating drug metabolites and its related toxicities. Additionally, medications that suppress respirations are either to be avoided or are given in small amounts and less often than the size of the body would otherwise dictate.

Seizures. Seizure precautions include nursing actions to protect the patient from injury (padded side rails, bed in low position) and to provide an open airway (oral airway, head turned to side without forcibly restraining the patient, suction equipment). If the patient is not intubated, oxygen would be administered via nasal cannula. Documentation of seizures

BOX 41-26 NURSING DIAGNOSIS AND MANAGEMENT

MYXEDEMA COMA

- Hypothermia related decreased thyroid hormone, p. 1050
- Inability to Sustain Spontaneous Ventilation related to respiratory fatigue or metabolic factors, p. 724
- Activity Intolerance related to prolonged immobility or deconditioning, p. 597
- Body Image Disturbance related to functional dependence on life-sustaining technolgy, p. 86
- Knowledge Deficit: Self-care of Hypothyroidism related to lack of previous exposure to information, p. 61 (see Patient Education Box 41-27)

includes onset, duration, and description of seizure activity.

Skin care. Patients with myxedema coma have rough, dry skin. Measures are taken to avoid skin breakdown related to decreased circulation and widespread edema. Soap is used sparingly, followed by an emollient. Frequent positioning minimizes pressure against capillary beds over bony prominences.

Elimination. Constipation is managed on a daily basis to avoid impaction. When permitted, food choices are to include sources of increased fiber, such as fresh fruits and vegetables. Fluids are encouraged as the hypovolemia is corrected and blood pressure stabilizes at normal. Daily doses of prunes, prune juice, and/or a stool softener may initiate frequent, soft formed stool. Enemas are to be avoided, as insertion of the rectal tube may stimulate the vagal nerve.

Cognition. Patients with myxedema coma have decreased comprehension and mental acuity. All instructions, procedures, and activities are to be explained slowly, with repetitions given as often as necessary.

Improvement in the patient's psycholgic, cardiopulmonary, and neurologic status plus T_4 and thyroid stimulating hormone laboratory values nearing normal are often used as hallmarks indicating accuracy of the thyroid hormone replacement therapy.

Patient education. Family members, as well as the patient experiencing myxedema coma, may go through a myriad of emotions with one constant: fear of the unknown. Before any teaching the nurse is to evaluate the family's ability to accept the patient's slowed thinking and decreased response time. The family may benefit from a referral to the hospital's social service department for assistance in dealing with the patient's neuropsychiatric symptoms.

All instructions given to the patient and/or family are to be given both verbally and in writing. In addition, a written copy of all schedules is given as a reference for home care before discharge. The nurse is to discuss the medication schedule and the frequency of the drug doses with the patient and family. Side effects of each drug are to be included. The patient and family are to know the side effects of drugs so that they can deal with them at home as well as know which signs or symptoms are to be reported to the health care provider. Over-the-counter medications are not to be taken unless the physician approves of the drug and dose.

The schedule of follow-up visits for laboratory tests are given to the family and/or patient before discharge. The patient and family need to know that the results of blood tests will determine whether daily medication dosages are to be changed or discontinued. A common schedule would be the FT_4 and thyroid stimulating hormone monitoring every 4 to 6 weeks.

The nurse provides the family with a list of hypothyroid signs and symptoms that need to be recognized by the family and referred to the physician. The list may include slow movements, slow deliberate speech, and an expressionless face. Difficulty swallowing, anorexia, and decreased urinary ouput are also to be included. The patient and family must also be alert to subtle signs of intolerance to cold. For example, the wearing of heavy clothing or several layers of clothing by the patient in a manner inconsistent with ambient temperatures may be an indication of an intolerance to reduced temperature that should be referred to the physician. Later signs of the disease that need immediate attention are difficulty breathing and changes in level of consciousness.

Skin care that includes frequent assessment, limited use of soaps, and liberal use of emollients is discussed.

The nurse discusses the treatment of constipation with the patient and family and offers practical home care interventions. Constipation, leading to impaction, is a serious problem for the patient with hypothyroidism. A schedule for toileting every day, perhaps after breakfast may help to establish the importance of the task of elimination. This schedule is based on the usual daily activity of the patient and family so as to assure its suitability and promote compliance. Patient's needs are to be attended to as soon as the urge is felt. Listings of foods high in fiber are to be given to the patient for daily choices. Liberal fluids, including juices and water, are taken with the physician's knowledge. See Patient Education Box 41-27 for more information.

BOX 41-27 PATIENT EDUCATION

MYXEDEMA COMA

- Acute phase
  - Explain reasons for admission to a critical care unit
- Predischarge
  - Assess knowledge level
  - Explain disease process of hypothyroidism
  - Self-care of hypothyroidism
  - Medications
    - Explain purpose, side effects, dosage, and how often to use
  - Signs and symptoms to report to a health care professional

REFERENCES

1. Stanford GG: The stress response to trauma and critical illness. In Gould KA, Toto KH, Hotter AN, editors: Endocrine and metabolic disturbances in the critically ill, *Crit Care Nurs Clin North Am* 6(4):693-702, 1994.
2. Waxman K: Physiologic response to injury. In Shoemaker WC and others, editors: *Textbook of critical care,* ed 3, Philadelphia, 1995, WB Saunders.
3. Modest GA: Cardiovascular risk factors: social determinants of cardiovascular disease. In Noble J and others, editors: *Textbook of primary care medicine,* ed 2, St Louis, 1996, Mosby.
4. Burr R: Neuroendocrinology. In Noble J and others, editors: *Textbook of primary care medicine,* ed 2, St Louis, 1996, Mosby.
5. *St. Anthony's DRG guidebook,* 1996, Reston, Va, 1996, St Anthony.
6. Bennett PH: Definition, diagnosis and classification of diabetes and impaired glucose intolerance. In Kahn C, Weir G, editors: *Joslin's diabetes mellitus,* ed 13, Philadelphia, 1994, Lea & Febiger.
7. American Diabetes Association: Clinical practice recommendations 1997, *Diabetes Care,* 20(suppl S1-S70), 1997.
8. Burch WM: *Endocrinology,* ed 3, Baltimore, 1994, William & Wilkins.
9. Malseed RT and others: *Pharmacology,* ed 4, Philadelphia, 1995, JB Lippincott.
10. Halperin JA and others, editors: *USP DI* ed 15, Rockville, Md, 1995, United States Pharmacopoeia.
11. Harris MI: Summary. In Harris MI and others, editors: *Diabetes in America,* National Diabetes Data Group, ed 2, NIH Publication, No. 95-1468, Washington, DC, 1995, National Institutes of Health, National Institutes of Diabetes and Digestive and Kidney Diseases.
12. Kitabchi AE, Fisher JN: Ketoacidosis and the hyperosmolar hyperglycemic non ketotic state. In Kahn C, Weir G, editors: *Joslins' diabetes mellitus,* ed 13, Philadelphia, 1994, Lea & Febiger.
13. Isselbacher KJ and others, editors: *Harrison's principles of internal medicine,* ed 13, New York, 1994, McGraw-Hill.
14. Karam JH, Forsham PH: Pancreatic hormones and diabetes mellitus. In Greenspan FS, Baxter JD, editors: *Basic and clinical endocrinology,* ed 4, Norwalk, Conn, 1994, Appleton & Lange.
15. Bhasin S, Tom L: Endocrine problems in the critically ill patient. In Bongard FS, Sue DY, editors: *Current critical care: diagnosis and treatment,* Norwalk, Conn, 1994, Appleton & Lange.
16. Ipp E: Diabetes mellitus and the critically ill patient. In Bongard FS, Sue DY, editors: *Current critical care: diagnosis and treatment,* Norwalk, Conn, 1994, Appleton & Lang.
17. Rudy DR, Tzagournis M: Endocrinology. In Rakel RE, eidtor: *Textbook of family practice,* ed 5, Philadelphia, 1995, WB Saunders.
18. Becker KL, editor: *Principles and practice of endocrinology and metabolism,* ed 2, Philadelphia, 1995, JB Lippincott.
19. Tierney LM, McPhee SJ, Papadakis MA, editors: *Current medical diagnosis and treatment,* Stamford, Conn, 1996, Appleton & Lange.
20. Shoemaker WC and others, editors: *Textbook of critical care,* ed 3, Philadelphia, 1995, WB Saunders.
21. Wannamethee SG, Perry IJ, Shaper AG: Hematocrit and risk of non insulin dependent diabetes mellitus, *Diabetes* 45:576-579, 1996.
22. Jones TL: From diabetic ketoacidosis to hyperglycemic hyperosmolar non ketotic syndrome, the spectrum of uncontrolled hyperglycemia in diabetes mellitus. In Gould KA, Toto KH, Hotter AN, editors: Endocrine & metabolic disturbances in the critically ill, *Crit Care Nurs Clin North Am* 6(4):703-721, 1994.
23. Genuth S: The endocrine system. In Berne RM, Levy MN, editors: *Physiology,* ed 3, St Louis, 1993, Mosby.
24. O'Donnell C: Patient and family education. In Urden LD, Lough ME, Stacy KM, editors: *Priorities in critical care nursing,* ed 2, St Louis, 1996, Mosby.
25. Bullock B, Rosendahl P: *Pathophysiology: adaptations and alterations in function,* ed 4, Philadelphia, 1996, JB Lippincott.
26. Tyrrell JB, Finding JW, Aron DC: Hypothalamus and pituitary. In Greenspan FS, Baxter JD, editors: *Basic and clinical endocrinology,* ed 4, Norwalk, Conn, 1994, Appleton & Lange.
27. Lubin M and others, editors: *Medical management of the surgical patient,* ed 3, Philadelphia, 1995, JB Lippincott.
28. Szerlip H and others: Sodium and water. In Noe DA, Rock RC, editors: *Laboratory medicine: the selection and interpretation of clinical laboratory studies,* Balitmore, 1994, Williams & Wilkins.
29. Ravel R: *Clinical laboratory medicine, clinical application of laboratory data,* ed 6, St Louis, 1995, Mosby.
30. Fischbach F: *A manual of laboratory and diagnostic tests,* ed 5, Philadelphia, 1996, JB Lippincott
31. Jordan CD and others: Massachusetts General hospital weekly clinical pathological exercises, case records of the Massachusetts General Hospital, Normal reference laboratory values, *N Engl J Med* 327:718-724 (Sept 3), 1992.
32. Chan PD, Winkle CR, Winkle PJ: *Current clinical strategies,* Fountain Valley, Calif, 1995, Current Clinical Strategies Publishing.
33. Guyton AC, Hall JE: *Textbook of medical physiology,* ed 9, Philadelphia, 1996, WB Saunders.
34. Batcheller J: Syndrome of inappropriate antidiuretic hormone secretion. In Gould KA, Toto KH, Hotter, AN, editors: Endocrine and metabolic disturbances in the critically ill, *Crit Care Nurs Clin North Am* 6(4):687-692, 1994.
35. Ganong WF: *Review of medical physiology,* ed 16, Norwalk, Conn, 1995, Appleton & Lange.
36. Talbot L: Physiologic changes. In Hogstel MO, editor: *Nursing care of the older adult,* ed 3, Albany, 1994, Delmar Publishers.
37. Schmitz T and others: A comparison of 5 methods of temperature measurement in febrile intensive care patients, *Am J Crit Care* 4(4):286-292, July 1995.
38. Koziol-McLain, J, Oman K, Edwards G: Ear temperatures: making research based clinical decisions, *J Emerg Nurs* 22(1):77-79, Feb 1996.

39. Porth CM, Hurwitz LS: Alterations in endocrine control of growth and metabolism. In Porth CM, editor: *Pathophysiology: concepts of altered health states,* ed 4, Philadelphia, 1994, JB Lippincott.
40. Davis KD, Lazar MA: Hypothyroidism. In Rakel RE, editor: *Conn's current therapy 1996,* Philadelphia, 1996, WB Saunders.
41. Becker DV and others: Optimal use of blood tests for assessment of thyroid function, (letter), JAMA 269(21):2736-2737, 1993.
42. Wartofsky L: Myxedema coma. In Braverman LE, Utiger RD, editors: *Werner and Ingbar's the thyroid,* ed 7, Philadelphia, 1996, Lippincott-Raven.

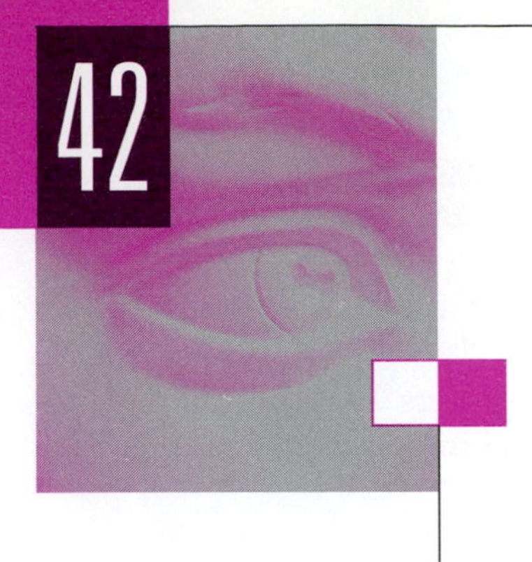

Endocrine Nursing Diagnosis and Management

THIS CHAPTER IS designed to supplement the preceding chapters in the *Endocrine Alterations* unit by integrating theoretic content into clinically applicable case studies and nursing management plans.

The case study is designed to illustrate clinical problem solving and patient care management occurring in actual patients. The case, reviewed retrospectively, demonstrates how medical and nursing diagnoses may be effectively used in critical care. The case study also demonstrates revisions to the plan of care and the nursing and medical management outcomes that are apt to occur during the course of a complicated hospitalization as the patient responds physiologically to treatment. Often in a short case anecdote, such as presented in the chapter, the clinical answer may appear to be obvious from the day of admission. In practice, however, critical care patient management is sometimes investigative and the "correct" diagnosis for an individual patient may not become apparent until midway in the hospitalization. Or a patient with an apparently straightforward diagnosis may develop an unexpected complication, and the plan of care and potential outcomes will then require revision. Many of the case studies demonstrate this principle.

The nursing management plans, which—unlike the case study—are not patient specific, provide a basis nurses can use to individualize care for their patients. In the previous *Endocrine Alterations* chapters, each medical diagnosis is assigned a Nursing Diagnosis and Management box. Using this box as a page guide, the reader can access relevant nursing management plans for each medical diagnosis. For example, nursing management of *hyperglycemic hyperosmotic nonketotic syndrome,* described on p. 1015, may involve several nursing diagnoses and management plans outlined in this chapter and in other Nursing Diagnosis and Management chapters. Specific examples are (1) *Decreased Cardiac Output related to alterations in preload,* on p. 590 and (2) *Anxiety related to threat to biologic, psychologic, and/or social integrity,* on p. 99. These examples highlight the interrelationship of the various physiologic systems in the body and the fact that pathology often has a multisystem impact in the critically ill.

Use of the case study and management plans can enhance the understanding and application of the *Endocrine* content in clinical practice.

CASE STUDY

ENDOCRINE

CLINICAL HISTORY

Ms. B is a 57-year-old woman who has been treated for Type I diabetes mellitus for 30 years. Family members report Ms. B is careful about her diet, checks her blood glucose frequently, and gives herself insulin every day.

CURRENT PROBLEMS

Ms. B has been complaining of flu-like symptoms with nausea, vomiting, and diarrhea for the past 3 days. Her family says that she seemed confused the previous evening and could not recognize her children. This morning the family had difficulty waking her.

Assessment findings included the following: height, 64 inches (5 ft, 4 in); weight, 47 kg (103 lb); mentation, obtunded; temperature (T), 97.2° F; pulse (P), 140; respiratory rate (RR), 40; blood pressure (BP), 80/60 mm Hg; fingerstick glucose, >400. (See Table 42-1, p. 1048, for other laboratory values.) Cardiac S_1 and S_2, within normal limits (WNL); no S_3 or S_4 or murmurs. Kussmaul's respirations; sweet breath odor. Skin was flushed, dry and warm; skin turgor >3 seconds at clavicle. Buccal membranes were dry, lips parched, and tongue furrowed. Bowel sounds were hyperactive; abdomen was soft and tender to touch with guarding behavior. Extremities were without cyanosis or edema. Pedal pulses were equal. Ms B was incontinent of a small amount of dark urine and approximately 50 ml diarrheal stool.

MEDICAL DIAGNOSES

Diabetic ketoacidosis (DKA) precipitated by gastroenteritis

Severe dehydration secondary to hyperosmolar status

NURSING DIAGNOSIS

Fluid Volume Deficit related to absolute loss

PLAN OF CARE

1. Reverse dehydration.
2. Restore insulin-glucagon ratio.
3. Treat and prevent circulatory collapse.
4. Replenish electrolytes.
5. Identify precipitating cause to prevent DKA from recurring.

MEDICAL AND NURSING MANAGEMENT AND PATIENT OUTCOME

Ms. B began receiving an intravenous infusion of 1000 ml 0.9% sodium chloride with 30 mEq potassium chloride per hour. A bolus of 14 units of human regular insulin was started intravenously (0.3 U/kg), and regular insulin was to be added to the primary container to deliver 5 U of human regular insulin per hour (0.1 U/kg). Ms. B was placed on NPO status and was given oxygen at 2 L/min per nasal cannula. Cardiac monitoring was initiated and revealed tachycardia. An indwelling catheter was inserted into the urinary bladder, and 600 ml of dark, concentrated urine was obtained. The intravenous solution was monitored by an electronic infusion pump to assure accuracy. As a precaution, containers of 5% dextrose and 50% dextrose intravenous solutions were available for immediate use should Ms. B's serum glucose level fall too rapidly and signs of hypoglycemia manifest. Ms. B required increased stimulation to evoke a response and was placed on her side in a low Fowler's position. Bedside fingerstick glucose tests were done every 30 minutes for the first 2 hours. Vital signs were taken every 15 minutes, at which time Ms. B's position in bed was slightly realigned to reduce pressure on the compromised skin tissues. (See Table 42-1, p. 1048, for other laboratory values.)

Kussmaul's respirations and fruity breath odor were assessed. Vital signs, especially BP, pulse characteristics, and hemodynamic findings, were monitored to assess for cardiac response to the rapid fluid replacement. Urine output was monitored hourly. Ms. B was assessed for circulatory overload, which could occur from such rapid rehydration; she was monitored for neck vein engorgement, sudden unexplained dyspnea, elevated central venous pressure and/or elevated pulmonary artery pressures, and moist lung sounds. Hydration assessment included temperature, skin moisture, and skin turgor.

CASE STUDY—CONT'D

ENDOCRINE

Ms. B's oral assessment and care included moist gauze pads to keep the oral membranes moistened and to prevent build-up of bacteria in the mouth. Her neurologic status was monitored and documented every 15 minutes for the first hour to determine the effects of the hyponatremia (because of osmotic diuresis) on the central nervous system. Nurses continually evaluated the extent of Ms. B's impaired thinking. Short words and sentences were used to give simple directions and provide reorientation to her immediate hospital surroundings.

During the first 2 hours, Ms. B showed dramatic improvement. The vigorous fluid replacement reversed the hypovolemia and diluted the relative blood osmolality. The continuous low-dose insulin therapy was used to transfer glucose from the blood stream to the cell receptor site, which reduced the need for fats to be broken down for energy. Respirations became easier because there was less carbonic acid in the blood stream to be blown off in the form of CO_2. In addition, a decrease in Kussmaul's respirations contributed to conservation of body fluid because less water was lost with each exhalation. Ms. B became more responsive and aware of her surroundings. Her level of consciousness was upgraded to lethargic. (See Table 42-1, p. 1048, for other laboratory values.)

She was no longer incontinent of stool, and bowel sounds returned to normal. Urine became more dilute. Serum sodium increased to 134 mEq/L, and blood pressure was 102/65. The intravenous solution was changed to 0.45% NaCl, and the flow rate was reduced to 500 ml/hr (1500 ml of NaCl had been absorbed at that time). The bicarbonate ion was reversing itself, and subsequently a rise in pH occurred as a result of adequate fluid and insulin therapy. Bicarbonate therapy was not required. Blood glucose levels were decreasing gradually because of the low-dose insulin replacement and because no signs of hypoglycemia were present. As the patient's level of consciousness improved and she had no difficulty swallowing, Ms. B was able to rinse her mouth for comfort. As the nausea subsided, the NPO order was changed and Ms. B took sips of water, which gradually supplemented the IV replacement fluids.

At 11 AM the fingerstick glucose level was 272 mg. According to the prescribed orders the IV solution was changed from 0.45% NaCl to 5% dextrose in 0.45% NaCl. The 30 mEq of KCl was added to the IV container, along with insulin to provide 5 U/hr. This change was made to prevent the glucose level from rapidly decreasing and precipitating hypoglycemia. The rate was set at 250 ml/hr. (See Table 42-1, p. 1048, for other laboratory values.)

At 12:30 PM Ms. B was alert and freely taking fluids by mouth. The serum glucose laboratory value was 226 mg/dL. At this time the IV insulin was no longer needed. BP was 129/70 mm Hg and indicated that subcutaneous insulin could be absorbed and distributed throughout the body. Human regular insulin, 5 U, was given subcutaneously. Ms. B was moving around in bed and asking if she could get up to go to the bathroom. (See Table 42-1, p. 1048, for other laboratory values.)

The remainder of Ms. B's clinical stay was uneventful. Once she was adequately hydrated and the blood osmolality returned to normal, the serum glucose levels returned to their pre-DKA status and were adequately controlled with subcutaneous injections of insulin. The blood pH continued a gradual rise to normal levels through fluid and insulin correction and without bicarbonate therapy. Postassium levels stayed within the normal range. Ms. B received discharge teaching to prevent this situation from recurring should she develop influenza or gastroenteritis again. It was recommended that she receive the influenza virus vaccine each season to minimize the course of the disease whenever she was exposed to the virus. Family members were included in the sessions, which included discussion of management of insulin doses when nausea is present and food cannot be consumed. In addition, the teaching plan for Ms. B and her family members included review of physical and emotional changes indicative of fluctuating glucose levels. Nursing instructions emphasized changes that must be brought to the attention of the health care practitioner, as well as steps that should be taken to avoid serious hyperglycemic or hypoglycemic complications.

TABLE 42-1 Ms. B's Laboratory Data

	8 AM	9 AM	10 AM	11 AM	11:30 AM	12:30 PM	1:30 PM
Mentation	Obtunded	Obtunded	Lethargic	Lethargic	Alert	Alert	Alert
Temperature (°F)	97.2	97.2	97.3	97.6	97.8	97.9	98.3
Pulse (/min)	140	140	138	128	123	120	113
Respiration (/min)	40	39	35	34	33	31	31
BP (mm Hg)	80/60	92/62	102/65	120/68	126/70	129/70	133/71
Urine ketones	4+	4+	4+	4+	3+	3+	2+
Plasma glucose (mg/dL)	460	350	290	272	250	226	200
Sodium (mEq/L)	129	133	134	135	136	136	138
Potassium (mEq/L)	4.5	4.3	4.1	3.9	3.9	3.8	3.7
Chloride (mEq/L)	96	98	99	99	100	100	101
Bicarbonate (mEq/L)	7.5	9.0	10.4	11.8	12.5	13.2	15
BUN (mEq/L)	34	32	31	30	29	29	28
Plasma ketones	4+	4+	4+	4+	4+	4+	4+
Pao_2 (mm Hg)	100	100	100	100	100	100	100
$Paco_2$ (mm Hg)	20	19.3	18.9	18.5	18.4	18.3	18.1
pH	7.19	7.23	7.26	7.29	7.3	7.31	7.33
Hgb (g/dL)	20	19.3	18.9	18.5	18.4	18.3	18.1
Hct (%/ml^3)	55.9	54.3	53.4	52.5	52.3	52.1	51.5
WBC (thousand/ml^3)	10.4	10.4	10.4	10.4	10.4	10.4	10.4

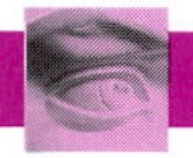

NURSING MANAGEMENT PLAN

FLUID VOLUME EXCESS

DEFINITION:

The state in which an individual experiences increased fluid retention and edema.

Fluid Volume Excess Related to Increased Secretion of ADH

DEFINING CHARACTERISTICS

- Weight gain *without* edema
- Hyponatremia (dilutional)
- Decreased urinary output
  Urinary osmolality above normal, exceeding plasma osmolality
- Urinary specific gravity >1.030
- Evidence of water intoxication:
  - Fatigue
  - Headache
  - Abdominal cramps
  - Altered level of consciousness
  - Diarrhea
  - Seizures

OUTCOME CRITERIA

- Weight returns to baseline.
- Serum sodium is 135-145 mEq/L.
- Urinary output is >30 ml/hr.
- Urinary osmolality is 200-800 mOsm/kg.
- Urinary specific gravity is 1.005-1.030.
- Patient has no evidence of water intoxication.

NURSING INTERVENTIONS AND *RATIONALE*

1. Monitor the assessment parameters listed under "Defining Characteristics." In addition, monitor patient closely for evidence of cardiac decompensation caused by excessive preload (i.e., elevated pulmonary artery diastolic pressure [PADP] or pulmonary artery wedge pressure [PAWP], tachycardia, lung congestion).
2. Anticipate administration of demeclocycline, lithium carbonate, furosemide, and/or narcotic agonists.
3. With physician's collaboration, administer intravenous hypertonic sodium chloride ***to temporarily correct hyponatremia.***
4. Weigh patient daily at same time in same clothing, pereferably with same scale.
5. Maintain fluid restriction.
6. Monitor hydration status.
7. Initiate seizure precautions ***because severe sodium deficit can result in seizures.***

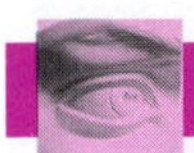

NURSING MANAGEMENT PLAN

FLUID VOLUME DEFICIT

DEFINITION:
The state in which an individual experiences vascular, cellular, or intracellular dehydration.

Fluid Volume Deficit Related to Decreased Secretion of ADH

DEFINING CHARACTERISTICS

- Polyuria (15 L/day)
- Serum sodium 145 mEq/L (particularly in patients who are not drinking to replace losses)
- Intense thirst
- Polydipsia (alert patients)
- Urinary specific gravity <1.005
- Urinary osmolality <300 mOsm/kg
- Plasma osmolality >300 mOsm/kg

OUTCOME CRITERIA

- Urinary volume, specific gravity, and osmolality are normal.
- Thirst is reduced.
- Plasma osmolality and serum sodium level are normal.

NURSING INTERVENTIONS AND *RATIONALE*

1. Monitor the assessment parameters listed under "Defining Characteristics." Additionally, monitor for signs of critical volume deficits (i.e., hypotension, fall in pulmonary artery pressures, tachycardia).
2. With physician's collaboration, administer intravenous electrolyte replacement solutions ***because critical electrolyte loss occurs along with water loss.*** Replace losses milliliter for milliliter plus 50 ml/hr for insensible losses. Avoid replacement of losses with intravenous dextrose solutions ***because of the risk of water intoxication.***
3. If patient is alert, encourage the patient to satisfy partially his or her replacement needs by drinking according to thirst. Caution should be observed regarding the patient's excessive ingestion of water (typically, the patient will crave iced water) ***because of the risk of water intoxication.***
4. With physician's collaboration, administer vasopressin intravenously, intramuscularly, or per the nasal route.
5. For patients after hypophysectomy, teach the administration of vasopressin and its reportable side and toxic effects, the monitoring of intake and output measurement, and the documentation of daily weights.

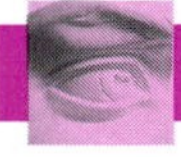

NURSING MANAGEMENT PLAN

HYPERTHERMIA

DEFINITION:
A state in which an individual's body temperature is elevated above his or her normal range.

Hyperthermia Related to Increased Thyroid Hormone

DEFINING CHARACTERISTICS

- Diaphoresis
- Hot, flushed skin
- Intolerance to heat
- Tachycardia
- Tachypnea

OUTCOME CRITERIA

- Temperature is normal.
- Heart rate is <100 beats/min.
- Respiratory effort is normal.
- Skin is warm, dry.

NURSING INTERVENTIONS AND *RATIONALE*

1. Assess temperature q 15 min
   - Obtain temperature via pulmonary arterial line
2. Provide a room with a cool environment, including the following:
   - Fan to circulate air
   - Lightweight bed coverings
   - Comfortable, nonrestrictive bed clothes
   - Tepid sponge bath to reduce heat by evaporation
   - Ice application to groin and axilla to increase heat loss at major blood vessels through conduction

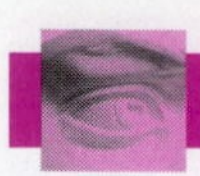

NURSING MANAGEMENT PLAN

HYPOTHERMIA

DEFINITION:

The state in which an individual's body temperature is reduced below normal range.

Hypothermia Related to Decreased Thyroid Hormone

DEFINING CHARACTERISTICS

- Complaints of "inability to stay warm": temperature between 80° F and 95° F
- Skin dry, cool to touch

OUTCOME CRITERIA

- Temperature is normal.
- Skin is warm and dry.

NURSING INTERVENTIONS AND *RATIONALE*

1. Warm blankets wrapped loosely around the patient—***passive rewarming is used to minimize heat loss; avoid rapid rewarming.***
2. Loosen clothing to ***avoid further vasodilation leading to hypotension and shock.***

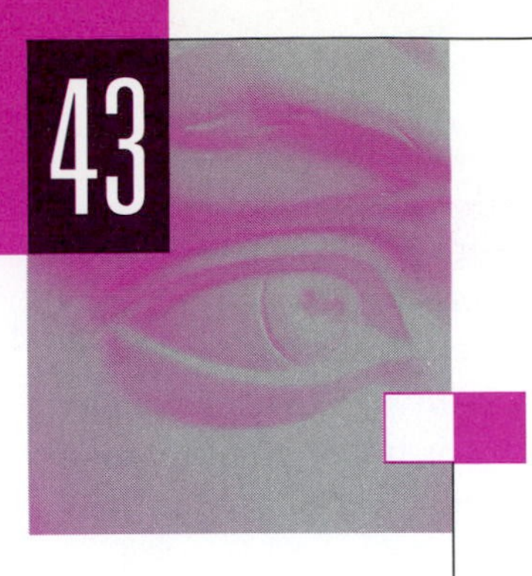

Trauma

TRAUMA IS A "neglected disease" in America. Traumatic injuries affect more than 50 million persons in the United States per year.[1] Trauma is the leading cause of death in the first four decades of life (ages 1 through 44 years).[2] Trauma is one of America's most expensive health problems. The cost to society, because of hospitalization and lost productivity, approaches $100 billion annually,[3] which represents approximately 40% of the health care dollars spent.[4] With these staggering costs, it is alarming that less than 4 cents of each federal research dollar is expended on trauma research.[4]

Injury as a result of trauma is no longer considered to be an "accident." The term *motor vehicle accident (MVA)* has been replaced with *motor vehicle crash (MVC),* and the term *accident* has been replaced with *unintentional injury.* Unintentional injury is no accident. Accident traditionally has implied an occurrence that is out of one's control;[5] however, unintentional injuries are occurrences related to risk-taking behaviors, actions, and decisions that usually involve alcohol.[2]

Over the past few decades major advances have been made in the management of patients with traumatic injuries, and significant improvements have been made in their care in both prehospital and emergency department settings. These improvements have affected critical care in that patients with complex, multisystem trauma are admitted to critical care units. These patients require complex nursing care. This chapter reviews nursing management of patients with traumatic injuries, particularly in the critical care setting.

MECHANISMS OF INJURY

Trauma occurs when an external force of energy impacts the body and causes structural or physiologic alterations, or "injuries." External forces can be radiation, electrical, thermal, chemical, or mechanical forms of energy. This chapter focuses on trauma from mechanical energy. Mechanical energy can produce either blunt or penetrating traumatic injuries. Knowledge of the mechanism of injury helps health care providers anticipate and predict potential internal injuries.

Blunt Trauma

Blunt trauma most often is seen with MVCs, contact sports, crush injuries, or falls. Injuries occur because of the forces sustained during a rapid change in velocity (deceleration). To estimate the amount of force a person would sustain in an MVC, multiply the person's weight by miles per hour of speed the vehicle was traveling.[6] A 130-pound woman in a vehicle traveling at 60 miles per hour that hits a brick wall, for example, would sustain 7800 pounds of force within milliseconds. As the body stops suddenly, tissues and organs continue to move forward. This sudden change in velocity causes injuries that result in lacerations or crush injuries of internal body structures.

Penetrating Trauma

Penetrating injuries occur with stabbings, firearms, or impalement of foreign objects, which penetrate the skin, with resultant damage to internal structures. Damage is created along the path of penetration. Penetrating injuries can be misleading inasmuch as the outside of the wound does not determine the extent of internal injury. Bullets can create internal cavities 5 to 30 times larger than the diameter of the bullet.[4]

Several factors determine the extent of damage sustained as a result of penetrating trauma. Different weapons cause different types of injuries. The severity of a gunshot wound depends on the type of gun, type of ammunition used, and the distance and angle from which the gun was fired. Pellets from a shotgun blast expand on impact and cause multiple injuries to internal structures. Handgun bullets, on the other hand, usually damage what is directly in the bullet's path. Once inside the body, the bullet can ricochet off bone and create further damage along its pathway. With penetrating stab wounds, factors that determine the extent of injury include type and length of object used, as well as the angle of insertion.

PHASES OF TRAUMA CARE

Care of trauma victims during wartime enhanced principles of triage and rapid transport of the injured to medical facilities.[7] The military experience has demonstrated that more lives can be saved by decreasing the time from injury to definitive care. It also has enhanced incentives and models for improvements in civilian trauma care, such as emergency medical service (EMS) systems and trauma care centers. The goal with critically injured patients is to minimize the time from initial insult to definitive care and to optimize prehospital care so that the patient arrives at the hospital alive.

Statistics demonstrate that deaths as a result of trauma occur in a trimodal distribution[4] (Figure 43-1). The first peak includes victims who die before medical attention can be provided. The second peak occurs within a few hours after injury. It is this peak that commonly is referred to as the *golden hour* for those critically injured. The golden hour is a 60-minute time frame that incorporates activation of the EMS system, stabilization in the prehospital setting, transportation to a medical facility, rapid resuscitation on arrival in the emergency department, and the provision of definitive care. Chance of survival increases if all these measures can be completed within the first hour after injury.[3] The third death peak occurs days to weeks after injury as a result of complications, including infection or multiple organ dysfunction syndrome. It is a nursing challenge to influence the quality of care the trauma patient receives in an attempt to "beat" the trimodal distribution of trauma deaths.

Nursing management of the patient with traumatic injuries begins the moment a call for help is received and continues until the patient's death or return to the community.[8] Care of the trauma patient is seen as a continuum that includes six phases: prehospital, hospital resuscitation, definitive care and operative phase, critical care, intermediate care, and rehabilitation.

Prehospital Resuscitation

The goal of prehospital care is immediate stabilization and transportation. Stabilization is accomplished through assessments and interventions related to airway, breathing, and circulation (ABCs). Once stabilized at the scene, the patient is transported to an appropriate medical facility by ground or air transport.

Emergency Department Resuscitation

The American College of Surgeons developed guidelines (Advanced Trauma Life Support [ATLS]) for rapid assessment, resuscitation, and definitive care for trauma patients in the emergency department.[4] A similar nursing model (Trauma Nurse Core Course [TNCC]) was developed by the Emergency Nurses' Association.[9] Both programs emphasize the need for a systematic approach to care of the trauma patient in the emergency department: primary survey, secondary survey to be conducted simultaneously with resuscitation, and definitive management.

Primary survey. On arrival of the trauma patient in the emergency department, the primary survey is initiated. During this assessment, life-threatening injuries are discovered and treated. The five steps in the primary survey comprise the ABCs, plus D and E—*D*, disability (mini-neurologic examination) and *E*, exposure (undress, with temperature control) (Table 43-1).

Airway. Airway is assessed for ineffective airway clearance and airway obstruction. The trauma patient is at risk for ineffective airway clearance, especially in the presence of altered consciousness, drugs and alcohol, and thoracic injuries.[4] Airway obstruction can be caused by foreign bodies, blood clots, or broken teeth. Airway assessment must incorporate cervical spine immobilization by either manual cervical immobilization or placement of a rigid cervical collar, with the head, neck, and body strapped to a spine board or stretcher. The cervical spine must be immobilized in all trauma patients until a cervical spinal cord injury has been definitively ruled out. If the airway is obstructed, foreign bodies are removed. In the presence of ineffective airway clearance, the airway is secured through intubation or cricothyrotomy.

Breathing. The patient is assessed for ineffective breathing patterns and impaired gas exchange. It is crucial to remember that an open, clear airway does not ensure adequate ventilation and gas exchange. Assessment includes chest wall integrity and respiratory rate, depth, and symmetry. Supplemental oxygen is used in all trauma patients.[4] Decreased breath sounds or alteration in chest wall integrity necessitate chest tube placement. Mechanical ventilation is used for

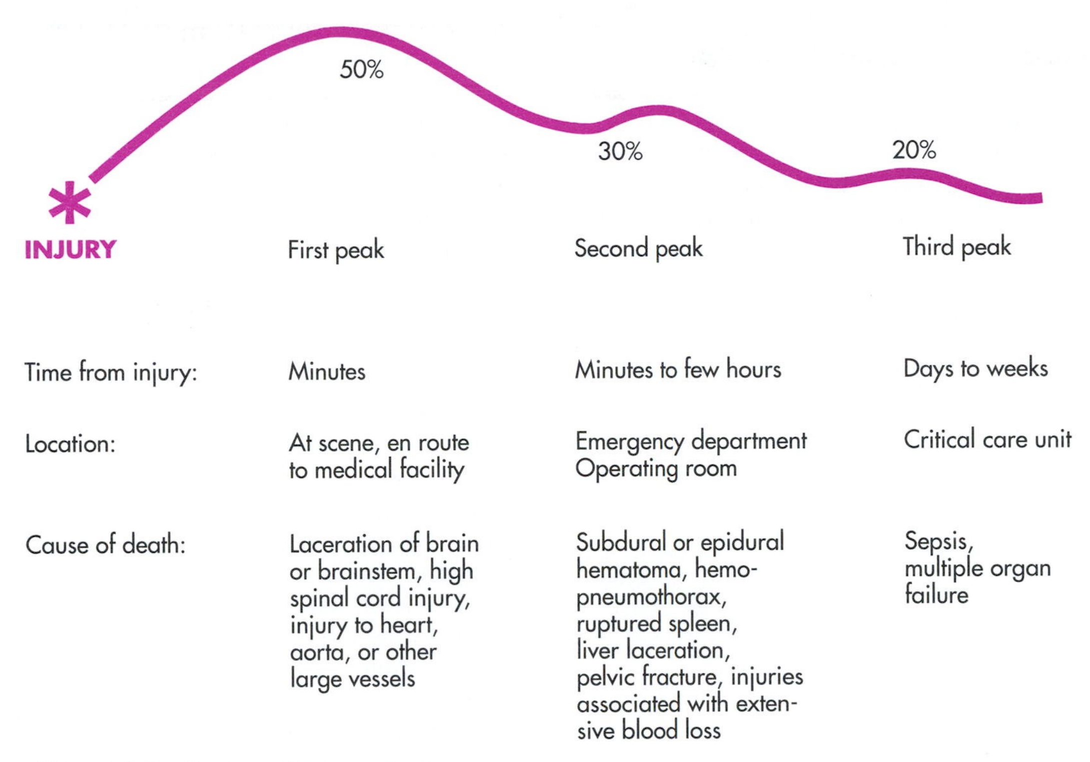

50%
30%
20%
INJURY
First peak
Second peak
Third peak
Time from injury:
Minutes
Minutes to few hours
Days to weeks
Location:
At scene, en route to medical facility
Emergency department
Operating room
Critical care unit
Cause of death:
Laceration of brain or brainstem, high spinal cord injury, injury to heart, aorta, or other large vessels
Subdural or epidural hematoma, hemo-pneumothorax, ruptured spleen, liver laceration, pelvic fracture, injuries associated with extensive blood loss
Sepsis, multiple organ failure

FIGURE 43-1. Trimodal distribution of trauma deaths.

patients with a loss of consciousness or ineffective breathing patterns, or both.

Circulation. After effective airway clearance, breathing patterns, and gas exchange have been ensured, the nurse assesses for alteration in cardiac output, alteration in tissue perfusion, and fluid volume deficit. External exsanguination is identified and controlled. Rapid assessment of the circulatory status includes assessment of level of consciousness, skin color, and pulse. Level of consciousness provides data on cerebral perfusion. Assessment of skin color can provide information about the patient's circulatory volume. Ominous signs of hypovolemia include ashen, gray, or white skin. Systemic blood pressure can be rapidly evaluated by use of the 60-70-80 method.[9] If a carotid pulse is palpable, the minimal systolic pressure is estimated to be 60 mm Hg. A palpable femoral pulse can represent a systolic pressure of 70 mm Hg, and a palpable radial pulse can represent a systolic pressure of 80 mm Hg. If a pulse is not present, advanced cardiac life support (ACLS) protocols are instituted (see Appendix C). Cardiac monitoring is initiated to assess for rhythm disturbances. Life-threatening dysrhythmias are treated according to ACLS protocols. Military antishock trousers (MAST) or a pneumatic antishock garment (PASG) may be used to raise the blood pressure; however, the use of these devices to increase blood pressure is controversial. Both devices encompass the lower extremities and the abdomen. When inflated, these garments increase systolic blood pressure by increasing peripheral vascular resistance and myocardial afterload.

Disability. Once airway, breathing, and circulation have been effectively managed, the nurse begins the fourth step of the primary survey: disability, *D*. During this step the nurse assesses the potential for injury by completing a brief neurologic assessment to establish the patient's level of consciousness and pupillary size and reaction. The AVPU method describes the patient's level of consciousness: *A*, *a*lert; *V*, responds to *v*erbal stimuli; *P*, responds to *p*ainful stimuli; and *U*, *u*nresponsive. A more detailed neurologic assessment is made during the secondary survey, discussed later.

Exposure. The final step in the primary survey is *E*, *e*xposure. All clothing is removed to facilitate a thorough examination of all body surfaces for the presence of injury. After all clothing is removed, it is imperative to cover and protect the patient from becoming hypothermic.

Resuscitation phase. After the primary survey the resuscitation phase begins. Hypovolemic shock is the most common type of shock that occurs in trauma patients.[4] Hemorrhage must be identified and treated rapidly. Vigorous intravenous (IV) fluid replacement

TABLE 43-1 **Primary Survey of the Trauma Patient**

Survey Component	Nursing Diagnosis	Nursing Assessment/Care
Airway	Airway clearance: Ineffective related to obstruction or actual injury	Look, listen, and feel Immobilize C-spine Position victim/patient: Supine Sitting Log roll Clear airway: Jaw thrust Chin lift Finger sweep Suctioning Airway devices: Oropharyngeal Nasopharynegeal Endotracheal tube Cricothyrotomy
Breathing	Breathing pattern: Ineffective related to actual injury Gas exchange: Impaired related to Actual injury or disrupted tissue perfusion	Assess for: Spontaneous breathing Respiratory rate, depth, and symmetry Chest wall integrity Administer high-glow oxygen Absent breathing: Intubate Positive-pressure ventilation Breathing but in effective: Assess and treat life-threatening conditions (e.g., tension pneumothorax, flail chest)
Circulation	Cardiac output, alteration in: Decreased related to actual injury Tissue perfusion, alteration in: Related to actual injury or shock Fluid volume deficit: Related to actual loss of circulating volume	Assess pulse: Quality Rate No pulse: Initiate BCLS Initiate ACLS Pulse but ineffective: Assess and treat life-threatening conditions (e.g., uncontrolled bleeding, shock) Two large-bore (14- or 16-gauge) IV catheters Fluid replacement ECG monitoring
Disability	Injury potential for: Trauma, spinal cord, and brain related to actual injury	Brief neurologic examination Eye opening Verbal response Motor response Pupils AVPU Glasgow Coma Scale
Exposure	N/A	To visualize the entire body for inspection, all clothing must be removed.

From Beaver BM: *Nurs Clin North Am* 25(1), 1990.

NURSING INTERVENTION CLASSIFICATIONS

BOX 43-1 Fluid Resuscitation

DEFINITION: Administering prescribed intravenous fluids rapidly

ACTIVITIES:
Obtain and maintain a large-bore IV
Collaborate with physicians to ensure administration of both crystalloids (e.g., normal saline and lactated Ringer's) and colloids (e.g., Hesban and Plasmanate), as appropriate
Administer IV fluids, as prescribed
Obtain blood specimens for crossmatching, as appropriate
Administer blood products, as prescribed
Monitor hemodynamic response
Monitor oxygen status
Monitor for fluid overload
Monitor output of various body fluids (e.g., urine, nasogastric drainage, and chest tube)
Monitor BUN, creatinine, total protein, and albumin levels
Monitor for pulmonary edema and third spacing

From McCloskey JC, Bulechek GM: *Nursing interventions classification,* ed 2, St Louis, 1996, Mosby.

is initiated (Box 43-1). Large-bore peripheral IV catheters (14 to 16 gauge) or a central venous catheter are inserted. Restoration of volume is accomplished through administration of crystalloid (lactated Ringer's solution, colloid (plasma or albumin), and/or blood products. During the initiation of IV lines, blood samples are drawn (Box 43-2). High-flow fluid warmers may be used to deliver warmed IV solutions at rates greater than 1000 ml/minute. If the patient remains unresponsive to bolus intravenous therapy, type-specific blood or O-negative blood may be administered.[4] Transfusion of autologous salvaged blood (autotransfusion) also may be used to replace intravascular volume and to provide oxygen-carrying capacity.

Gastric and urinary catheters are placed, unless contraindicated. Adequate resuscitation is assessed by monitoring for improvement in vital signs (including body temperature), arterial blood gas levels, and urinary output.

Secondary survey. The secondary survey begins when the primary survey is completed, resuscitation initiated, and the patient's ABCs are reassessed.[4] During the secondary survey each body region is thoroughly examined. The history is one of the most important aspects of the secondary survey. Often, head injury, shock, or the use of drugs or alcohol may preclude a good history, so the history must be pieced together from other sources. The prehospital providers (paramedics, emergency medical technicians [EMTs]) usually can provide most of the vital information pertaining to the accident. Specific information that must be elicited pertaining to the mechanism of injury is summarized in Box 43-3. This information can help predict internal injuries and facilitate rapid intervention. The patient's pertinent past history can be assessed by use of the mnemonic AMPLE: *a*llergies, *m*edications, *p*ast medical illnesses, *l*ast meal, and *e*vents immediately preceding the incident/environment related to the injury.

BOX 43-2 Serum Samples for Laboratory Studies to Obtain With IV Placement

Complete blood cell (CBC) count with differential
Electrolyte profile: sodium, potassium, chloride, carbon dioxide, glucose, urea, nitrogen, and creatinine
Coagulation parameters: prothrombin time (PT); partial thromboplastin time (PTT)
Type and screen (ABO compatibility)
Amylase
Ethanol
Liver function study (alanine aminotransferase—formerly SGPT)
Arterial blood gas (ABG)
Pregnancy test (for females of childbearing age)

During the secondary survey, the nurse ensures the completion of special procedures, such as an electrocardiogram (ECG); radiographic studies (chest, cervical spine, thorax, and pelvis); and peritoneal lavage. Throughout this survey the nurse continuously monitors the patient's vital signs and response to medical

BOX 43-3 History of Mechanism of Injury

PENETRATING TRAUMA

- Weapon used (handgun, shotgun, rifle, knife)
- Caliber of weapon
- Number of shots fired
- Gender of assailant
- Position of victim and assailant when injury occurred

BLUNT TRAUMA

- Length of fall
- MVC extrication time
- Ejection
- Location in automobile (passenger, driver, front seat, back seat)
- Restraint status (lapbelt, shoulder harness, or combination; unrestrained)
- Speed of automobile(s)/direction of impact
- Occupants (number and morbidity status)

BOX 43-4 Nursing Report From Referring Area

- Name
- Age
- Mechanism of injury/injuries sustained
- Diagnostic tests completed and results
- Any loss of consciousness and its duration
- Current Glasgow Coma Scale score
- Allergies
- Surgical procedures performed
- Established airway/mechanical ventilation settings
- Vital signs
- Serum laboratory tests (including blood alchohol and toxicology screen)
- IV access (field versus ED placement)
- Fluid replacement (colloid and crystalloid)
- Fluid loss (urine output, chest tube drainage, estimated intraoperative blood loss)
- Invasive hemodynamic values (if in place)
- Medications administered
- Past medical/surgical history
- Family members present, assessment of coping, assessment of knowledge of nature of injuries and treatment plan

Modified from Johnson KL: Critical care of the trauma patient. In Neff JA, Kidd PS, editors: *Trauma nursing: the art and science,* St Louis, 1993, Mosby.

therapies. Emotional support to the patient and family also is imperative.

Definitive Care/Operative Phase

Once the secondary survey has been completed, specific injuries usually have been diagnosed. Definitive care related to specific injuries is described throughout this chapter. Trauma, often referred to as a *surgical disease* because of the nature and extent of the injuries, usually requires operative management of injuries. After surgery, depending on the patient's status, a transfer to the critical care unit may be indicated.

Critical Care Phase

Critically ill trauma patients are admitted into the critical care unit (CCU) as direct transfers from the emergency department (ED) or operating room (OR). If surgery is required, the trauma patient is directly admitted to the CCU from the OR.[10,11]

Information the CCU nurse must obtain from the ED or OR nurse, or both, is summarized in Box 43-4. This information must be obtained before patient admission to the CCU to ensure availability of needed personnel, equipment, and supplies. This information also helps the CCU nurse to assess the impact of trauma resuscitation on the patient's CCU presentation and course. Box 43-5 summarizes the prehospital, ED, and OR resuscitative measures that can affect the trauma patient's care in the CCU.[12] Severe blood loss, circulatory dysfunction, and massive infusion of crystalloids or blood/blood products (greater than 10 units of whole blood or packed red blood cells or replacement of the patient's total blood volume in less than 24 hours) are associated with physiologic sequelae that present a multitude of problems for the trauma patient in the CCU. Massive volumes of fluid administration, such as required by trauma patients with major hemorrhage, are associated with hypothermia, coagulopathy, and metabolic acidosis.[13]

On the patient's arrival to the CCU, the nurse, using the primary and secondary surveys and resuscitative measures in accordance with ATLS and TNCC guidelines, assesses the trauma patient's status. The primary and secondary surveys of trauma assessment offer the critical care nurse a systematic method of assessing trauma patients for injuries and for the development of potential complications.[5] Priority nursing care during the critical care phase includes ongoing physical assessments and monitoring the patient's response to medical therapies. The CCU nurse constantly is aware that the third peak of the trimodal dis-

BOX 43-5 Aspects of Trauma Resuscitation That Affect the Patient's CCU Presentation and CCU Course

- Prolonged extrication time (gives an indication of the length of time the patient may have been hypotensive before medical care)
- Period of respiratory or cardiac arrest with a total loss of tissue perfusion
- Length of time the patient was hypotensive or hypovolemic
- Length of time the patient was hypothermic
- Blood loss and/or massive fluid resuscitation resulting in a low hematocrit value
- Time on the backboard, which potentiates the risk of sacral and occipital breakdown
- Number of units of blood received (gives an indication of the potential for development of acute respiratory distress syndrome [ARDS])

Modified from Johnson KL: Critical care of the trauma patient. In Neff JA, Kidd PS, editors: *Trauma nursing: the art and science,* St Louis, 1993, Mosby.

tribution of trauma deaths occurs in the CCU setting as a result of complications, including acute respiratory distress syndrome (ARDS), sepsis, prolonged shock states, and multiple organ dysfunction syndrome. Ongoing nursing assessments are imperative for early detection of complications.

One of the most important nursing roles is assessment of the balance between oxygen delivery and oxygen demand. Oxygen delivery must be optimized to prevent further system damage. Assessment of circulatory status includes the use of noninvasive and invasive techniques. (∞Cardiovascular Clinical Assessment, p. 355.)

Tissue hypoxemia, which is a threat to the trauma patient, results from a variety of factors. Box 43-6 lists these factors, as summarized by Von Reuden.[14] Prevention and treatment of hypoxemia depend on accurate assessment of the adequacy of pulmonary gas exchange, oxygen transport, and cellular oxygen utilization. The use of supranormal levels of oxygen delivery ($\geq$600 ml/min/m^2) may increase survival after shock in trauma patients.[15] This practice is based on the belief that physiologic shock perpetuates an oxygen debt that increases oxygen needs after a traumatic event.[16]

Frequent and thorough nursing assessments of all body systems are important because these assessments are the cornerstone to the management of the critically ill trauma patient. The nurse can detect subtle changes and facilitate the implementation of timely therapeutic interventions to prevent complications frequently associated with trauma. Interventions that increase oxygen delivery and decrease oxygen consumption are essential. The nurse must be knowledgeable about specific organ injuries, as well as their associated sequelae.

SPECIFIC TRAUMA INJURIES

Head Injuries

At least 2 million persons incur head injuries each year in the United States, and more than 400,000 patients with head injuries are admitted to hospitals, approximately half of whom were involved in motor vehicle crashes.[17] Approximately 50% of all trauma deaths are associated with head injury, and more than 60% of all vehicular trauma deaths are a result of head injury.[4]

Mechanism of Injury

Head injuries occur when mechanical forces are transmitted to brain tissue. Mechanisms of injury include penetrating or blunt trauma to the head. Penetrating trauma can result from the penetration of a foreign object (e.g., bullet) that causes direct damage to cerebral tissue. Blunt trauma can be the result of deceleration, acceleration, or rotational forces. Deceleration causes the brain to crash against the skull after it has hit something (e.g., the dashboard of a car). Acceleration injuries occur when the brain has been hit by something (e.g., a baseball bat). In many instances, head injury can be caused by both acceleration and deceleration. Acceleration injuries occur when the skull is hit by a force that causes the brain to move forward to the point of impact, and then as the brain reverses direction and hits the other side of the skull, deceleration injuries occur.

Pathophysiology

Review of the pathophysiology of head injury can be divided into two categories: primary injury (that which occurs on impact) and secondary injury (that which occurs as a result of the original trauma). It is important that the critical care nurse understands this pathophysiology, because the goals of CCU care are to support the patient to allow maximum recovery from the primary brain injury and to reverse/prevent secondary injuries from occurring.[18]

Primary injury. The primary injury occurs at the time of impact as a result of the dynamic forces of acceleration-deceleration or rotation. Primary injuries include

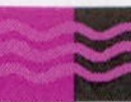

RESEARCH ABSTRACT

Risk factors of adolescent and young adult trauma victims.

Redeker NS and others: *Am J Crit Care* 4(5):370, 1995.

PURPOSE

Despite recent advances in trauma care, little attention has been given to the antecedents and behaviors associated with trauma. Evidence is growing that unintentional and intentional injuries are closely related to risk-taking behaviors and developmental, environmental, social, and psychological variables. Strategies that focus on reducing risk-taking behaviors may decrease repeated trauma. The purpose of this study was to describe demographic, social, environmental, psychological, and developmental antecedents and risk-taking behaviors and to examine their relationships to the types of trauma and rate of trauma recidivism in adolescents and young adults in an urban trauma center.

DESIGN

Qualitative research design using the Trauma Risk Factor Interview Schedule, the Adolescent Risk-Taking Instrument, and the Brief Anger/Aggression Questionnaire.

SAMPLE

The study consisted of 100 adolescent and young adult (ages 15–30 years) trauma patients admitted to the trauma floor of an urban level I trauma center. Subjects were predominantly black (75%) and male (84%). The mean age was 23.4 (SD = 4.0). Of the sample, 57% reported education levels less than 12 years, 25% graduated from high school, and 18% reported 13 or more years of education. The majority of the sample experienced intentional injury: firearm wounds, stab wounds, violent blunt trauma; other causes of trauma were motor vehicle crashes and falls. Twenty-seven had injuries to more than one body part; single injuries were to the abdomen (n = 19), lower extremity (n = 14), and chest (n = 12). Forty-five subjects had been injured at least once in the past—46% of the past injuries were firearm wounds, 13% were stab wounds, and 22% resulted from motor vehicle crashes.

INSTRUMENTS

A Trauma Risk Factor Interview Schedule was developed by the study's investigators through a review of the trauma and problem behavior literature. The schedule was used to obtain data on demographics; social network; environment; and risk-taking behaviors, including substance abuse, risky driving practices, and violence-prone behaviors. Subjects were asked to report how often in the past 3 months they had engaged in each of the behaviors. The Adolescent Risk-Taking Instrument was used to measure perceived risk-taking from a developmental perspective. The Brief Anger/Aggression Questionnaire was used to measure overtly expressed anger characterized by generalized irritability and a tendency to act in an aggressive and violent fashion.

PROCEDURE

Interviews were conducted by one of two investigators in a private patient care area. Medical records were reviewed for clinical data.

RESULTS

Of the sample, 89% experienced trauma related to interpersonal violence, including firearm injuries, stab wounds, and blunt trauma. Male gender unemployment, past arrest, low levels of spirituality, and high levels of anger/aggression and thrill-seeking accounted for 25% of the variance in the number of risk-taking behaviors. Factors such as male gender, past arrest, and no psychological counseling distinguished subjects with firearm-related injuries from subjects with other types of injury. Use of alcohol on weekdays, past arrest, and high education levels were associated with trauma recidivism, explaining 14% of the variance.

DISCUSSION/IMPLICATIONS

This study suggests the importance of trauma centers as sites for initiating trauma risk-reduction strategies. Clinical assessment tools need to be developed to screen trauma patients for trauma-related—risk-taking behaviors that are modifiable. Blood alcohol levels and toxicology screens need to be used as cues to refer patients for drug and alcohol counseling. The relationships between male gender, past crime-victim status, past arrest, lower autonomy, weapon use, involvement in fights, and firearm injury emphasize the need for interventions that address the reciprocal nature of violence and victimization. Networks for referral of at-risk trauma patients to community programs that provide job training and education must also be developed. The investigators suggest that health care professionals need to be advocates for social policies designed to reduce the devastation caused by intentional and unintentional injury.

BOX 43-6 Factors That Contribute to Tissue Hypoxia in the Trauma Patient

- Shifts to the left of the oxyhemoglobin dissociation curve (can be secondary to infusion of large volumes of banked blood, hypocarbia or alkalosis, or hypothermia)
- Reduced hemoglobin (secondary to hemorrhage)
- Reduced cardiac output (in the presence of cardiovascular insults)
- Impaired cellular oxygen consumption (associated with metabolic alterations of sepsis)
- Increased metabolic demands (associated with the stress response to injury)

From Johnson KL: Critical care of the trauma patient. In Neff JA, Kidd PS, editors: *Trauma nursing: the art and science,* St Louis, 1993, Mosby.

contusion, laceration, shearing injuries, or hemorrhage. Primary injury may be mild, with little or no neurologic damage, or severe, with major tissue damage.

Secondary injury. Secondary injury can be caused by further physiologic events that occur after the primary injury. Secondary injury can be caused by hypoxia, hypercapnia, hypotension, cerebral edema, or sustained hypertension. Beyond causing injury to tissue, each of these factors also contributes to significant increases in intracranial pressure (ICP). (∞Assessment of Intracranial Pressure, p. 821)

Hypoxia produces secondary injury through two mechanisms. Tissue ischemia occurs in the area inadequately oxygenated, and the cells of the ischemic area become edematous. Extreme vasodilation of the cerebral vasculature occurs in an attempt to supply oxygen to the cerebral tissue. This increase in blood volume increases intracranial volume and ICP.

Hypercapnia is a powerful vasodilator. Most often caused by hypoventilation in an unconscious patient, hypercapnia results in cerebral vasodilation and increased cerebral blood volume and ICP.

Significant hypotension causes inadequate perfusion to neural tissue. It is important to note that hypotension rarely is associated with head injury. If a trauma patient is unconscious and hypotensive, an aggressive assessment of the chest, abdomen, and pelvis is performed to rule out internal injuries.

Cerebral edema occurs as a result of the changes in the cellular environment caused by contusion, loss of autoregulation, and increased permeability of the blood-brain barrier. Cerebral edema can be focal as it localizes around the area of contusion (just as tissue edema occurs in other parts of the body in response to injury) or diffuse as a result of hypotension or hypoxia. The extent of cerebral edema can be minimized by controlling the other aspects of secondary injury, such as oxygenation, ventilation, and blood pressure.

Initial hypertension in the patient with severe head injury is common. As a result of the loss of autoregulation, increased blood pressure results in increased intracranial blood volume and ICP. Every effort must be made to control hypertension to prevent the secondary injury caused by increased ICP. (∞Management of Intracranial Pressure, p. 826.)

The effects of increases in intracranial pressure may be varied. As pressure increases inside the enclosed vault of the skull, cerebral perfusion decreases, which leads to further compromise of the intracranial contents. The effects of increasing pressure and decreasing perfusion precipitate a downward spiral of events. (∞Management of Intracranial Pressure, p. 826.)

Classification

Injuries of the brain are described by the functional changes or losses that occur. Some of the major functional abnormalities seen in head injury are described here.

Skull fractures. Skull fractures are common, but they do not by themselves cause neurologic deficits. Skull fractures can be classified as open (dura is torn) or closed (dura is not torn), or they can be classified as those of the vault or those of the base. Common vault fractures occur in the parietal and temporal regions. Basilar skull fractures usually are not visible on conventional skull films. Assessment findings may include cerebral spinal fluid otorrhea or rhinorrhea, Battle's sign (ecchymosis overlying the mastoid process), or "raccoon eyes" (subconjunctival and periorbital ecchymosis).

The significance of a skull fracture is that it identifies the patient with a higher probability of having or developing an intracranial hematoma. For this reason, all patients with skull fractures are hospitalized for observation.[4] Open skull fractures require surgical intervention to remove bony fragments and to close the dura. The major complications of basilar skull fractures are cranial nerve injury and leakage of cerebrospinal fluid (CSF). CSF leakage may result in a fistula, which increases the possibility of bacterial contamination and resultant meningitis. Because fistula formation may be delayed, patients with a basilar skull fracture are admitted to the hospital for observation and possible surgical intervention.

Concussion. A concussion is a brain injury accompanied by a brief loss of neurologic function, especially loss of consciousness.[4] If loss of consciousness occurs, it may last for seconds to an hour. The neurologic dysfunctions include confusion, disorientation, and sometimes a period of posttraumatic amnesia. Other clinical manifestations that occur after concussion are headache, dizziness, nausea, irritability, inability to concentrate, impaired memory, and fatigue. The diagnosis of concussion is based on the loss of consciousness inasmuch as the brain remains structurally intact despite functional impairment. Patients with a history of 5 or more minutes of loss of consciousness usually are admitted to the hospital for a 24-hour observation period.[4]

Contusion. Contusion, or bruising of the brain, usually is related to acceleration-deceleration injuries, which result in hemorrhage into the superficial parenchyma, often the frontal and temporal lobes. Frontal or temporal contusions can be seen in a coup-contrecoup mechanism of injury (Figure 43-2). Coup injury affects the cerebral tissue directly under the point of impact. Contrecoup injury occurs in a line directly opposite the point of impact.

The clinical manifestations of contusion are related to the location of the contusion, the degree of contusion, and the presence of associated lesions. Contusions can be small, in which localized areas of dysfunction result in a focal neurologic deficit. Larger contusions can evolve over 2 to 3 days after injury as a result of edema and further hemorrhaging. A large contusion can produce a mass effect that can cause a significant increase in ICP.

Contusions of the tips of the temporal lobe are a common occurrence and are of particular concern. Because the inner aspects of the temporal lobe surround the opening in the tentorium where the midbrain enters the cerebrum, edema in this area can cause rapid deterioration of the patient's condition and can lead to herniation. Because of the location, this deterioration can occur with little or no warning at a deceptively low ICP.

Diagnosis of contusion is made by computed tomography (CT) scan. If the CT scan indicates contusion, especially in the temporal area, the nurse must pay particular attention to neurologic assessments and look for subtle changes in pupillary signs or vital signs, irrespective of a stable ICP.

Medical management of cerebral contusions may consist of medical or surgical therapies. Because a contusion can progress over 3 to 5 days after injury, secondary injury may occur. If contusions are small, focal, or multiple, they are treated medically with serial neurologic assessments and possibly ICP monitoring. Larger contusions that produce considerable mass effect require surgical intervention to prevent the increased edema and intracranial pressure as the contusion matures.[4] Outcome of cerebral contusion varies, depending on the location and the degree of contusion.

Hematomas. Hematomas resulting from head injury form a mass lesion and lead to increased ICP. Three types of hematomas are discussed here (Figure 43-3). The first two hematomas, epidural and subdural, are extraparenchymal (outside of brain tissue) and produce injury by pressure effect and displacement of intracranial contents. The third type of hematoma, intracerebral, directly damages neural tissue and can produce further injury as a result of pressure and displacement of intracranial contents.

Epidural hematoma. Epidural hematoma (EDH), which is a collection of blood between the inner table of the skull and the outermost layer of the dura, most frequently is associated with skull fractures and middle meningeal artery laceration. A blow to the head that causes a linear skull fracture on the lateral surface of the head may tear the middle meningeal artery. As the artery bleeds, it pulls the dura away from the skull, creating a pouch that expands into the intracranial space.

The incidence of EDH is relatively low. EDH can occur as a result of low-impact injuries (such as falls) or high-impact injuries (such as motor vehicle crashes). EDH occurs from trauma to the skull and meninges rather than from the acceleration-deceleration forces seen in other types of head trauma.

The classic clinical manifestations of EDH include brief loss of consciousness followed by a period of lucidity that may last up to 12 hours. This lucid period is followed by a progressive deterioration in level of consciousness and the development of hemiparesis on the opposite side. A dilated and fixed pupil on the same side as the impact area is a hallmark sign of EDH.[4] The patient may complain of a severe, localized headache and may be sleepy. Diagnosis of EDH is based on clinical symptoms and evidence of a collection of epidural blood identified on CT scan. Treatment of EDH involves surgical intervention to remove the blood and to cauterize the bleeding vessels. Outcome is directly related to the patient's status preoperatively. For patients not in coma, mortality is very low; for those in light coma, mortality is 9%; and for patients in deep coma, mortality is 20%.[5]

Subdural hematoma. Subdural hematoma (SDH), which is the accumulation of blood between the dura and underlying arachnoid membrane, most often is

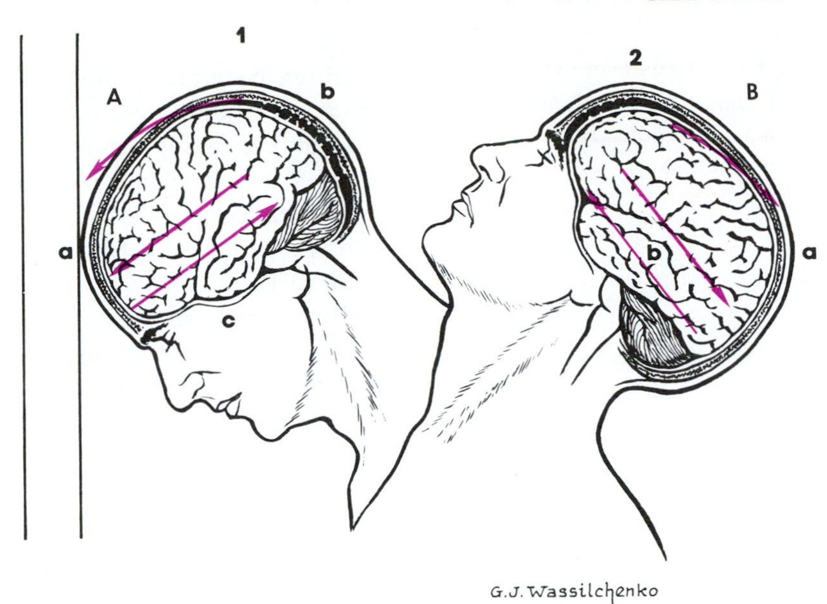

FIGURE 43-2. Coup and contrecoup head injury after blunt trauma. **A,** Coup injury: impact against object. *a,* Site of impact and direct trauma to brain. *b,* Shearing of subdural veins. *c,* Trauma to base of brain. **B,** Contrecoup injury: impact within skull. *a,* Site of impact from brain hitting opposite side of skull. *b,* Shearing forces throughout brain. These injuries occur in one continuous motion—the head strikes the wall (coup), then rebounds (contrecoup).

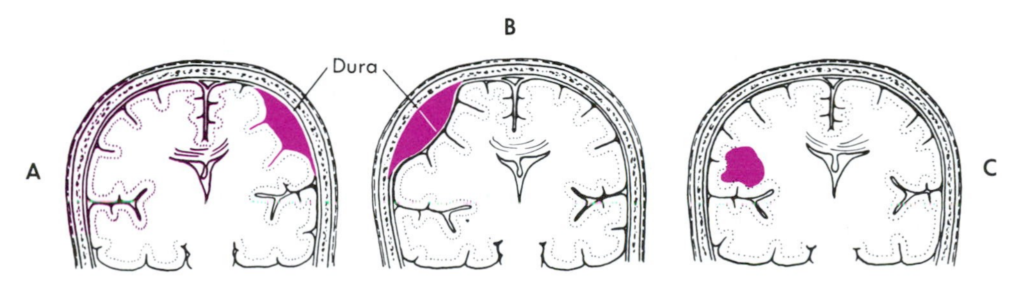

FIGURE 43-3. Types of cerebral hematomas. **A,** Epidural hematoma. **B,** Subdural hematoma. **C,** Intracerebral hematoma.

related to a rupture in the bridging veins between the brain and the dura.[4] Acceleration/deceleration and rotational forces are the major causes of SDH, which often is associated with cerebral contusions and intracerebral hemorrhage.

The three types of SDH are based on the timeframe from injury to clinical symptoms: acute, subacute, and chronic. Table 43-2 summarizes the time interval and presentation for each type of SDH.[19] Acute SHDs are hematomas that are clinically symptomatic in the first 48 hours after injury. The clinical presentation of acute SDH is determined by the severity of injury to the underlying brain at the time of impact and the rapidity of accumulation of blood in the subdural space.[20] In other situations the patient has a lucid period before deterioration. Careful observation for deterioration in level of consciousness or lateralizing signs, such as inequality of pupils or motor movements, is essential. Surgical intervention may include craniectomy, craniotomy, or burr hole evacuation. SDH results in a mortality of 22%, which rises to 50% with injuries to other body systems.[20]

Subacute SDHs are hematomas that develop symptomatically 2 days to 2 weeks after trauma. In subacute hematomas the expansion of the hematoma occurs at a rate slower than that in acute SDH; therefore it takes longer for symptoms to become obvious. Clinical deterioration with subacute SDH usually is slower than that with acute SDH, but treatment by surgical intervention, when appropriate, is the same.

Chronic subdural hematoma is the term used when symptoms appear 2 weeks or more after injury. Most patients with chronic SDH usually are elderly or in late middle age. Many have a history of alcoholism, and some are on a regimen of anticoagulation therapy.

The pathophysiology of chronic SDH is slightly different from that of acute SDH. The initial hemorrhage

TABLE 43-2 Classification of Subdural Hematomas

Type	Time Interval	Symptoms
Acute	Within 48 hr	Headache, drowsiness, agitation, confusion, deterioration in LOC, fixed and ipsilateral pupil dilation, contralateral hemiparesis **or** Profound coma
Subacute	2 days to 2 wk	Similar to acute SDH except that symptoms appear more slowly
Chronic	2 wk to months	Progressive lethargy, absent-mindedness, headache, vomiting, seizures, ipsilateral pupil dilation, or contralateral hemiparesis

LOC, Loss of consciousness.

is not sufficient to produce clinical signs of increasing pressure. Within 2 weeks, a vascular membrane encases the clot and the hematoma slowly enlarges. Once the hematoma becomes large enough to exert pressure on cerebral contents, symptoms appear.

Clinical manifestations of chronic SDH are insidious. The patient may report a variety of symptoms, such as lethargy, absent-mindedness, headache, vomiting, stiff neck, and photophobia, and show signs of transient ischemic attack, seizures, pupillary changes, or hemiparesis. Because history of trauma often is not significant enough to be recalled, chronic SDH seldom is seen as an initial diagnosis. CT scan evaluation can confirm the diagnosis of chronic SDH.

If surgical intervention is required, evacuation of the chronic SDH may occur by craniotomy, burr holes, or catheter drainage. Burr hole placement or catheter drainage involves drilling a hole in the skull over the site of the chronic SDH and draining the fluid. Drains or catheters are left in place for at least 24 hours to facilitate total drainage. Outcome after chronic SDH evacuation is variable. Return of neurologic status often depends on the degree of neurologic dysfunction before removal. Because this condition is most common in the elderly or debilitated patient, recovery is a slow process. Recurrence of chronic SDH is not infrequent.

Intracerebral hematoma. Intracerebral hematoma (ICH) results when there is bleeding within cerebral tissue. Traumatic causes of ICH include depressed skull fractures, penetrating injuries (bullet, knife), or sudden acceleration/deceleration motion. The ICH acts as a rapidly expanding lesion, and the mortality is high,[66] however, late ICH into the necrotic center of a contused area also is possible. Sudden clinical deterioration of a patient 6 to 10 days after trauma may be the result of ICH.

Medical management of ICH may include surgical or nonsurgical management. Generally it is believed that hemorrhages that do not cause significant ICP problems should be treated nonsurgically. Over time, the hemorrhage may be reabsorbed. If significant problems with ICP occur as a result of the ICH producing a mass effect, surgical removal is necessary. Outcome from ICH depends greatly on the location of the hemorrhage. Size, mass effect, and displacement of other intracranial structures also affect the outcome. ICH results in a mortality between 25% and 72%.[20]

Missile injuries. Missile injuries are caused by objects that penetrate the skull to produce a significant focal damage but little acceleration/deceleration or rotational injury. The injury may be depressed, penetrating, or perforating (Figure 43-4). Depressed injuries are caused by fractures of the skull, with penetration of bone into cerebral tissue. Penetrating injury is caused by a missile that enters the cranial cavity but does not exit. A low-velocity penetrating injury (knife) may involve only focal damage and no loss of consciousness. A high-velocity missile (bullet) can produce shock waves that are transmitted throughout the brain, in addition to injury caused by the bullet. Perforating injuries are missile injuries that enter and then exit the brain. Perforating injuries have much less ricochet effect but are still responsible for significant injury.

Risk of infection and cerebral abscess is a concern in missile injuries. If fragments of the missile are embedded within the brain, careful consideration of the location and risk of increasing neurologic deficit is weighed against the risk of abscess or infection. The outcome after missile injury is based on the degree of penetration and the location of the injury, as well as the velocity of the missile.

Diffuse axonal injury. Diffuse axonal injury (DAI) covers a wide range of brain dysfunction caused by acceleration/deceleration and rotational forces. This diagnosis usually is reserved for severe dysfunction. Cerebral concussion is the least severe form of diffuse axonal injury. DAI describes prolonged coma from the time of injury that is not the result of mass lesions or ischemia.

The pathophysiology of DAI is related to the stretching and tearing of axons as a result of move-

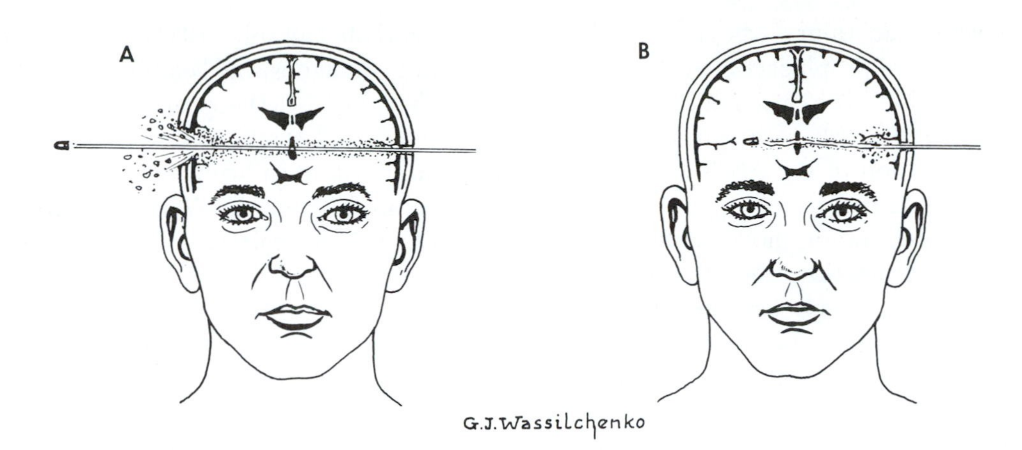

FIGURE 43-4. Bullet wounds of the head. Bullet wound or other penetrating missile wounds cause an open (compound) skull fracture and damage to brain tissue. Shock wave effects are transmitted throughout the brain. **A,** Perforating injury. **B,** Penetrating injury.

ment of the brain inside the cranium at the time of impact. The stretching and tearing of axons result in microscopic lesions throughout the brain, but especially deep within cerebral tissue and the base of the cerebrum. Disruption of axonal transmission of impulses results in loss of consciousness. Unless surrounding tissue areas are significantly injured, causing small hemorrhages, DAI is not visible on CT scan. The patient remains in a deep coma, often with decerebrate or decorticate posturing and autonomic dysfunction, including hyperthermia, hypertension, and diaphoresis.

Treatment of DAI includes support of vital functions and maintenance of ICP within normal limits. The outcome after severe DAI is poor because of the extensive dysfunction of cerebral pathways. DAI occurs in 44% of all coma-producing head injuries, with an overall mortality of 33%, but in its most severe form, mortality can be 50%.[4]

Assessment

The neurologic assessment is the most important tool for evaluating the patient with a severe head injury, because it can indicate severity of injury, provide prognostic information, and can dictate the speed with which further evaluation and treatment must proceed.[21] The cornerstone of the neurologic assessment is the Glasgow Coma Scale (GCS). To assist with the initial assessment, head injuries are divided into three descriptive categories on the basis of the patient's GCS score and length of the unconscious state.

Degree of injury

Mild injury. Mild head injury is described as a GCS score of 13 to 15, with a loss of consciousness that lasts up to 15 minutes. Patients with mild injury often are seen in the emergency department and discharged home with a family member who is instructed to evaluate the patient routinely and to bring the patient back to the hospital if any further neurologic symptoms appear.

Moderate injury. Moderate head injury is described as a GCS score of 9 to 12, with a loss of consciousness for up to 6 hours. Patients with this type of head injury usually are hospitalized. They are at high risk for deterioration from increasing cerebral edema and ICP, and therefore serial clinical assessments are an important function of the nurse. Hemodynamic and ICP monitoring and ventilatory support often are not required in this group unless other systemic injuries make them necessary. A CT scan usually is performed on admission. Repeat CT scans are indicated if the patient's neurologic status deteriorates.

Severe injury. Patients with a GCS score of 8 or less after resuscitation or those who deteriorate to that level within 48 hours of admission have a severe head injury.[22] Patients with severe head injury often receive ventilatory support along with ICP and hemodynamic monitoring. A CT scan is performed to rule out any mass lesions that can be surgically removed. Patients are placed in a critical care setting for continual assessment, monitoring, and management.

Nursing assessment. As in all traumatic injuries, the evaluation of the ABCs (airway, breathing, and circulation) is the first step in the assessment of the head-injured patient in the critical care unit. These assessments are particularly important in head injury because of secondary injury that can occur as a result of hypoxia, hypoventilation, and hypoperfusion.

A patient with severe head injury who is breathing spontaneously may require prophylactic endotracheal or nasotracheal intubation with mechanical ventilatory support to reduce the risk of hypoxia and hypercapnia. After stabilization of the ABCs is ensured, a neurologic assessment is performed.

Level of consciousness, motor movements, pupillary response, respiratory function, and vital signs are all part of a complete neurologic assessment in the patient with severe head injury. Level of consciousness can be elicited to assess wakefulness. Consciousness is assessed by obtaining the patient's response to verbal and painful stimuli. Determination of orientation to person, place, and time assesses mental alertness. Pupils are assessed for size, shape, equality, and reactivity. Asymmetry must be reported immediately. Pupils are also assessed for constriction to a light source (parasympathetic innervation) or dilation (sympathetic innervation). Because parasympathetic fibers are present in the brainstem, pupils that are slow to react to light may indicate a brainstem injury. A "blown" pupil can be caused by compression of the third ocular nerve or transtentorial herniation. Bilateral fixed pupils can indicate midbrain involvement. (∞Neurological Clinical Assessment, p. 763.)

Neurologic assessments are ongoing throughout the patient's critical care stay as part of the initial shift assessment and as part of ongoing assessments to detect subtle deteriorations. Serial assessments include monitoring of hemodynamic status and ICP monitoring. The use of muscle relaxants and sedation for ICP control may mask neurologic signs in the patient with severe head injury. In these situations, observations for changes in pupils and vital signs become extremely important.

Diagnostic procedures. The cornerstone of diagnostic procedures for evaluation of head injuries is the CT scan.[21] The CT scan is a rapid, noninvasive procedure that can provide invaluable information about the presence of mass lesions and cerebral edema. Serial CT scans may be used over a period of several days to assess areas of contusion and ischemia and to detect delayed hematomas.[22] A nurse must always remain with a head-injured patient during the CT scan to provide continued observation and monitoring during transport and scanning. Transporting the patient, moving the patient from the bed to the CT table, and positioning the head flat during the CT scan are all stressful events and could cause severe increases in ICP. Continuous monitoring allows for rapid intervention.

Electrophysiology studies can aid in ongoing assessments of neurologic function. Evoked potentials and electroencephalograph (EEG) are becoming widely used in the diagnosis of head injuries. Magnetic resonance imaging (MRI) appears to be useful in detecting hematomas and cerebral edema, and use of this diagnostic tool will most likely increase in the future when MRI becomes compatible with mechanical life support systems.[22] (∞Neurological Diagnostic Studies, p. 779.)

Medical Management

Surgical management. If a lesion, identified by CT scan, is causing a shift of intracranial contents or increasing ICP, surgical intervention is necessary. A craniotomy is performed to remove the EDH, SDH, or large ICH. Occasionally, if an area of contusion is large, hemorrhagic, and associated with an elevated ICP, a craniotomy for removal of the contused area may be performed to relieve pressure and prevent herniation. Patients who have had surgery for penetrating head trauma have a 25% incidence of post-traumatic seizures, and therefore these patients should receive anticonvulsants.[23]

Nonsurgical management. Nonsurgical management includes management of ICP; maintenance of adequate cerebral circulation and oxygenation; and treatment of any complications, such as pneumonia or infection. Medical management can include drainage of CSF through a ventricular catheter, use of diuretics, and/or administration of high-dose barbiturate therapy. (∞Management of Intracranial Hypertension, p. 826.)

Nursing Management

Nursing diagnoses and management for the patient with cerebral trauma are listed in Box 43-7. Priority nursing goals include stabilization of vital signs, prevention of further injury, and reduction of increased ICP. Ongoing nursing assessments are the cornerstone to the care of patients with head injuries. Such assessments are the primary mechanism for determining secondary brain injury from cerebral edema and increased ICP. In addition to astute neurologic assessments, it is critical to monitor ventilatory support, fluid and electrolyte balance, and nutrition. (∞Nursing Management of Intracranial Pressure, p. 826.)

SPINAL CORD INJURIES

Approximately 10,000 persons annually in the United States sustain permanent spinal cord injury,[24] and among these 60% to 80% are young adult men between 16 and 18 years old.[25] Of those who survive, about half have quadriplegia and half, paraplegia.[26]

BOX 43-7 NURSING DIAGNOSIS AND MANAGEMENT

CEREBRAL TRAUMA

- Risk for Aspiration risk factors: impaired laryngeal sensation or reflex; impaired pharyngeal peristalsis or tongue function; impaired laryngeal closure or elevation; increased gastric volume; decreased lower esophageal sphincter pressure, p. 727
- Impaired Gas Exchange related to ventilation/perfusion mismatching p. 725
- Altered Nutrition: Less Than Body Requirements related to lack of exogenous nutrients and increased metabolic demand, p. 165
- Body Image Disturbance related to actual change in body structure, function, or appearance, p. 87
- Powerlessness related to lack of control over current situation, p. 89
- Decreased Adaptive Capacity: Intracranial related to failure of normal compensatory mechanisms, p. 843

Motor vehicle crashes are the most common cause of spinal cord injury, with half of those injuries occurring in persons between the ages 15 and 25 years.[27]

Mechanism of Injury

The type of injury sustained depends on the mechanism of injury. Mechanisms of injury can include hyperflexion, hyperextension, rotation, axial loading (vertical compression), and missile or penetrating injuries.

Hyperflexion. Hyperflexion injury most often is seen in the cervical area, especially at the level of C5 to C6, because this is the most mobile portion of the cervical spine. This type of injury most frequently is caused by sudden deceleration motion, as in head-on collisions. Injury occurs from compression of the cord as a result of fracture fragments or dislocation of the vertebral bodies. Instability of the spinal column occurs because of the rupture or tearing of the posterior muscles and ligaments.

Hyperextension. Hyperextension injuries involve backward and downward motion of the head. With this injury, often seen in rear-end collisions or diving accidents, the spinal cord itself is stretched and distorted. Neurologic deficits associated with this injury often are caused by contusion and ischemia of the cord without significant bony involvement. A mild form of hyperextension is the *whiplash* injury.

Rotation. Rotation injuries often occur in conjunction with a flexion or extension injury. Severe rotation of the neck or body results in tearing of the posterior ligaments and displacement (rotation) of the spinal column.

Axial loading. Axial loading, or vertical compression, injuries occur from vertical force along the spinal cord. This most commonly is seen in a fall from a height in which the person lands on the feet or buttocks. Compression injuries cause burst fractures of the vertebral body that often send bony fragments into the spinal canal or directly into the spinal cord (Figure 43-5).

Penetrating injuries. Penetrating injury to the spinal cord can be caused by a bullet, knife, or any other object that penetrates the cord. These types of injury cause permanent damage by anatomically transecting the spinal cord.

Pathophysiology

Spinal cord injuries are the result of a mechanical force that disrupts neurologic tissue or its vascular supply, or both. Much like the pathophysiology of head injuries, a primary injury causes a chain of secondary events in response to the injury. Spinal cord damage appears to be the result of these secondary events, which include hemorrhage, vascular damage, structural changes, and subsequent biochemical alterations.

Several events after a spinal cord injury lead to spinal cord ischemia and loss of neurologic function. A cascade of events is initiated by a sudden flux of calcium from extracellular spaces to intracellular spaces. This cascade of events is summarized in Figure 43-6.[27]

Functional injury of the spinal cord. Functional injury of the spinal cord refers to the degree of disruption of normal spinal cord function. SCIs are first classified as complete or incomplete and then are further divided into functional injuries (Box 43-8).

Complete injury. Complete SCI results in a total loss of sensory and motor function below the level of injury. Regardless of the mechanism of injury, the result is a complete dissection of the spinal cord and its neurochemical pathways, resulting in one of two conditions: quadriplegia or paraplegia.

Quadriplegia. Injuries in the cervical spine region result in quadriplegia. Residual muscle function depends on the specific cervical segments involved. Cervical injuries that occur above C6 result in complete quadriplegia, whereas injuries below C6 produce incomplete quadriplegia with some potential for independence in activities of daily living.[24]

Paraplegia. A complete injury in the thoracolumbar region results in paraplegia. Thoracic L1 and L2 injuries produce paraplegia with variable innervation to intercostal and abdominal muscles.

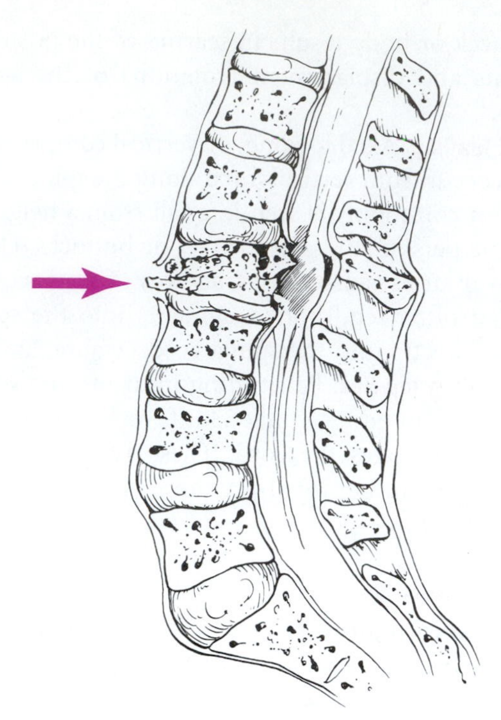

FIGURE 43-5. Spinal cord compression burst injuries. Compression injuries cause burst fractures of the vertebral body that often send bony fragments into the spinal canal or directly into the spinal cord. (From Long BC, Phipps WJ, Cassmeyer VL: *Medical-surgical nursing: a nursing process approach,* ed 3, St Louis, 1993, Mosby.)

Incomplete injury. Incomplete SCI results in a mixed loss of voluntary motor activity and sensation below the level of the lesion. Incomplete SCI exists if any function remains below the level of injury. Incomplete injuries can result in one of a variety of syndromes, which are classified according to the degree of motor and sensory loss below the level of injury. Some of the more common syndromes are described here.

Brown-Séquard syndrome. This syndrome is associated with a physiologic transverse hemisection of the cord. Injury to one side of the spinal cord produces loss of voluntary motor control on the same side of the injury, with accompanying loss of pain and temperature on the opposite side. Functionally, the side of the body with the best motor control has little or no sensation, whereas the side of the body with sensation has little or no motor control.

Central cord syndrome. Central cord syndrome is associated with cervical hyperextension/flexion injury. This injury produces a motor and sensory deficit more pronounced in the upper extremities than in the lower extremities. Varying degrees of bowel and bladder dysfunction may be present. This syndrome can result from contusion, compression, or hemorrhage of the gray matter of the cord.

Anterior cord syndrome. This syndrome is associated with injury to the anterior gray horn cells (motor), the spinothalamic tracts (pain), and the corticospinal tracts (temperature). The result is a loss of motor function, as well as loss of the sensations of pain and temperature below the level of injury. However, below the level of injury, sensations of touch, position, sense, pressure, and vibrations remain intact. Anterior cord syndrome most often is caused by flexion injuries or acute herniation of an intervertebral disk.

Posterior cord syndrome. This syndrome is associated with cervical hyperextension. Injury results in the loss of light touch and proprioception below the level of injury. Motor function and sensation of pain and temperature remain intact.

Spinal shock. Spinal shock is a condition that can occur shortly after traumatic injury to the spinal cord. Spinal shock is the complete loss of all normal reflex activity below the level of injury.[4] Manifestations of spinal shock include bradycardia and hypotension. The intensity of spinal shock is influenced by the level of injury, and the duration of this shock state can persist for up to 1 month after injury. Blood pressure support may be required with the use of sympathomimetic drugs. Because hypotension is a problem, the nurse must be cautious when repositioning a patient in bed, because orthostatic blood pressure changes can occur and further decrease spinal cord blood flow.[28] (∞Neurogenic Shock, p. 1109.)

Autonomic dysreflexia. Autonomic dysreflexia, or autonomic hyperreflexia, is a life-threatening complication that occurs frequently (83% of quadraplegics) in SCI.[29] This condition is caused by a massive sympathetic response to a noxious stimuli (full bladder, line insertions, fecal impaction), which results in bradycardia, hypertension, facial flushing, and headache. A severe vasoconstriction can occur, causing systolic blood pressure to be greater than 200 mm Hg and diastolic blood pressure to reach 130 mm Hg; therefore prompt recognition is critical to the patient's survival.[29] Treatment is aimed at alleviating the noxious stimuli. If symptoms persist, pharmacologic vasodilating drugs (nitroglycerin, nifedipine, hydralazine) can be administered to reduce blood pressure. Prevention of autonomic dysreflexia is imperative and can be accomplished through the use a good bowel and bladder program.

Assessment

Assessment of the patient with a known or suspected SCI must include stabilization of the spinal cord. *All* trauma patients must be protected from further spinal cord damage until presence of spinal cord

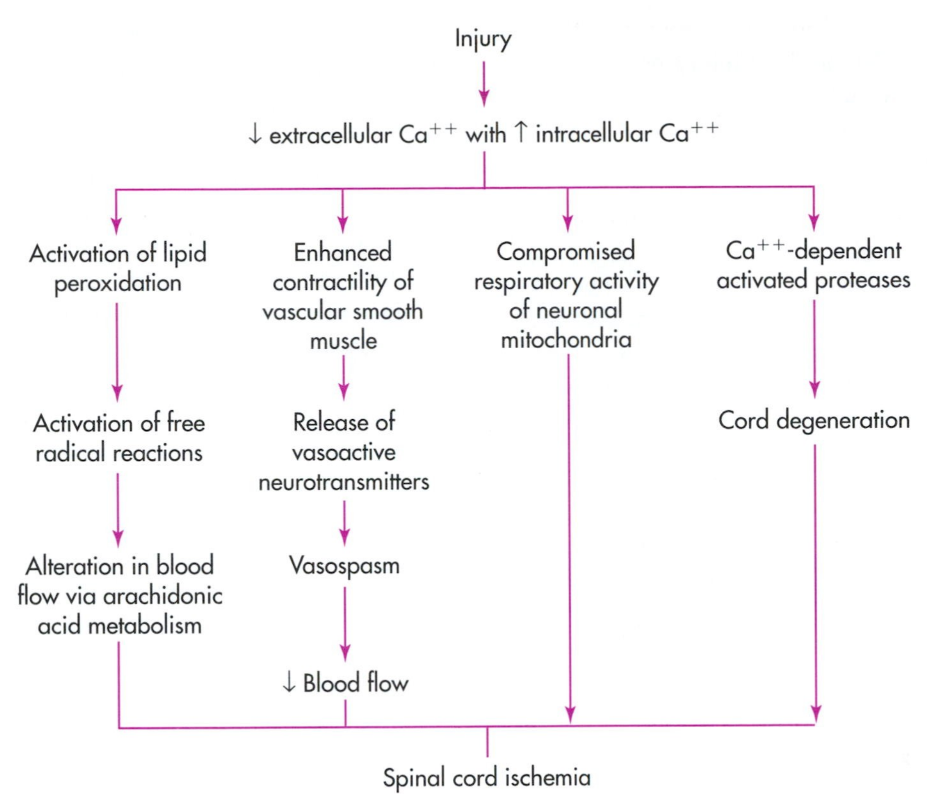

FIGURE 43-6. Schematic design of pathophysiologic events after spinal cord injury. Several events after traumatic injury to the spinal cord lead to cord ischemia and loss of neurologic function.

BOX 43-8 Classification of Spinal Cord Injuries

COMPLETE INJURY

Quadriplegia
Paraplegia

INCOMPLETE INJURY

Brown-Séquard syndrome
Central cord syndrome
Anterior cord syndrome
Posterior cord syndrome

injury is ruled out. Stabilization in the CCU includes bedrest and a cervical collar.[29]

Airway. Assessment of ABCs is essential to ensure optimal oxygenation and perfusion to all vital organs, including the spinal cord, inasmuch as recovery of spinal cord tissue depends partly on adequate oxygen and blood supply.[24] Complete cardiovascular and respiratory assessments are essential to the patient's survival and prognosis. The primary assessment begins with an evaluation of airway clearance. In an unresponsive person an oral airway is inserted while the patient's neck is maintained in a neutral position. The patient must undergo intubation before severe hypoxia can occur, which could further damage the spinal cord. Blind nasotracheal intubation generally is agreed to be the preferred route for establishing an artificial airway in the patient with an SCI.[30] Oral endotracheal intubation is contraindicated because of the degree of cervical spine manipulation required. The airway is further protected from aspiration by a nasogastric tube.

Breathing. Assessment of breathing patterns and gas exchange is made after an airway has been secured. The level of injury dictates the degree of altered breathing patterns and gas exchange. Because complete injuries above the C3 level result in paralysis of the diaphragm,[31] patients with these injuries require ventilatory assistance. Kocan[31] described the effects of SCI on the respiratory process (Table 43-3), which affects almost all patients with SCI.

Circulation. Assessment of cardiac output and tissue perfusion is imperative not only to detect life-threatening injuries, but to promote recovery of the injured spinal cord tissue, which depends in part on adequate perfusion of oxygenated blood.[24] The patient with SCI is at high risk for developing alterations in cardiac output and tissue perfusion because the

TABLE 43-3 Effects of Spinal Cord Injury on Ventilatory Function

Injury Level	Respiratory Function	Comment
Complete, above C3	Paralysis of diaphragm	Unable to sustain ventilation without mechanical assistance
C3 to C5	Varying degrees of diaphragm dysfunction	Generally able to be weaned from mechanical ventilation
C6 to T11	Intercostal muscles lost or impaired Abdominal muscles lost or impaired	Reduced inspiratory ability Paradoxical breathing patterns Diminished chest mobility
Below T12	Ventilation not affected	Ineffective cough

cardiovascular system is subjected to a variety of serious and potential physiologic alterations, including dysrhythmias, cardiac arrest, orthostatic hypotension, emboli, and thrombophlebitis.[24]

In spinal shock, the cardiovascular regulatory mechanisms are lost. Patients with SCI above T5 may have profound spinal shock as a result of interruption of the sympathetic nervous system and loss of vasoconstrictor response below the level of the injury.[24]

The patient with SCI is assessed for adequate tissue perfusion by means of both invasive and noninvasive hemodynamic monitoring techniques. Cardiac monitoring is required to detect bradycardia and other dysrhythmias that occur in response to reflex vagus activity mediated by the dominant parasympathetic nervous system, as well as changes in cardiac rhythm as a result of hypothermia or hypoxia.

The critical care nurse assesses for autonomic dysreflexia as spastic movements replace flaccidity. Signs of autonomic dysreflexia include acute onset of cephalgia, hypertension, bradycardia, diaphoresis, and flushing above the level of injury. Immediate medical intervention is required to prevent cerebral hemorrhage, seizures, and acute pulmonary edema. Frequent causes of autonomic dysreflexia include a distended bowel or bladder. Patency of urinary catheters is routinely assessed. Routine nursing assessments include bowel elimination to aid in early detection of fecal impaction.

Neurologic. The initial neurologic assessment may not be an accurate indication of eventual motor and sensory loss because of spinal shock.[24] It focuses on the rapid and accurate identification of present, absent, or impaired functioning of the motor, sensory, and reflex systems that coordinate and regulate vital functions. A detailed motor and sensory examination includes the assessment of all 32 spinal nerves for evidence of dysfunction. Carefully mapped pathways for the sensory portion of the spinal nerves, termed *dermatomes,* can assist in localizing the functional level of injury (see Figure 25-25). Initial findings must be performed correctly and thoroughly documented in detail so that subsequent serial assessments can rapidly identify deterioration. A complete spinal cord assessment must be documented at least every 4 hours during the critical care phase.[32]

Diagnostic procedures. Diagnostic radiographic evaluations can identify the severity of damage to the spinal cord. Initial evaluation includes anteroposterior and lateral views for all areas of the spinal cord. Films of all seven cervical vertebrae and the top of T1 must be obtained to rule out cervicothoracic junction injury.[33] Flexion and extension views can identify subtle ligamentous injuries. CT scan, tomograms, myelography, and MRI also may be used in the diagnostic process. (∞Neurologic Diagnostic Procedures, p. 779.)

Medical Management

After assessment and diagnosis of the SCI, medical management begins. The primary treatment goal is to preserve remaining neurologic function. Medical interventions are divided into pharmacologic, surgical, and nonsurgical interventions.

Pharmacologic management. After years of intensive research, high-dose methylprednisolone has been shown to improve neurologic outcome at 6 weeks and 6 months after spinal cord injury if administered within 8 hours of injury.[34] Dosing guidelines are summarized in Box 43-9.[12] Methylprednisolone directly affects the changes that occur within the spinal cord after injury, primarily by preventing posttraumatic spinal cord ischemia, improving energy metabolism, restoring extracellular calcium, and improving nerve impulse conduction.[27]

Surgical management. Surgical intervention provides spinal column stability in the presence of an unstable injury. Unstable injuries include disrupted ligaments and tendons, as well as a vertebral column that cannot maintain normal alignment. Identification and immobilization of unstable injuries are particularly important for the patient with incomplete neurologic

BOX 43-9 Administration of IV Methylprednisolone for Spinal Cord Injury

Based on drug concentration of 62.5 mg/ml:
1. Administer bolus dose 30 mg/kg IV over 15 minutes.
2. Pause for 45 minutes (administer IV fluid to keep vein open).
3. Begin maintenance dose at 5.4 mg/kg/hr IV for 23 hours.
4. Terminate drug administration 24 hours after bolus dose.

deficit. Without adequate stabilization, movement and dislocation of the vertebral column could cause a complete neurologic deficit. A variety of surgical procedures may be performed to achieve decompression and stabilization.

Laminectomy. This procedure is the removal of the lamina of the vertebral ring to allow decompression and removal of bony fragments or disk material from the spinal canal.

Spinal fusion. This procedure entails the surgical fusion of two to six vertebral elements to provide stability and to prevent motion. Fusion is accomplished through the use of bone parts or bone chips taken from the iliac crest or by use of wire or acrylic glue.

Rodding. This procedure stabilizes and realigns larger segments of the spinal column by means of a variety of rodding procedures, such as Harrington rods. The rods are attached by screws and glue to the posterior elements of the spinal column. These types of procedures most often are performed to stabilize the thoracolumbar area.

Nonsurgical management. If the injury to the spinal cord is stable, nonsurgical management is the treatment of choice. Nonsurgical management for cervical and thoracolumbar injuries is discussed separately.

Cervical injury. Management of cervical injuries involves the immobilization of the fracture site and realignment of any dislocation. This is accomplished through skeletal traction that involves the use of two-point tongs, which are inserted into the skull through shallow burr holes and are connected to traction weights. Several types of cervical tongs are used. Gardner-Wells and Crutchfield tongs are the most common. These tongs can be applied at the bedside with the use of a local anesthetic.

After the procedure, the patient can be immobilized on a kinetic therapy bed or a regular bed. The kinetic therapy bed is the most popular method used for cervical immobilization because it maintains spinal column alignment while providing constant turning motion to reduce pulmonary and skin breakdown. Use of cervical skeletal traction on a regular bed makes it difficult to provide adequate care to the pulmonary system and skin because of the extensive degree of immobility.

After adequate realignment of the spinal column has occurred through skeletal traction, a halo traction brace often is applied. The halo vest consists of a metal ring secured to the skull with two occipital and two temporal screws. Steel bars anchor the screws to the vest to provide cervical immobilization (Figure 43-7). The halo traction brace immobilizes the cervical spine, which allows the patient to ambulate and participate in self-care.

Thoracolumbar injury. Nonsurgical management of the patient with a thoracolumbar injury also involves immobilization. Skeletal traction may be used in high thoracic injury. For the most part, misalignment of the spinal canal does not occur in stable injuries of the thoracolumbar spine. Immobilization to allow fractures to heal is accomplished by bedrest (with bed flat) and the use of a plastic or fiberglass jacket, a body cast, or a brace.

Nursing Management

Nursing diagnoses and management for the patient with spinal cord injury are summarized in Box 43-10. The goal during the critical care phase is to prevent life-threatening complications while maximizing the functioning of all organ systems. Nursing interventions are aimed at preventing secondary damage to the spinal cord and managing the cardiovascular and respiratory complications of the neurologic deficit.[32] Because almost all body systems are affected by SCI, nursing management also must include interventions that optimize nutrition, elimination, skin integrity, and mobility. Prevention of complications that can delay the patient's rehabilitation is one of the goals of critical care.[32] Refer to page 1093 for the nursing management of dysreflexia. In addition, patients with SCI have complex psychosocial needs that require a great deal of emotional support from the critical care nurse. Numerous nursing diagnoses apply to the provision of quality care for the SCI patient in the critical care unit (see Box 43-10).

Cardiovascular. The risk for cardiovascular instability is especially profound in patients with SCI at the C3 to C5 levels, although cardiovascular alterations can occur with most injuries above T6.[35] Patients with SCI

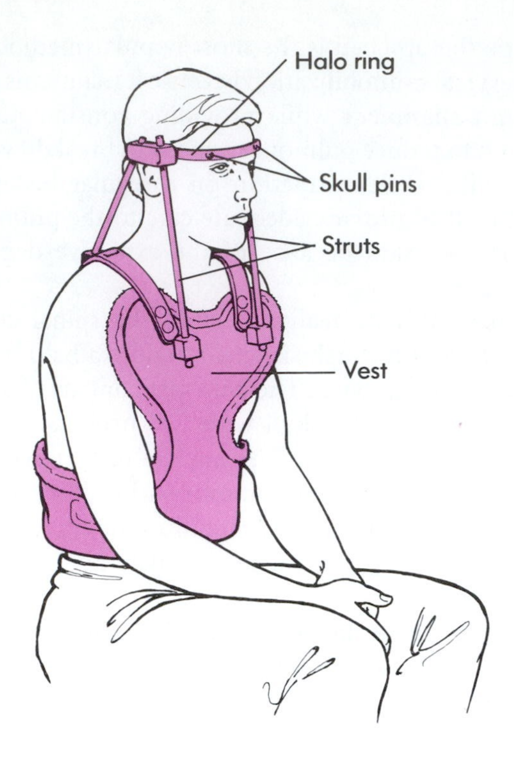

FIGURE 43-7. Halo vest. The halo traction brace immobilizes the cervical spine, which allows the patient to ambulate and participate in self-care.

BOX 43-10 NURSING DIAGNOSIS AND MANAGEMENT

SPINAL CORD INJURY

- Decreased Cardiac Output related to sympathetic blockade, p. 1118
- Dysreflexia related to excessive autonomic response to certain noxious stimuli (e.g., distended bladder, distended bowel, skin irritation) occurring in patients with cervical or high thoracic (T7 or above) spinal cord injury, p. 1093
- Impaired Gas Exchange related to alveolar hypoventilation, p. 726
- Impaired Gas Exchange related to ventilation/perfusion mismatching p. 725
- Risk for Aspiration risk factors: impaired laryngeal sensation or reflex; impaired laryngeal closure or elevation; increased gastric volume; decreased lower esophageal sphincter pressure, p. 727
- Body Image Disturbance related to actual change in body structure, function, or appearance, p. 87
- Ineffective Individual Coping related to situational crisis and personal vulnerability, p. 95

usually can tolerate a systolic blood pressure of 90 mm Hg.[24] Alteration in tissue perfusion secondary to hypotension may require the administration of IV fluids. Blood pressure is usually not restored by administration of IV fluids, and thus aggressive attempts to treat the hypotension may result in fluid overload.[4] Astute assessment of fluid volume is required, however, because pulmonary edema is a threat to SCI patients. Pulmonary artery catheterization may be required to assess for this complication. Once fluid volume status has been optimized, inotropic or vasopressor support, or both, may be implemented.

Because of the SCI patient's dependence on the environment for temperature control (poikilothermy), judicious use of heat or cold for therapeutic or comfort measures is required. Profound changes in body temperature must be avoided. Hypothermia can produce bradydysrhythmias and sinus arrest. Symptomatic bradydysrhythmias can be treated with inotropic drugs (isoproterenol), temporary transvenous or transcutaneous pacing, or propantheline.[35]

Pulmonary. Pulmonary complications are the most common cause of mortality in SCI patients.[36] Initial and ongoing nursing assessments of respiratory status are imperative for identifying actual or potential impairment in ventilation. These include observation of respiratory rate and rhythm, observation of symmetry of chest expansion and use of accessory muscles, inspection of quantity and character of secretions, and auscultation of breath sounds. Judicious use of serial arterial blood gas (ABG) values provides information on the adequacy of gas exchange.

Ineffective Airway Clearance is a particular problem for the SCI patient as a result of hypoventilation (paralysis of respiratory muscles), increased bronchial secretions, and atelectasis secondary to decreased cough. Frequent suctioning for airway clearance is required. Caution must be used with vigorous suctioning because the unopposed vagus nerve, when stimulated, can cause profound bradycardia.[29] Bradycardia exacerbated by hypoxia is likely to develop in patients with cervical SCI. Use of hyperventilation breaths with 100% oxygen before suctioning may help. Chest percussion and drainage facilitate removal of secretions. Kinetic therapy beds, which can rotate up to 60 degrees on each side, can provide continual postural drainage and mobilization of secretions.

Impaired Gas Exchange can occur in the SCI patient as a result of hypoventilation (paralysis of respiratory muscles), increased bronchial secretions that interfere with adequate gas diffusion, shunting secondary to atelectasis and associated pulmonary injuries, and pulmonary complications (pulmonary embolism). Nursing interventions are directed at improving and maintaining adequate gas exchange. Deep vein thrombosis (DVT) prophylaxis includes passive range-of-motion exercises, sequential compression stockings, subcutaneous heparin, and kinetic therapy. Because of the loss of sensation, assessment of Homans' sign is not applicable to the SCI patient. Serial calf measurements done once or twice a day may detect DVT, however, the ultimate value of these measurements in detecting DVT is not clear.

Depending on the level of SCI, the patient's breathing patterns may be ineffective. Intubation and mechanical ventilation may be required if the patient's respiratory rate is greater than 30 breaths/minute, there is evidence of aspiration, or the vital capacity is less than 500 ml.[29] Approximately 20% to 30% of patients with SCI require mechanical ventilatory support, although patients with lesions at the C4 level or lower generally are able to be weaned from the ventilator. Weaning can be a complex process, however, because of physical requirements of the diaphragm and the psychologic effects of the fear of the inability to breathe. Weaning usually can be accomplished by slowly increasing the length of time the patient spends off the ventilator. The patient is taken off the ventilator, and a T-piece is used for a period. Then the patient is placed back on the ventilator for "rest" in the assist/control mode, rather than the intermittent mandatory ventilation mode. Setbacks are common. If reintubation is required, neuromuscular blocking agents may be used. The critical care nurse must be aware that succinylcholine (Suxamethonium) never must be administered to an SCI patient any time after 72 hours after injury. Use of this depolarizing agent can produce hyperkalemic arrest. Weaning requires a well-coordinated approach planned by the nurse, physician, respiratory therapist, and patient. (∞ Invasive Mechanical Ventilation, p. 703.)

The SCI patient is at risk for aspiration. With injuries at T6 or above, a depressed cough reflex will inhibit coughing of aspirated material. Decreased gastric motility can result in retention of gastric secretions or tube feeding residuals. If possible, the head of the patient's bed is elevated. Enteral tube feedings administered via the small intestine can help reduce the risk of aspiration as a result of delayed gastric emptying.

Maximizing mobility and skin integrity. Nursing management of the SCI patient with impaired mobility should focus on four areas: (1) maintaining correct spinal alignment, (2) assessing for improvement or deterioration in condition, (3) facilitating progressive mobility, and (4) preventing complications of decreased mobility.[37] Once unstable fractures have been stabilized by medical intervention, nursing management can enhance spinal stability by the use of specific immobilization beds and by ensuring proper spinal alignment. Range-of-motion exercises are initiated as soon as the spine has been stabilized. Nursing management of the patient in a halo vest includes inspection of pins and traction for security, correct positioning and turning (traction bars or the halo ring must never be used to lift or reposition the patient), placement of wrenches on the front of the vest in case of cardiac arrest, and maintenance of skin integrity inside the halo vest.

Interventions to maintain skin integrity are started on admission to the critical care unit. Thorough skin assessments, regular turning, repositioning, meticulous skin care, and special mattresses can aid in preventing decubitus ulcers. Decubitus ulcers can cause extensive necrosis and sepsis, which will interfere or even prevent the patient's recovery and rehabilitation.[24]

Elimination. Initially after SCI, bowel and bladder tone are flaccid. Urinary retention occurs, and insertion of an indwelling urinary catheter is required. This prevents bladder stretching and overdistention, which could permanently injure the muscular wall of the bladder and prevent the return of spastic bladder control. An intermittent catheter program must be instituted early. An example of such a program is summarized in Box 43-11.[29] A bowel program to prevent fecal impaction and encourage normal, regular bowel function must be instituted.

Maximizing psychosocial adaptation. Nursing management of the patient with SCI must include the provision of dedicated emotional support. In the critical care unit, the patient and family experience anxiety, grief, denial, anger, frustration, and hopelessness because long-term neurologic deficits remain unknown. Nursing interventions include the promotion of coping mechanisms, support systems, and adaptive skills. Simple, accurate, and consistent information can alleviate fear and anxiety. The patient's anger may be expressed by demanding behavior, for which realistic limit setting and establishment of contracts may be helpful. Feelings of powerlessness may be reduced by including the patient and family in care and decision making. Further psychosocial support can be given by social workers, occupational therapists, psychiatric clinical nurse specialists, and pastors.

MAXILLOFACIAL INJURIES

Trauma to the face results in complex physiologic and psychologic sequelae. Vital functions that depend

BOX 43-11 Intermittent Catheter Program for Spinal Cord Injury

- Fluid restriction—200 ml every 2 hours at first, with intermittent catheterization every 4 hours.
- If urine volumes are ≤200 ml, decrease frequency of catheterization to every 6 hours.
- If urine volumes are ≥500 ml, increase frequency of catheterization and/or more fluid restriction.

on facial integrity include mastication; deglutination; perception of the environment (vision, hearing, speech, olfaction); and respiration. The face also represents a direct link to self and to expression by playing a major role in personal identity, appearance, and communication. Consequently, maxillofacial trauma has the potential to produce long-term sequelae, with emotional, sensory, and disfigurement implications. Facial injuries, are common because of the exposed position of the head.

Mechanism of Injury

Maxillofacial injury results from blunt or penetrating trauma. Blunt trauma may occur from motor vehicle, industrial or athletic accidents, violent blows to the head, or falls. Penetrating maxillofacial trauma is less common; causes include bullets or stabbings. High-velocity forces (caused by MVCs or firearms) to the maxillofacial region tend to be multiple and often are more life threatening than are injuries caused by low-velocity forces (falls, fists). Associated injuries may include concussion, skull fracture, rhinorrhea, spinal cord injury, and fractures of other bones.

Pathophysiology

The facial skeleton serves as an energy-absorbing shield to protect the brain, spinal cord, eyes, and pharynx. Nasal bones, the zygoma, and the mandibular condyle are the most susceptible to fracture.[38] Bullet wounds can be life threatening because of hemorrhage and airway obstruction. Maxillofacial trauma can result in soft tissue injury ranging from abrasions to destruction of most of the face, as well as maxillofacial skeletal fractures. This section is limited to the discussion of maxillofacial skeletal injuries.

Maxillofacial skeletal injuries. Fractures of the maxilla are diagnosed according to Le Fort's classification. Le Fort's fractures are classified into three broad categories, depending on the level of the fracture (Figure 43-8). The most common, Le Fort I, consists of horizontal fractures in which the entire maxillary arch moves separately from the upper facial skeleton. Le Fort II fractures are an extension of Le Fort I and involve the orbit, ethmoid, and nasal bones. Le Fort III fractures are associated with craniofacial disruption. Cerebrospinal fluid frequently leaks with these fractures.

Assessment

Assessment of the ABCs is once again critical. Patients with maxillofacial trauma are especially prone to Ineffective Airway Clearance, Fluid Volume Deficit related to hemorrhage, and Risk for Injury Life-threatening complications associated with maxillofacial trauma include airway obstruction, aspiration, and hemorrhage.[38]

Airway clearance. Patients with maxillofacial trauma are at risk for ineffective airway clearance. Edema, hemorrhage, foreign objects, vomit, broken teeth, or bone fragments can obstruct the airway. The mouth and oral pharynx must be inspected. An artificial airway may be required. An oral endotracheal tube is used unless there is a laryngeal fracture. Nasal intubation is contraindicated in the presence of facial fractures because of the risk of passing the tube into the cranium. If endotracheal intubation is unsuccessful, a cricothyrotomy may be indicated. Midface fractures may require a tracheostomy, because the mouth is wired shut and massive edema can obstruct the nose. The airway must be further protected from aspiration by an orogastric tube. Nasogastric tubes are contraindicated in the presence of facial fractures because of the risk of passing the tube into the cranium.

Fluid volume deficit. Patients with maxillofacial trauma are at risk for fluid volume deficit related to massive hemorrhage as a result of bleeding from the ethmoid or maxillary sinuses. Effective tamponade can occur with digital pressure, manual fracture reduction, or nasal packing. Intravenously administered fluids are given to correct the fluid volume deficit.

Risk for injury. Maxillofacial trauma frequently is associated with cervical spinal cord injury. An altered level of consciousness in the presence of maxillofacial fractures strongly suggests neurotrauma. Fractures involving the cranium and dura mater may enable oral bacterial flora to enter CSF, placing the patient at risk for meningitis. Nasal and auditory canals must be inspected for discharge. The *ring test* is performed to determine whether the drainage is CSF. This can be done by placing the drainage on a paper towel. If a double ring is formed when the fluid dries, the fluid is con-

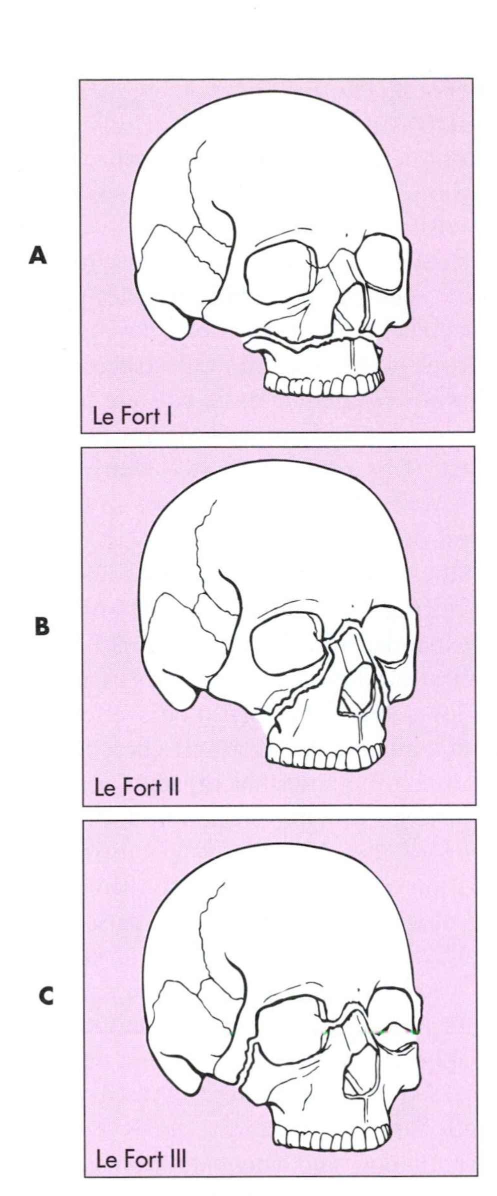

FIGURE 43-8. Fractures of the maxilla are diagnosed according to Le Fort's classification, which consists of three broad categories based on the level of the fracture. **A,** Le Fort I; **B,** Le Fort II; **C,** Le Fort III.

sidered to be CSF. The drainage also can be tested for glucose inasmuch as CSF has a high glucose content.

Diagnostic procedures. Special radiographic views are required for accurate diagnosis of maxillofacial fractures. Full maxillofacial fracture radiographic views include posteroanterior, lateral, lateral oblique, panorex, and tomograms.

Medical Management

Le Fort fractures require reduction by use of direct wiring or fixation devices. Some fractures can be reduced and immobilized immediately by the application of arch bars or intramaxillary fixation (wire) with the use of local anesthesia. Facial fractures (except mandibular fractures) can be repaired surgically up to 10 days after injury.[39]

Nursing Management

Nursing diagnoses and management for the patient with maxillofacial trauma are summarized in Box 43-12. Nursing interventions are directed toward the nursing diagnoses for the patient with maxillofacial trauma. Nursing management of the patient with jaw wires requires interventions aimed at protecting the airway by reducing the risk of emesis and aspiration. Proper orogastric tube functioning must be ensured. Antiemetics may be administered. Unless contraindicated, the head of the bed is elevated 30 degrees. If vomiting occurs, the patient is placed in a side or forward position and oral/nasal suctioning is used. Wire cutters must be available at the bedside in case the vomit cannot clear the wires and occludes the airway. Although this seldom is necessary, the principle in cutting the wires is to cut the vertical attachments, not the horizontal ones.[40]

THORACIC INJURIES

Thoracic injuries involve trauma to the chest wall, lungs, heart, great vessels, and esophagus. Thoracic trauma accounts for 20% to 25% of all traumatic deaths.[41] Most deaths caused by pulmonary trauma occur after the patient reaches the hospital. Thoracic trauma most commonly is the result of a violent crime or MVC.

Mechanism of Injury

Blunt thoracic trauma. Blunt trauma to the chest most frequently is caused by MVCs or falls. The underlying mechanism of injury tends to be a combination of acceleration/deceleration injury and direct transfer mechanics, such as a crush injury. Varying mechanisms of blunt trauma are associated with specific injury patterns. After head-on collisions, drivers have a higher frequency of injury than do back-seat passengers because the driver comes in contact with the steering assembly. Severe thoracic injuries frequently are seen in patients who are unrestrained. Falls from greater than 20 feet are associated with thoracic injury.

Penetrating thoracic injuries. The penetrating object determines the damage sustained from penetrating thoracic trauma. Low-velocity weapons (.22-caliber gun, knife) usually damage only what is in the weapon's direct path. Of particular concern, however, are stab wounds that involve the anterior chest wall between

BOX 43-12 NURSING DIAGNOSIS AND MANAGEMENT

MAXILLOFACIAL TRAUMA

- Risk for Aspiration risk factors: impaired pharyngeal peristalsis or tongue function; impaired laryngeal sensation or reflex; impaired laryngeal closure or elevation, p. 727
- Fluid Volume Deficit related to absolute loss, p. 914
- Altered Nutrition: Less Than Body Requirements related to lack of exogenous nutrients and increased metabolic demands, p. 165
- Acute Pain related to transmission and perception of cutaneous, visceral, muscular, or ischemic impulses, p. 197

the midclavicular lines, Louis's angle, and the epigastric region inasmuch as these wounds are likely to have entered the mediastinum, heart, and/or the great vessels.[42] High-velocity weapons (rifle, shotgun, or .38 caliber gun) produce more serious injuries. These weapons are associated with massive energy transfer and tissue destruction. Pellets from a shotgun blast cause further damage by expanding and causing multiple injuries.

Specific Thoracic Traumatic Injuries

Chest wall injuries

Rib fractures. Interruption of a single rib is the most minor and the most common chest wall injury associated with blunt thoracic trauma.[43] Fractures of certain ribs or multiple ribs can be more serious. Fractures of certain ribs are associated with more underlying life-threatening injuries. Fractures of the first and second ribs are associated with intrathoracic vascular injuries (brachial plexus, great vessels). Fractures of the seventh through tenth ribs are associated with liver or spleen injuries. The pain of rib fractures can be aggravated by movement associated with respiratory excursion. As a result, the patient often splints, takes shallow breaths, and refuses to cough, which can result in atelectasis and pneumonia.

Localized pain that increases with respiration or that is elicited by rib compression may indicate rib fractures. Definitive diagnosis can be made with a chest film. Nursing diagnoses may include Pain, Ineffective Airway Clearance, Ineffective Breathing Pattern, and Impaired Gas Exchange. Interventions include aggressive pulmonary physiotherapy and pain control to improve chest expansion efforts and gas exchange. Intercostal nerve blocks and thoracic epidural analgesia may be used to assist with pain control. External splints are not recommended because they further limit chest wall expansion and may add to atelectasis. The patient's preexisting pulmonary status may dictate the course of recovery. The major concern with rib fractures is the associated underlying injuries.

Flail chest. Flail chest, caused by blunt trauma, disrupts the continuity of chest wall structures. A flail chest occurs when three or more ribs are fractured in two or more places and are no longer attached to the thoracic cage. This results in a free-floating segment of the chest wall. This segment moves independently from the rest of the thorax and results in paradoxical chest wall movement during the respiratory cycle (Figure 43-9). During inspiration the intact portion of the chest wall expands while the injured part is sucked in. During expiration the chest wall moves in and the flail segment moves out. The physiologic effects of impaired chest wall motion of a flail chest include decreased tidal volume and vital capacity and impaired cough, which lead to hypoventilation and atelectasis.

Inspection of the chest reveals paradoxical movement. Palpation of the chest may indicate crepitus and tenderness near fractured ribs. The patient may be cyanotic and, if conscious, complain of shortness of breath. As a result of splinting the flail segment may not always be evident initially in the conscious patient. Nursing diagnoses for the patient with a flail chest include Decreased Cardiac Output, Impaired Gas Exchange, and Pain. Interventions focus on ensuring adequate ventilation and adequate pain control, administering oxygen, and accurately assessing fluid balance. A pulmonary contusion beneath the flail can cause capillary leakage of fluid. This, in combination with fluid volume excess, can precipitate ARDS. Diuretics also may be used to limit interstitial fluid accumulation. Progressive respiratory failure is treated with intubation and mechanical ventilatory support. The patient with a flail chest also must be observed for dysrhythmias. This is especially important with anterior flail chest because of the possibility of underlying cardiac damage.[44]

Ruptured diaphragm. Diaphragmatic rupture is a frequently missed diagnosis in trauma patients because of the subtle and nospecific symptoms this injury produces. The mechanism of injury appears to be a rapid rise in intraabdominal pressure as a result of compression force applied to the lower part of the chest or upper region of the abdomen. This injury can occur when a person is thrown forward over the tip of the steering wheel in a high-speed deceleration acci-

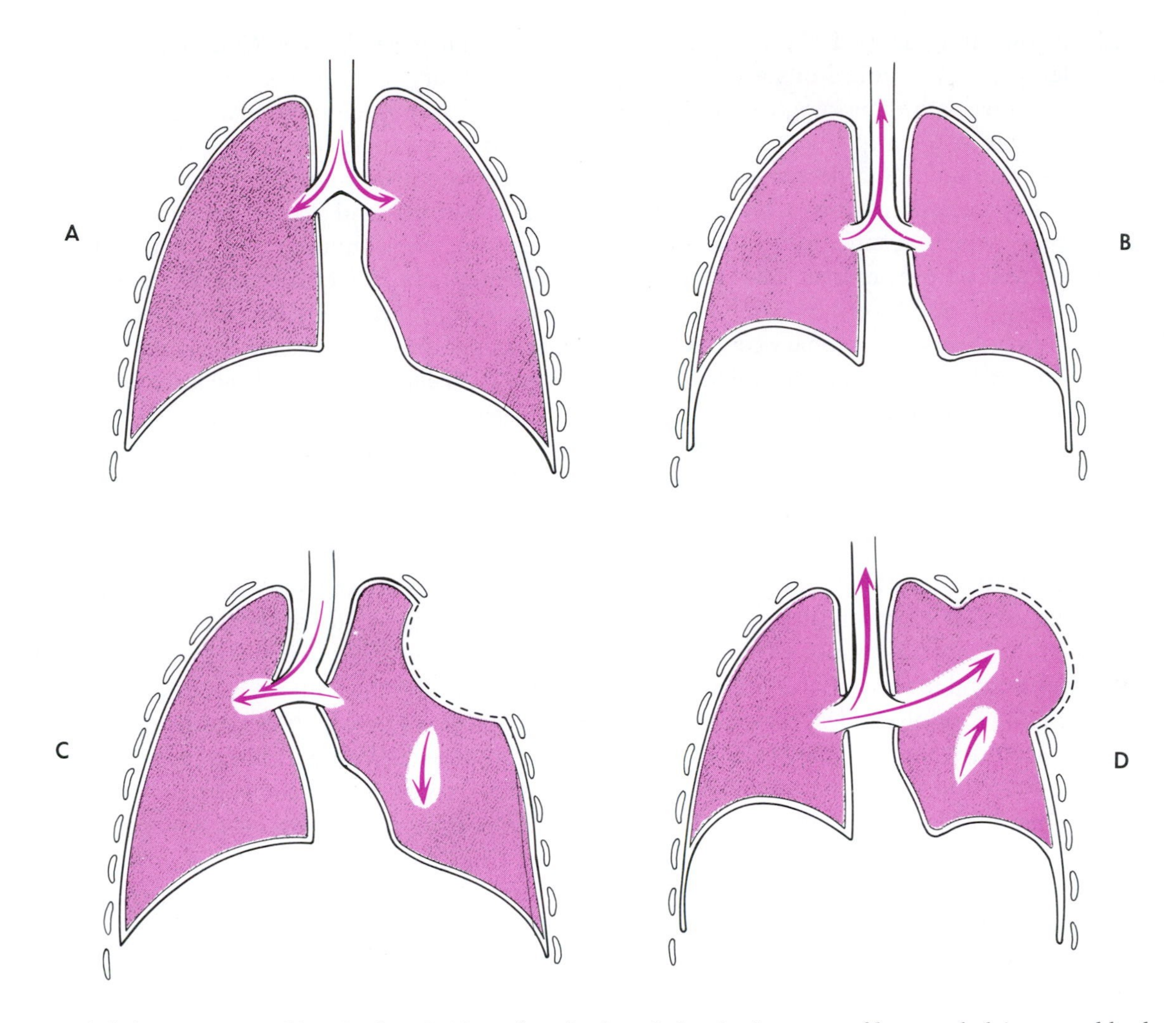

FIGURE 43-9. Flail chest. **A,** Normal inspiration. **B,** Normal expiration. **C,** Inspiration: area of lung underlying unstable chest wall sucks in on inspiration. **D,** Same area balloons out on expiration. Note movement of mediastinum toward opposite lung on inspiration. (From Long BC, Phipps WJ, Cassmeyer VL: *Medical-surgical nursing: a nursing process approach,* ed 3, St Louis, 1993, Mosby.)

dent. The force can cause the diaphragm, which offers little resistance, to rupture or tear. Abdominal viscera then can gradually enter the thoracic cavity, moving from the positive pressure of the abdomen to the negative pressure in the thorax. The stomach and colon are the most commonly herniated viscera.[45] Diaphragmatic rupture can be life-threatening. Massive herniation of abdominal contents into the thoracic cavity can compress the lungs and mediastinum, which then hampers venous return and leads to decreased cardiac output. In addition, herniated bowel can become strangulated and perforate.

Diaphragmatic herniation may produce significant compromise and changes in respiratory effort. Auscultation of bowel sounds in the chest or unilateral breath sounds may indicate a ruptured diaphragm. The patient may complain of shoulder pain, shortness of breath, or abdominal tenderness. The chest film findings may be normal in 25% to 30% of cases.[45] An abnormal finding often reveals the tip of a nasogastric tube above the diaphragm, a unilaterally elevated hemidiaphragm, a hollow or solid mass above the diaphragm, and a shift of the mediastinum away from the affected side. Treatment of a ruptured diaphragm includes its immediate repair.

Pulmonary injuries

Pulmonary contusion. A pulmonary contusion is fundamentally a bruise of the lung. Pulmonary contusion is frequently associated with blunt trauma and other chest injuries such as rib fractures and flail chest. Pulmonary contusions can occur unilaterally or bilaterally. A contusion occurs initially as a hemorrhage followed by alveolar and interstitial edema. The edema can remain rather localized in the contused area or can spread to other lung areas. Inflammation affects alveolar-capillary units. As more units are affected by inflammation, further pathophysiologic events can occur, including decreased compliance, increased pulmonary vascular resistance, and decreased pulmonary blood flow. These processes result in a ventilation/perfusion imbalance, which results in hypoxemia and poor ventilation that progresses over a 24- to 48-hour period.

Clinical manifestations of pulmonary contusion may take up to 24 to 48 hours to develop. Inspections of the chest wall may reveal ecchymosis at the site of impact. Moist rales may be noted in the contused lung. A cough may be present with blood-tinged sputum. Abnormal lung function can be detected by systemic arterial hypoxemia. The diagnosis is made primarily by chest x-ray consistent with pulmonary infiltrate corresponding to the area of external chest impact that is manifested within 12 to 24 hours of injury.[46] Pulmonary contusions tend to worsen over a 24 to 48 hour period and then slowly resolve unless complications occur (infection, ARDS).[46] Nursing diagnoses for the patient with pulmonary contusions may include Impaired Gas Exchange, Risk for Infection, Acute Pain, Decreased Tissue Perfusion, and Ineffective Airway Clearance.

Aggressive respiratory care is the cornerstone for care of nonintubated patients with pulmonary contusion.[46] Interventions include ambulation, deep-breathing exercises, turning, and incentive spirometry. Chest physiotherapy is not tolerated if there are co-existing rib fractures. Aggressive removal of airway secretions is important to avoid infection and to improve ventilation. Patients with unilateral contusions are placed with the injured side up and uninjured side down ("down with the good lung"). Patients with severe contusions may continue to show decompensation despite aggressive nursing management. Respiratory acidosis, increases in peak airway pressures, and increased work of breathing may require endotracheal intubation and mechanical ventilation with positive end-expiratory pressure (PEEP). Patients with significant pulmonary contusion may require nonconventional modes of ventilation, including synchronous independent lung ventilation (SILV), high frequency jet ventilation, and pressure controlled ventilation with permissive hypercapnia.[46] Because pulmonary injury can produce pulmonary interstitial edema, aggressive IV fluid administration must be avoided. If aggressive fluid resuscitation is required to improve cardiac output, the pulmonary artery wedge pressure must be maintained at approximately 15 mm Hg.[46] Adequate pain control is accomplished with administration of opiates or intercostal nerve blocks. Complications resulting from pulmonary contusions include pneumonia, ARDS, lung abscesses, emphysema, and pulmonary embolism. Despite advances in trauma and critical care, the mortality rate from pulmonary contusion is 15%, and factors that portend a poor outcome include shock, coexisting head injury, flail chest, falls from heights greater than 20 feet, advanced age, and preexisting disease (coronary artery disease, chronic obstructive pulmonary disease). (∞Acute Respiratory Distress Syndrome, p 660; Pneumonia, p 663; Pulmonary Embolism, p 668; Pain Management, p 180.)

Tension pneumothorax. A tension pneumothorax usually is caused by an injury that perforates the chest wall or pleural space. Air flows into the pleural space with inspiration and becomes trapped. As pressure in the pleural space increases, the lung on the injured side collapses and causes the mediastinum to shift to the opposite side. (Figure 43-10). As pressure continues to build, the shift exerts pressure on the heart and thoracic aorta, which results in decreased venous return and decreased cardiac output. Tissue perfusion with oxygenated blood is further hampered because the collapsed lung cannot participate in ventilation.

Clinical manifestations of a pneumothorax include dyspnea or sudden chest pain extending to the shoulders. Tracheal deviation will be noted as the trachea shifts away from the injured side. On the injured side, breath sounds can be decreased or absent. Neck vein distention, cyanosis, and respiratory distress also may be present. Percussion of the chest reveals a hyperresonant sound caused by the trapped air. Diagnosis of tension pneumothorax is made by clinical assessment. There is no time for a chest film inasmuch as this potentially lethal condition must be treated immediately. A large-bore (14-gauge) needle or chest tube is inserted into the affected lung. This procedure allows immediate release of air from the pleural space. A hissing sound is heard as the tension pneumothorax is converted to a simple pneumothorax. Nursing diagnoses for a patient with a tension pneumothorax include Decreased Cardiac Output and Impaired Gas Exchange.

Open pneumothorax. An open pneumothorax, or "sucking chest wound," usually is caused by penetrating trauma. Open communication between the atmosphere and intrathoracic pressure results in immediate lung deflation. Air moves in and out of the hole in the chest, producing a sucking sound heard on inspiration.

An open pneumothorax produces the same symptoms as does a tension pneumothorax. In addition,

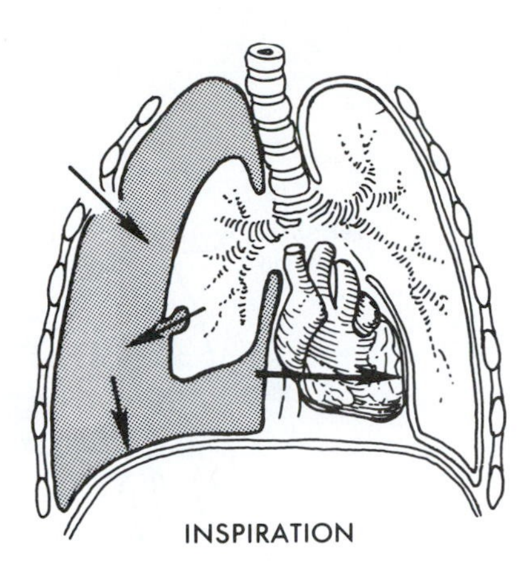

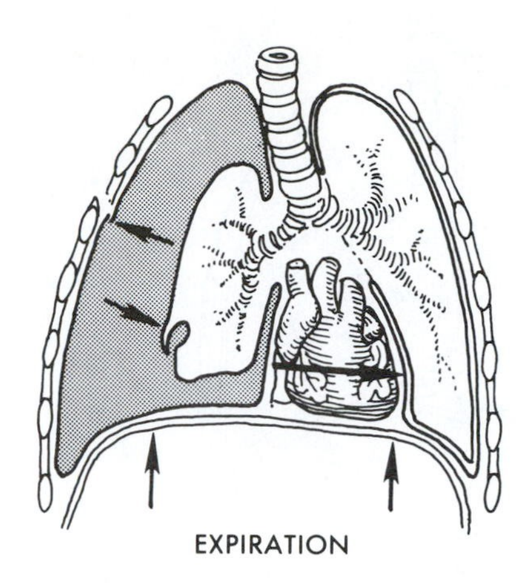

FIGURE 43-10. A tension pneumothorax usually is caused by an injury that perforates the chest wall or pleural space. Air flows into the pleural space with inspiration and becomes trapped. As pressure in the pleural space increases, the lung on the injured side collapses and causes the mediastinum to shift to the opposite side. (From Rosen P and others: *Emergency medicine: concepts and clinical practice,* ed 3, St Louis, 1992, Mosby.)

subcutaneous emphysema may be palpated around the wound. Patients with an open pneumothorax have some degree of alteration in cardiac output and gas exchange unless treated immediately. The wound must be occluded at once. A dressing of petrolatum (Vaseline) gauze, plastic wrap, or any other occlusive substance must be applied. The dressing is applied at the end of expiration and with only three sides taped to the skin surface. This allows the fourth side to act as a valve so that the open pneumothorax does not become a tension pneumothorax. Definitive management includes placement of a chest tube. Surgical intervention may be required to close the wound.

Hemothorax. Blunt or penetrating thoracic trauma can cause bleeding into the pleural space to produce a hemothorax (Figure 43-11). A massive hemothorax can cause a blood loss of more than 1500 m.[4] The source of bleeding may be the intercostal or internal mammary arteries, lungs, heart, or great vessels. Increasing intrapleural pressure results in a decrease in vital capacity. Increasing vascular blood loss into the pleural space causes decreased venous return and decreased cardiac output.

Assessment findings for patients with a hemothorax include hypovolemic shock and decreased breath sounds in the injured lung. With hemothorax, the neck veins are collapsed and the trachea is at midline. Massive hemothorax can be diagnosed on the basis of clinical manifestations of hypotension associated with the absence of breath sounds and/or dullness to percussion on one side of the chest.[4] Nursing diagnoses for a patient with a hemothorax include Fluid Volume Deficit, with resulting Decreased Cardiac Output, and

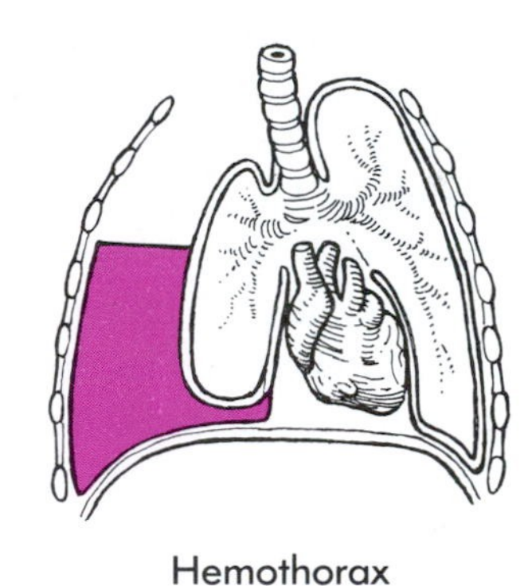

FIGURE 43-11. Blunt or penetrating thoracic trauma can cause bleeding into the pleural space to form a hemothorax.

Impaired Gas Exchange. This life-threatening condition must be treated immediately. Resuscitation with IV fluids is initiated to treat the hypovolemic shock. A chest tube is placed on the affected side to allow drainage of blood. An autotransfusion device can be attached to the chest tube collection chamber. Thoracotomy may be required for patients with significant bleeding (more than 1500 ml) and patients who have sustained deep, penetrating lung injuries; intercostal artery injuries; or injuries to major cardiovascular structures.[47]

Cardiac injuries

Penetrating cardiac injuries. Penetrating cardiac trauma can occur from mechanical injuries as a result of bullets, knives, or impalements. The chest wall offers little protection to the heart from penetrating trauma. The most common site of injury is the right ventricle because of its anterior position. Mortality

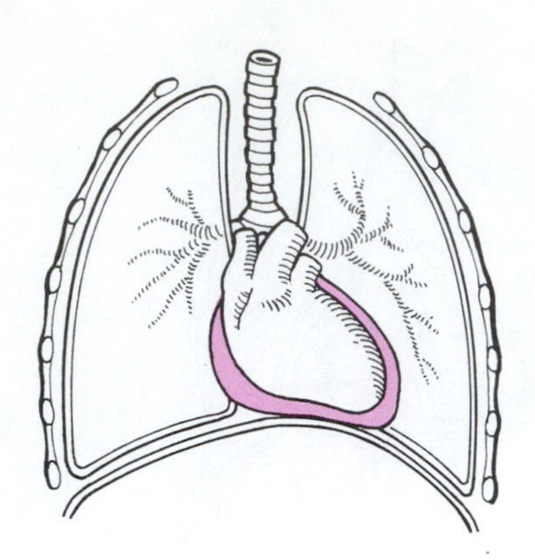

FIGURE 43-12. Cardiac tamponade is the progressive accumulation of blood in the pericardial sac.

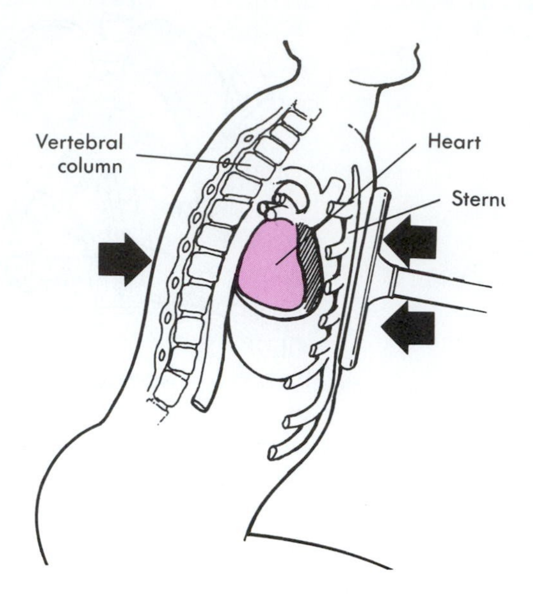

FIGURE 43-13. Blunt cardiac trauma. Sudden acceleration (as from contact with the steering wheel) can cause the heart to be thrown against the sternum.

from penetrating trauma to the heart is high. Prehospital mortality for penetrating cardiac injuries is 75%, and most deaths occur within 4 or 5 minutes after injury as a result of exsanguination or tamponade.[48]

Cardiac tamponade. Cardiac tamponade is the progressive accumulation of blood in the pericardial sac (Figure 43-12). With cardiac tamponade a progressive accumulation of blood, 120 to 150 ml, increases the intracardial pressure and compresses the atria and ventricles. Increased intracardial pressures lead to decreased venous return and decreased filling pressure, which lead to decreased cardiac output, myocardial hypoxia, cardiac failure, and cardiogenic shock.

Classic assessment findings associated with cardiac tamponade are termed *Beck's triad*—presence of elevated central venous pressure with neck vein distension, muffled heart sounds, and pulsus paradoxus. An ECG may reveal tachycardia with altered QRS complexes. The major nursing diagnosis for this injury is Decreased Cardiac Output. Immediate treatment is required to remove the accumulation of fluid in the pericardial sac. Pericardiocentesis involves the aspiration of fluid from the pericardium by use of a large-bore needle. The inherent risk in this procedure is potential laceration of the coronary artery. Other approaches include surgical procedures, such as thoracotomy or median sternotomy. The goal of these procedures is to locate and control the source of bleeding.

Blunt cardiac injuries. The most common causes of blunt cardiac trauma include high-speed MVCs, direct blows to the chest, and falls. The heart, because of its mobility and its location between the sternum and thoracic vertebrae, is susceptible to blunt traumatic injury. Sudden acceleration (as from contact with the steering wheel) can cause the heart to be thrown against the sternum (Figure 43-13). Sudden deceleration can cause the heart to be thrown against the thoracic vertebrae by a direct blow to the chest (baseball, animal kick, fall). Myocardial contusion is one of the most common injuries sustained as a result of blunt cardiac trauma.

Myocardial contusion. Myocardial cell injury results from the contusion. Histologically, contusions exhibit well-demarcated zones of hemorrhage, which are well-confined to the site of injury, as opposed to a more widespread pattern, as seen with infarction.[49] If the contusion is large enough and has resulted in a large area of myonecrosis, the patient may experience the same complications as those of an acute myocardial infarction. The right ventricle most often is affected because of its proximity to the sternum.

Diagnosis of myocardial contusion continues to be an area of controversy. Assessment findings associated with myocardial contusion depend on the extent and location of myocardial injury. The patient may be symptom-free or complain of dyspnea and precordial pain that is similar to that of angina, except that it typically is not relieved by nitroglycerin. If the contusion is large enough to affect cardiac output, hypotension may be present.

The initial ECG performed in the emergency room (ER) is a sensitive and specific diagnostic test that can detect real and potential cardiac morbidity following blunt chest trauma.[49] High risk patients (older than 65 years or patients with coronary artery disease) may be screened with additional ECGs over several days for the possibility of "late" myocardial infarctions. There are no "classic" ECG abnormalities seen with myocardial confusion, although the most prevalent abnormalities include PVCs and AV blocks.[49] Creatinine phosphokinase-myocardial band (CPK-MB) serum assays may be used in the diagnosis of myocardial contusion; however, they have severe limitations. CPK-MB values can be elevated in the patient with multiple trauma from crush injuries and injuries to skeletal muscle, lung, pancreas, liver, and gastrointestinal tissues. The level of CPK-MB considered diagnostic of myocardial confusion has not been determined.[49] CPK-MP isoenzyme levels may be obtained on the patient's admission to the ER and then every 6 to 8 hours for 24 hours to assess for the degree of myocardial damage.[50] Two-dimensional echocardiography (ECHO) can be used to determine structural abnormalities in pump failure, cardiac tamponade, and apical thrombi.[49]

Patients with isolated blunt chest trauma rarely require CCU care. Most require short-term monitoring in a telemetry setting. CCU care may be required for elderly patients, those with extensive cardiac histories, and those with significant multisystem trauma.[49] Medical management of these patients is aimed at preventing and treating complications. This may include the administration of antidysrhythmic medications, treatment of acute heart failure, insertion of a temporary pacemaker to control heart block, or the use of intraaortic balloon pump for severe cardiac failure.[48] (∞Temporary Pacemakers, p. 529; Intraaortic Balloon Pump, p. 567.)

Nursing diagnoses for the patient with a myocardial contusion include Decreased Cardiac Output, Altered Coronary Tissue Perfusion, and Acute Pain. Nursing interventions include: (1) monitor for dysrhythmia presence/development, (2) monitor for alteration in myocardial perfusion, (3) assess for signs and symptoms of right heart failure, and (4) promote patient comfort.[51] Ongoing assessments are imperative inasmuch as clinical manifestations usually appear hours after the injury. Assessment of fluid and electrolyte balance is imperative to ensure adequate cardiac output and myocardial conduction. (∞Cardiac Enzymes, p. 381; Twelve-Lead ECG Analysis, p. 392; Myocardial Infarction, p. 490.)

ABDOMINAL INJURIES

Abdominal injury accounts for 10% of trauma fatalities in the United States.[52] Abdominal injuries frequently are associated with multisystem trauma. Injuries to the abdomen are the result of blunt or penetrating trauma. Two major life-threatening conditions that occur after abdominal trauma are hemorrhage and hollow viscus perforation with its associated peritonitis.

Mechanism of Injury

Blunt trauma. Blunt abdominal injuries are common. They result most frequently from MVCs, falls, and assaults. The spleen is the most commonly injured organ in blunt trauma and ranks second to the liver as the source of life-threatening abdominal injury.[53] In MVCs, abdominal injury is more likely to occur when a vehicle is struck from the side. In the passenger position of the front seat, hepatic injury is likely when the point of impact is on the same side as the passenger. A driver is likely to sustain injury to the spleen when the impact is on the driver's side. Seat belts, which substantially reduce morbidity and mortality, also are associated with causing bladder and bowel rupture.[52] Pedestrians hit by motor vehicles are at risk for serious abdominal injuries. Blunt trauma to the thorax can produce injuries to the liver, spleen, and diaphragm. In spinal cord injury, large abdominal arteries and veins can be injured. Deceleration and direct forces can produce retroperitoneal hematomas. Blunt abdominal injuries often are hidden and are more likely to be fatal than are penetrating abdominal injuries.

Penetrating trauma. Penetrating abdominal trauma generally is caused by knives or bullets. The danger of penetrating abdominal trauma is that the outside appearance of the wound does not determine the extent of internal injury. The most commonly injured organs from knife wounds are the liver, spleen, diaphragm, and colon.[54] Gunshot wounds to the abdomen usually are more serious than are stab wounds. A bullet destroys tissue along its path. Once inside the abdomen, a bullet can travel in erratic paths and ricochet off bone. Death from penetrating injuries depends on the injury to major vascular structures and resultant intraabdominal hemorrhage.

Assessment

The initial assessment of the trauma patient, whether in the emergency department or the critical care unit, follows the primary and secondary survey techniques as outlined by ATLS and TNCC guidelines. Specific assessment findings associated with abdominal trauma are reviewed here.

Physical assessment. The location of entry and exit sites associated with penetrating trauma are assessed and documented. Inspection of the patient's abdomen may reveal purplish discoloration of the flanks or umbilicus (Cullen's sign), which is indicative of blood in the abdominal wall. Ecchymosis in the flank area (Grey Turner's sign) may indicate retroperitoneal bleeding or a possible fracture of the pancreas. A hematoma in the flank area is suggestive of renal injury. A distended abdomen may indicate the accumulation of blood, fluid, or gas secondary to a perforated organ or ruptured blood vessel. Serial measurement of abdominal girths can be helpful. The increase of abdominal girth by 1 inch can indicate intraabdominal accumulation of 500 to 1000 ml of blood.[55] Auscultation of the abdomen may reveal friction rubs over the liver or spleen and may indicate rupture. The abdomen is assessed for rebound tenderness and rigidity. Presence of these assessment findings indicates peritoneal inflammation. Referred pain to the left shoulder (Kehr's sign) may indicate a ruptured spleen or irritation of the diaphragm from bile or other material in the peritoneum. Subcutaneous emphysema palpated on the abdomen suggests free air as a result of a ruptured bowel.

Diagnostic procedures. Insertion of a nasogastric tube and urinary catheter serves as a useful diagnostic and therapeutic aid. A nasogastric tube can decompress the stomach, and the contents can be checked for blood. Urine obtained from the urinary catheter can be tested for the presence of blood.

Serial laboratory test results may be nonspecific for the patient with abdominal trauma. A serum amylase determination can detect pancreatic injuries. Initial leukocytosis can suggest splenic or hepatic injury. Because of hemoconcentration, hemoglobin and hematocrit results may not reflect actual values. Serial values are more valuable in diagnosing abdominal injuries.

Diagnostic peritoneal lavage (DPL) can exclude or confirm the presence of intraabdominal injury with a high accuracy rate. DPL is indicated for trauma patients with equivocal abdominal findings on physical assessment or for patients who are not alert and oriented enough to provide accurate information or cannot respond appropriately to physical asessments.[56] After the patient's bladder has been emptied, a small incision is made in the abdomen through the skin and into the peritoneum. A small catheter is inserted (Figure 43-14). If frank blood is encountered, intraabdominal injury is obvious and the patient is taken immediately to the (OR). If gross blood is not initially encountered, a liter of fluid (lactated Ringer's or 0.9% normal saline) is infused through the catheter into the abdomen. The IV bag is then placed in a dependent position and allowed to drain. The drainage fluid is sent to the laboratory for analysis. Positive DPL results signal intraabdominal trauma and usually necessitate surgical intervention (Box 43-13).

Abdominal CT scanning can detect retroperitoneal hemorrhage, can localize specific site(s) of abdominal injury, and can determine the relative severity of intraperitoneal or retroperitoneal hemorrhage.[56]

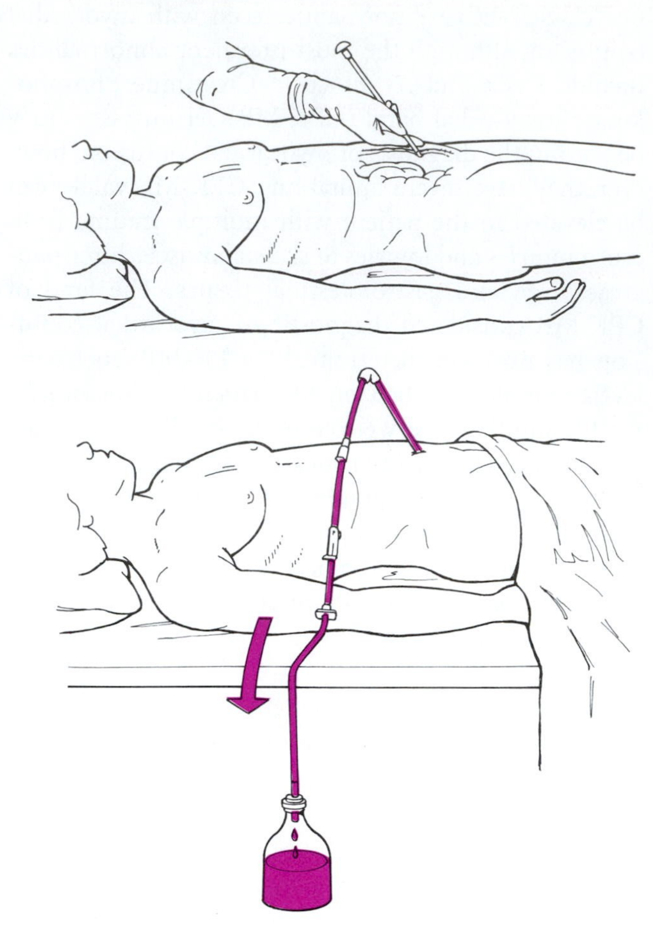

FIGURE 43-14. Diagnostic peritoneal lavage (DPL) can exclude or confirm the presence of intraabdominal injury with a high accuracy rate.

Combined Abdominal Organ Injuries

Patients with multivisceral injuries may require surgical intervention that uses somewhat nontraditional techniques, referred to as "damage control" or "planned reoperation." Planned reoperation is a strategy designed to reinstitute hemodynamic stability before anatomy reconstruction. There are three phases to this treatment strategy: initial operation, CCU resuscitation, and planned reoperation.[57] The initial operation occurs shortly after ER initial assessment and resuscitation. The goal of the operative procedure is to control bleeding and prevent spillage of intestinal content or urine into the peritoneal cavity and to rapidly close the abdominal cavity.[58] The duration of this initial operation is kept to a minimum. Hypothemia induced by an open visceral cavity in conjunction with massive blood transfusion can lead to coagulopathy and continued bleeding, which results in shock and metabolic acidosis. The triad of hypother-

BOX 43-13 Positive Diagnostic Peritoneal Lavage Results

- Red blood cell count: 100,000/mm^3
- White blood cell count: 500/mm^3
- Amylase: 175 U/dL
- Presence of blood, stool, bile, bacteria

mia, coagulopathy, and acidosis creates a self-propagating cycle that can eventually lead to an irreversible physiologic insult.[58] The initial operation must be completed quickly to terminate this self-propagating cycle. Reconstruction and formal closure of the wound are not completed at this time. The patient is transferred to the CCU.

The goal of the CCU phase of this strategy is to continue aggressive resuscitation and correct hypothermia, coagulopathy, and acidosis. The patient's first few hours in the CCU are labor intensive.[58] Active rewarming techniques, described in Box 43-14, are used to correct hypothermia. Warmed IV solutions are administered to patients with a temperature equal to or less than 35° C.[49] The patient is warmed 0.5° C/hr, and his or her temperature is assessed every 30 to 60 minutes.[49] Coagulation factors and platelets may be given to correct coagulopathies. An $S\bar{v}O_2$ pulmonary artery catheter may be used to guide fluid resuscitation, inotropic support, and oxygenation to prevent further development of acidosis. (∞Continuous Monitoring of Mixed Venous Oxygen Saturation $S\bar{v}O_2$, p. 471.)

The patient is assessed for additional complications, including ongoing hemorrhage and abdominal compartment syndrome. Abdominal compartment syndrome is a condition in which increased pressure within the abdominal cavity compromises circulation, resulting in ischemia and necrosis of tissues and organs within the abdominal cavity. The increased pressure can be caused by bleeding, ileus, visceral edema, or a noncompliant abdominal wall. Increased abdominal cavity pressure can impinge on diaphragmatic excursion and can also affect ventilation. Clinical manifestations of abdominal compartment syndrome include hypotension, oliguria, tense abdominal distention, and impaired ventilatory function.[58] Treatment consist of decompression, either in the CCU or in the OR.[59]

Once the patient is hemodynamically stable, and the triangle of hypothermia, coagulopathy, and acidosis

BOX 43-14 Active Rewarming Techniques

- Administer high volumes of IV fluid with high-volume fluid administration devices that have a pump and compressor capable of administering warmed (35–38°C) volumes at high flow rates.
- Warm IV solutions: microwave 1 L of normal saline solution on high for 1 minute; shake bag well; check temperature by folding bag over thermometer; repeat until desired solution temperature is 35–38°C.
- Administer blood with blood warming devices.
- Raise ambient temperature of room; keep patient covered.
- Warm inspired air with ventilator cascade.
- Use heat lamps or other external warming devices carefully.

From Christensen MA, Sutton KR: *Am J Crit Care* 2:28, 1993.

has been corrected, the patient is taken back to the OR for the planned operation. This usually occurs within 48 hours of the initial operation. It is during this phase that definitive repairs and wound closure are made. Postoperatively, the patient is transported back to the CCU for continued care, which is usually not as labor intensive as the initial CCU phase.

Specific Organ Injuries

Physical assessment findings, DPL, and CT scanning aid in making a diagnosis of specific abdominal organ injury. The medical and nursing management vary according to specific organ injuries. Liver, spleen, bowel, and pancreatic injuries, which are seen more commonly, are discussed here.

Liver injuries. The liver is the primary organ injured in penetrating trauma and the second most commonly injured organ in blunt trauma. Detection of liver injury, as with all intraabdominal injury, is accomplished through the use of physical assessment and DPL or CT scan. The severity of liver injuries is graded to provide a mechanism for determining the amount of trauma sustained by that organ, the care needed, and possible outcomes (Table 43-4). Until recently, most liver injuries required operative repair to accomplish hemostasis and healing. Recent evidence supports that patients who have sustained blunt liver injuries who are hemodynamically stable and do not require ongoing blood transfusions for their liver injury may be amenable to nonoperative treatment.[60] Patients with penetrating or blunt liver trauma who are hemodynamically unstable usually

TABLE 43-4 Liver Injury Scale (1994 Revision)

Grade*		Injury Descrition
I	Hematoma	Subcapsular, <10% surface area
	Laceration	Capsular tear, <1 cm parenchymal depth
II	Hematoma	Subcapsular, 10%-50% surface area; intraparenchymal <10 cm in diameter
	Laceration	Capsular tear, 1-3 cm parenchymal depth, <10 cm in length
III	Hematoma	Subcapsular, >50% surface area or expanding; ruptured subcapsular or parenchymal hematoma; intraparenchymal hematoma >10 cm or expanding
	Laceration	>3 cm parenchymal depth
IV	Laceration	Parenchymal disruption involving 25%-75% of hepatic lobe or 1-3 Couinaud's segments within a single lobe
V	Laceration	Parenchymal disruption involving >75% of hepatic lobe or >3 Couinaud's segments within a single lobe
	Vascular	Juxtahepatic venous injuries (i.e., retrohepatic vena cava/central major hepatic veins)
	Vascular	Hepatic avulsion

Modified from Moore EE and others: *Surg Clin North Am* 74:295, 1995.
*Advance one grade for multiple injuries up to Grade III.

require surgical intervention to correct the defect. Resection of the devitalized tissue is required for massive injuries. Hemorrhage is common with liver injuries, and ligation of the hepatic arteries or veins may be required to control hemorrhage. Drains may be placed intraoperatively to drain areas of blood and to prevent hematomas. Care of the patient with severe liver injuries can be challenging for the critical care nurse. Lack of hemodynamic stability can result from hemorrhage and hypovolemic shock, leading to fluid volume deficit, decreased cardiac output, and decreased tissue perfusion. Combinations of crystalloid and colloid IV solutions may be used to correct hypovolemia. Fresh frozen plasma, platelets, and cryoprecipitate may be administered to correct coagulopathies. A crucial nursing responsibility is to monitor the patient's response to medical therapies. Continued hemodynamic instability (hypotension, decreased cardiac output) in spite of aggressive medical intervention may indicate continued hemorrhage, in which case an exploratory laparotomy may be required to determine and correct the source of bleeding. The patient's postoperative CCU course may be complicated by coagulopathy, acidosis, and/or hypothermia. Jaundice may occur and be a sign of hepatic dysfunction, but more commonly it is related to resorption of hematomas, breakdown of transfused blood, or mild hepatic dysfunction.[61]

Spleen injuries. The spleen is the organ most commonly injured by blunt abdominal trauma and is second to the liver as a source of life-threatening hemorrhage. Spleen injuries, like liver injuries, are graded for determining the amount of trauma sustained, the care needed, and possible outcomes (Table 43-5). The treatment of an injured spleen is controversial because of the spleen's importance in preventing infection. Hemodynamically stable patients may be monitored in the critical care unit by means of serial hematocrit values and vital signs. Progressive deterioration may indicate the need for operative management. Patients who exhibit with hemodynamic instability require operative intervention with splenectomy, partial splenectomy, or splenorraphy. Patients who have had a splenectomy are at risk for the development of overwhelming postsplenectomy sepsis with streptococcal pneumonia. These patients require polyvalent pneumococcal vaccine (Pneumovax) to help promote immunity against most pneumococcal bacteria. Patients with isolated spleen injuries that require surgical intervention rarely are admitted to the critical care unit. Complications after splenic trauma include wound infection; sepsis; subdiaphragmatic abscess; and fistulas of the colon, pancreas, and stomach.

Intestinal injuries. Intestinal injuries can result from blunt or penetrating trauma. Regardless of mechanism of injury, intestinal contents (bile, stool, enzymes, bacteria) leak into the peritoneum and cause peritonitis. Surgical resection and repair are required. The patient's postoperative course is dictated by the amount of spillage of intestinal contents. The patient is observed for signs of sepsis and abscess or fistula formation.

Pancreatic injuries. Pancreatic injury rarely occurs alone. Death is related directly to the number of associated injuries. Penetrating wounds that cause injury to the pancreas require immediate surgical intervention. The diagnosis of pancreatic injury as a result of blunt trauma is difficult. Elevated serum amylase levels may not occur for 24 hours or more after injury. Diagnostic CT findings of pancreatic edema and fluid

TABLE 43-5 Spleen Injury Scale (1994 Revision)

	Grade*	Injury Description
I	Hematoma	Subcapsular, <10% surface area
	Laceration	Capsular tear, <1 cm parenchymal depth
II	Hematoma	Subcapsular, 10%-50% surface area; intraparenchymal <5 cm in diameter
	Laceration	Capsular tear: 1-3 cm parenchymal depth, which does not involve a trabecular vessel
III	Hematoma	Subcapsular, >50% surface area or expanding; ruptured subcapsular or parenchymal hematoma; intraparenchymal hematoma >5 cm or expanding
	Laceration	>3 cm parenchymal depth or involving trabecular vessels
IV	Laceration	Laceration involving segmental or hilar vessels producing major devascularization (>25% of spleen)
V	Laceration	Completely shattered spleen
	Vascular	Hilar vascular injury that devascularizes spleen

Modified from Moore EE and others: *Surg Clin North Am* 74:295, 1995.
*Advance one grade for multiple injuries up to Grade III.

may not develop for 24 to 48 hours after injury. Surgical intervention is required if there is any question of pancreatic injury. Postoperatively the patient must be assessed for complications of pancreatitis, pancreatic fistulas and pseudocysts, intraabdominal abscesses, and pancreatic insufficiency. Serial glucose and amylase levels are monitored. Meticulous skin care around drainage tube insertion sites is necessary to prevent breakdown from pancreatic enzymes. Displacement of intraoperatively placed drainage tubes must be brought to the physician's attention immediately.

GENITOURINARY INJURIES

Trauma to the genitourinary (GU) tract seldom occurs as an isolated injury. An associated GU injury must be suspected in any patient with penetrating trauma to the torso; pelvic fracture; blunt trauma to the lower chest or flank; contusions, hematoma, or tenderness over the flank, lower abdomen, or perineum; genital swelling or discoloration; blood at the urethral meatus; hematuria after Foley catheter placement; or difficulty with micturation.[62]

Mechanism of Injury

GU injuries, like all other traumatic injuries, can result from blunt or penetrating trauma. Blunt GU trauma can be caused by deceleration injuries, and penetrating injuries can occur with stabbings or gunshot wounds to the abdomen or back.

Assessment. Evaluation of GU trauma begins after the primary survey has been conducted and immediate life-threatening conditions have been effectively managed. The conscious patient may complain of flank pain or colic pain. Rebound tenderness can be elicited if intraperitoneal extravasation of urine has occurred. Inspection may reveal abdominal contusions, developing hematomas, and blood at the urethral meatus. Bluish discoloration of the flanks may indicate retroperitoneal bleeding, whereas perineal discoloration may indicate a pelvic fracture and possible bladder or urethral injury. Auscultation of an abdominal bruit can signify renal vascular injury. Results of serum laboratory tests are nonspecific for GU trauma, although blood urea nitrogen (BUN) and creatinine levels are obtained initially and monitored intermittently for trends. Hematuria is the most common assessment finding with GU trauma; however, the absence of gross or microscopic hematuria does not exclude a urinary tract injury.[62]

Specific Genitourinary Injuries

Renal trauma. Most renal trauma is caused by blunt trauma, resulting in contusions or lacerations without urinary extravasation. Renal injuries are graded for determining the amount of trauma sustained, the care need, and possible outcomes (Table 43-6). CT scan is the most accurate modality available for staging renal injuries because it can assess the extent of parenchymal laceration, urine extravasation, surrounding hemorrhage, and the presence of vascular injury.[62] Contusions and minor lacerations can usually be treated with observation whereas major lacerations and vascular injuries require operative intervention.[62] Postoperative complications can include infection, hemorrhage, infarction, extravasation, calcification, acute tubular necrosis, and hypertension.

Ureteral trauma. Injury to the ureters is the least common result of trauma to the GU tract because the ureters are protected anteriorly by the abdominal contents and musculature and posteriorly by the psoas muscle. The patient with ureteral trauma may complain of flank pain, and hematuria may be a presenting symptom. As in renal trauma, the degree of hematuria is not indicative of the severity of injury. A "missed" ureteral injury can result in intraperitoneal

TABLE 43-6 Kidney Injury Scale

	Grade*	Injury Description
I	Contusion	Microscopic or gross hematuria, urologic studies normal
	Hematoma	
II	Hematoma	Subcapsular, nonexpanding without parenchymal laceration
		Nonexpanding perirenal hematoma confined to renal retroperitoneum
	Laceration	<1.0 cm parenchymal depth of renal cortex without urinary extravasation
III	Laceration	<1.0 cm parenchymal depth of renal cortex without collecting system rupture or urinary extravasation
IV	Laceration	Parenchymal laceration extending through the renal cortex, medulla, and collecting system
	Vascular	Main renal artery or vein injury with contained hemorrhage
V	Laceration	Completely shattered kidney
	Vascular	Avulsion of renal hilum, which devascularizes kidney

Modified from Moore EE and others: *Surg Clin North Am* 75:299, 1995.
*Advance one grade for multiple injuries up to Grade III.

extravasation and produce peritoneal signs. Ureteral injuries are surgically repaired.

Bladder trauma. Most bladder injuries are the result of blunt trauma. Bladder injuries are classified as contusions, extraperitoneal ruptures, intraperitoneal ruptures, or combined injuries. The type of injury that occurs depends not only on the location and strength of the blunt force, but also on the volume of urine in the bladder at the time of injury.[63] Urinary extravasation is the hallmark sign of a ruptured bladder. Definitive diagnosis of bladder rupture is made by means of cystographic examination.

Nursing Management

Nursing diagnoses that can be applicable in caring for a patient with GU trauma include Altered Tissue Perfusion, Pain, Risk for Infection, and Risk for Fluid Volume Deficit.

After the patient is admitted to the critical care unit, the nurse makes an assessment according to ATLS and TNCC guidelines. Once the patient's condition has stabilized, nursing management of postoperative renal trauma is similar to that for GU surgery. The primary nursing interventions include assessment for hemorrhage, maintenance of fluid and electrolyte balance, and maintenance of patency of drains and tubes. Measurement of urinary output includes drainage from the urinary catheter and the nephrostomy or suprapubic tubes. Drainage from these areas is recorded separately. Urine output is measured hourly until bloody drainage and clots have cleared. Renal function is assessed by monitoring serum BUN and creatinine levels.

PELVIC FRACTURES

The pelvis is a ring-shaped structure composed of the hip bones, sacrum, and coccyx. Because the pelvis protects the lower urinary tract and major blood vessels and nerves of the lower extremities, pelvic trauma can result in life-threatening urologic and neurologic dysfunction and in hemorrhage.[64]

Mechanism of Injury

Blunt trauma to the pelvis can be caused by MVCs, falls, or a crushing accident. Most pelvic injuries involve fractures, with or without damage to underlying tissues. Pelvic injuries frequently are associated with motorcycle accidents and accidents that involve pedestrians and vehicles. Any patient who has been projected from a vehicle must be suspected of having a pelvic fracture.

Assessment

Signs of pelvic fracture include perineal ecchymosis (testicular or labial) indicating extravasation of urine or blood, pain on palpation or "rocking" of the iliac crests, lower limb paresis or hypesthesia, hematuria, and shortening of a lower extremity.

An anteroposterior x-ray film of the pelvis permits classification of a fracture as stable or unstable. Stable fractures usually are breaks in the pelvic ring, sacrum, or coccyx, with no displacement. Unstable fractures are breaks that occur in more than one place or in the acetabulum.

Classification of Pelvic Fractures

Minor. Minor pelvic fractures include breaks of individual bones without a break in continuity of the pelvic ring, or a single break in the pelvic ring.

Major. Major pelvic fractures involve double breaks in the pelvic ring. These fractures commonly are seen in patients in the critical care unit with multiple trauma. The condition of patients with posterior pelvic fractures is very unstable. The nearby iliac arteries frequently are damaged and can cause massive internal bleeding.

Straddle fracture

The four-ramus, or "straddle," fracture consists of bilateral fractures of the superior and inferior pubic rami. With this fracture comes a high incidence of associated injuries, especially lower urinary tract injuries.

Malgaigne's hemipelvis fracture dislocation. This fracture includes a variety of fracture patterns that have three separate injury components (Box 43-15). These fractures always are unstable and the result of severe trauma.

Open fractures. Open pelvic fractures involve an open wound with direct communication between the pelvic fractures and the buttocks, perineum, groin, pubis, or lower flank. The open wound allows contamination. Mortality rates from open pelvic fractures may exceed 50%.[4]

BOX 43-15 Malgaigne's Pelvic Fractures

Fracture patterns are characterized by three separate injury components:

1. Double vertical breaks in the pelvic ring
2. Anterior break, including fractures of pubic bone, ischial rami, and/or disruption of the pubic symphysis
3. Posterior break, posterior to hip joint; may involve fractures of ilium, or sacrum, and/or disruption of the sacroiliac joint

Medical Management

The priority of the medical management of pelvic fractures is to prevent or to control life-threatening hemorrhage. The use of the pneumatic antishock garment (PASG) has been advocated for stabilization of a hemodynamically unstable patient with pelvic and/or femur fractures.[5] Hemorrhage also may be controlled by placement of an external fixator device or use of therapeutic angiography for embolization of the lacerated vessel.

Almost every patient with a massive open pelvic fracture requires an exploratory laparotomy to treat intraabdominal injuries. A diverting colostomy is performed to prevent ongoing contamination of the pelvic wound from feces.[4] If there are no obvious intraabdominal injuries, the pelvis is stabilized.

Definitive management of pelvic fracture may include placement of internal or external fixation devices. External fixation allows pelvic stabilization until the patient can tolerate surgical open reduction and internal fixation. Using fluoroscopy, the physician inserts two or three pins percutaneously into each iliac crest. The pins are then attached to a rigid metal frame. Patients with fractures of the symphysis pubis, sacroiliac joints, iliac wings, or acetabulum usually undergo open reduction with internal fixation (ORIF).[64] ORIF occurs after bleeding has been controlled, and adequate hemodynamic stability has been achieved. In this procedure the surgeon reduces the fractures with contoured plates and screws. Blood loss from pelvic fractures may exceed 6 U.[4]

Nursing Management

Initial assessment of the patient with a pelvic fracture in the critical care unit proceeds according to ATLS and TNCC guidelines. Nursing diagnoses include Altered Tissue Perfusion, Pain, Risk for Infection, and Risk for Injury.

Massive blood loss contributes to alteration in tissue perfusion. On the patient's admission to the critical care unit, hemodynamic instability, with abnormal coagulation factors, may be present. Interventions include intravenously administered crystalloid and colloid fluids. Accurate assessment of fluid balance and tissue perfusion may require pulmonary artery catheter placement. The nurse must ensure that an appropriate amount of blood remains cross-matched and available if needed. Adequate oxygenation is assessed by means of pulse oximetry and systemic mixed venous oxygen saturation and by monitoring serial hematocrit and hemoglobin levels.

Pelvic fractures can be extremely painful. Nursing interventions include measures to ensure adequate pain control. The patient with pelvic fractures is at risk for infection because of associated injuries and external fixation. Contamination of the pelvic cavity can occur with associated intestinal or GU injuries, or both. Nursing management of external fixation insertion sites is directed at preventing infection. Most institutions have protocols for pin care that require strict compliance.

Risk for injury is secondary to neurovascular compromise, development of compartment syndrome, fat embolism syndrome, and wound infection. These syndromes are discussed in further detail later in this chapter. Routine nursing assessments include neurovascular assessments of the lower extremities. Neurovascular complications are most common with posterior fractures and in any patient who has been treated with PASG. Neurologic injury as a result of pelvic fracture usually is temporary and lasts less than 3 weeks.[64] Open pelvic fractures may necessitate repeated wound debridement in the OR. Aggressive nutrition, fluid, and appropriate antibiotic therapies are imperative. Patients with open pelvic fractures usually have a prolonged critical care course, with varying degrees of complications.

LOWER EXTREMITY ORTHOPEDIC INJURIES

The patient with only orthopedic injuries rarely is admitted to a critical care unit. However, the critical care nurse often encounters a multiple trauma patient who also has sustained lower extremity orthopedic trauma. The critical care nurse must be knowledgeable about orthopedic trauma, mechanism of injury, medical management, and nursing management.

Classification of Fractures

Orthopedic injury frequently occurs as a result of an MVC or a fall. A fracture is caused when a force exceeds the elasticity of the bone.

The classification of fractures is broad and depends on whether there is communication between the bone and outside the body. A closed or simple fracture does not expose the bone to the external environment. An open or compound fracture exposes bone to the external environment. The fracture can be complete, in which at least two pieces of bone are completely separated. A *greenstick* fracture occurs if bone is still hinged on one side. A comminuted fracture is one in which there are three or more fragments of bone. Comminuted fractures often occur as a result of crushing forces that cause the bone to collapse on itself.

Mechanism of Injury

In an MVC the knees of an unrestrained front-seat passenger can impact the dashboard with approximately 4500 pounds of force.[65] The force of this impact can result in posterior fracture-dislocation of the hip, fracture of the femoral shaft, or patellar injury. Lateral collisions can cause injury to the trochanter and head of the femur. Rotational injuries can occur when the vehicle spins.

Assessment

A fracture site is assessed for pain and tenderness, loss of function, deformity, discoloration, altered position, abnormal mobility, crepitus (caused by bone fragments), and neurovascular dysfunction.[65]

Medical Management

Early management and treatment of musculoskeletal trauma, "resuscitative orthopedics," results in fewer complications of musculoskeletal injuries.[66] The major goals of resuscitative orthopedics are prompt hemorrhage control, early management of large wound defects, and reduction and stabilization of fractures.

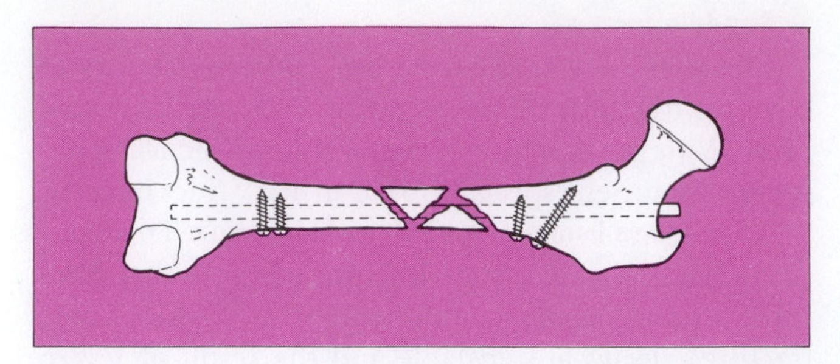

FIGURE 43-15. Interlocking nails can be used for internal fracture fixation.

Orthopedic injuries can be treated with or without surgical fixation. Nonsurgical fixation can be accomplished by aligning the bone fragments in as nearly an anatomic position as possible, then immobilizing the area. Immobilization can be performed internally by use of rods, plates, screws, or wires (Figure 43-15) or externally by the application of an external device (Figure 43-16). External devices, however, increasingly are being viewed as a temporary method of fracture stabilization in the patient with multiple traumatic injuries.

Nursing Management

Nursing management of the patient with orthopedic injuries depends on the method of fracture reduction. Nursing diagnoses include Impaired Physical Mobility, Impaired Skin Integrity, Altered Tissue Perfusion, and Pain.

Nursing interventions focus on assisting the patient to attain the highest level of mobility possible while injuries are healing. Proper position of splints must be ensured. Depending on other system injuries, the patient is encouraged to ambulate as soon as possible to prevent complications associated with immobility. If the patient is unable to get out of bed, a trapeze can be added to the bed frame to assist with mobility in bed.

The patient with orthopedic injuries can have impaired skin integrity as a result of compound fractures. Meticulous wound care is required. Because of their susceptibility to pressure ulcer development, all patients with orthopedic trauma are at risk for impaired skin integrity. A patient in traction cannot be completely turned off his or her back. Skin breakdown caused by the pressure of casts and splints can occur, for example, on the heels of a patient with fractures of the lower extremities and hips. Pillows placed un-

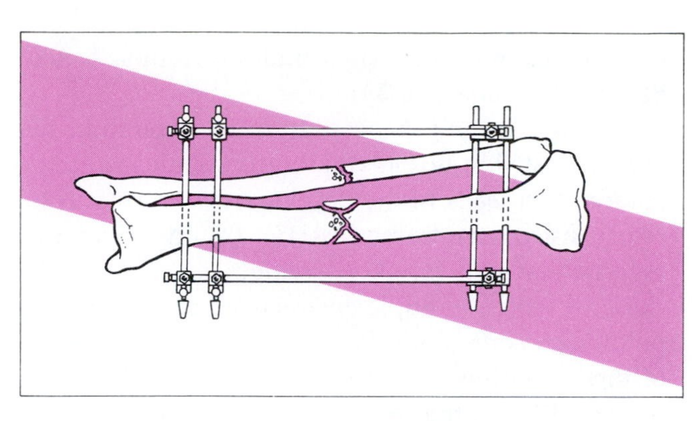

FIGURE 43-16. External fracture fixation promotes stabilization of the fracture as a temporary measure.

der the legs can free the heels of such pressure. Turning the patient on a regular schedule is imperative.

Neurovascular assessments of extremities are critical. Irreversible neurovascular injury can occur in as little as 6 hours as a result of compression of casts or immobilization devices.[65] Assessments are completed on both extremities, and the two sides are compared. Assessments of tissue perfusion include capillary refill, presence of edema and pain, palpation of temperature and pulses, and evaluation of sense of touch and mobility. Capillary refill in the toes should occur within 2 seconds, and pulses should be present by palpation or Doppler examination. The patient with lower extremity fractures is particularly at risk for alteration in tissue perfusion secondary to compartment syndrome. Frequent neurovascular assessments lead to early diagnoses and management of this limb-threatening condition. Orthopedic injuries can produce severe pain. Nursing interventions must ensure adequate pain control.

COMPLICATIONS OF TRAUMA

In the trimodal distribution of trauma deaths, the third peak of death often occurs in the critical care unit as a result of complications days to weeks after the initial injury. Ongoing nursing assessments are imperative for early detection of complications frequently associated with traumatic injuries. A single complication adds an average of 2 days to hospital length of stay in addition to the associated costs of treating the complication.[67] A postoperative infection has been reported to add an average cost of $12,000 to the cost of patient care.[68]

HYPERMETABOLISM

When individuals sustain traumatic injury, there is a predictable metabolic response characterized by hypermetabolism, hypercatabolism, and hyperglycemia.[69] Because of these unique metabolic demands, nutritional support in the trauma patient must be initiated within 24 to 72 hours after injury to prevent respiratory failure, disruption of gastrointestinal mucosal integrity, muscle breakdown, poor wound healing, progressive weakness, immune suppression, multiple organ dysfunction syndrome, and possible death. Inadequate nutritional support can impair trauma patients' ability to respond to the stress of injury and repair. Preinjury nutritional status significantly affects the trauma patient's ability to respond to stress. Energy expenditure and specific substrate requirements must be individually determined on a daily basis initially and then less frequently (one or two times/week) as the acute stress subsides; this is best determined by indirect calorimetry.[69] (∞Systemic Inflammatory Response Syndrome, p. 1121; Multiple Organ Dysfunction Syndrome, p. 1124.)

After initial assessment, the route of administration is determined. Despite the absence of bowel sounds, current recommendations suggest that nutrients be delivered beyond the stomach (past the pyloric sphincter) into the duodenum or jejunum within the first 24 to 48 hours after injury.[69] Many trauma surgeons place feeding tubes during surgery or under fluoroscopy or endoscopy to ensure proper positioning. When full nutritional support is not possible with enteral feeding, parenteral feeding may be initiated, but generally it is believed that "if the gut works, use it."

INFECTION

Infection remains a major source of mortality and morbidity in critical care units. Of trauma patients who survive longer than 3 days, infection is a frequent cause of death.[70] The trauma patient is at risk for infection because of contaminated wounds, invasive therapeutic and diagnostic catheters, intubation and mechanical ventilation, host susceptibility, and the critical care environment. Nursing management must include interventions to decrease and eliminate the trauma patient's risk of infection.

The patient with multiple trauma is at risk for infection because of host susceptibility (including preexisting medical conditions) and the adverse effect of trauma on the immune system. Systemic inflammatory response syndrome (SIRS) (see chapter 45) often follows traumatic injury because it is triggered by tissue injury and hypoxia.[71] Corticosteroids, released as a stress response to trauma, further suppress the inflammatory reaction and depress humoral and cell-mediated immunity. The physiologic and psychologic stress produced by trauma increases metabolic rate and oxygen consumption. As a result of shock, the compromised cardiovascular system cannot meet all these cellular demands. The patient who has had a splenectomy for splenic trauma is further compromised by a loss of T cells. (∞Systemic Inflammatory Response Syndrome, p. 1121.)

Wound contamination poses an infective risk to the trauma patient, especially with injuries resulting from deep or penetrating trauma. Exogenous bacteria (from the external environment) can enter through open wounds. Exogenous bacteria can be introduced by dirt, grass, and debris inoculated into the wound at the time of injury, or they can be introduced by personnel during wound care. Endogenous bacteria (from the internal environment) can be released as a result of gastrointestinal or genitourinary perforation, which spills bacteria into the internal environment. Meticulous wound care is essential. The goals of wound care include minimizing infective risks, removing dead and devitalized tissue, allowing for wound drainage, and promoting wound epithelialization and contraction. Wound healing also is accomplished through interventions that promote tissue perfusion of well-oxygenated blood and that ensure adequate nutritional support for wound healing.

SEPSIS

The patient with multiple injuries is especially at risk for overwhelming infections and sepsis. The source of sepsis in the trauma patient can be invasive therapeutic and diagnostic catheters or wound contamination with exogenous or endogenous bacteria. The source of the septic nidus must be promptly evaluated. Gram's stain and cultures of blood, urine, sputum, invasive catheters, and wounds are obtained.

Overwhelming infection can culminate through a cascade of events into septic shock. Decreased tissue perfusion can lead to cellular death. Bacterial endotoxins initiate myriad events that produce cellular and humoral immune defects and an impairment of cellular oxygen use. (∞Septic Shock, p. 1111.)

PULMONARY COMPLICATIONS

Respiratory Failure

Trauma to the pulmonary system is likely to result in complications through respiratory failure. This is particularly true if the patient was involved in a high-speed MVC, suffered major blunt trauma, experienced a mean arterial pressure of less than 60 mm Hg for a period of time, had 20% or more of blood volume replaced, or experienced a decrease in level of consciousness. Respiratory insufficiency is one of the most common complications after multiple trauma. (∞Acute Respiratory Failure, p. 655.)

Etiologic factors in posttraumatic respiratory failure[72] are listed in Box 43-16. Posttraumatic respiratory failure often leads to the development of acute respiratory distress syndrome (ARDS). Trauma patients are especially at risk for the development of ARDS because of sepsis, multiple emergency transfusions, and pulmonary contusions. The presence of more than one of these conditions significantly increases the risk for ARDS. ARDS in the trauma patient can develop 24-72 hours after initial injury and is associated with a PaO_2/FIO_2 ratio of less than 200, decreased lung compliance, and diffuse pulmonary infiltrates.[16] (∞Acute Respiratory Distress Syndrome, p. 660.)

Pulmonary Embolism

Pulmonary embolism (PE) occurs in 4% to 22% of all trauma patients. All trauma patients face the greatest risk for developing a PE in the first 2 weeks after injury. Those who are at high risk for developing a PE include patients with spinal cord injury, pelvic fracture, and lower extremity fracture with delayed orthopedic fixation. Prevention of PE begins with prevention of deep vein thrombosis, although only 35% to 50% of patients who develop PE have a clinically significant DVT.[73] High risk patients may be assessed for PE with continuous pulse oximetry. Sudden, unexplained, prolonged desaturations may indicate PE. Definitive diagnosis is usually made by pulmonary arteriography or a ventilation/perfusion scan. Treatment may consist of anticoagulation and/or placement of a vena caval filter. (∞Pulmonary Embolus, p. 668.)

Fat Embolism Syndrome

Fat embolism syndrome (FES) can occur as a complication of orthopedic trauma. The syndrome is characterized by pulmonary system dysfunction. FES appears to develop as a result of fat droplets that leak from fractured bone and embolize to the lungs. The droplets are broken down into free fatty acids that are toxic to the pulmonary microvascular membranes. Damage of these membranes results in edema, inactivation of surfactant, and atelectasis. Fat droplets further activate a coagulation cascade that results in thrombocytopenia. The lung becomes highly edematous and hemorrhagic. The clinical presentation is almost indistinguishable from ARDS. High pulmonary pressures can lead to increased left atrial pressures and decreased cardiac output, which further accentuates lung dysfunction. Early stabilization of unstable extremity fractures may limit the seeding of fat droplets into the pulmonary system. It has been demonstrated

BOX 43-16 Etiologic Factors in Posttraumatic Respiratory Failure and ARDS

- Pneumonia
  - Aspiration
  - Bacterial
  - Viral
- Blunt thoracic trauma
- Fat or amniotic fluid embolism
- Shock
  - Hypovolemic
  - Septic
  - Cardiogenic
- Pulmonary embolism
- Pancreatitis
- Near-drowning

that early fixation of long bone fractures significantly decreases the incidence of fat embolism syndrome and death from pulmonary insufficiency.[74]

PAIN

Relief of pain is a major component in the care of trauma patients. An issue that frequently complicates pain management is the high incidence of substance abusers who sustain traumatic injury. Active drug abusers may require higher-than-usual doses of opioids. Patient-controlled analgesia, when used with adequate safeguards, is appropriate in all trauma patients, including those with a substance abuse history.[75] (∞Pain Management, p. 180.)

GASTROINTESTINAL COMPLICATIONS

Hemorrhage

Life-threatening gastrointestinal (GI) bleeding as a result of stress ulcerations is infrequent but associated with high mortality. The patient with multiple traumatic injuries is particularly at risk for developing this complication. The pathophysiology of stress ulceration is thought to be caused by a variety of factors, including mucosal barrier breakdown, decreased mucosal blood flow, increased intraluminal acid, decreased epithelial regeneration, and lowered intramural pH. Prevention of stress ulcer development is accomplished through the use of histimine$_2$ antagonists, antacids and sucralfate. (∞Acute Gastrointestinal Hemorrhage, p. 945.)

Acalculous Cholecystitis

Prolonged critical illness predisposes the patient to bile stasis, biliary sludge development, and eventual cystic duct obstruction. Acalculous cholecystitis is inflammation of the gallbladder without evidence of gallstones. Several risk factors for acalculous cholecystitis are present in the patient with traumatic injuries—volume depletion, prolonged GI rest, morphine administration, ventilatory support, multiple transfusions, and infected wounds.[72] Diagnosis is difficult because the manifestations are similar to other posttraumatic complications. The patient's only symptoms may be unexplained leukocytosis and fever. Right upper quadrant pain is difficult to elicit from an unconscious patient, and diagnosis often is prompted by a high index of suspicion. Surgical intervention (cholecystectomy or cholecystostomy) usually is required.

RENAL COMPLICATIONS

Renal Failure

Assessment and ongoing monitoring of renal function are critical to the survival of the trauma patient. The etiology of posttraumatic renal failure is complex and may involve a variety of factors, as listed in Box 43-17.

Prevention of renal failure is the best treatment and begins with ensuring adequate renal perfusion. Serial assessments of BUN and creatinine levels commonly are used to evaluate renal function. Urine output as a measurement to determine renal function can be misleading because posttraumatic renal insufficiency can manifest as nonoliguric renal failure. Despite an adequate urine volume, the kidneys fail to remove metabolic wastes. Patients with nonoliguric renal failure, however, have a better chance of survival than do patients with oliguric renal failure.[76] Progressive renal failure requires prompt diagnosis and treatment. (∞Acute Renal Failure, p. 877.)

Myoglobinuria

Patients with a crush injury are susceptible to the development of myoglobinuria, with subsequent secondary renal failure. Crush injuries can result in arterial trauma. Loss of arterial blood flow, particularly to the extremities, results in the loss of oxygen transport to distal tissues and ischemia. This initiates a cascade of events that leads to the necrosis of skeletal muscle cells. As cells die, intracellular contents—particularly potassium and myoglobin—are released. Myoglobin, which is the muscular pigment, is a large molecule. As it circulates in the cardiovascular system, it causes acute renal tubular blockade and subsequent renal failure. Myoglobinuria frequently develops within 6 hours after injury. Signs of myoglobinuria include dark red or burgundy urine and decreasing urine output. Definitive diagnosis is made through serial testing of the urine for myoglobin.

BOX 43-17 Etiologic Factors in Posttraumatic Renal Failure

- Preexisting disease
  - Hypertension
  - Diabetes
  - Chronic renal insufficiency
  - Chronic liver disease
- Prolonged shock states
- Profound acidosis
- SIRS/reperfusion injury
- Abdominal compartment syndrome
- Muscle ischemia; myoglobinuria
- Microemboli
- Nephrotoxic drugs
- Radiocontrast dye

Recognition of patients at risk for the development of myoglobinuria is imperative to its prevention. Such prevention includes early external immobilization of fractures and early serial urine testing for myoglobin.

Once myoglobinuria is diagnosed, treatment is aimed at prevention of subsequent renal failure. Aggressive administration of intravenous fluids increases renal blood flow and decreases the concentration of nephrotoxic pigments. Continuous infusion of mannitol and sodium bicarbonate ($NaHCO_3$) maybe used, although this regimen is controversial.[77] Mannitol and $NaHCO_3$ are thought to alkalinize the urine and prevent myoglobin crystallization in the renal tubules. Acetazolamide (Diamox) may be given to prevent systemic alkalemia that may be caused by the continuous $NaHCO_3$ infusion. Nursing management is directed toward achievement of fluid and electrolyte balance. Assessment parameters may include maintaining urine output greater than or equal to 100 ml/hr and maintaining urine pH greater than or equal to 7.0.[77]

VASCULAR COMPLICATIONS

Compartment Syndrome

Compartment syndrome is a condition in which increased pressure within a limited space compromises circulation, resulting in ischemia and necrosis of tissues within that space. Among those at high risk for the development of compartment syndrome are patients with lower extremity trauma, including fractures, penetrating trauma, vascular ruptures, massive tissue injuries, or venous obstruction.

Clinical manifestations of compartment syndrome include obvious swelling and tightness of an extremity, paresis, and pain of the affected extremity. Diminished pulses and decreased capillary refill do not reliably identify compartment syndrome because they may be intact until after irreversible changes have occured. Elevated intracompartmental pressures confirm the diagnosis. The treatment can consist of simple interventions, such as removing an occlusive dressing, to more complex interventions, including a fasciotomy. Meticulous wound care after fasciotomy is imperative to prevent wound infection.

Venous Thromboembolism

Despite improvements in the care of the trauma patient, venous thromboembolism remains a significant source of morbidity and mortality in trauma patients.[28] Trauma patients are at risk for developing venous thrombosis because of endothelial injury, coagulopathy, immobility, and bedrest. Trauma patients are at the greatest risk for developing thromboembolism early in their hospitalization. Physical assessment for thromboembolism is the least-reliable method of detecting thromboembolism.[28] Venous thrombosis is best diagnosed with venography, impedance plethysmography (IPG), or ultrasonography. Venous thrombosis prophylaxis traditionally consists of low-dose subcutaneous heparin (5000 U every 12 hours) and/or compression boots.

MISSED INJURY

Nursing assessment of the multiple injury patient in the critical care unit may reveal missed diseases or missed injuries. Missed "diseases" may include preexisting undiagnosed medical illnesses, such as endocrine disorders (diabetes, hypothyroidism); myocardial infarction; hypertension; respiratory insufficiency; renal insufficiency; or malnutrition.

Occasionally injuries may not be diagnosed in the precritical care phases. Injuries can be subtle or masked, preventing accurate diagnosis. In the critical care unit, a missed injury may be suspected if the patient fails to show appropriate response to medical or surgical intervention. Change in the character of drainage from wounds or catheters may represent biliary or duodenal injuries. Hypotension and a falling hematocrit level despite aggressive fluid administration may indicate an expanding hematoma. Pelvic or peritoneal abscesses may develop in patients with missed rectal injuries.[72]

The critical care nurse must be alert to the possibility of a missed injury, especially when the patient does not appear to be responding appropriately to interventions. The physician must be notified immediately because potential complications of infection and hemorrhage can be life threatening.

MULTIPLE ORGAN DYSFUNCTION SYNDROME

Multiple organ dysfunction syndrome (MODS) is a clinical syndrome of progressive dysfunction of organ systems. Trauma patients are at high risk for SIRS and MODS because of circulatory shock with tissue hypoxemia, tissue injury, and infection.[16] Organ dysfunction can be the result of "primary MODS," which is caused by direct traumatic injury such as that which occurs with acute lung dysfunction because of pulmonary contusion. Organ dysfunction that occurs latently in the trauma patient's CCU course, "secondary MODS," results from uncontrolled systemic inflammation with resultant organ dysfunction. Trauma patients may experience both primary and secondary MODS. Treatment is aimed at controlling or eliminating the source of inflammation, maintenance of oxygen delivery and consumption, nutritional and metabolic support for individual organs, and effective pain control.[16] (∞Multiple Organ Dysfunction Syndrome, p. 1124.)

CASE STUDY

TRAUMA

CLINICAL HISTORY

Mr. J is a 32-year-old man who was driving home from a Super Bowl party. He hit a patch of ice and lost control of his car, hitting a guard rail and a tree. He was not wearing a seat belt. The emergency medical technicians at the scene reported a prolonged extrication time of 45 minutes.

CURRENT PROBLEMS

On arrival to the ED Mr. J's vital signs were BP, 88/56 mm Hg HR, 130/min; respirations, 24/min; temperature, 94°F. His respirations were shallow and his airway patent, but he had diminished breath sounds on the left side. Subcutaneous air was present from the left nipple line to the left upper abdominal quadrant. A chest tube was inserted, and after placement, breath sounds were audible bilaterally. He was placed on 40% O_2 by face mask. His skin was cold and clammy. Two peripheral 16-gauge intravenous (IV) infusions were initiated, and with use of a fluid warmer, he was given lactated Ringer's (LR) solution at a wide-open rate. The neurologic examination showed pupils equal, react to light and accommodation (PERLA) at 5 mm, and Mr. J was combative and disoriented to place and time. He had an obvious open fracture of his left lower extremity. His areterial blood gas (ABG) values revealed metabolic acidosis. Other pertinent laboratory values included hematocrit (Hct), 28%; hemoglobin (Hgb), 10 g/dL; alcohol (ETOH) level, 0.13; and normal urinalysis results. A Foley catheter was inserted, which yielded 100 ml clear yellow urine. A diagnostic peritoneal lavage (DPL) was performed, and findings were positive. X-ray films revealed fractures of the fifth to tenth left ribs, comminuted fracture of the left tibia, and normal cervical spinal alignment. A head computed tomography (CT) scan showed negative findings.

After 3 L of LR and 2 U of blood Mr. J remained hypotensive and was taken to the operating room (OR). During surgery the exploratory laparotomy revealed a ruptured spleen. A splenectomy and placement of an external fixation device were performed in the OR. Intraoperatively, Mr. J required 15 L of fluid (10 L crystalloid, 5 L colloid) to maintain a mean arterial pressure (MAP) > 70 mm Hg. He remained hypothermic and was then transported to the trauma critical care unit (CCU).

MEDICAL DIAGNOSES

Ruptured spleen, status post (SP) splenectomy
Tension pneumothorax, SP chest tube placement
Fracture of fifth through tenth ribs on left side
Comminuted fracture of left tibia

NURSING DIAGNOSES

Fluid Volume Deficit related to absolute loss: intraoperative blood

Ineffective Breathing Pattern related to decreased lung expansion

Hypothermia related to exposure to cold environment, trauma, or damage to the hypothalamus

Risk for Infection risk factors: altered integumentary system, invasive surgical procedures, presence of invasive lines, immobility, traumatic injuries, and stress

Acute Pain related to transmission and perception of cutaneous, visceral, muscular, or ischemic impulses

PLAN OF CARE

1. Admit to trauma CCU.
2. Continue to monitor fluid status and oxygenation by insertion of an oximetrix pulmonary artery catheter.
3. Monitor serial Hct level, ABG values, and coagulation factors.
4. Maintain MAP > 70 mm Hg.
5. Continue with mechanical ventilation, and monitor pneumothorax.
6. Treat hypothermia with warmed blankets and warmed IV fluids.
7. Monitor urine output.
8. Obtain clear thoracic and lumbar spinal films.

NURSING MANAGEMENT PLAN

DYSREFLEXIA

DEFINITION

The state in which in individual with a spinal cord injury at T7 or above experiences a life-threatening uninhibited sympathetic response of the nervous system to a noxious stimulus.

Dysreflexia Related to Excessive Autonomic Response to Certain Noxious Stimuli (e.g., Distended Bladder, Distended Bowel, Skin Irritation) Occurring in Patients with Cervical or High Thoracic (T7 or above) Spinal Cord Injury

DEFINING CHARACTERISTICS

NOTE: Anyone who has had dysreflexia knows how his or her body responds. Listen to the patient.

Major

- Paroxysmal hypertension (sudden periodic elevated blood pressure [BP] greater than 20 mm Hg above patient's normal BP); for many spinal cord injury patients, a normal BP may be only 90/60 mm Hg
- Bradycardia (most common; pulse rate < 60 beats/minute) or tachycardia (pulse rate > 100 beats/minute)
- Diaphoresis (above the injury)
- Facial flushing
- Pallor (below the injury)
- Pounding headache (a diffuse pain in different portions of the head and not confined to any nerve distribution area)

Minor

- Nasal congestion
- Engorgement of temporal and neck vessels
- Conjunctival congestion
- Chills without fever
- Pilomotor erection (goose bumps) below the injury
- Blurred vision
- Chest pain
- Metallic taste in mouth
- Horner's syndrome (constriction of the pupil, partial ptosis of the eyelid, enophthalmos, and sometimes loss of sweating over the affected side of the face)

OUTCOME CRITERIA

- BP has returned to patient's norm.
- Pulse rate is > 60 or < 100 beats/minute (or within patient's norm).
- Headache is absent.
- Nasal stuffiness, sweating, and flushing above level of injury are absent.
- Chills, goose bumps, and pallor below level of injury are absent.
- Patient verbalizes causes, prevention, symptoms, and treatment of condition.

NURSING INTERVENTIONS AND *RATIONALE*

1. Continue to monitor the assessment parameters listed under "Defining Characteristics."
2. Place patient on cardiac monitor, and assess for bradycardia, tachycardia, or other dysrhythmias. ***Disturbances of cardiac rate and rhythm can occur because of autonomic dysfunction associated with dysreflexia.***
3. Do not leave patient alone. One nurse monitors the BP and patient status every 3 to 5 minutes while another provides treatment.
4. Place patient's head of bed to upright position ***to decrease BP and promote cerebral venous return.***
5. Remove any support stockings or abdominal binder ***to reduce venous return.***
6. Investigate for and remove offending cause of dysreflexia.
   a. Bladder
      - If catheter not in place, immediately catheterize patient.
      - Lubricate catheter with lidocaine jelly before insertion.
      - Drain 500 ml of urine, and recheck BP.
      - If BP still elevated, drain another 500 ml of urine.
      - If BP declines after the bladder is empty, serial BP must be monitored closely ***because the bladder can go into severe contractions causing hypertension to recur.*** With physician's collaboration, instill 30 ml tetracaine through the catheter ***to decrease the flow of impulses from the bladder.***
      - If indwelling catheter in place, check for kinks or granular sediment that may indicate occlusion.
      - If plugged catheter is suspected, irrigate it gently with no more than 30 ml of sterile normal saline solution. If the bladder is in tetany, fluid will go in but will not drain out.
      - If unable to irrigate catheter, remove it, and prepare to reinsert a new catheter: proceed with its lubrication, drainage, and observation as previously stated.
      - Atropine is sometimes administered ***to relieve bladder tetany.***

Continued

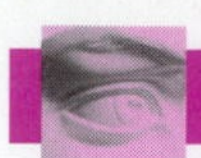

NURSING MANAGEMENT PLAN—CONT'D

Dysreflexia Related to Excessive Autonomic Response to Certain Noxious Stimuli (e.g., Distended Bladder, Distended Bowel, Skin Irritation) Occurring in Patients with Cervical or High Thoracic (T7 or above) Spinal Cord Injury

NURSING INTERVENTIONS AND *RATIONALE*—cont'd

b. Bowel
- Using glove lubricated with anesthetic ointment, check rectum for fecal impaction.
- If impaction is felt, ***to decrease flow of impulses from bowel,*** insert anesthetic ointment into rectum 10 minutes before manual removal of impaction.
- A low, hypertonic enema or a suppository may be given ***to assist bowel evacuation.***

c. Skin
- Loosen clothing or bed linens as indicated.
- Inspect skin for pimples, boils, pressure sores, and ingrown toenails and treat as indicated.

7. If symptoms of dysreflexia do not subside, have available the intravenous (IV) solutions and antihypertensive drugs of the physician's choosing (e.g., hydralazine, nifedipine, phentolamine, diazoxide, sodium nitroprusside). Administer medications and monitor their effectiveness. Assess BP, pulse, and subjective and objective signs and symptoms.
8. Instruct patient about causes, symptoms, treatment, and prevention of dysreflexia.
9. Encourage patient to carry medical bracelet or informational card to present to medical personnel in the event dysreflexia may be developing.

REFERENCES

1. Runge J: The cost of injury, *Emerg Med Clin North Am* 11:241, 1993.
2. National Safety Council: *Accident facts,* Itasca, Ill, 1994, National Safety Council.
3. Shackford SR: The evolution of modern trauma care, *Surg Clin North Am* 75:147, 1995.
4. American College of Surgeons: *Advanced trauma life support,* ed 5, Chicago, 1993, American College of Surgeons.
5. Keenan K: The role of nursing assessment of traumatic events in sudden injury, illness and death, *Crit Care Nurs Clin North Am* 7:483, 1995.
6. Robertson L: Motor vehicles, *Pediatr Clin North Am* 32:87, 1985.
7. Trimble P, Wallack D: Trauma nursing: past, present and future, *Md Med J* 37(7):547, 1988.
8. Cordonna V: *Trauma reference manual,* Baltimore, 1985, Brady Communications.
9. Emergency Nurses Association: *Trauma nursing care course instructor manual,* Chicago, 1987, Award Printing.
10. Boggs RL: Multiple system trauma: nursing implications, *J Adv Med Surg Nurs* 2(1):1, 1989.
11. Meyer AA, Trunkey DD: Critical care as an integral part of trauma care, *Crit Care Nurs Clin North Am* 2(4):673, 1986.
12. Bracken MB and others: Methylprednisolone or naloxone treatment after spinal cord injury: one year follow up data, *J Neurosurg* 76:23, 1992.
13. Von Reuden KT, Dunham CM: Sequelae of massive fluid resuscitation in trauma patients, *Crit Care Nurs Clin North Am* 6:463, 1994.
14. Von Reuden KT: Cardiopulmonary assessment of the critically ill trauma patient, *Crit Care Nurs Clin North Am* 1(1):33, 1989.
15. Yu M, Levy MM, Smith P: Effect of maximizing oxygen delivery on morbidity and mortality in critically ill patients: a prospective, randomized, controlled study, *Crit Care Med* 21:830, 1993.
16. Fitzsimmons L: Consequences of trauma: systemic inflammation and multiple organ dysfunction, *Crit Care Nurse Q* 17(2):74, 1994.
17. Gennarelli TA: Triage of head injured patients. In Trunkey DD, Lewis FR, editors: *Current therapy of trauma,* ed 3, Philadelphia, 1991, BC Decker.
18. Andrews BT: The intensive care management of patients with head injury. In Andrews BT, editor: *Neurosurgical intensive care,* New York, 1993, McGraw-Hill.
19. Ammons AM: Cerebral injuries and intracranial hemorrhages as a result of trauma, *Nurs Clin North Am* 25(1):23, 1990.
20. Stand PE: Diagnostic and therapeutic concerns in head injured patients, *J Am Acad Phys Assist* 1(2):112, 1988.
21. Valadka AB: Evaluating and monitoring head injury: jugular bulb and non-invasive CNS monitoring. Proceedings from trauma and critical care 1996, American College of Surgery Western States Committee on Trauma, 1996.
22. Walleck-Jastremski CA: Traumatic brain injury: assessment and treatment, *Crit Care Nurse Clin North Am* 6:472, 1994.
23. Ward JD and others: Penetrating head injury, *Crit Care Nurse Q* 17(1):79, 1994.

24. Hughes MC: Critical care nursing for the patient with a spinal cord injury, *Crit Care Nurs Clin North Am* 2(1):33, 1990.
25. Walker M: Acute spinal cord injury, *N Engl J Med* 324:1885, 1991.
26. Hickey JV: *The clinical practice of neurological and neurosurgical nursing,* ed 3, Philadelphia, 1992, JB Lippincott.
27. Nayduch D, Lee A, Butler D: High dose methylprednisolone after acute spinal cord injury, *Crit Care Nurse* 14(4):69, 1994.
28. Rogers FB: Venous thromboembolism in trauma patients, *Surg Clin North Am* 75:279, 1995.
29. Nolan S: Current trends in the management of acute spinal cord injury, *Crit Care Nurse Q* 17(1):64, 1994.
30. Kidd PS: Emergency department management of spinal cord injury, *Crit Care Nurs Clin North Am* 2(3):349, 1990.
31. Kocan MJ: Pulmonary considerations in the critical care phase, *Crit Care Nurs Clin North Am* 2(3):369, 1990.
32. Walleck CA: Neurologic considerations in the critical care phase, *Crit Care Nurs Clin North Am* 2(3):357, 1990.
33. Richmond TS: Spinal cord injury, *Nurs Clin North Am* 25(1):57, 1990.
34. Bracken MB and others: A randomized controlled trial of methylprednisolone or naloxone in the treatment of acute spinal cord injury, *N Engl J Med* 322:1405, 1990.
35. Schwenker D: Cardiovascular considerations in the acute care phase, *Crit Care Nurs Clin North Am* 2(3):363, 1990.
36. Yarcony GM and others: Neuromuscular stimulation in spinal cord injury II: prevention of secondary complications, *Arch Phys Med Rehabil* 73:195, 1992.
37. Metcalf JA: Acute phase management of persons with injury: a nursing diagnosis perspective, *Nurs Clin North Am* 21:589, 1986.
38. Barot LR: Maxillofacial trauma, *Top Emerg Med* 13(4):17, 1991.
39. Walton RL, Bunkis J, Borah GL: Maxillofacial trauma. In Trunkey DD, Lewis FR, editors: *Current therapy of trauma,* ed 3, Philadelphia, 1991, BC Decker.
40. Lower J: Maxillofacial trauma, *Nurs Clin North Am* 21(4):511, 1986.
41. Johnson SB, Kearney PK, Smith MD: Echocardiography in the evaluation of thoracic trauma, *Surg Clin North Am* 75:193, 1995.
42. Ross SE, Cernaianu AC: Epidemiology of thoracic injuries: mechanisms of injury and pathophysiology, *Top Emerg Med* 12(1):1, 1990.
43. Hammond SG: Chest injuries in the trauma patient, *Nurs Clin North Am* 25(1):35, 1990.
44. Gough JE, Allison EJ, Faju VP: Flail chest: management and implications for emergency nurses, *J Emerg Nurs* 13(6):330, 1987.
45. Andrew L: Difficult diagnoses in blunt thoraco-abdominal trauma, *J Emerg Nurs* 15(5):399, 1989 .
46. Moore FA, Haenel JB, Moore EE: Blunt pulmonary injury. In Maull and others, editors: *Advances in trauma and critical care,* vol 8, St Louis, 1993, Mosby.
47. Wall MJ: Pulmonary tractotomy. Proceedings from trauma and critical care 1996, American College of Surgery Western States Committee on Trauma, 1996.
48. Feliciano DV, Mattox KL: The heart. In Trunkey DD, Lewis FR, editors: *Current therapy of trauma,* ed 3, Philadelphia, 1991, BC Decker.
49. Christensen MA, Sutton KR: Myocardial contusion: new concepts in diagnosis and management, *Am J Crit Care* 2:28, 1993.
50. Bartlett R: Myocardial contusion, *DCCN* 10(3):133, 1991.
51. Daleiden A: Clinical manifestations of blunt cardiac injury: a challenge to the critical care practitioner, *Crit Care Nurse Q* 17(2):13, 1994.
52. Merrill CR, Sparger G: Current thoughts on blunt abdominal trauma, *Top Emerg Med* 12(2):21, 1990.
53. Carrico CJ: The spleen. In Trunkey DD, Lewis FR, editors: *Current therapy of trauma,* ed 3, Philadelphia, 1991, BC Decker
54. Wagner MM: The patient with abdominal injuries, *Nurs Clin North Am* 25(1):45, 1990.
55. Shoemaker W, Ayers S, Grenvick A: *Textbook of critical care,* ed 2, Philadelphia, 1988, WB Saunders.
56. Wachtel T: Critical care concepts in the management of abdominal trauma, *Crit Care Nurse Q* 17(2):34, 1994.
57. Hirshberg A, Mattox KL: Planned reoperation for severe trauma, *Ann Surg* 222:3, 1995.
58. Hirshberg A: Damage control surgery for trauma. Proceedings from trauma and critical care 1996, American College of Surgery Western States Committee on Trauma, 1996.
59. Morris JA and others: The staged celiotomy in trauma: issues in unpacking and reconstruction, *Ann Surg* 217:576, 1993.
60. Pacher HL and others: The status of nonoperative management of blunt hepatic injuries in 1995: a multicenter experience with 404 patients, *J Trauma* 40(1)31-38, 1996.
61. Jaggers J, Feliciano PD: Hepatic trauma. In Maull and others, editors: *Advances in trauma and critical care,* vol 8, St Louis, 1993, Mosby.
62. Cyer HG: Emergency center evaluation of urologic trauma. Proceedings from trauma and critical care 1996, American College of Surgery Western States Committee on Trauma, 1996.
63. Frevele G: Urinary tract injuries due to blunt abdominal trauma, *Phys Assist* 13(2):123, 1989.
64. Ruhl JM: Pelvic trauma, *RN* July:50 1991.
65. Herron DG, Nance J: Emergency department management of patients with orthopedic fractures resulting from motor vehicle accidents, *Nurs Clin North Am* 25(1):71, 1990.
66. Childs SA: Musculoskeletal trauma: implications for critical care nursing practice *Crit Care Nurs Clin North Am* 6:483, 1994.
67. Mitchell FL: Trauma center effectiveness: people, policies and policing. Proceedings from trauma and critical care 1996, American College of Surgery Western States Committee on Trauma, 1996.

68. Shulkin DJ and others: The economic impact of infections: an analysis of hospital costs and charges in surgical patients with cancer, *Arch Surg* 128:449, 1993.
69. Stamatos CA, Reed E: Nutritional needs of trauma patients: challenges, barriers, solutions, *Crit Care Nurse Clin North Am* 6:501, 1994.
70. Martin MT: Wound management and infection control after trauma: implications for the intensive care setting, *Crit Care Nurs Q* 11(2):43, 1988.
71. American College of Chest Physicians/Society of Critical Care Medicine Consensus Conference Committee: Definitions for sepsis and organ failure and guidelines for the use of innovative therapies in sepsis, *Crit Care Med* 20:6, 1992.
72. Langdale L, Schecter WP: Critical care complications in the trauma patient, *Crit Care Clin North Am* 2(4):839, 1986.
73. Brathwaite C and others: Continuous pulse oximetry and the diagnosis of pulmonary embolism in critically ill trauma patients, *J Trauma* 33:528, 1992.
74. Slye D: Orthopedic complications, *Nurs Clin North Am* 26:113, 1991.
75. Acute Pain Management Guidelines Panel: *Acute pain management: operative or medical procedures and trauma clinical practice guidelines,* AHCPR Pub No. 92-0032, 1992, Rockville, Md, Agency for Health Care Policy and Research, Public Health Service, U.S. Department of Health and Human Services.
76. Mackersie RC: Renal replacement therapy. Proceedings from trauma and critical care 1996, American College of Surgery Western States Committee on Trauma, 1996.
77. Cheney P: Early management and physiologic changes in crush injury, *Crit Care Nurse Q* 17(2):62, 1994.

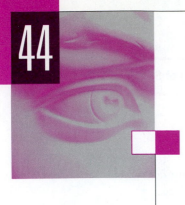

44

Shock

SHOCK IS AN acute, widespread process of impaired tissue perfusion that results in cellular, metabolic, and hemodynamic derangements. Impaired tissue perfusion occurs when an imbalance develops between cellular oxygen supply and cellular oxygen demand. This imbalance can occur for a variety of reasons and eventually results in cellular dysfunction and death. This chapter presents an overview of the general shock response, or shock syndrome, followed by a discussion of the different shock states.

SHOCK SYNDROME

Description

Shock is a complex pathophysiologic process that often results in multiple organ dysfunction syndrome (MODS) and death. All types of shock eventually result in impaired tissue perfusion and the development of acute circulatory failure or shock syndrome. Shock syndrome is a generalized systemic response to inadequate tissue perfusion.[1] It consists of four different stages: initial, compensatory, progressive, and refractory. Progression through each stage varies with the patient's prior condition, duration of initiating event, response to therapy, and correction of underlying cause.[2]

Etiology

Shock can be classified as hypovolemic, cardiogenic, or distributive, depending on the pathophysiologic cause. Hypovolemic shock results from a loss of circulating or intravascular volume. Cardiogenic shock results from the impaired ability of the heart to pump. Distributive shock results from maldistribution of circulating blood volume and can be further classified as septic, anaphylactic, and neurogenic. Septic shock is the result of microorganisms entering the body. Anaphylactic shock is the result of a severe antibody-antigen reaction. Neurogenic shock is the result of the loss of sympathetic tone.[3,4]

Pathophysiology

During the initial stage, cardiac output (CO) is decreased and tissue perfusion is impaired. As the blood supply to the cells decreases, the cells switch from aerobic to anaerobic metabolism as a source of energy. Anaerobic metabolism produces small amounts of energy but large amounts of lactic acid. Lactic acidemia quickly develops and causes more cellular damage.[2,5]

During the compensatory stage, an attempt is made by the body's homeostatic mechanisms to improve tissue perfusion. The compensatory mechanisms are mediated by the sympathetic nervous system (SNS) and consist of neural, hormonal, and chemical responses. Neural compensation includes an increase in heart rate (HR) and contractility, arterial and venous vasoconstriction, and shunting of blood to the vital organs. Hormonal compensation includes activation of the renin response and stimulation of the anterior pituitary and adrenal medulla. Activation of the renin response results in the production of angiotensin II, which causes vasoconstriction and the release of aldosterone and antidiuretic hormone (ADH), leading to sodium and water retention. Stimulation of the anterior pituitary results in the secretion of adrenocorticotropic hormone (ACTH), which in turn stimulates the adrenal cortex to produce glucocorticoids, causing a rise in blood glucose levels. Stimulation of the adrenal medulla causes the release of epinephrine and norepinephrine, which further enhance the compensatory mechanisms. Chemical compensation includes hyperventilation to neutralize lactic acidosis.[2,5]

During the progressive stage, the compensatory mechanisms start to fail and the shock cycle is perpetuated. At the cellular level, the small amount of energy created by anaerobic metabolism is not enough to keep the cell functional, and irreversible damage begins to occur. The sodium-potassium pump in the cell membrane fails, causing the cell and its organelles to swell. Cellular energy production comes to a complete halt as the mitochondria swell and rupture. At this point the problem becomes one of oxygen utilization instead of oxygen delivery. Even if the cell were to receive more oxygen, it would be unable to use it because of damage to the mitochondria. The cell's digestive organelles swell, resulting in leakage of destructive enzymes into the cell. Autodigestion occurs with ensuing cell death.[5]

Every system in the body is affected by this process (Box 44-1). Cardiac dysfunction develops as a result of myocardial hypoperfusion, lactic acidosis, and the release of myocardial depressant factor (MDF). MDF is a substance that is released from the pancreas as it becomes ischemic. Ventricular failure eventually occurs, further perpetuating the entire process. Central nervous system (CNS) dysfunction develops as a result of cerebral hypoperfusion, leading to failure of the SNS, cardiac and respiratory depression, and thermoregulatory failure. SNS failure in turn results in vasodilation, pooling of blood in the capillaries, increased capillary membrane permeability, and the formation of microemboli. Hematologic dysfunction occurs as a result of hypotension, hypoxemia, acidosis, and stasis of capillary blood flow. Disseminated intravascular coagulation (DIC) eventually develops. Pulmonary dysfunction occurs as a result of increased pulmonary capillary membrane permeability, pulmonary microemboli, and pulmonary vasoconstriction. Ventilatory failure and acute respiratory distress syndrome (ARDS) eventually develop. Renal dysfunction develops as a result of renal vasoconstriction and renal hypoperfusion, leading to acute tubular necrosis (ATN). Gastrointestinal dysfunction occurs as a result of splanchnic vasoconstriction and splanchnic hypoperfusion, leading to failure of the gut organs. Failure of the gut organs results in the release of gram-negative bacteria, which further perpetuates the entire shock syndrome.[6]

During the refractory stage, shock becomes unresponsive to therapy and is considered irreversible. As the individual organ systems die, *MODS,* defined as failure of two or more body systems, occurs. Death is the final outcome.[2] Regardless of etiologic factors, death occurs from impaired tissue perfusion because of the failure of the circulation to meet the oxygen needs of the cell.[7] (∞Multiple Organ Dysfunction Syndrome, p. 1124.)

BOX 44-1 Consequences of Shock

- Cardiovascular
  - Ventricular failure
- Neurologic
  - Sympathetic nervous system dysfunction
  - Cardiac and respiratory depression
  - Thermoregulatory failure
  - Coma
- Pulmonary
  - Acute respiratory failure
  - Acute respiratory distress syndrome (ARDS)
- Renal
  - Acute tubular necrosis (ATN)
- Hematologic
  - Disseminated intravascular coagulation (DIC)
- Gastrointestinal
  - Gastrointestinal tract failure
  - Hepatic failure
  - Pancreatic failure

Assessment and Diagnosis

The patient with a systolic blood pressure (SBP) less than 90 mm Hg that is accompanied by either tachycardia or bradycardia and altered mental status is considered to be in a shock state.[8] Clinical manifestations will differ, though, according to underlying cause and the stage of the shock and are related to both the cause and the patient's response to shock.[9] (See individual shock sections in this chapter for a discussion of clinical assessment and diagnosis of the patient in shock.)

Medical Management

The major focus of the treatment of shock is the improvement and preservation of tissue perfusion. Adequate tissue perfusion depends on an adequate supply of oxygen being transported to the tissues and the cell's ability to use it. Oxygen transport is influenced by pulmonary gas exchange, CO, and hemoglobin level. Oxygen utilization is influenced by the internal metabolic environment. Management of the patient in shock focuses on supporting oxygen transport and oxygen utilization.[1,7]

Adequate pulmonary gas exchange is critical to oxygen transport. Establishing and maintaining an adequate airway are the first steps in ensuring adequate oxygenation. Once the airway is patent, emphasis is placed on improving ventilation and oxygenation. Therapies include administration of supplemental oxygen and mechanical ventilatory support.[5,8,10]

An adequate CO and hemoglobin level are crucial to oxygen transport. CO depends on HR, preload, afterload, and contractility. A variety of fluids and drugs are used to manipulate these parameters. The types of fluids used include both crystalloids and colloids. The categories of drugs used include vasoconstrictors, vasodilators, positive inotropic agents, and antidysrhythmic agents.[5,8] (∞Cardiac Output, p. 348.)

Fluid administration, which is indicated for decreased preload related to intravascular volume depletion, can be accomplished by use of either a crystalloid or colloid solution, or both. Crystalloids are balanced electrolyte solutions that may be hypotonic, isotonic, or hypertonic. Examples of crystalloid solutions are normal saline, lactated Ringer's solution, and 5% dextrose in water. Colloids are protein- or starch-containing solutions. Examples of colloid solutions are blood and blood components and pharmaceutic plasma expanders, such as hetastarch, dextran, and mannitol. The choice of fluid depends on the situation. Advantages of colloids include faster restoration of intravascular volume and use of smaller amounts. Colloids stay in the intravascular space as opposed to crystalloids, which readily leak into the extravascular space. Disadvantages include expense, allergic reactions, and difficulties in typing and cross-matching blood. Colloids also can leak out of damaged capillaries and cause a variety of additional problems, particularly in the lungs.[5,10–13] Blood is used to augment oxygen transport if the patient's hemoglobin level is low.[1]

Vasoconstrictor agents are used to increase afterload by increasing the systemic vascular resistance (SVR) and improving the patient's blood pressure level. Vasodilator agents are used to decrease preload or afterload, or both, by decreasing venous return and SVR. Positive inotropic agents are used to increase contractility. Antidysrhythmic agents are used to influence HR. Box 44-2 provides examples of each of these agents.[5,10,14] (∞Cardiovascular Drugs, p. 574.)

BOX 44-2 Examples of the Different Agents Used in the Treatment of Shock

VASOCONSTRICTOR AGENTS

Epinephrine (Adrenalin)
Norepinephrine (Leyophed)
Alpha-range dopamine (Intropin)
Metaraminol (Aramine)
Phenylephrine (Neo-Synephrine)
Ephedrine

VASODILATOR AGENTS

Nitroprusside (Nipride, Nitropress)
Nitroglycerin (Nitrol, Tridil)
Hydralazine (Apresoline)
Labetalol (Normodyne, Trandate)

INOTROPIC AGENTS

Beta-range dopamine (Intropin)
Dobutamine (Dobutrex)
Amrinone (Inocor)
Epinephrine (Adrenalin)
Isoproterenol (Isuprel)
Norepinephrine (Levophed)
Digoxin (Lanoxin)

ANTIDYSRHYTHMIC AGENTS

Lidocaine (Xylocaine)
Bretylium (Bretylol)
Procainamide (Promestyl)
Labetalol (Normodyne, Trandate)
Verapamil (Calan, Isoptin)
Esmolol (Brevibloc)
Diltiazem (Cardizem)

An optimal metabolic environment is very important to oxygen utilization. Once the oxygen is delivered to the cells, they have to be able to use it. The major metabolic derangement seen in shock is lactic acidosis. Interventions to correct lactic acidosis include correcting the cause; reestablishing perfusion; inducing hyperventilation; and in severe cases, administering sodium bicarbonate.[15] The role of sodium bicarbonate in the treatment of acidosis is controversial because of the associated risks of using it, and it is usually reserved for severe cases that are refractory to other treatments. These risks include a rebound increase in lactic acid production; development of a hyperosmolar state; and fluid overload resulting from excessive sodium, shifting of the oxyhemoglobin dissociation curve to the left; and rapid cellular electrolyte shifts.[16]

The patient also must begin receiving nutritional support therapy. The type of nutritional supplementation initiated varies according to the cause of shock and is tailored to the individual patient's need, as indicated by the underlying condition and laboratory data. The enteral route generally is preferred over the parenteral.[17]

Nursing Management

The nursing management of a patient in shock is a complex and challenging responsibility. It requires an in-depth understanding of the pathophysiology of the disease and the anticipated effects of each intervention, as well as a solid understanding of the nursing process.[18] (Individual shock sections in this chapter contain separate discussions of specific interventions for the patient in shock.)

The psychosocial needs of the patient and family dealing with shock are extremely important. These needs, which differ with each patient and family, are based on situational, familial, and patient-centered variables. Nursing interventions for psychosocial problems include providing information on patient status, explaining procedures and routines, supporting the family, encouraging the expression of feelings, facilitating problem solving and decision making, involving the family in the patient's care, and establishing contacts with necessary resources.[19]

HYPOVOLEMIC SHOCK

Description

Hypovolemic shock occurs from inadequate fluid volume in the intravascular space. The lack of adequate circulating volume leads to decreased tissue perfusion and initiation of the general shock response. Hypovolemic shock is the most commonly occurring form of shock.[2,13]

Etiology

Hypovolemic shock can result from either absolute or relative hypovolemia. Absolute hypovolemia occurs when there is an external loss of fluid from the body including whole blood, plasma, or any other bodily fluid. Relative hypovolemia occurs when there is an internal shifting of fluid from the intravascular space to the extravascular space. This can result from a loss in intravascular integrity, increased capillary membrane permeability, or decreased colloidal osmotic pressure (Box 44-3).[2,13]

Pathophysiology

Hypovolemia results in a loss of circulating fluid volume. A decrease in circulating volume leads to a decrease in venous return, which in turn results in a decrease in end-diastolic volume, or preload. Preload is a major determinant of stroke volume (SV) and CO. A decrease in preload results in a decrease in SV and CO. The decrease in CO leads to inadequate cellular oxygen supply and impaired tissue perfusion (Figure 44-1).[2,13]

BOX 44-3 Etiologic Factors in Hypovolemic Shock

ABSOLUTE

- Loss of whole blood
  - Trauma
  - Surgery
  - Gastrointestinal bleeding
- Loss of plasma
  - Thermal injuries
  - Large lesions
- Loss of other bodily fluids
  - Severe vomiting
  - Severe diarrhea
  - Massive diuresis

RELATIVE

- Loss of intravascular integrity
  - Ruptured spleen
  - Long bone or pelvic fractures
  - Hemorrhagic pancreatitis
  - Hemothorax or hemoperitoneum
  - Arterial dissection
- Increased capillary membrane permeability
  - Sepsis
  - Anaphylaxis
  - Thermal injuries
- Decreased colloidal osmotic pressure
  - Severe sodium depletion
  - Hypopituitarism
  - Cirrhosis
  - Intestinal obstruction

Assessment and Diagnosis

The clinical manifestations of hypovolemic shock vary, depending on the severity of fluid loss and the patient's ability to compensate for it. The first, or initial, stage occurs with a fluid volume loss up to 15%, or an actual volume loss up to 750 ml. Compensatory mechanisms maintain CO, and the patient appears symptom-free.[4,11,13]

The second, or compensatory, stage occurs with a fluid volume loss of 15% to 30%, or an actual volume loss of 750 to 1500 ml.[11] CO falls, resulting in the initiation of a variety of compensatory responses. The HR increases in response to increased SNS stimulation. The pulse pressure (PP) narrows as the diastolic blood pressure increases because of vasoconstriction. Respiratory rate (RR) and depth increase in an attempt to improve oxygenation. Arterial blood gas (ABG) specimens drawn during this phase reveal respiratory

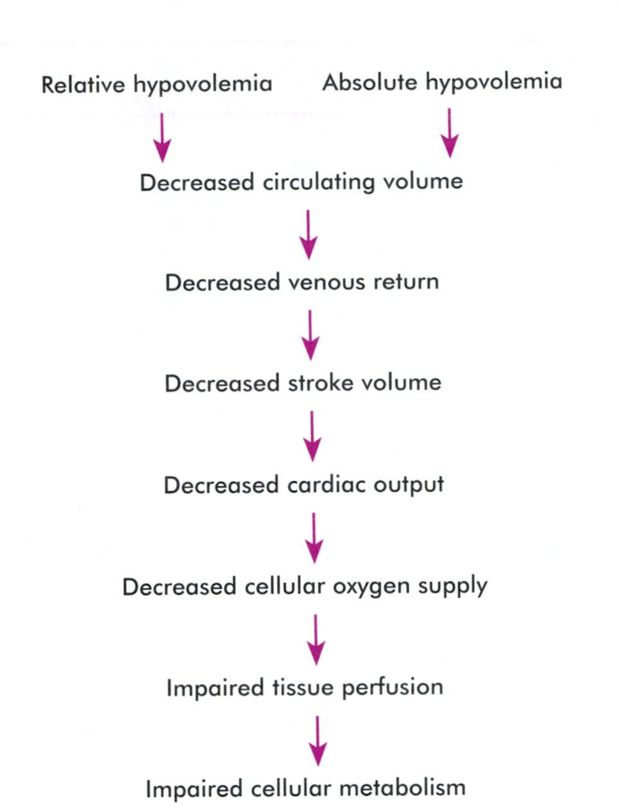

FIGURE 44-1. The pathophysiology of hypovolemic shock.

alkalosis and hypoxemia, as evidenced by low $Pa{CO_2}$ and low $Pa{O_2}$ levels, respectively. Urine output (UO) starts to decline as renal perfusion decreases. Urine sodium decreases, whereas urine osmolarity and specific gravity increase as the kidneys start to conserve sodium and water. The patient's skin becomes pale and cool, with delayed capillary refill because of peripheral vasoconstriction. Jugular veins appear flat as a result of decreased venous return. Decreased cerebral perfusion causes a change in level of consciousness (LOC). The patient may appear disoriented, confused, restless, anxious, or irritable.[9,11,13]

The third, or progressive, stage occurs with a fluid volume loss of 30% to 40%, or an actual volume loss of 1500 to 2000 ml.[11] The compensatory mechanisms become overwhelmed, and impaired tissue perfusion develops. The HR continues to increase, and dysrhythmias develop as myocardial ischemia ensues. Respiratory distress occurs as the pulmonary system deteriorates. ABG values during this phase reveal respiratory and metabolic acidosis and hypoxemia, as evidenced by high $Pa{CO_2}$, low bicarbonate (HCO_3^-), and low $Pa{O_2}$ levels, respectively. Decreased renal perfusion results in the development of oliguria. Blood urea nitrogen (BUN) and serum creatinine levels start to rise as the kidneys begin to fail. The patient's skin becomes ashen, cold, and clammy, with marked delayed capillary refill. The patient appears lethargic as cerebral perfusion decreases and LOC continues to deteriorate.[9,11,13]

The fourth, or refractory, stage occurs with a fluid volume loss of greater than 40%, or an actual volume loss of more than 2000 ml.[11] The compensatory mechanisms completely deteriorate, and organ failure occurs. Severe tachycardia and hypotension ensue. Peripheral pulses are absent, and because of marked peripheral vasoconstriction, capillary refill does not occur. The skin appears cyanotic, mottled, and extremely diaphoretic. The patient becomes unresponsive, and a variety of clinical manifestations associated with failure of the different body systems develop.[11,13]

Assessment of the hemodynamic parameters of a patient in hypovolemic shock reveals a decreased CO and cardiac index (CI). Loss of circulation volume leads to a decrease in venous return to the heart, which results in a decrease in the preload of the right and left ventricles. This is evidenced by a decline in the right atrial pressure (RAP) and pulmonary artery wedge pressure (PAWP). Vasoconstriction of the arterial system results in an increase in the afterload of the heart, as evidenced by an increase in the SVR.[9,13]

Medical Management

Treatment of the patient in hypovolemic shock requires an aggressive approach. The major goals of therapy are to correct the cause of the hypovolemia and to restore tissue perfusion. This approach includes identifying and stopping the source of fluid loss and vigorously administering fluid to replace circulating volume.[20] Fluid administration can be accomplished with either a crystalloid or a colloid solution, or both. The type of solution used usually depends on the type of fluid lost.[10–13]

Another therapy available for assisting with resuscitation of the patient in hypovolemic shock is autotransfusion. Autotransfusion is the collection and administration of the patient's own blood. It has been particularly useful in managing the patient in hypovolemic shock caused by chest trauma and hemorrhage.[21]

Nursing Management

Prevention of hypovolemic shock is one of the primary responsibilities of the nurse in the critical care area. Preventive measures include the identification of patients at risk and constant assessment of patients' fluid balance. Accurate monitoring of intake and output and daily weights are essential components of preventive nursing management. Early identification and treatment result in decreased mortality.[22]

The patient in hypovolemic shock may have any number of nursing diagnoses, depending on the progression of the process (Box 44-4). Nursing interventions include minimizing fluid loss, enhancing volume replacement, and monitoring the patient's response to care.

Measures to minimize fluid loss include limiting blood sampling, observing intravenous lines for accidental disconnection, and applying direct pressure to bleeding sites. Measures to enhance volume replacement include insertion of large-diameter peripheral intravenous catheters; rapid administration of prescribed fluids; and positioning the patient with the legs elevated, trunk flat, and head and shoulders above the chest. In addition, monitoring the patient for clinical manifestations of fluid overload is critical to preventing further problems.

BOX 44-4 NURSING DIAGNOSIS AND MANAGEMENT

HYPOVOLEMIC SHOCK

- Fluid Volume Deficit related to absolute loss, p. 914
- Fluid Volume Deficit related to relative loss, p. 915
- Decreased Cardiac Output related to alterations in preload, p. 590
- Altered Nutrition: Less Than Body Requirements related to increased metabolic demands or lack of exogenous nutrients, p. 165
- Risk for Infection, p. 1119
- Anxiety related to threat to biologic, psychologic, and/or social integrity, p. 99
- Ineffective Family Coping related to critically ill family member, p. 97

CARDIOGENIC SHOCK

Description

Cardiogenic shock is the result of failure of the heart to pump blood forward effectively. It can occur with dysfunction of either the right or the left ventricle, or both. The lack of adequate pumping function leads to decreased tissue perfusion and initiation of the general shock response.[3,23] It occurs in approximately 7% to 10% of patients with an acute myocardial infarction (MI), and the mortality rate is 65% to 90%.[23]

Etiology

Cardiogenic shock can result from primary ventricular ischemia, structural problems, and dysrhythmias.[23] The most common cause is acute MI resulting in the loss of 40% or more of the functional myocardium. The damage to the myocardium may occur after one massive MI, or it may be cumulative as a result of several smaller MIs.[3,23,24] Structural problems of the cardiopulmonary system and dysrhythmias also may cause cardiogenic shock if they disrupt the forward motion of the blood through the heart (Box 44-5).[2,23,24]

BOX 44-5 Etiologic Factors in Cardiogenic Shock

- Primary ventricular ischemia
  - Acute myocardial infarction
  - Cardiopulmonary arrest
  - Open heart surgery
- Structural problems
  - Septal rupture
  - Papillary muscle rupture
  - Free wall rupture
  - Ventricular aneurysm
  - Cardiomyopathies
    - Congestive
    - Hypertrophic
    - Restrictive
  - Intracardiac tumor
  - Pulmonary embolus
  - Atrial thrombus
  - Valvular dysfunction
  - Acute myocarditis
  - Cardiac tamponade
  - Myocardial contusion
- Dysrhythmias
  - Bradydysrhythmias
  - Tachydysrhythmias

Pathophysiology

Cardiogenic shock results from the impaired ability of the ventricle to pump blood forward, which leads to a decrease in SV and an increase in the blood left in the ventricle at the end of systole. The decrease in SV results in a decrease in CO, which leads to decreased cellular oxygen supply and impaired tissue perfusion. When the underlying problem involves the left ventricle, the increase in end-systolic volume results in the backup of blood into the pulmonary system and the subsequent development of pulmonary edema. Pulmonary edema causes impaired gas exchange and decreased oxygenation of the arterial blood, which further impairs tissue perfusion (Figure 44-2). Death may result from cardiopulmonary collapse.[3,23,24]

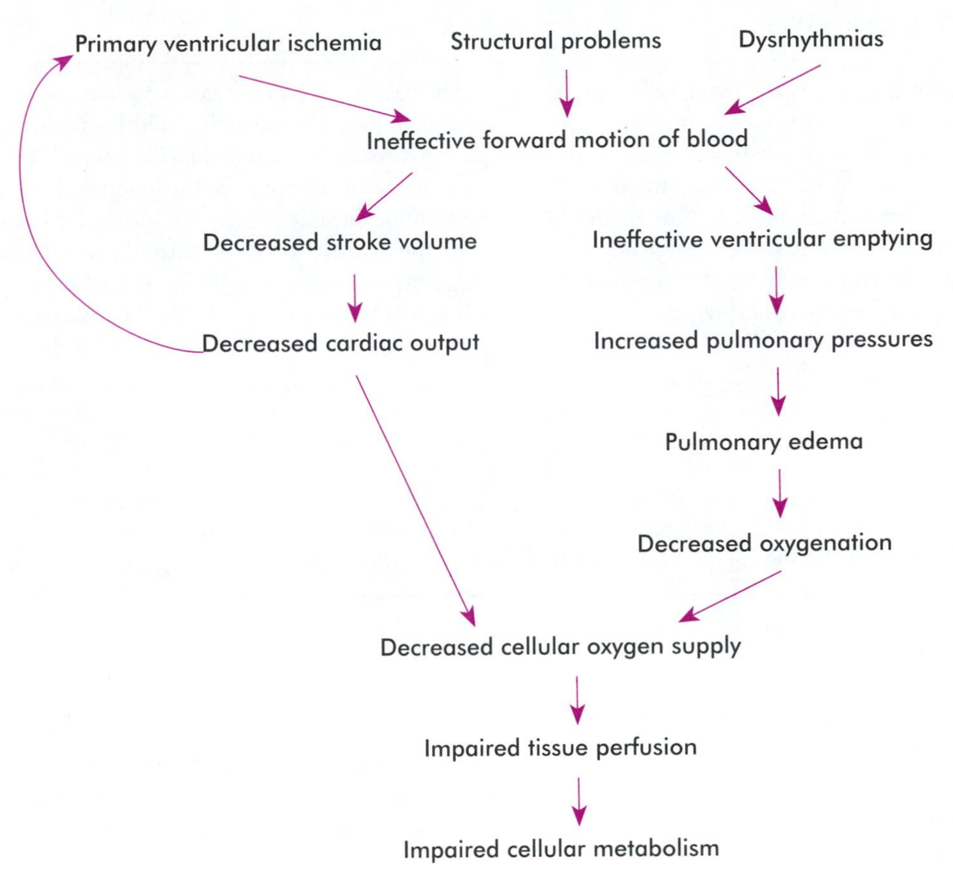

FIGURE 44-2. The pathophysiology of cardiogenic shock.

Assessment and Diagnosis

A variety of clinical manifestations occur in the patient in cardiogenic shock, depending on etiologic factors in pump failure, the patient's underlying medical status, and the severity of the shock state. Some clinical manifestations are caused by failure of the heart as a pump, whereas many relate to the overall shock response (Box 44-6).

Initially the clinical manifestations relate to the decline in CO. These signs and symptoms include SBP less than 90 mm Hg; decreased sensorium; cool, pale, moist skin; and UO less than 30 ml/hour. The patient also may complain of chest pain. Once the compensatory mechanisms are activated, tachycardia develops to compensate for the fall in CO. A weak, thready pulse develops, and heart sounds may reveal a diminished first heart sound (S_1) and second heart sound (S_2) as a result of the decrease in contractility. The respiratory rate increases to improve oxygenation. ABG values at this time indicate respiratory alkalosis, as evidenced by a decrease in $Paco_2$. Urinalysis findings demonstrate a decrease in urine sodium and an increase in urine osmolarity and specific gravity as the kidneys start to conserve sodium and water. The patient also may experience a variety of dysrhythmias, depending on the underlying problem.[9,23]

In the patient with left ventricular failure a variety of additional clinical manifestations may be seen. Auscultation of the lungs may disclose crackles and rhonchi, indicating the development of pulmonary edema. Hypoxemia occurs, as evidenced by a fall in Pao_2 as measured by ABG values. Heart sounds may reveal a third heart sound (S_3) and a fourth heart sound (S_4). If right ventricular failure occurs, jugular venous distention may become evident.[24]

Once the compensatory mechanisms become overwhelmed and impaired tissue perfusion develops, a variety of other clinical manifestations appear. Myocardial ischemia progresses, as evidenced by continued increases in HR, dysrhythmias, and chest pain. The pulmonary system starts to deteriorate, which leads to respiratory distress. ABG values during this phase reveal respiratory and metabolic acidosis and hypoxemia, as indicated by high $Paco_2$, low HCO_3^-, and low

LEGAL REVIEW

The Living Will

One type of advance directive is the living will, which typically is a signed, written, witnessed statement that explains the patient's preferences about withholding or withdrawing life-sustaining treatment at the time of terminal illness. This document is part of the medical record. The patient must be advised to periodically review his or her living will. In some states this is required by law, or the effect of the will is void. Living wills may be revoked at any time.

The vast majority of states have living will statutes; all states have pending legislation. The limitations to life-sustaining treatment and terminal illness are being revised in many state statutes to make the living will more compatible with the durable power of attorney for health care.

In the absence of state statute, the will must clearly define life-sustaining treatment and address whether nutrition and hydration are among the measures to be withheld or withdrawn and under what conditions.

See Choice in Dying: *A living will,* New York, Choice in Dying, 200 Varick Street, New York, 10014; Choice in Dying: *Questions and answers about the living will,* New York, Choice in Dying, 200 Varick Street, New York, 10014; Collins E, Weber D: *The complete guide to living wills,* New York, 1991, Bantam Books; Crisham P: Living wills—controversy and certainty, *J Prof Nurs* 6(6):321, 1990; Emanuel L: Beyond the living will, *Harv Med Sch Health Letter* 15(8):4, 1990; *In Re Estate of Greenspan,* 558 N.E.2d 1194 (Ill. 1990); *In Re Peter,* 529 A.2d 419 (N.J. 1987); Killian WH: Knowledge of living will laws essential, *Am Nurse* 22(7):33, 1990; Ney CA: Living wills: the ethical dilemmas, *Crit Care Nurse* 9(8):20, 1989.

BOX 44-6 Clinical Manifestations of Cardiogenic Shock

Systolic blood pressure <90 mm/Hg
Heart rate >100 beats/min
Weak, thready pulse
Diminished heart sounds
Change in sensorium
Cool, pale, moist skin
Urine output <30 ml/hr
Chest pain
Dysrhythmias
Tachypnea
Crackles
Decreased cardiac output
Cardiac index <2.2 L/min/m^2
Increased pulmonary artery wedge pressure
Increased right atrial pressure
Increased systemic vascular resistance

PaO_2 levels, respectively. Renal failure occurs, as exhibited by the development of anuria and increases in BUN and serum creatinine levels. Cerebral hypoperfusion manifests as decreasing LOC.[23]

Assessment of the hemodynamic parameters of a patient in cardiogenic shock reveals a decreased CO and a CI less than 2.2 L/min/m^2.[24] Inadequate pumping action leads to a decrease in SV, which results in an increase in the left ventricular end-diastolic pressure (LVEDP). This is reflected in an increase in the PAWP. Compensatory vasoconstriction results in an increase in the afterload of the heart, as evidenced by an increase in the SVR. If right ventricular failure is present, the RAP also will be increased.[9,24]

Medical Management

Treatment of the patient in cardiogenic shock requires an aggressive approach. The major goals of therapy are to treat the underlying cause, enhance the effectiveness of the pump, and improve tissue perfusion. This approach includes identifying the etiologic factors of pump failure and administering pharmacologic agents to enhance CO. Inotropic agents are used to increase contractility, whereas vasodilating agents and diuretics are used for afterload and preload reduction, respectively. Antidysrhythmic agents are used to suppress or control dysrhythmias that can affect CO.[10,25]

Once the cause of pump failure has been identified, measures are taken to correct the problem if possible. If the problem is related to an acute MI, measures are taken to increase myocardial oxygen supply and decrease myocardial oxygen demand. Therapies to increase myocardial oxygen supply include supplemental oxygen; intubation and mechanical ventilation; and coronary artery vasodilator agents, such as nitroglycerin. In addition, thrombolytic agents, coronary angioplasty, intracoronary stents, or coronary artery bypass surgery may also be used. Therapies to decrease myocardial demand include activity restrictions, analgesics, and sedatives.[10,24]

Two other therapies available to improve the effectiveness of the pumping action of the heart are the intraaortic balloon pump (IABP) and the ventricular assist device (VAD). The IABP is a temporary measure to decrease myocardial workload by improving myocardial supply and decreasing myocardial demand. It achieves this goal by improving coronary artery perfusion and reducing left ventricular afterload. The VAD is a temporary external pump that takes the place of the patient's ventricle, allowing it to heal.[24] (∞Mechanical Circulatory Assist Devices, p. 567.)

Nursing Management

Prevention of cardiogenic shock is one of the primary responsibilities of the nurse in the critical care area. Preventive measures include the identification of patients at risk and constant assessment of the patient's cardiopulmonary status.[22] Patients who require IABP therapy need to be observed frequently for complications. Complications include emboli formation, infection, rupture of the aorta, thrombocytopenia, improper balloon placement, bleeding, improper timing of the balloon, balloon rupture, and circulatory compromise of the cannulated extremity.[26]

The patient in cardiogenic shock may have any number of nursing diagnoses depending on the progression of the process (Box 44-7). Nursing interventions include limiting myocardial oxygen consumption, enhancing myocardial oxygen supply, and monitoring the patient's response to care.

Measures to limit myocardial oxygen consumption include administering analgesics and sedatives, positioning the patient for comfort, limiting activities, offering support to reduce anxiety, providing a calm and quiet environment, and teaching the patient about his or her condition. Measures to enhance oxygen myocardial supply include administering supplemental oxygen, monitoring the patient's respiratory status, and administering prescribed medications.

BOX 44-7 NURSING DIAGNOSIS AND MANAGEMENT

CARDIOGENIC SHOCK

- Altered Myocardial Tissue Perfusion related to acute myocardial ischemia, p. 595
- Decreased Cardiac Output related to alterations in contractility, p. 592
- Decreased Cardiac Output related to alterations in heart rate, p. 593
- Altered Nutrition: Less Than Body Requirements related to increased metabolic demands or lack of exogenous nutrients, p. 165
- Risk for Infection, p. 1119
- Body Image Disturbance related to functional dependence on life-sustaining technology, p. 86
- Ineffective Family Coping related to critically ill family member, p. 97

ANAPHYLACTIC SHOCK

Description

Anaphylactic shock, a type of distributive shock, is the result of an immediate hypersensitivity reaction. It is a life-threatening event that requires prompt intervention. The severe antibody-antigen response leads to decreased tissue perfusion and initiation of the general shock response.[2,27–29]

Etiology

Anaphylactic shock is caused by an antibody-antigen response. Almost any substance can cause a hypersensitivity reaction (Box 44-8). These substances, known as *antigens,* can be introduced by injection or ingestion or through the skin or respiratory tract. A number of antigens have been identified that can cause a reaction in a hypersensitive person. This list includes foods, food additives, diagnostic agents, biologic agents, environmental agents, drugs, and venoms (Box 44-9).[3,28,29]

Anaphylactic reactions can be either IgE-mediated or non–IgE-mediated responses. IgE is an antibody that is formed as part of the immune response. The first time an antigen enters the body, an antibody IgE, specific for the antigen, is formed. The antigen-specific IgE antibody is then stored by attachment to mast cells and basophils. This initial contact with the antigen is known as a *primary immune response.* The next time the antigen enters the body, the preformed IgE antibody reacts with it and a secondary immune response occurs. This reaction triggers the release of biochemical mediators from the mast cells and basophils and initiates the cascade of events that precipitate anaphylactic shock.[3,28,29]

Some anaphylactic reactions are non–IgE-mediated responses in that they occur in the absence of activation of IgE antibodies. These responses occur as a result of direct activation of the mast cells to release biochemical mediators. Direct activation of mast cells can be triggered by humoral mediators, such as the complement system and the coagulation-fibrinolytic system. In addition, biochemical mediators can be released as a direct or indirect response to many drugs. This type of reaction is known as *anaphylactoid reaction.* Anaphylactoid reactions are produced in persons not previously sensitized and can occur with the first exposure to an antigen.[28,29]

BOX 44-8 Etiologic Factors in Anaphylactic Shock

Foods
- Eggs and milk
- Fish and shellfish
- Nuts and seeds
- Legumes and cereals
- Citrus fruits
- Chocolate
- Strawberries
- Tomatoes
- Other

Food additives
- Food coloring
- Preservatives

Diagnostic agents
- Iodinated contrast dye
- Sulfobromophthalein (Bromsulphalein) (BSP)
- Dehydrocholic acid (Decholin)
- Iopanoic acid (Telepaque)

Biologic agents
- Blood and blood components
- Insulin and other hormones
- Gamma globulin
- Seminal plasma
- Enzymes
- Vaccines and antitoxins

Environmental agents
- Pollens, molds, and spores
- Sunlight
- Animal hair

Drugs
- Antibiotics
- Aspirin
- Narcotics
- Dextran
- Vitamins
- Local anesthetic agents
- Muscle relaxants
- Barbiturates
- Other

Venoms
- Bees and wasps
- Snakes
- Jellyfish
- Spiders
- Deer flies
- Fire ants

Pathophysiology

The antibody-antigen response (immunologic stimulation) or the direct triggering (nonimmunologic activation) of the mast cells results in the release of biochemical mediators. These mediators include histamine, eosinophilic chemotactic factor of anaphylaxis (ECF-A), neutrophilic chemotactic factor of anaphylaxis (NCF-A), proteinases, heparin, serotonin, leukotrienes (formerly known as slow-reacting substance of anaphylaxis), prostaglandins, and platelet-activating factor. The activation of the biochemical mediators causes vasodilation; increased capillary permeability; bronchoconstriction; excessive mucus secretion; coronary vasoconstriction; inflammation; cutaneous reactions; and constriction of the smooth muscle in the intestinal wall, bladder, and uterus. Coronary vasoconstriction causes severe myocardial depression. Cutaneous reactions cause stimulation of nerve endings followed by itching and pain.[29]

ECF-A promotes chemotaxis of eosinophils, thus facilitating the movement of eosinophils into the area. During allergic reactions, eosinophils phagocytose the antibody-antigen complex and other inflammatory debris and release enzymes that inhibit vasoactive mediators, such as histamine and leukotrienes. In addition, secondary mediators are produced that either enhance or inhibit the already released biochemical mediators. Bradykinin, a secondary mediator, increases capillary permeability, facilitates vasodilation, and contracts smooth muscles.[29]

Peripheral vasodilation results in decreased venous return. Increased capillary membrane permeability results in the loss of intravascular volume and the development of relative hypovolemia. Decreased venous return results in decreased end-diastolic volume and SV. The decline in SV leads to a fall in CO and impaired tissue perfusion. Death may result from airway obstruction or cardiovascular collapse (Figure 44-3).[3,27-29]

Assessment and Diagnosis

Anaphylactic shock is a severe systemic reaction that can affect any number of organ systems. A variety of clinical manifestations occur in the patient in anaphylactic shock, depending on the extent of multisystem involvement. The symptoms usually start to appear within minutes of exposure to the antigen, peak within 15 to 30 minutes, and resolve over the next several hours (Box 44-10).[28]

BOX 44-9 Latex Allergies

Latex is the milky sap of the rubber tree *Hevea brasilliensis.* It is treated with preservatives, accelerators, stabilizers, and antioxidants to make a more elastic, stable rubber. Reactions to products containing latex can be triggered by either the latex protein or by an additive used in the manufacturing process.

Latex reactions can be classified into three different categories: irritation (nonallergic inflammation occurring when the skin is abraded), delayed hypersensitivity (non–IgE-mediated response to the chemical agents added during the manufacturing process), or immediate sensitivity (IgE-mediated response to latex proteins). Although the overall prevalence of latex allergy in the general population is only 1%, it is much higher (28%–67%) in selected groups, such as patients with neural tube defects (spinal bifida, myelomeningocele, lipomyelomeningocele) or congenital urologic disorders; those who have undergone multiple surgeries or who have a history of allergy to anesthetic drugs; and health care, rubber industry, or glove manufacturing plant workers.

Five routes of exposure to latex proteins have resulted in systemic reactions: cutaneous (contact with moist skin); mucous membranes (mouth, vagina, urethra, or rectum); internal tissue (during surgery and other invasive procedures); intravascular; and inhalation (exposure to anesthesia equipment or endotracheal tubes or through the aerosolization of glove powder). It has been postulated that the latex allergen adheres to the cornstarch or powder that coats the gloves and is released into the air with the manipulation of rubber gloves.

The American Academy of Allergy and Immunology has published guidelines for providing care to persons with latex allergy. All persons at risk for latex allergy must have a careful history taken and must complete a standardized latex allergy questionnaire. A history suggestive of reactivity to latex includes local swelling or itching after blowing up balloons, dental examinations, contact with rubber gloves, vaginal or rectal examinations, using condoms or diaphragms, and contact with other rubber products. Other historical information that may suggest increased risk of latex allergy includes hand eczema; previous, unexplained anaphylaxis; oral itching after eating bananas, chestnuts, kiwis, and avocados; and multiple surgical procedures in infancy. Patients at high risk must be offered clinical testing for latex allergy.

The patient with a latex allergy must be cared for in a latex-free environment—that is, an environment in which there are no latex gloves used and no direct patient contact with other devices containing latex.[30,31]

The cutaneous effects usually appear first and include pruritus, generalized erythema, urticaria, and angioedema. Commonly seen on the face and in the oral cavity and lower pharynx, angioedema develops as a result of fluid leaking into the interstitial space. The patient may appear restless, uneasy, apprehensive, and anxious and complain of being warm. Respiratory effects include the development of laryngeal edema, bronchoconstriction, and mucus plugs. Clinical manifestations of laryngeal edema include inspiratory stridor, hoarseness, a sensation of fullness or a lump in the throat, and dysphagia. Bronchoconstriction causes dyspnea, wheezing, and chest tightness.[9,29–31] In addition, gastrointestinal and genitourinary manifestations may develop as a result of smooth muscle contraction. These include vomiting, diarrhea, cramping, abdominal pain, urinary incontinence, and vaginal bleeding.[27–29]

As the anaphylactic reaction progresses, hypotension and reflex tachycardia develop. This occurs in response to massive vasodilation and loss of circulating volume. Jugular veins appear flat as right ventricular end-diastolic volume is decreased. The eventual outcome is circulatory failure and shock.[9,27–29] The patient's level of consciousness may deteriorate to unresponsiveness.[29]

Assessment of the hemodynamic parameters of a patient in anaphylactic shock reveals a decreased CO and CI. Venous vasodilation and massive volume loss lead to a decrease in preload, which results in a decline in the RAP and PAWP. Vasodilation of the arterial system results in a decrease in the afterload of the heart, as evidenced by a decrease in the SVR.[9]

Medical Management

Treatment of anaphylactic shock requires an immediate and direct approach. The goals of therapy are to remove the offending antigen, reverse the effects of the biochemical mediators, and promote adequate tissue perfusion. When the hypersensitivity reaction occurs as a result of administration of medications, dye, blood, or blood products, the infusion must be immediately discontinued. Many times it is not possible to remove the antigen because it is unknown or has already entered the patient's system.[28]

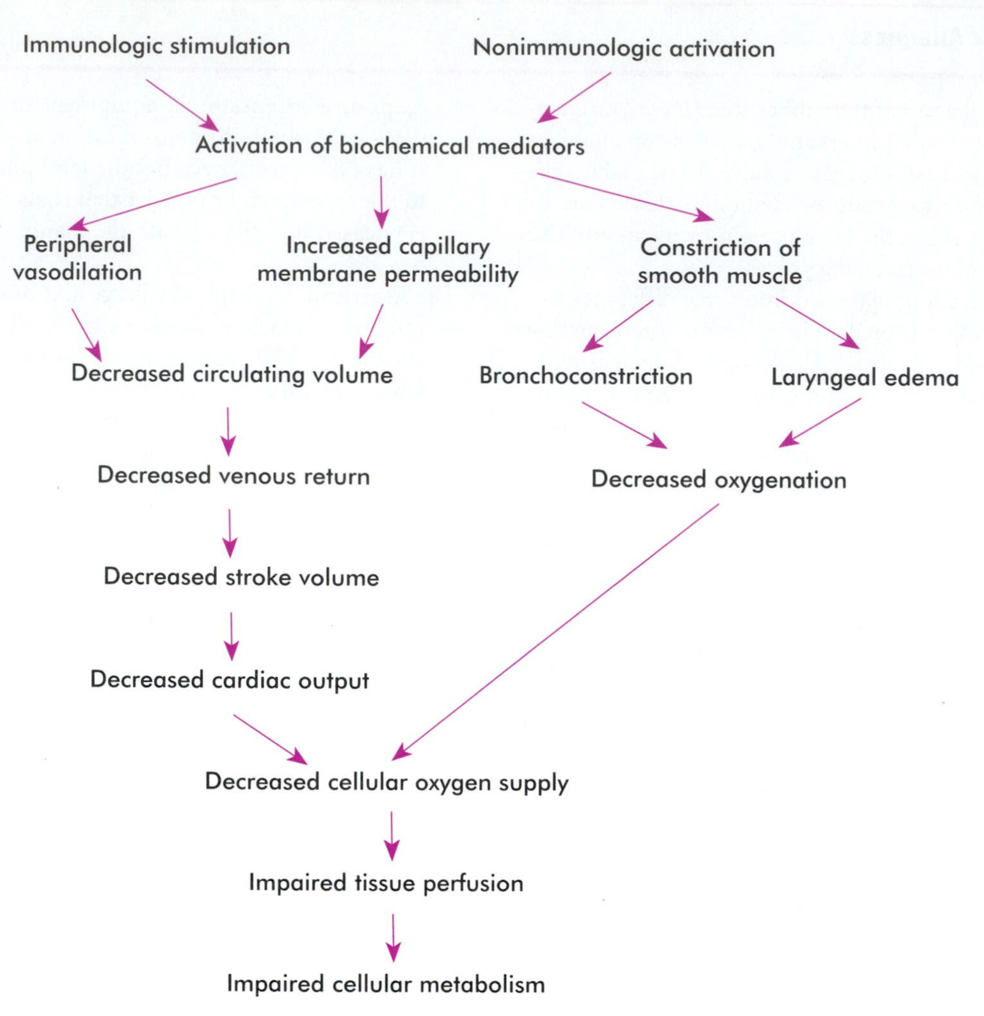

FIGURE 44-3. The pathophysiology of anaphylactic shock.

Reversal of the effects of the biochemical mediators involves the preservation and support of the patient's airway, ventilation, and circulation. This is accomplished through oxygen therapy, intubation, mechanical ventilation, and administration of drugs and fluids. Epinephrine is given to promote bronchodilation and vasoconstriction and to inhibit further release of biochemical mediators.[28,32] It usually is administered intravenously or via endotracheal tube. The dose is 0.1 mg/kg of 1:10,000 dilution IV over at least 3 to 5 minutes or 10 ml of 1:10,000 dilution endotracheally. Diphenhydramine (Benadryl), 1 to 2 mg/kg IV every 6 to 8 hours, is used to block the histamine response. Corticosteroids may also be given with the goal of preventing a delayed reaction and stabilizing capillary membranes.[32] Fluid replacement is accomplished by use of either a crystalloid or colloid solution. In addition, positive inotropic agents and vasoconstrictor agents may be necessary to reverse the effects of myocardial depression and vasodilation.[10,27,28,32]

Nursing Management

Prevention of anaphylactic shock is one of the primary responsibilities of the nurse in the critical care area. Preventive measures include the identification of patients at risk and cautious assessment of the patients' response to the administration of drugs, blood, and blood products. A complete and accurate history of the patient's allergies is an essential component of preventive nursing management. In addition to a list of the allergies, a detailed description of the type of response for each one must be obtained.[22]

The patient in anaphylactic shock may have any number of nursing diagnoses, depending on the progression of the process (Box 44-11). Nursing interventions include facilitating ventilation, enhancing volume replacement, promoting comfort, and monitoring the patient's response to care.

Measures to facilitate ventilation include positioning the patient to assist with breathing and instructing the patient to breathe slowly and deeply. Measures to enhance volume replacement include inserting large-

BOX 44-10 Clinical Manifestations of Anaphylactic Shock

Cardiovascular
- Hypotension
- Tachycardia

Respiratory
- Lump in throat
- Dysphagia
- Hoarseness
- Stridor
- Wheezing
- Rales and rhonchi

Cutaneous
- Pruritus
- Erythema
- Urticaria
- Angioedema

Neurologic
- Restlessness
- Uneasiness
- Apprehension
- Anxiety
- Decreased level of consciousness

Gastrointestinal
- Nausea
- Vomiting
- Diarrhea

Genitourinary
- Incontinence
- Vaginal bleeding

Subjective complaints
- Sensation of warmth
- Dyspnea
- Abdominal cramping and pain
- Itching

Hemodynamic parameters
- Decreased cardiac output (CO)
- Decreased cardiac index (CI)
- Decreased right atrial pressure (RAP)
- Decreased pulmonary artery wedge pressure (PAWP)
- Decreased systemic vascular resistance (SVR)

diameter peripheral intravenous catheters; rapidly administering prescribed fluids; and positioning the patient with the legs elevated, trunk flat, and head and shoulders above the chest. Measures to promote comfort include administering medications to relieve itching; applying warm soaks to skin; and, if necessary, covering the patient's hands to discourage scratching. In addition, observing the patient for clinical manifestations of a delayed reaction is critical to preventing further problems.

BOX 44-11 NURSING DIAGNOSIS AND MANAGEMENT

ANAPHYLACTIC SHOCK

- Fluid Volume Deficit related to relative loss, p. 915
- Decreased Cardiac Output related to alterations in preload, p. 590
- Decreased Cardiac Output related to alterations in afterload, p. 592
- Ineffective Breathing Pattern related to decreased lung expansion, p. 723
- Impaired Gas Exchange related to ventilation/perfusion mismatching or intrapulmonary shunting, p. 725
- Altered Nutrition: Less Than Body Requirements related to increased metabolic demands or lack of exogenous nutrients, p. 165
- Risk for Infection, p. 1119
- Ineffective Individual Coping related to situational crisis and personal vulnerability, p. 95
- Ineffective Family Coping related to critically ill family member, p. 97

NEUROGENIC SHOCK

Description

Neurogenic shock, a type of distributive shock, is the result of the loss or suppression of sympathetic tone. Its onset is within minutes, and it may last for days, weeks, or months depending on the cause.[33] The lack of sympathetic tone leads to decreased tissue perfusion and initiation of the general shock response. Neurogenic shock is the rarest form of shock.[3,34]

Etiology

Neurogenic shock can be caused by anything that disrupts the SNS. The problem can occur as the result of interrupted impulse transmission or blockage of sympathetic outflow from the vasomotor center in the brain.[3,34] The most common cause is a spinal cord injury above the level of T6; this is also known as *spinal shock*.[35] Other causes include spinal anesthesia, drugs, emotional stress, pain, and CNS dysfunction.[3] (∞Spinal Cord Injuries, p. 1064.)

Pathophysiology

Loss of sympathetic tone results in massive peripheral vasodilation, inhibition of the baroreceptor response, and impaired thermoregulation. Arterial vasodilation leads to a decrease in SVR and a fall in blood pressure. Venous vasodilation leads to decreased venous return because of pooling of blood in the venous circuit. A decreased venous return results in a decrease in end-diastolic volume, or preload. A decrease in preload results in a decrease in SV and CO, and relative hypovolemia develops. The fall in blood pressure and CO leads to inadequate or impaired tissue perfusion.[33,35] Inhibition of the baroreceptor response results in loss of compensatory reflex tachycardia. The HR does not increase to compensate for the fall in CO, which further compromises tissue perfusion.[36] Impaired thermoregulation occurs because of loss of vasomotor tone in the cutaneous blood vessels that dilate and constrict to maintain body temperature. The patient becomes poikilothermic, or dependent on the environment for temperature regulation (Figure 44-4).[33,36]

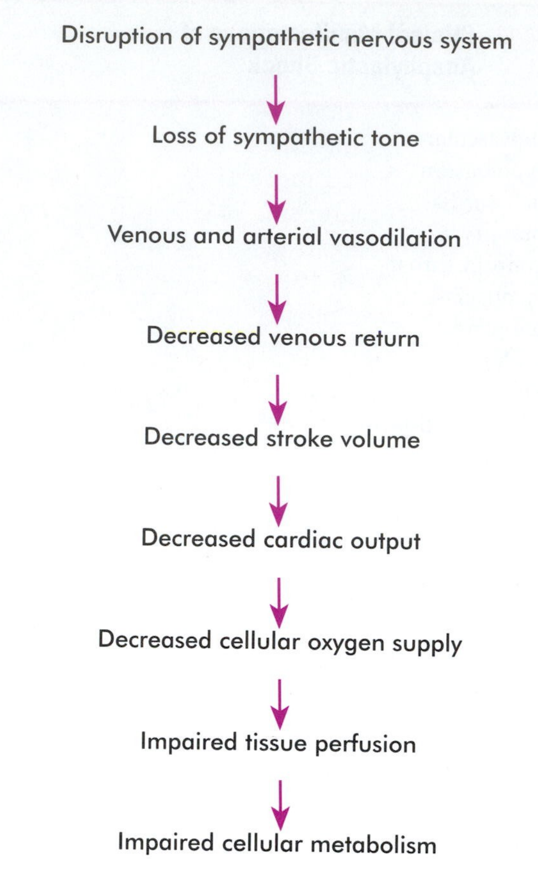

FIGURE 44-4. The pathophysiology of neurogenic shock.

Assessment and Diagnosis

The patient in neurogenic shock usually exhibits hypotension; bradycardia; hypothermia; and warm, dry skin. The decreased blood pressure results from massive peripheral vasodilation. The decreased HR is caused by inhibition of the baroreceptor response and unopposed parasympathetic control of the heart. Hypothermia occurs from uncontrolled heat loss peripherally. The warm, dry skin occurs as a consequence of pooling of blood in the extremities and loss of vasomotor control in surface vessels of the skin that control heat loss.[33,35]

Assessment of the hemodynamic parameters of a patient in neurogenic shock reveals a decreased CO and CI. Venous vasodilation leads to a decrease in preload, which results in a decline in the RAP and PAWP. Vasodilation of the arterial system causes a decrease in the afterload of the heart, as evidenced by a decrease in the SVR.[34]

Medical Management

Treatment of neurogenic shock requires a careful approach. The goals of therapy are to treat or remove the cause, prevent cardiovascular instability, and promote optimal tissue perfusion. Cardiovascular instability can occur from hypovolemia, hypothermia, hypoxia, and dysrhythmias. Specific treatments are aimed at preventing or correcting these problems as they occur.

Hypovolemia is treated with careful fluid resuscitation. The minimal amount of fluid is administered to ensure adequate tissue perfusion. Volume replacement is initiated for an SBP lower than 90 mm Hg, a urine output less than 30 ml/hour, or changes in mental status that indicate decreased cerebral tissue perfusion. The patient is carefully observed for evidence of fluid overload.[35] Vasopressors may be used as necessary to maintain blood pressure and organ perfusion.[34]

Hypothermia is treated with warming measures and environmental temperature regulation. The goal is to maintain normothermia and avoid large swings in the patient's body temperature.[36]

The treatment of hypoxia varies with the underlying cause. Chest wall paralysis, retained secretions, pulmonary edema, and suctioning contribute to the development of hypoxia. Management of this problem may include ventilatory support, vigorous pulmonary hygiene, and supplemental oxygen. Continuous pulse oximetry monitoring also may be helpful in recognizing hypoxia early, before complications arise. The major dysrhythmia seen in neurogenic shock is bradycardia, which is treated with atropine.[33,36]

Nursing Management

Prevention of neurogenic shock is one of the primary responsibilities of the nurse in the critical care area. This includes the identification of patients at risk and constant assessment of the neurologic status. Vigilant immobilization of spinal cord injuries and slight elevation of the patient's head of bed after spinal anesthesia are essential components of preventive nursing management. Early identification allows for early treatment and decreased mortality.[22]

The patient in neurogenic shock may have any number of nursing diagnoses, depending on the progression of the process (Box 44-12). Nursing interventions include treating hypovolemia, maintaining normothermia, preventing hypoxia, and monitoring for dysrhythmias.

Venous pooling in the lower extremities promotes the formation of deep vein thrombosis (DVT), which can result in a pulmonary embolism. All patients at risk for DVT begin receiving prophylaxis therapy. DVT prophylatic measures include monitoring calf and thigh measurements, passive range of motion, application of antiembolic stockings and/or sequential pneumatic stockings, and administration of prescribed anticoagulation therapy.

BOX 44-12 NURSING DIAGNOSIS AND MANAGEMENT

NEUROGENIC SHOCK

- Fluid Volume Deficit related to relative loss, p. 915
- Decreased Cardiac Output related to sympathetic blockade, p. 1118
- Hypothermia related to exposure to cold environment, trauma, or damage to the hypothalamus, p. 324
- Altered Nutrition: Less Than Body Requirements related to increased metabolic demands or lack of exogenous nutrients, p. 165
- Risk for Infection, p. 1119
- Anxiety related to threat to biologic, psychologic, and/or social integrity, p. 99
- Ineffective Family Coping related to critically ill family member, p. 97

SEPTIC SHOCK

Description

Septic shock, a form of distributive shock, occurs when microorganisms invade the body. The primary mechanism of this type of shock is the maldistribution of blood flow to the tissues, with some areas being overperfused and others being underperfused.[4,37] The incidence of sepsis is estimated at more than 400,000 cases annually in the United States, with the mortality rate for septic shock being estimated between 40% and 60%.[38]

A variety of terms may be used to describe the condition the patient with an infection experiences. In 1991, at the American College of Chest Physicians/Society of Critical Care Medicine Consensus Conference, definitions were developed to describe to these conditions (Box 44-13).[39] This discussion focuses only on septic shock.

Etiology

Septic shock is caused by a wide variety of microorganisms including gram-negative and gram-positive aerobes, anaerobes, fungi, and viruses. The source of these microorganisms is varied. Exogenous sources include the hospital environment and members of the health care team. Endogenous sources include the patient's skin, gastrointestinal (GI) tract, respiratory tract, and genitourinary tract. Gram-negative bacteria are responsible for more than half of the cases of septic shock.[5,38,40,41] Toxic shock syndrome is an example of gram-positive shock resulting from *Staphylococcus aureus* (Box 44-14).[42]

Sepsis and septic shock are associated with a wide variety of intrinsic and extrinsic precipitating factors (Box 44-15). All these factors interfere directly or indirectly with the body's anatomic and physiologic defense mechanisms. Several of the intrinsic factors are not modifiable or are very difficult to control. Several of the extrinsic factors may be required for diagnosis and management. All critically ill patients are therefore at risk for the development of septic shock.[38,41,42]

Pathophysiology

Septic shock is a complex systemic response that is initiated when a microorganism enters the body and stimulates the inflammatory/immune system. Shed protein fragments and the release of toxins and other substances from the microorganism activate the plasma enzyme cascades (complement, kallikrein/kinin, coagulation and fibrinolytic factors) as well as platelets, neutrophils, and macrophages. In addition, the toxins damage the endothelial cells. Once activated these systems and cells release a variety of mediators that target various organs throughout the body.[41,43,44]

These mediators initiate a chain of complex interactions that are controlled by numerous feedback mechanisms. Eventually the immune system is overwhelmed, the feedback mechanisms fail, and a process that was designed to protect the body actually harms the body.[5,43] Once the mediators are activated a variety of physiologic and pathophysiologic events occur that affect capillary membrane permeability, clotting,

BOX 44-13 Definitions for Sepsis and Organ Failure

Infection = microbial phenomenon characterized by an inflammatory response to the presence of microorganisms or the invasion of normally sterile host tissue by those organisms.

Bacteremia = the presence of viable bacteria in the blood.

Systemic inflammatory response syndrome (SIRS) = the systemic inflammatory response to a variety of severe clinical insults. The response is manifested by two or more of the following conditions: (1) temperature > 38° C or < 36° C; (2) heart rate > 90 beats per minute; (3) respiratory rate > 20 breaths per minute or $Paco_2$ < 32 mm Hg; and (4) white blood cell count > 12,000/cu mm, < 4,000/cu mm, or > 10% immature (band) forms.

Sepsis = the systemic response to infection, manifested by two or more of the following conditions as a result of infection: (1) temperature > 38° C or > 36° C; (2) heart rate > 90 beats per minute; (3) respiratory rate > 20 breaths per minute or $Paco_2$ < 32 mm Hg; and (4) white blood cell count > 12,000/cu mm, < 4,000/cu mm, or > 10% immature (band) forms.

Severe sepsis = sepsis associated with organ dysfunction, hypoperfusion, or hypotension. Hypoperfusion and perfusion abnormalities may include, but are not limited to, lactic acidosis, oliguria, or an acute alteration in mental status.

Septic shock = sepsis-induced with hypotension despite adequate fluid resuscitation along with the presence of perfusion abnormalities that may include, but are not limited to, lactic acidosis, oliguria, or an acute alteration in mental status. Patients who are receiving inotropic or vasopressor agents may not be hypotensive at the time that perfusion abnormalities are measured.

Sepsis-induced hypotension = a systolic blood pressure <90 mm Hg or a reduction of ≥40 mm Hg from baseline in the absence of other causes for hypotension

Multiple organ dysfunction syndrome (MODS) = presence of altered organ function in an acutely ill patient such that homeostasis cannot be maintained without intervention.

From American College of Chest Physicians/Society of Critical Care Medicine Consensus Conference Committee: *Crit Care Med* 20:864, 1992.

the distribution of blood flow to the tissues and organs, and the metabolic state of the body. Subsequently a systemic imbalance between cellular oxygen supply and demand develops that results in cellular hypoxia, damage, and death (Figure 44-5).[5,38,44]

Damage to the endothelial cells results in continued activation of the mediators, increased capillary membrane permeability, and the formation of microemboli. This leads to disruption of blood flow to the tissues, more endothelial cell damage, and further propagation of the septic process.[43,44]

Activation of the central nervous and endocrine systems also occurs as part of the primary response to invading microorganisms. This activation leads to stimulation of the SNS and the release of ACTH. These events trigger the release of epinephrine, norepinephrine, glucocorticoids, aldosterone, glucagon, and renin, which results in the development of a hypermetabolic state and further contributes to the vasoconstriction of the renal, pulmonary, and splanchnic beds. Activation of the CNS also causes the release of endogenous opiates that are believed to cause vasodilation and to decrease myocardial contractility.[45]

Once the initial sequence of events is triggered, a series of pathophysiologic responses occur that eventually culminate in the maldistribution of circulating blood volume. These responses include massive peripheral vasodilation, microemboli formation, selective vasoconstriction, and increased capillary membrane permeability.[5,44] The maldistribution of circulating blood volume eventually results in decreased cellular oxygen supply.[37,41]

Massive peripheral vasodilation results in the development of relative hypovolemia and decreased tissue perfusion. Microemboli formation leads to decreased tissue perfusion and further endothelial cell damage. Selective vasoconstriction results in decreased tissue perfusion of the kidneys, lungs, and gastrointestinal organs, with eventual system dysfunction. Increased capillary membrane permeability promotes fluid loss from the intravascular space and potentiates the relative hypovolemic effect induced by the massive peripheral vasodilation. The formation of microemboli also is exacerbated because of the increased viscosity of the blood left in the intravascular space.[5,38,41,44]

The maldistribution of circulating blood volume decreases the amount of oxygen delivered to the cells. This situation leads to a number of cellular derangements that ultimately result in cellular death. The hypermetabolic state created by activation of the CNS and the endocrine system further enhances the situation by increasing the oxygen demands of the cells.

A number of metabolic derangements occur as a result of CNS and endocrine system activation. A hypermetabolic state develops that increases cellular oxygen demand and contributes to cellular hypoxia. Lactic acid is produced as a result of anaerobic metabolism. Glucocorticoids, ACTH, epinephrine, and

BOX 44-14 Toxic Shock Syndrome

Toxic shock syndrome (TSS) is a form of septic shock that was first identified in 1978. TSS is a potentially lethal syndrome that is caused by a toxin-producing strain of the gram-positive bacteria *Staphylococcus aureus.* Although often associated with menstruating females who use tampons, it has been reported in males, children, and nonmenstruating females.

The syndrome starts with bacterial colonization or infection of a site. The bacteria release a toxin that is absorbed into the blood stream and circulated to the rest of the body. Once into the blood stream the septic cascade is initiated and septic shock develops.

A few features distinguish TSS. Initially the patient may have flulike symptoms, such as high fever, headache, vomiting, diarrhea, hyperactive bowel sounds, abdominal pain, arthralgia, myalgia, and malaise. The mucous membranes become hyperemic, and pharyngitis, conjunctivitis, vaginitis, and strawberry tongue may develop. In addition, a diffuse erythematous macular rash develops, which progresses to desquamation of the skin in 7 to 10 days. Blood cultures may be negative for bacteremia.

The circulating toxins can also affect the renal, hepatic, hemopoietic, and neurologic systems. Dysfunction of these systems may manifest as elevated levels of blood urea nitrogen (BUN), creatinine, lactic dehydrogenase (LDH), aspartate aminotransferase (AST), bilirubin, and alkaline phosphatase, as well as a decline in platelets. The patient may appear disoriented, confused, and agitated.

Treatment of TSS is essentially the same as the treatment of septic shock. Definitive measures are aimed at identifying the cause of the infection. Supportive measures include administering fluid, antibiotics, and vasoactive agents; treating the fever; and protecting the patient. Generally the acute phase lasts from 2 to 5 days.[44]

glucagon are all catabolic hormones that are released as part of this response. These hormones favor the use of fats and proteins over glucose for energy production.[45]

The hypermetabolic state also increases the cellular metabolic needs. Increased glucose requirements in conjunction with the high level of catabolic hormones result in the limited ability of the cells to use glucose as a substrate for energy production. This causes glucose intolerance, hyperglycemia, relative insulin resistance, and the use of fat for energy (lipolysis). The relative insulin resistance causes the body to produce more insulin, which inhibits the use of fat as an energy substrate. This promotes the use of protein as an energy substrate and catabolism of protein stores in the visceral organs and skeletal muscles.[46]

Assessment and Diagnosis

The patient in septic shock may exhibit a variety of clinical manifestations (Box 44-16). During the initial stage, massive vasodilation occurs in both the venous and arterial beds. Dilation of the venous system leads to a decrease in venous return to the heart, which results in a decrease in the preload of the right and left ventricles. This is evidenced by a decline in the RAP and PAWP. Dilation of the arterial system results in a decrease in the afterload of the heart, as evidenced by a decrease in the SVR. The patient's blood pressure falls in response to the reduction in preload and afterload. The patient's skin becomes pink, warm, and flushed as a result of the massive vasodilation.[9,38,41,44]

BOX 44-15 Precipitating Factors Associated With Septic Shock

INTRINSIC FACTORS

Extremes of age
Co-existing diseases
- Malignancies
- Burns
- Acquired immunodeficiency syndrome (AIDS)
- Diabetes
- Substance abuse
- Dysfunction of one or more of the major body systems

Malnutrition

EXTRINSIC FACTORS

Invasive devices
Drug therapy
Fluid therapy
Surgical and traumatic wounds
Surgical and invasive diagnostic procedures
Immunosuppressive therapy

The HR rises to compensate for the hypotension and in response to increased metabolic, SNS, and adrenal gland stimulation. This results in a normal to high CO and CI. The PP widens as the diastolic blood pressure decreases because of the vasodilation, and the SBP increases because of the elevated CO. A full,

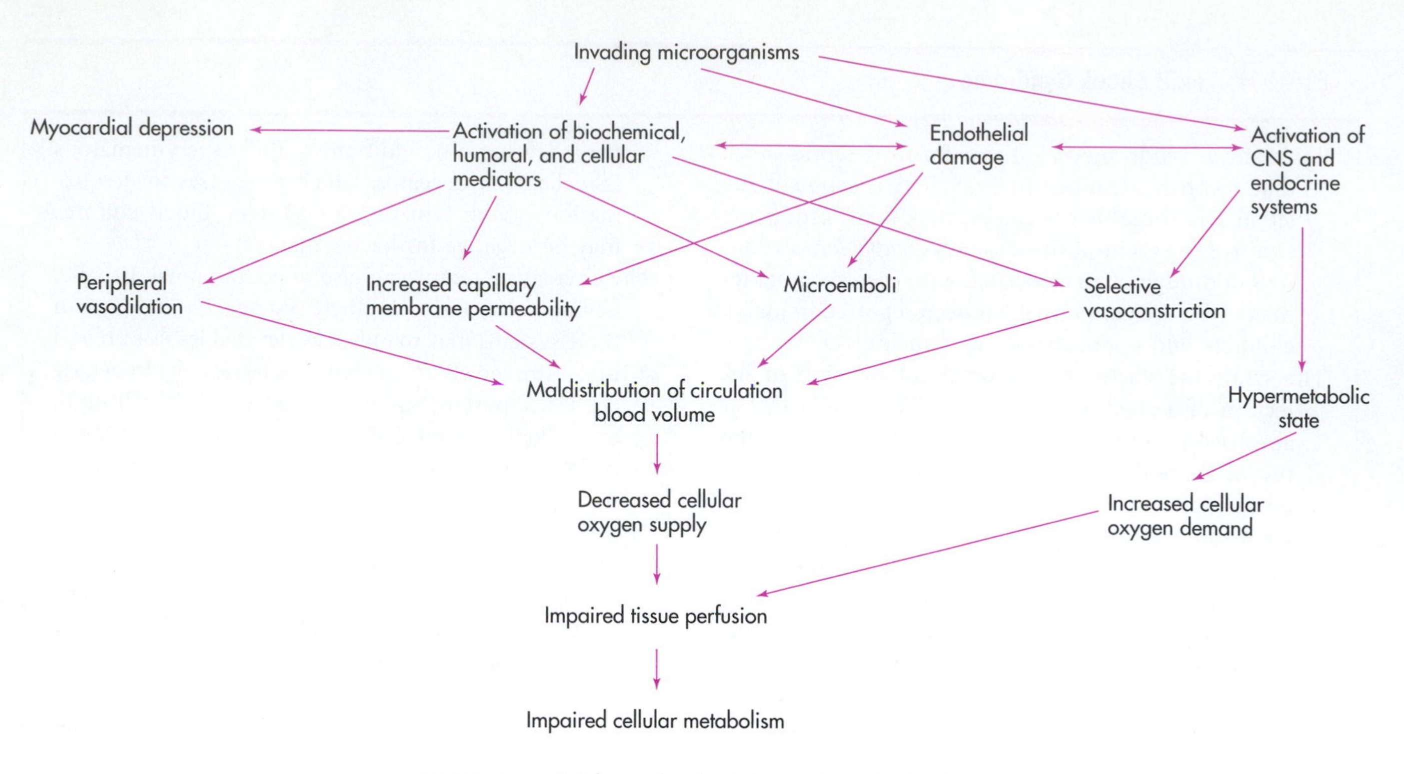

FIGURE 44-5. The pathophysiology of septic shock.

bounding pulse develops. Myocardial contractility is decreased, as evidenced by a decline in the left ventricular stroke work index (LVSWI), an effect of myocardial depression factor.[9,41,47]

In the lungs, ventilation/perfusion mismatching develops as a result of pulmonary vasoconstriction and the formation of pulmonary microemboli. Hypoxemia occurs, and the RR increases to compensate for the lack of oxygen. Crackles develop as increased pulmonary capillary membrane permeability leads to pulmonary interstitial edema.[38]

Level of consciousness starts to change as a result of decreased cerebral perfusion, immune mediator activation, hyperthermia, and lactic acidosis. The patient may appear disoriented, confused, combative, or lethargic. Urine output declines because of decreased perfusion of the kidneys. The patient's temperature is elevated in response to pyrogens released from the invading microorganisms, immune mediator activation, and increased metabolic activity.[9,38,41]

Arterial blood gas values during this phase reveal respiratory alkalosis, hypoxemia, and metabolic acidosis. This is demonstrated by low PaO_2, low $PaCO_2$, and low HCO_3^-, levels, respectively. The respiratory alkalosis is caused by the patient's increased RR. As the patient becomes fatigued the RR decreases and the $PaCO_2$ increases, resulting in respiratory acidosis. The metabolic acidosis is the result of lack of oxygen to the cells and the development of lactic acidemia. The mixed venous oxygen saturation (SvO_2) is increased because of maldistribution of the circulating blood volume and impaired cellular metabolism.[38]

The white blood cell (WBC) count is elevated as part of the immune response to the invading microorganisms. In addition, the white blood cell differential reveals an increase in immature neutrophils (shift to the left). This occurs because the body has to mobilize increasing numbers of WBCs to fight the infection.[41] Increased serum glucose also occurs as part of the hypermetabolic response and the development of insulin resistance.[46] As impaired tissue perfusion develops, a variety of other clinical manifestations appear, indicating the development of MODS.[38]

Medical Management

Treatment of the patient in septic shock requires a multifaceted approach. The goals of treatment are to control the infection, reverse the pathophysiologic responses, and promote metabolic support. This approach includes identifying and treating the infection, supporting the cardiovascular system and enhancing tissue perfusion, and initiating nutritional therapy. In addition, dysfunction of the individual organ systems must be prevented.

BOX 44-16 Clinical Manifestations of Septic Shock

Increased heart rate
Decreased blood pressure
Wide pulse pressure
Full, bounding pulse
Pink, warm, flushed skin
Increased respiratory rate (early)/decreased respiratory rate (late)
Crackles
Change in sensorium
Decreased urine output
Increased temperature
Increased cardiac output and cardiac index
Decreased systemic vascular resistance
Decreased right atrial pressure
Decreased pulmonary artery wedge pressure
Decreased left ventricular stroke work index
Decreased PaO_2
Decreased $PaCO_2$ (early)/increased $PaCO_2$ (late)
Decreased HCO_3^-
Increased mixed venous oxygen saturation (SvO_2)

One of the first measures that must be taken in the treatment of septic shock is finding and eradicating the cause of the infection. Blood, urine, sputum, and wound cultures are obtained to find the location of the infection. Antibiotic therapy is initiated as soon as possible. If the microorganism is unknown, a broad-spectrum antibiotic is administered. Once the microorganism is identified, an antibiotic more specific to the microorganism is started. Administration of antibiotics can be particularly hazardous in gram-negative shock because more endotoxin is released from the cell walls when the microorganisms die. This further aggravates the entire septic process. Surgical intervention to debride infected or necrotic tissue or to drain abscesses also may be necessary to facilitate removal of the septic source.[47]

Another important measure in the treatment of septic shock is supporting the cardiovascular system and enhancing tissue perfusion. Specific interventions are aimed at increasing cellular oxygen supply and decreasing cellular oxygen demand. These treatments include administration of fluids and vasoconstrictor and positive inotropic agents, as well as ventilatory support, temperature control, and reversal of acidosis.[41,47]

Aggressive fluid administration to augment intravascular volume and increase preload is very important during the initial phase. Crystalloids or colloids may be used depending on the patient's condition. The amount of fluid that is administered may vary, but generally the goal is to restore the patient's PAWP to the 15 to 18 mm Hg range. The administration of vasoconstrictor agents is indicated to reverse the massive peripheral vasodilation. These agents help increase the SVR and augment the patient's blood pressure. Positive inotropic agents are used to increase contractility and treat myocardial depression. All these medications are titrated to the patient's response.[41,47]

To optimize oxygenation and ventilation, intubation and mechanical ventilation are required. Ventilator settings are adjusted to provide the patient with a PaO_2 greater than 70 mm Hg and a pH within the normal range. Temperature control also is necessary to decrease the metabolic demands created by hyperthermia. Antipyretic agents and cooling measures often are used.[41,47]

The initiation of nutritional therapy is critical in the management of the patient in septic shock. The goal is to improve the patient's overall nutritional status, enhance the immune system, and promote wound healing. The ideal nutritional supplement for the patient in septic shock must be high in protein because of the metabolic derangements that develop in the hypermetabolic state. The amount of protein calories given depends on the patient's nitrogen balance. In early sepsis the mix of nonprotein calories may be divided evenly between carbohydrates and fats. In the later stages, significant alterations in fat metabolism occur and the lipid content must be limited to 10% to 15% of the total nonprotein calories. The lipid emulsion must contain long-chain fatty acid triglycerides for their protein sparing effects.[47]

Studies are now being conducted with drugs that are believed to block or alter the effects of the immune mediators. These include cyclooxygenase inhibitors, platelet-activating factor antagonists, pentoxifylline, antioxidants, N-acetylcysteine, naloxone, and bradykinin antagonists. Although these therapies have demonstrated positive results in animals, their efficacy in humans needs to be more extensively tested.[48] Corticosteriods have also been extensively studied in the management of sepsis. They have been found to be of no benefit to the patient and may actually be harmful.[49]

Nursing Management

Prevention of septic shock is one of the primary responsibilities of the nurse in the critical care area. These measures include the identification of patients at risk and reduction of their exposure to invading microorganisms. Handwashing, aseptic technique, and an understanding of how microorganisms can invade the body are essential components of preventive nursing management. Early identification allows for early treatment and decreased mortality.[22]

The patient in septic shock may have any number of nursing diagnoses depending on the progression of the process (Box 44-17). Nursing interventions include administering prescribed antibiotics, fluids, and vasoactive agents; preventing the development of concomitant infections; observing for complications of nutritional therapy; and monitoring the patient's response to care. Continual observation to detect subtle changes indicating the progression of the septic process is also very important.

BOX 44-17 NURSING DIAGNOSIS AND MANAGEMENT

SEPTIC SHOCK

- Fluid Volume Deficit related to relative loss, p. 915
- Decreased Cardiac Output related to alterations in preload, p. 590
- Decreased Cardiac Output related to alterations in afterload, p. 592
- Decreased Cardiac Output related to alterations in contractility, p. 592
- Impaired Gas Exchange related to ventilation/perfusion mismatching or intrapulmonary shunting, p. 725
- Altered Nutrition: Less Than Body Requirements related to increased metabolic demands or lack of exogenous nutrients, p. 165
- Risk for Infection, p. 1119
- Anxiety related to threat to biologic, psychologic, and/or social integrity, p. 99
- Ineffective Family Coping related to critically ill family member, p. 97

CASE STUDY

SHOCK

CLINICAL HISTORY

Mr. H is a 27-year-old man born with a neural tube defect and a neurogenic bladder. Shortly after birth, he underwent a meningomyelocele repair with a ventriculoperitoneal (VP) shunt placement. During the following years, Mr. H underwent six major surgeries, all of which were fairly uneventful. However, when he was 17 years old, while undergoing a surgical release of his lower leg contractures, Mr. H suddenly became hypotensive, tachycardiac, and developed a lower extremity rash and wheezing. The anesthesiologist was able to reverse this episode with the administration of fluids and ephedrine. The reaction was attributed to an allergic reaction to cefazolin (Kefzol); 500 mg IV had been administered 30 minutes before the event.

CURRENT PROBLEMS

On this admission Mr. H is taken to the operating room for an anterior spinal release. After 30 minutes of surgery, Mr. H develops generalized erythema, severe hypotension, tachycardia, wheezing, and hypoxemia, despite being ventilated with 100% oxygen. His jugular veins appear flat. Fluid resuscitation is initiated, epinephrine is administered, surgery is terminated, and Mr. H is transferred to the critical care unit on a ventilator. Upon arrival in the unit, Mr. H's vital signs are as follows: blood pressure (BP), 76/45; heart rate (HR), 145 (sinus tachycardia); temperature (T), 97°F; and urine output, 35 ml/hr. Ventilation is continued at a rate of 8 (assist/control mode), tidal volume of 1000 ml, FIO_2 of 100%, and positive end-expiratory pressure (PEEP) of 5 cm H_2O. Breath sounds reveal wheezing over both lung fields. His arterial blood gas values are: PaO_2, 70 mm Hg; $PaCO_2$, 37 mm Hg; pH, 7.30; HCO_3^-, 19 mEq/L; SaO_2, 92%.

CASE STUDY—CONT'D

SHOCK

MEDICAL DIAGNOSIS

Anaphylactic shock

NURSING DIAGNOSES

Fluid Volume Deficit related to relative loss

Decreased Cardiac Output related to alterations in preload

Decreased Cardiac Output related to alterations in afterload

Impaired Gas Exchange related to ventilation/perfusion mismatching

Risk for Altered Tissue Perfusion (cerebral, cardiopulmonary, renal, gastrointestinal, peripheral)

PLAN OF CARE

1. Collaborate with the physician regarding the administration of fluids, vasoactive agents, and bronchodilators.
2. Implement measures to optimize oxygenation and ventilation, including positioning, preventing desaturation and secretion retention, and facilitating secretion removal.
3. Monitor the patient for signs of inadequate tissue perfusion (decreased level of consciousness, dysrhythmias, myocardial ischemia, worsening hypoxemia, decreased urine output, elevated blood urea nitrogen and creatinine, elevated bilirubin, and lactic acidosis).

MEDICAL AND NURSING MANAGEMENT AND PATIENT OUTCOME

Initially it is unclear what caused the anaphylactic reaction. Mr. H is given fluid boluses and started on a dopamine drip, which is titrated to 12 μg/kg/min to keep his systolic BP greater than 90 mm Hg. A beta$_2$ agonist aerosol, diphenhydramine (Benadryl), and a corticosteroid are also started. A pulmonary artery (PA) catheter is inserted, and Mr. H's hemodynamic values are: right atrial pressure (RAP), 3 mm Hg; pulmonary artery wedge pressure (PAWP), 5 mm Hg; cardiac output (CO), 3.4 L/min; cardiac index (CI), 1.8 L/min/m^2; and systemic vascular resistance (SVR), 650. A dobutamine drip is initiated and titrated to 4.5 μg/kg/min to maintain a CI greater than 2.0 L/min/m^2. Throughout the day Mr. H continues to have low filling pressures, persistent vasodilation, and wheezing, despite the discontinuation of all suspected offending agents and aggressive treatment. A thorough review of his history reveals that Mr. H is at high risk for an allergy to latex.

MEDICAL DIAGNOSIS

Latex allergy

NURSING DIAGNOSES

Risk for Injury risk factor: Latex products

Anxiety related to threat to biologic, psychologic, and/or social integrity

Knowledge Deficit: Discharge Regimen related to lack of previous exposure to information

REVISED PLAN OF CARE

1. Provide the patient with a latex-free environment:
   - Post *Latex Allergy/Precaution* signs on patient's door and medical record.
   - Survey the environment and remove all latex products.
   - Wear vinyl or nonlatex gloves when performing care.
   - Read package labels to determine whether products contain rubber or latex before using them on the patient.
   - Remove rubber tops of vials before drawing up medications.
   - Avoid patient contact with bladder and tubing of the blood pressure cuff or stethoscope tubing.
   - Apply rubber tourniquets over cloth only.
   - Tape (with silk tape) rubber ports on IV tubing so they cannot be used.
   - Use stopcocks to administer medications and piggyback IV lines.
   - Develop a latex-free cart with nonlatex supplies stocked on it and a list of substitution items.

Continued

CASE STUDY—CONT'D

SHOCK

REVISED PLAN OF CARE—cont'd

2. Decrease anxiety by providing orientation and education to environment and illness, supporting existing coping mechanisms, speaking slowly and calmly, removing excess stimulation, and promoting presence of comforting significant other.
3. Educate patient and family about latex allergy and its etiologies and treatment, focusing on prevention and treatment.

MEDICAL AND NURSING MANAGEMENT AND PATIENT OUTCOME

All latex products are removed, and Mr. H is placed in a latex-free environment. Over the next 24 hours, Mr. H becomes awake and alert, his vital signs stabilize, and his symptoms are quickly reversed. The remainder of Mr. H's stay in the critical care unit is uneventful. Weaning from the dopamine drip and mechanical ventilation is accomplished. Mr. H is transferred to the intermediate care unit where discharge teaching regarding latex allergy is initiated. His surgery is rescheduled for 3 weeks later.

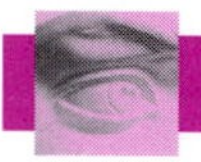

NURSING MANAGEMENT PLAN

DECREASED CARDIAC OUTPUT

DEFINITION:

The state in which the blood pumped by an individual's heart is sufficiently reduced to the extent that it is inadequate to meet the needs of the body's tissues.

Decreased Cardiac Output Related to Sympathetic Blockade

DEFINING CHARACTERISTICS

- Decreased cardiac output (CO) and cardiac index (CI)
- Systolic blood pressure (SBP) < 90 mm Hg or below patient's baseline
- Decreased right atrial pressure (RAP) and pulmonary artery wedge pressure (PAWP)
- Decreased systemic vascular resistance (SVR)
- Bradycardia
- Cardiac dysrhythmias
- Postural hypotension

OUTCOME CRITERIA

- CO and CI are within normal limits.
- SBP 90 mm Hg or returns to baseline.
- RAP and PAWP are within normal limits.
- SVR is within normal limits.
- Sinus rhythm.
- Dysrhythmias are absent.
- Fainting or dizziness with position change is absent.

NURSING INTERVENTIONS AND *RATIONALE*

1. Implement measures to prevent episodes of postural hypotension.
   - Change patient's position slowly ***to allow the cardiovascular system time to compensate.***
   - Apply antiembolic stockings ***to promote venous return.***
   - Perform range-of-motion exercises every 2 hours ***to prevent venous pooling.***
   - Collaborate with the physician and physical therapist regarding the use of a tilt table ***to progress the patient from supine to upright position.***
2. Collaborate with the physician regarding the administration of the following:
   - Crystalloids and/or colloids ***to increase the patient's circulating volume, which increases stroke volume and subsequently cardiac output.***
   - Vasopressors if fluids are ineffective ***to constrict the patient's vascular system, which increases resistance and subsequently blood pressure.***
3. Monitor cardiac rhythm for bradycardia and/or dysrhythmias, ***which can further decrease cardiac output.***
4. Avoid any activity that can stimulate the vagal response ***because bradycardia can result.***
5. Treat symptomatic bradycardia and symptomatic dysrhythmias according to unit's emergency protocol or Advanced Cardiac Life Support (ACLS) guidelines.

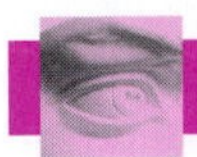

NURSING MANAGEMENT PLAN

RISK FOR INFECTION

DEFINITION:

The state in which an individual is at increased risk for being invaded by pathogenic organisms.

RISK FACTORS

- Inadequate primary defenses (broken skin, traumatized tissue, decreased ciliary action, stasis of body fluids, change in pH secretions, altered peristalsis)
- Inadequate secondary defenses (decreased hemoglobin, leukopenia, suppressed inflammatory/immune response)
- Immunocompromise
- Inadequate acquired immunity
- Tissue destruction and increased environmental exposure
- Chronic disease
- Invasive procedures
- Malnutrition
- Pharmaceutical agents (antibiotics, steroids)

OUTCOME CRITERIA

- Total lymphocyte count is > 2000 mm³.
- White blood cell count is within normal limits.
- Temperature is within normal limits.
- Blood, urine, wound, and sputum cultures are negative.

NURSING INTERVENTIONS AND *RATIONALE*

1. Wash hands before and after patient care ***to reduce the transmission of microorganisms.***
2. Use aseptic technique for insertion or manipulation of invasive monitoring devices, intravenous lines, and urinary drainage catheters ***to maintain sterility of environment.***
3. Use aseptic technique for dressing changes ***to prevent contamination of wounds or insertion sites.***
4. Change any line placed under emergent conditions within 24 hours ***since aseptic technique is usually breeched during an emergency.***
5. Collaborate with the physician to change any dressing that is saturated with blood or drainage ***since these are mediums for microorganism growth.***
6. Minimize use of stopcocks and maintain caps on all stopcock ports ***to reduce the ports of entry for microorganisms.***
7. Avoid the use of nasogastric tubes, nasal endotracheal tubes, and nasopharyngeal suctioning in the patient with a suspected cerebrospinal fluid leak ***to decrease the incidence of central nervous system infection.***
8. Change ventilator circuits with humidifiers no more than every 48 hours ***to avoid introducing microorganisms into the system.***
9. Use disposable sterile scissors, forceps, and hemostats ***to reduce the transmission of microorganisms.***
10. Maintain a closed urinary drainage system ***to decrease incidence of urinary infections.***
11. Protect all access device sites from potential sources of contamination (nasogastric reflux, draining wounds, ostomies, sputum).
12. Refrigerate parenteral nutrition solutions and open enteral nutrition formulas before use ***to inhibit bacterial growth.***
13. Perform daily inspection of all invasive devices for signs of infection.

REFERENCES

1. Barone JE, Snyder AB: Treatment strategies in shock: use of oxygen transport measurement, *Heart Lung* 20:81, 1991.
2. Rice V: Shock, a clinical syndrome: an update. II. The stages of shock, *Crit Care Nurse* 11(5):74, 1991.
3. Rice V: Shock, a clinical syndrome: an update. I. An overview of shock, *Crit Care Nurse* 11(4):20, 1991
4. Houston MC: Pathophysiology of shock, *Crit Care Nurs Clin North Am* 2:143, 1990.
5. Astiz ME, Rackow EC, Weil MH: Pathophysiology and treatment of circulatory shock, *Crit Care Clin* 9:183, 1993.
6. McMahon K: Multiple organ failure: the final complication of critical illness, *Crit Care Nurse* 15(6):20, 1995.
7. Shoemaker WC: Pathophysiology, monitoring and therapy of circulatory problems, *Crit Care Nurs Clin North Am* 6:295, 1994.
8. Nawas YN, Balk RA: General approach to shock, *Clin Geriatr Med* 10:185, 1994.
9. Summers G: The clinical and hemodynamic presentation of the shock patient, *Crit Care Nurs Clin North Am* 2:161, 1990.
10. Rice V: Shock, a clinical syndrome: an update. III. Therapeutic management, *Crit Care Nurse* 11(6):34, 1991.

11. Sommers MS: Fluid resuscitation following multiple trauma, *Crit Care Nurse* 10(10):74, 1990.
12. Kuhn MM: Colloids vs crystalloids, *Crit Care Nurse* 11(5):37, 1991.
13. Daleiden A: Pathophysiology and treatment of hemorrhagic shock during the early postoperative period, *Crit Care Nurs Q* 16:45, 1993.
14. Burns KM: Vasoactive drug therapy in shock, *Crit Care Nurs Clin North Am* 2:167, 1990.
15. Lorenz A: Lactic acidosis: a nursing challenge, *Crit Care Nurse* 9(4):64, 1989.
16. Arieff AI: Managing metabolic acidosis: update on the sodium bicarbonate controversy, *J Crit Illness* 8:224, 1993.
17. Kuhn MM: Nutritional support for the shock patient, *Crit Care Nurs Clin North Am* 2:201, 1990.
18. Lancaster LE, Rice V: Nursing care planning: overview and application to the patient in shock, *Crit Care Nurs Clin North Am* 2:279, 1990.
19. Jillings CR: Shock: psychosocial needs of the patient and family, *Crit Care Nurs Clin North Am* 2:325, 1990.
20. Britt LD and others: Priorities in the management of profound shock, *Surg Clin North Am* 76:645, 1996.
21. Blansfield J: Emergency autotransfusion in hypovolemia, *Crit Care Nurs Clin North Am* 2:195, 1990.
22. Rice V: Shock, a clinical syndrome: an update. IV. Nursing care of the shock patient, *Crit Care Nurse* 11(7):28, 1991.
23. Chatterjee K and others: Gaining ground on cardiogenic shock, *Patient Care* 28(15):24, 1994.
24. Alpert JS, Becker RC: Mechanisms and management of cardiogenic shock, *Crit Care Clin* 9:205, 1993.
25. Zaloga GP and others: Pharmacologic cardiovascular support, *Crit Care Clin* 9:335, 1993.
26. Schott KE: Intra-aortic balloon counterpulsation as a therapy for shock, *Crit Care Nurs Clin North Am* 2:187, 1990.
27. Crnkovick DJ, Carlson RW: Anaphylaxis: an organized approach to management and prevention, *J Crit Illness* 8:332, 1993.
28. Atkinson TP, Kaliner MA: Anaphylaxis, *Med Clin North Am* 76:841, 1992.
29. Mackan MD: Managing the patient with anaphylaxis. I. Mechanisms and manifestations, *Emer Med* 27(2):68, 1995.
30. Sussman GL, Beezhold DH: Allergy to latex rubber, *Ann Intern Med* 122:43, 1995
31. Steelman VM: Latex allergy precautions, *Nurs Clin North Am* 30:457, 1995.
32. Mackan MD: Managing the patient with anaphylaxis. II. Therapeutic strategies, *Emer Med* 27(3):20, 1995.
33. Schwenker D: Cardiovascular considerations in the critical care phase, *Crit Care Nurs Clin North Am* 2:363, 1990.
34. Walleck CA: Neurological considerations in the critical care phase, *Crit Care Nurs Clin North Am* 2:357, 1990.
35. Atkinson PP, Atkinson JLD: Spinal shock, *Mayo Clin Proc* 71:384, 1996.
36. Kidd PS: Emergency management of spinal cord injuries, *Crit Care Nurs Clin North Am* 2:349, 1990.
37. Vincent JL, Van Der Linden P: Septic shock: particular type of acute circulatory failure, *Crit Care Med* 18:S70, 1990.
38. Hazinski MF and others: Epidemiology, pathophysiology and clinical presentation of gram-negative sepsis, *Am J Crit Care* 2:224, 1993.
39. American College of Chest Physicians/Society of Critical Care Medicine Consensus Conference Committee: Definitions for sepsis and organ failure and guidelines for the use of innovative therapies in sepsis, *Crit Care Med* 20:864, 1992.
40. Hoyt NJ: Preventing septic shock: infection control in the intensive care unit, *Crit Care Nurs Clin North Am* 2:287, 1990.
41. Rackow EC, Astiz ME: Mechanisms and management of septic shock, *Crit Care Clin* 9:219, 1993.
42. Creehan PA: Toxic shock syndrome: an opportunity for nursing intervention, *J Obstet Gynecol Neonatal Nurs* 24:557, 1995.
43. Secor VH: The inflammatory/immune response in critical illness: role of the systemic inflammatory response syndrome, *Crit Care Nurs Clin North Am* 6:251, 1994.
44. Crowley SR: The pathogenesis of septic shock, *Heart Lung* 25:124, 1996.
45. Lawler DA: Hormonal response in sepsis, *Crit Care Nurs Clin North Am* 6:265, 1994.
46. Ackerman MH, Evans NJ, Ecklund MM: Systemic inflammatory response syndrome, sepsis, and nutritional support, *Crit Care Nurs Clin North Am* 6:321, 1994.
47. Wiessner WH, Casey LC, Zbilut JP: Treatment of sepsis and septic shock: a review, *Heart Lung* 24:380, 1995
48. Weikert LF, Bernard GR: Pharmacotherapy of sepsis, *Clin Chest Med* 17:289, 1996.
49. Cronin L and others: Corticosteroid treatment for sepsis: a critical appraisal and meta-analysis of the literature, *Crit Care Med* 23:1430, 1995.

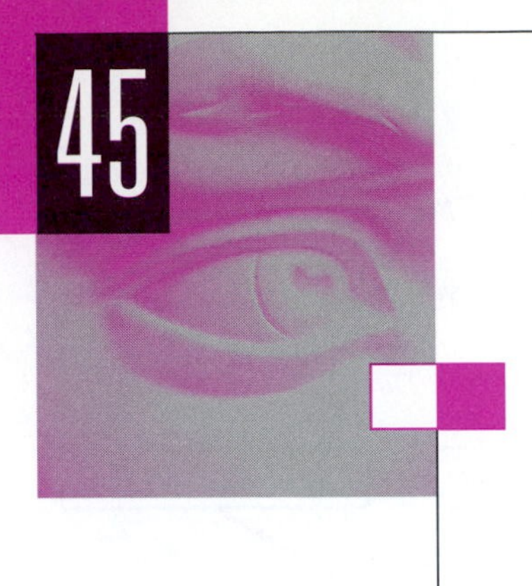

Systemic Inflammatory Response Syndrome and Multiple Organ Dysfunction Syndrome

ADVANCED CARDIOPULMONARY LIFE support techniques and technology have allowed for the survival of some critically ill or injured patients who previously would have died of an initial insult, such as trauma, infection, shock, or other acute processes. However, continued patient survival and long-term quality of life is threatened by two clinical syndromes, systemic inflammatory response syndrome (SIRS) and multiple organ multiple organ dysfunction syndrome (MODS), that may result in death or profound disability. SIRS is characterized by generalized systemic inflammation in organs remote from an initial insult. MODS results from SIRS and pertains to progressive physiologic failure of several interdependent organ systems.[1–4]

In 1992 the American College of Chest Physicians and the Society of Critical Care Medicine proposed a framework to describe the interrelationships among the systemic inflammatory response, sepsis, bacteremia, and infection (Figure 45-1), and multiple organ dysfunction (Figure 45-2).[5,6] New terminology was proposed to describe the clinical manifestations of SIRS, and its relationship to sepsis, and MODS. Critical care professionals were urged to standardize terminology used in diagnosis, intervention, and research protocols.[5,6] In the past, terms such as *multiple systems organ failure, multiple organ failure syndrome,* and *progressive* or *sequential organ failure* were used to describe clinical syndromes of organ failure in critically ill patients. Because these terms imply organ failure rather than the dynamic process of organ dysfunction, the name of the syndrome was changed to *multiple organ dysfunction syndrome.*[5,6]

This chapter provides information regarding the pathogenesis of SIRS and MODS. Current clinical management, investigational therapies, and appropriate nursing diagnoses are addressed.

THE INFLAMMATORY RESPONSE

Acute inflammation is a biochemical and cellular process that occurs in vascularized tissue in response to an insult or invasion.[7] During inflammation the body creates a lethal micro environment to localize the injury and kill microorganisms. Normally the inflammatory process is contained within a restricted environment. If not contained, a systemic widespread response, SIRS, occurs that is deleterious to organ function.[7–9] Fortunately, the body normally has a complex system of checks and balances to localize inflammation.

Local Inflammatory Response

The acute inflammatory response is a self-limiting (generally 8 to 10 days), nonspecific response that usually occurs in an identical manner regardless of the cause. The response generally starts within seconds of the insult. Cell injury or death initiates the acute inflammatory response. Cellular injury may result from trauma, hypoxia, and microorganisms.[7]

Mediators, facilitators of the local inflammatory response, are housed in the circulatory system and enhance the movement of plasma and blood cells from the circulation into the tissue around the injury. Mediators of the vascular response include leukocytes; plasma protein cascades (complement, coagulation, kinin/kallikrein); platelets; and other inflammatory biochemicals, such as arachidonic acid (AA) metabolites (e.g., prostaglandins, interleukins, tumor necrosis factor).[7]

Vascular response. The local vascular effects of inflammation start immediately and sustain increased vascular permeability that lasts through acute inflammation. Several mechanisms are operable. Arterioles near the injury constrict briefly, then dilate to increase blood flow to the injured area and allow exudation of

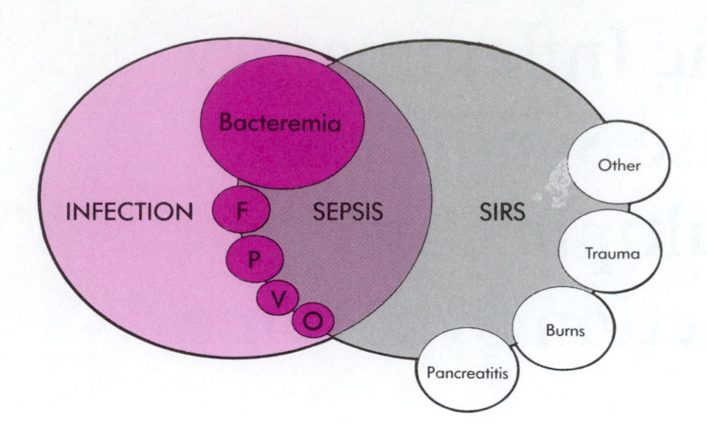

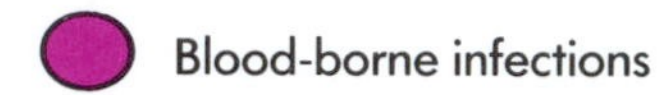

F Fungemia
P Parasitemia
V Viremia
O Other

FIGURE 45-1. Interrelationships among systemic inflammatory response syndrome (SIRS), sepsis, and infection. (From American College of Chest Physicians/Society of Critical Care Medicine Consensus Conference Committee: Definitions for sepsis and organ failure and guidelines for the use of innovative therapies in sepsis, *Crit Care Med* 20:865, 1992.)

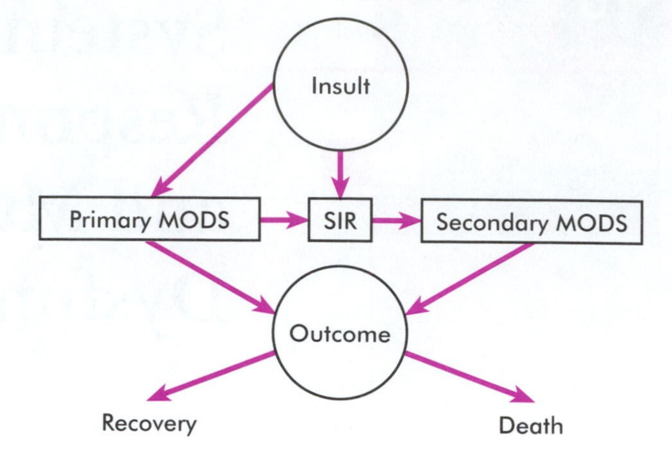

FIGURE 45-2. Different causes and results of primary and secondary multiple organ dysfunction syndrome (MODS). *SIR,* systemic inflammatory response. (From American College of Chest Physicians/Society of Critical Care Medicine Consensus Conference Committee: Definitions for sepsis and organ failure and guidelines for the use of innovative therapies in sepsis, *Crit Care Med* 20:868, 1992.)

plasma and cells into tissues. Exudation causes interstitial edema and slows the microcirculation, making it more viscous. Concurrently, mediators such as bradykinin stimulate capillary and venule endothelial cells to retract, creating spaces at junctions between cells. Endothelial cell retraction allows leukocytes to squeeze out of the cell. The net effect is the movement of blood cells and plasma proteins into the inflamed tissue.[7]

Neutrophil response. Neutrophils engage in four functions related to inflammation: margination, diapedesis, chemotaxis, and phagocytosis. Many neutrophils normally adhere to the inside of blood vessel walls until needed (margination). On activation, neutrophils move to the area of injury by squeezing through the pores of blood vessels (diapedesis), are attracted to microbials or debris by chemical substances (chemotaxis), phagocytose bacteria or cellular debris, and then die. Monocytes and macrophages perform similar functions in a later stage of the inflammatory process.[7]

Plasma protein response. Three major plasma protein systems—the complement, coagulation, and kinin/kallikrein systems—participate in the acute inflammatory response. The complement system, a complex cascade of more than 20 serum proteins, is involved in inflammatory and immune processes that destroy bacteria and contribute to vascular changes. Eleven principal proteins, labeled C1 to C9, have been identified. Activation of the complement cascade occurs through the classic pathway in response to an antigen/antibody complex or through an alternate pathway by exposure to polysaccharide from bacterial cell walls. The terminal pathway for both the classic and alternate pathways results in lysis of the target cell. The effects of complement during inflammation are outlined in Box 45-1.[7]

The kinin/kallikrein system controls vascular tone and permeability and is activated by stimulation of the plasma kinin cascade. Hageman factor (Factor XII) of the coagulation cascade is also directly involved in kinin activation. Kinins are biochemicals that are controlled by kinases, enzymes present in the plasma and tissues. The end result of kinin activation is the production of bradykinin. Bradykinin has profound effects, including vasodilation at low doses, pain, extravascular smooth muscle contraction, increased vascular permeability, and leukocyte chemotaxis. Bradykinin facilitates endothelial retraction and increased vascular permeability, processes involved in acute inflammation.[7]

The coagulation system traps bacteria in injured tissue and works with platelets to control excessive bleeding. The human body normally maintains a balance

BOX 45-1 Actions of Complement During Inflammation

Opsonization/phagocytosis
Lysis of invading cell membranes
Agglutination
Neutralization of viruses
Chemotaxis
Activation of mast cells
Inflammatory effects:
- Increased hyperemia
- Increased capillary leakage
- Increased protein coagulation in tissues

between clot formation (thrombosis), which is needed to minimize blood loss and to repair wounds, and clot lysis (fibrinolysis), which maintains the patency of blood vessels.[10,11] The coagulation system is a plasma protein system that, like the complement cascade, can be activated through two pathways. The intrinsic pathway is activated when the Hageman factor contacts damaged vessel endothelial cells. The extrinsic pathway is activated by damaged tissue. Both pathways converge at Factor X and proceed to fibrin polymerization and clot formation. Thirteen plasma proteins (Factors I to XIII), produced primarily in the liver, participate in the coagulation cascade. The fibrinolytic system lyses fibrin clots through the actions of proteolytic and lysosomal enzymes. Plasmin splits fibrin and fibrinogen into fibrin degradation products; consequently the clots dissolve. It is this delicate balance between thrombin and plasmin in the circulation that maintains normal coagulation and lysis during the inflammatory process. The end result of these complex interactions is a lesion that is ready to heal.[7,10,11]

Normally, complex systems work together to limit and localize the inflammatory response, thus limiting and confining the potentially destructive effects of uncontrolled mediator activity. Antiproteases, circulating albumin, vitamins C and E, red blood cells, and phagocytic cells limit the inflammatory response by inhibiting proteolytic enzyme activity, scavenging toxic oxygen metabolites, and removing the stimulus by phagocytosis.[8,9,12]

Systemic inflammatory response. The systemic inflammatory response, a continuous process, is an abnormal host response characterized by generalized inflammation in organs remote from the initial insult.[1] SIRS pertains to the widespread inflammation or clinical responses to inflammation occurring in patients with a variety of insults. Clinical conditions and manifestations associated with SIRS are listed in Box 45-2. These insults produce similar or identical systemic inflammatory responses, even in the absence of infection. SIRS is present when two or more of four clinical manifestations are present in the high risk patient. Manifestations of SIRS must represent an acute alteration from the patient's normal baseline and must not be related to other causes (e.g., neutropenia from chemotherapy or leukopenia). When SIRS is a result of infection, the term *sepsis* is used. Organ dysfunction or failure, such as acute lung injury, acute renal failure, and MODS, are complications of SIRS.[5,6]

BOX 45-2 Clinical Conditions and Manifestations Associated With Systemic Inflammatory Response Syndrome (SIRS)

CLINICAL CONDITIONS

Infection
Infection of vascular structures (heart and lungs)
Pancreatitis
Ischemia
Multiple trauma with massive tissue injury
Hemorrhagic shock
Immune-mediated organ injury
Exogenous administration of tumor necrosis factor or other cytokines
Aspiration of gastric contents
Massive transfusion
Host defense abnormalities

CLINICAL MANIFESTATIONS

Temperature $< 38°$ C or $> 36°$ C
Heart rate > 90 beats/min
Respiratory rate > 20 breaths/min or $Pa_{CO_2} < 32$ torr
WBC $> 12{,}000$ cells/mm^3 or < 4000 cells/mm^3 or $>$ 10% immature (band) forms

When SIRS is not contained, several consequences may occur that lead to organ dysfunction, including intense, uncontrolled activation of inflammatory cells (neutrophils, macrophages, lymphocytes); direct damage of vascular endothelium; disruption of immune cell function; persistent hypermetabolism; and maldistribution of circulatory volume to organ systems.[1,2,8,9] Consequently, inflammation becomes a systemic self-perpetuating process that is inadequately controlled and results in organ dysfunction.[7–9,12,13]

However, not all patients develop MODS from SIRS. The development of MODS appears to be associated with failure to control the source of inflammation or infection, a persistent perfusion, flow-dependent oxygen consumption (VO_2), or the continued presence of necrotic tissue.[14]

MULTIPLE ORGAN DYSFUNCTION SYNDROME

MODS results from progressive physiologic failure of several interdependent organ systems. It is defined as the "presence of altered organ function in an acutely ill patient such that homeostasis cannot be maintained without intervention."[5] Dysfunction of one organ may amplify dysfunction in another. Organ dysfunction may be absolute or relative and occurs over varying time periods. MODS is the major cause of morbidity in the critically ill patient and may account for up to 80% of all mortalities in the critical care unit. MODS is a leading cause of late mortality after trauma.

Incidence

Lack of consensus regarding acceptable definitions for organ dysfunction, the number of organs involved, and the duration of organ dysfunction has hampered an accurate account of organ dysfunction in critically ill patients. About 7% to 15% of critically ill patients experience dysfunction in at least two organ systems. Patient outcome is directly related to the number of organs that fail. Failure of three or more organs is associated with a 90% to 95% mortality rate.[15]

High Risk Patients

Although various patient populations are at risk for organ dysfunction, trauma patients are particularly vulnerable because they frequently experience prolonged episodes of circulatory shock with tissue hypoxemia, tissue injury, and infection.[4] Other high risk patients include those who have experienced a shock episode associated with a ruptured aneurysm, acute pancreatitis, sepsis, burns, or surgical complications.[2,4,16] Patients age 65 years and older are at increased risk secondary to their decreased organ reserve.[4]

Clinical Course and Progression

Organ dysfunction may be a direct consequence of the insult (primary MODS) or can manifest latently and involve organs not directly affected in the initial insult (secondary MODS) (see Figure 45-2). Patients can experience both primary and secondary MODS.

Primary MODS. Primary MODS "directly results from a well-defined insult in which organ dysfunction occurs early and is directly attributed to the insult itself."[5] Direct insults initially cause localized inflammatory responses. Examples of primary MODS include the immediate consequences of trauma, such as pulmonary contusion, pulmonary dysfunction after aspiration or inhalation injury, and renal dysfunction as a result of rhabdomyolysis or emergency aortic surgery.[5,6] Primary MODS generally results in one of three patient outcomes: recovery, a stable hypermetabolic state (limited SIRS), or death.[15]

Secondary MODS. Secondary MODS is a consequence of widespread systemic inflammation that results in dysfunction of organs not involved in the initial insult.[5,6] The focus of the following discussion pertains to the relationship between SIRS and secondary MODS.

Secondary MODS develops latently after a variety of insults. The early impairment of organs normally involved in immunoregulatory function, such as the liver and gastrointestinal (GI) tract, intensifies the host response to an insult.[4,8,9,13]

SIRS/sepsis is a common initiating event in the development of secondary MODS. Severe sepsis appears to initiate a period of circulatory instability and relative physiologic shock that perpetuates an inflammatory focus and resultant organ damage. Noninfectious stimuli (inflammation, perfusion deficit, or dead tissue) also initiate similar cellular consequences. Physiologic shock may create a tissue oxygen debt that sets the stage for activation of SIRS and MODS.[17] (∞Septic Shock, p. 1111).

The definitive clinical course of secondary MODS has not been completely identified. Clinical observations suggest that organ dysfunction may occur in a progressive pattern; however, organs may fail simultaneously.[2,4,10,13,18] Renal dysfunction, for example, may occur concurrently with hepatic dysfunction. The lungs generally are the first major organs affected. After the initial insult and resuscitation, patients develop a persistent hypermetabolism, a metabolic consequence of sustained systemic inflammation and physiologic stress, followed closely by pulmonary dysfunction, manifested as acute respiratory distress syndrome (ARDS).

Hypermetabolism accompanies SIRS but may not occur immediately after insult. Hypermetabolism generally lasts for 14 to 21 days. During hypermetabolism, changes occur in cellular anabolic and catabolic function, resulting in autocatabolism. Autocatabolism manifests as a severe decrease in lean body mass, severe weight loss, anergy, and increased cardiac output and VO_2. The patient experiences profound alterations in carbohydrate, protein, and fat metabolism.[19] Concurrently, GI, hepatic, and immunologic dysfunction may occur, which intensifies the SIRS. Clinical manifestations of cardiovascular instability and central nervous system dysfunction may be present. Ongoing perfusion deficits and septic foci continue to perpetuate SIRS. About 25% to 40% of patients die during hypermetabolism.[16] The development of renal and hepatic failure is a preterminal event in MODS.[16] Patients with decreased physiologic organ reserve may manifest signs and symptoms of organ dysfunction earlier than previously healthy patients.[17] Survivors may develop generalized polyneuropathy and a chronic form of pulmonary disease from ARDS, complicating recovery.[3] These patients often require prolonged, expensive rehabilitation.

Pathophysiological Mechanisms

Secondary MODS results from altered regulation of the patient's acute immune and inflammatory responses. Dysregulation, or failure to control the host inflammatory response, leads to the excessive production of inflammatory cells and biochemical mediators that cause widespread damage to vascular endothelium and organ damage.[20] The critically ill patient's compromised immune state also fosters an environment conducive to organ failure.

Mediators. The inflammatory and immune responses implicated in SIRS and MODS are mediated by certain cells and biochemicals that in turn affect cellular activity. As outlined in Box 45-3, mediators associated with SIRS and MODS can be classified as either inflammatory cells, plasma protein systems, or inflammatory biochemicals. Activation of one mediator often leads to activation of another. Plasma levels are not always indicative of cellular levels. The biologic activity of inflammatory cells, biochemical mediators, and plasma protein systems and how they work in concert to cause SIRS and MODS are not yet totally defined.

Inflammatory Cells. Neutrophils, macrophages, monocytes, mast cells, platelets, and endothelial cells are inflammatory cells that mediate SIRS through their production of cytokines (biochemical mediators). Along with proinflammatory biochemicals released from damaged or necrotic tissue and circulating catecholamines (stress response), these inflammatory cells create a hypermetabolic state, cause maldistribution of circulatory volume, and alter inflammatory and immune function.[20]

Neutrophils. During SIRS and MODS, neutrophils overreact systemically and damage normal cells, in addition to killing bacteria. Specifically, neutrophils adhere to vascular endothelium and release cytotoxic biochemicals including platelet activating factor (PAF), AA metabolites, and toxic oxygen metabolites.[2,4,8,9,12,16] These substances cause tissue damage, vascular injury, edema, thrombosis, and hemorrhage in multiple organ systems. During SIRS/sepsis, neutrophilic function also is modulated by other circulating mediators that intensify its inflammatory response.[20]

Monocytes and macrophages. Monocytes and macrophages normally perform three major functions relative to inflammation: antigen processing and presentation, bacterial phagocytosis, and mediator production. Monocytes and macrophages detect, process, and present antigen to lymphocytes for initiation of the humoral and cellular components of the lymphocytic immune response. Macrophages play a significant role in organ injury by producing oxygen metabolites, initiating procoagulant activity, and releasing interleukin-1 (IL-1) and tumor necrosis factor (TNF). Both TNF and IL-1 then stimulate neutrophils and lymphocytes to activate the AA cascade. AA metabolites are vasoactive and cause vascular instability and altered organ blood flow.[20,21]

BOX 45-3 Inflammatory Mediators Associated With SIRS and MODS

INFLAMMATORY CELLS

Neutrophils
Macrophages/monocytes
Mast
Endothelial

BIOCHEMICAL MEDIATORS

Interleukins
Tumor necrosis factor
Platelet activating factor
Arachidonic acid metabolites
- Prostaglandins
- Leukotrienes
- Thromboxanes

Oxygen radicals
- Superoxide radical
- Hydroxyl radical
- Hydrogen peroxide

Proteases

PLASMA PROTEIN SYSTEMS

Complement
Kinin/kallikrein
Coagulation

In the lungs, alveolar macrophages produce toxic oxygen metabolites and proteolytic enzymes that destroy alveolar epithelial cells. The role of macrophages and monocytes in organ dysfunction is most directly linked to their production of TNF and IL-1.[7,22,23]

Mast cells. Mast cells are found in all body tissues, especially those adjacent to blood vessels. As tissue-based cells, mast cells produce mediators that have both systemic and local effects. Endotoxin, direct cellular injury, complement proteins (C3a and C5a), and bradykinin stimulate the release of mast cell mediators. Mediators from mast cells include histamine, proteases, heparin, TNF, select AA metabolites, and PAF.[12]

Lymphocytes. Lymphocytes adhere to and sequester in the microvascular endothelium. Stimulated T and B lymphocytes produce cytokines such as IL-1 and IL-2, which in turn activate other inflammatory cells.[12]

Endothelial cells. Endothelial cells line the entire vascular system. Normally, there is little interaction between the endothelium and leukocytes. However, during SIRS, endothelial cells become targets for leukocyte-derived mediators. In addition, endothelial cells manufacture chemotactic agents that attract neutrophils to areas of inflammation and endothelial injury. Collectively, these processes cause widespread endothelial destruction and vascular permeability, a key element in SIRS/sepsis. Inflammatory mediators that cause endothelial damage include endotoxin, TNF, IL-1, and PAF. These mediators also recruit and activate neutrophils and activate complement and perpetuate destruction of the endothelium.[20]

Endothelial cells also produce and maintain equilibrium endothelin (a vasoconstrictor), endothelial-derived relaxant factor, and nitric oxide (a vasodilator). An alteration in this balance leads to vascular instability, vasodilation, and perfusion abnormalities commonly seen in patients with SIRS/sepsis. Endothelial damage results in the production of procoagulants, such as PAF, plasminogen-activating inhibitor, angiotensin II and prostacyclin (AA metabolite) and in the development of a procoagulant state, leading to thrombin in the microvasculature.[20]

Biochemical mediators. Multiple biochemical inflammatory mediators play a role in SIRS and MODS, including proteases, TNF, interleukins, PAF, AA metabolites, and oxygen metabolites. TNF, IL-1, and interluekin-6 (IL-6) appear to be the most important cytokines associated with SIRS and MODS.

Toxic oxygen metabolites. Toxic oxygen metabolites are produced in excessive amounts during critical illness and have been implicated in MODS. Oxygen metabolites are normally produced as the result of many physiologic processes. However, the body has numerous antioxidant and enzyme systems to convert free oxygen radicals to nontoxic substances to prevent tissue injury. Excessive oxygen metabolites cause lipid peroxidation and damage to the cell membrane, activate the complement and coagulation cascades, and cause deoxyribonucleic acid (DNA) damage.[24] Inflammatory neutrophils cause tissue injury by producing excessive numbers of toxic oxygen metabolites. For example, toxic oxygen metabolites produced by neutrophils cause lung injury in ARDS.

Reperfusion organ injury is partially attributed to excessive toxic oxygen metabolites. During reperfusion, severe tissue injury follows the massive production of oxygen free radicals. The organs most susceptible to injury include the small intestines, liver, lungs, muscles, heart, brain, stomach, and skin. In the future, antioxidant drug therapy may be effective in preventing organ dysfunction.[21]

Tumor necrosis factor. TNF, also known as *cachectin*, is a mononuclear phagocyte and T lymphocyte-derived cytokine that is produced in response to endotoxin, tissue injury, viral agents, and interleukins. When present in excessive amounts, TNF causes widespread destruction in most organ systems and is responsible for the pathophysiologic changes in SIRS/sepsis and gram-negative shock, including fever, hypotension, decreased organ perfusion, and increased capillary permeability. TNF may precipitate organ injury by causing generalized endothelial injury, fibrin deposition, and a procoagulant state. TNF causes disseminated intravascular coagulopathy (DIC); interstitial pneumonitis; acute tubular necrosis (ATN); and necrosis of the GI tract, liver, and adrenal glands. TNF stimulates AA metabolism, the clotting cascade, and the production of PAF. Metabolically, excessive TNF causes hyperglycemia that progresses to hypoglycemia and hypertriglyceridemia. The destructive effects of TNF are exacerbated by AA metabolites and stress hormones.[20,22,23,25] The biologic effects of TNF are numerous and are outlined in Box 45-4.

Interleukins. The interleukins are a class of cytokines that have similar biologic responses to those of TNF, and both work similarly. At this time there are 14 known interleukins. Interleukin-1 (IL-1) has two known forms that cause organ dysfunction synergistically. However, the effects of TNF are more destructive.

Interleukins are produced primarily by monophagocytic and endothelial cells. Macrophages secrete substantial amounts of IL-1, whereas less is secreted by endothelial cells, epithelial cells, neutrophils, and B lymphocytes. IL-1 causes vascular congestion, capillary leakage, and increased coagulation associated

BOX 45-4 Select Effects of Tumor Necrosis Factor and Interleukin-1

VASCULAR

Endothelial permeability
Increased procoagulant activity
Local vasodilation
Release of platelet activating factor (PAF)
Release of endothelial cytokines
Disseminated intravascular coagulation (DIC)
Leukocyte adherence

HEMATOLOGIC

Chemotaxis
Release of leukocyte AA metabolites
Initial neutropenia
Stimulation of polymorphonuclear leukocytes

HEPATIC

Increased triglycerides caused by suppression of lipoprotein lipase
Decreased synthesis of plasma proteins: albumin and transferrin
Increased synthesis of acute phase proteins
Production of complement components
Synthesis of clotting factors

CENTRAL NERVOUS SYSTEM

Prostaglandin release in the brain
Fever
Headache
Anorexia

CARDIOVASCULAR SYSTEM

Tachycardia
Increased cardiac output
Decreased systemic vascular resistance
Hypotension

Modified from Zimmerman JJ, Ringer TV: *Crit Care Clin* 8:163, 1992.

with SIRS/sepsis. Like TNF, IL-1 has profound vascular endothelial effects. IL-1 stimulates the production of procoagulants by endothelial cells, increases catabolism of muscle tissue, and causes neutrophilia. Cardiovascular and inflammatory effects commonly include hypotension, fever, tachycardia, diarrhea, acute lung injury, leukopenia, platelet aggregation, and disseminated intravascular coagulation.[20,22] IL-1 and other immune cells enhance the production of IL-2, which amplifies the cardiovascular responses. IL-6 is a glycoprotein released by lymphocytes, macrophages, and fibroblasts; it mediates the acute phase response to injury and stimulates the proliferation of B cells.

Platelet activating factor. PAF is a lipid that attaches to cell membrane phospholipids and is released from inflammatory and immune cells in response to a multitude of factors or stimuli that also initiate AA metabolism. PAF is released by platelets, mast cells, monocytes, macrophages, neutrophils, and endothelial cells. PAF has widespread effects on the heart, vascular system, coagulation, platelets, and the lungs. Effects of PAF include platelet aggregation, with resultant microvascular stasis and ischemia in the microvascular bed; platelet release of serotonin, which increases vascular permeability; and increased vasoconstriction from increased production of thromboxane A_2 and AA metabolite.[20]

Arachidonic acid metabolites. AA is a highly metabolic fatty acid that is a precursor of many biologically active substances known as *eicosanoids.* Select eicosanoids are implicated in the pathogenesis of SIRS and MODS. Eicosanoids contribute to organ failure by altering vascular reactivity and permeability and by fostering the accumulation and activation of inflammatory cells.[22–24,26–29]

Activation of the AA cascade by hypoxia, ischemia, endotoxin, catecholamines, and tissue injury produces metabolites from both the cyclooxygenase and lipooxygenase pathways. AA metabolites produced via the cyclooxygenase pathway are called *prostaglandins* (PG) and *thromboxanes* (Tx), whereas those from the lipooxygenase pathway are called *leukotrienes* (LT). AA metabolites have profound effects on vasculature and cause vascular instability and maldistribution of blood flow. Eicosanoids (such as PGH_2 and PGF_2, TxA_2 and TxB_2) and leukotrienes LTD_4, LTC_4, and LTE_4, are vasoconstrictors. In contrast, some eicosanoids have vasodilatory properties. All leukotrienes and TxA_2 enhance capillary membrane permeability and increase vascular leakage. TxA_2, PGH_2, and PGF_2 are potent platelet aggregators.[26–29]

Proteases. Proteases are proteolytic (protein-digesting) enzymes released from inflammatory cells. Proteases digest tissue and can cause significant parenchymal damage. Neutrophils in the lung, for example, produce proteases that destroy lung tissue. In the GI tract, protease-induced mucosal injuries occur.[13]

Complement. Complement is directly implicated in SIRS and MODS. Complement activation occurs in response to endotoxin and TNF. Circulating complement concentrations are greatly increased in patients with SIRS/sepsis. ARDS patients may have a functional deficiency in a C5a inhibitor called *chemotactic factor inactivator.*[21]

Organ-Specific Manifestations

Secondary MODS is a systemic disease with organ-specific manifestations. Organ dysfunction is influenced by numerous factors, including organ host defense function, response time to the injury, metabolic requirements, organ vasculature response to vasoactive drugs, and organ sensitivity to damage and physiologic reserve. The responses of the GI, hepatobiliary, cardiovascular, pulmonary, renal, and coagulation systems are discussed in the following text. Clinical manifestations of organ dysfunction are outlined in Box 45-5.

Gastrointestinal dysfunction. The GI tract plays an important role in MODS. GI organs normally have immunoregulatory functions. Consequently, GI dysfunction amplifies SIRS and gut damage, which may lead to bacterial translocation and endogenous endotoxemia.[7–9,12,13]

Three specific mechanisms link the GI tract and latent organ dysfunction. First, hypoperfusion and/or shocklike states damage the normal GI mucosa barrier. The GI tract is extremely vulnerable to oxygen metabolite–induced reperfusion injury. Endothelial injury and GI lesions occur in response to mediator-induced tissue damage. In addition, ischemic events and the absence of feedings can disrupt the normal metabolism of the gastric/intestinal lumen and the normal protective function of the gut barrier.[13,20]

Second, the translocation of normal GI bacteria via a "leaky gut" into the systemic circulation initiates and perpetuates an inflammatory focus in the critically ill patient. The GI tract harbors organisms that present an inflammatory focus when translocated from the gut into the portal circulation and inadequately cleared by the liver. Hepatic macrophages respond to the presence of enteric organisms by producing tissue-damaging amounts of TNF. Bacterial translocation has been associated with paralytic ileus and drugs commonly used in the critically ill patient, including antibiotics, antacids, and histamine blockers.[13]

The third mechanism linking the GI tract and organ dysfunction is colonization. The oropharynx of the critically ill patient becomes colonized with potentially pathogenic organisms from the GI tract. Pulmonary aspiration of colonized sputum presents an inflammatory focus. Antacids, $histamine_2$ antagonists, and antibiotics also increase colonization of the upper GI tract.[13,30] (∞Pneumonia, p. 663.)

Hepatobiliary dysfunction. The liver plays a vital role in host homeostasis related to the acute inflammatory response. In addition, the liver responds to SIRS by selectively changing carbohydrate (CHO), fat, and protein metabolism. Consequently, hepatic dysfunction after a critical insult threatens the patient's survival.

The liver normally controls the inflammatory response by several mechanisms. Kupffer's cells, which are hepatic macrophages, detoxify substances that might normally induce systemic inflammation, as well as vasoactive substances that cause hemodynamic instability. Failure to detoxify gram-negative bacteria translocated from the GI tract causes endotoxemia, perpetuates SIRS, and may lead to MODS. Additionally, the liver produces proteins and antiproteases to control the inflammatory response; however, hepatic dysfunction limits this response.[8,9]

The liver and gallbladder are extremely vulnerable to ischemic injury. Ischemic hepatitis occurs after a prolonged period of physiologic shock and is associated with centrilobular hepatocellular necrosis. The degree of hepatic damage is related directly to the severity and duration of the shock episode. Terms such as *shock liver* and *posttraumatic hepatic insufficiency* have been used to describe ischemic hepatitis. Both anoxic and reperfusion injury damage hepatocytes and the vascular endothelium.[31] Patients at high risk for ischemic hepatitis after a hypotensive event include those with a history of cardiac failure and/or cardiac dysrhythmias. Clinical manifestations of hepatic insufficiency are evident 1 to 2 days after the insult. Jaundice and transient elevations in serum transaminase and bilirubin levels occur. Hyperbilirubinemia results from hepatocyte anoxic injury and an increased production of bilirubin from the hemoglobin catabolism. Ischemic hepatitis may either resolve spontaneously or progress to fulminant hepatic failure. Although ischemic hepatitis is not a life-threatening complication, it can contribute to patient morbidity and mortality as a component of MODS.[31] Researchers have recently proposed that serum bilirubin is a valid indicator of hepatic dysfunction in MODS because it significantly differentiates MODS survivors from nonsurvivors.[32] (∞Fulminant Hepatic Failure, p. 962.)

Acalculous cholecystitis manifests 3 to 4 weeks after an insult. Its pathogenesis is unclear but may be related to ischemic reperfusion injury, narcotics, and cystic duct obstruction as a result of hyperviscous bile. Mediator-induced gallbladder dysfunction associated with acalculous cholecystitis may be related to the release of TxA_2 and leukotrienes (vasoactive substances) into the microcirculation in response to a damaged endothelium, aggregated platelets, and neutrophils. Clinical manifestations of acalculous cholecystitis may mimic acute cholecystitis with gallstones. Patients may demonstrate vague symptoms, however, includ-

BOX 45-5 Clinical Manifestations of Organ Dysfunction

GASTROINTESTINAL

Abdominal distention
Intolerance to enteral feedings
Paralytic ileus
Upper/lower GI bleeding
Diarrhea
Ischemic colitis
Mucosal ulceration
Decreased bowel sounds
Bacterial overgrowth in stool

LIVER

Jaundice
Increased serum bilirubin (hyperbilirubinemia)
Increased liver enzymes (AST, ALT, LDH, alkaline phosphatase)
Increased serum ammonia
Decreased serum albumin
Decreased serum transferrin

GALLBLADDER

Right upper quadrant tenderness/pain
Abdominal distention
Unexplained fever
Decreased bowel sounds

METABOLIC/NUTRITIONAL

Decreased lean body mass
Muscle wasting
Severe weight loss
Negative nitrogen balance
Hyperglycemia
Hypertriglyceridemia
Increased serum lactate
Decreased serum albumin, serum transferrin, prealbumin
Decreased retinol-binding protein

IMMUNE

Infection
Decreased lymphocyte count
Anergy

PULMONARY

Tachypnea
ARDS pattern of respiratory failure (dyspnea, patchy infiltrates, refractory hypoxemia, respiratory acidosis, abnormal O_2indexes)
Pulmonary hypertension

RENAL

Increased serum creatinine, BUN levels
Oliguria, anuria, or polyuria consistent with prerenal azotemia or acute tubular necrosis
Urinary indexes consistent with prerenal azotemia or acute tubular necrosis

CARDIOVASCULAR

Hyperdynamic

Decreased pulmonary capillary wedge pressure
Decreased systemic vascular resistance
Decreased right atrial pressure
Decreased left ventricular stroke work index
Increased oxygen consumption
Increased cardiac output, cardiac index, heart rate

Hypodynamic

Increased systemic vascular resistance
Increased right atrial pressure
Increased left ventricular stroke work index
Decreased oxygen delivery and consumption
Decreased cardiac output and cardiac index

CENTRAL-NERVOUS SYSTEM

Lethargy
Altered level of consciousness
Fever
Hepatic encephalopathy

Coagulation/Hematologic

Thrombocytopenia
DIC pattern

AST, Aspartate aminotransferase; *ALT,* alanine aminotransferase; *LDH,* lactate dehydrogenase.

ing right upper quadrant pain and tenderness. Critical to the detection of acalculous cholecystitis is the recognition of abdominal distention, unexplained fever, loss of bowel sounds, and a sudden deterioration in the patient's condition. About 50% of patients with acalculous cholecystitis have gallbladder gangrene, and 10% have gallbladder perforation. Consequently, a cholecystectomy may be performed.[33]

Hypermetabolism accompanies SIRS and is commonly referred to as the "metabolic response to injury."

During hypermetabolism and SIRS, the liver perpetuates select changes in metabolism including increased gluconeogenesis, glucogenesis, lipogenesis, and increased production of acute phase reactant proteins. Concurrently, the liver decreases synthesis of proteins, particularly albumin and transferrin. This metabolic response is partially mediated by IL-1, TNF, select AA metabolites, and the stress hormones.[18]

Pulmonary dysfunction. The lungs, a frequent and early target organ for mediator-induced injury, are usually the first organs affected in secondary MODS. Acute pulmonary dysfunction in secondary MODS manifests as ARDS. Patients who develop MODS generally develop ARDS; however, not all patients with ARDS develop secondary MODS. ARDS patients who develop SIRS/sepsis concurrently with acute respiratory failure are at the greatest risk for MODS.[2]

ARDS generally occurs 24 to 72 hours after the initial insult. Patients initially exhibit a low-grade fever, tachycardia, dyspnea, and mental confusion. As dyspnea, hypoxemia, and the work of breathing increase, intubation and mechanical ventilation are required. Pulmonary function is acutely disrupted, resulting in refractory hypoxemia secondary to intrapulmonary shunting, decreased pulmonary compliance, altered airway mechanics, and radiographic evidence of noncardiogenic pulmonary edema. ARDS is also associated with severe hypermetabolism equated to running an 8-minute mile, 24 hours a day, 7 days a week.[14]

Mediators associated with ARDS include AA metabolites, toxic oxygen metabolites, proteases, TNF, PAF, and interleukins.[1,3] Intense mediator activity damages the pulmonary vascular endothelium and the alveolar epithelium, resulting in surfactant deficiency, mild pulmonary hypertension, and increased lung water (noncardiogenic pulmonary edema) resulting from increased pulmonary capillary permeability. Pulmonary hypertension and hypoxic pulmonary vasoconstriction occur secondary to loss of the vascular bed.

Attempts to quantify the severity of pulmonary dysfunction in ARDS has led to the development of an acute lung injury scoring system. Variables included in the score are chest x-ray findings, the magnitude of hypoxemia using the PaO_2/FIO_2 ratio, pulmonary compliance during mechanical ventilation, and the use of positive end-expiratory pressure (PEEP) with mechanical ventilation. The total score is intended to provide an index of pulmonary dysfunction.[34] Attempts to predict outcome in MODS patients and quantify the magnitude of pulmonary dysfunction using scoring systems are ongoing. (∞Acute Respiratory Distress Syndrome, p. 660.)

Renal dysfunction. Acute renal failure is a common manifestation of MODS. The kidney is highly vulnerable to reperfusion injury. Consequently, renal ischemic-reperfusion injury may be a major cause of renal dysfunction in MODS. The patient may demonstrate oliguria or anuria secondary to decreased renal perfusion and relative hypovolemia. The condition may become refractory to diuretics, fluid challenges, and dopamine. Additional signs and symptoms include azotemia, decreased creatinine clearance, abnormal renal indices, and fluid and electrolyte imbalances. Prerenal oliguria may progress to acute tubular necrosis, necessitating hemodialysis or other renal therapies. The frequent use of nephrotoxic drugs during critical illness also intensifies the risk of renal failure.[35] Researchers have proposed that the serum creatinine is a valid indicator of renal function because it significantly differentiates MODS survivors from nonsurvivors.[32] (∞Acute Renal Failure, p. 877.)

Cardiovascular dysfunction. The initial cardiovascular response in SIRS/sepsis is myocardial depression; decreased right atrial pressure and systemic vascular resistance (SVR); and increased venous capacitance, VO_2, cardiac output (CO), and heart rate (HR). Despite an increased CO, myocardial depression occurs and is accompanied by decreased SVR, increased HR, and ventricular dilation. These compensatory mechanisms help maintain CO during the early phase of SIRS/sepsis. An inability to increase CO in response to a low SVR may indicate myocardial failure or inadequate fluid resuscitation and is associated with increased mortality. VO_2 may be twice as normal and may be flow-dependent. Mediators implicated in the hyperdynamic response include bradykinin, select AA metabolites, PAF, endogenous opioids, and beta-adrenergic stimulators.[4,36–38]

As MODS progresses, cardiac failure develops. Cardiac dysfunction is characterized by ventricular dilation, decreased diastolic compliance, and decreased systolic contractile function. Cardiovascular function becomes vasopressor-dependent. Cardiac failure may be caused by immune mediators; TNF; acidosis; or myocardial depressant factor (MDF), a substance secreted by the pancreas. TNF has a myocardial-depressant effect and is associated with myocardial depression during septic shock.[39] Myocardial depression is exacerbated by myocardial hypoperfusion from a low CO state and persistent lactic acidosis. Cardiogenic shock and biventricular failure occur and lead to death. (∞Cardiogenic Shock, p. 1102.)

Coagulation system dysfunction. Failure of the coagulation system manifests as disseminated intravascular coagulation. DIC results in simultaneous microvascular clotting and hemorrhage in organ systems because of the depletion of clotting factors and excessive fibrinolysis. As depicted in Figure 45-3, cell injury and damage to the endothelium initiate the intrinsic or extrinsic coagulation pathways. The endothelium is closely involved in DIC. Several relationships have been proposed. Endotoxins may roughen and expose the endothelial lining of blood vessels and consequently stimulate clotting. Low-flow states during hypotensive episodes may damage vessel endothelium and release tissue thromboplastin, with subsequent activation of the extrinsic pathway. A variety of clinical conditions, such as trauma, burns, and radiographic procedures, also can cause damage to the local endothelium and activation of the intrinsic coagulation pathway.[10,11]

DIC is a complex, consumptive coagulopathy that occurs in patients with a variety of disorders, including sepsis, tissue injury, and shock, and is an overstimulation of the normal coagulation process. Thrombosis and fibrinolysis are magnified to life-threatening proportions. The initial alteration in DIC is a generalized state of systemic hypercoagulation that produces organ ischemia. All organs, particularly the skin, lungs, and kidneys, are involved.[10,11] The thrombotic clinical manifestations of DIC are presented in Box 45-6.

Hemorrhage is the second pathophysiologic alteration in DIC. The lysis of clots (fibrinolysis) normally is initiated by the coagulation cascade. The intensity of the thrombosis enhances an equally intense lysis; however, clot lyse cannot effectively maintain blood vessel patency. As depicted in Figure 45-3, the production of fibrin split products exerts further anticoagulant effects, and hemorrhage ensues. Clotting factors, platelets, fibrinogen, and thrombin are consumed in large quantities during the thrombosis. Consequently, coagulation substances are depleted. The hemorrhagic signs and symptoms of DIC are presented in Box 45-6.

The abnormal clotting studies in patients with DIC may indicate thrombocytopenia; prolonged clotting times; depressed levels of clotting factors, particularly Factor VII; and fibrinogen/fibrin and high levels of breakdown products of fibrinogen and fibrin (fibrin degradation products, D-dimer). Medical management of DIC includes immediate treatment of the underlying cause; transfusion of blood products, such as red blood cells, platelets, and fresh frozen plasma, to correct the clotting factor deficiencies; and cryoprecipitate to treat hypofibrinogenemia. The use of heparin therapy in DIC remains controversial. Heparin must be used with caution; however, it is contraindicated in patients with bleeding in critical areas such as the cranium. Antifibrinolytic agents may be used concurrently with heparin therapy but generally are contraindicated because of the risk of thrombotic complications. Strict adherence to bleeding precautions is essential to minimize tissue and vascular trauma.[10,11]

Nursing Management of High Risk Patients

Caring for the high risk SIRS/MODS patient requires astute assessments to detect early organ manifestations of this syndrome. Patients who continue to experience sites of inflammation, septic foci, and inadequate tissue perfusion may be at higher risk. Nursing diagnoses applicable to this patient population are outlined in Box 45-7.

The MODS patient requires interdisciplinary collaboration in clinical management, including prevention and treatment of infection, maintenance of tissue oxygenation, nutritional/metabolic support, and support for individual organs.[2,4,35,40] The use of investigational therapies may be part of the patient's clinical management.

Prevention, detection, and treatment of infection. Elimination of the source of inflammation or infection can reduce mortality.[16] Therefore surgical procedures such as early fracture stabilization, removal of infected organs or tissue, and burn excision may be helpful in limiting the inflammatory response. Appropriate antibiotics are needed if the focus cannot be removed surgically. Patients are assessed closely for infection. Subtle expressions of infection warrant investigation. Risk for Infection is a highly relevant nursing diagnosis during this time period. Nursing management includes strict adherence to standards of practice to prevent infection. Practices related to infection control with invasive hemodynamic monitoring, urinary catheters, endotracheal tubes, intracranial pressure monitoring devices, total parenteral nutrition, and wound care must be stringent to prevent further infection.

Despite compliance with meticulous infection control practices, critically ill patients may "infect" themselves. As previously noted, bacterial contamination of the highly vulnerable respiratory tract and pneumonia can result from the colonization of GI tract bacteria. New approaches to infection control have been proposed, including selective decontamination of the GI tract with enteral antibiotics to prevent nosocomial infections, topical antibiotics in the oral pharynx to prevent colonization, monoclonal antibodies against

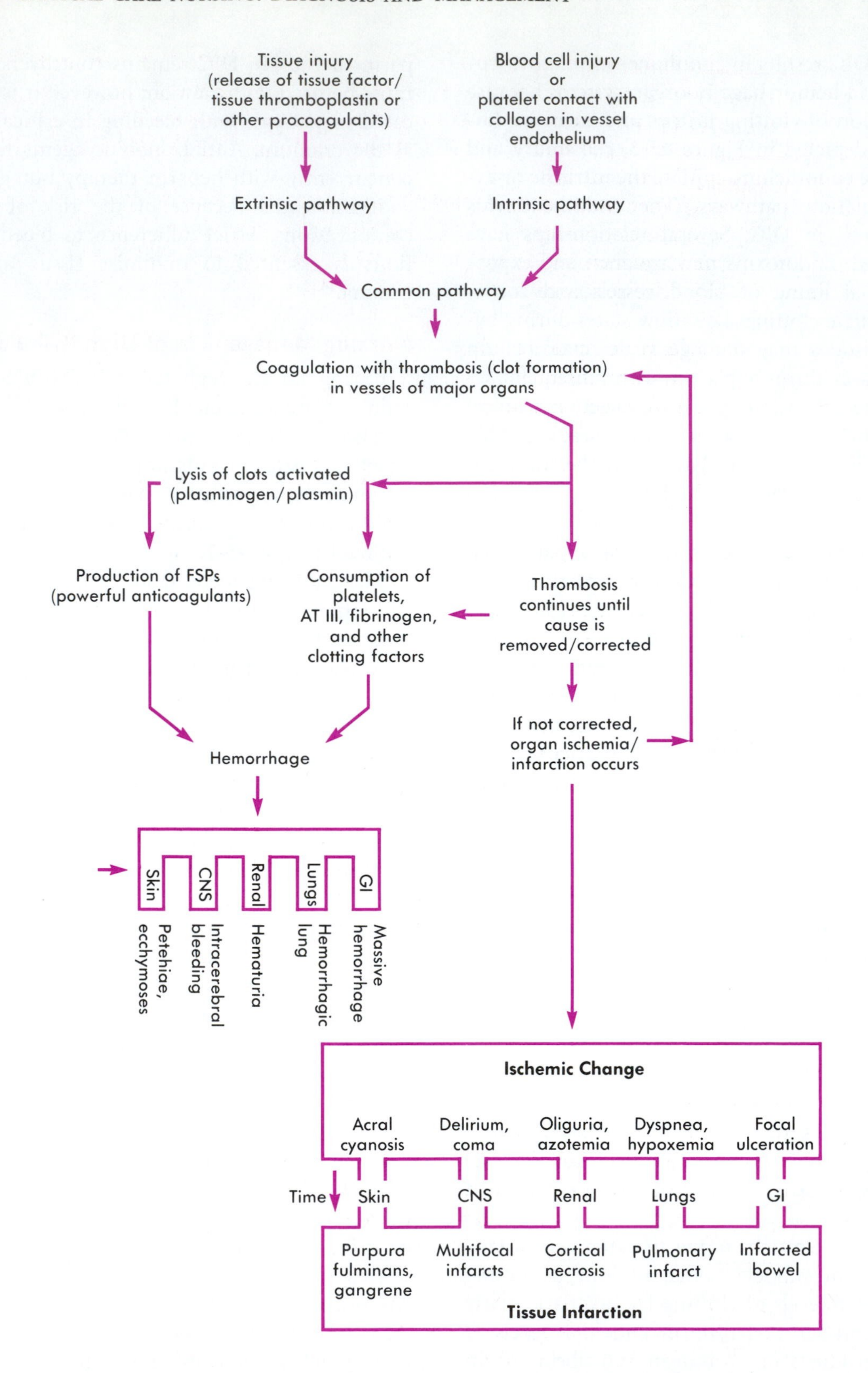

FIGURE 45-3. Pathophysiology of DIC. Lysis of clots (fibrinolysis) is a natural consequence of and is activated by coagulation. It is intensified in patients with DIC. DIC is termed a *consumptive coagulopathy.* During thrombosis, clotting factors are used to form clots. During fibrinolysis, clotting factors are destroyed inside the clot. The end result is a depletion of coagulation substances. *FSP,* Fibrin split products or fibrin degradation products. (Modified from Carr M: Disseminated intravascular coagulation: pathogenesis, diagnosis, and therapy, *J Emer Med* 5:316, 1987.)

BOX 45-6 Clinical Manifestations of Disseminated Intravascular Coagulation

THROMBOTIC CLINICAL MANIFESTATIONS

Skin involvement
Red, indurated areas along vessel wall
Purpura fulminans (diffuse skin infarction)
Acral cyanosis
Necrosis of fingers, toes, nose, and genitalia
Cool, pale extremities with mottling, cyanosis, or edema
Renal involvement
Renal failure
Cerebral infarcts or hemorrhage
Focal neurologic deficits (e.g., hemiplegia or loss of vision)
Nonspecific changes (e.g., altered loss of consciousness, confusion, headache, or seizures)
Bowel infarction
Melena, hematemesis, abdominal distention, or absent or hyperactive bowel sounds
Thrombophlebitis
Pulmonary embolism

HEMORRHAGIC CLINICAL MANIFESTATIONS

Spontaneous hemorrhage into body cavities and skin surfaces
Classic symptom of oozing or bleeding from invasive-line insertion sites or from body orifices.
Bleeding from body orifices such as the rectum, vagina, urethra, nose, and ears, as well as from the lung and gastrointestinal tract
Petechiae, purpura, or ecchymosis
Gingival, nasal, or scleral hemorrhage on physical examination
Hemorrhaging into all body cavities, including the abdomen, retroperitoneal space, cranium, and thorax

BOX 45-7 NURSING DIAGNOSIS AND MANAGEMENT

MULTIPLE ORGAN DYSFUNCTION SYNDROME

- Decreased Cardiac Output related to alterations in preload, p. 590
- Decreased Cardiac Output related to alterations in afterload, p. 592
- Decreased Cardiac Output related to alterations in contractility, p. 592
- Impaired Gas Exchange related to ventilation/perfusion mismatching or intrapulmonary shunting, p. 725
- Altered Renal Tissue Perfusion related to decreased renal blood flow, p. 916
- Altered Myocardial Tissue Perfusion related to acute myocardial ischemia, p. 595
- Altered Nutrition: Less Than Body Requirements related to increased metabolic demands or lack of exogenous nutrients, p. 165
- Risk for Infection, p. 1119
- Acute Pain related to transmission and perception of cutaneous, visceral, muscular, or ischemic impulses, p. 197
- Acute Confusion related to sensory overload, sensory deprivation, and sleep pattern disturbance, p. 90
- Anxiety related to threat to biologic, psychologic, and or social integrity, p. 99
- Ineffective Family Coping related to critically ill family member, p. 97

endotoxin, and passive antibody protection.[16,25] Gut decontamination and prevention of oral pharyngeal colonization reduce the incidence of infection; however, morbidity from MODS is not significantly affected.[30]

New approaches to infection and inflammation control currently are being investigated, including immunotherapy. Immunotherapy is antibody therapy that lessens the SIRS to microbes (antiinflammatory immunotherapy) and is based on the principle that antibodies directed against endotoxin can prevent the endotoxin from stimulating SIRS.[41]

Maintenance of tissue oxygenation. Normally, under steady state conditions, VO_2 is relatively constant and independent of oxygen delivery (DO_2) unless delivery becomes severely impaired. The relationship is termed *supply-independent oxygen consumption.* VO_2 is about 25% of DO_2. Consequently a percentage of oxygen is not used (physiologic reserve).

SIRS/MODS patients often develop supply-dependent oxygen consumption in which VO_2 becomes dependent on DO_2, rather than demand, at a normal or high DO_2. When VO_2 does not equal demand a tissue oxygen debt develops, subjecting organs to failure.

Hypoperfusion and resultant organ hypoxemia frequently occur in patients at high risk for MODS, subjecting essential organs to failure. Therefore effective fluid resuscitation and early recognition of flow-dependent VO_2 is essential. Patients at risk for MODS require pulmonary artery catheterization, frequent measurements of DO_2 and VO_2, and arterial lactate levels to guide therapy. Arterial lactate levels provide

LEGAL REVIEW 

Confidentiality and Disclosure of Human Immunodeficiency Virus and Acquired Immunodeficiency Syndrome Patient Information

Physicians, nurses, and other pertinent hospital employees have a duty to maintain the confidentiality of medical records and patient communications. This duty is derived broadly from the privilege doctrine. There is ethical privilege for both physicians and nurses. In every state there is statutory privilege (duty of confidentiality) between physicians and patients; a minority of states have codified the nurse-patient privilege. Every institution has policies and procedures regarding nurse-patient confidentiality, and the nurse must be familiar with them. Finally, the common law theories of invasion of privacy, breach of confidential relationship, professional malpractice, breach of contract, and defamation have been advanced to impose liability on health care professionals who disclose medical information.

Exceptions to the privilege include implicit or explicit waiver by the patient of the right to confidentiality; legal discovery procedures; court order and subpoena; and government agency requests for vital statistics, communicable disease data, abuse data, and wounds of violence. The scope of the privilege duty involves the balancing of the patient's right to privacy and confidentiality with other public or private interests, including the right to know.

In the following cases, the Washington Supreme Court ordered the blood bank to disclose the identity of the donor of transfused blood who was infected with the human immunodeficiency virus (HIV). However, the Maryland Appeals Court held that a patient with acquired immunodeficiency syndrome (AIDS) was entitled to anonymity in his lawsuit against a hospital for violation of the confidentiality of his medical record and invasion of privacy. Several states have enacted statutes specifically addressing confidentiality and AIDS or HIV patient data.

See *The AIDS epidemic: private rights and the public interest,* Boston, 1989, Beacon Press; *AIDS and ethics,* New York, 1991, Columbia University Press; Bureau of National Affairs: *AIDS in the workplace: resource material,* ed 3, Washington, DC, 1989, Bureau of National Affairs; *Doe v Puget Sound Blood Center,* No 56236-9 (Wash Sup Ct, Nov 14, 1991); *Doe v Shady Grove Adventist Hosp,* No. 1058 (Md Ct Spec App, Nov 27, 1991); *HIV/AIDS: a guide to nursing care,* ed 2, Philadelphia, 1992, WB Saunders; Jarvis AM: *AIDS law in a nutshell,* St Paul, 1991, West Publishing; Lambda Legal Defense and Education Fund, Inc: *AIDS legal guide: a professional resource on AIDS-related legal issues and discrimination,* ed 2, New York, 1990, The Fund; Pratt RJ: *AIDS: a strategy for nursing care,* ed 3, London, 1991, Edward Arnold.

information regarding the severity of impaired perfusion and the presence of lactic acidosis[15] and differ significantly in MODS survivors and nonsurvivors. Failure to maintain adequate oxygenation to vital organs results in organ dysfunction. Despite adequate DO_2, VO_2 may not meet the needs of the body during MODS.

Patients with ARDS and sepsis frequently manifest supply-dependent oxygen consumption and are unable to use oxygen appropriately despite normal delivery.[36,37,42,43] Possible causes of this flow-dependent VO_2 include abnormal mitochondrial function, redistribution of blood flow to organs, decreased SVR (secondary to prostaglandins), maldistribution of blood flow, microembolization, and capillary obstruction.[40,42]

Interventions that decrease oxygen demand and increase oxygen delivery are essential. Decreasing oxygen demand may be accomplished by sedation, mechanical ventilation, temperature and pain control, and rest. DO_2 may be increased by maintaining normal hematocrit and PaO_2 levels, using PEEP, increasing preload or myocardial contractility to enhance CO, or reducing afterload to increase CO. Many critical care clinicians advocate the maintenance of a supranormal DO_2 to increase VO_2; however, this therapeutic measure has not significantly improved survival, except in select groups of trauma patients.[14]

Nutritional/metabolic support. Hypermetabolism in SIRS/MODS results in profound weight loss, cachexia, and loss of organ function. The goal of nutritional support is the preservation of organ structure and function. Although nutritional support may not alter the course of organ dysfunction, it prevents generalized nutritional deficiencies and preserves gut integrity. The enteral route is preferable to parenteral support.[15,44] Enteral feedings are given distal to the pylorus to prevent pulmonary aspiration. Enteral feedings may limit bacterial translocation. In addition to early nutritional support the pharmacologic properties of enteral feeding formulas may limit SIRS for select critical care populations. Supplementation of enteral feedings with glutamine and arginine may be beneficial. Enteral feedings with omega-3 fatty acids may lessen SIRS.[44-47]

Recent guidelines have been proposed regarding nutritional support during SIRS for trauma patients. Patients are to receive 25 to 30 kcal/kg/day, with 3 to 5 g/kg/day as glucose. The respiratory quotient is monitored and maintained under 0.9. Long-chain polyunsaturated fatty acids (less than 1.5 g/kg/day) and amino acids (1.5 mg/kg/day) are given. Fat emulsions are limited to 0.5 to 1 g/kg/day to prevent iatrogenic immunosuppression associated with lipids and fat overload syndromes. Plasma transferrin and prealbumin levels are used to monitor hepatic protein synthesis.[16] Efficient protein use must be assessed via nitrogen balance studies. (∞Metabolic Response to Starvation and Stress, p. 123).

EXPERIMENTAL PHARMACOLOGIC APPROACHES IN SIRS AND MODS

Organ-specific interventions have not been highly effective in improving survival in MODS. Although organ-specific therapies such as mechanical ventilation and hemodialysis are needed for immediate survival, future medical management must target and control the effects of mediators that cause SIRS and MODS. Animal model studies continue to provide information regarding the efficacy of drugs that prevent organ dysfunction. Several experimental drugs and agents are currently being tested in human clinical trials. However, the initial enthusiasm about inflammatory therapies has been dampened, with many clinical trials reporting negative findings.

As previously described, endothelial cells are common targets for inflammatory mediators; consequently, endothelial cell protection is a primary goal in pharmacologic management. Endothelial cell protection against the effects of inflammatory cells and mediators may include therapeutic agents that act as neutrophil inhibitors, white blood cell (WBC) adherence inhibitors, antioxidants, eicosanoid modulators, PAF inhibitors, and monoclonal antibodies aimed at cytokines and cell surface receptors. Monoclonal antibodies are antibodies that have specific antigens as targets and a constant binding affinity.[43]

Drugs that inhibit neutrophil function theoretically hold great promise in the treatment of SIRS and MODS. As previously noted, endotoxin, TNF, IL-1, and PAF cause endothelial damage and activate neutrophils. Subsequently activated neutrophils release destructive mediators. TNF also activates complement, a process that ultimately affects neutrophils. Proinflammatory effects also are mediated through the lipooxygenase and cyclooxygenase pathways. Drugs that inhibit neutrophil function may be beneficial in SIRS and are listed in Box 45-8. As immunomodulators, these drugs moderate neutrophil-induced injury in endothelial cells. Specifically, pentoxifylline reduces the adhesiveness of activated neutrophils to the endothelium and the release of toxic oxygen metabolites and lysosomal enzymes and inhibits neutrophil activation by endotoxin, TNF, and IL-1. Current data regarding the effectiveness of pentoxifylline in humans with SIRS/sepsis are limited. Adenosine, another potential neutrophil inhibitor, reduces granulocyte adherence, inhibits superoxide ion formation, limits the effects of reperfusion injury, and protects endothelial cells.[43]

BOX 45-8 Experimental Pharmacologic Approaches in SIRS and MODS

- Neutrophil inhibitors (pentoxifylline, adenosine, aminophylline, terbutaline, dibutyl-cAMP, caffeine, forskolin)
- WBC adherence inhibitors
- Antioxidants/oxygen radical scavengers
- Arachidonic acid metabolite modulators
  - Monoclonal antibodies to phospholipase A_2
  - Cyclooxygenase inhibitors (ibuprofen, indomethacin)
  - Thromboxane synthetase inhibitors
  - Thromboxane receptor blockers
  - Lipooxygenase inhibitors
  - Leukotrienes antagonists
- PAF inhibitors
- Monoclonal antibodies to decrease adhesion of neutrophils to the endothelium
- Protease inhibitors
- Modulation of macrophage function (n-3 polyunsaturated fatty acids)
- Stimulation of lymphocyte function (arginine, n-3 polyunsaturated fatty acids)
- Antiendorphin therapy
- Antihistamines
- Glucocorticoids

Naturally occurring substances, including some interleukins, inhibit the adherence of neutrophils to the endothelium. Monoclonal antibodies may be available to decrease the adhesion of neutrophils to the endothelium. Antioxidants, drugs that scavenge oxygen radicals or bind free oxygen radicals, and protease inhibitors may be effective in SIRS/sepsis.[43]

Eicosanoid modulation involves the use of pharmacologic agents to negate the destructive effects of AA metabolites. Agents that may inhibit the release or destructive activity of AA metabolites are listed in Box 45-8. The effectiveness of these agents in modulating the response to sepsis is under investigation. In contrast to AA metabolites that have damaging effects, the administration of PGI-1 may be effective in limiting the systemic inflammatory response because of its local vasodilatory effects and antiplatelet properties.[48]

Other therapies that have been investigated include antiendorphin therapy with SIRS/sepsis patients. No scientific evidence exists that endorphin neutralization with naloxone benefits patients with sepsis or multiple organ involvement. In some patients, however, naloxone has pressor effects.[41,49] Other investigational therapies that have not demonstrated significant effects in limiting SIRS include those using antihistamines and glucocorticoids.[21]

Recent investigational emphasis has been placed on anticytokine therapy in the treatment of SIRS and MODS. Several cytokines play an important role in uncontrolled inflammation, including TNF-alpha and IL-1. Therefore TNF-alpha inhibitors, anti-TNF–alpha antibody agents, and IL-1 receptor antagonists may demonstrate efficacy in the future. In addition, anticomplement therapy may be effective in attenuating complement activation in septic patients.[48] It is highly likely that a combination of drugs may be needed to suppress SIRS and to prevent MODS.

CASE STUDY

MULTIPLE ORGAN DYSFUNCTION SYNDROME

CLINICAL HISTORY

Mr. H is a 38-year-old white, well-nourished construction worker who sustained abdominal injuries and a liver laceration that required surgical intervention (exploratory laparotomy, repair of liver laceration, splenectomy) after volume resuscitation in the field and emergency room. His previous medical history reveals no chronic health problems. He is, however, a 20 pack/year smoker.

CURRENT PROBLEMS

During the immediate postoperative period (days 1 and 2), extubation occurred. Mr. H was lethargic but oriented and hemodynamically stable, with mild volume depletion (as evidenced by measured and derived hemodynamic data from the pulmonary artery catheter). He required low-flow nasal oxygen (2 L/min) to maintain a PaO_2 of 75 mm Hg and an O_2 saturation above 95% (assessed continuously via pulse oximetry). Despite his relatively stable hemodynamic profile, he was tachycardic (sinus) and mildly tachypneic (respiratory rate, 26 breaths/min), with diminished breath sounds at both bases. He comprehended and was able to use patient controlled analgesia (PCA) but frequently awakened anxious and in pain. Urine output was low but adequate for intravenous intake; skin and extremities were cool to the touch, and core temperature was 37° C. Mr. H's abdomen was distended, with absent bowel sounds. A nasogastric tube was draining small amounts of dark green drainage. His surgical wound was well approximated, with no redness or drainage. Laboratory data revealed normochromic normocytic anemia (hemoglobin, 9.8 g/dL; hematocrit, 25%), leukocytosis (white blood cell [WBC] count, 13,000 mm^3), and an elevated serum lactate level. Arterial blood gas (ABG) values indicated a primary respiratory alkalosis and metabolic acidosis. Serum potassium levels were high; consequently all potassium was removed from intravenous fluids.

MEDICAL DIAGNOSES

Abdominal trauma requiring exploratory laparotomy repair of liver laceration

Systemic inflammatory response syndrome secondary to multiple trauma

NURSING DIAGNOSES

Acute Pain related to transmission and perception of cutaneous, visceral, muscular, or ischemic impulses

Ineffective Breathing Pattern related to decreased lung expansion

Fluid Volume Deficit related to absolute loss

Risk for Infection

Anxiety related to threat to biologic, psychologic, and/or social integrity

Risk for Altered Tissue Perfusion (Cerebral, Cardiopulmonary, Renal, Gastrointestinal, Peripheral)

PLAN OF CARE

1. Minimize proinflammatory stimuli, such as perfusion deficits, hypoxia, hypotension, and bacteria, that further activate the systemic inflammatory response.
2. Maintain optimal pulmonary function by aggressive use of incentive spirometry, turning, and effective pain control.
3. Optimize tissue perfusion and oxygen transport and delivery to organ systems.
4. Monitor closely for clinical manifestations of SIRS and progression to organ dysfunction.

Continued

CASE STUDY—CONT'D

MULTIPLE ORGAN DYSFUNCTION SYNDROME

MEDICAL AND NURSING MANAGEMENT AND PATIENT OUTCOME

Despite his relatively stable clinical status during the first 2 postoperative days, on day 3 Mr. H was becoming progressively more tachycardic, tachypneic, and anxious. He required 100% oxygen via face mask. Chest film results demonstrated widespread alveolar opacification consistent with acute respiratory distress syndrome (ARDS). ABG values revealed refractory hypoxemia, with high anion gap primary metabolic acidosis and respiratory acidosis. Consequently, oral intubation and volume-cycled mechanical ventilation were used. Positive end-expiratory pressure (PEEP) at 10 cm H_2O was added incrementally to maximize oxygenation without compromising cardiac output and oxygen delivery. Measures of static and dynamic lung compliance were consistent with decreasing lung compliance; oxygen indexes and derived shunt calculations demonstrated severe ventilation/perfusion mismatching. Hemodynamic data continued to show a hyperdynamic cardiovascular profile. ABG values remained unchanged. Energy expenditure as measured with use of a metabolic cart demonstrated hypermetabolism, with increased oxygen consumption and carbon dioxide production. Enteral nutrition via a small-bore jejunal feeding tubing was attempted without success; consequently, total parenteral nutrition (TPN) was started at 25 to 30 kcal/kg/day via a newly placed internal jugular catheter. Appropriate fat supplementation also was provided.

MEDICAL DIAGNOSIS

Acute respiratory distress syndrome

NURSING DIAGNOSES

Impaired Gas Exchange related to ventilation/perfusion mismatching and intrapulmonary shunting

Altered Nutrition: Less Than Body Requirements related to lack of exogenous nutrients and increased metabolic demand

Body Image Disturbance related to functional dependence on life-sustaining technology

MEDICAL AND NURSING MANAGEMENT AND PATIENT OUTCOME

On days 6 and 7 Mr. H remained intubated and required 100% O_2 to maintain a PaO_2 of 70 mm Hg. Core temperature was 38.4° C and WBC count 18,000/mm^3 with a shift to the left. However, blood, urine, and wound cultures were negative. Despite the aggressive administration of diuretics (furosemide and mannitol), Mr. H was oliguric and azotemic, with renal indexes consistent with acute tubular necrosis. Serum creatinine and blood urea nitrogen (BUN) levels were approaching the need for hemodialysis. His level of consciousness was difficult to evaluate because paralytic agents and narcotics had been used to facilitate effective mechanical ventilation. Since admission, Mr. H had lost 8 pounds. His condition was highly catabolic, hyperglycemic, and in a negative nitrogen balance. Visceral protein (serum albumin, transferrin, prealbumin) levels were low despite nutritional and metabolic support. Hepatic function was altered as evidenced by elevated serum bilirubin, aspartate aminotransferase (AST), alanine aminotransferase (ALT), and lactate dehydrogenase (LDH) levels; clinical jaundice was evident. Mr. H's abdomen was distended, and bowel sounds were absent. He was unresponsive to all noxious stimuli and no longer required paralytics or narcotics for effective ventilation. Cardiovascular function was dependent on vasoactive drugs (dopamine at 10 μg/kg/min) to maintain a subnormal cardiac output. Mr. H's family was notified of his grave prognosis. They were angry and grief stricken.

MEDICAL DIAGNOSIS

Multiple organ dysfunction syndrome secondary to pulmonary, renal, and liver dysfunction

NURSING DIAGNOSES

Decreased Cardiac Output related to alterations in contractility

Decreased Cardiac Output related to alterations in preload

Decreased Cardiac Output related to alterations in afterload

Altered Renal Tissue Perfusion related to decreased renal blood flow

Altered Myocardial Tissue Perfusion related to decreased myocardial blood flow

Ineffective Family Coping related to critically ill family member

REFERENCES

1. Bone RC: Toward a theory regarding the pathogenesis of the systemic inflammatory response syndrome: what we do and do not know about cytokine regulation, *Crit Care Med* 24:163, 1996.
2. Cerra FB: The multiple organ failure syndrome, *Hosp Pract* 25(15):169, 1990.
3. Knaus WA, Wagner DP: Multiple systems organ failure: epidemiology and prognosis, *Crit Care Clin* 5:221, 1989.
4. Matuschak GM: Multiple systems organ failure: clinical expression, pathogenesis, and therapy. In Hall JB, Schmidt GA, Wood LD, editors: *Principles of critical care,* New York, 1992, McGraw-Hill.
5. American College of Chest Physicians/Society of Critical Care Medicine Consensus Conference Committee: Definitions for sepsis and organ failure and guidelines for the use of innovative therapies in sepsis, *Crit Care Med* 20:864, 1992.
6. Bone RC, Sprung CL, Sibbald WJ: Definitions for sepsis and organ failure, *Crit Care Med* 20:724, 1992.
7. Rote NS: Inflammation. In McCance KL, Huether SE, editors: *Pathophysiology: the biological basis for disease in adults and children,* ed 2, St Louis, 1994, Mosby.
8. Pinsky MR: Multiple systems organ failure: malignant intravascular inflammation, *Crit Care Clin* 5:195, 1989.
9. Pinsky MR, Matuschak GM: Multiple systems organ failure: failure of host defense homeostasis, *Crit Care Clin* 5:199, 1989.
10. Bell TN: Disseminated intravascular coagulation and shock, *Crit Care Nurs Clin* 2:255, 1990.
11. Guyton AC: *Textbook of medical physiology,* ed 9, Philadelphia, 1996, WB Saunders.
12. Yurt RW, Lowry SF: Role of the macrophage and endogenous mediators in multiple organ failure. In Deitch EA, editor: *Multiple organ failure: pathophysiology and basic concepts of therapy,* New York, 1990, Thieme Medical.
13. Deitch EA: Gut failure: its role in the multiple organ failure syndrome. In Deitch EA, editor: *Multiple organ failure: pathophysiology and basic concepts of therapy,* New York, 1990, Thieme Medical.
14. Bishop M and others: Prospective trial of supranormal values in severely traumatized patients, *Crit Care Med* 20:S93, 1992 (abstract).
15. Cipolle MD, Pasquale MD, Cerra F: Secondary organ dysfunction from clinical perspective to molecular mediators, *Crit Care Clin* 8:261, 1993.
16. Cerra FB: The syndrome of hypermetabolism and multiple systems organ failure. In Hall JB, Schmidt GA, Wood LD, editors: *Principles of critical care,* New York, 1992, McGraw-Hill.
17. Waxman K: Postoperative multiple organ failure, *Crit Care Clin* 3:429, 1987.
18. Cerra FB: Hypermetabolism-organ failure syndrome: a metabolic response to injury, *Crit Care Clin* 5:289, 1989.
19. Cerra FB: Nutritional pharmacology: its role in the hypermetabolism-organ failure syndrome, *Crit Care Med* 18:S154, 1990.
20. Zimmerman JJ, Ringer TV: Inflammatory host responses in sepsis, *Crit Care Clin* 8:163, 1992.
21. Bone RC: Inhibitors of complement and neutrophils: a critical evaluation of their role in the treatment of sepsis, *Crit Care Med* 20:891, 1992.
22. Damas P and others: Tumor necrosis factor and interleukin-1 serum levels during severe sepsis in humans, *Crit Care Med* 17:975, 1989.
23. Demets JM and others: Plasma tumor necrosis factor and mortality in critically ill septic patients, *Crit Care Med* 17:489, 1989.
24. Nahum A, Sznajder JI: Role of free radicals in critical illness. In Hall JB, Schmidt GA, Wood LD, editors: *Principles of critical care,* New York, 1992, McGraw-Hill.
25. Beutler B: Cachectin in tissue injury, shock, and related states, *Crit Care Clin* 5:353, 1989.
26. Bernard GR: Cyclooxygenase inhibition, *Crit Care Rep* 1:193, 1990.
27. Bone RC: Phospholipids and their inhibitors: a critical evaluation of their role in the treatment of sepsis, *Crit Care Med* 20:884, 1992.
28. Petrak RA, Balk RA, Bone RC: Prostaglandins, cyclo-oxygenase inhibitors, and thromboxane synthetase inhibitors in the pathogenesis of multiple systems organ failure, *Crit Care Clin* 5:303, 1989.
29. Sprague RS and others: Proposed role of leukotrienes in the pathophysiology of multiple systems organ failure, *Crit Care Clin* 4:315, 1989.
30. van Saene HK, Stoutenbeek CC, Stoller JK: Selective decontamination of the digestive tract in the intensive care unit: current status and future prospects, *Crit Care Med* 20:691, 1992.
31. Vickers SM, Bailey RW, Bulkley GB: Ischemic hepatitis. In Marston A and others, editors: *Splanchnic ischemia and multiple organ failure,* St Louis, 1989, Mosby.
32. Marshall JC and others: Multiple organs dysfunction score: a reliable descriptor of a complex clinical outcome, *Crit Care Med* 23:1638, 1995.
33. Haglund UH, Arvidsson D: Acute acalculous cholecystitis. In Marston A and others, editors: *Splanchnic ischemia and multiple organ failure,* St Louis, 1989, Mosby.
34. Murray JF and others: An expanded definition of the adult respiratory distress syndrome, *Am Rev Respir Dis* 138:720, 1988.
35. Gamelli RL, Silver GM: Acute renal failure. In Deitch EA, editor: *Multiple organ failure: pathophysiology and basic concepts of therapy,* New York, 1990, Thieme Medical.
36. Berstern A, Sibbald WJ: Circulatory disturbances in multiple systems organ failure, *Crit Care Clin* 5:233, 1989.
37. Shoemaker WC, Kram HB, Appel PL: Therapy of shock based on pathophysiology, monitoring, and outcome prediction, *Crit Care Med* 18:S19, 1990.
38. Vincent JL, De Backer D: Initial management of circulatory shock as prevention of MSOF, *Crit Care Clin* 5:369, 1989.
39. Kumar A and others: Tumor necrosis factor produces depression of myocardial cell contraction in vitro, *Crit Care Med* 20:S52, 1992 (abstract).

40. Macho JR, Luce JM: Rational approach to the management of multiple systems organ failure, *Crit Care Clin* 5:379, 1989.
41. Sheagren JN: Mechanism-oriented therapy for multiple systems organ failure, *Crit Care Clin* 5:393, 1989.
42. Feustel PJ and others: Oxygen delivery and consumption in head-injured and multiple trauma patients, *J Trauma* 30:30, 1990.
43. Edwards JD: Use of survivors' cardiopulmonary values as therapeutic goals in septic shock, *Crit Care Med* 17:1098, 1989.
44. Lehman S: Nutritional support in the hypermetabolic patient, *Crit Care Nurs Clin North Am* 5:97, 1993.
45. Daly JM, Lieberman MD, Goldfine L: Enteral nutrition with supplemental arginine, RNA, and omega-3 fatty acids in patients after operation: immunologic, metabolic and clinical outcome, *Surg* 112:56, 1992.
46. Keithley J, Eisenberg P: The significance of enteral nutrition in the intensive care unit patient, *Crit Care Nurs Clin North Am* 5:23, 1993.
47. Moore FA, Felicano DV, Andrassy RJ: Early enteral feeding compared with parenteral reduces postoperative septic complications, *Ann Surg* 216:172, 1992.
48. Hudson LD: New therapies for ARDS, *Chest* 108:79S, 1995.
49. Hacksaw KV, Parker GA, Roberts JW: Naloxone in septic shock, *Crit Care Med* 18:47, 1990.

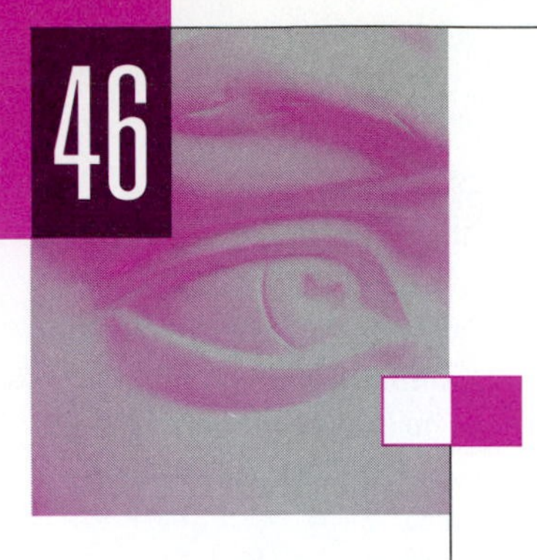

46 Burns

SOME AUTHORITIES ESTIMATE that 75% of all burn injuries could be prevented with reasonable caution and adherence to safety measures. The nurse can play an active role in preventing fires and burns by promoting legislation and teaching safety practices. Many programs and organizations are dedicated to the prevention of burn injury; yet 2.5 million Americans each year require medical attention for burns.[1] Approximately 100,000 thermally injured patients are hospitalized annually, of whom 12,000 will die annually. Great advances have been made in the care of burn patients. Fifty years ago in an otherwise healthy adult, a 30% total body surface area burn was associated with a 50% mortality rate; whereas today an 80% total body surface area burn carries the same mortality. Fifty years ago the leading cause of in-hospital deaths was associated with burn shock. Today, with improvements in fluid resuscitation, the leading cause of in-hospital deaths is associated with late infectious complications.[2]

To provide comprehensive, holistic care for burn patients, close collaboration is required among members of the multidisciplinary team. This burn team comprises nurses, physicians, physical therapists, occupational therapists, recreational therapists, nutritionists, psychologists, social workers, family, and spiritual support staff members. The burn patient is characterized as the universal trauma model. The patient's response to a major burn injury is dramatic and involves multisystem alterations. Knowledge of local and systemic changes associated with patient needs is essential, which places extraordinary demands on the nurse in burn practice who must be both a specialist and a broadly based generalist.[3]

The purpose of this chapter is to provide a basic understanding of the complexities of burn care and the patient's response to burn injury.

ANATOMY AND FUNCTIONS OF THE SKIN

The skin is the largest organ of the human body, ranging from 0.2 m^2 in the newborn to more than 2 m^2 in the adult. The integumentary system consists of two major layers: the epidermis and the dermis (Figure 46-1).

The outermost layer of epidermis varies from 0.07 to 0.12 mm in thickness, with the deepest layer found on the soles of the feet and palms of the hand. The epidermis is composed of dead, cornified cells that act as a tough protective barrier against the environment. From the surface inward the five layers are stratum corneum, stratum lucidum, stratum granulosum, stratum spinosum, and stratum basale. The second, thicker layer, the dermis, ranges from 1 to 2 mm in thickness and lies below the epidermis. The dermis is composed of two layers: the papillary layer next to the stratum basale and the reticular layer. The dermis, composed primarily of connective tissue and collagenous fiber bundles, provides nutritional support to the epidermis. The dermis contains the blood vessels; sweat and sebaceous glands; hair follicles; nerves to the skin and capillaries that nourish the avascular epidermis; and sensory fibers for pain, touch, and temperature. Mast cells in the connective tissue perform the functions of secretion, phagocytosis, and production of fibroblasts. Beneath the dermis is the hypodermis, which contains the fat, smooth muscle, and areolar tissue. The hypodermis acts as a heat insulator, shock absorber, and nutritional depot.

The skin provides functions crucial to human survival. These functions include maintenance of body temperature; barrier to evaporative water loss; metabolic activity (vitamin D production); protection against the environment through the sensations of touch, pressure, and pain; overall cosmetic appearance; and other functions that remain unknown.

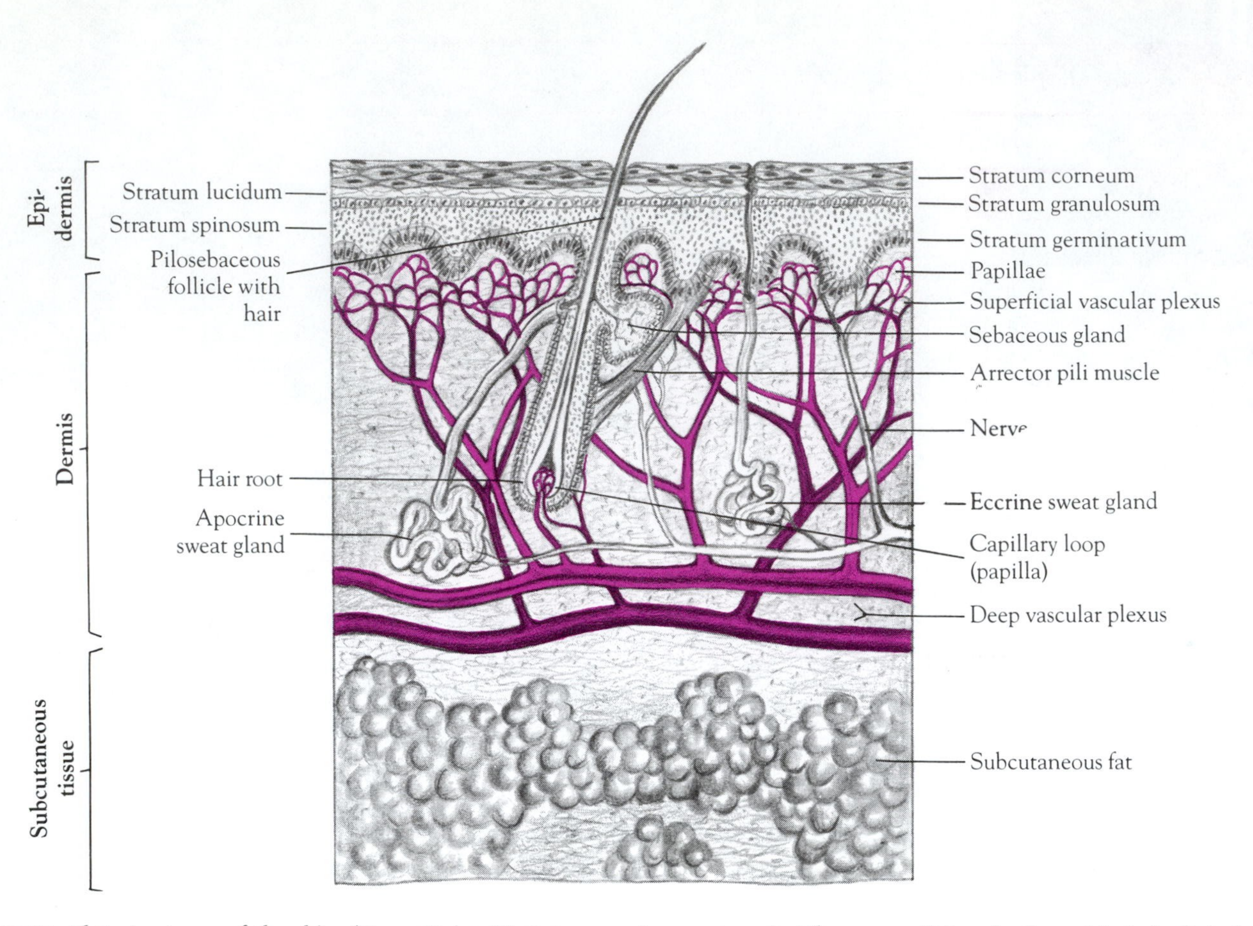

FIGURE 46-1. Anatomy of the skin. (From Dains JE: Integumentary system. In Thompson JM and others: *Mosby's clinical nursing,* ed 4, St Louis, 1997, Mosby.)

PATHOPHYSIOLOGY AND ETIOLOGY OF BURN INJURY

A burn is an injury resulting in tissue loss or damage. Injury to tissue can be caused by exposure to thermal, electrical, chemical, and/or radiation sources. Injury to the tissue is determined by the temperature or causticity of the burning agent and duration of tissue contact with the source.

At the cellular level the burning agent produces a dilation of the capillaries and small vessels, thus increasing the capillary permeability. Plasma seeps out into the surrounding tissue, producing blisters and edema. The type, duration, and intensity of the burn affect the amount and extent of fluid loss. This progressive fluid loss in major burns results in significant intravascular fluid volume deficit. The pathophysiology response to injury is twofold. Early postinjury organ hypoperfusion develops as a result of low cardiac output, and increased peripheral vascular resistance develops because of the normal neurohormonal response to trauma.

The clinical course of a burn injury comprises three phases: the resuscitative phase, acute care phase, and the rehabilitative phase. The resuscitative phase begins with the initial hemodynamic response to the injury and lasts until capillary integrity is restored and the repletion of plasma volume by fluid replacement occurs. The acute phase begins with the onset of diuresis of fluid mobilized from the interstitial space and ends with the closure of the burn wound. The rehabilitative phase begins on the patient's admission to the hospital, with correction of functional deficits and scar management being major considerations. The rehabilitative phase may last from months to years depending on the severity of injury.

CLASSIFICATION OF BURN INJURIES

Burns are classified primarily according to the size and depth of the injury (Table 46-1). The type and location of the burn, as well as the patient's age and medical history, however, are significant considera-

TABLE 46-1 Burn Classifications by the American Burn Association

Injury Severity	Identifying Criteria	Recommended Treatment Facility
Minor burns	Partial thickness of 1 ≤5% TBSA	Emergency rooms—outpatients
Moderate burns	No full thickness	General hospital or may be outpatients
Major burns	No involvement of eyes or ears	Burn unit or center
	Partial thickness of 15%-25% TBSA	
	Full thickness of <10% TBSA not involving the hands, face, eyes, ears, feet, or genitalia	
	Partial thickness of >25% TBSA	
	Full thickness of >10% TBSA	
	True electrical injuries	
	Injury to hands, face, eyes, ears, feet, or genitalia	
	Concomitant injuries (e.g., inhalation injury, fractures, or other trauma)	
	High risk patients (e.g., <2 years old, >50 years old, or with preexisting condition)	

From Trunkey DD and Lewis FR: *Current therapy of trauma,* Philadelphia 1991, BC Decker.
TBSA, Total body surface area.

tions. Recognition of the magnitude of burn injury, which is based on the depth, size, and prior health of the host, is of crucial importance in the overall care plan. Decisions concerning complete patient management are based on this assessment. Patient age and the burn size are the cardinal determinants of survival.[4–6]

Size of Injury

Several different methods can be used to estimate the size of the burn area. A quick and easy method is the *rule of nines,* which often is used in the prehospital setting for initial triage of the burn patient (Figure 46-2). With this method the adult body is divided into surface areas of 9%. This method is modified in infants and very small children. In the adult, the head and the anterior and posterior surfaces of the trunk are each 18%, each arm is 9%, each leg is 18%, and the perineum is 1%.

In the hospital setting the Lund and Browder method (Figure 46-3) is the most accurate and accepted method for determining the percentage of burn. Surface area measurements are assigned to each body part in terms of the age of the patient. Therefore this method is highly recommended for use with children younger than 10 years because it corrects for smaller surface areas of the lower extremities. It also is used for adult burn victims because it provides additional accuracy.

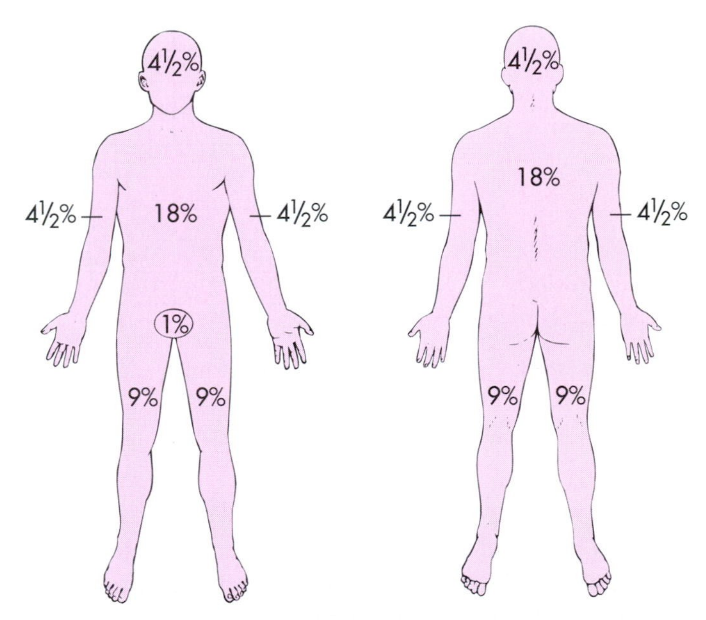

FIGURE 46-2. Estimation of adult burn injury: rule of nines. **A,** Anterior view. **B,** Posterior view. (From Dains JE: Integumentary system. In Thompson JM and others: *Mosby's clinical nursing,* ed 4, St Louis, 1997, Mosby.)

Small and scattered areas of burns can be calculated by using the principle that the palmar surface of the victim's hand represents 1% of the total body surface area (TBSA).

Berkow's method also is used to estimate burn size for infants and children because it accounts for the

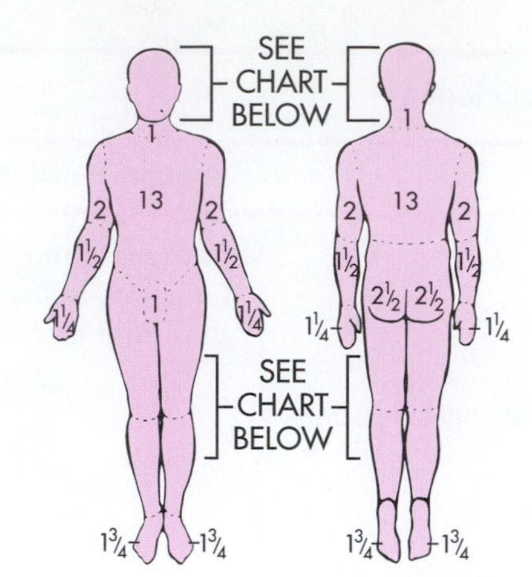

AGE: ________
SEX: ________
WEIGHT: ________
HEIGHT: ________

AERA	Inf.	1-4	5-9	10-14	15	Adult	Part.	Full	Total	Donor areas
HEAD	19	17	13	11	9	7				
NECK	2	2	2	2	2	2				
ANT. TRUNK	13	13	13	13	13	13				
POST. TRUNK	13	13	13	13	13	13				
R. BUTTOCK	2½	2½	2½	2½	2½	2½				
L. BUTTOCK	2½	2½	2½	2½	2½	2½				
GENITALIA	1	1	1	1	1	1				
R.U. ARM	4	4	4	4	4	4				
L.U. ARM	4	4	4	4	4	4				
R.L. ARM	3	3	3	3	3	3				
L.L. ARM	3	3	3	3	3	3				
R. HAND	2½	2½	2½	2½	2½	2½				
L. HAND	2½	2½	2½	2½	2½	2½				
R. THIGH	5½	6½	8	8½	9	9½				
L. THIGH	5½	6½	8	8½	9	9½				
R. LEG	5	5	5½	6	6½	7				
L. LEG	5	5	5½	6	6½	7				
R. FOOT	3½	3½	3½	3½	3½	3½				
L. FOOT	3½	3½	3½	3½	3½	3½				
						TOTAL				

FIGURE 46-3. Lund and Browder's burn estimate diagram. (Modified from Cardona VD: *Trauma nursing from resuscitation through rehabilitation,* Philadelphia, 1995, WB Saunders.)

proportionate growth. (This method requires special charts provided by the National Burn Institute, which are not always available in local hospitals but may be at hand in a designated burn center.)

Depth of Injury

Traditionally, burn depth has been classified in degrees of injury based on the amount of injured epidermis or dermis, or both (i.e., first-, second-, or third-degree burns). These terms, however, are not descriptive of the burn surface.

Currently, burns are classified as *partial thickness* and *full thickness.* These descriptions are based on the surface appearance of the wound. Partial thickness includes first and second degree. Full thickness includes third degree. Partial-thickness burns are further classified as *superficial, moderate,* and *deep dermal partial-thickness burns.* Wound assessment involves recognition of the depth of injury and size of burn.

A *superficial partial-thickness burn (first degree)* involves only the first two or three of the five layers of the epidermis. Superficial partial-thickness wounds are characterized by erythema and mild discomfort. Pain, the chief symptom, usually resolves in 48 to 72 hours. Common examples of these burn injuries are sunburns and minor steam burns that occur while a person is cooking. Generally, these wounds heal in 2 to 7 days and usually do not require medical intervention aside from pain relief and oral fluids.

A *moderate partial-thickness burn (second degree)* involves the upper third of the dermis. These burns usually are caused by brief contact with flames, hot liquid, or exposure to dilute chemicals. Superficial second-degree burns are characterized by a light- to bright red or mottled appearance. These wounds may appear wet and weeping, may contain bullae, and are extremely painful and sensitive to air currents. The microvessels that perfuse this area are injured, and permeability is increased, resulting in the leakage of large amounts of plasma into the interstitium. This fluid, in turn, lifts off the thin damaged epidermis, causing blister formation. Despite the loss of the entire basal layer of the epidermis, a burn of this depth will heal in 7 to 21 days. Minimal scarring can be expected. Moderately deep partial-thickness wounds commonly take 4 to 6 weeks to heal.

A *deep dermal partial-thickness burn* (second degree) involves the entire epidermal layer and part of the dermis. These burns often result from contact with hot liquids, solids, and intense radiant energy. A deep dermal partial-thickness burn generally is not characterized by blister formation. Only a modest plasma surface leakage occurs because of severe impairment in blood supply. The wound surface usually is red, with white areas in deeper parts, and blanching follows capillary refill. The appearance of the deep dermal wound changes over time. Dermal necrosis, along with surface coagulated protein, turns the wound white to yellow. These wounds have a prolonged healing time. They can heal spontaneously as the epidermal elements germinate and migrate until the epidermal surface is restored. This process of healing by epithelialization can take up to 6 weeks. Left untreated, these wounds can heal primarily with unstable epithelium, late hypertrophic scarring, and marked contracture formation. The treatment of choice is surgical excision and skin grafting. Partial-thickness injuries can become full-thickness injuries if they become infected, if blood supply is diminished, or if further trauma occurs to the site.

A *full-thickness burn (third degree)* involves destruction of all the layers of the skin down to and including the subcutaneous tissue. The subcutaneous tissue is composed of adipose tissue, includes the hair follicles and sweat glands, and is poorly vascularized. A full-thickness burn appears pale white or charred, red or brown, and leathery. At first, a full-thickness burn may resemble a partial-thickness burn. The surface of the burn may be dry, and if the skin is broken, fat may be exposed. Full-thickness burns usually are painless and insensitive to palpation. All epithelial elements are destroyed; therefore the wound will not heal by reepithelialization. Wound closure of small full-thickness burns (less than a 4 cm area) can be achieved with healing by contraction. All other full-thickness wounds require skin grafting for closure. Extensive full-thickness wounds leave the patient extremely susceptible to infections, fluid and electrolyte imbalances, alterations in thermoregulation, and metabolic disturbances.

The exact depth of many burn wounds cannot be clearly defined on the first inspection. A major difficulty is distinguishing deep-dermal from full-thickness injury. Burn wounds may evolve over time and require frequent reassessment. Special consideration must always be given to very young and elderly patients because of their thin dermal layer. Burn injuries in these age groups may be more severe than they initially appear.[7]

At the same time that assessment for wound depth occurs, the total percentage, or TBSA, of the burn is calculated by means of either the rule of nines or the Lund and Browder chart. This calculation provides the basis for determining the amount of fluid required for treatment. Typically, only second- and third-degree burns are used to estimate the patient's fluid requirements.

Zones of Injury

Thermal burns are additionally classified into three concentric zones of injury—the central zone being the site of most severe damage and the peripheral zone being the site of the least damaged. In the middle, usually the site of greatest heat transfer, is the zone of coagulation where irreversible skin death occurs. This zone is surrounded by the zone of stasis, which is characterized by a pronounced inflammatory reaction. This is a potentially salvageable area; however, it can be converted by infection or inadequate resuscitation into a full-thickness injury. The outermost area is the zone of hyperemia, where there is minimal cell involvement and where early spontaneous recovery occurs.[6]

Types of Injury

Thermal burns. The most common type of burn is a thermal burn caused by steam, scalds, contact with heat, and fire injuries. The most common age-groups involved are toddlers (2 to 4 years), for whom scalds are the most common cause, and young adults (17 to 25 years, usually male), for whom the most common cause is flammable liquid. Structural fires account for fewer than 5% of hospital admissions but are responsible for more than 45% of burn-related deaths.[1]

Electrical burns. Electrical and lightning injuries result in 1000 deaths per year in the United States. The incidence of electrical burn injury is 17 times greater in males. Electrical burns can be caused by low-voltage (alternating) current or high-voltage (alternating or direct) current. Common situations that may increase the risk for electrical injuries include occupational exposure and accidents involving household current. Lightning causes death in approximately 25% of those injured, and permanent sequelae in about 75%.[8]

Chemical burns. Chemical burns are caused by acids and alkalies. Alkalies commonly result in more severe injuries than do acid burns. Acids and alkali agents are found in household substances, such as liquid concrete. The concentration of the chemical agent and the duration of exposure are the key factors that determine the extent and depth of damage. Time must not be wasted in looking for the specific neutralizing agents because the injury is related directly to the concentration of the chemical and the duration of the exposure; also, the heat of neutralization can extend the injury. Tar and asphalt burns are serious and rather common injuries.[1,4] Approximately 70% of chemical burns occur to the hands.

Radiation burns. Burns associated with radiation exposure are uncommon. Radiation burns usually are localized and indicate high radiation doses to the affected area. Radiation burns may appear identical to thermal burns. The major difference is the time between exposure and clinical manifestation—days to weeks depending on the level of the dose. Radiation injury can occur with exposure to industrial equipment, such as accelerators and cyclotrons, and equipment used for medical treatment.

Location of Injury

Location of injury can be a determining factor in differentiating a minor burn from a major burn. According to triage criteria (Box 46-1), burns on the face, hands, feet, and perineum are considered major burns. These involve functional areas of the body and often require specialized intervention. Injuries to these areas can result in significant long-term morbidity, both from impaired function and altered appearance.

Patient Age and History

Age and history are significant determinants of survival. Patients considered most at risk are those younger than 2 years and those older than 60 years. History of inhalation injury, electrical burns, and all burns complicated by trauma and fractures—considered major injuries—significantly increases mortality. Obtaining a past medical history is important, particularly a history relating to cardiac, pulmonary, and renal disorders, as well as diabetes and central nervous system disorders. (∞Cardiac History, p. 355; Pulmonary History, p. 625; Renal History, p. 865; Endocrine History, p. 990; Neurologic History, p. 763.)

BOX 46-1 Triage Criteria for Burn Patients

Minor burn injury: can be treated initially on outpatient basis
1. Second-degree burn
   a. Less than 15% of body surface in adult
   b. Less than 10% of body surface in child
2. Third-degree burn
   a. Less than 2% of body surface

Moderate uncomplicated burn injury: usually requires hospitalization (general hospital with experience in burn care or specialized burn treatment facility)
1. Second-degree burn
   a. 15%–20% of body surface in adult
   b. 10%–20% of body surface in child
2. Third-degree burn
   a. 2%–10% of body surface

Major burn injury: requires hospitalization in a specialized burn treatment facility
1. Second-degree burn
   a. More than 25% of body surface in adult
   b. More than 20% of body surface in child
2. Third-degree burn
   a. More than 10% of body surface
3. Smaller burns with complicating features
   a. Extremes of age: less than 5 or more than 60
   b. Burns of hands, face, perineum, feet
   c. Chronic alcoholism or drug addiction
   d. Inhalation injury
   e. Significant preexisting disease (e.g., diabetes mellitus)
   f. Associated trauma
   g. Unreliable home environment for small children
   h. Child abuse

From Shires GT, *Principles of trauma care,* New York, 1985, McGraw-Hill.

INITIAL EMERGENCY BURN MANAGEMENT

The goals of acute care of the patient with thermal injuries are to save life, minimize disability, and prepare the patient for definitive care. The burn injury may involve multiple organ systems, and the approach to the injured patient must be expeditious and methodic in identifying problems and establishing priorities of care.[9]

The resuscitation phase begins immediately after the burn insult has occurred; therefore the nurse is concerned with patient management at the scene until admission to an appropriate medical facility and preparation for care of the burn injury can occur. As with any major trauma, the first hour is crucial but the first 24 to 36 hours also are vitally important in burn patient management. This time interval has a major impact on the patient's survival and ultimate rehabilitation.

Obtaining a history of the nature of the injury is extremely valuable in management. Water heater, propane gas, grain elevator, and other types of explosions frequently throw the patient some distance and may result in concomitant orthopedic, neurologic, and/or internal trauma. It is valuable to know the specific agents involved if the burns are chemical. It also helps to know what was burned or inhaled and how long the patient was exposed to superheated air. A detailed patient history is important and must include the mechanism of injury, patient's age, location and size of burn, type and amount of fluid already administered, known allergies, status of tetanus immunization, and significant past medical history. All rings, watches, and jewelry are removed from injured limbs to avoid a tourniquet effect when edema occurs as a result of fluid shifts and fluid resuscitation.

Airway Management

The first priority of emergency burn care is to secure and protect the airway. If there is any possibility of underlying cervical instability, cervical precautions must be initiated.[9] For patients with facial burns or exposure to an enclosed space of fire, or both, a high index of suspicion exists for inhalation injury. Carbon monoxide poisoning or intoxication is associated with high mortality. Carboxyhemoglobin levels are obtained, and oxygen therapy is continued until levels are no longer toxic. All patients with major burns or suspected inhalation injury are initially administered 100% oxygen.[10] The nurse must continue to observe the patient for clinical manifestations of impaired oxygenation, such as tachypnea, agitation, anxiety, and upper airway obstruction (e.g., hoarseness, stridor, and wheezing). Early intubation may save the life of the patient who has an inhalation injury, since it may be impossible to perform this procedure later, when edema has obstructed the larynx. (∞Artificial Airways, p 692.)

Circulatory Management

At this point, the extent and depth of the burn are assessed. The extent of TBSA of the burn is calculated for estimation of fluid resuscitation requirements (see Table 46-1); the Parkland formula is the most widely used method of calculation. Burn shock is caused by the loss of fluid from the vascular compartment into the area of injury, resulting in hypovolemia. Therefore the larger the percentage of burn, the greater the potential for development of shock. Lactated Ringer's solution is infused via large-bore cannula (16 gauge or larger) in a peripheral vein. Lactated Ringer's (LR) solution, an isotonic crystalloid, is the most popular resuscitation fluid. Lactated Ringer's solution given in large amounts can restore cardiac output toward normal in most patients. It is preferred to normal saline because it most closely matches extracellular fluid. Because isotonic salt solutions generate no difference in osmotic pressure between plasma and interstitial space, the entire extracellular space must be expanded to replace intravascular losses. The Parkland formula is as follows:

4 ml LR × kilogram × BSA* burn =
24-hour fluid resuscitation

In the first 8 hours after injury, half the calculated amount of fluid is administered to the patient; 25% is given in the second 8 hours and 25% in the third 8 hours. It is important to remember that calculated fluid requirements are guidelines. Fluid resuscitation is a dynamic process. The rate of fluid administration is adjusted according to the individual's response, which is determined by monitoring urine output, heart rate, blood pressure, and level of consciousness. Meticulous attention to detail is imperative to ensure that patients are neither underresuscitated nor overresuscitated. Underresuscitation may result in inadequate organ perfusion and the potential for wound conversion from partial to full thickness. Overresuscitation may lead to severe pulmonary edema; excessive wound edema causing a decrease in perfusion of unburned tissue in the distal portions of the extremities, or edema impeding perfusion of the zone of stasis, causing wound conversion.[5,10]

Renal Management

If fluid resuscitation is inadequate, acute renal failure may occur. A Foley catheter is placed to monitor renal perfusion and the effectiveness of fluid resuscitation. The nurse measures urine output hourly. Adequate urine output is 0.5 to 1 ml/kg/hour in adults and 1 ml/kg/hour in children.[5,10] (∞Acute Renal Failure, p 877.)

Gastrointestinal Management

Patients with burns of more than 20% BSA are prone to gastric dilation as a result of paralytic ileus. Nasogastric tubes are placed in these patients to prevent abdominal distention, emesis, and potential aspiration. This decrease in gastrointestinal function is caused by a combination of the effects of hypovolemia

*Body surface area

RESEARCH ABSTRACT

Effect of relaxation and music on postoperative pain: a review.

Good M: *J Adv Nurs* 24:905, 1996.

PURPOSE

The purpose of this review was to summarize and critique studies on the effectiveness of relaxation and music on postoperative pain. Specifically, four questions were asked: (1) What relaxation and music interventions for relief of postoperative pain have been studied? (2) What theories are used to study the effects of relaxation and music on postoperative pain? (3) Do the results show relaxation and music to be effective in reducing postoperative pain? (4) What methodologic issues may confound the inferences of the studies?

DESIGN

Integrative review of the literature.

SAMPLE

All published research studies from 1966 to 1995 on the use of relaxation techniques and/or music to reduce acute pain after surgery on adults were included in the review. The sample consisted of 21 studies from medical and nursing journals.

PROCEDURE

A survey instrument to document the data points of the study was developed by the investigator. The investigator read each study and documented the data on the survey instrument. Studies were arranged into three groups: (1) randomized studies; (2) nonrandomized studies; and (3) preexperimental studies that had no control group. Information on variables thought most likely to affect the validity of the results was also included in the listing.

RESULTS

Effectiveness was found in 6 of the 12 studies in which sensory pain was measured, 10 of the 13 studies in which reported affective pain was measured, 4 of the 7 studies in which reported unidimensional pain was measured, all 4 of the studies in which observed pain was measured, and 5 of the 15 studies in which opioid intake was measured. In the majority of the studies, investigators tested individual interventions in resting patients after a variety of abdominal surgeries. The gate control theory was used most frequently as the basis for the studies. The majority of the studies used immediate posttests (n = 11), did not establish the pretest equivalence of groups (n = 17), did not provide practice (n = 16), and did not control for time since medication (n = 14). ANOVA and *t*-tests were used in seven studies; there was no consistency in data analysis.

DISCUSSION/IMPLICATIONS

The finding suggest that relaxation and music were effective in providing relief in the majority of studies concerning affective pain and concerning reported and observed unidimensional pain, but were not effective in the majority of studies concerning opioid intake. These studies included 12 different kinds of surgical procedures; pain may have differed in these studies. In the studies, a variety of relaxation and music interventions were used and tested for postoperative pain relief. Treatment conditions and interventions varied in both number and type. Not every study investigator measured both the sensory and affective components of pain. Several methodologic issues were identified that related to sample size and to inconsistency in control of extraneous variables and actual focus of intervention. More rigorous methods and further research are needed to clarify the mixed results from these various studies. Although research findings are inconclusive, there are implications for nursing practice in the areas of nonpharmacologic interventions, such as relaxation and music. These low risk interventions can enhance pain relief in some patients and can easily be incorporated into nursing practice.

---

and the neurologic and endocrine response to injury. Gastrointestinal activity usually returns in 24 to 48 hours. Gastric prophylaxis is initiated since burn patients are prone to stress ulcers. (∞Stress Ulcers, p 945.)

Pain Management

Burn injuries are very painful so pain management must be addressed early and frequently reassessed to determine adequacy of interventions. Intravenous opiates are indicated, which are titrated against effect. Intramuscular or subcutaneous injections must not be administered since absorption by these routes is unpredictable because of the fluid shifts that occur with burn injury.[11] (∞Pain, p 169.)

Extremity Pulse Assessment

Edema formation may cause neurovascular compromise to the extremities; frequent assessments are necessary to evaluate pulses, skin color, capillary refill, and sensation. Arterial circulation is at greatest risk with circumferential burns. If not corrected, reduced arterial flow will result in ischemia and necrosis. The Doppler flow probe maybe one of the best ways to evaluate compromise. An escharotomy may be required to restore arterial circulation and to allow for further swelling. The escharotomy can be performed at the bedside with a sterile field and scalpel. Care must be taken to avoid major nerves, vessels, and tendons. The incision extends through the length of the eschar, over joints and down to the subcutaneous fat. The incision is placed laterally or medially on the extremity. If a single incision does not restore circulation, then bilateral incisions are required (Figure 46-4).[4,6]

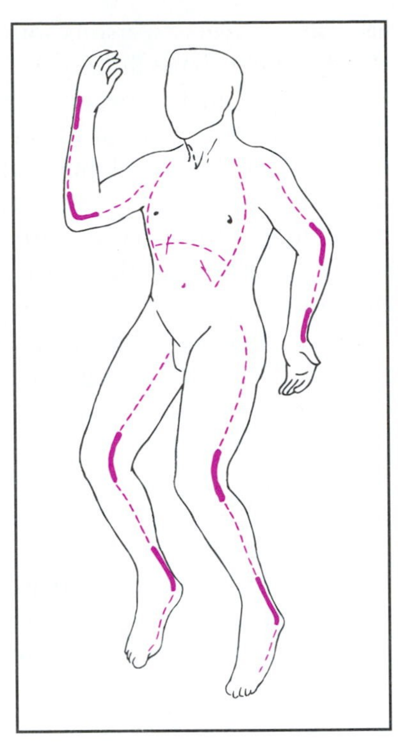

FIGURE 46-4. Preferred sites of escharotomy-incisions. (From Ahrens T, Prentice D: *Critical Care Certification Preparation and Review,* Norwalk, Conn, 1993, Appleton & Lange.)

Laboratory Assessment

Initial laboratory studies are performed: hematocrit, electrolytes, blood urea nitrogen, urinalysis, and chest roentgenogram. Special situations warrant arterial blood gas, carboxyhemoglobin, and alcohol and drug screens. An electrocardiogram (ECG) is obtained for all patients with electrical burns or preexisting cardiac problems.

Wound Care

After the wounds have been assessed, topical antimicrobial therapy is not a priority during emergency care. The wounds, however, must be covered with clean, dry dressings or sheets. Every attempt must be made to keep the patient warm because of the high risk of hypothermia.

Burn Center Referral

After initial treatment and stabilization at an emergency department, referral to a burn center is considered. By definition a burn center must be capable of delivering all therapy required, including rehabilitation, and must perform personnel training and burn research.[1] Patients meeting the criteria for referral require the expertise of a multidisciplinary team. The United States and Canada are divided into 12 regions, each with one or more tertiary burn care centers. Referring hospitals must always contact the burn center in their region.[1]

SPECIAL MANAGEMENT CONSIDERATIONS

Inhalation Injury

Inhalation injury can occur either in the presence or the absence of cutaneous injury. Inhalation injuries are highly associated with burns sustained in a closed space. Smoke inhalation accounts for 20% to 30% of burn center admissions and 60% to 70% of burn center fatalities. For any given severity of skin burns, inhalation injury doubles the mortality rate.[12] Inhalation injury appears in three basic forms, alone or in combination: carbon monoxide poisoning, direct heat injury, and/or chemical damage. There are three distinguishing types of inhalation injury: carbon monoxide poisoning, upper airway injury, and lower airway injury. Immediate measures to save the life of the burn patient include management of the airway. The burn patient may exhibit few if any signs of airway distress; however, thermal injury to the airway must be anticipated if there are facial burns, singed eyebrows and nasal hair, carbon deposits in the oropharynx, carbonaceous sputum, or if the history suggests confinement in a burning environment. Any of these findings indicates acute inhalation injury and requires immediate and definitive care. To prevent the necessity of tracheostomy or cricothyrotomy, the use of early intubation and respiratory support must be considered before tracheal edema occurs. Inhalation injury predisposes the patient to the development of pneumonia and acute respiratory distress syndrome (ARDS).[12,13] The occurrence of inhalation injury with cutaneous burns increases the fluid requirements during resuscitation more than would be predicted by the cutaneous burn alone. (∞Acute Respiratory Distress Syndrome, p 660.)

Carbon monoxide poisoning. Persons found dead at the scene of a fire often have little or no cutaneous thermal injury but have died of carbon monoxide poisoning. Carbon monoxide is a colorless, odorless, and tasteless gas. It binds with hemoglobin at the expense of hemoglobin's oxygen-carrying capacity, and the affinity of hemoglobin molecules for carbon monoxide is approximately 200 times that for oxygen. Carboxyhemoglobin binds poorly with oxygen, reducing the oxygen-carrying capacity of blood and causing hypoxia. The major clinical manifestations of severe carbon monoxide poisoning are related to the central nervous system and the heart. Measurement of arterial oxygen tension is of no value, because oxygen tension may be quite high in the presence of a dangerously low oxygen content of carbon monoxide-saturated hemoglobin. Remember that the pulse oximeter cannot distinguish between oxyhemoglobin and carboxyhemoglobin, thus making it unreliable during initial stages of carbon monoxide poisoning. Arterial blood must be drawn to accurately assess the level of hemoglobin oxygen saturation. The most reliable treatment of carbon monoxide poisoning consists of 100% oxygen administration by a tight-fitting mask or endotracheal tube if the patient is unresponsive. Normal carboxyhemoglobin levels are less than 2%. Carboxyhemoglobin levels of 40% to 60% frequently produce unresponsiveness or obtundation; levels of 15% to 40% may manifest central nervous system dysfunction of varying degrees; and levels of 10% to 15% often are found in cigarette smokers and rarely are symptomatic.

Upper airway injury. Burns of the upper respiratory tract include those involving the pharynx, larynx, glottis, trachea, and larger bronchi. Injuries are caused either by direct heat or by chemical inflammation and necrosis. Except for rare events, respiratory injury is confined to the upper airway. The heat exchange capability is so efficient that most heat absorption and damage occur in the pharynx and larynx above the true vocal cords.

Heat damage often is severe enough to cause upper airway destruction, which also may cause airway obstruction at any time during the resuscitation. Caution is taken for patients with severe hypovolemia, because supraglottic edema may be delayed until fluid resuscitation is under way. Patients must be monitored for hoarseness, stridor, audible air-flow turbulence, and the production of carbonaceous sputum.

Lower airway injury. Heated air rarely causes lower airway injury. If it does, it usually is associated with death at the scene. Lower airway injuries also may be caused by chemical damage to mucosal surfaces. Tracheobronchitis with severe spasm and wheezing may occur in the first minutes to hours after injury. The most accurate method of documenting lower airway injury is the xenon-ventilation perfusion lung scan. Prolonged retention or symmetry of washout of the radioisotope indicates pulmonary parenchymal injury on the side of the retained emissions. Treatment is largely symptomatic. The fiberoptic bronchoscope is used both in the diagnosis and in the management of inhalation injury associated with complications.[13] The burn surgeon diagnoses inhalation injury by bronchoscopic examination. The onset of symptoms is so unpredictable with possible smoke inhalation that patients at risk must be closely observed for at least 24 to 48 hours.

Nonthermal Burns

Chemical burns. In the past, the irrigation of acid, alkali, and organic compound burns with neutralizing solutions was recommended to limit the extent and depth of chemical burns. Neutralizing agents, however, may cause reactions that are exothermic (i.e., produce heat) thereby increasing the extent and depth of the burn. It also is possible that the neutralizing agent is not immediately known nor available. Therefore the use of large amounts of water to flush the area is recommended. Alkali burns of the eyes require continuous irrigation for many hours after the injury. Once the chemical agent as been diluted, a more individualized treatment can be initiated to reduce systemic absorption of the toxin.

Phenol burns are first diluted, and then the skin is wiped quickly with polyethylene glycol or vegetable oil to decrease the severity of the burn. Areas exposed to hydrofluoric acid must also be copiously irrigated with water; the burned area then can be treated with 2.5% calcium gluconate gel. The patient may need calcium gluconate replacements because the fluoride ion precipitates serum calcium, causing hypocalcemia. White phosphorous can ignite if kept dry; therefore wounds must be covered with a moist dressing.

After a tar or asphalt injury, the removal of tar or asphalt is best accomplished with the use of bacitracin or Neosporin ointment. The tar must not be peeled off because of potential damage to the involved hair and skin (Figure 46-5). There is no real advantage to early tar removal; it may result only in greater pain and discomfort. Thus patients usually find delayed removal acceptable. Daily wound care, consisting of debridement of loose skin and tar, followed by application of an antibiotic-containing emollient, is preferable. All chemical wounds

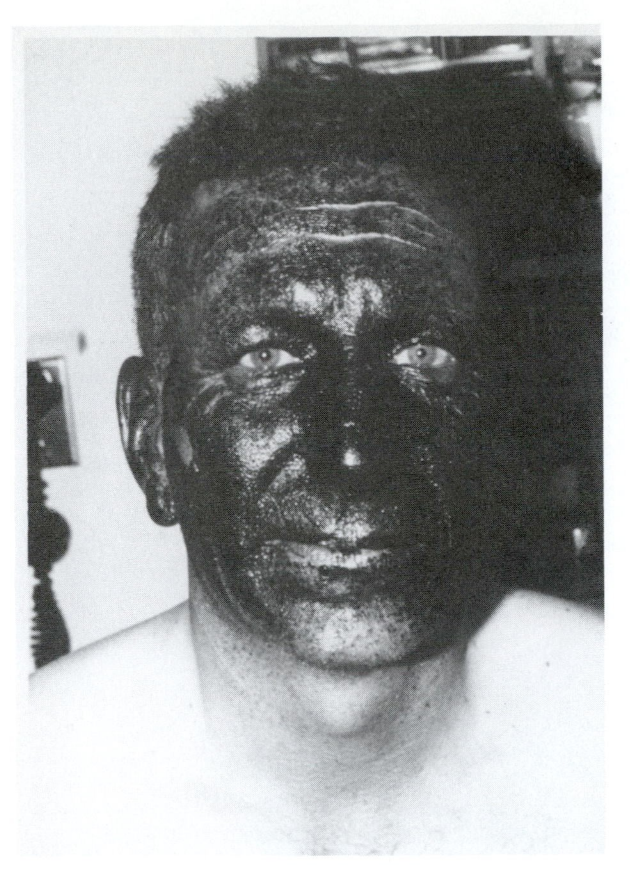

FIGURE 46-5. Tar burn to the face.

are treated with appropriate topical therapy once the chemical has been diluted, neutralized, or removed.[1]

Electrical burns. In electrical burns, the type and voltage of the circuit, resistance, pathway of transmission through the body, and duration of contact are considered in determining the amount of damage sustained. Frequently in these situations the rescuer also may be injured if he or she becomes part of the electrical circuit. The rescuer must disconnect the electrical source to break the circuit or must know how to avoid becoming part of the circuit. The use of appropriately insulated equipment that diverts the circuit elsewhere is essential. Extreme caution must be used in the rescue of victims.

Electricity always travels toward the ground. It travels most quickly through the circulatory system, then through the nerves, muscles, the integumentary system, and finally bone. Electrical burns frequently are much more serious than their surface appearance suggests. As the electrical current passes through the body, it damages the inner tissues and may leave little evidence of a burn on the skin surface (Figure 46-6).

The electrical burn process can result in a profound alteration in acid-base balance and the production of myoglobinuria, which poses a serious threat to renal functioning. Fluid resuscitation for the electrical burn patient does not correlate with the Parkland formula, and the fluid is adjusted according to the patient's urine output. If myoglobin is present in the urine, a urine output of 100 to 150 ml/hour is established until the urine is clear of all gross pigment. Myoglobin is a normal constituent of muscle; with extensive muscle destruction it is released into the circulatory system and filtered by the kidneys. It can be highly toxic and can lead to intrinsic renal failure.

In the presence of hemoglobinuria, one must assume that myoglobinuria and acidosis are present. Sodium bicarbonate may be administered to bring the pH level into normal range, to correct a documented acidosis, and/or to alkalize urine to promote myoglobin excretion. Mannitol also may be administered intravenously until the qualitative myoglobinuria disappears. A baseline ECG and cardiac enzyme levels are obtained while the patient is in the emergency department. The following are criteria for the cardiac monitoring of patients:

- A history of loss of consciousness or cardiac arrest
- Documentation of cardiac dysrhythmia at the scene of the accident or in the emergency department
- Abnormal ECG findings on admission
- Large TBSA burns
- Very young or elderly persons

Other burn patients may be admitted to nonmonitored settings and observed closely. Cardiac dysrhythmias must be treated promptly, and a protocol to rule out myocardial infarction must be followed.[8]

BURN NURSING DIAGNOSIS AND MANAGEMENT

Management of the patient with burn injuries can be divided into three phases: resuscitation, acute care, and rehabilitation. Each phase is unique and has its own set of actual and potential problems.

The resuscitation phase takes place immediately after injury until the onset of spontaneous diuresis, the hallmark that demonstrates the capillaries have regained their integrity. The major focus of the acute phase that follows is wound healing, wound closure, and prevention of infection and other complications. The rehabilitation phase overlaps the acute phase and may continue for up to 2 years after the burn injury. The rehabilitation phase focuses on support for adequate wound healing, prevention of scarring and contractures, and psychologic support of the patient and family.[14] (∞Chapter 5 p. 63.)

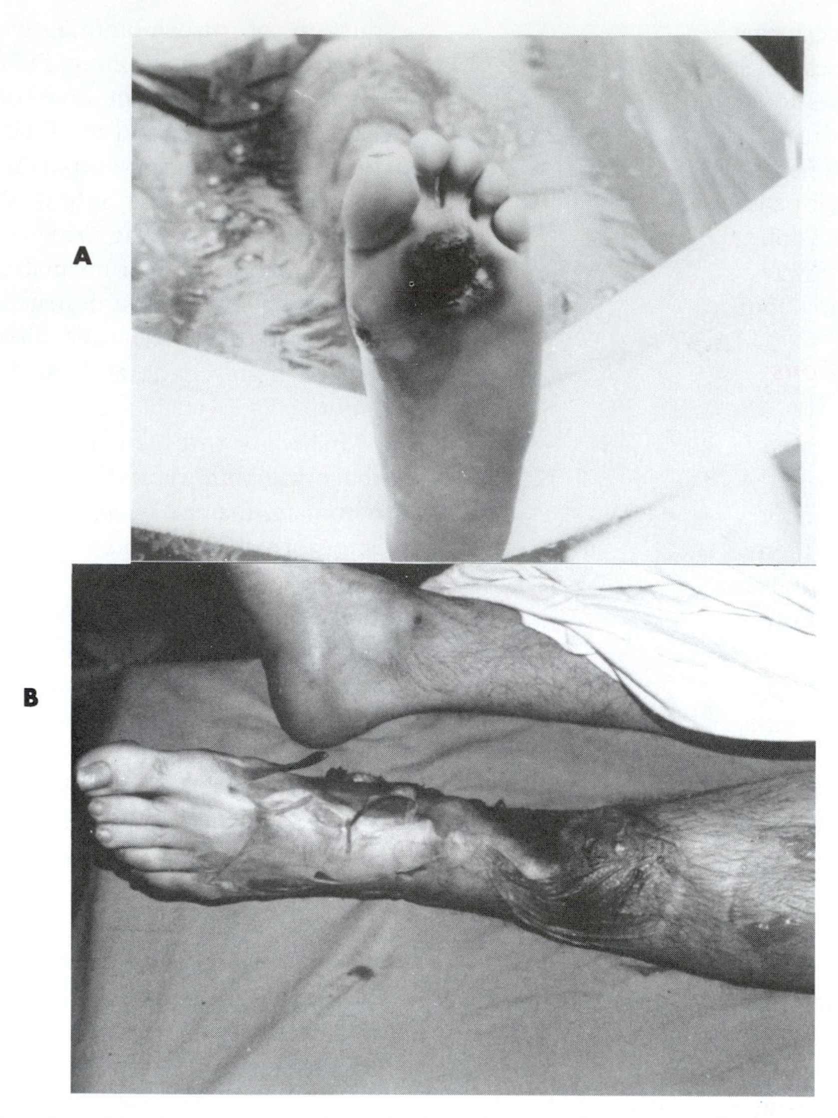

FIGURE 46-6. A, Exit site of electrical burn on sole of foot. **B,** Same leg several days later, illustrating extension of tissue damage after the injury.

RESUSCITATION PHASE

The resuscitation phase, or shock phase, of burn injury is characterized by cardiopulmonary instability, life-threatening airway and breathing problems, and hypovolemia. Every organ is involved in the physiologic response that occurs with thermal injury of greater than 20% TBSA. The magnitude of this pathophysiologic response is proportional to the extent of cutaneous injury, which is maximal when approximately 60% of the TBSA is burned.[15,16]

After thermal injury, a marked increase in capillary hydrostatic pressure occurs in the injured tissue early in the postinjury phase. Later, an increase in capillary permeability occurs, which returns toward normal during the latter half of the first 24 hours after injury. A marked increase in peripheral vascular resistance, accompanied by a decrease in cardiac output, is one of the earliest manifestations of the systemic effects of thermal injury. Organ hypoperfusion develops as a result of low cardiac output and increased peripheral vascular resistance caused by the normal neurohormonal response to trauma. With adequate volume repletion, hemodynamic functions improve, and as plasma volume increases, cardiac output rises, resulting in a hyperdynamic state and overall increase in organ perfusion.

These initial changes appear to be unrelated to hypovolemia and have been attributed to neurogenic and humoral effects.[4] These alterations result in the formation of edema within the wound. This progressive loss of fluid may result in significant intravascular fluid volume deficit. With adequate volume repletion, hemodynamic performance improves, and as plasma volume increases during the second 24 hours, cardiac output increases to supernormal levels, characteristic of the hypermetabolic response to injury. (∞Systemic Inflammatory Response Syndrome, p 1121.)

The goal of the shock phase is to maintain vital organ function and perfusion. Emergent interventions for inhalation injury, airway management, and hypovolemia are concurrently addressed.

Oxygenation Alterations

Forty to fifty years ago, burn shock accounted for most burn deaths, followed in more recent years by burn wound sepsis. Currently, inhalation injuries have emerged as the most common cause of death in burn patients. The degree of thermal injury is not an indication of presence or absence of inhalation injury.[12] Three separate oxygenation complications are associated with smoke inhalation during the resuscitation phase: *carbon monoxide poisoning, upper airway obstruction,* and *chemical pneumonitis.* Early diagnosis of inhalation injuries is vital to minimize complications and to decrease the mortality rate.

The assessment of a patient for inhalation injury includes the following parameters: physical assessment (singed facial hairs, mucosal burns of nose or mouth, carbonaceous sputum); arterial blood gas analysis; carboxyhemoglobin levels; chest radiography; flexible fiberoptic bronchoscopy; xenon-133 lung scan; and pulmonary function tests.[12,13] Nursing actions include the following:

- Assess breath sounds, as well as the rate and quality of respirations, and document.
- Administer oxygen as prescribed.
- Monitor carboxyhemoglobin levels.
- Assess and document pulmonary secretions.
- Provide suction as needed.
- Observe for signs of airway obstruction (e.g., stridor, wheezing, hoarseness, crackles).
- Prepare for endotracheal intubation and mechanical ventilation.

Impaired gas exchange. The most common pulmonary burn complication is carbon monoxide poisoning. Inhalation of carbon monoxide, a by-product of the incomplete combustion of carbon, results in its bonding to available hemoglobin, producing carboxyhemoglobin (HbCO), which effectively decreases oxygen saturation of hemoglobin.

Symptoms associated with carbon monoxide poisoning include headache, dizziness, nausea, vomiting, dyspnea, and confusion. In severe cases, carbon monoxide poisoning may lead to myocardial ischemia and central nervous system complications caused by lowered oxygen delivery and the already compromised circulatory system. The shortage of oxygen at the tissue level is worsened by a leftward shift of the oxyhemoglobin dissociation curve so that the oxygen on the hemoglobin is not readily given up to the cells. Early signs of carbon monoxide poisoning may include tachycardia, tachypnea, confusion, and lightheadedness. As the level of carbon monoxide rises, the patient demonstrates cherry red skin and membranes and a decreased level of responsiveness, which may progress to unresponsiveness and respiratory failure.

The treatment of choice is high-flow oxygen administered at 100% through a nonrebreathing mask or endotracheal intubation. The half-life of carbon monoxide in the body is 4 hours at room air (21% oxygen), 2 hours at 40% oxygen, and 60 to 80 minutes at 100% oxygen. The half-life of carbon monoxide is 30 minutes in a hyperbaric oxygen chamber at three times the atmospheric pressure. Currently the use of hyperbaric oxygen is not recommended for most burn patients.

Chemical pneumonitis is caused by inhalation of the by-products of combustion of substances such as those in burning cotton, aldehydes, oxides of sulfur, and nitrogen. Burning polyvinylchloride yields at least 75 potentially toxic compounds, including hydrochloric acid and carbon monoxide. Within 5 days after a burn, ARDS frequently develops in patients with chemical pneumonitis, with the chief manifestation being hypoxemia refractory to oxygen therapy.[13] Early signs include increased pH, decreased partial pressure of carbon dioxide ($PaCO_2$), and an increased respiratory rate. Ventilatory support with the use of positive end-expiratory pressure (PEEP) is the treatment of choice. (∞Acute Respiratory Distress Syndrome, p 660.)

Ineffective airway clearance. Laryngeal swelling and upper airway obstruction generally occur 4 to 6 hours after the burn injury. Endotracheal intubation must be accomplished early because this simple procedure can become extremely difficult in the presence of laryngeal edema. Generally, however, time to intervene is available after obtaining the history and transporting the patient to the primary hospital. Edema may continue to develop for 72 hours after the burn incident. The patient who has not initially undergone intubation must be carefully monitored during this critical period.

The prediction of an upper airway obstruction is based on consideration of the following variables: extent of injury to the face and neck, the presence of blisters on or redness of the posterior pharynx, signs of singed nasal hair, increased carboxyhemoglobin levels, increased rate and decreased depth of breathing, hoarseness (which indicates a significant decrease in the diameter of the airway), increased amount of sputum, and the circumstances of the burn event (i.e., whether it occurred in an enclosed space and/or if it involved superheated gases or steam). Only steam has a heat-carrying capacity many times that of dry air and is capable of overwhelming the extremely efficient heat-dissipating capabilities of the upper airway.

Extubation must occur only if these patients can meet extubation criteria: awake level of consciousness, intact cough and gag reflexes, inspiratory effort greater than −25, vital capacity of 10 ml/kg, and decreased volume and tenacity of the sputum. Resolution of airway edema can be assessed by deflating the endotracheal cuff and observing the patient for the ability to breathe around the endotracheal tube. (∞Airway Management, p 695.)

Laryngospasm is another complication that, although not commonly seen, must be addressed. It generally is brought on by airway irritation secondary to inhalation of noxious agents.

Ineffective breathing pattern. Circumferential full-thickness burns to the chest wall can lead to restriction of chest wall expansion and decreased compliance. Decreased compliance requires higher ventilatory pressures to provide the patient with adequate tidal volumes. In the patient who has not undergone intubation, clinical manifestations include rapid, shallow respirations; poor chest wall excursion; and severe agitation. Patients receiving mechanical ventilation will demonstrate rising peak airway pressure.

Escharotomies must immediately be performed to increase compliance, leading to improved ventilation. These incisions generally are made down the lateral sides of the chest, and if necessary they are connected with an incision across the abdomen.

Fluid Resuscitation

As mentioned, current resuscitation protocols emphasize fluid delivery rates based on the extent of burn and the patient's weight. Therefore a weight measured in kilograms must be obtained on the patient's admission. The extent of the burn is calculated by using one of the methods previously described. Although several formulas exist, the Parkland formula remains the one most commonly used by burn centers around the country (Table 46-2).

Ideally, the capillary leak seals approximately 24 hours after the injury, making it possible to give colloid without leakage of protein into the interstitium. Colloid deficits are replaced in the next 24 hours with salt-free albumin or fresh frozen plasma, at 0.3 to 0.5 ml/kg/% TBSA burn. In addition, 5% dextrose solution is given to replace evaporative losses, and the amount is adjusted according to the patient's serum sodium level.

Fluid volume deficit. Tissue damage that occurs after the burn insult is complicated by the physiologic effects of the burn. Coagulation factors are affected, protein is denatured, and cellular content is ionized. These factors, coupled with the dilation of capillaries and small vessels, lead to increased capillary permeability and fluid shifts from the intravascular space to the interstitial space. The lymphatic system, which normally would carry away the increased interstitial fluid, may be damaged or overloaded and unable to function to its normal capacity.

In addition to the protein and electrolyte shift, there is an increased insensible water loss. In the healthy adult this loss is estimated at 35 to 50 ml/hour. The burn patient's insensible water loss may be as much as 300 to 3000 ml. This increase may be related to temperature elevation, tracheostomy, and the size of the burn.

Burn shock is proportional to the extent and depth of injury. The loss of plasma begins almost immediately after the injury and reaches its peak within the first 48 hours. Fluid volume deficit must be addressed during the first 24 to 36 hours of the resuscitation phase.

Several formulas are used to guide fluid resuscitation, each with its advantages and disadvantages (see Table 46-2). The formulas differ primarily in terms of administration, volume, and sodium content. Lactated Ringer's solution is the crystalloid solution of choice because of its physiologic similarity to the composition of extracellular fluid. Whichever fluid resuscitation formula is used, it is only a guideline. The actual amount of fluid given to any patient must be based on that individual's response.

Desired clinical responses to fluid resuscitation include a urinary output of 0.5 to 1 ml/kg/hour; a pulse rate less than 120/minute; blood pressure in normal to high ranges; a central venous pressure less than 12 cm H_2O or a pulmonary artery wedge pressure less than 18 mm Hg; clear lung sounds; clear sensorium; and the absence of intestinal events, such as nausea and paralytic ileus. Heart rate, blood pressure, and central venous pressure values are not always accurate or reliable predictors of successful fluid resuscitation.

Potassium and sodium, the two electrolytes of concern during the resuscitation period, must be monitored carefully until the wounds are healed. *Hyperkalemia* can occur during this phase because of the release of potassium from damaged cells; metabolic

TABLE 46-2 Formulas for Fluid Replacement/Resuscitation

	Evans Formula	Brooke Formula	Modified Brooke Formula	Artz Formula	Parkland Formula	Hypertonic Formula
First 24 hours:						
Electrolyte solution	Normal saline	Ringer's lactate	Ringer's lactate	Ringer's lactate	Ringer's lactate	Hypertonic lactated saline (sodium, 250 mEq/liter)
ml/kg/% burned	1.0	1.5	2.0	3.0	4.0	Rate based on urine output of 70 ml/hr in adults
Colloid	1 ml whole blood plasma, or plasma expanders/kg/% burn	0.5 ml/kg% burn	None	None	None	None
Free water (D_5W)	2000 ml	2000 ml	None	None	None	None
Second 24 hours:	One-half first 24 hour dose; same amount D_5W	One-half first 24 hour dose; same amount D_5W	D_5W and colloid	D_5W and colloid	Only D_5W to maintain urine output; colloid, 0.5 to 2 liters	Continued at rate to maintain urine output >30 ml

From Wachtel, Kahn, & Frank: *Current topics in burn care,* Gaithersburg, Md, 1983, Aspen.

acidosis; and/or impaired renal function secondary to hemoglobinuria, myoglobinuria, or decreased renal perfusion. The patient must be assessed for the clinical manifestations of hyperkalemia. Treatment includes correction of acidosis. During the resuscitation phase, however, it is not recommended to use cation-exchange resins or intravenously administered insulin and hypertonic dextrose to transport potassium back into the cell.

Hypokalemia also can occur during the resuscitation phase because of the massive loss of fluids and electrolytes through the burn wounds or because of hemodilution. During the acute phase it may be related to hemodilution; inadequate replacement; loss associated with diuresis, diarrhea, vomiting, nasogastric drainage, and long hydrotherapy sessions; and/or the shift of potassium from the intravascular space to the cell after the acidosis has been corrected. Nursing interventions include treating nausea and vomiting, limiting hydrotherapy sessions, preventing fluid volume excess, and monitoring potassium replacement.

Hyponatremia is not uncommon during the resuscitation phase because of the loss of sodium through the burn wound, the shift of fluid into the interstitial space, vomiting, nasogastric drainage, diarrhea, and/or the use of hypotonic salt solutions during the early phase of resuscitation. During this phase it may be necessary to monitor serum sodium levels every 2 to 4 hours. Hyponatremia also may occur during the acute phase because of hemodilution and loss through the wound, lengthy hydrotherapy sessions, and excessive diuresis resulting from the fluid shift back into the intravascular space. Interventions are followed for treating nausea and vomiting, hydrotherapy sessions are limited, and consideration is given to the intravenous replacement of sodium. During diuresis, which occurs during the acute phase, restricting free water intake usually is the only required intervention to increase the serum sodium.

Risk for Infection

Preventing infection in the burn patient is a true challenge and involves complex decision making. Infection is the most common cause of death after burn injury.

There has been considerable discussion in recent years about the type of isolation precautions to use with burn patients. Hand washing and the use of gowns, gloves, and masks alone are effective in controlling contamination and infection the in adult patient with burns. Significant contributors to infection are auto contamination from exogenous sources. Cross-contamination by direct contact is the most significant source of infection and subsequent cause of sepsis.[17]

Proper hand-washing technique cannot be overemphasized. Nurses must wash their hands and change gloves when moving from area to area on the same patient. For example, after changing the chest dressing, which may be contaminated with sputum from the tracheostomy, hands must be washed and gloves changed before the nurse moves to the legs. Gowns, gloves, and masks must be changed and hands washed before caring for a different patient.

Whichever precautions are used, it is vital that everyone coming in contact with the patient (including the family and visitors) be knowledgeable about the standard for infection control and that it be strictly followed by all. Precautions must have sound rationale and must not increase the workload or the frustration of the burn team. Otherwise, compliance and consistent application of the standard will not occur, thus increasing the risk of infection and sepsis for the burn patient.

Tissue Perfusion

Altered renal tissue perfusion. Urinalysis to determine the myoglobin level is performed early in burn care. Myoglobinuria can be detected grossly by a dark, port wine color of the urine. Myoglobin is extremely toxic to the kidneys and can cause massive tubular destruction. It is best treated with rapid fluid administration and forced diuresis with mannitol, an osmotic diuretic. The goal is an hourly urinary output that is at least double the general recommendations to flush the tubules. All other diuretics are avoided because they will deplete the already compromised intravascular volume.

Maintaining and monitoring the renal system are vital in burn patient management. Impairment of the renal system may be related to hemoglobinuria, myoglobinuria, hypoperfusion, and hypovolemia. Urinary output must be monitored every hour for the first 48 to 72 hours, and specific gravity values are used to determine adequacy of hydration status and renal competency. Urinary glucose is monitored, as are urinary sodium, creatinine, and blood urea nitrogen (BUN) levels. Use of a Foley catheter is appropriate for the first 48 to 72 hours. Because of the tremendous risk of infection related to indwelling catheters, they are removed as soon as possible. Leaving the catheter in place may be necessary if perineal burns are involved. Oliguria usually is related to inadequate fluid resuscitation but may be associated with acute renal failure. Other signs of renal failure include increasing creatinine, BUN, phosphorus, and potassium levels; excessive weight gain; excessive edema; elevated blood pressure; lethargy; and confusion. (∞Acute Renal Failure, p. 877.)

The presence of glucose in the urine causes osmotic diuresis, which does not necessarily reflect the patient's volume status and may, in fact, suggest the need for additional fluid to make up for the compensatory mechanism.

Altered cerebral tissue perfusion. The patient's neurologic status is assessed frequently during the first few days. Changes may be related to an associated head injury that occurred with the burn, hypoperfusion related to hypovolemia, hypoxemia associated with inadequate ventilation, carbon monoxide poisoning, and/or electrolyte imbalances. Patients with electrical burns or major thermal burns may have peripheral neurologic injuries, which may not become evident for several days after the injury. The neurologic assessment includes use of the *Glasgow Coma Scale,* detailed in Chapter 26. It is not unusual for the patient to be agitated, restless, and extremely anxious during the emergent phase of burn injury as a result of hypovolemia, pain, and/or the fear of disfigurement or even death. The possibility of neurologic involvement, however, must not be overlooked. Maintaining an adequate mean arterial pressure is essential to ensure adequate cerebral perfusion pressure.

Altered peripheral tissue perfusion. Altered peripheral tissue perfusion results from third spacing of fluid during the resuscitation phase, which restricts blood flow to extremities. As hypovolemia ensues, vasoconstriction increases, which can be potentiated by the loss of body temperature. Peripheral tissue perfusion must be monitored carefully in all burn patients, as discussed earlier. Burned and unburned areas are carefully assessed for warmth, color, and peripheral pulses. Capillary refill time should be less than 2 seconds. Any clinical manifestation of diminished systemic tissue perfusion must be reported immediately. Nursing actions are taken to minimize any compromise of peripheral circulation. Care must be taken to avoid excessive fluid resuscitation and to not position the patient in a way that compromises blood flow, such as crossing legs, pillows under knees, or dependent positioning. If possible, elevate the limbs to decrease the peripheral edema by enhancing venous return.[5]

Monitoring the peripheral circulation is vital in the burn patient with circumferential full-thickness burns of the extremities. The resulting edema may severely compromise the venous system and then the arterial system. Neurovascular integrity of extremities with circumferential burns must be assessed every hour for the first 24 to 48 hours using the "six p's:" *pulselessness, pallor, pain, paresthesia, paralysis,* and *poikilothermy.* The use of a Doppler flow meter may be necessary. Loss of pulses may be a late sign of compromised vascular flow. If any other changes are noted, the physician must be notified immediately. Numbness and paresthesia can occur in 30 minutes of loss of pulses. Irreversible nerve ischemia resulting in a loss of function may begin after 12 to 24 hours.

A most unfortunate scenario results when the patient's reports of ischemic pain and paresthesia in a circumferentially burned extremity go unheeded and neurovascular compromise is allowed to persist. Sensory nerve fibers become damaged and altered sensations cease, which may be misinterpreted as improvement in neurovascular status. Permanent disability and quite possible loss of limb are eventual outcomes.

Extremities can be put through passive range-of-motion exercises to reduce edema. This, however, may not be a sufficient intervention to improve circulation. An escharotomy may become necessary to allow the underlying tissue to expand. In deeper wounds a fasciotomy, which involves incision of the fascia, may be necessary.

Altered gastrointestinal tissue perfusion. Paralytic ileus is a common gastrointestinal (GI) complication during resuscitation or when sepsis develops. The abdomen and the bowel sounds must be assessed every 2 hours during the initial phase and every 4 hours thereafter. If clinical manifestations of a paralytic ileus occur, all oral intake is withheld and a nasogastric tube inserted, using low to medium suction.

A paralytic ileus can be related to hypokalemia, the sympathetic response to severe trauma, and/or decreased tissue perfusion related to hypovolemia. (∞Intestinal Obstruction, p. 958.)

A stress ulcer (Curling's) may develop as a result of decreased tissue perfusion to the GI tract, a change in the quantity or quality of mucus (which has a pH of 1), and/or an increase in gastric acid secretion resulting from the stress response. Gastric acid should be maintained above pH 5 through the administration of antacids or H_2 blockers to prevent the development of these ulcers. The patient must be carefully monitored for GI bleeding. All stools and gastric content are tested for occult blood. The patient must be observed for epigastric discomfort of fullness, decreased blood pressure, or increased pulse. (∞Acute Gastrointestinal Hemorrhage, p. 945.)

Invasive Monitoring

The decision to use invasive techniques requires careful consideration of the potential risk factors and how the data collected will influence the course of treatment. Invasive monitoring certainly must be considered if treatment seems ineffective or if complicating factors occur, such as severe respiratory involvement; major life-threatening injuries; head injuries; pneumothorax; or preexisting medical conditions such as chronic obstructive pulmonary disease (COPD), congestive heart failure, and renal failure.[18]

During the past 10 years invasive cardiovascular monitoring has become commonplace. This procedure includes direct measurement of central venous pressure, pulmonary artery pressure, arterial pressure, core temperature, cardiac output, systemic vascular resistance, and pulmonary vascular resistance. The use of *arterial lines* is considered if data about serial and frequent arterial blood gas values are required for respiratory management or if vasoactive drugs are being titrated. *Central venous catheters* often are required for fluid resuscitation in the early stages to deliver the massive amount of fluids required. The physician placing these catheters considers where the burns are located and the purpose of the catheter. It is preferable not to insert these catheters through burns. It may be appropriate to use a multilumen catheter that can serve for fluid resuscitation and maintenance, antibiotic therapy, and vasoactive drugs. The risks involved include the increased chance of infection, potential for pneumothorax, and difficulty with the procedure if hypovolemia is present. (∞Bedside Hemodynamic Monitoring, p. 442)

Pulmonary artery catheters are placed only when necessary for optimal care. They may be absolutely essential to the survival of the septic patient despite the risks involved. Pulmonary artery catheters can provide data about pulmonary artery wedge pressure (PAWP), cardiac output, systemic and pulmonary vascular resistance, core temperature, and oxygen saturation. (∞Pulmonary Artery Pressure Monitoring, p. 459.)

These catheters require meticulous care. Strict guidelines must be established and monitored. Catheters are inserted under sterile conditions, and the dressings are changed under the same conditions. Since infection is such a major concern, all invasive catheters are removed as early as possible.[17]

Hypothermia

The patient with extensive burn injury is at high risk for hypothermia. Hypothermia is especially problematic during initial treatment, during hydrotherapy, and immediately after surgery. Heat is lost through open burn wounds by means of evaporation and radiation. The patient's core temperature must be maintained at 99.6° to 101°F. Thermoregulation is a nursing challenge. Heat shields/lamps, hypothermia blankets, and fluid warmers can be individually or simultaneously used to maintain body temperature.

Laboratory Assessment

Laboratory assessment is another important aspect of burn care. Because of the invasive nature of drawing blood, it is done only if absolutely indicated. Consideration must be given to the age of the patient, the size of the burn, the time since injury, and any underlying disease process.

White blood cell (WBC) counts usually are monitored for elevation, a sign of sepsis. It is not unusual, however, for the WBC count to fall below 5000 mm^3 within 48 hours after injury. It may drop even lower—1500 to 2000 mm^3—with the use of silver sulfadiazine. If the WBC count stays in this range for more than 12 hours, the use of a different topical agent is recommended. The WBC count generally will become normal again. At this point the use of silver sulfadiazine can be tested again by applying it to a small area. If the WBC count does not drop again within 12 hours, the use of silver can be sulfadiazine resumed. In practice, discontinuation of silver sulfadiazine in not common but must be considered if the WBC count continues to fall.

ACUTE CARE PHASE

The acute care phase of burn management begins after resuscitation and lasts until complete wound closure is achieved. The early postresuscitation phase is a period of transition from the shock phase to the hypermetabolic phase. Major cardiopulmonary and wound changes occur that substantially alter the manner of patient care from that during resuscitation. In general, cardiopulmonary stability is optimal during this period because wound inflammation and infection have not developed. Hypermetabolic changes, however, may become complicated with the onset of wound infection and sepsis. Early wound excision and skin grafting procedures, local wound care, nutritional support, and infection control characterize this phase. (∞Septic Shock, p. 1111.)

Critical care nurses play a major role in promoting the healing process. Nurses, as skilled clinicians of the burn team, provide daily wound assessment, hydrotherapy, debridement, preoperative and postoperative management, and pain management. Appropriate treatment results in critical differences in patient care and outcomes. Immediately after injury, the body responds by initiating a series of physiologic changes to restore skin integrity. These physiologic changes include the inflammatory phase, the proliferative phase, and the maturation phase.

The inflammatory phase. The inflammatory phase begins immediately after injury. This period is characterized by vascular changes and cellular activity. Changes in the severed vessels occur in an attempt to wall the wound off from the external environment. Platelets, activated as a result of vessel wall injury, aggregate; blood coagulation is initiated; and in larger vessels, smooth muscle tissue contraction occurs, resulting in reduction in the diameter of the vessel lumen. These brief but important compensatory mechanisms serve to protect the entire organism from excessive blood loss and increased exposure to bacterial contamination. As vasodilation occurs, there is an increase in vascular permeability and increased blood supply to the wound site. As extravascular volume increases, signs of erythema, edema, and tenderness become apparent. Granulocytes invade the wound within 24 hours and initiate the phagocytosis of necrotic tissue and bacteria. Fibroblasts migrate to the wound and multiply, producing a bed of collagen. This phase of healing lasts from the moment of injury to day 3 or 4 after the traumatic event.[15]

The proliferative phase. This phase of healing occurs approximately 4 to 20 days after injury. The key cell in this phase of healing, the fibroblast, rapidly synthesizes collagen. Collagen synthesis provides the needed strength for a healing wound. Epithelial cells migrate across the wound bed. Once these cells contact each other, the wound is covered. This process is known as *epithelialization.* Myofibroblasts also play a role in healing by pulling down the wound edge toward the center in an effort to close the wound; this process is known as *wound contraction.*

The maturation phase. This phase of healing occurs from approximately 20 days after injury to longer than 1 year after injury. During this period the wound develops tensile strength as collagen deposits form scar tissue. Regardless of how well collagen realigns itself, the tissue of the wound will never regain the degree of strength or intactness inherent in uninjured tissue. Over time, scar tissue matures and becomes smaller and less bulky, and pigmentation returns.

Impaired Tissue Integrity

Management of the burn wound is the top priority after the resuscitation phase. The depth of the burn wound is the principal determinant of wound management. Expedient closure of the wounds decreases the potential for multiple complications, such as fluid and electrolyte imbalances, loss of proteins and nitrogen, and infection. The major goal of burn wound care is to close the wound. Several objectives must be met for optimal wound closure: to control infection through meticulous cleansing and debridement, to promote reepithelization, and to prepare the wound for grafting. Other goals are to reduce scarring and contracture formation and to provide patient comfort with appropriate psychologic support and pharmacologic intervention.

Wound cleansing. A variety of equally appropriate methods can be used to cleanse burn wounds (e.g., sterile normal saline at the bedside or tap water in a hydrotherapy room). Generally, a mild antimicrobial cleansing agent is used, such as chlorhexidine (Hibiclens). Wounds are gently rinsed and patted dry before application of topical agents. Hydrotherapy facilitates the removal of debris and loose eschar. Daily cleansing and inspection of the wound and remaining skin integrity are performed for assessment of healing and local infection. Generally this therapy is performed once or twice daily and must last no longer than 20 to 30 minutes per session. Pain management and measures to reduce hypothermia are used. Patients must receive adequate premedication with analgesics, narcotics, and/or sedatives. Morphine, the drug of choice, is administered intravenously and titrated to effect. The patient's vital signs are carefully monitored during this time, especially body temperature and blood pressure. Mechanical debridement with scissors and forceps can be performed during these treatments. Total immersion is not as popular as it once was. Currently, spray tables and specially designed upright and chair showers are being used. The force of the spray assists in the removal of topical agents and debridement.[4,6]

Wound debridement. Debridement has two major aims: (1) removal of tissue contaminated by foreign bodies and bacteria, thus protecting patients from invasive infection; and (2) removal of devitalized tissue. There are three types of debridement:

- Mechanical
- Enzymatic
- Surgical

Eschar is the nonviable tissue that forms after the burn injury. This tissue has no blood supply. Therefore polymorphonuclear leukocytes, antibodies, and systemic antibodies cannot reach these areas. Eschar provides an excellent medium for bacterial growth; thus it is vital that the burn wounds be cleansed daily and loose eschar debrided as necessary.

Mechanical debridement involves the use of scissors and forceps to gently lift and to trim loose, necrotic tissue. This procedure is performed by experienced professional nurses and physicians. Sterile gauze also may be used in the form of a wet-to-dry or wet-to-wet dressing to further debride the wound bed. Enzymatic debridement involves the topical application of proteolytic substances to the wound bed. These agents are useful in softening eschar and dissolving devitalized tissue. They promote the separation of eschar, which can lead to earlier wound closure. Surgical debridement employs the use of two techniques; tangential excision and fascial excision. Tangential excision involves sequentially excising the eschar down to bleeding, viable tissue and then placing a split-thickness skin graft over the wound. Fascial excision is used when the wounds are particularly deep and the fat does not appear viable. Split-thickness skin grafts are harvested at approximately twelve thousandths of an inch in thickness by means of a dermatome. It is now commonly recommended that if a burn wound will not heal in 10 to 14 days, excision should be undertaken to improve functional and cosmetic results, to decrease in-hospital time, and to reduce the cost of burn care.[6] Surgical intervention with split-thickness skin grafts often yields a better cosmetic result than does the natural healing process with deep partial- and full-thickness injuries.

This surgical debridement technique may begin as early as 3 to 5 days after the burn insult when hemodynamic stability has been achieved. It involves excision of full-thickness tissue down to freely bleeding and viable tissue. The area that has been excised is immediately grafted with autografts or temporary biologic or synthetic dressings. This procedure is not without risk because the blood loss can be significant (up to 200 ml/% of burn tissue removed). Typically, excision procedures are limited to 20% of the body surface or 2 hours of operating time. In patients with massive burns, excision procedures are commonly staged, requiring the patient to return to the operating room every 2 to 3 days until all wounds have been excised. This technique helps avoid excessive transfusions and limits the physiologic stress.[6]

After cleansing and mechanical or enzymatic debridement has been performed, burn wounds are managed in one of three methods. The *open method* involves leaving the burn open with only a topical agent applied. Advantages to this method are (1) the wound can be easily assessed, (2) there are no dressings that would limit range of motion, and (3) the risk of diminishing circulation is decreased. There are, however, several disadvantages to the open method, including the need for strict isolation techniques. In addition, patients may experience more discomfort with this method because the wound is exposed to air currents and environmental temperatures.

The *semiopen method* consists of covering the wound with topical antimicrobial agents and then applying a thin layer of gauze and netting material to keep the antimicrobial agent in place.

The *closed method* of management generally consists of the application of topical agents covered with gauze or a nonadherent dressing (e.g., Adaptic, Xeroform) followed by a woven gauze dressing (e.g., Kerlix) to secure the dressing in place. Advantages to this method include (1) greater ease for patient mobility and (2) the decreased likelihood that the agent will be wiped off with movement. Disadvantages of this method include (1) the amount of nursing time required to change these dressings, (2) the inability to assess the wound directly, and (3) the increased risk of impaired peripheral circulation.[4]

Topical Antibiotic Therapy

Burn injuries destroy the function of the skin's protective mechanism, including that of the sebaceous glands. Sebaceous glands normally secrete sebum, which contains fatty acids, including oleic acid. In addition to lubricating the skin, sebum is believed to help destroy some microorganisms, such as streptococci and some strains of staphylococci. In addition, serum is lost from damaged capillaries, providing a rich nutritional medium for bacterial colonization. Topical antibiotic agents are used to control this colonization.

Effective antibacterial agents should control colonization so that specimens for wound biopsy reflect fewer than 10^{-4} microorganisms per gram of tissue. More than 10^{-4} microorganisms per gram of tissue make control of wound sepsis with topical antibiotics questionable. Consideration must then be given to parenteral therapy. Topical antibiotics selected must meet the following criteria: side effects are minimal; resistant strains will not develop with use; application must be easy and rapid; and use must be relatively economical. Currently the most commonly used topical antibiotics are silver sulfadiazine (Silvadene), bacitracin ointment, 0.5% silver nitrate solution, and mafenide acetate (Sulfamylon).

Silver sulfadiazine is a broad-spectrum antimicrobial agent that has bactericidal action against many gram-negative and gram-positive bacteria. It does not penetrate eschar as readily as mafenide acetate. Its application, however, is much more comfortable for the patient. A frequent side effect of silver sulfadiazine is leukopenia, which may develop 24 to 72 hours after application. Silver sulfadiazine is indicated for use with partial- and full-thickness wounds. Bacitracin ointment is a topical agent applied to superficial burns and facial burns; 0.5% silver nitrate is indicated for use with patients who are sensitive to sulfa drugs. It is applied two or three times daily in the form of saturated dressings. This agent does not penetrate eschar and may cause severe electrolyte imbalances. Silver nitrate possesses a broad-spectrum antimicrobial property. It ideally is used early in the postburn course before establishment of a heavy population of bacterial organisms. Mafenide acetate penetrates through burn eschar and is bacteriostatic against many gram-negative and gram-positive organisms. Its application generally is uncomfortable for the patient. It routinely is used for coverage of wounds involving anatomic areas that contain cartilage. Metabolic acidosis that results from use of mafenide acetate is not uncommon. The patient must be observed closely for hyperventilation (Table 46-3).

Factors Affecting Healing of the Burn Wound

For a short period after injury the burn wound is sterile. If topical antimicrobial therapy is not initiated in a timely fashion, bacteria will contaminate the surface of the wound within 48 hours. The sources of contamination are many and include the patient's endogenous flora found on the skin, the upper respiratory tract, and the gastrointestinal tract. Exogenous flora found in the patient care setting include bacteria carried by staff members and the environment. Patient-specific factors, as distinct from local wound factors,

TABLE 46-3 Topical Antimicrobial Agents

Agent	Advantages	Disadvantages	Implications
Silver sulfadiazine	Painless application Broad spectrum Easy application Rare sensitivities	May produce transient leukopenia Minimal penetration of eschar Some gram-negative species resistant	Monitor complete blood count Observe wounds for subeschar infection Monitor culture reports
Mafenide acetate	Broad spectrum Easy application Penetrates eschar	Painful application Promotes acid-base imbalance Frequent sensitivities	Administer adequate analgesia Monitor arterial blood gases Observe for hyperventilation Monitor for rashes
Nystatin	Painless application Specific efficacy Transparent	Specific efficacy No eschar penetration	Monitor cultures for growth of nonsensitive organisms Monitor wounds for subeschar infection
Bacitracin, Polysporin	Painless application Nonirritating Transparent May be used on nonburn wounds	No eschar penetration	Monitor wounds for subeschar infection
Silver nitrate (0.5% solution)	Painless application Broad spectrum Rare sensitivity	No eschar penetration Electrolyte imbalances Discolors the wound and environment Must be kept moist	Observe wounds for subeschar infections Monitor serum potassium and sodium Protect floor and bed Wear plastic apron to protect clothing
Povidone-iodine	Broad spectrum	Painful application Systemically absorbed Requires frequent reapplication Discolors wounds	Administer adequate analgesia Monitor thyroid function Protect environment
Gentamicin	Painless application Broad spectrum	Ototoxic; nephrotoxic Encourages the development of resistant organisms	Monitor serum levels Monitor renal function Monitor eighth cranial nerve function Monitor culture reports for sensitivities

From Trunkey DD, Lewis FR, *Current therapy of trauma,* Philadelphia 1991, BC Decker.

that predispose the patient to infection include age, diabetes, steroid therapy, extreme obesity, severe malnutrition, and infections in remote sites. Because both wound healing and clinical infection are inflammatory responses, it is essential to differentiate between normal wound inflammation in the presence of colonization of microorganisms and that of invading organisms. In diagnosing infection, the importance of microbiologic results must be evaluated in conjunction with clinical findings such as excessive erythema, edema, pain, and purulence. Generally, clinical findings in conjunction with burn wound biopsy results are the hallmark determinants of wound sepsis.

Autograft

An autograft is a skin graft harvested from a healthy, uninjured donor site and placed over a clean excised burn wound on the same individual to provide permanent coverage of the wound. Autografts are the only grafts that provide permanent wound coverage. Preferred sites for obtaining these grafts are the thighs, back, and abdomen. Grafts, however, can be harvested from almost anywhere on the body. Surgical excision is performed to mechanically remove necrotic tissue from the burn wound. As previously discussed, excision is performed tangentially or fascially. Sheets of the patient's epidermis and a partial layer of the dermis are harvested with use of a dermatome. These grafts are referred to as *split thickness* and can be applied to the wound bed as a sheet or in meshed form (Figure 46-7). The split-thickness skin graft can be meshed $1^1/_2$:1 to 4:1 in a mesher and then placed on the wounds.[6] This meshing maneuver prevents serum accumulation under the graft and permits coverage of a larger surface area than its original surface. Grafts that are placed on the face, neck, lower portions of the arms, and hands generally are sheet grafts. Grafts that are meshed can cover more area but may not produce the cosmetic appearance desired and therefore usually are placed on areas generally covered by clothing.

Autografting usually is performed in the operating room. The grafts can be secured with sutures, fibrin glue, or staples. Fine mesh gauze impregnated with an emollient is placed over the graft; covered with a heavy gauze dressing; and secured to the patient with or without a splint, depending on the anatomic area of the graft. Great care must be taken not to disturb the graft. The dressings are removed by trained nursing professionals, routinely on postoperative day 5 for assessment.[6] Secure graft adherence must occur in 48 to 72 hours. Autograft sites are assessed for adherence, presence of infection, and closure of interstices. Nursing management during the postoperative period includes proper positioning, splinting, and pain management.

Care of the donor site is equally important because it represents a wound similar to that of a partial-thickness injury. Donor sites can be covered with many different types of dressings. Fine mesh gauze can be applied and exposed to heat until dried. The gauze is then trimmed as it separates from the healing donor site over the next 10 days. This technique can cause discomfort, especially with motion or stretching. A thin polyurethane film dressing is permeable to oxygen and water vapor, therefore maintaining a moist surface over the donor site. The technique is less painful and is associated with faster healing.[6,19]

Burn Wound Closure

The primary goal of burn wound management is wound closing during the acute phase. Many methods are available to achieve this goal. Creative attempts have been initiated to establish a skin substitute that permanently closes the wound in a cosmetically acceptable fashion. Temporary skin substitutes may be used but to date do not provide permanent wound closure. These materials temporarily restore the protective barrier that the skin provides naturally. Skin substitutes can be used until the patient's own skin is available for harvesting.

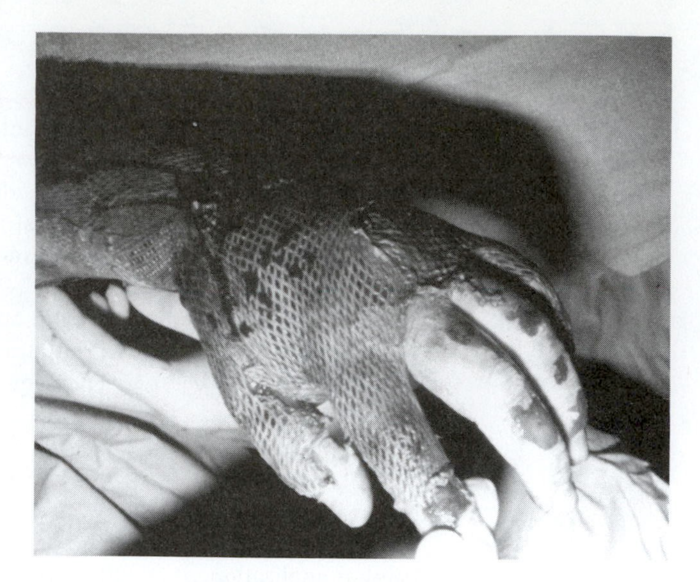

FIGURE 46-7. Meshed autograft.

Skin substitutes may be biologic or synthetic. Biologic substitutes include homograft (allograft) and heterograft (xenograft skin) techniques.

Biologic skin substitutes

Homograft (allograft). Homograft skin can be obtained from live or deceased donors (cadaver skin). The homograft is harvested from cadaver skin and with advances in cryopreservation can be frozen and stored in a tissue bank. It is possible to transmit disease through the application of a homograft; therefore tissue banks must adhere to strict guidelines. Before application, homograft skin is tested for a variety of transmittable diseases, including the human immunodeficiency virus (HIV) and hepatitis B surface antigens. Homograft skin can be used as biologic dressing for debridement applied at the bedside or a temporary wound coverage on excised burn wounds. The patient's wound readily accepts the homograft. Vascular ingrowth occurs, and the homograft seals the wound and protects it from bacterial invasion; however, it is rejected approximately 2 weeks after its application. Allografts must be handled and applied very carefully. They must be placed with the shiny surface down and must be wrinkle-free. They must neither overlap each other nor lap over infected areas or uninjured areas. The grafts can be dressed with a nonadherent agent that usually is not changed for 24 to 48 hours (Figure 46-8).

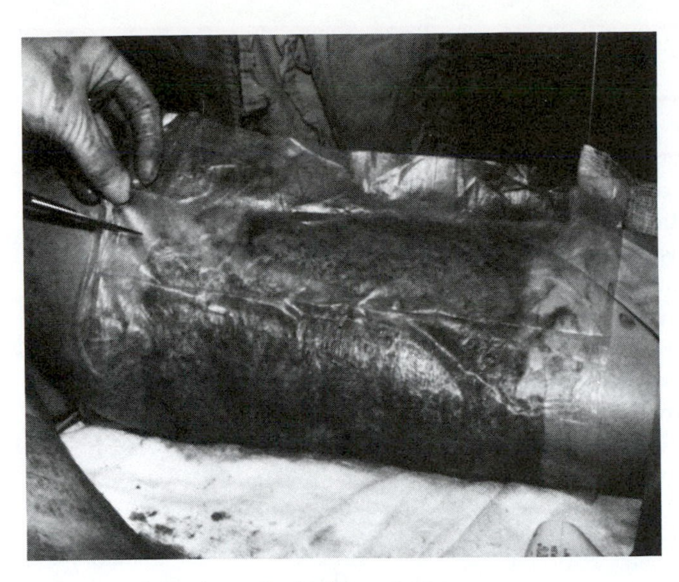

FIGURE 46-8. Biosynthetic skin substitute.

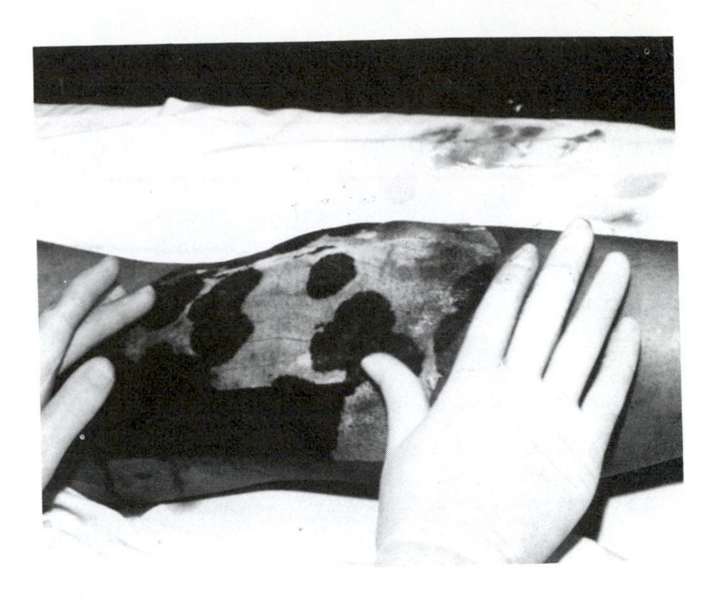

FIGURE 46-9. Xenograft (pigskin).

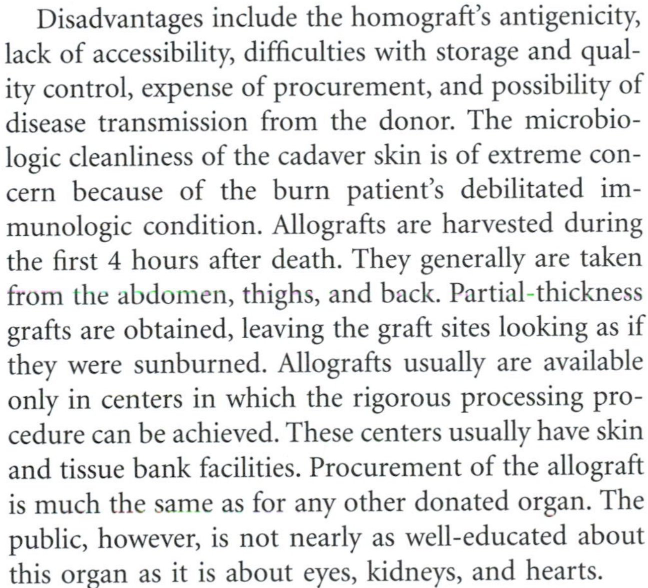

Disadvantages include the homograft's antigenicity, lack of accessibility, difficulties with storage and quality control, expense of procurement, and possibility of disease transmission from the donor. The microbiologic cleanliness of the cadaver skin is of extreme concern because of the burn patient's debilitated immunologic condition. Allografts are harvested during the first 4 hours after death. They generally are taken from the abdomen, thighs, and back. Partial-thickness grafts are obtained, leaving the graft sites looking as if they were sunburned. Allografts usually are available only in centers in which the rigorous processing procedure can be achieved. These centers usually have skin and tissue bank facilities. Procurement of the allograft is much the same as for any other donated organ. The public, however, is not nearly as well-educated about this organ as it is about eyes, kidneys, and hearts.

Heterograft (xenograft). The xenograft, or heterograft, is a graft transferred between two different species to provide temporary wound coverage. The most common and widely accepted xenograft is pigskin (porcine). Pigskin is available in frozen and shelf forms, with each type having a much longer storage life than the allograft. Depending on how the pigskin was prepared, it can have a shelf life of 1 month to 1 year. The pigskin is packaged in a variety of ways and in various sizes. It can be treated with silver sulfadiazine and can be meshed or nonmeshed. Pigskin can be used for temporary coverage of full- and partial-thickness wounds, burn wounds, and donor sites. It meets many of the ideal skin substitute properties mentioned previously. It has two disadvantages, however; it is antigenic, and it has the potential for digestion by the wound collagenase, possibly leading to infection.

Pigskin is applied in the same manner as allograft (Figure 46-9). If the pigskin is frozen, it is thawed in a warm saline-solution bath. If it has been treated with silver sulfadiazine, it is thawed in water. The pigskin is placed on the wound with the dermal side down (the dermal side faces the center of the roll) and may be distinguished by its tendency to curl toward the dermal surface when held up at one end. Shelf-stored pigskin may be applied with either side to the wound. Once the pigskin is in place, it may be dressed with antibacterial-impregnated dressings or other forms of dressings. Pigskin usually is removed in 3 to 4 days. If sloughing or purulent drainage occurs, the xenograft is removed (Table 46-4).

Synthetic skin. The lack of available donor sites for major burn injury often delays wound closure. In an effort to minimize infection and to promote healing, many attempts have been made to develop skin substitutes that will seal the wound in a cosmetically acceptable fashion. This goal has yet to be achieved. A technique that involves the growth and subsequent graft placement of cultured epithelial autografts has become an important adjunct to treatment of burn wounds. Biopsy specimens obtained from areas of unburned skin are minced and trypsin crystallized to reduce the epithelial layers to single cells. This mixture of single cells is placed in a flask that contains growth medium. During the primary culture, which takes from 8 to 10 days, the surface area will expand to 50 to 70 times the size of the initial biopsy specimens. The cells are again separated into single cells and

TABLE 46-4 Types of Grafts

Graft	Usage	Advantages	Disadvantages
Autograft	Provides permanent coverage of burn wounds Used in sheets or meshed form	Permanent coverage Nonantigenic Least expensive Meshing allows a small amount of tissue to cover a large area	Lack of available donor sites, which may delay wound coverage Donor sites are painful partial-thickness wounds Must be done in surgical suite
Homograft (allograft)	Temporary wound coverage	Can be placed at bedside or in operating room Allows for vascularization over deep wound Provides better control over bacterial growth than xenograft	Possibility of disease transmission Antigenic; body rejects in approximately 2 weeks Not readily available to all burn centers Expensive Requires rigorous quality controls
Heterograph (xenograft)	Temporary wound coverage	Longer shelf life than allograft Can be meshed or nonmeshed Comes in a variety of sizes	Antigenic; body rejects in 3 to 4 days Potential for digestion by wound collagenase, thus leading to increased chance of infection

replated in culture medium. Between days 10 and 12, those cells become confluent and are approximately three to eight cell layers thick in the flask. These confluent sheets of cultured epithelial cells are attached to a gauze backing and placed on the wound.[6]

The cultured epidermal sheets appear to have limited effectiveness. The take of these tissues decreased by approximately two thirds by 28 days and appears to be inversely proportional to the extent of the burn.[6]

Synthetic skin dressings. The use of synthetic skin substitutes has gained popularity throughout the United States during the past 5 to 10 years. Synthetic skin dressings include a deluge of products currently available on the market, and they are composed of a variety of materials. These products can be characterized as nonsynthetic gauze (scarlet red, Xeroform), synthetic and semisynthetic polymers (Op-Site, Biobrane), and synthetic and semisynthetic hydrocolloid polymers (DuoDerm).

Each dressing has specific indications for use. Skin barrier substitutes must possess several properties to accomplish their desired effect as a temporary wound covering to protect the granulating tissue and/or to preserve a clean, viable wound surface for future autografting (Box 46-2). The most important property of these materials is adherence so that the skin substitute can simulate the function of the skin. Adherence must be uniform to prevent fluid accumulation beneath the surface of the substitute, which could lead to bacterial proliferation. For application of skin substitutes, the wound must be clean and ideally have a bacterial count of less than 10^5 organisms per gram of tissue. The burn wound must be free from eschar, and hemostasis must be present. Both eschar and blood provide an excellent medium for bacterial proliferation, and the presence of blood may interfere with adherence. The surface is cleaned and rinsed with saline solution, and the skin substitutes must be applied according to established procedures by means of sterile techniques.[6]

Scarlet red and Xeroform. Scarlet red, which is a fine mesh gauze impregnated with a blend of lanolin, olive oil, and petroleum, is used primarily over the donor sites. It possesses many of the ideal skin substitute properties; however, it has several serious disadvantages. It causes red stains on clothing and linen and can cause discomfort related to the way the material dries, hardens, stretches, and pulls underlying skin.

BOX 46-2 Ideal Properties of Skin Substitutes

- Adherence
- Minimal discomfort or pain
- Easy application and removal
- Intact bacterial barrier
- Shelf storage capability
- Inexpensive in relation to alternatives
- Nonantigenic
- Similar to normal skin in transport of water vapor
- Nontoxic
- Elastic
- Hemostatic
- Decreased protein and electrolyte loss
- Enhanced natural healing processes

Xeroform is a fine mesh gauze that contains 3% bismuth tribromphenate in a petrolatum blend. It, too, generally is used on donor sites. Xeroform has no major disadvantages and possesses many of the ideal skin substitute properties. Application is easy, and it does not have the disadvantages of scarlet red. As the donor site heals, the edges of the scarlet red and Xeroform loosen and may be trimmed. These dressings must not be removed forcibly, because this would interfere with the reepithelialization process.

The disadvantages of using gauze on burn sites include delayed healing times and increased pain.

Biosynthetic dressing. Biobrane is a semipermeable biosynthetic temporary wound dressing. It is composed of nylon and Silastic membrane combined with a collagen derivative. It also can be used on several types of wounds, including partial- and full-thickness burns and wounds, granulating wounds, donor sites, and over split-thickness grafts.

Biobrane has many of the properties of an ideal skin substitute. It has two advantages that other skin substitutes do not share. Biosynthetic skin has elasticity in all directions and conforms well to surfaces that are difficult to dress, such as breast, joints, and axilla. Also, because of its porosity, it allows the passage of some topical antibiotics, such as silver sulfadiazine, to penetrate its membrane, reducing the bacterial count of the burn wound. Biosynthetic skin may be applied after daily cleaning at the bedside or in the operating room. It is applied with the dull or nylon mesh side facing the wound. It can be held in place with sutures, staples, steri-strips, or stent. If fluid accumulates under the biosynthetic skin, it may be slit and the fluid expressed. If a large amount of fluid accumulates, the biosynthetic skin is removed and replaced. Biosynthetic skin initially adheres to the wound fibrin, which binds to the collagen and nylon backing of the material. Later the cells migrate into the nylon mesh and further bind to the wound.

Polyurethane film. Polyurethane film is a semiocclusive dressing that is impermeable to bacteria and liquid. Polyurethane film is used primarily in the coverage of donor sites, but some practitioners report using it over some partial-thickness burn wounds. Polyurethane film dressings possess many of the properties of an ideal skin substitute. However, fluid can collect under the dressing in large quantities. When fluid collects, it often leaks and decreases the adherence of the dressing. The fluid can be removed with a needle and syringe; however, the needle puncture must be patched with a small piece of polyurethane film. The wound exudate trapped under the dressing may provide a physiologic milieu that enhances healing.

Polyurethane film has an adhesive side that is designed to adhere to normal skin adjacent to the wound. It generally takes two persons to apply large pieces of polyurethane film because of its tendency to wrinkle and stick to itself. The dressing may be further secured with an elastic wrap or netting material.

Hydrocolloid dressings. DuoDerm is an oxygen-impermeable, occlusive hydrocolloid dressing. It is composed of an outer layer of polyurethane foam and an inner layer of hydrocolloid polymer complex. Hydrocolloid dressings are indicated for use on donor sites and partial-thickness wounds. The dressing does not adhere to the wound bed; therefore it does not damage new epithelium and decreases pain. Historically, bacterial proliferation has been feared with the use of occlusive dressings. To date clinical investigations have revealed colonization but not clinical infection.

Dressings are applied to donor sites in the operating room after cleansing of partial-thickness wounds at the bedside. The adhesive side is applied to the wound bed. Disadvantages of using hydrocolloid dressings include large amounts of exudate, odor, and an inability to visualize the wound bed. Advantages include rapid healing times and decreased pain, and because the dressing is self-adhesive, staples are not required (Table 46-5).

Closed burn wound care. Two to six weeks after wound closure, a problem with the formation of tiny water blisters frequently occurs. These blisters usually open and heal without incident in 3 to 5 days. These areas must be kept clean with mild soap and covered with a bland ointment. For 6 to 8 weeks, a mild nonalcohol-based skin cream is applied every 4 hours to

TABLE 46-5 Synthetic Skin Dressings

Dressing	Usage	Advantages	Disadvantages
Cultured epithelial autograft	Provides skin when limited skin available	Can expand available skin	Takes approximately 2 weeks to grow Very expensive Limited take
Nonsynthetic gauze (scarlet red, Xeroform)	Donor sites	Easy application Inexpensive Scarlet red can help provide hemostasis	Stains clothing and linens (scarlet red) Painful during drying Delayed healing times Inability to visualize wound Damage to epithelium if pulled off early
Synthetic and semisynthetic polymers (Biosynthetic, polyurethane film, hydrocolloid polymers, hydrogel sheeting, calcium alginate)	Biosynthetic Temporary wound dressing on variety of wounds (partial- and full-thickness burns, granulating wounds, donor sites, and over split-thickness skin grafts) Polyurethane film Donor site Hydrocolloid polymers Donor sites and partial-thickness wounds Hydrogel sheeting Donor sites and partial-thickness wounds Calcium alginate Donor sites and partial-thickness wounds	Biosynthethic Elasticity in all directions Conforms to difficult surfaces Allows some topical antibiotic penetration Applied at bedside or in operating room Less painful Polyurethane film Impermeable to fluid and bacteria Provides moist wound healing Less painful Able to visualize wound Easier removal of fluid accumulated under dressing Hydrocolloid polymers and hydrogel sheeting No damage to new epithelium Decreased pain Can be placed at bedside or in operating room Faster healing tissue Calcium alginate Assists in achieving hemostasis	Biosynthetic Expensive Must be split to allow for fluid drainage Inability to visualize wound Polyurethane film Fluid collection can cause decreased adherence of dressing Must have normal skin adjacent to wound for dressing adherence Difficult to apply in large pieces Must have hemostasis before application Hydrocolloid polymers, hydrogel sheeting, and calcium alginate Possibility of bacterial proliferation Inability to visualize wound Large amount of exudate and odor (hydrocolloid polymer)

these areas to lubricate the skin until natural lubrication occurs. Pruritus is common in the maturing burn wound. Patients can be relieved of this discomfort by the administration of an antipruritic agent, such as diphenhydramine hydrochloride or hydroxyzine, and by the application of moisturizing creams.

Another concern in burn wound healing is the prevention or reduction of hypertrophic scarring. Its prevention or reduction depends on the timely application of uniform pressure. Hypertrophic scarring can be controlled with the use of tubular support bandages applied within 5 to 7 days after the graft. Bandages are available in a variety of sizes and have the advantage of applying pressure to selected body areas while allowing the remaining burned area to heal sufficiently. They are also readily available for immediate use during the wait for the commercial manufacture of the customized elastic pressure garment for long-term use, which can take up to 3 or 4 weeks.

Tubular support bandages apply tension in the medium range of 10 to 20 mm Hg. Tensions lower than this do not exert adequate pressure to control scarring, and higher tensions tend to cause edema in the distal parts of the extremities and may be too abra-

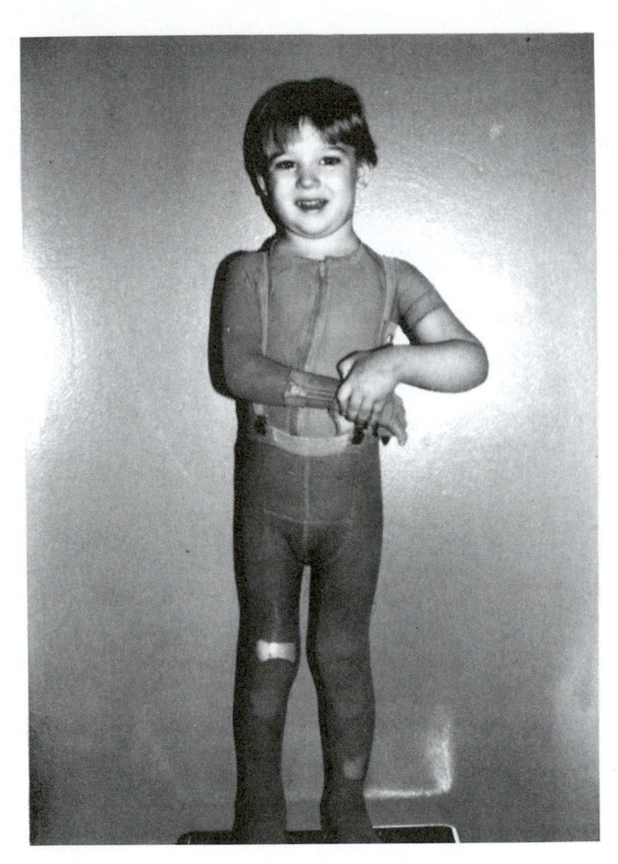

FIGURE 46-10. Custom-made elastic pressure garment.

sive to newly grafted skin. Tension can be elevated if needed by placing silicone foam under the tubular support bandages over areas such as the axilla and knees.

Custom-made elastic pressure garments generally are worn for 6 months to 1 year after grafting. It is important to assess the patient for pressure points during this time as weight is gained and as children grow (Figure 46-10). It also is necessary to assess the garment for elasticity; with many washings over time, this property may be decreased.

Acute Pain

Pain is an individualized and subjective phenomenon. It comprises both physiologic and psychologic aspects. Pain after burn injury is significant. Physiologic changes associated with pain include the damage or exposure of the nerve endings within a partial-thickness burn and donor sites, range of motion of the affected limbs, tightening scar tissue, and/or extensive and frequent treatments for debridement. Other pain-producing interventions include arterial punctures; chest physical therapy; injections; and use of nasogastric tubes, suction, and pressure garments. Loss of control, forced dependence, loneliness, and separation from home and family can all contribute to anxiety, which heightens the patient's perception of the pain. The patient's fears abound in thoughts of disfigurement and loss of love, function, and job. The psychologic experience or subjective component may be related to past experiences, anxiety, and altered coping mechanisms. Attention to the psychologic component of the patient's pain may lead to very useful strategies in decreasing perceived pain. If possible, how the patient has responded in the past to pain and which interventions, if any, were successful in relieving pain must be determined.

Patients with partial-thickness burns experience a great deal of discomfort. The slightest air current to the surface of the burn may stimulate pain. Covering wounds with topical agents, dressings, and linen significantly decreases the pain. The nerve endings that have been completely destroyed by full-thickness burns are initially insensate until they regenerate. It is a common misconception that these wounds are painless. Patients may experience deep somatic pain from ischemia or inflammation. It is unlikely that all wounds will be full thickness. Wound edges, as they transition to less severely burned areas, will be hypersensitive.[11,15]

Pain continues even after healing, with some patients describing the itching, tingling, and parasthesias as equally discomforting as the initial injury. Parasthesias can last 1 year or more after injury. It may be a false assumption to believe burn pain decreases over time.[11]

The burn patient confronts pain on a daily basis for many weeks. Pharmacotherapy is the mainstay for analgesia in burn patients. Inadequate pain management is a problem in many burn units because of the fear of opioid side effects and opioid addiction and the lack of pain evaluation and/or lack of treatment protocols. Initially after burn injury, narcotics are administered intravenously in small doses and titrated to effect. The constant background pain may be addressed with the use of a patient-controlled analgesia device. Once hemodynamic stability has occurred and gastrointestinal function has returned, oral narcotics can be useful. Additional premedication and analgesics will be necessary during therapeutic procedures. The nurse must be flexible with dosing and assess the effectiveness by using a numerical or visual analog scale.

Nonpharmacologic techniques, such as imagery, hypnosis, distraction, and methods adapted from some of the popular childbirth techniques, can be effective in reducing anxiety and the pain experience. Giving the patient some management control also can reduce the anxiety and the pain experience. The perception of pain often is increased in the patient who is anxious and lacks control of the situation.[20]

Treatment strategies are individualized. Failure to adequately treat pain can increase burn hypermetabolism, result in loss of confidence between the burn team and patient, and lead to the development of psychiatric disorders. Assess and discuss on a regular basis the patient's psychologic status. Avoid using psychotropics for analgesia and narcotics for anxiety and depression.[11]

Altered Nutrition: Less Than Body Requirements

The basic metabolic rate of a burn patient may be elevated 40% to 100% above the normal rate, depending on the amount of BSA involved. The metabolic rate is influenced by the amount of protein and albumin lost through the wounds, the catabolic response associated with stress and other associated injuries, fluid loss, fever, infection, immobility, gender, and the height and weight of the patient before the injury.[16] The goal in nutritional management of the burn patient is to provide adequate calories to prevent starvation and to enhance wound healing. To achieve this goal, nutritional support is imperative, and the reduction of energy demand also is vital. Every effort should be made to reduce the release of catecholamines, which increase metabolic rate. Release of catecholamine stores is stimulated by pain, fear, anxiety, and cold. Appropriate interventions for each of these stimuli must be performed.

The use of enteral and oral routes is preferred in the management of burn patients. Caloric requirements are calculated on the basis of the size of the burn; the age, height, and weight of the patient; and the stress factors. Protein and caloric requirements of each patient are highly individualized and are assessed daily. The daily protein requirement for the burn patient is elevated in light of a negative nitrogen balance. The daily protein requirement may increase to two to four times the normal 0.8 g/kg of body weight. Carbohydrates and fat are used for energy and to spare proteins required for wound healing. Daily caloric intake can be 2 to 20 times higher than normal. Vitamins and minerals generally are given in doses higher than normal. Serum iron, zinc, calcium, phosphate, and potassium values are monitored and supplements given as indicated.[16]

REHABILITATION PHASE

The rehabilitation phase is one of recuperation and healing, both physically and emotionally. The patient is not acutely ill but may or may not be ready for discharge. This phase can last several years. The patient may require extensive reconstructive surgery. Psychologically, the patient focuses on attaining specific personal goals related to achieving as much preburn function as possible.[14] Minor and major accomplishments must be praised. This phase is characterized by scar management techniques and by physical and occupational therapy. The burn team and the patient prepare for the transition to the outside world. The use of group therapy is a valuable tool used at many burn centers. Patients, family members, and health care providers express ideas and feelings. Many times burn patients establish priorities and make realistic decisions about their lives. Staff intervention during this phase is primarily one of support.

Impaired Physical Mobility

Tremendous advances have been made during the past 10 to 15 years in the physical care of the burn patient. The survival rate of patients with full-thickness burns greater than 40% of TBSA has increased significantly. Currently, survival of patients with burns greater than 90% of TBSA is not impossible. As patients with larger and deeper burns survive, the challenge to maintain their optimal mobility and cosmetic appearance has been met with increased success. It is imperative that rehabilitation needs are addressed early in burn care. Nursing prescriptions for range-of-motion exercises, positioning, splinting, ambulation, and activities of daily living are initiated within the first 48 hours of hospitalization.

Contracture may develop after a burn injury because of a variety of factors: the extent, depth, location, and configuration of the burn; the position of comfort the patient most frequently assumes; the relative underlying muscle strength; and the patient's motivation and compliance. Positioning the affected body parts in *antideformity positions* is vital. Frequent change of position also is important and may need to be performed as frequently as every hour. Burn patients are at greater risk for the development of pressure sores than the general hospital population, as well as the possible conversion of their partial-thickness burns to full-thickness burns.

Splints can be used to prevent and/or correct contracture or to immobilize joints after grafting (Figure 46-11). If splints are used, they must be checked daily for proper fit and effectiveness. Splints that are used to immobilize body parts after grafting must be left on at all times except to assess the graft site for pressure points every shift. Splints to correct severe contracture may be off for 2 hours per shift to allow burn

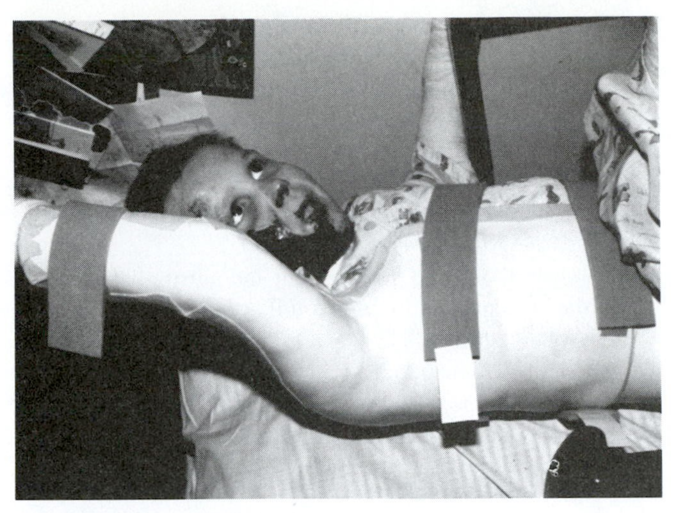

FIGURE 46-11. Splinting in the antideformity position.

BOX 46-3 NURSING DIAGNOSIS AND MANAGEMENT

BURN INJURY

- Impaired Gas Exchange related to ventilation/perfusion mismatching, p. 725
- Ineffective Airway Clearance related to excessive secretions or abnormal viscosity of mucus, p. 722
- Fluid Volume Deficit related to relative loss, p. 915
- Risk for Infection risk factors: invasive lines, immunodeficiencies, p. 598
- Acute confusion related to sensory overload, sensory deprivation, sleep-pattern disturbance, p. 90
- Body Image Disturbance related to actual change in body structure, function, or appearance, p. 87
- Powerlessness related to physical deterioration despite compliance, p. 89

care and range-of-motion exercises. Mild contracture may be in splints for 4 hours and out of splints for 4 hours to promote exercise and mobility.

Active exercise is encouraged and is preferred, although active-assisted or gentle-passive exercises also may be an important part of the rehabilitation program. Active exercise maintains muscle mass, aids in restoring protein structures within the muscle tissue, aids in venous and lymphatic return, and reduces the risk of pulmonary embolus and deep vein thrombosis. Patient tolerance must be carefully evaluated. The number of repetitions will be proportional to the degree of anticipated contracture and the patient's tolerance. Anticipation of the patient's pain also must be carefully considered. Before range-of-motion exercises and activities of daily living are performed, the need for pain medication must be assessed.[7] Nursing diagnoses and management for the burn patient is summarized in Box 46-3.

Outpatient Burn Care

Outpatient burn care must be considered for minor burns. It is cost-effective and removes the potential for a wound infection from endemic, drug-resistant microorganisms within the hospital environment. The hospital environment also changes many of the self-care routines, such as diet, family contact, hygiene, and coping mechanisms. Patients considered for outpatient burn care, however, must be screened carefully. Nursing evaluation of the patient or family, or both, includes consideration of motivation, willingness to participate in care, ability to understand and perform the necessary procedures, potential aversions to wound care or dressing changes, and reliability of transportation. Medical considerations include hemodynamic stabilization, nutritional status, fluid and electrolyte balance, adequate pain control, and ruling out any complications.[21]

In general, small burns must be washed daily with a mild soap and water, and a bland ointment and/or synthetic antimicrobial agent can be applied and held in place with dressings. Initially these wounds must be monitored daily and then on a weekly basis until the wound begins to reepithelialize. Generally, if epithelialization of these wounds has not occurred in 2 to 3 weeks, use of primary excision and grafting must be considered.

To check for evidence of scarring, partial-thickness injuries must be monitored until the epithelialization has occurred. If scarring occurs, compression dressings must be fitted and worn until the wound becomes quiescent, which requires 12 to 18 months.

STRESSORS OF BURN NURSING

Burn units are fascinating environments in which to work. They offer the fast-paced, high-technology atmosphere of any critical care setting; the complexity of advanced nursing management; and the dynamics of an interdisciplinary, collaborative model of practice. All these elements combined, however, contribute to a potentially stressful work environment for the nurse. The physical environment can be a difficult one in which to work for a variety of reasons. The amount of equipment necessary to maintain the patient can be overwhelming and can limit the work space dramatically. The temperature of the room generally is kept at approximately 85°F and can get much warmer, depending on the amount of equipment in the room. Odors vary and can be very unpleasant. Noise levels within a unit also are distressing. These variables exact a physical toll on nursing staff members. The decision to specialize in burn nursing is a meaningful one, an important one; this decision, however, also must be an informed one. Self-care and care of other nurses are just as important issues as the care of the patient and his or her significant other.

In addition, there are patient care complexities unique to burn nursing. The daily hydrotherapy treatments and dressing changes are extremely stressful for both the nurse and the patient. The nursing management of patients' pain is a complex issue in burn care and is one that contributes significantly to the stress level of nurses who specialize in burn injuries. The psychodynamics associated with the patient's burn injury experience are just that - *dynamic* - and require constant, high-level nursing assessment and intervention.

REFERENCES

1. Nebraska Burn Institute: *Advanced burn life support (ABLS) course* (first rev), Lincoln, 1990, The Institute.
2. Saffle JR, Davis B, Williams P: Recent outcomes in the treatment of burn injury in the United States: a report from the American Burn Association patient registry, *J Burn Care Rehabil* 16:219, 1995.
3. Demling RH: The advantage of the burn team approach, *J Burn Care Rehabil* 16:569, 1995.
4. Duncan D, Driscall D: Burn wound management, *Crit Care Clinics North Am* 3(2):199, 1991.
5. Burgess M: Initial management of a patient with extensive burn injury, *Crit Care Clinics North Am* 3(2):165, 1991.
6. Pruitt BA: Burn wound. In Cameron JL, editor: *Current surgical therapy,* ed 5, St Louis, 1995, Mosby.
7. Cadier MA, Shakespeare PG: Burns in octogenarians, *Burns* 21:200, 1995.
8. Carleton S: Cardiac problems associated with electrical injury, *Cardiol Clin* 13:263, 1995.
9. Shaw A and others: Early management of large burns, *Br J Hos Med* 53(6):247, 1995.
10. Goodwin CW: Fluid management and nutritional support of the burn patient. In Cameron JL, editor: *Current surgical therapy,* ed 5, St Louis, 1995, Mosby.
11. Laterjet J, Choinere M: Pain in burn patients, *Burns* 21:344, 1995.
12. Darling GE and others: Pulmonary complications in inhalation injuries with associated cutaneous burn, *J Trauma* 40:83, 1996.
13. Masanes MJ and others: Fiberoptic bronchoscopy for the early diagnosis of subglottal inhalation injury: comparative value in the assessment of prognosis, *J Trauma* 36:59, 1994.
14. Partridge J, Robinson E: Psychological and social aspects of burns, *Burns* 21:453, 1995.
15. Arturson G: Pathophysiology of the burn wound macological treatment, *Burns* 22:255, 1996.
16. Deitch E: Nutritional support of the burn patient, *Crit Care Clin* 11:735, 1995.
17. Wurtz R and others: Nosocomial infections in a burn intensive care unit, *Burns* 21:181, 1995.
18. Carleton S: Cardiac problems associated with burns, *Cardiol Clin* 13:257, 1995.
19. Hansbrough W: Nursing care of donor site wounds, *J Burn Care Rehabil* 16:337, 1995.
20. Patterson DR: Non-opioid based approaches to burn pain, *J Burn Care Rehabil* 116:372, 1995.
21. Bolinger B: Burn care in the home, *J Wound, Ostomy, Continence Nurs* 22(3):122, 1995.

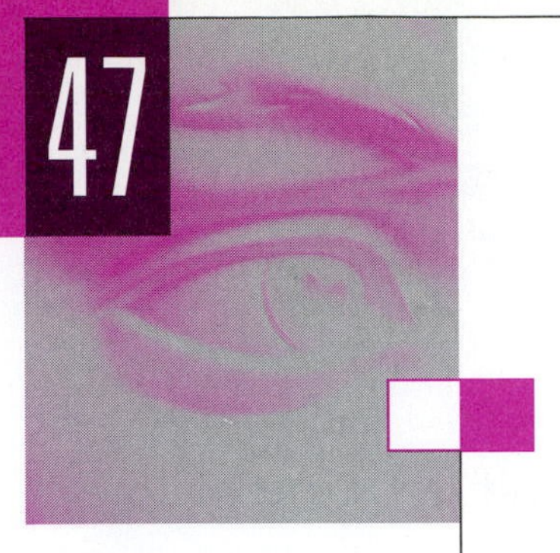

47 Transplantation

MAJOR ADVANCES IN transplantation have been achieved since the first cadaver organ transplants in the 1960s. Today transplantation has become an accepted form of therapy for end-stage organ failure. The field of transplantation is highly specialized and requires expert teams of surgeons, immunologists, and medical and nurse specialists to achieve successful outcomes.

Many problems are yet to be solved in the field of transplantation. Organs are a scarce commodity, and a lack of available organs restricts the availability of transplantation for many individuals. Safe and efficacious control of the immune system remains elusive. Rejection and infection as a result of immunosuppression persist as the major causes of death in recipients. Chronic rejection is still not well-understood. This type of rejection results in eventual graft failure and limits long-term survival in many types of organ recipients.

This chapter overviews the specialized areas of solid organ transplantation, the immune system, and current therapies to prevent rejection.

IMMUNOLOGY OF TRANSPLANT REJECTION

Organ transplantation has become a commonly practiced procedure for end-stage cardiac, pulmonary, hepatic, renal, and pancreatic disease. Major advances have been made in organ procurement and preservation, surgical techniques, and identifying and treating rejection. The ultimate long-term success of any organ transplant depends on the immune system's tolerance of the transplanted graft. Virtually every body cell carries distinctive molecules that enable the immune system to distinguish self from nonself. When nonself is recognized, a normally functioning immune system is designed to eliminate the foreign invader. Tolerance of the transplanted organ can be achieved only by suppressing or regulating this normal immune response to the foreign organ.

To understand the principles of immunosuppressive therapy, it is important to have some understanding of the cells of the immune system, the immune response, and the process of organ rejection.

Immune Mechanism

Whenever the body is confronted with any substance that is nonself, a primary immune response is elicited. There are three phases to each *primary* immune response: (1) recognition of the substance as nonself, (2) proliferation of immunocompetent cells, and (3) the effector phase or action against the foreign substance. During this primary response, immunologic memory is established and any subsequent encounter with the same substance will provide a more rapid and intense immune response. Subsequent encounters are termed *secondary immune responses.*

An antigen is a substance that is capable of eliciting an immune response. Each cell has antigens on its surface that are genetically predetermined by a series of linked genes known as the *major histocompatibility complex* (MHC). If tissue from one person is transplanted into a genetically different person, the antigens on the transplanted tissue cells are immediately recognized as nonself and rejection occurs. MHC determines the antigens to which the immune system should respond. The human MHC is called *human leukocyte antigen* (HLA) because these markers were first discovered on lymphocytes. The HLA gene complex is located on chromosome number 6. Each chromosome contains four loci: HLA-A, -B, -C, and -D. More than 150 antigens have been recognized in the

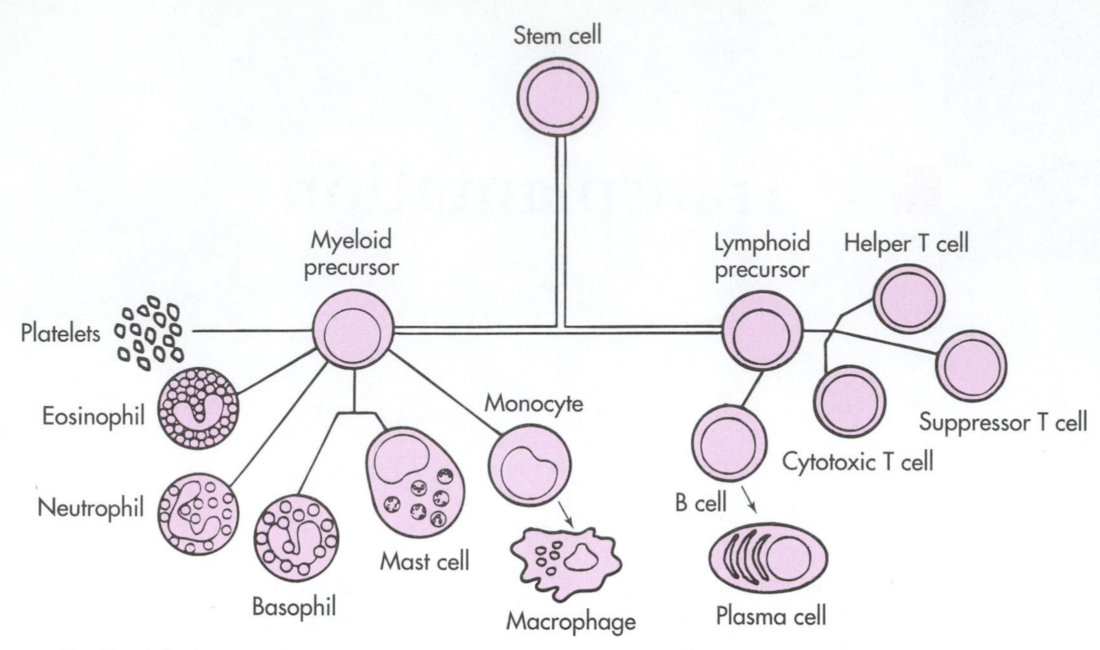

FIGURE 47-1. All cells of the immune system originate from stem cells in the bone marrow. (From Schindler LW: *Understanding the immune system,* NIH Publ No 90-529, Bethesda, MD, 1990, US Department of Health and Human Services.)

HLA system: 23 on the A locus, 52 on the B locus, 11 on the C locus, and 61 on the D locus.[1] Because a potential for millions of different arrangements of these antigens exists, the chances of finding a donor organ with the same histocompatibility genes as a recipient are virtually impossible unless donor and recipient are identical twins.

HLA antigens are divided into three classes of antigens. Class I antigens are present on almost all body cells and are thus the markers of self. The Class II antigens are present on B lymphocytes, macrophages, and other cells responsible for presenting foreign antigen to the immune system and inducing the immune response. Class III antigens include some red blood cell antigens and complement.

Cells of the Immune System

The immune system houses a vast number of cells responsible for general defense and very specific immune responses. Only a few cells of each specificity are stored. When a specific antigen appears, those few cells are stimulated to multiply and mount a response to the foreign antigen. Immune cells are originally produced in the bone marrow as stem cells. Their descendants become either lymphocytes or phagocytes (Figure 47-1).

There are two major classes of lymphocytes: B cells and T cells. B cells remain in the bone marrow to complete their maturation. The T cells migrate to the thymus gland where they mature. In the thymus, T cells acquire the ability to distinguish self from nonself. Once mature, some B and T cells are housed in the lymph nodes, whereas others circulate in the blood and lymph system.

Humoral immunity is mediated by B cells. They are responsible for the production of antibody or immunoglobulin. When a B cell encounters an antigen to which it is specifically coded to respond, the B cell enlarges, divides, and differentiates into a plasma cell. It is the plasma cell that actually produces and secretes antigen-specific antibody (Figure 47-2). Once exposed to an antigen, the immune system retains a memory of that antigen. Subsequent exposure stimulates the B cell memory cells, resulting in a rapid mobilization of antibody-secreting cells. Antibodies work in several ways, but their primary purpose is to mark an antigen for destruction by the immune system. Other antibodies are capable of neutralizing toxins produced by bacteria or can trigger the release of serum proteins known as *complement.*

Cell-mediated immunity is determined by T cells that are specifically sensitized. Approximately 65% to 80% of all lymphocytes are T cells, of which there are three basic types.

Cytotoxic T cells are cells capable of killing invading cells. Their primary role is to rid the body of cells

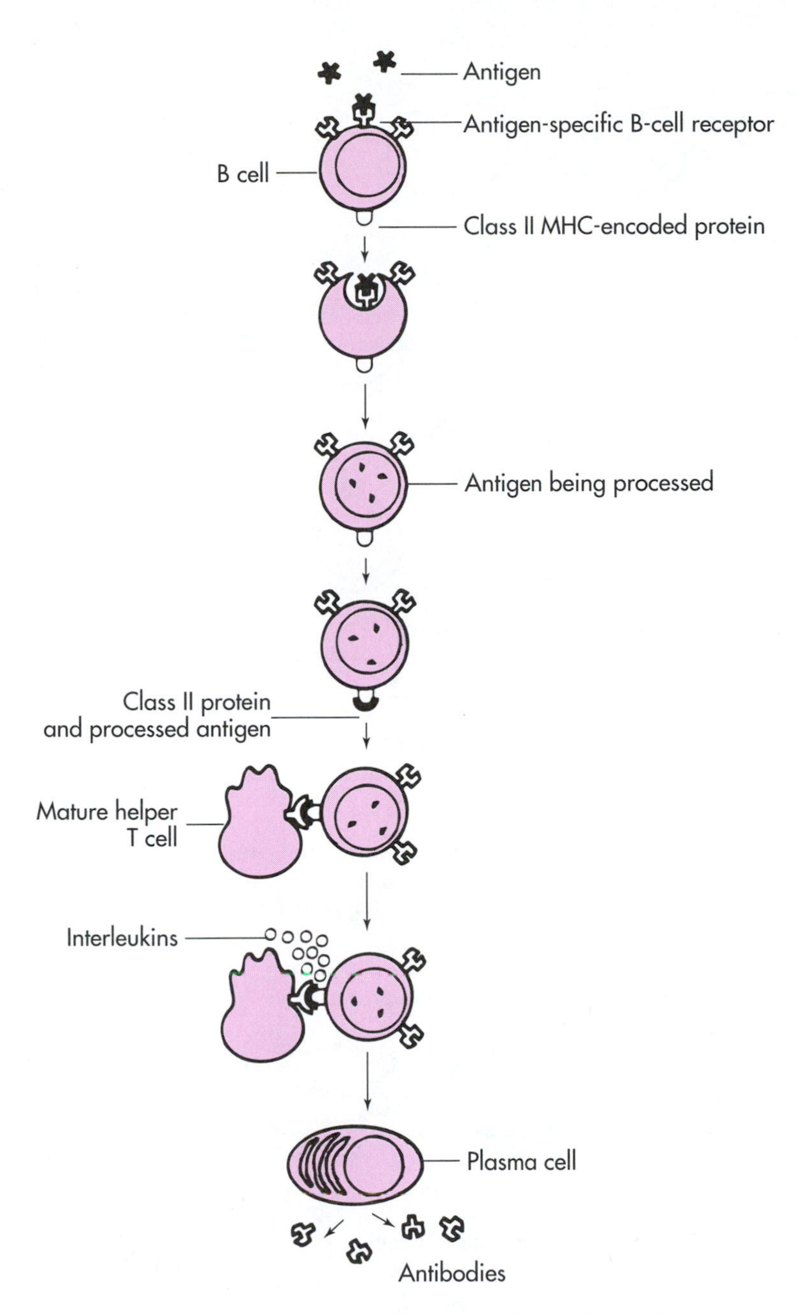

FIGURE 47-2. Foreign antigen is processed by the B cell and displayed with its MHC Class II antigen (protein), which attracts helper T cells. The release of interleukins by the helper T cell stimulates differentiation of the B cell into a plasma cell, which begins to produce antibody. (From Schindler LW: *Understanding the immune system,* NIH Publ No 90-629, Bethesda, MD, 1990, US Department of Health and Human Services.)

that have become infected; transformed by cancer; or are nonself, as in the case of transplanted tissue. They also are called *T8* or *CD8 lymphocytes,* referring to a marker that distinguishes cytotoxic T cells from other T cells. Cytotoxic T cells are activated by macrophages that present the foreign antigen to immature cytotoxic T cells. With the assistance of the helper T cell and its release of chemical mediators, the cytotoxic T cell matures and kills foreign cells that carry that specific antigen (Figure 47-3).

Helper T cells up-regulate the immune response by stimulating B cells to differentiate into plasma cells and begin antibody production, by activating cytotoxic T cells, and by stimulating natural killer cells and macrophages. Helper T cells are identified by their T4 or CD4 marker. Figure 47-4 illustrates the process

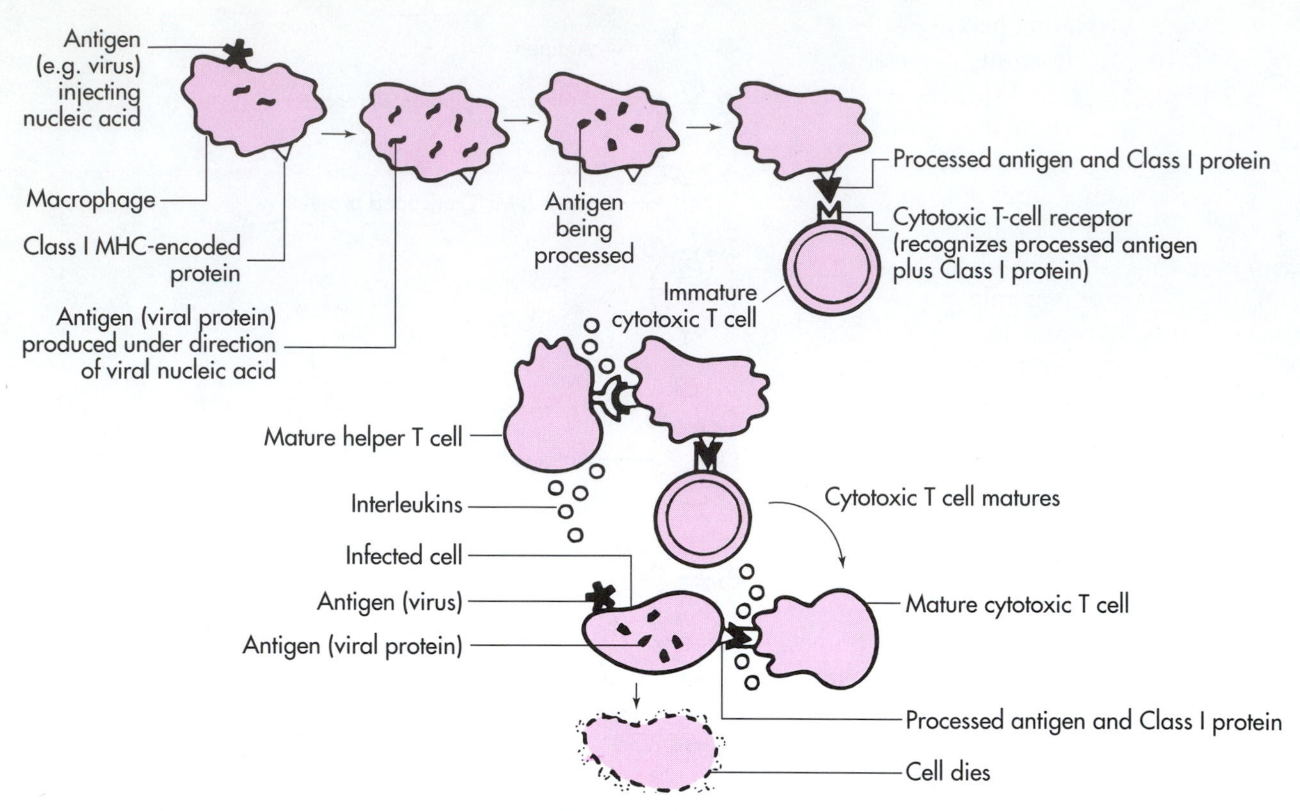

FIGURE 47-3. The macrophage presents MCH Class I antigen (protein) and processed antigen from the foreign organism to the cytotoxic and helper T cell. Aided by the helper T cell, the cytotoxic T cell matures and kills the foreign cell. (From Schindler LW: *Understanding the immune system,* NIH Publ No 90-629, Bethesda, MD, 1990, US Department of Health and Human Services.)

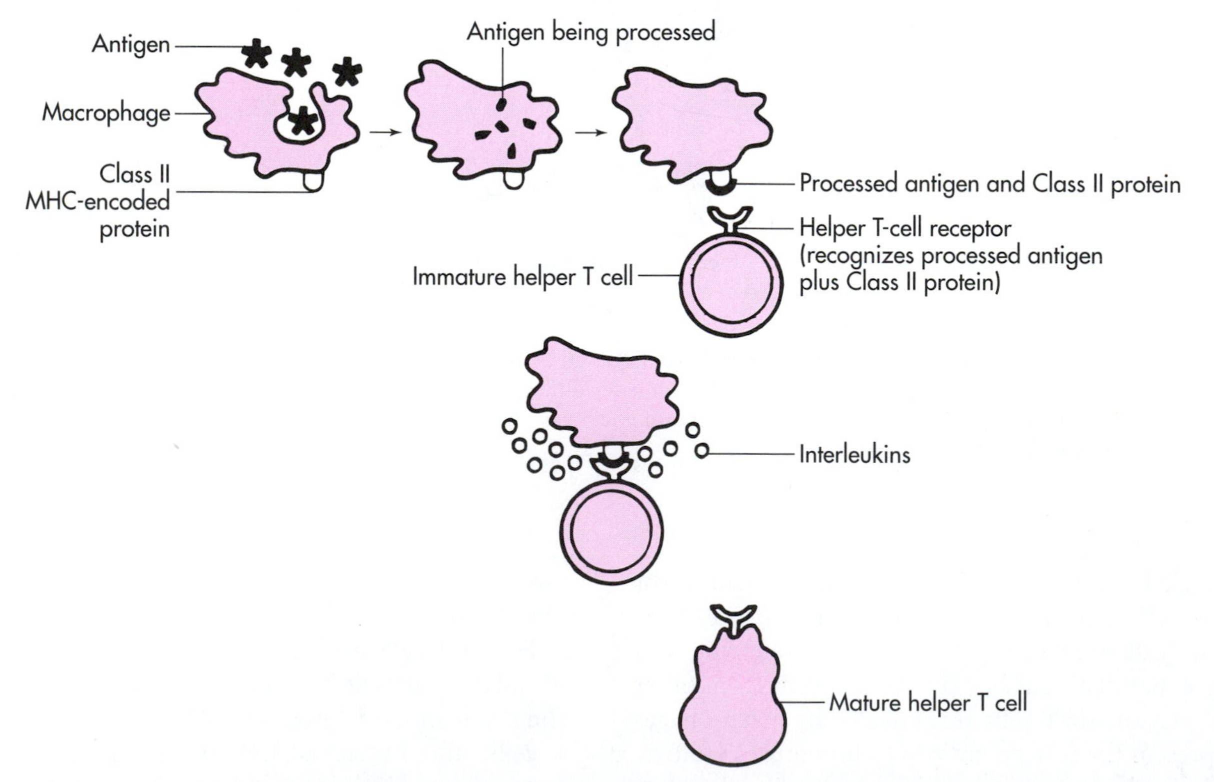

FIGURE 47-4. The helper T cell is activated by the presence of processed antigen in combination with the Class II antigen (protein) on the surface of a macrophage. It matures with the stimulus from interleukins. (From Schindler LW: *Understanding the immune system,* NIH Publ No 90-629, Bethesda, MD, 1990, US Department of Health and Human Services.)

responsible for activating helper T cells. Macrophages are responsible for presenting processed antigen to the immature helper T cells. With the assistance of chemical mediators released by the macrophage, the helper T cell matures and begins to activate other cells of the immune system previously described.

A third type of T cell is the suppressor T cell. These cells suppress or down-regulate the immune response. They play an important role in keeping the immune response controlled and in turning off the response once the antigenic threat is no longer present.

Natural killer cells represent another type of lymphocyte. These cells are not targeted for any specific antigen but will attack and destroy any cell that is identified as nonself. Natural killer cells contain granules filled with potent chemicals that are released when the natural killer cell binds to the targeted nonself cell. These chemicals are capable of lysing the cell membrane and causing the cell's death.

Phagocytes are a major category of immune cells capable of destroying alien cells. Critical phagocytes include monocytes, macrophages, neutrophils, eosinophils, and basophils. Table 47-1 outlines the primary function of these cells. Macrophages are vitally important to the immune response because of their role in "presenting" the antigen to the helper and cytotoxic T cells. This presentation alerts the T cells to the presence of antigen. Macrophages also produce chemical regulators that stimulate the maturation of helper and cytotoxic T cells.

As just described, chemical substances are released by macrophages, helper T cells, and cytotoxic T cells, which allows these immune cells to communicate with each other. These substances provide a network of soluble, low–molecular-weight peptides called *cytokines*, or more specifically, *interleukins*.[2] Interleukins are capable of activating or suppressing the proliferation of lymphocyte subsets. Several different types of interleukins with specific functions have been identified, but researchers are just beginning to understand the role that interleukins play in modulating the immune response.

An important system in the immune response is complement. Complement consists of a series of 25 proteins, which, when activated, develop into a powerful enzyme capable of lysing alien cell walls. Complement is triggered by the presence of antibody bound to an alien cell or antigen (antigen-antibody complex). Complement also stimulates basophils, attracts neutrophils, and coats alien cells to make them more attractive to phagocytes. The latter action is referred to as *opsonization.*

TABLE 47-1 Phagocytes and Their Functions

Phagocyte	Function
Monocytes	Migrate from blood tissues to become macrophages
Macrophages	Scavenger cells in tissues Present antigen to T cells Secrete enzymes, complement proteins, and immune regulatory factors (cytokines) Activated by lymphokines
Neutrophils	Contain granules capable of destroying alien organisms Key role in inflammatory reactions
Eosinophils	Contain granules capable of destroying alien organisms Weaker phagocyte
Basophils	Contain granules capable of destroying alien organisms Key role in allergic reaction

Graft Rejection

Rejection of any transplanted organ occurs when the transplanted tissue is recognized as nonself by the immune system. Cellular-mediated rejection occurs when HLA Class II antigens, displayed on donor cells, activate helper T cells that promote the expansion of cytotoxic T cells and recruitment of macrophages into the transplanted tissue. Natural killer cells also begin to attack any cell with foreign HLA Class I antigens. As a result, the transplanted organ becomes infiltrated with these cells, which proceed to destroy the foreign graft tissue.

At the same time, antibody-mediated or humoral-mediated rejection occurs as antigen-antibody complexes form. These complexes also are present in the transplanted organ and release complement that is capable of cell destruction. Complement plays a role in recruiting basophils and tissue-destroying neutrophils to the site. Antibody also coats the foreign cells, making them more attractive to macrophages.

Graft rejection can occur at different time intervals and has different injury patterns. There are three different types of rejection patterns: hyperacute rejection, acute rejection, and chronic rejection. Hyperacute rejection occurs within hours after transplantation and results in immediate graft failure. The primary mechanism triggering this response is activation of humoral-mediated rejection. Such an immediate response by the immune system is caused by the presence of preformed reactive antibodies resulting from previous exposure to antigens. Presensitization can be the result of previous blood transfusions, multiple pregnancies, or previous organ transplants.[3] Transplanting an organ from a donor with an incompatible blood type can have the same effect. Hyperacute rejection is prevented by testing for the presence of preformed antibodies in the recipient and by selecting donors with compatible blood types. Acute rejection occurs weeks to months after transplantation. Class I or II antigens on the cells of the transplanted graft activate cellular-mediated rejection. Chronic rejection occurs at varying times after transplantation and progresses for years until ultimate deterioration of the transplanted organ. Chronic rejection is the result of both humoral- and cellular-mediated immune responses. Chronic inflammation results in diffuse scarring of tissue and stenosis of the vasculature of the organ. Lack of blood supply leads to ischemia and necrosis of tissue. Chronic lung rejection results in small airway destruction, and chronic liver rejection causes diminution of bile ducts.

Immunosuppressive Therapy

Immunosuppressive protocols vary among institutions and with specific organ transplants. The primary goal of all protocols is to suppress the activity of helper and cytotoxic T cells. Therapy ideally interferes with the secretion of interleukins, which stimulate the immune response. The five most common agents used for immunosuppression include cyclosporine, corticosteroids, azathioprine, muromonab-CD3, and antithymocyte preparations. Table 47-2 summarizes the adverse effects of these drugs. Absolute care must be taken to monitor the effectiveness of drug therapy and to minimize unnecessarily high doses of these agents, which could predispose patients to greater risks for infection or malignancy.

Cyclosporine. Graft survival has improved dramatically since the introduction of cyclosporine. Its primary action seems to be inhibition of cytotoxic T cell generation.[4–6] It also interferes with the secretion of interleukins by helper T cells and the ability for cytotoxic T cells to respond to interleukins. Interleukin secretion by macrophages also is impaired. Because cyclosporine is specifically targeted for T cells, the patient's immune system is not totally impaired and some ability to protect the body from infection is preserved. T cells play a major role in providing protection from viral infections; thus cyclosporine's interference with T cell function prevents full immunologic competence against viral infection.[7]

Corticosteroids. Corticosteroids (IV methylprednisolone [Solu-Medrol] and oral prednisone) have complex and diverse effects on the immune system. They are used both for maintenance therapy and to treat acute rejection. The antiinflammatory actions of steroids provide important protection of the transplanted organ from permanent damage from the rejection process. As a maintenance therapy, steroids impair the sensitivity of T cells to antigen, decrease the proliferation of sensitized T cells, and impair the production of interleukins. Steroids also decrease macrophage mobility. Chronic steroid therapy is associated with numerous adverse effects and predisposes the patient to an increased risk of infection (see Table 47-2). A primary goal of therapy is to titrate the drug dose to as minimal a level as possible.

Azathioprine. Azathioprine (Imuran) is an antimetabolite that interferes with the purine synthesis necessary for the production of antibodies. Purine synthesis also is necessary for the synthesis of nucleic acids in rapidly proliferating cells, such as the cells of the immune system. Azathioprine is used as a maintenance drug to prevent the activation and rapid proliferation of T cells responding to an antigen. A common adverse effect is the suppression of other rapidly proliferating cells, resulting in leukopenia, thrombocytopenia, and anemia. The dose of the drug is adjusted to keep the white blood cell count between 3000 and 5000 cells/mm^3, thus protecting the patient from an increased risk of infection. The actual minimum acceptable white blood cell count varies with institutional preferences and type of organ transplant.

Muromonab-CD3. Muromonab-CD3 (Orthoclone OKT3) was one of the first drugs introduced to target distinct subpopulations of T cells. The drug is a monoclonal antibody produced in mice to specifically target cells with the T3 surface antigen found on mature T cells. Orthoclone OKT3 removes these cells from circulation by forming antibody-antigen complexes. Orthoclone OKT3 also interferes with T cell recognition of foreign antigen, which renders the T cells incapable of responding.[5,8] The drug is used as induction therapy by some centers to eliminate T cell response for the first 2 weeks after transplantation. Other centers use it to treat and reverse a severe rejection episode. Because it is an animal protein, antibodies against the drug develop in some patients. For that reason it cannot be used repeatedly in patients with sensitivity. Its adverse effects seem to be caused by the massive destruction of T cells, resulting in fever, general malaise, and rigors.[8] Reactions usually subside

TABLE 47-2 Immunosuppressive Drugs Used in Organ Transplantation in Adult Patients

Drug	Dosage*	Actions	Special Considerations
Azathioprine	Titrate to WBC between 3000-6000 cells/mm^3	Inhibits purine synthesis	Monitor for bone marrow depression
Cyclosporine (Neoral) Oral solution and gelation capsules	Standard dose range (organ specific): 14-18 mg/kg/day (liver transplant) 10-14 mg/kg/day (kidney transplant) Tapered to 5-10 mg/kg/day 5-10 mg/kg/day (heart transplant) Dosage split bid Therapeutic range: 100-400 μg/L in blood 50-200 μg/L in plasma	Suppresses T lymphocytes	Hold for elevated levels Watch for nephrotoxicity, HTN, hepatotoxity, tremors, and seizures Watch for drugs that exhibit nephrotoxic synergy: (i.e., gentamicin, tobramycin, vancomycin, amphotericin B, ketoconazole, cimetidine, and ranitidine)
Tacrolimus (Prograf, FK506)	0.1-0.3 mg/kg/day Dosage split bid Therapeutic range: 5-20 μg/L in blood 0.1-5 μg/L in plasma	Inhibition of interleukin release	Nephrotoxicity with high doses Hyperkalemia
Mycophenolate mofetil (Cellcept)	2-3 g/day split bid	Similar to azathioprine but less toxic	Increased blood level concentrations when used with other drugs excreted via the renal tubules
Muromonab-CD3 (Orthoclone OKT3)	5 mg/day for 10-14 days	Suppresses circulating T lymphocytes	Watch for reactions Pretreatment for initial doses with: Acetaminophen (Tylenol) Diphenhydramine (Benadryl) Hydrocortisone, 50 mg for first dose
Prednisone	1 mg/kg/day Tapered to 0.3 mg/kg/day or off, if tolerated	Suppresses inflammatory response	Tapered to as low a dose as tolerated Dose is increased with rejection
RATG	2.5 mg/kg for 1-7 days May be given daily initially then qod	Suppresses circulating T lymphocytes	Used in lung transplants for induction therapy Used as rescue therapy for other transplants Watch for reactions Pretreatment may be used

*These dosage ranges are general guidelines. Significant variations in dosages occur based on institutional practices, other drugs being used in combination, transplant type, and patient response to the drugs.
HTN, Hypertension; *RATG*, rabbit-antithymocyte globulin.

with subsequent doses. As the T cell population declines, the severity of the reaction diminishes. Orthoclone OKT3 usually is administered for 14 days and then stopped.

Antithymocyte preparations. Antithymocyte preparations are made by injecting human thymocytes into an animal, usually a horse, rabbit, or goat. The animal produces antibody in response to the foreign human antigen. Antibody to human thymocytes can then be extracted from the serum of the animal. The same process can be used to obtain antilymphocyte preparations. Antibody preparations are made with serum or globulin. If globulin is produced, globulin molecules are extracted from the animal serum.[7] Many centers make their own preparations. Only two preparations are commercially available in the United States, and they are made from horse serum. Depending on the protocol of the institution and the type of organ transplant, antithymocyte or antilymphocyte preparations may be given as part of induction therapy or may be used only to treat rejection. The duration of therapy is typically around 7 days but may be shorter or longer, depending on institutional preference. Administration of the drug depletes circulating T cells and reduces the proliferative function of the T cells. As with Orthoclone OKT3, patients are subject to reactions from the release of pyrogens during the massive T cell lysis, as well as to the foreign animal protein contained in the preparation. Orthoclone OKT3, antilymphocyte, and antithymocyte preparations are referred to as *cytolytic drugs*. Use of cytolytic drugs has been associated with an increased incidence of malignancy. This increased incidence is most likely caused by the suppression of cytotoxic T cells, which play an important role in identifying and eliminating cancer cells. For that reason, many centers use these drugs only to reverse rejections that are unresponsive to conventional treatment with increased corticosteroid.

FK506. FK506 is an immunosuppressant first released for human clinical trials in February 1989 for use in liver transplant patients.[9] Since that time, trials have been completed with recipients of heart, lung and kidney transplants.[10,11] The immunologic action of FK506 is mediated through the inhibition of a specific type of interleukin release (interleukin-2).[12] FK506 has been shown to have fewer side effects than cyclosporine and is used in place of cyclosporine in the immunosuppressive regimen. If cyclosporine has been used in a patient, the recommendation is that before the first dose of FK506 is administered, cyclosporine be discontinued for a minimum of 24 hours to prevent synergistic side effects. These effects include hypertensive episodes and body rash.[9]

Initially, intravenously administered FK506 is given during the perioperative period and then every 12 hours. The dose is adjusted according to the patient's liver chemistry findings, blood levels, and the degree to which the drug is tolerated. On the basis of these factors, dosing schedules can be varied, and some patients may not require the drug on a 12-hour regimen or even on a daily basis. Conversion to oral administration occurs when patients are able to tolerate oral intake.

Side effects are encountered most frequently with intravenous administration. These untoward effects include headaches, nausea, and vomiting.[12] Hyperkalemia associated with low aldosterone and renin levels has occurred and may require treatment with potassium-restricted diets. FK506 does not appear to be as nephrotoxic as cyclosporine, nor does it cause hypertension. Other adverse effects include neurotoxicity and glucose intolerance. Unlike cyclosporine, FK-506 does not cause hypertrichosis, gingival hyperplasia, or facial dysmorphism.[12] Also, patients receiving FK506 tend to require lower doses of azathioprine and corticosteroids long-term. All of these factors may improve the quality of life for transplant recipients.

Mycophenolate mofetil (RS-61443). Mycophenolate mofetil (RS-61443), a drug recently added to the pharmacologic armory of many immunosuppressive protocols, is a derivative of mycophenolic acid. Mycophenolic acid is a fermentation product of several *Penicillium* species.[13] Mycophenolate mofetil inhibits inosine monophosphate dehydrogenase, which is a key enzyme in the de novo pathway of purine synthesis.[13,14] Therefore it is a potent inhibitor of the proliferative responses of T and B lymphocytes.[13] This inhibition also disrupts antibody formation and the generation of cytotoxic T cells. It effectively suppresses both cellular- and humoral-mediated immunity. The mechanism of action is similar to that of azathioprine except that mycophenolate mofetil selectively inhibits T and B cells. Global bone marrow suppression is not seen with mycophenolate mofetil.[8] Clinical immunosuppression can thus be obtained without increased susceptibility to bacterial and fungal infections.[13]

In animal studies, long-term heart recipients had a lower incidence and severity of proliferative arteriopathy seen with chronic rejection.[13,15] The drug may have an effect in reducing mechanisms that are thought to participate in the smooth muscle cell proliferation that causes concentric intimal thickening, resulting in obliterative arteriopathy of transplanted organs.

In clinical trials, doses vary from 100 mg/day to 3500 mg/day administered orally in conjunction with cyclosprine and corticosteriods.[13] Responses to the drug are dose-dependent. Preliminary data suggest that the fewest episodes of rejection occur in patients receiving doses of at least 200 mg/day. Doses of greater than 2000 mg/day are considered rescue doses. Side effects consist mainly of gastrointestinal symptoms such as nausea, vomiting, ileus, and gastritis.[8,13]

Many research centers are now substituting azathioprine with mycophenolate mofetil to avoid the leukopenia, thrombocytopenia, and anemia associated with the bone marrow suppression that can occur with azathioprine. Mycophenolate mofetil may offer better protection against rejection without placing the recipient at increased risk for infection.

Risk of infection. A major adverse effect of all immunosuppressive drugs is an increased risk for infection. Patients on a multiple drug regimen that is administered at high doses are at greatest risk. Few patients complete their first year of immunosuppressive therapy without an episode of infection. It is important for the clinician to be astute and look for subtle signs of infection. Infections can be treated successfully if clinicians are vigilant, if patients are taught to recognize signs of possible infection, and if aggressive treatment is started early. The nursing management plan at the end of this chapter outlines important interventions for treatment of infection (p. 1216).

HEART TRANSPLANTATION

Laboratory research and development of tissue and organ transplantation were initiated in 1904 when Guthrie and Carrel began their investigations of whole organ transplant at the University of Chicago. Initial studies of heart rejection were described as early as 1914 by Frank C. Mann at the Mayo Clinic. It was not until the mid-1940s that Russian researchers Demikhov and Sinitsyn successfully transplanted heart-lung blocks in dogs. Later, heart transplantation was achieved, again in a dog, with a survival of 32 days. Early years of research focused on heterotopic (transplanting a heart as an augmentation to the native heart) transplant because of the unavailability of cardiopulmonary bypass. The first heart preservation techniques evolved in the mid-1950s, coinciding with the advent of the cardiopulmonary bypass. These developments opened the door for investigations of orthotopic (replacement of the heart in the native position) transplantation in animals. In 1960 Lower and Shumway first reported the surgical technique of orthotopic transplantation in dogs, with a maximum survival of 2 weeks without immunosuppression. The same team recognized the validity of using the electrocardiogram to detect rejection, which resulted in longer survival.[16]

The first human heart transplantion was performed at the University of Capetown in 1967 by Dr. Christian Barnard, with the patient surviving 18 days. In 1968 Shumway performed the first transplant in the United States at Stanford University. Heart transplant procedures dramatically grew in number for the first few years and then rapidly declined because of poor results. It was not until 1972 to 1974 that clinical survival improved and interest regenerated. The development of the endomyocardial biopsy in 1972 was a major milestone in the detection of allograft rejection. In addition, the introduction of T cell-specific agents, such as rabbit antithymocyte globulin, and the ability of laboratories to measure specific T cells (rosette counts) contributed to an increase in 1-year survival by approximately 20% of patients. In 1981 the immunosuppressive drug cyclosporine was introduced in the clinical setting, improving survival by about 20% at 1 year. Once again the number of transplant procedures grew rapidly.[16]

Indications and Selection

General candidate criteria for heart transplantation is a life expectancy of only 6 to 12 months because of end-stage cardiac disease.[16] Common causes of such conditions are cardiomyopathy of various origins (idiopathic, viral, valvular) and coronary artery disease.[17] Other less common etiologic factors include severe heart failure resulting from chemotherapy, radiation treatment, myocardial tumor, and complex congenital defects. Many centers grade the severity of heart failure by the New York Heart Association (NYHA) functional classification (Table 47-3), which is based on the amount of exertion required to cause symptoms. Although most patients fall into the category of NYHA Class IV, the condition of some is graded Class III because of recent recompensation.[17]

Heart transplantation is covered under diagnostic-related group (DRG) 103. The anticipated length of stay is 39.1 days.[18]

In addition to satisfying medical criteria, patients generally are evaluated for the presence of familial or social support; absence of chemical dependence; and commitment to adhering to a strict, lifelong medical regimen and follow-up.

Specific contraindications to cardiac transplantation are listed in Box 47-1. The age range in heart transplantation is from the neonatal period to approximately 65 years; upper age limits vary among transplant institutions. Preexisting malignancy has been an absolute contraindication because of the potential for recurring cancer or development of second cancers as a result of therapeutic immunosuppression. Some centers, however, consider cured, nonmetastatic malignancies as a relative contraindication.[19,20] Severe liver and kidney dysfunctions that are not reversible by an increase in cardiac output are contraindications for transplantation.[17] Diabetes mellitus (DM) was once an absolute contraindication because steroid administration can cause exacerbation of the condition. With good medical management, however, hyperglycemia can be controlled.

It also was believed that diabetic persons would incur an increased risk for infectious complications. Currently, however, DM is considered a relative contraindication if the hyperglycemia is adequately treated, because it has been demonstrated that the early survival rates of patients with DM are equal to those without DM.[21–23] If patients have active infections, transplantation is delayed until the infections are cleared. Recent pulmonary infarctions increase the risk for postoperative infection and complicate oxygenation and ventilation. Thus a recent history of infarction often precludes transplantation.

LEGAL REVIEW

Organ Transplantation

Among the most rapid developments in medical technology has been the evolution of organ transplantation, which raises many legal issues. Of major import are the issues of supply and demand, rationing and allocation, cost and reimbursement, locating organ donors, organs from live donors, and confidentiality and access to donor-donee data.

Critical care nurses are involved in the process of organ procurement for donation and transplantation, as well as the care of the organ donee–that is, the recipient. Federal and state statutes and regulations govern this area of health care delivery.

Federal law has established a national system of organ donation and procurement for the purpose of maximizing supply to meet increasing demand but simultaneously prohibiting the sale of organs. It is unlawful for any person to knowingly acquire, receive, or otherwise transfer any human organ for valuable consideration for use in human transplantation if the transfer affects interstate commerce. Violations of this law can result in substantial fines and incarceration.

Because there is a paucity of available organs for donation, a need exists for rationing and allocation. The purpose and intent of the Uniform Anatomical Gift Act (UAGA) are to establish the legal framework for cadaveric organ donation and to locate donors for organ transplantation; each state has adopted a variation of this uniform statute. Generally, the law provides that any adult of sound mind may donate any part or all of his or her body. In most states this individual decision cannot be overruled by a family member after death. In some states, however, family members can reverse this bequest. State law also specifies who may donate, who may receive the anatomic gift, and how the gift is made. In addition, state law includes restrictions. The physician who certifies or determines the time of death, for example, may not participate in the removal or transplantation of organs.

To increase the availability of organs, state and federal laws and regulations have been passed that require hospitals to ask patients or their family members about organ donation. At the federal level, hospitals receiving Medicare or Medicaid funding must establish written protocols for the identification of potential donors. Under state law hospitals establish policies addressing the request for organ donations. These policies must specify clearly the nurse's duties and responsibilities in organ procurement.

The major legal problem surrounding live donors arises when the potential donor is a minor or is incompetent. The courts have reached various decisions in these cases. In some jurisdictions the courts have adopted the substituted judgment rule. In others, the courts have rejected this doctrine and have adopted in its place the rule that the guardian must act, if at all, in the best interests of the guardian's ward, who is the potential donor.

Other legal issues have arisen, for example, questions about the right of access of a person in need of an organ to a hospital's records of the identities of potential donors. In the Iowa case cited in the footnote, the court held that the records of potential donors were confidential.

See Bouressa Fr G, O'Mara RJ: Ethical dilemmas in organ procurement and donation, *Crit Care Nurs Q* 10(2):37, 1987; *Guardianship of Pescinski,* 226 NW2d 180 (Wis 1975); *Head v Colloton,* 331 NW2d 870 (Iowa 1983); National Organ Transplant Act (NOTA). PL 98-507 (1984); 42 USCA Sec 274(e) (1986); O'Connell DA: Ethical implications of organ transplantation, *Crit Care Nurs Q* 13(4):1, 1991; Smith SL: *AACN tissue and organ transplantation: implications for professional nursing practice,* St Louis, 1990, Mosby; *Strunk v Strunk,* 445 SW2d 145 (Ky App 1969); Uniform Anatomical Gift Act (UAGA), 8A Uniform Law Acts [ULA] (1983).

The active waiting list is prioritized by acuity, length of time on the list, ABO blood group, and weight. Distribution of organs is regulated by a regional, state, and national network organized and managed by the federal government. Acuity is determined by a patient's need for inotropic support or mechanical assist devices. Patients requiring this degree of assistance are listed as *status one.* All other heart transplant candidates are listed as *status two.*

Surgical Procedure

The standard surgical procedure has changed little since its development by Lower and Shumway.[24] A standard median sternotomy is used, the great vessels are cannulated, and cardiopulmonary bypass (CPB) is instituted after anticoagulation with standard hypothermic technique. Continuous topical cold saline solution at 4° C is used to protect the myocardium from ischemia. The donor heart is prepared by interconnecting the pulmonary veins to form a single left atrial cuff and by trimming the aorta and pulmonary artery to fit the recipient's anatomy. All of the recipient's heart is removed except the posterior walls of the atria that contain the orifices of the pulmonary veins and vena cava, which minimizes the need for multiple anastomoses. Three major anastomoses are performed be-

TABLE 47-3 New York Heart Association Functional Classification of Heart Disease

Class	Physical Manifestation
I	No limitation of physical activity. No dyspnea, fatigue, or palpitation with ordinary physical activity.
II	Slight limitation of physical activity. These patients have fatigue, palpitations, and dyspnea with ordinary physical activity but are comfortable at rest.
III	Marked limitation of activity. Less than ordinary physical activity results in symptoms, but patients are comfortable at rest.
IV	Symptoms are present at rest, and any physical exertion exacerbates the symptoms.

BOX 47-1 Contraindications to Heart Transplantation

- Advanced age
- Significant systemic or multisystem disease
- Fixed severe pulmonary hypertension
- Active infection
- Recent pulmonary infarction
- Cachexia or obesity
- Psychiatric illness
- Drug or alcohol abuse

tween the donor heart and recipient's native atrial remnant. These include the anastomoses and connection of the atria, the aorta, and the pulmonary artery, in that order[24] (Figure 47-5). Atrial and ventricular epicardial pacing wires are placed before sternal closure, in the event pacing is needed in the postoperative period.

The native atrial remnant remains innervated by the parasympathetic and sympathetic nerve fibers from the autonomic nervous system (ANS). The donor heart, however, is now denervated, resulting in a faster resting heart rate of 90 to 100 beats/minute. The rate of the transplanted heart is the normal intrinsic rate generated by the donor sinoatrial (SA) node located in the right atria. Even though the donor SA paces the heart, the remnant native atria will have a separate rate of conduction influenced by the ANS. Manipulation of the atria during surgery and edema around the suture line can cause conduction disturbances that may result in postoperative bradycardia.

Postoperative Medical and Nursing Management

Immediate postoperative management of the transplant recipient is similar to that of patients undergoing other heart surgery procedures. Nursing care of the transplant recipient involves several nursing diagnoses, as listed in Box 47-2. The most frequently used diagnosis is decreased cardiac output (CO). Possible causes for a decrease in CO are dysrhythmia, hypothermia, myocardial depression, tamponade, and rejection.

Variables that influence myocardial performance are prolonged ischemic times (time from excision of heart from the donor to removal of the aortic cross clamp after the implant to the recipient), reperfusion injury, and hypothermia. Dysrhythmias may occur as a result of myocardial irritation, local ischemia, edema around the atrial suture line, and disruption of the SA nodal blood supply.[25] An electrocardiogram abnormality unique to the transplanted heart is the presence of a second P wave, generated by the native SA node left in the atrial cuff. Because this impulse does not cross the suture line, it is capable of conducting only through the remnant of the native recipient atria.

Isoproterenol, a powerful beta-adrenergic antagonist, is the agent most commonly used in the postoperative period for chronotropic (heart rate) support. Its chronotropic and vasodilator properties effectively sustain heart rate, increase CO, and decrease pulmonary vascular resistance (PVR). PVR may be increased as a result of preexisting left ventricular failure and may be a cause of transient right ventricular dysfunction in the newly transplanted heart. Dopamine is the most frequently used drug for inotropic support in the postoperative period. Usually, within 48 hours, the inotropic support drugs can be gradually discontinued, and the need for isoproterenol decreases as the heart begins to maintain its normal intrinsic rate of 100 beats/minute. Temporary pacing is required only occasionally, and fewer than 10% of transplant patients require a permanent pacemaker implant.[25]

Cardiac tamponade generally does not occur with greater frequency in transplantation than in other cardiac surgeries, but it may occur insidiously as a result of an enlarged pericardial sac from longstanding cardiomyopathy.[26] Patients who have had chronic right ventricular failure, subsequent liver enlargement, and abnormal coagulation studies may benefit from preoperative administration of fresh plasma or fresh frozen plasma (FFP). Plasma contains most clotting factors and is indicated for liver dysfunction. Administration of plasma may decrease the risk of bleeding and tamponade.[27]

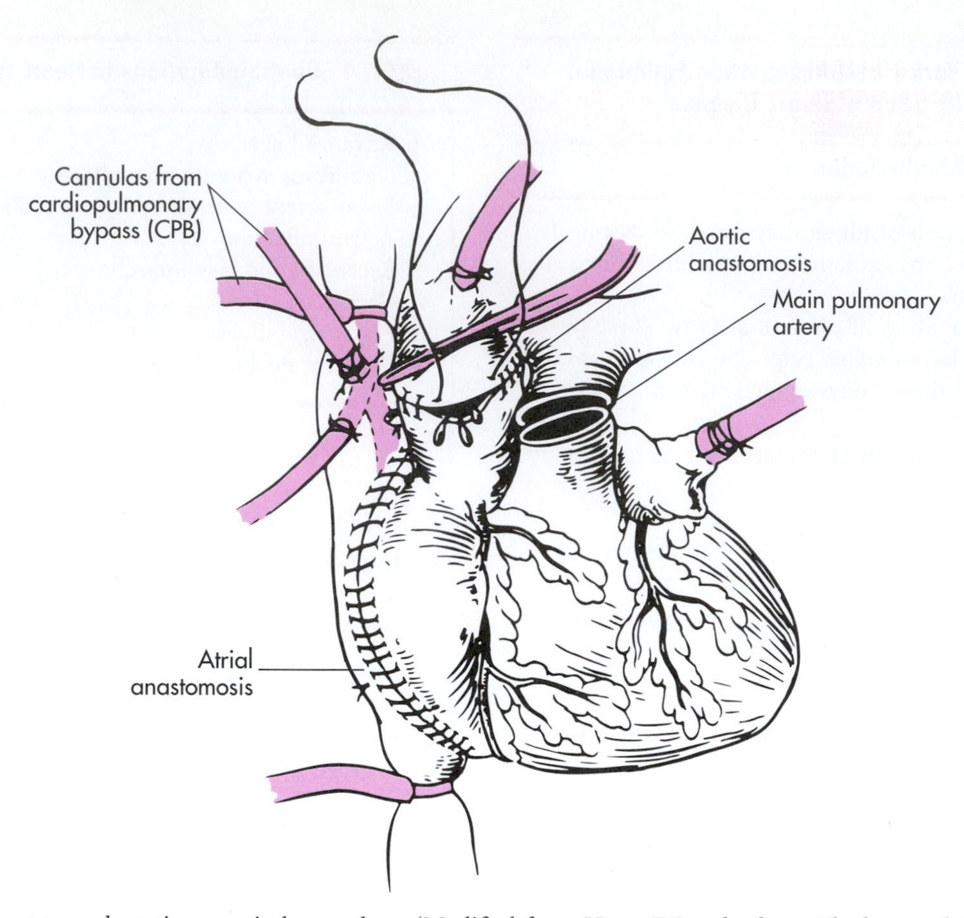

FIGURE 47-5. Heart transplantation: surgical procedure. (Modified from Hurst JW and others: *The heart,* ed 7, New York, 1990, McGraw-Hill.)

Rejection surveillance. Rejection is the most common etiologic factor responsible for causing low CO for the first 3 months after transplantation.[26] Hyperacute rejection occurs only in the immediate postoperative period. It is a rare complication that necessitates retransplantation for survival. Acute rejection occurs most frequently in the first 3 to 6 months after transplantation. Diagnosis of rejection is determined by endomyocardial biopsy. Biopsy specimens are obtained by inserting a bioptome percutaneously through the right internal jugular vein, advancing it through the right atrium to the right ventricle with the aid of fluoroscopy or echocardiography. Four to five samples of myocardial tissue are obtained from the interventricular septum. The samples are microscopically evaluated for interstitial and perivascular infiltration. Cardiac biopsies are graded according to the severity of the interstitial infiltration of lymphocytes. Many large transplant centers follow the international grading system introduced in 1990. This standardized cardiac biopsy grading scale ranges from 0 to 4 (Box 47-3).[28] Surveillance for rejection is performed on a weekly basis for the first 4 to 6 weeks. The frequency of surveillance gradually is decreased relative to the patient's rejection history. A major but rare complication of biopsy is ventricular perforation, resulting in cardiac tamponade. This emergency situation may require open heart surgical repair. Pneumothorax may result from the perforation of the visceral pleura during cannulation of the jugular vein. Clinical manifestations are a sudden onset of sharp pain in the affected side and dyspnea. Many institutions require transplant patients to undergo biopsy monitoring for the rest of their lives.

Treatment of the initial and second rejection episodes requires intravenously administered methylprednisolone (Solu-Medrol). Recurrent rejection is treated with various pharmacologic agents, depending on the institution. Orthoclone OKT3, a monoclonal antibody, commonly is used for recurrent rejection. It also is used as an induction immunosuppressive agent for the first 10 to 14 days after surgery. If Orthoclone OKT3 is being used for a second time, the patient must be tested for the presence of antibodies. Antibodies

BOX 47-2 NURSING DIAGNOSIS AND MANAGEMENT

HEART TRANSPLANTATION

- Decreased Cardiac Output related to alterations in preload, p. 590
- Decreased Cardiac Output related to alterations in afterload, p. 592
- Decreased Cardiac output related to alterations in heart rate, p. 593
- Risk for Infection risk factor: immunosuppressive drugs required to prevent rejection of transplanted organ, p. 1216
- Body Image Disturbance related to actual change in body structure, function, or appearance, p. 87
- Anxiety related to threat to biologic, psychologic, and/or social integrity p 99
- Activity Intolerance related to prolonged immobility or deconditioning, p. 597
- Knowledge Deficit: Posttransplant Self-care Regimen, immunosuppressive drugs, cardiac drugs, diuretics, and clinical manifestations of infection related to lack of previous exposure to information, p. 61

may contraindicate use of Orthoclone OKT3. Other agents used for recurrent rejection are polyclonal antibodies, such as antilymphocyte globulin (ALG) or antithymocyte globulin (ATG). Salvage therapy for persistent rejection that has not responded to conventional immunosuppression, multiple steroid boluses, or anti-T cell antibodies consists of total lymphoid irradiation (TLI). Low-dose ionizing radiation is used to treat the lymphoid tissue. Areas exposed to radiation are the axilla, sternum, clavicle, paraaorta, ilium, inguinofemoral lymph nodes, and the spleen.[29]

Infection surveillance. Infection surveillance is a high priority for the immunocompromised person. It is well-known that immunosuppression predisposes the patient to infection by a multitude of opportunistic pathogens, which cannot easily be prevented with infection control. Development of infection is encountered most frequently in the early postoperative period when immunosuppression is maximized. Infection is the leading cause of death during this period (up to 2 years after surgery).[24,30] Great care must be taken to use aseptic technique for all intravenous line and dressing changes. Centers differ widely in protective practices regarding the transplant recipient. Some use reverse isolation, whereas others put transplant recipients in rooms with other patients and simply use universal precautions.

BOX 47-3 Standardized Cardiac Biopsy Grading

GRADE	NOMENCLATURE
0	No acute rejection [AR]
1A	Focal, mild AR
1B	Diffuse, mild AR
2	Focal, moderate AR
3A	Multifocal aggressive, low moderate AR
3B	Diffuse borderline, severe AR
4	Diffuse aggressive, severe AR

Any development of fever is aggressively pursued by systematic blood, wound, and respiratory tract cultures, chest x-ray films, and observation. Because steroids are known to suppress the body's inflammatory reaction, a temperature generally is considered significant at 38° C. Nurses must be suspicious of any new productive cough, dry cough, change in type of secretions, or change in chest roentgenogram findings.

Cytomegalovirus (CMV) is a particular threat to transplant recipients. CMV is a herpes virus that can produce latent infection that persists throughout life; approximately 50% of the general population is infected. The virus can be transmitted through organ and blood product donation; thus the transplantation from a CMV-seropositive donor to a CMV-seronegative recipient poses the highest risk to the recipient for acquiring a primary infection. An antiviral agent, ganciclovir, can inhibit viral replication and ameliorate symptoms and thus is used in the prophylaxis and treatment of CMV infections.[31,32] In addition, CMV immune globulin (CMVIG) is being used increasingly for the prevention of primary CMV disease and for treatment of CMV disease.[32-35]

Long-Term Considerations

Chronic immunosuppression results in significant morbidity. Steroid administration can result in osteoporosis, avascular necrosis of joints, fragile skin, and obesity. Cyclosporine can induce renal insufficiency, excessive hair growth, gingival hyperplasia, tremor, and hypertension that requires pharmacologic control. Azathioprine can be hepatotoxic. Concomitant use of these immunosuppressants also leaves patients more susceptible to malignancies and late infections (see Table 47-2).

Accelerated graft atherosclerosis (AGAS), or coronary artery disease in the transplanted heart, is a major cause of late morbidity and mortality.[36] AGAS is a diffuse and rapidly progressive type of coronary artery disease that causes concentric narrowing of the coronary arteries. Because the lesions are not discrete, they are not amenable to angioplasty or bypass grafting.[36] The etiology of AGAS remains unclear, but chronic rejection likely plays a role.[37] Patients with denervated hearts usually cannot feel anginal pain; although recent literature reports evidence of reinnervation and subsequent chest pain.[38] More often, their symptoms are ischemic injury, heart failure, or sudden death. The disease is recognized initially by angiographic screening and, later in the course of the disease, by the presence of silent infarctions on electrocardiogram. Many patients may have the disease and demonstrate no clinical sequelae.[36] The only therapy for advanced AGAS is retransplantation.

In general, heart transplant recipients report being highly satisfied with their quality of life.[39-42] Fewer than 35% return to full-time employment, but many who are able to work cannot find suitable employment because of employers' concerns about liability, lack of health insurance, and the need to qualify for medical disability.[42,43]

In 1995 there were 2359 cardiac transplants performed in the United States. In the same year 3468 persons were registered on waiting lists.[44] The number of cardiac transplants performed is greatly influenced by the limited donor pool. Current 1-year survival for heart transplant recipients, as reported by the United Network for Organ Sharing,[44] is 85%.

HEART AND LUNG TRANSPLANTATION

Heart and lung transplantation research has been built on the foundation established by heart transplantation through years of laboratory investigation. The first attempts at heart-lung transplantation in humans were in 1968 by Cooly and his associates, with a 14-hour survival; in 1969 by Lellehei, which produced a survival of several days; and in 1971 by Barnard, whose patient survived for 23 days. Interest in the procedure gained momentum with the introduction of cyclosporine, because it permitted the delay of high-dose steroid therapy (its use impaired bronchial healing and favored early postoperative infections). In 1981 at Stanford University, Bruce Rietz performed the first heart-lung transplant resulting in long-term survival; the patient lived for more than 5 years.

Heart and lung transplantation, now in its third decade, currently is the therapy of choice for some cardiac and cardiopulmonary diseases. Research and laboratory investigations continue in the development of new immunosuppressants, preservation solutions, and techniques. Recent advances have led to single-lung and double-lung transplantation, lobar lung transplantation, and single-lung transplantation with cardiac repair.

Heart lung transplantation is covered under DRG 103. This is the same DRG as heart transplantation, and the anticipated length of stay is 39.1 days.[18]

Indications and Selection

Heart-lung transplantation (HLT) is an established treatment for selected patients with irreversible, progressively disabling end-stage cardiopulmonary and pulmonary disease.[45-47] Transplantation usually is offered to patients as an option when life expectancy is limited to 15 to 24 months.[45,46] Patients are evaluated and listed earlier than are heart transplant recipients because of the paucity of heart-lung donors and the inevitable long wait for transplantation.

Specific etiologic factors in pulmonary disease can be grouped according to the type of lung abnormality. Categories are pulmonary vascular disease, obstructive lung disease and restrictive lung disease,[45,46] Box 47-4 lists indications for heart-lung transplantation. Optional lung transplantation, such as single- and bilateral- or double-lung transplantation, is discussed in a later section.

HLT is the operation of choice for patients whose pulmonary disease process has irreversibly disabled the heart. HLT is considered the preferential procedure because transplantation of the entire heart-lung block eliminates having to separate the pulmonary artery and veins, avoiding subsequent reanastomoses and thus decreasing bleeding complications. However, in the case of disease processes in which the heart is judged to be only temporarily dysfunctional and can be expected to regain adequate function after the transplantation of a healthy lung or lungs, the native heart may be left in place[46,48] and a single- or double-lung transplant performed. Another option is to transplant the heart-lung block into such an individual and then donate the native heart to another recipient, which is referred to as the *domino procedure.*

The evaluation of HLT candidates is similar to that for heart transplant recipients with respect to patient commitment to compliance with a strict lifelong medical regimen. Contraindications to HLT are listed in Box 47-5. Systematic disease, active extrapulmonary infection, and other organ diseases are absolute contraindications. Cachexia and obesity are obstacles that can be eliminated by nutritional support and weight

BOX 47-4 Heart-Lung Transplantation Indications

Pulmonary vascular disease
- Primary pulmonary hypertension
- Eisenmenger's syndrome
- Cardiomyopathy with pulmonary hypertension

Obstructive lung disease
- Emphysema—idiopathic
- Emphysema—alpha$_1$-antitrypsin deficiency
- Cystic fibrosis
- Bronchiectasis
- Posttransplant obliterative bronchiolitis

Restrictive lung disease
- Idiopathic pulmonary fibrosis
- Sarcoidosis
- Lymphangiomyomatosis

BOX 47-5 Absolute and Relative Contraindications to Heart-Lung Transplantation

ABSOLUTE CONTRAINDICATIONS

Significant systemic or multisystem disease
Active extrapulmonary infection
Cachexia or obesity
Current cigarette smoking
Psychiatric illness
Drug or alcohol abuse

RELATIVE CONTRAINDICATIONS

Corticosteroid therapy
Previous cardiothoracic surgery

reduction. Truncal obesity is especially undesirable because it significantly decreases diaphragmatic excursion, hinders postoperative mobilization, and may complicate recovery.[45] Preoperative use of corticosteroids has been implicated as a cause of tracheal and bronchial dehiscence in the early postoperative period.[45,46] Prior cardiothoracic surgery is a relative contraindication because of the risk of bleeding associated with the presence of pleural adhesions.[45] Removal of the native lung may precipitate pleural bleeding in the posterior pleural space, which can be particularly difficult to control because of location.[49]

Surgical Procedure

Success of HLT depends in part on selection and procurement of suitable donor organs. The lungs are particularly difficult to procure because they are vulnerable to complications related to brain death. Prolonged mechanical ventilation is required, which increases the risk of infection. Any infection generally precludes donation. Neurogenic pulmonary edema also may damage the lungs, making their donation impossible. Lungs have a limited ischemic time of about 4 hours, which limits the geographic area for donor procurement.[49] Lung preservation has improved, and distant procurement with 2 to 3 hours transport time has increased the donor pool.[50]

Before the removal of the heart-lung block, alprostadil (prostaglandin E_1) (PGE_1) is administered gradually until a systemic effect is achieved. PGE_1 is used to ensure complete pulmonary vasodilation for uniform cooling and distribution of pulmonoplegia.[50,51]

The operative procedure for the recipient is through a median sternotomy or a bilateral thoracosternotomy (clam shell) incision. The patient is heparinized and placed on cardiopulmonary bypass, and the heart is excised.[52] Care is used to ensure the preservation of the recipient's phrenic, vagus, and laryngeal nerves. The bronchus is divided, and the lungs are removed separately to decrease the risk of nerve damage. The donor heart and lungs are implanted as a block. The heart is put into the orthotopic position and anastomosed to the native aorta and remnant recipient atria. The tracheal anastomosis is performed just above the level of the carina[51] (Figure 47-6).

Postoperative Medical and Nursing Management

Immediate postoperative care of the heart-lung transplant recipient is similar to that used for the heart transplant recipient. Several nursing diagnoses are associated with care of heart-lung transplant recipient, as listed in Box 47-6. The most common complication is bleeding. Patients who have been cyanotic often have large bronchial vessels that cross behind the trachea and tend to be a source of bleeding. Control of bleeding at this site is difficult because of the location. Patients who have had previous thoracic surgery require more surgical dissection because of scarring and therefore achieve hemostasis with more difficulty. Careful monitoring of bleeding and maintenance of the patency and function of mediastinal and pleural chest tubes are essential. Bleeding of greater than 100 to 200 ml/hour for more than 3 hours with normal coagulation studies is cause for concern. If bleeding of this nature persists, reexploration of the chest

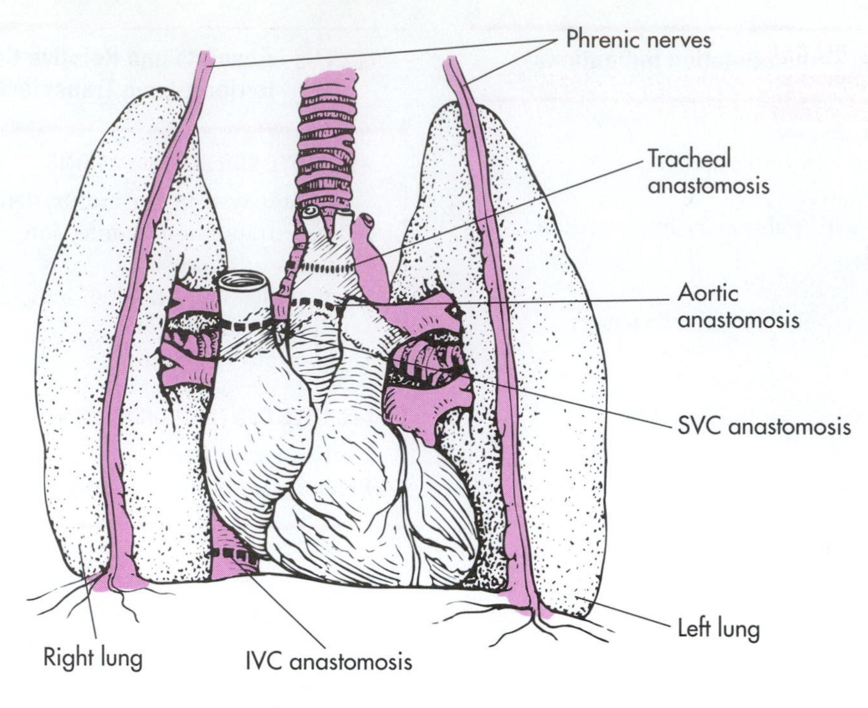

FIGURE 47-6. Heart-lung transplantation: surgical procedure. (Modified from Reitz BA and others: Heart and lung transplantation, *J Thorac and Cardiovasc Surg* 80(3):360, 1980.

usually is indicated. The transplanted lung is susceptible to fluid overload because of the disruption of pulmonary lymphatics and the increase in extravascular lung water that is common after lung transplantation.[46] Replacement of blood loss with crystalloid or colloid therapy must be used carefully to minimize the risk of fluid overload of the transplanted lungs and the development of acute respiratory distress syndrome (ARDS). (∞ARDS, p. 660.)

Patients are maintained on mechanical ventilation to support oxygenation for 12 to 48 hours. At least 5 mm Hg of positive end-expiratory pressure (PEEP) is used routinely to prevent atelectasis. Endotracheal tube placement is monitored by auscultation and chest x-ray evaluation. It must be well-secured and movement minimized to protect the tracheal anastomosis. In addition, suctioning must be gentle, and, to avoid disruption of the suture line, the suction catheter is not advanced beyond the end of the tube. Small amounts of bloody secretions can be expected with suctioning, but overt hemoptysis can be a sign of dehiscence, which requires immediate attention. Patients are weaned from ventilatory support as soon as possible. The longer the period of intubation, the higher the risk of pneumonia.[46] After extubation, patients are encouraged to cough, deep-breathe, and ambulate at the bedside.

Pharmacologic support is similar to that used for heart transplantation. Isoproterenol is given to augment heart rate, and dopamine is used for inotropic support and renal vasodilation. Additional inotropic support is achieved with epinephrine if necessary. PGE_1 is administered primarily for pulmonary vasodilation, and sodium nitroprusside is given for its systemic vasodilatory properties. (∞Cardiac Drugs: Inotropic Vasodilators, p. 577.)

Immunosuppression. Initial immunosuppression usually does not include the use of methylprednisone. A single dose of methylprednisone usually is given in the operating room, and maintenance dosing begins within the first 2 weeks. The use of methylprednisone in the immediate postoperative period varies with institution. Daily steroid use is avoided for the first 2 to 3 weeks because of the deleterious effects on wound healing, especially the tracheal anastomosis.

Infection surveillance. Surveillance for infection and rejection in the HLT recipient is accomplished by bronchoscopy. This is performed initially at clinically determined or set intervals to monitor the tracheal anastomosis for evidence of healing, to obtain bronchoalveolar lavage washings for appropriate cultures, and to take biopsy specimens for the diagnosis of rejection. Bronchoscopic examination provides visual

BOX 47-6 NURSING DIAGNOSIS AND MANAGEMENT

HEART-LUNG TRANSPLANTATION

- Ineffective Airway Clearance related to excessive secretions or abnormal viscosity of mucus, p. 722
- Ineffective Breathing Pattern related to decreased lung expansion, p. 723
- Impaired Gas Exchange related to ventilation/perfusion mismatching or intrapulmonary shunting, p. 725
- Decreased Cardiac Output related to alterations in preload, p 590
- Decreased Cardiac Output related to alterations in afterload, p. 592
- Decreased Cardiac Output related to alterations in heart rate, p. 593
- Risk for Infection risk factor: immunosuppressive drugs required to prevent rejection of transplanted organ, p. 1216
- Body Image Disturbance related to actual change in body structure, function, or appearance, p. 87
- Anxiety related to threat to biologic, psychologic, and/or social integrity, p. 99
- Knowledge Deficit: Posttransplant Self-care Regimen, immunosuppressive drugs, cardiopulmonary drugs, diuretics, and clinical manifestations of infection related to lack of previous exposure to information, p. 61

evidence of tracheal anastomosis healing, which can determine the introduction of maintenance corticosteroids to the immunosuppressive regimen.[53]

As in the heart transplant recipient, presence of fever is an indication for aggressive evaluation. Sèrial chest roentgenograms are used to monitor for infiltrates. It is difficult, however, to distinguish infection from rejection by means of chest roentgenograms. Radiographic changes are used with other clinical evidence, the including $Pa{O_2}$ level, O_2 saturation, presence or absence of fever, and culture reports, to determine the course of action. Documented infections are treated with appropriate antibiotics.

Rejection surveillance. Rejection, which can be definitively diagnosed only by transbronchial biopsy, is graded by histologic findings of acute and chronic lung rejection (Box 47-7).[54] Pulmonary rejection is treated either by augmentation of immunosuppression or by pulses of intravenously administered corticosteroid. Augmentation may be in the form of increasing the cyclosporine dose to achieve a higher cyclosporine level, and/or increasing the azathioprine to lower the white blood cell (WBC) count, and/or increasing the

BOX 47-7 Standardized Pulmonary Biopsy Grading

GRADE	NOMENCLATURE
0	No significant abnormality
1	Minimal acute rejection (AR)
2	Mild AR
3	Moderate AR
4	Severe AR

maintenance prednisone dose slightly. Pulsing is the method of administering large doses of corticosteroids over a relatively short period of time. A common pulse of steroid is 1 g of Solu-Medrol every day for 3 consecutive days. Quick resolution of radiographic changes after the administration of steroid pulses provides a retrospective confirmation of the diagnosis of rejection. Procedural complications after bronchoscopic examination are a transient fever, fall in the $Pa{O_2}$ level, infection, and pneumothorax. Chest x-ray examination must follow each bronchoscopy to rule out pneumothorax.

Pulmonary function testing is a noninvasive method of assessing lung function and the presence of rejection. Lung denervation does not adversely affect the control of ventilation, at rest or during exercise.[55] Pulmonary function testing uses a wide range of parameters to measure the function of the lung at rest and during exercise. The functions are measured in percentages based on weight, gender, and age. The focus is usually on forced expiratory volume in 1 second (FEV_1), forced vital capacity (FVC), forced expiratory flow rate between 25% and 75% of FVC (FEF 25% to 75%), and the measurement of arterial blood gases. These functions are sensitive to slight changes in oxygenation and ventilation caused by infection or rejection. Acute changes in pulmonary function test (PFT) results and in $Pa{O_2}$ are indications for transbronchial biopsy.[53]

Heart rejection occurs less often in the HLT recipient. Thus endomyocardial biopsy is performed less often[56]; when required, the procedure is similar to that in the heart transplant recipient.

Long-Term Considerations

Chronic immunosuppression in the HLT patient carries the same consequences as it does in the heart transplant recipient. Accelerated graft atherosclerosis can be a late complication in HLT patients and follows a course similar to that in the heart recipient. A

BOX 47-8 Features of Obliterative Bronchiolitis

- Rapid rate of development; several months to 1 to 2 years
- Bronchitic symptoms followed by early development of dyspnea
- Distinct infiltrative component on chest film
- Severe obstructive and restrictive disease
- Decreased total lung capacity
- Largely irreversible with bronchodilator

major long-term complication in the pulmonary transplant patient is obliterative bronchiolitis (OB). Obliterative bronchiolitis is an inflammatory disorder of the small airways, which leads to obstruction and destruction of pulmonary bronchioles.[57] Features of obliterative bronchiolitis are listed in Box 47-8. Obliterative bronchiolitis may represent a manifestation of chronic pulmonary allograft rejection.[58] The only treatment for end-stage obliterative bronchiolitis is retransplantation. Retransplantation in the HLT group carries a high risk for complications related to infection, delayed healing as a result of steroids, renal insufficiency related to chronic cyclosporine use, and bleeding from scarring from the previous surgery.

CMV is also a significant threat to the lung transplant recipient. Prophalaxis and treatment of CMV disease is similar to that for heart recipients, however, institutions vary regarding anti-CMV agents and duration of prophylaxis and treatment.[31–34]

Heart-lung transplantation has increased annually for 10 years. In 1995 69 HLTs were performed in the United States. The number of patients listed as candidates in the same year was cited as 208.[44] National 1-year survival for HLT was 60.8%,[44] which closely parallels international survival rates. The limited donor pool remains the major factor limiting the number of HLTs performed.

SINGLE- AND DOUBLE-LUNG TRANSPLANTATION

Single-lung transplantation (SLT) is an alternative to HLT in a select group of patients. Transplant teams have explored, modified, and successfully pursued the development of pulmonary transplantation. Indications for single-lung ransplantation are similar to those listed for HLT, with some exceptions. Pulmonary diseases that typically are associated with chronic lung infections, such as cystic fibrosis and bronchiectasis, require transplantation of both lungs because of the risk of cross contamination. In addition, severe cardiac disease mandates heart replacement.[45] Thorough evaluation of cardiac function is essential to the success of SLT. Contraindications to SLT parallel those for HLT (see Box 47-4). Advantages to SLT are better use of donor resources, decreased operative risks, and decreased short- and long-term complications (Box 47-9).

BOX 47-9 Advantages of Single-Lung Transplantation

- One lung donor provides organs for two lung recipients
- Increased donor availability
- Decreased recipient waiting time
- Decreased need for intraoperative cardiopulmonary bypass
- Potential shorter recovery and hospital stay
- Preservation of native heart
- Heart rejection avoided
- Accelerated graft atherosclerosis not as prevalent

Single-lung transplantation is covered under DRG 75: major chest procedures. The anticipated length of stay is 12.4 days.[18]

Surgical Procedure

Considerations in choosing lung transplantation include the specific disease process, the need for cardiac repair, and donor availability. Transplantation contralateral to a previous thoracotomy is preferable to avoid adhesions that require further surgical dissection.[45] The left lung is preferred because it is easier to expose and has a longer left main bronchus. The longer bronchus gives the surgeon more flexibility in trimming the suture site as needed for anastomosis.[59] If there is a significant disproportion of ventilation and perfusion to one side, then transplantation of the worse side may be the preferred option.[46]

Use of cardiopulmonary bypass (CPB) depends on the disease process. Patients with pulmonary hypertension usually require CPB, whereas patients with pulmonary fibrosis or emphysema do not.[59] Surgical intervention first requires the removal of the diseased lung. The pulmonary artery is then divided, and the pulmonary vein is mobilized. Donor and recipient arteries are trimmed to suitable lengths, and an end-to-end anastomosis is performed. Bronchial anasto-

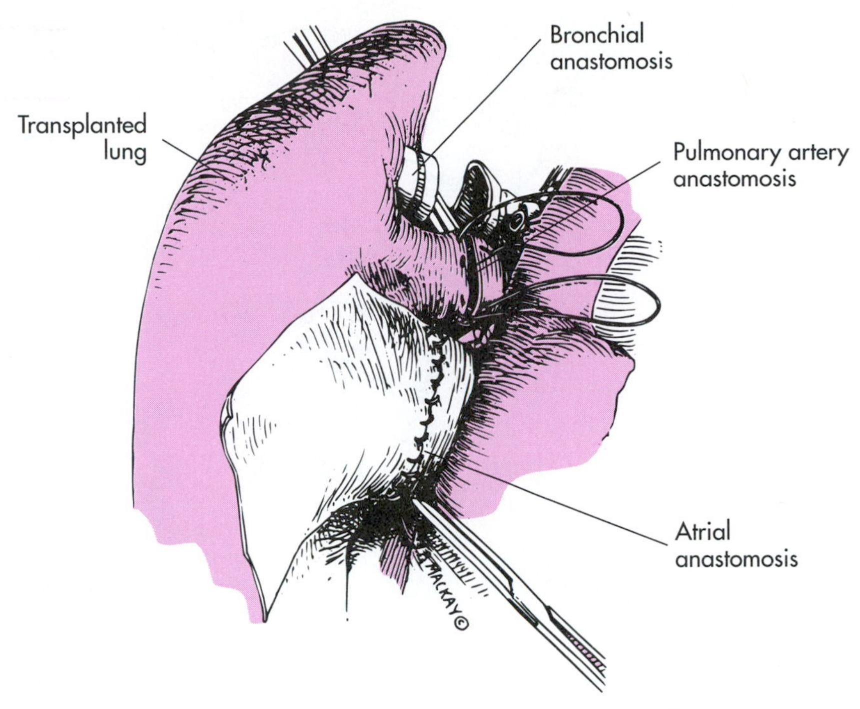

FIGURE 47-7. Single-lung transplant: surgical procedure. (Modified from Baumgartner WA, Reitz BA, Achuff SC, editors: *Heart and heart-lung transplantation,* Philadelphia, 1990, WB Saunders.)

mosis is performed with a running suture. After the atrial clamp is slowly removed, the patient is assessed for bleeding[46,59] (Figure 47-7). In some transplant centers the omentum is brought through the diaphragm from the abdomen and is wrapped around the bronchus for added stability of the anastomosis and increased vascular supply. Disadvantages of this maneuver include a larger incision and involvement of the abdominal cavity.[46]

Lung volume reduction is a relatively new surgical procedure that may be an option for lung transplant candidates. Although the procedure does not result in better lung function than from transplantation, it does avoid immunosuppression- and transplant-related complications. It may be an early option for patients who may require lung transplant in the future.[59,60]

Double- or Bilateral-Lung Transplant

A double-lung transplant may be performed for clinical conditions such as cystic fibrosis, pulmonary fibrosis or bronchiectasis. In these situations the native heart remains healthy but the lungs are diseased. The surgical technique involves removal of the heart-lung block from the donor. The heart is transplanted into one recipient (see Figure 47-5), and the lungs are transplanted into another recipient (Figure 47-8). The surgical anastomosis sites are the back wall of the atria (the back wall of the left atrium contains the four pulmonary vein orifices), the trachea, and the main pulmonary artery.

Double-lung transplant is covered under DRG 75: major chest procedures. The anticipated length of stay is 12.4 days.[18]

Postoperative Medical and Nursing Management

Postoperative care of the single/double lung transplant recipient is similar to that of HLT patients, as described in the previous discussion. Several nursing diagnosis are associated with care of the single and double lung transplant patient, as listed in Box 47-10. SLT patients generally require mechanical ventilation of shorter duration. Less bleeding can be anticipated because of the brevity of the surgical procedure. A single pleural chest tube usually is sufficient for drainage. A pulmonary artery catheter may be used to measure right ventricular response when significant ventilation/perfusion (V/Q) mismatch occurs. In the event of elevated pulmonary artery pressures, pharmacologic vasodilation or afterload reduction can be instituted. Patients with pulmonary hypertension potentially may have a greater V/Q mismatch, resulting in larger A-aO_2 gradients.[59]

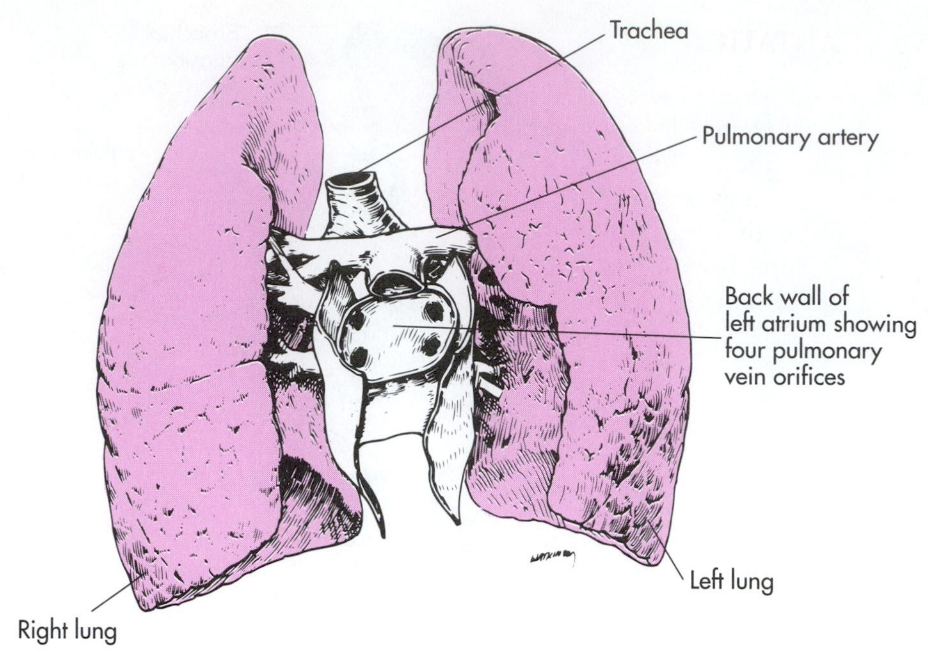

FIGURE 47-8. Double-lung transplant graft before implantation into a recipient. (Modified from Baumgartner WA, Reitz BA, Achuff SC, editors: *Heart and heart-lung transplantation,* Philadelphia, 1990, WB Saunders.)

BOX 47-10 NURSING DIAGNOSIS AND MANAGEMENT

SINGLE- AND DOUBLE-LUNG TRANSPLANTATION

- Ineffective Airway Clearance related to excessive secretions or abnormal viscosity of mucus, p. 722
- Impaired Gas Exchange related to ventilation/perfusion mismatching or intrapulmonary shunting, p. 725
- Risk for Infection risk factors: immunosuppressive drugs required to prevent rejection of transplanted organ, p. 1216
- Body Image Disturbance related to actual change in body structure, function, or appearance, p. 87
- Anxiety related to threat to biologic, psychologic, and/or social integrity, p. 99
- Knowledge Deficit: Posttransplant Self-care Regimen, immunosuppressive drugs, cardiopulmonary drugs, diuretics, and clinical manifestations of infection related to lack of previous exposure to information p. 61

Immunosuppression for lung recipients is essentially the same as that for HLT patients. Initiation of steroids depends on institutional preference and healing of the bronchial anastomosis.

Surveillance of rejection and infection is similar to that in HLT. Pulmonary function testing is not initiated until the second or third week postoperatively to allow for surgical recovery.[62] Decreased lung function because of fluid shifts, microatelectasis, and splinting from incisional pain would interfere with accurate testing. Unlike HLT, in unilateral lung transplantation the transplanted lung functions in parallel with the native lung, which can be expected to retain any pathology.[61] The patient must be measured by a comparison with his or her own baseline and not with normal standards. This concept also can be applied to the immediate postoperative period of intubation during the evaluation of arterial blood gases. Oxygenation and ventilation occur in both the diseased and transplanted lungs, and parameters for evaluation need to be adjusted accordingly. Clinically, SLT recipients function as well as other patients with only one lung. With physical exertion, some patients may complain of shortness of breath. A combination of chest roentgenogram, bronchoscopic examination, and pulmonary function testing is used in the detection and diagnosis of rejection and infection.

Long-term outcome for lung transplant parallels that for HLT. One-year survival for patients with SLT is quoted at 71.6% (+/-1.0)[44] as a national figure. International statistics compare equally. In 1995, 1,923 SLT candidates were listed with the United Network for Organ Sharing (UNOS) and 863 patients received transplants.[29]

LIVER TRANSPLANTATION

Liver transplantation was first attempted in canine models in the 1950s. The outcomes were unsuccessful because of technical complications, infection, and graft failure.[63,64] The effort to improve surgical technique continued, and successful liver transplantation in dogs was achieved several years later by both Moore and others,[65,66] and Starzl and others.[67] In 1963 Starzl and colleagues performed the first human liver transplant operation.[68] Although the patient died intraoperatively, this attempt pioneered the possibility of liver transplantation in human beings.

The first successful human liver transplant was performed in 1967, also by Starzl and his co-workers,[69] in a patient with malignant hepatoma. The patient survived 1 year before succumbing to recurrent disease. Patient 1-year survival rates in the late 1960s and throughout the 1970s remained less than 50% despite continued improvements in the surgical techniques. These early attempts were hindered by difficulty of the surgery, poor methods of organ preservation, and inadequate immunosuppression.

Cyclosporine clinical trials began in 1979 and revolutionized liver transplantation. One-year survival rates in the early 1980s increased to 70% and higher.[70,71] This improvement in survival rates prompted the National Institutes of Health (NIH) to declare that liver transplantation was no longer experimental, but rather an accepted therapeutic modality for patients with end-stage liver disease.[72] This position statement by the NIH resulted in an increase in the number of liver transplant centers worldwide and in the number of liver transplants as well. Each year more liver transplants are being performed than in the previous year. According to United Network of Organ Sharing, in the United States less than 200 liver transplants were performed in 1983, more than 1000 in 1987,[73] more than 2000 in 1989, and more than 3600 in 1994.[74]

Indications and Selection

Liver transplantation must be considered for any patient who suffers from irreversible acute or chronic liver disease that is progressive and has no therapy of established efficacy. Diseases of the liver may be categorized as chronic, vascular, fulminant or subfulminant, inborn errors of metabolism, and hepatic malignancies. Box 47-11 lists diseases seen in patients undergoing liver transplantation. These are not all inclusive but the most common. As of 1995, in the United States, the most prevalent indications for liver transplantation in adults were alcoholic cirrhosis and chronic viral hepatitis (B and C), which accounted for more than 47% of the cases.[75] In the pediatric population, biliary atresia and metabolic disorders account for more than 70% of the diseases leading to transplantation.[75]

Candidate selection is an important aspect of transplantation. Given the shortage of available organs, the transplant team must have a reasonable assurance of a successful outcome. Timing of transplantation is of utmost importance. The patient must not be so ill as to be unable to survive the surgery but is experiencing deterioration in the quality of life. In general, liver transplantation is not be offered to those persons who (1) would not likely survive major surgery; (2) would not survive the effects of long-term immunosuppression; (3) have a disease that is likely to recur quickly and fatally after transplantation; or (4) are not willing to comply with long-term, sometimes even difficult

BOX 47-11 Diseases Commonly Treated With Liver Transplantation

- Cholestatic liver diseases
  - Biliary atresia
  - Primary sclerosing cholangitis
  - Primary biliary cirrhosis
- Chronic hepatocellular diseases
  - Viral hepatitis (types A, B, C, D, E)
  - Alcoholic liver disease (Läennec's)
  - Autoimmune hepatitis
  - Cryptogenic cirrhosis
  - Drug-induced liver disease
- Vascular diseases
  - Budd-Chiari syndrome
  - Venoocclusive disease
- Fulminant and subfulminant hepatic failure
  - Viral hepatitis (types A, B, C, D, E)
  - Drug-induced (acetaminophen, isoniazid overdoses)
  - Fulminant Wilson's disease
- Inborn metabolic disorders
  - Wilson's disease
  - Alpha$_1$-antitrypsin deficiency
  - Hemochromatosis
  - Tyrosinemia
  - Glycogen storage disease, Types I and II
- Primary hepatic malignancies
  - Hepatocellular carcinoma
  - Hemangioendothelioma
  - Hepatoblastoma

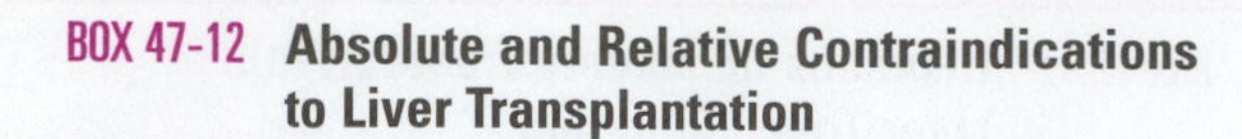

BOX 47-12 Absolute and Relative Contraindications to Liver Transplantation

ABSOLUTE

Brain death
Metastatic malignancies
Extrahepatic malignancy
Active drug or alcohol abuse
Advanced cardiopulmonary disease
Acquired immune deficiency syndrome
Extrahepatic sepsis

RELATIVE

Physiologic age
Advanced renal disease
Multiple hepatic malignancies
Moderate cardiopulmonary disease
Peripheral vascular disease
Psychosocial behaviors indicating noncompliance to medical regimens

and demanding medical regimens. The absolute contraindications in Box 47-12, fall under these four considerations.

Having one relative contraindication may not rule out transplantation, but having several may predict poor outcome. Chronologic age is less important than physiologic age. Reports of transplantation in the older population conclude with favorable results.[76] Certain diseases can recur after transplantation, such as viral hepatitis,[77,78] sclerosing cholangitis,[79] biliary malignancies,[80] and others. In the case of viral hepatitis, serologic indicators of replication of virus are followed closely. In the presence of aggressively replicating virus, and in certain malignancies, it is in the patient's best interest not to proceed to transplantation because it would actually hasten his or her demise. Multicenter protocols are important in evaluating outcomes and efficacies when performing transplantations in patients with diseases that recur. The decision to offer liver transplantation to any patient must be based on evaluation criteria, which vary among institutions and which will be modified as advances in technical ability, immunosuppression, and perioperative management continue.

Liver transplant is covered under DRG 480. The anticipated length of stay is 31.2 days.[18]

Recipient evaluation. The candidate for liver transplant undergoes a thorough evaluation to determine the etiology and severity of the liver disease, to establish the need for transplantation versus others interventions, and to identify objective indications and contraindications. Evaluation begins with a carefully elicited patient history (Box 47-13). A comprehensive approach includes laboratory, radiographic, and diagnostic testing and multidisciplinary consultations (Box 47-14). Not every patient undergoes every test and consult. Careful history taking and a good physical examination will direct the initial diagnostic testing. For instance, a patient with a past history of malignancy would undergo extensive testing to rule out metastases, whereas a patient with fulminant hepatic failure may have a more abbreviated work up that is focused on determining etiology and potential for hepatic recovery.

BOX 47-13 Pretransplant Patient History

Risk factors for viral hepatitis:

Transfusions, IV drug abuse, tattoos, other parenteral exposure

Family history of liver disease

Associated disorders:

Hypothyroidism, osteoporosis, infertility, arthritis

Onset, duration, and description of symptoms/complications:

Jaundice, lethargy, bleeding disorders, pruritus, confusion, ascites, edema, melanotic stools, abdominal pain, bone pain or fractures, chronic diarrhea, gynecomastia (in men), amenorrhea

Current and past medical histories:

Hospitalizations, surgeries

Social history:

Exposure to alcohol, drugs, toxins, use of tobacco products

Status of immunizations

During the work up, the candidate and his or her support systems are evaluated by the entire transplant team: the surgeon, hepatologist, nurse coordinator, social worker, dietitian, and financial counselor. Other services, such as cardiology, nephrology, psychiatry, gynecology, anesthesia, infectious disease, endocrinology, hematology, rheumatology, and oral surgery or dentistry may also be included in the evaluation. Ideally, all immunizations are brought up to date in an attempt

BOX 47-14 Sample of a Pretransplant Evaluation for Liver Transplantation

Laboratory tests:
- Blood: liver function profiles: transaminases (AST, ALT, GGT); alkaline phosphatase; bilirubin; albumin; prothrombin time; partial thromboplastin time; clotting factors; cholesterol; triglycerides
- Renal function profile with electrolytes: blood urea nitrogen, creatinine, sodium, potassium, carbon dioxide, chloride
- Hematology: CBC, reticulocytes, eosinophile sedimentation rate
- Thyroid function: T_3RIA; T_4RIA; thyroid stimulating hormone; T_4, T_3 uptake
- Serologies for hepatic viruses and other infectious diseases: viral hepatitis (A, B, C, D, E); cytomegalovirus, Epstein-Barr virus, herpes I and II, parvovirus, RPR, HIV
- Blood type and antibody screen
- Immunologic profiles: antinuclear antibody; antimitochondrial antibody; anti-smooth muscle antibody; immunoglobulins (A, G, M)
- Nutritional profiles: vitamin levels (A, D, E, B_{12}, folate); iron studies with ferritin
- Tumor markers: alpha-fetoprotein, CEA, PSA, CA 19-9
- Miscellaneous: ceruloplasmin, alpha$_1$-antitrypsin level and phenotype
- Urine: 24-hour protein and electrolytes, cultures, creatinine clearance, urinalysis, copper
- Stool: ova, cysts, parasites, occult blood, 48-hour fecal fats, cultures
- Gastrointestinal work up: endoscopy, colonoscopy, endoscopic retrograde cholangiopancreatography, liver biopsy
- Pulmonary profile: arterial blood gases, pulmonary function studies
- Radiographic and diagnostic tests: chest x-ray, ultrasound of liver including vascular
- Other optional tests: Doppler studies; sinus x-ray; computerized tomography (abdomen, chest, head); electrocardiogram; echocardiogram; cardiac stress test; cardiac catheterization; mammogram; peripheral vascular studies; carotid ultrasound; abdominal angiography; percutaneous cholangiogram; bone mineral density

AST, Aspartate transaminase; *ALT,* alanine aminotransferase; *GGT,* γ-glutamyltransferase; *T_3RIA*; serum triiodothyronine (T_3); *T_4RIA*, serum triiodothyronine (T_4); *RPR,* rapid plasma reagin; *CEA,* carcinoembryonic agents; *PSA,* prostate-specific antigen; *CA 19-9,* investigational cancer antigen.

to minimize postoperative infections. The patient and family receive education regarding the evaluation, transplant waiting list, surgery, postoperative management including immunosuppression, and long-term follow-up. At the conclusion of the evaluation, one of several outcomes is possible: (1) the patient is deemed a transplant candidate, (2) the patient is not a candidate, or (3) the patient may be a candidate some time in the future if certain criteria are met. These criteria may be of a physical nature (i.e., it is too early in the disease process to list now, in which case the patient will be followed at certain intervals). The criteria may also be of a psychosocial nature (i.e., the patient must attend a formal rehabilitation program or undergo treatment of depression).

After candidacy has been determined and the patient is ready for transplantation, his or her social security number is entered into the national computer system operated by UNOS. Status on the list is determined by objective criteria based on blood type, weight, patient urgency, and time on the list. Now, one of the most difficult phases begins—the waiting period. It is not possible to anticipate when an appropriate organ will become available. Thus the patient may feel his or her life is being put "on hold." Because of the shortage of donors, it is not uncommon for the patient in the critical care unit to die awaiting transplantation; this is especially true for pediatric recipients. And knowing that another must die so that he or she may live can cause feelings of guilt as the patient hopes for a liver to become available. In addition, the patient with end-stage liver disease knows that the only alternative to transplant is death. It is therefore important for the patient and family to receive ongoing psychosocial assessment and to attend pretransplant support groups, which are available at most transplant centers.

Pretransplant phase. The patient with end-stage liver disease awaiting transplant may be one of the most challenging to care for in the critical care unit. Hepatic encephalopathy, coagulopathies, portal hypertension, severe fluid and electrolyte imbalances, cardiac compromise, and renal deterioration are not uncommon. Frequent mental status assessments are important in determining continued candidacy for transplant. Hepatic encephalopathy may improve with administration of antibiotics and laxatives or may proceed to Stage IV coma, in which case diagnostic studies may be needed to evaluate the possibility of intracranial bleed. Patients who have chronic liver disease also have nutritional deficits. They require supplements of the fat-soluble vitamins (A, D, E, and K), may be on protein restrictions to reduce serum ammonia levels, and may experience severe muscle wasting.

Consequences of portal hypertension must be corrected. Gastrointestinal hemorrhage from varices may respond to administration of propranolol or sclerotherapy. Patients with massive ascites usually have total body fluid overload but are intravascularly contracted and require sodium restriction and administration of colloidal fluids, such as albumin, along with diuretics. Careful documentation of fluid intake and output, daily weights, and frequent vital signs is needed to monitor fluid status. Ascites may require paracentesis or, if refractory to all other treatments, surgery (LeVeen or Denver shunts). Portal hypertension may be reduced by transjugular intrahepatic portosystemic shunting (TIPS) in interventional radiology. If this is unsuccessful, the patient may need to undergo surgical intervention with a vascular shunt created between the portacaval system and the mesangial, splenic, or renal vascular systems.

Spontaneous bacterial peritonitis (SBP) can be manifested in the end-stage liver patient by an acute demise in the hepatic and renal function, accompanied by fever, abdominal pain, and hepatic encephalopathy. Paracentesis will show increased white blood cells with or without a positive fluid culture. Patients are treated aggressively with antibiotics and are temporarily deferred from transplantation during treatment for and recovery from SBP.

Determining donor suitability. The two criteria necessary for matching a donor liver to a recipient are blood type and body size. Human lymphocyte antigen (HLA) tissue typing is not used in the matching of donor livers because this has not been shown to significantly affect patient outcomes. Donors are carefully screened for infectious diseases and metastatic carcinomas because these can be transmitted to the recipient. The transplant center is notified by an Organ Procurement Organization (a regional agency that is a member of UNOS) that a liver is available. If the organ is accepted, the patient is contacted by the transplant team. In very urgent situations the donor blood type may not be compatible with the recipient's, for example, an A donor and an O recipient. Despite this incompatibility, liver transplantation can be successful. There may be some early postoperative complications, such as mild hemolysis, but long-term follow-up of patients with ABO incompatibility has been favorable.[81]

Once a donor liver becomes available, it is necessary to expedite the preoperative preparation of the recipient. The use of University of Wisconsin (UW) preservation solution has allowed for longer cold ischemia time (the length of time an organ is removed from the donor, flushed, and packed in ice). However, some statistics have shown that cold ischemia times of greater than 12 hours correlated with increased recipient morbidity and mortality.[82]

Surgical Procedure

Liver transplant surgery is lengthy and technically difficult, often lasting 8 to 12 hours. The procedure involves the combined efforts of surgeons; anesthesiologists; nurse anesthetists; operating room nurses and technicians; perfusionists; and personnel from the blood bank and laboratory and radiology departments, to name a few. The patient is taken to the operating room for anesthesia induction, insertion of large bore intravenous catheters that allow high-volume fluid infusion, and insertion of a pulmonary artery catheter for hemodynamic monitoring. Other devices such as an arterial line, a nasogastric tube, and a urinary drainage catheter are also inserted. The patient is positioned on the operating room table in such a way as to minimize pressure that may cause ischemia and chronic injury to tissue and peripheral nerves.

The surgery can be divided into three stages: (1) recipient hepatectomy, (2) vascular anastomoses with donor liver, and (3) biliary anastomosis. The longest and most difficult part of the surgery is removal of the native liver, stage 1. It is complicated even more by coagulopathies, adhesions, portal hypertension, and venous collaterals. Before completion of this stage the patient may be put on venovenous bypass (Figure 47-9). A centrifugal pump cycles the blood out via iliac and portal vein cannulas and returns it to the central circulation via the axillary or subclavian vein. Bypass accomplishes (1) improved perfusion of intestines, kidneys, and lower extremities by decreasing engorgement of blood in these organs; (2) improved hemodynamic stability by improving venous return and therefore cardiac output; and (3) fewer bleeding complications during the anhepatic phase. Other advances in surgical techniques, anesthesia, and fluid management have improved enough to warrant not using venovenous bypass on all transplants. Patients not put on bypass may have slower return of intestinal function.

Stage 2 comprises the four vascular anastomoses: suprahepatic inferior vena cava, infrahepatic vena cava, hepatic artery, and portal vein. Venovenous bypass is removed after the infrahepatic vena caval anastomosis and before the hepatic artery anastomosis.

Stage 3, biliary anastomosis, can be achieved in two ways: choledochojejunostomy (bile duct to jejunum)

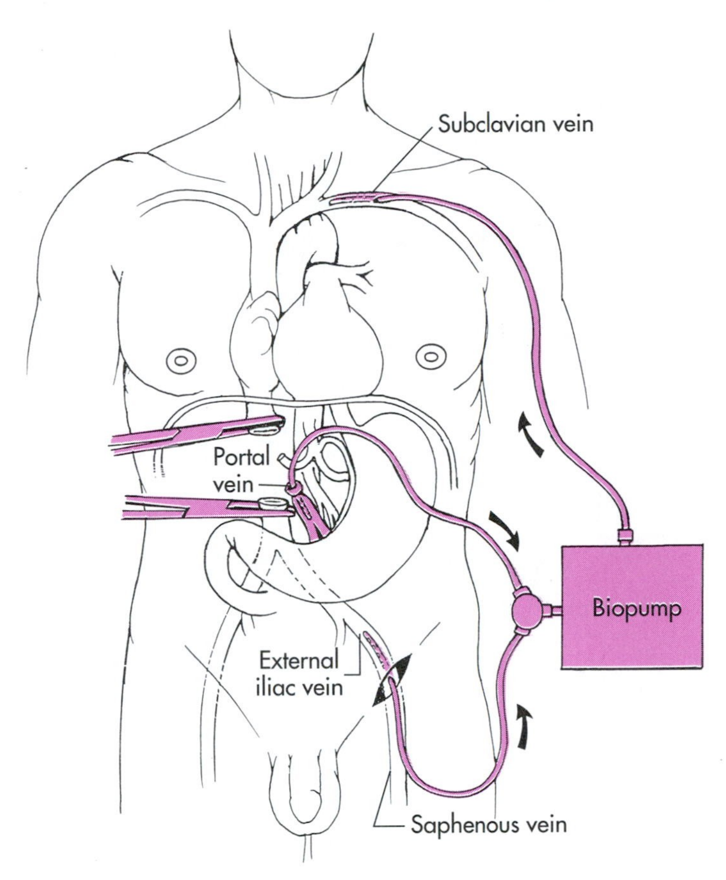

FIGURE 47-9. Venovenous bypass during removal of the native liver. The portal and iliac veins are cannulated and blood is circulated via a centrifugal pump to the subclavian vein.

and choledochocholedochostomy (bile duct to bile duct). Choledochojejunostomy is done in patients with diseased bile ducts such as those with biliary atresia or sclerosing cholangitis. It is also known as a Roux-en-Y procedure and is shown in Figure 47-10. The choledochocholedochostomy is performed when the patient has a healthy and intact common bile duct and is shown in Figure 47-11. The patient returns from surgery with or without an external stent or T-tube. These tubes are connected to a bag into which bile drains. Patients who do not have external stents may have an internal stent inserted across the biliary anastomosis. Eventually, the internal stent moves and is passed with the stool.

Postoperative Medical and Nursing Management

The common nursing diagnoses associated with liver transplantation are listed in Box 47-15. The patient arrives in the critical care unit unreversed from anesthesia. Immediate goals include (1) reestablishment of normal body temperature, (2) hemodynamic stabilization, and (3) maintenance of an effective airway. Postoperative hypothermia is common after an orthotopic liver transplant (OLT). The critical care nurse must achieve rewarming safely by methods such as using warming blankets, heating lamps, and head covers. Hemodynamic stabilization is a particular challenge, because the patient may arrive hypervolemic, euvolemic, or hypovolemic and also be hypersensitive or hypotensive. Assessment of total body fluids versus intravascular fluid status is important. Accurate measurements of hemodynamic function, such as arterial blood pressure, peripheral blood pressure, central venous pressure (CVP) pulmonary artery pressure (PAP), pulmonary artery wedge pressure (PAWP), urinary output, drains, and bile totals, are done frequently to assess true volume status. Choice of replacement fluid and pharmacologic agent for correcting volume and blood pressure abnormalities is transplant-center specific. These protocols vary as to use of albumin or fresh frozen plasma and use of intravenous renal dose dopamine or prostaglandin, as well as other agents and solutions. But the goals are all the same: optimize tissue perfusion and deliver oxygen to all tissues, especially the newly transplanted graft.

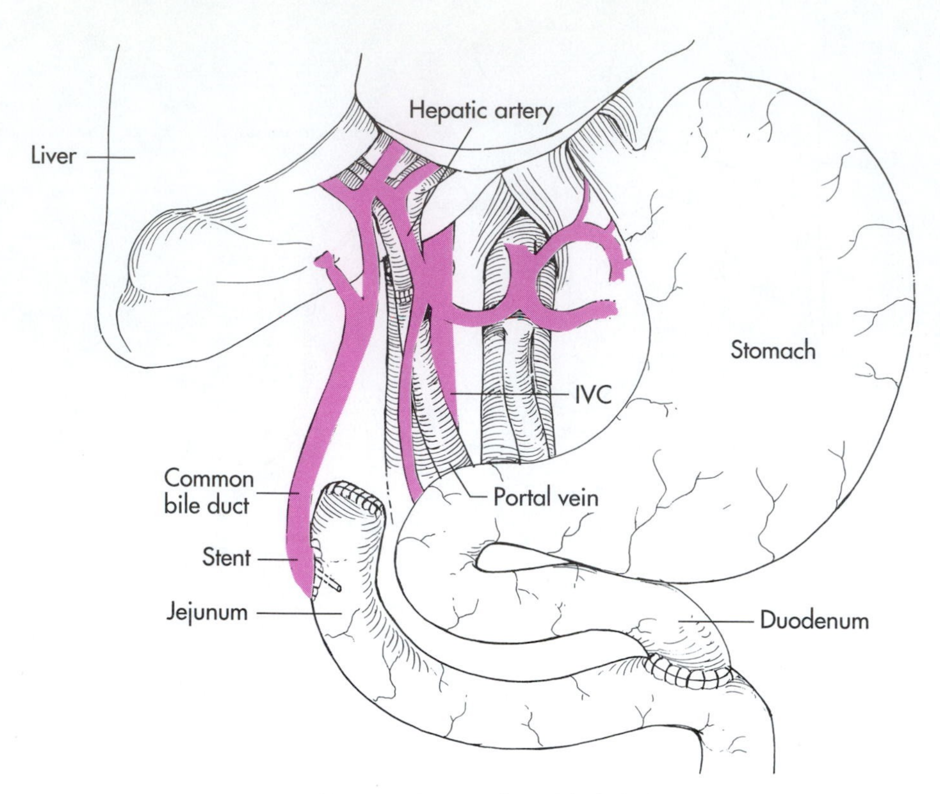

FIGURE 47-10. Roux-en-Y procedure (choledochojejunostomy).

Electrolyte abnormalities can occur after OLT. Disturbances in potassium and magnesium are common. High serum levels are usually associated with renal impairment; low levels can be the result of drug side effects, such as diuretic therapy. The patient may also be hypernatremic or hyponatremic, which will complicate correction of volume status and replacement fluids.

Ventilatory support of the patient is maintained until anesthesia has been cleared by the new liver and the patient awakens. Frequent measurement of arterial blood gas levels, continuous pulse oximetry, and assessment of breath sounds are needed. The patient may require changes in ventilatory settings, suctioning to remove secretions, or administration of pharmacologic agents to correct acid-base imbalances. Pulmonary complications are common, as listed in Box 47-16. After extubation, patients must be encouraged to perform incentive spirometry exercises and to turn, cough, and deep breathe frequently to help prevent atelectasis and pneumonia. Respiratory treatments with bronchodilators, prophylactic antimicrobials, and chest physiotherapy may also be used.

Management of coagulopathies is important in the early postoperative phase. Characterization and careful measurement of drain lines and drainage from incisions are needed along with other nursing assessments of blood loss, such as signs of hypovolemia, tachypnea, tachycardia, or poor peripheral oxygenation. A sudden increase in measurement of abdominal girth, sanguineous nasogastric output, and black tarry stools are hallmarks of bleeding problems and must be reported immediately. Laboratory monitoring to assess blood loss and coagulopathies includes hematocrit, hemoglobin, platelet count, prothrombin time, partial thromboplastin time, fibrinogen, and fibrin split products. Reversal of coagulopathies is done judiciously with consideration for the potential to thrombose newly anastomosed blood vessels in the liver. Blood products, such as platelets, fresh frozen plasma and specific factors, can be given along with pharmacologic agents such as vitamin K.

Neurologic assessment of the patient is important in the early postoperative phase to determine mental status and graft function. Patients who preoperatively were encephalopathic will generally be slower to clear mentally. But with good hepatic function, the patient should be alert and oriented within 1 to 2 days. Neurologic assessment can also be influenced by certain pharmacologic agents, including the immunosuppressants, which can cause both peripheral and central neurologic side effects. The critical care nurse must al-

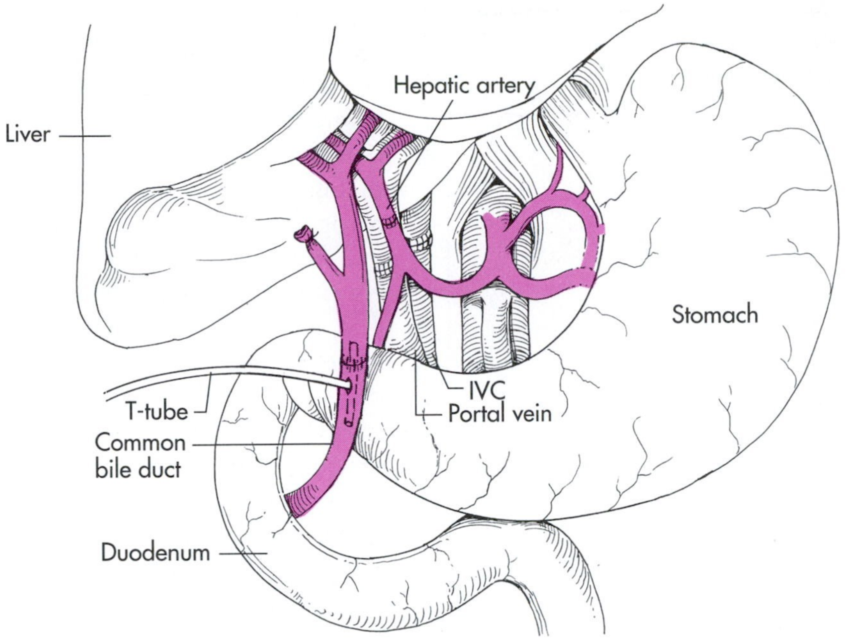

FIGURE 47-11. Choledocholedochostomy procedure.

BOX 47-15 NURSING DIAGNOSIS AND MANAGEMENT

LIVER TRANSPLANTATION

- Risk for Infection risk factor: immunosuppressive drugs required to prevent rejection of the transplanted liver, p. 1216
- Altered Nutrition: Less Than Body Requirements related to lack of exogenous nutrients or increased metabolic demand, p. 165
- Fluid Volume Deficit related to absolute loss, p. 914
- Body Image Disturbance related to actual change in body, structure, function or appearance, p. 87
- Anxiety related to threat to biologic, psychologic, and/or social integrity, p. 99
- Knowledge Deficit: Posttransplant Self-care Regimen, immunosuppressive drugs and clinical manifestations of infection related to lack of previous exposure to information, p. 61

ways be aware of the potential for intracranial bleeds in a patient who has coagulopathies, serum sodium imbalances, and hemodynamic instability. All of these can interfere with pain management, since pharmacologic agents can mask deterioration in mental status. Medications to relieve pain are administered, but other non-pharmacologic nursing interventions must also be used.

Renal function can be altered after a liver transplant because of acute tubular necrosis, intrinsic renal disease, or poor hepatic function. Some studies estimate 21% to 73% of OLT patients develop renal failure.[83] Patients are managed with attention to fluid and electrolyte imbalances; avoidance of nephrotoxic drugs; and occasionally, ultrafiltration or hemodialysis. With good hepatic function, renal function usually improves.

Immunosuppressive therapy places the transplant patient at an increased risk of infection. Infectious complications continue to be the leading cause of death in the OLT patient,[84-87] and the potential for infection is greatest when patients receive high doses of immunosuppressants. Good handwashing techniques and universal precautions must be practiced by all persons who come into contact with the transplantation patient throughout the hospitalization. Infections are treated with appropriate antimicrobials specific to the invading organism. Prophylactic therapies are commonly used as well.[88]

Careful attention to any external biliary drain line is important. Biliary complications can occur after OLT.[89] The critical care nurse documents color, character, and amount of biliary drainage and reports any changes. Biliary and other complications after OLT are listed in Box 47-16.

Posttransplant assessment of hepatic function. Serum aspartate aminotransferase (AST) (formerly SGOT), alanine aminotransferase (ALT) (formerly SGPT),

BOX 47-16 Common Complications After Liver Transplant

PULMONARY COMPLICATIONS

Pleural effusion
Pulmonary edema
Pneumonia
Pneumothorax or hemothorax
Atelectasis
Paralysis of right diaphragm

BILIARY COMPLICATIONS

Leaks
Strictures
Obstruction
Infection (cholangitis)
Breakdown of anastomosis

GASTROINTESTINAL COMPLICATIONS

Bleeding/ulceration
Infections (cytomegalovirus, *Candida*, *Clostridium difficile*)
Bowel perforations

VASCULAR COMPLICATIONS

Hepatic artery thrombosis
Portal vein thrombosis
Vena caval thrombosis
Peripheral and/or central line sepsis
Hepatic vein thrombosis

alkaline phosphatase, and gamma glutamyltransferase (GGT), serum bilirubin, and prothrombin times are the standard laboratory measures used to follow graft function. In the first few postoperative days, the serum levels may continue to rise before peaking and subsequently falling. The patient with suspected primary nonfunction of the graft will continue to demonstrate (1) hemodynamic instability, (2) progressive renal deterioration, (3) increasing coagulopathies and serum liver function laboratory tests, (4) hypoglycemia, (5) continued ventilatory dependency, and (6) an inability to awaken from anesthesia. Continued nonfunction of the graft will necessitate relisting the patient for another donor liver. If the patient is expected to be intubated longer than several days, total parenteral nutrition may be started.

Early signs of optimal graft function include improving renal function, mental alertness, a high to normal serum glucose, and early extubation. The serum ALT, AST, GGT, and alkaline phosphatase may peak on the third or fourth day but will subsequently decrease thereafter. The serum bilirubin may take 1 week before beginning to fall, and may have a mild elevation when the biliary drainage tube is clamped. Early mobilization and physical therapy are encouraged. The nasogastric tube is removed when its output is minimal, bowel sounds return, and the patient is extubated. Nutrition may begin orally or by feeding tube. The diet is slowly advanced as tolerated. Central line catheters and arterial lines are removed. The urinary catheter is removed as soon as the patient is awake enough to be continent. Drain lines are removed as drainage outputs become minimal. As the patient begins to participate in self-care, plans are made to transfer the patient out of the critical care unit to the transplant nursing unit.

During the post-critical care unit phase, laboratory data and vital signs continue to be monitored on a routine basis. Increasing levels of physical therapy are encouraged, diet is advanced, and much of the nurse's effort is directed at patient education and discharge planning. Discharge booklets are helpful in the education process. It is important for the patient to learn how to self-administer medications, monitor vital signs, care for incision and T-tube (if present), prevent infections, and identify problems that must promptly receive medical attention. Since it is not uncommon for patients to be discharged within 2 weeks after an OLT, it is important for discharge instructions to begin as soon as the patient is mentally alert. Patients discharged early may require home health nurse referrals to assist with follow-up of incisional care, intravenous therapies, and more.

Rejection surveillance. Acute rejection in OLT is a cellular-mediated event and is suspected any time the serum liver function laboratory tests become elevated over the previous levels. Sometimes the patient also exhibits fever, a drop in bile output (if a T-tube is still connected to a drainage bag), and a change in the color and viscosity of the bile. At first the patient may not have any other physical symptoms, but eventually malaise may occur and the urine may darken and stools become clay-colored. With the onset of an elevation in laboratory levels, a liver biopsy is usually scheduled. Acute rejection can occur anytime after transplant, but most commonly it occurs in the first few months and even as early as 1 week. The majority of liver transplant patients experience at least one acute rejection episode. Treatment of acute rejection requires increasing immunosuppression (i.e., steroids, monoclonal or polyclonal antilymphocyte antibodies, or other newer pharmacologic agents). Immunosuppressant protocols vary from center to center and are usually very successful at reversing acute rejection.[90]

Chronic rejection is a humoral event and is progressive and nonreversible. Chronic rejection in a liver transplant patient usually requires retransplantation if the patient is still considered a candidate.

Long-Term Follow-Up

Unless the OLT patient lives in the same city, after discharge from the hospital, he or she usually remains in the immediate area of the transplant center before returning home. During this period the patient may be followed by a home health nurse and is also seen in clinic several times a week by the transplant team. Continued serologic testing is done to monitor graft function, to determine blood levels of certain immunosuppressive agents, and to monitor for postoperative complications. While many of these complications can be managed successfully in the outpatient setting, readmissions do occur. Since rejections, readmissions, grieving for the donor, and pharmacologic side effects can create anxiety for the family and the patient, they are encouraged to attend transplant support groups if offered by the center. Once patients do return home, they are encouraged to resume a close relationship with their local primary care physician and gastroenterologist.[91] Because of the proliferation in the number of liver transplants being performed, it is not unreasonable for these patients to be admitted to a nontertiary care hospital for management of some long-term posttransplant complications. Thus even nurses who work for hospitals that do not perform transplants may have the opportunity to care for these patients.

Liver transplant patients need long-term follow-up for hypertension,[83] renal insufficiency,[83] biliary[80] and infectious complications,[92] and malignancies.[93] Early intervention affects both quality and length of life. Financial concerns are a major source of stress in this patient population. The largest group of transplant recipients are those who have suffered from some type of chronic liver disease. They often are disabled for some length of time before transplant and have already experienced financial stressors related to illness. As these patients live longer with liver transplants, issues of insurability, continued disability, and even the ability to obtain work need to be addressed.[94]

Future of Liver Transplant

Transplant offers hope for survival, but at considerable expense. Many insurance providers, including Medicare, provide partial reimbursement for liver transplantation. The costs, however, can be staggering. Liver transplant surgery has been reported to be the single most costly procedure in health care.[95] In this age of managed health care it becomes a challenge for institutions to provide this labor-intensive, life-saving procedure economically. In attempts to control costs and optimize outcomes, insurance companies are designating "centers of excellence." This will mean more patients will travel some distances to receive transplants. As competition for the health care dollar increases, workloads and the character of the work itself will change. Nurses need to remain in the forefront, providing research for cost-effective health care techniques.[96]

Clinical trials are seeking to identify new drugs and to define treatment protocols.[97] With increasing choices of therapies, drugs will be selected for patients in whom other immunosuppressive therapies fail or for patients who develop severe side effects.[98] Studies on tolerance and chimerism[99,100] may also influence future immunosuppressive protocols.

Attention also is being focused on ways to increase the number and availability of donor organs. Reduced-size organs are a common occurrence.[101] Studies are exploring the roles of xenografts and bioartificial liver devices used to support the patient awaiting a homograft.[102,103] The use of living related donors will continue.[104] Recipient selection criteria will also continue to be redefined as statistics related to long-term outcomes become available.[105] As recipients live longer and healthier lives, the issue of reproduction will become more common.[100] There are many factors that will influence the future of liver transplantation. Box 47-17 lists some of the factors influencing the future of liver transplantation.

KIDNEY TRANSPLANTATION

In 1954 a team of surgeons led by Dr. Joseph Murray performed a successful renal transplant between identical (monozygotic) twins at Peter Bent Brigham Hospital in Boston. Although transplantation had been attempted since the beginning of the 20th century, this landmark event marked the potential for renal transplantation as a treatment for end-stage renal disease (ESRD).[107] Improved surgical techniques and better understanding of the immune system have resulted in renal transplantation becoming the treatment of choice for many individuals rather than an experimental procedure. In 1991, 8597 cadaveric renal transplants and 3210 living related renal transplants were performed.[108] Not only is transplantation the most

BOX 47-17 Factors Influencing the Future of Liver Transplantation

- Cost-effective management of the patient
- Donor shortage
- Donor allocation
- Advances in organ recovery and preservation
- Advances in surgical techniques
- Advances in perioperative management
- Advances in immunobiology and immunosuppression
- Advances in antimicrobial therapies
- Innovative uses of partial organs and marginal donor organs
- Xenografts
- Timing of transplantation in relationship to the disease process
- Access to care issues as they relate to insurability and coverage of recipient
- Cost of immunosuppression

cost-effective treatment for ESRD; it also offers successful transplant recipients an improved quality of life and increased activity levels compared with other forms of ESRD treatments.[109,110]

In the early years of renal transplantation, information was limited about the immune system and long-term effects of immunosuppressive medications. High dosages of these medications led to liver malfunction, facial disfigurement, severe osteoporosis, cancer, and fatal infections. During the 1970s, procedures such as total body irradiation, splenectomy, and depleting the lymphatic system of lymphocytes through thoracic duct drainage were used to modify the immune system of kidney transplant recipients. It was hoped that these procedures would permit administration of lower doses of immunosuppressive medications. The complications of these procedures, however, including severe infections, have prevented these treatments from becoming routine in transplantation today.[111] Preconditioning recipients with blood transfusions before transplantation was begun in the late 1970s. This practice has decreased in recent years because of the success of new immunosuppressive medications in prolonging graft survival.[112]

Indications and Selection

Because of the broad range of diseases that can lead to ESRD, the potential transplant recipient must undergo extensive evaluation to determine whether transplantation is a viable treatment option. Box 47-18, lists

BOX 47-18 Evaluation Testing for Kidney Transplantation

Laboratory tests

- SMA-23, CBC with differential, RPR, HBsAg and HBsAb (anti-HBS), HLA typing
- HIV, HCVAB and HTLVI antibody, CMV, EBV, HSV and VZV titers, fasting lipid profile and PSA
- Platelet count, PT, PTT, HLA typing, urine for urinalysis and C&S (if patient is receiving peritoneal dialysis, then the peritoneal fluid must also be sent for C&S and AFB)

Roentgenograms

- Posteroanterior (PA) and lateral chest films
- Mammogram for women older than 35 years

Renal ultrasound

- 12-lead electrocardiogram (ECG)

Thallium scan

- Age 45 years or older
- Diabetes mellitus
- Abnormal ECG findings
- History of angina or myocardial infarction

Noninvasive vascular studies

- Diabetes mellitus

Consultations

- Psychiatry, urology, transplant nephrology, social services, nursing, gynecology for female patients. Financial counseling

SMA Sequential Multiple Analyzer; *RPR,* rapid plasma reagin; *HBsAg,* hepatitis B surface antigen; *HBsAb,* hepatitis B surface antigen antibody; *HLA,* human leukocyte antigens; *HCVAB,* hepatitis C virus antibody; *HTLVI,* human T-cell leukemia virus; *CMV,* cytomegalovirus; *EBV,* Epstein-Barr virus; *HSV,* herpes virus; *VZV,* varicella-zoster virus; *PSA,* prostatic specific antigen; *PT,* prothrombin time; *PTT,* partial thromboplastin time; *C&S,* culture and sensitivity; *AFB,* acid-fast bacillus.

the laboratory tests and diagnostic studies most often performed during an evaluation. Specific findings that would contraindicate transplantation are listed in Box 47-19. Because ESRD affects many of the body's systems, many patients who are evaluated have abnormal findings, which must be assessed on an individual basis. If active infection is present, the evaluation may need to be resumed when the infection is controlled. An extensive cardiac evaluation may be needed, including possible angioplasty or coronary

BOX 47-19 Contraindications to Kidney Transplantation

Active infections, including active HIV, tuberculosis, or systemic infections
Active vasculitis/glomerulonephritis: lupus, Wegener's granulomatosis, Goodpasture's syndrome
Advanced cardiopulmonary disease
Persons at high risk for surgery (e.g., advanced chronic obstructive pulmonary disease [COPD], obesity)
Malignancy
Active IV drug use
Noncompliance with medical course of therapy
Mental incompetence
Positive T-cell lymphocytotoxic crossmatch

BOX 47-20 Evaluation Testing for Living Kidney Donors

Laboratory test

SMA-23, CBC with differential, RPR, HBsAg and HBsAb (anti-HBS), HLA typing, HTLVI antibody, HCV antibody, HIV, amylase, CMV, EBV, HSV, and VZV titers, platelet count, PT, PTT, urine for urinalysis and C&S, 24-hr urine collection for creatinine clearance, serum creatinine, and protein

Roentgenograms

PA and lateral chest films

12-lead electrocardiogram (ECG)

Renal scan

Renal arteriogram

Consultations

Psychiatry, urology, transplant nephrology, social services, nursing, gynecology for female donors, and financial counseling

SMA, Sequential Multiple Aanalyzer; *RPR,* rapid plasma reagin; *HBsAg,* hepatitis B surface antigen,*HBsAB,* hepatitis B surface antigen antibody; *HTLVI,* human T-cell leukemia virus; *HCV,* hepatitis C antibody; *CMV,* cytomegalovirus; *EBV,* Epstein-Barr virus; *HSV,* herpesvirus; *VZV,* varicella-zoster virus; *PT,* prothrombin time; *PTT,* partial thromboplastin time; *C&S,* culture and sensitivity; *PA,* posteroanterior.

artery bypass surgery before a patient is considered a candidate. Some individuals who are overweight are recommended for transplantation on the condition that they lose weight to decrease surgical risk. Smokers, especially those with diabetes or chronic obstructive pulmonary disease (COPD), are strongly advised to quit smoking. Individuals with malignancies that have been in remission for 2 to 5 years, depending on the type of malignancy, may be considered as candidates. Persons with ESRD as a result of active vasculitis or glomerulonephritis, or both, may be considered when the disease process becomes inactive. Individuals with substance abuse problems are required to have treatment, and close substance screening is required for an appropriate amount of time to monitor compliance. Persons who are noncompliant with their medical treatment also may be given time to improve their compliance before transplantation occurs. Persons with severe learning deficits, mental retardation, or other processes that may alter their mental status may be considered for transplantation if there is strong, consistent support from a family member or significant other.

Once transplantation is considered as a possible treatment, the potential recipient must either be placed on the UNOS waiting list for a cadaveric donation or receive a kidney from a living related donor. Several factors are considered in allocation of cadaveric kidneys, including blood type, degree of HLA match between the donor and recipient, the length of time the patient has been on the waiting list, and the proximity of the organ to the patient.[113] The supply of cadaveric organs does not meet the demand of the number of persons on the waiting list. To avoid this wait, a living donor may be considered. A living donor must be evaluated to rule out surgical risks and to consider any medical risk in having one kidney. Box 47-20 lists the tests required in evaluation of a potential living donor. There has been some concern over whether the use of living donors is justified. If, however, there is no perceived risk to the donor and the organ is freely given, most transplant centers will use a living donor.

Kidney transplant is covered under DRG 302. The anticipated length of stay is 14.0 days.[18]

Surgical Procedure

When the kidney is harvested, the ureter, renal vein, and renal artery are dissected. If the kidney is taken from a living donor, the organ is flushed with an iced solution to remove formed blood elements. It is then taken to the recipient's operating room for transplantation. When the kidney is taken from a cadaveric donor, the organ is flushed with a hyperosmolar, hyperkalemic, and hypothermic preservation solution

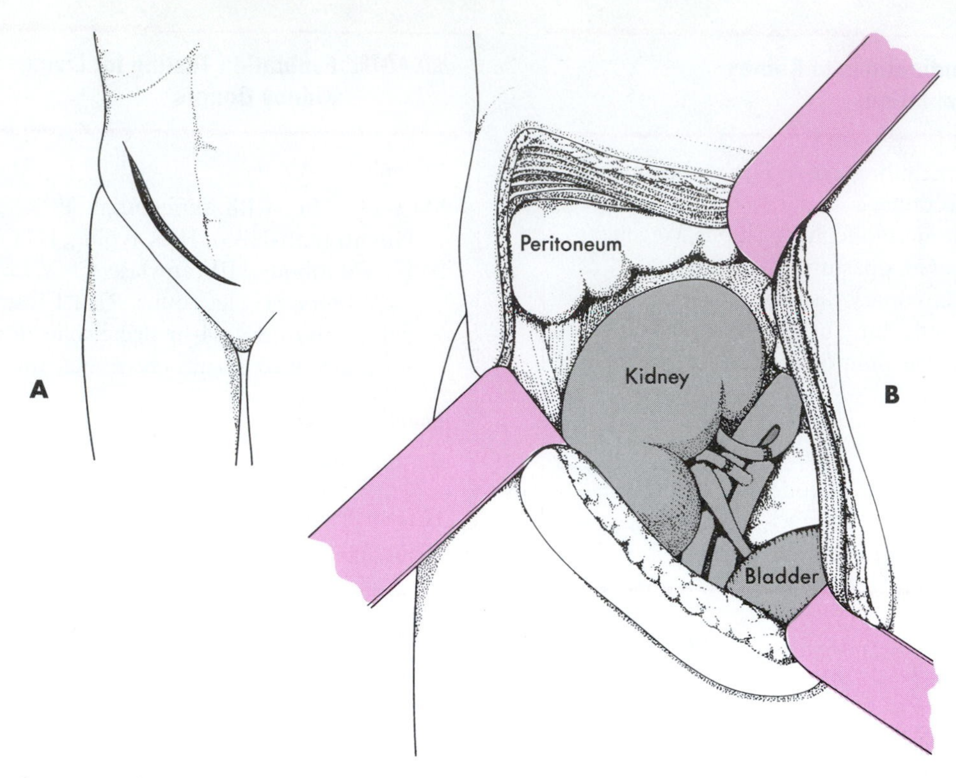

FIGURE 47-12. Placement of the renal graft into iliac fossa. **A,** The incision depicted is for the right side of the abdomen, representing graft implantation in the right iliac fossa. **B,** The iliac vessels are exposed. (Modified from Smith SL: *AACN tissue and organ transplantation: implications for professional nursing practice,* St Louis, 1990, Mosby.)

and then placed in an iced solution. Once the kidney is in this hypothermic solution, metabolism is slowed and the organ may be preserved for up to 48 hours. To decrease the potential for acute tubular necrosis (ATN), most centers attempt to transplant the organ as soon as possible.

After the patient is anesthetized, a urinary catheter is inserted and irrigated with a sterile antibiotic fluid.[114] A curved incision is made just above the symphysis pubis that extends to the iliac crest. The transplanted kidney is placed in the extraperitoneal site of either the right or left iliac fossa (Figure 47-12). The muscles and facia are divided, and the peritoneum is freed and retracted medially, exposing the iliac vessels.[114] The renal artery is anastomosed end-to-end to the external iliac artery, and the vein is sutured end-to-side to the external iliac vein. If the aortic cuff is recovered from a cadaveric donation, a Carrel patch may be used to attach the renal artery end-to-side to the external iliac artery. Examples of potential anastomoses can be seen in Figure 47-13.

During the surgery a CVP of 8 to 16 mm Hg must be maintained. Systolic blood pressure at or above preoperative levels also is recommended.[114] This is necessary to ensure adequate reperfusion of the transplanted kidney.

Once revascularization is completed, the ureteral anastomosis is begun, with the most common being the ureteroneocystostomy. This involves making an incision into the dome of the bladder. After the donor ureter is tunneled through the recipient's mucosal layer of the bladder, it is sutured end-to-side into the mucosal opening.[114] (Figure 47-14). With each bladder contraction the tunnel prevents reflux by acting as a one-way valve, thus reducing the potential for bladder contamination.[114] If the recipient has had multiple bladder surgeries or has a history of infections, a ureteroureterostomy may be performed. This involves an anastomosis of the donor ureter to the recipient's ureter.

Postoperative Medical and Nursing Management

Depending on the transplant center's protocol, the recipient is transferred either to a critical care unit or the transplant nursing unit after surgery. Regardless of where the patient begins recovery, close monitoring is needed. A knowledge of surgical postoperative care, renal function, and immunosuppression is necessary to detect any complications. An immediate response to complications ensures graft, and possibly patient,

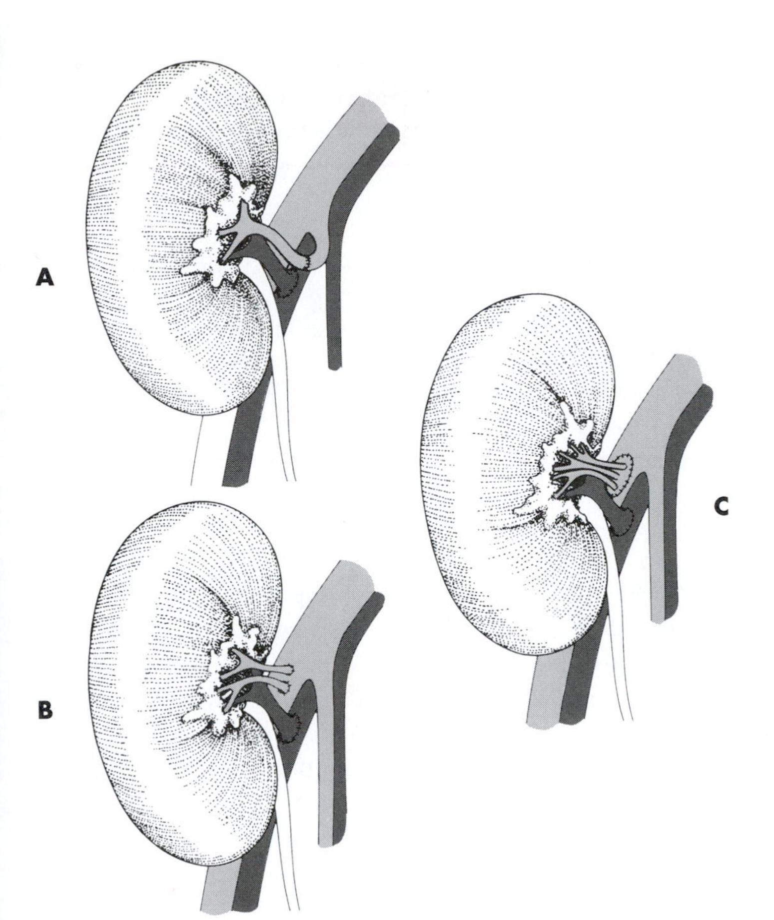

FIGURE 47-13. Anastomosis of the renal artery to the iliac artery. **A,** Single renal artery to internal iliac artery and renal vein to external iliac vein. **B,** Multiple renal arteries to external iliac artery. **C,** Carrel patch containing multiple renal arteries to external iliac artery. (From Smith SL: *AACN tissue and organ transplantation: implications for professional nursing practice,* St Louis, 1990, Mosby. Redrawn from Whelchel JD: Renal transportation. In Grabar GB, editor: *Anesthesia for renal transplantation,* vol 14, Norwell, Mass, 1987, Cluwer Academic Publishers.)

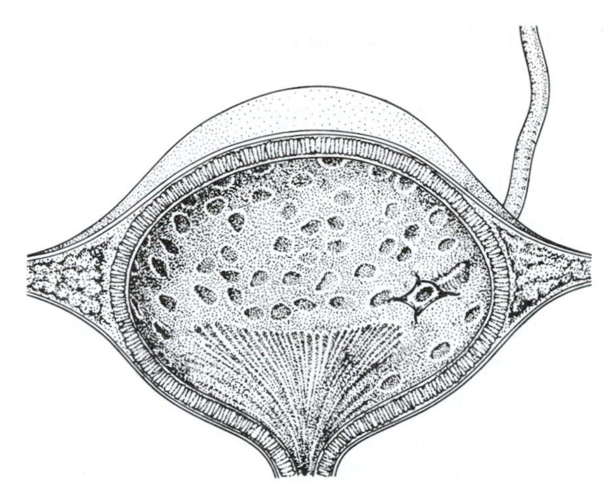

FIGURE 47-14. Ureteroneocystostomy reconstruction of the urinary tract. The donor ureter is passed through a posterior bladder wall tunnel and anastomosed to the bladder mucosa. (From Smith SL: *AACN tissue and organ transplantation: implications for professional nursing practice,* St Louis, 1990, Mosby. Redrawn from Whelchel JD: Renal transportation. In Grabar GB, editor: *Anesthesia for renal transplantation,* vol 14, Norwell, Mass, 1987, Cluwer Academic Publishers.)

survival.[115] Several nursing diagnoses are associated with care of the kidney transplant recipient, as listed in Box 47-21.

If the graft is functioning well, the patient may become dehydrated or hypotensive as a result of diuresis. Adequate hydration and blood pressure are necessary to ensure adequate blood flow to the transplanted organ. Inadequate blood flow may cause ATN and, if uncorrected, possible graft failure.[116] The amount of urine output may vary as a result of factors such as cold ischemia time or administration of diuretics. Therefore intravenous (IV) fluid replacement of 1 ml for each milliliter of urine may be indicated. However, a limit on total fluid given each hour is necessary to avoid complications of fluid overload.

BOX 47-21 NURSING DIAGNOSIS AND MANAGEMENT

KIDNEY TRANSPLANTATION

- Fluid Volume Deficit related to absolute loss, p. 914
- Altered Renal Tissue Perfusion related to decreased renal blood flow, p. 916
- Risk for Infection risk factor: immunosuppressive drugs to prevent rejection of the transplanted kidney, p. 1216
- Body Image Disturbance related to actual change in body structure, function or appearance, p. 87
- Anxiety related to threat to biologic, psychologic, and/or social integrity, p. 99
- Knowledge Deficit: Posttransplant Self-care Regimen, immunosuppressive drugs and clinical manifestations related to lack of previous exposure to information, p. 61

The patient's CVP must not fall below 4 mm Hg, and the systolic blood pressure must remain above 110 mm Hg.[115] Albumin may be needed to maintain these levels in the event of extensive diuresis. Noninvasive monitoring of fluid status includes accurate recording of intake and output; daily weights; and assessment of skin turgor, sacral edema, and jugular venous distention.

Monitoring of serum electrolyte levels is required every 4 to 6 hours for the first 24 hours. Blood urea nitrogen (BUN) and serum creatinine levels are needed to monitor graft function. A steady decline of these levels is seen as graft function improves. Hypokalemia may occur if there is excessive diuresis, and hyperkalemia may occur if the graft is not functioning well. Both require assessment of frequent potassium levels, and cardiac monitoring sometimes is indicated. Steroid-induced hyperglycemia is a potential complication. If this occurs, an insulin drip is necessary in the immediate postoperative phase. When the patient's condition becomes stable, obtaining daily serum electrolyte levels is adequate for monitoring graft function.

Because of the surgical anastomoses that involve the renal artery and vein, there is potential for hemorrhage and thrombosis. Frequent serum hematocrit (Hct) measurements are obtained. Any drainage or swelling at the incision site or a sudden drop in blood pressure or Hct level must alert the nurse to possible hemorrhage. In addition, leakage at the bladder anastomosis can occur, resulting in decreased urine output or leakage of urine from the incision. In the immunosuppressed patient a urine leak can lead to life-threatening peritonitis. These complications must be surgically corrected as soon as possible.

Renal transplant patients are immunocompromised to prevent rejection, which also places them at an increased risk for infections. All dressing changes are performed with use of aseptic technique, and any unnecessary IV line must be discontinued. Any fever or elevation in white blood cell count is a cause for concern, and blood and urine cultures must be obtained. Not only are these patients susceptible to wound and urinary tract infections, they are at risk for opportunistic infections. As the patient recovers from surgery, the importance of good hand washing and hygiene, as well as the recognition of the clinical manifestations of infection, must be stressed. See the nursing management plan on p. 1216 for additional information on infection control.

After transplantation, many of the dietary restrictions of ESRD are no longer necessary. Patients are instructed to include enough protein in their diets to promote healing. With the increased potential for weight gain resulting from steroid use, patients are also instructed to follow a low-salt, low-fat, low-cholesterol diet. Recipients are weighed at each clinic visit to monitor weight gain and obtain any needed information regarding diet and exercise.

In the present era of managed care it is important to remember that the length of hospital stay for posttransplant recipients is becoming shorter and shorter. As soon as patients are medically stable, they are being discharged to housing near the transplant center or to home. Each insurance company has different conditions for hospital benefits, medication coverage, and clinic visits. It is important that social workers and financial counselors discuss these issues with recipients before and after transplantation to ensure that transplantation is a viable and affordable treatment option.

BOX 47-22 Kidney Transplantation Clinical Manifestations of Rejection

- Tenderness at graft site
- Decrease in urine output
- Sudden increase in weight: 3 to 5 pounds in a 24-hour period
- Edema—usually begins in hands and feet
- Elevated temperature
- Elevated serum creatinine above the individual's baseline

In addition, during their hospitalization, patients are taught the clinical manifestations of rejection (Box 47-22), record keeping of laboratory values and vital signs, and the importance of compliance with the posttransplant regimen. Many centers start recipients on a self-medication program before discharge. Frequent clinic visits during the first 3 to 6 months are needed to monitor progress and to adjust medications. As the patient progresses, a schedule is established for routine laboratory tests and clinic visits to ensure long-term success of the transplant.[115]

Long-Term Considerations

As with any transplant patient, rejection is always a possibility. If rejection is suspected, a biopsy specimen of the kidney will determine which medication is indicated for treatment. This can be an emotionally charged time for the patient. The uncertainty of graft survival and concerns regarding the possible return to dialysis are areas that need to be discussed with patients and their significant others. Frequent outpatient monitoring after a rejection episode is necessary until graft function is determined to be stable.

The future of renal transplantation lies in the improvement of immunosuppressive medications. As cyclosporine increased the graft survival of transplanted organs in the 1980s, future medications may lead to effective immunosuppression with fewer side effects. Many organizations also are investigating methods to improve organ donation. An increase in donation, combined with improved immunosuppression, can enhance the quality of life for thousands of individuals waiting for a transplant each year.

PANCREAS TRANSPLANTATION

The devastating effects of insulin-dependent diabetes mellitus (IDDM) are well-documented.[116] Providing the diabetic person with a functioning pancreas, thus eliminating the need for insulin and, it is hoped, reducing the complications of the disease, are the goals of pancreatic transplantation. Many years of experimentation and research led to the first human pancreas transplant in 1966 at the University of Minnesota. The patient, who had diabetic uremia, received a simultaneous renal-pancreas transplant. Unfortunately, sepsis and rejection proved fatal 2 months after the procedure.[117]

During the 1960s and 1970s the progress in pancreas transplantation was slow and relatively unsuccessful. This was because of difficulties involving organ grafting, management of exocrine graft function, and immunosuppression. In the 1980s, however, with improved surgical technique and the use of medications such as cyclosporine, the success rate of this procedure improved. In 1995, 914 simultaneous renal-pancreas transplants and 110 pancreas transplants were performed.[108]

Pancreas transplant is covered under DRGs 191 and 192: pancreas, liver, and shunt procedures. The anticipated length of stay ranges from 9.8 to 18.2 days. The longer length of stay (DRG 191) is for patients with complications.[18]

Indications and Selection

Persons with diabetes who are considered for pancreas transplantation must undergo a thorough medical evaluation. Systems that are adversely affected by IDDM are examined closely. Because of the effects of diabetes on the cardiovascular system and the extensive surgical procedures involved, a complete cardiac evaluation is necessary.[118] Extensive vascular studies are required to ensure adequate vascularization of the graft. Nerve conduction studies are needed to evaluate neuropathy. Depending on the type of surgical technique used, urologic and bladder function testing may be needed to evaluate possible difficulties with a bladder anastomosis. An endocrinologist evaluates the patient and decides appropriate endocrine function tests. If the pancreas is to be transplanted simultaneously with another organ, the patient must complete all the evaluation procedures required for the additional organ, including the psychologic evaluation.

Because of diabetic glomerular nephropathy resulting in ESRD, many candidates for pancreas transplant often are candidates for renal transplant. Many programs perform simultaneous renal-pancreas transplants. Combined renal-pancreas transplants have a 1-year graft survival rate of approximately 80%.[119] Diabetic persons with a successful pancreas or renal-pancreas transplant report a higher quality of life after transplantation.[110,120] Regardless of whether the transplant program performs single-pancreas or combined renal-pancreas transplantation, the surgery is performed if the projected benefits outweigh the risks of the procedure.[118,121]

Surgical Procedure

Transplantation of the pancreas may involve islet cell transplantation, segmental transplantation, or whole organ transplantation. Regardless of the type of surgery performed, the native pancreas is left intact for continued exocrine function. The purpose of a pancreas transplant is to replace the endocrine function (insulin production). Islet cell transplantation involves isolation and extraction of endocrine cells from a donor, which are then inoculated into the recipient. Once isolated the islet cells can be injected into the portal vein and carried to the liver, placed under the kidney capsule, or placed intraperitoneally.[122] The complications to this procedure include an inadequate amount of cell mass, damage of the cells, and rejection. Success with this procedure is limited, and research is continuing to improve the technique and immunosuppression involved.

Segmental transplantation involves grafting the body and tail of the donor pancreas. The segmental pancreas can be recovered from either a cadaveric or a living donor, although pancreas transplantation involving a living donor remains controversial. The success rates between the whole and segmental organ transplantation are comparable, although whole organ transplantation is performed more often than segmental organ transplantation. The advantages of whole organ transplantation include a larger mass of islet cells and adequate vessel perfusion.[123]

When the pancreas is recovered for whole organ transplantation, the superior mesenteric and splenic arteries also are procured. A 5 cm to 8 cm segment of the duodenum is resected, which assists in handling the organ and, depending on the surgical technique, may be used for surgical drainage. Once the pancreas is recovered, the cold ischemic time is 18 to 24 hours.[119]

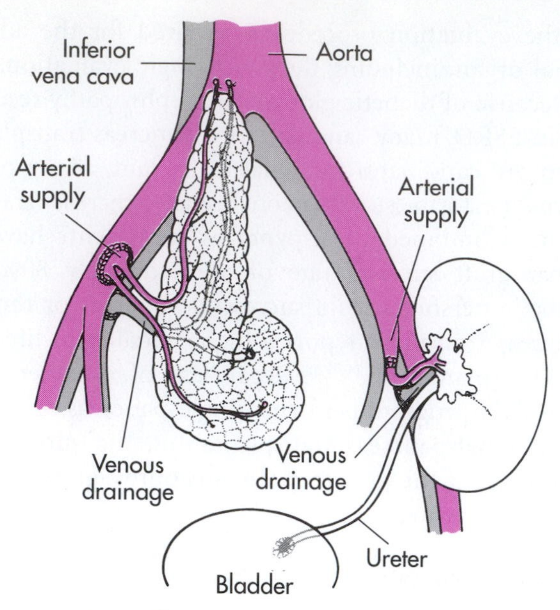

FIGURE 47-15. Placement of organs during simultaneous kidney pancreas transplant. (Modified from Smith SL: *AACN tissue and organ transplantation: implications for professional nursing practice,* St Louis, 1990, Mosby.)

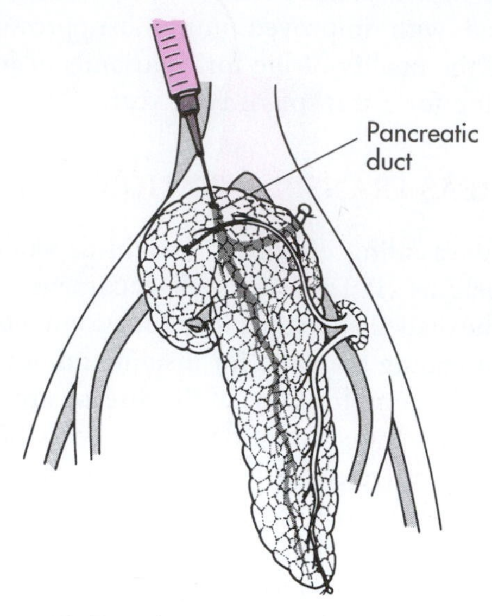

FIGURE 47-16. Exocrine mangagement by ductal injection. (Modified from Smith SL: *AACN tissue and organ transplantation: implications for professional nursing practice,* St Louis, 1990, Mosby.)

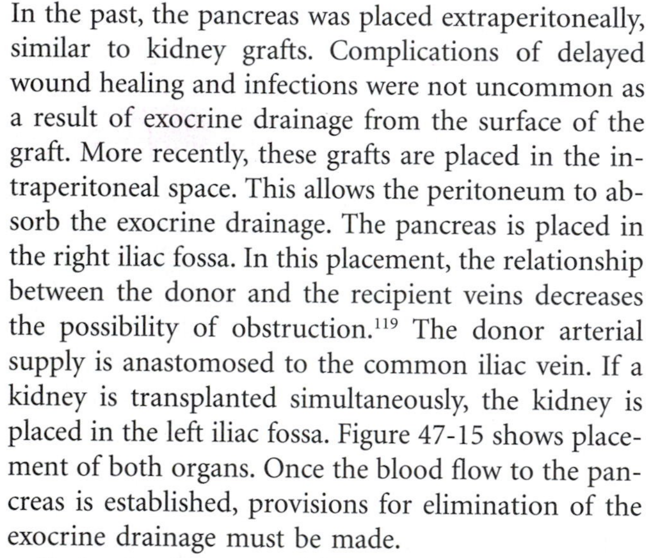
In the past, the pancreas was placed extraperitoneally, similar to kidney grafts. Complications of delayed wound healing and infections were not uncommon as a result of exocrine drainage from the surface of the graft. More recently, these grafts are placed in the intraperitoneal space. This allows the peritoneum to absorb the exocrine drainage. The pancreas is placed in the right iliac fossa. In this placement, the relationship between the donor and the recipient veins decreases the possibility of obstruction.[119] The donor arterial supply is anastomosed to the common iliac vein. If a kidney is transplanted simultaneously, the kidney is placed in the left iliac fossa. Figure 47-15 shows placement of both organs. Once the blood flow to the pancreas is established, provisions for elimination of the exocrine drainage must be made.

Endocrine function of the transplanted pancreas is all that is needed to eliminate the need for insulin therapy. In most cases there is adequate exocrine function (digestive enzymes) of the native pancreas, thus creating a need for elimination of the exocrine function of the transplanted graft. Management of these digestive enzymes has proved to be the surgical challenge of this procedure. Over the years the three most common techniques that have developed are ductal occlusion, enteric drainage, and urinary diversion.

Ductal occlusion involves injecting a polymer substance into the main pancreatic duct (Figure 47-16). This injection causes hardening and occlusion of the duct. Although there are short-term complications, such as leakage and wound infection, the major concerns are the potential for long-term complications. Fibrosis resulting from the injection may involve the islet cells and ultimately cause graft failure.

Anastomosing the graft to a Roux-en-Y loop of recipient jejunum is the second method of eliminating exocrine drainage (Figure 47-17). This method of enteric drainage, pancreaticojejunostomy, is used if both endocrine and exocrine function is desired from the transplanted pancreas or if there is an indication that urinary diversion is not appropriate, such as in the presence of chronic bladder dysfunction.[124] The reabsorption of the pancreatic enzymes creates fewer metabolic imbalances; however, the inability to monitor enzyme secretion eliminates a method of detecting graft dysfunction or rejection; therefore serum creatinine levels in renal-pancreas recipients must be monitored closely.[125]

The third technique, which manages exocrine drainage by urinary diversion, is termed *pancreaticoduodenocystostomy.* This technique involves anastomosing the pancreas to the recipient's bladder. A portion of the donor duodenum is recovered with the pancreas and is sutured into place as a conduit for drainage (Figure 47-18). Adequate bladder function is necessary if this technique is to be successful. Complications of this procedure include ulceration and cystitis resulting from duodenal irritation by the pancreatic enzymes. If a simultaneous renal-pancreas transplant is performed, there may be leakage because of the mul-

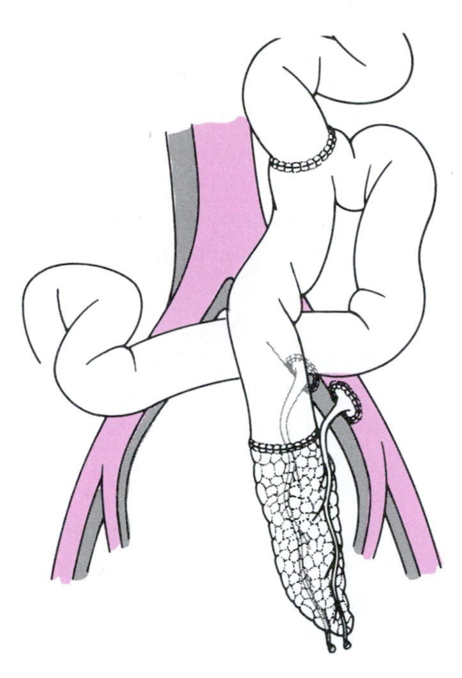

FIGURE 47-17. Exocrine management by enteric drainage (Roux-en-Y jejunum). (Modified from Smith SL: *AACN tissue and organ transplantation: implications for professional nursing practice*, St Louis, 1990, Mosby.)

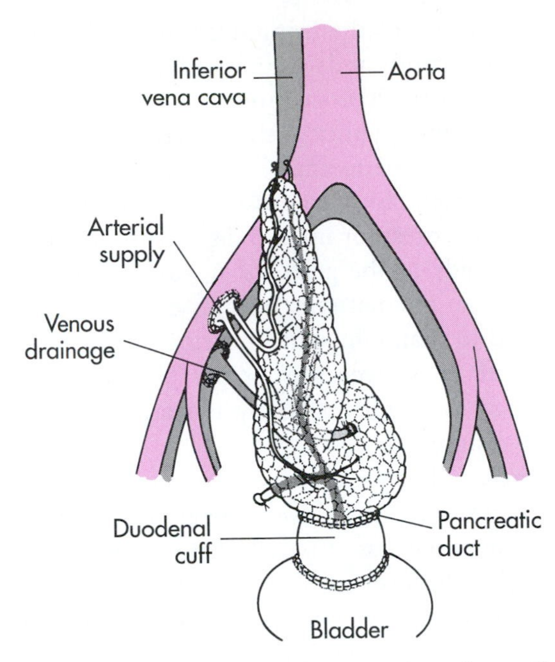

FIGURE 47-18. Exocrine management by urinary diversion. (Modified from Smith SL: *AACN tissue and organ transplantation: implications for professional nursing practice*, St Louis, 1990, Mosby.)

tiple bladder anastomoses.[125] Also, there is a significant amount of sodium and bicarbonate lost in the urine. Patients who have this procedure are at high risk for hypotension and metabolic acidosis. Daily oral sodium bicarbonate replacement is necessary, and intravenous hydration sometimes is needed. Despite the potential complications of this procedure, several advantages are noteworthy. The incidence of fistulas is decreased as a result of inactivation of pancreatic enzymes in the urine. The main advantage of this procedure is the ability to evaluate pancreatic function by monitoring urinary amylase levels. A decrease in urinary amylase has proved to be one of the earliest indicators of graft dysfunction and rejection.[125]

Postoperative Medical and Nursing Management

After surgery the patient is taken to the critical care unit. Although these patients have a functioning pancreas, they are at increased risk for surgical complications because of the long-term adverse effects of diabetes. Oxygenation, hemodynamics, and cardiac status are monitored closely. Many nursing diagnoses are associated with care of the pancreas transplant recipient, as listed in Box 47-23. If a simultaneous renal transplant has been performed, fluid and electrolyte management is indicated, including fluid replacement; recording intake and output; and monitoring potassium, BUN, and serum creatinine levels. A nasogastric tube usually is in place for 24 to 48 hours after surgery. The patient also may be receiving a continuous insulin infusion to rest the graft. Frequent monitoring of blood glucose levels is needed, and the infusion is discontinued as soon as

BOX 47-23 NURSING DIAGNOSIS AND MANAGEMENT

PANCREAS TRANSPLANTATION

- Risk for Infection risk factor: immunosuppressive drugs required to prevent rejection of pancreas, p. 1216
- Altered Nutrition: Less Than Body Requirements related to lack of exogenous nutrients and increased metabolic demand, p. 165
- Body Image Disturbance related to actual change in body structure, function, or appearance, p. 87
- Anxiety related to threat to biologic, psychologic, and/or social integrity, p. 99
- Activity Intolerance related to prolonged immobility or deconditioning, p. 597
- Knowledge Deficit: Posttransplant Self-care Regimen, immunosuppressive drugs and clinical manifestation of infection related to lack of previous exposure to information, p. 61
- If simultaneous kidney-pancreas transplant has been performed see Box 47-22

possible. Because of the immunosuppressed status of these patients, good hand washing and aseptic technique are necessary with all procedures.

Because of the fragility of the pancreas and the delicate anastomosis performed in this surgery, these patients are at high risk for graft thrombosis. Activity is restricted to bedrest for up to 5 days, with no hip flexion on the side of the graft for up to 7 days. Gentle log rolling, an air mattress, and an overhead trapeze are needed to maintain skin integrity. Low-molecular weight dextran is given during this time to decrease blood viscosity. Aspirin therapy is started when oral intake is resumed.

If there has been a urinary diversion for exocrine management, the potential for metabolic acidosis exists because of the loss of bicarbonate in the urine. Intravenously administered bicarbonate replacement is given until oral replacement is possible. The increased loss of sodium in the urine predisposes this patient to dehydration and hypotension. Hematuria also may occur because of the anastomosis, and cystitis may occur. Careful urinary irrigation may be required.

Rejection surveillance. Rejection in this patient population may be difficult to detect. Serum amylase levels have not proved effective in monitoring graft function, and blood glucose levels seem to become elevated only in the late phases of rejection. A decrease in urine amylase in patients with urinary diversions has proved to be an indicator of rejection.[125] During the postoperative stay, urine amylase collections are obtained every 12 to 24 hours. If a simultaneous renal-pancreas transplant has been performed, a rise in the serum creatinine level also is useful in diagnosing rejection. In these cases, because of the fragility of the pancreas, a renal biopsy specimen may be obtained to determine rejection and treatment. If the transplant is a single organ, a computed tomography (CT) scan–directed biopsy of the pancreas may be indicated.

Long-Term Considerations

As with all transplant patients, postoperative care includes educating the patient regarding compliance and record keeping. Patients may be required to check their blood glucose levels at home. Blood pressure monitoring is necessary after discharge to detect the development of hypotension. Outpatient 24-hour urine collections are obtained to monitor urinary amylase levels. If recipients have normal blood glucose levels they must follow a low-sodium, low-fat, low-cholesterol diet. At first, frequent clinic visits are needed to monitor progress and adjust medications. As the patient progresses, a schedule is established for routine laboratory tests and clinic visits to ensure long-term success of the transplant.

Although islet cell transplantation remains investigational, ongoing research continues in this area.[126] In the future this procedure may offer a nonsurgical method of transplantation. Continued improvement of surgical technique, immunosuppressive medications, and organ donation will offer an insulin-free treatment option and may one day be the most effective form of treatment available for diabetes.

CASE STUDY

HEART TRANSPLANTATION

CLINICAL HISTORY

AB is a 58-year-old man who is diagnosed with ischemic cardiomyopathy. He has been accepted as a transplant candidate and is currently waiting in the coronary care unit.

CURRENT PROBLEMS

AB is receiving 8 μg/kg/min of dopamine; 12 μg/kg/min of dobutamine; 2 μg/kg/min of nitroglycerin; and a heparin drip of 50 units/hour. He has been intubated and mechanically ventilated for 48 hours. His nutrition is being supported with hyperalimentation. He has been anorexic for the past 3 weeks, and his weight had dropped from 78 kg to 70 kg. Current cardiac index (CI) ranges from 2.0 to 2.3 L/min/m². Serum creatinine is 1.7 mg/dL. During the ensuing 24 hours, a suitable heart is obtained. The operation proceeded without incident. Six hours after his return to the critical care unit, he is mechanically ventilated with an FIO_2 of 50% and a rate of 10 breaths/min. His blood pressure (BP) is 102/52 mm Hg (mean 68), heart rate (HR), 78; pulmonary artery pressure (PAP), 40/18 mm Hg (wedge 17 mm Hg); central venous pressure (CVP), 15 mm Hg. His most recent CI is 2.2 L/min/m². Hourly urine output for the past 2 hours averages 40 ml/hr. Peripheral pulses are present, but his legs are cool to touch from feet to knees. His temperature is 36.2° C (core). Chest tube drainage averages 25–35 ml/hr over the last 2 hours.

Hemodynamic support consists of dopamine at 3 μg/kg/min; sodium nitroprusside at 0.5 μg/kg/min; nitroglycerin at 1 μg/kg/min; and isoproterenol is hanging (ready to infuse), but currently is turned off.

MEDICAL DIAGNOSIS

Orthotopic heart transplant

NURSING DIAGNOSES

Decreased Cardiac Output related to alterations in preload

Decreased Cardiac Output related to alterations in afterload

Hypothermia related to exposure to cold environment (decreased temperature intraoperatively and cardiopulmonary bypass)

PLAN OF CARE

1. Initiate inotropic and chronotropic support with isoproterenol.
2. Monitor for improvement in CI.
3. Monitor for HR greater than 115 beats/min.
4. Consult with physician about need for standby pacemaker; obtain parameters.
5. Monitor for any new-onset dysrhythmia

MEDICAL AND NURSING MANAGEMENT AND PATIENT OUTCOME

Over the next 2 hours CI increased to 3.1 L/min/m² after initiating isoproterenol at 3 μg/min. HR was then 100 beats/min. Urine output ranged from 50 to 60 ml/hr. The patient received his first postoperative dose of methylprednisolone (125 mg) and an IV cyclosporine dose of 50 mg, which continued bid. He was extubated 16 hours after admission and placed on 40% oxygen by mask. He was oriented and moved all extremities. He received a total of 90 mg of cyclosporine IV. His first cyclosporine level was 220 ng/ml. At 18 hours postoperatively his serum creatinine level was 2.5 mg/dL with a urine output decreased to 35 ml/hr. A later 12-hour urine creatinine clearance revealed a clearance of 40 ml/hr. The patient had a very weak cough, but fairly clear lung fields. He refused clear liquids. Sodium nitroprusside and nitroglycerin were weaned off.

MEDICAL DIAGNOSIS

Orthotopic heart transplant

NURSING DIAGNOSES

Impaired Gas Exchange related to alveolar hypoventilation

Altered Nutrition: Less than Body Requirements related to lack of exogenous nutrients and increased metabolic demand

Continued

CASE STUDY—CONT'D

HEART TRANSPLANTATION

REVISED PLAN OF CARE

1. Consult with physician about adjusting or holding cyclosporine.
2. Monitor for clinical manifestations of fluid volume excess.
3. Monitor for elevations in potassium.
4. Monitor for changes in respiratory pattern, rate, and character and quality of chest expansion and cough.
5. Evaluate breath sounds every 2 to 4 hours.
6. Mobilize patient as soon as possible.
7. Consult with physician about possible need for respiratory therapy treatments.
8. Consult with physician about need to augment nutrition via enteral feedings if patient unable or uninterested in taking nutrition by mouth.
9. Monitor cyclosporine level.

MEDICAL AND NURSING MANAGEMENT AND PATIENT OUTCOME

The cyclosporine dose was held for 36 hours. By postoperative day 3 the patient's cyclosporine level fell to 150 ng/ml with a serum creatinine level of 2.1 mg/dL. Oral cyclosporine was instituted at a dose of 25 mg bid and was to be gradually increased according to the cyclosporine level. Oral prednisone and azathioprine were begun after extubation. An inability to take in adequate nutrition led to a prescription for supplementary Ensure taken between meals. By day 3 AB was ambulating in his room with the assistance of physical therapy. His ability to clear secretions with a stronger cough maintained clear lung fields. Isoproterenol was weaned off, and he consistently maintained a HR of 90 to 100 beats/min with a CI of 3.2 L/min/m². He was transferred to the intermediate critical care unit on 2 μg/kg/min of dopamine for renal perfusion. At that point minimal teaching had been done.

MEDICAL DIAGNOSIS

Orthotopic heart transplant

NURSING DIAGNOSES

Knowledge Deficit: Dietary Needs, Medications, Reportable Symptoms related to lack of previous exposure to information

Altered Nutrition: Less Than Body Requirements related to lack of exogenous nutrients and increased metabolic demand

REVISED PLAN OF CARE

1. Continue instruction and activity progression with the assistance of physical therapy.
2. Obtain a dietary consult to increase caloric intake.
3. Encourage spouse to suggest favorite foods and bring in favorite foods from home.
4. Begin teaching patient and spouse about care regimen at home, medications, and side effects to watch for.
5. Teach patient about clinical manifestations of infection.

MEDICAL AND NURSING MANAGEMENT AND PATIENT OUTCOME

AB underwent endomyocardial biopsy at day 7. The results indicated no evidence of rejection. His appetite improved, and he took in adequate nutrition without supplements. He was able to cycle on a stationary bicycle for 15 minutes with some resistance. His BP was 165/95 mm Hg. His cyclosporine level stabilized at 200 ng/ml with a dose of 40 mg bid. AB and his spouse demonstrated a knowledge of medications, side effects, and clinical manifestations of infection. The patient administered his own medications without error.

MEDICAL DIAGNOSES

Orthotopic heart transplant
Hypertension related to cyclosporine

NURSING DIAGNOSIS

Knowledge Deficit: Instruction on Home Monitoring of Blood Pressure related to lack of previous exposure to information

REVISED PLAN OF CARE

1. Consult with physician about the need for antihypertensive medication.
2. Teach patient and spouse how to take blood pressure.
3. Acquire equipment so that patient can take his blood pressure at home.

CASE STUDY—CONT'D

HEART TRANSPLANTATION

MEDICAL AND NURSING MANAGEMENT AND PATIENT OUTCOME

AB was started on captopril, which controlled his blood pressure by postoperative day 9. He and his spouse demonstrated their ability to accurately measure his blood pressure. AB was discharged on postoperative day 10 with a stethoscope and sphygmomanometer, confident that he could manage his own health outside the hospital.

CASE STUDY

LIVER TRANSPLANTATION

CLINICAL HISTORY

Mr. B is a 20-year-old man who was diagnosed with primary sclerosing cholangitis 6 years ago. This disease is characterized by progressive narrowing of the bile ducts, which prevents the normal outflow of bile from the liver. Cirrhosis is the result of prolonged cholestasis. Mr. B has successfully completed evaluation and is followed at regular intervals through the outpatient clinic.

CURRENT PROBLEMS

After undergoing orthotopic liver transplantation, Mr. B arrives in the critical care unit directly from the operating room. He is mechanically ventilated at a rate of 12 breaths/min with an FIO_2 of 60%. He has a pulmonary artery catheter, which indicates a core temperature of 35.5° C. Other initial vital signs are a blood pressure (BP) of 150/95 mm Hg; pulse (P), 70; pulmonary artery pressure (PAP), 45/25 mm Hg; pulmonary artery wedge pressure (PAWP), 16 mm Hg; and central venous pressure (CVP), 12 mm Hg. His cardiac output (CO) is 5 L/min with a cardiac index (CI) of 2.2 L/min/m^2. He has an indwelling urinary catheter. Urine output during the first hour totals 160 ml. Initial arterial blood gases (ABGs) reveal a PaO_2 of 100; $PaCO_2$, 32; pH, 7.49; and O_2 saturation, 99%. Serum liver enzyme levels show marked elevations, which often occur as a result of manipulation of the graft during procurement and transplantation (harvest injury).

MEDICAL DIAGNOSIS

Orthotopic liver transplant

NURSING DIAGNOSES

Hypothermia related to exposure to cold environment

Impaired Gas Exchange related to ventilation/perfusion mismatching or intrapulmonary shunting

PLAN OF CARE

1. Use rewarming techniques.
2. Wean mechanical ventilations.
3. Begin immunosuppressive medications.

MEDICAL AND NURSING MANAGEMENT AND PATIENT OUTCOME

Warm blankets and a head cover were applied to the patient, and a heating lamp was positioned 3 feet from the thorax. The ventilator was weaned to 8 respirations/min after satisfactory ABGs were obtained with each decrease in ventilator rate. The patient remained anesthetized. Two hours after admission, the vital signs were as follows: BP, 105/60 mm Hg; P, 108; PAP, 20/8 mm Hg; PAWP, 6 mm Hg; CVP, 4 mm Hg; CO, 7.2 L/min; CI, 3.3 L/min/m^2. The urine output for the last hour totaled 20 ml. Core temperature rose to 37° C.

MEDICAL DIAGNOSIS

Orthotopic liver transplant

NURSING DIAGNOSES

Fluid Volume Deficit related to relative loss

Decreased Cardiac Output related to alterations in preload

Continued

CASE STUDY—CONT'D

LIVER TRANSPLANTATION

REVISED PLAN OF CARE

1. Infuse 250 ml of 5% albumin over 1 hour.
2. Remove warming apparatus—cover patient with one sheet and blanket.

MEDICAL AND NURSING MANAGEMENT AND PATIENT OUTCOME

After the revised plan of care was instituted, Mr. B's blood pressure rose to 130/75 mm Hg and his pulse returned to 70 bpm. Other measurements were as follows: PAP, 30/12 mm Hg; PAWP, 10 mm Hg; CVP, 7 mm Hg; CO, 6 L/min. His core temperature remained at 37° C. Fifteen hours after surgery, the patient was awake and alert. Successful weaning from the ventilator allowed extubation. The patient was placed on 40% oxygen by face mask, and ABGs were monitored every 6 to 8 hours. Other vital signs remained stable.

MEDICAL DIAGNOSIS

Orthotopic liver transplant

NURSING DIAGNOSIS

Ineffective Breathing Pattern related to decreased lung expansion

REVISED PLAN OF CARE

1. Institute mobilization—assist patient out of bed three times daily.
2. Incorporate aspects of self-care with activities of daily living.
3. Facilitate vigorous deep-breathing regimen q 2 hours.
4. Assist with incentive spirometry q 2 hours.
5. Advance diet to full liquids/regular diet.

MEDICAL AND NURSING MANAGEMENT AND PATIENT OUTCOME

On the second postoperative day, the route of oxygen administration was changed to nasal cannula. The nurse auscultated bowel sounds in all four quadrants. The nasogastric (NG) tube was removed, and the patient began to sip clear liquids. Liver enzyme values were decreasing appropriately, and other laboratory values were stable. Urine output and vital signs also were stable. On the fourth postoperative day, the pulmonary artery catheter was removed, and a multilumened central venous catheter was inserted. All unnecessary peripheral intravenous lines were removed.

On the fifth postoperative day, Mr. B's temperature spiked to 39° C. His pulse was 130; BP, 110/55 mm Hg; and respiratory rate (RR), 34/min. His central venous pressure dropped to 4 mm Hg.

MEDICAL DIAGNOSIS

Orthotopic liver transplant

NURSING DIAGNOSES

Risk for Infection risk factor: immunosuppressive drugs required to prevent rejection of liver

Ineffective Breathing Pattern related to decreased lung expansion

REVISED PLAN OF CARE

1. Culture blood, urine, and sputum for bacterial, fungal, and viral organisms (culture bile from T tube in appropriate patients).
2. Remove and culture indwelling IV catheters.
3. Institute measures to decrease body temperature.
4. Administer antibiotics.
5. Obtain abdominal computed tomography (CT) scan if all cultures are negative.

MEDICAL AND NURSING MANAGEMENT AND PATIENT OUTCOME

On day 6, preliminary blood culture results revealed enterococcus. Mr. B's antibiotic regimen was tailored to combat the specific organism. His temperature decreased to 37.5° C. His pulse decreased to 76, and his BP was 140/88 mm Hg. His liver enzymes continued to decrease over the next day to the following levels: aspartate transaminase (AST) (formerly SGOT), 123 U/L; alanine aminotransferase (ALT) (formerly SGPT), 94 U/L; γ-glutamyltransferase, (GGT), 174 IU/L; and alkaline phosphatase, 14 U/L. His total bilirubin was 2.5 dL (normal ranges from 0.1 to 1.1 mg/dL).

CASE STUDY—CONT'D

LIVER TRANSPLANTATION

MEDICAL AND NURSING MANAGEMENT AND PATIENT OUTCOME—cont'd

By the seventh postoperative day Mr. B was taking a regular diet, ambulating small distances, and performing most activities of daily living (ADLs). He began to learn how to self-administer his oral medications. One of his abdominal drains was discontinued, and the remaining two others, were draining minimal amounts of serosanguineous drainage. His urinary catheter was discontinued. On day 8 he was transferred to the floor.

Mr. B continued to learn aspects of self-care on the general nursing unit. He participated in physical and occupational therapy for muscle strengthening. He attended posttransplant support groups. On day 14, Mr. B's liver enzymes were as follows: AST, 160 U/L; ALT, 156 U/L; GGT, 230 IU/L; and alkaline phosphatase, 223 U/L. He underwent a percutaneous liver biopsy under ultrasound guidance. The biopsy revealed moderate acute cellular rejection.

MEDICAL DIAGNOSES

Orthotopic liver transplant
Acute cellular rejection (moderate)

NURSING DIAGNOSES

Anxiety related to threat to biologic integrity
Knowledge Deficit: Dietary Needs, Medications, Reportable Symptoms related to lack of previous exposure to information

REVISED PLAN OF CARE

1. Administer IV bolus of methylprednisolone (Solu-Medrol) 500 mg.
2. Administer oral prednisone as follows:
   80 mg/day for 2 days; then
   60 mg/day for 2 days; then
   40 mg/day for 2 days; then
   20 mg/day maintenance dose thereafter.
3. Measure blood glucose levels twice daily.
4. Begin teaching patient and spouse about self-care regimen, medications, and side effects.

MEDICAL AND NURSING MANAGEMENT AND PATIENT OUTCOME

During the treatment Mr. B's blood glucose levels elevated in response to the extra doses of steroids. He required subcutaneous regular insulin coverage to maintain normal blood glucose levels during the steroid cycle. During the treatment Mr. B's enzymes decreased. On day 20, they reached normal levels and his blood glucose levels again were normal. By this time he had learned all aspects of self-care. By day 23, Mr. B's blood pressure trended up to 160/98 mm Hg and remained elevated. He learned that this is a common side effect of both cyclosporine and prednisone; antihypertensive medication was begun. He learned how to monitor his own blood pressure measurements. On day 26, a discharge conference was held for Mr. B. He went home the following day.

CASE STUDY

KIDNEY-PANCREAS TRANSPLANTATION

CLINICAL HISTORY

Mr. G is a 36-year-old man with a 20-year history of insulin-dependent diabetes mellitus (IDDM). Complications from the diabetes include retinopathy, neuropathy, and end-stage renal disease (ESRD). He has been on continuous ambulatory peritoneal dialysis (CAPD) for 18 months. He has undergone a simultaneous kidney-pancreas transplant and arrives to the critical care unit in stable condition.

CURRENT PROBLEMS

On admission to the critical care unit Mr. G had a serum creatinine of 14.3 mg/dL; hematocrit (Hct), 26%; and blood glucose level, 100 mg/dL. He had a nasogastric (NG) tube connected to continuous low pressure wall suction; 4 L oxygen per nasal cannula; and a right triple-lumen central line was present with the following fluids infusing: milliliter per milliliter replacement fluid of normal saline (NS) (did not exceed 300 ml/hr), low-molecular dextran infused at 20 ml/hr, and an insulin drip. An abdominal midline dressing was dry and intact. A urinary catheter was in place and drained approximately 200 ml of slightly blood-tinged urine each hour. Mr. G was on bedrest with no hip flexion. Continuous 12-hour urine specimens were collected to monitor urinary amylase levels. His blood pressure was stable at 130/70 mm Hg; central venous pressure (CVP) remained at 7 mm Hg.

MEDICAL DIAGNOSIS

Kidney-pancreas transplant

NURSING DIAGNOSES

Risk for Infection risk factor: immunosuppressive drugs required to prevent rejection of kidney and pancreas
Fluid Volume Deficit related to absolute loss
Impaired Gas Exchange related to alveolar hypoventilation
Altered Nutrition: Less Than Body Requirements related to lack of exogenous nutrients or increased metabolic demand

PLAN OF CARE

1. Maintain aseptic technique with all lines/catheters.
2. Accurately measure and record intake and output, and continuously monitor volume status.
3. Assist patient with incentive spirometery q 2 hours.
4. Administer pain medication as needed for adequate relief.

MEDICAL AND NURSING MANAGEMENT AND PATIENT OUTCOME

Over the first 5 postoperative days, Mr. G's creatinine decreased to 1.3 mg/dL. Urinary amylase levels remained at approximately 40,000 U/ml. He began to have positive bowel sounds, and his NG tube was discontinued. He tolerated liquids well. His blood glucose was stable with values between 50 and 120 mg/dL. On day 3 he was transferred to the general transplant unit. On day 5 Mr. G began to ambulate and ask questions regarding his medications. He was tolerating a low-sodium, low-fat diet without difficulty.

MEDICAL DIAGNOSIS

Kidney-pancreas transplant

NURSING DIAGNOSES

Activity Intolerance related to prolonged immobility or deconditioning
Knowledge Deficit: Medications, interpretation of laboratory values related to lack of previous exposure to information

REVISED PLAN OF CARE

1. Assist in increasing activity as tolerated.
2. Incorporate activities of daily living and self-care into daily activity.
3. Begin self-medication program; teach patient regarding laboratory values.

CASE STUDY—CONT'D

KIDNEY-PANCREAS TRANSPLANTATION

MEDICAL AND NURSING MANAGEMENT AND PATIENT OUTCOME

By day 10 Mr. G had a stable creatinine that ranged from 1.3 to 1.5 mg/dL Blood glucose values were stable, and he did not require any insulin. A cystoscopy revealed healing sutures, and the urinary catheter was removed. On day 12 Mr. G's white blood cell (WBC) count had climbed from 7.8 to 15.7 mm^3 He had orthostatic hypotension with blood pressures (BPs) of 138/80 mm Hg, lying; 110/70 mm Hg, sitting; and 80/50 mm Hg, standing. His temperature ranged between 99 and 100.6° F. He complained of dizziness when he first stood, but otherwise he felt well. An infection was suspected. Blood, throat, urine, and cytomegalovirus (CMV) cultures were obtained. On postoperative day 19, Mr. G was transferred back to the critical care unit with a temperature of 102° F, WBC count of 7.8 to 15.7 mm^3, and a blood pressure of 90/50 mm Hg, supine.

MEDICAL DIAGNOSIS

Kidney-pancreas transplant

NURSING DIAGNOSES

Risk for Infection risk factor: immunosuppressive drugs required to prevent rejection of kidney and pancreas

Activity Intolerance related to prolonged immobility or deconditioning

REVISED PLAN OF CARE

1. Use aseptic technique with all lines and catheters.
2. Administer fluids IV and by mouth (PO).
3. Closely monitor blood pressure. Maintain systolic BP >100 mm Hg.
4. Reassure patient of need for close monitoring to ensure his well-being.

MEDICAL AND NURSING MANAGEMENT AND PATIENT OUTCOME

Mr. G's blood cultures showed that he had a *Staphylococcus* infection. After treatment with appropriate antibiotics and aggressive fluid replacement, Mr. G became afebrile and maintained a stable blood pressure range of 120–130s/70–80s mm Hg. However, over the next 48 hours his creatinine rose from 1.3 to 1.7 mg/dL despite hydration. Also, his urine amylase levels decreased from 30,210 to 12,620 U/ml. His blood glucose levels remained stable. Rejection was suspected, and a renal biopsy was obtained. The biopsy revealed acute rejection (mild).

MEDICAL DIAGNOSES

Kidney-pancreas transplant

Post-*Staphylcoccus* infection

Acute rejection (mild)

NURSING DIAGNOSES

Risk for Infection risk factor: immunosuppressive drugs required to prevent rejection of kidney and pancreas

Anxiety related to threat to biologic, psychologic, and/or social integrity

Knowledge Deficit: Self-care Regimen related to lack of previous exposure to information

REVISED PLAN OF CARE

1. Use aseptic technique with all lines and catheters.
2. Discuss patient's concerns regarding this rejection episode.
3. Continue teaching patient about self-care regimen, medications, and side-effects.

MEDICAL AND NURSING MANAGEMENT AND PATIENT OUTCOME

Mr. G was treated with IV methylprednisolone (Solu-Medrol). By the third treatment day his creatinine was 1.4 mg/dL, and his urinary amylase was 40,700 U/ml. He was transferred to the general transplant unit. He continued to improve and became very knowledgeable regarding medications, laboratory values, symptoms of rejection, physical limitations, diet, and clinic appointments. On postoperative day 17 he was discharged home.

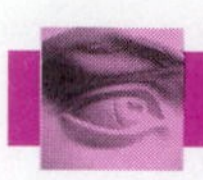

NURSING MANAGEMENT PLAN

RISK FOR INFECTION

DEFINITION:

The state in which an individual is at increased risk for being invaded by pathogenic organisms.

Risk for Infection Risk Factor: Immunosuppressive Drugs Required to Prevent Rejection of Transplanted Organ

DEFINING CHARACTERISTICS

- Temperature >38° C or persistent temperature >37.5° C
- Leukocytosis or leukopenia
- Infiltrate on chest x-ray film
- Cough (may be nonproductive)
- Redness, pain, tenderness, or drainage over wounds or IV access sites
- Positive blood, urine, or sputum cultures
- Specific manifestations related to site of infection (e.g., decreased PaO_2 with lung infection)

OUTCOME CRITERIA

- Temperature is normal.
- Chest film is clear.
- No clinical signs of infection are present.
- Wounds are healing normally.
- All cultures are negative.
- Patient is knowledgeable about clinical manifestations of infection and when to seek medical care.

NURSING INTERVENTIONS AND *RATIONALE*

1. Monitor for temperature elevation > 37.5° C, and report elevations to physician.
2. Obtain blood, urine, and sputum cultures for temperature elevations > 38° C ***inasmuch as elevation likely is caused by bacteremia or bladder or pulmonary infection.***
3. Auscultate breath sounds at least every 6 hours. ***Pulmonary infection is the most common type of infection, and changes in breath sounds might be an early indication.***
4. Inspect wounds at least every 8 hours for redness, swelling, and/or drainage, ***which may indicate infection.***
5. Inspect overall skin integrity and oral mucosa for signs of breakdown, ***which place the patient at risk of infection.***
6. Notify physician of any new onset cough. ***Even a nonproductive cough may indicate pulmonary infection.***
7. Monitor white blood cell count daily, and report leukocytosis or sudden development of leukopenia, ***which may indicate an infectious process.***
8. Protect patient from exposure to any staff or family member with contagious lesions (e.g., herpes simplex) or respiratory infections.
9. Evaluate nutritional status, and suggest augmentation of nutritional intake as necessary ***to prevent debilitation and increased susceptibility to infection.***
10. Encourage physician to remove invasive lines and catheters as soon as possible ***to decrease potential portals of entry.***
11. Teach patient the clinical manifestations of infection. ***A knowledgeable patient will seek medical attention promptly, which will result in earlier treatment and a decreased risk that an infection will become life threatening.***

REFERENCES

1. Bartucci MR, Seller MC: The immunology of transplant rejection. In Sigardson-Poor KM, Haggerty LM, editors: *Nursing care of the transplant patient,* Philadelphia, 1990, WB Saunders.
2. Bierer BE: Immunosuppressive agents targeting T-cell activation pathways. In Sollinger H, Przepiorka D, editors: *Recent developments in transplantation medicine, vol 1. New immunosuppressant drugs,* Glenview, Ill, 1994, Physicians & Scientists Publishing.
3. Colling EG, Hubbell EA: Immunologic aspects of organ transplantation. In Williams BAH, Grady KL, Sandiford-Guttebiel DM, editors: *Organ transplantation,* New York, 1991, Springer.
4. Morris RE: Overview of immunosuppressive drugs for transplantation: Where are we? How did we get here? And where are we going? *Clinical Transplantation* 7:138, 1993.
5. Payne JL: Immune modification and complications of immunosuppression, *Crit Care Nurs Clin North Am* 4:43, 1992.
6. Schreiber SL, Crabtree GR: The mechanism of action of cyclosporin A and FK506, *Immunol Today* 13:136, 1992.
7. Crandell B: Immunosuppression. In Sigardson-Poor KM, Haggerty LM, editors: *Nursing care of the transplant recipient,* Philadelphia, 1990, WB Saunders.

8. White-Williams C: Immunosuppressive therapy following cardiac transplantation, *Crit Care Nurs Q* 16:1, 1993.
9. Staschak SM, Zamberlan K: Recent development: FK506. In Sigardson-Poor KM, Haggerty LM, editors: *Nursing care of the transplant recipient,* Philadelphia, 1990, WB Saunders.
10. Armitage JM and others: Clinical trial of FK506 immunosuppression in adult cardiac transplantation, *Ann Thoracic Surg* 54:205, 1992.
11. Griffith BP and others: Prospective randomized trial of FK506 versus cyclosporin after human pulmonary transplantation, *Transplantation* 57:848, 1994.
12. Przepiorka D: Tacrolimus: Preclinical and clinical experience. In Sollinger H, Przepiorka D, editors: *Recent developments in transplantation medicine, vol 1. New immunosuppressant drugs,* Glenview, Ill, 1994, Physicians & Scientists Publishing.
13. Young CJ, Sollinger H: Mycophenolate mofetil (RS-61443). In Sollinger H, Przepiorka D, editors: *Recent developments in transplantation medicine, vol 1. New immunosuppressant drugs,* Glenview, Ill, 1994, Physicians & Scientists Publishing.
14. Allison AC, Eugui EM, Sollinger HW: Mycophenolate mofetil (RS-61443): mechanisms of action and effects in transplantation, *Transplant Reviews* 7:129, 1993.
15. Morris RE: New immunosuppressive molecules for control of organ transplant rejection. In Williams BAH, Sandiford-Guttenbiel DM, editors: *Trends in organ transplantation,* New York, 1996, Springer.
16. Reitz B: The history of heart and heart-lung transplantation. In Baumgartner WA, Reitz BA, Achuff SC, editors: *Heart and heart-lung transplantation,* Philadelphia, 1990, WB Saunders.
17. Losse B: Indications and selection criteria for cardiac transplantation, *Thorac Cardiovasc Surg* 38:276, 1990.
18. St. Anthony: *DRA Guidebook,* 1996, St. Anthony's Publishing, Reston Va.
19. Dillon TA and others: Cardiac transplantation in patients with preexisting malignancies, *Transplantation* 52:82, 1991.
20. Edwards BS and others: Cardiac transplantation in patients with preexisting neoplastic diseases, *Am J Cardiol* 65:501, 1990.
21. Badellino NM and others: Cardiac transplantation in diabetic patients, *Transplant Proc* 22:2384, 1990.
22. Ladowski JS and others: Heart transplantation in diabetic recipients, *Transplantation* 49:303, 1990.
23. Rhenman MJ and others: Diabetics and heart transplantation, *J Heart Transplant* 7:356, 1988.
24. Hurst JW and others: *The heart,* ed 7, New York, 1990, McGraw-Hill.
25. Dibiase A and others: Frequency and mechanism of bradycardia in cardiac transplant recipients and need for pacemakers, *Am J Cardiol* 67:1385, 1991.
26. Whitman GR, Hicks LE: Major nursing diagnoses following cardiac transplantation, *J Cardiovasc Nurs* 2:1, 1988.
27. Masoorli ST, Piercy S: A lifesaving guide to blood products, *RN* 47:32, 1984.
28. Billingham ME and others: A working formulation for the standardization of nomenclature in the diagnosis of heart and lung rejection: heart rejection study group, *J Heart Lung Transplant* 9:587, 1990.
29. Hunt SA and others: Total lymphoid irradiation for treatment of intractable cardiac allograft rejection, *J Heart Lung Transplant* 10:211, 1991.
30. Futterman LG: Cardiac transplantation: a comprehensive nursing perspective. II. *Heart Lung* 17:631, 1988.
31. Merigan TC and others: A controlled trial of ganciclovir to prevent cytomegalovirus disease after heart transplantation, *N Engl J Med* 326:1182, 1992.
32. Patel R and others: Cytomegalovirus prophylaxis in solid organ transplant recipients, *Transplantation* 61:1279, 1996.
33. Snydman DR and others: Final analysis of primary cytomegalovirus disease prevention in renal transplant recipients with a cytomegalovirus-immune globulin: comparison of the randomized and open label trials, *Transplant Proc* 23:1357, 1991.
34. George MJ and others: Use of ganciclovir plus cytomegalovirus immune globulin to treat CMV pneumonia in orthotopic liver transplant recipients, *Transplant Proc* 25:22, 1993.
35. *Cytomegalovirus infections in the immunocompromised transplant patient: diagnosis and treatment* (special symposium review), San Francisco, 1991, Professional Healthcare Communications.
36. Gao S and others: Accelerated coronary vascular disease in the heart transplant patient: coronary arteriographic findings, *J Am Coll Cardiol* 12:334, 1988.
37. Sharples LD and others: Risk factor analysis for the major hazards following heart transplantation, rejection, infection and coronary occlusive disease, *Transplantation* 52:244, 1991.
38. Stark RP, McGinn AL, Wilson RF: Chest pain in cardiac transplant recipients, *N Engl J Med* 324:1791, 1991.
39. Decampli WM and others: Characteristics of patients surviving more than ten years after cardiac transplantation, *J Thoracic Cardiovasc Surg* 109: 1103, 1995.
40. Lough ME and others: Impact of symptom frequency and symptom distress on self-reported quality of life in heart transplant recipients, *Heart Lung* 16:193, 1987.
41. Packa RD: Quality of life of adults after a heart transplant, *J Cardiovasc Nurs* 13:12, 1989.
42. Evans RW and others: *The national heart transplantation study:* final report, Seattle, 1984, Battelle Human Affairs Research Centers.
43. Lough ME: Quality of life issues following heart transplantation, *Prog Cardiovasc Nurs* 1:17, 1986.
44. United Network for Organ Sharing, based on UNOS OPTN/Scientific Registry data as of May 13, 1996.

45. Marshall SE and others: Selection and evaluation of recipients for heart-lung and lung transplantation, *Chest* 98:1488, 1990.
46. Egan TM, Kaiser LR, Cooper JD: Lung transplantation, *Curr Probl Surg* 10:673, 1989.
47. Hutter JA: Heart-lung transplantation : better use of resources, *Am J Med* 85:4, 1988.
48. Klepetko W and others: Domino transplantation of heart-lung and heart: an approach to overcome the scarcity of donor organs, *J Heart Lung Transplant* 10:129, 1991.
49. Theodore J, Lewiston N: Lung transplantation comes of age, *N Engl J Med* 322:772, 1990.
50. Hakim M and others: Selection and procurement of combined heart and lung grafts for transplantation, *J Thorac Cardiovasc Surg* 95:474, 1988.
51. Starnes VA: Heart-lung transplantation: an overview, *Cardiol Clin* 8:159, 1990.
52. Starnes VA and others: Cystic fibrosis: target population for lung transplantation in North America in the 1990's, *J Thorac Cardiovasc Surg* 103 (5):1008, 1992.
53. Valentine VG and others: Clinical diagnosis in heart and lung allograft rejection. In Solez K, Racusen LC, Billingham ME, editors: *Solid organ transplant rejection,* New York, 1996, Marcel Dekker.
54. Yousem SA and others: A working formulation for the standardization of nomenclature in the diagnosis of heart and lung rejection: lung rejection study group, *J Heart Lung Transplant* 9:593, 1990.
55. Theodore J: Pulmonary function in the uncomplicated human transplanted lung, *ACP* 2:301, 1987.
56. Baldwin JC: Comparison of cardiac rejection in heart and heart-lung transplantation, *J Heart Transplant* 6:352, 1987.
57. Theodore J, Starnes VA, Lewiston NJ: Obliterative bronchiolitis, *Clin Chest Med* 11:309, 1990.
58. Glanville AR and others: Obliterative bronchiolitis after heart-lung transplantation: apparent arrest by augmented immunosuppression, *Ann Intern Med* 107:300, 1987.
59. Starnes VA and others: Current trends in lung transplantation: lobar transplantation and expanded use of single lungs, *J Thorac Cardiovasc Surg* 104:1060, 1992.
60. Cooper JD and others: Bilateral pneumectomy (volume reduction) for chronic obstructive pulmonary disease, *J Thoracic Cardiovasc Surg* 109:106, 1995.
61. Gaissert HA and others: Comparison of early functional results after volume reduction or lung transplantation for chronic obstructive pulmonary disease, *J Thoracic Cardiovasc Surg* 111:296, 1996.
62. Marshall SE and others: Prospective analysis of serial pulmonary function studies, transbronchial biopsies in single-lung transplant recipients, *Transplant Proc* 23:12 1991.
63. Welch CS: A note on transplantation of the whole liver in dogs, *Transplant Bulletin* 2(2):54, 1955.
64. Cannon GA: Organs, *Transplant Bulletin* 3(1):7, 1956 (communication).
65. Moore FD and others: One-stage homotransplantation of the liver following total hepatectomy in dogs, *Transplant Bulletin* 6:103, 1959.
66. Moore FD and others: Experimental whole organ transplantation of the liver and of the spleen, *Ann Surg* 152(3):374, 1960.
67. Starzl TE and others: Reconstructive problems in canine homotransplantation with special reference to the postoperative role of hepatic vein flow, *Surg Gynecol Obstet* 11:733, 1960.
68. Starzl TE and others: Homotransplantation of the liver in humans, *Surg Gynecol Obstet* 117(6):659, 1963.
69. Starzl TE and others: Orthotopic homotransplantation the human liver, *Ann Surg* 168(3):392, 1968.
70. Cosimi AB: Update on liver transplantation, *Transplant Proc* 23(4):2083, 1991.
71. Starzl TE and others: Liver transplantation with the use of cyclosporin A and prednisone, *N Engl J Med* 305:266, 1981.
72. National Institutes of Health: National Institutes of Health Consensus Development Conference Statement: liver transplantation—June 20–23, 1983, *Hepatology* 4(1S): 107S, 1984.
73. United Network for Organ Sharing: *UNOS Annual Report,* 1988, Richmond, Va , United Network for Organ Sharing.
74. United Network for Organ Sharing: *UNOS Update* 12(3), March 1996.
75. Wiesner R: Current indications, contraindications, and timing for liver transplantation. In Busuttil RW, Klintmalm GB, editors: *Transplantation of the liver,* Philadelphia, 1996, WB Saunders.
76. Bilbao I and others: Liver transplantation in patients over 60 years of age, *Transplant Proc* 27(4): 2337, 1995.
77. Lake JR: Transplantation for chronic viral hepatitis. In Busuttil RW, Klintmalm GB, editors: *Transplantation of the liver,* Philadelphia, 1996, WB Saunders:
78. Harren P and others: Incidence and treatment of recurrent hepatitis C after liver transplantation, *J Transplant Coordination* 6:24, 1996.
79. Crippen J: Transplantation for sclerosing cholangitis. In Busuttil RW, Klintmalm GB, editors: *Transplantation of the liver,* Philadelphia, 1996, WB Saunders.
80. Porayko MK, Kondo M, Steers JL: Liver transplantation: late complications of the biliary tract and their management, *Semin Liver Dis* 15:139, 1995.
81. Farges O and others: Long-term results of ABO-incompatible liver transplantation, *Transplant Proc* 27:1701, 1995.
82. Nuño J and others: Is liver transplantation an emergency or an elective surgical procedure? Analysis of risk factors related to early mortality in 139 liver transplant recipients, *Transplant Proc* 27:2321, 1995.
83. Monsour HP Jr and others: Renal insufficiency and hypertension as long-term complications in liver transplantation, *Semin Liver Dis* 15(2):123, 1995.

84. Garcia-Valdecasas JC and others: Risk factors for severe bacterial infection after liver transplantation, *Transplant Proc* 27:2334, 1995.
85. Kanj SS and others: Cytomegalovirus infection following liver transplantation: review of the literature, *Clin Infect Dis* 22:537, 1996.
86. Rubin R: Infection in the organ transplant recipient. In Rubin RH, Young LS, editors: *Clinical approach to infection in the compromised host,* New York, 1994, Plenum Medical Book Co.
87. Winston D, Emmanouilides C, Busuttil RW: Infections in liver transplant recipients, *Clin Infect Dis* 21:1077, 1995.
88. Basgoz N, Rubin RH: Antimicrobial prophylaxis in patients undergoing solid organ transplantation. In Remington JS, Swartz MN, editors: *Current clinical topics in infectious diseases,* vol 15, New York, 1995, Blackwell Science.
89. Balsells J, and others: Evaluation of biliary complications in liver transplant without biliary drainage, *Transplant Proc* 27:2339, 1995.
90. Makowka L, Sher L: *Orthobiotech handbook of organ transplantation,* Austin, 1995, RG Landes.
91. Zetterman RK, McCashland TM: Long-term follow-up of the orthotopic liver transplatation patient, *Semin Liver Dis* 15:173, 1995.
92. Dominquez EA: Long-term infectious complications of liver transplantation, *Semin Liver Dis* 15(2):133, 1995.
93. Tan-Shalaby J, Temero M: Malignancies after transplantation: a comparative review, *Semin Liver Dis* 15:156, 1995.
94. Thomas DJ: The lived experience of people with liver transplants, *J Transplant Coordination* 5:65, 1995.
95. Morrissey M, Rustand L: Financial consideration in liver transplantation. In Busuttil RW, Klintmalm GB, editors: *Transplantation of the liver,* Philadelphia, 1996, WB Saunders.
96. Whiteman K and others: The effect of continuous lateral rotation therapy on pulmonary complications in liver transplant, *Am J Crit Care* 4(2):133, 1995.
97. Przepiorka D: New immunosuppressive drugs. In Sollinger H, Przepiorka D, editors. *Recent developments in transplantation medication,* vol. 1. *New immunosuppressant drugs,* Glenview, Ill, 1994, Physicians and Scientists Publishers.
98. Guy E and others: Immunosuppression conversion for relief of side effects, *Transplant Proc* 26:3235, 1994.
99. Dahmen U and others: The role of antibodies in liver graft-induced tolerance in mice: passive transfer of serum and effect of recipient B-cell depletion, *Transplant Proc* 27:511, 1995.
100. Demetris AJ and others: The liver allograft, chronic (ductopenic) rejection, and microchimerism: what can they teach us? *Transplant Proc* 27:67, 1995.
101. Cacciarelli TV and others: Impact of reduced-size liver transplantation on rejection and liver allograft outcome in the pediatric population, *Transplant Proc* 27:1239, 1995.
102. Cramer DV: The use of xenografts for acute hepatic failure, *Transplant Proc* 27:80, 1995.
103. Makowka L and others: The use of a pig liver xenograft for temporary support of a patient with fulminant hepatic failure, *Transplantation* 59:1654, 1995.
104. Heffron T: Living related liver transplantation, *Semin Liver Dis* 15:165, 1995.
105. Slapak G and others: Biochemical and histologic study of long-term liver transplant survivors, *Transplant Proc* 27(1):1228, 1995.
106. Fleschler RG, Sala DJ: Pregnancy after organ transplantation, *J Obstet Gynecol Neonatal Nurs* 24:413, 1995.
107. Gutkind L: *Many sleepless nights,* New York, 1988, WW Norton.
108. Data Source: United Network for Organ Sharing (UNOS), 1996, Richmond, Va.
109. Yoshimura N and others: Quality of life in renal transplant recipients treated with cyclosporine in comparison with hemodialysis maintenance, *Trans Proc* 26(5):2542, 1994.
110. Zeher CL, Gross CR: Comparisons of quality of life between pancreas/kidney and kidney transplant recipients: one year out, *Trans Proc* 26:508, 1994.
111. Perryman JP, Stillerman PU: Kidney transplantation. In Smith SL, editor: *AACN tissue and organ transplantation: implications for professional nursing practice,* St Louis, 1990, Mosby.
112. Evans RW and others: Immunosuppressive therapy as a determinant of transplantation outcomes, *Transplantation* 55:1297, 1993.
113. United Network of Organ Sharing (UNOS) by-laws and policies, 1994, Richmond, Va.
114. Bry W, Warvariv V, Levin B: Kidney transplantation. In Makowka L, Sher L, editors: *Orthobiotech handbook of organ transplantation,* Austin, 1995, RG Landes.
115. Cunningham NH, Boeter S, Windham S: Renal transplantation, *Crit Care Nurs Clin North Am* 4(1):79, 1992.
116. The Diabetes Control and Complications Trial Research Group: The effects of intensive treatment of diabetes on the development and progression of long term complications in insulin-dependent diabetes mellitus, *N Engl J Med* 329(14):759, 1993.
117. Wills BG, Post CL: Pancreas transplantation. In Smith SL, editor: *AACN tissue and organ transplantation: implications for professional nursing practice,* St. Louis, 1990, Mosby.
118. Manske CL, Wang Y, Thomas W: Mortality of cadaveric kidney transplantation in diabetic patients, *Lancet* 346:1658, 1995.
119. Henry M: Pancreas transplantation. In Makowka L, Sher L, editors: *Orthobiotech handbook of transplantation,* Austin, 1995, RG Landes.
120. Zehr PS and others: Impact of pancreas transplantation on quality of life of diabetic renal transplant recipients, *Trans Proc* 26(2):520, 1994.

121. Remuzzi G, Ruggenenti P, Mauer SM: Pancreas and kidney/pancreas transplants: experimental medicine or real improvement? *Lancet* 343:27, 1994.
122. Robertson RP: Pancreatic and islet transplantation for diabetes—cures or curiosities? *N Engl J Med* 326(26):1861, 1992.
123. Grewel HP and others: Risk factors for post implantation pancreatitis and pancreatic thrombosis in pancreas transplant recipients, *Transplantation* 56:609, 1992.
124. Gaber AO and others: Pancreas transplantation with portal venous and enteric drainage eliminates hyperinsulinemia and reduces postoperative complications, *Trans Proc* 25(1):1176, 1993.
125. Trusler LA: Simultaneous kidney-pancreas transplantation, *Crit Care Nurs North Am* 4(1):89, 1992.
126. Warnuck GL, Rajotte RV: Human pancreatic islet transplantation, *Transplant Rev* 6:1995, 1992.

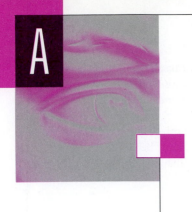

North American Nursing Diagnosis Association's (NANDA) Taxonomy

Pattern 1: Exchanging

1.1.2.1 Altered Nutrition: More Than Body Requirements
1.1.2.2 Altered Nutrition: Less Than Body Requirements
1.1.2.3 Altered Nutrition: Risk for More Than Body Requirements
1.2.1.1 Risk for Infection
1.2.2.1 Risk for Altered Body Temperature
1.2.2.2 Hypothermia
1.2.2.3 Hyperthermia
1.2.2.4 Ineffective Thermoregulation
1.2.3.1 Dysreflexia
1.3.1.1 Constipation
1.3.1.1.1 Perceived Constipation
1.3.1.1.2 Colonic Constipation
1.3.1.2 Diarrhea
1.3.1.3 Bowel Incontinence
1.3.2 Altered Urinary Elimination
1.3.2.1.1 Stress Incontinence
1.3.2.1.2 Reflex Incontinence
1.3.2.1.3 Urge Incontinence
1.3.2.1.4 Functional Incontinence
1.3.2.1.5 Total Incontinence
1.3.2.2 Urinary Retention
1.4.1.1 Altered (Specify Type) Tissue Perfusion (Renal, Cerebral, Cardiopulmonary, Gastrointestinal, Peripheral)
1.4.1.2.1 Fluid Volume Excess
1.4.1.2.2.1 Fluid Volume Deficit
1.4.1.2.2.2 Risk for Fluid Volume Deficit
1.4.2.1 Decreased Cardiac Output
1.5.1.1 Impaired Gas Exchange
1.5.1.2 Ineffective Airway Clearance
1.5.1.3 Ineffective Breathing Pattern
1.5.1.3.1 Inability to Sustain Spontaneous Ventilation
1.5.1.3.2 Dysfunctional Ventilatory Weaning Response (DVWR)
1.6.1 Risk for Injury
1.6.1.1 Risk for Suffocation
1.6.1.2 Risk for Poisoning
1.6.1.3 Risk for Trauma
1.6.1.4 Risk for Aspiration
1.6.1.5 Risk for Disuse Syndrome
1.6.2 Altered Protection
1.6.2.1 Impaired Tissue Integrity
1.6.2.1.1 Altered Oral Mucous Membrane
1.6.2.1.2.1 Impaired Skin Integrity
1.6.2.1.2.2 Risk for Impaired Skin Integrity
1.7.1 Decreased Adaptive Capacity: Intracranial
1.8 Energy Field Disturbance

Pattern 2: Communicating

2.1.1.1 Impaired Verbal Communication

Pattern 3: Relating

3.1.1 Impaired Social Interaction
3.1.2 Social Isolation
3.1.3 Risk for Loneliness
3.2.1 Altered Role Performance
3.2.1.1.1 Altered Parenting
3.2.1.1.2 Risk for Altered Parenting
3.2.1.1.2.1 Risk for Altered Parent/Infant/Child Attachment
3.2.1.2.1 Sexual Dysfunction
3.2.2 Altered Family Processes
3.2.2.1 Caregiver Role Strain
3.2.2.2 Risk for Caregiver Role Strain
3.2.2.3.1 Altered Family Processes: Alcoholism
3.2.3.1 Parental Role Conflict
3.3 Altered Sexuality Patterns

*From North American Nursing Diagnosis Association: *NANDA nursing diagnoses: definitions and classification,* 1995–1996, Philadelphia, 1994, The Association.

Pattern 4: Valuing

4.1.1 Spiritual Distress (Distress of the Human Spirit)
4.2 Potential for Enhanced Spiritual Well–Being

Pattern 5: Choosing

5.1.1.1 Ineffective Individual Coping
5.1.1.1.1 Impaired Adjustment
5.1.1.1.2 Defensive Coping
5.1.1.1.3 Ineffective Denial
5.1.2.1.1 Ineffective Family Coping: Disabling
5.1.2.1.2 Ineffective Family Coping: Compromised
5.1.2.2 Family Coping: Potential for Growth
5.1.3.1 Potential for Enhanced Community Coping
5.1.3.2 Ineffective Community Coping
5.2.1 Ineffective Management of Therapeutic Regimen (Individuals)
5.2.1.1 Noncompliance (Specify)
5.2.2 Ineffective Management of Therapeutic Regimen: Families
5.2.3 Ineffective Management of Therapeutic Regimen: Community
5.2.4 Effective Management of Therapeutic Regimen: Individual
5.3.1.1 Decisional Conflict (Specify)
5.4 Health-Seeking Behaviors (Specify)

Pattern 6: Moving

6.1.1.1 Impaired Physical Mobility
6.1.1.1.1 Risk for Peripheral Neurovascular Dysfunction
6.1.1.1.2 Risk for Perioperative Positioning Injury
6.1.1.2 Activity Intolerance
6.1.1.2.1 Fatigue
6.1.1.3 Risk for Activity Intolerance
6.2.1 Sleep Pattern Disturbance
6.3.1.1 Diversional Activity Deficit
6.4.1.1 Impaired Home Maintenance Management
6.4.2 Altered Health Maintenance
6.5.1 Feeding Self-Care Deficit
6.5.1.1 Impaired Swallowing
6.5.1.2 Ineffective Breastfeeding
6.5.1.2.1 Interrupted Breastfeeding
6.5.1.3 Effective Breastfeeding
6.5.1.4 Ineffective Infant Feeding Pattern
6.5.2 Bathing/Hygiene Self-Care Deficit
6.5.3 Dressing/Grooming Self-Care Deficit
6.5.4 Toileting Self-Care Deficit
6.6 Altered Growth and Development
6.7 Relocation Stress Syndrome
6.8.1 Risk for Disorganized Infant Behavior
6.8.2 Disorganized Infant Behavior
6.8.3 Potential for Enhanced Organized Infant Behavior

Pattern 7: Perceiving

7.1.1 Body Image Disturbance
7.1.2 Self-Esteem Disturbance
7.1.2.1 Chronic Low Self-Esteem
7.1.2.2 Situational Low Self-Esteem
7.1.3 Personal Identity Disturbance
7.2 Sensory/Perceptual Alterations (Specify) (Visual, Auditory, Kinesthetic, Gustatory, Tactile, Olfactory)
7.2.1.1 Unilateral Neglect
7.3.1 Hopelessness
7.3.2 Powerlessness

Pattern 8: Knowing

8.1.1 Knowledge Deficit (Specify)
8.2.1 Impaired Environmental Interpretation Syndrome
8.2.2 Acute Confusion
8.2.3 Chronic Confusion
8.3 Altered Thought Processes
8.3.1 Impaired Memory

Pattern 9: Feeling

9.1.1 Pain
9.1.1.1 Chronic Pain
9.2.1.1 Dysfunctional Grieving
9.2.1.2 Anticipatory Grieving
9.2.2 Risk for Violence: Self-Directed or Directed at Others
9.2.2.1 Risk for Self-Mutilation
9.2.3 Post-Trauma Response
9.2.3.1 Rape-Trauma Syndrome
9.2.3.1.1 Rape-Trauma Syndrome: Compound Reaction
9.2.3.1.2 Rape-Trauma Syndrome: Silent Reaction
9.3.1 Anxiety
9.3.2 Fear

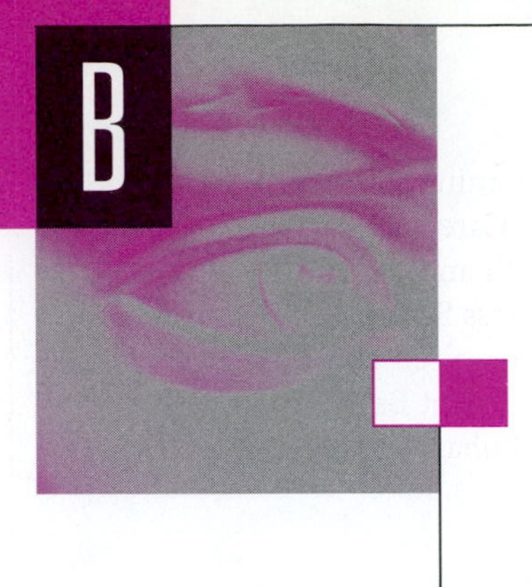

Nursing Interventions Classification (NIC) Taxonomy

The Nursing Interventions Classification (NIC) is a comprehensive, standardized language used to describe the treatments that nurses perform. Developed by a research team at the University of Iowa, this clinical tool standardizes and defines the knowledge base for nursing curricula and practice; communicates the nature of nursing; and facilitates the appropriate selection of nursing interventions for nurses, including practicing nurses, nursing students, nursing administrators and faculty.

The following is a taxonomy of the Nursing Interventions Classification in McCloskey JC, Bulechek GM: *Nursing interventions classification (NIC)*, ed 2, St Louis, 1996, Mosby.

NIC TAXONOMY

	Domain 1	Domain 2	Domain 3	Domain 4	Domain 5	Domain 6
LEVEL 1 DOMAINS	**1. Physiological: Basic** Care that supports physical functioning	**2. Physiological: Complex** Care that supports homeostatic regulation	**3. Behavioral** Care that supports psychosocial functioning and facilitates life-style changes	**4. Safety** Care that supports protection against harm	**5. Family** Care that supports the family unit	**6. Health System** Care that supports effective use of the health care delivery system
LEVEL 2 CLASSES	A *Activity and Exercise Management:* Interventions to organize or assist with physical activity and energy conservation and expenditure B *Elimination Management:* Interventions to establish and maintain regular bowel and urinary elimination patterns and manage complications due to altered patterns C *Immobility Management:* Interventions to manage restricted body movement and the sequelae D *Nutrition Support:* Interventions to modify or maintain nutritional status E *Physical Comfort Promotion:* Interventions to promote comfort using physical techniques F *Self-Care Facilitation:* Interventions to provide or assist with routine activities of daily living	G *Electrolyte and Acid-Base Management:* Interventions to regulate electrolyte/acid base balance and prevent complications H *Drug Management:* Interventions to facilitate desired effects of pharmacological agents I *Neurologic Management:* Interventions to optimize neurologic functions J *Perioperative Care:* Interventions to provide care before, during, and immediately after surgery K *Respiratory Management:* Interventions to promote airway patency and gas exchange L *Skin/Wound Management:* Interventions to maintain or restore tissue integrity M *Thermoregulation:* Interventions to maintain body temperature within a normal range N *Tissue Perfusion Management:* Interventions to optimize circulation of blood and fluids to the tissue	O *Behavior Therapy:* Interventions to reinforce or promote desirable behaviors or alter undesirable behaviors. P *Cognitive Therapy:* Interventions to reinforce or promote desirable cognitive functioning or alter undesirable cognitive functioning Q *Communication Enhancement:* Interventions to facilitate delivering and receiving verbal and nonverbal messages R *Coping Assistance:* Interventions to assist another to build on own strengths, to adapt to a change in function, or to achieve a higher level of function S *Patient Education:* Interventions to facilitate learning T *Psychological Comfort Promotion:* Interventions to promote comfort using psychological techniques	U *Crisis Management:* Interventions to provide immediate short-term help in both psychological and physiological crises V *Risk Management:* Interventions to initiate risk-reduction activities and continue monitoring risks over time	W *Childbearing Care:* Interventions to assist in understanding and coping with the psychological and physiological changes during the childbearing period X *Lifespan Care:* Interventions to facilitate family unit functioning and promote the health and welfare of family members throughout the lifespan	Y *Health System Mediation:* Interventions to facilitate the interface between patient/family and the health care system a *Health System Management:* Interventions to provide and enhance support services for the delivery of care b *Information Management:* Interventions to facilitate communication among health care providers

LEVEL 1 DOMAINS	1. PHYSIOLOGICAL: BASIC Care that Supports Physical Functioning					
LEVEL 2 CLASSES	A **Activity and Exercise Management** Interventions to organize or assist with physical activity and energy conservation and expenditure	B **Elimination Management** Interventions to establish and maintain regular bowel and urinary elimination patterns and manage complications due to altered patterns	C **Immobility Management** Interventions to manage restricted body movement and the sequelae	D **Nutrition Support** Interventions to modify or maintain nutritional status	E **Physical Comfort Promotion** Interventions to promote comfort using physical techniques	F **Self-Care Facilitation** Interventions to provide or assist with routine activities of daily living
LEVEL 3 INTERVENTIONS	0140 Body Mechanics Promotion 0180 Energy Management 0200 Exercise Promotion 0202 Exercise Promotion: Stretching 0221 Exercise Therapy: Ambulation 0222 Exercise Therapy: Balance 0224 Exercise Therapy: Joint Mobility 0226 Exercise Therapy: Muscle Control 5612 Teaching: Prescribed Activity/Exercise **S*** **0100 to 0399**	0410 Bowel Incontinence Care 0412 Bowel Incontinence Care: Encopresis **X** 0420 Bowel Irrigation 0430 Bowel Management 0440 Bowel Training 0450 Constipation/Impaction Management 0460 Diarrhea Management 0470 Flatulence Reduction 0480 Ostomy Care **L** 0490 Rectal Prolapse Management 0550 Bladder Irrigation 0560 Pelvic Floor Exercise 1876 Tube Care: Urinary 0570 Urinary Bladder Training 0580 Urinary Catheterization 0582 Urinary Catheterization: Intermittent 0590 Urinary Elimination Management 0600 Urinary Habit Training 0610 Urinary Incontinence Care 0612 Urinary Incontinence Care: Enuresis **X** 0620 Urinary Retention Care 1804 Self-Care Assistance: Toileting **F** **0400 to 0699**	0740 Bed Rest Care 0762 Cast Care: Maintenance 0764 Cast Care: Wet 6580 Physical Restraint **V** 0840 Positioning 0846 Positioning: Wheelchair 0910 Splinting 0940 Traction/Immobilization Care 0960 Transport **0700 to 0999**	1020 Diet Staging 1030 Eating Disorders Management 1050 Feeding **F** 1056 Enteral Tube Feeding 1080 Gastrointestinal Intubation 1100 Nutrition Management 1120 Nutrition Therapy 5246 Nutritional Counseling 1160 Nutritional Monitoring 1803 Self-Care Assistance: Feeding **F** 1860 Swallowing Therapy **F** 5614 Teaching: Prescribed Diet **S** 1200 Total Parenteral Nutrition (TPN) Administration **G** 1874 Tube Care: Gastrointestinal 1240 Weight Gain Assistance 1260 Weight Management 1280 Weight Reduction Assistance **1000 to 1299**	1320 Acupressure 1340 Cutaneous Stimulation 6482 Environmental Management: Comfort 1380 Heat/Cold Application 1400 Pain Management 1460 Progressive Muscle Relaxation 1480 Simple Massage 5465 Therapeutic Touch 1540 Transcutaneous Electrical Nerve Stimulation (TENS) **1300 to 1599**	1610 Bathing 1620 Contact Lens Care 1630 Dressing 1640 Ear Care 1650 Eye Care 1050 Feeding **D** 1660 Foot Care 1670 Hair Care 1680 Nail Care 1710 Oral Health Maintenance 1720 Oral Health Promotion 1730 Oral Health Restoration 1750 Perineal Care 1770 Postmortem Care 1780 Prosthesis Care 1800 Self-Care Assistance 1801 Self-Care Assistance: Bathing/Hygiene 1802 Self-Care Assistance: Dressing/Grooming 1803 Self-Care Assistance: Feeding **D** 1804 Self-Care Assistance: Toileting **B** 1850 Sleep Enhancement 1860 Swallowing Therapy **D** 1870 Tube Care **1600 to 1899**

*Letter indicates another class where the intervention is also included.

Continued

LEVEL 1 DOMAINS	**2. PHYSIOLOGICAL: COMPLEX** Care that Supports Homeostatic Regulation			
LEVEL 2 CLASSES	G **Electrolyte and Acid-Base Management** Interventions to regulate electrolyte/acid base balance and prevent complications	H **Drug Management** Interventions to facilitate desired effects of pharmacological agents	I **Neurologic Management** Interventions to optimize neurologic function	J **Perioperative Care** Interventions to provide care before, during, and immediately after surgery
LEVEL 3 INTERVENTIONS	1910 Acid-Base Management 1911 Acid-Base Management: Metabolic Acidosis 1912 Acid-Base Management: Metabolic Alkalosis 1913 Acid-Base Management: Respiratory Acidosis **K*** 1914 Acid-Base Management: Respiratory Alkalosis **K** 1920 Acid-Base Monitoring 2000 Electrolyte Management 2001 Electrolyte Management: Hypercalcemia 2002 Electrolyte Management: Hyperkalemia 2003 Electrolyte Management: Hypermagnesemia 2004 Electrolyte Management: Hypernatremia 2005 Electrolyte Management: Hyperphosphatemia 2006 Electrolyte Management: Hypocalcemia 2007 Electrolyte Management: Hypokalemia 2008 Electrolyte Management: Hypomagnesemia 2009 Electrolyte Management: Hyponatremia 2010 Electrolyte Management: Hypophosphatemia 2020 Electrolyte Monitoring 2080 Fluid/Electrolyte Management **N** 2100 Hemodialysis Therapy 2120 Hyperglycemia Management 2130 Hypoglycemia Management 2150 Peritoneal Dialysis Therapy 4232 Phlebotomy: Arterial Blood Sample **N** 1200 Total Parenteral Nutrition (TPN) Administration **D**	2210 Analgesic Administration 2214 Analgesic Administration: Intraspinal 2840 Anesthesia Administration **J** 2240 Chemotherapy Management **S** 2260 Conscious Sedation 2300 Medication Administration 2301 Medication Administration: Enteral 2302 Medication Administration: Interpleural 2303 Medication Administration: Intraosseous 2304 Medication Administration: Oral 2305 Medication Administration: Parenteral 2306 Medication Administration: Topical 2307 Medication Administration: Ventricular Reservoir 2380 Medication Management 2390 Medication Prescribing 2400 Patient-Controlled Analgesia (PCA) Assistance 5616 Teaching: Prescribed Medication **S** 2440 Venous Access Devices (VAD) Maintenance **N**	2540 Cerebral Edema Management 2550 Cerebral Perfusion Promotion 2560 Dysreflexia Management 2590 Intracranial Pressure (ICP) Monitoring 2620 Neurologic Monitoring 2660 Peripheral Sensation Management 0844 Positioning: Neurologic 2680 Seizure Management **V** 2690 Seizure Precautions 2720 Subarachnoid Hemorrhage Precautions 1878 Tube Care: Ventriculostomy/Lumbar Drain 2760 Unilateral Neglect Management	2840 Anesthesia Administration **H** 2860 Autotransfusion **N** 6545 Infection Control: Intraoperative 0842 Positioning: Intraoperative 2870 Postanesthesia Care 2880 Preoperative Coordination **Y** 2900 Surgical Assistance 2920 Surgical Precautions **V** 2930 Surgical Preparation 5610 Teaching: Preoperative **S** 3902 Temperature Regulation: Intraoperative **M**
	1900 to 2199	**2200 to 2499**	**2500 to 2799**	**2800 to 3099**

*Letter indicates another class where the intervention is also included.

LEVEL 1 DOMAINS	**2. PHYSIOLOGICAL: COMPLEX** Care that Supports Homeostatic Regulation—Cont'd			
LEVEL 2 CLASSES	K **Respiratory Management** Interventions to promote airway patency and gas exchange	L **Skin/Wound Management** Interventions to maintain or restore tissue integrity	M **Thermoregulation** Interventions to maintain body temperature within a normal range	N **Tissue Perfusion Management** Interventions to optimize circulation of blood and fluids to the tissue
LEVEL 3 INTERVENTIONS	1913 Acid-Base Management: Respiratory Acidosis **G** 1914 Acid-Base Management: Respiratory Alkalosis **G** 3120 Airway Insertion and Stabilization 3140 Airway Management 3160 Airway Suctioning 3180 Artificial Airway Management 3200 Aspiration Precautions **V** 3230 Chest Physiotherapy 3250 Cough Enhancement 4106 Embolus Care: Pulmonary **N** 3270 Endotracheal Extubation 3300 Mechanical Ventilation 3310 Mechanical Ventilatory Weaning 3320 Oxygen Therapy 3350 Respiratory Monitoring 1872 Tube Care: Chest 3390 Ventilation Assistance	3420 Amputation Care 3440 Incision Site Care 3460 Leech Therapy 0480 Ostomy Care **B** 3500 Pressure Management 3520 Pressure Ulcer Care 3540 Pressure Ulcer Prevention **V** 3584 Skin Care: Topical Treatments 3590 Skin Surveillance 3620 Suturing 3660 Wound Care 3662 Wound Care: Closed Drainage 3680 Wound Irrigation	3740 Fever Treatment 3780 Heat Exposure Treatment 3800 Hypothermia Treatment 3840 Malignant Hyperthermia Precautions **U** 3900 Temperature Regulation 3902 Temperature Regulation: Intraoperative J	2860 Autotransfusion **J** 4010 Bleeding Precautions 4020 Bleeding Reduction 4021 Bleeding Reduction: Antepartum Uterus **W** 4022 Bleeding Reduction: Gastrointestinal 4024 Bleeding Reduction: Nasal 4026 Bleeding Reduction: Postpartum Uterus **W** 4028 Bleeding Reduction: Wound 4030 Blood Products Administration 4040 Cardiac Care 4044 Cardiac Care: Acute 4046 Cardiac Care: Rehabilitative 4050 Cardiac Precautions 4060 Circulatory Care 4064 Circulatory Care: Mechanical Assist Device 4070 Circulatory Precautions 4090 Dysrhythmia Management 4104 Embolus Care: Peripheral 4106 Embolus Care: Pulmonary **K** 4110 Embolus Precautions 2080 Fluid/Electrolyte Management **G** 4120 Fluid Management 4130 Fluid Monitoring 4140 Fluid Resuscitation 4150 Hemodynamic Regulation 4160 Hemorrhage Control 4170 Hypervolemia Management 4180 Hypovolemia Management 4190 Intravenous (IV) Insertion 4200 Intravenous (IV) Therapy 4210 Invasive Hemodynamic Monitoring 4220 Peripherally Inserted Central (PIC) Catheter Care 4232 Phlebotomy: Arterial Blood Sample **G** 4234 Phlebotomy: Blood Unit Acquisition 4238 Phlebotomy: Venous Blood Sample 4250 Shock Management 4254 Shock Management: Cardiac 4256 Shock Management: Vasogenic 4258 Shock Management: Volume 4260 Shock Prevention 2440 Venous Access Devices (VAD) Maintenance **H**
	3100 to 3399	**3400 to 3699**	**3700 to 3999**	**4000 to 4299**

Continued

LEVEL 1 DOMAINS	**3. BEHAVIORAL** Care that Supports Psychosocial Functioning and Facilitates Life-style Changes					
LEVEL 2 CLASSES	O **Behavior Therapy** Interventions to reinforce or promote desirable behaviors or alter undesirable behaviors	P **Cognitive Therapy** Interventions to reinforce or promote desirable cognitive functioning or alter undesirable cognitive functioning	Q **Communication Enhancement** Interventions to facilitate delivering and receiving verbal and nonverbal messages	R **Coping Assistance** Interventions to assist another to build on own strengths, adapt to a change in function, or to achieve a higher level of function	S **Patient Education** Interventions to facilitate learning	T **Psychological Comfort Promotion** Interventions to promote comfort using psychological techniques
LEVEL 3 INTERVENTIONS	4310 Activity Therapy 4320 Animal-Assisted Therapy **Q*** 4330 Art Therapy **Q** 4340 Assertiveness Training 4350 Behavior Management 4352 Behavior Management: Overactivity/Inattention 4354 Behavior Management: Self-Harm 4356 Behavior Management: Sexual 4360 Behavior Modification 4362 Behavior Modification: Social Skills 4370 Impulse Control Training 4380 Limit Setting 4390 Milieu Therapy 4400 Music Therapy **Q** 4410 Mutual Goal Setting 4420 Patient Contracting 4430 Play Therapy **Q** 4470 Self-Modification Assistance 4480 Self-Responsibility Facilitation 4490 Smoking Cessation Assistance 4500 Substance Use Prevention 4510 Substance Use Treatment 4512 Substance Use Treatment: Alcohol Withdrawal 4514 Substance Use Treatment: Drug Withdrawal 4516 Substance Use Treatment: Overdose	4640 Anger Control Assistance 4680 Bibliotherapy 4700 Cognitive Restructuring 4720 Cognitive Stimulation 5520 Learning Facilitation **S** 5540 Learning Readiness Enhancement **S** 4760 Memory Training 4820 Reality Orientation 4860 Reminiscence Therapy	4920 Active Listening 4320 Animal-Assisted Therapy **O** 4330 Art Therapy **O** 4974 Communication Enhancement: Hearing Deficit 4976 Communication Enhancement: Speech Deficit 4978 Communication Enhancement: Visual Deficit 5000 Complex Relationship Building 4400 Music Therapy **O** 4430 Play Therapy **O** 5100 Socialization Enhancement	5210 Anticipatory Guidance **W** 5220 Body Image Enhancement 5230 Coping Enhancement 5240 Counseling 5242 Genetic Counseling **W** 5248 Sexual Counseling 6160 Crisis Intervention **U** 5250 Decision-Making Support **Y** 5260 Dying Care 5270 Emotional Support 5290 Grief Work Facilitation 5294 Grief Work Facilitation: Perinatal Death **W** 5300 Guilt Work Facilitation 5310 Hope Instillation 5320 Humor 5330 Mood Management 5340 Presence 5360 Recreation Therapy 5370 Role Enhancement **X** 5380 Security Enhancement 5390 Self-Awareness Enhancement 5400 Self-Esteem Enhancement 5420 Spiritual Support 5430 Support Group 5440 Support System Enhancement 5450 Therapy Group 5460 Touch 5470 Truth Telling 5480 Values Clarification	2240 Chemotherapy Management **H** 6784 Family Planning: Contraception **W** 5510 Health Education 5520 Learning Facilitation **P** 5540 Learning Readiness Enhancement **P** 5562 Parent Education: Adolescent **X** 5564 Parent Education: Childbearing Family **W** 5566 Parent Education: Childrearing Family **X** 5580 Preparatory Sensory Information 5602 Teaching: Disease Process 5604 Teaching: Group 5606 Teaching: Individual 5608 Teaching: Infant Care **W** 5610 Teaching: Preoperative **J** 5612 Teaching: Prescribed Activity/Exercise **A** 5614 Teaching: Prescribed Diet **D** 5616 Teaching: Prescribed Medication **H** 5618 Teaching: Procedure/Treatment 5620 Teaching: Psychomotor Skill 5622 Teaching: Safe Sex 5624 Teaching: Sexuality	5820 Anxiety Reduction 5840 Autogenic Training 5860 Biofeedback 5880 Calming Technique 5900 Distraction 5920 Hypnosis 5960 Meditation 6000 Simple Guided Imagery 6040 Simple Relaxation Therapy
	4300 to 4599	**4600 to 4899**	**4900 to 5199**	**5200 to 5499**	**5500 to 5799**	**5800 to 6099**

*Letter indicates another class where the intervention is also included.

LEVEL 1 DOMAINS	**4. SAFETY** **Care that Supports Protection against Harm**	
LEVEL 2 CLASSES	**U Crisis Management** Interventions to provide immediate short-term help in both psychological and physiological crises	**V Risk Management** Interventions to initiate risk-reduction activities and continue monitoring risks over time
LEVEL 3 INTERVENTIONS	6140 Code Management 6160 Crisis Intervention **R*** 6200 Emergency Care 6240 First Aid 3840 Malignant Hyperthermia Precautions **M** 6260 Organ Procurement 6300 Rape-Trauma Treatment 6320 Resuscitation 6340 Suicide Prevention **V** 6360 Triage	6400 Abuse Protection 6402 Abuse Protection: Child 6404 Abuse Protection: Elder 6410 Allergy Management 6420 Area Restriction 3200 Aspiration Precautions **K** 6440 Delirium Management 6450 Delusion Management 6460 Dementia Management 6470 Elopement Precautions 6480 Environmental Management 6484 Environmental Management: Community 6486 Environmental Management: Safety 6487 Environmental Management: Violence Prevention 6489 Environmental Management: Worker Safety 6490 Fall Prevention 6500 Fire-Setting Precautions 6510 Hallucination Management 6520 Health Screening 6530 Immunization/Vaccination Administration 6540 Infection Control 6550 Infection Protection 6560 Laser Precautions 6570 Latex Precautions 6580 Physical Restraint **C** 6590 Pneumatic Tourniquet Precautions 3540 Pressure Ulcer Prevention **L** 6600 Radiation Therapy Management 6610 Risk Identification 6630 Seclusion 2680 Seizure Management **I** 6340 Suicide Prevention **U** 2920 Surgical Precautions **J** 6650 Surveillance 6654 Surveillance: Safety 6680 Vital Signs Monitoring
	6100 to 6399	**6400 to 6699**

Continued

LEVEL 1 DOMAINS	**5. FAMILY** Care that Supports the Family Unit	
LEVEL 2 CLASSES	**W Childbearing Care** Interventions to assist in understanding and coping with the psychological and physiological changes during the childbearing period	**X Lifespan Care** Interventions to facilitate family unit functioning and promote the health and welfare of family members throughout the lifespan
LEVEL 3 INTERVENTIONS	6700 Amnioinfusion 5210 Anticipatory Guidance **R*** 6710 Attachment Promotion 6720 Birthing 4021 Bleeding Reduction: Antepartum Uterus **N** 4026 Bleeding Reduction: Postpartum Uterus **N** 1052 Bottle Feeding 1054 Breastfeeding Assistance 6750 Cesarean Section Care 6760 Childbirth Preparation 6771 Electronic Fetal Monitoring: Antepartum 6772 Electronic Fetal Monitoring: Intrapartum 6481 Environmental Management: Attachment Process 7104 Family Integrity Promotion: Childbearing Family 6784 Family Planning: Contraception **S** 6786 Family Planning: Infertility 6788 Family Planning: Unplanned Pregnancy 5242 Genetic Counseling **R** 5294 Grief Work Facilitation: Perinatal Death **R** 6800 High-Risk Pregnancy Care 6820 Infant Care 6830 Intrapartal Care 6834 Intrapartal Care: High-Risk Delivery 6840 Kangaroo Care 6850 Labor Induction 6860 Labor Suppression 5244 Lactation Counseling 6870 Lactation Suppression 6880 Newborn Care 6890 Newborn Monitoring 6900 Nonnutritive Sucking 5564 Parent Education: Childbearing Family **S** 6924 Phototherapy: Neonate 6930 Postpartal Care 5247 Preconception Counseling 6950 Pregnancy Termination Care 6960 Prenatal Care 7886 Reproductive Technology Management 6972 Resuscitation: Fetus 6974 Resuscitation: Neonate 6612 Risk Identification: Childbearing Family 6656 Surveillance: Late Pregnancy 5608 Teaching: Infant Care **S** 1875 Tube Care: Umbilical Line 6982 Ultrasonography: Limited Obstetric **6700 to 6999**	0412 Bowel Incontinence Care: Encopresis **B** 7040 Caregiver Support 7050 Developmental Enhancement 7100 Family Integrity Promotion 7110 Family Involvement 7120 Family Mobilization 7130 Family Process Maintenance 7140 Family Support 7150 Family Therapy 7160 Fertility Preservation 7180 Home Maintenance Assistance 7200 Normalization Promotion 5562 Parent Education: Adolescent **S** 5566 Parent Education: Childrearing Family **S** 7260 Respite Care 5370 Role Enhancement **R** 7280 Sibling Support 0612 Urinary Incontinence Care: Enuresis **B** **7000 to 7299**

*Letter indicates another class where the intervention is also included.

LEVEL 1 DOMAINS	**6. HEALTH SYSTEM** **Care that Supports Effective Use of the Health Care Delivery System**		
LEVEL 2 CLASSES	**Y Health System Mediation** Interventions to facilitate the interface between patient/family and the health care system	**a Health System Management** Interventions to provide and enhance support services for the delivery of care	**b Information Management** Interventions to facilitate communication among health care providers
LEVEL 3 INTERVENTIONS	7310 Admission Care 7330 Culture Brokerage 5250 Decision-Making Support **R*** 7370 Discharge Planning 7400 Health System Guidance 7410 Insurance Authorization 7440 Pass Facilitation 7460 Patient Rights Protection 2880 Preoperative Coordination **J** 7500 Sustenance Support 7560 Visitation Facilitation	7610 Bedside Laboratory Testing 7620 Controlled Substance Checking 7640 Critical Path Development 7650 Delegation 7660 Emergency Cart Checking 7680 Examination Assistance 7690 Laboratory Data Interpretation 7700 Peer Review 7710 Physician Support 7722 Preceptor: Employee 7726 Preceptor: Student 7760 Product Evaluation 7800 Quality Monitoring 7820 Specimen Management 7830 Staff Supervision 7840 Supply Management 7880 Technology Management	7920 Documentation 7960 Health Care Information Exchange 7970 Health Policy Monitoring 7980 Incident Reporting 8020 Multidisciplinary Care Conference 8060 Order Transcription 8100 Referral 8120 Research Data Collection 8140 Shift Report 8180 Telephone Consultation
	7300 to 7599	**7600 to 7899**	**7900 to 8199**

C

Advanced Cardiac Life Support (ACLS) Guidelines

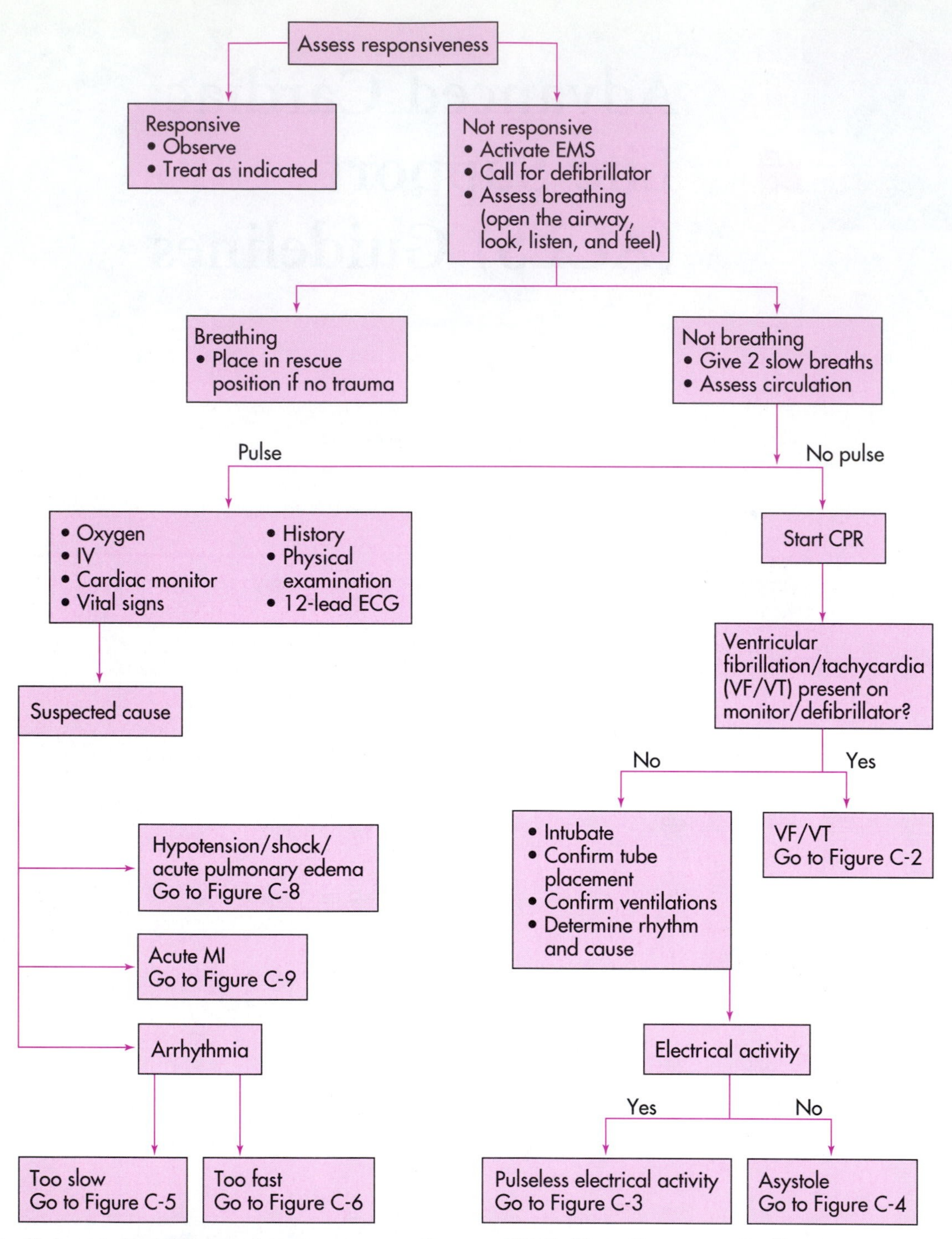

FIGURE C-1. Universal algorithm for adult emergency cardiac care (ECC). (From Emergency Cardiac Care Committees and Subcommittees, American Heart Association: Guidelines for cardiopulmonary resuscitation and emergency care III: Adult advanced cardiac life support, *JAMA* 268(16):2216, 1992.)

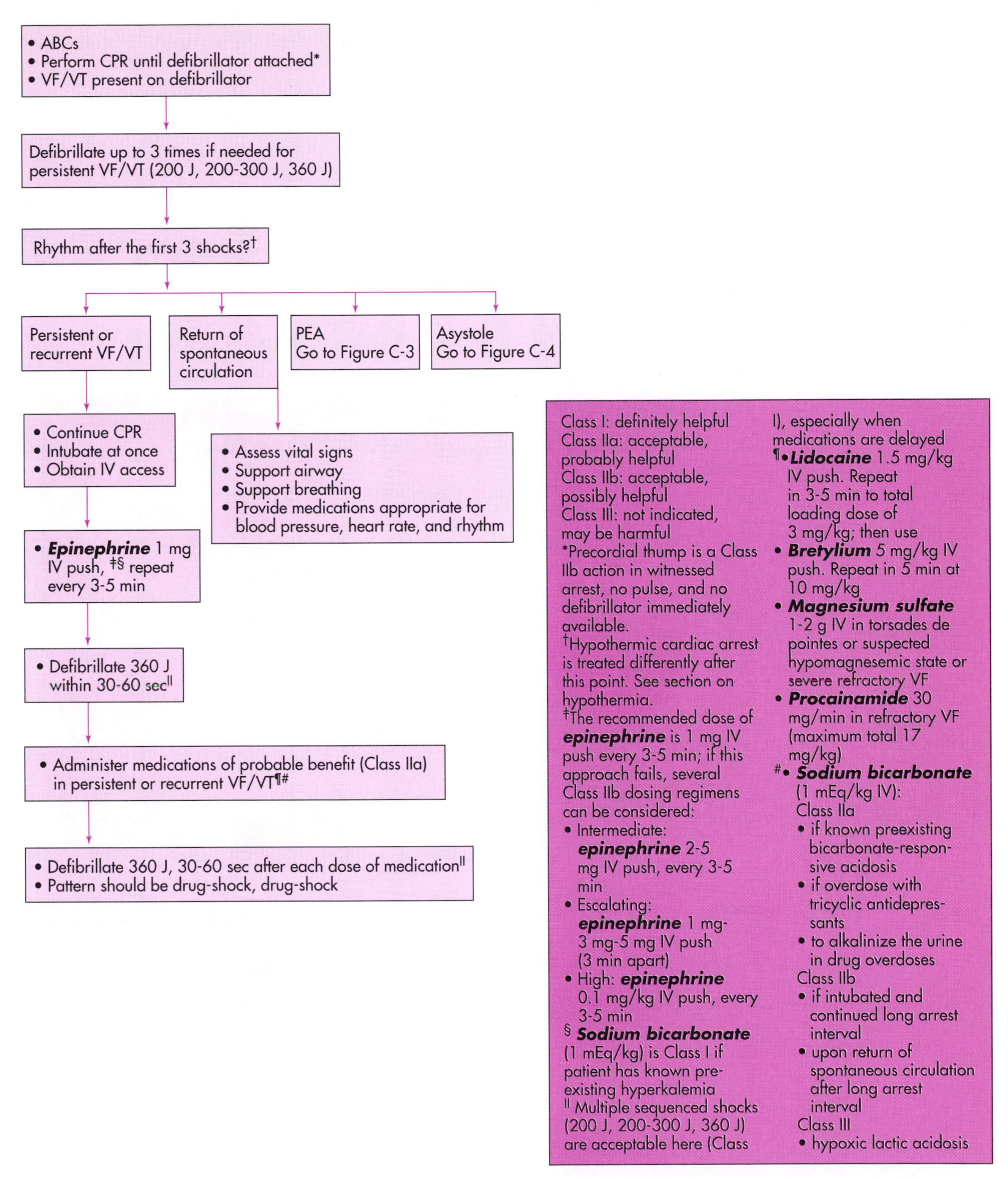

FIGURE C-2. Algorithm for ventricular fibrillation and pulseless ventricular tachycardia (VF/VT). (From Emergency Cardiac Care Committees and Subcommittees, American Heart Association: Guidelines for cardiopulmonary resuscitation and emergency care III: Adult advanced cardiac life support, *JAMA* 268(16):2217, 1992.)

PEA includes
- Electromechanical dissociation (EMD)
- Pseudo-EMD
- Idioventricular rhythms
- Ventricular escape rhythms
- Bradyasystolic rhythms
- Postdefibrillation idioventricular rhythms

- Continue CPR
- Intubate at once
- Obtain IV access
- Assess blood flow using Doppler ultrasound

↓

Consider possible causes
(Parentheses = possible therapies and treatments)
- Hypovolemia (volume infusion)
- Hypoxia (ventilation)
- Cardiac tamponade (pericardiocentesis)
- Tension pneumothorax (needle decompression)
- Hypothermia (see hypothermia algorithm, Figure C-11)
- Massive pulmonary embolism (surgery, *thrombolytics*)
- Drug overdoses such as tricyclics, digitalis, β-blockers, calcium channel blockers
- Hyperkalemia*
- Acidosis†
- Massive acute myocardial infarction (go to Figure C-9)

↓

- ***Epinephrine*** 1 mg IV push, *‡repeat every 3-5 min

↓

- If absolute bradycardia (<60 beats/min) or relative bradycardia, give ***atropine*** 1 mg IV
- Repeat every 3-5 min up to a total of 0.4 mg/kg§

Class I: definitely helpful
Class IIa: acceptable, probably helpful
Class IIb: acceptable, possibly helpful
Class III: not indicated, may be harmful

****Sodium bicarbonate*** 1 mEq/kg is Class I if patient has known preexisting hyperkalemia.

†***Sodium bicarbonate*** 1mEq/kg:
Class IIa
- if known preexisting bicarbonate-responsive acidosis
- if overdose with tricyclic antidepressants
- to alkalinize the urine in drug overdoses

Class IIb
- if Intubated and long arrest interval
- upon return of spontaneous circulation after long arrest interval

Class III
- hypoxic lactic acidosis

‡The recommended doses of ***epinephrine*** is 1 mg IV push every 3-5 min. If this approach fails, several Class IIb dosing regimens can be considered.
- Intermediate: ***epinephrine*** 2-5 mg IV push every 3-5 min
- Escalating: ***epinephrine*** 1 mg-3 mg-5 mg IV push (3 min apart)
- High: ***epinephrine*** 0.1 mg/kg IV push every 3-5 min

§Shorter ***atropine*** dosing intervals are possibly helpful in cardiac arrest (Class IIb).

FIGURE C-3. Algorithm for pulseless electrical activity (PEA) (electromechanical dissociation [EMD]). (From Emergency Cardiac Care Committees and Subcommittees, American Heart Association: Guidelines for cardiopulmonary resuscitation and emergency care III: Adult advanced cardiac life support, *JAMA* 268(16):2219, 1992.)

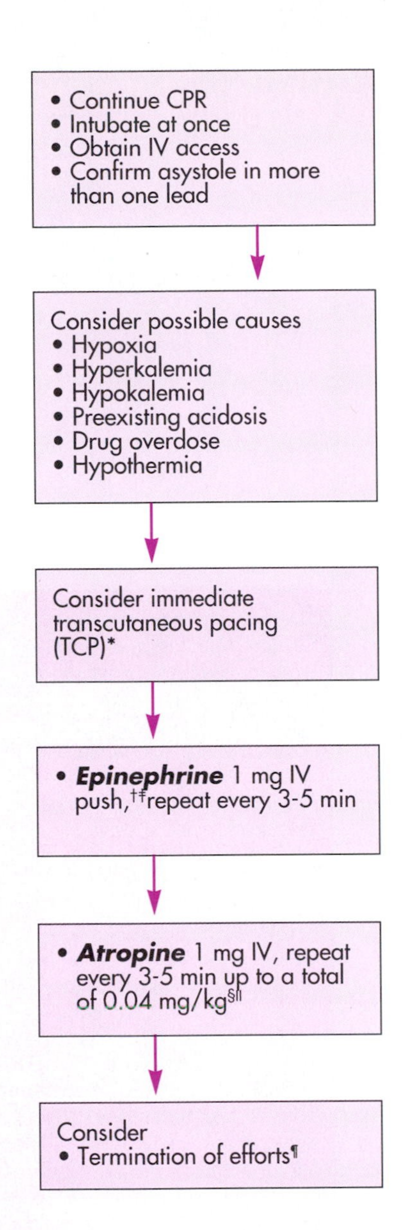

• Continue CPR
• Intubate at once
• Obtain IV access
• Confirm asystole in more than one lead
Consider possible causes
• Hypoxia
• Hyperkalemia
• Hypokalemia
• Preexisting acidosis
• Drug overdose
• Hypothermia
Consider immediate transcutaneous pacing (TCP)*
• Epinephrine 1 mg IV push,†‡ repeat every 3-5 min
• Atropine 1 mg IV, repeat every 3-5 min up to a total of 0.04 mg/kg§||
Consider
• Termination of efforts¶

Class I: definitely helpful
Class IIa: acceptable, probably helpful
Class IIb: acceptable, possibly helpful
Class III: not indicated, may be harmful

*TCP is a Class IIb intervention. Lack of success may be due to delays in pacing. To be effective TCP must be performed early, simultaneously with drugs. Evidence does not support routine use of TCP for asystole.

†The recommended dose of ***epinephrine*** is 1 mg IV push every 3-5 min. If this approach fails, several Class IIb dosing regimens can be considered:
- Intermediate: ***epinephrine*** 2-5 mg IV push every 3-5 min
- Escalating: ***epinephrine*** 1 mg-3 mg-5 mg IV push, (3 min apart)
- High: ***epinephrine*** 0.1 mg/kg IV push every 3-5 min

‡***Sodium bicarbonate*** 1 mEq/kg is Class I if patient has known preexisting hyperkalemia.

§Shorter ***atropine*** dosing intervals are Class IIb in asystolic arrest.

||***Sodium bicarbonate*** 1 mEq/kg:
Class IIa
- if known preexisting bicarbonate-responsive acidosis
- if overdose with tricyclic antidepressants
- to alkalinize the urine in drug overdoses

Class IIb
- if intubated and continued long arrest interval
- upon return of spontaneous circulation after long arrest interval

Class III
- hypoxic lactic acidosis

¶If patient remains in asystole or other agonal rhythms after successful intubation and initial medications and no reversible causes are identified, consider termination of resuscitative efforts by a physician. Consider interval since arrest.

FIGURE C-4. Asystole treatment algorithm. (From Emergency Cardiac Care Committees and Subcommittees, American Heart Association: Guidelines for cardiopulmonary resuscitation and emergency care III: Adult advanced cardiac life support, *JAMA* 268(16):2220, 1992.)

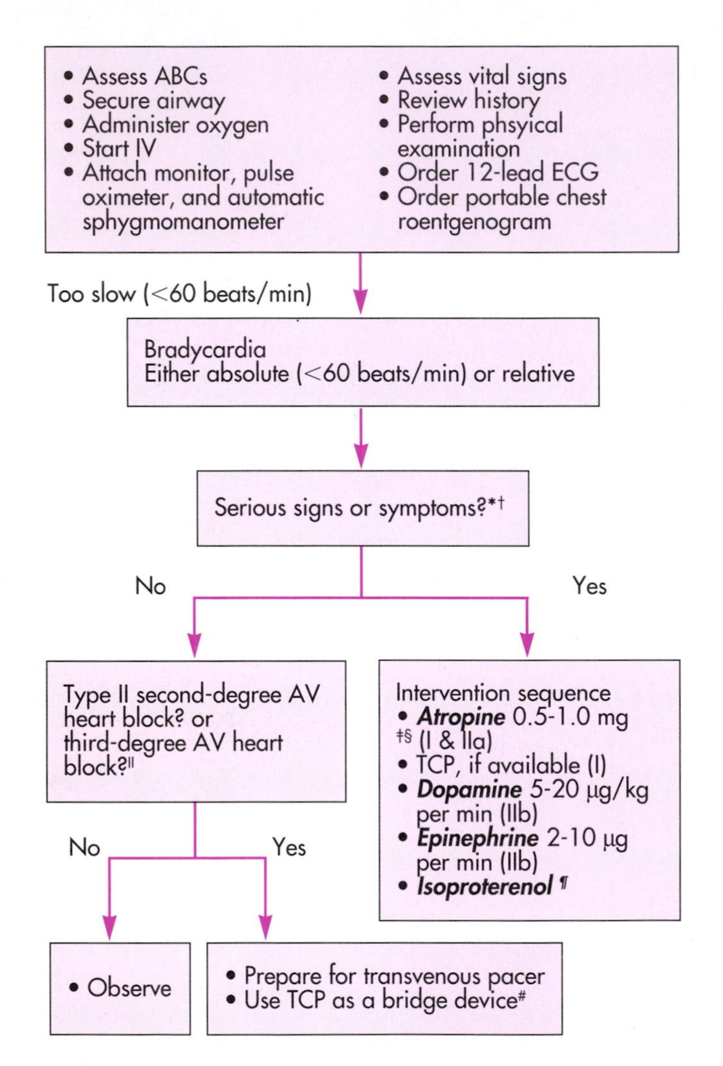

*Serious signs or symptoms must be related to the slow rate. Clinical Manifestations include:
symptoms (chest pains, shortness of breath, decreased level of consciousness) and
signs (low BP, shock, pulmonary congestion, CHF, acute MI)
†Do not delay TCP while awaiting IV access or for ***atropine*** to take effect if patient is symptomatic.
‡Denervated transplanted hearts will not respond to ***atropine.*** Go at once to pacing, ***catecholamine*** infusion, or both.
§***Atropine*** should be given at repeat doses in 3-5 min up to total of 0.04 mb/kg. Consider shorter dosing intervals in severe clinical conditions. It has been suggested that atropine should be used with caution in atrioventricular (AV) block at the His-Purkinie level (type II AV block and new third-degree block with wide QRS complexes) (Class IIb)
||Never treat third-degree heart block plus ventricular escape beats with ***lidocaine.***
¶***Isoproterenol*** should be used, if at all, with extreme caution. At low doses it is Class IIb (probably helpful); at higher doses it is Class III (harmful).

FIGURE C-5. Bradycardia algorithm (with the patient not in cardiac arrest). (From Emergency Cardiac Care Committees and Subcommittees, American Heart Association: Guidelines for cardiopulmonary resuscitation and emergency care III: Adult advanced cardiac life support, *JAMA* 268(16):2221, 1992.)

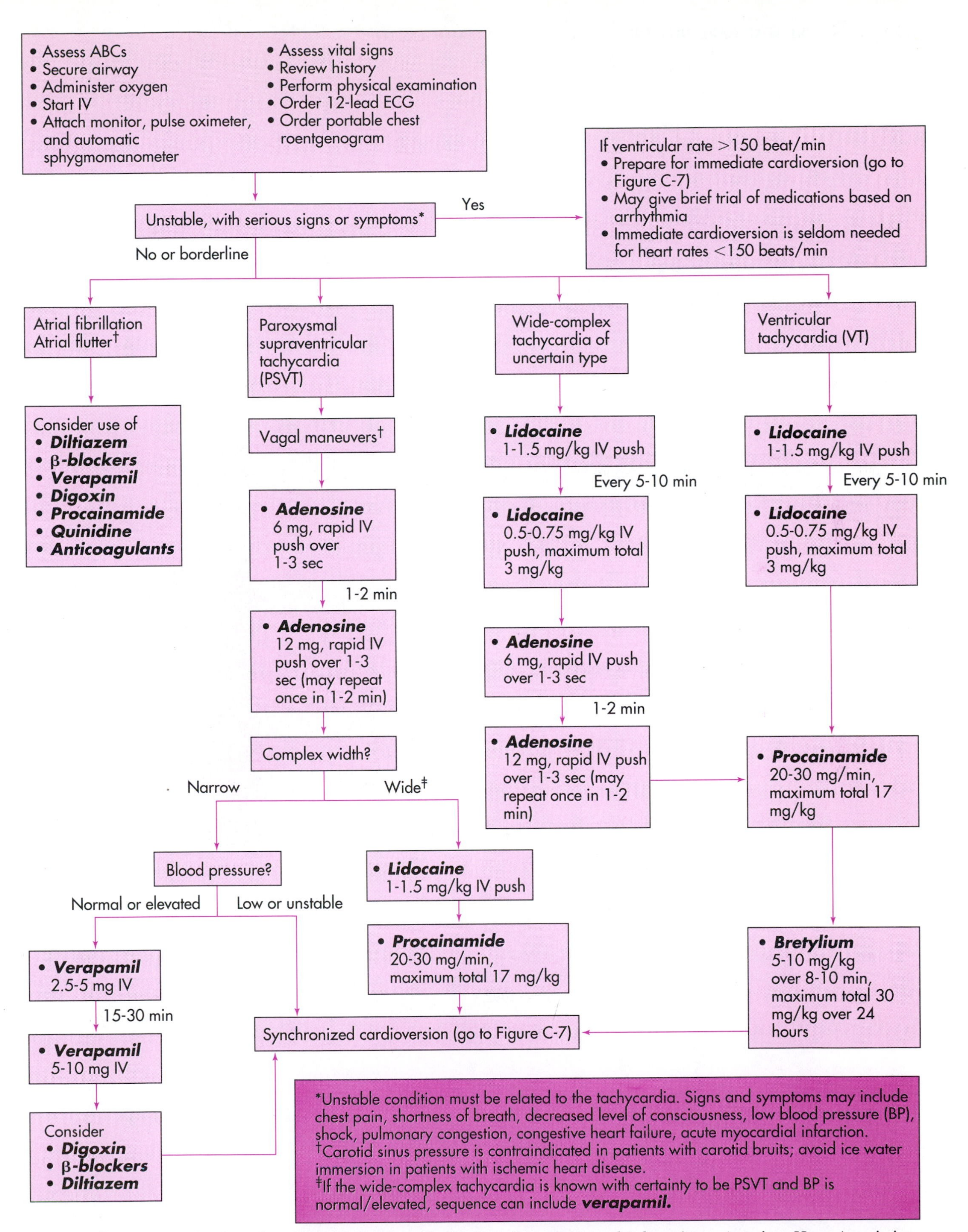

FIGURE C-6. Tachycardia algorithm. (From Emergency Cardiac Care Committees and Subcomittees, American Heart Association: Guidelines for cardiopulmonary resuscitation and emergency care III: Adult advanced cardiac life support, *JAMA* 268(16):2223, 1992.)

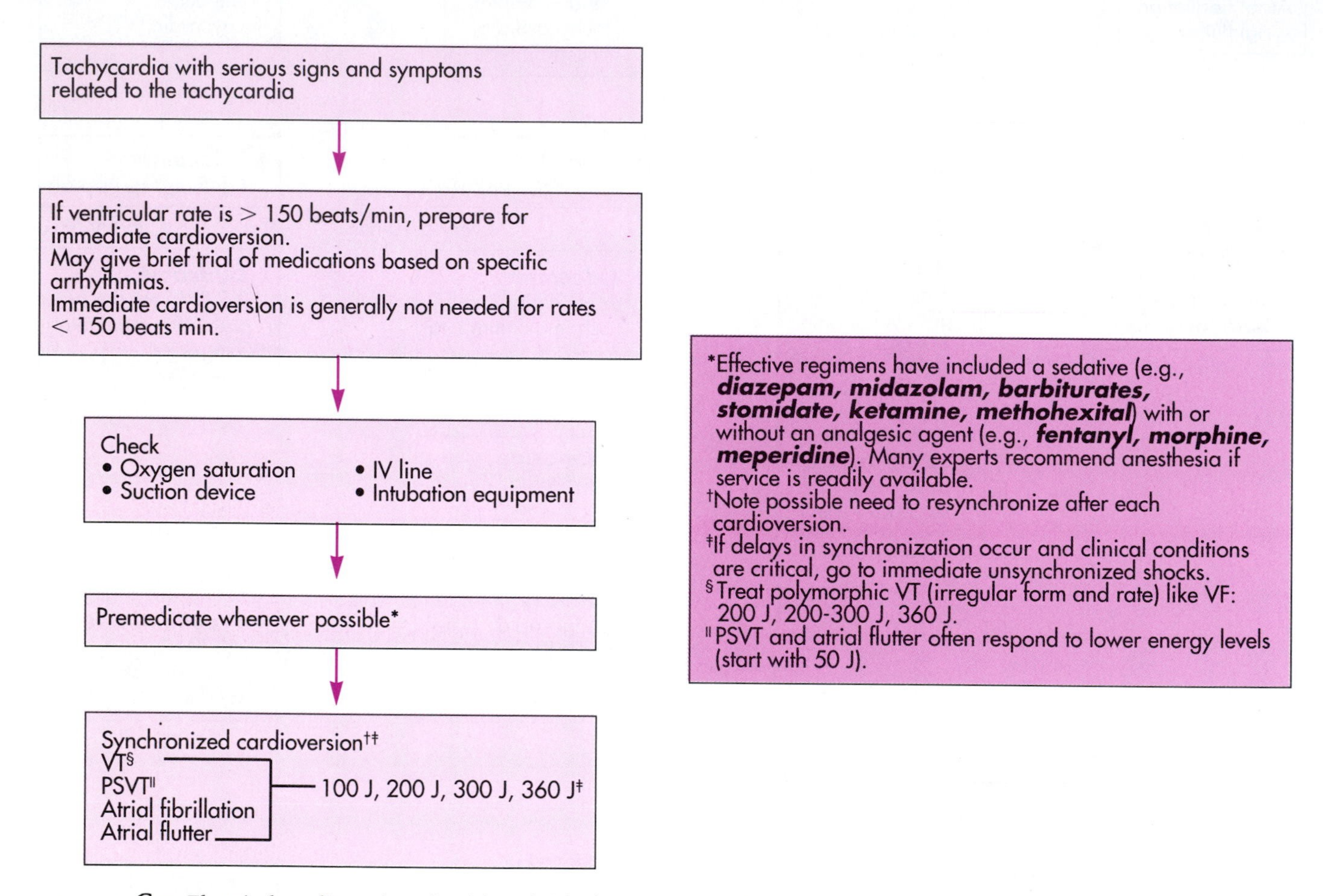

Tachycardia with serious signs and symptoms related to the tachycardia
If ventricular rate is > 150 beats/min, prepare for immediate cardioversion.
May give brief trial of medications based on specific arrhythmias.
Immediate cardioversion is generally not needed for rates < 150 beats min.
Check
• Oxygen saturation
• Suction device
• IV line
• Intubation equipment
Premedicate whenever possible*
Synchronized cardioversion†‡
VT§
PSVT‖
Atrial fibrillation
Atrial flutter
100 J, 200 J, 300 J, 360 J‡
*Effective regimens have included a sedative (e.g., diazepam, midazolam, barbiturates, stomidate, ketamine, methohexital) with or without an analgesic agent (e.g., fentanyl, morphine, meperidine). Many experts recommend anesthesia if service is readily available.
†Note possible need to resynchronize after each cardioversion.
‡If delays in synchronization occur and clinical conditions are critical, go to immediate unsynchronized shocks.
§Treat polymorphic VT (irregular form and rate) like VF: 200 J, 200-300 J, 360 J.
‖PSVT and atrial flutter often respond to lower energy levels (start with 50 J).

FIGURE C-7. Electrical cardioversion algorithm (with the patient not in cardiac arrest). (From Emergency Cardiac Care Committees and Subcommittees, American Heart Association: Guidelines for cardiopulmonary resuscitation and emergency care III: Adult advanced cardiac life support, *JAMA* 268(16):2224, 1992.)

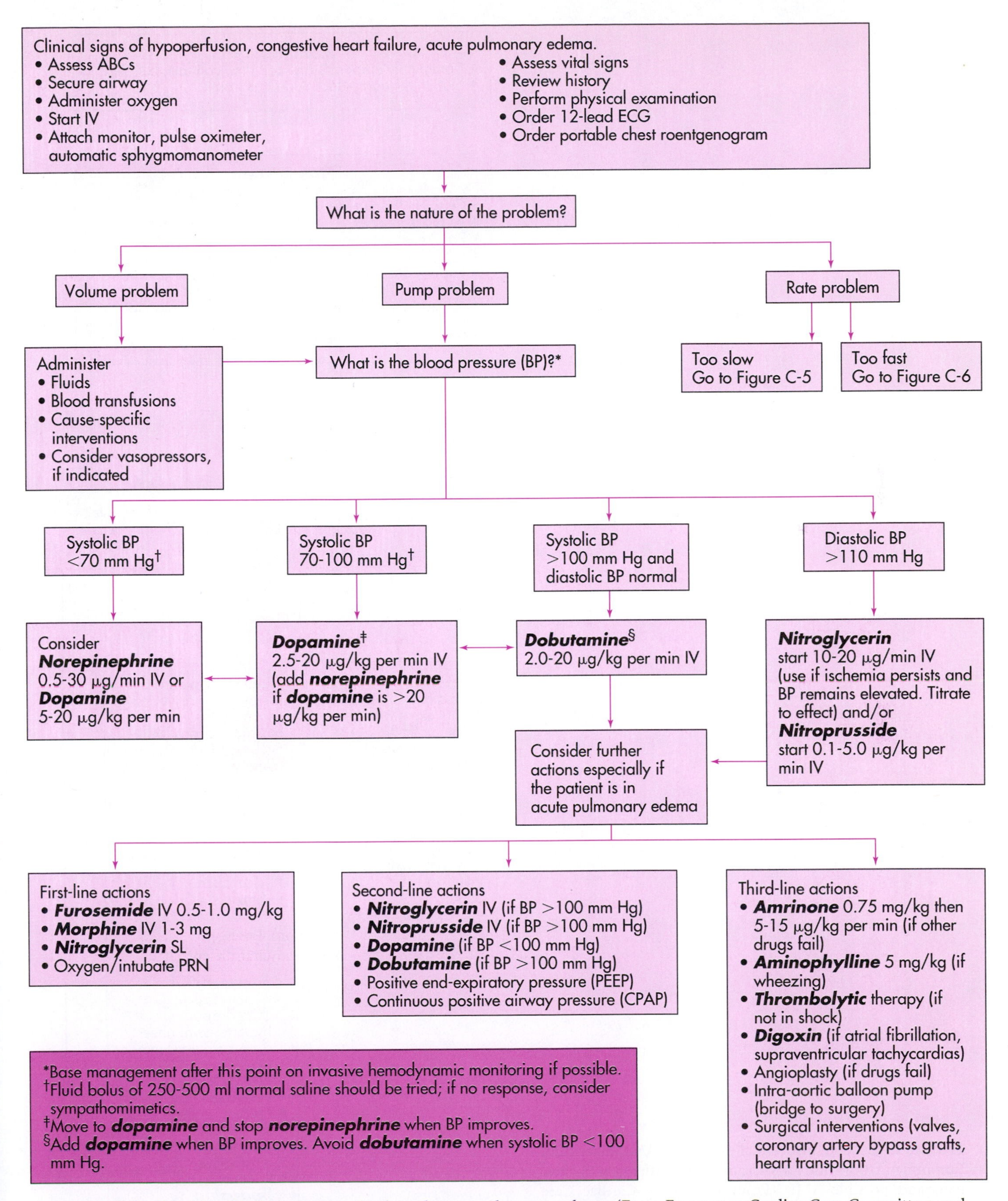

FIGURE C-8. Algorithm for hypotension, shock, and acute pulmonary edema. (From Emergency Cardiac Care Committees and Subcommittees, American Heart Association: Guidelines for cardiopulmonary resuscitation and emergency care III: Adult advanced cardiac life support, *JAMA* 268(16):2227, 1992.)

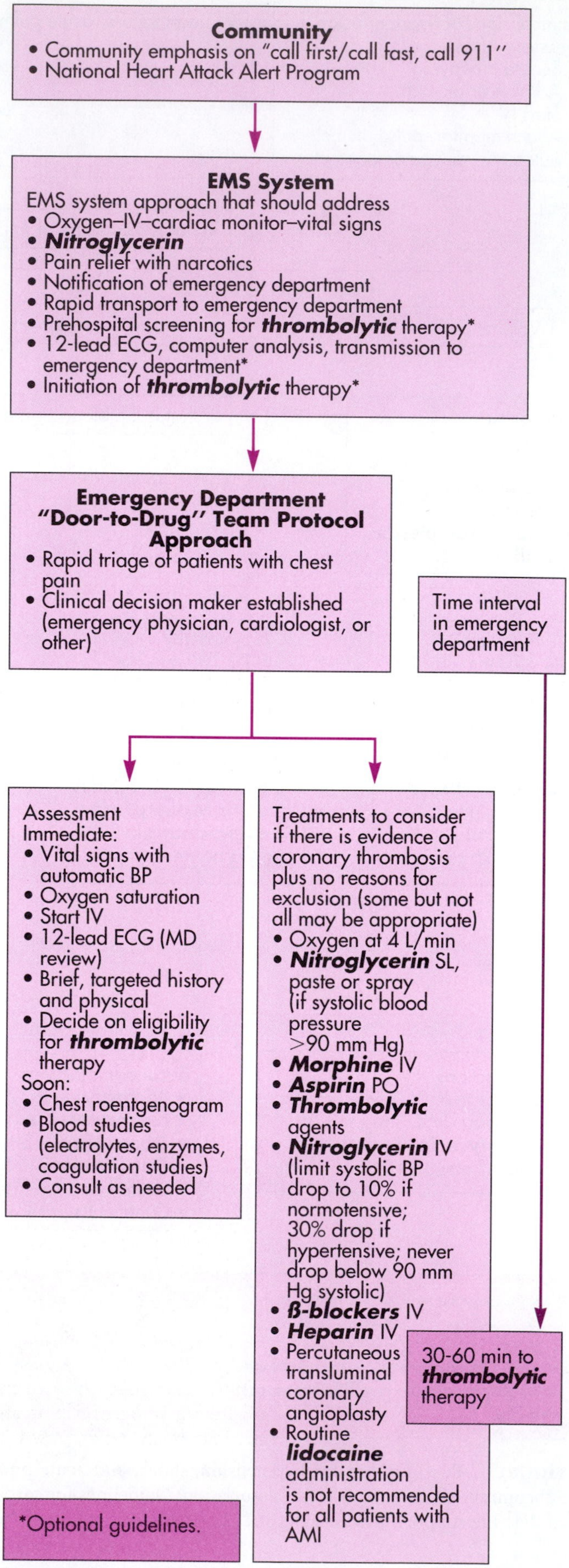

Community
- Community emphasis on "call first/call fast, call 911"
- National Heart Attack Alert Program

↓

EMS System
EMS system approach that should address
- Oxygen–IV–cardiac monitor–vital signs
- ***Nitroglycerin***
- Pain relief with narcotics
- Notification of emergency department
- Rapid transport to emergency department
- Prehospital screening for ***thrombolytic*** therapy*
- 12-lead ECG, computer analysis, transmission to emergency department*
- Initiation of ***thrombolytic*** therapy*

↓

Emergency Department "Door-to-Drug" Team Protocol Approach
- Rapid triage of patients with chest pain
- Clinical decision maker established (emergency physician, cardiologist, or other)

Time interval in emergency department

Assessment
Immediate:
- Vital signs with automatic BP
- Oxygen saturation
- Start IV
- 12-lead ECG (MD review)
- Brief, targeted history and physical
- Decide on eligibility for ***thrombolytic*** therapy

Soon:
- Chest roentgenogram
- Blood studies (electrolytes, enzymes, coagulation studies)
- Consult as needed

Treatments to consider if there is evidence of coronary thrombosis plus no reasons for exclusion (some but not all may be appropriate)
- Oxygen at 4 L/min
- ***Nitroglycerin*** SL, paste or spray (if systolic blood pressure >90 mm Hg)
- ***Morphine*** IV
- ***Aspirin*** PO
- ***Thrombolytic*** agents
- ***Nitroglycerin*** IV (limit systolic BP drop to 10% if normotensive; 30% drop if hypertensive; never drop below 90 mm Hg systolic)
- ***ß-blockers*** IV
- ***Heparin*** IV
- Percutaneous transluminal coronary angioplasty
- Routine ***lidocaine*** administration is not recommended for all patients with AMI

30-60 min to ***thrombolytic*** therapy

*Optional guidelines.

FIGURE C-9. Acute myocardial infarction (AMI) algorithm. Recommendations for early treatment of patients with chest pain and possible AMI. (From Emergency Cardiac Care Committees and Subcommittees, American Heart Association: Guidelines for cardiopulmonary resuscitation and emergency care III: Adult advanced cardiac life support, *JAMA* 268(16):2230, 1992.)

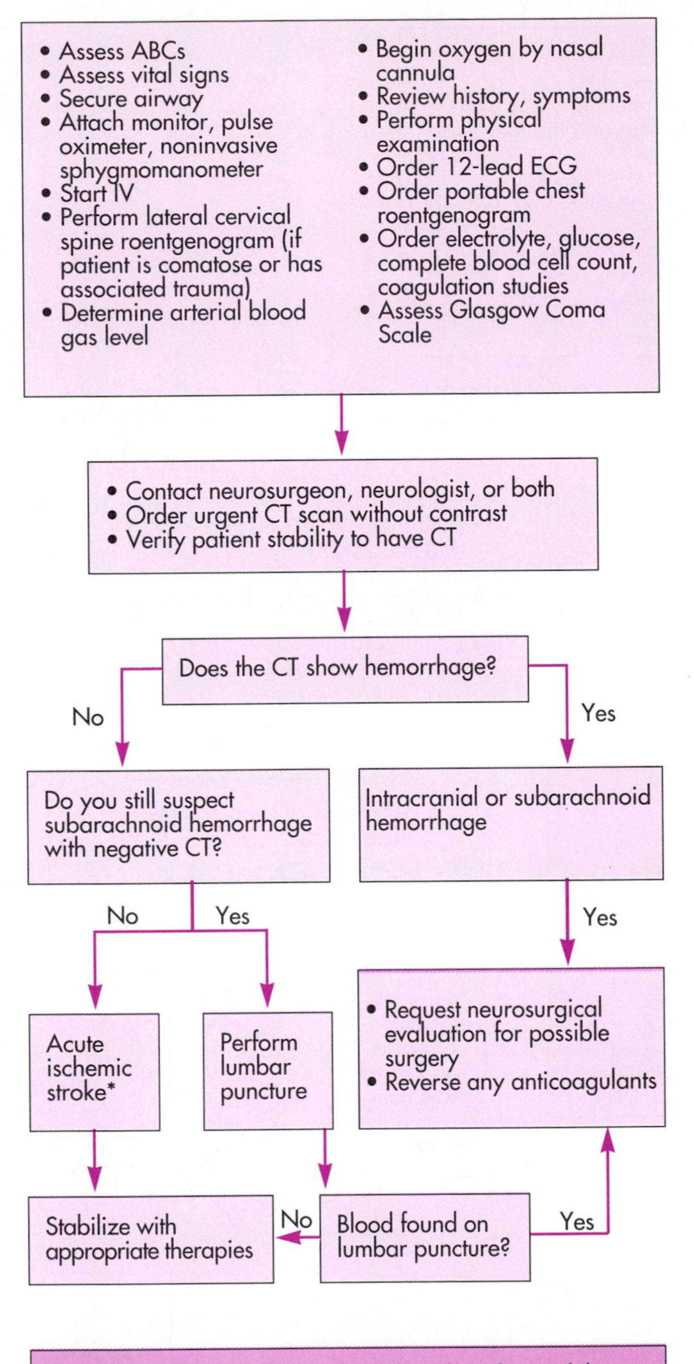
• Assess ABCs
• Assess vital signs
• Secure airway
• Attach monitor, pulse oximeter, noninvasive sphygmomanometer
• Start IV
• Perform lateral cervical spine roentgenogram (if patient is comatose or has associated trauma)
• Determine arterial blood gas level
• Begin oxygen by nasal cannula
• Review history, symptoms
• Perform physical examination
• Order 12-lead ECG
• Order portable chest roentgenogram
• Order electrolyte, glucose, complete blood cell count, coagulation studies
• Assess Glasgow Coma Scale
• Contact neurosurgeon, neurologist, or both
• Order urgent CT scan without contrast
• Verify patient stability to have CT
Does the CT show hemorrhage?
No
Yes
Do you still suspect subarachnoid hemorrhage with negative CT?
Intracranial or subarachnoid hemorrhage
No
Yes
Yes
Acute ischemic stroke*
Perform lumbar puncture
• Request neurosurgical evaluation for possible surgery
• Reverse any anticoagulants
Stabilize with appropriate therapies
No
Blood found on lumbar puncture?
Yes
*The detailed management of acute stroke is beyond the scope of the ACLS program. Management of cardiovascular emergencies in stroke victims is similar to the management in other patients. Never forget, however, that acute stroke can coexist with acute cardiovascular problems.

FIGURE C-10. Algorithm for initial evaluation of suspected stroke. (From Emergency Cardiac Care Committees and Subcommittees, American Heart Association: Guidelines for cardiopulmonary resuscitation and emergency care IV: Special resuscitation situations, *JAMA* 268(16):2243, 1992.)

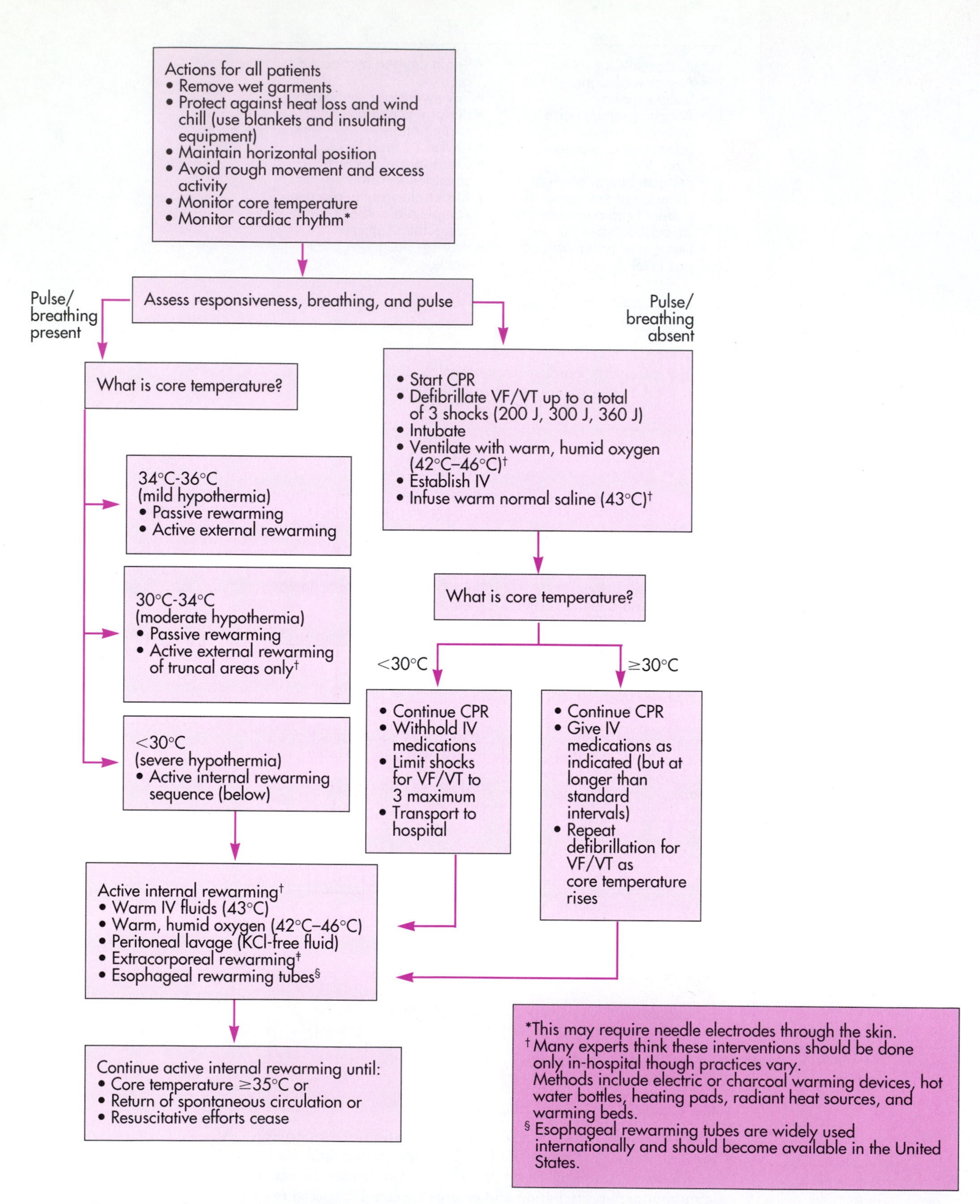

FIGURE C-11. Algorithm for treatment of hypothermia. (From Emergency Cardiac Care Committees and Subcommittees, American Heart Association: Guidelines for cardiopulmonary resuscitation and emergency care IV: Special resuscitation situations, *JAMA* 268(16):2245, 1992.)

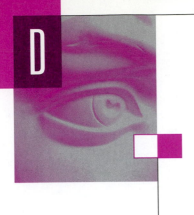

Physiologic Formulas for Critical Care

HEMODYNAMIC FORMULAS

Mean (Systemic) Arterial Pressure (MAP)

$$\text{SMAP} = \frac{(\text{Diastolic} \times 2) + (\text{Systolic} \times 1)}{3}$$

Systemic Vascular Resistance (SVR)

$$\frac{\text{MAP} - \text{RAP}}{\text{CO}} = \text{SVR in units}$$
(Normal range 10-18 units)

$$\frac{\text{MAP} - \text{RAP}}{\text{CO}} \times 80 = \text{SVR in dynes/sec/cm}^{-5}$$
(Normal range 800-1400 dynes/sec/cm^{-5})

Systemic Vascular Resistance Index (SVRI)

$$\frac{\text{MAP} - \text{RAP}}{\text{CI}} \times 80 = \text{SVR in dynes/sec/cm}^{-5}/\text{m}^2$$
(Normal range 2000-2400 dynes/sec/cm^{-5})

Pulmonary Vascular Resistance (PVR)

$$\frac{\text{PAP mean} - \text{RAP}}{\text{CO}} = \text{PVR in units}$$
(Normal range 1.2-3.0 units)

$$\frac{\text{PAP mean} - \text{RAP}}{\text{CO} \times 80} = \text{PVR in dynes/sec/cm}^{-5}$$
(Normal range 100-250 dynes/sec/cm^{-5})

Pulmonary Vascular Resistance Index (PVRI)

$$\frac{\text{PAP mean} - \text{PAWP}}{\text{CI}} \times 80 = \text{PVR in dynes/sec/cm}^{-5}/\text{m}^2$$
(Normal range 225-315 dynes/sec/cm^{-5}/m^2)

RAP, Right atrial pressure; *CO,* cardiac output; *CI,* cardiac index; *SV,* stroke volume; *HR,* heart rate; *PAP* mean, pulmonary artery mean pressure; *PAWP,* pulmonary artery wedge pressure; *BSA,* body surface area; *MAP,* mean arterial pressure.

Left Cardiac Work Index (LCWI)

Step 1. $\text{MAP} \times \text{CO} \times 0.0136 = \text{LCW}$

Step 2. $\frac{\text{LCW}}{\text{BSA}} = \text{LCWI}$ (Normal range 3.4-4.2 kg-m/m^2)

Left Ventricular Stroke Work Index (LVSWI)

Step 1. $\text{MAP} \times \text{SV} \times 0.0136 = \text{LVSW}$

Step 2. $\frac{\text{LVSW}}{\text{BSA}} = \text{LVSW}$ (Normal range 50-62 g-m/m^2)

Right Cardiac Work Index (RCWI)

Step 1. $\text{PAP mean} \times \text{CO} \times 0.0136 = \text{RCW}$

Step 2. $\frac{\text{RCW}}{\text{BSA}} = \text{RCWI}$ (Normal range 0.54-0.66 kg-m/m^2)

Right Ventricular Stroke Work Index (RVSWI)

Step 1. $\text{PAP mean} \times \text{SV} \times 0.0136 = \text{RVSW}$

Step 2. $\frac{\text{RVSW}}{\text{BSA}} = \text{RVSWI}$ (Normal range 7.9-9.7 g-m/m^2)

Corrected QT Interval (QTc)

$$\frac{\text{QT}}{\sqrt{\text{RR}}} = \text{QTc}$$

Body Surface Area

Many hemodynamic formulas can be *indexed* or adjusted to body size by use of a BSA nomogram (Figure D-1). To calculate BSA:

1. Obtain height and weight.
2. Mark height on the left scale and weight on the right scale.
3. Draw a straight line between the two points marked on the nomogram.

The number where the line crosses the middle scale is the BSA value.

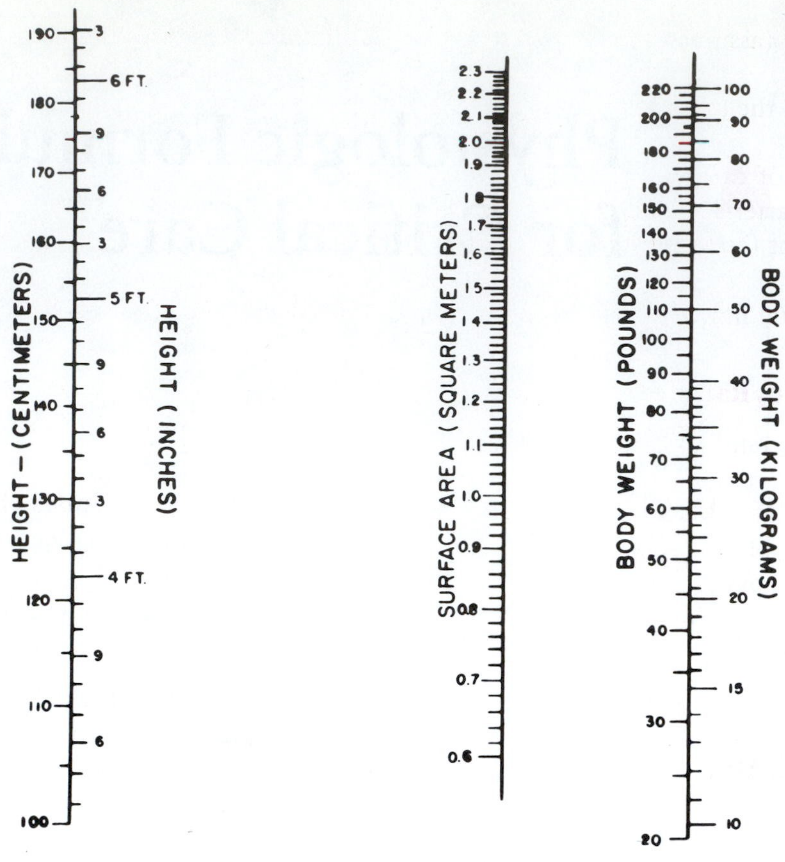

FIGURE D-1. Body surface area (BSA) nomogram.

PULMONARY FORMULAS

Calculation of the Shunt Equation (Qs/Qt)

$$\frac{Qs}{Qt} = \frac{Cco_2 - Cao_2}{Cco_2 - Cvo_2}$$

Cco_2 = Capillary oxygen content (calculated value)
Cao_2 = Arterial oxygen content (calculated value)
Cvo_2 = Venous oxygen content (calculated value)

Normal range is less than 5.90.

Calculation of the Capillary Oxygen Content (Cco_2)

$$Cco_2 = (Hgb \times 1.34^{*} \times Sco_2) + (Pco_2 \times 0.003^{\dagger})$$

Hgb = hemoglobin (measured via laboratory sample or arterial blood gas)
Sco_2 = pulmonary capillary oxygen saturation
Pco_2 = partial pressure of oxygen in capillary blood

There is no established normal value.

Calculation of Arterial Oxygen Content (Cao_2)

$$Cao_2 = (Hgb \times 1.34 \times Sao_2) + (0.003^{\dagger} \times Pao_2)$$

Hgb = hemoglobin (measured via laboratory sample or arterial blood gas)
Sao_2 = arterial oxygen saturation (measured via arterial blood gas)
Pao_2 = partial pressure of oxygen in arterial blood (measured via arterial blood gas)

Normal value is 20 ml/100 ml

Calculation of Venous Oxygen Content (Cvo_2)

$$Cvo_2 = (Hgb \times 1.34^{*} \times Svo_2) + (0.003^{\dagger} \times Pvo_2)$$

Hgb = hemoglobin (measured via laboratory sample or arterial blood gas)
Svo_2 = mixed venous oxygen saturation (measured via mixed venous blood gas)
Pvo_2 = partial pressure of oxygen in mixed venous blood (measured via mixed venous blood gas)

Normal value is 15 ml/100 ml

Calculation of Alveolar Pressure of Oxygen (PAo_2)

$$PAo_2 = FIo_2 \times (Pb - PH_2O) - Paco_2/RQ$$

FIo_2 - fraction of inspired oxygen (obtained from oxygen settings)

*1.34 is a constant used because each gram of hemoglobin will carry 1.34 ml oxygen. Actually, if the hemoglobin is chemically pure (rare), each gram is capable of carrying 1.39 ml of oxygen. Because most hemoglobin has impurities, 1.34 is the accepted constant.
†1.003 is a constant used because 0.003 ml of oxygen will dissolve in each 100 ml of blood.

Pb - barometric pressure (assumed to be 760 mm Hg at sea level)
PH_2O - water pressure in the lungs (assumed to be 47 mm Hg)
$PaCO_2$ - partial pressure of carbon dioxide in arterial blood (measured via arterial blood gas)
RQ - respiratory quotient (assumed to be 0.8)

Normal range is 60 to 100 mm Hg

Calculation of PaO_2/FIO_2 Ratio

$$PaO_2/FIO_2 \text{ ratio} = \frac{PaO_2}{FIO_2}$$

PaO_2 - partial pressure of oxygen in arterial blood (measured via arterial blood gas)
FIO_2 - fraction of inspired oxygen (obtained from oxygen settings)

Normal range is greater than 286

Calculation of Arterial/Alveolar Ratio

$$PaO_2/PAO_2 \text{ ratio} = \frac{PaO_2}{PAO_2}$$

PaO_2 - partial pressure of oxygen in arterial blood (measured via arterial blood gas)
PAO_2 - partial pressure of oxygen in alveoli (calculated value)

Normal range is greater than 60%

Calculation of Alveolar-Arterial Gradient

$$P(A\text{-}a)O_2 = PAO_2 - PaO_2$$

PAO_2 - partial pressure of oxygen in alveoli (calculated value)
PaO_2 - partial pressure of oxygen in arterial blood (measured via arterial blood gas)

Normal range is 0 to 20 mm Hg

Calculation of the Dead Space Equation (V_D/V_T)

$$\frac{V_D}{V_T} = \frac{PaCO_2 - PetCO_2}{PaCO_2}$$

$PaCO_2$ - partial pressure of carbon dioxide in arterial blood (measured via arterial blood gas)
$PetCO_2$ - partial pressure of carbon dioxide in exhaled gas (measured via end-tidal CO_2 monitor)

Normal range is 0.2 to 0.4 (20% to 40%)

Calculation of Anion Gap

$$\text{Anion Gap} = Na^+ - (Cl^- + HCO_3^-)$$

Na^+ - sodium (measured via laboratory sample)
Cl^- - chloride (measured via laboratory sample)
HCO_3^- - bicarbonate (measured via laboratory sample)

Normal range is 1 to 12 mEq/L

Calculation of Static Compliance (C_{ST})

(This value is calculated on mechanically ventilated patients.)

$$C_{ST} = \frac{V_T}{PP - PEEP}$$

V_T - tidal volume (obtained from ventilator)
PP - plateau pressure (measured via ventilator)
PEEP - positive end-expiratory pressure (obtained from ventilator)

Normal value is greater than 50 ml/cm H_2O

Calculation of Dynamic Compliance (C_{DY}) (also called characteristic)

(This value is calculated on mechanically ventilated patients.)

$$C_{DY} = \frac{V_T}{PIP - PEEP}$$

V_T - tidal volume (obtained from ventilator)
PIP - peak inspiratory pressure (obtained from ventilator)
PEEP - positive end-expiratory pressure (obtained from ventilator)

Normal value is 40 to 50 ml/cm H_2O

NEUROLOGIC FORMULAS

Calculation of Cerebral Perfusion Pressure (CPP)

$$CPP = MAP - ICP$$

MAP - mean arterial pressure (measured via arterial line or blood pressure cuff)
ICP - intracranial pressure (measured via intracranial pressure monitoring device)

Normal range is 60 to 150 mm Hg

Calculation of Arteriojugular Oxygen Difference ($AJDO_2$)

$$AJDO_2 = (SaO_2 - SjO_2) \times 1.34^* \times Hgb$$

*1.34 is a constant used because each gram of hemoglobin will carry 1.34 ml oxygen. Actually, if the hemoglobin is chemically pure (rare), each gram is capable of carrying 1.39 ml of oxygen. Because most hemoglobin has impurities, 1.34 is the accepted constant.

SaO_2 - arterial oxygen saturation (measured via arterial blood gas)
SjO_2 - jugular venous saturation (measured via jugular bulb catheter or jugular blood gas)
Hgb = hemoglobin (measured via blood sample or arterial blood gas)

Normal range is 5.0 to 7.0 vol%

ENDOCRINE FORMULAS

Serum Osmolality

$$\text{Serum Osmolality} = 2(Na^+ + K^+) + \frac{\text{glucose mg/dL}}{18} + \frac{\text{BUN mg/dL}}{2.8}$$

BUN - blood urea nitrogen

Normal range is dependent on substance measured

Estimated Fluid Volume Deficit in Liters

$$\frac{0.6\ (\text{kg/weight}) \times ([\text{measured serum sodium}] - 140)}{140}$$

Normal range is dependent on substance measured

RENAL FORMULA

Clearance

$$\text{Clearance} = U \times \left(\frac{V}{P}\right)$$

U = concentration of substance in urine
V = time
P = concentration of substance in plasma

Normal range is dependent on substance measured

NUTRITIONAL FORMULAS*

Formulas for Estimating Caloric Needs

Step 1. Calculate basal energy expenditure (BEE). This is the energy needed for basic life processes such as respiratory function and maintenance of body temperature.

Women: BEE = 795 + 7.18 × weight (kg)
Men: BEE = 879 + 10.20 × weight (kg)

Step 2. Multiply by an appropriate stress factor to meet the needs of the ill or injured patient (see the following table). If the patient has more than one stress present (e.g., burn and pneumonia), use only the stress factor for the highest level of stress.

Type of Stress	Multiply the Value Obtained in Step 2 By
Fever	1 + 0.13/ C elevation above normal (or 0.07/° F)
Pneumonia	1.2
Major injury	1.3
Severe sepsis, burn of 15%-30% of body surface area (BSA)	1.5
Burn of 31%-49% BSA content (calculated value)	1.5–2.0
Burn ≥ 50% BSA	1.8–2.1

*Deitch EA: *Crit Care Clin* 11:735, 1995; Owen OE and others: *Am J Clin Nutr* 4:1, 1986; Owen OE and others: *Am J Clin Nutr* 46:875, 1987; Garrel DR, Jobin N, de Jonge LH: *Nutr Clin Prac* 11:99, 1996.

Estimating Protein Needs

Protein needs vary with degree of malnutrition and stress.

Condition	Multiply Desirable Body Weight (kg) By
Healthy individual or well-nourished elective surgery patient	0.8-1.0 g protein
Malnourished or catabolic state (e.g., sepsis, major injury)	1.2 to 2+ g protein
Burns	
15%-30% BSA	1.5 g protein
31%-49% BSA	1.5-2.0 g protein
≥ 50% BSA	2.0-2.5 g protein

Example of Calculation of Calorie and Protein Needs

A 28-year-old female patient has a fracture of the left femur and burns of 40% of her BSA after an automobile accident. Her height is 1.65 m (5′5″) and her weight is 59.1 kg (130 lb).

Energy needs

1. BEE = 795 + 7.18 × 59.1 = 1219 calories/day
2. Energy needs for injury = 1219 calories × 1.75 = 2133 calories/day

Protein needs

Protein needs = 59.1 kg × 1.75 g = 103 g/day

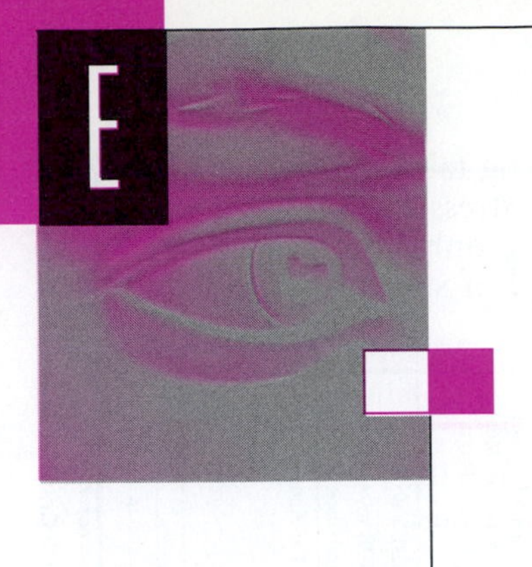

Interdisciplinary Plans of Care*

*These pathways are only guidelines. Patient care will vary, depending on their individual needs.

Butterworth
HEALTH SYSTEM
Grand Rapids, MI 49503

STROKE CLINICAL PATH

(ICD-9: 434; DRG 14)

This pathway is only a guideline. Patient care will vary on their individual needs. Refer to Guidelines for Care and Education Record of the Patient with Stroke.

General Demographics:
___ Gender Admit From:
___ Age ___ Home
___ Race ___ Ext. Care

Admission Findings:
BP__________
Blood Sugar______
EKG __________
Swallow Assessment
(Note on tool on back)

Stroke Severity: _______
(See Barthel Index on back)

Known Risk Factors:
___ Hx. of Prev. Stroke
___ Hx. of Prev. TIA(s)
___ Hx. of HTN
___ Hx. of DM
___ Hx. of A.Fib.
___ Smoking

Stroke Type:
___ Thrombotic
___ Cardioembolic
___ Hemorrhagic
___ Other (_________)

Location of Stroke:
R L Ant. Cerebral Cortex
R L Mid. Cerebral Cortex
R L Post. Cerebral Cortex
R L Subcortical Area
R L Cerebellum
R L Brainstem

Timing of Events:
___ Time of Symptom Awareness
*** First Medical Care Contact
___ Phys. Office ___ ED
*** Mode of Transportation
___ Ambulance
___ Car; driven by another/self
___ Time of Arrival in ED
___ Time of CT
*** Type of Treatment
___ Anticoagulation (___ Time started)
___ Antiplatelet Therapy
___ Thrombolytic Therapy
___ Research Protocol (_____________)

Discharge:
Stroke Severity *(See Barthel Index on back)*:___________
Disposition: ___Home ___Home w/ Support ___Acute Rehab ___Sub-Acute Rehab ___Extended Care ___Death
"Avoidable Days": _______ and Reason: __________________ *(Completed by MSW or UM)*

Stamp with addressograph

Please fill in dates and check all boxes that are completed. "NA" over those boxes not applicable. Leave blank those boxes not yet completed. Document reason in "exceptions" grid on back. Sign at bottom of column.

Dates	Emergency Dept.	Day #1	Day #2	Day #3	Day #4	Day #5	Outcomes ✓ if met by DC
Discharge Planning		☐ MSW: Eval. Pt/Fam. Social Support ☐ MSW: Eval. Financial/Insurance Status	☐ Rehab Team: Develop Rehab and/or Disposition Plan ☐ MSW: Contact Approp. DC Site/Service	☐ Rehab. Facility Intake Eval.	☐ MSW: Verify DC Plan ☐ Rehab Team: Report to DC Site/Service	☐ Discharge as Planned	☐ DC by Day #5 ☐ Disposition (See above)
Teaching (see Education Record)	☐ Need for Admission	☐ See Education Record (Videos & Booklets, Safety, & Mobility)	☐ Treatment/Rehab Plan/Goal ☐ Nutrition/Diet Needs (e.g. assist, safety) ☐ See Ed.Record (Coping, ↓ Risk & Recur)	☐ See Ed. Record (Self-Care/ ADL Adapt/Compens. Skills)	☐ See Ed. Record	☐ See Education Record	☐ Covered all items on Ed. Record
Consults	☐ Consider Neurologist	☐ Consider PT ☐ Consider OT ☐ Consider SLP	☐ Consider Stroke Rehab Team Evaluation ☐ Consider Dietitian -- if albumin <3.0, enteral feedings, or poor intake				
Treatments	☐ Consider Oxygen ☐ Consider IV Hydration	☐ Wean Oxygen per O_2 Protocol ☐ Basic Aspiration Precautions *(see back)* ☐ DC Maintenance IV if good PO intake (Δ to Saline Lock if no heparin infus.) ☐ Bowel Mgmt per Stroke Guideline ☐ Bladder Mgmt per Stroke Guideline ☐ Calf & thigh measurements	☐ Wean O_2 per Protocol ☐ Basic Aspiration Precautions ☐ DC IV site(if adeq. PO intake, Ø Hep/ study infus, or diag.study needing IV site) ☐ Bowel Mgmt per Stroke Guideline ☐ Bladder Mgmt per Stroke Guideline	☐ Wean O_2 per Protocol ☐ Basic Aspiration Precautions ☐ Bowel Mgmt per Guideline ☐ Bladder Mgmt per Guide.	☐ Wean O_2 per Protocol ☐ Basic Aspiration Prec. ☐ Bowel Mgmt per Guide. ☐ Bladder Mgmt per Guide ☐ Calf & thigh measurements	☐ O_2 per Protocol ☐ Basic Asp. Prec ☐ Bowel per Guide. ☐ Bladder per Guide.	☐ Ø Oxygen at DC ☐ ØPneumonia ☐ Ø Bowel Const/Incont ☐ Ø Bladder Incont/UTI
Medications	☐ Consider Research Protocol(If < 8° symp.) ☐ Consider Anticoag (Heparin Infusion) ☐ Consider TPA(if<3°)	☐ Subq Heparin for DVT Prophylaxis ☐ Consider Anticoagulation Therapy ☐ Consider Antiplatelet Therapy ☐ Bld. Sugar Mgmt if > 200 ☐ Treat A.Fib. if present	☐ Subq. Heparin for DVT Pryphylaxis ☐ Consider Starting Coumadin ☐ Cont. Antiplatelet Therapy ☐ BS Mgmt if > 200 ☐ Cont. A.Fib. Therapy	☐ Subq. Heparin ☐ Cont. Heparin/Coumadin ☐ Cont. Antiplatelet Therapy ☐ BS Manage. if > 200 ☐ Con. A.Fib. Therapy	☐ Subq. Heparin ☐ Consider DCing Heparin ☐ Cont. Antiplatelet Therapy ☐ BS Mgmt if > 200 ☐ Cont. A.Fib. Therapy	☐ Subq. Heparin ☐ Cont. Coumadin ☐ Cont. Antiplat. Tx. ☐ BS Mgmt if >200 ☐ Cont. A.Fib. Tx.	☐ Ø DVT/PE ☐ Ø ↓ in BP > 15% of MAP ☐ Ø BS > 240 ☐ Ø A.Fib at DC
Diet	☐ Dysphagia Screen by RN *(see back)*	☐ Dysphagia Screen by RN *(see back)* ☐ Diet as appropriate: ___Supervised DysphasiaIV, Liquid D ___TF; Oral Motor Assessment	☐ Diet as appropriate: ___ Dysphagia IV Liquid D ___ Supervised Meals ___Tube Feedings ☐ Consider PEG if still unsafe to swallow	☐ Diet as appropriate: ___Dysphagia IV Liquid D ___Supervised Meals ___Tube Feedings	☐ Diet as appropriate: ___ DysphagiaIV Liquid D ___ Supervised Meals ___Tube Feedings	☐ Diet as approp. ___ Dysph.IV Liq.D ___ Supervis. Meals ___Tube Feedings	☐ Ø Aspiration ☐ Nutritional needs met
Activity	☐ Bedrest	☐ ADL's w/assist as needed ☐ OOB w/assist 2-4 x day ☐ Ambulation w/assist as needed	☐ ADL's w/assist as needed ☐ OOB w/assist 2-4 x day ☐ Ambulation w/assist as needed	☐ ADL's w/assist as needed ☐ OOB w/assist 2-4 x day ☐ Ambulate w/assist as need	☐ ADL's w/assist as needed ☐ OOB w/assist 2-4 x day ☐ Ambulate w/assist as need	☐ ADL's w/ Assist ☐ OOB w/ Assist ☐ Ambulate w/ Assist	☐ Ø Falls ☐ Ø Skin Breakdown
Tests	☐ CT of Brain ☐ EKG ☐ Chem Profile, CBC, PT, PTT	☐ Consider Echocardiogram ☐ Consider Carotid Doppler ☐ PT/PTT if on Anticoag. Therapy ☐ If <55y/o eval Other Coags,TEE,Angio	☐ Chest X-Ray if Rehab/Disposition Plan involves another facility ☐ PT/PTT if on Anticoag Tx	☐ Consider Repeat CT ☐ PT/PTT if on Anticoag Tx	☐ PT/PTT if Anticoag Tx	☐ PT if Anticoag Tx	☐ If Anticoag Tx, to target range w/in 24 hours
Signatures (Name, Title, & Time)	________ ________	________ ________	________ ________	________ ________	________ ________	________ ________	________ ________

This report is prepared pursuant to but not limited to (P.A.368 of 1978). This report is a review function and as such is confidential and shall be used only for the purpose provided by law and shall not be a public record and shall not be available for court subpoena.

R:\NURSING\PATHS\STROKE.DOC 12/24/96 2:09 PM ©Butterworth Hospital (616-391-1276) XO2757 **Return to Mail Code 16 when completed**

FIGURE E-1. Stroke clinical path. *(Courtesy Butterworth Health System, Grand Rapids, Mich.)*

(Adm/Disch) **Barthel Index (Patient's Total Score** Adm: Disc:)

___/___ Feeding (Independent-10; Needs food cut-5; Dependent-0)
___/___ Bed ↔ Chair (Independent-15; Min Assist-10; Able to sit but Max Assist w/ Transfer-5; Dependent-0)
___/___ Personal Toilet *(Face, teeth, hair)* (Independent-5; Dependent 0)
___/___ Toileting *(Getting on & off; handling clothing, wiping & flushing)* (Independent-10; Some Assist-5; Dependent-0)
___/___ Bathing (Independent-5; Dependent-0)
___/___ Walking *(or wheelchair if unable to walk)* (Independent for 50 yds-15; Needs Assist for 50 yds-10; Wheelchair for 50 yds-5; dependent-0)
___/___ Stairs (Independent-10; With Assist-5; Unable-0)
___/___ Dressing *(Includes buttons, zippers, & shoelaces)* (Independent-10; With Assist-5; Dependent-0)
___/___ Bowel Control (Continent-10; Occasional Incont-5; Incontinent-0)
___/___ Bladder Control (Continent-10; Occasional Incont-5; Incont.-0)

Blood Pressure Management in Stroke

1. **Consider not treating pt. until BP > 210/110** (for 3 consecutive readings, 15" apart; need pressure to perfuse brain).
2. **Treat BP conservatively; try not to ↓ MAP > 10%** (Mean Arterial Pressure [2SBP + 1DBP] ÷ 3).
3. **Report a sustained ↑/↓ BP of 20% from baseline** (BP swings can neutralize autoregulation ∴ ↓ perfusion to ischemic brain).

Recommended Treatment for Atrial Fibrillation

★ **A.Fib is a major risk factor for stroke** (clots that form in the heart may be released into cerebrovascular circulation)

Treatment Recommendations:

1. **Digoxin** (PO or IV) usually first line
2. Progress to diltiazem, nifedipine, and/or cardioversion
3. If persistant A. Fib. -- Warfarin (unless contraindicated)

Dysphagia(Swallowing Safety) Screen

1. Before PO intake, RN to complete (w/in 8° admit).
2. Check all of the following ("✓" if present):

A.___ Any facial weakness
___ Incomplete oral closure
___ Drooling
___ Unable to protrude tongue
___ Unable to move tongue side-to-side
___ Speech that is unclear or difficult to understand

B. Ask patient to take a drink of water; then assess for:
___ Coughing during or shortly after swallowing
___ Takes more than 1 swallow to empty mouth
___ "Wet voice" after swallow
___ "Wet" lung sounds after swallow

*** **"Unsafe" is 3 or more items from part "A" or any from part "B" -- refer to physician's orders (NPO, TF's per dietitian, oral motor eval)**

3. The RN will reassess for dysphagia before any PO food/fluids/meds if their conditions changes signif.

Basic Aspiration Precautions

1. **Head of Bed ↑ 30° at all times.**
2. **Remind pt to cough & deep breath 10 times Q2°& PRN WA.**
3. **Oral Care at least BID.**
4. **Do not use straws** (cause airway to open during swallow).
5. **Ensure pt fully awake & sitting upright before eating or drinking.**
6. **Decrease environmental stim. (noise, distractions, etc) during eating/drinking.**
7. **Encourage pt** (visitor) **to NOT talk while eating.**
8. **Encourage pt to completely empty mouth before taking another bite/drink** (may help to set down the cup/spoon/fork).

Bowel & Bladder Managment

(from Stroke Guideline of Care & Imprinted Orders)

1. **Maintain adequate hydration** (2,000-2,5000cc/day)
2. **Toilet the pt vis BR or BSC If at all possible.**
3. **Bowel Managment:**
   a. Assess bowel function at least QD.
      → Notify physician if no BS present
   b. Toilet 30" after each meal (reflex strongest)
   c. High fiber diet; juice or fruit with each meal
   d. If no BM within 48° of admission (& BS present):
      → Pericolace 100mg PO BID
   e. If no BM within 96° of admission (& BS present):
      → Check for impaction & digitally evacuate
      → Follow with cleansing enema
   f. If diarrhea:
      → Same as "e"
      → If continues, notify physician
      → If continues & incontinent, use fecal collector
4. **Bladder Management:**
   a. Assess bladder function & urine output Qshift.
   b. If incontinent, toilet Q2° during day & Q4° at nite
   c. If no UO x 8°, palpate & percuss for bladder
   d. If bladder distended:
      → st. cath Q4-6° to keep bladder volume < 400cc.
   e. If pt starts voiding:
      → continue w/ post-void cath (5-15" after void) until volume consitantly <100cc
   f. If urine cloudy, foul smelling, or pt c/o dysuria:
      → Urine for UA (with C&S if > 5 WBCs)
      → If UA shows > 100,000 organisms: Call physician
   g. If foley: → DC 24° after admission.
      → Secure to thigh with leg strap/tape.

Instructions: Please indicate any significant variances from the pathway in the boxes to the right. Write in the variance code, the date the variance occurred, comments and your initials. Your comments for improving the care for this population or the pathways format are appreciated.

CODES FOR COMMON VARIANCES:

Code	Issue
787.2	Insufficient PO Intake (Due to poor swallowing)
P3	Signif. Others Not Available for Teaching
P6	ICU Stay (Due to Neurological/General Status)
P15	NPO (Why???)
P16	Concurrent Complex Medical Issues (e.g.: DM, CAD, Resp)

Code	Issue
P23	Insufficient PO Intake (Due to poor endurance)
P24	Activity Intolerance
S5	Discharge Facility; Delay in Discharge/Transfer
S6	PT Services Not Available
S7	OT Services Not Available

Code	Issue
S8	MSW Services Not Available
S17	Discharge Plan Change (due to Δ in patient status)
S23	Intubation/Ventilation (due to Respiratory Status)
S26	Awaiting PEG Placement
S27	Discharge Facility; Delay in Evaluation
S28	SLP Services Not Available

Pathway Variance/Exception	Date	Comments	Initials

Ideas for improving care for this population:	Ideas for improving format of this pathway:

This report is prepared pursuant to but not limited to (P.A.368 of 1978). This report is a review function and as such is confidential and shall be used only for the purpose provided by law and shall not be a public record and shall not be available for court subpoena.

R:\NURSING\PATHS\STROKE.DOC 12/24/96 2:09 PM ©Butterworth Hospital (616-391-1276) XO2757 **Return to Mail Code 16 when completed**

FIGURE E-1. Cont'd.

Butterworth
HEALTH SYSTEM

Grand Rapids, MI 49503

Please fill in dates and check all boxes that apply, write NA over boxes that do not apply.

MYOCARDIAL INFARCTION CLINICAL PATH
(DRG 121 & 122)

This pathway is only a guideline. Patient care will vary based on their individual needs. Refer to Guidelines of Care and Education Record for Patient with Coronary Artery Disease.

___ R/O MI

Stamp with addressograph

Length of stay will vary for each patient. Pathway is based on average stay. Less complicated and younger patients may have shorter than average length of stays. Some patients may stay longer than the average if their condition is more severe.

Dates→							
	ED	Day 1	Day 2	Day 3	Day 4	Day 5	OUTCOMES
Consults	☐ Primary Care Physician ☐ Cardiologist ☐ MSW if crisis situation ☐ MCCS Resident	☐ Cardiac Rehab/PT ☐ Cardiac Rehab/RN ☐ Dietitian ☐ MSW (see back)	☐MSW	☐Cardiac Rehab Phase II			☐Follow up appointment is arranged in cardiac rehab program (see Rehab pathway)
Assessment and Intervention	☐ H&P ☐ 2-3 IV lines/Thrombolytic ☐ O2 ☐ ECG Monitor ☐Cath/PTCA	☐Imprinted orders ☐O2 ☐ECG Monitor	☐ Daily weight if S & S of CHF ☐ D/C O2 per protocol ☐ECG Monitor	☐Daily weight if S & S of CHF ☐Functional Capacity test ☐ECG Monitor	☐ Cardiac cath/Site checks ☐Daily weight if S & S of CHF ☐ DC Monitor	☐Daily weight if S & S of CHF	☐ NSR ☐ No evidence of chest pain ☐ No evidence of CHF
Medications	☐ ASA (if not prehosp) ☐ NTG sl ☐ NTG IV ☐ TPA bolus/gtt ☐ Heparin bolus/gtt ☐ B Blocker	☐ ASA(if not given in ED) ☐ NTG IV ☐ Heparin IV ☐ B Blocker PO	☐ ASA ☐ PO Nitrates ☐ Heparin IV ☐ B Blocker PO ☐ ACE <40% EF	☐ ASA ☐ PO Nitrates ☐ Heparin IV ☐ B Blocker PO ☐ ACE <40% EF	☐ ASA ☐ PO Nitrates ☐ DC Heparin ☐ B Blocker ☐ ACE <40% EF	☐ ASA ☐ PO Nitrates ☐ B Blocker ☐ ACE <40% EF ☐Calcium Channel blocker post PTCA	☐ ASA ☐ PO Nitrates ☐ B Blocker ☐ ACE <40% EF ☐Calcium channel if post PTCA
Diet	☐ NPO/Cl. Liq	☐ ↓Chol/↓Fat ☐ NAS ☐ ADA	☐ ↓Chol/↓Fat ☐ NAS ☐ ADA	☐ ↓Chol/↓Fat ☐ NAS ☐ ADA	☐ ↓Chol/↓Fat ☐ NAS ☐ ADA		☐ Able to verbalize dietary modifications
Activity	☐ CBR.	☐ BR with BSC ☐ Dangle ☐ Bed bath	☐Partial bath ☐Up in chair ☐Short walks/hall bid ☐BRP	☐Self bathe ☐Walk in hall prn	☐HEP ☐Shower before discharge		☐ ADL's without chest pain. ☐ Able to demonstrate HEP ☐Able to verbalize activity guidelines
Tests	☐ STAT 12 Lead ECG ☐ Port CXR ☐ Cardiac Enzymes	☐ 12 Lead ECG ☐ Chem Profile add-on ☐ PTT q6h/nomogram ☐ Cardiac Enzymes Series ☐ Fasting Lipid Profile 1st a.m.	☐ 12 Lead ECG ☐ Pulse Ox ☐ PTT/Nomogram	☐ PTT	☐PTT/DC when Heparin DC ☐Intervention: PTCA__________(date) STENT__________(date) Athrectomy________(date) Surgery __________(date)		☐ Diagnostic studies within normal for this patient
Smoking Status		☐Counseling re: smoking ☐ Non smoker	☐Counseling re:smoking	☐Counseling re: smoking	☐Counseling re: smoking	☐Counseling re: smoking	☐Able to verbalize plan for Smoking Cessation
Education (See Ed Rec)	☐ Brief explanation of Diagnosis. ☐ S&S to report to staff	☐ Reinforce per Ed Rec	☐ Reinforce per Ed Rec ☐ Orient to 4S	☐ Reinforce per Ed Rec	☐ Reinforce per Ed Rec	☐Reinforce per Ed Rec	☐ Able to verbalize actions for recurrent chest pain ☐Able to verbalize medication administration, dose & action
Discharge							☐ Able to verbalize discharge plan.
Signatures (Name And Time)	________ ________	________ ________	________ ________	________ ________	________ ________	________ ________	________ ________

MSW Screening	Preventive/Rehabilitation Services Screening
• excessive anxiety • depressed mood/affect	Patient must be functionally and mentally able to participate in rehabilitation program and also have one of the following: • MI

This report is prepared pursuant to but not limited to (P.A.368 of 1978). This report is a review function and as such is confidential and shall be used only for the purpose provided by law and shall not be a public record and shall not be available for court subpoena.

R:\NURSING\PATHS\MI.DOC 1/15/97 10:00 AM ©Butterworth Hospital (616-391-1276) XO2132 **Return to Mail Code 16 when completed**

FIGURE E-2. Myocardial infarction clinical path. *(Courtesy Butterworth Health System, Grand Rapids, Mich.)*

• caregiver of a dependent spouse • socially isolated/limited support system • inadequate financial resources to meet needs • referral to ECF	• Interventional procedure • Pre-coronary artery bypass surgery • documented coronary artery disease

Instructions: Please indicate any significant variances from the pathway in the boxes to the right. Write in the variance code, the date the variance occurred, comments and your initials. Your comments for improving the care for this population or the pathways format are appreciated.

CODES FOR COMMON VARIANCES:

Code	Issue	Code	Issue	Code	Issue	Code	Issue
300.00	Anxiety	787.91	Diarrhea	P1	Lives alone/lack of home support	S1	Pathway documentation incomplete
285.1	Anemia	780.6	Fever/FUO	P2	Pt education not complete	S2	Imprinted Orders not used
427.9	Arrhythmia	998.1	Hemorrhage	P3	Family not available	S3	Discharge instructions not used
518.0	Atelectasis	560.1	Ileus	P4	Grieving	S5	Discharge facility delay
427.0	CHF	788.2	Inability to void/urinary retention	P6	Unexpected transfer to ICU	S6	Delay in PT consult
785.51	Cardiogenic shock	787.02	Nausea	P7	Not advancing diet intake	S8	Delay in MSW consult
786.50	Chest pain	451.19	PE	P8	Abnormal lab values	S9	Delay in dietitian consult
564.0	Constipation	410.91	Ventricular rupture	P24	Activity intolerance	S10	Other
293.9	Confusion	787.01	Vomiting	P25	Inadequate pain control		
453.8	DVT			P26	IABP		
				P29	Skin breakdown		
				P33	Infection, other (specify)		

Pathway Variance/ Exception Code	Date	Comments	Initials

Ideas for improving care for this population:	Ideas for improving format of this pathway:

This report is prepared pursuant to but not limited to (P.A.368 of 1978). This report is a review function and as such is confidential and shall be used only for the purpose provided by law and shall not be a public record and shall not be available for court subpoena.

R:\NURSING\PATHS\MI.DOC 1/15/97 10:00 AM ©Butterworth Hospital (616-391-1276) XO2132 **Return to Mail Code 16 when completed**

FIGURE E-2. Cont'd.

Butterworth
HEALTH SYSTEM
Grand Rapids, MI 49503

Please fill in dates and check all boxes that apply, write NA over boxes that do not apply.

CAROTID ENDARTERECTOMY
CLINICAL PATH
ICD-9: 38.12

This pathway is only a guideline. Patient care will vary on their individual needs. Refer to Guidelines of Care and Education Record for the Carotid Endarterectomy Patient

Stamp with addressograph

Length of stay will vary for each patient. Pathway is based on average stay. Less complicated and younger patients may have shorter than average length of stays. Som patients may stay longer than the average if their condition is more severe.

DATE							
	OFFICE	PAT	DOS-BOC-OR	DOS-PACU	DOS-4S	POD 1	OUTCOMES
CONSULTS	Prior to PAT visit send to BOC: • copy of H&P if not to be done in PAT • consults done/to be done • copy of any diagnostic studies(ie angio, EKG, etc)	☐ARN - anesthesia method ☐Dietary consult ☐MSW if following are IDd; • excessive anxiety • depressed mood/affect • caregiver of depend spouse • socially isolated/limited sup syst • inadeq. financial resources				☐Neuro rehab is CVA occurred ☐Start CVA path if needed	
ASSESSMENTS AND INTERVENTIONS		☐H&P dictated / on chart ☐Diagnostic studies on chart ☐Initiate Braden Risk Assess. & note score on profile	Pre-op ☐H&P, angio report, old records on chart & sent to OR ☐Mark operative site Intra-op ☐IV placed ☐Hardline monitor ☐JP drain placed ☐Arterial line placed	☐Neuro assessment ☐JP to self suction ☐D/C arterial line ☐Straight cath PRN ☐Wean O2	☐Telemetry ☐Straight cath PRN ☐Wean O2	☐D/C IV ☐D/C telemetry ☐D/C JP ☐O2 off	☐Neuro checks are stable ☐Incision healing without complications
MEDICATIONS	☐Cont. ASA	☐Patients meds pre-op ☐Cont ASA	☐Pre-op ☐Apply Nitropaste ☐PO anti-HTN given ☐Intra-op ☐Ancef IV given ☐Dextran started ☐Nipride given	☐Nitropaste (Reapply in PACU if needed) ☐Ancef IV given ☐Dextran cont. ☐Wean off nipride ☐SL/IV anti-HTN given PRN ☐Analgesic given		☐ASA QD started ☐D/C Ancef ☐D/C dextran	☐BP controlled by oral meds
DIET	☐Pts. usual diet	☐Instruct NPO per anes guideline	☐NPO per anesthesia guidleines		☐Sips of liquids	☐Resume pre-op diet	☐Diet intake is adeq to meet needs
ACTIVITY	☐Ambulatory	☐Usual activity for patient		☐Bedrest	☐Bedrest; BSC or stand to void	☐Ambulatory	☐Performs ADLs
TESTS		☐Chem profile ☐Lytes ☐CBC ☐EKG ☐CXR	☐Glucose if diabetic	☐USG Q4H	☐USG Q4H	☐D/C USG after Dextran D/C	
EDUCATION	☐Per Education Record	☐Per Education Record ☐Carotid book ☐Seen by surgeon's clinical RN	Pre-op ☐Per Education Record ☐Orient pt. OR ☐Family to waiting area	☐Per Education Record	☐Per Education Record	☐Per Education Record	☐Educational goals met (per Education Record)
DISCHARGE	☐Anticipated LOS ☐Return to work ☐ I mo. post-op MD visit ☐No driving x 2 wks						
SIGNATURES							

This report is prepared pursuant to but not limited to (P.A.368 of 1978). This report is a review function and as such is confidential and shall be used only for the purpose provided by law and shall not be a public record and shall not be available for court subpoena.
R:\NURSING\PATHS\CEA.DOC 12/23/96 7:42 AM ©Butterworth Hospital (616-391-1276) X02195 Return to Mail Code 16 when completed

FIGURE E-3. Carotid endarterectomy clinical path. *(Courtesy Butterworth Health System, Grand Rapids, Mich.)*

Instructions: Please indicate any significant variances from the pathway in the boxes to the right. Write in the variance code, the date the variance occurred, comments and your initials. Your comments for improving the care for this population or the pathways format are appreciated.

CODES FOR COMMON VARIANCES:

Code	Issue	Code	Issue	Code	Issue	Code	Issue
285.1	Anemia	401.9	Hypertension	P2	Pt education not complete	S1	Pathway documentation incomplete
427.9	Arrhythmia	458.9	Hypotension	P3	Family not available	S2	Imprinted Orders not used
436	CVA (start CVA pathway)	788.2	Inability to void/urinary retention	P6	Unexpected transfer to ICU	S3	Discharge instructions not used
786.50	Chest pain	787.02	Nausea	P7	Not advancing diet intake	S9	Delay in dietitian consult
293.9	Confusion	998.5	Surgical wound infection	P8	Abnormal lab values	S10	Other
564.0	Constipation	787.01	Vomiting	P25	Inadequate pain control		
998.1	Hematoma			P33	Infection, other (specify)		

Pathway Variance/ Exception Code	Date	Comments	Initials

Ideas for improving care for this population:	Ideas for improving format of this pathway:

This report is prepared pursuant to but not limited to (P.A.368 of 1978). This report is a review function and as such is confidential and shall be used only for the purpose provided by law and shall not be a public record and shall not be available for court subpoena.

R:\NURSING\PATHS\CEA.DOC 12/23/96 7:42 AM ©Butterworth Hospital (616-391-1276) X02195 Return to Mail Code 16 when completed

FIGURE E-3. Cont'd.

DARTMOUTH-HITCHCOCK MEDICAL CENTER CRITICAL PATH: CARDIAC SURGERY - PART 1

ADDRESSOGRAPH

VARIANCE NOTES

CT ICU VARIANCES

Date	Initials	
______	☐	Hemodynamic instability
______	☐	Heart rate >120
______	☐	Prolonged intubation
______	☐	Intensive pulmonary hygiene needs
______	☐	Nausea
______	☐	Inability to progress activity per protocol
______	☐	Added diagnostic tests
______	☐	L5 border
______	☐	Patient removed from path

CATEGORY	PRE-OP DATE: ______	SURGERY DATE: ______ ADMIT TIME TO CTICU: ______	POD 1 DATE: ______	POD 2 DATE: ______	THE PATIENT MAY BE TRANSFERRED OUT OF CTICU WHEN:	PERTINENT CTICU HISTORY AND STATUS AT TRANSFER:
Cardiac Status	Admission vital signs	ECG monitoring Epicardial pacing wire care Hemodynamic monitoring per standards of care TPR and B.P. per standard of care; report if T > 38.5	→ (continued)		☐ Resting heart rate >60 and <120/min. ☐ No life threatening arrhythmias ☐ Angina free ☐ Systolic B.P. >90 but <160 mmHg ☐ No central monitoring lines	Vital signs: Rhythm:
Respiratory Status	☐ Anesthesia consult ☐ O_2 on way to OR	ET suction prn ☐ Initiate weaning protocol after 1st ABG ☐ O_2 via face mask to NP; wean as long as $SpO_2 \geq 90\%$ Continuous SpO_2 monitoring CDB, incentive spirometer q. 1-2h. Chest P.T.	→ (continued)		☐ Extubated ☐ Resting $SpO_2 \geq 90\%$ on NP O_2 ☐ $SpO_2 \geq 85\%$ on O_2 with activity ☐ Effective cough and airway clearance	O_2 requirement: Lung sounds: SpO_2 on room air:
Nutrition / Elimination	Usual home diet NPO after midnight	NG / orogastric tube NPO	☐ Remove NG/orogastric tube Diet consult to evaluate for high protein supplements Clear liquids after extubation and when bowels sounds present	Diet consult if intubated > 24 hrs		Diet: Bowel sounds:
Wound/ Sternum	☐ Hibiclens shower / bath	Chest tubes to 10cm H_2O pressure Dry, sterile dressings to incisions	Remove incision dressings at 24 hrs Betadine to incisions b.i.d. ☐ Remove chest tubes per protocol			Incisions:
Fluid Status	Weigh q.d. SDP: Weigh AM of surgery	→ (continued) Foley to constant drainage I & O until transfer IV fluids per protocol Autotransfusion per protocol	→ (continued) Cap IV at transfer	☐ Remove Foley in AM		DTV: Edema: Weight:
Activity	Up ad lib	Initiate activity progression per protocol	Up in chair t.i.d. March in place 25-30 times Walk to bathroom; walk 1 min. assisted after mediastinal tubes out & on ICCU Monitor ECG, P, & SpO_2 with timed walks on ICCU Advance ADLs as appropriate		☐ Up in chair for 1 hour	Activity:
Medications	p.o. H_2 blocker if ordered hs sedation Usual cardiac medications Check allergies Meds on call to OR	Meds per protocol: Morphine IV prn; Antibiotic IV Versed IV prn; Demerol IV prn KCl per protocol Vasoactive IV meds per order & protocol After extubation & when bowel sounds present: p.o. analgesic q. 3-4h. prn p.o. H_2 blocker Insulin IV drip for diabetic per protocol	→ (continued) ASA 81 mg p.o. q.d. (none if mechanical valve) Consider diuretic until pre-op weight ☐ If mechanical valve, consider anticoagulation → (continued) ☐ Evaluate to restart pre-op meds		☐ No continuous cardiac drips	Pain control: Last pain med: ☐ Antibiotics complete
Diagnostic Tests	Room air SpO_2 ______ EKG, PA & LAT chest x-ray, and blood tests per anesthesia guidelines Fasting glucose per fingerstick for diabetics immediately before surgery	AP portable chest x-ray post-op EKG post-op Post-op labs per protocol	☐ AP portable chest x-ray after chest tubes out Hgb / HCT, K+, glucose			Last K+:
Education	Share plan of care ☐ Patient/family view pre-op video ☐ Give pre-op booklet ☐ Discuss with patient/family Pre-op orders Pain management post-op Sensory/perceptual changes post-op Weight gain & anasarca ☐ Patient can demonstrate C & IB ☐ Patient can demonstrate use of I.S. ☐ Offer "Patient Progress Record After Open Heart Surgery" pathway Sign consent forms	→ (continued)	→ (continued) Encourage/assist patient to update "Patient Progress Record After Open Heart Surgery" Explain usual care activities to patient	→ (continued)		Other:
Psychosocial & Discharge Planning	☐ Patient / Family Services evaluation Chaplain consult as needed	Call referring MD			☐ Plan of care individualized ☐ CT ICU data completed on NNECVDSG Data Collection Form	

DARTMOUTH-HITCHCOCK MEDICAL CENTER CRITICAL PATH: CARDIAC SURGERY - PART II

ADDRESSOGRAPH

VARIANCE NOTES

ICCU VARIANCES

Date	Initials	Variance	Date	Initials	Variance	Date	Initials	Variance
____	☐	Hemodynamic instability	____	☐	Wound infection	____	☐	Added diagnostic tests
____	☐	R/O MI	____	☐	Slow activity progression	____	☐	Delayed discharge due to home/family issue
____	☐	Atrial fibrillation	____	☐	Delirium	____	☐	Patient removed from path
____	☐	Bradycardia requiring pacing	____	☐	CVA			
____	☐	Ventricular arrhythmias	____	☐	Prolonged telemetry			
____	☐	Slow respiratory progression	____	☐	Prolonged oxygen therapy			
____	☐	Nausea	____	☐	Prolonged chest tubes			

CATEGORY	POD:___ DATE:___	POD:___ DATE:___	POD:___ DATE:___	POD:___ DATE:___	POD:___ DATE:___
Cardiac Status	Epicardial pacing wire care Check P, R and B.P. q. 4h. for 24h. and then q. shift ECG monitoring	☐ Pacing wires out or ☐ clipped if on Coumadin when off telemetry > 24h → ☐ DC ECG monitoring 24h. after transfer if rhythm stable	→ →	→ →	→ →
Respiratory Status	O_2 via face mask to NP; wean as long as O_2 sat ≥ 90% SpO_2 q.d. at rest CDB, Incentive spirometer q. 1-2h. W.A.	→ ☐ NP 4L ☐ 2L ☐ None → →	→ ☐ NP 4L ☐ 2L ☐ None → →	→ ☐ NP 4L ☐ 2L ☐ None → →	☐ O_2 off → →
Nutrition/Elimination	Progress to regular diet when bowel sounds present; no concentrated sweets for diabetics Diet consult for discharge diet information	☐ →	☐ → ☐ Diet information given on low cholesterol, low saturated fat, moderation in salt diet	☐ →	☐ →
Wound/Sternum	Betadine to incisions b.i.d. Remove chest tubes Remove sternal and leg dressings at 24 hrs Check temperature q. 4h. for 24h., then q. shift; If T>38.5 call HO Ace wraps in figure 8 to legs if leg incision	→ Remove chest tube dressing 24h. after tubes out → →	→ ☐ Chest tube site sutures out → →	→ → →	→ → →
Fluid Status	Weigh q.d. ☐ Remove Foley POD 2 in AM Capped IV	→ →	→ →	→ ☐ Discontinue capped IV if off telemetry >24 h	→ →
Activity	Cardiac Surgery Exercise Class (if L5 border arrange with ICCU) Walk continuously, increase 1-3 min./day Walked ________min. Once walking 5 min. and off O_2, go up and down stairs Monitor P with timed walks Monitor SpO_2 with timed walks until off O_2 and O_2 sat ≥ 90% Flexibility exercises b.i.d. Advance ADLs as appropriate Encourage patient to walk ad lib when able When in chair position "toes above the nose" if leg incision P.T. consult	→ → Walked ________min. → → → → → → →	→ → Walked ________min. → → → → → → →	→ → Walked ________min. → → → → → → → Shower after pacing wires out →	→ → Walked ________min. → → → → → → → →
Medications	Consider diuretic until pre-op weight ASA 81 mg p.o. q.d. Colace 100 mg b.i.d. MOM 15 ml if no BM p.o. analgesic q. 3-4h. prn p.o. H_2 blocker	→ → → Dulcolax suppository if no BM → ☐ Evaluate to restart pre-op meds →	→ → → Fleets enema if no BM → ☐ Pain controlled by p.o. analgesic	→ → → → →	→ → → → Write prescriptions →
Diagnostic Tests	☐ AP portable chest x-ray after chest tubes out ☐ Potassium POD 2		☐ CBC, lytes, BUN, creatinine ☐ Review POD 4 labs	☐ PA and LAT chest x-ray ☐ EKG	
Education	☐ Give post-op Heartlines packet and review If valve include: ☐ Bacterial Endocarditis prophylaxis ☐ Medic Alert ☐ Coumadin ☐ Patient/family watch homegoing videotape prior to discharge Explain usual care activities to patient Teach patient daily in order to meet discharge outcomes Share plan of care Offer patient a "Patient Progress Record After Open Heart Surgery"	☐ Patient/family watch nutrition video on TV → ☐ Cardiac Rehab consult for risk factor modification Encourage/assist patient to update "Patient Progress Record After Open Heart Surgery" → → → →	→ → → → → →	→ → ☐ Discuss bacterial endocarditis prophylaxis with appropriate patients ☐ Discuss anticoagulation, precautions, & follow-up plan with appropriate patients →	→ → → → → →
Psychosocial & Discharge Planning			Patient/Family Services re-evaluation	→ ☐ Cardiac Rehabilitation referral	→

F703 (REV. 2/96)

Continued

FIGURE E-4. Cont'd.

POD: ____ DATE: ______
POD: ____ DATE: ______
POD: ____ DATE: ______
POD: ____ DATE: ______
POD: ____ DATE: ______

DARTMOUTH-HITCHCOCK MEDICAL CENTER

One Medical Center Drive
Lebanon, NH 03756
(603) 650-7390

THE PATIENT MAY BE DISCHARGED WHEN:

Cardiac status is stable. Stability is defined for the patient by:
- ☐ Resting heart rate >60 and <100/min. for 24h.
- ☐ NSR for 24h. determined by ECG or telemetry.
- ☐ Off ECG monitoring.
- ☐ Angina free. Pulse: ______
- ☐ Systolic B.P. >90 but <160 mmHg.
- ☐ No pacing wires for 24h. B.P.: ______
- ☐ Temperature is <38° tympanically for 24h.

Rhythm: ______

Oxygen saturation is ≥90% on room air during a 5 min. walk.

Respiratory rate: ______

Lung sounds at Disc: ______

- ☐ Resumed eating normal foods.
- ☐ Had a bowel movement. Last BM: ______

Diet: ______
Comprehension: ☐ Denies Need
☐ Excellent ☐ Very Good ☐ Good ☐ Fair ☐ Poor

- ☐ The wound shows no sign of infection.
- ☐ Chest tube site sutures are out.
- ☐ The sternum is stable.

Describe incisions: ______

Temperature: ______

☐ No gross pitting edema.

Weight: ______

- ☐ Can walk unassisted and continuously for 5 min.
- ☐ Can walk up and down one flight of stairs.

Walked ______ min.
Walked ______ min.
Walked ______ min.

These activities are accomplished:
- ☐ without pulse increasing more than 25 beats/min. above resting level.
- ☐ with pulse returning to resting level in 3 min.
- ☐ with O_2 sat ≥90% on room air.
- ☐ with no dizziness or lightheadedness.
- ☐ with no angina.

ADLS are evaluated.

	Admit	Disc
Feeding	____	____
Bathing	____	____
Toileting	____	____
Dressing	____	____

Key
0 Independent
1 Uses equipment or devices
2 Needs assistance or supervision
3 Needs assistance and special equipment
4 Dependent; does not participate

- ☐ The medications have been reviewed by the intern or nurse practitioner to determine necessity and accessibility.
- ☐ The prescriptions have been written.

The following tests are performed and reviewed:
- ☐ Chest x-ray - one PA and lateral must be done, reviewed by a physician, and judged to be satisfactory within 4 days of discharge.
- ☐ WBC <15,000 and falling within 4 days of discharge.
- ☐ K+ ≥ 4.0 mmol/L within 4 days of discharge.
- ☐ ECG performed during post-op period.
- ☐ Hgb ≥8 G/dl within 4 days of discharge.
- ☐ If mechanical valve INR > ______ & < ______

Latest INR ______
Date ______

Can demonstrate knowledge of the following:
- ☐ wound care, sternal healing
- ☐ exercise plan
- ☐ pain management
- ☐ warning signs and actions to take
- ☐ psychological adaptations
- ☐ DHMC person or local physician to call with problems
- ☐ follow up care/appointments.
- ☐ activities/rest
- ☐ medication regimen
- ☐ diet
- ☐ risk factor modification
- ☐ Patient able to massage scar.
- ☐ Patient able to count pulse with exercise.
- ☐ Patient has received medication pamphlets, Med Card, Med Schedule.

- ☐ VNA called
- ☐ If mechanical valve, arrange PT follow-up with referring MD

- ☐ Pt. and the family feel pt. is ready.
- ☐ There is a specific person(s) identified who will assist with meals, transportation, personal care and home maintenance.
- ☐ Adequate shelter is assured.

Admit Date: ______
Allergies: ______
Age: ______
Past Medical History: ______

ADDRESSOGRAPH

Address: ______
Telephone: ______

Functional Deficits/Limitations: ______

Psycho/Social History: ______

Admission Medications: ______

Cath Data: ______

Admission / Pre-Op: wt: ______ ht: ______ TPR: ______ B.P.: ______

Surgical Procedure: ______ Date of Surgery: ______

Surgeon: ______ Cardiologist: ______

REFERRAL FOR CONTINUING HEALTH CARE AT HOME NA ☐

Home health orders: ☐ 2x/wk x 2 wk and prn ☐ Other

Check incisions, cardiopulmonary status, vital signs, effectiveness of meds, and rehabilitation progress.

PT/INR follow-up: ______

Other: ______

HOME HEALTH AGENCY/FACILITY

Name: ______

Telephone: ______ FAX: ______

Insurance: ______

Discharge Planning Nurse: ______

Transferred to home health agency: ☐ Pt. is homebound: ☐

Routine discharge instructions provided: ☐ 4 week F/U appt. to be mailed to pt. ☐

DURABLE MEDICAL EQUIPMENT

Vendor: ______

Telephone: ______

Equipment: ______

MEDICATIONS

I understand and have been given a copy of discharge instructions. I authorize DHMC to make a home health referral for continued care, if necessary, as ordered above.

Patient/Agent: ______

Discharging Nurse: ______ Disc. Date: ______

Physician: ______ Disc. Time: ______

FIGURE E-4. Cont'd.

Butterworth
HEALTH SYSTEM

Grand Rapids, MI 49503

Please fill in dates and check all boxes that apply

LOWER EXTREMITY RE-VASCULARIZATION
(ICD-9: 39.29)

This pathway is only a guideline. Patient care will vary on their individual needs. Refer to Guidelines of Care and Education Record for the Lower Extremilty Arterial Insufficiency/Revascularization Patient

Stamp form with addressograph

Length of stay will vary for each patient. Pathway is based on average stay. Less complicated and younger patients may have shorter than average length of stays. Some patients may stay longer than the average if their condition is more severe.

DATE												
	OFFICE	PRE-OP / PAT	DOS / BOC	DOS / OR	DOS / PACU	DOS / 4S	POD 1	POD 2	POD 3	POD 4	POD 5-6	OUTCOMES
CONSULTS	Prior to PAT visit send to BOC: • copy of H&P if not to be done in PAT • consults done/to be done • copy of any diagnostic studies(ie angio, EKG, etc)	☐ Anesthesia (epidural) ☐ Dietitian if following are ID'd • Wt loss>10% of usual wt • albumin < 3.0 gm/dl • transferrin < 170 mg/dl • pre-albumin < 18 mg/dl • < 50-75% of PO intake f 3-5 days • inability to self feed, chew or swallow food ☐ ET if wound present, photograph wounds ☐ Home health care ☐ PT if following are ID'd; • impaired mobility/ROM • orthotic/support needs ☐ MSW if following are IDd,; • excessive anxiety • depressed mood/affect • caregiver of depend spouse • socially isolated/limited suppport • inadeq. financial resources					Reassess need for • PT • MSW • Dietitian • Home Health				☐ ET photograph wounds ☐ Dressing change with home health care	☐ Follow up appointment is arranged ☐ Home health care arranged
ASSESSMENT AND INTERVENTION		☐ H&P dictated / on chart ☐ Diagnostic studies on chart ☐ Initiate Braden Risk Assess. & note score on profile ☐ Initiate skin interventions according to algorhythm ☐ Waffle boots for inpatients ☐ Enema in PM before surgery ☐ Hibiclens scrub X 2 before surgery ☐ Wound care per POC	☐ H&P, angio report, old records on chart & sent to OR ☐ Mark operative site ☐ AM admits - measure for waffle boots, note size on pre-op orders & deliver to PACU In PACU ☐ IV placed ☐ Epidural placed	☐ Position for pressure relief ☐ Gel pad on table ☐ Epidural placed ☐ Perip IV placed ☐ Foley placed	☐ Assess pressure points ☐ Pressure relief measures ☐ Apply waffle boots ☐ Vasc checks ☐ Wean O2 ☐ I&O	☐ Assess pressure points ☐ Pressure relief measures ☐ Waffle boots on ☐ Telemetry ☐ Foley → drg ☐ Wean O2 per protocol ☐ Wound care per POC	☐ Assess pressure points ☐ Pressure relief measures ☐ Waffle boots on ☐ Weigh QD ☐ Consider Δ IV to IIV ☐ D/C O2 ☐ Wound care	☐ Assess pressure points ☐ Pressure relief measures ☐ Waffle boots on ☐ Weigh QD ☐ D/CTelemetry ☐ Wound care	☐ Assess pressure points ☐ Pressure relief measures ☐ Waffle boots on ☐ Weigh QD ☐ D/C epidural ☐ D/C IIV & foley after epidural out ☐ Straight cath PRN ☐ Wound care	☐ Assess pressure points ☐ Pressure relief measures ☐ Waffle boots on ☐ Weigh QD ☐ D/C I&O ☐ Wound care	☐ Assess pressure points ☐ Pressure relief measures ☐ Waffle boots on ☐ Weigh QD ☐ Wound care ☐ Pt/fam does incis / wound care	☐ No preventable areas of breakdown ☐ Incisions healing without problems ☐ Pt physiologically stable AEB • afebrile • RA SpO2>90% ☐ Pt/fam does incis / wound care
MEDICATIONS	☐ Pts. usual meds	☐ D/C oral anticoagulent 2 days per-op ☐ Heparin drip (inpts only)	☐ D/C heparin 6 hrs pre-op ☐ Apply nitropaste ☐ IV antibiotic (Ancef) given I hour pre-op		☐ IV Antibiotic ☐ Re-apply nitropaste if needed ☐ Epidural mgt.	☐ Nitropaste ☐ Verify plans for anticoagulation if not specified		☐ PO analgesic after epidural out			☐ D/C IV Antibiotic	☐ Pt. understands D/C medications
DIET	☐ Pts. usual diet	☐ NPO per anesthesia guidelines	☐ NPO after MN		☐ Ice chips		☐ Clear liquids, advance as tol	☐ Usual diet				☐ Diet is adequate to meet pt. needs
ACTIVITY	☐ Usual activity for pt.				☐ Bedrest ☐ Legs in neutral / vascular position	☐ Bedrest ☐ Legs in neutral / vascular position	☐ Chair ☐ Legs in neutral / vascular position	☐ Chair; ambulate as tolerated				☐ Able to perform ADLs / tolerates ambulation
TESTS		☐ CBC,Chem 7,lytes,Pre-albumin,PT/PTT ☐ CCMS with C & S if WBC > 5 ☐ ECG ☐ PA & Lat CXR in radiology ☐ T & screen 3U PRBCs	☐ PT/PTT 4 hours after heparin D/C'd ☐ PT/PTT in AM DOS if pt. has been taking anticoagulants within past 5 days									☐ Diagnostic studies within norms for pt.

This report is prepared pursuant to but not limited to (P.A.368 of 1978). This report is a review function and as such is confidential and shall be used only for the purpose provided by law and shall not be a public record and shall not be available for court subpoena.

R:\NURSING\PATHS\LEAR.DOC 1/2/97 11:32 AM1/2/97 11:32 AM ©Butterworth Hospital (616-391-1276) XO2898 **Return to Mail Code 16 when completed**

Continued

FIGURE E-5. Lower extremity revascularization clinical path. *(Courtesy Butterworth Health System, Grand Rapids, Mich.)*

DATE												
	OFFICE	PRE-OP / PAT	DOS / BOC	DOS / OR	DOS / PACU	DOS / 4S	POD 1	POD 2	POD 3	POD 4	POD 5-6	OUTCOMES
EDUCATION	☐ Vascular booklet given ☐ OR time & potential for Δ	☐ Per Education Record ☐ Vascular booklet given ☐ Pre-op booklet ☐ Seen by surgeon's clinical RN		☐ Orient family to OR ☐ Family update	☐ See Ed Rec	☐ See Ed Rec	☐ See Ed Rec	☐ See Ed Rec	☐ See Ed Rec	☐ See Ed Rec ☐ Instruct pt/fam on wound care	☐ See Ed Rec ☐ Review D/C instruct	☐ Pt able to meet outcomes on Ed Rec
DISCHARGE	☐ ID pt. support sys	☐ Confirm avail post D/C sup sys										
SIGNATURES												

Instructions: Please indicate any significant variances from the pathway in the boxes to the right. Write in the variance code, the date the variance occurred, comments and your initials. Your comments for improving the care for this population or the pathways format are appreciated.

CODES FOR COMMON VARIANCES:

Code	Issue	Code	Issue	Code	Issue	Code	Issue
996.74	Acute arterial/graft closure	780.6	Fever/FUO	P1	Lives alone/lack of home support	S1	Pathway documentation incomplete
285.1	Anemia	401.9	HTN	P2	Pt education not complete	S2	Imprinted Orders not used
300.00	Anxiety	998.1	Hemorrhage	P3	Family not available	S3	Discharge instructions not used
427.9	Arrhythmia	560.1	Ileus	P4	Grieving	S5	Discharge facility delay
518.0	Atelectasis	788.20	Inability to void/urinary retention	P6	Unexpected transfer to ICU	S6	Delay in PT consult
786.50	Chest pain	787.07	Nausea	P7	Not advancing diet intake	S7	Delay in OT consult
293.9	Confusion	451.11	Post-op PE	P8	Abnormal lab values	S8	Delay in MSW consult
564.0	Constipation	998.5	Surgical wound infection	P9	Activity intolerance	S9	Delay in dietitian consult
453.8	DVT	787.01	Vomiting	P25	Inadequate pain control	S10	Other
787.91	Diarrhea			P29	Skin breakdown		
				P33	Infection, other (specify)		

Pathway Variance/ Exception Code	Date	Comments	Initials

Ideas for improving care for this population:

IDENTIFICATION OF ISCHEMIC ULCERS

- *Location*
- Between or on tips of toes
- Fingertips
- Around lateral malleolus
- *Characteristics*
- Even wound margins
- Gangrene or necrosis
- Deep, pale wound beds
- Painful
- Cellulitis

- *Assessment*
- Thin, shiny dry skin
- Loss of hair on ankle or foot
- Thickened toenails
- Pallor on elevation
- Rubor when dependent
- Cyanosis
- Decreased temperature
- Absent or diminished pulses

Ideas for improving format of this pathway:

ULCER

NO

- Wash QD w/ mild soap, rinse thoroughly
- Moisturize w/ non-irritating agent (ie Vaseline, Eucerin)
- Avoid agents with fragrance
- Avoid heating devices
- Use cotton socks
- Avoid constricting clothing
- Avoid crossing legs
- Relieve pressure points

YES

CLEAN

- Cleans with NSS
- Dry dressing (i.e. foam, gauze)
- Protect from injury
- **NO** occlusive dressings(i.e. duoderm)
- **NO** compression stockings (TEDs, SCDs)

DRY GANGRENE (eschar)

- Debridement is contraindicated
- **NO** dressing
- Keep dry
- Relive pressure
- Protect area (i.e. foam to ↓ friction)
- **NO** compression stockings

INFECTED

- Cleanse w/ NSS or as orders by MD
- Aerobic & anaerobic cultures
- Assess for S/S of infection
- R/O osteomylitis
- Debridement of necrotic tissue
- Oral/parenteral antibiotics
- **NO** occlusive dressing (i.e. duoderm)
- Topical dressing per MD order

This report is prepared pursuant to but not limited to (P.A.368 of 1978). This report is a review function and as such is confidential and shall be used only for the purpose provided by law and shall not be a public record and shall not be available for court subpoena.

R:\NURSING\PATHS\LEAR.DOC 1/2/97 11:32 AM1/2/97 11:32 AM ©Butterworth Hospital (616-391-1276) XO2898 **Return to Mail Code 16 when completed**

FIGURE E-5. Cont'd.

Butterworth
HEALTH SYSTEM

Grand Rapids, MI 49503

MAJOR TRAUMA CLINICAL PATH
(ISS>14)

This pathway is only a guideline. Patient care will vary on their individual needs. Refer to Guidelines for Care and Education Record of the Patient with Multiple Trauma

Stamp with addressograph

Please fill in dates and check all boxes that apply, write NA over boxes that do not apply.

Length of stay will vary for each patient. Pathway is based on average stay. Lesscomplicated and younger patients may my have shorter than average length of stays. Some patients may stay longer than the average if their condition is more severe.

DATES									
DAY	**ED RESUSCITATION PHASE**	**DAY 1**	**DAY 2**	**DAY 3 → EXTUBATED**	**POST EXTUBATION → TELEMETRY STATUS**	**TELEMETRY STATUS**	**MED-SURG STATUS → DISCHARGE**	**DAY BEFORE DISCHARGE**	**OUTCOMES**
CONSULTS	☐ Orthopedic ☐ Neurosurgery ☐ MSW ☐ Clergy See trauma flowsheet ATLS format	☐ Physiatry ☐ ET for wound prev/mgmt ☐ Neuroscience Rehab Coord ☐ Metabolic Service/Nutrition ☐ MSW ☐ PT/OT ☐ Speech path if any LOC ☐ Psych (if self inflicted injury) ☐ SMAST screen	☐ Nutrition consult for;: • wt loss>10% usual wt • albumin < 3.0 gm/dl • transferrin < 170 mg/dl • pre-albumin < 18 mg/dl • < 50-75 % of PO intake X 3-5 days • inability to self feed, chew or swallow food			☐ Re-evaluate need for consults listed in Day1 column	☐ Re-evaluate need for consults listed in Day1 column	☐ All consults have "signed off" on chart	
ASSESSMENT AND INTERVENTION	☐ Crystalloid - if ≥ 6L given &/or SBP < 90, consider giving PRBCs ☐ Blood - type specific &/or X matched ☐ Temp Q1H (warm fluids, heat lamp, room temp > 75°F, WarmTouch, ↑vent temp) ☐ ✓ rectal tone/prostate ☐ ✓ meatus, insert foley ☐ Neuro assess/GCS Q30" ☐ Cardiopulm assess ☐ ID skin injury (including entire back)	☐ Braden Risk Assess, initiate skin interventions according to algorhythm ☐ Δ field IV's within 24 hrs ☐ NG tube → WS ☐ Foley → drg. ☐ Establish vent weaning plan if intubated ☐ Antiembolic device applied ☐ Daily weight ☐ I&O ☐ ✓ skin under ED dsgs/splints/collars	☐ Daily weight ☐ I&O ☐ ✓ skin under splints/collars ☐ Review need for bowel program	☐ Daily weight ☐ I&O ☐ Re-evaluate wound prev/mgmt measures ☐ ✓ skin under splints/collars ☐ ✓ suture/staples & estimate removal date ☐ Establish pulmonary care/vent weaning plan ☐ Consider trach if vent weaning not progressing	☐ Daily Weight ☐ I&O ☐ Establish post-extubation pulmonary care plan ☐ Wean O_2 per protocol ☐ Re-evaluate need for: AL, foley, CVC, PAC, NG ☐ Re-evaluate freq of VS, neuro & CSM checks ☐ Re-evaluate bowel program	☐ Daily Weight ☐ I&O ☐ Braden Risk Assess ☐ Re-evaluate freq of VS, neuro & CSM checks ☐ D/C:CVC, foley, NG	☐ Daily weight ☐ I&O ☐ Braden Risk Assess ☐ Re-evaluate wound prev/mgmt measures ☐ Re-evaluate freq of VS, neuro & CSM checks ☐ Suture/staples removed	☐ Final Braden Risk Assess done ☐ All invasive lines out, if line left in rationale is documented ☐ Date/time of last void/BM documented	☐ Able to maintain airway ☐ Stabilization of fractures & dislocations ☐ No preventable areas of skin breakdown
MEDICATIONS	☐ Antibiotics ☐ Tetanus ☐ Pain meds	☐ Establish pain mgmt/sedation plan ☐ DVT/PE prophylaxis ☐ GI stress ulcer prophylaxis ☐ Bronchodilator protocol	☐ Re-evaluate need for antibiotics ☐ Consider bowel meds if no BM	☐ Re-evaluate pain mgmt/sedation needs in anticipation of vent weaning	☐ Wean from IV analgesics ☐ Re-evaluate • DVT/PE prophylaxis • GI stress ulcer prophylaxis	☐ PO/NG analgesics	☐ Consider coumadin therapy ☐ Pneumovax given	☐ Disch meds reviewed	☐ Effective pain control on PO analgesics X 24 hrs prior to discharge
DIET	☐ NPO	☐ Evaluate mode for nutrient delivery: PO/TF/PPN/TPN ☐ Nutrition goals ID'd ☐ Nutrition begun		☐ Consider PEG/PEJ if long term TF possible ☐ Consider TPN if PO/TF not tolerated	☐ Calorie count for first 24 hrs of PO diet		☐ Calorie count X 3 days	☐ Re-evaluate nutrition status	☐ Target nutrition goals met
ACTIVITY	☐ Remove/minimize time on back board ☐ BR, C-Spine precautions	☐ C-Spine cleared per guidelines ☐ Activity level established ☐ Plan for stabilization of Fx's	☐ OOB to cardiac chair ☐ PT/OT started		☐ Clarify wt bearing status ☐ OOB to regular chair ☐ Eval ADL performance		☐ Re-eval mobility ☐ Clarify wt bearing status	☐ Re-eval need for assistive device	☐ Performs ADL &/or assistance available
TESTS	☐ Radiographics ☐ DPL ☐ Heme test stool sample	☐ Establish need for daily lab tests, radiologic studies, etc	☐ Nutrition labs		☐ Re-evaluate need for routine labs & radiologic studies	☐ Re-evaluate need for routine labs & radiologic studies	☐ Re-evaluate need for routine labs & radiologic studies		
EDUCATION		☐ Per Ed Rec ☐ Family conference	☐ Per Ed Rec	☐ Per Ed Rec	☐ Per Ed Rec	☐ Per Ed Rec ☐ Family conf PRN	☐ Per Ed Rec	☐ Per Ed Rec	☐ Ed Rec goals met
DISCHARGE	☐ Evidence preservation	☐ Preliminary rehab plan developed			☐ Confirm payer status and available benefits ☐ Re-evaluate disch plan	☐ Contact rehab/Home Health/SNF center	☐ Re-eval disch plan	☐ Contact rehab/ home Health/SNF center	☐ Adeq support system/resources/ finances

Continued

This report is prepared pursuant to but not limited to (P.A.368 of 1978). This report is a review function and as such is confidential and shall be used only for the purpose provided by law and shall not be a public record and shall not be available for court subpoena.

R:\NURSING\PATHS\TRAUMA.DOC 12/2/96 10:16 AM ©Butterworth Hospital (616-391-1276) XO2968 **Return to Mail Code 16 when completed**

FIGURE E-6. Major trauma clinical path. *(Courtesy Butterworth Health System, Grand Rapids, Mich.)*

Instructions: Please indicate any significant variances from the pathway in the boxes to the right. Write in the variance code, the date the variance occurred, comments and your initials. Your comments for improving the care for this population or the pathways format are appreciated.

CODES FOR COMMON VARIANCES:

Code	Issue	Code	Issue	Code	Issue
285.9	Anemia	P1	Lives alone/lack of home support	S1	Pathway documentation incomplete
518	Atelectasis	P3	Family not available	S5	Discharge facility delay
286.9	Coagulopathy	P6	Unexpected transfer/readmit to ICU	S6	Delay in PT consult
298.9	Confusion	P7	Not advancing diet intake	S7	Delay in OT consult
787.91	Diarrhea	P9	Activity intolerance	S8	Delay in MSW consult
453.8	DVT/PE	P10	Inadequate pain control	S9	Delay in dietary consult
780.6	Fever/FUO	P16	Concurrent complex medical condition (CAD, DM, resp)	S23	Delay in weaning/extubation
998.1	Hemorrhage/hematoma	P29	Skin breakdown	S44	Delay consulting service
560.1	Ileus	P38	C-spine not cleared within 24 hrs		
787.2	Insufficient PO intake	P40	Reintubated		
486	Pneumonia	P41	O2 not weaned		
997.5	Renal complications	P42	Restrictions with positioning		
998.5	Surgical wound infection				

Pathway Variance/ Exception Code	Date	Comments	Initials

Ideas for improving care for this population:	Ideas for improving format of this pathway:

This report is prepared pursuant to but not limited to (P.A.368 of 1978). This report is a review function and as such is confidential and shall be used only for the purpose provided by law and shall not be a public record and shall not be available for court subpoena.

R:\NURSING\PATHS\TRAUMA.DOC 12/2/96 10:16 AM ©Butterworth Hospital (616-391-1276) XO2968 **Return to Mail Code 16 when completed**

FIGURE E-6. Cont'd.

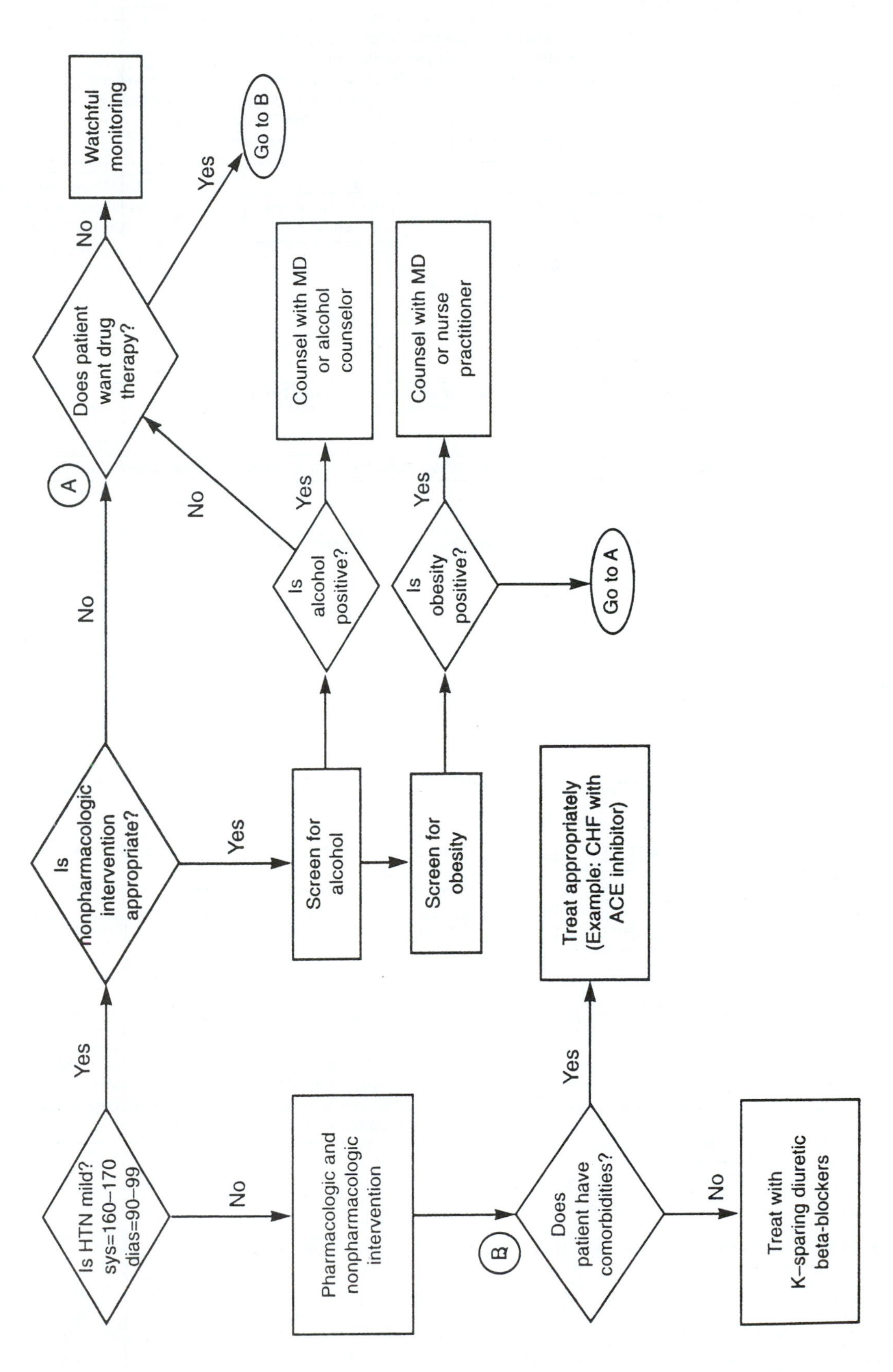

FIGURE E-7. Hypertension algorithm. *HTN,* Hypertension; *K,* potassium; *CHF,* congestive heart failure; *ACE,* angiotensin-converting enzyme; *MD,* physician. (From J *Qual Improve,* 22(11):749, 1994.)

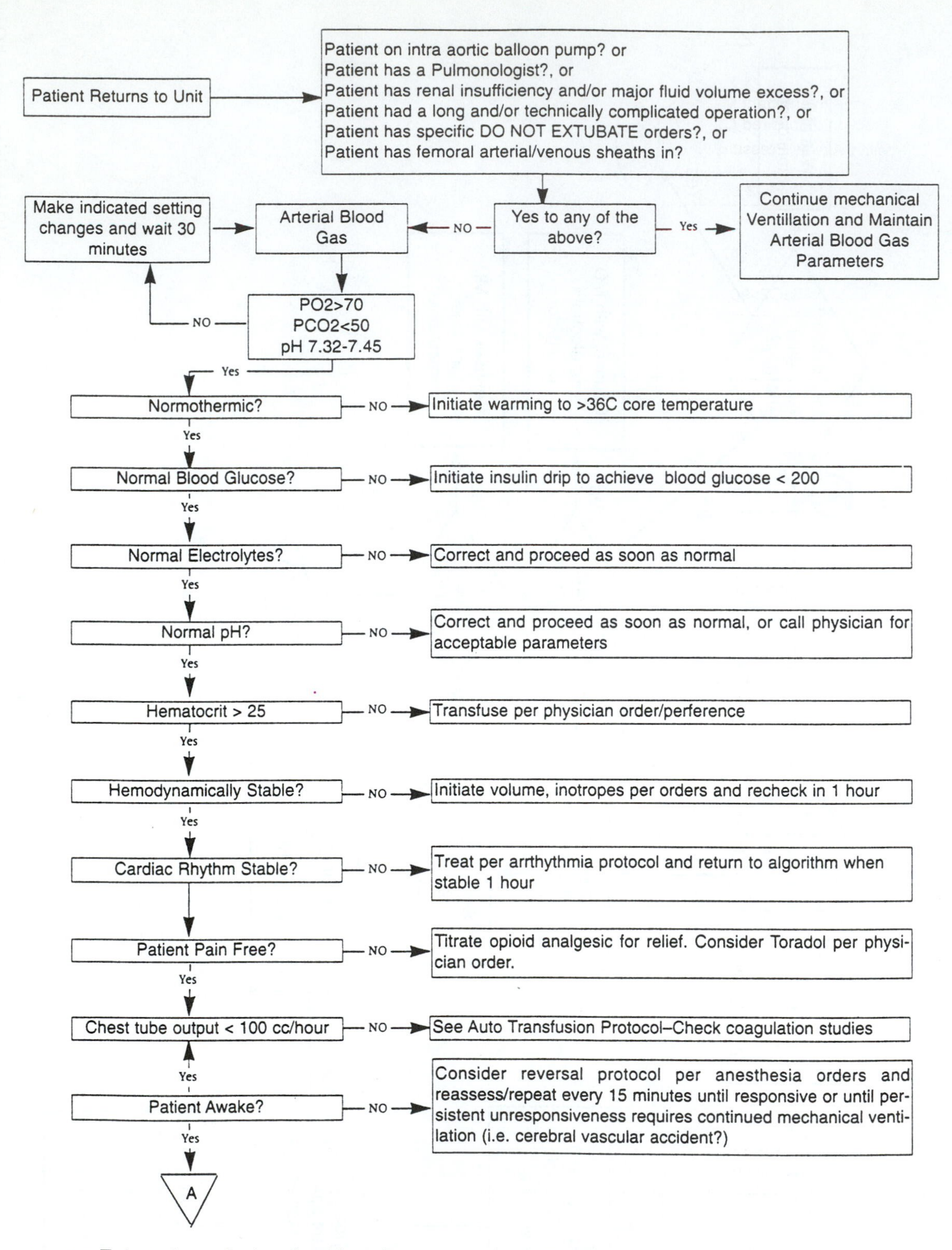

FIGURE E-8. Early extubation algorithm. (From *Heart Lung* 25(1):64, 1996.)

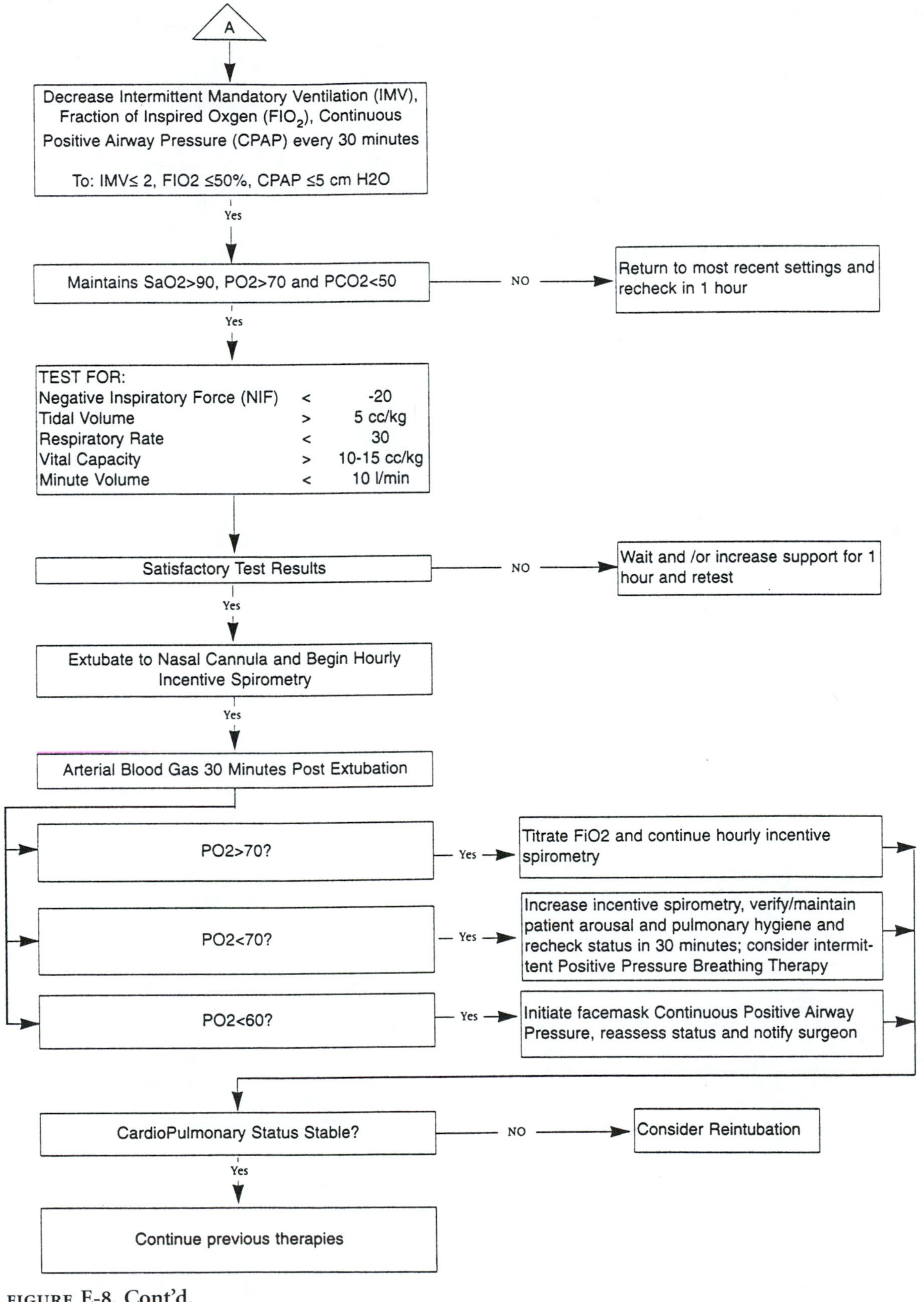

FIGURE E-8. Cont'd.

Index

A

A cell, glucagon and, 981
Aδ nerve fiber, 170-171
A wave, intracranial pressure, 825-826
Abandonment, 38
Abciximab, 554
ABCs; *see* Life support
Abdomen
  auscultation of, 933-934
  cardiovascular assessment and, 365
  common disorders of, 941-942
  palpation of, 935
  percussion of, 868-869, 934-935
  trauma to, 1079-1083
    in pregnancy, 265-266
Abdominal compartment syndrome, 1081
Abdominal distention, 1011
Abdominojugular reflux, 359-360
Abducens nerve, 745
  eye movement and, 770
Ablation, radiofrequency catheter, 414, 420
Abruptio placentae, 258
  trauma causing, 266
Abscess
  brain
    coma and, 791-792
    missile injury and, 1062
  cricoid, 697
Absent breath sounds, 632, 634
Absorption
  bowel resection and, 147
  colon and, 926
  drug, 281
  gastrointestinal, 924
  of lipids, 123
Absorption atelectasis, 692
Abstract thinking, 76
Abuse, elderly, 288-289
Acalculous cholecystitis, 1128-1129
Acarbose, 1005
Accelerated graft atherosclerosis, 1184
Accelerated idioventricular rhythm, 420
Accelerated junctional rhythm, 415
Acceleration injury, 1057
  thoracic, 1073
Accessory muscles
  age-related changes in, 277
  asthma and, 215
  of child, 206
  definition of, 604
Accessory nerve, spinal, 746
Accessory organs of digestion, 926-930
Accessory pathway, 335, 422
Accident; *see* Cerebrovascular accident; Vehicular accident
Acetaminophen, 227
Acetohexamide, 1004
Acetylcholine
  age-related changes in, 286
  neuromuscular blocking agent and, 304
Acetylcysteine, 714
Acid, aspiration lung disorder and, 667
Acid-base balance
  age-related changes in, 280
  electrical burn and, 1151
  ketoacidosis and, 1007
  kidney and, 855-856
  renal failure and, 886
Acid-base management, 10, 11
Acidemia, ketoacidosis; *see* Ketoacidosis
Acidosis
  blood gas assessment in, 644
  calcium and, 862
  cardiopulmonary arrest in child and, 224
  cerebral blood flow and, 821
  electrical burn and, 1151
  ketoacidosis and; *see* Ketoacidosis
  lactic, status asthmaticus and, 672
  obstructive sleep apnea and, 111
  respiratory failure and, 658
  thyrotoxic crisis and, 1033
Acinar cell of pancreas, 929
Acquired immunodeficiency syndrome
  blood shield statutes and, 516
  nutrition and, 152-155
  spiritual well-being and, 82
Actin filament, 342
Action potential, cardiac, 344-345
Activated coagulation time, 383
Activated partial thromboplastin time, 383
Active transport, 854
  fluid balance and, 858
  placental membranes and, 244
Activity
  cardiopulmonary dysfunction and, 596-597
  craniotomy and, 818
  deep vein thrombosis and, 522
  thoracic surgery and, 681
Acute renal failure, 877-878; *see also* Renal failure
Acute respiratory distress syndrome, 660-663
  flail chest and, 1074
  multiple organ dysfunction syndrome and, 1130
  oxygenation and, 1134
  pulmonary artery catheter and, 459
  shock and, 1098
Acute versus chronic heart failure, 503
Acyanotic heart defect, 219
Acyclovir
  nutrition-related effects of, 154
  renal failure and, 908
Adaptation
  to illness, 50-51, 52
  to stress, 65
Addiction, fear of, 179-180
Adenohypophysis, 982-983
Adenosine
  cardiovascular effects of, 576
  dosage and side effects of, 578
  echocardiography and, 436
Adenosine—cont'd
  multiple organ dysfunction syndrome and, 1135
Adenosine triphosphate
  active transport and, 854
  tubular necrosis and, 878-879
Adjunctive agent, opioid, 304
Administrative law, 38
Admission guidelines in critical care, 26
Adolescent, 235
Adrenal gland, stress response of, 1002
Adrenalin; *see* Epinephrine
Adrenergic system, heart failure and, 504
Adrenocorticotropic hormone, 748
  physiologic stress and, 124
  shock and, 1097
  sleep and, 106
Adult learning theory, 50
Adult respiratory distress syndrome, 660-663
  pregnancy and, 260
Advance directives, 44-46
Advanced life support
  cardiac
    guidelines for, C-1 to C-12
    in pregnancy, 254-255
  trauma, 1052-1056
Adventitia, 338
Adventitious breath sounds, 632
Advocate, nurse as, 28, 65-66
Aerosol mask, 691
Aerosol therapy, 699
Affect, 75
Afferent nerve fiber, 170-171, 733
Afterload, 350
  cardiac surgery and, 546-547
  heart failure and, 505, 506
  nursing management and, 591-592
  pulmonary artery pressure and, 462, 464
Age
  burn injury and, 1146
  coronary artery disease and, 483
  infarct, 402-403
  sleep changes and, 106-107
Aging, 271-292; *see also* Elderly patient
Agitation
  definition of, 188
  differential diagnosis of, 190
Agnosia, 809-810
Air embolism
  delayed arousal from anesthesia and, 321
  hemodynamic monitoring and, 452-453, 455-456
  parenteral nutrition and, 163
Air leak disorder, 673-677
Air passage, collateral, 608-609
Air-entrainment mask, 691
Airway
  anatomy of, 607-610
  artificial, 692-703
    endotracheal tube for, 693-695

Airway—cont'd
artificial—cont'd
nasopharyngeal, 692-693
oropharyngeal, 692-693
burn injury and, 1147, 1153-1154
conduction, 604-606
facial injury and, 1072
ineffective clearance of, 722-723
inhalation injury and, 1149-1150
neurologic disorder and, 772
obstructive sleep apnea and, 111
oxygen toxicity and, 692
in primary survey of trauma patient, 1052
spinal injury and, 1067, 1070
trauma in pregnancy and, 263
Airway management
in child, 207
with endotracheal or tracheostomy tube, 695, 699-703
Airway obstruction
in postanesthesia period, 312
respiratory syncytial virus and, 213
Airway pressure, continuous positive, 707
Akinetic mutism, 797
Alanine aminotransferase
cardiovascular alteration and, 381
values for, 937
Alarm, ventilator, 712
Albumin
calcium and, 861
liver and, 928
renal failure and, 882, 883, 884
renal function and, 873
Albuterol, 714
Alcohol
coma and, 792
pancreatitis and, 951
Aldactone, 905
Aldosterone, 1029
Algorithm
for atrial fibrillation, 16
definition of, 14-15
sedation, 190, 191-192
Alkali burn, 1150
Alkaline phosphatase, 937
Alkalosis
blood gas assessment in, 644
calcium and, 862
cerebral blood flow and, 821
respiratory, septic shock and, 1114
Allen test, 362, 445-446
Allergic reaction
anaphylactic, 1105-1109
to streptokinase, 562, 563
Allocation of resources, 25-26
Allograft for burn wound, 1162-1163
Alpha-adrenergic antagonist
characteristics of, 581-582
thyrotoxic crisis and, 1035
Alpha glucose inhibitors, 1005
Aluminum, 139
Alveolar cell, 692
Alveolar dead space, 619
Alveolar hypoventilation, 655, 726
sleep apnea and, 113-114
Alveolar macrophage, 610
Alveolar partial pressure, 298
Alveolar-arterial gradient, 646
Alveolar-capillary membrane, 611
Alveolar-capillary membrane—cont'd
diffusion and, 618
respiratory failure and, 656
Alveolus
age-related changes in, 278-279
anatomy of, 607-610
distended, 637
of infant, 206
in respiratory distress syndrome, 660
rupture of, 674
Ambulatory electrocardiography, 427-429
American Association of Critical Care Nurses
case management and, 67
definition of nursing practice of, 35
position statement of, 27
American Association of Pediatric Nurse Practitioners, 36
American Burn Association classification, 1143
American College of Critical Care Medicine, 194
American College of Obstetricians, 255-256
American Diabetes Association, 151
American Dietetic Association, 151
American Nurses Association, code of ethics of, 26
American Society of Anesthesiologists, 297, 298
Amikacin, 906
Amino acid
enteral nutrition and, 155
liver failure and, 143, 145, 147
metabolism of, 122
parenteral nutrition and, 161-162
in parenteral nutrition formula for child, 231
renal alterations and, 140
renal failure and, 143
Aminophylline
mechanical ventilation and, 715
for renal disorder, 905
Amiodarone, 576, 578
for supraventricular tachycardia, 414
Amitriptyline, 183
Amniotic fluid embolism, 261-262
Amobarbital, 108
Amphogen, 905
Amphotericin B
nutrition-related effects of, 154
renal failure and, 908
Ampicillin, 906
Amrinone, 579
Amylase
pancreatic function and, 937
pancreatitis and, 952
Anabolism
definition of, 980
insulin and, 979-980
Analgesic, 180-185
chest pain and, 489
myocardial infarction and, 499
nonopioid, 181
opioid; *see* Opioid
renal failure and, 909
sleep and, 108
thoracic surgery and, 681
Anaphylactic shock, 1105-1109
Anastomosis
arteriovenous fistula and, 887
pancreas transplant and, 1206
Anatomic shunt, bronchial, 612
Anemia, renal failure and, 886
Anesthesia, 297-326
agents for, 298-303
assessment preceding, 297-308
complications of, 312-326
cardiovascular, 315-317
nausea and vomiting as, 323-324
neurologic, 321-323
respiratory, 312-315
thermoregulatory, 317-321, 325-326
general, 297-304
intraspinal
characteristics of, 182
nursing interventions for, 186
intrathecal, 182, 184
neurologic disorder and, 835
neuromuscular blocking agent with, 303-304
postanesthesia care and, 308-312
stages of, 297-298
status asthmaticus and, 673
Aneurysm
aortic, 514-517
cerebral
subarachnoid hemorrhage and, 802, 803
surgery for, 805-806
ventricular, myocardial infarction and, 497
Anger of parents, 236-237
Angina
cardiac catheterization and, 439-440
catheter-related intervention and, 559
characteristics of, 488
patient education about, 491
types of, 486-487
Angiography
cerebral, 781-782
gastrointestinal disorder and, 936-937
in neurologic assessment, 782
Angioplasty
laser, 557
percutaneous transluminal coronary, 553-555
ST-segment monitoring and, 399-401
transluminal cerebral, 807
Angiotensin II, 855
Angiotensin-converting enzyme inhibitor
characteristics of, 580-582
elderly patient and, 283
heart failure and, 505
hypertensive crisis and, 524
renal failure and, 908
Anion, fluid balance and, 857
Anion gap, 645
renal function and, 872-873
Anisocoria, 769
Anistreplase, 565-566
Antacid, 971
Antagonist
alpha-adrenergic
characteristics of, 581-582
thyrotoxic crisis and, 1034
benzodiazepine, 300
H_2-receptor
dosage and actions of, 971
gastrointestinal disorder and, 970
renal failure and, 909
to interleukins, 1137-1138
neuromuscular blocking agent, 304, 307
opioid; *see* Naloxone
for sedative, 195
Anterior cerebral artery, 753

Anterior cerebral circulation, 753-754
Anterior cord syndrome, 1066
Anterior pituitary gland, 748, 982-983
Anterior wall myocardial infarction, 493, 494
Anterolateral myocardial infarction, 493
Anteroposterior diameter, 628
Anteroseptal myocardial infarction, 493
Anthropomorphic measurement, 125
  in evaluation of nutrition support, 165
Antibiotic
  for AIDS, 154
  for burn wound, 1160
  endocarditis and, 510
  liver failure and, 964
  meningitis in child and, 227
  pneumonia and, 666
  refusal of, for elderly patient, 288
  renal failure and, 906-907
Antibody
  heart transplant and, 1183-1184
  transplant rejection and, 1177-1178
Antibody-antigen response, 1105-1109
Anticholinergic agent
  mechanical ventilation and, 715
  respiratory failure and, 658
Anticipatory grief, 81
Anticoagulation
  deep vein thrombosis and, 522, 523
  heart failure and, 506
  in hemodialysis, 891
  ischemic stroke and, 836
  myocardial infarction and, 499
  pulmonary embolism and, 670
  in slow continuous ultrafiltration, 897
  ventricular assist device and, 573
Anticonvulsant agent, 226
  neurologic disorder and, 835
  pregnancy and, 266
  renal failure and, 909
Anticytokine therapy, 1137-1138
Antidiuretic hormone
  aging and, 276
  diabetes insipidus and; *see* Diabetes insipidus
  factors affecting, 985
  fluid and, 859, 1048-1049
  function of, 983
  hyperglycemic hyperosmolar nonketotic syndrome and, 1016
  hypersecretion of, 1027-1031
  hyposecretion of, 1021-1027
  inappropriate secretion of, 1027-1031
    craniotomy and, 816
    etiology of, 978-979
    patient history of, 993
  physiologic stress and, 124
  pituitary assessment and, 993-994
  recognition of disorder of, 989
  renal system and, 852
  shock and, 1097
  water intake and, 748
Antidysrhythmic drug
  classes of, 575-577
  premature ventricular contraction and, 418
  renal failure and, 909
  shock and, 1099
Antifibrinolytic agent, 806
Antifungal agent
  HIV infection and, 154
Antifungal agent—cont'd
  renal failure and, 908
Antigen, human leukocyte, 1171-1172
Antihypertensive agent
  cerebrovascular accident and, 801
  intracranial hemorrhage and, 808
  intracranial hypertension and, 829-830
  pregnancy and, 258
Antiplatelet therapy, 836
Antiprotozoal agent, 154
Antishock garment, 1085
Antithymocyte agent, 1177-1178
Antithyroid drug, 1035
Antiviral drug
  nutrition-related effects of, 154
  renal failure and, 908
Anuria
  multiple organ dysfunction syndrome and, 1130
  tubular necrosis and, 879
Anxiety
  in child, 234-235
  coronary artery disease and, 485, 489
  definition of, 188
  emergence delirium and, 322
  nursing management plan for, 99-100
  in parents of ill child, 236
  pathophysiology of, 188-190
  sedation for, 188-195; *see also* Sedation
  status asthmaticus in child and, 214
Aorta
  atherosclerosis of, 514-517
  coarctation of, 253
  Marfan's syndrome and, 253
Aortic dissection, 515-517
Aortic stenosis, 252, 511, 512
Aortic valve
  anatomy of, 334
  regurgitation and, 511-513
  surgery on, 542-543
Aphasia
  cerebrovascular accident and, 810-811
  nursing management of, 844-845
Apical impulse, 360, 364
Apnea
  in child, 206, 214-216
    seizures and, 225-226
  sleep
    central, 113-114
    obstructive, 110-113
Apparent life-threatening event, 214-215
Appendicitis, 941
Apraxia, 810
Aqueduct of Sylvius, 738
Arachidonic acid metabolite, 1127
Arachnoid membrane, 738, 756, 758
ARDS, 660-663
Arginine, 155
Aromatic amino acid, 143, 145
Arousal
  assessment of, 763
  persistent vegetative state and, 795-798
  postanesthesia, 321
Arrhythmia; *see* Dysrhythmia
Arterial blood gases; *see* Blood gases
Arterial perfusion, decreased, 448
Arterial pressure
  mean; *see* Mean arterial pressure
Arterial pressure—cont'd
  partial
    carbon dioxide; *see also* Carbon dioxide, partial pressure of
    inhalation anesthetics and, 298
    oxygen; *see also* Oxygen, partial pressure of
Arterial pressure waveform, 446-447
Arterial pulse
  auscultation of, 362
  peripheral vascular disease and, 519
Arterial system, 337-338
Arteriography, coronary, 438-440
Arteriojugular oxygen difference, 823
Arteriole, 338
Arteriosclerosis, 276
  diabetes and, 151
Arteriovenous fistula, 887
Arteriovenous graft, 887-888
Arteriovenous hemodialysis, continuous, 897-898
Arteriovenous hemofiltration, 897
  protein and, 140
Arteriovenous malformation
  subarachnoid hemorrhage and, 802, 803-804
  surgery for, 806
Arteriovenous shunt, 887
Artery
  angiography and; *see* Angiography
  carotid, 519-521
  celiac, 921
  cerebral, 753-754, 755
    arteriovenous malformation and, 803-804
  of colon, 925
  coronary, 336
    bypass surgery on, 541-542
    disease of, 483-490
  femoral, gastrointestinal angiography and, 938
  gastroduodenal, 923
  gastroepiploic, 542
  intraarterial blood pressure monitoring and, 444-445
  of liver, 926
  pancreatic, 929
  peripheral vascular disease and, 517-519
  pulmonary; *see* Pulmonary artery *entries*
  renal, 849-850
  spinal, 761, 762
  tracheoinnominate fistula and, 699
Artifact, pacing, 536-538
Artificial airway, 692-703; *see also* Airway, artificial
Ascending pain pathway, 171-172
Ascites, 868-869
Aspartate aminotransferase
  cardiovascular alteration and, 381
  values for, 937
Asphalt burn, 1150
Aspiration
  enteral nutrition and, 160
  nasogastric tube and, 706
  of pneumothorax, 675
  in postanesthesia period, 314
  prevention of, 668
  risk for, 727
  spinal injury and, 1071
  tube feeding and, 156
Aspiration lung disorder, 667-668
Aspiration pneumonia, 665

Aspirin
coronary stent and, 557
ischemic stroke and, 836
myocardial infarction and, 499
neurologic disorder and, 835
thyrotoxicosis and, 1033
Assault, 36-37
Assessment
of abdominal trauma, 1079-1080
of anaphylaxis, 1106-1107
of asthma, 215, 635
cardiovascular, 355-374, 377-383; *see also* Cardiovascular system, assessment of
coping, 80
of facial injury, 1072-1073
of genitourinary injury, 1083
of head injury, 1063-1064
of intracranial pressure, 821-826
neurologic, 763-777; *see also* Neurologic assessment
in nursing process, 4-5
nutritional status, 124-128
orthopedic injury and, 1087
pain, 176-177
in patient teaching, 50
perianesthesia, 304-308
pulmonary, 625-639; *see also* Respiratory alteration, assessment of
renal, 865-876
in renal failure, 879-886
of septic shock, 1113-1114
spinal injury, 1066-1068
Assist-control ventilation, 707
Association of Operating Room Nurses, 36
Associative area of temporal lobe, 752
Asterixis, 964
Asthma
assessment of, 215, 635
in child, 213-214
pregnancy and, 260
Astroglia, 735
Asymmetry of chest movement, 629
Asynchrony
patient-ventilator, 706
ventilator-patient, in child, 210-211
Asystole, in child, 224
Atelectasis
absorption, 692
assessment findings in, 636
oxygen toxicity and, 692
thoracic surgery and, 680
Atenolol, 908
Atherectomy, directional coronary, 555
Atherosclerosis, 336
accelerated graft, 1184-1185
aortic, 514-517
atherectomy for, 555
myocardial infarction and, 490-491
peripheral vascular disease and, 518
Atovaquone, 154
Atrial catheter, left, 386
Atrial contraction, premature, 409-410
Atrial dysrhythmia, 409-414; *see also* Atrium
fibrillation as, algorithm for, 16
myocardial infarction and, 496
Atrial electrocardiogram, 530
Atrial fibrillation, 412, 413-414
Atrial flutter, 411-412
multifocal tachycardia, 411, 412
Atrial kick, 348
Atrial natriuretic factor, 352-353
Atrial natriuretic peptide, 859-860
Atrial pacing wire, 531
Atrial pressure, left, 447
Atrial pressure monitoring, left, 456-457
Atrial refractory period on pacemaker, 535-536
Atrial septal defect, 252
Atrial waveform, right, 465-466
Atrioventricular block, 424-427
Atrioventricular control on pacemaker, 534-535
Atrioventricular heart block, 497
Atrioventricular node, 334-335
atrial flutter and, 412
cardiac surgery and, 549
conduction disturbance and, 424-427
drugs affecting, 578
effects of, 576
premature atrial contraction and, 409
Atrioventricular synchrony, 533
Atrioventricular valve, 333-334
Atrium
anatomy of, 332-333
drugs affecting, 578
right, pulmonary artery pressure and, 465
tricuspid valve stenosis and, 513
Atrophy, 518-519
Atropine
echocardiography and, 436
as neuromuscular blocking agent antagonist, 307
Auditory area of temporal lobe, 752
Auscultation
in cardiovascular assessment, 365-372
in gastrointestinal assessment, 933-934
landmarks for, 361
pancreatitis and, 952
in pulmonary assessment of, 632-633
renal function and, 867-868
Authorization for treatment, 42-43
Autograft for burn injury, 1159-1160, 1161-1162
Autonomic dysreflexia, 1066, 1068
Autonomic nervous system, 733
renal system and, 852
responses of, 748
Autonomy as ethical principle, 20-21
Autoregulation of cerebral blood flow, 821-822
Autotransfusion
cardiac surgery and, 547, 548
fetal, 249-250
hypovolemic shock and, 1101
Awareness, 763-764
in mental status examination, 75
persistent vegetative state and, 795-798
Axial loading, 1065
Axion, 734
Axis
hypothalamus-pituitary-thyroid, 984, 986
phlebostatic, 444
ventricular, 395-396
Axonal injury, diffuse, 1062-1063
Azathioprine
rejection and, 1183
transplant and, 1176, 1177
Azotemia
intrarenal, 877-878
Azotemia—cont'd
postrenal, 878
prerenal, 877
AZT; *see* Zidovudine

B

B lymphocyte, 1172, 1173
B wave, intracranial pressure, 826
Babinski reflex, 768-769
Bacitracin, for burn wound, 1161
Backward heart failure, 503
Bacteremia, endocarditis and, 509
Bacteria, urinary, 874
Bacterial endocarditis in child, 222-223
Bacterial infection; *see* Infection
Bacterial translocation, 155, 1128
Bainbridge reflex, 352
Baker tube, 966
Balloon, intraaortic, 567-571
Balloon angioplasty, 553-555
Balloon pump, intraaortic, chest x-ray and, 386-387
Balloon tamponade tube, esophagogastric, 966-968
Balloon valvuloplasty, 561
Band ligation, endoscopic variceal, 968
Bandage, tubular support, 1166-1167
Barbiturate
anesthesia with, 302
cardiac effects of, 315-316
delirium and, 76-77
intracranial hypertension and, 832
neurologic disorder and, 835
renal failure and, 909
sleep and, 108
Baroreceptor
age-related changes in, 274-275
heartbeat and, 352
Barotrauma
mechanical ventilation and, 706
pneumothorax and, 674, 675
Barrier
blood-brain, 739-740
to infection, in gastrointestinal system, 155
Basal ganglia, 749
Base excess or deficit, 645
Baseline distortion in electrocardiography, 391-392
Basement membrane, glomerular, 851
Basic life support, 254
Basilar artery, 754
Basilar skull fracture, 1059
Basophil, 1175
Battery, 37
Battery of pacemaker, 539
Battle's sign, 1059
Beck's triad, 1078
Beclomethasone, 715
Bedside hemodynamic monitoring, 442-444
Bedside monitoring
cerebral blood flow, 786
electrocardiographic, 397, 399
of mechanical ventilation, 709
pulmonary, 653-654
Bedside pulmonary function testing, 648-649
Behavior
hypothalamus and, 748

Behavior—cont'd
  in mental status examination, 75
  pain, 172, 174, 177
    in child, 233
Beneficence, 21-22
Benzodiazepine
  anesthesia with, 303
  characteristics of, 581
  sedation with, 193, 194
  sleep and, 108
Benzodiazepine antagonist, 300
Berkow method of estimating burn injury, 1143-1144
Best interests standard, 43
Beta-adrenergic agonist
  mechanical ventilation and, 714
  respiratory failure and, 658
  status asthmaticus and, 673
Beta-adrenergic blocking agent
  characteristics of, 575
  hypertensive crisis and, 524
  myocardial infarction and, 499-500
  renal failure and, 908
  thyrotoxic crisis and, 1035, 1037
Beta-endorphin, 174
Bicarbonate
  acid-base balance and, 642, 643
  cardiopulmonary arrest in child and, 224
  fetal effects of, 254-255
  ketoacidosis and, 1007, 1011
  kidney and, 856
  myoglobinuria and, 1090
  renal system and, 863
  shock and, 1099
  thyrotoxic crisis and, 1036
Bifascicular block, 405-406
Bigeminy, 417
Bilateral lung transplant, 1188-1189
Bile
  function of, 928-929
  pancreatitis and, 951
Bile salt
  function of, 928
  lipid metabolism and, 122
  nutrition and, 143
Biliary disorder, pancreatitis and, 951
Biliary stone, 941
Biliary system
  anatomy and physiology of, 928-929
  multiple organ dysfunction syndrome and, 1128-1130
Bilirubin
  function of, 928
  laboratory values for, 937
Biochemical data in nutritional assessment, 125
Biochemical mediator, inflammatory, 1126
Biologic skin substitute, 1162-1164
Bioprosthesis, cardiac valve, 543, 545
Biopsy
  liver, 939
  renal, 876
  synthetic skin and, 1163-1164
Biosynthetic dressing, 1165
Bipolar lead, pacemaker, 530
Bitolterol, 714
Biventricular assist device, 571
Bjork-Shiley prosthetic valve, 544
Bladder
  anatomy of, 849
  injury of, 1084
  innervation of, 852
Blade, endotracheal tube, 694
Bleeding
  angioplasty and, 555
  antidiuretic hormone and, 983
  cardiac surgery and, 547
  cerebrovascular accident and, 801, 809
  classification of blood loss from, 948
  continuous renal replacement therapy and, 900
  craniotomy and, 816
  disseminated intravascular coagulation and, 1133
  gastrointestinal, 945-950
    angiography and, 938
    description of, 945
    diagnosis of, 948
    etiology of, 945-946
    management of, 948-950
    pathophysiology of, 946-947
    renal failure and, 886
  heart-lung transplant and, 1185-1186
  hematoma and
    angioplasty and, 555
    epidural, 738, 1060
    head injury causing, 1060-1062
  hemodynamic monitoring and, 452
  hemothorax and, 1077
  intracranial, 807-808
    delayed arousal from anesthesia and, 321
    in pregnancy, 267
  in labor and delivery, 250-251
  liver failure and, 964
  liver injury and, 1082
  multiple organ dysfunction syndrome and, 1130-1131, 1132, 1133
  pelvic fracture and, 1085
  pulmonary embolism and, 671
  renal system and, 866
  subarachnoid hemorrhage and, 802-807
  thoracic surgery and, 679
  tracheostomy tube and, 698
Blink reflex, coma and, 794
Block
  atrioventricular, 424-427
  bifascicular, 405-406
Blood
  abdominal injury and, 1080
  bronchial circulation and, 612
  cardiac tamponade and, 1078
  hemodialysis and, 890-893
  liver and, digestion and, 926-927
  lumbar puncture and, 787-788
  peritoneal dialysis and, 904
  pituitary assessment and, 994
  renal clearance and, 854
  in urine, 875
Blood cell
  burn injury and, 1158
  chloride and, 863
  HELLP syndrome in pregnancy and, 256
  kidney and, 855
  myxedema and, 1040
  in postanesthesia period, 310
  renal failure and, anemia and, 886
  septic shock and, 1114
Blood cell—cont'd
  urine and, 874
Blood cells, cardiovascular alteration and, 382
Blood flow
  blood pressure and, 338-339
  cephalization of, 388
  cerebral
    age-related changes in, 286
    assessment of, 784-786
    cerebrovascular accident and, 801
    in child, 224-225
    intracranial pressure and, 821-822
  congenital heart defect and, 219
  decreased, 595-596
  inhalation anesthetics and, 298-299
  placental, 244-245
  trauma in pregnancy and, 263
  uterine, 247
Blood gases; *see also* Carbon dioxide, partial pressure of; Oxygen; partial pressure of
  hypovolemic shock and, 1100-1101
  procedure for, 641-644
  pulmonary edema and, 504
  respiratory distress syndrome and, 662
Blood pressure
  age-related changes in, 274-275
  autonomic dysreflexia and, 1066
  blood flow and, 338-339
  burn injury and, 1154
  cardiovascular assessment and, 366
  cerebrovascular accident and, 801
  in child, 218
  intraarterial, 444-450
    troubleshooting for, 452-454
  intracranial hypertension and, 829-830
  kidney and, 855
  measurement of, 341
  in perianesthesia assessment, 306
  pituitary assessment and, 992
  pregnancy and, 247
  rebleeding after subarachnoid hemorrhage, 804-805
  renal function and, 867-868
  septic shock and, 1113-1114
  spinal shock and, 1066
  trauma and, 1053
Blood shield statute, 516
Blood supply
  coronary, 336
  dura mater and, 737-738
  pulmonary, 610-612
Blood transfusion, blood shield statutes and, 516
Blood urea nitrogen
  azotemia and, 877
  cardiovascular alteration and, 381
  renal failure and, 880
  renal function and, 872
Blood volume
  burn injury and, 1154-1156
  in child, 221
  facial injury and, 1072-1073
  hyperglycemic hyperosmolar nonketotic syndrome and, 1016
  pregnancy and, 247
  renal system and, 866-867
  septic shock and, 1112
  shock and, 1097-1119; *see also* Shock
  trauma and, 1053

Blood-brain barrier, 739-740
inhalation anesthetics and, 298-299
osmotic diuretic and, 831
Blown pupil, 1064
Blunt trauma, 1051
abdominal, 1079
cardiac, 1078-1079
pelvic, 1084
thoracic, 1073
Body image disturbance, 68-69
nursing management plan for, 87-88
Body mass index, 125, 126
Body surface area, 1143
Body systems, 5
Body temperature; *see* Temperature
Body water, in child, 229
Body weight; *see* Weight
Bolt, subarachnoid, 823, 824
Bone
age-related changes in, 289
calcium and, 861
chest radiography and, 650
cranial, 737
fracture of, 994-995
facial, 1072
spinal, 755
Bone marrow transplantation, 83
Bowel, short, 147
Bowel elimination; *see also* Colon; Intestine; Small intestine
antidiuretic hormone and, 1031
myxedema and, 1040, 1042
spinal injury and, 1071
Bowel motility, 165
Bowel sounds
in gastrointestinal assessment, 933-934
intestinal obstruction and, 960
Bowman's capsule, 851
Brachial artery, 781
Bradycardia
calcium and, 380
in child, 222, 224
pacemaker for, 529; *see also* Pacemaker, cardiac
postanesthesia period and, 316
sinus, 408
nursing management and, 593
spinal injury and, 1070
Bradykinin
inflammation and, 1122
pain and, 176
Brain; *see also* Head injury
age-related changes in, 282, 285
anatomy of, 736-754
basal ganglia and, 749
brainstem and, 740
cerebellum and, 741, 743, 746
cerebrum and, 749-753
circulation of, 753-754, 755
cranial nerves and, 742-746
diencephalon and, 746-749
protective mechanisms of, 737-740
reticular formation and, 741
contusion of, 1060
diffuse axonal injury to, 1063
intracranial pressure and; *see* Intracranial pressure
missile injury of, 1062
persistent vegetative state and, 795-796
Brain—cont'd
protective mechanisms of, 737-740
radiography of, 779-784
Brain abscess
coma and, 791-792
missile injury and, 1062
Brain death
characteristics of, 797
in child, 228
definition of, 798
as legal issue, 776
Brain tumor
coma and, 791-792
craniotomy and, 814-818
Brainstem
anatomy of, 740
cerebrovascular accident and, 802
lumbar puncture and, 788
oculovestibular reflex and, 770
ventilation regulation and, 616
Brainstem auditory evoked response, 787
Branch block, bundle
electrocardiography and, 403-404
Branched-chain amino acids, 147
Breach of duty, 38-39
Breath sounds
asthma and, 215
conditions with, 634
normal and abnormal, 632
pneumonia and, 665, 666
Breathing
burn injury and, 1154
ineffective, 723-724
in infant, 205
in primary survey of trauma patient, 1052-1053
sleep apnea and, 110-114
spinal injury and, 1067, 1071
trauma in pregnancy and, 263
work of, 613-614
Breathing mechanics, bedside measurement of, 648
Breathlessness, heart failure and, 506
Bretylium
dosage and side effects of, 578
fetal effects of, 254
Broca's aphasia, 811
Broca's area, 752
cerebrovascular accident and, 810
Bromsulphalein, liver function and, 937
Bronchial sounds, 632, 633, 634
Bronchial tree, 605-606
Bronchiectasis, 636
Bronchiole
anatomy of, 606
electron micrograph of, 608
respiratory, 607
Bronchiolitis in child, 212-213
Bronchitis, 637
Bronchoalveolar lavage, 668
Bronchoconstriction
anaphylaxis and, 1107
pulmonary embolism and, 669
receptors and, 618
in respiratory distress syndrome, 660-661
Bronchodilator
mechanical ventilation and, 713
respiratory failure and, 658
status asthmaticus and, 672
Bronchophony, 633
Bronchoplastic reconstruction, 678
Bronchoscopy, 647
aspiration lung disorder and, 668
burn injury and, 1150
Bronchospasm
assessment findings in, 635
postanesthesia, 313-314
Bronchovesicular breath sounds, 633
Bronchus
anatomy of, 605-606
circulation in, 612
inhalation injury of, 1150
Brown-Séquard syndrome, 1066
Bruising of brain, 1060
Bruit, 367
Bullet trauma, head, 1057
Bullet wound, 1051-1052
cardiac, 1077-1078
of head, 1062
Bundle branch, 336
Bundle branch block
definition of, 403
electrocardiography and, 403-404
Bundle of His, 336
Bupivacaine, 183
Burn
chemical, 1150-1151
classification of, 1142-1146
electrical, 1151
inhalation injury and, 1149-1150
management of
acute care phase of, 1158-1168
emergency, 1146-1149
rehabilitation phase of, 1168-1169
resuscitation phase of, 1152-1158
nonthermal, 1150-1151
nursing management plan for, 85-100
pathophysiology of, 1142
self-esteem and, 70
skin functions and, 1141
stressors of nursing patient with, 1169-1170
Burn center referral, 1149
Butorphanol, 183
Butyrophenone, 302-303
Buxem, 905
Bypass
cardiopulmonary, 543, 545
minimally invasive, 549-550
coronary artery, 541-542

C

C nerve fiber, 170-171
pain and, somatic, 176
C wave, intracranial pressure, 826
Ca^{2+}-ATPase pump, 272-273
Cachectin; *see* Tumor necrosis factor
Cachexia, cardiac, 129-130
Calcitonin, 984
Calcium
cardiac electrical activity and, 346, 348
cardiovascular alteration and, 378-380
gastrointestinal disorder and, 144
osteoporosis and, 289
renal failure and, 142, 881, 885
renal system and, 861-862
short bowel syndrome and, 149

Calcium channel blocker
  characteristics of, 576, 580, 581
  elderly patient and, 283
  hypertensive crisis and, 525
  myocardial infarction and, 499-500
  neurologic disorder and, 835
  renal failure and, 908
  thyrotoxicosis and, 1034
Calcium gluconate for burn, 1150
Calculus, biliary, 941
Caloric test, cold, 770, 773
Calories, 140, 143
Calorimetry, indirect, 126
Calyx, renal, 849
Canals of Lambert, 608-609
Cancer; *see* Malignancy
Cannon wave, 456
Cantor tube, 966
CaO_2, 643-644
Capacitance vessel, 340
Capillary
  alveolar-capillary membrane and, 611
  oxygen toxicity and, 692
  peritoneal dialysis and, 899-900
  renal, 850
  venous circulation of brain and, 754
Capillary leak in burn injury, 1154
Capillary membrane, in respiratory distress syndrome, 660
Capillary refill, 362
Capnography, 653
Capsule, Bowman's, 851
Captain of ship, doctrine of, 41
Captopril
  characteristics of, 581
  renal failure and, 908
Carbohydrate
  diabetes and, 151-152
  insulin/glucagon ratio and, 981
  renal disorder and, 140
Carbohydrate metabolism, 121
Carbon dioxide
  capnography and, 653
  extracorporeal removal of, 715-716
  gas transport and, 622
  intramucosal pH monitoring and, 969
  ketoacidosis and, 1007
  neurologic disorder and, 771
  partial pressure of, 616-617
    acid-base balance and, 642
    age-related changes in, 277, 279
    asthma and, 215
    chemoreceptors and, 616-617
    intracranial pressure and, 822
    maternal hypoxia and, 259
    postoperative shivering and, 317-318
    pregnancy and, 248
    respiratory distress syndrome and, 662
    respiratory syncytial virus and, 213
    septic shock and, 1114
  pulmonary embolism and, 670
  respiration and, 618
  retention of, 692
  shock and, 1099
    hypovolemic, 1100
  trauma patient and, 1059
Carbon monoxide poisoning, 1150, 1153
Carbonic acid, kidney and, 856
Carboxyhemoglobin, 622
  burn injury and, 1153
  carbon monoxide poisoning and, 1150
Carboxypeptidase, 929-930
Cardiac advanced life support
  guidelines for, C-1 to C-12
  in pregnancy, 254-255
Cardiac arrhythmia suppression test, 419
Cardiac catheterization
  bleeding after, 434
  chest pain, 439-440
Cardiac contractility; *see* Contractility, cardiac
Cardiac cycle, 348, 349
Cardiac fiber, 342
Cardiac glycoside, 577
  elderly patient and, 283
Cardiac index, 871
Cardiac output
  age-related changes in, 274
    exercise and, 275
  in child, 221
  definition of, 447
  exercise electrocardiography and, 429
  heart and vessels and, 348, 350-351
  labor and delivery and, 251
  multiple organ dysfunction syndrome and, 1130
  nursing diagnosis and management for, 590-594
  pregnancy and, 248, 249
    mitral stenosis and, 252
  pulmonary artery pressure and, 460, 468-469
  respiratory distress syndrome and, 663
  shock and, 1097, 1118
    cardiogenic, 1102, 1104
    hypovolemic, 1100
    neurogenic, 1110
    septic, 1113-1114
  sinus tachycardia and, 409
  spinal injury and, 1067-1068
  valvular disease and, 514
  venous oxygen saturation and, 474
  venous system and, 340, 342
  ventricular tachycardia and, 420
Cardiac sphincter, 920
Cardiac surgery, 541-550; *see also* Surgery, cardiac
Cardiac tamponade, 1181
Cardiac valve
  anatomy of, 333-334
  balloon valvuloplasty and, 561
  disease of, 252, 510-514
    clinical features of, 512-513
    description of, 510-511
    etiology of, 511, 513
    management of, 513-514
    in pregnancy, 252
  pulmonary artery pressure and, 462
  surgery on, 542-543, 544
Cardiac wall rupture, 498
Cardiogenic shock, 1102-1105
  in child, 223
  pregnancy and, 254
  pulmonary artery catheter and, 459
Cardiomyopathy
  etiology of, 507-508
  peripartum, 253
  surgery for, 549
  types of, 507
  ventricular ectopy and, 417
Cardiomyoplasty, 549
Cardioplegia, 547
Cardiopulmonary arrest, in child, 224
Cardiopulmonary bypass, 543-545
  lung transplant and, 1188-1189
  minimally invasive, 549-550
  physiologic effects of, 546
Cardiopulmonary decompensation, 792
Cardiopulmonary resuscitation
  cognitive function after, 372
  pregnancy and, 254-255
Cardiovascular alteration; *see also* Cardiovascular system; Heart
  anaphylactic shock and, 1108
  atherosclerosis of aorta and, 514-517
  cardiogenic shock and, 1102-1105
  cardiomyopathy and, 507-508
  carotid artery disease and, 519-521
  catheter-based interventions for, 552-561; *see also* Catheter-based cardiac intervention
  cerebrovascular accident and, 801
  in child, 219-224
  clinical findings in, 373-374
  coronary artery disease as; *see also* Coronary artery disease
  coronary heart disease as, 483-490
  deep vein thrombosis and, 521-523
  diagnosis of, 377-482; *see also* Cardiovascular diagnostic procedure
  drug therapy for, 574-582
    antidysrhythmic, 574-577
    inotropic, 577-579
    vasodilator, 579-582
  dysrhythmia as; *see* Dysrhythmia
  electrical burn and, 1151
  electrocardiography for; *see* Electrocardiography
  endocarditis and, 508-510
  heart failure and, 502-507
  heart transplantation and, 1179-1184
  heart-lung transplantation and, 1184-1188
  hypertensive crisis and, 523-525
  mechanical ventilation causing, 706
  multiple organ dysfunction syndrome and, 1129, 1130
  myocardial infarction as, 490-501; *see also* Myocardial infarction
  myxedema and, 1039, 1041
  nursing diagnosis and management of, 585-597
    contractility and, 592
    heart rate alterations and, 593-594
    invasive monitoring device and, 597
    low cardiac output and, 590-594
    mobility and, 597
    myocardial ischemia and, 594-595
    peripheral blood flow and, 595-596
    physical assessment and, 586-587
    surgery and, 587-590
  nutrition and, 126, 128-133
  obstructive sleep apnea and, 111
  pacemaker for, 529-541; *see also* Pacemaker
  peripheral vascular disease and, 517-519
  postanesthesia, 315-317
  in pregnancy, 251-254
  pulmonary embolism and, 669
  septic shock and, 1113-1114
  shock and, 1098
  spinal injury and, 1069-1070

Cardiovascular alteration—cont'd
  status asthmaticus and, 672
  sudden death and, 501-502
  surgery for, 541-550; *see also* Cardiac surgery
  thoracic surgery and, 679-680
  thyrotoxic crisis and, 1034, 1037
  trauma causing, 1077-1079
  valvular, 510-514
  weaning from mechanical ventilation and, 685
Cardiovascular diagnostic procedure, 377-480; *see also* Cardiovascular alteration, nursing diagnosis and management of
  bedside hemodynamic monitoring, 442-444
  cardiac catheterization, 438-440
  case study of, 464-471, 476-480
  central venous pressure monitoring, 451, 453-456
  chest radiography, 384-389
  echocardiography, 430-436
  electrocardiography, 389-430; *see also* Electrocardiography
  electrophysiologic, 440-441
  head-up–tilt table test, 441
  intraarterial blood pressure monitoring, 444-450
  laboratory assessment, 377-384
    chemistry studies, 381-382
    electrolytes, 377-381
    hematologic studies, 382-383
    lipid studies, 383-384
  left arterial pressure monitoring, 456-457
  magnetic resonance imaging, 436-438
  mixed venous oxygen saturation and, 471, 474-480
  pulmonary artery pressure, 458-464
  thallium scan, 438
  troubleshooting, 452-453
Cardiovascular system; *see also* Heart; *other Cardiovascular entries*
  age-related changes in, 272-276, 292
    examination for, 289-290
  anatomy of, 331-344
  assessment of, 355-374
    auscultation in, 365-372
    history in, 355
    inspection in, 355-360
    laboratory, 377-383
    palpation in, 360-365
    percussion in, 365
  of child, 216-219
  circulation and
    coronary, 336-337
    systemic, 337-342
  drugs affecting, 908
  of heart, 331-336
  heart transplant and, 1179-1184
  high-dose barbiturate therapy and, 832
  labor and delivery and, 250-251
  neurologic assessment and, 773
  in perianesthesia assessment, 306
  physiology of, 344-354
  in pregnancy, 247-248
  renal failure and, 882-883
  renal function and, 867
  respiratory failure and, 657
  septic shock and, 1115
  sleep and, 104-105
  status asthmaticus and, 672
  trauma in pregnancy and, 265
Cardioverter defibrillator; *see* Defibrillator, cardioverter
Care management, 12
Care management tools, 13-15
Carina, 605
Carotid artery
  cerebral circulation and, 753
  circle of Willis and, 754
Carotid artery bruit, 367
Carotid artery disease, 519-521
  education about, 522
Carotid pulse, 363
Case management, 12, 67
Cast, urinary, 874, 875
Catabolism
  definition of, 980
  insulin and, 981
Catecholamine
  inotropic drug and, 577
  postanesthesia period and, 316
Catheter
  cardiovascular intervention with; *see* Catheter-based cardiovascular intervention
  central venous, 451, 453-455; *see also* Central venous *entries*
  cerebral angiography and, 781-782
  chest radiography and, 385-386, 651-652
  for dialysis, 886-887
  hemodynamic monitoring in child, 218-219
  intraarterial blood pressure monitoring and, 444-445
  intracranial pressure monitoring and, 824
  left atrial, 456-457
  parenteral nutrition and, 159, 161-162
  peritoneal dialysis and, 902, 904
  pulmonary artery; *see* Pulmonary artery *entries*
  urinary
    burn injury and, 1156
    spinal injury and, 1071
Catheter ablation, radiofrequency, 414, 420
Catheter-based cardiac intervention, 552-561
  atherectomy as, 555
  coronary stent as, 557
  indications for, 552-553
  intraaortic balloon pump as, 567-571
  laser angioplasty as, 557
  nursing management of, 557, 559
  patient education about, 559-561
  percutaneous transluminal coronary angioplasty as, 553-555
Catheterization, cardiac, bed rest after, 434
Catheter-related sepsis, 163
Cation, 857
Causation, 38-39
Cause, proximate, 39
Caustic burn, 1150
Cecal volvulus, 941
Cecum, 925
Cefazolin, 906
Cefotaxime, 906
Cefotetan, 907
Cefoxitin, 906
Ceftriaxone, 906
Celiac artery, stomach and, 921
Cell
  acinar, 929
  alveolar epithelial, 607-610
  blood, urine and, 874
Cell—cont'd
  burn injury and, 1142
  cardiac, 342-343
  endothelial
    inflammation and, 1126
    multiple organ dysfunction syndrome and, 1135
  epithelial
    alveolar, 607-610
    burn injury and, 1158-1159
    gastric, 921-922
    in urine, 875
  immune system, 1172-1175
  inflammatory, 1125-1126
  Kupffer's, 1128
  mast, 1125
  neuroglial, 734
  neuron and, 733-734
  red blood
    alveolar-capillary membrane and, 611
    chloride and, 863
    kidney and, 855
  shock and, 1098
  in urine, 875
Cell membrane, cardiac, 342
Cell-mediated immunity, 286; *see also* Immune system
Cellular debris in tubular necrosis, 878
Central apnea in child, 214
Central chemoreceptor, ventilation and, 616-617
Central cord syndrome, 1066
Central cyanosis, 357
  pulmonary assessment and, 627-628
Central herniation, 833-834
Central nervous system; *see* Nervous system; Neurologic *entries*
Central sleep apnea, 113-114
Central venous catheter
  burn injury and, 1157
  chest x-ray and, 384-385
  parenteral nutrition via, 159, 161-162
  renal function and, 870
Central venous pressure, 451-456
  antidiuretic hormone and, 1031
  definition of, 447
  positioning for, 444
  renal failure and, 883
  renal transplant and, 1203
  thyrotoxic crisis and, 1037
Central venous thrombosis, parenteral nutrition and, 163
Centrifugal ventricular assist device, 572
Cephalization of blood flow, 388
Cephalosporin, 906
Cerebellum, 741, 743, 746
Cerebral abscess; *see also* Cerebrum
  coma and, 791-792
  missile injury and, 1062
Cerebral aneurysm
  subarachnoid hemorrhage and, 802, 803
  surgery for, 805-806
Cerebral angiography, 781-782
Cerebral aqueduct, 738
Cerebral artery, 753
  arteriovenous malformation and, 803-804
Cerebral blood flow
  age-related changes in, 286
  assessment of, 784-786

Cerebral blood flow—cont'd
cerebrovascular accident and, 801
in child, 224-225
intracranial pressure and, 821-822
Cerebral cortex
anatomy of, 749
ventilation regulation and, 616
Cerebral edema
cerebrovascular accident and, 801
craniotomy and, 817
liver failure and, 963-964
management of, 828
trauma patient and, 1059
Cerebral hemisphere, 802, 809-811
Cerebral hemorrhage, 807-808
delayed arousal from anesthesia and, 321
in pregnancy, 267
Cerebral perfusion pressure, 822
in child, 224-225
Cerebral resuscitation, 834, 836
Cerebral tissue perfusion, burn injury and, 1156
Cerebral vasodilation, 829-830
Cerebral vasospasm, 806-807
Cerebrospinal fluid
age-related changes in, 282
arachnoid membrane and, 756, 758
blood-brain barrier and, 739-740
craniotomy and, 816-817
facial injury and, 1072-1073
intracranial pressure and, 822, 830-831; *see also* Intracranial pressure
lumbar puncture and, 787-788
meningitis and, 226
skull fracture and, 1059
subarachnoid hemorrhage and, 807
ventricular system and, 738-739
Cerebrovascular accident
carotid artery disease and, 521
incidence of, 798
intracranial hemorrhage and, 807-808
ischemic stroke and, 800-802
management of, 808-811
subarachnoid hemorrhage and, 802-807
Cerebrum
age-related changes in, 282, 285
anatomy of, 749-753
circulation of, 753-755
Cervical spinal injury, 1069
Chamber, cardiac, 332-333
Chemical burn, 1146, 1150-1151
Chemical pneumonitis, 1153
Chemoreceptor
heartbeat and, 352
ventilation and, 616-617
Chemotactic factor inactivator, 1127
Chemotherapy for AIDS, 154
Chest; *see also* Thoracic *entries*
flail, 1074
of infant, 206
injury to, 1073-1079
Chest movement, 629
Chest pain
angina and, 486-487, 488
history of, 626
myocardial infarction and, 494, 496
oxygen toxicity and, 692
pulmonary embolism and, 670
relief of, 489
Chest physiotherapy; *see also* Pulmonary care
pulmonary contusion and, 1076
sputum studies and, 646
Chest radiography; *see* Radiography, chest
Chest tube
cardiac surgery and, 547
hemothorax and, 1077
pneumothorax and, 675, 676-677
thoracic surgery and, 681
Chest wall
burn injury and, 1154
cardiovascular assessment and, 363-364
injury to, 1074-1075
pulmonary assessment and, 628
Chest x-ray; *see* Radiography, chest
Child, 205-237
cardiovascular system of, 216-224
gastrointestinal system of, 229-230
malnutrition in, 125
nervous system of, 224-228
pain management in, 230-232
psychosocial issues of, 232-237
respiratory alteration in, 205-216; *see also* Respiratory alteration, in child
Chloral hydrate, 108
Chlordiazepoxide, 108
Chloride
renal failure and, 882
renal system and, 862-863
Chlorpropamide, 1004
Cholecystitis
acalculous, 1128-1129
findings in, 942
Cholecystokinin, 923, 928-929
Cholesterol
aging and, 276
bile and, 929
characteristics of, 383
coronary artery disease and, 484
patient teaching about, 130-131
renal disorder and, 141
Chordae tendineae, 333
Chorionic gonadotropin, human, 246
Chronic access for dialysis, 886-887
Chronic illness
psychosocial alterations with, 82-83
sleep changes with, 107
Chronic pancreatitis, 950-952, 957-958
Chronic subdural hematoma, 1061-1062
Chronic versus acute heart failure, 503
Chylomicron, 122-123
Chyme
colon and, 926
small intestine and, 923-924
Chymotrypsin, 929-930
Cigarette smoking, 484
Cimetidine
dosage and actions of, 971
renal failure and, 909
Cingulate herniation, 834
Ciprofloxacin, 906
Circadian desynchronization, 107
nursing management plan for, 119
Circadian rhythm, 105, 106
Circle of Willis, 754
Circulation; *see also* Blood *entries*; Cardiovascular *entries*
burn injury and, 1147, 1149
Circulation—cont'd
cerebral, 753-755
coronary, 336-337
inflammatory mediators in, 1121-1122
peripheral, 353-354
in primary survey of trauma patient, 1053
pulmonary, 611-612
spinal injury and, 1067-1068
systemic, 337-342
Circulatory assist device, mechanical, 567-574
intraaortic balloon pump as, 567-571
ventricular, 571-574
Cisternal puncture, 788
CK-MB values, 381
Classification, nursing intervention, 9
Claudication, intermittent, 518
Cleaning of burn wound, 1159
Clearance
airway, burn injury and, 1153-1154
renal, 853-854
Clindamycin, 906
Clinical pathway, 13-14
Clonus, 767
Closed tracheal suction system, 701-702
Closed wound care, 1160, 1165-1166
Closed-circuit television, 57
Closure of burn wound, 1162-1167
Clot, in catheter, 452
Clotting factor; *see also* Coagulation
disseminated intravascular coagulation and, 1131
inflammation and, 1123
liver and, 928
Clubbing of nailbed, 357
Coagulation
abdominal injury and, 1081
cardiovascular alteration and, 382-383
disseminated intravascular
multiple organ dysfunction syndrome and, 1130-1131, 1132, 1133
pregnancy and, 258-259
shock and, 1098
hemodynamic monitoring and, 452
inflammation and, 1122-1123
liver function tests and, 937
liver transplant and, 1196
Coarctation of aorta, pregnancy and, 253
Coarse ventricular fibrillation, 421
Code
of ethics, 26, 28
five-letter pacemaker, 532-533, 534
Codeine
dosage and action of, 183
for pain, 181
renal failure and, 909
Cognitive appraisal of stress, 65
Cognitive function; *see also* Mental status
after cardiopulmonary resuscitation, 372
age-related changes in, 282
examination for, 290-291
delirium and, 74-75
examination for, 75-76
nursing management of, 76-77
Cold, in postanesthesia period, 312; *see also* Hypothermia
Cold caloric test, 770, 773
Cold stress in child, 225
Colitis, 942

Collagen, 278
Collapsed lung; *see* Pneumothorax
Collateral air passage, 608-609
Collecting duct, renal, 852
  reabsortion and, 853
Collecting tubule, 852
Colloid
  pelvic fracture and, 1085
  renal failure and, 883, 884
  shock and, 1099
Colon
  anatomy and physiology of, 924-926
  diverticulitis of, 942
  obstruction of, 958-962
Colonization, gastrointestinal, 1128
Color, skin
  asthma and, 215
  cardiovascular assessment and, 356-357
Color-flow Doppler echocardiography, 433
Coma, 791-795
  barbiturate-induced, 833
  characteristics of, 797
  description of, 791
  diagnosis of, 793
  etiology of, 791-793
  hyperglycemic hyperosmotic nonketotic, 151
  legal issues of, 776
  management of, 794-795
  myxedema, 979, 1038-1042
  pathophysiology of, 793
  persistent vegetative state versus, 796
Coma scale, Glasgow; *see* Glasgow Coma Scale
Commissural fiber, 749
Commissurotomy, 542
Committee, ethics
  institutional, 31
  nursing, 32
Communication
  aphasia and, 810-811, 844-845
  artificial airway and, 702-703
  locked-in syndrome and, 796
  in mental status examination, 75
  pain assessment and, 178
  risk management and, 41
Communication enhancement, 10
Community-acquired pneumonia, 663-667
Compartment, fluid, 856-857
Compartment syndrome
  abdominal, 1081
  pelvic fracture and, 1085-1086
  trauma and, 1090
Compensated pulmonary condition, 642-643
Compensatory mechanisms
  cardiogenic shock and, 1102-1103
  in heart failure, 503-504
  in shock, 1097-1098
Compensatory shunting in pulmonary
    embolism, 669
Complement, 1122, 1127
Complete heart block, 593
Compliance
  bedside measurement of, 648
  lung, 614
Complications
  of bronchoscopy, 647
  of cerebrovascular accident, 808-809
  in child
    extubation, 211
    head injury and, 228
Complications—cont'd
  in child—cont'd
    meningitis and, 227
  of craniotomy, 816-817
  of endocarditis, 510
  of endotracheal intubation, 694-697, 701
  of enteral tube nutrition, 160
  of high-dose barbiturate therapy, 832
  of hypertensive disease in pregnancy, 256
  of intraaortic balloon pump, 570
  of oxygen therapy, 689-692
  of pancreatitis, 958
  of parenteral nutrition, 163
  of peritoneal dialysis, 902-903, 904
  postanesthesia, 312-326; *see also* Anesthesia,
    complications of
  of respiratory failure, 656, 658
  of thoracentesis, 648
  of tracheostomy tube, 698
  of trauma, 1087-1091
Computed tomography
  abdominal injury and, 1080
  cerebrovascular accident and, 801
  coma and, 793
  contusion and, 1060
  gastrointestinal, 938-939
  head injury and, 1064
  ischemic stroke and, 836
  neurologic, 780
  pituitary gland and, 995
  renal, 876
  single photon emission, 786
Computer as teaching tool, 56
Concussion, 1060
Conditioned air, 604
Conducting airway, 604-606
Conduction system, cardiac, 334-336
Conference, ethics, 32
Confidentiality, 22-24
Confusion
  acute, 74-75
  discomfort and, 287
Congenital heart defect, 216, 219
Congestion, hepatic, 941
Congestive heart failure; *see* Heart failure
Conjugated bile salt, 143
Conjugated bilirubin, 928
Conscious sedation, 193-194
  nursing interventions for, 195
Consciousness
  asthma and, 215
  categories of, 764-765
  in child, 225
  coma and; *see* Coma
  components of, 763-764
  head injury and, 1064
  pain assessment and, 178-179
  rapid neurologic assessment and, 775
Consent, informed, 42-43
Consequentialism, 19-20
Consolidation, pneumonia with, 638
Constipation
  cultural factors in, 953-956
  diabetes insipidus and, 1025-1026
  enteral nutrition and, 161
  myxedema and, 1042
Constrictor, bronchiolar, 313
Contamination
  burn wound, 1160-1161
Contamination—cont'd
  food, AIDS and, 155
Continuous cardiac output measurement,
    470-471
Continuous electroencephalographic monitoring,
    786-787
Continuous monitoring of mixed venous oxygen
    saturation, 471, 474-480
Continuous positive airway pressure
  advantages/disadvantages of, 691
  child and, 208
  clinical applications for, 707
  obstructive sleep apnea and, 112
  for postanesthesia pulmonary edema, 314
  weaning from mechanical ventilation
    and, 684
Continuous recording system for
    electrocardiography, 427-428
Continuous renal replacement, 893-899
  complications of, 899
  indications for, 894-895
  management of, 899
  methods of
    arteriovenous hemodialysis, 897-898
    arteriovenous hemofiltration and, 897
    slow ultrafiltration, 895-897
    venovenous hemodialysis and, 898-899
Contraceptive, oral, 485
Contract, insurance, 41
Contract law, 36
Contractility, cardiac, 350-351
  cardiac surgery and, 547
  chemistry values affecting, 379
  heart failure and, 505
  nursing management and, 592
  pulmonary artery pressure and, 464
Contraction
  cardiac
    age-related changes in, 272-273
    premature atrial, 409-410
    premature ventricular, 416-422
  uterine, 249-250
Contracture, burn and, 1168-1169
Contrast medium
  angiography and, 781-782
  myelography and, 782-784
  renal failure and, 883
Control ventilation, 707
Controller of ventilation, 615
Contusion
  brain, 1060
  pulmonary, 1075-1076
Convoluted tubule
  distal, 852
  proximal, 851-852
Convulsion; *see* Seizure
Coordination of care, 3-16
  interdisciplinary planning and, 10,
    12-15
  nursing diagnosis and, 5-10
  nursing process and, 4-5
  nursing's role in health care and, 3-4
Coping, 78-82
  assessment of, 80
  assistance with, 10
  concept of, 78-79
  enhancement for, 80-82
  mechanisms of, 79-80
  nursing management plan for, 96-99

Coronary angioplasty, percutaneous transluminal, 553-555
ST-segment monitoring and, 399-401
Coronary arteriography, 438-440
Coronary artery bypass graft, 541-542
Coronary artery disease, 483-490
angina and, 486-489
catheter interventions for, 552-561
description of, 483
etiology of, 483
management of, 489-490
myocardial infarction and, 490
pathophysiology of, 485-486
risk factors for, 483-485
Coronary atherectomy, directional, 555-556
Coronary blood supply, 336
Coronary precautions, 489-490
Coronary stent, 557
Corporate liability, 41
Cortex
cerebral
anatomy of, 749
ventilation regulation and, 616
visual, 752
Cortical nephron, 850
Corticosteroid
anaphylaxis and, 1108
hyperglycemia and, 137
status asthmaticus and, 672
transplant and, 1176
Corticotropin-releasing hormone, 106
Cortisol
neurologic alterations and, 137
sleep and, 106
Costal margin, 629
Cough
postanesthesia, 309
pulmonary history of, 626
Coumadin; *see* Warfarin
CPK-MB, 1079
Crackles, 632
in child, 221
conditions with, 634
Cranial nerve
eye movement and, 769, 770
function of, 742-746
Guillain Barré syndrome and, 812
pons and, 740
Craniotomy, 814-818
for head injury, 1064
Creatine kinase, 566
Creatinine
kidney and, 855
renal function and, 872
urine and, 874
Creatinine phosphokinase-myocardial band, 1079
Cricoid abscess, 697
Crisis
hypertensive, 523-525
coma and, 792
thyroid, 995
thyrotoxic, 1031-1038
Critical care phase of trauma care, 1056-1057
Critical pathways, 67
Crohn's disease, 148
CRRT; *see* Continuous renal replacement therapy
Crush injury, 1089-1090
Cruzan, Nancy, 44-45
Cry, asthma and, 215
Crystalloid
burn injury and, 1154
pelvic fracture and, 1085
renal failure and, 883, 884
shock and, 1099
Cuff
blood pressure, 366
endotracheal tube, 699-700
Cuff blood pressure, 446
Cuff pressure, of endotracheal tube, 700, 701
Cuff-inflation technique for endotracheal tube, 700-701
Cuffing, peribronchial, 388
Cullen's sign, 952, 1079
Cultural factors
in death rituals, 799-800
in ethical decision-making, 940
pain and, 173, 179
in symptom management, 953-956
Culture, synthetic skin and, 1163-1164
Curling's ulcer; *see* Stress ulcer
Curve
oxygen dissociation, 621-622, 623
oxyhemoglobin dissociation, 248
volume-pressure, 821
Cushing's triad, 773
Cutaneous pain, 176
nursing management of, 197-199
Cyanosis
cardiovascular assessment and, 357
central, 627-628
in child, 221-222
Cyanotic heart defect, 219
Cycle
cardiac, 348, 349
sleep, 105-106
Cyclosporine
liver transplant and, 1191
rejection and, 1183
transplant and, 1176, 1177
Cytokine, 1125-1127
Cytomegalovirus, 1184
Cytotoxic T cell, 1172-1173

D

D cell, 981
Damages, 39
Damped waveform, 450
DDD cardiac pacing, 533, 534, 535-536
Dead fetus syndrome, 258-259
Dead space
alveolar, 619
equation for, 646
pulmonary embolism and, 669
Deafferentation pain, 176
Death
brain
characteristics of, 797
in child, 228
definition of, 798
as legal issue, 776
cultural differences and, 799-800
family coping with, 81
fetal
diabetic ketoacidosis and, 262
trauma causing, 266
ketoacidosis and, 1003
mechanical ventilation and, 686
Death—cont'd
removal of life support and, 785
rituals concerning, 799-800
sleep deprivation and, 109-110
subarachnoid hemorrhage and, 804
sudden
cardiac, 501
implantable cardioverter defibrillator and, 550
pregnancy and, 253
status asthmaticus in child and, 214
ventricular tachycardia and, 419
trauma causing, 1052
Debridement, burn injury and, 1159
Decannulation, artificial airway and, 703
Deceleration injury
of head, 1057
thoracic, 1073
Decision making, ethical, 28-32
Decompensation, cardiopulmonary, coma and, 792
Deconditioning, 597
Deconjugated bile salt, 143
Deep breathing
postanesthesia, 309
respiratory failure and, 659
thoracic surgery and, 680-681
Deep dermal partial-thickness burn, 1144, 1145
Deep sedation, 190, 193
Deep tendon reflex, 768
Deep vein thrombosis; *see* Thrombosis
Defamation, 38
Defibrillation
in child, 224
pain after, 177
Defibrillator
cardioverter, 550-552
atrial fibrillation and, 413-414
electrophysiology and, 440-441
tiered therapy, 419-420
ventricular tachycardia and, 419-420
Deficit, pulse, 448
Defining characteristics, 6-7
Dehydration
hyperglycemic hyperosmolar nonketotic syndrome and, 1018
ketoacidosis and, 1008-1009
peritoneal dialysis and, 904
thyrotoxic crisis and, 1036
Dehydration test, diabetes insipidus and, 1024-1025
Delayed arousal, postanesthesia, 321
Delayed drug clearance, 318
Delayed gastric emptying, 161
Delirium, 74-75
assessment of, 75
definition of, 188
emergence from anesthesia, 322-323
etiology of, 74-75
management of, 76-77, 189
plan for, 91-95
mental status examination for, 75-76
sleep deprivation and, 109-110
Demand pacemaker, 534
Dementia, 797
Demerol; *see* Meperidine
Demineralization, aging and, 289
Dendrite, 734
Dendritic spine, 282

Denial
  as coping mechanism, 79-80
  as reaction to illness, 51-52
Dentition, 288
Deontologic theory, 20
Deoxyribonucleic acid
  myocardial gene expression and, 273-274
  neuron and, 734
Dependence
  drug, 180
  excessive, 72
Depolarization, cardiac, 344-345, 389
Depression
  cultural factors in, 953-956
  major, 77
  respiratory
    opioid anesthesia and, 301-302
    in postanesthesia period, 315
Deprivation, sleep, 109-110
Dermatome, 759-760
Dermis, 1141
Desaturation
  obstructive sleep apnea and, 111
  respiratory failure and, 659
Descending pain pathway, 172, 174
Desflurane, 301
Desynchronization, circadian, 107, 119
Desynchronized sleep, 106
Detoxification, by liver, 928
Dexamethasone, 1034, 1035
Dextran, for renal failure, 884
Dextrose
  in parenteral nutrition formula for child, 231
  renal failure and, 884
Dextrose-amino acid solution, 161-162
Diabetes insipidus, 1021-1027
  case study of, 1043
  craniotomy and, 816
  description of, 1021-1022
  diagnosis of, 1024-1025
  etiology of, 978-979, 1022
  management of, 1025-1027
  pathophysiology of, 1022-1023
  patient history of, 993
Diabetes mellitus
  complications of, 991
  coronary artery disease and, 485
  non–insulin-dependent, case study of, 1003
  nutrition and, 149
  pancreas transplant and, 1205
  pregnancy and, 262
  types of, 1001, 1003
Diabetic ketoacidosis, 1003, 1006-1015; *see also* Ketoacidosis
Diagnosis, nursing, 5-7
Diagnosis related groups
  acute respiratory distress syndrome and, 660
  air leak disorder and, 673
  aspiration lung disorder and, 667
  cerebrovascular accident and, 800
  fulminant hepatic failure and, 962
  Guillain Barré syndrome and, 812
  intestinal obstruction and, 959
  mechanical circulatory assist device and, 567-568
  myxedema and, 1038
  pulmonary embolism and, 668
  status asthmaticus and, 671-672
Diagnosis related groups—cont'd
  thoracic surgery and, 677, 679
  valve surgery and, 543
Dialysis, 883-903
  body image disturbance and, 87-88
  continuous renal replacement and, 893-899
  hemodialysis, 890-893
    protein and, 138
  peritoneal
    complications of, 904
    glucose and, 140
    process of, 899-903
  psychosocial alterations and, 83-84
  vascular access for, 886-890
Dialyzer, hemodialysis, 891
Diaphragm
  age-related changes in, 277
  chest radiography and, 650-651
  of child, 206
  excursion of, 630-631
  inhalation and, 604
  rupture of, 1074-1075
Diarrhea
  cultural factors in, 953-956
  diabetes insipidus and, 1025-1026
  endocrine alterations and, 151
  enteral nutrition and, 160
Diastole, 446-447
Diastolic blood pressure, 339-340
Diastolic murmur, 370
Diastolic pressure, pulmonary artery, 463
Diazepam
  anesthesia with, 303
  conscious sedation with, 193
  dosage and action of, 183
  renal failure and, 909
  sleep and, 108
DIC; *see* Disseminated intravascular coagulation
Dicrotic wave, intracranial pressure, 825
Didanosine, 154
Diencephalon, 746-749
Diet; *see* Nutrition; Nutritional support
Diet history, 125-126
Diffuse axonal injury, 1062-1063
Diffusion
  fluid balance and, 858
  placental membranes and, 244
  respiration and, 618
Digestion
  accessory organs of, 926-930
  nutrient metabolism and, 121-124
  pancreas and, 929-930
  process of, 924
Digestive enzyme, 924
Digestive hormone, 923
  pancreas and, 930
Digital radiography, cardiovascular, 389
Digital subtraction angiography of brain, 782
Digitalis, 577
  ventricular ectopy and, 417-418
Digoxin
  cardiac contractility and, 350-351
  for child, 221
  dosage and side effects of, 578
  elderly patient and, 283
  medication card for, 58
  renal failure and, 909
Dihydropyridine, 581
Dilated bronchus, 636
Dilated cardiomyopathy, 507-508
Dilemma, ethical, 29-30
Diltiazem
  characteristics of, 581
  dosage and side effects of, 578
  effects of, 576
  elderly patient and, 283
Diminished breath sounds, 632, 634
Diphenhydramine, streptokinase allergy and, 562
2,3-Diphosphoglycerate, 624
Directional coronary atherectomy, 555-556
Disability, in trauma survey, 1053
Disbelief as reaction to illness, 51
Disc, intercalated, 342
Discharge guidelines in critical care, 26
Disk, intervertebral, 755-756, 757
Dislocation, Malgaigne's hemipelvis fracture, 1085
Disopyramide, 575
Disorientation, 65; *see also* Delirium
Dissection, aortic, 515-517
Disseminated intravascular coagulation
  multiple organ dysfunction syndrome and, 1130-1131, 1132, 1133
  pregnancy and, 258-259
  shock and, 1098
Distal renal tubule, 852, 853
Distention
  abdominal
    ketoacidosis and, 1011
    postanesthesia, 323, 324
  intestinal, 960
  jugular vein, 358-359
Distortion in electrocardiography, 391-392
Distress, spiritual, 82
Diuresis
  antidiuretic hormone disorder and, 1030
  hyperglycemic hyperosmolar nonketotic syndrome and, 1018
Diuretic
  diabetes insipidus and, 1026
  elderly patient and, 283
  heart failure and, 505
  hypertensive crisis and, 524
  intracranial hypertension and, 831-832
  neurologic disorder and, 835
  renal disorder and, 885, 905
Diuretic phase of tubular necrosis, 879
Diuril, 905
Diverticulitis, colonic, 942
DNA
  myocardial gene expression and, 273-274
  neuron and, 734
DNA virus, endocarditis and, 509
Dobutamine
  echocardiography and, 436
  effects of, 577-578
  physiologic effects of, 579
Doctrine, of *respondeat superior*, 40
Documentation, legal issues of, 1018
Doll's eyes, 770, 772
Donor, transplant; *see* Transplantation
Do-not-resuscitate orders, 44
Dopamine
  age-related changes in, 286
  effects of, 577
  myxedema and, 1041
  physiologic effects of, 579

Dopamine—cont'd
sleep and, 105-106
Dopaminergic agents, stress and, 190
Doppler ultrasound, cerebral, 784-786
Double-lung transplant, 1188-1190
Drainage
cerebrospinal fluid, 830-831
craniotomy and, 818
Drainage tube, mediastinal, 386
Dressing
for burn wound, 1160
biosynthetic, 1165
synthetic skin, 1164
craniotomy and, 818
Driving pressure of oxygen, 618
Droperidol, 303
Drug clearance, delayed, 318
Drug therapy
age-related changes in, 281-282
for AIDS, 154
antibiotic; *see* Antibiotic
antidiuretic hormone and, 985
antidiuretic hormone disorder and, 1030
antiemetic, 324
autonomic dysreflexia and, 1066
burn pain and, 1167
cardiogenic shock and, 1104
cardiomyopathy and, 508
cardiovascular
antidysrhythmic, 574-577
inotropic, 577-579
vasodilator, 579-582
delirium and, 74, 76-77
emergence, 322
diabetes insipidus and, 1026
diabetes mellitus and, 1004-1005
endocarditis and, 510
epilepsy in pregnancy and, 266
fear of addiction and, 179-180
fetal effects of, 243-244
for gastrointestinal disorder, 971
heart failure and, 505, 506
heart-lung transplant and, 1186
hyperglycemic hyperosmolar nonketotic syndrome and, 1016
hypertensive crisis and, 524
insulin affected by, 980
intracranial hemorrhage and, 808
intracranial hypertension and, 830-832
liver failure caused by, 963
malignant hyperthermia and, 320
mechanical ventilation and, 713-715
multiple organ dysfunction syndrome and, 1135, 1137-1138
myocardial infarction and, 499
myxedema and, 1041
nutrition and, 162
for pain, 180-185
delivery systems for, 182, 184-185
equianalgesia and, 184-185
nonopioid analgesics for, 181
nonsteroidal antiinflammatory drug for, 181-182
opioid analgesics for, 180-181
pneumonia and, 666
pregnancy and, advanced cardiac life support and, 254-255
for renal alteration, 903, 905-909
Drug therapy—cont'd
renal failure and, 883, 885, 903, 905-910
respiratory distress syndrome and, 663
respiratory failure and, 658
septic shock and, 1115
shock and, 1099
short bowel syndrome and, 148
sleep and, 107-108, 305
spinal injury and, 1068
status asthmaticus and, 672
subarachnoid hemorrhage and, 806
thyrotoxic crisis and, 1034, 1035
Drug-induced condition
pancreatitis as, 951
ventricular ectopy as, 417-418
Dry mouth, tube feeding and, 158
Duct
collecting, renal, 852
of Wirsung, 929
Ductal occlusion, pancreatic, 1206
Ductus arteriosus, 216
Duodenal ulcer
bleeding and, 945
findings in, 941
DuoDerm, 1164, 1165
Dura mater, 737
Duty
breach of, 38-39
definition of, 38
Dynamic compliance, bedside measurement of, 648
Dynorphin, 175
Dysconjugate eye movement, 770
Dysfunctional ventilatory weaning response, 728-729
Dyslexia, spatial, 810
Dysphagia
cerebrovascular accident and, 811
weight and, 137
Dyspnea
asthma and, 215
cultural factors in, 953-956
paroxysmal nocturnal, 504
Dysreflexia, autonomic, 1066, 1068
Dysrhythmia
atrial, 409-414
atrioventricular node and, 335-336
cardiac catheterization and, 440
cardiogenic shock and, 1102
causes of, 502
central venous pressure and, 456
in child, 222
drugs for, 574-577
ECG monitoring of, 399
elderly patient and, 274
heart transplantation and, 1181
hypomagnesemia and, 380-381
intraaortic balloon pump and, 570
monitoring of, 399
myocardial infarction and, 496
myxedema and, 1041
neurologic assessment and, 773
obstructive sleep apnea and, 111
pacemaker for, 529-530; *see also* Pacemaker, cardiac
postanesthesia period and, 316
postoperative, 545-546
potassium and, 377-378
Dysrhythmia—cont'd
renal failure and, 882-883
respiratory failure and, 658
sinus, 408, 409
surgery for, 549
ventricular, 415

E

Ecchymosis, 288-289
Echocardiography, 430-436
cerebrovascular accident and, 801
myocardial contusion and, 1079
Eclampsia, 255-256
Ectopic beat, ventricular, 416
Ectopic P wave, 409
Ectopy
premature ventricular contraction and, 416, 417
T wave and, 392
Edema
burn injury and, 1148-1149, 1154
cardiovascular assessment and, 357, 362-363
cerebral
cerebrovascular accident and, 801
craniotomy and, 817
liver failure and, 963-964
management of, 828
trauma patient and, 1059
laryngeal, 312-313
pulmonary
heart failure and, 504
postanesthesia, 314
thoracentesis and, 648
renal function and, 867
tracheal, 1149
Edrophonium, 307
Education
antidiuretic hormone and, 1031
cardiac catheterization and, 440
cardiovascular alteration and
angina and, 491
aortic dissection and, 517
cardiac surgery and, 549
cardiomyopathy and, 508, 509
carotid artery disease and, 522
catheter-related intervention and, 559
coronary artery disease and, 489
deep vein thrombosis and, 523
endocarditis and, 510, 511
exercise electrocardiography and, 430
heart failure and, 507
hypertensive crisis and, 525
implantable cardioverter defibrillator and, 552
intraaortic balloon pump and, 571
myocardial infarction and, 500-501
pacemaker and, 540
peripheral vascular disease and, 519, 520
thrombolytic therapy and, 567
valvular disease and, 514
cerebrovascular accident and, 811
continuous renal replacement therapy and, 899
diabetes insipidus and, 1027
echocardiography and, 436
endocrine disorder and, 1015
ethical, 31
Guillain Barré syndrome and, 814

Education—cont'd
hyperglycemic hyperosmolar nonketotic syndrome and, 1021
intestinal obstruction and, 963
myxedema and, 1042
nuclear magnetic resonance and, 438
nutrition
AIDS and, 154-155
for cardiovascular alteration, 130-131, 133
endocrine alterations and, 151-152
for gastrointestinal alterations, 148-149
for neurologic alteration, 137
renal disorder and, 143
for respiratory alterations, 135
pain, 187
pancreatitis and, 959
patient and family, 49-60
adult learning theory and, 50
content of, 49-50
readiness to learn and, 53
teaching plan for, 53-60
teaching-learning process and, 50-52
peritoneal dialysis and, 903
plan for, 53-60
pulmonary embolism and, 671
renal failure and, 886, 887
respiratory failure and, 655, 659, 660
sedation and, 196
status asthmaticus and, 673
thyrotoxic crisis and, 1037-1038
Effectors of ventilation, 616
Efferent nerve fiber, 733
Egg, cholesterol and, 131
Egophony, 633
Eicosanoid, 1127
modulation of, 1135, 1137
Eisenmenger's syndrome, 253
Ejection fraction, 348, 460-461
Elastase, pancreatitis and, 951
Elastic pressure garment for burn, 1167
Elastin, 278
Elderly patient, 271-292
cardiovascular system of, 272-276
central nervous system of, 282, 285-286
delirium in, 74
gastrointestinal system of, 280
immune system of, 286-287
liver of, 280-282
nursing diagnosis for, 292
physical examination of, 287-291
psychosocial alterations in, 83
renal system of, 279-280
respiratory system of, 276-279
self-esteem of, 70
studies on aging and, 271
Electric ventricular assist device, 572
Electrical activity, cardiac, 344-348
Electrical burn, 1145-1146, 1151
Electrical cardioversion, atrial fibrillation and, 413-414
Electrical nerve stimulation, transcutaneous, 184-185
Electrocardiography, 389-430
age-related changes in, 274
ambulatory, 427-429
baseline distortion in, 391-392
for bedside monitoring, 397, 399
bifascicular block and, 405-406
Electrocardiography—cont'd
bundle branch block and, 403-404
calcium and, 380
cardiac tamponade and, 1078
in child, 222
dysrhythmia and
atrial, 409-410, 411-414
atrioventricular, 424-427
interpretation of, 406
junctional, 414-415
tachycardia and, 410-411, 414, 422-424
ventricular, 415-422
dysrhythmia monitoring and, 399
exercise, 429-430
heart rate determination and, 406
hemiblock and, 405
hypertrophy and, 401
ischemia and infarction, 401-403
leads for, 389-391, 396-399
magnesium and, 380-381
monitor lead analysis and, 396
myocardial contusion and, 1078-1079
myocardial infarction and, 491-493
myxedema and, 1041
P wave and, 406
pacemaker and, 530
artifacts from, 536-538
paper for, 392
in perianesthesia assessment, 306
potassium and, 377-378
PR interval and, 406
pulmonary embolism and, 670
QRS complex, evaluation of, 406-407
rhythm determination and, 406
signal-averaged, 441
sinus rhythm and, 407-409
ST-segment monitoring and, 399-401
ventricular axis in, 395-396
ventricular conduction defects and, 403
waveforms in, 392-395
Electrode
electrocardiographic, 389
for implantable cardioverter defibrillator, 550
pacemaker, 530
microshock from, 539
Electroencephalography
in child, 226
head injury and, 1064
neurologic assessment and, 786-787
sleep and, 104
Electrolyte
anesthesia and, 308
bowel resection and, 147
burn injury and, 1154-1156
cardiovascular alteration and, 377-381
fluid balance and, 857
hyperglycemic hyperosmolar nonketotic syndrome and, 1020
intestinal obstruction and, 959-960
ketoacidosis and, 1008-1009, 1012-1013
liver failure and, 145
liver transplant and, 1196
osmotic diuretic and, 831
postanesthesia period and, 310, 321
renal system and, 860-863, 871
continuous renal replacement therapy and, 900
renal failure and, 143, 880, 881, 884-885, 886
Electrolyte—cont'd
thyrotoxic crisis and, 1037
in urine, 875
Electrolyte management, 10
Electromechanical dissociation, in child, 224
Electromyography, 104
Electrooculography, 104
Electrophysiology study, intracardiac, 440-441
Elemental enteral formula, 157
Elements of negligence and malpractice, 38-41
Elevation of head for neurologic deficit, 137
Elimination
antidiuretic hormone and, 1031
myxedema and, 1040, 1042
spinal injury and, 1071
Emancipated minor, 43
Embolectomy, pulmonary, 670
Embolism; *see also* Thrombosis
air
delayed arousal from anesthesia and, 321
hemodynamic monitoring and, 451-452, 452-453, 455-456
parenteral nutrition and, 163
amniotic fluid, 261-262
delayed arousal from anesthesia and, 321
fat, trauma and, 1088-1089
pregnancy and, 260-261
pulmonary; *see* Pulmonary embolism
Embolization
cerebral aneurysm and, 806
gastrointestinal bleeding and, 949
Embryonic stage of fetal development, 243
Emergency, subarachnoid hemorrhage as, 804
Emergency burn management, 1146-1149
Emergency Department Nurses Association, 36
Emergency department resuscitation, 1052-1056
Emission tomography, neurologic, 786
Emphysema, subcutaneous, 675
tracheostomy tube and, 698
Emptying, gastric
normal, 922
nutritional support and, 165
Emulsion, lipid, 162
Enalapril
characteristics of, 581
elderly patient and, 283
renal failure and, 908
Encephalitis, coma and, 793
Encephalopathy
hepatic, 963
hypertensive, 792
liver failure and, 146
oculovestibular reflex and, 770
End-diastolic pressure, left ventricular, 460
End-diastolic volume, left ventricular, 348
End-expiratory pressure, positive; *see* Positive end-expiratory pressure
Endocardial lead for defibrillator, 550
Endocarditis, 508-510
in child, 222-223
education about, 511
Endocardium, 331-332
Endocrine functions of pancreas, 930
Endocrine system
alterations in, 149-152
anatomy and physiology of, 977-987
hypothalamus and, 982
pancreas and, 979-982

Endocrine system—cont'd
  anatomy and physiology of—cont'd
    pituitary gland and, 982-983
    thyroid gland and, 982-987
  antidiuretic hormone and; *see* Antidiuretic hormone
  assessment and diagnostic procedures of, 989-999
    pancreas, 990-992
    pituitary, 992-995
    thyroid, 995-999
  diabetes insipidus and, 1021-1027
  diabetes mellitus and; *see* Diabetes insipidus; Diabetes mellitus
  diabetic ketoacidosis and, 1003-1015; *see also* Ketoacidosis
  hyperglycemic hyperosmolar nonketotic syndrome and, 1015-1021
  pancreas and, transplantation of, 1205-1208
  physiologic stress and, 123-124
  pituitary gland and; *see* Pituitary gland
  placenta and, 244, 246
  in pregnancy, 246-247
  septic shock and, 1112-1113
  thyroid gland and; *see* Thyroid *entries*
Endogenous pain modulation system, 172-173
Endorphin, 174
Endoscopic sclerotherapy, 968
Endoscopic variceal band ligation, 968
Endoscopy, 936
Endothelial cell
  inflammation and, 1126
  multiple organ dysfunction syndrome and, 1135
Endothelial injury, vascular, 669
Endotracheal intubation
  airway management with, 695, 699-703
  artificial airway and, 693-695
  burn injury and, 1153
  of child, 208-211
  extubation and, 704
  facial injury and, 1072
  mechanical ventilation and; *see* Mechanical ventilation
  postanesthesia laryngospasm and, 313
  sputum specimen and, 647
  status asthmaticus and, 672-673
End-stage hypothyroidism, 1040
End-stage liver disease, 1191-1199
End-stage renal disease, 1205-1208
End-tidal carbon dioxide, 653
Energy
  health care, 24
  thyrotoxic crisis and, 1032-1033
Enfamil, 230
Enkephalin, 174, 175
Enteral nutrition
  administration of, 155-159
  burn and, 1168
  complications of, 160
  endocrine alterations and, 149
  formulas for, 157
  multiple organ dysfunction syndrome and, 1134
  neurologic alteration and, 135
  nursing management of, 141, 158
  spinal injury and, 1071
Enterogastrone, 923
Entero-oxyntin, 923
Enterostomy, tube, 156
Environment, coronary artery disease and, 489
Environmental stressors, 52
Environmental trigger of malignant hyperthermia, 320
Enzyme
  cardiac, 381
  digestive, 924
  electrical burn and, 1151
  myocardial infarction and, 496
  oxygen-free radicals and, 691-692
  pancreatic, 149, 929-930, 951
Eosinophil, 1175
Eosinophilic chemotactic factor of anaphylaxis, 1106
Ependyma, 735
Epicardial pacing system of pacemaker, 530
Epicardial pacing wire, 531
Epicardium, 331
Epidermal sheet, cultured, 1164
Epidermis, 1141
Epidural analgesia, 184-185
Epidural hematoma, 738
Epidural monitor, 823-824
Epiglottis, 605
Epiglottitis, in newborn, 205
Epilepsy
  in child, 225-226
  pregnancy and, 266
Epinephrine
  anaphylaxis and, 1108
  for asystole in child, 224
  cardiovascular effects of, 578-579
  fetal effects of, 254
  hyperglycemic hyperosmolar nonketotic syndrome and, 1018
  neurologic alterations and, 137
  physiologic effects of, 579
Epithalamus, 748
Epithelial cell
  alveolar, 607-610, 612
  burn injury and, 1158-1159
  gastric, 921-922
  in urine, 875
Epogen, 905
Equation
  for dead space, 646
  Henderson-Hasselbalch, 969
  for intrapulmonary shunt, 645-646
Equianalgesia, 184
Equipment for hemodynamic monitoring, 442
Erythrocyte; *see* Red blood cells
Erythrocyte sedimentation rate, cardiovascular alteration and, 382
Erythrocyte-stimulating hormone, 905
Erythromycin, 907
Erythropoiesis, myxedema and, 1040
Erythropoietin
  kidney and, 855
  renal failure and, 886
Escalator, mucociliary, 606
Escape rhythm, junctional, 415
Eschar, 1159
Escharotomy, 1149
  breathing pattern and, 1154
Esmolol
  dosage and side effects of, 578
Esmolol—cont'd
  thyrotoxic crisis and, 1035
Esophageal varices
  management of, 949
  vasopressin for, 970
Esophagogastric balloon tamponade tube, 966-968
Esophagus
  age-related changes in, 280
  anatomy of, 920
  varices of, 946
Estrogen
  osteoporosis and, 289
  pregnancy and, 248
Ethical issues, cultural factors in, 940
Ethics, 19-32
  decision making and, 28-32
  definition of, 19
  medical futility as, 25-26
  morals and, 19
  nursing practice and, 26, 28
  principles of, 20-24
  theories of, 19-20
  withholding and withdrawing treatment and, 24-25
Ethics committee, institutional, 31
Ethnic differences; *see* Cultural factors
Etiologic/related factors, 6
Etomidate, 302
Evaluation in nursing process, 9-10
Evoked potentials, 787
Excitation-contraction coupling, 348
Excretion, drug, 281
Excursion
  diaphragmatic, 630-631
  respiratory, 629, 631
Exercise
  burn and, 1169
  coronary artery disease and, 485
  diabetes and, 152
  left ventricular function and, 275
  work of breathing and, 614
Exercise electrocardiography, 429-430
Exhalation, 604
Exocrine functions of pancreas, 929-930
Expiratory pressure, 648-649
Expiratory reserve volume, 649
Exposure in trauma survey, 1053
Express consent, 43
Expressive aphasia, 811
Extension, abnormal, 767-768
External fixation
  for extremity injury, 1086
  of pelvic fracture, 1085
External jugular vein, 358-359
Extracellular fluid, 857, 858-859
  bicarbonate and, 863
  magnesium and, 862
Extracorporeal carbon dioxide removal, 715-716
Extracorporeal membrane oxygenation, 715-716
Extracranial Doppler studies, 784
Extraocular movement, 770
Extremity
  cardiovascular assessment and, 357
  injury to, 1086-1087
    burn, 1157
Extremity pulse in burn injury, 1148-1149
Extrinsic control of peripheral circulation, 353-354

Extubation
burn injury and, 1154
cardiac surgery and, 547
in child, 211
endotracheal, 704
tracheostomy tube, 703
unintentional, 695
Exudative phase of respiratory distress syndrome, 661
Exudative stage of oxygen toxicity, 692
Eye
age-related changes in, 288
alkali burn of, 1150
Battle's sign and, 1059
cerebrovascular accident and, 810
coma and, 794
cranial nerves and, 742-743
doll's, 770, 772
head injury and, 1064
hypertensive crisis and, 792
neurologic assessment and, 769-770
sleep and, 104-105
Eyelid, coma and, 794

F

Face in cardiovascular assessment, 356-357
Face mask for oxygen therapy, 690
Face tent, 691
Facial injury, 1071-1073
Facilitated diffusion, 244
Falciform ligament of liver, 926
Fall, by child, 228
False neurotransmitter hypothesis, 143, 145
Falx cerebri, 737
Family
coping by, 80, 98-99
removal of life support and, 785
Family and patient education, 49-60; *see also* Education
Famotidine, 909
Fast-flush square wave test, 450
Fasting
lipids and, 123
metabolic response to, 123-124
Fat
bowel resection and, 147
cardiovascular alterations and, 130-131
insulin and, 981
metabolism of, 122-123
short bowel syndrome and, 148
steatorrhea and, 148-149
stool, 937
Fat embolism syndrome, 1088-1089
Fatigue
cultural factors in, 953-956
ineffective breathing pattern and, 724
Fatty acid
lipid metabolism and, 122-123
nutrition therapy and, 162
Feces; *see* Stool
Federal Tort Claims Act, 40
Feedback mechanism in septic shock, 1111-1112
Feeder artery, 803-804
Feeding tube in child, 230
Femoral artery
cardiac catheterization and, 439, 559-560
cerebral angiography and, 781
Femoral artery—cont'd
gastrointestinal angiography and, 938
Femoral artery bruit, 367
Femoral vein catheter for dialysis, 886
Fentanyl
dosage and action of, 183
for pain, 181
in child, 232
Fetal death
dead fetus syndrome, 258-259
diabetic ketoacidosis and, 262
Fetal development, 243-244
Fetal heart rate, 247
Fetus
basic life support and, 254
circulation of, 216
trauma to, 264, 266
Fever, postoperative, 319
Fiber
cardiac, 342
commissural, 749
myocardial, 346
nerve, 733
Fiberoptic bronchoscopy, 647
Fiberoptic catheter, 824
Fiberoptic endoscopy, 936
Fibrillation
atrial, 412, 413-414
algorithm for, 16
ventricular
in child, 224
definition of, 392
electrocardiography and, 420-422
sudden death from, 501
Fibrin, subarachnoid hemorrhage and, 806
Fibrosis, pulmonary, 639
Fidelity, 22-23
Fight-or-flight response, 65
Filament
actin, 342
myosin, 342
Film, polyurethane, 1165
Filter
continuous renal replacement therapy and, 900
vena caval, 670
Filtrate, renal, 852
Filtration rate, glomerular, 853-854
blood pressure and, 855
Fine ventricular fibrillation, 421
Fingerstick glucose test, 990-991
ketoacidosis and, 1008
Firearm injury; *see* Gunshot wound
First-degree atrioventricular block, 424
First-degree burn, 1144
Fistula
arteriovenous, 887
cerebrospinal fluid leakage and, 1059
tracheocutaneous, 699
tracheoesophageal, 699
tracheoinnominate artery, 699
Five-letter pacemaker code, 532-533, 534
Fixation
for extremity injury, 1086
of pelvic fracture, 1085
Fixed rate pacemaker, 534
FK506, 1177, 1178
Flail chest, 1074
Flap, liver, 964
Flexion, abnormal, 766, 767
Flow-cycled ventilator, 704
Fluazepam, 108
Fluconazole
nutrition-related effects of, 154
renal failure and, 908
Fluent aphasia, 811
Fluid; *see also* Blood volume; Dehydration
abdominal injury and, 1080
amniotic fluid embolism and, 261-262
anaphylaxis and, 1108
anesthesia and, 308
antidiuretic hormone and, 983
antidiuretic hormone disorder and, 1029, 1030
ascites and, 868-869
aspiration lung disorder and, 668
bowel resection and, 147
burn injury and, 1142, 1147, 1154-1156
cardiomyopathy and, 508
cerebral angiography and, 781
cerebrospinal; *see* Cerebrospinal fluid
continuous arteriovenous hemodialysis and, 898
continuous renal replacement therapy and, 900
craniotomy and, 816, 818
diabetes insipidus and, 1022-1023, 1025
edema and, 362-363
extracellular, 857, 858-859
bicarbonate and, 863
magnesium and, 862
facial injury and, 1072
gastrointestinal disorder and, 144
heart failure and, 129, 506
hemodialysis, 891
for hemodialysis, 892-893
hyperglycemic hyperosmolar nonketotic syndrome and, 1018, 1019-1020
intestinal obstruction and, 959-960
intracellular, 857, 858-859
magnesium and, 862
ketoacidosis and, 1006-1007, 1011-1012
kidney and, 856-859
liver failure and, 145
movement of, 858-859
myxedema and, 1041
neurogenic shock and, 1110
neurologic alterations and, 136
oxygen toxicity and, 692
pelvic fracture and, 1085
peritoneal dialysis and, 904
pituitary assessment and, 992-993
pleural, 602, 638
in postanesthesia period, 310
pulmonary contusion and, 1076
renal disorder and, 138, 140, 880, 882, 883-884, 885
renal function and, 869-870, 871
respiratory alterations and, 134, 135
septic shock and, 1115
shock and, 1099
hypovolemic, 1101
subarachnoid hemorrhage and, 807
thyrotoxic crisis and, 1037
total body water in child, 229
trauma patient and, 1055
valvular disease and, 514
Flumazenil
intravenous anesthetics and, 300

Flumazenil—cont'd
  sedation and, 195
Flunisolide, 715
Flutter, atrial, 411-412
Foam cuff tracheostomy tube, 701
Folic acid, 139
Follicle-stimulating hormone, 748
Fontanelle, 224-225
Food and Drug Administration
  drug use in pregnancy and, 245
  new or investigational devices and, 299
Food intake, hunger center and, 748
Food particle aspiration, 667
Food safety for AIDS patient, 155
Foramen
  of Luschka, 738
  of Magendie, 738
  of Monro, 738
Foramen ovale, 216
Force, peak inspiratory, 648
Forced expiratory volume
  age-related changes in, 279
  status asthmaticus in child and, 214
Forgetfulness, 290
Formalism, 20
Format for nursing diagnosis, 7
Formula
  for child, 229
  Parkland, 1147
    electrical burn and, 1151
  physiologic, D-1 to D-4
Forward heart failure, 503
Fossa, posterior, 737
Fracture
  classification of, 1086
  pelvic, 1084-1086
    in trauma, 266
  rib, 1074
  skull, 1059
    pituitary gland and, 994-995
Frameworks, assessment, 4-5
Free radical, oxygen
  neurologic alteration and, 834
  reperfusion organ injury and, 1126
Fremitus, tactile, 629-630, 631
Frequency response test, 450
Friction rub
  barotrauma and, 675
  pericardial, 371
  pleural, 632
    conditions with, 634
Frontal lobe of cerebrum, 750-751
Full-thickness burn, 1144
Fulminant hepatic failure, 962-965
Functional health pattern typology, 5
Functional residual capacity, 649
  age-related changes in, 279
  in postanesthesia period, 315
Furosemide
  hypertensive crisis and, 524
  intracranial hypertension and, 831-832
Fusion, spinal, 1069
Futility, medical, 25-26

G

Gallbladder
  anatomy of, 927
Gallbladder—cont'd
  function of, 928-929
  multiple organ dysfunction syndrome and, 1128-1129
Gallstone, 941
  pancreatitis and, 951
Gamma-aminobutyric acid
  age-related changes in, 286
  nonopioid anesthetic and, 300
Gancyclovir, 908
Ganglion, 734, 749
Gap, anion, 645
  renal function and, 872-873
Gap junction, 342
Garment
  antishock, pelvic fracture and, 1085
  elastic pressure, 1167
Gas, blood; *see* Blood gases
Gas exchange
  age-related changes in, 279
  burn injury and, 1153
  nursing management plan for, 725-728
  in respiratory decompensation, 625
  shock and, 1098-1099
  spinal injury and, 1070-1071
Gas transport, 620-624
Gastric acid
  burn injury and, 1157
  stimulation of, 936
Gastric distention, 323, 324
Gastric emptying
  in evaluation of nutrition support, 165
  normal, 922
Gastric lavage, 950
Gastric mucosa, 280
Gastric retention, 161
Gastric ulcer, 945
Gastric volume, 229
Gastric-inhibitory peptide, 923
Gastrin, 923
Gastroduodenal artery, 923
Gastroepiploic artery graft, 542, 544
Gastrointestinal alteration; *see also* Gastrointestinal system
  anaphylactic shock and, 1108
  assessment of, 931-936
  bleeding and, 945-950
  burn injury and, 1147-1148, 1157
  case history of, 974-975
  drugs for, 970-971
  injury causing, 1082
  intestinal obstruction as, 958-962
  liver failure and, 962-965
  management of, 965-971
    endoscopic sclerotherapy in, 968
    endoscopic variceal band ligation in, 968
    intubation and, 965-968
    pH monitoring and, 968-970
    transjugular intrahepatic portosystemic shunt and, 968
  mechanical ventilation causing, 706
  multiple organ dysfunction syndrome and, 1128, 1129
  nursing diagnosis and management of, 973-976
  nutrition and, 143-149
    assessment of, 143, 144-145
    education about, 148-149
    interventions for, 143, 145-148
Gastrointestinal alteration—cont'd
  pancreatitis as, 950-952, 957-958
  renal failure and, 886
  shock and, 1098
  swallowing disorder and, 976
  thyrotoxic crisis and, 1034
  trauma and, 1089
    in pregnancy, 265-266
Gastrointestinal intubation, 965-968
Gastrointestinal system
  age-related changes in, 280, 292
    examination for, 290
  anatomy and physiology of, 919-930
  assessment of, 931-936
    history in, 931, 932
    laboratory studies in, 935-936
    physical examination in, 931-935
  in child, 229-230
  enteral nutrition support and, 155
  pregnancy and, 248-249, 250
  respiratory failure and, 657
  role of brain and, 919
Gastrostomy, 156
Gavage feeding for child, 230
Gene expression, 273-274
General adaptation syndrome, 65
General anesthesia, 297-304
  agents for, 298-303
  neuromuscular blocking agent with, 303-304
  stages of, 297-298
  status asthmaticus and, 673
General inhibition syndrome, 65
Genitourinary system
  injury to, 1083-1084
  pregnancy and, 248-249
Gentamicin
  for burn wound, 1161
  renal failure and, 907
Geriatrics, 271-292; *see also* Elderly patient
Gland; *see also* Endocrine system
  pituitary; *see* Pituitary gland
  salivary, 919-920
  thyroid; *see* Thyroid *entries*
Glasgow Coma Scale
  burn injury and, 1156
  in child, 225
  head injury and, 1063
  in neurologic assessment, 765
Glimepiride, 1004
Glipizide, 1004
Global aphasia, 811
Globulin, thyroxine-binding
  drugs affecting, 999
  myxedema and, 1041
Glomerular filtration rate, 853-854
  age-related changes in, 279-280
  aging and, 276
  blood pressure and, 855
  pregnancy and, 248-249, 250
  tubular necrosis and, 879
Glomerulus
  reabsortion and, 853
  structure and function of, 850-851
  vascular anatomy of, 850
Glossopharyngeal nerve, 745
Glottis, 1150
Glove, burn injury and, 1156

Glucagon
  action of, 980
  function of, 981
  hyperglycemic hyperosmolar nonketotic syndrome and, 1016
  ketoacidosis, 1006
  physiologic stress and, 123
Glucocorticoid
  myxedema and, 1041
  physiologic stress and, 124
Gluconeogenesis, 121
  definition of, 980
  insulin and, 981
  ketoacidosis and, 1007
  protein metabolism and, 122
Glucose
  burn injury and, 1156
  carbohydrate metabolism and, 121
  corticosteroid and, 137
  glucagon and, 981
  hyperglycemia and, 151
  hyperglycemic hyperosmolar nonketotic syndrome and, 1015-1021
  hypoglycemia and, 151-152
  insulin production and, 979
  ketoacidosis and, 1006, 1008, 1009
    insulin and, 1012
  multiple organ dysfunction syndrome and, 1134-1135
  pancreatic assessment and, 990-991
  physiologic stress and, 123
  renal disorder and, 140
  septic shock and, 1113, 1114
  in urine, 875
Glucose intolerance, 157
Glucose oligosaccharide, 149
Glutamate, 286
Glutamide, 834
Glutamine, 155
Glyburide, 1004
Glycogen, 928
Glycogenolysis, 981
Glycopyrrolate, 307
Glycosuria, 249
Glycosylated hemoglobin, 991-992
Gonad, stress response of, 1002
Gonadotropin, human chorionic, 246
Good Samaritan laws, 40
Gown, burn injury and, 1156
Graft
  accelerated atherosclerosis of, 1184
  arteriovenous, 887-888
  burn injury and, 1159
  for burn wound, 1161-1163
  coronary artery bypass, 541-542
  rejection of, 1175-1176
Grand mal seizure, 767
Granulocyte, burn injury and, 1158
Gravity, ventilation/perfusion relationships and, 618-619, 620
Gray matter, 758
Grey Turner's sign, 952, 1079
Grief
  anticipatory, 81
  cultural differences in, 799-800
Growth hormone, 748
  nutrition therapy and, 162
  sleep and, 104
Guanethidine, 1035
Guided imagery in pain management, 186
Guillain Barré syndrome, 812-814
Guilt of parents of ill child, 236
Gunshot wound, 1051-1052
  in child, 228
  thoracic, 1073-1074

H

Halo traction, 87-88, 1069, 1071
Haloperidol
  anesthesia with, 302
  for delirium, 76
  sedation with, 194
Halothane
  effects of, 301
  vomiting and, 323
Hamman's sign, 675
Hancock II aortic valve, 544
Hand vein, 866
Hand-washing, burn injury and, 1156
Haustral segmentation, 923-924
HCO_3^-; *see* Bicarbonate ion
Head and neck examination in elderly, 288
Head injury, 1057-1064
  assessment of, 1063-1064
  in child, 225, 227-228
  classification of, 1059-1063
  high-dose barbiturate therapy and, 832
  management of, 1064
  mechanism of, 1057
  nursing diagnosis and management, 1064, 1065
  nutrition intervention and, 137
  pathophysiology of, 1057, 1059
  temperature fluctuation and, 829
Head up–tilt table test, 441-444
Headache, apnea and, 112
Healing, wound, 1088
  burn, 1160-1161
Health care energy, 24
Health system management, 10
Hearing, 288
Heart; *see also* Cardiovascular *entries*; Coronary *entries*; Myocardial *entries*; Myocardium
  age-related changes in, 272-276
    baroreceptor, 274-275
    exercise and, 275
    functional, 272-275
    hemodynamics and, 274
    morphologic, 272
    myocardial gene expression and, 273-274
  anatomy of, 331-336
    chambers of, 332-333
    conduction system of, 334-336
    layers of, 331-332
    structures of, 331
    valves of, 333-334
  auscultation of, 367
  blood supply of, 336-337
  dysrhythmia of; *see* Dysrhythmia
  high-dose barbiturate therapy and, 832
  injury of, 1077-1079
  mechanical ventilation and, 706
  myocardial infarction and, 490-501; *see also* Myocardial infarction
  myxedema and, 1041
Heart—cont'd
  pneumopericardium and, 676
  postanesthesia period and, 315-316
  pregnancy and, 247
  renal function and, 867
  shock and, 1098
  surgery on, 541-550; *see also* Cardiac surgery
  thyrotoxic crisis and, 1037
  transplantation of, 1179-1184
    case study of, 1209-1211
  trauma to, 1077-1079
  valvular disease of; *see* Cardiac valve
Heart block
  myocardial infarction and, 497
  nursing management and, 593
  pacemaker for, 529, 533; *see also* Pacemaker, cardiac
Heart defect, congenital, 219
Heart failure, 502-507
  chest radiography and, 388
  in child, 219, 221
  clinical findings in, 373-374
  complications of, 504
  description of, 502
  diagnosis of, 502-504
  management of, 505-507
  mechanical circulatory assist device for, 567-574
    intraaortic balloon pump as, 567-571
    ventricular, 571-574
  multiple organ dysfunction syndrome and, 1130
  nutrition intervention for, 129
    patient teaching about, 133
  pathophysiology of, 502
  pulmonary artery pressure and, 462
Heart murmur
  characteristics of, 369-371
  pregnancy and, 247
Heart rate
  age-related changes in, 274
  cardiac surgery and, 545-546
  in child, 218
  electrocardiography and, 406
  fetal, 247
  nursing management and, 593-594
  shock and, 1097
Heart sounds
  characteristics of, 367-368
  pregnancy and, 247
  renal function and, 867
Heart transplantation
  psychosocial alterations and, 84
  stress on spouse and, 568
Heartbeat, regulation of, 351-353
Heat injury; *see* Burn injury
Height, 125
Heimlich valve, 675
Helicobacter pylori, 945
Heliox, status asthmaticus and, 673
HELLP syndrome, 71
  definition of, 255
  management of, 256-258
Helper T cell, 1173-1175
Helplessness, learned, 72
Hematemesis, 948
Hematochezia, 948

Hematocrit
 hyperglycemic hyperosmolar nonketotic syndrome and, 1018
 obstructive sleep apnea and, 112
Hematoimmune alteration, 152-155
Hematologic disorder, 258-259
Hematologic studies
 cardiovascular alteration and, 382
Hematologic system
 liver and, 928
 nutrition assessment and, 127
Hematoma
 angioplasty and, 555
 epidural, 738, 1060
 intracerebral, 1062
 subdural, 1060-1062
Hematuria, 875
Hemianopia, homonymous, 810
Hemiblock, cardiac, 405
Hemipelvis fracture dislocation, Malgaigne's, 1085
Hemisphere, cerebral, 749-750
 cerebrovascular accident and, 802, 809-811
Hemoconcentration, 1016
Hemocystine, 484
Hemodialysis; *see also* Dialysis
 continuous arteriovenous, 897-898
 continuous venovenous, 898-899
 drugs affected by, 906-910
 intermittent, 899
 procedure for, 890-893
 protein and, 140
Hemodilution therapy, hypervolemic, hypertensive, 807
Hemodynamic monitoring, nursing interventions for, 445
Hemodynamic profile, 471, 472-473, 477-478
Hemodynamics
 age-related changes in, 274
 anaphylactic shock and, 1108
 aspiration lung disorder and, 668
 bedside monitoring of, 442-444
 cardiogenic shock and, 1103
 of child, 216-217
 coronary artery disease and, 485
 hypovolemic shock and, 1101
 liver and
  injury to, 1083
  liver failure and, 964
  transplant of, 1195
 in perianesthesia assessment, 306
 in postanesthesia period, 310-311
  dysrhythmia and, 316
 pregnancy and, 249
 pulmonary embolism and, 669
 renal failure and, 880, 882
 renal function and, 870-871
 thyrotoxic crisis and, 1037
Hemofiltration, arteriovenous
 continuous, 897
 protein and, 140
Hemoglobin
 abnormality of, 622
 alveolar-capillary membrane and, 611
 burn injury and, 1155
 fetal, 245
 glycosylated, 991-992
 oxygen saturation and, 643
Hemoglobin—cont'd
 renal function and, 873
 shock and, 1099
 venous oxygen saturation and, 474
Hemoglobinuria, electrical burn, 1151
Hemolysis, in HELLP syndrome, 256
Hemorrhage; *see* Bleeding
Hemorrhagic shock; *see* Shock
Hemostasis
 gastrointestinal bleeding and, 949
 thrombolytic therapy and, 563
Hemothorax, 1077
Henderson-Hasselbalch equation, 969
Henle's loop, 849, 852
Heparin
 bedside hemodynamic monitoring and, 442
 coronary stent and, 557
 deep vein thrombosis and, 522
 hemodialysis and, 891
 myocardial infarction and, 499
 pulmonary embolism and, 670
Hepatic coma, 793
Hepatic congestion, 941
Hepatic disorder; *see* Liver
Hepatic encephalopathy, 963, 964
Hepatitis
 clinical findings in, 941
 multiple organ dysfunction syndrome and, 1128
Hepatocellular necrosis, 962-965
Hering-Breuer reflex, 618
Hernia
 peritoneal dialysis and, 904
 strangulated, 941
Herniated disk, 756
Herniation
 brainstem, 788
 diaphragmatic, 1075
 intracerebral, 832-834
Hetastarch
 for renal failure, 884
 renal failure and, 883
Hexaxial reference system, 395
High density lipoprotein, 276
 characteristics of, 384
 coronary artery disease and, 484
High-frequency ventilation ventilation, 708
High-nitrogen enteral formula, 157
High-risk obstetrics, 243-268; *see also* Pregnancy
Hind brain, 741, 743, 746
Histamine, pain and, 176
History
 diet, 125-126
 neurologic, 763
 pulmonary, 625-627
 renal function and, 865
Holistic patient-centered care, 66
Home care, parenteral nutrition and, 149
Homeostasis
 hyperglycemic hyperosmolar nonketotic syndrome and, 1018
 shock and, 1097
Homograft for burn wound, 1162-1163
Homonymous hemianopia, 810
Homunculus, 751-752
Hope as coping mechanism, 80
Hopelessness, 72-74
Hormone; *see also* Endocrine *entries*
 antidiuretic; *see* Antidiuretic hormone
Hormone—cont'd
 digestive, 923
  pancreas and, 930
 insulin; *see* Insulin
 neurologic alterations and, 137
 pancreatic, 979-982
 physiologic stress and, 123-124
 pituitary, 748-749, 982-983
 pregnancy and, 246-247
 shock and, 1097
 thyroid; *see* Thyroid *entries*
 thyroid-stimulating; *see* Thyroid-stimulating hormone
Hospital-acquired pneumonia, 663-665
Houston's valve, 925
H_2-receptor antagonist
 dosage and actions of, 971
 gastrointestinal disorder and, 970
 renal failure and, 909
Hum, venous, 933-934
Human chorionic gonadotropin, placenta and, 246
Human immunodeficiency virus infection
 blood shield statutes and, 516
 nutrition and, 152-155
 Pneumocystis carinii pneumonia and, 664
Human leukocyte antigen, 1171-1172
Human placental lactogen, 246
Humidification
 artificial airway and, 695, 699
 for oxygen therapy, 691
 upper airway and, 604-605
Humoral immunity, 1172
Humoral-mediated immunity, 286
Hunger center, 748
Hyaline membrane, 661-662
Hydralazine, 258
Hydration
 antidiuretic hormone disorder and, 1031
 cerebral angiography and, 781
 in evaluation of nutrition support, 165
 ketoacidosis and, 1009, 1011
  skin assessment for, 1014
 pituitary assessment and, 992
Hydrocephalus, 807
Hydrocolloid dressing, 1165
Hydrofluoric acid, 1150
Hydromorphone
 dosage and action of, 183
 for pain, 181
Hydrophilic drug, 184
Hydrostatic pressure, 858
 tubular necrosis and, 878-879
Hydrotherapy for burn injury, 1170
Hyperbilirubinemia, 1128
Hypercalcemia
 cardiovascular alteration and, 380
 renal failure and, 881
Hypercapnia
 obstructive sleep apnea and, 111
 trauma patient and, 1059
Hypercarbia, 315
Hyperchloremia, 882
Hypercholesterolemia, 141; *see also* Cholesterol
Hyperextension, spinal, 1065
Hyperflexion, spinal, 1065
Hyperglycemia
 clinical manifestations of, 1012

Hyperglycemia—cont'd
insulin and, 981
ketoacidosis and, 1003, 1006-1007; *see also* Ketoacidosis
neurologic alteration and, 137
nutrition and, 151
parenteral nutrition and, 163
physiologic stress and, 124
somatostatin and, 981
Hyperglycemic hyperosmolar nonketotic syndrome
coma and, 151
description of, 1015-1016
diagnosis of, 1018-1019
etiology of, 978, 1015-1016
management of, 1019-1021
pathophysiology of, 1016-1018
Hyperkalemia
burn injury and, 1154-1155
cardiovascular alteration and, 377, 378
ketoacidosis and, 1009, 1013
renal failure and, 881, 885, 886
Hyperlipidemia, 484
Hypermagnesemia, 882
Hypermetabolism, 124
multiple organ failure and, 1124-1125
septic shock and, 1113
systemic inflammatory response syndrome and, 1129-1130
trauma and, 1087
Hypernatremia
osmotic diuretic and, 831
renal failure and, 881
Hyperosmolality, 1016
Hyperosmolar nonketotic coma, hyperglycemic, 151
Hyperoxaluria, 148
Hyperoxia, 691-692
Hyperphosphatemia, 882, 886
Hyperpnea, 618
Hyperreflexia, 1033
Hypersensitivity reaction, anaphylactic, 1105-1109
Hypersensitivity to pain, 169-170
Hypertension
aortic dissection and, 517
autonomic dysreflexia and, 1066
coronary artery disease and, 484
diabetes and, 151
intracranial; *see* Intracranial pressure
intracranial hemorrhage and, 808
neurologic assessment and, 773
nutrition intervention for, 128
patient teaching about, 131, 133
obstructive sleep apnea and, 111
postoperative, 316-317
in pregnancy, 255-258
pulmonary, 612
pregnancy and, 253
pulmonary embolism and, 670
in respiratory distress syndrome, 661-662
trauma patient and, 1059
Hypertensive, hypervolemic, hemodilution therapy, 807
Hypertensive crisis, 523-525
coma and, 792
Hypertensive encephalopathy, 792
Hyperthermia
malignant, management of, 325-326
postoperative, 318-319
thyrotoxic crisis and, 1036-1037
Hyperthyroidism
assessment of, 996
atrial fibrillation and, 414
diagnosis of, 996
etiology of, 979
hypothyroidism versus, 1039
patient history for, 997
thyrotoxic crisis and, 1031-1037
Hypertonic fluid, 858
Hypertonic solution, antidiuretic hormone and, 1031
Hypertriglyceridemia, 140-141
Hypertrophic, subaortic stenosis, 507
Hypertrophic cardiomyopathy, 507
Hypertrophic scarring, 1166
Hypertrophy, ventricular, 365
electrocardiography and, 400
heart failure and, 504
Hyperventilation
intracranial hypertension and, 829
pregnancy and, 248
Hypervolemia, 992
Hypervolemic, hypertensive, hemodilution therapy, 807
Hypnotic agent, 107-108
Hypoalbuminemia, 882
Hypocalcemia
cardiovascular alteration and, 380
renal failure and, 881
Hypocarbia, 670
Hypochloremia, 882
Hypodermis, 1141
Hypoglycemia
clinical manifestations of, 1012
hyperglycemic hyperosmolar nonketotic syndrome and, 1019
management of, 1013
nutrition and, 151-152
parenteral nutrition and, 163
Hypoglycemia agent, 1004-1005
Hypokalemia
burn injury and, 1155
cardiovascular alteration and, 377-378
ketoacidosis and, 1013
osmotic diuretic and, 831
renal failure and, 881
Hypomagnesemia
cardiovascular alteration and, 380-381
renal failure and, 882
Hyponatremia
antidiuretic hormone disorder and, 1029, 1030
burn injury and, 1155-1156
emergence delirium and, 322
ketoacidosis and, 1008, 1013
renal failure and, 881, 885, 886
subarachnoid hemorrhage and, 807
Hypoperfusion
gastrointestinal system and, 1128
liver failure and, 963
Hypopharyngeal sphincter, 920
Hypophosphatemia, 882
Hypophysis, 748; *see* Pituitary gland
Hypotension
anaphylaxis and, 1107
Hypotension—cont'd
continuous renal replacement therapy and, 900
delayed arousal from anesthesia and, 322
hypovolemic shock and, 1101
morphine causing, 181
neurologic assessment and, 773
pituitary assessment and, 992
postoperative, 317
pregnancy and, 247
sepsis-induced, 1112
spinal shock and, 1066
trauma patient and, 1059
Hypothalamus, 747
anatomy and physiology of, 982
diabetes insipidus and, 1022
Hypothalamus-pituitary-thyroid axis, 984, 986
Hypothermia
abdominal injury and, 1081
burn injury and, 1158
cardiac surgery and, 547
cardiopulmonary bypass and, 543, 545
intracranial hypertension and, 829
myxedema and, 1040, 1041
neurogenic shock and, 1110
postoperative, 317
management of, 324-325
thyroid hormone and, 1049
Hypothesis, Monro-Kellie, 821
Hypothyroidism
assessment of, 996
clinical manifestations of, 1039
diagnosis of, 995-996
myxedema and
coma and, 979, 1038-1042
diagnosis of, 996
patient history for, 997
patient history for, 997
Hypotonic fluid, 858
Hypoventilation
alveolar, 655, 726
neurologic disorder and, 771
in postanesthesia period, 315
prevention of, 659
Hypovolemia
antidiuretic hormone and, 983
burn injury and, 1156-1157
hyperglycemic hyperosmolar nonketotic syndrome and, 1017-1018
neurogenic shock and, 1110
renal failure and, 880, 882
renal function and, 871
trauma and, 1053
Hypovolemic shock, 1100-1102
in child, 223
pulmonary artery catheter and, 458
Hypoxemia
aspiration lung disorder and, 668
in child, 221-222
obstructive sleep apnea and, 111
partial pressure of arterial oxygen and, 641-642
pneumonia and, 665
in postanesthesia period, 314-315
respiratory failure and, 655, 656, 658
acidosis and, 658
trauma patient and, 1057
Hypoxia
emergence from anesthesia, 322
neurogenic shock and, 1110

Hypoxia—cont'd
pregnancy and, 259
in trauma patient, 1059
Hypoxic vasoconstriction
pulmonary hypertension and, 612
ventilation/perfusion relationships and, 619-620

I

Iatrogenic disorder
pneumonia as, 663-666
pneumothorax as, 674
Ibuprofen
dosage and action of, 183
renal failure and, 909
Ibutilide, 578
Identity change as reaction to illness, 52
Idioventricular rhythm, 420
Ileus, paralytic, burn injury and, 1157
Illness, stages of, 68
Imagery, guided, in pain management, 186
Imipenem, 907
Immobility
Guillain-Barré syndrome and, 813
management of, 10
Immune system
age-related changes in, 286-287
examination for, 291
anaphylaxis and, 1105-1109
gastrointestinal system and, 155
multiple organ dysfunction syndrome and, 1124, 1129
transplantation and, 1171-1179
Immunodeficiency; *see* Human immunodeficiency virus infection
Immunoglobulin
anaphylaxis and, 1105
Guillain Barré syndrome and, 813
Immunosuppression, 1176-1179
heart-lung transplant and, 1186, 1187-1188
liver transplant and, 1197
lung transplant and, 1190
renal transplant and, 1203
Implant
intravascular oxygenation and, 715-716
nuclear magnetic resonance and, 437
pacemaker as, 540
Implantable cardioverter defibrillator, 550-552
Implementation in nursing process, 9-10
Implied consent, 43
Incentive spirometry
respiratory failure and, 659
thoracic surgery and, 680-681
Independent lung ventilation, 707
Indeterminate axis, 395
Index
cardiac, 871
oxygen tension, 645-646
pulmonary vascular resistance, 448
right ventricular stroke work, 448
vascular resistance, 447
Indirect calorimetry, 126
Infant; *see also* Child
airway in, 205-206
malnutrition in, 125
Infarction, myocardial; *see also* Myocardial infarction
Infection
blood shield statutes and, 516
burn injury and, 1156
cardiac surgery and, 549
central venous pressure and, 456
continuous renal replacement therapy and, 900
endocarditis and, 508-510
gastrointestinal tract coloniztration and, 155
head injury in child and, 228
heart transplant and, 1184
heart-lung transplant and, 1186-1187
human immunodeficiency virus, 152-155
invasive monitoring device and, 597
liver failure and, 963
mechanical ventilation and, 706
meningitis, coma and, 792-793
missile injury and, 1062
multiple organ dysfunction syndrome and, 1131, 1133
pacemaker and, 539
pancreatic, 959; *see also* Pancreatitis
pelvic fracture and, 1085
peritoneal dialysis and, 904
pneumonia and, 663-667
prevention of, 666-667
renal failure and, 885
respiratory syncytial virus, 212-213
risk factors for, 1119
septic shock and, 1111-1115, 1117
in child, 223-224
splenectomy and, 1083
sputum studies and, 646-657
surveillance for, 1182
tracheostomy tube and, 698
transplant and, immunosuppression and, 1178-1179
trauma and, 1087-1088
urinary tract, in elderly, 287
ventricular assist device and, 574
wound, 1088
Inferior mesenteric artery, 925
Inferior vena cava, 670
Inferior wall myocardial infarction, 493, 494
Inflammation; *see also* Inflammatory response
bronchial, 637
burn injury and, 1158
endocarditis and, 508-510
Guillain Barré syndrome and, 812
multiple organ failure and, 1124; *see also* Multiple organ dysfunction syndrome
pancreatic, 950-952, 957-958
pericardial, myocardial infarction and, 498
pneumonia and, 663-667
respiratory syncytial virus and, 213
Inflammatory bowel disease, 148
Inflammatory response
definition of, 1112
local, 1121-1124
mediators in, 1125-1127
septic shock and, 1111
Informed consent, 42-43
Infratentorial herniation, 834
Infratentorial structure, 737
Infundibular stalk, 982
diabetes insipidus and, 1022
Infusion
opioid, 182
transpyloric feeding and, 149
Ingestion, mastication and, 919
Inhalation
aerosol, 699
respiratory muscles and, 603-604
Inhalation anesthetics, 298-300
Inhalation injury, 1149-1150
Injectate, temperature of, 469
Injury, 39
Inotropic drug, 577-579
cardiogenic shock and, 1104
for child, 221
shock and, 1099
Inservice education, ethical, 31
Inspection
in cardiovascular assessment, 355-360
in gastrointestinal assessment, 931-932
in pulmonary assessment, 627-629
in renal assessment, 866-867
Inspiration, sustained maximal, 309
Inspiratory capacity, 250
Inspiratory muscle
status asthmaticus and, 672
strength of, 648
Inspiratory pressure
bedside measurement of, 648-649
negative, 648-649
Inspiratory reserve volume, 649
age-related changes in, 279
Institutional ethics committee, 31
Insulin
action of, 980
functions of, 979-980
hyperglycemic hyperosmolar nonketotic syndrome and, 1015-1021
ketoacidosis and, 1003, 1006, 1009
nutrition and, 149
pancreatic assessment and, 990
physiologic stress and, 123
septic shock and, 1113
types of, 1010
Insulin pump, 1006
Insulin-dependent diabetes mellitus
characteristics of, 1001; *see also* Diabetes mellitus
nutrition and, 149
Insulin/glucose balance in ketoacidosis, 1012
Insulin-like growth factor, 162
Insurance, 41
Intake and output
pituitary assessment and, 993
renal function and, 869-870
Integumentary system; *see also* Skin
Intentional tort, 36
Intercalated disc, 342
Intercostal muscle of child, 206
Interdisciplinary plan of care, E-1 to E-16, 10, 12-15
Interleukins
age-related changes in, 286
antagonist to, 1137-1138
inflammation and, 1125-1127
Intermediate pituitary, 983
Intermittent claudication, 518
Intermittent hemodialysis, 899
Intermittent mandatory ventilation
in child, 210
synchronized, 662
weaning and, 684, 709

Intermittent mandatory ventilation—cont'd
  synchronous, 707
Intermittent recording system for electrocardiography, 428-429
Internal capsule of diencephalon, 749
Internal carotid artery
  cerebral circulation and, 753
  circle of Willis and, 754
Internal jugular vein, 359
Internal mammary artery graft, 541-542, 544
Inter-Society Commission for Heart Disease pacemaker codes, 532-533
Intervention, nursing, 8-9
  for sleep disturbance, 11
Interventional angiography, neurologic, 782
Intervertebral disk, 755-756, 757
Intestinal obstruction, 963
  management of, 958-962
Intestine
  injury to, 1082
  large, 924-926
  obstruction of, 958-962
  small, anatomy and physiology of, 922-924
Intima, 337-338
Intolerance, lactose, 121
Intoxication, coma and, 792
Intraabdominal pressure, trauma and, 1081
Intraaortic balloon pump, 567-571
  body image disturbance and, 87-88
  cardiogenic shock and, 1104-1105
  chest x-ray and, 386-387
Intraarterial blood pressure monitoring, 444-450
Intracardial pressure, cardiac tamponade and, 1078
Intracellular fluid, 857, 858-859
  magnesium and, 862
Intracerebral hematoma, 1062
Intracoronary stent, 557-559
Intracorporeal/extracorporeal gas exchange, 715-716
Intracranial hemorrhage, 807-808
  delayed arousal from anesthesia and, 321
  in pregnancy, 267
Intracranial pressure
  assessment of, 821-826
  cerebrovascular accident and, 809
  coma and, 793
  contusion and, 1060
  craniotomy and, 816, 818
  head injury and, 1063, 1064
  head injury in child and, 228
  intracranial hemorrhage and, 808
  lumbar puncture and, 788
  management of, 826-832
  rapid neurologic assessment and, 775
  trauma patient and, 1059
Intracranial pressure wave, 824
Intrahepatic portosystemic shunt, transjugular, 949, 968, 969
Intralobular vein of liver, 926-927
Intramucosal pH monitoring, 968-970
Intraoperative mapping, cardiac, 549
Intrapleural pressure, 602-603
Intrapulmonary pressure, 604
Intrapulmonary shunt, 619
  equation for, 645-646
  respiratory failure and, 656
Intrarenal azotemia, 877-878
Intrarenal failure, 883-884
Intraspinal anesthesia, 182
  nursing interventions for, 186
Intrathecal anesthesia, 182, 184
Intrathoracic pressure, 706
Intravascular coagulation, disseminated
  multiple organ dysfunction syndrome and, 1130-1131, 1132, 1133
  pregnancy and, 258-259
  shock and, 1098
Intravascular oxygenation, 715-716
Intravenous access, parenteral nutrition via, 159, 161-162
Intravenous anesthetic, 300-303
Intravenous fluid, trauma patient and, 1055
Intravenous pyelography, 876
Intravenous solution, for renal failure, 884
Intrinsic control of peripheral circulation, 353
Intropin; *see* Dopamine
Intubation
  artificial airway and, 692-703
  facial injury and, 1072
  intestinal obstruction and, 961-962
  nasogastric; *see* Nasogastric intubation
  procedure for, 965-968
  status asthmaticus and, 672
Invasion of privacy, 38
Invasive cardiac monitoring, 552-561
  burn injury and, 1157-1158
  nursing interventions for, 445
  nursing management for, 597
Inverse ratio ventilation, 662, 708
Involuntary nervous system, 733
Iodide, 1033-1034, 1035
Ionized calcium, 378, 861
Ipratropium, 715
Iron
  AIDS and, 153
  gastrointestinal disorder and, 144
  neurologic alterations and, 136
  renal disorder and, 138, 142
Irritant receptor, 618
Ischemia
  acute tubular necrosis and, 878
  cardiogenic shock and, 1102-1105
  cerebrovascular accident and, 800-802, 836
  hepatobiliary, 1128
  myocardial
    clinical findings in, 373-374
    electrocardiography and, 401-402
    infarction and, 491, 492
    intraaortic balloon pump and, 567-569
    nursing management and, 594-595
    pain of, 176
    postanesthesia period and, 316
    ST-segment monitoring and, 399
    ventricular ectopy and, 417
  pain from, 197-199
  silent, coronary artery, 487, 488
Ischemic stroke, 800-802, 836
Islets of Langerhans, 930
Isoetharine, 714
Isoflurane, 301
Isophane insulin, 1010
Isoproterenol
  cardiovascular effects of, 579
  physiologic effects of, 579
Isoproterol, heart transplant and, 1181
Isotonic fluid, 858
  hyperglycemic hyperosmolar nonketotic syndrome and, 1019

J

Jejunostomy, 156
Jejunum, 922
Jet nebulizer, 699
Jet ventilation, 708
Jitteriness in child, 226
Johnston tube, 966
Judgment in mental status examination, 76
Jugular bulb monitor, 823
Jugular vein, cardiovascular assessment and, 357-359
Junction, tight, 739
Junctional dysrhythmia, 414-415
Junctional escape rhythm, 415
Junctional rhythm, accelerated, 415
Justice as ethical principle, 25
Juxtaglomerular apparatus, 855
Juxtamedullary nephron, 850
  loop of Henle and, 852

K

Kallikrein, 951
Kallikrein-kinin system, 1122
K-complex, 103
Kerley lines, 388
Ketamine
  anesthesia with, 302
  cardiac effects of, 316
Ketoacid, 122
Ketoacidosis
  description of, 1003
  diagnosis of, 1008-1009
  etiology of, 978, 1006
  hyperglycemic hyperosmolar nonketotic syndrome versus, 1016
  management of, 1009, 1011-1015
  nutrition and, 151
  pathophysiology of, 1006-1008
  pregnancy and, 262
Ketoconazole
  nutrition-related effects of, 154
  renal failure and, 908
Ketone
  lipid metabolism and, 123
  testing for, 991
Ketonemia, 980
Ketonuria, 980
Ketorolac, 183
Ketosis, insulin and, 981
Kick, atrial, 332, 348
Kidney; *see also* Renal *entries*
  anatomy of, 849
  function of, 854-856
  percussion of, 868
  transplantation of, 1205-1208
    psychosocial alterations and, 83-84
Kidney-ureter-bladder imaging, 876
Killer cell, natural, 1175
Kinase, inflammation and, 1122
Kinetic therapy bed, 1069
Kinin, inflammation and, 1122
Knee injury, 1086

KUB imaging, 876
Kupffer's cell, 1128
Kussmaul's respiration, 771
  renal failure and, 882
Kwashiorkor, 126

L

Labetalol
  characteristics of, 581, 582
  hypertensive crisis and, 525
  pregnancy and, 258
Labetolol, 908
Labor and delivery, 249-251
Lactate, 834-835
Lactate dehydrogenase
  cardiovascular alteration and, 381-382
  values for, 937
Lactated Ringer's solution
  burn injury and, 1154
  renal failure and, 884
Lactic acidosis, 672
Lactose
  bowel resection and, 148
  intolerance to, 121
Lactulose, 964
Lambert's canals, 608-609
Laminar blood flow, 338-339
Laminectomy, 756
  spinal injury and, 1069
Landmark, thoracic, 361
Landry-Guillain Barré syndrome, 812-814
Language, 810-811
Large intestine; *see* Colon
Laryngospasm
  burn injury and, 1154
  postanesthesia, 313
Larynx
  edema of, 312-313
  of infant, 205, 206
  inhalation injury of, 1150
  stenosis of, 697
Laser angioplasty, 557
Lasix
  elderly patient and, 283
  for renal disorder, 905
Lateralizing sign, 768
Lavage
  aspiration lung disorder and, 668
  gastric, 950
  peritoneal, 1080
Law; *see* Legal issues
  Starling's, 460
Lazaroid, 834
Lead
  electrocardiographic, 389-391, 396-399
  implantable cardioverter defibrillator and, 550, 551
  pacemaker, 530
Leak
  cerebrospinal fluid, 816-817
  subarachnoid hemorrhage and, 804
Learned helplessness, 72
Learning, readiness to, 53
Learning theory, adult, 50
LeFort fracture, 1073
Left anterior descending artery, 541
Left atrial catheter, chest x-ray and, 386
Left atrial pressure, definition of, 447
Left atrial pressure monitoring, 456-457
Left bundle branch, 336
Left bundle branch block, electrocardiography and, 403-404
Left coronary artery, 336
Left heart failure, 503
Left internal mammary artery graft, 542
Left posterior hemiblock, 405
Left ventricle
  age-related changes in, 272, 275
  anatomy of, 332-333
  Starling's law and, 460
  status asthmaticus and, 672
Left ventricular assist device, 571
Left ventricular end-diastolic pressure, 460, 503
Left ventricular end-diastolic volume, 348
Left ventricular hypertrophy, 365
Left ventricular preload, 252
Legal doctrine, 39-41
Legal issues, 35-46
  licensing statutes and, 38
  medical records and, 1018
  negligence and malpractice as, 38-41
  neurologic status as, 776
  nurse practice acts as, 41-42
  overview of, 35-36
  patient care issues and, 42-46
  product liability as, 516
  tort liability as, 36-38
  transplantation as, 1180
Legislation, advanced nursing practice, 267
Leukocyte antigen, human, 1171-1172
Leukotreine, 1127
Level of consciousness; *see* Consciousness
Levothyroxine, 1041
Liability
  corporate, 41
  personal, 40
  products, 516
  theories of, 39-41
  tort, 36-37, 38
  vicarious, 40
Libel, 38
Licensing statute, 38
Lidocaine
  dosage and side effects of, 578
  elderly patient and, 283
  fetal effects of, 254
  intracranial hypertension and, 830
  neurologic disorder and, 835
  renal failure and, 909
Life support
  guidelines for, C-1 to C-12
  in pregnancy, 254-255
  removal of, 785
  trauma, 1052-1056
Ligament, falciform, of liver, 926
Ligation, endoscopic variceal band, 968
Light reflex, pupillary, 769
Light sedation, 190
Limbic lobe, 749, 753
Line, Kerley, 388
Linton tube, 966
Lipase
  pancreatic function and, 937
  pancreatitis and, 952
Lipid
  cardiovascular alteration and, 383-384
  insulin and, 981
  in parenteral nutrition formula for child, 231
Lipid emulsion for parenteral nutrition, 162
Lipid metabolism, 122-123
  cardiovascular alterations and, 131
  renal disorder and, 138
  respiratory disorder and, 133, 135
Lipophilic drug, epidural analgesia and, 184
Lipoprotein
  arteriosclerosis and, 276
  coronary artery disease and, 484
  types of, 383-384
Liquid, aspiration lung disorder and, 667
Liquid ventilation, partial, 716
Liver
  age-related changes in, 280-282, 292
  anatomy of, 926-927
  esophagogastric varices and, 946
  hepatitis and, 941
  injury of, 1081-1082
  lipid metabolism and, 123
  multiple organ dysfunction syndrome and, 1128-1130, 1129
  scan of, 939
  transplantation of, 1191-1199
    case study of, 1211-1213
    indications for, 1191-1194
    nutrition and, 147
    postoperative care for, 1195-1199
    procedure for, 1194-1195
    screening for, 965
Liver failure
  enteral formulas for, 157
  fulminant, 962-965
  nutrition intervention in, 143, 145
Liver function test, 937
  cardiovascular alteration and, 381
Living will, 1104
Lobe
  cerebral, 749-753
  of liver, 926, 927
  of lung, 601
Lobectomy, lung, 678
  postoperative management of, 680
Local anesthetic, 316
Local inflammatory response, 1121-1124
Locked-in state, 796
Long QT syndrome, 394-395
Loop diuretic
  intracranial hypertension and, 831-832
  neurologic disorder and, 835
  for renal disorder, 905
Loop of Henle, 849, 852
  reabsortion and, 853
Lorazepam
  anesthesia with, 303
  for delirium, 76
  sedation with, 194
Loss of consciousness; *see* Consciousness
Low density lipoprotein, 276
  characteristics of, 383-384
Lower airway
  of infant, 206
  inhalation injury of, 1150
Lower extremity
  cardiovascular assessment and, 357, 362

Lower extremity—cont'd
  injury to, 1086-1087
Lumbar puncture, 787-788
Lumen of pulmonary artery catheter, 465
Lund-Browder method of estimating burn injury, 1143
Lung; *see also* Pneumothorax; Pulmonary *entries*; Respiratory *entries*
  anatomy of, 601
  chest radiography and, 651
  circulation in, 612
  injury of, 1075-1077
  oxygen toxicity and, 692
  percussion of, 630
  renal function and, 867
  surgery on, 677-681
  transplantation of, 1188-1190
Lung transplantation, 1188-1190
Lung volume
  age-related changes in, 279
  bedside measurement of, 648
  definitions of, 649
Luschka's foramen, 738
Luteinizing hormone, 748
Lymphatic system
  pulmonary, 611-612
  of small intestine, 923
Lymphocyte
  immune system and, 1172-1175
  inflammation and, 1126
Lypressin, diabetes insipidus and, 1026
Lysis of clot, 1132
Lytic agent, 499; *see also* Thrombolytic therapy

M

Macrophage
  alveolar, 610
  function of, 1175
  inflammation and, 1125-1126
Mafenide acetate, 1161
Magnesium
  cardiovascular alteration and, 380-381
  cardiovascular system and, 577
  gastrointestinal disorder and, 144
  HELLP syndrome and, 257
  renal system and, 862, 882
  status asthmaticus and, 673
  supraventricular tachycardia and, 414
Magnetic resonance imaging
  cerebrovascular accident and, 801
  head injury and, 1064
  neurologic, 780-781
  pituitary gland and, 995
  renal, 876
Main-stem bronchus, 605-606
Major depression, 77
Major histocompatibility complex, 1171
Malformation, arteriovenous
  subarachnoid hemorrhage and, 802, 803-804
  surgery for, 806
Malgaigne's hemipelvis fracture dislocation, 1085
Malignancy
  AIDS and, 152
  antidiuretic hormone and, 1028
  brain, 780
    coma and, 791-792
    craniotomy for, 814-818
Malignancy—cont'd
  pain of, deafferentation, 176
  pulmonary embolism and, 669
Malignant hyperthermia, 319-321
  management of, 325-326
Malnutrition; *see also* Nutritional support
  cardiac cachexia and, 129-130
  in elderly, 287
  endocrine alteration and, 149
  immune system and, 287
  protein-calorie, 123
    causes of, 124
    clinical manifestations of, 126
  respiratory alterations and, 133
  significance of, 124
Malpractice, 37, 38-41
Mammary artery graft, 541-542, 544
Managing variances, 15
Mandatory ventilation, synchronized intermittent, 662
  weaning and, 684, 709
Mannitol
  electrical burn and, 1151
  intracranial hypertension and, 831
  neurologic disorder and, 835
  for renal disorder, 905
Manometry, 936
Marasmus, 126
Marfan's syndrome, 253
Mask, oxygen, 690-691
  for child, 208
  for sleep apnea
    central, 114
    obstructive, 112-113
Mast cell, 1125
Master's two-step exercise test, 429-430
Mastication, 919
Maturation phase in burn injury, 1159
Mature minor, 43
Maxillofacial injury, 1071-1073
Maximal expiratory pressure, 648-649
Maze procedure for dysrhythmia, 549
Mazicon; *see* Flumazenil
Mean arterial pressure, 340
  continuous renal replacement therapy and, 893-894
  definition of, 447
  intracranial pressure and, 822
  renal function and, 871
Mean pulmonary artery pressure, 463
Mean vector, 395
Mechanical cardiac valve, 543, 544, 545
Mechanical circulatory assist device, 567-574
  intraaortic balloon pump as, 567-571
  ventricular, 571-574
Mechanical ventilation
  in child, 209-211
  drug therapy with, 713-715
  heart-lung transplant and, 1186
  interaction between nurse and patient, 711
  invasive, 703-710
  long-term, 681-686
    description of, 681
    psychologic factors in, 681
    weaning from, 681-686
  modes of, 707-708
  noninvasive, 710-713
  nursing management plan for, 724-725
Mechanical ventilation—cont'd
  respiratory distress syndrome and, 662
  respiratory failure and, 658
  septic shock and, 1115
  spinal injury and, 1071
  status asthmaticus and, 672-673
  weaning from, 681-686, 706, 708-709
Mechanics of breathing, 648
Medial longitudinal fasciculus, 770
Mediastinal bleeding, postoperative, 547
Mediastinal drainage tube, 386
Mediastinal shift, 680
Mediastinum
  anatomy of, 601-602
  chest radiography and, 650
Mediator
  inflammatory, 1121
  multiple organ dysfunction syndrome and, 1125
  in septic shock, 1111-1112
Medical futility, 25-26
Medical practice, 42
Medical record, legal issues of, 1018
Medication card, format for, 58
Medication management, 10
Medium-chain triglyceride
  bowel resection and, 148
  hepatic failure and, 146
Medulla oblongata, 740
Melanocyte-stimulating hormone, 748
Melena, 948
Membrane
  alveolar-capillary, 611
    diffusion and, 618
  amniotic, 261-262
  arachnoid, 738, 756, 758
  basement, glomerular, 851
  capillary, 660
  cardiac cell, 342
  fluid compartment and, 856-857
  placental, 244-245
Memory, mental status and, 75-76
Meningeal artery, middle, 753
Meninges
  of brain, 737
  spinal, 756-758
Meningitis
  in child, 226-227
  coma and, 792-793
Meningococcal infection
  in child, 227
  coma and, 792-793
Mental status; *see also* Neurologic assessment
  changes in, 74-77
  craniotomy and, 818
  examination for, 75-76
  hypovolemic shock and, 1101
  ketoacidosis and, 1015
  myxedema and, 1042
  pain assessment and, 178-179
  renal failure and, 883
  renal function and, 871-872
  sleep deprivation and, 109-110
Meperidine
  cardiac effects of, 315-316
  dosage and action of, 183
  elderly patient and, 284
  for pain, 181
  renal failure and, 909

Mercury central venous pressure, 455
Mesenteric artery, 925
Meshed autograft, 1162
Messenger RNA, 272-273
Metabolic acidosis, 644
Metabolic alkalosis, 644
Metabolic disorder
  coma and, 792, 793
  liver failure and, 963
  respiratory patterns in, 771
  septic shock and, 1113
  thyrotoxic crisis and, 1032
  trauma and, 1087
  ventricular tachycardia and, 417
Metabolic response to injury, 1129-1130
Metabolic waste, 855
Metabolism
  bone, 861
  drug, 281
  intracranial pressure and, 822, 823
  myxedema and, 1038-1039
  nutrient, 121-124
  shock and, 1098
Metabolite, arachidonic acid, 1127
Metallic implant, 437
Metaproterenol, 714
Metformin, 1004
Methaqualone, 108
Methemoglobin, 622
Methimazole, 1033, 1035
Methylprednisolone
  heart transplant and, 1183
  spinal injury and, 1068
Methylxanthine, 905
Metoprolol, 908
Mezlocillin, 907
Microcirculation, 340
Microglia, 735
Microshock from pacemaker, 539
Microstructure of nervous system, 733-734
Midazolam
  anesthesia with, 303
  renal failure and, 909
  sedation with
    characteristics of, 194
    conscious, 193
    light, 190
  sleep and, 108
Midbrain, 740
Middle cerebral artery, 753
Middle meningeal artery, 737-738, 753
Miglitol, 1005
Miller-Abbott tube, 966
Milrinone, 579
Mind/body interactions, 64-65
Mineral, renal failure and, 143
Mineral deficiency, 126
  gastrointestinal alterations and, 149
Mineralocorticoid, 124
Minimal leak cuff-inflation technique, 700-701
Minimal occlusion volume cuff-inflation technique, 700-701
Minimally invasive bypass surgery, 549-550
Minnesota tube, 966
Minor, consent and, 43
Missed injury, 1090-1091
Missile injury, head, 1062
Mitochondria, 342
Mitral regurgitation, 542-543
  pulmonary artery pressure and, 462
Mitral valve, 333-334
  stenosis of, 252, 511, 512
    pulmonary artery pressure and, 462
Mixed valvular disease, 513
Mixed venous oxygen saturation, 471, 474-480
  partial pressure of arterial, 1114
M-mode echocardiography, 431
Mobility
  burn and, 1168-1169
  cardiomyopathy and, 508
  cardiovascular alteration and, 597
  Guillain Barré syndrome and, 813
  postanesthesia, 309
  spinal injury and, 1071
Mobitz type atrioventricular block, 424-427, 593
Moderate partial-thickness burn, 1145
Monitoring
  asthma and, 215
  cardiac, 396
  central venous pressure; *see* Central venous *entries*
  of intracranial pressure, 823
  intramucosal pH, 968-970
  jugular bulb, 823
  pulmonary, 653-654
  pulmonary artery pressure; *see* Pulmonary artery *entries*
Monoamine system, 175-176
Monocyte
  function of, 1175
  inflammation and, 1125
Monoglyceride, 122
Monro-Kellie hypothesis, 821
Monro's foramen, 738
Mood in mental status examination, 75
Moral, 19
Morphine
  dosage and action of, 183
  elderly patient and, 284
  heart failure and, 505
  myocardial infarction and, 499
  pain and, 180-181
    in child, 231-232
  sleep and, 108
Mortality; *see* Death
Motilin, 923
Motility
  colonic, 926
  esophageal, 280
  gastric, 922
  intestinal, 923-924
    in evaluation of nutrition support, 165
Motor aphasia, 811
Motor function, 765-769
  rapid, 777
Motor nerve fiber, 733
Motor speech center, 810
Motor strength, 768
Motor stroke, pure, 802
Motor vehicle accident
  abdominal trauma and, 1079
  orthopedic injury from, 1086
  respiratory failure and, 1088
  rupture of diaphragm and, 1074-1075
  thoracic injury and, 1073
Motor-strip function of cerebrum, 751-752
Mouth care
  ketoacidosis and, 1014
  postanesthesia, 312
Movement; *see also* Activity; Mobility
  levels of, 766-767
  of water, 858-859
Mucin, 280
Mucociliary escalator, 606
Mucolytic
  mechanical ventilation and, 714
  respiratory failure and, 658
Mucosa
  endotracheal intubation and, 696
  gastric, 921-922
    age-related changes in, 280
  intestinal, 923
    ulcer and, 945
Mucus, of colon, 925
Multifocal atrial tachycardia, 411, 412
Multiple organ dysfunction syndrome
  acute respiratory distress and, 660
  cardiovascular dysfunction in, 1130
  coagulation dysfunction in, 1130-1131, 1132-1135
  continuous renal replacement therapy and, 899
  definition of, 1112
  drug therapy for, 1135, 1137-1138
  gastrointestinal dysfunction in, 1128
  hepatobiliary dysfunction in, 1128-1130
  management of, 1131, 1133
  pathophysiology of, 1125-1127
  pulmonary artery catheter and, 458
  pulmonary dysfunction in, 1130
  renal dysfunction in, 1130
  shock and, 1097, 1098
  systemic inflammatory response syndrome and, 1123-1124
  trauma and, 1091
Multivisceral injury, 1080-1081
Murmur, heart
  characteristics of, 369-371
  pregnancy and, 247
Muromonab-CD3, 1176-1177
Muscle
  of colon, 925
  intercostal, of child, 206
  malignant hyperthermia and, 320
  myoglobinuria and, 1089-1090
  neuromuscular blocking agent and, 303-304
  respiratory
    age-related changes in, 277
    anatomy of, 603-604
    asthma and, 215
    of child, 206
    status asthmaticus and, 672
    strength of, 648-649
Muscle relaxant
  as vasodilator, 580, 581
  vomiting and, 323
Muscle-stretch reflex, 768
Muscular pain, 197-199
Musculoskeletal system, 289
Music therapy in pain management, 187, 1148
Mutism, akinetic, 797
Myasthenia gravis, 267-268
Mycophenolate mofentil, 1177, 1178
Myelin, 734
  Guillain Barré syndrome and, 812

Myelinated nerve fiber, 734
Myelography, 782-784
Myocardial cell, electrical activity of, 344-346
Myocardial depressant factor, 1098
Myocardial fiber, 346
Myocardial gene expression, 273-274
Myocardial infarction, 490-501
  cardiogenic shock and, 1102-1105
  clinical findings in, 373-374
  description of, 490
  dysrhythmia and, 496-497
  education about, 500-501
  electrocardiography and, 401-403
  enzymes and, 381-382
  etiology of, 490-491
  management of, 498-500
  mitral valve regurgitation and, 513
  murmurs associated with, 371
  nutrition intervention for, 128
    patient teaching about, 130
  pain of, 176
  pathophysiology of, 491-496
  pregnancy and, 253
  prevention of, 489
  structural complications after, 497-498
  ST-segment monitoring and, 399
  thrombolytic therapy after, 561-567; *see also* Thrombolytic therapy
Myocardial ischemia
  clinical findings in, 373-374
  nursing management and, 594-595
  postanesthesia period and, 316
  ST-segment monitoring and, 399
Myocardium
  age-related changes in, 272-274
  anatomy of, 331-332
  bypass surgery and, 541-542
  calcium and, 380
  contusion of, 1078-1079
  heart transplantation and, 1181
  high-dose barbiturate therapy and, 832
  multiple organ dysfunction syndrome and, 1130
  myxedema and, 1039-1040
  pulmonary artery pressure monitoring and, 461-462
  supply/demand balance in
    coronary artery disease and, 488-489
    myocardial infarction and, 500
Myofibril, 342
Myofibroblast, burn injury and, 1158-1159
Myoglobin
  burn injury and, 1156
    electrical, 1151
  trauma and, 1089-1090
  urine and, 874, 875
Myosin filament, 342
Myosin heavy chain, 273
Myxedema
  diagnosis of, 996
  patient history for, 997
Myxedema coma, 979, 1038-1042
  clinical manifestations of, 1039

N

Nadolol, 908
Nafcillin, 907
Nailbed, 357
Na^+-K^+-ATPase pump, 350-351
Naloxone
  opioid anesthesia and, 301-302
  patient-controlled analgesia and, 182
  in postanesthesia period, 315
  respiratory depression and, 180
  sedation and, 195
NANDA taxonomy, 5
Narcotic; *see* Opioid
Narrow QRS complex, 422
Nasal cannula, 690
Nasal continuous positive airway pressure, 112
Nasal injury, from intubation, 696
Nasal mask for apnea, 112-113, 114
Nasoduodenal tube, 156
Nasogastric intubation
  abdominal injury and, 1080
  aspiration and, 706
  burn injury and, 1147-1148
  facial injury and, 1072
  intestinal obstruction and, 961-962
  procedure for, 965-966
Nasogastric tonometer, 968-969
Nasojejunal tube, 156
Nasopharyngeal artificial airway, 692-693
Nasotracheal intubation, of child, 208-209
NASPE/BPEG generic code, 534
National Cholesterol Education Program, 130
Natriuretic peptide, atrial, 352-353, 859-860
Natural killer cell, 1175
Nausea and vomiting; *see* Vomiting
Nebulizer, 699
Neck
  in cardiovascular assessment, 357-358
  in elderly, 288
Necrosis
  hepatocellular, 962-965
  tubular, 878-879
Negative inspiratory pressure, 648-649
Negative-pressure ventilator, 703
Negligence, 37, 38-41
Neomycin, 964
Neostigmine
  as neuromuscular blocking antagonist, 304, 307
  vomiting and, 323
Nephrogenic diabetes insipidus, 1022
Nephron
  age-related changes in, 279-280
  loop of Henle and, 852
  structure and function of, 850
  urine formation and, 852-853
Nerve, cranial
  function of, 742-746
  Guillain Barré syndrome and, 812
  pons and, 740
Nerve fiber, 733
  age-related changes in, 285
Nerve stimulation, transcutaneous electrical, 184-185
Nerve stimulator, peripheral, 713
Nervous system; *see also* Brain; Neurologic *entries*
  age-related changes in, 282, 285-286, 292
    examination for, 290-291
  anatomy of, 733-761
    basal ganglia and, 749
    brain and, 736-754; *see also* Brain, anatomy of
Nervous system—cont'd
  anatomy of—cont'd
    brainstem and, 740
    cerebellum and, 741-743, 746
    cerebrum and, 749-754; *see also* Cerebrum
    cranial protective mechanisms and, 736-740
    diencephalon and, 746-749
    divisions and, 733
    microstructural, 733-736
    reticular formation and, 741
    spinal cord and, 754-762; *see also* Spinal cord
  antidiuretic hormone disorder and, 1030-1031
  central sleep apnea and, 113
  of child, 224-228
  colon and, 925-926
  emergence delirium and, 322
  glucose and, 980
  heartbeat regulation and, 351-353
  hypertensive crisis and, 523-524
  multiple organ dysfunction syndrome and, 1129
  myxedema and, 1040
  neurologic injury in pregnancy, 265
  pain and, 169-176; *see also* Pain
  in perianesthesia assessment, 306
  postanesthesia period and, 321-322
  REM sleep and, 104-105
  renal innervation and, 852
  respiratory failure and, 657
  septic shock and, 1112-1113
  shock and, 1097
  small intestine and, 923
  sympathetic; *see* Sympathetic nervous system
  thyrotoxic crisis and, 1034
  ventilation regulation and, 615-616
Neurocardiogenic syncope, 441
Neuroendocrine control, 982
Neurofibrillary body, 282
Neurogenic shock, 1109-1111
Neuroglia, 734
Neuroleptic malignant syndrome, 1112
Neurologic alteration, 791-818; *see also* Nervous system
  anaphylactic shock and, 1108
  antidiuretic hormone disorder and, 1030-1031
  aphasia and, nursing management of, 844-845
  assessment of; *see* Neurologic assessment
  brain death and, 798
  burn injury and, 1156
  cardiac surgery and, 547-548
  case study of, 839, 840-841
  cerebral resuscitation and, 834, 836
  cerebrovascular accident and, 798-811; *see also* Cerebrovascular accident
  coma and, 791-795
    hyperglycemic hyperosmotic nonketotic, 151
    legal issues and, 776
  craniotomy and, 814-818
  decreased adaptive capacity and, 842
  diagnosis of, 779-788
    cerebral blood flow studies in, 784-786
    electrophysiology in, 786-787
    lumbar puncture in, 787-788
    radiography for, 779-784
  drug therapy for, 835
  Guillain Barré syndrome and, 812-814
  hepatic encephalopathy and, 963, 964

Neurologic alteration—cont'd
  herniation syndromes and, 832-834
  hyperglycemic hyperosmolar nonketotic syndrome and, 1020
  hypertensive crisis and, 523-524, 525
  intracranial pressure and, 821-832; *see also* Intracranial pressure
  ketoacidosis and, 1015
  liver failure and, 965
  nursing management of, 839-846
  nutrition interventions for, 135-137
  pelvic fracture and, 1085
  persistent vegetative state and, 795-798
  pituitary assessment and, 993
  postanesthesia period and, 321-322
  in pregnancy, 266-268
    epilepsy and, 266
    intracranial hemorrhage and, 267
    myasthenia gravis and, 267-268
    trauma causing, 265
  renal failure and, 883
  respiratory failure and, 656
  thyrotoxic crisis and, 1034
  tissue perfusion and, 841
  unilateral neglect and, 843-844
Neurologic assessment, 763-777
  antidiuretic hormone disorder and, 1030-1031
  carotid artery disease and, 521
  eye movement in, 769-770
  head injury and, 1064
  history in, 763
  level of consciousness and, 763-765
  liver transplant and, 1196-1197
  motor function in, 765-769
  rapid, 774-775, 777
  respiratory patterns in, 771-772
  spinal injury and, 1068
  thyrotoxic crisis and, 1037
  vital signs in, 772-774
Neuromuscular blocking agent
  anesthesia and, 303-304
  delirium and, 77
  intracranial hypertension and, 829
  mechanical ventilation and, 713, 714
  respiratory failure and, 658
Neuromuscular disorder
  central sleep apnea and, 113
  respiratory failure and, 656
Neuron, 733-734
  age-related changes in, 282
  impulse conduction and, 734-736
Neurosecretory substance, 748
Neurotransmitter, 736
  age-related changes in, 285-286
  false neurotransmitter hypothesis and, 143, 145
  pain and, 172, 174, 175-176
    in child, 231
  sleep and, 105-106
Neurovascular assessment in orthopedic injury, 1087
Neutralizing agent for chemical burn, 1150
Neutrophil, 1175
  in inflammatory response, 1122, 1125
    drugs to inhibit, 1135
Neutrophilic chemotactic factor of anaphylaxis, 1106
Newborn, airway of, 205-206
Nicardipine, 581
Nifedipine
  characteristics of, 581
  elderly patient and, 283
  hypertensive crisis and, 525
  pregnancy and, 258
  renal failure and, 908
Nimodipine
  cerebral vasospasm and, 807
  neurologic disorder and, 835
Nitrate
  chest pain and, 489
  heart failure and, 505
Nitric oxide, respiratory distress syndrome and, 716
Nitrogen
  blood urea
    cardiovascular alteration and, 381
    renal function and, 872
  insulin and, 981
Nitrogen balance
  in nutrition assessment, 127
  protein metabolism and, 122
Nitroglycerin
  angina and, 489, 491
  catheter-related intervention and, 559
  characteristics of, 580
Nitroprusside
  characteristics of, 580, 581
  pregnancy and, 258
Nitrous oxide
  effects of, 301
  postanesthesia period and, 311
  vomiting and, 323
NK cell, 286
Nociception, 172
Nociceptor, postanesthesia period and, 311
Nocturnal dyspnea, paroxysmal, 504
Node
  atrioventricular; *see* Atrioventricular node
  sinoatrial, 334
  sinus, drugs affecting, 578
Node of Ranvier, 734
Nonbarbiturate anesthetic, 302
Nonconducted premature atrial contraction, 409
Nondepolarizing neuromuscular blocking agent, 304
Nonfluent aphasia, 811
Nonketotic coma, hyperosmolar hyperglycemic, 151
Nonmalfeasence, 22
Non–insulin-dependent diabetes mellitus
  case study of, 1003
  characteristics of, 1001, 1003
  nutrition and, 149
Nonopioid analgesic, 181
Nonopioid intravenous anesthetic, 300
Nonpacemaker action potential, 346-348
Non-Q wave myocardial infarction, 491-492
Non-rapid eye movement sleep, 103-104
  recovery sleep and, 110
  sleep deprivation and, 109
Nonrebreathing mask, 690
Nonsteroidal antiinflammatory drug, for pain, 181-182
Nonthermal burn, 1150-1151
Noradrenergic agent, stress and, 189
Norepinephrine
  age-related changes in, 286
Norepinephrine—cont'd
  cardiovascular effects of, 579
  neurologic alterations and, 137
  pain and, 175-176
  physiologic effects of, 579
North American Nursing Diagnosis Association, A-1 to A-2
  taxonomy of, 5
Nosocomial pneumonia, 663-664
  mechanical ventilation and, 706
Noxious stimulus, 766, 767
Nuclear magnetic resonance, 436-438
Nucleotidase, 937
Nucleus propulsus, 756
Nurse
  ethical decision making by, 28-29
  self-insurance and, 41
  stress in, 652
Nurse practice act, 38, 41-42
  nursing diagnosis and, 267
Nursing
  ethics as foundation of, 26
  paradigm of, 66
  role of, 3-4
Nursing diagnosis, 5-7
Nursing ethics committee, 32
Nursing intervention classification taxonomy, B-1 to B-10
Nursing management plan
  for knowledge deficit, 59-60
  for psychosocial alterations in burn patient, 85-100
Nursing process, 4-10
  assessment in, 4-5
  implementation in, 9-10
  nursing diagnosis in, 5-7
  outcome in, 7-8
  planning in, 8-9
Nutrient
  absorption of, 924
  liver and, 928
  metabolism of, 121-124
Nutrition, 121-165
  assessment of, 124-126
  cardiovascular alterations and, 126, 128-133
  endocrine alterations and, 149-152
  enteral, 155-159
    evaluation of, 164
    nursing management of, 141
  gastrointestinal alterations and, 143-149
  heart failure and, 506
  hematimmune alterations and, 152-155
  hunger center and, 748
  immune system and, 287
  neurologic alterations and, 135-137
  nursing management plan for, 165
  nutrient metabolism and, 121-124
  parenteral, 159-162
    complications of, 163
    evaluation of, 162
  pharmacology and, 162
  renal alterations and, 137-143
  respiratory alterations and, 133-135
  undernutrition and, 124
Nutritional support
  burn and, 1168
  Guillain Barré syndrome and, 813-814

Nutritional support—cont'd
multiple organ dysfunction syndrome and, 1134-1135
myxedema and, 1040
renal failure and, 885
respiratory distress syndrome and, 663
respiratory failure and, 659-660
septic shock and, 1115
shock and, 1099
trauma patient and, 1087
Nystagmus, 770
Nystatin
for burn wound, 1161
nutrition-related effects of, 154

O

Obesity
coronary artery disease and, 485
endocrine alterations and, 150-151
neurologic alterations and, 137
respiratory alterations and, 133-135
Obstetrics, 243-268; *see also* Pregnancy
Obstruction
airway
in postanesthesia period, 312
respiratory syncytial virus and, 213
of endotracheal tube, 696
intestinal, 958-962, 963
peritoneal dialysis and, 904
pyloric, 942
of tracheostomy tube, 698
Obstructive apnea, 110-113
in child, 214
Occipital lobe, 752
Occlusion
catheter, 163
of feeding tube, 161
myocardial infarction and, 490
peripheral vascular disease and, 518
Oculocephalic reflex, 770, 772
Oculomotor nerve, 743
neurologic assessment and, 769
Oculovestibular reflex, 770, 773
Oddi's sphincter, 929
OKT3, 1176-1177
heart transplant and, 1183-1184
Olfactory nerve, 742
Oligodendrolia, 735
Oliguria
burn injury and, 1156
HELLP syndrome in pregnancy and, 257
multiple organ dysfunction syndrome and, 1130
tubular necrosis and, 879
Omeprazole, 971
Open heart surgery, 541-550
Open pneumothorax, 1076-1077
Open wound care, 1160
Opiate receptor, 174, 175
Opioid
adjunctive, 304
in child, 232
delirium and, 76
elderly patient and, 284
endogenous, 174
as intravenous anesthetic, 300-303
nonsteroidal antiinflammatory drugs with, 181-182
Opioid—cont'd
pain and, in child, 231-232, 232
postanesthesia period and, 311
thoracic surgery and, 681
Optic chiasm, 810
Optic nerve, 742
Oral breathing of infant, 205
Oral contraceptive, 485
Oral nutrition; *see also* Nutrition
AIDS and, 153
burn and, 1168
neurologic alteration and, 135
supplementary, 156
Orders, do-not-resuscitate, 44
Organ failure, multiple; *see* Multiple organ dysfunction syndrome
Organ transplantation, 1171-1216; *see also* Transplantation
Orientation, 75
Oronasal breathing, 205
Oropharyngeal artificial airway, 692-693
Oropharyngeal suctioning, 668
Oropharynx, 665
Orthoclone, 1183-1184
Orthopedic injury, 1086-1087
Orthopnea, 504
Orthostatic hypotension, 992
Osmolality
antidiuretic hormone and, 983
definition of, 980
diabetes insipidus and, 1024
hyperglycemic hyperosmolar nonketotic syndrome and, 1016
pancreatic assessment and, 991
pituitary assessment and, 994
renal function and, 872
of urine, 874-875
Osmolite, 230
Osmosis
fluid balance and, 858
renal transport and, 854
Osmotic diuretic
intracranial hypertension and, 831
for renal disorder, 905
Osteoporosis, aging and, 289
Ostomy, 70
Outcome identification, 7-8
Outcome in nursing process, 7-8
Outcomes management, 12
Outpatient burn care, 1169
Output dial on pacemaker, 533
Oval pupil, 770
Overdamped waveform, 452
Overfeeding, respiratory alterations and, 133-135
Overhydration, 1012
Overload, volume, 1031
Oversensing by pacemaker, 536, 538
Overweight; *see* Obesity
Oxalate, 148
Oximetry, pulse, 653
Oxycodone, 181
dosage and action of, 183
Oxygen; *see also* Oxygen therapy; Oxygenation
arteriojugular oxygen difference and, 823
blood gas analysis and, 643-644
cardiogenic shock and, 1104
chest pain and, 489
complications of, 689-692
Oxygen—cont'd
delivery methods for, 689-692, 690-691
diffusion of, 618
fetal, 245
goals of therapy with, 689
obstructive sleep apnea and, 112
partial pressure of
age-related changes in, 277, 279
expected versus actual, 644-645
hypoxemia and, 641-642
intracranial pressure and, 822
maternal hypoxia and, 259
postoperative shivering and, 318
in postanesthesia period, 310
postoperative shivering and, 317-318
pregnancy and, 248
principles of therapy with, 689
pulmonary artery pressure and, 460
respiration and, 618
respiratory syncytial virus and, 213
shock and, 1098-1099
status asthmaticus and, 672
in child, 214
thyrotoxic crisis and, 1032, 1036
transport of, 620-621
trauma patient and, 1057, 1059
ventricular ectopy and, 417
Oxygen device, pediatric, 206-208, 209
Oxygen dissociation curve, 621-622, 623
Oxygen free radical
neurologic alteration and, 834
reperfusion organ injury and, 1126
Oxygen metabolite, toxic, 1126
Oxygen saturation
asthma and, 215
pulmonary alteration and, 643
Oxygen saturation, mixed venous, 471, 474-480
Oxygen tension index, 645-646
Oxygen therapy, 689-693
Oxygenation
air leak disorder and, 676
aspiration lung disorder and, 668
burn injury and, 1153
cerebral metabolism and, 823
intravascular, 715-716
multiple organ dysfunction syndrome and, 1133-1134
neurologic disorder and, 771
pneumonia and, 666
pulmonary embolism and, 671
respiratory distress syndrome and, 662
for respiratory failure, 656, 658
septic shock and, 1115
status asthmaticus and, 673
thoracic surgery and, 680
Oxygen-free radical, 691-692
Oxyhemoglobin dissociation curve, 248
Oxytocin, 983

P

P wave
analysis of, 392
atrioventricular block and, 426-427
cardiac pacing and, 533
evaluation of, 406
hypertrophy and, 401
potassium and, 377

P wave—cont'd
  premature atrial contraction and, 409-410
  sinus rhythm and, 408
Pacemaker
  atrioventricular block and, 427
  cardiac, 334-335
    permanent, 540-541
    temporary, 529-540
  indications for, 529-530
  nuclear magnetic resonance and, 437
  phrenic nerve, for sleep apnea, 113-114
Pacemaker action potential, 346-348
Pain, 169-199
  aging and, 286
  aortic dissection and, 517
  assessment of, 176-180
  burn injury and, 1157, 1167-1168
  chest; *see* Chest pain
  in child, 230-232
  craniotomy and, 818
  cultural factors in, 953-956
  deep vein thrombosis and, 522
  Guillain Barré syndrome and, 814
  management of, 180-188
    delivery methods for, 182, 184-185
    equianalgesia and, 185
    nonopioid analgesics for, 181
    nonpharmacologic, 185-188
    nonsteroidal antiinflammatory drugs for, 181-182
    opioid analgesics for, 180-181
  motor movement and, 766
  myocardial infarction and, 499, 500
  nursing management of, 197-199
  pancreatitis and, 952
  pelvic fracture and, 1085
  peripheral vascular disease and, 519
  peritoneal dialysis and, 904
  physiology of, 169-176
    central nervous system and, 171-176
    peripheral nervous system and, 169-171
  pneumothorax and, 675
  postanesthesia, 309
  postoperative, 310-311
    effect of relaxation and music on, 1148
    hypertension and, 317
  renal, 868
  rest, peripheral vascular disease and, 518
  rib fracture and, 1074
  self-report of, 232, 233
  thoracic surgery and, 681
  thrombolytic therapy and, 565
  trauma and, 1089
  types of, 176
Pain behavior, 172, 174, 177
  in child, 233
  cultural differences in, 173
Pallor, burn injury and, 1157
Palpation
  in cardiovascular system assessment, 360-365
  in gastrointestinal assessment, 935
  in pulmonary assessment, 629-630
  renal function and, 868
Pancreas
  anatomy and physiology of
    endocrine function and, 979-982
    gastrointestinal function and, 927, 929-930
  assessment of, 990-992
Pancreas—cont'd
  injury to, 1082-1083
  laboratory testing of, 937
  recognition of disorder of, 989
  stress response of, 1002
  transplantation of, 1205-1208
    case study of, 1213-1215
Pancreas transplantation, 1213-1215
Pancreatic polypeptide
  action of, 980
  function of, 982
Pancreaticoduodenocystotomy, 1206-1207
Pancreatitis
  complications of, 958
  findings in, 942, 952
  management of, 950-952, 957-958
  nutrition and, 149
Pancuronium, 714
Panic attack, agitation versus, 190
Paper, electrocardiographic, 392
Papillary layer of dermis, 1141
Papillary muscle, 333-334
  myocardial infarction and, 498
Paradoxic chest movement in infant, 206
Paradoxical sleep, 104-105
Paralysis
  burn injury and, 1157
  mechanical ventilation and, 713
  respiratory failure and, 658
Paralytic ileus, burn injury and, 1157
Paraplegia, 1065
  weight and, 137
Parasympathetic nervous system, 351
Parenchyma, alveolar, 278-279
Parenchymal damage, renal, 877-878
Parent of child, 234-237
Parenteral nutrition, total
  administration of, 159, 161-162
  AIDS and, 154
  bowel resection and, 148
  cardiac cachexia and, 129-130
  in child, 229-230
  education about, 149
  neurologic alteration and, 135, 137
  respiratory distress syndrome and, 663
  respiratory failure and, 659-660
Parenteral therapy, 1031
Paresthesia
  burn injury and, 1157
  Guillain Barré syndrome and, 812
  myxedema and, 1040
Parietal lobe, 752
  cerebrovascular accident and, 810
Parkland formula for burn patient, 1147
  electrical burn and, 1151
Parotid gland, 919-920
Paroxysmal atrial fibrillation, 414
Paroxysmal nocturnal dyspnea, 504
Paroxysmal supraventricular tachycardia, 410-411, 412
Pars intermedia, 983
Partial liquid ventilation, 716
Partial pressure
  of carbon dioxide; *see* Carbon dioxide, partial pressure of
  inhalation anesthetics and, 298
  of oxygen; *see* Oxygen, partial pressure of
Partial rebreathing mask, 690
Partial thromboplastin time
  cardiovascular alteration and, 383
  liver function and, 937
Partial-thickness burn, 1144
  pain of, 1167
Passage, collateral air, 608-609
Passive transport, 854
Passy-Muir valve, 703
Patent ductus arteriosus, 216
  in pregnancy, 252
Pathologic reflex, 768-769
Pathway
  accessory, 422
  clinical, 13-14
Patient advocate, nurse as, 28
Patient and family education, 49-60; *see also* Education
Patient Self-Determination Act, 44-46
Patient-controlled analgesia, 182
  nursing interventions for, 184
  thoracic surgery and, 681
Patient's right
  to accept or refuse treatment, 44
  to know, 49-50
Patient-ventilator asynchrony, 706
Peak expiratory flow rate
  asthma and, 215
  status asthmaticus in child and, 214
Peak inspiratory force, 648
Pectoriloquy, whispering, 633
PEEP; *see* Positive end-expiratory pressure
Peer review, 41
Pelvic trauma
  fracture and, 1084-1086
  in pregnancy, 265-266
Penetrating trauma, 1051-1052
  abdominal, 1079
  cardiac, 1077-1078
  facial, 1072
  of head, 1057, 1062
  pancreatic, 1082-1083
  in pregnancy, 265-266
  spinal, 1065
  thoracic, 1073-1074
Penicillin, 907
Pentamidine
  nutrition-related effects of, 154
  Pneumocystis carinii pneumonia and, 664
Pentazocine, 183
Pentobarbital
  intracranial hypertension and, 832
  sleep and, 108
Pentoxifylline, 1135
Peptic ulcer
  bleeding and, 945
  findings in, 942
Peptide
  atrial natriuretic, 859-860
  gastric-inhibitory, 923
Perception, 76
Percussion, in assessment
  cardiovascular, 365
  gastrointestinal, 934-935
  pulmonary, 630-632
  renal, 868-869
Percutaneous biopsy, liver, 939

Percutaneous transluminal coronary angioplasty, 553-555
  bleeding after, 559-560
  ST-segment monitoring and, 399-401
Perfluorocarbon, 716
Perforated ulcer
  duodenal, 941
  peptic, 942
Perforation of intraaortic balloon, 570
Perfusion
  burn injury and, 1156-1157
  decreased arterial, 448
  lung, 612
  nursing management and, 595-596
  orthopedic injury and, 1087
  reperfusion organ injury and, 1126
  respiratory distress syndrome and, 663
  spinal injury and, 1067-1068
  ventilation/perfusion relationships and, 618-620
Perfusion pressure
  cardiac, 446
  cerebral, 822
    in child, 224-225
Perianesthesia management; *see* Anesthesia
Peribronchial cuffing, 388
Pericardial friction rub, 371
Pericardiocentesis, 1078
Pericarditis
  clinical findings in, 373-374
  myocardial infarction and, 498
Pericardium, 331
Peripartum cardiomyopathy, 253
Peripheral chemoreceptor, 617-618
Peripheral circulation, 353-354
Peripheral ischemia, 570
Peripheral nerve stimulator, 713
Peripheral nervous system
  heartbeat and, 351
  pain and, 169-171
Peripheral tissue perfusion
  burn injury and, 1156-1157
  nursing management and, 595-596
Peripheral vascular disease, 517-519
  education about, 520
Peripheral vascular system, 275-276
Peristalsis
  aging and, 280
  esophageal, 920
  in small intestine, 923-924
Peritoneal dialysis
  complications of, 902-903, 904
  glucose and, 140
  process of, 899-903
Peritoneal lavage, 1080
Peritonitis, 904
Permanent pacemaker, 540, 541
Permeability
  burn injury and, 1154
  in respiratory distress syndrome, 660
Persantine, 436
Persistent vegetative state, 795-798
Personal liability, 40
PetCO_2, 653
pH
  aspiration lung disorder and, 667
  calcium and, 861
  intracranial pressure and, 822
pH—cont'd
  intramucosal monitoring of, 968-970
  pulmonary alteration and, 642-643
  tube feeding and, 158, 159
  of urine, 873, 874
Pharmacodynamics, 281-282
Pharmacokinetics
  age-related changes in, 281-282
  of inhalation anesthetics, 298-300
  pain in child and, 231-232
Pharmacology; *see* Drug therapy
Pharyngeal airway, 692-693
Pharynx
  anatomy of, 920
  inhalation injury of, 1150
  swallowing and, 920
Phenobarbital
  renal failure and, 909
  sleep and, 108
Phenol burn, 1150
Phentolamine, 581, 582
Phenylalkylamine, 581
Phenylephrine, 579
Phenytoin
  neurologic disorder and, 835
  renal failure and, 909
Phlebostatic axis, 444
Phonocardiogram, 433
Phosphate, renal function and, 862, 882, 885
Phosphodiesterase inhibitor, 579
Phospholipase A, 951
Phosphorus
  ketoacidosis and, 1009, 1011
  renal system and, 138, 142, 862, 885
Phrenic nerve pacemaker, 113-114
Physical comfort promotion, 10
Physical restraint for elderly patient, 284
Physiologic formula, D-1 to D-4
Physiologic shunting, 336
  bronchial, 612
Physiologic stressor, 50
Physiology, oxygen transport, 475
Physiology of sleep, 103-104
Physiotherapy, chest, 646; *see also* Pulmonary care
Physostigmine, 300
Pia mater, 738
Pickwickian syndrome, 110
Pigment, lipofuscin, 282, 285
Pigskin graft for burn wound, 1163
Pinocytosis, 244-245
Piperacillin, 907
Pitting edema, 362-363
  renal function and, 867
Pituitary gland
  anatomy of, 748-749, 982-983
  assessment of, 992-995
  diabetes insipidus and, 1022
  diagnostic procedures for, 994-995
  stress response of, 1002
Placenta, 244-246
Plaintiff, 39
Plan of care, interdisciplinary, 10, 12-15, E-1 to E-16
Planning in nursing process, 8-9
Plaque
  atherosclerotic, 336
  coronary artery disease and, 485-486
  myocardial infarction and, 490-491
  neuritic, 282, 285
Plasma
  heart transplantation and, 1180
  renal clearance and, 853
Plasma osmolality, 983
Plasma protein
  inflammation and, 1122-1123
  liver and, 928
Plasmapheresis, 813
Plateau wave, intracranial pressure, 825-826
Platelet
  HELLP syndrome in pregnancy and, 256-257
  myocardial infarction and, 499
  in postanesthesia period, 310
Platelet inhibitor, 835
Platelet-activating factor, 1127
Pleura
  air leak disorder and, 674
  anatomy of, 602-603
  respiratory failure and, 656
Pleural fluid, 638
Pleural friction rub, 632
  conditions with, 634
Pleural space, 651
Pneumatic antishock garment, 1085
Pneumatic ventricular assist device, 572
Pneumococcal vaccine, 1083
Pneumocystis carinii pneumonia, 664
Pneumomediastinum, 675
Pneumonectomy, 678
  postoperative management of, 680
Pneumonia, 663-667
  assessment findings in, 638
  coma and, 793
  craniotomy and, 817
  nosocomial, 664-665
    mechanical ventilation and, 706
  pregnancy and, 260
Pneumonitis, chemical, 1153
Pneumopericardium, tension, 676
Pneumothorax, 673-677
  assessment findings in, 639
  parenteral nutrition and, 163
  trauma and, 1076-1077
Poikilothermy, 1157
Point of maximal impulse, 360
Poisoning
  carbon monoxide, 1150, 1153
  coma and, 792
Polydipsia
  diabetes insipidus and, 1023
  ketoacidosis and, 1006-1007
Polymer, semisynthetic, 1164
Polymeric enteral formula, 157
Polypeptide, pancreatic, 980
Polysomnography, 112
Polysporin, 1161
Polyurethane film, 1165
Polyuria
  diabetes insipidus and, 1023
  ketoacidosis and, 1006-1007
Polyvinylchoride, burning of, 1153
Pons, 740
Portal vein
  liver and, 926
  pancreas and, 929
Portosystemic shunt, transjugular intrahepatic, 949, 968, 969

Positioning
aspiration lung disorder and, 668
burn and, 1168-1169
cardiovascular assessment and, 357
central venous pressure and, 455
for chest radiography, 384-385
craniotomy and, 817-818
for hemodynamic monitoring, 444
intracranial hypertension and, 827, 829
for neurologic radiography, 779-780
postanesthesia, 309
pulmonary artery pressure and, 468, 470
respiratory failure and, 658-659
thoracic surgery and, 680
Positive airway pressure, continuous, 707
Positive end-expiratory pressure
cardiac surgery and, 547
for child, 208
clinical applications for, 707
for postanesthesia pulmonary edema, 314
pulmonary artery pressure and, 468
respiratory distress syndrome and, 662
Positive-pressure ventilation
cardiovascular compromise and, 706
weaning and, 709
Positive-pressure ventilator, 703
Possum response, 65
Postanesthesia care, 309-312
Postanesthesia emergency, 312-326
Postcardiotomy psychosis, 548
Postconvulsion coma, 793
Posterior cerebral circulation, 753-754
Posterior cord syndrome, 1066
Posterior fossa, 737
Posterior hemiblock, left, 405
Posterior pituitary, 748-749, 983
Posterior wall myocardial infarction, 494
Postoperative pain, 310-311, 1148
hypertension and, 317
Postpartum period, 71
Postrenal azotemia, 878
Posttransplant hepatic function, 1197-1198
Potassium
burn injury and, 1154-1155
cardiac electrical activity and, 344
cardiovascular alteration and, 377
gastrointestinal disorder and, 145
ketoacidosis and, 1008-1009, 1011, 1012-1013
osmotic diuretic and, 831
renal disorder and, 139, 142, 860, 861, 881, 884-885, 886
Potassium iodide, 1035
Potentials, evoked, 787
Povidone-iodine for burn wound, 1161
Powerlessness, 71-72
nursing management plan for, 90
PR interval
atrial flutter and, 412
definition of, 393
evaluation of, 406
sinus rhythm and, 408
PR segment, 399-400
Practice act, nurse, 38, 41-42
nursing diagnosis and, 267
Practice guidelines, 15
Precapillary sphincter, 340
Precautions, coronary, 489-490
Precordium, auscultation of, 371
Predigested enteral formula, 157
Prednisone, transplant and, 1177
Preeclampsia
definition of, 255
disseminated intravascular coagulation and, 258
HELLP syndrome and, 257
Preembryonic stage of fetal development, 243
Prefrontal area of brain, 751
Pregnancy
cardiopulmonary resuscitation in, 254-255
diabetic ketoacidosis in, 262
disseminated intravascular coagulation and, 258-259
fetal development and, 243-244
heart disease in, 251-254
hypertension in, 255-258
neurologic disorder in, 266-268
physiologic alterations in, 246-251
placental development and, 244-246
pulmonary dysfunction in, 259-262
trauma in, 262-266
Pregnancy-induced hypertension, 256
Preload, 350
cardiac surgery and, 546
heart failure and, 505
mitral stenosis in pregnancy and, 252
nursing management and, 590-591
pulmonary artery pressure and, 460
Premature atrial contraction
definition of, 409-410
myocardial infarction and, 496
Premature ventricular contraction, 416-422
myocardial infarction and, 496-497
potassium and, 377
Premotor area of brain, 751
Prerenal azotemia, 877
Presbyesophagus, 280
Pressure
central venous; *see* Central venous *entries*
cerebral perfusion, 822
in child, 224-225
continuous positive airway; *see* Continuous positive airway pressure
cuff, of endotracheal tube, 700, 701
expiratory, 648-649
glomerulus and, 851
hydrostatic, 858
tubular necrosis and, 878-879
inspiratory, 648-649
intraabdominal, 1081
intracardial, 1078
intracranial; *see* Intracranial pressure
intrapleural, 602-603
intrapulmonary, 604
intrathoracic, 706
left atrial, 447, 456-457
left ventricular end-diastolic, 460
mean arterial; *see* Mean arterial pressure
negative inspiratory, 648-649
partial; *see* Carbon dioxide, partial pressure of; Oxygen, partial pressure of
perfusion, 446
positive end-expiratory; *see* Positive end-expiratory pressure
pulmonary artery; *see* Pulmonary artery *entries*
pulmonary artery wedge, 870-871
pulse, 446
Pressure support ventilation
in child, 211
clinical applications for, 707
volume-assured, 707
weaning and, 684
Pressure wave, intracranial, 824
Pressure-cycled ventilator, 704
Preweaning phase of mechanical ventilation, 682
Primary survey in resuscitation, 1052
Privacy
as ethical principle, 24
invasion of, 38
Procainamide, 575
dosage and side effects of, 578
elderly patient and, 283
renal failure and, 909
Process, nursing, 4-10
Products liability, 516
Prodysrhythmic effect of drug, 577
Professional organization, 35-36
Progesterone, 248
Programming of implantable cardioverter defibrillator, 552
Prolactin, 748
Proliferative phase of burn injury, 1158-1159
Proliferative stage of oxygen toxicity, 692
Prophylaxis
antibiotic, liver failure and, 964
pulmonary embolism and, 670
Propofol
anesthesia with, 302
cardiac effects of, 316
sedation with
characteristics of, 194
deep, 193
Propoxyphene, 183
Propranolol
dosage and side effects of, 578
renal failure and, 908
thyrotoxic crisis and, 1035
Propylthiouracil, 1033, 1035
Prosopagnosia, 810
Prostaglandins, 1127
kidney and, 855
Prosthetic valve, cardiac, 252, 542-543
Protease
inflammation and, 1127
pancreatitis and, 951
Protective mechanisms of brain, 737-740
Protein
burn injury and, 1154
fluid balance and, 859
insulin and, 981
liver and, 145-147, 928, 937
metabolism of, 121-122
renal system and, 138, 139-140, 142
urine and, 874
Protein-calorie malnutrition, 123
AIDS and, 152, 153
clinical manifestations of, 126
gastrointestinal disorder and, 144
neurologic alterations and, 137
renal disorder and, 138
respiratory alterations and, 134
Proteinuria, pregnancy and, 249
Prothrombin time
cardiovascular alteration and, 383
liver function and, 937

Protocol, 15
Protriptyline, obstructive sleep apnea and, 112
Proximal convoluted tubule, 851-852
  reabsortion and, 853
Proximate cause, 39
Pseudoaneurysm, 887
Psychogenic diabetes insipidus, 1022
Psychologic factors
  diabetes insipidus and, 1027
  mechanical ventilation and, 681
  myxedema and, 1040
  shock and, 1100
  spinal injury and, 1071
  weaning from mechanical ventilation and, 685
Psychologic stressor, 50-51
  intraaortic balloon pump and, 570-571
  sleep deprivation and, 109-110
Psychosis
  myxedema and, 1040
  postcardiotomy, 548
Psychosocial alterations, 63-100
  anesthesia and, 308-309
  body image disturbance and, 68-69
  in chronically ill, 82-83
  coping and, 78-82
  in elderly, 83
  hopelessness and, 72-74
  mental status changes and, 74-77
  nursing management plan for, 85-100
  powerlessness and, 71-72
  role performance and, 70-71
  self-concept and, 67-68
  self-esteem disturbance and, 69-70
  significance of, to nursing, 65-67
  stress and, mind/body interactions and, 64-65
  in transplant patient, 83-84
Psychosocial factors
  for child, 232-237
  craniotomy and, 815
  Guillain Barré syndrome and, 814
Pulmonary alteration; *see* Respiratory *entries*
Pulmonary artery catheter
  burn injury and, 1157-1158
  chest radiography and, 386, 651-652
Pulmonary artery pressure, 459-471
  antidiuretic hormone and, 1031
  definition of, 447
  diastolic, 462
  mean, 612
  positioning for, 444
  pulmonary circulation and, 611
  thyrotoxic crisis and, 1037
Pulmonary artery waveform, 463, 465-467
Pulmonary artery wedge pressure
  chest radiography and, 388
  positioning for, 444
  pulmonary artery diastolic pressure and, 462
  renal function and, 870-871, 883
  waveform interpretation of, 463
  waveform of, 467
Pulmonary blood flow, 219
Pulmonary capillary wedge pressure
  chest x-ray and, 388
  definition of, 447
Pulmonary care
  craniotomy and, 818
  myxedema and, 1040
  respiratory failure and, 659
Pulmonary care—cont'd
  sputum studies and, 646
Pulmonary edema
  heart failure and, 504
  postanesthesia, 314
  thoracentesis and, 648
Pulmonary embolism
  clinical findings in, 373-374
  description of, 668
  diagnosis of, 669-670
  education about, 671
  etiology of, 668-669
  management of, 668, 670-671
  pathophysiology of, 669
  pregnancy and, 260-261
  prevention of, 670, 671
  respiratory failure and, 658
  risk of, 522-523
  trauma and, 1088
Pulmonary fibrosis, 639
Pulmonary function testing
  age-related changes in, 277
  bedside, 648-649
  heart-lung transplant and, 1187
Pulmonary hypertension, 612
  pregnancy and, 253
  pulmonary embolism and, 670
  in respiratory distress syndrome, 661-662
Pulmonary system; *see* Respiratory *entries*
Pulmonary valve disease, 252
Pulmonary vascular resistance
  definition of, 448
  heart transplantation and, 1181
  pulmonary artery pressure and, 462, 464
Pulmonary vascular resistance index, 448
Pulmonary volumes, 250
Pulmonary-to-systemic shunting, 216
Pulmonic valve, 334
Pulmonic valve disease, 513
Pulse
  auscultation of, 362
  burn injury and, 1148-1149
  carotid, 363
  peripheral vascular disease and, 519
Pulse deficit, 448
Pulse generator of pacemaker, 530, 533-534
Pulse oximetry, 653
  neurogenic shock and, 1110
Pulse pressure, 446
  in perianesthesia assessment, 306
Pulse width on pacemaker, 535
Pulseless arrest in child, 224
Pulselessness, burn injury and, 1157
Pulsus paradoxus, 366, 450
Pump
  insulin, 1006
  intraaortic balloon, 568-571
    chest x-ray and, 386-387
  sodium, 860
Pump failure, cardiac, 1104-1105
Puncture
  cisternal, 788
  lumbar, 787-788
Pupil
  age-related changes in, 288
  head injury and, 1064
  in neurologic assessment, rapid, 775
  neurologic assessment and, 769
Pupil—cont'd
  persistent vegetative state and, 796
Pure motor or sensory stroke, 802
Pyelography, intravenous, 876
Pyloric obstruction, 942
Pyrexia, 1033
Pyrodistigmine, 307

Q

Q wave
  analysis of, 392
  infarction and, 402
QRS complex
  atrial flutter and, 412
  atrioventricular block and, 424-427
  bundle branch block and, 404
  evaluation of, 406-407
  explanation of, 392
  hemiblock and, 405
  paroxysmal supraventricular tachycardia and, 411
  premature ventricular contraction and, 416
  sinus rhythm and, 408
  ventricular axis and, 395-396
  ventricular tachycardia and, 420
  wide, 422-424
QT interval, 394
Quadrant of abdomen, 941-942
Quadriplegia, 1065
  weight and, 137
Quality assurance, 41
Quality of life, 24
Quinidine, 575

R

Racial differences in coronary artery disease, 484
Radial artery graft, 542, 544
Radiation burn, 1146
Radiation dose from radiologic studies, 245
Radical, oxygen free, 691-692
  reperfusion organ injury and, 1126
Radiofrequency catheter ablation, 414, 420
Radiofrequency current catheter ablation, 530
Radiography
  of brain, 779-784
  chest
    aspiration lung disorder and, 668
    barotrauma and, 675
    cardiovascular alteration and, 384-389
    diaphragmatic rupture and, 1075
    oxygen toxicity and, 692
    pulmonary alteration and, 650-652
    pulmonary embolism and, 670
    respiratory distress syndrome and, 662
  coma and, 793
  digital cardiovascular, 389
  gastrointestinal, 938
  pituitary gland and, 995
  radiation dose from, 245
  renal, 875-876, 880
  spinal, 782-784, 1068
Radionuclide imaging
  cardiovascular alteration and, 438
  thyroid, 997
  ventilation/perfusion, 649-650
Rales, 632, 634

Ranitidine
dosage and actions of, 971
renal failure and, 909
Ranson's criteria for pancreatitis, 951
Ranvier's node, 734
Rapid eye movement sleep, 104
recovery sleep and, 110
sleep deprivation and, 109
Rapid neurologic assessment, 774-775, 777
Rate control on pacemaker, 533
RATG, 1177
Reabsorption
in colon, 926
renal tubular, 854
Readiness to learn, 53
Reading level, 56, 57
Rebleeding after subarachnoid hemorrhage, 804-805
Rebreathing mask, 690
Receptive aphasia, 811
Receptor, opiate, 174, 175
Recoil, lung, 614
Recombinant plasminogen activator, 564
Record, medical, 1018
Recording system for electrocardiography, 427-429
Recovery phase of tubular necrosis, 879
Recovery sleep, 110
Rectum, 925
Red blood cells
alveolar-capillary membrane and, 611
cardiovascular alteration and, 382
chloride and, 863
HELLP syndrome in pregnancy and, 256
kidney and, 855
in postanesthesia period, 310
renal failure and, anemia and, 886
urine and, 874
Reexpansion pulmonary edema, 648
Referral to burn center, 1149
Reflex
Babinski, 768-769
Bainbridge, 352
baroreceptor, 274-275
blink, coma and, 794
Hering-Breuer, 618
in neurologic assessment, 768-769
oculocephalic, 770, 772
oculovestibular, 770, 773
spinal shock and, 1066
Reflux, abdominojugular, 359-360
Refusal of treatment, 44
antibiotic, for elderly patient, 288
Regression as coping mechanism, 79
Regurgitation
aortic valve, 511-513
mitral, 462
mitral valve, 511, 512
tricuspid valve, 513
Rehabilitation, burn and, 1168-1169
Rehydration
cardiac catheterization and, 439
diabetes insipidus and, 1025
hyperglycemic hyperosmolar nonketotic syndrome and, 1019
Rejection, transplant, 1171-1178
heart-lung, 1187
immune system and, 1171-1176
Rejection, transplant—cont'd
immunosuppressive therapy and, 1176-1179
surveillance for
heart, 1182-1183
liver, 1198-1199
pancreatic, 1208
Relaxation
pain management and, 186
postoperative pain and, 1148
Release-inhibiting factor, pituitary, 982
Religious belief, 80, 82, 799-800
Renal alteration, 877-916; *see also* Renal failure; Renal system
burn injury and, 1156
cardiac surgery and, 549
case study of, 912-914
continuous renal replacement and, 893-899
diabetes insipidus and, 1022
diagnosis of, 879-886
dialysis for, 883-903; *see also* Dialysis
drug therapy and, 903, 905-909
fluid volume and, 914-915
HELLP syndrome in pregnancy and, 257
hyperglycemic hyperosmolar nonketotic syndrome and, 1019
multiple organ dysfunction syndrome and, 1129, 1130
myxedema and, 1040
nursing diagnosis and management of, 911-916
nutrition and, 137-143, 885
tissue perfusion and, 916
trauma causing, 1083, 1089-1090
tubular necrosis as, 878-879
Renal artery, 849-850
Renal failure
anemia and, 886
anion gap and, 872-873
ascites and, 869
burn injury and, 1147
cardiovascular system and, 882-883
description of, 877
diagnosis of, 879-886
blood urea nitrogen and, 880
hemodynamics and, 880, 882
laboratory assessment in, 879-880
radiography and, 880
urinalysis in, 880
dialysis for, 886-903; *see also* Dialysis
drugs affected by, 903, 905-910
electrolytes and, 881-882, 884-885, 886
enteral formulas for, 157
etiology of, 877-878
fluid and, 870, 883-884, 885
infection and, 885
liver failure and, 964
management of, 883
multiple organ dysfunction syndrome and, 1130
nutrition and, 885
prevention of, 883
radiography and, 875-876
sediment in urine and, 875
trauma and, 1089
Renal replacement, continuous, 893-899
Renal system; *see also* Renal alteration
age-related changes in, 279-280, 292
examination for, 290
Renal system—cont'd
anatomy of, 847-863
macroscopic, 847
microscopic, 848-852
nervous system and, 852
vascular, 847-848
antidiuretic hormone and, 983
assessment of, 865-876
fluid and electrolytes and, 871
hemodynamics and, 870-871
history in, 865
intake and output in, 869-870
laboratory, 872-875
mental status and, 871-872
physical examination in, 865-869
radiographic, 875-876
weight and, 869
electrolyte balance and, 860-863
fluid balance and, 856-860
hypovolemic shock and, 1101
kidney function and, 854-856
pregnancy and, 248-249, 250
respiratory failure and, 657
urine formation and, 852-854
Renal transplantation, 1199-1205
case study of, 1213-1215
psychosocial alterations and, 83-84
transplantation of, case study of, 1213-1215
Renal tubule
reabsortion by, 853
secretion of, 854
Renin, blood pressure and, 855
Renin-angiotensin system
aging and, 276
fluid balance and, 859
heart failure and, 504
shock and, 1097
Reopro, 554
Reperfusion, after thrombolytic therapy, 566
Reperfusion organ injury, 1126
Repolarization, cardiac, 345-346, 389
Reproductive system in pregnancy, 247
trauma to, 266
Res ipsa loquitur, 39
Reserpine, 1035
Reserve volume, 649
Residual capacity, functional
age-related changes in, 279
in postanesthesia period, 315
Residual volume, 649
age-related changes in, 279
Resistance
insulin
ketoacidosis and, 1009, 1011
septic shock and, 1113
pulmonary vascular
definition of, 448
heart transplantation and, 1181
systemic vascular, 340
postanesthesia, 315
Resistance index, vascular, 447
Resources, allocation of, 25-26
Respiration
abnormal patterns of, 630
Kussmaul's, 771
renal failure and, 882
process of, 618
pulmonary artery pressure and, 468

Respiratory acidosis, 644
Respiratory alkalosis
  blood gas assessment in, 644
  septic shock and, 1114
Respiratory alteration, 601-729
  acute respiratory distress syndrome and; *see also* Respiratory distress
  adult respiratory distress syndrome as, 660-663
  air leak disorder as, 673-677
  anaphylaxis and, 1107, 1108
  anatomy and, 601-610
  antidiuretic hormone disorder and, 1028
  aspiration lung disorder as, 667-668
  assessment of, 625-639
    findings in, 633-639
    history in, 625-627
    physical examination in, 627-633
  burn injury and, 1154
  in child, 206-216
    anatomy and physiology of, 205-206
    apnea and, 214-215
    bronchiolitis and, 212-213
    endotracheal intubation and, 208-211
    oxygen devices for, 206-208
    respiratory syncytial virus and, 212-213
    status asthmaticus and, 213-214
    tracheotomy in, 211
  diagnosis of, 641-654
    arterial blood gases and, 641-645
    bedside monitoring and, 653-654
    bronchoscopy in, 647
    chest radiography and, 650-652
    dead space equation and, 646
    nursing management in, 652
    pulmonary function tests and, 648-649
    shunt equation for, 645-646
    sputum studies in, 646-647
    thoracentesis in, 647-648
    ventilation/perfusion scanning and, 649-650
  drug therapy for, 713-715
  enteral formulas for, 157
  heart-lung transplantation and, 1184-1188
  injury causing, 1075-1077
  ketoacidosis and, 1015
  lung transplantation and, 1188-1190
  management of
    artificial airway for, 692-703
    drug therapy for, 713-715
    mechanical ventilation for, 681-686; *see also* Mechanical ventilation
    new methods of, 715-716
    oxygen therapy in, 689-692
  multiple organ dysfunction syndrome and, 1129
  myxedema and, 1039-1040
  nursing diagnosis and management of, 719-729
    aspiration risk and, 727
    case study and, 720-722
    impaired gas exchange and, 725-726
    inability to sustain spontaneous ventilation and, 724-725
    ineffective airway clearance and, 722-723
    ineffective breathing pattern and, 723-724
    weaning and, 728-729
  nutrition intervention for, 133-135
  pancreatitis and, 958
  physiology and, 613-624
  pneumonia as, 663-667
  postanesthesia, 309-310
Respiratory alteration—cont'd
  in postanesthesia period, 312-315
  in pregnancy, 259-262
  pulmonary embolus as, 668-671
    clinical findings in, 373-374
    pregnancy and, 260-261
    risk of, 522-523
  renal failure and, 882-883
  respiratory failure as, 655-660
  septic shock and, 1114
  shock and, 1098
  sleep apnea and
    central, 113
    obstructive, 111
  spinal injury and, 1068, 1070-1071
  status asthmaticus as, 671-673
  thoracic surgery for, 677-681
  trauma and, 1075-1077, 1088-1089
    in pregnancy, 263, 265
  work of breathing and, 614
Respiratory depression; *see also* Respiratory alteration
  drug-related
    fear of, 180
    morphine and, 180
  opioid anesthesia and, 301-302
  in postanesthesia period, 315
Respiratory distress
  acute, 660-663
  flail chest and, 1074
  multiple organ dysfunction syndrome and, 1130
  oxygenation and, 1134
  pregnancy and, 260
  pulmonary artery catheter and, 459
  shock and, 1098
    hypovolemic, 1101
Respiratory effort, evaluation of, 628-629
Respiratory excursion, 629, 631
Respiratory failure, 655-660
  description of, 655
  etiology of, 655
  management of, 656, 658-660
  manifestations of, 657
  pathophysiology of, 655-656
  patient education about, 655
  pregnancy and, 260
  thoracic surgery and, 679
  trauma and, 1088
Respiratory management, 10
Respiratory mechanics of infant or child, 206
Respiratory muscle
  age-related changes in, 277
  asthma and, 215
  of child, 206
Respiratory patterns in neurologic assessment, 771-772
  rapid, 777
Respiratory rate
  asthma and, 215
  septic shock and, 1114
Respiratory syncytial virus, in child, 212-213
Respiratory system; *see also* Airway; Pulmonary *entries*
  age-related changes in, 276-279, 292
    examination for, 289-290
  anatomy of, 601-610
    blood and lymph supply of, 610-613
    conducting airways and, 604-606
Respiratory system—cont'd
  anatomy of—cont'd
    muscles of ventilation and, 603-604
    pleura and, 602-603
    respiratory airways and, 607-610
    thorax and, 601-604
  cardiac surgery and, 547
  of child, 205-216
    anatomy and physiology of, 205-206
  neurologic assessment and, 771-772, 773
  pancreatitis and, 958
  in perianesthesia assessment, 305-306
  physiology of
    gas transport and, 620-624
    respiration and, 618
    ventilation and, 613-618
    ventilation/perfusion relationships and, 618-620
  pregnancy and, 248
  renal failure and, 882-883
  renal function and, 867
  respiratory failure and, 657
  spinal injury and, 1068
Respondeat superior, doctrine of, 40
Rest
  heart failure and, 506
  thyrotoxic crisis and, 1037
Rest pain, peripheral vascular disease and, 518
Restenosis, angioplasty and, 555
Resting membrane potential, 344
Restraints for elderly patient, 284
Restrictive cardiomyopathy, 508
Restrictive lung disease, 615
Resuscitation
  cardiopulmonary, pregnancy and, 254-255
  cerebral, 834, 836
  of trauma patient, 1052-1056
Resuscitation bag, for child, 208
Resuscitation phase of burn injury management, 1151-1158
  fluid therapy and, 1154-1156
  hypothermia and, 1158
  infection risk and, 1156
  initial emergency, 1146-1149
  invasive monitoring and, 1157-1158
  laboratory assessment in, 1158
  oxygenation and, 1153-1154
  tissue perfusion and, 1156-1157
Resynchronization of sleep, 106
Retention, carbon dioxide, 692
Reteplase, 565
Reticular activating system, 741
Reticular formation, 741
Reticular layer of dermis, 1141
Reticulin, 278
Revascularization, myocardial, 541-542
Reversal agent
  benzodiazepine, 300
  for neuromuscular blocking agent, 304, 307
  opioid; *see* Naloxone
  in sedation, 195
Rewarming
  abdominal injury and, 1081
  postoperative hypothermia and, 318
Rhonchus, 632, 634
Rhythm, cardiac
  accelerated idioventricular, 420
  accelerated junctional, 415

Rhythm, cardiac—cont'd
description of, 406
idioventricular, 420
junctional escape, 415
sinus, 407-409
Rib
chest radiography and, 650
of child, 206
trauma in pregnancy and, 265
Rib fracture, 1074
Ribavirin, 213
Ribonucleic acid
age-related changes cardiac changes and, 272-273
myocardial gene expression and, 272, 273-274
neuron and, 734
Rifabutin, 154
Right
to accept or refuse treatment, 44
to know, 49-50
Right atrial waveform, 465-466
Right atrium, pulmonary artery pressure and, 465
Right bundle branch, 336
Right bundle branch block, 403-404
Right coronary artery, 336
Right heart failure, 502-503
Right internal mammary artery graft, 542
Right ventricle
anatomy of, 332
status asthmaticus and, 672
Right ventricular assist device, 573
Right ventricular myocardial infarction, 494
Right ventricular stroke work index, 448
Right ventricular waveform, 465-466
Rigidity in malignant hyperthermia, 320
Ring test, 1072-1073
Ringer's solution, lactated
burn injury and, 1154
renal failure and, 884
Risk factors
for cerebrovascular accident, 801
for coronary artery disease, 483-484
for infection, 1119
in nursing diagnosis, 7
for trauma, 1057
Risk management, 10, 41
RNA
age-related changes cardiac changes and, 272-273
myocardial gene expression and, 272, 273-274
neuron and, 734
RNA virus, endocarditis and, 509
Rod, spinal, 1069
Role performance, altered, 70-71
Rotary ventricular assist device, 573
Rotation injury of spine, 1065
Rotoblator device, 556
Rounds, ethics, 32
Route, cardiac pacing, 531-532
Roux-en-Y reconstruction, 1206
RS-61443, 1178
Rub, friction
barotrauma and, 675
pericardial, 371
pleural, 632, 634
Rule of nines, 1143
Rules of evidence, 39
Rupture
alveolar, 674
atherosclerotic plaque, 485-486
cardiac wall, 498
of cerebral aneurysm, 802, 803
of diaphragm, 1074-1075
of esophagogastric varices, 946
papillary muscle, 498

S

S_1 heart sound, 367
S_2 heart sound, 367
Safety
delirium and, 77
food, for AIDS patient, 155
St. Jude prosthetic valve, 544
Saline eyedrops, 794
Saline solution
antidiuretic hormone and, 1031
hyperglycemic hyperosmolar nonketotic syndrome and, 1019
renal failure and, 884
Salivation, 919-920
Salt
bile
function of, 928
nutrition and, 143
hypertension and, 128
Saltatory transmission, 735
Saphenous vein graft, 541-542, 544
Sarcolemma, 342
Sarcoplasmic reticulum, 342
Saturation, oxygen
arterial, 471, 474
mixed venous, 471, 474-480
pulmonary alteration and, 643
Scan
computed tomography; *see* Computed tomography
liver, 939
thyroid, 997
ventilation/perfusion, 649-650, 670
Scarlet red, 1164
Scarring, hypertrophic, 1166
Scavenger, 834
Scintillation, 649-650
Sclerotherapy, endoscopic, 968
Screening, nutritional, 124-128
Secobarbital, 108
Secondary survey in resuscitation, 1055-1056
Second-degree atrioventricular block, 424-426
Second-degree burn, 1145
Secretin, 923
pancreatic function and, 937
Secretion
gastric, 922
intestinal, 923
respiratory failure and, 659
Sedation
anxiety and, 188-190
definition of, 188
intracranial hypertension and, 829
levels of, 190, 193-195
respiratory failure and, 658
Sedative, 909
Sediment, in urine, 875
Segment, lung, 601
Segmental resection of lung, 678
Segmentation, Haustral, 923-924
Seizure
antidiuretic hormone disorder and, 1030-1031
in child, 225-226
coma and, 793
HELLP syndrome in pregnancy and, 257-258
intracranial hypertension and, 830
myxedema and, 1041-1042
in pregnancy, 266
types of, 767
Self-care, 888
cultural factors in, 953-956
Self-care facilitation, 10
Self-concept, altered, 67-68
Self-Determination Act, 44-46
Self-esteem disturbance, 69-70
nursing management plan for, 89
Self-insurance, 41
Sella turcica, 737, 982
Semilunar valve, 334
Semiopen wound care, 1160
Semisynthetic polymer, 1164
Sengstaken-Blaken tube, 966
Sensing malfunction of pacemaker, 536, 538
Sensitivity control on pacemaker, 533-534
Sensitivity threshold on pacemaker, 535
Sensor, ventilation, 616
Sensory aphasia, 811
Sensory function, 809-810
Sensory nerve fiber, 733
Sensory overload or deprivation, 91-95
Sensory stimulation for coma, 795
Sensory stroke, pure, 802
Sepsis
catheter-related, 163
definition of, 1112
enteral nutrition and, 155
multiple organ failure and, 1124
oxygenation and, 1134
splenectomy and, 1083
trauma and, 1088
Sepsis-induced hypotension, 1112
Septal defect, ventricular, 336
myocardial infarction and, 497-498
Septic abortion, 259
Septic shock, 1111-1115, 1117
in child, 223-224
definition of, 1112
pregnancy and, 254
pulmonary artery catheter and, 458
Serotonin
age-related changes in, 286
pain and, 174, 175-176
sleep and, 105-106
Serum lipid, cardiovascular alteration and, 383-384
Sevoflurane, 301
Shift, mediastinal, 680
Shifting of oxygen dissociation curve, 621-622, 623
Shivering, postoperative, 317-318
Shock, 1097-1119
anaphylactic, 1105-1109
burn, 1154
cardiac output and, 1118
cardiogenic, 1102-1105
case study of, 1116-1117

Shock—cont'd
in child, 223-224
definition of, 1112
description of, 1097
diagnosis of, 1098
etiology of, 1097
gastrointestinal system and, 1128
hypovolemic, 1100-1102
infection risk and, 1119
management of, 1098-1100
microshock from pacemaker, 539
neurogenic, 1109-1111
pathophysiology of, 1097-1098
pregnancy and, 253-254
pulmonary artery catheter and, 458, 459
septic, 1111-1115, 1117
spinal, 1066, 1109-1111
vasopressor and, 582
Shock phase of burn injury, 1151-1158
Short bowel syndrome, 147, 148-149
Shortness of breath
heart failure and, 504
pulmonary history of, 626
Shunt
arteriovenous, 887
intrapulmonary, 619, 645-646
respiratory failure and, 656
physiologic, 336
portosystemic transjugular intrahepatic, 968
pulmonary embolism and, 669
transjugular intrahepatic portosystemic, 949, 969
Sickle cell anemia, 622
Sigmoid colon, 924-925, 925
Sign
Battle's, 1059
Cullen's, 1079
Grey Turner's, 952, 1079
Hamman's, 675
lateralizing, 768
neurologic, 801
Signal-averaged electrocardiography, 441
Silent ischemia, coronary artery, 487, 488
Silicone catheter for peritoneal dialysis, 902
Silver sulfadiazine, 1158, 1161
Similac, 230
Single photon emission computed tomography, neurologic
alteration and, 786
Single-lung transplant, 1188-1190
Sinoatrial node, 334
Sinus
dura mater and, 737
venous circulation of brain and, 754
Sinus bradycardia, 408, 593
Sinus dysrhythmia, 408, 409
Sinus node, drugs affecting, 578
Sinus rhythm, 407-409
myocardial infarction and, 496
Sinus tachycardia, 408-409, 504
Sinusitis, 696
Sinusoid of liver, 926
SIRS; *see* Systemic inflammatory response syndrome
Skeletal muscle relaxant, anesthesia and, 303-304
Skin
age-related changes in, 288-289
anaphylaxis and, 1107, 1108
Skin—cont'd
anatomy of, 1141, 1142
burn injury to, 1141-1170; *see also* Burn
cardiovascular assessment and, 356-357
function of, 1141
gastrointestinal assessment and, 931, 933
heart failure and, 506
hyperglycemic hyperosmolar nonketotic syndrome and, 1020
hypovolemic shock and, 1101
ketoacidosis and, 1013-1014
myxedema and, 1038-1039, 1042
orthopedic injury and, 1086
peripheral vascular disease and, 518-519
renal failure and, 883
respiratory failure and, 657
septic shock and, 1113
spinal injury and, 1071
thyrotoxic crisis and, 1034
tube feeding and, 158
turgor of, 866-867
Skin substitute for burn wound, 1162-1166
Skin/wound management, 10
Skull film, 779-782
Skull fracture, 1059
pituitary gland and, 994-995
Slander, 38
Sleep
drugs affecting, 107-109, 305
persistent vegetative state and, 796
Sleep pattern disturbance, 103-119
age-related changes and, 106-107
apnea and, 110-114
assessment of, 114
case study of, 114-117
chronic illness and, 107
circadian desynchronization and, 107
delirium and, 74-75
drugs affecting, 107-109
interventions for, 11
intraaortic balloon pump and, 570-571
nursing management plan for, 91-95, 118-119
physiology and, 103-106
recovery sleep and, 110
sleep deprivation and, 109-110
thyrtotoxic crisis and, 1037
Sleeve resection of lung, 678
Small intestine
age-related changes in, 280
anatomy and physiology of, 922-923
digestion and absorption by, 924
obstruction of, 958-962
Smoke inhalation, 1149-1150
Smoking, coronary artery disease and, 484
Smooth muscle relaxant, 580, 581
Snoring, apnea and, 110, 113
Society of Critical Care Medicine, 194
Sociocultural stressors, 52
Sodium
antidiuretic hormone and, 983
antidiuretic hormone disorder and, 1029, 1030
burn injury and, 1154-1156
cardiac action potential and, 345-346
diabetes insipidus and, 1024-1025
emergence delirium and, 322
hypertension and, 128
ketoacidosis and, 1008, 1013
osmotic diuretic and, 831
Sodium—cont'd
renal disorder and, 138, 142, 860, 881, 885, 886
renin-angiotensin system and, 859
subarachnoid hemorrhage and, 807
urine and, 874
Sodium bicarbonate; *see* Bicarbonate
Sodium channel blocker, 575
Sodium iodide, 1035
Sodium nitroprusside
characteristics of, 580, 581
pregnancy and, 258
Sodium-potassium pump, 1098
Solute, renal tubule and, 851-852
Solution
antidiuretic hormone and, 1031
for continuous arteriovenous hemofiltration, 897
for continuous renal replacement, 897
for hemodialysis, 892-893
continuous venovenous, 899
hyperglycemic hyperosmolar nonketotic syndrome and, 1019
lactated Ringer's
burn injury and, 1154
renal failure and, 884
for parenteral nutrition, 161-162
for renal failure, 884
in slow continuous ultrafiltration, 897
Somatic nervous system, 733
Somatic pain, 176
Somatosensory evoked response, 787
Somatostatin
action of, 980
function of, 981
Sounds
bowel
in gastrointestinal assessment, 933-934
intestinal obstruction and, 960
breath
normal and abnormal, 632
pneumonia and, 665, 666
heart
characteristics of, 367-368
pregnancy and, 247
renal function and, 867
Space, pleural, 651
Spatial orientation, 810
Specific gravity of urine, 873-874
diabetes insipidus and, 1024
Speech
aphasia and, 810-811, 844-845
cerebrovascular accident and, 810-811
in mental status examination, 75
Sphincter
esophageal, 920
of Oddi, 929
precapillary, 340
Sphygmomanometer, 366
Spinal accessory nerve, 746
Spinal anesthesia, 182
vomiting and, 323
Spinal cord
anatomy of, 755-762
in cross section, 758, 761-762
intervertebral disk of, 755-756
meninges and, 756-758
protective mechanisms of, 755
spinal nerves and, 758
dermatomes and, 759-760

Spinal cord—cont'd
  injury to, 265, 1064-1071
    assessment of, 1066-1068
    management of, 1068-1071
    mechanism of, 1065
    pathophysiology of, 1065-1066
  respiratory failure and, 656
Spinal nerve, 758-760
Spinal shock, 1066, 1109-1111
Spindle, sleep, 103
Spine
  dendritic, 282
  radiography of, 782-784
Spiritual distress, 82
Spirometry
  respiratory failure and, 659
  thoracic surgery and, 680-681
Spleen injury, 942, 1082
Splenic vein, 921
Splint, burn and, 1168-1169
Split-thickness graft for burn wound, 1159, 1162
Sputum study, 646-657
ST segment
  definition of, 393
  monitoring of, 399-401
  myocardial ischemia and, 401-402
  thrombolytic therapy and, 566
Stab wound, 1062; *see also* Penetrating trauma
Stable angina, 486-487
Stages of adaptation to illness, 50-51
Stalk, infundibular, 982
  diabetes insipidus and, 1022
Staphylococcal infection
  endocarditis in child and, 222-223
  septic shock and, 1111
Starling's law of the heart, 460
Starr-Edwards prosthetic valve, 544
Starvation, 123-124; *see also* Malnutrition
Static compliance, 648
Status asthmaticus, 671-673
  in child, 213-214
Status epilepticus in child, 226
Statute
  brain death and, 776
  licensing, 38
Steatorrhea, 148
Stenosis
  aortic, 252, 511, 512
  endotracheal intubation and, 697
  idiopathic hypertrophic subaortic, 507
  mitral, 252, 511, 512
    pulmonary artery pressure and, 462
  tricuspid valve, 513
Stent, coronary, 557
Sterile technique, 1015
Steroid
  anaphylaxis and, 1108
  hyperglycemia and, 137
  liver and, 928
  mechanical ventilation and, 715
  status asthmaticus and, 672
  transplant and, 1176
Stimulation
  coma and, 795
  transcutaneous electrical nerve, for pain, 184-185
Stimulator, peripheral nerve, 713
Stimulus
  noxious, 766, 767
  reflex assessment and, 768-769
  verbal, 765-766
Stir-up regimen, postanesthesia, 312
Stomach; *see also* Gastric *entries*
  age-related changes in, 280
  anatomy of, 920-921
  distention of, 323, 324
Stone, biliary, 941
Stool
  blood in, 948
  in gastrointestinal assessment, 936
  pancreatic function and, 937
Storage, by liver, 928
Storm, thyroid, 1031-1038
Straddle fracture, 1085
Strangulated hernia, 941
Streamlined blood flow, 338-339
Strength
  age-related changes in, 290
  motor, 768
Streptococcal endocarditis, 222-223
Streptokinase, 562, 565
Stress
  anxiety and, 189-190
  cold, in child, 225
  coronary artery disease and, 485
  dopaminergic agents and, 190
  endocrine response to, 1001, 1002
  heart transplantation and, 568
  hyperglycemic hyperosmolar nonketotic syndrome and, 1015-1016
  metabolic response to, 123-124
  mind/body interactions and, 64-65
  in nurse, 652
    burn care and, 1169-1170
  organ transplantation and, 84
  pneumonia and, 665
  sleep deprivation and, 109
Stress testing
  echocardiography and, 436
  electrocardiographic, 429-430
Stress ulcer
  bleeding and, 945-946
  burn injury and, 1157
  craniotomy and, 817
Stressor, 50-52
Stroke, 798-811; *see also* Cerebrovascular accident
Stroke volume, 460
  in child, 221
  definition of, 447
Stroke work index, right ventricular, 448
Subaortic stenosis, idiopathic hypertrophic, 507
Subarachnoid bolt, 823, 824
Subarachnoid hemorrhage, 802-807
  arteriovenous malformation and, 803-804
  cerebral aneurysm and, 803
  description of, 802
  diagnosis of, 804
  etiology of, 802-803
  management of, 804
  rebleeding of, 804-806
  vasospasm and, 806-807
Subarachnoid opioid, 182, 183
Subclavian artery
  cerebral angiography and, 781
  cerebral circulation and, 753-754
Subclavian catheter for dialysis, 886-887
Subcutaneous emphysema, 675
  tracheostomy tube and, 698
Subdural hematoma, 1060-1062
Sublingual area assessment, 627
Submaxillary gland, 919
Subthalamus, 748
Subtraction angiography, digital, 782
Succinylcholine
  anesthesia and, 304
  cardiac effects of, 316
Sucking, 229
Sucralfate, 971
Suctioning
  aspiration lung disorder and, 668
  closed tracheal, 701-702
  endotracheal intubation and, 701
  tracheostomy tube and, 701
Sudden death; *see* Death, sudden
Suicide ideation, 76
Sulfamethoxazole, 907
Sulfamethoxazole-trimethoprim, 664
Superfical burn, 1144
Superficial partial-thickness burn, 1144
Superficial reflex, 768
Superior mesenteric artery, colon and, 925
Superior vena cava, central venous catheter in, 385-386
Superoxide dismutase, 834
Supersensitive state, 169-170
Supplemental oxygen device, pediatric, 206-208, 209
Suppression as coping mechanism, 79
Supratentorial herniation, 832-833
Supratentorial structure, 737
Supraventricular tachycardia
  characteristics of, 414
  in child, 222
  nursing management and, 594-595
  paroxysmal, 410-411, 412
Surfactant, 610
  respiratory distress syndrome and, 716
Surgery
  abdominal injury and, 1080-1081
  cardiac, 541-550
    angioplasty and, 554
    cardiopulmonary bypass, 543, 545
    coronary artery bypass and, 541-542
    education about, 549
    nursing management in, 587-590
    pacemaker after, 529; *see also* Pacemaker, cardiac
    patient education about, 549
    postoperative management after, 545-549
    recent advances in, 549-550
    valvular, 542-543, 544
  cardiac tamponade and, 1078
  craniotomy and, 814-818
  gastrointestinal bleeding and, 949
  head injury and, 1064
  intestinal obstruction and, 962
  liver failure and, 963
  pancreatic injury and, 1083
  pulmonary embolism and, 669, 670
  spinal injury and, 1068-1069
  splenectomy, 1083
  subarachnoid hemorrhage and, 805-806
  thoracic, 677-681
  transplant; *see* Transplantation

Surveillance, transplant
infection and, 1182, 1184
rejection and
heart, 1181-1182
liver, 1198-1199
pancreatic, 1208
Survey
primary, 1052
secondary, 1055-1056
Sustained maximal inspiration, postanesthesia, 309
Swallowing
cerebrovascular accident and, 811
esophagus and, 920
salivation and, 919
Sylvius' foramen, 738
Sympathetic nervous system
colon and, 925-926
eye movement and, 769
heartbeat and, 351-352
REM sleep and, 104-105
renal system and, 852
shock and, 1097
neurogenic, 1109
septic, 1112
small intestine and, 923
Sympathomimetic drug
effects of, 577
vasopressor and, 582
Synapse, 735-736
Synaptogenesis in elderly, 285
Synchronized intermittent mandatory ventilation, 662, 707
in child, 210
weaning and, 684, 709
Synchrony, atrioventricular, 533
Syncope, vasovagal, 441
Syncytium, functional, 342
Syndrome of inappropriate secretion of antidiuretic hormone; *see also* Antidiuretic hormone
Synthetic antidiuretic hormone test, 994
Synthetic skin, 1163-1164
Systemic blood supply to lung, 612
Systemic inflammatory response syndrome, 1123-1124; *see also* Multiple organ dysfunction syndrome
definition of, 1112
mediators in, 1125
Systemic vascular resistance; *see* Vascular resistance
Systole, 446-447
age-related changes in, 272
ventricular, 348
Systolic blood pressure, 339
Systolic murmur, 370
Systolic pressure
pulmonary artery, 463

T

T lymphocyte
age-related changes in, 286
immune system and, 1172-1175
T wave
analysis of, 392
myocardial ischemia and, 401-402
Tachycardia
anaphylaxis and, 1107
Tachycardia—cont'd
blood flow and, 337
hypovolemic shock and, 1101
implantable cardioverter defibrillator for, 550
junctional, 415
multifocal atrial, 411, 412
pacemaker for, 530
paroxysmal supraventricular, 410-411, 412
postanesthesia period and, 316
postoperative, 545-546
pulmonary embolism and, 670
sinus, 408-409
heart failure and, 504
supraventricular
characteristics of, 414
in child, 222
nursing management and, 594-595
surgery for, 549
thyrotoxic crisis and, 1032
ventricular
implantable cardioverter defibrillator for, 550
nursing management and, 594
sudden death from, 501
Tactile agnosia, 810
Tactile fremitus, 629-630, 631
"Talk and die" phenomenon, 225
Tamponade
cardiac, 1078
heart transplantation and, 1181
clinical findings in, 373-374
Tamponade tube, esophagogastric balloon, 966-968
Tar burn, 1150
Teaching; *see* Education
Teaching-learning process, 50-52
Technology, as resource, 24
Teleologic theory, 19-20
Television, closed-circuit, 57
Temperature
abdominal injury and, 1081
cardiac surgery and, 547
of injectate, 469
intracranial hypertension and, 829
myxedema and, 1040
neurogenic shock and, 1110
neurologic assessment and, 774
in perianesthesia assessment, 306-307
in postanesthesia period, 317-321
postanesthesia period and, 312
regulation of, 747
thyrotoxic crisis and, 1036-1037
ventilator and, 712
Temporal lobe, 752
uncal herniation and, 832-833
Temporary or borrowed servant, doctrine of, 41
Tension pneumopericardium, 676
Tension pneumothorax, 674, 675, 676, 1076
Tentorium, 737
Teratogenicity, drug, 243-244
Terbutaline, 714
Terminal respiratory unit, 607
Terminal weaning from mechanical ventilation, 686
Termination of treatment
persistent vegetative state and, 798
refusal of antibiotic for elderly patient and, 288
removal of life support and, 785
Tetralogy of Fallot, pregnancy and, 252-253
Thalamus, 746
Thallium scan, cardiovascular alteration and, 438
Thebesian system, 612
Thebesian vessel, 336
Theophylline, 715
Theory, ethical, 19-20
Thermal balance in perianesthesia assessment, 306, 308
Thermal burn; *see* Burn
Thermistor lumen of pulmonary artery catheter, 465
Thermoregulation; *see also* Temperature
cardiac surgery and, 547
in child, 225
myxedema and, 1040, 1041
postanesthesia period and, 317-321
thyrotoxic crisis and, 1034, 1036-1037
Thiamine, coma and, 792
Thiazide diuretic
diabetes insipidus and, 1026
for renal disorder, 905
Thiazolidinediones, 1005
Thinking process, 75
Thiopental
anesthesia with, 302
intracranial hypertension and, 832
Third-degree atrioventricular block, 426-427
Third-degree burn, 1145
Thirst, ketoacidosis and, 1006-1007
Thoracentesis, 647-648
Thoracic injury, 1073-1079
cardiac, 1077-1079
chest wall, 1074-1075
mechanism of, 1073-1074
pulmonary, 1075-1077
Thoracic surgery
complications of, 679-680
postoperative management after, 680-681
preoperative care in, 679
types of, 677-681
Thoracic wall, 277
Thoracolumbar injury, 1069
Thoracoscopy, 678
Thorax; *see also* Thoracic *entries*
anatomy of, 601-604
cardiovascular assessment and, 360, 363-364
percussion of, 630-632
respiratory failure and, 656
Three-beat run of ventricular tachycardia, 417
Three-dimensional echocardiography, 436
Threshold, of myocardial membrane, 344-345
Thromboembolism; *see* Embolism; Pulmonary embolism; Thrombosis
Thrombolytic therapy, 561-567
agents for, 562-566
cerebrovascular accident and, 802
eligibility criteria for, 562
ischemic stroke and, 836
management of, 566-567
patient education about, 567
pulmonary embolism and, 670
reperfusion and, 566
Thrombophlebitis, 363, 521
Thrombosis
cerebrovascular accident and, 800-802
clinical findings in, 373-374
disseminated intravascular coagulation and, 1133

Thrombosis—cont'd
- myocardial infarction and, 490
- pulmonary embolism and; *see* Pulmonary embolism
- venous, 363, 521-523
  - clinical findings in, 373-374
  - craniotomy and, 817
  - neurogenic shock and, 1111
  - parenteral nutrition and, 163
  - spinal injury and, 1071
  - trauma and, 1090

Thromboxane, 1127
Thromboxane A_2, 1127
Thyrocalcitonin; *see* Calcitonin
Thyroid gland
- cardiovascular alteration and, 381, 414
- description of, 982
- diagnostic procedures for, 995-999
- function of, 984-985
- hormones of, 985, 987
- hyperthermia and, 1049
- myxedema and
  - diagnosis of, 996
  - patient history for, 997
- myxedema coma and, 979, 1038-1042; *see also* Myxedema
- recognition of disorder of, 989
- stress response of, 1002
- thyroid crisis and, 979

Thyroid panel, 997, 998
Thyroid storm, 1031-1038
Thyroid-stimulating hormone
- drugs affecting, 999
- function of, 984, 985
- testing for, 996-997
- values of, 998

Thyrotoxic crisis, 1031-1038
- description of, 1031-1032
- diagnosis of, 1033
- etiology of, 1032
- management of, 1033-1038
- pathophysiology of, 1032-1033

Thyrotoxicosis, 996, 997
Thyrotropin-releasing hormone, 982
- function of, 985
- testing for, 997
- values of, 998

Thyroxine
- drugs affecting, 999
- function of, 984, 985
- thyroid crisis and, 996
- values of, 998

Thyroxine-binding globulin
- drugs affecting, 999
- myxedema and, 1041

Tidal volume, 649
Tiered therapy, cardiac, 419-420, 440-441
Tight junction, 739
Time-cycled ventilator, 704
Tirilazad, 834
Tissue perfusion; *see* Perfusion
Tissue plasminogen activator, 564-565
Tolazamide, 1004
Tolbutamide, 1004
Tolerance, drug, 180
Tong, cervical, 1069
Tongue
- of infant, 205

Tongue—cont'd
- pulmonary assessment and, 627

Tonicity of fluid, 858
Tonometer, nasogastric, 968-969
Tonsillectomy, 112
Tonus, 767
Tools
- for assessment of consciousness, 765
- care management, 13

Topical antibiotic for burn wound, 1160
Torsade de pointes, 380, 418
Tort liability, 36-38, 39
Total body water, in child, 229
Total cholesterol, 383
Total lung capacity, 649
Total parenteral nutrition; *see* Parenteral nutrition, total
Toxic acute tubular necrosis, 878
Toxic oxygen metabolite, 1126
Toxicity of oxygen therapy, 690-691
Toxin, liver failure caused by, 963
TP segment, 399
Trach mask, 691
Trachea
- anatomy of, 605
- edema of, 1149
- inhalation injury of, 1150
- in pulmonary assessment, 629
- surgery on, 678

Tracheal intubation, 647
Tracheal stenosis
- endotracheal intubation and, 697
- tracheostomy tube and, 698

Tracheal suction system, closed, 701-702
Tracheobronchial tree, circulation in, 612
Tracheocutaneous fistula, 699
Tracheoesophageal fistula
- endotracheal intubation and, 696
- tracheostomy tube and, 699

Tracheoinnominate artery fistula, 699
Tracheostomy tube
- airway management with, 695, 699-703
- complications of, 698
- extubation of, 703
- foam cuff, 701
- obstructive sleep apnea and, 112, 113

Tracheotomy in child, 211
Tracking variances, 15
Traction for spinal injury, 1069
Transcalvarial herniation, 834
Transcranial approach for craniotomy, 815
Transcranial Doppler studies, 784-786
Transcutaneous cardiac pacing, 531
Transcutaneous electrical nerve stimulation, 184-185
Transducer, for hemodynamic monitoring, 442-443
Transesophageal echocardiography, 414, 431, 432, 433-436
Transfer from critical care unit, teaching and, 57-59
Transfusion
- autotransfusion and, 547, 548
- blood shield statutes and, 516

Transient ischemic attack, 521
Transition in role status, 70
Transjugular intrahepatic portosystemic shunt, 949, 968, 969

Translocation, bacterial, 155, 1128
Transluminal cerebral angioplasty, 807
Transluminal coronary angioplasty, percutaneous, 553-555
- ST-segment monitoring and, 399-401

Transluminal extraction catheter, 556-557
Transmembrane potential, cardiac, 344
Transmembrane pressure in ultrafiltration, 891
Transmission, saltatory, 735
Transmural myocardial infarction, 491-492
Transplantation, 1171-1216
- heart, 1179-1184
  - case study of, 1209-1211
  - stress on spouse and, 569
- heart-lung, 1184-1188
- immunology of, 1171-1179
- liver, 1191-1199
  - case study of, 1211-1213
  - nutrition and, 147
  - screening for, 965
- lung, 1188-1190
- pancreatic, 1205-1208, 1213-1215
- psychosocial alterations and, 83-84
- renal, 1199-1205, 1213-1215

Transport
- active, 854
  - placental membranes and, 244
- gas, 620-624
- passive, 854

Transport physiology, oxygen, 475
Transpyloric feeding
- administration of, 156, 158
- endocrine alterations and, 149

Transsphenoidal approach for craniotomy, 815-816
Transtelephonic recording system for electrocardiography, 428-429
Transtentorial herniation, 833-834
Transthoracic echocardiography, 431-433
Transvenous electrode lead for defibrillator, 550
Transvenous endocardial pacing, 531-532
Transvenous pacing system of pacemaker, 530
Transverse tubule, 342
Trauma, 1051-1094
- abdominal, 1079-1083
- air leak disorder and, 674
- burn, nursing management plan for, 85-100
- case study of, 1092
- coma and, 791
- complications of, 1087-1091
- diabetes insipidus and, 1022
- dysreflexia and, 1093-1094
- in elderly, 83
- endotracheal intubation causing, 696
- genitourinary, 1083-1084
- head; *see* Head injury
- lower extremity, 1086-1087
- maxillofacial, 1071-1073
- mechanism of, 1051-1052
- missed, 1090-1091
- pelvic, 1084-1086
- phases of care for, 1052-1057
- pituitary gland and, 994-995
- pregnancy and, 262-266
- pulmonary embolism and, 669
- renal, 868
- risk factors for, 1057
- spinal cord, 1064-1071; *see also* Spinal cord
- thoracic, 1073-1079

Treadmill test, 429-430
Tree, tracheobronchial, 612
Triad
  Beck's, 1078
  Cushing's, neurologic assessment and, 773
  Virchow's, 521
Triamcinolone, 715
Triazolam, 108
Tricuspid valve, 333-334
  disease of, 252
  regurgitation of, 513
  stenosis of, 513
Trigeminal nerve, 744
Trigger
  for malignant hyperthermia, 320
  for status asthmaticus, 672
Triglyceride, 384
  metabolism of, 122-123
  renal disorder and, 140-141
Triiodothyronine
  drugs affecting, 999
  function of, 984, 985
  thyroid crisis and, 996
  values of, 998
Trimethoprim, 907
Trimethoprim-sulfamethoxazole, 154
Trochlear nerve
  cranial nerves and, 744
  eye movement and, 770
Troglitazone, 1005
Trust as coping mechanism, 80
Trypsin, 929-930
  pancreatitis and, 951
Trypsinogen, 929-930
T-tube
  humidification and, 691
  weaning from mechanical ventilation and, 684, 709
Tube
  chest
    cardiac surgery and, 547
    hemothorax and, 1077
    pneumothorax and, 675, 676-677
  chest radiography and, 384-385, 386, 651-652
  endotracheal; *see* Endotracheal intubation
  esophagogastric balloon tamponade, 966-968
  feeding, in child, 230
  nasogastric; *see* Nasogastric intubation
  tracheostomy, 695, 699-703
    obstructive sleep apnea and, 112, 113
Tube feeding
  administration of, 156, 158
  AIDS and, 154
  endocrine alterations and, 149
  neurologic alteration and, 135, 137
  spinal injury and, 1071
Tubular necrosis, 878-879
Tubular support bandage, 1166-1167
Tubule
  renal
    age-related changes in, 280
    anatomy of, 851-852
    reabsorption by, 853, 854
    secretion of, 854
  transverse, 342
Tumor; *see* Malignancy
Tumor necrosis factor
  inflammation and, 1125-1126, 1126
  inhibitors of, 1137-1138
Tumor necrosis factor—cont'd
  multiple organ dysfunction syndrome and, 1135
    heart and, 1130
Tunica
  of colon, 925
  of small intestine, 922-923
  of stomach, 921
Turgor, skin, 866-867
Turnover, protein, 122
Two-dimensional echocardiography, 431, 433
Two-stopcock blood sampling, 220
Typology, functional health pattern, 5

U

U wave, 377
Ulcer
  Cushing, 946
  duodenal, 941
  gastric, 970
  peptic
    bleeding and, 945
    findings in, 942
  stress
    bleeding and, 945-946
    burn injury and, 1157
    craniotomy and, 817
Ulcerative colitis, 942
Ultrafiltration
  definition of, 896-897
  in hemodialysis, 891
  slow continuous, 895-897
Ultrasonic nebulizer, 699
Ultrasound
  cerebral, 784-786
  echocardiography and, 430-436
  gastrointestinal, 938
Uncal herniation, 832-833
Uncompensated pulmonary condition, 642-643
Unconjugated bilirubin, 928
Unconsciousness; *see also* Neurologic assessment
  coma and; *see* Coma
  motor responses and, 767
  nutrition intervention and, 135, 137
  persistent vegetative state and, 795-798
  postanesthesia period and, 321
Underdamped waveform, 450
Undernutrition
  respiratory alterations and, 133
  significance of, 124
Undersensing by pacemaker, 536
Underweight, 149
Unintentional tort, 37-38
Unipolar lead, pacemaker, 530
Universal pacemaker, 534
Unmyelinated nerve fiber, 734
Unstable angina, 487
Upper airway
  anatomy of, 604-605
  burn injury and, 1153
  of child, 205-206
  inhalation injury of, 1150
  oxygen toxicity and, 692
Upper extremity, cardiovascular assessment and, 362
Urea
  kidney and, 855
  urine and, 874
Uremia, protein and, 138, 139
Ureter
  injury to, 1083-1084
  peristaltic action of, 849
Urinalysis
  components of, 873-875
  renal failure and, 880
Urinary creatinine, 127
Urinary tract infection in elderly, 287
Urine
  antidiuretic hormone disorder and, 1029, 1030
  burn injury and, 1156
  diabetes insipidus and, 1024
  formation of, 849, 852-854
  hypovolemic shock and, 1101
  ketoacidosis and, 1006-1007, 1008
  ketones in, 991
  loop of Henle and, 852
  multiple organ dysfunction syndrome and, 1130
  pancreatitis and, 952
  pituitary assessment and, 994
  spinal injury and, 1071
  thyrotoxic crisis and, 1034
Urokinase, 562, 564
Uterine contraction, 249-250
Uteroplacental insufficiency, 246
Uterus in pregnancy, 247
  trauma to, 266
Uvulopalatopharyngoplasty, 112, 113

V

Vaccine, pneumococcal, 1083
Vagus nerve, 746
Valium; *see* Diazepam
Valsalva maneuver
  coronary artery disease and, 489
  craniotomy and, 815
Valve
  cardiac; *see* Cardiac valve
  Heimlich, 675
  Houston's, 925
  Passy-Muir, 703
Valvuloplasty, balloon, 561
Vancomycin, 907
Variances, managing and tracking, 15
Variant angina, 487
Variceal band ligation, endoscopic, 968
Varices
  esophagogastric, 946
  management of, 949
  vasopressin for, 970
Vascular access for dialysis, 886-890
Vascular disease, peripheral, 517-519
Vascular endothelial injury, 669
Vascular lesion, coma and, 791
Vascular resistance, 340
  definition of, 447, 448
  neurogenic shock and, 1109-1110
  postanesthesia, 315
  pulmonary
    definition of, 448
    heart transplantation and, 1181
  pulmonary artery pressure and, 462, 464
Vascular resistance index, 447
  pulmonary, 448
Vascular steal syndrome, 887

Vascular system; *see also* Artery; Vein
  arteriovenous malformation and, 804
  esophagogastric varices and, 946
  inflammatory response and, 1121-1122
  of liver, 926
  pulmonary, 610-612
  renal, 849-850
  spinal, 761, 762
  trauma and, 1090
Vasoconstriction
  autonomic dysreflexia and, 1066
  hypoxic
    pulmonary hypertension and, 612
    ventilation/perfusion relationships and, 619-620
  postoperative hypothermia and, 318
Vasoconstrictor, shock and, 1099
Vasodilation
  anaphylaxis and, 1107
  inflammatory phase in burn injury, 1158
  intracranial hypertension and, 829-830
  neurogenic shock and, 1109-1110
  septic shock and, 1112
Vasodilator, 579-582
  shock and, 1099
Vasopressin
  diabetes insipidus and, 1026
  dosage and actions of, 971
  gastrointestinal bleeding and, 949, 970
Vasopressor, 582
  myxedema and, 1041
Vasospasm, cerebral, 806-807
Vasovagal syncope, 441
Vector, mean, 395
Vegetative state
  characteristics of, 797
  persistent, 776, 795-798
Vehicular accident
  abdominal trauma and, 1079
  orthopedic injury from, 1086
  respiratory failure and, 1088
  rupture of diaphragm and, 1074-1075
  thoracic injury and, 1073
Vein
  hand, 866
  jugular, 357-359
  of liver, 926-927
  pancreas and, 929
  splenic, 921
Vena cava, central venous catheter in, 385-386
Vena caval filter, 670
Venous blood, 612
Venous catheter, central
  parenteral nutrition via, 159, 161-162
  renal function and, 870
Venous circulation of brain, 754
Venous disease, 517
Venous hum, 933-934
Venous oxygen saturation, mixed, 471, 474-480
Venous pressure, central, 451-456; *see also* Central venous *entries*
Venous stasis, 669
Venous system, 340-341
Venous thrombosis; *see* Thrombosis, venous
Venous vasodilation in anaphylaxis, 1107
Venovenous hemodialysis, continuous, 898-899
Ventilation, 613-618
  air leak disorder and, 676
Ventilation—cont'd
  anaphylaxis and, 1108
  aspiration lung disorder and, 668
  mechanical; *see* Mechanical ventilation
  partial liquid, 716
  pneumonia and, 666
  positive-pressure
    cardiovascular compromise and, 706
    weaning and, 709
  pulmonary embolism and, 671
  pulmonary volumes and, 614-615
  regulation of, 615-618
  respiratory failure and, 658
  status asthmaticus and, 673
  synchronized intermittent mandatory, 707
    in child, 210
    weaning from mechanical ventilation and, 684, 709
  thoracic surgery and, 680
  work of breathing and, 613-614
Ventilation/perfusion relationship, 618-620
  capnography and, 653
  lung transplant and, 1189
  pneumonia and, 665
  in postanesthesia period, 315
  respiratory failure and, 665-666
Ventilation/perfusion scan, 649-650
  pulmonary embolism and, 670
Ventilator
  alarms on, 712
  body image disturbance and, 87-88
  complications of, 704, 706
  modes of, 704
  settings on, 704, 708
  types of, 703-704, 705
Ventilator-associated pneumonia, 663-664
Ventilator-patient asynchrony, in child, 210-211
Ventricle
  anatomy of, 332-333
  cerebral, 282
  drugs affecting, 578
  heart failure and, 502-503
  left, Starling's law and, 460
  status asthmaticus and, 672
Ventricular aneurysm, 497
Ventricular assist device, 571-574
Ventricular axis, 395-396
Ventricular conduction defect, 403
Ventricular contraction, premature, 416-422
Ventricular dysrhythmia, 415-424
  myocardial infarction and, 496-497
  potassium and, 377
Ventricular ectopy, 545-546
Ventricular end-diastolic pressure, left, 460
Ventricular end-diastolic volume, left, 348
Ventricular fibrillation
  in child, 224
  definition of, 392
  electrocardiography and, 420-422
  sudden death from, 501
Ventricular hypertrophy
  electrocardiography and, 400
  heart failure and, 504
  left, 365
Ventricular ischemia, 1102
Ventricular pacing wire, 531
Ventricular preload, left, 252
Ventricular septal defect, 336
  myocardial infarction and, 497-498
  in pregnancy, 252
Ventricular stroke work index, right, 448
Ventricular system of brain, 738
Ventricular systole, 348
Ventricular tachycardia, 419, 420
  implantable cardioverter defibrillator for, 550
  nursing management and, 594
  sudden death from, 501
Ventricular waveform, right, 465-466
Ventriculostomy, 823
Ventriculostomy catheter, 823, 824
Venturi mask, 691
Veracity as ethical principle, 22
Verapamil
  characteristics of, 581
  dosage and side effects of, 578
  elderly patient and, 283
  renal failure and, 908
  thyrotoxicosis and, 1034
Verbal communication, impaired, 810-811, 844-845
Verbal stimulus, 765-766
Vercuronium, 714
Vermis, 741, 743, 746
Versed; *see* Midazolam
Vertebral artery, 753-754
Vertebral column, 755; *see also* Spinal cord
Vertical compression injury of spine, 1065
Very low density lipoprotein, 276, 384
  coronary artery disease and, 484
Vesicular breath sounds, 633
Vestibular nerve, eye movement and, 770
Viability of fetus, 244
Vicarious liability, 40
Videotape, educational, 57
Villus
  arachnoid, 738
  of small intestine, 923
Viral infection
  endocarditis and, 509
  human immunodeficiency, 152-155
  pneumonia as, 664
  respiratory syncytial virus, 212-213
Virchow's triad, 521
Virus, heart transplant and, 1184
Visceral pain, 176
  nursing management of, 197-199
Visual cortex, 752
Visual evoked responses, 787
Visual field defect, 810
Visual object agnosia, 810
Vital capacity
  pregnancy and, 248
  weaning from mechanical ventilation and, 706, 708
Vital signs
  intracranial hemorrhage and, 808
  in neurologic assessment, 772-774
    rapid, 777
  sleep and, 105
Vitamin
  B_{12}, AIDS and, 153
  D, 855
  deficiency of, 126
    neurologic alterations and, 137
  gastrointestinal system and, 145, 149

Vitamin—cont'd
K, 266
renal disorder and, 139, 142-143
Vivactil, 112
Volume
blood; *see* Blood volume
expiratory reserve, 649
inspiratory reserve, 649
left ventricular end-diastolic, 348
lung
age-related changes in, 279
definitions of, 649
in pregnancy, 250
stroke, 447, 460
Volume overload, 1031, 1048-1049
Volume-assured pressure support ventilation, 707
Volume-cycled ventilator, 704, 705
Volume-pressure curve, 821
Voluntary nervous system, 733
Volvulus, 941
Vomiting
craniotomy and, 818
cultural factors in, 953-956
endocrine alterations and, 151
hematemesis, 948
mechanical ventilation causing, 706
postanesthesia, 323-324
subarachnoid hemorrhage and, 804

W

Wakefulness, 795-798
Wall, chest, 1154
Warfarin
deep vein thrombosis and, 522
ischemic stroke and, 836
pulmonary embolism and, 670
Warning leak in subarachnoid hemorrhage, 804
Washout, 566
Waste, elimination of, 855
Water; *see also* Fluid
diabetes insipidus and, 1022-1023
for hemodialysis, 892-893
movement of, 858-859
renin-angiotensin system and, 859
total body, in child, 229
Water central venous pressure, 455
Water deprivation test
diabetes insipidus and, 1024
in pituitary assessment, 994
Water intake, control of, 748
Water load test, 994
Waterhouse-Friderichsen syndrome, 227
Water's view, 779
Wave
P; *see* P wave
T; *see* T wave
U, 377
Wave, intracranial pressure, 824
Waveform
central venous pressure, 456
damped, 450
electrocardiographic, 392-395
hemodynamic monitoring and, 453
intracranial pressure, 824-825
left atrial pressure, 457
overdamped, 452
pulmonary artery, 463, 465-467
underdamped, 450, 452
Weakness
Guillain Barré syndrome and, 812
myasthenia gravis and, 267-268
Weaning
from intraaortic balloon pump, 571
from mechanical ventilation
in child, 211
dysfunctional, 728-729
method of, 681-686, 706, 708-709
spinal injury and, 1071
from ventricular assist device, 574
Wedge pressure
pulmonary artery
positioning for, 444
pulmonary artery diastolic pressure and, 462
renal function and, 870-871, 883
waveform interpretation of, 463
waveform of, 467
pulmonary capillary, 462
chest x-ray and, 388
definition of, 447
Wedge resection of lung, 678
Weight
anthropomorphic measurements and, 125
cardiovascular alterations and, 130
cardiovascular assessment and, 356-357
in evaluation of nutrition support, 165
myxedema and, 1040
pituitary assessment and, 992-993
renal system and, 869, 882, 883
respiratory alterations and, 133, 1314
Wenckebach pattern, 593
Wernicke's aphasia, 811
Wernicke's area, 752
cerebrovascular accident and, 810
Wheeze, 632, 634
Whispering pectoriloquy, 633
White blood cells
burn injury and, 1158
cardiovascular alteration and, 382
septic shock and, 1114
urine and, 874
White matter, 758, 760
Wide QRS complex, 422-424
Will, living, 1104
Willis' circle, 754
Wire, chest radiography and, 651-652
Wirsung's duct, 929
Withholding or withdrawing treatment, 24-25
AACN policy statement on, 27
Wolff-Parkinson-White syndrome, 422, 440
Work index, right ventricular stroke, 448
Work of breathing, 613-614
Wound care, 10
burn injury and, 1149, 1159-1160
chemical burn and, 1150-1151
Wound infection
tracheostomy tube and, 698
trauma and, 1088

X

Xanthine
mechanical ventilation and, 715
respiratory failure and, 658
Xenograft for burn wound, 1163
Xenon washout technique, 784
Xeroform, 1165
D-Xylose, 936

Z

Z band, 342
Zalcitabine, nutrition-related effects of, 154
Zidovudine, nutrition-related effects of, 154
Zinc
AIDS and, 153
gastrointestinal disorder and, 145
neurologic alterations and, 136
renal disorder and, 138
renal failure and, 142
Zone of burn injury, 1145
Zone of ischemia in myocardial infarction, 491, 492